How does the eye see? Why do we ingest food? How does the brain retain images? Why do our bodies grow, mature, age, contract diseases, sustain injuries, become stronger when we exercise, become fatter when we eat too much, require sleep every 16 hours, and eventually die and decay?

The *Oxford Companion to the Body* is a comprehensive resource for anyone who has questions about the fantastic machine that is the human body. Written in clear, straightforward language for the serious researcher or the curious reader, this information-packed reference book incorporates the latest research in evolutionary biology and medical technology. *The Oxford Companion to the Body* surveys every major system, examining their development, processes, and functions—along with the diseases and disorders that can affect them. Over 150 illustrations—many of them in full colour—help make the incredibly complex workings of the human body understandable to the layperson.

This fascinating and authoritative guide covers every aspect of the human body. *The Oxford Companion to the Body* includes over 1000 concise and readable alphabetical entries, from addiction and Adam's Rib to witchcraft and X-rays, written by 350 expert contributors. Interwoven with this coverage of anatomical science are entertaining and informative articles on social and religious attitudes toward the body, its decoration and mutilation throughout history, the ceremonies and myths that surround it, and its significance for artists, writers, and philosophers.

This remarkable compendium includes essays on Body Language and Brain Death, Freckles and Frostbite, Potty Training and

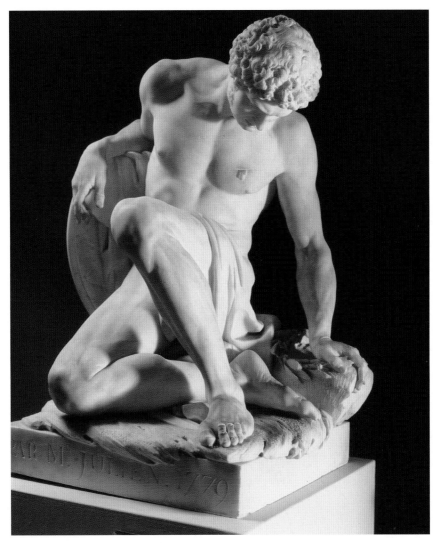

Dying Gladiator, (marble, 1779, by Pierre Julien (1731–1804). The Art Archive/Musée du Louvre, Paris/Dagli Orti (A)

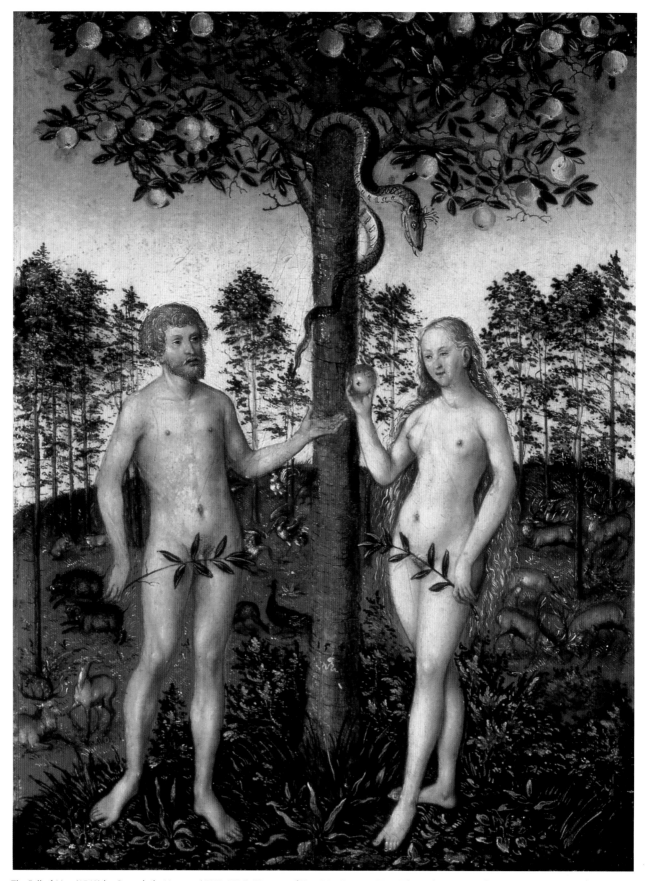

The Fall of Man (1549) by Cranach the Younger (1515–1586). Museum of Fine Arts, Houston, Texas/The Bridgeman Art Library.

The Oxford Companion to
The Body

Editors
Colin Blakemore and Sheila Jennett

Section editors
Alan Cuthbert
Roy Porter
Londa Schiebinger
Tom Sears
Tilli Tansey

Published by

OXFORD
UNIVERSITY PRESS

with the generous support of
THE PHYSIOLOGICAL SOCIETY

OXFORD

UNIVERSITY PRESS

Great Clarendon Street, Oxford OX2 6DP

Oxford University Press is a department of the University of Oxford.
It furthers the University's objective of excellence in research, scholarship,
and education by publishing worldwide in

Oxford New York

Athens Auckland Bangkok Bogotá Buenos Aires Cape Town
Chennai Dar es Salaam Delhi Florence Hong Kong Istanbul Karachi
Kolkata Kuala Lumpur Madrid Melbourne Mexico City Mumbai Nairobi
Paris São Paulo Shanghai Singapore Taipei Tokyo Toronto Warsaw

with associated companies in Berlin Ibadan

Published in the United States
by Oxford University Press Inc., New York

British Library Cataloguing in Publication Data

Data available

Library of Congress Cataloguing in Publication Data

ISBN 0 19 852403 X

10 9 8 7 6 5 4 3 2 1

Typeset in Minion
by EXPO Holdings, Malaysia
Printed in Great Britain
on acid-free paper by
Butler & Tanner, Frome, Somerset

Preface

We are our bodies. The evolution of humanity is the adaptation of bodies. Bodies are the tangible material of being. Bodies contain us, restrain us, perplex us, attract us, disgust us. They are the objects of most of the thoughts and actions of human beings. Scientists, writers, artists and poets are bodies with a mission. It is no surprise that the mission has centred so intensely on the body itself. This book is a celebration of the achievements of those who have pursued that mission.

The book was conceived a decade ago, as a twinkle in the eye of Vanessa Whitting, then an editor at Oxford University Press. But at that stage, the pressure of other commitments and the magnitude of the task dissuaded us from taking it on. Conception turned into gestation a few years later, when, quite independently, the Physiological Society—a professional organization, established in the 1870s to represent biological scientists involved in research into the mysteries of bodily function—offered to support the production of *The Oxford Companion to the Body*. The involvement of the Physiological Society, with its great influence and authority in the biomedical world, brought new impetus to the proposal. It became an offer we couldn't refuse.

The Physiological Society had originally imagined this *Companion* as a way of bringing the wonders and excitement of the science of physiology to a broad audience. But, it happily acceded to our view that the book should embrace the 'art' of the human body—cultural, mythological, religious, historical and artistic perspectives—as well as the science.

People must always have been fascinated by their bodies and the bodies of other people. But never has the human body been a focus of such intense interest from so many perspectives as it now is, at the start of the twenty-first century. Not just in the graphic and plastic arts, but in sociology and psychology, in literature and women's studies, in philosophy and archaeology, in film and sport, the body is a topic of analysis and enquiry. The march of genetics, spurred on by the completion of the Human Genome Project, is leading us to deeper understanding of the fundamental machinery of our cells and organs, as well as new insights into the basis of variation of body and mind among the human population. But the new genetics also makes us question what it is to be a person, how our experiences interact with our inheritance to build our bodies and our minds, and what fundamental limits there are to the ability of the human body to adapt, survive, heal, and achieve.

To do any kind of justice to such a universe of disciplines, we had to recruit an Editorial Board with expertise covering the humanities as well as the whole range of physiological and medical sciences. The first job of that Board was the lateral-thinking, stream-of-consciousness task of devising the list of over 1000 headwords that fill this encyclopaedic volume. It made for amusing meetings. From conception to resurrection; from kiss to orgasm; from codpieces to pubic wigs; from blood clotting to blood letting; from fasting to farting. All human life is here!

The diversity of topics and of the professional backgrounds of the more than 350 experts who contributed articles for this *Companion*, inevitably precluded total uniformity of style and presentation. But we hope that editing has produced some sense of coherence. We set as our ultimate goal the seamless blending of science and humanities, and many of the more extended entries have come close to this. The encyclopaedic arrangement that characterizes Oxford Companions prevented close grouping of related topics, except by alphabetical accident. For this we make no apology. Rather, we hope that the resulting contiguity of sometimes surprising neighbours on the pages may delight the casual reader as much as the chronic browser.

In no way is this book intended to be a popular guide to health, or a dictionary of illnesses and their treatments. In the scientifically based entries, the focus is mainly on normal bodily function, although general categories of disease, and a few medical conditions and abnormalities of great consequence in medical or social history are represented. Included also are historical and contemporary approaches to diagnosis and treatment, in the contexts of different cultures and religions, and of 'complementary' therapies, as well as medical practice based on the 'conventional' clinical sciences. For more specific reference to medicine in all its aspects, readers are referred to the *Oxford Illustrated Companion to Medicine*.

It has been our aim that each entry should as far as possible be self-contained—readable without the need for recourse to other information—although cross-references do point to related topics. It follows that a degree of overlap among entries has been inevitable and acceptable, sometimes with similar information presented from different viewpoints. Where matters of fact are concerned, the reader should not find major contradictions. Matters of interpretation, outlook and opinion, on the other hand, may be personal to the individual authors or the groups to which they belong, and are not necessarily endorsed by the editors.

Oxford   CB
Glasgow   SJ
August 2001

Acknowledgments

Producing an Oxford Companion is a mammoth undertaking, involving and depending on the great breadth of experience of Oxford University Press. We thank all those at the Press who were midwives for the birth of this volume. In particular, we are grateful to the original editor, Vanessa Whitting, her successor Susan Harrison, Beth Knight, who bridged a gap in charge of day-to-day progress, and finally Richard Lawrence and Gill Watts who expedited its completion, with the diligent assistance of Anna Campbell. Emma Chapman dealt valiantly with the huge task of copy-editing. Debbie Sutcliffe, as picture editor, identified and obtained illustrations from many sources, and oversaw the design and production of the colour plates from artwork by Halli Verrinder. James Dobson of the Technical Graphics Department prepared many of the illustrations, and dealt patiently with requests for amendments. Finally in the approach to publication, Elisabeth Pickard prepared the index and Jane Kirby of Science and Medicine Marketing was in charge of promoting the book.

Without the initiative of the Physiological Society and its support for this project, the book would never have been born. Kwabena Appenteng, then Chairman of the Publications Committee, and John Widdicombe, the former Treasurer of the Society, were closely involved, together with other members of the Society's Committee, in the early planning and the pledge of sponsorship. John's successor, Philip Harrison, and the administrative staff of the Society, have maintained this support, and provided facilities for editorial meetings.

Jeannie Wallace, who was recruited and supported by the Physiological Society to assist the editors, gave invaluable assistance in commissioning and correspondence with authors, the receipt of the entries, storing information and generally acting as a friendly link between the editors and the Press.

The members of the Editorial Board are grateful to their many colleagues who agreed to contribute or helped in other ways with the preparation of this volume. Particular thanks for assistance are due to Daphne Christie, from Tilli Tansey, to Frieda Hauser, from Roy Porter, and to Sue Brooks, from Colin Blakemore.

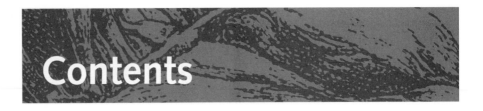

Contents

Plates appear at the end of the book

Note to the reader

Some will go first to the index, pinpointing an item of particular interest, either because they would like to know about it, or because they are curious to see how it is handled here. Some will simply flick through the pages and settle randomly on a title that stirs their interest, or perhaps an illustration that catches their eye. A systematic few might even start here, looking first for guidance on how best to use the book.

For the sake of those few, and maybe for the retrospective consultation of the many, interested in, or at worst frustrated by, any eccentricities in the presentation, we offer these explanations.

The alphabetically arranged titles are referred to as **headwords**, and the text of each is an *entry*. It will be obvious that entries vary greatly in length. The very shortest are dictionary-type definitions; the longest are reviews of the subject—but still brief by the standard of knowledge of the respective experts. They have been written for the reader who may have little prior familiarity with the topic, or perhaps with its technical vocabulary. Each entry has been designed as far as possible to stand alone, so that in most cases it is not necessary to read others that provide related information—although the strategy of following cross-references may be the ideal way to explore a subject of interest. Guidance to such cross-references is provided in two ways. Within each entry SMALL CAPITALS highlight other relevant headwords; and at the foot the entry, major relevant words; and at the foot the entry, major relevant

headwords are listed under '*See also*'. If there is a relevant anatomical illustration in the colour plate section, the plate number also appears here. The shortest entries, which offer only summaries or define terms, direct the reader (under '*See*') to more extensive treatment of the topic under different headwords. In addition there is a detailed index, where readers may seek reference to subjects that do not appear as headwords, but may well be covered in a different guise.

The majority of the longer entries provide a list of '*Further reading*' recommended by the author. These lists are not intended to give full reference to sources used or quoted by the author (although some may do so), but rather to suggest books or articles that expand on the topic and that should be accessible to the non-specialist reader.

The list of contributors provides details of authors and their affiliations. The shortest entries, which generally do not involve personal expertise or opinion are attributed to the provider by initials only. With this exception, the full names of authors and co-authors appear at the foot of their entries. In instances where more than one author is named, each has contributed a separate component from a different background, and has accepted collation of their material by the editors, so that, for instance, cultural and scientific aspects are combined under the common headword.

Contributors

Phillip Aaronson Department of Pharmacology, Guy's, King's and St Thomas' Hospitals, UK

Anne Abichou Altrincham, UK

J Hume Adams Institute of Neurological Sciences, University of Glasgow, UK

Michael Adler Department of Sexually Transmitted Diseases, Royal Free and University College Medical School, London, UK

Garland Allen Department of Biology, Washington University in St Louis, USA

Praveen Anand Department of Neurology, Hammersmith Hospital, UK

Josephine Arendt School of Biomedical and Life Sciences, University of Surrey, UK

William Arens Department of Anthropology, State University of New York, Stony Brook, USA

David Armstrong Department of General Practice, King's College London, UK

David M Armstrong Department of Physiology, School of Medical Sciences, University of Bristol, UK

Vic Armstrong Church Hill, Berkshire, UK

Frances Ashcroft University Laboratory of Physiology, University of Oxford, UK

H F Augstein Süddeutsche Zeitung, Munich, Germany

Anne Ballinger Digestive Diseases Research Centre, St Bartholomew's and the Royal London School of Medicine and Dentistry, UK

Duncan Banks Department of Biological Sciences, The Open University, UK

Jeffrey Barker Department of Philosophy, Albright College, USA

Graham Barnes Department of Optometry and Neuroscience, University of Manchester Institute of Science and Technology, UK

Amanda Barrow Archive, London, UK

Joan Bassey School of Biomedical Sciences, Queen's Medical Centre, Nottingham, UK

Ron H Baxendale Institute of Biomedical and Life Sciences, University of Glasgow, UK

Daniel Beaver Department of History, Pennsylvania State University, USA

Dominic Beer Institute of Psychiatry and Guy's, King's and St Thomas' Hospitals, London, and Oxleas NHS Trust, Bexley, UK

G Bentley Institute of Orthopaedics, Royal National Orthopaedic Hospital, UK

John Bidmead Department of Urogynaecology, King's College Hospital, UK

Sandra Billington Department of Theatre, Film and Television Studies, University of Glasgow, UK

Sue M Black Human Identification Centre, Department of Forensic Medicine and Science, University of Glasgow, UK

Susan Blackmore Bristol, UK

Andrée Blakemore Oxford, UK

Colin Blakemore University Laboratory of Physiology, University of Oxford, UK

Sarah-Jayne Blakemore INSERM Unit 280, Lyon, France

Martin Blanchard University College London, UK

Lyn A Blanchfield Department of History, Binghamton University, NY, USA

Stuart Blume Vakgroep Wetenschapsdynamica, Amsterdam, The Netherlands

Iain Boal Department of Geography, University of California at Berkeley, USA

Michael Bond Department of Psychological Medicine, University of Glasgow, UK

Kelvin Boos Royal Sussex County Hospital, UK

Christopher Booth Wellcome Trust Centre for the History of Medicine at University College London, UK

Marian A Borde The Industrial Society, Glasgow, UK

Claus Bossen New Ways of Working, Aarhus University, Denmark

Anthony Bottoms Department of Criminology, University of Cambridge, UK

Jonathan Boulton Department of History, University of Notre Dame, USA

Joanna Bourke School of History, Classics and Archaeology, Birkbeck College, UK

David Bowyer Department of Pathology, University of Cambridge, UK

Iain Boyle Royal College of Physicians and Surgeons of Glasgow, UK

James Bradley Wellcome Unit for the History of Medicine, University of Glasgow, UK

Alan G Brown Preclinical Veterinary Department, University of Edinburgh, UK

Donald C Brown Department of Reproductive and Developmental Sciences, University of Edinburgh, UK

Daniel Brownstein Consortium for the Humanities, University of California, Los Angeles, USA

Mark J Buckley Department of Experimental Psychology, University of Oxford, UK

Arnold Burgen Downing College, University of Cambridge, UK

Arthur M Butt Centre for Neuroscience Research, King's College London, UK

Brian Callingham Department of Pharmacology, University of Cambridge, UK

Gemma A Calvert University Laboratory of Physiology, University of Oxford, UK

Jane Caplan Department of History, Bryn Mawr College, USA

Linda Cardozo Department of Urogynaecology, King's College Hospital, London, UK

John Carson Department of History, University of Michigan, USA

Kumkum Chatterjee Department of History, Pennsylvania State University, USA

Ian Christie School of Art, Film and Visual Media, Birkbeck College, University of London, UK

Stuart Clark Department of History, University of Wales Swansea, UK

Constance Classen Department of Sociology and Anthropology, Concordia University, Canada

Martin Clayton The Print Room, The Royal Library, Windsor Castle, UK

Forrester Cockburn Department of Child Health, University of Glasgow, UK

Richard Coker London School of Hygiene and Tropical Medicine, London, UK

Lawrence I Conrad Asia-Africa Institute, University of Hamburg, Germany

Cary L Cooper Manchester School of Management, University of Manchester Institute of Science and Technology, UK

Kate Cooper Department of History, University of Manchester, UK

Michael Corballis Department of Psychology, University of Auckland, New Zealand

Paul Corballis Center for Cognitive Neuroscience, Dartmouth College, USA

Gary Cross Department of History, Pennsylvania State University, USA

Valerie Cumming London, UK

Alan W Cuthbert Department of Medicine, University of Cambridge, UK

Ann Dally Wellcome Trust Centre for the History of Medicine at University College London, UK

Alan Dangour Department of Biological Anthropology, University of Cambridge, UK

J K Davidson Formerly, Department of Radiology, Western Infirmary and Garnavel General Hospitals, Glasgow, UK

Jane W Davidson Department of Music, University of Sheffield, UK

Luke Davidson London, UK

Angharad Puw Davies Department of Medical Microbiology, Royal Free Hospital, London, UK

Robbie E Davis-Floyd Department of Anthropology, University of Texas, USA

Ruth Day Department of Neurology and Child Development, Royal Hospital for Sick Children, Glasgow, UK

Jan M A de Vries Loyola Marymount University, Los Angeles, USA, and Trinity College, University of Dublin, Republic of Ireland

Anthony Dickinson Department of Experimental Psychology, University of Cambridge, UK

Graham Dockray Department of Physiology, University of Liverpool, UK

Brian Dolan Wellcome Unit for the History of Medicine at the University of East Anglia, UK

Julia Douthwaite Department of Romance Languages, University of Notre Dame, USA

Ian Dowbiggin Department of History, University of Prince Edward Island, Canada

Alice Domurat Dreger Lyman Briggs School, Michigan State University, USA

Sarah Dunant London, UK

J V G A Durnin Department of Human Nutrition, University of Glasgow, UK

Kirsten Dwight Wray, Lancashire, UK

Michael Edward Department of Dermatology, University of Glasgow, UK

Michael Edwardson Department of Pharmacology, University of Cambridge, UK

Paul Ekman Department of Psychiatry, University of California, San Francisco, USA

Hugh Y Elder Institute of Biomedical and Life Sciences, University of Glasgow, UK

David Elliott Haslemere, Surrey, UK

Harold Ellis Human Sciences Research, Guy's, King's and St Thomas' School of Biomedical Sciences, London, UK

Susanna Elm Department of History, University of California at Berkeley, USA

John Ernsting Human Physiology and Aerospace Medicine Group, Guy's, King's and St Thomas' School of Biomedical Sciences, London, UK

Dylan Evans Department of Philosophy, King's College London, UK

Martin Evans Cardiff School of Biosciences, University of Cardiff, UK

Thomas J Evans Royal Hospital for Sick Children, Glasgow, UK

Pasi Falk Department of Sociology, University of Helsinki, Finland

Lynne Fallwell Department of History, Pennsylvania State University, USA

Tai-Ping Fan Department of Pharmacology, University of Cambridge, UK

Patricia Fara Clare College, University of Cambridge, UK

Liam Farrell Crossmaglen Health Centre, County Armagh, UK

Michael J G Farthing Faculty of Medicine, University of Glasgow, UK

Peter Fells Moorfields Eye Hospital, London, UK

William R Ferrell Centre for Rheumatic Diseases and Institute of Biomedical and Life Sciences, University of Glasgow, UK

Maureen Flynn Department of History, Hobart and William Smith Colleges, USA

Robert Foley Department of Biological Anthropology, University of Cambridge, UK

Mary L Forsling Neuroendocrine Laboratories, Guy's, King's and St Thomas' School of Medicine, London, UK

Susan Foster Department of Dance, University of California at Riverside, USA

Alan Fox Department of Philosophy, University of Delaware, USA

Silvia Frenk London, UK

Chris Frith Wellcome Department of Cognitive Neurology, Institute of Neurology at University College London, UK

Uta Frith Institute of Cognitive Neuroscience, University College London, UK

Simon Gandevia Prince of Wales Medical Research Institute, Prince of Wales Hospital, Sydney, Australia

Laurence Garey Faculty of Medicine, UAE University, United Arab Emirates

Alan Gauld School of Psychology, University of Nottingham, UK

Michael Gazzaniga Center for Cognitive Neuroscience, Dartmouth College, USA

Faye Getz Rickmansworth, Hertfordshire, UK

Sander L Gilman Humanities Laboratory, College of Liberal Arts and Sciences at the College of Medicine, University of Illinois, USA

Anne Glazier St Ives, UK

Peter J Goadsby Institute of Neurology, The National Hospital for Neurology and Neurosurgery, London, UK

Victor Goh Hng Hang Department of Obstetrics and Gynaecology, National University Hospital, Singapore

Alex Goldbloom Wellcome Trust Centre for the History of Medicine at University College London, UK

Frank St C Golden Institute of Biomedical and Biomolecular Sciences, Department of Sport and Exercise Science, University of Portsmouth, UK

Janet Golden Department of History, Rutgers University, New Jersey, USA

Christopher Goodey London, UK

Sarah Goodfellow Department of History, Pennsylvania State University, USA

Mark Gosbee Wellcome Trust Centre for the History of Medicine at University College London, UK

George R Gray Victoria Infirmary, Glasgow, UK

Emily Green Los Angeles, USA

Richard L Gregory Department of Psychology, University of Bristol, UK

Abe Guz National Heart and Lung Institute at Charing Cross, Imperial College School of Medicine, London, UK

Roger Hainsworth Institute of Cardiovascular Research, University of Leeds, UK

Lesley A Hall Archives and Manuscripts, Wellcome Library for the History and Understanding of Medicine, London, UK

Nicola Hall The British Reflexology Association, UK

David N Hamilton Transplant Unit, Western Infirmary, Glasgow, UK

Anne Hardy Wellcome Trust Centre for the History of Medicine at University College London, UK

Tim Hargreave Department of Urology, Western General Hospital, Edinburgh, UK

Mark Harries Department of Respiratory Medicine, Northwick Park and St Mark's NHS Trust, Harrow, UK

Bernard Harris Department of Sociology and Social Policy, University of Southampton, UK

J D Harrison National Radiological Protection Board, Chilton, UK

Adam Hart-Davis Bristol, UK

Lucy Hartley Department of English, University of Southampton, UK

Natsu Hattori Wellcome Trust Centre for the History of Medicine at University College London, UK

Debra Hawhee Department of English, University of Illinois at Urbana-Champaign, USA

Alastair Hay Molecular Epidemiology Unit, University of Leeds, UK

Stephen Haylock City of London Police, London, UK

Rhodri Hayward Wellcome Unit for the History of Medicine in the School of History at the University of East Anglia, UK

Suzette Heald Department of Human Sciences, Brunel University, UK

Steven Heine Department of History, Pennsylvania State University, USA

Graeme Henderson Department of Pharmacology, University of Bristol, UK

John Henderson Wellcome Trust Centre for the History of Medicine at University College London, UK

Mike Hepworth Department of Sociology, University of Aberdeen, UK

Joe Herbert Department of Anatomy, University of Cambridge, UK

Rebecca Herzig Women's Studies Program, Bates College, USA

Andrew Hextall Department of Obstetrics and Gynaecology, Hammersmith Hospital, UK

Robin Hiley Department of Pharmacology, University of Cambridge, UK

Stephen B Hladky Department of Pharmacology, University of Cambridge, UK

J Allan Hobson Laboratory of Neurophysiology, Harvard Medical School, USA

Stuart Hogarth London, UK

Anne Hollander New York, USA

Elizabeth Hollander Oakland, CA, USA

Amy Hollywood Department of Religion, Dartmouth College, USA

Oliver Holmes Institute of Biomedical and Life Sciences, University of Glasgow, UK

Nick Hopwood Department of History and Philosophy of Science, University of Cambridge, UK

L S Illis Department of Neurology, Southampton General Hospital, UK

Roger Ingham Department of Speech and Hearing Sciences, University of California at Santa Barbara, USA

Leslie L Iversen University Department of Pharmacology, University of Oxford, UK

Christina Jarvis Department of English, State University of New York at Fredonia, USA

John G R Jefferys Division of Neuroscience, University of Birmingham, UK

Bryan Jennett Institute of Neurological Sciences, University of Glasgow, UK

Sheila Jennett Institute of Biomedical and Life Sciences, University of Glasgow, UK

Maggy Jennings RSPCA Research Animals Department, Horsham, UK

Claudia Jeschke Hochschule fur Musik, Cologne, Germany

Caroline Jones Art History Department, Boston University, USA

Robert Jones School of English, University of Leeds, UK

Stuart Judge University Laboratory of Physiology, University of Oxford, UK

W R Keatinge Department of Physiology, Queen Mary and Westfield College, UK

Christopher Kelnar Department of Reproductive and Developmental Sciences, University of Edinburgh, UK

Áine Kennedy Celtic Health Connection, Glasgow, UK

Gavin N C Kenny University Department of Anaesthesia, Glasgow Royal Infirmary, UK

Tim Key ICRF Cancer Epidemiology Unit, Radcliffe Infirmary, University of Oxford, UK

Vik Khullar Division of Paediatrics, Obstetrics and Gynaecology, Imperial College London, UK

Andrew King University Laboratory of Physiology, University of Oxford, UK

Helen King Departments of Classics and History, University of Reading, UK

Tom Kirkwood Wolfson Research Centre, Newcastle General Hospital, UK

Henry C Kitchener Academic Unit of Obstetrics and Gynaecology and Reproductive Health Care at St Mary's Hospital, Manchester, UK

Jill Kraye The Warburg Institute, University of London, UK

Prem Kumar Department of Physiology, University of Birmingham, UK

Peter J Kyberd Department of Cybernetics, University of Reading, UK

Gary Laderman Department of Religion, Emory University, USA

Joe Langford Ergonomics Society, Loughborough, UK

David Langstroth Cardiff, UK

Gerry Larkin School of Social Sciences and Law, Sheffield Hallam University, UK

Charles D Laughlin Department of Sociology and Anthropology, Carleton University, Ottawa, Canada

Susan Lawrence Department of History, University of Iowa, USA

R N Lemon Sobell Department of Neurophysiology, Institute of Neurology, University College London, UK

Paul Lerner Department of History, University of Southern California, USA

Lisa Lieberman Department of History, Dickinson College, USA

Roger W A Linden Clinical Craniofacial Biology Research Unit, King's College London, UK

Evan L Lloyd Edinburgh, UK

Stephen Lock Formerly, British Medical Journal, UK

Marjorie Lorch Applied Linguistics, School of Languages, Linguistics and Culture, Birkbeck College, UK

Chris Lote Division of Medical Science, University of Birmingham Medical School, UK

Christopher Lowe Institute of Biotechnology, University of Cambridge, UK

Margaret A Lowe Department of History, Bridgewater State College, USA

Dan Lusthaus Department of Religion, University of Missouri, USA

Fiona Macdonald Wellcome Trust Centre for the History of Medicine at University College London, UK

Ian A Macdonald Department of Physiology and Pharmacology at Queen's Medical Centre, Nottingham, UK

Niall G MacFarlane Institute of Biomedical and Life Sciences, University of Glasgow, UK

Rona MacKie Department of Dermatology, University of Glasgow, UK

Malcolm Macnaughton Department of Obstetrics and Gynaecology, University of Glasgow, UK

Laurie Maguire Magdalen College, University of Oxford, UK

Vishy Mahadevan Royal College of Surgeons, London, UK

Gin S Malhi Mood Disorders Unit, University of New South Wales, Australia

Nick J Marshall Department of Immunology and Molecular Pathology, University College London, UK

Peter Martin Hamburger Institut für Sozialforschung, Germany

C J Mathias Neurovascular Medicine Unit, St Mary's, Imperial College School of Science, Technology and Medicine, and Autonomic Unit, National Hospital and Institute of Neurology, University College London, UK

Keith Matthews Department of Pharmacology, University of Cambridge, UK

Paul M Matthews Centre for the Functional Magnetic Resonance Imaging of the Brain, John Radcliffe Hospital, Oxford, UK

Ron J Maughan Department of Biomedical Sciences, University Medical School, Aberdeen, UK

Sheryl McCurdy Center for Health Promotion and Prevention Research, University of Texas – Houston School of Public Health, USA

A Colin McDougall Radley, UK

Heather McHold Connecticut, USA

Manya McMahon British Chiropractic Association, Reading, UK

Paul Mellars Department of Archaeology, University of Cambridge, UK

Mark Micale Department of History, University of Illinois, USA

Meredith Michaels Department of Philosophy, Smith College, USA

David J Miller Institute of Biomedical and Life Sciences, University of Glasgow, UK

Tasha Miller The Society of Teachers of the Alexander Technique, UK

J D Mollon Department of Experimental Psychology, University of Cambridge, UK

John Morrison Department of Physiology and Pharmacology, UAE University, United Arab Emirates

Javier Moscoso Department of History of Science, Harvard University, USA

Marie Mulvey-Roberts School of English, The University of the West of England, UK

Ruth Murrell-Lagnado Department of Pharmacology, University of Cambridge, UK

J Neilson Department of Obstetrics and Gynaecology, University of Liverpool, UK

J Newsom-Davis Department of Clinical Neurology, University of Oxford, UK

Malcolm Nicolson Wellcome Unit for the History of Medicine, University of Glasgow, UK

Isak Niehaus Department of Social Anthropology, University of Witwatersrand, South Africa

Kate Norberg Department of History, University of California, USA

Moira O'Brien Department of Anatomy, Trinity College, Dublin, Republic of Ireland

Brian O'Callaghan Department of Continuing Education, University of Reading, UK

P J O'Dwyer University Department of Surgery, Glasgow Western Infirmary, UK

Eric T Olson Churchill College, University of Cambridge, UK

Robin Orchardson Institute of Biomedical and Life Sciences, University of Glasgow, UK

Andrew Packard Stazione Zoologica, Naples, Italy

Kim Pelis Department of Medical History, Uniformed Services University, USA

Martin Pernick Department of History, University of Michigan, USA

Anthony L Podberscek Department of Clinical Veterinary Medicine, University of Cambridge, UK

Dorothy Porter Department of History, Birkbeck College, UK

Roy Porter Wellcome Trust Centre for the History of Medicine at University College London, UK

Jane E Preston Institute of Gerontology, King's College London, UK

Ashley E Pryor Department of Philosophy and Women's Studies, University of Toledo, Ohio, USA

Benjamin S Pryor Department of Philosophy, University of Toledo, Ohio, USA

John Pultz Department of Art History, University of Kansas, USA

V S Ramachandran Department of Psychology, University of California at San Diego, USA

S S Ratnam Department of Obstetrics and Gynaecology, National University Hospital, Singapore

Arup Ray Plastic Surgery Unit, Canniesburn Hospital, Glasgow, UK

Daniel Reid Formerly, Scottish Centre for Infection and Environmental Health, Glasgow, UK

Ruth Richardson London, UK

Stephen M Riordan Department of Gastroenterology, The Prince of Wales Hospital, Sydney, Australia

T D M Roberts Formerly, University of Glasgow, UK

Barbara J Rolls Nutrition Department, Pennsylvania State University, USA

Edmund T Rolls Department of Experimental Psychology, University of Oxford, UK

Herman Roodenburg Meertens Instituut, Amsterdam, The Netherlands

Noliwe Rooks African American Studies Program, Princeton University, USA

David Rosner Mailman School of Public Health, Columbia University, USA

John A S Ross Department of Environmental and Occupational Medicine, University of Aberdeen Medical School, UK

Martin Rossor Institute of Neurology at the National Hospital for Neurology, London, UK

John Rothwell Sobell Department of Neurophysiology, Institute of Neurology, London, UK

Nancy J Rothwell School of Biological Sciences, University of Manchester, UK

George Rousseau Department of English, De Montfort University, Leicester, UK

Roy A Ruddle Informatics Research Institute, School of Computing, University of Leeds, UK

Janina Safran Department of History, Pennsylvania State University, USA

Mike Saks Faculty of Health and Community Studies, De Montfort University, Leicester, UK

G Samuel Department of Sociology and Anthropology, University of Newcastle, NSW, Australia

Craig Saper Department of English, University of Pennsylvania, USA

Richard D Saunders National Radiological Protection Board, Chilton, UK

Peter Savundra Department of Audiological Medicine, Northwick Park Hospital, Harrow, UK

Francesco Scaravilli Department of Neuropathology, Institute of Neurology, London, UK

Londa Schiebinger Department of History, Pennsylvania State University, USA

Martin Schwellnus Sports Science Institute of South Africa, Newlands, S. Africa

Tom Sears Division of Physiology, King's College London, UK

Malcolm Segal Guy's, King's and St Thomas' School of Biomedical Sciences, King's College London, UK

Kerry Segrave Vancouver, B.C., Canada

Chandak Sengoopta Centre for the History of Science, Technology and Medicine, University of Manchester, UK

Shiladitya Sengupta Department of Pharmacology, University of Cambridge, UK

Sonu Shamdasani Wellcome Trust Centre for the History of Medicine at University College London, UK

N C Craig Sharp Department of Sports Sciences, Brunel University, UK

J A Sharpe Department of History, University of York, UK

Jane Shaw New College, University of Oxford, UK

Mary D Sheriff Department of Art, University of North Carolina at Chapel Hill, USA

Michael Shortland Unit for History and Philosophy of Science, University of Sydney, Australia

David Shotton Department of Zoology, University of Oxford, UK

David Shuker Department of Chemistry, The Open University, UK

G A Smith Victoria Infirmary, Glasgow, UK

Virginia Smith London, UK

Greg Smits Department of History, Pennsylvania State University, USA

John Springhall School of History and International Affairs, University of Ulster, UK

Neil C Spurway Centre for Exercise Science and Medicine, University of Glasgow and British Association for Sport and Exercise Science, UK

Magi Sque School of Nursing and Midwifery, University of Southampton, UK

John W Stather National Radiological Protection Board, Chilton, UK

Christine Stevenson Department of History of Art, University of Reading, UK

J R Stradling Oxford Centre for Respiratory Medicine, Churchill Hospital, Oxford, UK

Claudia Swan Department of Art History, Northwestern University, USA

E M (Tilli) Tansey Wellcome Trust Centre for the History of Medicine at University College London, UK

C W Taylor Department of Pharmacology, University of Cambridge, UK

S G Taylor Western Infirmary, Glasgow, UK

Allan Thexton Division of Physiology, Kings College London, UK

Betsy Thom School of Social Science, Middlesex University, UK

Michael J Tipton Institute of Biomedical and Biomolecular Sciences, Department of Sport and Exercise Science, University of Portsmouth, UK

P Tobias Department of Anatomy, University of Witwatersrand, South Africa

Graeme Tobyn Hereford, UK

Sylvana Tomaselli Hughes Hall and St John's College, University of Cambridge, UK

Philip Toozs-Hobson Department of Urogynaecology, Birmingham Hospital for Women and Children, UK

Roger D Traub Division of Neuroscience, University of Birmingham, UK

Mike Tripp West Ewell, Surrey, UK

William Tyldesley Liverpool, UK

Jennifer Aydelott Utman Department of Experimental Psychology, University of Oxford, UK

Jyotsna Vaid Department of Psychology, Texas A & M University, USA

Wray Vamplew Department of Sports Studies, University of Stirling, UK

Julie Vedder Department of English, West Virginia University, USA

Angela Vincent Neurosciences Group of the Institute of Molecular Medicine, John Radcliffe Hospital, Oxford, UK

Keir Waddington School of History and Archaeology, Cardiff University, UK

E Geoffrey Walsh University of Edinburgh, UK

Tony Walter Department of Sociology, University of Reading, UK

Jeremy P T Ward Department of Medicine and Allergy, Guy's, King's and St Thomas' School of Medicine, London, UK

Michael J Waring Department of Pharmacology, University of Cambridge, UK

Dylan Warren-Davis Murwillumbah, New South Wales, Australia

Katherine D Watson Wolfson College, University of Oxford, UK

Andrew Wear Wellcome Trust Centre for the History of Medicine at University College London, UK

David J Weatherall Weatherall Institute of Molecular Medicine, John Radcliffe Hospital, Oxford, UK

Mark Weatherall Department of Neurology, Radcliffe Infirmary, Oxford, UK

Karol K. Weaver Department of History, Purdue University, USA

Andrew Webber Churchill College, University of Cambridge, UK

Paul Weindling Wellcome Unit for the History of Medicine, Humanities Research Centre at Oxford Brookes University, UK

John B West Department of Medicine, University of California at San Diego, USA

David J Wheatley University Department of Cardiac Surgery, Glasgow Royal Infirmary, Glasgow, UK

M J Wheeler Department of Chemical Pathology, St Thomas' Hospital, London, UK

Brian J Whipp Department of Physiology, St Georges Hospital Medical School, London, UK

Saffron A Whitehead Department of Physiology, St Georges Hospital Medical School, London, UK

David J Whitfield The Ergonomics Society, Loughborough, UK

John Widdicombe Guy's, King's and St Thomas' School of Biomedical Science, London, UK

Jacqueline Wilkie Luther College, Iowa, USA

Lise Wilkinson Wellcome Trust Centre for the History of Medicine at University College London, UK

Adrian J Williams Respiratory Unit and Sleep Disorders Centre, St Thomas' Hospital, London, UK

Caroyln Williams Department of English, University of Reading, UK

Roger Williams Institute of Hepatology, University College London, UK

Jan Wilson Oxford, UK

A Winter Crosshouse Hospital, Kilmarnock, UK

Roger Woledge UCL Institute of Human Performance, Royal National Orthopaedic Hospital Trust, Stanmore, UK

Roderick Woods Department of Physiology, University of Cambridge, UK

Marilyn Yalom Institute for Research on Women and Gender, Stanford University, USA

Christopher Yeo Department of Anatomy and Developmental Biology, University College London, UK

Archie Young Department of Clinical and Surgical Sciences, University of Edinburgh, UK

Kristen Zacharias Department of Philosophy, Albright College, USA

Amy B. Zavatsky Department of Engineering Science, University of Oxford, UK

David Zuck History of Anaesthesia Society, London, UK

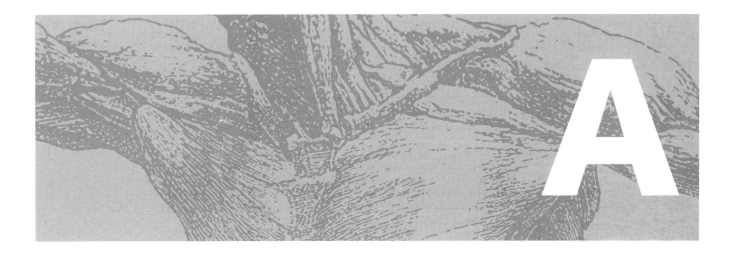

Abdomen The proper anatomical term for what is known colloquially as the belly, or as the 'STOMACH', especially when localizing an ache or pain. The abdomen is roofed by the diaphragm, which separates it from the *thorax* (chest). At the front and sides is the abdominal wall, of skin, fat and muscle, and at the back, the spine (*vertebral column*); this whole compartment is the *abdominal cavity*. 'Cavity' suggests an empty space, which it is not. It is completely filled with the *abdominal organs*: the stomach and intestines; the LIVER, GALL BLADDER, PANCREAS, SPLEEN, and KIDNEYS. These are all covered by a thin membrane, continuous with that which also lines the inside of the abdominal wall (PERITONEUM). This encloses the peritoneal 'cavity' that normally contains only a film of fluid. The abdominal cavity and its peritoneal lining are continuous below with those of the pelvis.   S.J.

See ALIMENTARY SYSTEM; PERITONEUM; PLATE 1.

Abortion means the end of a PREGNANCY before the FETUS can survive. It may be either spontaneous — when it is also known as *miscarriage* — or induced, when it is a deliberate termination of pregnancy.

Spontaneous abortion

Spontaneous abortion is defined in the UK as a pregnancy loss occurring before 24 completed weeks of pregnancy. Approximately 50–70% of pregnancies end in spontaneous abortion. Most of these losses are unrecognized because they occur before or at the time of the next expected menstrual period. About 15–20% of clinically diagnosed pregnancies are lost by 16 weeks. Recurrent abortion, defined as the loss of three or more consecutive pregnancies, occurs in 0.5–1% of pregnant women. Causes of spontaneous abortion may relate to the fetus, the PLACENTA, or the UTERUS. Genetic factors, developmental problems, placental problems, and infection are known causes, but in a quarter of all spontaneous abortions the cause is unknown. This may be due to lack of ability to investigate these cases.

It is generally accepted that 50% of all recognized pregnancy losses in the first 3 months are due to a genetic abnormality. Abnormalities of the placenta have probably greater importance than is realized, but information on this aspect is scanty. A number of organisms have been associated with spontaneous abortion, such as listeria, brucella infection from animals, and the rubella virus. In isolated instances fetal or placental infection with various organisms may result in spontaneous abortion, but there is no evidence of their involvement in a recurrent problem. Some cases of recurrent abortion are due to congenital abnormalities of the uterus and these may be corrected surgically; 70–80% of women with the most frequent abnormalities have successful pregnancies following surgery.

Spontaneous abortion may become evident clinically either as '*threatened*' or '*inevitable*'. A threatened abortion is said to occur when a woman bleeds from the uterus before 24 weeks of pregnancy. There are three possible outcomes: the bleeding may settle and the pregnancy continue; the fetus may die but be retained in the uterus (confirmed by an ultrasound examination) and this is known as a 'missed' abortion; a missed abortion may proceed to an inevitable abortion, with continued or intensified bleeding and expulsion of the products of conception. Bleeding may be severe, causing SHOCK; in some cases this is life-threatening and BLOOD TRANSFUSION may be required. Death occurs in a few cases where medical care is poor or absent. In the UK the death rate is of the order of 12.5 per million pregnancies.

If the pregnancy is expelled intact the abortion is said to be 'complete', but this is rare in the first 3 months of pregnancy. More commonly some material is left behind and only when it is removed surgically will bleeding cease. If this is not done, bleeding may continue and the uterus become infected, with serious consequences for the woman. Rarely in developed countries, but commonly in underdeveloped regions and where abortion laws are restrictive, infection occurs and abortion is a well-recognized cause of maternal death.

The emotional effects of an abortion vary greatly. A majority of women have feelings of depression, and there is usually associated fear and anxiety caused by the pain and bleeding and the uncertainty as to the cause. Reaction to abortion as a bereavement means that women require to grieve after the event. Often the intensity of the emotional reaction is not appreciated by the carers or by friends or relatives. Health workers should help the woman to express her grief. Women who have experienced such loss require considerable reassurance and support in a subsequent pregnancy.

Recurrent spontaneous abortion

Recurrent spontaneous abortion is a particularly distressing condition and there is very limited understanding of its causes. Genetic factors such as parental chromosome abnormalities are a major known cause which should be looked for. Anatomical factors such as uterine abnormalities account for perhaps 10–15% of recurrent loss. Hormonal factors, such as deficient production of PROGESTERONE, which is important for the maintenance of early pregnancy, are also cited — but evidence for such causes is scanty.

In some cases an immune response is mounted by the mother against the pregnancy, causing its demise. Chronic maternal disease such as diabetes and kidney disease may also be associated. SMOKING and alcohol consumption have been linked to recurrent abortion but there is no hard evidence for this.

In the case of genetic abnormalities, genetic counselling is advisable and if, for example, the abnormality is traced to the male partner, insemination of the woman with sperm from a donor (*donor insemination*, DI) may be a possible solution. An abnormally shaped uterus can be corrected by surgery. Hormonal therapy has not proved successful. In the case of an immunological cause, immunotherapy has been helpful, and in some women with no ascertainable cause

1

psychotherapy has been of value. In the event intervention may not be the best answer and it may be just as successful to wait and see.

Induced abortion: termination of pregnancy

The study of induced abortion, especially where abortion is illegal, is a major challenge in the contexts of reproductive health and women's rights.

At the International Conference on Population and Development in Cairo in 1994 the following statement was made: 'Since unsafe abortion is a major threat to the health and lives of women, research to understand and better address the determinants and consequences should be promoted'. The conference also recognized that unsafe abortion was a world-wide public health problem and agreed that each country should legislate to solve the problem. In developed countries like the UK where abortion is readily available the related mortality is extremely low — less than 1 per 100 000 procedures. In less optimal settings where women are only able to find unsafe abortion, mortality is high. World-wide, estimates vary from a minimum of 50 000 up to 150 000 abortion-related deaths per annum.

Experience from many countries confirms that permissive legislation on abortion does not increase the abortion rate: it only determines whether it is performed under safe or unsafe conditions. The restrictive legislation which some countries have, for cultural or religious reasons, prevents a reduction in the death rate and health hazards of abortion.

In the UK restrictive legislation was still in place in 1938 — the year when Mr Alec Bourne, an eminent London gynaecologist, terminated a woman's pregnancy which had resulted from rape. He was reported for this criminal offence and was prosecuted. The judge allowed the mental health of the woman to be taken into account and Bourne was acquitted, marking a changing attitude to abortion in the UK. In 1967 the Abortion Act legalized abortion under certain circumstances, and amendments were made in 1990. Currently the Act permits termination of pregnancy if two doctors:

> are of the opinion in good faith a) that the pregnancy has not exceeded its twenty-fourth week and that the continuance of the pregnancy would involve risk, greater than if the pregnancy were terminated, of injury to the physical or mental health of the pregnant woman or any existing children of her family; or b) that the termination is necessary to prevent grave permanent injury to the physical or mental health of the pregnant woman; or c) that the continuance of the pregnancy would involve risk to the life of the pregnant woman, greater than if the pregnancy were terminated; or d) that there is a substantial risk that if the child were born it would suffer from such physical or mental abnormalities as to be seriously handicapped.

It is essential that a woman who seeks abortion receive proper counselling. If she wishes her partner to be involved he may be, but this is not mandatory. This involves giving the woman as much information as possible after a medical, social, and family history has been obtained: information regarding the methods of termination, their risks, and their benefits, and alternative courses of action such as adoption, and also advice which may help to determine her real wishes. All is designed to help her to reach a decision. Certain high risk groups require special counselling: teenagers; those with genetic factor risks; cases of sexual abuse; and those seeking late terminations or repeated terminations.

Most terminations are done in the first 3 months of pregnancy. At this stage it is done surgically under an anaesthetic, by dilating the cervix and removing the pregnancy by suction or by forceps. Alternatively, up to 8 weeks or so, termination using drugs is possible, and is now common. A choice may therefore be offered. In 85% of early cases no further treatment is required as the abortion is complete. Where it is not complete surgery is required.

After 3 months it is usual to use a method of termination by administration of PROSTAGLANDINS. These drugs cause contractions of the uterus and the fetus and placenta are expelled.

Complications which may occur are bleeding, perforation of the uterus, tearing of the cervix, and sepsis — but these are rare when the procedure is properly performed. Where abortion is performed in unsafe circumstances these complications are common and have serious consequences.

Abortion has been regarded in some countries as a method of birth control. This should not be so. Abortion services should include advice on CONTRACEPTION and the better this advice is the less often will abortion be resorted to.

MALCOLM MACNAUGHTON

See also ANTENATAL DEVELOPMENT; CONTRACEPTION; PREGNANCY.

Abortion: historical and social aspects

For many centuries women finding themselves pregnant have endeavoured to implement retroactive birth control by means of abortion. This practice was often occluded from legal and medical eyes, information being passed on within a female oral subculture. However manuscripts survive from a range of historical periods which record numerous substances reputed to be abortifacients, though some are also highly toxic to the woman; and various practices have also been believed to induce miscarriage. For many centuries the law only concerned itself with pregnancy subsequent to 'quickening'. This traditional distinction and the persistent conceptualization by women of the problem as 'bringing on' menstruation, suggest that women did not experience pregnancy as an absolute, either/or, state.

The law, however, at least in Europe and North America, increasingly formulated the ending of all pregnancy as abortion, possibly reflecting developing medical ability in accurate, early recognition of conception. In England and Wales abortion initially became a statutory offence in 1803 under Lord Ellenborough's Act, at a time when the medical profession was increasingly concerning itself with previously woman-controlled areas such as obstetrics, and desirous of differentiating the medical man from the irregular practitioner. The concept of 'unlawful' abortion enabled medical practitioners to claim a right to use their clinical judgement over 'lawful' therapeutic abortion. Induced abortion, pre-antibiotics, was a significant cause of female mortality and morbidity, although many 'back street' operators were not lacking in skill. It was largely married women who patronized these, since they could more readily pass off miscarriages without need of concealment. The 'Female Pills' widely purveyed in the later nineteenth and early twentieth centuries were a successful commercial racket, with little in the way of effective ingredients.

Laws on the availability of surgical abortion have varied widely from nation to nation: medical expertise may be privileged over unlicensed operators, or operations even by regular practitioners regarded as a crime. Though legally condemned, abortion has frequently been available to those with the right contacts and able to pay. While certain religious groups, especially Roman Catholics, have strongly condemned abortion, such condemnation has not universally prevented women from seeking it. The role of popular feeling and debate has been influential in altering the law: in Britain the important legal case of Rex v. Bourne, 1938, establishing a common-law precedent for abortion on the grounds of a woman's mental, not merely physical, health, took place in the context of widespread debate and agitation for reform of the law. In the US, however, there was no such climate of opinion, and similarly idealistic and concerned abortionists paid the full legal penalty.

Abortion became legalized in many countries during the late 1960s and early 1970s. Unfortunately the overt inscription of the right to abortion in law (as opposed to something performed, if at all, within the privileged secrecy of the doctor/patient encounter) has provoked a vigorous 'backlash', particularly violent in the US. There is little evidence that abortions would be fewer if illegal; only more dangerous, and the availability of the operation more erratic and inequitable.

LESLEY A. HALL

Accommodation Optical instruments (such as microscopes, cameras, and some telescopes) work by passing light through the curved surfaces of lenses, where the light is bent (refracted) to bring it to focus at a particular point (e.g. on the film of a camera). Their power depends on the tightness of curvature of these surfaces. To adjust focus for targets at different distances, most optical devices move one or more of their lenses closer to or further from the focusing point. The human EYE contains several refractive surfaces, but it alters focus or 'accommodates' largely by changing the curvature of one of them — the front surface of the lens inside the eye. The more curved this is, the more powerful the lens becomes, focusing the eye on closer objects. And when the lens flattens, the eye focuses on more distant objects.

This is not the only way of focusing an eye. In chickens, accommodation is produced partly by changing the curvature of the cornea itself. Animals that move between air and water have a special problem, because immersion in water greatly reduces the optical power of the cornea (as anyone who has opened their eyes under water knows). Diving birds gain the extra focusing power that they need under water by squeezing the lens forward into the aperture of the very tough iris, which greatly increases the curvature of the front surface.

The lens of the human eye is a stiff gel of transparent protein, inside an elastic capsule. It is held in place by fine, elastic *zonular fibres*, which run from the equator of the lens to the muscular *ciliary body*, which runs around the inner wall of the eyeball, just behind the iris. Accommodation is controlled by the *ciliary muscle* inside the ciliary body, which encircles the lens. This muscle, which is of the 'smooth' type, is controlled by fibres of the parasympathetic division of the AUTONOMIC NERVOUS SYSTEM. When the ciliary muscle contracts, it does not squeeze the lens directly but reduces the tension of the zonular fibres, which relaxes the tension on the capsule of the lens, causing it to assume a more spherical shape, hence increasing the curvature of its front surface.

Accommodation can be prevented with eye drops containing the drug ATROPINE (*belladonna* — originally extracted from the plant deadly nightshade), which blocks the contraction of the ciliary muscle. The nerve cells that command accommodation (and pupil constriction) are in a small structure in the mid brain called the Edinger–Westphal nucleus, close to many of the cells that direct EYE MOVEMENTS.

With the exception of the first few months of life, when accommodation is not fully functional, accommodation becomes progressively less effective with age, with the ability to change lens power falling to zero at an age of about 50 years. This loss of accommodation, or *presbyopia*, is believed to be caused by changes in the stiffness of the lens proteins, rather than changes in ciliary muscle strength, or in lens size, which increases throughout life. With its accommodation frozen, the eye becomes like a cheap fixed-focus camera, which relies on the depth of field produced by a small aperture to give reasonable focus at different distances. Older people have most difficulty reading fine print (because they have to hold it far away to focus it), especially in dim illumination, when the pupil dilates and the depth of field decreases. Interestingly, people becoming presbyotic do not usually complain that things actually look blurred when held too close, but that what should be black and white looks grey.

The optical quality of the human eye is far from perfect. The great German physicist, Hermann von Helmholtz, once remarked that if he were offered an instrument with such defects by a manufacturer he would send it back — but that he was gladly hanging on to his own eyes, with all their shortcomings! One striking defect, or 'aberration', of the eye is that it does not focus light of different wavelengths in the same plane. If deep red is in sharp focus, violet will be somewhat de-focused, and vice versa. Interestingly enough, the retinal cones that are most sensitive to blue– violet light are very few and far between compared with those that are most sensitive in the yellow–green part of the spectrum (the so-called 'green' and 'red' cones), and are absent in the central *fovea* (the part of the retina that we point towards things when we look directly at them). Perhaps this is an adaptation to the impossibility of focusing all wavelengths at the same time.   STUART JUDGE

See also ATROPINE; AUTONOMIC NERVOUS SYSTEM; COLOUR BLINDNESS; EYE; REFRACTIVE ERRORS; SMOOTH MUSCLE.

Acetylcholine

Acetylcholine is a NEUROTRANSMITTER released from nerve endings (terminals) in both the peripheral and the central nervous systems. It is synthesized within the nerve terminal from choline, taken up from the tissue fluid into the nerve ending by a specialized transport mechanism. The ENZYME necessary for this synthesis (*choline acetyltransferase*) is formed in the nerve cell body and passes down the axon to its end, carried in the *axoplasmic flow*, the slow movement of intracellular substance (*cytoplasm*). Acetylcholine is stored in the nerve terminal, sequestered in small vesicles awaiting release.

When a nerve ACTION POTENTIAL reaches and invades the nerve terminal, a shower of acetylcholine vesicles is released into the junction (SYNAPSE) between the nerve terminal and the 'effector' cell which the nerve activates. This may be another nerve cell or a muscle or gland cell. Thus electrical signals are converted to chemical signals, allowing messages to be passed between nerve cells or between nerve cells and non-nerve cells. This process is termed 'chemical neurotransmission' and was first demonstrated, for nerves to the heart, by the German pharmacologist Loewi in 1921. Chemical transmission involving acetylcholine is known as 'cholinergic'.

Acetylcholine acts as a transmitter between motor nerves and the fibres of skeletal muscle at all NEUROMUSCULAR JUNCTIONS. At this type of synapse, the nerve terminal is closely opposed to the cell membrane of a muscle fibre at the so-called motor end plate. On release, acetylcholine acts almost instantly, to cause a sequence of chemical and physical events (starting with depolarization of the motor endplate) which cause contraction of the muscle fibre. This is exactly what is required for voluntary muscles in which a rapid response to a command is required. The action of acetylcholine is terminated rapidly, in around 10 milliseconds; an enzyme (*cholinesterase*) breaks the transmitter down into choline and an acetate ion. The choline is then available for re-uptake into the nerve terminal.

These same principles apply to cholinergic transmission at sites other than neuromuscular junctions, although the structure of the synapses differs. In the AUTONOMIC NERVOUS SYSTEM these include nerve-to-nerve synapses at the relay stations (*ganglia*) in both the sympathetic and the parasympathetic divisions, and the endings of parasympathetic nerve fibres on non-voluntary (*smooth*) muscle, the heart, and

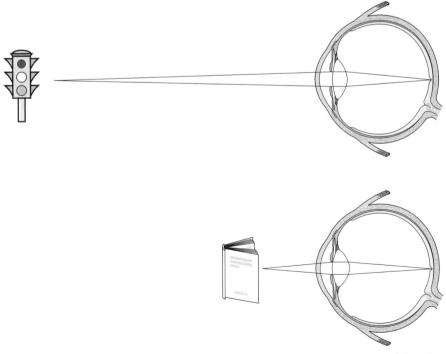

To focus on a nearby object, as when reading, the front surface of the lens becomes more curved than when looking at a distant object.

glandular cells; in response to activation of this nerve supply, smooth muscle contracts (notably in the gut), the frequency of heart beat is slowed, and glands secrete. Acetylcholine is also an important transmitter at many sites in the BRAIN at nerve-to-nerve synapses.

To understand how acetylcholine brings about a variety of effects in different cells it is necessary to understand MEMBRANE RECEPTORS. In *post-synaptic membranes* (those of the cells on which the nerve fibres terminate) there are many different sorts of receptors and some are receptors for acetylcholine. These are protein molecules that react specifically with acetylcholine in a reversible fashion. It is the complex of receptor combined with acetylcholine which brings about a biophysical reaction, resulting in the response from the receptive cell. Two major types of acetylcholine receptors exist in the membranes of cells. The type in skeletal muscle is known as '*nicotinic*'; in glands, smooth muscle, and the heart they are '*muscarinic*'; and there are some of each type in the brain. These terms are used because nicotine mimics the action of acetylcholine at nicotinic receptors, whereas muscarine, an alkaloid from the mushroom *Amanita muscaria*, mimics the action of acetylcholine at the muscarinic receptors. ALAN W. CUTHBERT

See also AUTONOMIC NERVOUS SYSTEM; NEUROTRANSMITTERS.

Achilles' heel

The 'Achilles' heel' is one's weak point, and is named for the only part of the body of the Greek hero Achilles which was vulnerable. The son of King Peleus of Thessaly and the shape-changing nymph Thetis, Achilles is the central character of Homer's great poem, the *Iliad*.

The weakness of the heel, or more accurately the tendon, of Achilles derives from the story of the unsuccessful attempt by his mother Thetis to make Achilles invulnerable. This seems to be a late addition to his biography, first found in the first-century AD Roman poet Statius. When he was still a child, and against the wishes of Peleus, Thetis held her son by the heel and dipped him in the waters of the river Styx which flows through the underworld; it was in this heel that he was to receive the wound from a poisoned arrow, which killed him. Earlier versions, while omitting this story, have another variation on the theme of the mother desperately trying to preserve her son; Thetis is said to have hidden Achilles at the court of King Lycomedes on Scyros, where he was disguised as a girl. Despite this disguise, he fell in love with the king's daughter — who bore him a son, Neoptolemus — and he was discovered by a party of Greeks sent to find him and take him with the army to Troy. In Homer, Achilles is always aware that he will die young, a premonition heightened by the death of his beloved friend Patroclus; the circumstances of his own death at the hands of the Trojan prince Paris, aided by the god Apollo, are also predicted in Homer.

The *Iliad* covers just a few weeks of the tenth year of the long period over which the Greek forces laid siege to the city of Troy. It is the 'Wrath of Achilles' — his anger at losing his slave concubine, Briseis, to Agamemnon — which forms the theme of the *Iliad*. Achilles responds to this loss by sulking in his tent, withdrawing his forces — the Myrmidons — from the combined Greek army. In terms of simple military success, Achilles is 'the best of the Achaeans', or Greeks, but he takes the heroic code of honour to extremes. For example, while revenge was a perfectly acceptable part of the code, the Greeks considered that there were limits to what counted as acceptable acts of revenge; yet when he kills the Trojan Hector, Achilles slits Hector's 'Achilles' tendons' then uses leather thongs to tie him to his chariot before proceeding to drive round the walls of Troy, watched by an audience of horrified Trojans that includes Hector's mother and father. As a final indignity, Achilles throws what is left of Hector's corpse to the dogs, but the goddess Aphrodite keeps them away. This behaviour is explicitly labelled as 'shameful' by Homer, and eventually Hector's remains are returned to the Trojans for proper burial.

In anatomical terms, 'Achilles' tendon' survives as an alternative to the formal name of *tendo calcaneus* for the thick tendon which links the calf muscles to the heel bone (the *calcaneum* from the Latin for heel). Though very far from weak, the tendon can sometimes be vulnerable to rupture during vigorous sporting activity.
HELEN KING

See PLATE 5.

See also ANKLE; FEET.

Acid–base homeostasis

All living things depend on water. Life consists of a highly complex series of chemical reactions occurring in aqueous media. Among the most important factors in the composition of these fluids are the concentrations of *hydrogen* ions and *hydroxide* ions, which determine the acidity or alkalinity of the fluid. The maintenance of suitable concentrations of these ions is called acid–base homeostasis.

The cells of the most primitive marine organisms are bathed directly by the sea. The environment of such cells is very variable, being at the mercy of the tides and winds. As evolution proceeded, organisms walled off some of this watery environment and took it as their own, to provide a specialized fluid surrounding the cells. This fluid is thus, in evolutionary terms, the 'sea within us'; it is called the *extracellular fluid*, to distinguish it from the fluid inside cells, the *intracellular fluid*. In higher animals, the extracellular fluid is further subdivided into that in the circulating blood (the *plasma*, in which the blood corpuscles are suspended) and that which is outside the walls of the blood vessels (the *interstitial fluid*, filling the interstices between the body's cells). There is continuous interchange of fluid across the walls of capillaries between the interstitial fluid and the blood plasma; this serves to mix the extracellular fluid. Small molecules and ions in solution move freely between the components of the extracellular fluid.

As animals became more advanced, control mechanisms evolved to minimize changes in the composition of the extracellular fluid, thereby providing a stable environment for the cells of the body. The importance of this was first recognized by the French physiologist Claude BERNARD (1813–78), who described the extracellular fluid as the '*milieu intérieur*' or the 'internal environment' of the body. The tendency of the body to stabilize the composition of the extracellular fluid is called HOMEOSTASIS, which means 'staying similar'. Such stability had to be achieved before higher animals could evolve. In the words of Joseph Barcroft (1938), 'To look for high intellectual development in a milieu whose properties have not become stabilized is to seek music amongst the crashings of a rudimentary wireless or the ripple patterns on the surface of the stormy Atlantic.'

Water, then, is the substrate of life. Most standard laboratory solvents act merely as vehicles and take no part in chemical reactions between chemicals dissolved in them (the solutes). Water has the remarkable property of itself participating in many of the chemical reactions that occur in it; this is because water molecules show a very weak tendency to dissociate into hydrogen ions and hydroxide ions, according to the chemical reaction:

Reaction 1

$$H_2O \rightleftharpoons H^+ + OH^-$$

| water molecule | hydrogen ion | hydroxide ion |

This chemical reaction demonstrates that, in pure water, hydrogen ions and hydroxide ions are present in equal concentrations; thus pure water is said to be *neutral*. When there are solutes present, the solution is also called neutral if the concentrations of hydrogen and hydroxide ions are the same. However, a solution is *acid* if the concentration of hydrogen ions exceeds that of hydroxide ions and *alkaline* if the concentration of hydroxide ions exceeds that of the hydrogen ions.

A hydrogen ion is a *proton* — a hydrogen atom that has lost its electron. An acid is a chemical that releases protons; it is called a *proton donor*. A base, which is a chemical that takes up protons, is known as a *proton acceptor*. If an acid is added to an equal amount of base, the protons released by the acid are all taken up by the base and the resulting solution is neutral.

Acid and base production in the body

Various chemical reactions in the body produce acids and bases: if they are simultaneously generated in equal amounts they will chemically combine and neutralize each other. If production of one or other predominates, then body fluids tend to become acid or alkaline. If the acid or base is produced continuously, a steady state can be maintained only when production is matched by the elimination of the excess acid or base from the body.

CARBON DIOXIDE is produced as one of the main end products of the aerobic METABOLISM of energy-yielding chemicals derived from the food that we eat. Carbon dioxide is not itself an acid, but in aqueous solution it reacts with water to yield hydrogen ions and bicarbonate ions, according to the chemical reaction:

Reaction 2

$$CO_2 + H_2O \rightleftharpoons H^+ + HCO_3^-$$

carbon dioxide — water — hydrogen ion — bicarbonate ion

Metabolizing cells continuously liberate carbon dioxide, and therefore acid, into our body fluids. The carbon dioxide diffuses to the blood, where a little remains dissolved but most is chemically combined. When the blood reaches the LUNGS the carbon dioxide is released and diffuses out of the blood into the gas in the alveoli of the lungs. The refreshing of the alveolar gas by breathing results in the carbon dioxide being expelled from the body and into the atmosphere. Since carbon dioxide can be eliminated as a gas, it is called a *volatile acid*. All other acids in the body are called *non-volatile acids*, or *fixed acids*.

Non-volatile acids. When a healthy person exercises maximally, the exercising muscles cannot obtain all the energy that they need by aerobic metabolism (using oxygen) and must in addition metabolize anaerobically (i.e. without oxygen). This results in the breakdown of glucose to *lactic acid*, via a series of chemical reactions that release energy but do not require oxygen. This is a normal physiological situation in which excess non-volatile acid is released into the body fluids. The excess acid is subsequently taken up from the blood by the liver where most of the lactic acid is reconverted to glucose.

Hydrogen ions are produced as an end product of the oxidation of sulphur-containing AMINO ACIDS derived from proteins in the diet; this yields sulphuric acid. The metabolism of phospholipids, nucleic acids, and other phosphorus-containing chemicals yields phosphoric acid. Certain organic acids are formed during the metabolism of carbohydrates and fats; normally these acids are further oxidized to carbon dioxide and water, but in certain circumstances they may accumulate.

A pathological example is *diabetes mellitus*, which has been called 'starvation in the presence of plenty'. Here, although the concentration of glucose in the blood is high, the tissues are unable to metabolize it properly. Instead of using glucose, the body derives energy from excessive breakdown of lipids to yield so-called *ketone bodies*, including aceto-acetic and β-hydroxybutyric acids. An excess of these fixed acids accumulates in the body.

Surplus alkali accumulates when a person persistently vomits gastric contents. Acid is secreted into the gastric contents by cells in the wall of the stomach as part of the digestive process. This secretion of acid is accompanied by an equal movement of alkali from the acid-secreting cells in the opposite direction into the body fluids, so loss of acid in vomitus results in a surplus of alkali in the body.

Defence of hydrogen ion concentration. The body has several lines of defence to accommodate surplus acid or base. The extracellular fluid, the contents of the cells, and BONE all provide chemical *buffering*. A buffer is a system of chemicals that combines with an excess of hydrogen ions or hydroxide ions. Buffering therefore tends to stabilize the hydrogen ion concentration. It minimizes changes but does not alter the total acid or base load in the body. The final disposal of surplus fixed acid or base may be via metabolic pathways in the body, as described for lactic acid in the healthy exercising person. If such mechanisms are not available, then the excess acid or base must be expelled from the body, via the lungs and KIDNEYS — the homeostatic processes of respiratory compensation and renal compensation.

Respiratory compensation. The aeration of the lungs influences the hydrogen ion concentration of the blood by regulating the amount of carbon dioxide expelled from the body into the atmosphere. Other things being equal, an increase in the volume of air breathed in and out leads to a washing-out of carbon dioxide from the body, and hence a lowering of the hydrogen ion concentration of the body. In reaction 2, the concentration of carbon dioxide falls so the reaction is driven to the left, with a reduction in the number of hydrogen ions in the body. Conversely, a reduction of breathing results in a rise in hydrogen ion concentration in the body.

In a healthy person, the concentration of carbon dioxide in the arterial blood is usually held constant by appropriate aeration of the lungs. The depth and rate of breathing are controlled by special centres in the brain, which influence the nerves that cause contraction and relaxation of the muscles of respiration. In a person with a surplus of fixed acid in the body, such as in maximal muscular exercise or in uncontrolled diabetes mellitus, the shift towards acidity (detected by CHEMORECEPTORS — specialized sensory structures) stimulates breathing. As a result, the concentration of carbon dioxide falls below normal. This in effect removes some of the excess hydrogen ions. In this way breathing can help to bring the hydrogen ion concentration back towards normal, despite the excess of fixed acid in the body. This is *respiratory compensation*.

Renal compensation. Whereas the lungs regulate the amount of *volatile acid* (carbon dioxide) in the body, the kidneys regulate other acids and bases by excreting acidic or alkaline urine. In healthy people on a mixed diet, although the food itself is neutral, its metabolism releases an excess of non-volatile acid, and the kidneys must match this by excreting acidic urine as a normal necessity. The food of vegetarians yields an excess of base and the urine of healthy vegetarians is alkaline.

In patients with renal damage the contribution of the kidneys is compromised; a feature of renal failure, in a person on a mixed diet, is an accumulation of acid in the body.

The hydrogen ion concentration in aqueous solutions

One way of expressing the concentration of a substance is in moles of the substance per litre of solution. A mole of a substance is its molecular weight in grams. For hydrogen ions, the concentration is conventionally described as a *pH* value: the pH is the negative logarithm of the hydrogen ion concentration expressed in moles per litre. As the hydrogen ion concentration of a solution becomes higher, its pH becomes lower — more acidic. In a neutral solution at a temperature of 25°C, the hydrogen ion concentration is 10^{-7} moles per litre, or 100 nanomoles/litre (1 nanomole = 10^{-9} mole). This corresponds to a pH value of 7.0. In a neutral solution at 37°C, the hydrogen ion concentration is 157 nanomoles/litre. In the arterial blood plasma of a normal person at rest, the hydrogen ion concentration usually lies in the range 35 to 45 nanomoles/litre, with an average of 40. The hydrogen ion concentration of plasma is therefore normally about a quarter of that for a neutral solution at body temperature. A rise in plasma hydrogen ion concentration towards that of a neutral solution will result in death in most people. By contrast, the hydrogen ion concentration of the intracellular fluid is normally close to that of a neutral solution.

The range of hydrogen ion concentration in disease

In persons with acid–base disorders, hydrogen ion concentration may be as low as 20 or as high as 80 nanomoles/litre, this being the usually tolerable range for survival. Thus a 4-fold range is compatible with life. This is a much larger variation than the range tolerated for certain other chemicals, for instance sodium ions, chloride ions, and water itself. For short periods of time, it is possible for the hydrogen ion concentration to go beyond these limits, particularly on the acid side.

Enzymes and hydrogen ion concentration. Ultimately the regulation of hydrogen ion concentration is important in keeping conditions ideal for the biological catalysts, ENZYMES. These enzymes are essential for the chemical processes of life, both inside cells and in the extracellular fluids. Enzymes consist of complex protein molecules: there are sites on these molecules that attract and release hydrogen ions. Enzymic activity depends on the molecule being in the correct state of ionization; if an enzyme is associated with an excess of hydrogen ions or has lost many hydrogen ions, its enzymic activity is reduced or abolished. This is why enzymes operate optimally at a given hydrogen ion concentration. Enzymes on the surfaces of cells, which are bathed in extracellular fluid, operate optimally at the hydrogen ion concentration of extracellular fluid. Intracellular enzymes operate optimally at the hydrogen ion concentration of intracellular fluid.

Effects of disturbances of hydrogen ion concentration. In disease states, deviation from normal hydrogen ion concentration usually occurs in association with other serious pathological processes, and it may be difficult to specify the effects of altered hydrogen ion concentration alone. With a high hydrogen ion concentration, there is a widespread relaxation of SMOOTH MUSCLE, including the muscle in the walls of BLOOD VESSELS: this results in a severe drop in arterial blood pressure, with circulatory collapse. When elevation of hydrogen ion concentration is prolonged, minerals are leached from bones, causing them to become weak mechanically; the condition of OSTEOPOROSIS.

A low hydrogen ion concentration occurs as a result of overbreathing, in which carbon dioxide is blown off excessively in the lungs. The condition occurs in certain otherwise normal people who overbreathe as a reaction to stress. A reduction in hydrogen ion concentration unveils sites on protein molecules that attract positive ions. Other positive ions then tend to attach to these binding sites instead of hydrogen ions. An ion of importance in this respect is calcium; a lowering of hydrogen ions leads to a lowering of the concentration in the body fluids of calcium ions, the condition of *hypocalcaemia*. This leads to an increase in the excitability of nerve fibres, resulting in the occurrence of spontaneous action potentials. These cause *hypocalcaemic tetany* — involuntary uncoordinated contractions of skeletal muscles — bizarre subjective sensations, and numbness.

The balance of hydrogen and hydroxide ions influences our bodily functions out of all proportion to the minute concentrations of these ions in biological fluids. The adverse effects arising from disturbances of hydrogen ion concentration are due to interference with the normal harmonious interaction of the many thousands of enzymes on which life depends.

OLIVER HOLMES

Further reading

Holmes, O. (1993). *Human acid–base physiology.* Chapman and Hall Medical, London.

See also BODY FLUIDS; CARBON DIOXIDE; ENZYMES; HOMEOSTASIS; HYPERVENTILATION; KIDNEYS; RESPIRATION.

Acrobatics The specialized art of jumping, tumbling, and balancing, requiring agility and skilful control of the body. The word derives from the Greek *akrobatos*, which may be translated 'walking on tiptoe', but which literally means 'to go to the highest point' (*akros*: highest; *batos*, from the verb for 'to go'). While the etymology is Greek, the performing art of acrobatics has roots in ancient Chinese culture, where it emerged in tribal rituals related to daily activities. Work, intertribal relations, and religious sacrifices all had their own corresponding

acrobatic movements as the art developed alongside music, song, and dance. Acrobatics has maintained its status as a spectacular bodily art; complex gymnastic feats are now often performed with apparatus such as balls, unicycles, trampolines, tightropes, and trapezes.

DEBRA HAWHEE

Action potentials govern our lives. These are the electrical signals that are transmitted along our NERVE and MUSCLE fibres. They are essential for the communication of information to, from, and within the BRAIN. Your ability to read this page and to understand its message, to laugh and cry, to think and feel, to see and hear, and to move your muscles, depends on action potentials.

Each action potential (also called an impulse or 'spike') is a transient change in the voltage (electrical potential) across the CELL MEMBRANE. In nerve fibres, action potentials are brief (lasting less than 1 millisecond) and are said to be 'all-or-nothing', because they always have pretty much the same amplitude (voltage change), regardless of the intensity of the stimulus that sets them off. Without the capacity to produce these voltage pulses, a nerve could not transmit information over more than a very short distance, because they are such poor electrical conductors that a voltage change at one point rapidly decays as it spreads away from that point. Action potentials are, therefore, essential for signals to be sent over long distances without loss. The use of all-or-nothing pulses means that information has to be coded in *digital* form (in terms of the frequency of the impulses) rather than in *analogue* form (variation in amplitude). The frequency of nerve impulses varies with the signal strength — for example, with the intensity of sound in the case of the auditory nerves, or with the amount of pressure on the skin for cutaneous nerve fibres. The stronger the stimulus, the greater the number of action potentials per second, up to a normal maximum of a few hundred per second. A similar strategy (frequency coding rather than amplitude coding) is used by engineers to send light signals along fibre optic cables.

All cells, including nerve and muscle cells, have an electrical gradient across their cell membranes, with the inside of the cell being negative with respect to the outside at rest. This is known as the *resting potential*, and it is due to the unequal distribution of salts in the intracellular and extracellular fluids. Potassium ions are more concentrated inside the cell, while sodium ions are higher in concentration outside. Left to themselves, these ion concentrations would tend to equalize out: if the cell membrane were to be punctured, potassium would diffuse out of the cell, while sodium would move in, until eventually their intracellular and extracellular concentrations would equilibrate. This does not happen, however, because the cell membrane itself is impermeable to ions like sodium and potassium. Instead, the movement of ions across the membrane is restricted to tiny pores, known as ION

CHANNELS, whose opening and closing is tightly controlled. At rest, the sodium channels are closed, but some potassium channels are open. Potassium ions therefore tend to move out of the cell down their concentration gradient, and because they are positively charged, this makes the inside of the cell around 70–80 mV more negative than the outside. The whole system is then roughly in balance, because the negativity inside tends to resist further efflux of potassium ions. There is, however, a very slight leakage of sodium ions into the cell. Over the long run, this is opposed by so-called *sodium pumps* — protein molecules in the membrane that use energy to push sodium ions out of the cell, in exchange for potassium ions moving in. This quite complex equilibrium is, then, the origin of the resting potential.

By the beginning of the twentieth century, physiologists had discovered that the action potential involves a temporary *reversal* of the electrical gradient across the nerve cell membrane — the inside of the cell rapidly becomes positive (*depolarization*) and then equally rapidly reverts to its negative resting state (*repolarization*). Studies of the giant axon of the squid (the motor nerve that connects to the muscles of propulsion), by Alan Hodgkin and Andrew Huxley in the Marine Biological Laboratories at Plymouth, England, in the 1940s, showed that this is due to time-dependent changes in the permeability of the cell membrane to sodium and potassium ions. World War II broke out before they could write up their results and it was not until 1952 that they published a series of seminal papers that were to win them the NOBEL PRIZE in 1963. Subsequently, a new technique (*patch clamping*), invented by the German physiologists Erwin Neher and Bert Sakmann (also Nobel Prize winners, in 1991), provided insight into the molecular actions of the ion channels that underlie the action potential.

Action potentials can be triggered by any local depolarization of a nerve that exceeds a certain threshold (usually about 10 mV but sometimes up to 50 mV). In the laboratory, brief electrical stimulation can be employed to set off an action potential at any point in a nerve or muscle fibre. However, in normal circumstances, impulses are usually initiated only in SENSE ORGANS and in the *axon hillock* — the point at which the nerve axon emerges from the cell body of a neuron. In SENSORY RECEPTORS, physical or chemical stimulation triggers changes in the membrane that result in local depolarization. In the cell body, depolarization occurs when an excitatory NEUROTRANSMITTER is released by the terminals of nerve fibres ending in synapses on the cell. The local depolarization directly influences specialized ion channels, producing an initial opening of 'voltage-gated' sodium channels, followed shortly afterwards by opening of voltage-gated potassium channels. Because the sodium channels open more quickly than the potassium channels there is an initial inward flow of sodium ions. The positive charge that they carry produces a *further* membrane depolarization, which activates additional sodium channels, so depolarizing the membrane even further. This explosive reaction causes the rapid initial phase of the impulse, reversing the internal potential.

The amplitude of the action potential (which is typically more than a tenth of a volt) is limited by two processes. First, the sodium channels enter a specialized closed state known as the inactivated state, which curtails the depolarizing flow of sodium ions. Secondly, voltage-gated potassium channels open and the resulting outward potassium current returns the membrane potential to its resting level. The changes in potential that make up an action potential involve the movement of very small numbers of sodium and potassium ions, but, in the long run, the ion concentration gradients would degrade unless restored by the sodium–potassium pump.

Other kinds of ions, flowing through their own specialized channels, may contribute to the action potentials of nerve and muscle fibres. For example, calcium entry plays a part in the action potentials of heart muscle, and chloride flow is important in the electrical activity of skeletal muscle. As might be expected, mutations in the genes that encode ion channel proteins produce a range of nerve and muscle diseases in man. These include EPILEPSY, cardiac conduction abnormalities, and the muscle disorders known as myotonias.

Nerve axons come in two varieties: *myelinated* and *unmyelinated*. MYELIN is a fatty sheath that surrounds the myelinated fibres and allows faster transmission of nerve impulses. Action potentials race along myelinated nerve fibres at rates of up to 100 metres/second or more, but can barely manage 1 metre/second in many unmyelinated fibres. The rate at which action potentials are transmitted also depends on temperature, and conduction slows down when the nerve is cooled. This explains why your fingers have difficulty in buttoning your jacket on a frosty morning and why 'cold-blooded' animals like insects and lizards, which do not maintain a constant body temperature, move around more slowly in the cold.   FRANCES ASHCROFT

Further reading
Hodgkin, A. L. (1963). *The conduction of the nervous impulse.* Liverpool University Press.

See also SENSORY RECEPTORS; REFRACTORY PERIOD; SYNAPSE.

Acupuncture is perhaps most helpfully defined in general as the insertion of one or more needles into the body with therapeutic intent. The advantage of this wide definition is that it covers the many current different variants of this ancient practice, without being specifically tied to any one of them. At the broadest level, the most critical difference of approach lies between classical Oriental forms of acupuncture and those rooted more in modern Western biomedicine. Most of the main differences in practice are based on this dichotomy, although there

are significant distinctions both between and within these two traditions, in terms of such issues as the model used to explain the operation of acupuncture and the scope of its practice. There are also debates in both traditions about the number and location of the acupuncture points themselves.

What is not in dispute, however, is that acupuncture has a history spanning well over 2000 years, taking its origin from ancient China. One of the oldest known books on acupuncture here is the Yellow Emperor's classic of internal medicine (the *Nei Jing*), which is held to date back many hundreds of years BC. From China, acupuncture spread to such local cultural areas

as Korea and Japan, where it became incorporated into mainstream medicine by the seventh and eighth centuries AD. By the sixteenth and seventeenth centuries knowledge of it had reached Europe, mainly through missionaries and ships' surgeons who had witnessed its use in the East, but who had only a rudimentary understanding of its operation.

In the early nineteenth century it began to be practised by a number of doctors in Britain and the US. It went into something of a decline in most countries in the Western world thereafter — and even, briefly, in China in the modernization period under the Kuomintang in the first half of the twentieth century. However, the

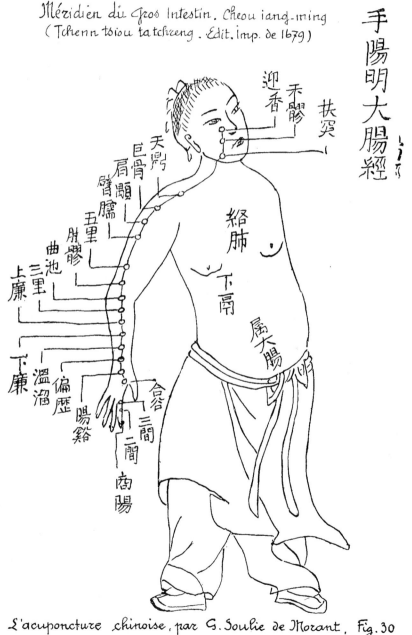

Chinese acupuncture points showing the meridian of the large intestine. Mary Evans Picture Library.

advent of 'ping-pong' diplomacy between China and the West in the first half of the 1970s, associated with dramatic television pictures of open-heart surgery being carried out by the Chinese with the use of 'acupuncture anaesthesia', led to spiralling public interest. This interest has continued to grow in both medical and non-medical circles up to the present day, alongside other complementary and alternative therapies—resulting in increasing numbers of acupuncturists and its widespread employment in the West in pain clinics and other settings.

In its classic application within traditional Chinese medicine, acupuncture is seen as being underpinned by the interplay of yin and yang; disease is seen as deriving from the disequilibrium of such opposing forces. In this conceptualization, drawing on Taoist philosophy, acupuncture treatment for the sick is used to correct imbalances and to maintain equilibrium in the healthy to prevent illness. This involves manipulating the patient's *Qi*, the life force, by stimulating needles strategically placed at selected acupuncture points which lie on the 12 main *meridians* that run along the body and connect with central internal organs. Typically, the needles are placed in sites at a distance from the condition itself. In this frame of reference — and as employed in China and many other Oriental societies — acupuncture is seen as something of a panacea, which can deal with a wide range of disorders spanning from asthma and ulcers to depression and angina.

Acupuncture, though, is characteristically used very differently in Western biomedicine — mainly as a more narrowly defined remedy for pain and for addictions of various kinds. The traditional Chinese philosophies about acupuncture are usually seen as problematic within this framework, not least because there is no consistent correspondence between biomedical conceptions of the physical structures of the body and the classical acupuncture points and the meridians along which they are held to run. Indeed, within more Westernized approaches, needling often occurs *in situ* rather than at a distance. Other explanations of its operation have also typically been sought by Western doctors, generally based on neurophysiology. Initially the 'gate-control' theory was widely adopted, centred on the notion that the stimulation of the larger nerve fibres can block pain. More recently, however, emphasis has shifted to the notion that endorphins — opiates of a type naturally produced by the body — are released by acupuncture, thus giving rise to its analgesic effects. However, neither theory adequately explains the long-term relief of chronic pain nor the wider therapeutic effects traditionally claimed for acupuncture.

From a conventional Western perspective, many studies of acupuncture to date have been methodologically unsound — although its proponents might point to the difficulties of evaluating its efficacy through randomized trials in view of its holistic, classical Oriental origins. Current evidence based on trials of its efficacy in treating pain is growing, though, even if rigorous trials of acupuncture for other disorders are few and far between and are not always supportive of the claimed benefits. Another important issue in the West is the regulation of acupuncture practice and whether it should be formally restricted either to doctors or to those appropriately trained in acupuncture, given that it is an invasive technique. In untutored hands, acupuncture has occasionally given rise to a number of complications, such as Hepatitis B and AIDS, and the puncturing of the heart and lungs, which carry potentially fatal consequences.

It should be stressed in conclusion that, even as discussed here, there are difficulties in clearly defining the boundaries of acupuncture. There are, for example, associated forms of treatment which do not employ needles, but which use acupuncture points. These range from the traditional application of finger pressure, through shiatsu and the burning of a herb, moxa, at such points, to the stimulation of acupuncture points using electrodes, as with techniques such as TENS (*transcutaneous electrical nerve stimulation*) in modern medical practice. Equally, there are surgical techniques, like suturing and the injection of medicinal substances, that are closer to the definition of acupuncture in so far as they involve needles, but are not conventionally regarded as such. Notwithstanding these definitional issues, though, acupuncture in both its traditional and modern forms looks as if it will continue to be important in the foreseeable future in both the contemporary Western and Eastern worlds, where it is being subjected to increasing use and scientific study.   MIKE SAKS

Further reading

Lewith, G., Kenyon, J., and Lewis, P. (1996). *Complementary medicine: an integrated approach.* Oxford University Press.

Lu Gwei-Djen and Needham, J. (1980). *Celestial lancets: a history and rationale of acupuncture and moxa.* Cambridge University Press.

Mole, P. (1992). *Acupuncture: energy balancing for body, mind and spirit.* Element, Longmead.

Saks, M. (1995). *Professions and the public interest: medical power, altruism and alternative medicine.* Routledge, London.

Adam's rib In the second account of the creation of humankind in Genesis (2: 21–3), Eve or 'woman' was formed from the rib (or 'side') of Adam (that is, 'man') while he was in a deep sleep. In this account woman was created as a counterpart to man, for it was not good for man to be alone (Genesis 2: 18). God split Adam in two, and thus woman was the other half of man; this suggests the creation of an androgynous Adam initially which came to be split into 'man' and 'woman'. By contrast, the first account of the creation of humankind, in Genesis 1: 26–30, has 'Adam' divided into two human beings, male and female, from the beginning: 'And God created the adam in His image, in the image of God, He created him, male and female, He created them.' These two humans have dominion over the earth.

The second creation account, in which Eve was formed from Adam's rib, is clearly not just an account of woman born of man, but rather of Adam split into two. Nevertheless, it has been used as biblical evidence to justify the subordination of woman within both Judaism and Christianity (especially when coupled with the story related in Genesis 3, in which Eve was tempted by the serpent, and in turn tempted Adam, to eat the fruit and disobey God; her punishment was pain in childbirth and subordination to her husband, along with expulsion from the Garden of Eden with Adam). This story may have jibed well with Galenic and Aristotlean views of the female body as an inferior version of the male body, rather than a separate 'sex' — scientific views which prevailed until the eighteenth century in the West. By contrast, modern scientific views, based on the sequence of embryological developments, see the female as the norm of humankind, and male anatomical difference as a modification of the female.

The creation of Eve from Adam's rib was a popular visual image in medieval church and cathedral sculpture. In modern culture 'Adam's rib' is a phrase sometimes used to represent the battle of the sexes, as illustrated by the 1950 film of that title. Spencer Tracy and Katherine Hepburn star as married lawyers on opposite sides of the courtroom, in the trial of a woman charged with the attempted murder of the lover of her philandering husband, and, as a result, battling each other in the minefield of sexual politics not only at work but also at home.

In Judaism, according to a midrash, Eve was God's second attempt at creating woman. Lilith, God's first attempt, had left man after only a short time because of a dispute with him about her equality, which she was unwilling to forgo. She flew away and vanished into the air. She, like Adam, was made out of the dust of the ground, and she derived her rights from their identical origin.

In Islam, Eve is not mentioned by name in the Quran, but rather only as Adam's wife. However, various legends, probably of Rabbinic and Syriac origin, refer to Hawwa (the Arabic for Eve) by name and describe her creation from Adam's rib, the punishment both she and Adam received, and their travels over the earth, including pilgrimage to Mecca, where they are both said to be buried.

JANE SHAW

See also CREATION MYTHS.

Addiction The consumption of any psychoactive drug, legal or illegal, can be thought of as comprising three stages: *use, abuse,* and *addiction.* Initially the user may consume the drug simply to obtain the resulting pleasurable or other beneficial effects. If use of the drug then escalates to the point where it is interfering with the ability of the user to function normally, use may turn into abuse, and if drug consumption increases further the user may become addicted. People can also become addicted to other pleasurable activities, including gambling, computer games, exercise, surfing the Internet, or sex.

The terms 'abuse' and 'addiction', however, have been defined and re-defined over the years. Addiction used to be a term used to describe only those conditions in which terminating use leads to unpleasant physical signs of withdrawal. These are particularly prominent in regular users of such 'hard drugs' as heroin and cocaine, and in alcoholics. The most commonly accepted current modern system of diagnosis is that published by the American Psychiatric Association, in the *Diagnostic and Statistical Manual of Mental Disorders (DSM-IV)*, (Washington DC, 1994). This uses the term *substance dependence* instead of 'addiction' and defines it as follows:

DSM-IV Criteria for Substance Dependence (American Psychiatric Association, 1994) A maladaptive pattern of substance abuse, leading to clinically significant impairment or distress, as manifested by three (or more) of the following, occurring at any time in the same 12-month period:

(1) *Tolerance, as defined by either of the following:*

  (a) *A need for markedly increased amount of the substance to achieve intoxication or desired effect.*

  (b) *Markedly diminished effect with continued use of the same amount of the substance.*

(2) *Withdrawal, as defined by either of the following:*

  (a) *The characteristic withdrawal syndrome for the substance.*

  (b) *The same (or a closely related) substance is taken to relieve or avoid withdrawal symptoms.*

(3) *The substance is often taken in larger amounts or over a longer period than was intended.*

(4) *There is a persistent desire or unsuccessful efforts to cut down or control substance use.*

(5) *A great deal of time is spent in activities to obtain the substance (e.g. visiting multiple doctors or driving long distances), use the substance (e.g. chain-smoking), or recover from its effects.*

(6) *Important social, occupational, or recreational activities are given up or reduced because of substance use.*

(7) *The substance use is continued despite knowledge of having a persistent or recurrent physical or psychological problem that is likely to have been caused or exacerbated by the substance (e.g. current cocaine use despite recognition of cocaine-induced depression or continued drinking despite recognition that an ulcer was made worse by alcohol consumption).*

This new way of thinking about drug-dependence is significantly different from much of the earlier work in this field. It means that neither physical dependence nor tolerance need necessarily be present to make the diagnosis of 'substance dependence'. The diagnosis can be made simply on the grounds of psychological dependence. This removes, for example, some of the confusion from previous debates over whether tobacco smoking is 'addictive'. Even though it does not lead to tolerance or physical dependence, smokers find it very difficult to quit, as do many gamblers, athletes, and surfers of the Internet.   LESLIE L. IVERSEN

See also ALCOHOLISM; DRUG ABUSE; NICOTINE; SMOKING.

Adenosine triphosphate (ATP):

sometimes called 'the spark of life'. Any bodily movement powered by voluntary or involuntary muscle; other cellular movements such as the migration of white blood cells; the swimming of sperm; and even the contraction of hair cells in the inner ear need a supply of free energy. But so too does the transport of molecules from one body compartment to another, and the synthesis of all biomolecules required for growth, repair, or maintenance of bodily functions. ATP is an energy-rich molecule, which releases free energy when it is broken down to either ADP (*adenosine diphosphate*) or AMP (*adenosine monophosphate*). This reaction is usually stimulated by enzymes collectively called ATP-ases. Even a sedentary adult breaks down 40 kg/day of ATP and the rate of consumption rises to 0.5 kg/minute during strenuous exercise. But cells do not store large amounts of ATP, so it must be continually replenished. The energy that must be put back to reconstruct ATP from ADP is supplied by the oxidation (burning) of foods.   ALAN W. CUTHBERT

Adolescence

The period of transition from childhood to adulthood. Although sometimes described as beginning in parallel with FERTILITY or PUBERTY and ending with maturity and independence, adolescence has a very variable and imprecise duration. The onset of adolescence cannot be pinpointed in physiological terms, although it is influenced by the same SEX HORMONES and refers to the same general period as physical sexual development. It represents a complex and sometimes disturbing psychological transition, accompanying the requirement for the accepted social behaviour of the particular adult culture.   S.J.

See DEVELOPMENT AND GROWTH; MENARCHE; PUBERTY.

Adrenal glands

There are two adrenal glands, one sitting on top of each of the KIDNEYS. They are pyramidal in shape and weigh about 4 g each. Their presence was recognized as early as the late sixteenth century, but it was not until 1805 that Cuvier reported that the adrenal was made up of two regions, the cortex on the outside and an inner medulla. Fifty years later, a Guy's Hospital physician, Thomas Addison, showed that the adrenal glands were necessary for life, by identifying them as the site of damage in a previously mysterious and ultimately fatal illness, which became known as Addison's disease.

The adrenal cortex is known now to have three distinct regions: the *zona glomerulosa*, *zone fasciculata*, and *zona reticularis*. The first of these regions produces the steroid *aldosterone*, while another steroid hormone, *cortisol*, is produced by the other two regions. The cells which make up all of these regions are full of lipid droplets containing CHOLESTEROL, which can be converted into the steroid hormones.

Aldosterone, by acting on the kidneys, controls the SALT content of the body — by which means it also indirectly controls the blood pressure. The amount of aldosterone produced is controlled by other substances, including a protein from the kidney known as *renin*. Specialized cells in the kidney, which form the *juxtaglomerular apparatus*, are very sensitive to changes in BLOOD PRESSURE — well placed for this function by being wrapped around arterioles. If there is a fall in blood pressure, for example when getting out of bed in the morning, this is sensed by these cells and they respond by increasing the amount of renin put out into the bloodstream. Renin is an enzyme that converts the protein *angiotensinogen* to angiotensin I which is converted to angiotensin II. This in turn stimulates more aldosterone to be produced by the adrenal cortex; the aldosterone acts on the kidneys to retain more *salt*, and the salt is followed by *water*; both the salt and the water are reabsorbed into the blood and the resulting increase in the volume of the blood helps to restore the blood pressure to normal. Abnormally high production of aldosterone (*hyperaldosteronism*) causes excessive retention of salt and water in the body. This results in OEDEMA and high blood pressure. If insufficient aldosterone is produced (*hypoaldosteronism*) there is a loss of water and salt which causes a fall in blood pressure, heart and kidney abnormalities, and general weakness.

Cortisol acts on cells in many tissues in the body and influences general METABOLISM, BLOOD PRESSURE, and appetite. The amount of cortisol produced is controlled by another hormone, *adrenocorticotrophic hormone* (ACTH), secreted by the PITUITARY gland. This secretion in turn is controlled by *corticotrophin-releasing hormone* (CRH) from the hypothalamus. CRH secretion responds to signals from elsewhere in the brain, but both CRH and ACTH secretion are also influenced by the amount of cortisol in the blood. A major stimulus to this whole sequence of hormone secretions is STRESS. The biggest increase in the amount of cortisol produced by the adrenal glands is seen during surgery, although modern anaesthetics minimize the increase. Anxiety such as waiting for the beginning of a race or examinations also causes an increase in cortisol production. Cortisol is therefore a key component of the 'fight or flight' reaction of the individual in moments of crisis. The condition of cortisol excess is known as *Cushing's syndrome* after Harvey Cushing, the American neurosurgeon who, in 1932, described a condition associated with obesity and stretch marks (*striae*) around the abdomen, a round rosy face, hypertension, muscle weakness, diabetes, and increased hair growth on the face and body. These changes are attributable mainly to the action of cortisol on fat and protein in the body, although the growth of hair is due to an excess of the weak androgenic steroids also produced by the adrenal cortex. The features of this condition are associated with the presence of high levels of cortisol in the blood over a long period; it can be due either to overstimulation of the adrenal cortex by an excessive secretion of ACTH from a tumour of the anterior pituitary (the context in which Cushing encountered it), or to an abnormal growth of cortisol-secreting tissue in the adrenals themselves. Prolonged medication with corticosteroids can also mimic the syndrome.

Abnormally *low* levels of cortisol (*hypocortisolism*), result in a general feeling of being unwell, with tiredness, vomiting, nausea, and weight loss. A person in this condition is unable to cope with stress and liable to collapse with relatively minor injury or insult. Because there is insufficient cortisol in the blood to inhibit the secretion of ACTH, this hormone is produced in very high amounts and causes the skin to become dark or 'bronzed'.

There can be loss of secretion of both cortisol and aldosterone if there is destruction of the adrenal glands by tumour or infection. This condition is known as *Addison's disease*, following its elegant description by Thomas Addison in 1855.

The adrenal medulla makes up about 10% of the substance of the adrenal glands and is essentially and developmentally a part of the sympathetic division of the autonomic nervous system. It consists of 'chromaffin cells' (so named because of their affinity for chromium) and their main product is ADRENALINE (also known as *epinephrine*), which is involved in the fight or flight reaction along with cortisol. More adrenaline is produced in times of stress, by the stimulating action of sympathetic nerves directly upon the chromaffin cells. Adrenaline was the first hormone to be discovered, in 1894 — an event which encouraged the search for similar chemical mediators in the body, and led to the creation of the specialty of *endocrinology*. Unlike cortisol, which is produced exclusively in the adrenal cortex, adrenaline is produced in other parts of the body, including the brain, as well as in the adrenal medulla. Like cortisol, adrenaline has widespread actions at many sites in the body, including the heart, lungs, and blood vessels, facilitating an increase in the supply of nutrients and oxygen. It also redeploys necessary fuels very rapidly, in readiness for immediate action if required: acting for example in the liver to enhance the release of glucose into the blood. However, because adrenaline is produced in other areas of the body, removing the medulla does not seem to be a critical threat to life, though there does seem to be benefit in having adrenaline produced from the medulla at times of acute stress. NORADRENALINE (norepinephrine), better known and most important as a neurotransmitter at sympathetic nerve endings, is also secreted by the medulla, along with adrenaline, but in much smaller amounts.

None of the adrenal hormones are released at a constant rate, but in amounts which change in response to various stimuli throughout the day. In addition, in the case of cortisol and to a certain extent aldosterone, there is a gradual change of background levels in the blood over each 24-hour period. This pattern of release is called a circadian rhythm, and is linked to the sleep–wake cycle of the individual — the 'BODY CLOCK'. In the normal individual the greatest amounts of cortisol are released at about 8 o'clock in the morning; the level in the blood gradually falls during the day so that the lowest levels are found at about midnight. ACTH also shows a circadian rhythm reaching maximum levels in the blood just before those of cortisol. The circadian rhythm of aldosterone is of much smaller amplitude than that of cortisol. Changing the times a person is asleep or awake will change the pattern of secretion; if shift workers sleep during the day and are awake at night then the circadian rhythm will be displaced by about 12 hours, with the highest blood levels of cortisol occurring in the early evening and the lowest levels about mid-day. Similar changes occur when travelling across time zones. The shift in the circadian rhythm occurs gradually over a period of several days

Corticosteroid therapy

Treatment of a variety of conditions by synthetic corticosteroids became common from the latter half of the twentieth century. They have been invaluable in suppressing adverse reactions to curative drugs, such as in the treatment of tuberculosis and other life-threatening illnesses; also in controlling inflammatory and allergic conditions, notably rheumatoid arthritis, asthma, and some skin diseases. It follows, however, from the normal control of cortisol secretion, that when the level of corticosteroids in the blood is deliberately raised by medication, the secretion of ACTH from the pituitary is suppressed. This becomes a problem if treatment is suddenly withdrawn, leaving the person liable to collapse under stress because there is no ACTH to stimulate the adrenal glands to produce their own cortisol.   M. WHEELER

See PLATE 7.

See also AUTONOMIC NERVOUS SYSTEM; BODY CLOCK; BODY FLUIDS; STEROIDS.

Adrenaline (also called *epinephrine*), along with *noradrenaline* (*norepinephrine*) and *dopamine*, are CATECHOLAMINES (substances containing a dihydroxy phenyl grouping with the hydroxy groups in adjacent positions). All three are released at some nerve terminals to act as NEUROTRANSMITTERS, but adrenaline is also found in the *adrenal medulla* and in *chromaffin cells* and can be released from these sites into the circulating blood to have effects throughout the body. Adrenaline is synthesized in the adrenal medulla by the methylation of noradrenaline, and both compounds are released from the gland together. Release of adrenal medullary catecholamines is caused by stressful stimuli, acting via the sympathetic nervous system in the so-called flight, fright, and fight phenomenon. Release of adrenaline prepares the individual to deal with the stress; heart rate and force are increased, blood pressure rises, and blood flow to the skeletal and cardiac muscles is increased, while blood flow to the less essential areas (e.g. gut, skin) is decreased. Adrenaline also mobilizes glycogen energy stores from the liver to increase blood glucose.   ALAN W. CUTHBERT.

See also ADRENAL GLANDS; AUTONOMIC NERVOUS SYSTEM.

Aerobic as applied to METABOLISM in cells of the body, or in microorganisms, means *oxygen-utilizing*. Aerobic metabolism occurs in most animal cells, and depends upon the presence of mitochondria, in which the key chemical processes take place. Aerobic bacteria inhabit the body surface and orifices — they do not have mitochondria. Aerobic excercise is that which is sustainable in balance with oxygen intake — for example, a 10 km race, or any milder rhythmic exercise.   N.C.S.

See METABOLISM.

Aerobics Programmed rhythmic exercises, typically performed to music in sessions lasting the order of 30 min, at an intensity requiring the heart and respiratory rates to be high throughout most of the period but never maximal; original concept defined in numerical terms by Cooper in the 1960s. Contrast the more general physiological adjective 'AEROBIC'.   N.C.S.

See EXERCISE.

Aesthetics is the branch of philosophy which deals with the nature of art and of artistic judgment. Some of the central questions of aesthetics focus on the beautiful: under what circumstances it may be said to exist, what criteria are to be used to judge the beautiful, and whether or not these criteria apply equally to literature and music.

There are two traditional views concerning what constitutes aesthetic values. The first finds beauty to be objective, that is, inherent in the entity itself. The second position holds that beauty is subjective, in that it depends on the attitude of the observer. Immanuel Kant argued that judgments of taste, as he called aesthetic judgments, rest on feelings, which, though subjective, have universal validity. The instrumental theory of value, an extension of subjectivism, holds that the value of art consists in its capacity to produce an aesthetic experience.   KRISTEN L. ZACHARIAS

See also ART AND THE BODY; BEAUTY.

Ageing

Why ageing occurs

Ageing affects all parts of the body and leads to increasing frailty, a declining capacity to respond to stress, increasing incidence of age-related diseases, and eventually, death. Why the body should undergo this spectrum of degenerative changes, when it is equipped with sophisticated mechanisms for self-maintenance and repair, is a question that has long puzzled biologists.

Animals in the wild do not usually live long enough to show obvious signs of ageing; they tend to die young from extrinsic hazards such as infection, starvation, or being killed by a predator. Because Darwinian fitness is strongly governed by the survival and reproductive success of young animals, genetic factors that promote growth and fecundity in early life are favoured by natural selection, even though these same factors may bring deleterious consequences later on. Thus, ageing is thought to result from trade-offs. In effect, late survival is sacrificed for reproduction.

An important trade-off is that which concerns the allocation of metabolic resources, especially energy, between activities of growth, maintenance, and reproduction. Each of these activities is metabolically expensive. Natural selection requires only enough maintenance for the body remain in sound condition through the normal life expectancy in the natural ('wild') environment. This concept is known as the 'disposable soma' theory, the soma consisting of all those parts of body which do not form a part of the reproductive cell lineage, or germ-line (the germ-line must of course be maintained to a high standard, else the reproductive lineage would die out over successive generations).

Evolution theory therefore supports the view that ageing arises principally through the gradual accumulation of random (or stochastic) faults in somatic cells and tissues. This is not to deny the importance of genetic factors in specifying longevity. Genes determine the levels of action of key maintenance systems, like DNA repair, and genes affect hereditary predisposition to a wide range of age-related diseases. However, it is no longer thought plausible that ageing, such as occurs in a species like Homo sapiens, is programmed through mechanisms which exist for the specific purpose of causing death.

Ageing at the cellular level

Our understanding of cellular aspects of ageing is focused on how cells change during the course of the life span, on the mechanisms that underly these changes, and on how changes at the cell level may affect the functions of tissues and organs. As yet our knowledge of these matters is far from complete.

Cell replicative senescence Much research on cell ageing has concerned the phenomenon of cell replicative senescence. Cells from many tissues can be propagated *in vitro* (in culture outside the body) and normal cells grown in this way have finite replicative life spans. The cell type most commonly studied is the *fibroblast*, a constituent of connective tissue, which grows readily in culture. After as many as 60 cell divisions, the growth rate of fibroblast cultures slows down, the cells stop dividing, and eventually they will die.

This phenomenon has been widely regarded as a manifestation of ageing at the cell level. Three lines of evidence support this view: (i) a negative correlation has been reported between the number of cell divisions that a culture can achieve, and the age of the cell donor (Fig. 1); (ii) cells from short-lived mammalian species undergo fewer divisions in culture than cells from long-lived species; (iii) cells from human subjects with Werner's syndrome, a genetic condition showing an approximately two-fold acceleration of many features of ageing, undergo markedly fewer divisions than cells from normal age-matched controls (Fig. 1).

Intriguingly, cells grown from malignant tumours or cells treated with cancer-causing chemicals or viruses often grow without limit. Such cultures are said to have been 'immortalized'. Because of this connection between cell immortalization and cancer, some suggest that cell replicative senescence may be primarily an anti-cancer mechanism, a 'fail-safe' device to

arrest the growth of abnormal cells. However, this hypothesis remains controversial.

Ageing of cells in vivo Within the living body, cells age in very different ways, associated with the proliferative status of the tissues in which they are found. Some cells such as neurons and muscle cells are 'post-mitotic' from birth, meaning that they can no longer divide. Ageing changes lead either to loss of cell function or even to cell death. By the time that such changes affect significant numbers of cells within an organ they will have important and probably irreversible effects on its function. Other tissues such as the covering and lining layers (*epithelia*) in skin and gut, or the blood-forming (*haemopoietic*) system, depend upon rapid cell proliferation and turnover for their proper function. In these highly proliferative systems, the responsibility for maintenance of homeostasis can be traced to small numbers of pluripotent stem cells. Stem cells themselves divide at a low rate but they give rise to rapidly dividing, differentiated cells which undergo considerable clonal expansion. The ageing of stem cells has so far been little studied because of the intrinsic difficulty of working with these cells. Recently, however, it has been found that epithelial stem cells in the small intestine of the mouse show important functional changes with age, being more likely to undergo cell death (*apoptosis*) when subjected to low doses of ionizing radiation, and less able to regenerate the tissue after damage.

Between the extremes of post-mitotic organs (e.g. the brain) and highly proliferative tissues (e.g. the gut wall), there are many tissues where cell division occurs when and where it is required for ongoing homeostasis. It is from these kinds of tissues that cells are most easily grown in culture. However, in spite of the evidence (see above) that cell replicative senescence is a manifestation of ageing at the cell level, the normal ageing of these tissues *in vivo* is not thought to be caused directly by the exhaustion of cell replicative capacity. Even cultures from centenarians are capable of ample proliferation. Nevertheless, it is possible that, with advancing age, growing numbers of individual cells do reach the end of their capacity for division and may contribute to a decline in cell renewal. A biochemical marker known as *senescent β-galactosidase*, which characterizes cells that have reached the end of their replicative capacity *in vitro*, can be detected in small numbers of cells *in vivo*, and the number of such cells increases with age.

Mechanisms of cell ageing There are many kinds of damage that might affect a cell and contribute to its ageing. Chief among these are (i) damage and mutation affecting genetic information (DNA); (ii) accumulation of aberrant proteins due to errors in protein synthesis or processing, heat denaturation, or other damage; (iii) damage to subcellular organelles, particularly mitochondria; (iv) damage to membranes. The mechanisms responsible for these kinds of damage include a variety of intrinsic and extrinsic

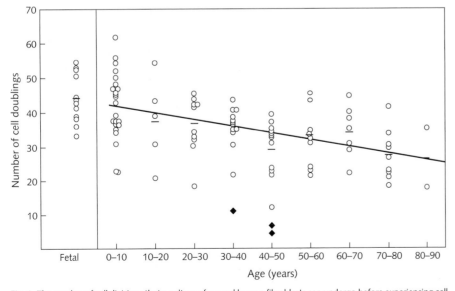

Fig. 1 The number of cell divisions that a culture of normal human fibroblasts can undergo before experiencing cell replicative senescence declines, on average, with the age of the cell donor, as shown by the fitted line. Each data point is for cells cultured from a different donor. The circles correspond to normal subjects. The 3 diamonds show results for cells grown from individuals with Werner's syndrome, a genetic condition of accelerated ageing.

stressors such as reactive oxygen species (including free radicals) and heat, as well as mistakes in the synthesis and processing of macromolecules. Cell ageing is likely to be due to a combination of all of these processes, with the cell being protected by a network of defence and repair mechanisms.

A special mechanism implicated in the replicative senescence of cultured cells is the progressive shortening of *telomeres* (structures at the ends of chromosomes), which is due to the shutting off of the enzyme *telomerase* in somatic tissues. Telomerase acts in germ cells to maintain telomeres at a constant length, and the enzyme is often found to be reactivated in immortal cell lines and in cancers. The extent to which telomere shortening contributes to cell ageing as a causal factor *in vivo* remains to be determined.

Physiological functions

Ageing and 'normality' In adulthood, increasing age is accompanied by a progressive decline in the function of most physiological systems. Contrary to the uniformity implied by the expression 'the elderly', however, there are considerable differences between elderly individuals, as a result of the broad age range, interindividual differences in the rate of deterioration, and a rising prevalence of chronic diseases. For example, some elderly people have exceedingly limited physical abilities whereas others are capable of performances which are better than those of many young adults.

Subject selection is thus a crucial issue in any gerontological study. Some investigations will require subjects who are representative of their contemporaries, with a typical complement of chronic disorders and medication. Other studies might require highly selected subjects who, although atypical, are free of disease, free of risk factors for subclinical disease, and free of medication.

The rising prevalence of chronic pathologies complicates any attempt to determine the rate (or the cellular mechanism) of the age-related decline in a physiological function. It is not even clear how often it is valid to distinguish between 'ageing' and diseases associated with old age. (In osteoporosis, for example, the boundary between ageing and disease is especially indistinct.) Nevertheless, it is clear that in many organs the loss of function is largely attributable to the loss of functioning cells, even in the absence of overt disease.

Physiological decline and loss of safety margins As one ages, the decline in physiological functions may not be immediately apparent, the individual living successfully without testing the function of any system to its limit. All the time, however, the safety margins between maximal function and critical threshold levels of function are being eroded.

Examples include the decline of *bone mineral content* (towards a threshold for likelihood of fracture), of *glomerular filtration rate* (towards a threshold for susceptibility to clinical renal

failure), of *renal tubular function* (towards a threshold for clinically important susceptibility to dehydration), of *hepatic function* (towards a threshold for toxic accumulation following conventional 'young adult' doses of common medications), or of *lower limb strength* (towards a series of thresholds for aspects of independent everyday mobility). These changes in function are mainly due to an age-related loss of functioning cells, the residual tissue continuing to function normally. Some others, however, are due more to qualitative changes, such as increasing stiffness of the chest wall (increasing the rate at which oxygen must be consumed just to meet the needs of the respiratory muscles) or decreasing sensitivity of tissues to circulating catecholamines (reducing maximal heart rate, for example).

The loss of spare capacity also lowers the maximal extent to which an individual can respond to an environmental or situational challenge, and thus limits their ability to meet that challenge. Such impairments of homoeostasis are usually the result of effector organs functioning less successfully. In some cases, however, it seems to be the control mechanisms which are affected. For example, after water deprivation, older people are less thirsty and drink less than young adults. Similarly, some elderly people appear to show a blunted sense of thermal discomfort in a cold environment.

The ability to balance this precarious situation is central to the skills of the physician specializing in the management of illness in elderly people. The geriatric physician recognizes that, in an elderly person, an apparently minor illness must often be treated with great urgency, before it suddenly becomes life-threatening. Similarly, an elderly patient demands much greater precision in prescribing, as the margin between the wanted and unwanted effects of medications becomes narrower.

Muscle and physical performance

The loss of muscle (*muscular cachexia*, or *sarcopenia*) is a good example of the age-related loss of functioning cells and of the resulting loss of functional safety margins (Fig. 2). Sarcopenia is central to the declining physical ability, increasing fatiguability, and progressive frailty of old age. It begins in middle age, proceeds at approximately 1% per year, and impairs all aspects of muscle function. Much of the loss is due to the loss of contractile muscle cells (muscle fibres) — probably resulting from a slowly progressive and incompletely compensated denervation — and is unrelated to habitual activity. The loss of muscle fibres may also be due to impaired regeneration of muscle after damage. A variable degree of shrinkage of some of the surviving muscle fibres also contributes to the loss of active muscle tissue and may reflect individual variation in habitual activity. Although most of the weakness is directly attributable to the reduced muscle mass, older muscle may also be weak for its size.

The age-related loss of muscle performance is greater than the loss of body weight. This has important implications for gait and mobility, especially for women, as they have a lower percentage of their body weight as muscle than men of the same age. In the English National Fitness Survey, nearly half of all women (compared with 15% of men) aged 70 to 74 had a power/weight ratio below the value at which they could still be confident of managing a 30 cm step without using a hand rail. The loss of muscle, together with changes in cardiovascular function, also limits the ability to perform endurance (*aerobic*) exercise, so that many elderly people (especially women) are unable to perform some everyday activities in comfort and without fatigue. For example, in the English National Fitness Survey, 80% of women (but only 35% of men) aged 70 to 74 had an aerobic power/weight ratio such that they would be unable to walk comfortably at 3 miles per hour.

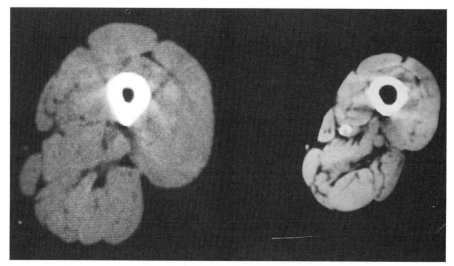

Fig. 2 Cross-sectional images at mid-thigh (by computed tomography) from a healthy woman in her twenties and a healthy woman in her eighties, to the same magnification. Reproduced, with permission, from Ebrahim, S. and Kalache, A. (ed.) (1996). *Epidemiology of old age*. BMJ Publications, London.

Muscle also acts as a crucial, dynamic metabolic store during severe illness. If the acute event is severe or prolonged, the elderly person's greatly diminished muscle mass may no longer be adequate as a source of materials for tissue repair and of cellular fuels for immune competence.

An octogenarian's remaining muscle, however, still shows a normal response to physical training. The improvements are equivalent to 10–20 years' 'rejuvenation'. STRENGTH TRAINING may also provoke valuable enlargement of remaining muscle fibres although the underlying, progressive, age-associated reduction in the number of muscle fibres appears to continue.

TOM KIRKWOOD

ARCHIE YOUNG

Further reading

Concar, D. (1996). Death of old age. *New Scientist*, **150**(2035), 24–9.

Kennie, D. C., Dinan, S., and Young, A. (1998). Health promotion and physical activity. In *Textbook of geriatric medicine and gerontology*, (ed. J. Brocklehurst, R. Tallis and H. Fillit). Churchill Livingstone, London.

Kirkwood, T. B. L. (1996). Human senescence. *BioEssays*, **18**(12) 1009–16.

Kirkwood, T. B. L. (1999). *Time of our Lives: the Science of Human Ageing*. Weidenfeld and Nicolson, London; Oxford University Press, New York.

Woodhouse, K., Williams, R., Macmahon, D., Archer-Jones, P., Kennedy, R., and Main, A. (ed.) (1997). *Services for people who are elderly: addressing the balance*. An NHS Health Advisory Service Thematic Review. HMSO, Norwich.

Aggression has been defined as a behaviour characterized by the intention of inflicting unpleasant stimulation on another individual — but this underestimates its subtlety and omits some important features. It is well known that aggression is not a simple, single category of behaviour. Several classifications of aggression have been proposed, some more elaborate than others. Aggression, unlike some other behaviours, has no biological function or purpose in isolation. Aggressive interactions occur mostly as part of some other pattern of behaviour; for example, as a strategy to achieve sexual goals or access to preferred foods. More generally they form part of the process whereby individuals define their position in the social groups to which they belong, and hence ensure access to restricted resources without the need for constant conflict — a form of social control. However, this does not rule out the possibility that the performance of aggressive acts can itself be rewarding.

Distinctions have been made between different types of aggression, largely on the basis of the context in which it occurs or the stimuli that provoke it: (i) inter-male, or inter-female (territorial, social conflict, etc.); (ii) maternal; (iii) self defence; and (iv) infanticide. Aggression towards members of the same species has been divided more simply into 'offence' and 'defence'. Predation, the hunting of other species, is sometimes included in discussions of aggressive behaviour, but is more properly classed as feeding behaviour.

Human aggression has been separated into 'emotional' aggression, carried out by people with the main intention of harming someone, and 'instrumental' aggression, with some other objective, such as to obtain something rewarding, rather than specifically to injure a victim. In general, both the form of the aggressive act and the context in which it occurs have to be taken into account.

Social factors

Most species, including human beings, live in social groups whose structure affects access by individuals to items in short supply — such as food, mates, or shelter. Direct aggressive confrontation may be used to determine which individual has priority, but it is more usual that animals come to know, through a process of social learning, who is likely to win in such an encounter. This determines their strategy, and also gives the group its dominance structure. Animals, or people, low in the hierarchy may not challenge those higher in the scale, presumably because of the cost in terms of potential injury. This mechanism of social control, based on previous aggressive interactions, functions to reduce aggression; but it does have potent effects on individuals. If it is to be effective, social control by hierarchy requires extremely sophisticated neural processing; indeed, there are those who claim that the primary function of the human brain is to facilitate social interaction.

Gender influences

There are marked individual and gender-related differences in aggression. In most mammalian species aggression is more common between males than between females. Exposure of the brain to TESTOSTERONE in the womb may alter infant behaviour: young males show more aggressive-like play than females. Testosterone may also sensitize the individual to the later effects of the same hormones: for example, increasing the likelihood of adult aggressive behaviour, particularly in the context of competition for desirable, but limited, resources. However, giving excess testosterone to men has had rather inconspicuous effects on their aggressive behaviour or tendencies (including thoughts), though levels of testosterone in the saliva have been shown to correlate positively with violent crimes in male prison inmates. But social status also alters testosterone, so the relation between individual differences in aggressivity and testosterone may be indirect. A variety of studies, in both human and non-human primates, has shown that social 'STRESS' (that is, demands made by the social or working environment) lowers testosterone and that 'dominant' males have higher levels. However, injecting 'subordinate' monkeys with testosterone does not improve their position in the hierarchy, or make them more aggressive.

Aggression is not a male prerogative. It also occurs in females, particularly when they need to defend their young. For example, lactating rats are highly aggressive to intruding males (rather than females). In this context, different hormones may play a role. This aggressive reaction seems to depend upon suckling, and has the obvious biological function of protecting the young. Testosterone given to lactating females actually reduces their aggressive reaction to males.

Are specific parts of the brain involved in aggression?

Since much of aggression in the biological world is part of another behaviour, it is difficult to separate those areas of the brain responsible for the underlying behaviour (getting food, winning mates, etc.) from those associated with the particular behavioural strategy of aggression to achieve these ends. It has been known for many years that damage to a part of the brain called the *amygdala* results in 'tameness' and reduced aggression. The amygdala is part of the LIMBIC SYSTEM, a set of brain structures particularly concerned with survival, adaptation, and the defence of the body against the metabolic or social demands that constitute stress. The amygdala is closely involved in the ability of the brain to classify stimuli in a motivationally and emotionally meaningful way. Its role is not, therefore, restricted to aggression, but this along with many other behaviours is dependent on proper functioning of this part of the brain. Human cases are known in which disturbances of the amygdala have led to inappropriate or excessive aggression.

Another area of the brain implicated in aggression is the HYPOTHALAMUS. Lesions or stimulation in several areas of the hypothalamus have altered aggressive interactions. The hypothalamus is implicated in other behaviours. For example, part of it has well-established roles in sexual and maternal behaviour, and is prominently involved in the regulation of feeding and drinking. Bearing in mind the relation between aggression and other categories of adaptive behaviour, it is clear that there is still uncertainty about the exact role of the hypothalamus in aggression, and whether this can be truly separated from its other adaptive and homeostatic functions. Nevertheless, there are well-documented cases describing humans with tumours in the particular parts of the hypothalamus who became highly aggressive, responding with aggression to stimuli they would have previously considered only annoying. 'Sedative' surgical interventions, involving the hypothalamus, have been used in the treatment of aggressive patients.

We have seen that aggression forms an important part of social regulation and social interaction. This is known to involve the cortex of the frontal lobes of the brain. The frontal cortex is also intimately connected with both the amygdala and the hypothalamus and is therefore in a position to influence these other brain centres that control aggression. This behaviour can occur as a feature of frontal lobe damage in man.

Patients with damage in one region of the frontal cortex react impulsively, without planning or taking into account the consequences of their behaviour; they are irritable and have short tempers, responding to minor provocation. But the frontal cortex is a complex area of the brain, and it is still not very clear whether particular parts may have distinct roles in aggression.

Are there specific aggression-related chemicals in the brain?

The brain is a chemical machine, and the recognition that different parts can be defined by the chemical transmitters that they use offers a different perspective. In humans, changes in the level and metabolism of SEROTONIN have been correlated with affective behaviour in general and more specifically with aggressive behaviour. Serotonin has become the major focus of biological studies of suicidal behaviour (defined as 'self-aggression') and impulsive aggressive behaviour in humans. An association has been reported between low serotonin concentration in the brain and impulsive, destructive behaviours, particularly when aggression and violence are involved. Studies in animals show that a wide range of aggressive behaviours are sensitive to manipulations of the serotonergic system. Depletion of brain serotonin increases aggression. Conversely, serotonergic-enhancing drugs, such as the specific serotonin-uptake inhibitors (SSRIs), reduce aggression. A class of drugs acting on serotonin are known as 'serenics'; these reduce aggression.

But serotonin is not the only neurochemical implicated in aggression. Animal studies suggest that increasing brain DOPAMINE activity creates a state in which they are more prepared to respond aggressively to stimuli in the environment. Antagonists of dopamine receptors are the most frequently used therapeutic agents in the management of violent patients. However, dopamine has important roles in generalized behavioural categories such as reward or punishment; this may be the real reason why it contributes to the display of aggression.

Hyperactivity of NORADRENALINE in the brain has been found to correlate with aggressive behaviour in humans, and noradrenergic receptor blockade is clinically useful in its treatment. This is supported by the effects on aggressive behaviours in isolated mice of drugs that modify noradrenaline activity in the brain.

Many PEPTIDES are found in the brain, particularly in the limbic system, that act as neurotransmitters. One of these, *corticotrophin releasing factor*, is present throughout the limbic system. It has an important role in organizing the co-ordinated response to stress; this includes behaviour, hormones, and the emergency - systems regulating the cardiovascular and other autonomic responses. It may also increase aggression. *Vasopressin* (first known as a pituitary hormone) is another peptide found in the limbic system, and microinjections of this into the hypothalamus and amygdala increased offensive aggression in rodents. Although alterations in several peptides, as well as other

substances, are known to change aggression, no single one so far has been specifically associated with this behaviour. Clearly, given the current preoccupation with understanding and controlling aggression in man, the existence of such compounds, should they be proved, would be most important.

The complexity of aggression — the behaviour pattern, the contexts in which it occurs, and the uses to which it is put — means that there can never be a single, definable system underlying it. Nevertheless, attempts should continue to define aggression more precisely, since this offers not only greater understanding of the relation between this behaviour and others but also direct help to those who try to control undesirable aggression in either animals or humans.

J. HERBERT

Further reading
Albert, D. J., Walsh, M. L., and Jonik, R. H. (1993). Aggression in humans: what is its biological foundation? *Neuroscience and Biobehavioural Reviews*, **17**, 405–25.

Archer, J. (1988). *Behavioural biology of aggression.* Cambridge University Press.

Valzellli, L. (1981). *Psychobiology of aggression and violence.* Raven Press Books, New York.

See also HORMONES; PEPTIDES; SEROTONIN; VIOLENCE.

Albino

Albino *dondo* (Spanish), *blafard* (French), and *Kakerlak* (a derisive Dutch word that also means 'cockroach') are all terms used for human beings who have a total or partial lack of the pigment MELANIN in the SKIN, HAIR, and EYES as well as in some internal sites. It is an incurable congenital condition, due in its total form to absence of the enzyme *tyrosinase*, which is required for melanin to be synthesized in specialized cells — the *melanocytes*. Failure of transfer of pigment from melanocytes to its normal destinations accounts for less severe *albinism*.

The skin of such individuals is usually pale pink or milky white. The hair (including body hair, beard, eyebrows, and eyelashes) is extremely fine and silky, and yellowish-white, substantially different from the snow-white associated with old age. The eyes have a dull, despondent look; the irises are pale grey or pink; the pupils appear bright red, because light falls on the blood vessels of the retina (normally concealed by pigment) in the depth of the eyes. Since a lack of pigment leaves albinos defenseless against both ultraviolet rays and light, they are subject to severe *photophobia* and *heliophobia* (fear of light and the sun) from birth on. Like 'spears' the sun would 'fling his flaring beams', the poet John Milton — who some have suggested suffered from albinism — declared, and cried in torment: 'How I hate thy beams!' And indeed bright daylight hurts the eyes of an albino, for without pigment the iris is translucent so that light penetrates it as well as entering the pupil, flooding the retina with unbearable brightness. Albinos regularly turn their heads to the side and roll their

eyes in a circular motion in an attempt to find a favourable axis of sight; they suffer from rapid NYSTAGMUS (an oscillatory motion of the eyeball), and blink constantly. Light becomes tolerable only with the onset of twilight, when smaller quantities penetrate the iris, so that vision is more or less normalized. Albinos feel especially good — or so it would appear — and can see best on starlit nights and by the light of the moon, which is probably the reason why the native peoples in Central America called them 'moon eyes' or 'children of the moon'. These problems are associated with defective binocular vision and a comparable difficulty in locating sounds, due to abnormally-arranged nerve pathways from the eyes and inner ears to the brain. Whilst the lack of pigment protection for the eyes is the greatest discomfort, it is the unprotected skin which is the greatest hazard, because of the high risk of skin cancer as well as of minor irritation. The claim occasionally advanced that albinism is linked with a lack of intelligence cannot be proved, whereas psychological problems resulting from difficulties of living with a lack of melanin may very well be common.

Despite a few early references, for example by the Roman naturalist Pliny (23–79 CE), until the end of the seventeenth century albinos in Europe were generally regarded as belonging to no special category, but were taken simply as extremely blond and pale people who were strangely shy of light. Only in connection with the fierce debate about the nature and origin of human skin colour, which arose against the background of European colonization and the transatlantic slave trade, were 'albinos' (a word taken from the Portuguese) 'discovered', so to speak, and for the next 150 years they were the object of an attention that went far beyond any medical interest. An albino displayed in Paris in 1744 at an *exhibition célèbre* cast such a spell over the public that even Voltaire wrote an extensive description of the case. In England two 'piebald niggers' (*Nègres mouchetés, Elsterneger*) — black men who suffered from 'partial albinism' (*vitiligo* or *leukoderma*) — became a great sensation: George Alexander Gratton, a little boy exhibited at the Bartholomew Fair in London, 'was covered with a diversity of [white] spots'; the other, John Richardson Primrose Bobey, born in Jamaica in 1744, was presented as a 'white-spotted Negro'. The reason for such extraordinary interest lay in the fact that albinos could be brought forward as an excellent piece of evidence for both proving and disproving the most important theories about the origin and nature of skin colour.

Abbé Demanet (died *c.* 1786), a scholar who had travelled in Africa, and the natural scientist Comte de Buffon (1707–88), declared that albinos were most common among 'coloured' peoples in Earth's humid and hot equatorial zones: on various islands in the Pacific, among the Papuans of New Guinea, on Ambon, on Nias west of Sumatra, and in Biafra and Luanda, as well as among American aborigines on the isthmus of Panama. They concluded therefore that the skin colour of all human beings must originally have been 'white', but that under extreme conditions some individuals then experienced an 'accidental' (and later inheritable) 'degenerative colouration'. To be sure, they could not explain why, for example, the sun which had burned one person black did not do so with others who lived in the same environment. The surgeon Claude-Nicolas Le Cat (1700–68) from Rouen therefore considered albinos as a previously unrecognized and unique 'species' of human being, whose existence 'was due neither to the climate, nor the sun, nor a mixture [of other races]', as he wrote in his *Treatise on the Color of the Human Skin in General, and on that of Negroes in Particular, and of the Metamorphosis of the one Color into the Other, Whether by Birth or by Accident.* Voltaire even considered whether the albino might not be the missing link between man and beast so eagerly sought by the natural philosophers of the period; and working from that premise the author of the article *Nègres* in Diderot's *Encyclopédie* posed the question of whether 'white Negroes' (*Leucaethiopes*) might not be the progeny of white women and orangutans. It is no wonder, then, that in his *Systema naturae* Carl von Linné (1707–78) ultimately saw the albino, whom he called *Homo nocturnus*, as closely related to the Troglodytes, the Forest Man (*Homo sylvestris*), and the Orangutan.

At the beginning of the twentieth century, Mendelian genetics, at least for the most part, put a halt to such learned racial discrimination by defining albinism as a genetic defect that results in a mutation: the permanent, inheritable, and pathological alteration of a healthy organism. Thereafter only the National Socialists and their scientific henchmen (race theoreticians like Erwin Baur, Eugen Fischer, and Fritz Lenz) kept alive the traditional view of albinos as 'half-animal' and 'subhuman'. Nazi ideology welcomed the fact that as far back as the age of Milton albinos were maligned as 'effeminate' (in much the same way as homosexuals) on the basis of their weak constitutions and the colour of their skin — and that even the poet himself had been mocked by his fellow students at Cambridge as 'The Lady of Christ's College'. It may be thanks solely to the Allied victory over Germany that albinos did not ultimately fall victim to the Nazi programmes of euthanasia.   PETER MARTIN

Further reading

Pearson, K., Nettleship, E. and Usher, C. H. (1911–13). *A monograph of Albinism in Man*, (3 vols). Draper's Company Research Memoirs, London.

Sarasin, F. (1936). Die Anschauungen der Völker über den Albinismus. *Schweizerisches Archiv für Volkskunde*, **34**, 198–233.

See also EYES; PIGMENTATION; SKIN COLOUR.

Alcoholism

The term 'alcoholism' was first used by a Swedish professor of medicine, Magnus Huss (1807–90), to mean poisoning by alcohol. Huss distinguished between two types of alcoholism. *Acute alcoholism* was a result of the temporary effects of alcohol taken within a short period of time — drunkenness and intoxication; *chronic alcoholism* was a pathological condition caused by the habitual use of alcoholic beverages in poisonous amounts over a long period of time. Using case studies to illustrate the condition of chronic alcoholism, Huss provided the first systematic description of the physical damage caused by excessive drinking. This first use of the term 'alcoholism' in 1852 emerged from a combination of specific historical circumstances within which changes in perceptions of excessive alcohol consumption were taking place.

Prior to the nineteenth century, symptoms and problems related to '*habitual drunkenness*', or excessive alcohol use, were known and recorded, but habitual drunkards were seen as morally weak or criminal, rather than suffering from an illness or a disease. Public concern revolved around drunkards' moral attitudes and social behaviours, which were regarded as licentious, sinful, or criminal, punishable by a period in the stocks, whipping, or fines — or by the eternal damnation preached in fiery sermons. On the whole, however, the dominant social response to drunkenness was tolerance and social disapproval; heavy drinking was not, in itself, regarded as a problem. The emergence of a new understanding of habitual drunkenness (or *inebriety*) as a disease was led by medical and psychiatric practitioners at the beginning of the nineteenth century, most notably by Benjamin Rush (1745–1813) in America and Thomas Trotter (1760–1832) in Scotland. According to some historians, it was Rush who provided the first clearly developed modern conception of *alcohol addiction*. This included the idea of gradual and progressive addiction; bouts of drunkenness characterized by an inability to refrain from alcohol; the description of the condition as a 'disease'; and total abstinence as the cure. For the first time, 'treatment' became a possible option in responding to the harm associated with habitual drunkenness. Throughout the nineteenth century efforts were made to provide more scientific descriptions of the disease and its cure, leading, in 1901, to the use of the term 'alcohol addiction' to describe the inability to give up harmful drinking.

Twentieth century developments

During the first half of the twentieth century interest in alcoholism and the alcoholic waned. Prohibition in America and changing social conditions and consumption patterns in Britain drew attention towards control of the substance and away from the disease and its treatment. But with the repeal of prohibition in America, any attempt to address problems associated with drinking had to be concerned with the behaviour of individuals rather than with the consumption patterns of the nation or the nature of the substance itself. In post-prohibition America and, later, in post war Britain, the freedom of the majority to drink as they pleased was paramount. The nineteenth century temperance approach, which had inveighed against the dangers of alcohol itself, was now rejected as moralistic and unscientific and the focus of attention was, once again, on the *disease of alcoholism*.

The 'new' disease approach to alcoholism started in America and was led by three linked groups, often referred to as the '*alcoholism movement*': a research group established at the Yale Centre for Alcohol Studies; Alcoholics Anonymous (AA) (a self-help group which was set up in 1935), and the National Committee for Education on Alcoholism (later the National Council on Alcoholism), which became the leading voluntary organization offering alcoholism treatment. The 'alcoholism movement' quickly spread to Britain and subsequently throughout the world.

In essence there was little difference between descriptions of the disease in Rush's work and later use of the term. The main objectives in labelling it as the 'new' approach to alcoholism were practical and political rather than based on any 'scientific' discovery. On the practical side was the desire to gain a better deal for people suffering from alcoholism. Promoting the disease concept was part of a strategy to combat the stigma and prejudice that hindered alcoholics and their families from seeking help and that was a barrier to securing the interest and involvement of the helping professions. On the political side, the concept served as a device to unite diverse interests, including the alcohol industry, because the focus was on a few unfortunate individuals rather than on the drinking habits of the majority.

The strategy was successful. The disease theory was accepted by the American Medical Association in 1956 and by a number of influential doctors and voluntary groups in Britain over the course of the 1950s and 60s. In the early 1950s, the World Health Organization formally declared its support and provided a definition of 'alcoholism' which noted that alcoholics were excessive drinkers, dependent on alcohol to the extent that they suffered noticeable mental disturbance or interference with bodily or mental health, interpersonal relations, and economic functioning. They were people who required treatment.

As in the previous century, there was continuing interest in refining the disease concept and in producing classifications or 'typologies of drinkers'. The most famous typology was derived from the research of E. M. Jellinek, a member of the Yale Centre for Alcohol Studies and a consultant to the WHO during the 1950s. Influenced strongly by AA philosophy, Jellinek distinguished between five different types of alcoholism. Only two types (*Gamma* and *Delta*) were diseases because, in his view, they were addictions in the pharmacological sense that physical dependence on alcohol was present and too sudden cessation of alcohol use would result in withdrawal symptoms. The defining characteristics of Gamma and Delta alcoholism were: acquired increased tissue tolerance; adaptive cell metabolism; withdrawal and craving; and loss of control (Gamma alcoholism) or an inability to abstain (Delta alcoholism). Typically, Gamma alcoholics drank mainly in bouts and were often drunk; Delta alcoholics drank regularly to achieve a blood alcohol level at which they felt comfortable, usually without getting drunk. According to Jellinek, 'alcoholics' were those who suffered from Gamma or Delta forms of alcoholism. Other forms of alcoholism were considered to be symptomatic, the dependence on alcohol being psychological without the presence of physiological addiction; individuals in those groups were not, therefore, alcoholics.

Alcohol dependence and related disabilities

Jellinek's classification has continued to have a significant influence over beliefs about alcoholism and about appropriate treatment approaches for alcoholics. But the ambiguities in the terms led to repeated efforts to clarify the concepts, resulting eventually in the substitution of 'alcoholism' with the term 'alcohol-dependence syndrome', approved by the World Health Assembly in 1976 and incorporated, three years later, into the International Classification of Diseases as a new medical diagnosis. One important feature of the syndrome is that it includes both psychological and physiological dependence. It has seven elements: subjective awareness of the compulsion to drink; narrowing of the drinking repertoire (drinking becomes predominantly a response to the need to avoid withdrawal so that daily intake becomes 'scheduled'); primacy of drinking (drinking becomes more important than any other activity); altered tolerance to alcohol; repeated withdrawal symptoms; relief or avoidance of withdrawal symptoms by further drinking; reinstatement after abstinence (return to the drinking pattern established before abstinence, which can happen very quickly after starting to drink again).

At the same time as the alcohol dependence syndrome emerged as a new concept, a WHO group were formulating criteria for the identification and classification of *alcohol-related disabilities*. The report, published in 1977, described the range of mental, physical, and social disabilities related to alcohol use and emphasized that there were degrees of disabilities. It was not only the 'alcoholic' or alcohol-dependent person who was adversely affected by alcohol; damage might be incurred even if the individual was neither dependent nor an excessive drinker.

The emphasis on degrees of disability related to alcohol use rather than dependence is significant since it signalled changes in perceptions of the nature of the alcohol problem. The notion that 'alcoholics' suffering from a 'disease' were different from the remainder of the population was no longer generally accepted (although some groups still base their therapeutic approaches on disease theories). By the 1980s, many people preferred the term 'problem drinking', which covered a continuum of drinking harms, from relatively minor harm, such as behaving in socially embarrassing ways when drunk, missing work because of a hangover, or suffering a fall when drinking, to the severe harms associated with excessive and dependent drinking. Problem drinking was not a disease; it was a 'learned behaviour', and anyone who drank was at risk of becoming alcohol dependent. Concern now focused on the much greater number of people drinking above recommended levels, or in ways likely to incur harm to themselves, to other people, or to the wider community.

Today, the term 'alcoholism' and 'alcoholic' are regarded by many people as stigmatizing labels which are unhelpful in developing appropriate responses to alcohol-related harms. But their continuing use by some groups indicates the co-existence of alternative beliefs about the nature of harmful alcohol use and of different approaches to helping those who become 'problem drinkers' or 'alcoholics'. BETSY THOM

Further reading

Heather, N. and Robertson, I. (1997). *Problem drinking: the new approach*, (3rd edn). Oxford University Press.

See also ADDICTION; DISEASE; DRUG ABUSE.

Alexander Technique

Frederick Matthias Alexander (1869–1955) was an Australian actor and Shakespearean reciter who suffered persistent loss of voice during performance. Although the treatments prescribed by his doctor, combined with rest, succeeded in restoring his voice, this was only a temporary solution. The problem returned as soon as he went back on the stage. Alexander put it to his doctor that the cause must lie in the way he was using his voice, in something that he was doing. Although the doctor agreed, he couldn't say what was wrong. Alexander decided, therefore, to find out for himself.

Over a period of years, beginning in about 1892, Alexander made careful observations of himself and experimented with the way in which he spoke. He did this with nothing more elaborate than a simple arrangement of mirrors. He discovered a pattern of habits which were putting a strain on his larynx and which were responsible for his vocal problems. Through his efforts to change his habits and restore his voice to its proper functioning, he discovered a great deal about human co-ordination and created the method which is taught today as the Alexander Technique.

The particular habits which were the source of Alexander's problem included the tendency to pull his head back and down upon his spine, depress his larynx, and gasp in air through the mouth. These habits were not difficult to discover, though he had not noticed them before. What was really difficult however, was to change them. His repeated failures forced him to reconsider some common and basic assumptions about how the human organism works.

One such assumption was the idea that specific habits can be dealt with separately. Alexander discovered, to the contrary, that specific habits are inseparable from the whole. The way he used his head, neck, larynx, and his breathing were all tied up with everything else he was doing. He found that the solution was to change the way he co-ordinated his action as a whole. When he improved the quality of his co-ordination, the specific habits improved as a consequence. This illustrates the principle of *psycho-physical unity*, which is central to the Alexander Technique. The individual always acts as a whole, which includes all mental and physical processes.

Alexander also had to reconsider his reliance on the sense of feeling. For he saw that at critical moments he was not doing what he felt he was doing. Even though he felt he was speaking without pulling back his head, the mirror showed otherwise. He had discovered *unreliable sensory appreciation*. He learned that to change his habits he had to rely on reasoning, for the sense of feeling only enables the repetition of familiar, habitual actions. It could not guide him into a new experience. In the Alexander Technique, you maintain a series of thoughts to direct your co-ordination, rather than relying on the sense of feeling.

The Alexander Technique is a method you can use to change your habitual patterns of co-ordination. It is a skill which you can apply in any circumstance. The first step is *inhibition*, which is the refusal to act immediately. The second step is *direction*, which involves thinking of the optimum pattern of co-ordination. This optimum pattern consists of a certain relationship between head, neck, back, and limbs, which is referred to as the *primary control*. The third step is to make a conscious choice, whether to go ahead with the original intention, do nothing at all, or do something different. These procedures must be unpacked and expanded with the help of a teacher in order for them to be accurately understood.

The improvements in Alexander's voice, and in his health in general, were striking. He was soon in great demand to teach his technique to other actors and singers. As they learned to correct their habits of co-ordination on a general basis, they too experienced greater control in performance and an improvement in functioning in all areas. Poor co-ordination and the chronic strain it entails is associated with problems as diverse as backache, migraine, arthritis, digestive disturbances, circulatory disturbances, breathing disorders, acne, eczema, insomnia, anxiety, neurosis, and depression. When he saw that improvements in co-ordination led to corresponding improvements in health, that *use determines functioning*, Alexander realized that he had discovered something more important than vocal development, and gave up the stage to devote himself to teaching full time. In 1904 Alexander came to London, armed with letters of introduction from prominent Sydney doctors and specialists who urged him to seek wider recognition. Later he also took his technique to the U.S. Between 1914 and 1924 he spent half of his time there and half of his time in London.

The Alexander Technique is fundamentally educative, in that people learn to improve the way in which they use themselves in any activity. They learn a skill which gives them greater control over themselves. Yet, as Alexander discovered with his first pupils, it is very difficult for people to put this into practice with only a verbal explanation. He evolved a way of putting his hands on people to guide them away from their fixed habits and into a better co-ordination. This use of the hands is often misunderstood. It is not therapeutic, but is instructive for the student who is learning to put the technique into practice. Alexander also discovered that individual attention was of utmost importance. Lessons in the Alexander Technique are given on a one to one basis.

The Alexander Technique is often grouped with alternative therapies. However, it is neither a therapy, nor is it alternative. It is founded on the same scientific process of investigation as any orthodox practice. It is based on the evidence, not yet fully appreciated by modern medicine, that our psycho-physical habits in the daily activities of life play a significant part in determining our state of health and performance.

The Society of Teachers of the Alexander Technique in London, and affiliated societies in other countries, oversee and certify the training of teachers, who must undergo a 3-year practical training programme. Teachers are increasingly accepted in scientific and medical circles, for even though the technique represents an approach to human problems which is new and challenging, it does not conflict with any established anatomical or physiological principles. When Nikolaas Timbergen won the Nobel Prize for Physiology or Medicine in 1973 he devoted a portion of his oration to praise the value of Alexander's technique, and to confirm its scientific standing.   TASHA MILLER
        DAVID LANGSTROTH

Further reading

Alexander, F. M. (1985 [1932]). *The use of the self*. Gollancz, London.

Barlow, W. (1973). *The Alexander Principle*. Gollancz, London.

See also MIND–BODY INTERACTION; MOVEMENT, CONTROL OF.

Alimentary system
The alimentary system is responsible for the breakdown of food into its component parts, and for the absorption of the products into the body. The system consists of a tube running from the mouth to the anus that is variously known as the alimentary tract, digestive tract, gastrointestinal tract, or gut. The salivary glands, LIVER, GALL BLADDER, and PANCREAS are distinct organs, but they are intimately associated with the alimentary tract and pass juices into it that are required for digestion.

The inner lining of the gastrointestinal tract (the *mucosa*) is covered by a layer of cells, the EPITHELIUM that performs the separate processes of secretion and absorption. The movement of gut contents from one region to the next is achieved by two layers of SMOOTH MUSCLE

(circular and longitudinal) that lie outside the mucosa and that contract and relax in co-ordinated patterns. Between the mucosa and muscle layers lies the *submucosa*, which is rich in blood vessels and connective tissue. Different regions of the digestive tract are concerned with storage, secretion, the processes of food digestion, absorption, and the elimination of waste products. All regions of the gut have a capacity for the renewal of mucosal cells, and for protection against toxic or damaging agents. The various functions of the gut are co-ordinated by neurons, hormones, and local (*paracrine*) regulatory molecules.

The conversion of food into a form suitable for digestion is helped by cooking, which may also destroy toxins and microorganisms. The initial steps of digestion occur in the mouth where the ENZYME amylase, which is present in SALIVA, breaks down starch. Mixing of saliva and food is aided by mastication or chewing, which also prepares an appropriately-sized 'bolus' of food for SWALLOWING. The secretion of saliva is prompted by the presence of food in the mouth. Slightly acidic solutions are strong salivary stimulants, which might explain why a twist of lemon is perceived as a valuable addition to aperitifs.

The process of swallowing involves raising the larynx to close off the respiratory tract. The progression of a bolus of food down the OESOPHAGUS is aided by a muscular reflex, *peristalsis*, consisting of a wave of relaxation to accommodate the bolus followed by a wave of contraction pushing it ahead. Peristaltic movements are co-ordinated by neurons within the oesophagus and connecting it to the brain. The lower part of the oesophagus is separated from the stomach by a sphincter, the *lower oesophageal sphincter*, which relaxes to allow food to pass through. This sphincter normally prevents acid from the stomach entering the oesophagus. Failure of this mechanism is one cause of the sensation known as heartburn, and if persistent leads to chronic inflammation: *oesophagitis*.

Stomach

The adjective '*gastric*' applies to all things pertaining to the stomach. The stomach stores food prior to delivery to the small intestine, initiates the digestion of protein, and secretes hydrochloric acid, which destroys many microorganisms. Hydrochloric acid in gastric juice was identified by the physician-chemist William Prout in the 1820s. Important early observations on human gastric digestion were made at about the same time by William Beaumont on his patient, the Canadian trapper Alexis St Martin, who had survived a gun-shot wound leaving him with a permanent hole, or fistula, connecting the stomach with the exterior of the upper left side of the abdomen. Beaumont recorded over 100 separate experiments in which he directly observed gastric function in this subject concluding, in one experiment, '… I am confident, generally speaking, that venison is the most digestible of any diet …'

Proteins in the stomach are broken down to *polypeptides* by the enzyme *pepsin*, which works best in acidic environments and is produced by 'chief', or '*zymogen*', cells in the gastric mucosa. Separate specialized cells, the *parietal cells*, secrete hydrochloric acid. The concentration of hydrogen ions in gastric juice is about a million times higher than in blood. The gastric epithelium therefore maintains one of the steepest concentration gradients of an electrolyte in the body. The secretion of acid against this gradient requires energy. It is achieved by a protein known as the *proton pump* (or, more precisely, the $H^+/K^+ATPase$) that exchanges intracellular hydrogen ions for extracellular potassium using energy provided by the breakdown of ATP (adenosine 5′-triphosphate).

The Russian physiologist I. P. PAVLOV identified three phases in the control of acid secretion during digestion — the cephalic, gastric, and intestinal phases. The thought, smell, or taste of food stimulate acid secretion in the cephalic phase. In humans up to 50% of maximum acid secretion by the stomach can be evoked by this kind of stimulation. The gastric phase is initiated by the presence of food in the stomach, and the intestinal phase by food in the intestine. At the cellular level, acid secretion is controlled by ACETYLCHOLINE released from mucosal nerve endings, by the gastric hormone GASTRIN, and by the local regulator histamine released from cells adjacent to parietal cells. Parietal cells, which also secrete a protein (*intrinsic factor*) essential for the absorption of vitamin B12, are lost by an autoimmune process in the condition of pernicious ANAEMIA — which is characterized by a failure to produce acid and intrinsic factor, leading to vitamin B12 deficiency.

The stomach converts food to a sludge-like consistency (*chyme*) suitable for further digestion in the small intestine. The rate of emptying of chyme from the stomach varies with the composition of the meal. Fat-rich meals empty more slowly than carbohydrate-rich meals. Indigestible solids empty more slowly than liquids or semi-solid meals. The rate of emptying is determined by pressure differences between the stomach and duodenum, by the resistance to flow across the muscular band (the *pyloric sphincter*) separating the two organs, and by a pumping action of the last part of the stomach. Gastric emptying is regulated by signals arising from the duodenum, which therefore itself determines the rate at which it receives chyme.

The intestines

The small intestine is the primary site of digestion and absorption. It is a tube approximately 20 feet long consisting of three regions; the duodenum, jejunum, and ileum. Gastric acid entering the duodenum is neutralized by bicarbonate secreted by the pancreas, which also secretes a wide variety of digestive enzymes. The major classes of pancreatic enzymes are *proteases*, which convert protein to polypeptides, peptides, and then amino acids; *amylase*, which completes the breakdown of starch; and *lipase*, which converts fats (triglyceride) to glycerol and fatty acids. The digestion of fat also requires *bile salts*, delivered to the duodenum in BILE from the liver, via the gall bladder. The final stages of digestion are completed both within epithelial cells of the small intestine and by enzymes on their surface; for example peptides may be converted to amino acids within these cells, and sucrose is converted to glucose and fructose by a membrane-bound enzyme, sucrase–isomaltase.

The lining of the small intestine is folded into finger-like projections, the *villi* (each 0.5– 0.8 mm long), and deeper glands, the *crypts*. The immensely increased surface area provided by the villi aids absorption. Substances move between the gut lumen and the blood both by passing through epithelial cells (the *transcellular route*) and by passing between them (the *paracellular route*). Water also moves by these routes along osmotic gradients. Absorption of the products of digestion is mediated by a series of specific 'transport proteins'. Amino acids and peptides, sugars, and inorganic ions are often moved from the lumen into intestinal cells against a concentration gradient. The energy required for this transport is provided by gradients of sodium or hydrogen ions. The sodium gradient in particular is generated by sodium pumps located on the surface membrane of epithelial cells facing the bloodstream, which lower intracellular sodium. The conditions are thereby created for sodium in the intestinal lumen to move down its concentration gradient into the cells carrying nutrients with it.

Nutrient digestion and absorption is largely completed in the jejunum. In the ileum, there is further absorption of water, electrolytes, remaining nutrients, and also bile salts which are returned to the liver for re-use. The residue then passes to the large intestine, or colon, for the final steps of water and electrolyte absorption, and for storage of the waste products prior to their discharge when socially appropriate (defecation).

Approximately 9 litres of fluid enter the human small intestine each day, some from ingested food and liquids, and more from the secretions of the salivary glands, stomach, pancreas, liver, and the small intestine itself. The jejunum and ileum each account for the reabsorption of about 45% of fluid and sodium chloride. The remainder is delivered to the colon, where all but about 100 ml is reabsorbed. The colon has the capacity to absorb up to 1.5 litres of fluid per day. When greater volumes arrive from the small intestine the excess is lost in faeces as DIARRHOEA. Although the small intestine is a net absorptive organ, the crypt cells secrete water and sodium chloride. This secretion may be stimulated by toxins generated by microorganisms; one example is cholera toxin, which is responsible for the secretory diarrhoea of cholera. Watery diarrhoea therefore happens when intestinal secretions overwhelm the capacity of the small and large intestines to absorb water and electrolytes. Absorption may be aided by oral administration of solutions consisting of sodium chloride and glucose which engage multiple transport processes. This treatment, *oral rehydration therapy*, has proved valuable in treating patients with infectious diarrhoea, particularly in Third World countries where access to medical services is limited.

Within the gut there is a rich diversity of MICROORGANISMS, many of which are beneficial although some are potentially pathogenic. The colon typically contains very large numbers of microorganisms: approximately 1013 individual organisms, and up to 200 different types. The small intestine and stomach are usually relatively free of microorganisms. An important exception is *Helicobacter pylori* which is found in the stomach in approximately 50% of people.

Many microorganisms within the gastrointestinal tract are able to convert the otherwise indigestible components of food, particularly plant cell walls, into forms suitable for absorption. In ruminant species (cow, sheep) a modified part of the stomach functions as a fermentation chamber where microorganisms digest the non-starch polysaccharides which make up plant fibre into short chain FATTY ACIDS which are readily absorbed. In other species (e.g. horse, elephant), an expanded region of the first part of the large intestine, the caecum, serves a similar function.

Protection and renewal

Many substances present in the gut lumen are potentially damaging, such as gastric acid, ingested noxious molecules, and microorganisms. To counteract these forces, the gut has an elaborate range of protective mechanisms. Gastric acid is resisted by special properties of the surface membrane of mucosal cells, tight connections between cells, good blood flow, and the local production of bicarbonate and mucus gel that lies on the epithelial surface. Breakdown of these mechanisms may lead to the formation of a *peptic ulcer*. The protective barrier is reduced by aspirin and other non-steroidal anti-inflammatory drugs; this is an important side-effect which limits the use of these compounds. Drugs that inhibit acid secretion are widely used. Some (the *proton pump inhibitors*, e.g. omeprazole) block the pump that transports acid into the stomach, others block the site at which histamine acts on parietal cells (the *H2 receptor antagonists*: cimetidine, ranitidine). The presence of *Helicobacter pylori* in the stomach is associated with peptic ulcer disease, and also with cancer of the stomach. Its recognition and its elimination by antibiotic therapy has provided a major advance in the management of peptic ulcer in the 1990s.

The gastrointestinal tract is well endowed with cells of the IMMUNE SYSTEM, which are important in protection against pathogenic microorganisms and antigens. Malfunction of this system is a factor in inflammatory bowel diseases (Crohn's disease and ulcerative colitis). In addition some components of food may trigger an immune response, for example in coeliac disease there is an intolerance to the protein component of wheat, gliadin.

Epithelial cells of the alimentary tract are subject to continuous wear and tear and so must be regularly replaced. In the small intestine, epithelial cells are generated in the crypts, then migrate up the villi and are lost at the tip. This process takes about three days. During migration cells differentiate into particular types. Cell renewal in the mucosa occurs similarly throughout the gut. Damage to the DNA within dividing cells may disrupt mechanisms that regulate this process, leading to accumulation of mutated forms of genes and development of tumours, particularly in the colon and stomach, which are common sites for cancer.

Nerves and hormones

The gut possesses its own nervous system which can function independently of the central nervous system. The gut and brain do engage each other in two-way communication, but, with exceptions such as swallowing and defecation, the functions of the alimentary system are not under voluntary control. Moreover, the normal processes of digestion do not involve consciousness, even though expressions of the sensations attributed to digestion are commonplace (*gut feelings*, etc.).

The main nerve trunks linking the gastrointestinal tract and the central nervous system are known as the VAGUS and *splanchnic* nerves. In both cases, separate nerve fibres communicate from the gut to the central nervous system, and in the opposite direction. Splanchnic nerve fibres communicating to the central nervous system respond to noxious stimuli, leading to perceptions of pain or discomfort. The sensitivity of these nerves can be modified, for example by inflammation, so that otherwise innocuous stimuli may be perceived as painful. Nerve fibres running from the central nervous system to the gut are part of the AUTONOMIC NERVOUS SYSTEM. In general, alimentary processes are activated by the 'parasympathetic' component of this system via the vagus nerves, and are quietened by the 'sympathetic' component via the splanchic nerve. Both vagus and splanchnic nerves influence digestion via neurons located within the gut wall. However, because gut neurons can also function independently of the remainder of the autonomic nervous system, they are often considered to represent a third division of this system, the 'enteric' component.

The control of digestion depends on interactions between enteric neurons and a system of hormones produced by, and acting on, the gut. The pancreas-stimulating hormone, *secretin*, was the first hormone to be discovered (by W. M. Bayliss and E. H. Starling in London in 1902). At the turn of the twentieth century, ideas of how digestion might be controlled were dominated by Pavlov who emphasized the role of the nerves supplying the gut. However, Bayliss and Starling observed that acid in the small intestine of an anaesthetized dog stimulated a flow of pancreatic juice even after all nerves to the intestine had been cut. They reasoned that a messenger molecule might be secreted by the intestine into the bloodstream and conveyed by this route to the pancreas. They then found that such a substance could be recovered by extraction from the intestinal mucosa. They called the active factor secretin, and they showed that it stimulated a flow of pancreatic juice when injected into the bloodstream. The word *hormone* (from the Greek: to rouse or set in motion) was later introduced by Starling in recognition of this novel mechanism of action.

The gut hormones are produced by specialised epithelial cells, the gut endocrine cells, each with a characteristic distribution. Endocrine cells in the stomach, including the *gastrin* or 'G' cells, are mainly responsible for regulating acid secretion. Endocrine cells in the duodenum and jejunum produce secretin, which stimulates water and bicarbonate secretion by the pancreas, and CHOLECYSTOKININ, which stimulates pancreatic enzyme secretion and gall bladder contraction, and which inhibits gastric emptying and food intake. Hormones produced in the ileum and colon (peptide YY, neurotensin, glucagon-like peptides-I and -II) mediate a phenomenon sometimes called the 'ileal brake', by which functions occurring in upper regions of the gut are inhibited, including food intake.

Digestion and fasting

The time taken to digest a meal depends on its composition. Fat-rich meals take longer to digest than those rich in protein or carbohydrate. There is considerable variation between individuals, but representative times to complete the progression from mouth to anus are about 55 hours in UK men, and 72 hours in women. Gastric digestion is completed in 2–3 hours, and small intestinal digestion in about 6 hours, so that the time spent in the colon is around 50–60 hours.

During FASTING, or between meals, the gastrointestinal tract is not completely quiescent. Cell debris and microorganisms continue to accumulate during fasting, necessitating a mechanism to maintain the health of the gut. Approximately 12 hours after the last meal, strong waves of contraction start in the stomach and then progress the full length of the gut carrying accumulated debris forwards. These contractions are sometimes called house-keeping movements, or more accurately the 'migrating myoelectric complex'. They start every 90 minutes, and take approximately 90 min to move the full length of the gut; as one finishes in the colon the next starts in the stomach. They cease on feeding.

GRAHAM DOCKRAY

Further reading

The British Digestive Foundation (PO Box 251, Edgware, Middlesex, HA8 6HG) can provide information on a range of diseases of the alimentary tract.

Johnson, L. R. (1997). *Gastrointestinal physiology*, (5th edn), Mosby Year Book Inc., St Louis, Missouri.

See PLATE 7.

See also APPENDIX; BILE; CONSTIPATION; DEFECATION; DIARRHOEA; FAECES; GALL BLADDER; GASTRIN; HERNIA; INDIGESTION; LIVER; PANCREAS; SALIVA; VOMITING.

Allergy

Every spring and summer, many people suffer from hay fever, a very common form of allergy. The symptoms include itchy eyes, sneezing, and congested nostrils. Most of these symptoms can be controlled by antihistamine or steroid nasal spray. Unfortunately, in some forms of allergy, violent reactions may take place leading to serious or even fatal consequences — *anaphylactic shock* — as seen in allergies to seafood, nuts, or certain drugs such as penicillin.

In the realm of immunology, substances that cause immune responses or allergic reactions are known as antigens. Specific antigens that provoke an allergic reaction are called allergens. Typical allergens include pollens, house-dust mites, animal dander, bacteria, foods, drugs, and chemicals. At present, we do not know why, in similar amounts and circumstances, these substances are harmless to most people but can cause health hazards in others. Avoidance of known allergens is the best protection against such reactions.

In the IMMUNE SYSTEM several mechanisms have been evolved to protect the body against antigens. Prominent among these are the lymphocytes, white blood cells that are specialised to react to specific antigens. There are two kinds of lymphocytes — B cells and T cells. B cells produce antibodies, which are proteins that bind to and destroy or neutralize antigens. T cells do not produce antibodies; instead, they produce *cytokines* — soluble molecules mediating interaction between cells. T cells also bind directly to an antigen and initiate an attack on it by 'presenting' parts of it to B cells, to stimulate antibody production.

Allergic reactions

Depending on whether the antigen triggers a response by B cells or T cells, allergic (*hypersensitivity*) reactions can have immediate or delayed effects. They are classified as Type I, II, III, and IV. Type I, II, and III allergic reactions are the products of B cell stimulation, and, as a result of antibody–antigen responses, these reactions take immediate effect. Different types of reaction may occur together — for example, in asthma, bronchial reactions to allergens show both an immediate and a late-phase response.

Type I reactions, which include hay fever and insect venom allergy, involve the class of antibodies known as *immunoglobulin E* (IgE). IgE molecules are bound to *mast cells*, which are found in connective tissue. When enough antigen has bound with the IgE antibodies, the mast cells release granules of histamine and heparin and produce other substances that cause inflammation. These potent chemicals dilate blood vessels and constrict bronchial air passages. Histamine is responsible for the visible symptoms of an allergic attack, such as running nose, wheezing, and tissue swelling. Antihistamines or

steroid nasal spray are often used to give temporary relief. An alternative treatment is desensitization, in which increasing amounts of the antigen are injected over a period of time until the sufferer no longer experiences an allergic response.

In severe allergic reactions, 'complement' fragments (*anaphylatoxins*) — proteins circulating in the blood — stimulate a more massive release of substances from mast cells which dilate blood vessels and constrict bronchioles. This sequence of events results in the collapse of the circulatory system, together with respiratory symptoms, leading to a potentially fatal reaction — anaphylactic shock.

Drug allergy is a hypersensitivity reaction to therapeutic agents. It occurs occasionally on second exposure to a drug against which an individual has already produced antibodies. It remains to be established why some drugs rarely cause allergic reactions (e.g. tetracyclines, digitalis), while others frequently provoke them (e.g. penicillin, phenytoin).

The mechanisms of immune activation in drug allergy are similar to antibody responses to foreign molecules, especially proteins, that enter the body. Although drug molecules are too small to be antigenic by themselves, they can conjugate to body proteins and elicit an immune response. Symptoms vary with the drug and the sensitivity of the affected person, but include, as separate reactions, hives (urticaria), serum sickness, and, sometimes, anaphylaxis. Several drugs can successfully counteract these allergic symptoms (antihistamines, cromolyn, and corticosteroids) — but at present, the best way to combat drug allergy is to identify the offending drug and to observe a lifelong avoidance of that particular compound and its derivatives.

Type II reactions involve different immunoglobulins, known as IgG or IgM, which are antibodies against antigens on the surface of certain 'target' cells or in their immediate environment. These antigens may be natural components of healthy cells, or they may be extrinsic components induced by drugs or infectious microbes. The resulting antigen–antibody complex activates the complement system: a series of potent enzymes that destroy the target cell. An example of Type II reactions is *autoimmune haemolytic anaemia*. In patients with this condition, antibodies destroy their own red blood cells, leading to anaemia.

Type III reactions result when the antigen–antibody complexes (*immune complexes*) become deposited on the walls of the small blood vessels. Normally, PHAGOCYTES remove immune complexes effectively. However, if this mechanism is overloaded, the immune complexes persist and are eventually deposited in a range of tissues and organs. These complexes then trigger the complement system, resulting in damage to blood vessels and inflammation; an example is *glomerulonephritis*, when the 'filtering' components of the kidneys are affected.

Type IV allergic reactions are the only ones that involve delayed hypersensitivity. These reactions are caused by the actions of T cells. Here the antigens are trapped inside *macrophages* and cannot be cleared. T cells are then activated to produce cytokines, which mediate a range of inflammatory responses. In contrast to the rapid responses mediated by B-cell antibodies, T cells take longer to accumulate at the site where the antigen is present. Thus the allergic responses are delayed and appear 12 to 24 hours or more after exposure to an appropriate antigen. Contact dermatitis is one example, in which the skin responds to allergens such as nickel and rubber accelerators. These substances penetrate the skin and become linked to a carrier protein, capable of producing allergic reactions.

Hypersensitivity involving T-cell-mediated immunity occurs also in some chronic diseases due to infectious agents such as the mycobacteria that cause leprosy and tuberculosis, and parasitic worms such as schistosomiasis.

Organ TRANSPLANTATION (of kidney, heart, or lungs, respectively) is increasingly used to save patients with renal failure, cardiac failure, or cystic fibrosis. Unfortunately, T cells of the recipients can recognize and respond to foreign antigens of the grafts, leading to their eventual destruction. Immunosuppressive drugs such as steroids and cyclosporin are successful in preventing rejection. However, these drugs do not work specifically against the particular unwanted functions of macrophages or T-cells, and may reduce the patients' resistance to infections.   TAI-PING FAN

See also AUTOIMMUNE DISEASE; PHAGOCYTES; THYMUS.

Alopecia The medical term for baldness. Well known, and varying in onset, in the course of ageing. It also occurs, less irrevocably, due to skin damage or disease or to the side-effects of chemotherapy or radiotherapy in the treatment of cancer. The cells at the base of the hair follicles of the scalp, which normally keep on manufacturing new keratinous substance to add to the root of the hair, die or cease to function; the hair therefore falls out and is not replaced, until or unless that cellular function is restored. Alopecia may extend beyond the scalp to other body hair. *Alopecia areata* is a chronic condition of patchy baldness.   S.J.

See BALDNESS; HAIR; SKIN.

Altitude There is no precise definition of high altitude. However, many people feel lightheaded and have other symptoms if they ascend from near sea level to 3000 metres (about 10 000 feet). Some individuals are affected at as low as 2000 metres. Nearly 140 million people live at altitudes above 2500 metres (about 8000 feet). Substantial numbers live permanently at altitudes as high as 4500 metres in the Peruvian Andes, and caretakers of a mine in Chile have lived at nearly 6000 metres. The highest point on Earth is the summit of Mt. Everest (8848 metres), and well-

acclimatized climbers can just reach that altitude without using supplementary oxygen.

The two regions of the world with the largest high-altitude populations are the South American Andes and the Tibetan plateau. It is estimated that between 10 and 17 million people live at over 2500 metres in the Andes, and that over 50 000 people in Peru reside above 4000 metres. Lhasa, in Tibet, altitude 3658 metres, has over 130 000 inhabitants. Other parts of the world with substantial high-altitude populations include Central and North America, Europe, Russia, Africa, and Indonesia.

It is useful to divide people at high altitude into two groups; those who live there permanently ('highlanders') and those who have moved up temporarily from sea level ('lowlanders'). Lowlanders who go to high altitude undergo a process known as acclimatization, which greatly assists them in tolerating the high altitude. Some permanent residents who have been at high altitude for generations have probably undergone true Darwinian adaptation. Many features of acclimatization and adaptation are similar, but there are some differences.

Altitude and oxygen
High altitude provides physiological and medical challenges because the amount of oxygen in the air

is reduced. As we go higher, the barometric pressure falls, for the same reason as, when we are submerged deeper in water, the pressure rises. Indeed, Torricelli, who invented the mercury barometer in the mid-seventeenth century, stated, 'We live submerged at the bottom of an ocean of the element air, which by unquestioned experiments is known to have weight.' For example, if we go to an altitude of about 5800 metres, the pressure falls to half the normal sea level value of 760 mm Hg (1013 millibars or hectopascals). At the summit of Mt. Everest the pressure is about one-third of the sea level value. Since oxygen accounts for one-fifth of the volume of the air, and this fraction does not alter with altitude, the pressure of oxygen decreases proportionally with the total barometric pressure. A decrease in this 'partial pressure' of oxygen in the lungs results in a decrease in the amount of oxygen in the blood — the state of oxygen shortage, or HYPOXIA. This hypoxia is responsible for almost all the physiological changes and the potential medical problems that occur at high altitude.

The relationship between barometric pressure and altitude is not the same over the whole surface of the globe. Because of the warming of the atmosphere by the sun near the Equator, the column of air is higher there, and therefore the barometric pressure at any given altitude is higher than at the poles. These differences are

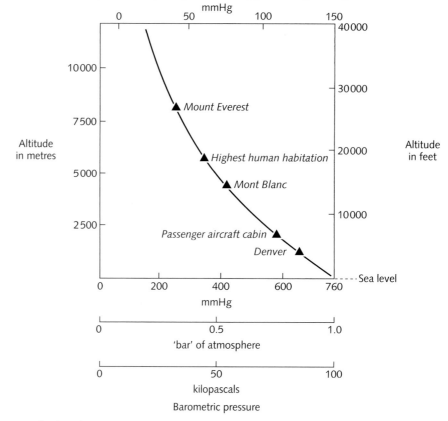

Fig. 1 Altitude and oxygen pressures. Modified, with author's approval, from J. B. West *Respiratory physiology — the essentials*. 6th edition, Lippincott Williams and Wilkins, Philadelphia, 2000.

important to the mountain climber. For example, it can be shown that if Mt. Everest were at the latitude of Mt. McKinley (Denali) in Alaska, which is 60° N, the summit would in effect be over 950 metres (3000 feet) higher because the barometric pressure at high altitude at latitudes far from the Equator is so much lower. This would make it impossible to climb the mountain without supplementary oxygen. On the other hand, the use of the International Civil Aviation Organization (ICAO) Standard Atmosphere (often used to calibrate altimeters) considerably underestimates the barometric pressure on the summit of Everest: the severity of hypoxia was therefore overestimated in some predictions based on this method in the past.

Acclimatization

The role of acclimatization in enabling lowlanders to tolerate high altitude is critical; indeed it is one of the classical examples of how the human body can adapt to hostile conditions. A normal person who is acutely exposed to the barometric pressure of the summit of Mt. Everest in a low-pressure chamber will lose consciousness within 2 or 3 minutes, but with the advantages of acclimatization, many climbers have now reached the summit without supplementary oxygen.

The most important feature of acclimatization to high altitude is an increase in the rate and depth of BREATHING. The product of the volume of each breath multiplied by the frequency of breathing is known as the total ventilation. The increase in ventilation is brought about by stimulation of CHEMORECEPTORS by the low oxygen pressure in the arterial blood. A chemoreceptor is a specialized tissue which responds to its environment by sending nerve impulses to the brain. In order for a climber to reach the Everest summit, he must increase his ventilation some 5-fold. Anecdotal evidence of this comes from tape recordings of climbers on the summit; they are so short of breath that they need to breathe after every two or three words! The reason why the increase in ventilation is so important is that it raises the pressure of oxygen in the alveoli in the depths of the lung, where the exchange between the air and blood takes place. At the same time, the increase in ventilation greatly reduces the pressure of carbon dioxide in the lungs and in the blood.

The extent to which people increase their breathing when they go to high altitude depends on their genetic make-up: some increase it much more than others. There is some evidence that climbers who have a poor ventilatory response to hypoxia tolerate very high altitudes badly. A test for this can be administered at sea level by giving people a low-oxygen mixture to breathe.

Interestingly, many people who are born at high altitude have a relatively low ventilatory response to hypoxia. This seems to be paradoxical, although it may protect them from periodic breathing during sleep (see below). It may be that these permanent residents have other adaptations at the tissue level which are not yet understood.

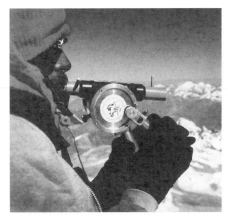

Fig. 2 Dr Christopher Pizzo taking samples of air from his lungs while sitting on the summit of Mt. Everest during the course of the 1981 American Medical Research Expedition to Everest. Photograph by Yong Tenzing Sherpa.

Another feature of acclimatization is an increase in the concentration of red cells in the blood. For example, a permanent resident at 4600 metres in the Peruvian Andes typically has a 30% increase in red cell concentration. This *polycythaemia* increases the oxygen carrying capacity of the blood. However, the value of polycythaemia in the acclimatization process is not as clear as it was once thought to be. Severe polycythaemia increases the viscosity of the blood and probably leads to problems with unloading oxygen from the blood to the tissues. Some permanent residents of the Andes can actually do more physical work when the concentration of red cells in their blood is reduced by bloodletting.

The mechanism responsible for polycythaemia is the release of the hormone *erythropoietin* from the kidney as a result of the shortage of oxygen there. The erythropoietin then stimulates the production of red blood cells by the bone marrow. The evolutionary pressure for the development of this mechanism probably occurred at sea level, promoting survival after injury, because blood loss also causes inadequacy of oxygen supply. It may be that its value as an adaptation to high altitude has been overemphasized.

The CARDIAC OUTPUT increases with acute hypoxia, compensating for the shortage of oxygen in the blood by increasing the rate of blood supply, but in acclimatized subjects it returns to the sea level value. Other features of acclimatization include an increase in the concentration of capillaries in peripheral tissues, and increases in the amount of oxidative ENZYMES within cells. It is likely that some of the acclimatization processes at the cellular level have not yet been discovered.

Many features of the adaptation of permanent residents to high altitude are similar to those of acclimatization. Interestingly, there is some evidence that Tibetans have progressed further in the adaptation process than Andeans, consistent with the much longer period that they have spent at

high altitude. Features that suggest better adaptation include less polycythaemia, greater ventilation, lower pressures in the pulmonary circulation, and an apparent lower incidence of '*chronic mountain sickness*' (see below). However, this is an active area of research and there is some controversy.

Mount Everest

One of the great sagas of this century has been the ascent of Mt. Everest without supplementary oxygen. In 1920 the mountaineer–physiologist Alexander Kellas predicted that it could be done if the technical difficulties were not too great. During the 1924 British expedition to Everest, E. F. Norton climbed to within 300 metres of the summit without supplementary oxygen, but in the 1930s several physiological studies suggested that the summit could not be reached. It was not until 1978, 54 years after Norton, that the last 300 metres were conquered by Messner and Habeler.

The critical factors on the summit are the barometric pressure, the extent of the increase in the climber's ventilation, and his maximal oxygen uptake. The first measurements of these were obtained by the American Medical Research Expedition to Everest in 1981 (Fig. 2). In 1985 a simulated climb in a low-pressure chamber, Operation Everest II, greatly clarified the physiological adaptations at extreme altitudes, particularly in the pulmonary circulation and skeletal muscle. For example, the resistance of the pulmonary circulation was greatly increased at very high altitudes, because hypoxia constricted the blood vessels. Also, muscle biopsies showed an increase in the concentration of capillaries because the muscle fibres became thinner.

Altitude sickness

Various forms of altitude sickness are recognized. Newcomers to high altitude frequently complain of headache, fatigue, dizziness, palpitations, nausea, loss of appetite, and insomnia. This is known as *acute mountain sickness*, and usually resolves after 2 or 3 days at medium altitudes. It is probably caused by the combination of the low oxygen and the *alkalosis* in the blood resulting from the reduced pressure of carbon dioxide. Administration of the drug *acetazolamide* reduces the incidence of acute mountain sickness.

A more severe illness is *high-altitude pulmonary oedema*, in which the capillaries in the lung are damaged and leak high-protein fluid into the alveolar spaces. The damage is due to high pressures in the pulmonary circulation, which develop in response to the hypoxia. This potentially fatal condition is best treated by taking the patient down to a lower altitude as rapidly as possible, though oxygen is given if this is available. An even more serious problem is *high-altitude cerebral oedema* due to leakage of fluid into the brain tissues. Again, descent is by far the best treatment. Long-term residents at high altitude sometimes develop an ill-defined syndrome characterized by fatigue, reduced ability to exercise, very low levels of oxygen in the blood, and marked polycythaemia. This is called *chronic mountain sickness*, and again descent is the best treatment if this is practicable.

Newcomers to high altitude often complain that the most distressing period is during the night when they try to sleep. *Periodic breathing* frequently occurs. This is characterized by a gradual waxing and then waning of breathing movements, and often there is a period of no breathing at all (*apnea*) which may last for 10 sec or more. Sometimes people wake up at the end of the apneic period feeling smothered. Treatment with acetazolamide reduces the incidence and severity of periodic breathing. Permanent residents of high altitude who have a reduced ventilatory response to hypoxia develop less periodic breathing.

Factors other than hypoxia

All of the physiological and medical problems of going to high altitude described above have their root in the low partial pressure of oxygen in the air. This is an inevitable consequence of going to high altitude unless, of course, supplementary oxygen is breathed. However there are other potentially hostile factors at high altitude. One is cold. The air temperature falls at the rate of about 1 °C for every 150 metres of altitude. The effects of cold can of course be mitigated by warm clothing and shelter, but if there is a high wind the resulting chill factor makes it impossible to climb at great altitudes.

Another potential problem results from the low absolute humidity of the air because of the low temperatures. Climbers frequently become dehydrated because they lose a great deal of water vapour as a result of their high ventilation, and it is difficult to obtain water by melting snow. Solar radiation is increased at high altitude because of reduced absorption by the thinner atmosphere, and reflection of the sun from snow. Ionizing radiation, for example by cosmic rays, is also increased because of the thinner atmosphere.

Working at high altitude

Recently there has been a large increase in commercial and scientific facilities, such as mines and telescopes, at very high altitudes. Much of this development has taken place in the Andes, particularly in north Chile. As an example, the Collahuasi copper mine at an altitude of 4500 metres was being greatly expanded in the late 1990s. The workers live at sea level and are taken by bus up to the mine in a few hours, where they spend the next seven days working. They are then taken down to their families at sea level for seven days, and the cycle continues indefinitely. This cycling raises many physiological and medical problems which are poorly understood as yet. Another example is a new radiotelescope being planned for an altitude of 5000 metres in north Chile. The workers will live at an altitude of about 2400 metres and commute up to the telescope each day.

An interesting innovation is the addition of oxygen to the air conditioning in these facilities, in dormitories, offices, conference rooms, laboratories, and even in the cabins of large trucks and mechanical shovels. Every 1% of enrichment (for example increasing the oxygen concentration from 21% to 22%) is equivalent to reducing the altitude by 300 metres. Five per cent oxygen enrichment in a mine at 4500 metres could therefore reduce the equivalent altitude to 3000 metres, which is much more easily tolerated. Oxygen enrichment has become feasible because large amounts of oxygen can easily be produced from air by oxygen concentrators, and also because liquid oxygen is relatively inexpensive. The potential value of this proactive approach to dealing with the hypoxia of high altitude is still being clarified.   JOHN B. WEST

Further reading
Ward, M. P., Milledge, J. S., and West, J. B. (2000). *High altitude medicine and physiology*, (3rd edn). Arnold, London.

West, J. B. (1985). *Everest — the testing place*. McGraw-Hill, New York.

See also FLYING; HYPOXIA; OXYGEN.

Amazons A legendary nation of female warriors, supposedly of Caucasian origin, living in Pontus near the shore of the Euxine Sea. The distinctiveness of the fabled Amazons lay in their being an all-female tribe who destroyed the right breasts of girls at puberty so as to permit them to draw a bow more easily – hence their Greek name: *mazon* (breast), and *a* (no). According to Herodotus they formed a separate realm under the government of their queen, their capital being Themiscyra in Cappadocia on the banks of the River Thermodon. From there they were said to carry out warlike raids into Scythia, Thrace, the coasts of Asia Minor, and the Aegean islands, penetrating as far as Arabia, Syria, and Egypt.

No men were permitted to live in their territory, but once a year, to prevent them from dying out, they visited the neighbouring Gargareans and formed temporary sexual unions. Such male children as resulted were either put to death or sent back to their fathers; but the daughters were kept, brought up by their mothers, and trained in agriculture, hunting, and fighting.

These legendary Amazons appear in several Greek fables. The *Iliad* tells us that they invaded Lycia, but were defeated by Bellerophon. According to Virgil they attacked the Phrygians, who were assisted by Priam, though later they took his side against the Greeks, under the Amazon queen Penthesileia, who was killed by Achilles. One of the labours imposed on Heracles (the Roman Hercules) was to gain possession of the girdle of the Amazonian queen, Hippolyte. Hercules' companion, Theseus, ravished Princess Antiope, Hippolyte's sister. The Amazons also crop up at the time of Alexander the Great, and Pompey was said to have come across them in Mithridates' army. The deities they worshipped were Ares (whom they saw as a god of war of

Thracian origin), and Artemis — not the Greek goddess but the Asiatic deity.

The origin of the story of the Amazons has been widely disputed. Many have argued that they were purely a mythical people; but others assume some kind of historical foundation. It has been suggested that, with the spread of geographical knowledge, travellers brought back reports of tribes, on the very borders of the known world, ruled by women who fulfilled duties elsewhere judged as unique to men. Hence belief grew in the Amazons as a nation of female warriors, organized and governed entirely by women. The fact that Heracles and Theseus, the two famous heroes of Greek mythology, are credited with the conquest of the Amazons has been taken by some to suggest that the Amazons were mythical representations of the perils that beset the Greeks on the coasts of Asia Minor. Alternatively the Amazon legend may represent the struggle between Greek culture and native barbarism, or the perennial travellers' tale of an upside-down world, or — a Freudian explanation — basic misogynistic fears.

In works of art, fighting between Amazons and Greeks is represented as similar to combats between Greeks and centaurs. Their arms were the bow, spear, and axe, a crescent-shaped shield, called *pelta*, and (in early art) a helmet — the original model in the Greek mind apparently being the goddess Athena. In later art they approach the style of Artemis, wearing flimsy attire, hitched up for speed. On still later painted vases, their dress is distinctively Persian — close-fitting trousers and a high cap called the *kidaris*. The battle between Theseus and the Amazons is a favoured subject on temple friezes, vases and sarcophagus reliefs; at Athens it was represented on the shield of the statue of Athena Parthenos.

Since classical times, 'amazonian' has been widely applied as an epithet to barbarous women or self-sufficient groups of women who eschew the company of males.   ROY PORTER

Amino acids are the building blocks of PROTEINS. They are so named because all have a basic amino group (–NH$_2$) and an acidic carboxyl group (–COOH). PEPTIDES, polypeptides, and proteins are formed from strings of amino acids joined together by the formation of peptide bonds. All proteins are formed from combinations of only 20 different amino acids, whether the proteins derive from bacteria or from man.

Amino acids are described as essential or non-essential. The non-essential ones can be synthesized in the body but the essential amino acids are those which must be present in the diet (phenylalanine, valine, tryptophan, threonine, lysine, leucine, isoleucine, and methionine). If any one of these amino acids is missing from the diet then many proteins which include this essential component cannot be synthesized. Consequently many other amino acids cannot then be used; they are broken down (deaminated) and the nitrogen is excreted as urea and creatinine, leading to a negative nitrogen balance, as more

Apache Native American coming-of-age ceremony, entailing blessing with pollen. Martha Cooper/Still Pictures.

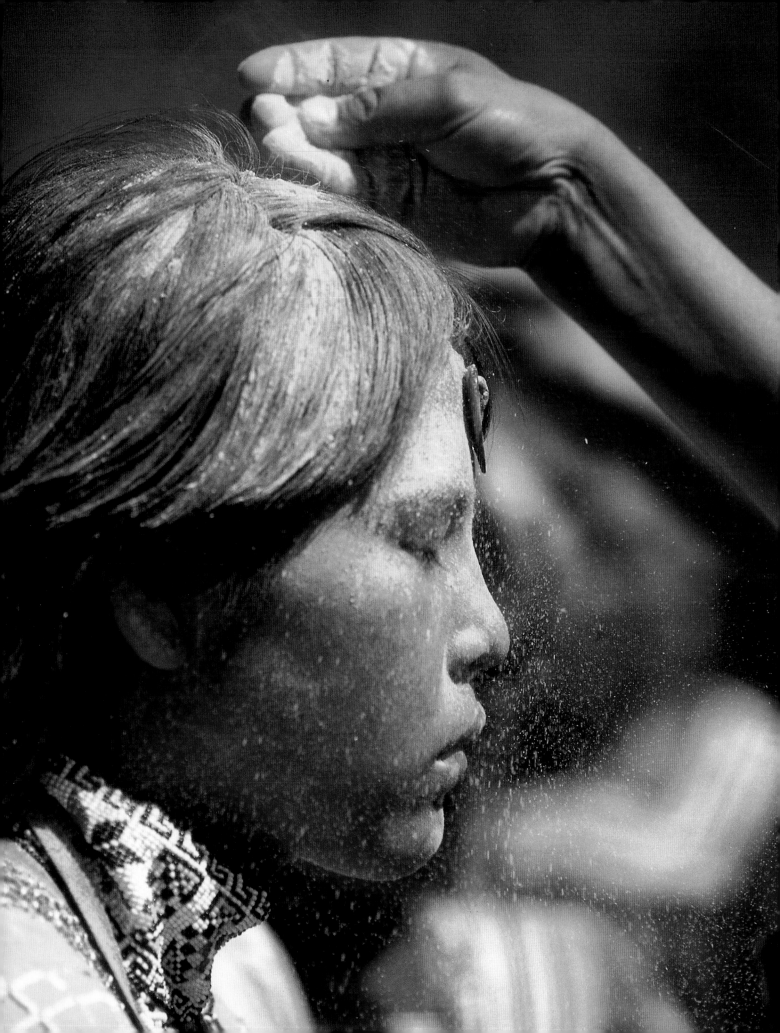

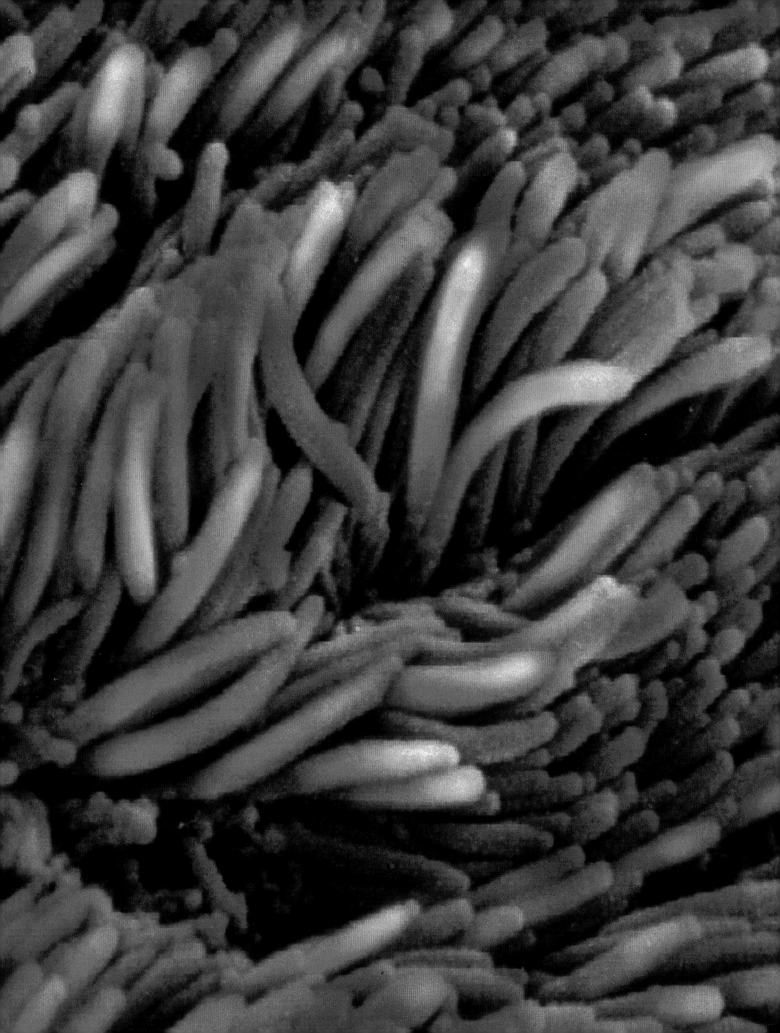

nitrogen is excreted than is taken in as dietary protein.

The adult body cannot absorb whole proteins from the gut, although young babies are able to absorb antibodies, which are proteins, from mother's milk; this provides passive immunity for the first year or so of life. The digestive processes break down dietary protein to amino acids and small peptides (two or more linked amino acids). Carriers, specific for a single amino acid or a group of similar amino acids, are present in the cells lining the intestine and are responsible for the specific uptake into these cells. Some dipeptides (and maybe tripeptides) also have specialized carrier molecules for uptake in the intestine, and the final stage of their digestion to amino acids takes place in these epithelial cells themselves. Thence they move into the circulating blood; thus amino acids from the diet enter the body's amino acid pool, mixing with other amino acids derived from the breakdown of body proteins in the continual turnover associated with growth, repair, and renewal of tissues. Cells of the different tissues take up selectively from the blood whichever amino acids they need for synthesis of their own proteins. The circulating amino acids gained from digestion are in no great danger of excretion via the kidneys: they are filtered at the glomeruli but are mostly reabsorbed into the blood as they pass down the kidney tubules.

Finally, how is the dietary intake of protein linked to the need for amino acids, particularly the essential ones? The linkage need not be a strong one, as connections exist between the metabolism of amino acids and the metabolism of fats and carbohydrates. Further, there can be conversion of one amino acid to another, at least for the non-essential amino acids. These *transamination* reactions are common in tissues that have been damaged, as repair and resynthesis take place. Thus after a myocardial infarction the level of the relevant enzymes — *transaminases* — rises in the blood, and this measurement is used for diagnostic purposes. Excess amino acids are subject to *oxidative deamination*: the amino group is removed and excreted as nitrogen products and the residue converted either to a ketone body, called acetoacetic acid (one of the products also of fat metabolism), or to products readily converted to glucose. Amino acids are therefore divided into *ketogenic* or *gluconeogenic* (conversion to glucose) types.

Nitrogen losses in the urine may be greater than the nitrogen intake in the diet (negative nitrogen balance) not only when the essential amino acids are missing, but also when the calorie intake is adequate but the overall protein content of the diet is too low; this occurs in *kwashiorkor*, common in poorly nourished children. If the diet is inadequate in calories as well as deficient in protein, body proteins are broken down to form glucose for energy. This can be prevented by giving glucose, which is thus said to be 'protein-sparing'.   ALAN W. CUTHBERT

See also PEPTIDES; PROTEINS.

Amnesia We forget almost everything that we have, at some time, briefly remembered. Think of all the telephone numbers you have kept in mind between looking in the directory and dialling the number; of all the people and places you once knew for a few minutes but have now mostly forgotten; of every meal that you have eaten, which you could have described in detail the same day, but could not possibly remember now. Given the overwhelming flood of information that pours into our brains each day, forgetting most things is just as important as remembering some.

On the other hand, forgetfulness can become an illness, an incapacitating inability to remember things, which is called amnesia. Amnesia occurs in many situations — after head injuries, in Alzheimer's disease, and, to some extent, in all old people. But it has mainly been studied in particular patients with profound impairments of MEMORY, despite otherwise normal cognitive ability and intelligence. These patients are said to have the amnesic syndrome, whose characteristics include: (i) *severe anterograde amnesia*: poor retention of new information, exhibited by difficulty in spontaneously recalling words and objects, in recognizing faces (unless they are very familiar), and in learning associations between words or things; (ii) *retrograde amnesia*: poor recollection of previously established memories (such as knowledge of one's childhood, and even such things as one's own name). In general, the retrograde component of clinical amnesia is less severe than the anterograde, and may be limited to a period of months or years prior to the onset of the amnesia. In some way, ancient memories are more robust than newer ones, and can persist even when new, conscious long-term memories cannot be formed.

Despite these defects in long-term memory, patients with clinical amnesia have relatively normal short-term memory span (as measured by the ability immediately to recall a list of digits). Indeed, amnesic patients are able to engage in normal conversation and recall current information so long as it is continually 'rehearsed'. But after just a few seconds of distraction, they may forget not only what has been said but even whether they have met the person they were talking to moments before.

Not all forms of long-term learning are impaired. Motor skills (such as typing on a keyboard or driving a car) learnt prior to the onset of the illness are unaffected, and patients show residual abilities to learn new motor skills (even though they are not consciously aware of having done the motor task before). Other simple forms of memory also persist, including classical conditioning (the kind of simple learning shown by PAVLOV's dogs when they salivated to the sound of a bell after it had been rung a few times before the presentation of food). The common denominator between the forms of learning still exhibited by amnesic patients is that they can all be mediated without the need for recollection of past experience: they involve what has been called *procedural learning* (the learning of skills) or *implicit learning* (unconscious learning).

The vast majority of amnesic patients are chronic alcoholics, suffering from *Korsakoff's syndrome*. This is due to diffuse brain damage, predominately to lower parts of the cerebral hemispheres (principally the mamillary bodies and dorso-medial nucleus of the THALAMUS), although there is also frequently degeneration of the frontal lobes of the CEREBRAL CORTEX. The gradual deterioration of mental function is probably due to the toxic effects of alcohol, combined with thiamine deficiency. In addition to profound memory impairments, Korsakoff patients also exhibit a range of impairments shared by patients with damage to the frontal lobes, such as lack of insight into their own deficits, confabulation (inventing explanations for their difficulties), and impairments on tests of card sorting. Due to the multiple sites of damage and the diffuse nature of the brain damage it is hard to draw firm conclusions from Korsakoff patients about which particular structures in the brain contribute to memory.

Discrete damage to the brain, especially to parts of the interior surface of the temporal lobes of the cerebral hemispheres, can also cause profound anterograde amnesia. The classical example of this devastating condition is the patient known by his initials, H. M., who underwent surgery to remove the inner parts of the temporal lobe on both sides, to relieve intractable epilepsy, and has subsequently suffered deep amnesia for decades. This part of the brain includes specialized regions of cerebral cortex called the hippocampus and the amygdala, which are thought to be involved in the laying down of memories. Unfortunately this vital part of the brain seems to be particularly vulnerable: it is relatively easily damaged by hypoxia (for instance during surgical operations in which blood supply to the brain is compromised), by the degenerative changes that occur in Alzheimer's disease, and by infection in herpes simplex encephalitis. All of these conditions can produce pronounced amnesia.

Although intensively studied and extensively documented in a small group of select patients, the classical amnesic syndrome may not be completely typical of most people with amnesia. The extent of retrograde amnesia for personal recollections of the past is particularly hard to assess in the absence of any independent verification. The amount of retrograde amnesia in H. M., for example, may have been grossly underestimated. It has even been argued that there may not be a single amnesic syndrome, since patients with temporal lobe damage tend to forget information rapidly, whereas Korsakoff patients, given enough training, are able to retain information over longer periods of time.

Because of the complexity of clinical syndromes, most of our present understanding of which neural systems contribute to normal learning and memory have come from the study of animals, especially of animal 'models' of

Cilia on cells of the mucous membrane in the nose. BSIP VEM/Science Photo Library.

human amnesia. It was initially believed that combined damage to the hippocampus and amygdala was necessary to produce severe anterograde amnesia, and the hippocampus in particular became the supposed seat of '*episodic*' (personal, conscious) memory. However, this view has been challenged by the discovery that damage to a neighbouring region, the rhinal cortex, which underlies the hippocampus and amygdala, was necessary and sufficient to produce memory impairments.

Behavioural studies on monkeys, analysing the effect of circumscribed damage to specific regions in the inner part of the temporal lobe, have identified several dissociable, interacting memory structures. Much research effort is presently focused on ascertaining the role of these different components. For example, current research has called into question the traditionally accepted role of the hippocampus in episodic memory and suggests instead that this structure may play a more restricted role in the memory of places, which then contributes to a broader neural memory system. Other components of this system include the amygdala, now believed to be involved in remembering whether particular stimuli are associated with rewarding or punishing events. Another important nearby structure is the perirhinal cortex, which appears to be specialized for processing knowledge about objects. The nerve fibres of the white matter within the temporal lobe, known as the temporal stem, have also been implicated in memory. However the temporal lobe is by no means the only structure involved in human learning and memory. Communication between the temporal lobe and the frontal lobe is also important and this interaction occurs via multiple routes. In fact, neither the hippocampus, amygdala, perirhinal cortex, temporal stem, nor any other single structure in the temporal lobe when damaged on its own results in dense amnesia. But this does occur when the majority of the routes by which the temporal lobe can interact with the frontal lobe are interrupted.

Detailed structural imaging of the brain of H. M., through magnetic resonance imaging (MRI), has recently confirmed the extent of bilateral damage sustained by each of the temporal lobe structures in H. M., and this has been interpreted in terms of the understanding gained from the study of animals. The damage in H. M. is entirely consistent with the predictions from animal studies — one indication of the usefulness of these models in understanding the neural systems underlying normal human learning and memory.　　　　　　　MARK BUCKLEY

Further reading

Bolhuis, J. J.(2000). *Brain, perception, memory: advances in cognitive neuroscience*. Oxford University Press, Oxford.

Eysenck, M. W. (1995). *Cognitive psychology: a student's handbook*, (3rd edn). Erlbaum, Hove.

See also BRAIN; CEREBRAL CORTEX; HYPOTHALAMUS; LIMBIC SYSTEM; MEMORY.

Amniocentesis Removal of fluid from the amniotic cavity. This is accomplished by passing a long, fine needle through the abdominal wall and through the underlying wall of the pregnant uterus, and aspirating a sample into a syringe. The purpose is to obtain stray cells shed from the fetus into the fluid, which can provide evidence of genetic abnormalities, especially Down's syndrome. Because the risk of conceiving such an infant increases with age, amniocentesis is commonly advised at about 16 weeks of pregnancy in any mother over about 35. The procedure is combined with ultrasound scanning, which allows the fetus, the placenta, and the needle to be visualized, and damage thus avoided. There is a very small risk of inducing miscarriage (less than 1% in good hands). Preliminary tests on the mother's blood may indicate how strongly amniocentesis is to be advised.　　　　　　　　　　　　S.J.

See ANTENATAL DEVELOPMENT; CONGENITAL ABNORMALITIES; PREGNANCY; ULTRASOUND.

Amputation The word 'amputation' derives from the Latin *ambi* — around — and *putare* — to prune or lop. The word can be applied to the removal of any part of the body, but it is usually restricted to removal of part of a limb, unless the word is qualified, as in 'amputation of the nose'. Children born with an absent part of a limb are often said to have a congenital amputation.

The amputation of a limb represents one of the earliest forms of SURGERY and was performed for severely damaged arms and legs in both war and peace over many centuries. In the days before anaesthesia, speed was of the essence; the surgeon would cut through the flesh of the limb with a single sweep of the knife and then divide the bone with a few strokes of the saw. Haemorrhage was dealt with by the crude technique of cauterization of the stump, using boiling oil or a red-hot iron, until Ambroise Paré (1510–90), a French military surgeon, showed that tying of the blood vessels was a far safer and much kinder method. In modern surgical amputations, skin flaps are raised, the soft tissues carefully divided, blood vessels tied, the bone divided, the soft tissues and then skin carefully sutured, and the stump bandaged to produce a relatively aesthetic appearance.

The indications for amputation of a limb include severe injury, where the blood supply to the limb has been hopelessly damaged; severe infection following injury (particularly gas gangrene); malignant tumours of bone or of the adjacent soft tissues; and occasionally the removal of a hopelessly deformed arm or leg. In peacetime, however, by far the commonest indication is gangrene due to severe arterial disease, usually arteriosclerotic or diabetic in origin, and not infrequently from a combination of these two conditions.

With modern surgical techniques, the limb that was once doomed to amputation can often be saved. Whereas at one time damage to the main limb artery in a fracture or a missile injury usually meant loss of the arm or leg, reconstructive arterial surgery can now often repair the damaged vessel, often by means of an interposed graft of a vein taken from the superficial tissues of the leg. For example, surgeons in Northern Ireland have become experts at reconstruction of the popliteal vessels behind the knee destroyed in terrorist 'knee capping' punishments with salvage of the leg in almost every case.

Severe arterial disease of the leg arteries is common and once inevitably led to amputation. Fortunately, this again may be overcome by a bypass of the obstructed segment of the artery, using the patient's own vein or a synthetic graft. In other cases, the diseased artery can be opened and cored out, in the operation of *endarterectomy*. Alternatively, the narrowed, stenosed segment can be dilated by a catheter which carries an inflatable balloon, inserted above the segment and guided to it under X-ray.

Limbs that once had to be removed due to a tumour can now sometimes be preserved by removing the bone growth itself and replacing the missing segment by means of a metal prosthesis.

When amputation is necessary, rehabilitation of the amputee is an important adjunct to management. The crude artificial limbs of the past — the amputee kneeling on a peg leg, or a purely cosmetic and non-functional upper limb prosthesis — have now been replaced by very sophisticated devices. For lower limb amputees lightweight limbs with ingenious 'joints' allow a below-knee amputee to walk normally, and even engage in various exercises, such as running in Olympic-style events. Above-knee prostheses are more of a problem, but a 'knee joint' with a locking device enables efficient walking to be carried out. An upper limb prosthesis may be fitted with pulleys activated by the shoulder girdle muscles, which enable activation of an artificial gripping 'hand' and a functioning 'elbow'. These devices, ingenious though they are, can only be made to be effective if used by an enthusiastic and motivated patient trained by a dedicated team of orthopaedic surgeons, physiotherapists, and limb makers; these are combined in the modern speciality of orthotics.　　　HAROLD ELLIS

See also PHANTOM LIMB; PROSTHESES.

Anaemia The main task of red blood cells is to transport OXYGEN bound to HAEMOGLOBIN from the lungs to the tissues. Anaemia is a condition in which the circulating red cell mass is insufficient to serve this function normally. It is usually defined by measuring the haemoglobin level in the BLOOD. Because of the wide range of haemoglobin values at different ages and in different populations the definition of anaemia involves the adoption of arbitrary criteria. The World Health Organization recommends that anaemia should be considered to exist in adults with haemoglobin levels lower than 13 grams per decilitre (g/dl) (males) or 12 g/dl (females). Children aged 6 months to 6 years are considered to be anaemic if their haemoglobin levels are below 11 g/dl, and those 6–14 years, below 12 g/dl.

At haemoglobin values not less than 8–9 g/dl, compensatory mechanisms involving subtle changes in the chemistry of the red cell are brought into play, such that adequate oxygenation of the tissues is maintained and there may be no symptoms. However, even at this moderately reduced haemoglobin level it has been found that the ability to work and carry out day-to-day activities is impaired. Below 8 g/dl, further compensatory mechanisms are required, including an increased cardiac output: faster heart rate and greater volume of blood pumped out at each beat. At less than 5 g/dl even these mechanisms fail to maintain oxygenation of the organs and tissues; there are symptoms and signs of oxygen deprivation and, eventually, of HEART FAILURE. These include lethargy, shortness of breath, pallor, a rapid bounding pulse, accumulation of fluid in the tissues (OEDEMA), buzzing in the ears (TINNITUS), visual disturbances, and chest pain due to reduced oxygen delivery to the heart muscle.

Anaemia is an important world health problem. It is estimated that it affects 47% of all women, 59% of pregnant women, and 26% of men in the developing world. In the richer, developed countries, it affects approximately 10% of women and 3% of men at some time during their lives.

Anaemia results either from defective production of red blood cells and their contents, or from their increased rate of destruction or loss from the body. Most forms of anaemia are acquired during a person's lifetime. There are also some inherited varieties but, with the exception of the genetic disorders of haemoglobin, these are extremely rare.

Red cells are the products of precursors that proliferate in the bone marrow and develop through a series of stages to produce mature forms. The commonest cause of anaemia is defective proliferation and maturation due to *iron deficiency*, because iron is a necessary component of the haemoglobin molecule. In the developing countries this is normally the result of poor diet, often combined with blood loss due to parasitic infection, particularly hookworm. In richer countries iron deficiency may also be due to diet, or to chronic bleeding. Common causes include duodenal ulcers, haemorrhoids, bowel cancer, and uterine bleeding. Heavy or even normal menstrual blood loss may be a cause if there is not adequate iron in the diet. Iron deficiency anaemias are described as *hypochromic* and *microcytic*, meaning that the red blood cells are pale and small.

As well as iron, red cell production also requires certain VITAMINS, particularly B$_{12}$ and folic acid. Their deficiency results in a failure of red cell maturation, with the production of large, immature red cells that are called macrocytes; hence anaemias of this type are called *macrocytic*. Vitamin B$_{12}$ deficiency usually

follows autoimmune (self-destructive) damage to the stomach, leading to the defective production of *intrinsic factor*, a protein that is required for its absorption. Occasionally it results from dietary deficiency, but only in total vegetarians (VEGANS), because it is present only in animal sources. Because vitamin B$_{12}$ is also required for the normal function of the nervous system, the resulting disease, *pernicious anaemia* is characterized by neurological disturbances as well as profound anaemia. Folic acid deficiency may be nutritional or due to disease of the small bowel — coeliac disease for example — leading to its defective absorption. This also causes a macrocytic anaemia, but without the neurological features of vitamin B$_{12}$ deficiency.

Anaemia may also result from defective proliferation of red cell precursors. This may follow the action of drugs or toxins that damage the bone marrow, causing *aplastic anaemia* or infiltration of the marrow with neoplastic (cancer) cells, usually those associated with different forms of leukaemia.

Normally, red cells survive in the circulation for about 120 days, when they are disrupted by *haemolysis*, and their chemical components recycled. Anaemia can occur if their survival time is shortened, such that replacement cannot keep up with destruction. These *haemolytic anaemias* may be due to inherited abnormalities of the red cell membrane, of the cells' internal chemical pathways, or of haemoglobin; or they may develop because of production of antibodies that destroy red cells, or by damage to the microscopic blood vessels, which has the same effect. Genetic defects of the red cell membrane may cause the red cells to assume a spherical rather than a biconcave shape, or alter their configuration to an elliptical form. Inherited abnormalities involving the chemistry of the red cell are rarer. The only common anaemia of this type is due to the deficiency of an enzyme called glucose-6-phosphate dehydrogenase. This disorder, which affects millions of people world-wide, results in a haemolytic anaemia in response to a variety of drugs.

By far the most widespread genetic forms of anaemia are those that involve the structure or synthesis of haemoglobin. The commonest structural abnormality is *sickle cell anaemia*, in which an inherited defect in the structure of globin makes red cells assume a sickle shape when the oxygen tension of the blood falls; sickled cells are prematurely destroyed, causing a haemolytic anaemia. The commonest genetic disorders of haemoglobin are the *thalassaemias*; diseases due to the defective synthesis of the α or β chains of haemoglobin. Some forms of thalassaemia cause profound anaemia due to ineffective red cell production; they affect hundreds of thousands of children throughout the Mediterranean region, the Middle East, Indian subcontinent, and South-east Asia.

MARK WEATHERALL
D.J. WEATHERALL

See also BLOOD.

Anaerobic Applying to METABOLISM in the cells of the body, or to micro-organisms, this means functioning without oxygen. Examples include anaerobic glycolysis: the pathway of hexose breakdown from glucose 6-phosphate to lactate in muscle, and the main component of the metabolism of red blood cells, which have no mitochondria. Anaerobic bacteria inhabit the lower part of the intestines. Applying to EXERCISE: more intense than can be maintained in balance with oxygen intake, aerobic pathways being insufficient to supply energy at the required rate (though they always contribute as well) — as in a 200-metre sprint.   N.C.S.

See EXERCISE; LACTATE THRESHOLD; METABOLISM.

Anaesthesia, general The idea of deliberately inducing unconsciousness to avoid the pain of an operation must have been a strange one to our forebears: *ether*, one of the earliest anaesthetics, had been known and available for some 300 years before it was used, and Humphry Davy, in 1800, had suggested NITROUS OXIDE (laughing gas) for this purpose. Following the not entirely satisfactory introduction of nitrous oxide by the American dentist Horace Wells (1815–48) in Hertford, Connecticut, in December 1844, the first successful public administration of ether anaesthesia for a surgical operation was demonstrated by his colleague W. T. G. Morton (1819–68), on 16 October 1846, at the Massachusetts General Hospital, Boston. The news was brought to England by steam ship, and the first ether anaesthetic for a surgical operation in London was administered at University College Hospital on 21 December.

In England the practice of anaesthesia was established on a firm foundation of basic science by John Snow (1813–58), who devised inhalers which allowed him to know and control the strength of the vapour that the patient was breathing. The psychological barrier having been broken, the unpleasant and irritating ether was replaced within a year by the pleasanter and more potent *chloroform*, introduced primarily to relieve the pains of labour by the Scottish obstetrician James Young Simpson (1811–70). Other vapours were soon tried, but with less success. Although the inception of general anaesthesia at this particular time is attributed by some historians to the development of a greater sense of empathy with one's fellows, citing in support of this thesis the many humanitarian reforms of the early Victorian period, it has to be pointed out that general anaesthesia originated not in Great Britain, but in the US, where the climate was quite different. Morton, who tried to patent the process, was motivated by the desire to emulate the entrepreneurial success of other Americans who had become extremely wealthy in a very short time. It is significant that both Wells and Morton were specifically looking for a means of rendering dental extractions pain free.

The spread of the practice of anaesthesia across the globe has been traced assiduously in recent years, but research has shown also that its availability tended to be restricted by financial considerations. The operation for club foot, without an anaesthetic, described vividly by Flaubert, son of a surgeon, in his novel *Madame Bovary*, was not a rarity in real life, and as late as 1893 some English Poor Law institutions were being criticized for not providing anaesthesia for surgical operations. But John Snow was called in 1853, and again in 1857, to administer chloroform to Queen Victoria in childbirth.

Snow introduced quantitative methods into anaesthesia. He recorded the amount used in each case, attempted to measure in animals the blood level of ether and chloroform required for surgical anaesthesia, and established that the potency of an anaesthetic agent is inversely related to its solubility in the blood. At his death his mantle fell on Joseph Clover (1825–82), who devoted his life to making anaesthesia safer. The photograph below, well known to anaesthetists, shows him demonstrating the induction of chloroform anaesthesia with a finger on the patient's pulse. He was involved in reintroducing nitrous oxide into anaesthetic practice during the late 1860s, and devised a number of apparatuses, one of which, the famous Clover inhaler, remained in use, in its various modifications, for many years.

Following Clover's death, British anaesthesia settled into a state of complacency and inertia, until stirred out of it towards the turn of the century by the physiologist A. D. Waller (1856–1922). Concerned by the steadily increasing number of deaths attributed to chloroform, Waller advocated limitation of the concentration being inhaled, and stimulated the design of several 'dosimetric' apparatuses. But the peripatetic anaesthetist, who generally gave his hospital services free, and

travelled from one nursing home, or even private house, to another, to earn his living, had little enthusiasm for anything which could not be carried in his pocket or his top hat. Hence the popularity of the 'rag and bottle' widely used for chloroform.

In 1910 Frederick Hewitt, the leader of the specialty, pointed out that whereas it was illegal to sell alcohol without a licence, anyone, even a hospital porter or the surgeon's coachman, could, and did, administer anaesthetics. But his attempt to get the practice of anaesthesia restricted to the medically qualified received no support from the then Home Secretary, Winston Churchill, and to this day there is no specific legislation on the subject. In the 1890s Hewitt designed a nitrous oxide apparatus which remained in use in casualty departments and dental surgeries for the next 40 years. The gas flowed to the face mask via a large rubber reservoir bag and a three-way valve. The routine was to administer pure nitrous oxide until the patient was deep blue, then allow one breath of air via the valve, or two if the patient was twitching, then settle down to three breaths of gas to one of air.

The Great War brought with it the Boyle's machine, a name now generically applied to most anaesthetic apparatuses. Copied by H. E. G. Boyle (1875–1941) of St Bartholomew's Hospital from an American apparatus, this incorporated cylinders of nitrous oxide and oxygen, a flowmeter, and vaporizers for ether and chloroform, all mounted on a trolley. The vapour mixture flowed to the patient via a reservoir bag, delivery tube, expiratory valve (the breathing circuit), and a face mask.

The Great War also put many possible developments into abeyance, and during the 1920s the lead passed to the US. The 1930s saw the introduction of new inhalational agents, notably *cyclopropane*, so potent that it could be given with a high percentage of oxygen, and as a result valuable for the developing surgery for lung disease. The decade saw also the spread of 'mechanization', deplored by some, the increasing use of Boyle's-type machines to replace the 'art' of dripping ether or chloroform onto a gauze-covered wire mask. Also, rather tentatively at first, came the introduction of drugs which could be given by intravenous injection to induce unconsciousness rapidly and avoid the unpleasantness of an inhalational induction. This, together with the development of methods that involved passing a tube through the larynx into the trachea to prevent obstruction of the air passages during operations on the nose and throat, and to allow control of respiration during surgery of the lungs, required the anaesthetist to learn a range of new skills. This did not come easily to the older generation.

The 1930s also saw a drive, led by Lucy Baldwin, wife of the then Prime Minister, towards the improvement of pain relief in midwifery. The Minnitt apparatus, devised by R. J. Minnitt (1890–1974) of Liverpool in 1934, supplied a mixture of nitrous oxide and air, and was approved by

the Central Midwives Board for use by midwives without medical supervision. Another important development, which stemmed from the generosity of Lord Nuffield, was the establishment in the University of Oxford of an academic research and teaching department with its own professor, the first in the UK.

Anaesthesia developed rapidly during the second half of the 1940s, both in techniques and standards. During World War II many doctors were trained as anaesthetists in the Forces, and found hospital appointments on demobilization, during the run-up to the establishment of the National Health Service in 1948, so expertise became much more widely spread. Until the late 1940s, outside the major teaching hospitals, the great majority of general anaesthetics were given by self-trained general practitioners who had learned the easy way, and by dentists usually working dangerously on their own.

The introduction in 1946 of the relaxant drugs — derived from CURARE, the South American arrow poison — dramatically changed the techniques of anaesthesia. One of the problems was always to secure relaxation of the muscles, particularly in abdominal surgery, where the sensitiveness of the viscera tended to produce spasm of the abdominal muscles, causing the intestines to be heaved out, and the surgeon to complain about the moving target. The older inhalational anaesthetics affected every cell in the body. Their safe use depended on the nervous system being more susceptible than the remainder. This could be relied on in a healthy person, but not, for example, where there was a diseased heart. But now, rather than soaking the whole body with ether, with the postoperative sequelae of prolonged nausea and vomiting, it was possible to aim at specific pharmacological targets, so the concept of the 'anaesthetic triad' was developed, using one drug to produce unconsciousness, another for analgesia, and a third for muscular relaxation. Paralyzing the muscles required that the anaesthetist take over the ventilation of the patient's lungs, and this resulted in the development of automatic ventilators, the forerunners of today's LIFE SUPPORT machines. The expertise so learned brought anaesthetists to the care of the seriously injured or ill, and thence to involvement in the development and staffing of intensive care units. Expertise in performing nerve blocks with local anaesthetics led to the treatment of severe and chronic PAIN, and the establishment of pain clinics, a movement which started during the 1960s. A third development during the same period was the growth of the obstetric epidural analgesia service.

The work of the anaesthetist has been greatly aided, and the safety of the patient greatly improved, by the introduction of sterile disposable equipment — at first, syringes and needles, which removed the need to keep in one's waistcoat pocket a small sharpening stone (an *Arkansas slip*), and a fine wire, for removing hooked points and blood clots from non-disposable needles which were repeatedly resterilized and reused.

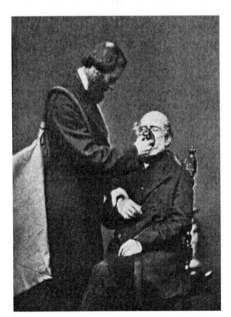

Joseph Clover, demonstrating the induction of chloroform anaesthesia, 1862

More and more items, even entire breathing circuits, and complete sterile packs for the induction of epidural anaesthesia, have become available in disposable versions, minimizing the risk of infection being transferred from one patient to another.

Another major development, commencing in the 1970s, has been the increasing availability of apparatus which allows the anaesthetist to monitor routinely not only the patient's pulse rate, blood pressure, and electrocardiogram, but also such physiological parameters as the oxygen and carbon dioxide levels in the blood. This, together with the measurement of blood loss during operations, provides an early warning of possible problems. The new generation of inhalational and intravenous agents, which are rapidly removed from the body leaving no hangover, has greatly improved patient comfort and safety.

From the earliest days the British pioneers set the trend for safety, and self audit has been a continuing feature of anaesthesia. Several commissions of enquiry were set up by the profession from the 1860s on, and the tradition has been continued by the Association of Anaesthetists, which participates very actively in the establishment of the fruitful and continuing confidential enquiry into perioperative deaths (NCEPOD).

The older anaesthetists regarded their technique as an art, learned by trial and error. Today it is still an art, but established on a firm foundation of science, and in the UK has its own academic body to establish standards, supervise training, and conduct examinations for its own higher qualification, the Fellowship of the Royal College of Anaesthetists (FRCA).   DAVID ZUCK

Further reading

Duncum, B. (1994, 1947). *The development of inhalation anaesthesia.* Royal Society of Medicine Press, London (1994). Oxford University Press (1947).

Rushman, G. B., *et al.* (1996). *A short history of anaesthesia.* Butterworth-Heinemann, Oxford.

Thomas, K. B. (1975). *The development of anaesthetic apparatus.* Blackwell, Oxford.

Thorwald, J. (1961, 1957). *The century of the surgeon.* Thames and Hudson, London (1957). Pan Books (1961).

See also ANAESTHESIA, LOCAL; ANAESTHETIC MECHANISMS; SURGERY.

Anaesthesia, local

Early attempts to relieve the PAIN of operations were by the application of cold, notably during the retreat of Napoleon's army from Moscow in 1812, and by pressure on main nerves. Not until COCAINE was isolated from the South American coca leaf, by Albert Niemann at Gottingen University in 1860, did a drug become available that would effectively block impulses travelling along nerves — though even then its anaesthetic application was not immediately appreciated. The numbing effect on the mouth of chewing coca leaves was well known, and this action of the pure drug on the tongue was soon confirmed. It was known to Sigmund Freud (1856–1939), who thought cocaine might be the antidote to morphine addiction. The potential of cocaine as a local anaesthetic was eventually realized in 1884, when Carl Koller, a young Viennese doctor who was looking for a means of preventing the pain of eye operations without general anaesthesia and its after-effects, applied it to his own tongue. His report of successful trials on animals and people created a sensation, and the use of cocaine spread rapidly, from surface application to injection under the skin and around main nerves.

The method was taken up enthusiastically on the continent of Europe and in the US, but not in the UK, where general anaesthesia reigned supreme. In America, by the end of the 1880s, the leading exponent, the surgeon W. S. Halstead, had become a cocaine addict as the result of self-experimentation, and although eventually cured, he suffered a sad change of personality.

Injection of cocaine solution in the region of the SPINAL CORD by the New York neurologist Leonard Corning in 1885 opened the way for *spinal anaesthesia.* The deliberate introduction of a needle through the *dura*, the thick membrane which surrounds the spinal cord, and the injection of cocaine solution into the CEREBROSPINAL FLUID which bathes it, was first performed by the German surgeon August Bier in 1898. The patient was judged unfit for a general anaesthetic, and the profound anaesthesia of the legs which ensued allowed Bier to remove several segments of infected bone. Spinal anaesthesia was taken up, again enthusiastically, in the US, and its application gradually spread to abdominal operations. But cocaine is a very toxic drug, and there were a number of deaths from overdose. The search for less dangerous substitutes was soon on, culminating in the synthesis of *amylocaine* (stovaine), used specifically for spinal anaesthesia, in 1904, and *novocaine* (procaine), with more general applications, in 1905.

Spinal anaesthesia was a boon for the surgeon. Since he could make the injection himself it freed him from reliance on another practitioner to administer a general anaesthetic. It allowed him to operate on patients who were unfit for general anaesthesia, and since it relaxed the muscles it provided better operating conditions, a more level playing field, so to speak, than he could expect from the often inexpertly administered ether or chloroform. Fall of blood pressure was an undesirable side-effect — very unpleasant for the patient, and treated by tilting the operating table head-down, but not unwelcome to the surgeon, because it reduced bleeding.

As the patients were conscious during the operation, American surgeons in the 1920s attempted to distract their attention by encouraging them to listen to the radio or a Victrola through earphones, to converse, to sing, or, if it did not interfere with the operation, to smoke. The distraction most effectively employed by the surgeon G. P. Pitkin of New Jersey was what he called his psychoanaesthetist, described by him as an auburn-haired vamp who made the patient wish the operation would go on for ever, as long as she would only stay with him.

Spinal anaesthesia was often followed by headache, due to leakage of fluid through the needle puncture, and it was found that this could be avoided if the solution was injected outside the dural membrane — extradural, or *epidural anaesthesia.* The injection could be made either through an opening in the sacrum at the base of the spine (a '*caudal block*', very useful for operations such as haemorrhoids, or for relieving the pain of childbirth), or higher up the spine, depending on the operation. The discovery that a low epidural could relieve LABOUR pains without affecting the strength of uterine contractions led to the popularization of the method during childbirth. Inserting a fine catheter through a needle, so that repeated doses could be given, brought the added advantage that if operative intervention such as forceps or CAESAREAN SECTION became necessary the means of anaesthesia was already installed.

Extradural methods received a boost, and spinals a severe blow, with the publication of a paper by the American neurologist Foster Kennedy and his colleagues in 1950, in which it was claimed that every spinal injection left some pathological changes around the cord. This was augmented by a case which hit the headlines in 1947: two successive patients on an operating list had suffered permanent paralysis of the lower limbs after spinal anaesthesia. Although the anaesthetist was exonerated when the case came to court, and Kennedy's allegations of spinal damage in all cases was resoundingly refuted, the worry remained, and spinal anaesthesia was not practised again to any great extent in the UK until the 1980s. By then the availability of sterile disposable equipment, and a new generation of drugs, allowed a new generation of anaesthetists to restore this valuable technique to its rightful place. Local anaesthesia, either by widespread infiltration or aimed to block particular nerves, is now widely used for day surgery, and also to provide postoperative pain relief.   DAVID ZUCK

Further reading

Rushman, G. B., Davies, N. J. H., and Atkinson, R. S. (1996). *A short history of anaesthesia.* Butterworth-Heinemann, London.

Thorwald, J. (1960). *The triumph of surgery.* Thames and Hudson, London.

Anaesthetic mechanisms

General anaesthetics are among the most useful, the most dangerous, the least specific, and the least understood of the major drugs. They are useful because they allow surgery without sensation or any memory of the trauma or pain. They are dangerous because the dose that can kill is not much larger than the dose needed for anaesthesia. They are non-specific in that substances ranging from the noble gas xenon to barbiturates and steroids can produce general anaesthesia, and furthermore in that general anaesthetics affect many functions. Finally, the mechanisms of anaesthetic action are still not known and we also do not know which of the actions are critical to allow surgery.

Anaesthesia can be defined as 'the reversible, non-specific suppression of organized function in a living system' (Meyer 1937). Clinical or general anaesthesia is only one example — but it is the example of overwhelming practical importance. Surgery requires: loss of consciousness, prevention of any memory of the trauma (amnesia), pain relief (analgesia), and muscle relaxation. All of this must be achieved without stopping the heart and with ventilation of the lungs maintained — either by leaving normal breathing unaffected, or artificially. Most general anaesthetics are capable of producing the desired combination of effects, but only at precisely controlled concentrations. In early days, the dose of chloroform or of ether had to be sufficient to achieve all the required effects, but in modern practice the anaesthetic drug is used only to produce the loss of consciousness and amnesia. Pain relief and relaxation of muscles, which would require higher and hence more dangerous concentrations of the anaesthetic, are usually secured by using more specific analgesics and muscle relaxants. The relaxants suppress normal breathing, so patients must be artificially ventilated.

The physiologist and the clinician have tended to approach the study of general anaesthesia by asking two questions: where do general anaesthetics act, and which function do they suppress? Suggestions for regions of the brain that could be the site of action have included the BRAIN STEM reticular formation, the CEREBRAL CORTEX, and the thalamus. When SENSORY RECEPTORS are stimulated there are electrical responses that can be observed in the cortex. Anaesthetics applied at clinical concentrations to certain layers of the cortex, or to relay cells in the thalamus, delay the appearance of the responses and reduce their amplitudes. In one view anaesthetics 'turn a valve' shutting off the sensory input to the cortex.

ACTION POTENTIAL propagation in nerve fibres, release of NEUROTRANSMITTERS, and the responses of nerve cells to them, have all been suggested as the critical function that anaesthetics must suppress. Long distance communication in the nervous system occurs via 'all-or-none' action potentials which are designed to be reliable. High concentrations of anaesthetics can be shown experimentally to block these action potentials — but the levels required would be lethal in a patient. Subtler effects can be observed at the SYNAPSES where nerve cells come into contact with each other. Here communication occurs by release of chemicals — the neurotransmitters — which then act on the receptor sites of other nerve cells to stimulate their activity. At many synapses the transmitters are now known. Two of these have been proposed as playing critical roles in general anaesthesia: glutamate produces excitation of the cells it acts upon, and some anaesthetics decrease this excitatory effect;

by contrast, GABA (gamma-aminobutyric acid) tends to inhibit electrical activity in the cells it acts on, and many anaesthetics potentiate this effect. It is proposed that by increasing an inhibitory effect, the level of activity in many portions of the nervous system can be reduced, which might very plausibly be a mechanism for general anaesthesia. Interaction with GABA receptors is virtually certain to be an important effect in the general anaesthesia produced by the barbiturates, certain steroids, and the benzodiazepines (drugs related to valium).

Physical chemists and pharmacologists, on the other hand, fascinated by the wide range of effects produced by anaesthetics, have been more concerned with different but closely-related questions that could be crucial for the development of more effective and safer anaesthetics: what are the molecular properties of the anaesthetic receptors or targets on cell membranes? And what are the properties that make a molecule a potent anaesthetic?

How do we characterize anaesthetics and their receptors when all that is known initially is that an effect is produced? There are two main approaches: determination of the relation between the chemical structure of the anaesthetics and their activity, and the measurement of binding of the anaesthetics to preparations which might contain the targets on which they act. About the only firm rules for the structure of anaesthetics are that they must be primarily hydrophobic (not soluble in water but soluble in lipids) and that the molecules must not be too large. The largest anaesthetic drugs are similar in size to cofactors for proteins and to the steroid lipids that form part of the structure of membranes. Because so many substances can satisfy these requirements, structure–activity relations have not been very helpful, and attention has been concentrated on the alternative approach.

A common method is to compare the potency of a drug at producing an effect with its binding to tissues, to homogenates of tissues, or to models that might contain the receptors (or at least sites that look like the receptors). Where possible, similar studies are carried out for every type of receptor. To apply this method, two key types of experiment must be performed. First, the dose or concentration needed to produce the effect must be determined. Given the great variety of effects produced by anaesthetics, many different effects or end points can and have been used — including the suppression of light flashes by fireflies (see later), the increased survival of red blood cells made to swell by exposure to dilute solutions, and the prevention of convulsions in deep sea divers. However, the two most commonly employed measures have been the loss of righting reflex in animals and loss of flinching response to surgical incision in people. If goldfish are released in tanks containing a range of concentrations of the alcohols, from ethanol through octanol, the concentration of the alcohol at which 50% of the goldfish lose the ability to keep upright and to swim can be determined. Now remember one

important property of anaesthesia is that it is reversible (the patient must survive!) — so after the test, if the goldfish are put back into clean water they quickly recover. A common technique for measuring the righting reflex in mice is a rolling cage very much like the exercise wheels often provided for pet gerbils. The difference is that here the wheel is made to turn and the mouse must respond to stay upright. In this instance, as in most clinical use of anaesthetics, the anaesthetic is added as a gas or vapour.

Regardless of the end point chosen to indicate that the anaesthetic has taken effect, the experimental data for the first type of experiment are then a list of the concentrations, either in the water or in the air inhaled, at which a variety of anaesthetics produce equal effect — the C_{an}. An anaesthetic which produces an effect at a lower concentration is said to be more potent. Thus for a series of anaesthetics applied in the same way, potency is defined as the reciprocal of the concentration, $1/C_{an}$.

The second key experiment is measurement of the amount bound. The principles are the same as for any type of drug, but there is an important difference. Most useful drugs, other than anaesthetics, bind with high affinity to specific cell membrane receptors. With a little luck in the choice of preparation, if measurements are repeated first for very low concentrations of drug and then for increasing concentrations, at first the amount bound increases, but it then reaches an apparent limit as the specific sites become saturated — that is, when there are no more free sites to allow more drug to bind. When this pattern is seen, the interaction between the drug and the site can be described by the concentration required for half-maximal binding. But for anaesthetics the binding is weak and no saturation is seen. Binding increases linearly with the applied concentration of the drug, and the amount that is bound depends only on the partition (or distribution) coefficient — the ratio of concentration of the drug in the chosen preparation to its concentration in the water or air used to deliver it. The higher this coefficient is, the lower the concentration that is required to reach a chosen level of binding. In other words, if different anaesthetics are applied by the same route until each produces the same amount bound, the concentration of each that is required is inversely proportional to its own partition coefficient. Many different preparations have been used in the binding experiments, ranging from simple solvents, like octanol and olive oil, to lipid vesicles, the membranes of red blood cells, and specific proteins.

One of the most striking and famous correlations in biology was first reported in 1901 by Meyer and by Overton, who found that anaesthetic potency was directly proportional to the partition into olive oil. Very similar results can be obtained in the goldfish experiment described above. In 1937 K. H. Meyer restated this result in a way which more clearly draws out its significance:

[Anaesthesia] commences when any chemically indifferent substance has achieved a certain molar concentration in the lipoids of the cell. This concentration depends on the nature of the animal or cell, but is independent of [the anaesthetic].

Lipoids are the *hydrophobic* parts of a cell (the CELL MEMBRANES including the lipid bilayers and the proteins embedded in them). Meyer's rule, that anaesthetic effect depends solely on how many anaesthetic molecules are bound to the lipoids, does not explain anaesthesia, but it does tell us that the site of action is strongly hydrophobic; this almost certainly implies that anaesthetics act within membranes.

Theories for the mechanism of action have tended to divide into two groups: anaesthetics alter some physical property of the lipid membranes, which in turn alters the function of the proteins which form the ion channels in the membranes; or anaesthetics bind directly to membrane proteins and alter their function. This question remains unresolved, very possibly because the correct answer is both — but to varying degrees for different anaesthetics.

There are many aspects of cell membrane structure and function that anaesthetics could change and that could in turn alter nerve cell excitability. Proposals have included membrane volume expansion, changes in thickness of the membrane, changes in its tension, or changes in its fluidity. Perhaps the most important reason why many people favoured theories involving indirect effects, such as changes in fluidity, was that they 'explained' the need for anaesthetics to be hydrophobic — but work on fireflies showed that interactions directly with proteins could also 'explain' this need. Fireflies are found in the eastern US. On warm early summer evenings, they fly about emitting flashes of light from their tails. Presumably the purpose is to attract a mate, though it often also attracts small kids with jars. The flashes of light are produced by a change in the form of the molecules of the protein *luciferase*. Light emission from luciferase is inhibited by anaesthetics at concentrations that are remarkably close to those needed to produce general anaesthesia. The anaesthetics bind in a hydrophobic pocket which is the normal binding site for a necessary cofactor. These data lead to two important conclusions. Firstly, we must not take the models too seriously. None would claim that there is firefly luciferase in our brains any more than anyone would claim that we have pools of olive oil in our brains. Thus none are claiming that binding to a pocket in this particular protein or partitioning into a pool of olive oil is responsible for all anaesthetic effects. But — and this is the second point — since one such pocket has been found, there may well be others, and binding in these pockets may be the key factor in clinical general anaesthesia. It will be interesting indeed if membrane proteins turn out to have such hydrophobic pockets. Perhaps the binding sites for barbiturates and steroids on the GABA

receptors are examples waiting for a more complete molecular description.

S. B. HLADKY

See also MEMBRANE RECEPTORS.

Analgesia In contrast to *anaesthesia*, which signifies loss of feeling — including such sensations as heat and cold, consciousness being optional — the *Oxford English Dictionary* defines *analgesia* as insensibility to pain; painlessness. In medical terms anaesthesia would imply the total relief of pain which is necessary for a surgical operation, while analgesia would provide a varying amount of relief for a painful condition. This difference is laboured here because of inconsistency in the use of the words by anaesthetists, for some of whom *anaesthesia* implies loss of consciousness — hence the insistence on the usage *local* (and *regional*, and *spinal*) *analgesia* rather than local anaesthesia. However, it is common to speak in the same breath about spinal anaesthesia and epidural analgesia, while the patch of skin insensitivity that results from cutaneous nerve damage is invariably referred to as anaesthesia. Since painlessness is the normal condition, *analgesia* here will refer to the relief of pain, acute or chronic, and the subject will be considered from its anatomical, physiological, pharmacological, and psychological aspects.

The anatomical approach implies the relief of pain by surgery or by injection. Nerve compression, which may occur at several sites, most commonly the sciatica that results from disc protrusion in the spinal canal, or the carpal tunnel syndrome at the wrist, can be cured by operation; and, rarely, severe intractable pain, such as trigeminal neuralgia, which affects the face, may, as a last resort, be treated by division or destruction of the appropriate nerve. Analgesia may also be produced by the injection of a local anaesthetic, generally into the epidural space around the SPINAL CORD, for the relief of pain in childbirth, or when analgesia is required for some days after an operation, or after a major injury which involves fractures of the ribs.

Two recent advances in the understanding of the physiological mechanisms of pain and its suppression have suggested new approaches to pain relief, and have explained the efficacy of some very old methods. The *gate control theory* of pain, first proposed in 1965 by Patrick Wall (physiologist at University College, London) and Ronald Melzack, has given rise to the use of transcutaneous electrical nerve stimulation (TENS) by means of a small battery-operated apparatus, to produce analgesia. This involves the electrical stimulation of nerves at or adjacent to the painful region, which enter the spinal cord at about the same level. It has been used with some effect for the treatment of chronic pain, and to produce relief during childbirth. The gate control theory also offers a physiological explanation for the efficacy of such psychology-laden folk remedies as rubbing the offending part; the application of cold or of counterirritants such as

camphor; cupping; and moxibustion (the burning of small piles of moxa, the common mugwort, on the skin, to produce a blister).

The discovery in 1973 of opiate receptors in the central nervous system led to the search for, and discovery of, endogenous analgesic substances, the ENDORPHINS a year later, the assumption of the scientists having been that the receptors must be there for a physiological purpose. The release of these hormones at times of stress explains the phenomenon that pain may not be felt until some considerable time after the injury — the legendary footballer who continues to play with a broken leg, for example. This observation of delayed pain in the wounded, described by the Harvard anesthesiologist Henry Beecher (1907–76) during the 1943 North Africa campaign, was already well-known to earlier army surgeons. Richard Wiseman (1622–76), caring for the injured during the English Civil War, advised that wounds should be cleaned and dressed as soon as possible, before pain began to be felt. The discovery of endorphins has given rise to hopes that analgesics with more specific sites of action than OPIATES, and without their undesirable side-effects such as constipation, respiratory depression, and addiction, might be synthesized. Both the gate control theory and endorphin release have been invoked in attempts to give physiological respectability to acupuncture for the relief of pain.

The greatest part of pain relief, however, is dependent on pharmacological agents. The relief of acute, intermittent pain, such as during childbirth or DENTISTRY, can be achieved rapidly and effectively by the intermittent inhalation of an analgesic gas or vapour: NITROUS OXIDE, or until recently, when it was judged too expensive to manufacture in pure form, *trichlorethylene* (trilene). Otherwise pain relief involves the administration, either by mouth or by injection, of analgesic drugs. These come in gradations of effectiveness, and with different mechanisms of action, which make them more appropriate either for acute or chronic requirements. The basis of the most potent analgesics is still the opiates. *Opium*, the dried juice of the poppy seed capsule, is one of the oldest drugs known. It was mentioned by Homer, and by Aristotle, but until 1805, when the German apothecary Friedrich Wilhelm Sertürner (1783–1841) prepared pure crystals of the active principle — to which the French scientist Gay-Lussac gave the name *morphine* — it was available only as a crude, unstandardized preparation. Sertürner's researches opened the door to the isolation of many alkaloids, and eventually to the synthesis of morphine derivatives such as *diamorphine* (heroin), and *codeine*.

During the 1980s two methods of administration developed which made the patient less dependent on the attention of others; the battery operated syringe pump and electronic, fail-safe, patient-controlled systems. The first may be used when there is the need to provide continuous analgesia in advanced cancer, and the second to relieve pain postoperatively.

Of the milder analgesics, *salicylic acid* was isolated from willow bark, and its acetyl derivative, better known as ASPIRIN, was prepared in 1897, and was hailed as a wonder drug for its analgesic and antipyretic (fever-controlling) properties. During the first half of the twentieth century it was used for the control of both acute pain and chronic inflammatory conditions such as rheumatic fever. For acute use it has largely been replaced by *paracetamol*, which came on the market in 1953 and has generally proved a safer analgesic, certainly in children.

Drugs used for the control of long-standing pain include the *non-steroidal anti-inflammatory drugs* (NSAIDS). The first of these, *ibuprofen*, resulted from the screening of more than one thousand compounds in the laboratories of Boots of Nottingham, and was patented in 1964. Since then a number of non-steroidals effective in chronic conditions, such as rheumatoid arthritis, have been synthesized, and have been found effective also in relieving postoperative pain. They, and also acetylsalicylic acid, act by preventing the synthesis of PROSTAGLANDINS, which are to a large extent the cause of the pain, swelling, redness, and fever characteristic of inflammation.

States of 'altered consciousness', HYPNOSIS, autohypnosis, euphoria, and psychosomatic conditions such as HYSTERIA, may be accompanied by insensitivity to pain. Hypnosis has been used successfully for obstetric pain relief, and has even been able to produce the profound analgesia necessary for surgical operations, but it is a very time-consuming process. However, even such a simple measure as relieving ANXIETY can be effective in reducing the severity of pain. Who has not experienced the relief which comes from just making an appointment with the doctor or dentist? In recent years an attempt has been made to relieve psychologically certain — mercifully rare — states of chronic pain that are not susceptible to relief by any of the conventional methods. Often no anatomical or pathological cause can be found, and the condition becomes all-absorbing and is characterized by a state of alienation from ordinary everyday life. Attempts to produce relief have invoked research into medical anthropology — into, for example, the trance-like state which may be entered into to relieve the pain of certain INITIATION RITES. Another approach has been to attempt to dissociate the physical pain from the sufferer's response to it, involving an attempt to rebuild a life around the pain. While much abstruse philosophy has been written about the theory behind this movement, essentially it involves listening to the sufferer, taking his symptoms seriously, and finding some means of taking his mind off them.   DAVID ZUCK

Further reading

Melzack, R. and Wall, P. (1992). *The challenge of pain*. Penguin Books, Harmondsworth.

Rey, R. (1998). *The history of pain*. Harvard University Press, Cambridge, MA.

Sneader, W. (1985). *Drug discovery — the evolution of modern medicines*. Wiley, Chichester.

See also OPIATES AND OPOID DRUGS; PAIN.

Anatomy The word 'anatomy' derives from the Greek *ana* (up) and *tome* (a cutting) — hence 'DISSECTION' — and it can be defined as the science of the structure of a body learned by dissection. The word can thus be applied to any structure, and we can talk about the anatomy of a plant, an insect, or even a machine, but here the term will be restricted to the structure of the human being.

Since earliest times, man may have been curious about the inner structure and workings of his body. Certainly the ancient Egyptians, in performing mummification, which involved preliminary removal of the viscera, would have gained considerable information about the organs of the chest and abdomen. However, the practitioners of this art were not medical, and there is little evidence that the doctors of those times derived any knowledge from this potentially rich source of anatomical material. The first recorded school of anatomy, where dissection of the human body was performed, was in Alexandria, and it flourished between the first century BC and the second century AD. Here two Greeks, Herophilus and Erasistratus, were celebrated for their experience of anatomy acquired by the dissection of condemned criminals, and they described many structures of the human body. Herophilus recognized the brain as the central organ of the nervous system and the seat of intelligence, thus reversing the view of Aristotle, the Greek philosopher, of the primacy of the heart. Erasistratus observed the convolutions of the brain, noted that they were more marked in man than in lower animals, and associated this complexity with the higher intelligence of man. He also described the main parts of the brain, its coverings, and its cavities, the ventricles.

The most celebrated anatomist of the ancient world was undoubtedly GALEN (129–216 AD). Born in Pergamon in Asia Minor, he studied in Smyrna and Alexandria before settling in Rome. He studied the human skeleton in Alexandria, but by then human dissection had virtually ceased, and much of his anatomy was based on animal studies.

Although Galen made many contributions to the subject, his work on bones and muscles being particularly good, and although many of the anatomical terms still in use today have their roots in his work, he also made errors and misinterpretations in his findings. In spite of this, his writings were regarded as definitive and beyond criticism over the next 1300 years. As a simple example, he described the kidneys as being lobulated, as they are in cattle, when the most casual glance would have shown that they are smooth in man. His statement that blood passed through pores between the left and right side of the heart again could have been refuted by simple observation. To make matters worse, continued copying of his writings and translations from one language to another led to further mistakes and faults creeping into his texts.

During the Middle Ages, human dissection was frowned upon by the Church. In the late fifteenth and early sixteenth centuries, a revival of learning and, with it, of anatomical observation took place, especially in Italy and more particularly in the University of Padua. It was there that a revolution in anatomy took place with the publication, in 1543, by Andreas VESALIUS, then aged only 28, of his book *De Fabrica Corporis Humani* (The Structure of the Human Body). This was based on his personal observations of his own human dissections, and of studies of the human skeleton. It contained magnificent illustrations, taken directly from his dissections, which could be used today in any modern textbook of anatomy.

Over the next centuries dissection of the human body became a standard part of the training of medical students. Indeed, it provided more or less the only scientific subject in the curriculum. However, because of religious and social attitudes surrounding the acquisition of bodies, and because of the unpleasant nature of dissection on unpreserved and often decomposing material, both anatomy and practitioners followed a somewhat chequered course. Anatomies were usually made in winter months, when the process of putrefaction was delayed, and the timing in England was also made to correspond with the assizes, when the bodies of executed criminals would be available. The legitimate sources of bodies — executed criminals and unclaimed corpses of paupers — were often inadequate for the increasing numbers of medical schools and of medical students. In Britain in particular, there was the scandal of the grave robbers (or 'resurrectionists' as they were called), who would dig up a body shortly after burial and sell it to an anatomy school. Relatives would sit up, armed, at night to protect the grave, or secure the graves with iron cages known as 'mort-safes'. Sometimes, indeed, because of the chronic shortage of bodies, criminals would resort to murder to obtain their material, as in the infamous case of BURKE AND HARE in Edinburgh, who committed no less than 16 murders. Hare turned King's evidence, but Burke was hanged and afterwards publicly dissected. The scandal of this case undoubtedly led to the Anatomy Act of 1832, which licensed premises for dissection and made legal the provision of bodies from workhouses or elsewhere which were unclaimed. The anatomy school was responsible for the subsequent burial or cremation of the body according to the religion of the deceased. These regulations have gradually been replaced by the bequests of individuals of their bodies for anatomical purposes after death so that today, in the UK, virtually all bodies are received at anatomy departments by these means.

The techniques of anatomical studies were improved by the injection of coloured materials into blood vessels and lymphatics, and by methods of embalming and preserving the body. Formalin, discovered in 1868 by Von Hoffman, rapidly replaced other preservative agents, and remains the basis of modern preservation methods.

The development of simple microscopes in the seventeenth century founded the important science of *microscopic anatomy*. A pioneer in this field was Malpighi, whose extensive studies demonstrated the blood capillaries, thus finally establishing the anatomical basis of the circulation of the blood. He also described red blood corpuscles, and the structure of the skin and of many other tissues. The modern achromatic compound microscope was invented in 1878, and it was this instrument that added the extra dimension of the microscopic study of tissues to anatomical teaching.

With the advent of anaesthesia in 1846, and the introduction of antiseptic surgery as a result of the work of Lister in 1867, the vistas of surgery were greatly increased and, with them, the importance of a detailed knowledge of anatomy to the surgeon. To most students, however, anatomical teaching was something of a sterile test of memory, with emphasis on exact topographical details of the finer ramifications of nerves and blood vessels. In the twentieth century, particularly in its second half, the subject of anatomy became much wider and of a more practical nature. It is true to say that there is little interest today in 'pure' topographical anatomy. The detailed mapping of the human body is now fully documented and is to be found in the major textbooks. Indeed, the name of *Gray's Anatomy*, the standard text, has passed into popular parlance. However, in its various sub-divisions, the subject is thriving and the most important of these need some separate descriptions.

Topographic anatomy

In this, the body is studied by regions rather than by organs. This is of importance to the surgeon who exposes different planes after the skin incision and who, of course, must be perfectly familiar with structures as he explores the limbs and body cavities. Once the sole preserve of the surgeon, this field has acquired immense significance today for the radiologist (see below). In this respect cross-sectional topographic anatomy has come into its own.

Endoscopic anatomy

With the development of fibreoptic instruments, the body's tubes and cavities are now being explored in life. The detailed anatomy, for example, of the bronchial tree as seen through the bronchoscope is now of great importance. The introduction of laparoscopic and thoracoscopic instruments to explore and operate in the abdomen and thorax respectively has also opened new vistas as surgeons require to learn their anatomical landmarks through these approaches.

Surface (living) anatomy

From the practical point of view, every medical practitioner needs to know the detailed structure of the tissues beneath the skin of his patient. This forms an important part of the teaching of medical students, who can practise on themselves the identification of bones, landmarks, muscles, and arterial pulses; the palpation of normal structures through the intact skin; and the range of movement of the joints.

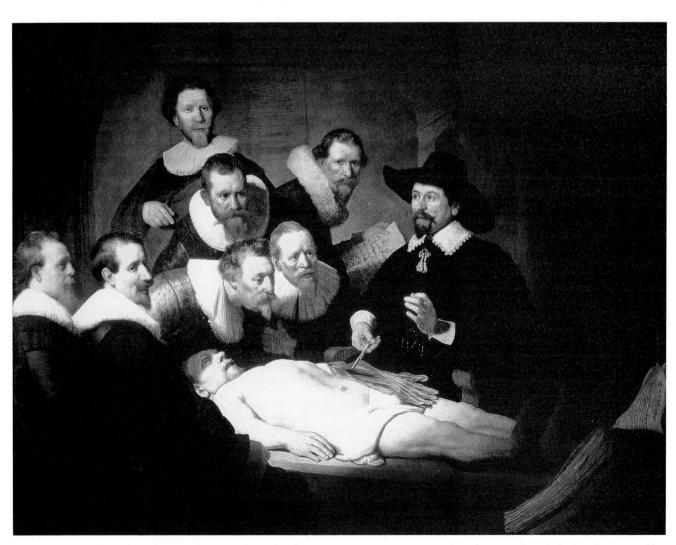

The Anatomy Lesson of Dr Nicolaes Tulp, 1632 (oil on canvas) by Rembrandt Harmensz. van Rijn (1606–69). Mauritshuis, The Hague, The Netherlands/Bridgeman Art Library.

Radiological and imaging anatomy

The discovery by Röntgen of X-RAYS a century ago opened new vistas of anatomical study. This was enhanced by the development of radiological techniques to outline viscera, for example by injecting radio-opaque solutions into blood vessels (*angiography*) or by swallowing barium paste in order to demonstrate the oesophagus and stomach. More recently, other IMAGING TECHNIQUES, which include ultrasonography, computerized tomography, and, in particular, magnetic resonance imaging, have provided unrivalled information of three-dimensional anatomy in the living body. Indeed, today, the radiologist must possess a detailed knowledge of anatomy that certainly rivals that of his surgical colleagues.

Embryological anatomy

The complex changes in the growing fetus are studied because much of adult anatomy can only be understood by appreciating its prenatal development. More and more has been learned about the underlying causes of the numerous CONGENITAL ABNORMALITIES that may arise as aberrations of normal development.

Microscopic anatomy is of fundamental importance in the understanding of pathological changes, and has advanced with the introduction of electron microscopy, which enables the finest details of the cells to be studied at an *ultramicroscopic* magnification of several thousands.

Kinesiology, the study of joint and limb movement, has developed into a subject of immense importance, together with biomechanics and *orthotics* (the study and use of artificial limbs). Here, research has an immediate application in orthopaedic practice, for the study of joint prostheses, the measurement of forces acting on the skeleton, and choosing the strength of materials utilized in reconstructive surgery; also for the analysis of the causes of failures of artificial joint implants, or of the materials used in internal fixation of fractures.

Neuroanatomy, the study of the brain, spinal cord, and nerves, forms an important part of the battery of approaches needed for neurobiological exploration, which today is complemented by physiology, pharmacology, molecular biology, and dynamic whole brain imaging.

All these topics are of obvious importance in the various expanding fields of medicine, but anatomy also impinges on other sciences. Examples are *comparative anatomy* — the comparison of structures in different animals and species; *palaeoanatomy* — the study of ancient remains — mainly, of course, of bones; and *physical anthropology* — the study of the different human races.

A recent development has been the appearance of a complete, sectioned human body appearing on the World Wide Web. The Visible Human Project presents transverse CT, MRI and cryosection images of two complete human cadavers, one male and one female, at an average

of 1 mm intervals. These allow three-dimensional constructions to be 'visualized' from any angle on the computer screen.

Anatomy is thus a subject which encompasses a great variety of endeavours characterized by the study of the organization of the human body, and which impinges on many other sciences. In teaching anatomy to medical students, dissection of the cadaver remains fundamental, but the student also studies living, imaging, microscopic, and embryological anatomy. Anatomy forms an essential part of the scientific basis of medicine. All those concerned with disorders of the human body must start from a background of knowledge of its normal macroscopic and microscopic structure.   HAROLD ELLIS

See also DISSECTION; GRAY, HENRY.

Androgens The family of closely related steroid hormones associated mainly with development and maintenance of male sexual function and bodily characteristics. Androgens are made in the TESTES, and the chief member of the group is TESTOSTERONE; but they are also made in small quantities in the ADRENAL GLANDS in both sexes, and during the sequence of steroid synthesis in the ovaries which leads to the end product of oestrogens. As well as the essential function of SPERM formation in the testes, androgens promote hairiness and muscular development.   S.J.

See SEX HORMONES; STEROIDS; TESTES.

Angels From the Greek '*angelos*', meaning messenger, angels are seen as intermediaries between heaven and earth. This notion of angel as messenger is found particularly in the monotheistic religions (for in polytheistic religions, gods and goddesses often arrive in person to deliver messages), and was initially developed in the first major monotheistic religion, Zoroastrianism. In Judaism, stories of angels occur throughout the Hebrew scriptures, and speculation about the nature of angels is found in the Talmud. Christianity inherited its ideas about angels from Judaism, and significantly developed them, especially in the Middle Ages. In Islam, angels appear in the Koran, and are important figures to Mohammed, as when Djibril (Gabriel) contacted the Prophet and dictated the Koran to him, and conducted him to heaven on the Night Journey. In some Islamic areas of the world, angels — many with unusual names — are important in popular Islamic practices, many of which may be rooted in the pre-Islamic religion of those areas. In recent years, angels have come to be very important in the (primarily North American) New Age religious movement.

There has been considerable debate as to whether angels can be said to have bodies. In the Christian tradition, Jesus' statement in Luke 20:36, that human beings, after our RESURRECTION, will be 'like the angels' is important but not necessarily clarifying. Given that there have been differences of opinion in the Christian tradition about whether our resurrection will be bodily, this

passage in Luke can be seen to attribute embodiment to angels — or not to. Origen (c. 185–c. 254) suggested that angels have a subtle or ethereal body, and this opinion continued to be held into the Middle Ages by philosophers such as the twelfth-century Duns Scotus. However, this view was challenged by Thomas Aquinas in the thirteenth century, who argued that intellect is above sense, and therefore some creatures must be incorporeal and comprehensible by the intellect only. Angels are such incorporeal creatures and are purely spiritual, as suggested, for example, in Psalm 104:4, which affirms that God 'makes his angels spirits'. Aquinas saw angels not as belonging to a single species, but each as having its own separate substance and species.

Aquinas also argued that angels are incorruptible, and indeed the general opinion within the church, in the Middle Ages, was that angels are perfect and therefore in no danger of sinning, unlike human beings who are, of course, sinful by nature. Indeed, even Lucifer, like all the angels, was created in a state of grace. Aquinas suggested that Lucifer impiously exercised the free will with which all angels are endowed, and hence fell from grace. (This accords with the traditional story in Christianity, of Lucifer, jealous of God, leading a rebellion of angels against the heavenly order, and thereby being thrown out of heaven; he continued to wage war against God in his creation, Earth — as, for example, in the Garden of Eden.) Origen argued that angels were created with free will, and some eventually migrated away from God, some taking on human form, and those who migrated the furthest becoming demons. Another story of fallen angels is found in the apocalyptic Book of Enoch, in which a group of angels lusted after human women, and thus fell when they left their heavenly abode to have sexual intercourse with those women.

Despite his views on the 'spirit' nature of angels, Aquinas agreed that angels can, visiting the earthly realm, assume bodies, as in the case of the angels who visited Abraham in Genesis 18. There are numerous examples, in the scriptures of the main monotheistic religions, in fiction, in film, and in the writings of the twentieth-century New Age movement, of angels assuming bodily form when they come to earth. There are many such embodied angels in the Hebrew scriptures and New Testament, two of the most well-known examples being the angel who wrestles with Jacob (Genesis 32), and the angel Gabriel, who visited Mary to announce the birth of Jesus — the Annunciation (Luke 1:26–38). A number of popular films in the twentieth century played on the idea of angels taking human bodily form when they come to earth. The most famous, perhaps, is the aptly named Clarence Oddbody, the kind but rather bumbling angel (odd in his angelic body because, as he is a second-class angel, he has no wings yet) who comes to earth to help George Bailey, in Frank Capra's film, *It's a Wonderful Life* (1946), giving him the gift of reliving events as if he had never been born. Oddbody plays the familiar role of guardian angel. The notion that each person has a guardian angel to guide them is found in numerous religious traditions, but has been developed especially in Christianity; Aquinas, for example, suggested that each person has a guardian close to hand throughout life. The theme of the guardian angel taking human bodily form is also found in *The Bishop's Wife* (1947), in which Cary Grant plays a suave and soothing angel, Dudley, sent to the aid of an absent-minded Episcopalian bishop, his family, and his friends. Wim Wenders' 1988 film, *Wings of Desire*, explores the idea of an angel, Ganz — one of many watching life in Berlin from a distance — who wishes not merely to assume bodily form, but to experience earthly life as humans do, after falling in love with a circus performer. Wenders takes the trope of the fall of angels onto earth, and gives it an unusual twist by suggesting that redemption occurs with a descent into physicality. Embodied angels on earth play an important part in many New Age recovery stories and narratives of NEAR-DEATH EXPERIENCES: much New Age literature, such as the *Angel Times*, a magazine begun in 1994 in the USA, explores these themes.

The gender of angels has been debated. Angels have most often been considered androgynous, or to be neither distinctly female or male, or to combine both genders. Jesus' statement in the Gospel of Matthew may be evidence for this sort of view within the Christian tradition: 'At the resurrection men and women do not marry; they are like angels in heaven' (Matthew 22: 30). Thus angels are generally portrayed in paintings and sculpture as of indistinct gender, or in a pre-pubescent human form. Angels are therefore by default often thought of as male, although the archangel Gabriel — one of the two highest ranking angels in Judaism, Christianity, and Islam — is commonly thought to be female, and depicted as such, at least within Christianity.

Wings are perhaps the most distinctive symbol of the angel 'body' and represent swiftness, power, and spirit. However, the notion of angels as winged creatures is not scriptural, but, rather, was developed in the Middle Ages. Depictions of winged angels first occurred in the fourth century. Indeed, in the early (pre-fourth-century) Church, figures such as wanderers with a staff and young men clothed in simple tunics may represent angels, as in the wall paintings of the Priscilla catacomb in Rome. The depiction of angels as '*putti*' — small children's heads with wings — became popular in the Renaissance. At the same time, artists came to paint more angels as female. Angels are almost always shown as young, for they are changeless, so time does not exist for them. They enjoy perpetual youth.

JANE SHAW

Animal magnetism An umbrella term covering a diverse set of practices, animal magnetism refers most often to the therapeutic methods originally developed in late-eighteenth-century France by Franz Mesmer (1734–1815) and his followers; more generally, it signifies the sympathetic attraction between people. Animal magnetizers generally claimed to effect cures for chronic ailments by their ability to redistribute the magnetic or nervous fluid circulating through a patient's body, frequently inducing a trance-like somnambulistic state. Magnetized patients might be impervious to pain, obey the magnetizer's suggestions, or display abnormal abilities. Like other currently discredited treatments, animal magnetism is too easily dismissed as charlatanry, and episodes must be considered within their cultural context. Its recurrent popularity derived from its apparently successful cures, its close relationship to other contemporary medical and scientific ideas, and its resonances with political and social interests.

Mesmer initially treated patients by strapping magnets to their bodies, but after arriving in Paris in 1778, he gradually moved away from this literal application to a more metaphorical vision of a universal magnetic fluid. The central feature attracting wealthy patrons to his fashionable, music-filled salon was the *baquet*, a large, oaken tub filled with magnetic materials, magnetized water, and aromatic herbs. Clients — predominantly women — sucked up its healing magnetic powers by holding protruding iron bars and wrapping ropes round afflicted limbs. Mesmer also treated patients individually, passing his hands around them while gazing intently into their eyes to achieve healing crises which resembled fits or trances. Leading to accusations of sexual misconduct, this technique was proclaimed to redirect and unblock the flow of universal magnetic fluid through the body — reflecting contemporary medical insistence on restoring natural circulation and equilibrium.

After a few lucrative years of intense popularity, Mesmer himself was discredited by a governmental enquiry, but his followers developed and propagated his methods. Often spreading through masonic and occultist networks, versions of mesmerism flourished throughout Revolutionary France, appealing particularly to radicals seeking a democratic scientific medicine. Adherents transmitted it to Germany, where, in the early nineteenth century, a more mystical and less therapeutic animal magnetism emerged, as part of a Romantic fascination with visionary states and paranormal powers also articulated by some English poets. Animal magnetism continued to become increasingly popular in France, and during the 1830s was exported to the US, where it was adopted by progressive reformers often associated with spiritualism, and to Britain.

Animal magnetism had been briefly popular in London during the 1780s, but was revived by theatrical demonstrators and progressive early Victorian medical men such as the university professor John Elliotson. Particularly after the dramatic and well-publicized cure of the journalist Harriet Martineau, interest escalated amongst the intellectual élite in therapeutic mesmerism and its use as an anaesthetic during surgery. Like PHRENOLOGY, animal magnetism held appeal as a radical alternative which could be practised outside professional institutions, but was effectively suppressed by the scientific and medical establishment. PATRICIA FARA

Animals in research Animals are widely used in the biomedical sciences, for purposes ranging from studying the functions of human and animal bodies and the nature of disease, to toxicological testing to assess the safety of both medical and non-medical products. Their use in science has a long and well-documented history, as has the philosophical debate over such use (see, for example, *Vivisection in Historical Perspective*, edited by N. A. Rupke). A few points will be mentioned briefly here to put this in context with the present day situation.

Animal experiments were described in ancient Greece and Rome. The author of the Hippocratic text (around 350 BC), for example, describes cutting the throat of pigs to observe the mechanism of swallowing. GALEN, (129–216 AD) the most renowned physician of the Hellenic period, used pigs to demonstrate the effects of severance of various nerves. Even toxicity tests were performed by King Mithridates of Persia (132–63 AD) on both humans and animals to learn more about poisons and their antidotes.

The disciplines of anatomy and physiology were keenly pursued from the Renaissance period onwards, with studies largely based on the dissection of living animals. Some of the most influential figures during this period were Andreas VESALIUS (1514–64), who dissected monkeys, pigs, and goats; William HARVEY (1578–1657), well known for his discovery of the circulation of the blood through live dissection; and René Descartes (1596–1650), the French scientist/philosopher.

From the mid-1880s science, and particularly physiology, increasingly used animal experimentation as a major 'tool'. The French physiologist Francois Magendie (1783–1855) and his pupil Claude BERNARD (1813–78) performed thousands of experiments on animals, with Bernard subsequently becoming known as the 'father of modern medicine'. These early experiments on animals caused great suffering. Either there were no anaesthetics, or they were not used, so living, conscious animals were cut up (literally vivisected) with no consideration for what they experienced in terms of pain or suffering. Descartes, in fact, expressed the view that animals were like machines and did not feel 'real' pain, and that their lack of rational awareness meant that such pain was morally unimportant.

As interest in science and medicine developed, so the use of animals became an integral part of the research method in many scientific disciplines. It remains so as we have moved into the twenty-first century. The developing scientific use of animals, however, has been accompanied by doubts and concerns, both about the morality of such use (particularly once more was learned about animals and their ability to suffer) and the validity of experiments with regard to the information they provided and its application to human medicine. Until the second half of the eighteenth century, proponents of such views came mainly from the disciplines of philosophy and the arts and, to a lesser extent, the sciences. However, after this time 'vivisection' entered into both public and political debate, at first in the UK, much later elsewhere. The use of animals in experiments is now one of the most contentious issues of debate within the public arena.

Legislative controls

Until the nineteenth century there were no controls anywhere in the world on what could be done to animals in experiments, other than that exerted by the moral consciousness of the scientists themselves, or of their critics. However, once the issue became of public and political concern, legislation soon followed, and in 1876 the first law governing the use of animals in experiments — the Cruelty to Animals Act 1876 — was introduced in the UK. This Act applied to '*experiments calculated to give pain to vertebrates*'. It established the Home Office as the controlling authority and required premises where experiments were carried out to be registered and subject to '*random and unannounced inspection by Home Office Inspectors*'. Individual researchers had to be licenced and provide an Annual Return of the numbers of experiments performed under the Act. A special certificate was required to work on cats, dogs, horses, or mules, reflecting additional public concern about such animals. This legislation remained in force until 1986, when it was replaced with the more stringent Animals (Scientific Procedures) Act 1986 (ASPA). There are now at least 20 countries worldwide with legislation regulating experiments on animals.

The UK Animals (Scientific Procedures) Act 1986 — how it operates. The ASPA regulates '*any experimental or other scientific procedures applied to a protected animal which may have the effect of causing that animal pain, suffering, distress or lasting harm*'. It covers all vertebrate species and one invertebrate, *Octopus vulgaris*. Mammals and birds are covered from halfway through their gestation or incubation period; fish and amphibians from the time at which they become capable of independent feeding.

The Act is based on a three-tier licensing system, administered by the Home Office through a team of Inspectors qualified in medicine or veterinary science. The establishment where procedures on animals are carried out must have a licence (the *Certificate of Designation*), as must the research project (the *Project licence*), and the individuals carrying out experiments or procedures (the *Personal licence*).

Further provisions include the need for two people to be appointed at each establishment (the *Named Veterinary Surgeon* and the *Named Animal Care and Welfare Officer*) who have statutory responsibility for overseeing the animals' health and daily care. The person who has overall responsibility for the establishment itself is appointed as the Certificate Holder.

Standards of animal husbandry and care are defined in Home Office Codes of Practice issued under the Act. These represent minimum standards — although they are often wrongly interpreted as providing guidelines on best practice.

There is also the provision for a statutory committee (the Animal Procedures Committee (APC)) to provide independent advice to the Secretary of State about matters of particular concern relating to the Act; the use of animals for testing cosmetics and the use of primates, for example. There are currently 24 members of the APC, drawn from various disciplines including science, animal protection, philosophy, and law.

The ASPA requires that a certain amount of information be made available within the public domain. Each year the Home Office collects and publishes statistics on the numbers and species of animals used. A limited amount of information on the purposes for which animals are used is also published, including categorization of the scientific disciplines (e.g. immunology, physiology, microbiology) and whether or not the use was to satisfy a national or international regulatory requirement (for example regarding the safety assessment of chemicals). In addition a summary of the work of the APC is made public through the Committee's annual report. This information, though welcome, is insufficient to gain a full understanding of what is done to animals, the reason for animal use, and the amount they suffer in the name of science. Nevertheless, the UK is the only country to provide this level of information.

Facts and figures from the Home Office statistics.

Types of animal used in research and testing Animals are used as 'models' of humans and/or of other animals in a wide range of scientific disciplines. In broad terms these relate to: the study and treatment of human and animal diseases and disorders, gaining fundamental knowledge in the biological sciences, and the assessment of the safety (or level of risk) of chemicals and non-medical products such as pesticides, agricultural chemicals, food additives, and household products. A considerable amount of animal use (about 80% in the case of dogs) is actually carried out to satisfy international regulatory laws or guidelines on the safety of human and veterinary medicines and other non-medical products. Other uses defined under the Act include breeding for genetic defects or modified genes, the diagnosis of disease, and in education and training. By far the greatest proportion of animals are used in fundamental and applied medical research.

Number of animals The number of animals used annually in the UK is currently around 2.6 million. The figure world-wide has been estimated to be over 41 million, but it is impossible to be more accurate than this, since most countries do not collect detailed (or any) statistics.

Trends The number of animals used in the UK has decreased steadily over the last 25 years. The numbers rose from the late 1940s when statistics were first recorded, reaching a peak of 5.5 million in 1971. The decrease in animal use results from a number of interrelated factors, including changing trends in scientific research, the high costs of using animals, and changes in attitudes to animals and their welfare in general.

The decrease in numbers levelled out in the mid-1990s, then in 1998 the UK statistics showed a slight rise. This was due to developments in genetic engineering with the use of genetically modified animals rising by 14% between 1998 and 1999. Genetic engineering is a rapidly developing science with applications in many different scientific disciplines, so this increase in animal use is likely to continue.

Species of animal A wide range of vertebrate and invertebrate animal species are used in biomedical research, but only vertebrates, and one species of invertebrate (*Octopus vulgaris*), are regulated by the ASPA. Of vertebrates, by far the largest number used according to the most recent figures (for 1999) are mice and rats (63% and 21% respectively of the total). Birds accounted for 4%, fish for nearly 5%, guinea-pigs just over 2% and rabbits 1%. Dogs, cats and primates taken together accounted for about 0.3%; however, this still represents a lot of individual animals: 5933 dogs, 683 cats and 3191 primates. Other species of animals used include hamsters, gerbils, ferrets, horses, cattle, sheep, pigs, goats, reptiles, and amphibians.

In the UK most of the common laboratory species, including rodents, rabbits, dogs, cats, and primates, have to be bred specifically for research purposes and obtained from Government-licensed breeders and suppliers. Some (for example dogs, primates, and certain strains of genetically-engineered rodents) may be imported if they are not available in the UK, but this too requires Government licence.

Ethical issues

The philosophical arguments over the use of animals are well documented. In society as a whole there is a spectrum of views on whether animal experiments are acceptable. There is a controversial public debate encompassing arguments regarding the morality of using animals and the perceived scientific validity and potential benefit of animal experiments. At one end of the spectrum of views are those who consider all animal experiments to be immoral whether or not they can be shown to have benefit (to humans or other animals). At the other are those who consider few experiments to be unjustified if they benefit humans in any way. People express a variety of views within these extremes, depending on their overall view of the human–animal relationship, their understanding of the overall purpose of the work and its perceived benefit, the nature of the experiments, the amount of suffering caused, and the species of animal.

The use of animals in experiments undoubtedly presents a complex ethical dilemma. In medical research, for example, animals are used as 'models' of diseases that cause a considerable amount of human suffering. It is irrational to suppose that animals do not suffer similarly in such studies. Thus, there is clearly a conflict of interests between the individual animals who will suffer pain or distress and who are usually killed at the conclusion of the experiment, and the benefits of the research — whether these apply to medicine and science in general, the public, individual scientists, industry, or indeed other animals. From an animal welfare point of view, it is important for all those directly or indirectly involved with animal use, and who directly or indirectly benefit from it, to recognize this and to try to minimize the impact on animals.

One problem with how the debate is presented in public, particularly relating to the issue of the scientific validity of experiments, is that the arguments are usually put in absolute terms: it is stated that animal experiments have, or have not, contributed to medical advances. Selected examples are provided to support each view. But the situation is not that simple. Animals are used for many different purposes, not all of them intended to have a medical application (acquisition of knowledge is an acceptable benefit under ASPA), and each area of use has its particular scientific, animal welfare, and moral questions. The use of selective arguments can often mask, and thus prevent constructive discussion of, underlying issues of animal welfare and the need to critically assess the necessity and justification for individual animal experiments in practice.

How ethical views are interpreted and incorporated into the ASPA The Act is utilitarian, in that it operates from the basic assumption that animal experiments can have benefit, and a benefit that justifies causing animals harm, which it then sets out to minimize and regulate. The fundamental ethical question of whether, and in what circumstances, an animal can be used for a scientific purpose is addressed by the 'cost benefit' assessment that must be carried out prior to granting a project licence. The costs to animals (the adverse effects) must be weighed against the potential benefits that are likely to result.

The definition of benefit under the Act is very wide and includes: protecting or improving human and animal health and safety, protecting the environment, and increasing scientific knowledge. The costs and benefits are set out in the project licence application, which is first assessed by the local Ethical Review Process (ERP) before being submitted to the Home Office Inspectorate for review on behalf of the Secretary of State. The system of local ethical review was introduced in 1999 to act as an adjunct to the Home Office Inspectorate in an attempt to improve implementation of the legislation. The aim is to provide a *local* framework '*to ensure that all animal use in an establishment is carefully considered and justified and that proper account is taken of all opportunities for reduction, refinement and replacement*'.

The costs to animals used to be interpreted as solely relating to the adverse effects of a procedure. However, it is increasingly recognized that the full costs for the animals are much greater, with the sourcing, transport, husbandry, handling and care, and euthanasia all contributing significantly to the overall impact on the animal. Primates, for example, may undergo journeys of up to 60 hours, and be housed in cages quite inappropriate to their social and behavioural needs, before they are even used in an experimental procedure, and this needs to be taken into account in any assessment of the justification for using them.

Ethics also have a practical component: as well as allowing decisions on *whether* an animal is used, they should also encompass consideration of *how* in practice animals are treated. In this context, reduction of animal suffering and improvement of welfare are duties both explicit and implicit in the Act, requiring adherence not only to the letter of the law, but also to its spirit. A major guiding principle is the '3Rs' principle of humane experimental technique set out over 40 years ago by Russell and Burch. They believed that humane experimental technique was integral to good science. They proposed that scientists should wherever possible *replace* animals with humane alternatives, *reduce* the number of animals in an experiment to a minimum consistent with obtaining good statistical data, and *refine* techniques to minimize suffering. The provision of husbandry systems that meet both the behavioural and the physiological needs of the animals is another practical consideration that should be given high priority alongside the scientific objective of the project. The 3Rs are now widely accepted as a means not only of reducing the impact of experiments on animals but also of improving the quality of the science. Indeed, UK and EU legislation requires scientists to use alternatives to living animals if available.

Difficult decision The cost–benefit assessment is widely claimed to ensure that animals are only used when there will be a 'benefit' which is 'necessary and justified'. However, necessity and justification are subjective concepts, as too is benefit, and all can be interpreted in very different ways by different people, at different times, in different situations, cultures, and contexts. In practice it is difficult to know how to weigh such disparate units as a known harm versus a potential benefit. In recognition of this, there have been several ethical schemes developed to try to help people think through the factors which are important in making their judgements.

The introduction of the Ethical Review Process will widen the review of projects to include more members of each establishment that carries out animal experiments. There is also provision for including 'lay' members in the process, and this will be an evolving concept in the coming years.

In conclusion

The prevailing view within the biomedical sciences is that animal research has led to medical and veterinary advances and will continue to do so. However, this use of animals leads to a serious conflict between the needs of laboratory animals and those of humans and other animals, with all the attendant moral and ethical dilemmas that this entails.

The use of animals in experiments is a privilege not a right, and the necessity and justification for using them should always be critically evaluated on a case by case basis. Care and consideration for animals should be a basic principle within science. There needs to be a proactive approach, which should go beyond the bare minimum legal requirements, giving animals and their welfare high priority. Where animals continue to be used, the aim should always be to minimize that use, to minimize or avoid harms to animals, to maximize the potential benefits of the research, and to ensure that these benefits are applied in practice.

MAGGY JENNINGS

Further reading

Regan, T. and Singer, P. (1989). *Animal rights and human obligations*, (2nd edn). Prentice Hall, New Jersey.

Rupke, N. A. (ed.) (1987). *Vivisection in historical perspective.* Croom Helm, US.

Russell, W. M. S. and Burch, R. L. (1959). *The principles of humane experimental technique.* Methuen, London.

Smith, J. A. and Boyd, K. M. (eds) (1991). *Lives in the balance: the ethics of using animals in research.* Oxford University Press, Oxford.

Ankle The bones which constitute the ankle are the two long bones of the lower leg (*tibia* and *fibula*), which articulate with a short ankle bone called the *talus*. This is an 'uniaxial', or hinge, joint, which allows flexion and extension movements. In the case of the ankle these movements are called *dorsiflexion* (sole of the foot up) and *plantarflexion* (foot down) respectively. Plantarflexion is achieved by the calf muscles (*gastrocnemius* and *soleus*), which form a large strong tendon (*Achilles tendon*) which inserts into the bone of the heel (*calcaneum*). This tendon is not uncommonly a site of injury in athletes. Dorsiflexion is achieved by muscles at the front of the lower leg (*peroneal muscles*), and damage to their nerve supply can result in 'foot drop' — an inability to lift the end of the foot requiring higher lifting of the knee during walking. The joints below the ankle (*sub-talar* joints) permit movements of the sole of the foot inward (*inversion*) and outwards (*eversion*), which are important when walking on uneven surfaces. A common problem is 'going over' or twisting the ankle, often occurring when walking on uneven ground. This can result in injury ranging from a minor sprain (tearing of some fibres of a ligament) through to complete rupture of ankle ligaments, sometimes also accompanied by fracture of the lower end of the tibia or fibula. Sprains and fractures are often followed by swelling of the soft tissues in the injured area, due to fluid leaking from blood vessels at the site of injury, and also bruising ('black and blue' discolouration of the skin) due to blood leaking from torn vessels.

WILLIAM R. FERRELL

See also FEET; JOINTS; SKELETON.

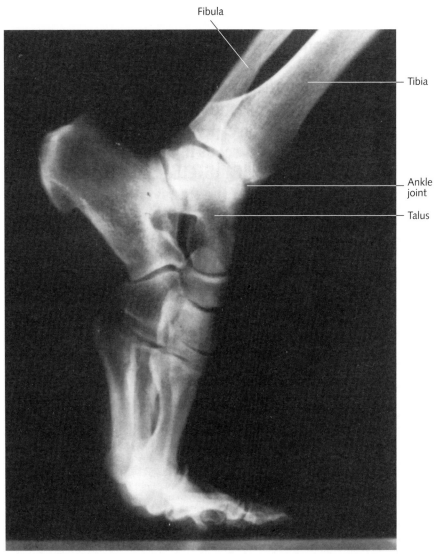

Fibula

Tibia

Ankle joint

Talus

X-ray of the foot in 'tiptoe', showing the ankle joint. Reproduced, with permission, from *Cunningham's textbook of anatomy*, (12th edn), Oxford University Press.

Antenatal development

The embryonic period of human antenatal development starts with fusion of the SPERM and egg. Fertilization occurs in the FALLOPIAN TUBE, usually within 12 hours of the release of the egg from the ovary ('ovulation'). The chromosomes of mother and father intermingle, and shortly afterwards, the first cell division takes place. By the time that implantation takes place in the uterus a week later, the 'conceptus' contains around 100 cells and is called a 'blastocyst'. Following implantation, an 'embryonic disk' becomes distinct from the other cells, and at 3 weeks after CONCEPTION, or one week after the first missed menstrual period, this becomes a definable embryo. (Other cellular components of the conceptus will form the amniotic sac, the UMBILICAL CORD, and part of the PLACENTA). The early embryo contains a *notochord* from which the spine develops, and the three germ layers from which all tissues and organs develop:

the *ectoderm*, which gives rise to skin and nervous tissue; the *mesoderm*, which gives rise to muscles, muscular coats of the various tubular structures, connective tissues, and blood vessels; and the *endoderm*, which gives rise to the linings of the lungs and digestive tract and the glandular parts of organs like the liver and pancreas.

As the notochord develops, the overlying ectoderm thickens to form the neural plate which subsequently folds and fuses to form the *neural tube*: this will become the brain and spinal cord. Disturbances in this process may produce some of the more common CONGENITAL ABNORMALITIES: the neural tube defects. These include *anencephaly*, in which the brain and skull are missing, and *spina bifida*, in which the spinal cord is both abnormal and usually uncovered by skin. Neural tube defects are most common in Celtic populations of Western Europe and it is now known that the risk of these serious defects can be minimized if the

mother takes the vitamin, *folic acid*, before and during early pregnancy. They can also be diagnosed by ULTRASOUND examination later during pregnancy.

Between the fourth and eighth week after conception, most of the major organ systems start to form in the embryo, although it is very much later before these start to function properly. The process of *embryogenesis* is highly complex. Major advances are now taking place in our understanding of the genetic control of the cell migrations, cell proliferation, and programmed cell death ('*apoptosis*') that need to happen in a highly co-ordinated fashion over a short time-scale for the successful development of an individual. Many of these insights have emerged from study of the fruitfly, *Drosophila*.

From around 5 weeks after conception and 7 weeks after the mother's last menstrual period, it becomes possible to identify the embryo on an ultrasound scan. As the pregnancy advances, more and more detail can be seen so that, by 18 weeks, normality can be confirmed — or many subtle abnormalities can be identified. Around 15% of pregnancies miscarry, usually in the early weeks of pregnancy. The majority of these unsuccessful pregnancies have abnormal numbers of chromosomes, notably one extra, one too few, or a full extra complement. Many of these pregnancies are clearly abnormal on ultrasound examination long before the miscarriage occurs. Conversely, many women who have bled in early pregnancy can be reassured by normal ultrasound findings that their pregnancy is likely to continue.

Ultrasound has been a pivotal development in our ability to study the unborn child. The technique developed from the pioneering studies, in the 1950s and 1960s, of Ian Donald, Professor of Obstetrics and Gynaecology in Glasgow. He applied to human imaging the technology used to detect flaws in metal in engineering works. Now all maternity units in developed countries rely extensively on ultrasound imaging to monitor the growth and development of the fetus.

The fetal period of antenatal development starts 9 weeks after fertilization, when the major organs have been formed and the embryo has reached 33 mm length from the crown of the head to the rump. It is characterized by rapid growth and, in the later stages, by maturing function of the different organ systems.

Throughout the pregnancy the fetus obtains nutrients and oxygen from the mother's blood, by transfer in the placenta to its own umbilical cord blood, and it excretes waste products of metabolism by the same route in reverse. In the great majority of instances, the fetus progresses normally to maturity, and is born at full term with fully functional organs, becoming a healthy neonate and infant.

There can, however, be damage during development due to a variety of *teratogens*, collectively defined as any agent or factor that when present during prenatal life produces a permanent alteration in form or function in the offspring. This can be a chemical, drug, infectious, or physical agent, or a maternal condition.

The fetus is less vulnerable than the embryo to these extraneous damaging agents, although infections such as syphilis or toxoplasmosis can cause serious damage in later pregnancy.

Fetal alcohol syndrome
The effects on the fetus of maternal ingestion of alcohol were first described in Europe in 1968. World-wide studies have now revealed a consistent picture of prenatal and postnatal growth deficiency with microcephaly (undersized head), mental handicap, a characteristic facial appearance, and heart abnormalities. The microcephaly is secondary to the disordered brain development resulting from alcohol exposure. Typical facial features include narrow eyes, flat nasal bridge, underdeveloped jaw, and thin upper lip. Speech, language, and behavioural problems, including severe hyperactivity and attention deficit disorders, contribute to the learning disabilities characteristically found in these children. Fetal alcohol syndrome (FAS) is estimated to occur in 30–40% of pregnant women who consume 3 oz (85 ml) of absolute alcohol per day. Large but lesser degrees of alcohol consumption are associated with intrauterine growth retardation, learning difficulties, and hyperactive behaviour. During the neonatal period the infant may show jitteriness and poor feeding similar to those features found with misuse of other substances. The term 'alcohol-related birth defects' is now used to reflect the range of anomalies associated with alcohol consumption during pregnancy.

Drug addiction has effects in pregnancy that include miscarriage, fetal malformation (genitourinary), fetal growth retardation, liver damage, ante-partum haemorrhage, fetal distress in labour, prematurity, and brain damage. After birth the infant is difficult to feed, jittery, and may have long-term problems from defective development of the nervous system. COCAINE usage is an increasing problem world-wide, resulting in vasoconstriction and hypertension in both the mother and the fetus. Attributed effects on the fetus include limb reduction, cerebrovascular accidents, and long-term neurobehavioural disorders.

Amphetamines, like cocaine, are psychomotor stimulants, previously used primarily by those involved in sports and entertainment to enhance performance. They potentiate the action of noradrenaline, dopamine, and serotonin but, unlike cocaine, they appear to exert their central nervous system effects primarily by enhancing the release of neurotransmitters from presynaptic neurones. In children born to addicted mothers cardiovascular malformations have been described, and these children subsequently exhibit disturbed behaviour including hyperactivity, aggressiveness, and sleep disturbances. In New York city the proportion of women in the known addicted population rose from 14% in

1968 to 25% in 1973 and was expected to be 40% in 1995. In the US women make up approximately 30% of the drug treatment hospital admissions and 25% of the alcohol treatment admissions. In addition to the side effects produced by alcohol, nicotine, and prescription drugs, there are major problems now arising from the abuse of amphetamines, heroin, and cocaine. With the emergence of cocaine, especially in its 'crack' or smoked form, there has been an alarming increase in the incidence of fetal exposure to the drug. Studies in the US indicate that 10–15% of major urban area newborn births are affected by cocaine use. A majority of women who use cocaine during pregnancy are 'poly drug' users and take alcohol, marijuana, and heroin in addition to the cocaine.

Premature labour is a major threat to the fetus, when it is born before its organs have matured sufficiently to ensure survival outside the uterus. However, modern neonatal intensive care does allow the survival of many premature babies that would have perished in the past. The lungs are the most critical organs. Their maturity can be accelerated by giving the mother high doses of corticosteroids if premature delivery can be anticipated — a highly effective treatment that emerged from the pioneering work of Liggins in New Zealand to explore the mechanisms of labour in sheep. After birth, the very premature baby usually requires artificial ventilation, and with intensive care some 90% of babies survive after delivery as early as 28 weeks. Survival may occur even from birth at 24 weeks, but this is uncommon.

Other *low birthweight* babies are not premature, but are small because of poor growth, usually as result of poor function of the placenta. The babies may be born to women who are heavy smokers, or who have disorders of their blood vessels, notably high blood pressure. These babies are malnourished and are prone to asphyxia before and during labour. They often require to be delivered before the time that natural labour would occur.   JIM NEILSON
                                FORRESTER COCKBURN

See also ABORTION; CONGENITAL ABNORMALITIES; PLACENTA; PREGNANCY.

Anthropology

Embracing nature and the cosmos, the philosophical thinking of classical antiquity did not consider anthropology, the 'science of man', as a subject independent of the greater ontological context. Yet the problems set out in those days were to shape inquiry in later centuries. Were ideas innate or acquired? How did body and soul communicate with the outside world? How did progress come about? And how was it possible that there were varying types of men?

Within Christendom, in the period from the decline of the Roman Empire until the Renaissance all knowledge of mankind was believed to reside in the religious doctrines. The bases of anthropological curiosity were

established during the sixteenth century. By the end of the eighteenth century the subject was systematically treated. Subsequently it developed into a science, diversifying into social, physical, and linguistic anthropology; ethnology; ethnography; archaeology; and other sub-disciplines.

In a literal translation of the Greek term, René Descartes (1596–1650) and Gottfried Wilhelm von Leibniz (1646–1716) spoke of '*doctrina de homine*': Descartes applied the mechanistic philosophy to the natural realm; considering all animals — including mankind in its physical respects — as machines, he showed that human nature was open to scientific investigation. Leibniz built upon the theory of the 'GREAT CHAIN OF BEING', situating mankind on an uninterrupted ascending scale that led from the realm of the mineral, through lesser organisms, to mankind, and thence to heavenly creatures. Man's place in nature was thus fixed — until the end of the eighteenth century, when the theory came into disrepute.

At that time, anthropology stood on three legs. Dealing with the individual, medicine told people how to be legislators of their personal bodily constitutions; cultural and political philosophers, by contrast, treating society, inquired into the historical laws governing the growth of civilization; naturalists, finally, devised natural systems which assigned mankind a place among their fellow creatures. Yet philosophers were increasingly occupied not just with the uniqueness of mankind, but also with the classification of human varieties and the question of how physical and psychological differences had been engendered.

In 1594, Otto Casmann had determined anthropology as a science accounting for the dual nature of man as a physical and spiritual being. Reiterating the point, Chambers' *Cyclopaedia* (1727–51) stated that anthropology 'includes the consideration both of the human body and soul'. Eighteenth-century Germany has been credited with exploring human nature in this vein, thus putting anthropology as a science in its own right on the map. In his *Anthropologie für Ärzte und Weltweise* ('Anthropology for Doctors and Savants', 1772), Ernst Platner stressed that it was the task of the anthropologists to investigate the relationships between, and mutual influences of, body and soul. The idea struck a chord with minds dwelling in pre-Romantic complexities of thought.

Eighteenth-century Germany knew three different approaches to the subject: anthropology was treated (i) as part of theoretical philosophy; (ii) as part of psychological investigations; and (iii) as one among several empirical sciences dealing with mankind. Immanuel Kant's *Anthropologie in pragmatischer Hinsicht* ('Anthropology in a pragmatic understanding', 1798), aiming to scrutinize the framework of the human soul from an empirical viewpoint, belongs to the second category. As the *Penny Cyclopedia* put it in the 1830s, this perspective did not turn on 'the investigation of what nature makes of man', but on the question 'what man, as a free agent, either makes, or can and ought to make of himself'. The third approach was pursued in various ways. It was here that writers throughout Europe departed from the assumption of the psychological and physiological unity of mankind: physiologists and anatomists, in particular, attempted to differentiate between varying human types.

Physical anthropology, as it was to be called, took its starting point from the dissatisfaction with previous attempts to depict man's place in nature. In 1735 the Swedish naturalist Carolus Linnaeus set down a taxonomy of nature (*Systema naturae*). Considering hands and feet as equal units, he subsumed several sorts of men under the common name of 'quadrupeds', including the mythical, ape-like 'Troglodytes' as well as humans properly speaking. Himself a pious Protestant, Linnaeus was later accused of having devalued man's special role. In order to defend mankind against the Cartesian suspicion that they were no better than reasoning animals, Johann Friedrich Blumenbach (1752–1840) came up with a new category that applied solely to humans: bimana — the two-handed. On the basis of his examination of skulls, he distinguished five different human varieties. Numerous alternative classifications were put forward by Oliver Goldsmith, John Hunter, Immanuel Kant, Johann Gottfried Herder, Buffon, Georges Cuvier, Julien-Joseph Virey, Louis-Antoine Desmouslins, and many others.

In *The Order of Things* (1970), Michel Foucault famously characterized eighteenth-century science as descriptive. Discussing the anthropology of French Enlightenment philosophers, Michel Duchet has, however, shown that the quest for causes was equally characteristic of eighteenth-century anthropology. In France, its purpose was not unanimously regarded as the theory of body and soul. Pierre-Jean-Georges Cabanis (1757–1808) and A. L. C. Destutt de Tracy (1754–1836) — followers of Condillac's philosophy of the mind — argued that medicine and morals were two branches of the same science, but the influential school of Paul-Joseph Barthez (1734–1806) stressed that the science of man was only another name for general physiology. In France the 'physical' was widely seen to be opposed to the 'moral'. A reconciliation was brought about once anthropology was established as a science. Until the second half of the nineteenth century it was dominated by PHRENOLOGY, which soon became the paramount technique of determining physiological as well as psychological racial traits.

The eighteenth century had not distinguished between anthropological and ethnological enquiries, the latter forming part of the physical history of man. In the early nineteenth century that changed. The new science of ethnology concentrated on the description of different peoples. Its early students tended to believe in the unity of mankind, using historical linguistics to trace genealogical links, while until the mid century physical anthropology was rather the domain of those who thought that mankind was made up of several species or races of man. One of the scholars whose works contributed much to the development of an antagonism between anthropology and ethnology was the doctor James Cowles Prichard. On account of his philanthropic outlooks and his strong belief in the truth of Genesis, he was fervently opposed to the theory of race. His *Researches into the Physical History of Mankind* (1836–47, 3rd edn) aimed to delineate the genealogical links between all human races. Praised as the founder of British ethnology, he himself referred the origins of the science to Blumenbach, whom others cherished as the father of anthropology. The parallel in France was Georges Louis Leclerc, Comte de Buffon (1707–88). Nowadays, adulating the fathers of a particular discipline has given way to a more historical perspective.

During the nineteenth century, anthropological institutions were set up in many countries, the *Société Ethnologique de Paris* being founded in 1839. In London, the Ethnological Society was established in 1843, and the Anthropological Society in 1863 — modelled on Paul Broca's *Société Anthropologique de Paris* that had opened its doors four years previously. The first German institute, Rudolf Virchow's *Berliner Gesellschaft für Anthropologie*, dated from 1869. Initially, the discipline was dominated by physical anthropology. Craniology — or phrenology — was the core of all ANTHROPOMETRY, as the form of the skull seemed to permit inferences on mental faculties. The polygenist Paul Broca became the dominant figure in the field.

Physical anthropology did not necessarily imply RACISM, as the example of the liberal Rudolf Virchow proved. Not least thanks to his influence, German physical anthropology between 1860 and 1890 — unlike that in America, France, and Austria — was adamantly anti-racist. Darwinian biological determinism was rejected in favour of neo-Lamarckian theories and the belief that PHYSIOGNOMY was subject to cultural influences. This changed towards the end of the century, when a turn to evolutionist Darwinian theory and German nationalism drove German anthropology towards racialism. Physical yielded to biological anthropology. Craniology was replaced by Mendelism and biometry. The latter, a brainchild of Francis Galton and Karl Pearson, held sway throughout the Western world. Eugenic theories and the urges to implement policies of 'public hygiene' and race hygiene began to thrive.

These international developments notwithstanding, in Britain and America anthropology also took a course of its own. A universalizing form of cultural philosophy had been pursued during the age of Enlightenment. From the 1860s the threads were taken up by scholars like Edward B. Tylor, James G. Frazer, and Lewis Henry Morgan, once the theory of EVOLUTION gained ground. As in the eighteenth century, human development was seen as progress from ape-like rudeness to civilization, this time within the framework of Darwinism. Classical Victorian evolutionism regarded the archaically living Tasmanian Aborigines — who were dying out before their very eyes — as the living representatives of the early Stone Age. Not until 1911 did the American Franz Boas — a former pupil of Virchow, who adhered to the theory of cultural diffusionism and was interested in linguistic differentiation — criticize the evolutionist view of anthropology in his *The Mind of Primitive Man*. In the same year, the Englishman William Rivers discarded evolutionism in favour of diffusionist theories to explain the historical spread of customs and belief systems. Bronislaw Malinowski, A. R. Radcliffe-Brown, and others, by contrast, followed a functional approach, pursued by Emile Durkheim and Marcel Mauss (and later resumed by Claude Lévi-Strauss). A pluralist and relativist methodology was introduced.

The 'revolutionary' reaction against evolutionary anthropology brought about a dehistoricization of the subject. Descriptive ethnography and field work found many adherents, some researchers depicting foreign peoples in the tradition of the 'noble savage' — Lucien Lévy-Bruhl's notion of a particular 'primitive mentality' (*Mentalité primitive*, 1922) formed part of that tendency. The French philosopher Maurice Merleau-Ponty was not only an ardent proponent of existentialist philosophy, but also formulated ideas on bodily behaviour and perception which stimulated interest in the phenomenology of the body. Marxist theory, being based on a developmental philosophy, brought new acumen to evolutionism. Latterly, functional anthropology has been criticized by advocates of a more historically-oriented position. In any case, the multi-faceted nature of the discipline, which inquires into the evolution from *Australopithecus* to *Homo sapiens* as well as into functions and the development of myths and rites, hardly instills the impression that one method alone will suffice to answer all anthropological problems.

H. F. AUGSTEIN

Further reading

Leaf, M. (1979). *Man, mind and science: a history of anthropology*. Columbia University Press, New York.

Slotkin, J. S. (ed.) (1965). *Readings in early anthropology*. Methuen, London.

Stocking, G. (1987). *Victorian anthropology*. Free Press, New York.

See also CRANIOMETRY; EVOLUTION, HUMAN; PHRENOLOGY; SKULL.

Anthropometry

According to James Tanner, formerly Professor of Child Health at the University of London, 'anthropometry was born not of medicine or science, but of the arts, impregnated by the spirit of Pythagorean philosophy. Painters and sculptors needed instruction about the relative proportions of legs and trunk, shoulders and hips, eyes and forehead, so that they could more easily go about what we might nowadays consider the mundane occupation of making life-like images'. The earliest recorded attempt in the West to study the development of the human form for medical or scientific purposes appears to have been made by the German physician, Johann Sigismund Elsholtz (1623–88), as part of an enquiry into the relationship between body proportions and the incidence of disease. During the nineteenth century, the term 'anthropometry' was promoted and popularized by such writers as Adolphe Quetelet (1796–1874), Charles Roberts (d. 1901), and Paul Topinard (1830–1911). Topinard defined the study of anthropometry as the systematic measurement of the different parts of the human body in order to determine their respective proportions not only at different ages, but also 'in the human races, so as to distinguish them and establish their relations to each other' (quoted in Spencer 1997, p. 80).

As this brief history indicates, the origins of the science of anthropometry can be traced in a number of different ways. One of the earliest spurs to development in the modern era was the study of human growth, as indicated by the famous series of measurements conducted on his son by Count Philibert Guéneau de Montbeillard (1720–1785), and published by Georges-Louis Leclerc Buffon (1707–88) in the fourth *Supplement* to his *Natural History* (1777). The development of anthropometry was also influenced by the development of physical anthropology and the search for evidence of 'racial' variations. During the second half of the nineteenth century, several researchers, including the Austrian physician, Karl Scherzer (1821–1903), conducted investigations into the physical measurements of supposedly 'primitive' peoples, and the British anthropologist, John Beddoe (1826–1911), assembled information on the height, weight, and other characteristics of the different 'races' of the British Isles. The development of anthropometry was also closely bound up with research into the health and physical condition of people living under different social and economic conditions. Tanner quotes the French physician, Louis-René Villermé (1782–1863), as noting that

> Human height becomes greater and growth takes place more rapidly, other things being equal, in proportion as the country is richer, comfort more general, houses, clothes and nourishment better, and labour, fatigue and privation during infancy and youth less; in other words, the circumstances which accompany poverty delay the age at which complete stature is reached and stunt adult height.

Although it is important to recognize the scientific reasons for the growth of interest in anthropometry, one should also acknowledge the fact that many of the measurements made of human beings in the past were conducted for more immediate and, perhaps, less exalted reasons. With the exception of skeletal evidence, most of the information which we now possess about the heights of people in the more distant past has come from measurements made of soldiers at the time of recruitment. One of the reasons for measuring soldiers was to discover whether they met the Army's minimum height standards, but other groups, such as convicts, slaves, and indentured servants, were measured so that they could be identified more readily in the event of escape. By the nineteenth and twentieth centuries, increasing interest was being shown in the measurement of children. Some of the earliest measurements, such as those made by the British factory surgeons, were designed to establish whether the children were old enough to be employed; others were intended to establish the children's fitness for physical education.

The subject of anthropometry is of considerable interest to historians, not only because of its intellectual importance, but also because of the capacity of anthropometric measurements to shed new light on the health and well-being of past generations. In 1969, the French historian, Emmanuel Le Roy Ladurie (b. 1929), showed that there was a close relationship between the average height of soldiers who were recruited by the French army in 1868, and their level of literacy. This work provided the initial stepping-stone for the development of a new field of historical enquiry, known as anthropometric history, in both Europe and the US. Some of the leading examples of this new field include Robert Fogel's work on the average heights of native-born white males in the US; Richard Steckel's investigations into the heights of American slaves; Roderick Floud, Kenneth Wachter, and Annabel Gregory's examination of the heights of British soldiers; and John Komlos' study of the heights of Austro-Hungarian soldiers under the Hapsburg monarchy.

The investigations conducted by historians, physical anthropologists, human biologists, and others have generated a vast amount of data on the history of human height, weight, and body proportions over the course of the last two centuries. It is now apparent that the average height of human beings in most parts of the world is significantly greater than that of their forebears 100–200 years ago. The extent of these changes is a further indication of the overwhelming importance of social and economic factors in determining average height, and the relatively minor role played by 'racial' differences. At the same time, it is also clear that some populations have experienced greater increases in height than others, and that there are still substantial variations in the heights of people living on different parts of the globe. The persistence of these variations highlights the need for further improvements in standards of diet and sanitation in order to ensure that all children have the opportunity to achieve their full growth potential in the future.

Anthropometry in the twentieth century included estimation of the ration of fat to lean body mass — important in the study of ENERGY BALANCE and OBESITY — by measurement of body density or skinfold thicknesses, and more recently by the application of technologies such as MAGNETIC RESONANCE imaging and radioisotope studies.

BERNARD HARRIS

Further reading

Eveleth, P. B. and Tanner, J. M. (1990). *Worldwide variation in human growth.* Cambridge University Press.

Harris, B. (1994). Health, height and history: an overview of recent developments in anthropometric history. *Social History of Medicine,* 7, 297–320.

Spencer, F. ed. (1997). *History of physical anthropology.* Garland, New York and London.

Tanner, J. M. (1981). *A history of the study of human growth.* Cambridge University Press, Cambridge.

See also ANTHROPOLOGY; ENERGY BALANCE; OBESITY; PHRENOLOGY.

Anthropomorphism

Anthropomorphism can refer to the representation of the gods in human form or, more generally, to the attribution of human characteristics to animals or to inanimate objects. In both cases it can be seen as a statement of human superiority — everything else that there is must be just like us — or as an attempt to understand that to which we have no direct cognitive access, by imagining it to behave just like us.

The gods of many ancient societies were thoroughly anthropomorphized, both in their form and in their familial and social relationships; for example, as presented in the Homeric poems which were familiar throughout the ancient Mediterranean world, they get drunk, marry, quarrel, and make up just like people. The Greeks solved the problem of how, in this case, the gods are any different from us by attributing to them alone the features of being 'immortal and ageless'. Either the cause or the effect of these two (usually related) features lies in a different diet: the diet of the gods consists of nectar and 'ambrosia', which literally means 'immortal', and this leads to a different fluid flowing in their bodies. The Greeks called this fluid *ichor*. In classical myth, the anthropomorphic nature of the gods meant that gods and mortals were thought to be fully capable of interbreeding, although the gods could also take on forms other than their human ones by METAMORPHOSIS. However, immortality and agelessness continued to be the prerogative of the gods; neither the children of mixed unions, nor mortals who were especially precious to the gods, could share them. For example, the mortal Tithonos was loved by Eos, goddess of dawn, and was granted the power to ask for anything he wanted. He asked for immortality, but forgot to mention agelessness, so that he grew older and older until all that was left of his physical self was his voice.

The body of a god may function sexually just like a mortal body, and Greek mythology included the difficult labour of the female Titan, Leto, in which she gave birth to the twin deities Apollo and Artemis — the first-born child Artemis helping to deliver her own brother.

One consequence of imagining the gods in human form, so that in art the only way to tell which figures are divine may be their representation on a larger scale, is that it can make it easier to believe that some humans may really be gods.

This was a feature of the Mediterranean world before Alexander the Great decided that his mother's stories of having been impregnated by a god in the form of a snake conveyed divine status on him. The idea that a man could show himself to be a god by achieving something which was impossible for a mere mortal, such as conquest of a large proportion of the known world, meant that subsequent great generals could hint at such a status for themselves. From the third century BC, there was increased contact with Egypt, where for many centuries anthropomorphic representations of the gods had existed alongside the belief in the divinity of the ruler. This fuelled belief in the possession of divinity by certain humans, culminating in the cult of the living emperor in the Roman world.

Christianity, in common with the Islamic and Jewish traditions, generally avoids anthropomorphism, but still proposes that connections between the divine world and the human world can result in the birth of a child who is divine, as well as representing God the Father in art as a benign patriarch.

The attribution of human — particularly emotional or mental — characteristics to animals, or even to inanimate objects, has a long history, from Aesop's fables to fairy tales such as 'Goldilocks and the three bears' and on to Beatrix Potter. Pleading with one's computer or cajoling one's temperamental car can be variations on this theme. The whole animal kingdom can be anthropomorphized, with the lion as 'King of the beasts', or the hive as a 'Queen' bee running her obedient 'workers'. The 'politics' of such an animal world then act as a commentary on our own, with the animal representing the 'natural' way of acting. Additionally, individual species — such as the 'wily' fox — can be given a dominant anthropomorphic character trait; this enables different valuations to be placed on each species, and on each trait, within a given social context.

HELEN KING

See also GREEKS; METAMORPHOSIS; REPRODUCTION MYTHS; TITAN.

Antibiotics

Antibiotics have come to be regarded in the minds of most people as substances used to combat infection. In fact they are both more and less than that; *more* because they are increasingly important in the chemotherapy of cancer, and *less* because not all drugs used to treat microbial infections are actually antibiotics. Antibiotics are substances of natural origin, and their name derives from the ecological relationship between the organism which produces them and the microbe or living tissue whose growth is inhibited by them: *antibiosis* — the exact antithesis of *symbiosis* (living together for mutual benefit). Antibiosis as a biological phenomenon was known in the nineteenth century, but the scientific term 'antibiotic' was only coined much later, after the young physician Alexander Fleming (later Sir Alexander) had made his seminal observations which led to the discovery of penicillin and ushered in the era of modern chemotherapy. As the story goes, in 1929 Fleming was working at St Mary's Hospital in Paddington with cultures of pathogenic bacteria (staphylococci), when one day there blew in through the partially open window of his laboratory above Praed Street a fungal spore, which landed on one of his agar plates and grew up to produce a large clump of the mould. For an ordinary microbiologist this could have been regarded as a minor inconvenience, the sort of contamination which happens from time to time if one is not super-meticulous about sterile precautions, and calls for nothing more demanding than the disposal of the contaminated plate and inoculation of a fresh one. To his credit, Fleming noticed that not only was the growth of the bacteria inhibited in the vicinity of the mould, but the colonies of staphylococci were actually disappearing or *lysing*. He showed that the effect was due to a substance secreted by the mould, and attempted to purify it — but it proved unstable.

It took the outbreak of World War II to galvanize the scientific community into action and exploit the discovery of penicillin for widespread clinical benefit. The problems of producing the material on an industrial scale were solved, and for the first time many infectious diseases were brought under effective control. But not all. In general, infections caused by 'Gram positive' bacteria (categorized by Gram's staining process) proved curable by penicillin, but treatment of those caused by 'Gram negative' organisms (such as dysentery, cholera, and the like) had to await the discovery of other antibiotics by screening methods which are still largely in use today. *Streptomycin*, *tetracyclines*, and numerous *macrolide* ('large-ring') *antibiotics* were found whose activities complemented those of penicillin. In parallel with screening approaches the chemists succeeded in creating a whole family of semi-synthetic derivatives of penicillin (generically known as β-lactam antibiotics, because they all contain the essential 4-membered β-lactam ring). These semi-synthetic drugs have extended the antibacterial spectrum of 'natural' penicillin, and have helped to counter the emergence of antibiotic-resistant strains of pathogenic bacteria.

Antibiotics work by selectively inhibiting processes which are peculiar to microbial cells, often ones associated with a unique structural feature, enzyme, or organelle not present in human cells. A prime example is the bacterial cell wall, the composition of which is unique in several respects. Penicillins are selectively toxic because they mimic a particular dipeptide sequence present in cell wall precursors. This molecular mimicry inactivates a crucial enzyme needed to form cross-links between the peptidoglycan chains which impart mechanical strength to the bacterial cell wall. Other antibiotics prevent protein synthesis in the bacterial cell, or inactivate enzymes concerned with the complicated processes of nucleotide and nucleic acid biosynthesis.

M. J. WARING

See also CHEMOTHERAPY; INFECTION.

Anxiety

Anxiety is an emotional state, represented by a feeling of dread, apprehension, or fear. In humans, this can be defined by description using language; in animals, it must be inferred from behavioural observations. Tests of anxiety in man are thus based on self report, and these may be divided into features that characterize the person's temperament ('*trait*' anxiety) or that describe a current emotional state ('*state*' anxiety). In animals, it is inferred by the animal's response to an anxiety-provoking situation such as a threatening environment. Distinctions between anxiety and other emotional states, such as fear or even 'arousal', are not always clear. Also, there are close associations between cognition and EMOTION: man has the capacity not only to know, but also to respond emotionally to what he knows.

However, anxiety is not only a behavioural phenomenon. Characteristic autonomic changes take place, typically including increased heart rate and/or blood pressure. There is also marked endocrine activation, particularly increased secretion of the adrenal hormones ADRENALINE (and NORADRENALINE) and *cortisol* (the 'STRESS' hormone). There has been much discussion of how far these 'peripheral' events can actually induce emotional states such as anxiety, or are part of the body's response to those states. Current opinion puts most emphasis on 'central' instigation (by neural mechanisms), though it may be true that accentuated autonomic activity can elicit emotional states, especially when there is a perceived rationale for such activity — '*cognitive labelling*'. Persistent changes in certain hormones (for example, cortisol) may alter the ability of an individual to respond anxiously to provoking stimuli.

Biologically, anxiety has a prime function in adapting to, or avoiding, threatening situations. In animals, one of many ways of inducing such a presumed response would be by pairing a neutral stimulus (say, a light) with a consequent aversive stimulus (such as a footshock). After several such pairings, presentation of the light alone will result in the behavioural and physiological features of anxiety. Similar features can be elicited by exposing animals to situations that they find naturally threatening, such as strange surroundings, or physical peril. This implies that a state of high anxiety is aversive — borne out in humans by the demand for drugs that reduce it, and in animals by showing that they will work to reduce their anxiety levels. Because animals and people find anxiety aversive, they will avoid those circumstances that give rise to it, and hence the threat itself. 'Fear' can be substituted for 'anxiety' in many of these contexts.

Anxiety can, therefore, be the result of stimuli which are naturally threatening (for example the response of a rat to the presence of a cat), those that have been associated with previous danger (the surroundings where the cat is found), or stimuli that are not in themselves threatening, but have become so because of a learned association between them and subsequent discomfort or threat.

Clinically, if significant or disabling levels of anxiety occur without there being sufficient apparent cause, either current or past, then the patient is said to suffer from an *anxiety disorder*. These disorders can be 'global', or generalized, in those people who have high levels of anxiety without evident provoking events; or they can be 'specific', where high anxiety is induced by circumstances which, for most people, would not be considered *anxiogenic* (such as open spaces, spiders, meeting people) — these are sometimes termed 'phobias'. In some cases, anxiety occurs in sudden waves ('*panic attacks*'). Anxiety may also occur as part of another medical condition, or as one result of a drug of abuse or a medication. *Post-traumatic stress disorder* is a particular form of anxious attack provoked by involuntary recall of a previously life-threatening episode (usually triggered by some salient stimulus; for example the sound of a helicopter in those traumatized by war). Psychoanalytical theory has been much concerned with the causes and meaning of individual differences in anxiety.

Attempts have been made to define particular parts of the brain that may be responsible both for physiological or pathological anxiety. There is general agreement that damage to the *amygdala* can reduce anxiety, both that which is a response to 'natural' stimuli and that generated by learned associations. The amygdala (or *amygdaloid complex*, or *nucleus*) is a collection of grey matter that is part of the limbic system, situated in each temporal lobe of the brain, between the cerebral cortex and the hypothalamus. It consists of a number of sub-components (*nuclei*), and some evidence is emerging that different nuclei in the amygdala may play defined roles in certain forms of anxiety. Electrical or chemical stimulation of the amygdala may induce anxiety-like states. There are those who think that the principal or only role of the amygdala is to generate fear or anxiety-like states, but it is more likely that this is one special case of a more general role for this part of the brain. Humans with congenital damage to the amygdala may also have difficulty, for example, in recognizing emotionality, such as fear, in others, or the emotional content of stories.

Scans of the brain by *magnetic resonance imaging* (MRI) show that the amygdala is activated by stimuli that induce or represent emotional states, including fear or anxiety. However, MRI and other imaging techniques have also shown many other parts of the brain to be activated in anxiety states, depending on the condition being studied, or the way in which anxiety is generated; these include parts of the cortex of the frontal lobes, known to be involved in emotional responses, and closely associated cortical areas. There are many connections between the amygdala and these areas of cortex. There is some evidence in the human brain for asymmetry in the role of the frontal cortex: the right side may be particularly important in aversive emotional states such as anxiety.

A number of chemical systems in the brain have been implicated in anxiety. The discovery that the *benzodiazepine* drugs (e.g. librium, valium) had major and quite specific anxiety-reducing (*anxiolytic*) effects on both humans and experimental animals prompted the search for chemicals in the brain that might regulate anxiety levels. Benzodiazepines act by antagonizing the neurotransmitter *GABA* (γ-aminobutyric acid), a compound widely used by nerve cells in the brain to inhibit the activity of other nerve cells. Why this should result in a specific effect on anxiety remains an enigma. At one time, many millions of prescriptions for benzodiazepines were written each year, but it has now become apparent that persistent use may have undesirable side effects, including rebound anxiety once they are discontinued. They nevertheless remain a staple treatment for anxiety disorders. Drugs acting on other systems also have clinically useful anxiolytic effects; these include drugs that modify the action in the brain of *serotonin* or of *noradrenaline*. Both serotonin and noradrenaline are activated in the brain by anxiety-inducing circumstances.

More recently, certain *peptides* in the brain have been shown to be involved in anxiety. One is *corticotrophin-releasing factor* (CRF). This peptide, when infused into the brain of an experimental animal, results in anxiety-like behaviour, as well as the other physiological signs of anxiety. CRF acts on specific receptors on neuronal cell membranes in the brain. These have been shown to be responsible for its anxiogenic actions, because drugs that block CRF1 receptors, or animals that are bred without these receptors (*CRF1R-deficient transgenic mice*), show reduced anxiety. CRF antagonists may, therefore, be the precursors of a new generation of anti-anxiety drugs. However, CRF has other behavioural effects, including actions on food intake and sexual behaviour, and it remains to be established whether other categories of receptors are responsible for these various roles. It is also not clear whether anxiety disorders can be related to inappropriate amounts of these normal neuropeptides, or to the presence of abnormal molecules.   J. HERBERT

Further reading

Davis, M. (1992). The role of the amygdala in fear and anxiety. *Annual Review of Neuroscience*, 15, 353–75.

Le Doux, J. E. (1995). Emotion: clues from the brain. *Annual Review of Psychology*, 46, 209–35.

LeDoux, J. E. (1998). *The emotional brain*. Weidenfeld and Nicolson, London.

See also CONDITIONING; PEPTIDES; MEMBRANE RECEPTORS; STRESS.

Ape man The term 'ape man' is usually applied to a creature that is a member of the human family, but shows in addition features which do not occur in modern humans but are common in apes (such as chimpanzees and gorillas). The overall effect is of a creature whose anatomy is a blend of ape-like and human-like features and, in some metrical traits, is intermediate between apes and humans. The opposite concept, that of man ape or anthropoid ape, is applied to apes which show some features, anatomical and behavioural, which incline them towards humans.

We encounter the term 'ape man' in its Greek version, *Pithecanthropus*, in the writings of Ernst Haeckel (1834–1919), who was one of Charles Darwin's great supporters in Germany during the nineteenth century. Haeckel enthusiastically constructed genealogies of living things and posited the former existence of a primate which was intermediate in form between anthropoid apes and *Homo sapiens* (modern humans). To this hypothecated 'missing link' Haeckel in 1867 gave the name *Pithecanthropus*, years before such a creature was found. In the early 1890s, remains deemed to show such intermediate characteristics were recovered by Eugene Dubois at Trinil in Java (Indonesia); in 1894, with a nice historical sense, Dubois resurrected the old name and called the Javanese species *Pithecanthropus erectus*.

The anatomical traits shown by the Trinil specimen, and other examples subsequently found in Java, China, and north and east Africa, included a brain size (reflected in the capacity of the SKULL) which was intermediate between the small brains of apes and the large brains of modern humans; smaller cheek teeth than those of apes but not as small as in modern humans; and the absence of a bony chin, as in apes, in contrast with the chin at the front of the mandible in modern humans.

Thus, 'ape man' — or its Greek equivalent — was originally applied to a kind of hominid or member of the human family; some people use the term for members of that group to the present, whilst, for others, that species is now known as *Homo erectus*.

From 1925 onwards, a much more ape-like hominid came to light in Africa. These creatures had small brain-sizes like apes, and large premolar and molar teeth, yet their canine teeth were small and they walked bipedally. They are regarded as hominids. These African early hominids were called by Raymond Dart *Australopithecus*. It is to this group of ancient hominids that the term 'ape man' is most commonly applied today, but the term is informal or colloquial. Many would therefore dismiss it as being imprecise, while others continue to find it useful to dub these small-brained members of the human family. It certainly rolls off the tongue far more easily than the formal technical name, *Australopithecus*!

In evolutionary terms, 'ape man' refers to a stage in hominid development represented by a primate which is inferred to have arisen from an apeish origin and structure, and has acquired some critical features that align it with later hominids.   P. TOBIAS

See also BIPEDALISM; EVOLUTION, HUMAN.

Aphrodisiacs the name applied to substances producing sexual desire. It is doubtful whether any such substances exist; rather, substances are known which promote sexual activity if the desire is present. The search for and promotion of substances with presumed aphrodisiac activity is of ancient origin. The Roman empress Livia (58 BC–29 AD) used Spanish Fly to doctor the food of other members of the Imperial family, in the hope of promoting sexual indiscretions which could then be used for political advantage. In 1772, the Marquis de Sade laced sweets with Spanish Fly to give to young women. Toxic effects followed and the Marquis was eventually brought to trial for poisoning. Spanish Fly refers to beautiful, iridescent green insects, *Cantharis vesicatoria*, which contain cantharidin, which is both a vesicant (causes blisters) and a DIURETIC. The dried beetles were simply ground to a powder and used to adulterate food or drink to be consumed by the victim. Cantharidin was quite useful for the removal of warts, but its use as an aphrodisiac probably relates to the irritation caused to the genito-urinary tract, especially the URETHRA, so that victims become more aware of their sexual organs. Rhinoceros horn has been considered through the ages to have magical properties, either fashioned into objects or powdered and consumed. Cups made of rhino horn were expected to protect the drinker against poison, and powdered horn was reputed to be useful for many disease states, including IMPOTENCE, and for promotion of sexual activity. Any effects of rhino horn are almost certainly placebo effects, of which scarcity, improbability, and high cost play a part. Trade in rhino horn is now banned world wide. The MANDRAKE root is also reputed to have aphrodisiac properties.

A number of foods are reputed to have aphrodisiac properties, including asparagus, caviar, eel, garlic, ginseng, honey, lobster, oysters, peaches, and truffles. Many of these foods are exotic, and any effect they have on sexual desire is more likely due to the setting in which they are presented.

In much of the above account the receivers of the supposed aphrodisiac were unaware what was being offered to them. In recent times therapeutic strategies have been developed to assist those who have sexual desire but lack the ability to perform. Male impotence affects large numbers of men from age 40 onwards, because of the inability to maintain an ERECTION. In some instances, for example paraplegics, the nerve pathways from the brain to the penis are interrupted, so that desire cannot lead to an erection. A breakthrough in understanding occurred when it was realized that, to obtain an erection, the penile muscles, especially of the blood vessels, need to relax. This allows the blood spaces to fill causing swelling, the resulting tumescence compressing the veins, preventing venous drainage. Papaverine and phenoxybenzamine, an α-adrenoceptor blocking drug, were amongst the first to be used. The former is a spasmolytic, (a smooth muscle relaxant), whereas phenoxybenzamine prevents vasoconstriction by blocking the effects of sympathetic vasoconstriction and so allowing the filling of the blood spaces. For the latter an intact sympathetic outflow is needed. These agents have widespread activity throughout the body and therefore have to be injected, locally, into the penis. An alternative approach is to increase levels of cyclic AMP locally in the penis, again causing muscle relaxation. This has been achieved by using an inhibitor of phosphodiesterase (which breaks down cyclic AMP). The penile tissue is particularly rich in a particular phosphodiesterase, PDE5, so a specific inhibitor of PDE5 was developed which can be taken orally, namely sildenafil citrate (Viagra). An erection is obtained only when sexual stimulation is present; the drug is therefore useful in male erectile dysfunction, but only if other pathways are intact. Whether phenoxybenzamine or sildenafil should be described as aphrodisiacs is arguable.

Finally, a word about alcohol. In Macbeth, Shakespeare wrote of alcohol 'Lechery it provokes and improvokes. It provokes the desire but takes away the performance.' Clearly alcohol reduces inhibitions, causing Ogden Nash to note 'Candy is dandy, but liquor is quicker.' Scientific research has shown alcohol raises testosterone levels in women — a hormone linked to LIBIDO in both sexes.

A great variety of odours have been found to increase penile blood flow, including liquorice, lavender, and pumpkin pie.

ALAN W. CUTHBERT

See also IMPOTENCE; LIBIDO; SEX HORMONES.

Apoplexy In modern usage, apoplexy and STROKE are synonymous terms, referring to sudden and lasting impairment of brain function caused by obstruction of or haemorrhage from the cerebral blood vessels. Cerebrovascular disease is characterized by dramatic physical effects, high mortality, and serious long-term morbidity. Several ancient Greek medical authors, including Hippocrates and GALEN, wrote on 'apoplexy', leaving careful descriptions of its clinical characteristics. There has, moreover, long been an appreciation that the study of the disorders of the brain might shed light on the nature of mental processes.

The roots of our understanding of the cerebrovascular circulation in disease may be found in the work of the seventeenth-century Swiss physician and anatomist, Johannes Wepfer, who was the first to propose, on the basis of post-mortem examination, that cerebral haemorrhage was a cause of apoplexy. He also suggested that the disorder could arise if the arteries supplying the brain were occluded by blood clots. Apoplexy, in Wepfer's usage, was a wider concept than the modern category of stroke, including cases caused by disease of the cervical arteries. This explains his belief that the damage caused by apoplexy could impair function on both sides of the body.

Apoplexy cases, with their obvious and circumscribed brain lesions, were of great interest to the early pathological anatomists. In eighteenth-century Italy, Giovanni Morgagni demonstrated conclusively that damage within a cerebral hemisphere produced PARALYSIS on the opposite side of the body. In the nineteenth century, the study of stroke lesions played a major role in the localization of specific functions to particular sites within the brain: the French surgeon Paul Broca, for example, correlated loss of SPEECH with localized damage to the base of the third frontal convolution of the left hemisphere. Stroke lesions are generally more discrete and more stable throughout the remaining life of the subject than other forms of damage to the human brain. Experiments upon animal brains can shed little light on the human characteristics of language, personality, and creativity. Strokes thus have functioned, for neuroscientists and psychologists, as 'natural experiments' on the human brain.

As well as being physically handicapped, stroke victims often suffer severe psychological effects. The prognosis of stroke has long been regarded very pessimistically indeed. The Hippocratic dictum that 'It is impossible to cure a severe attack of apoplexy and difficult to cure a mild one' may be found often reiterated in twentieth-century medical textbooks. However, in the last decade, a mood of greater optimism has emerged. This was first stimulated by developments in stroke rehabilitation, which confirmed the possibility of functional improvement. Also, increased understanding of the pattern of occurrence and the causes of cerebrovascular disease has stimulated interest in the prevention of stroke, with attention being given to the risks of SMOKING, HYPERTENSION, and cardiac disease.

MALCOLM NICOLSON

See also STROKE.

Appendix The appendix is more correctly known as the '*vermiform appendix*', meaning worm-like. It is present only in man, certain anthropoid apes, and the wombat (a nocturnal, burrowing Australian marsupial). Many herbivores are provided with a comparable, but larger structure, in which bacterial breakdown of cellulose, the main constituent of cell walls in plant fibre, takes place. In man the appendix is thought to represent a vestigial organ — one that remains in diminished form after it has ceased, in evolutionary terms, to have any significant function.

The appendix is a short, blind-ended tube arising from the caecum, the first part of the large intestine, within the lower right part of the abdominal cavity. In about half the population, the appendix is '*retrocaecal*' — behind the caecum; in most cases, it is mobile within the abdominal cavity, suspended from the rest of the bowel by a sling-like fold of tissue (a *mesentery*), which has the artery to the appendix running in its free edge. The appendix first appears in the fetus at about 6 weeks of development, being initially high up in the abdomen but later descending to its final position. Approximately 1 in 100 000 people are born without an appendix — and very rarely there are two. The appendix is typically 6–9 cm long, but the length varies considerably, from 2 to 30 cm; on average it is 0.5 cm longer in the male than in the female. It is longer in the child than in the adult and shrinks further after mid life. The internal diameter of the appendix is described as wide enough to admit a matchstick, but this lumen may be partially or completely obliterated after middle age. The structure of the tube is basically the same as that of the large intestine: it has an outer muscular coat lined by a much-folded lining (*mucosa*). It also has aggregates of lymphoid tissue within its walls, which may replace the muscle coat in places.

The appendix in man is medically important because of its propensity to become inflamed in the condition known as *acute appendicitis*. In this condition, the appendix becomes swollen and the wall fills with inflammatory cells. The process may be initiated by blockage with material from the bowel. If this inflammatory process is allowed to continue, the appendix will become gangrenous and perforate, leading to peritonitis. Acute appendicitis is the most common cause of intra-abdominal infection in developed countries and appendicectomy is the most commonly performed emergency surgical operation. It is less common in developing countries where the diet contains significantly more fibre than our own. In the UK, 1.9 females and 1.5 males per thousand of the population each year get acute appendicitis and have their appendix removed. At the current rate, one in every 6 or 7 people will eventually undergo appendicectomy, even though the incidence of acute appendicitis in the UK has decreased by 50% since the 1970s. The mortality from acute appendicitis has also fallen dramatically, due to a number of factors including better general nutrition, earlier presentation to hospital, and improved anaesthetics. Post-operative problems, such as wound infection, have also become rarer due to the widespread use of antibiotics before surgery. Although appendicitis can occur at any age, it is commonest between 8 and 14 years. It is rare in the elderly and in infants below the age of 2. The cardinal sign of appendicitis is abdominal pain, which is often rather vague and poorly localized initially. As the inflammatory process proceeds, however, the pain usually localizes to the right side of the lower abdomen over the site of the appendix. There is tenderness over the appendix, often accompanied by a slight fever, a facial flush, and a rapid pulse. Despite this apparently typical picture the diagnosis is often difficult to make, particularly in females in whom gynaecological problems are also common and may closely mimic appendicitis. A percentage of appendices removed prove to be normal when examined under the microscope.

The first record of what may have been appendicitis was made by Aretaios around the third century AD. Though the appendix appeared in the anatomical drawings of LEONARDO DA VINCI from 1492, it was not until 1521 that it was described by an Italian anatomist, Berengario da Carpi. While there is some debate as to who first removed an appendix in England, the first deliberate appendicectomy for acute appendicitis was undertaken by a gynaecologist, Robert Lawson Tait, in May 1880 in Birmingham. The patient recovered. Prior to this Claudius Amyand, physician to Queen Anne, in 1736 successfully removed an acutely inflamed appendix from inside the hernial sac of a young boy.

A. WINTER
P. J. O'DWYER

Further reading
Knut, H., (ed.) (1989). *The illustrated history of surgery*. Harold Starke, London.

See PLATE 1

See also ALIMENTARY SYSTEM.

Armour any form of covering employed to protect some or all of the body from physical assaults. Although armour has most commonly been worn by warriors and soldiers in military contexts, it has also been used by athletes in various forms of sport, and has more recently come to be employed by police officers when dealing with rioters, terrorists, and heavily armed offenders. The use and form of armour has been related both to the types of weapons employed by expected adversaries and to the techniques available for its manufacture, but wealth and the general availability of suitable materials have tended to play a greater role in determining whether and what quantity of armour is worn. Although some of its elements developed earlier in Mesopotamia, full body armour was apparently first used by Mycenaean Greek charioteers in the last few centuries of the Bronze Age. It only came into general use in regions of south-central Europe, south-west Asia, and northern Africa at the beginning of the Iron Age around 1150 BC, with a revolution in military tactics involving the use of a long, slashing sword.

Armour came to be made up of a number of distinct elements, protecting different parts of the body. The oldest and by far the most widespread element is the *shield*. Though they varied greatly in size and shape from one society to the next and over time in many individual societies, shields were normally constructed of wicker, wood, leather, or plywood covered with leather. In Latin Europe after *c.* 1450 the use of a shield was largely abandoned, though a small, round form continued to be used by some infantry units into the seventeenth century. More recently, large, oblong shields have been adopted by riot police in several countries.

The shield differed from all of the later elements of armour in being held *before* the body like a weapon rather than worn *on* the body like a garment. The oldest type of body armour seems to have been the *helmet*, designed to deflect blows to the head. Though adopted for use in Mesopotamia in the third millennium BC, helmets were rare before the military revolution of the twelfth century BC. From that time onward, metal helmets were worn by soldiers, regardless of rank. Until approximately 1200 AD, most helmets were roughly **hemispherical** or **conical**, and some covered only the upper half of the head. Many helmets, however, had projections of plate covering the back of the neck, the cheeks, the nose, or (more rarely) the whole face, while others had some form of flexible **curtain** suspended from the lower rim, and sometimes joined at the front to form an *aventail*. Sometimes the projections were extended downwards to the point where they produced the nearly cylindrical form seen in the Corinthian helmet of the eighth century BC. The fully cylindrical form of helmet, or *great helm*, however — covering all of the neck as well as the head, and pierced only with slits for seeing and holes for breathing — was peculiar to Latin Christendom between *c.* 1220 and *c.* 1540. Like other forms of body armour, metal helmets were generally abandoned in Latin Europe around 1660, but were revived around 1810 for units of heavy cavalry and dragoons, and are still worn by such units on formal occasions. More utilitarian forms of helmet were adopted for military use during World War I, and are still worn in all armed forces today.

Helmets were normally worn along with some form of armour for the *torso*, often extended to cover at least the upper arms and thighs; armour for the lower arms, legs, hands, and feet was usually separate, and less commonly used. The most primitive armour for the torso was composed principally of a flexible continuous material, such as the layers of linen, glued together to form a relatively stiff material, that was standard in Greek armies from 600 to 200 BC. Torso armour could also consist of a fabric covered with small, flat pieces of metal: abutting hollow discs (*ring armour*), overlapping scales (*scale armour*), or *lames* (flat, narrow, rectangular metal plates roughly the size of playing cards) sewn or (in *brigandine armour*) riveted between the layers. Scale armour was the most successful form, and continued in use until 1100.

A second type of torso armour was composed of discontinuous fabric. It was made up entirely of small, connected pieces of metal or some other hard substance. *Lamellar* armour consisted of small narrow lames pierced at the top and bottom and tied together vertically with cords in many abutting or upwardly overlapping rows. Lamellar armour was common in most of the West, the Byzantine Empire, and much of Islam, from the early Iron Age to the fifteenth century, and continued in use in eastern Asia, especially Japan, until the nineteenth century. From about 200 BC, however, discontinuous-fabric armour increasingly took the superior form of small rings of iron wire interlinked on all sides to form the purely metallic fabric eventually called *mail* (*not* chain-mail). Invented by the Celts or Scyths of eastern Europe, this **mail armour** gradually displaced all other types in western Europe and was later worn under plate armour until about 1500. Mail armour for the torso typically took the form of a loose **tunic** whose lower hem fell somewhere between the hips and the knees. It might be sleeveless or have sleeves falling anywhere from the upper arm to the lower wrist; later versions often ended in mittens. By 1066 it also had a hood or *coif* of the same material, attached directly or (later) separate and worn over the tunic with a short cape covering the shoulders.

The oldest form of *plate-armour* for the body is known as *curve-plate* armour, as it was constructed mainly of large and strongly curved metal plates. The oldest subtype took the form of semi-cylindrical plates of various widths, constituting either *tubular-plate* armour — of the sort employed by charioteers in Mycenaean Greece — or *banded* armour — especially popular among the Parthians and the Romans of the early Empire. A second subtype of plate armour took the form of *moulded-plate* armour and came into general use at the beginning of the Iron Age around 1150 BC, but was at first largely restricted to armour for the lower leg, now called *greaves*. Around 800 BC a form of moulded armour for the body was adopted, consisting of two large plates abutting one another under the arms, and covering everything from the neck to the top of the hips. This combination of *breastplate* and *backplate* (now called a *cuirass*) was worn principally by princes and the higher officers of most armies from that time down to around 400 AD, and often took the form now called the *muscled cuirass*, which imitated the natural musculature of the torso. In the fourteenth century a new form of cuirass, unmuscled and bulbous, would be created by the armourers, in which large plates were sewn inside a fabric poncho in the fashion of brigandine armour. A fully articulated steel cuirass continued in use in heavy cavalry units until c. 1660, and in many units until 1914. In the British army the steel cuirass was abandoned in 1660 but revived for élite cavalry units in 1817–21, and is still worn on parade today.

Armour for the *lower legs* was roughly coeval with that for the torso. Leg-armour was also made of the same variety of materials in the same variety of constructions, but was not nearly so general in its use. The moulded-plate **greaves** widely adopted in the twelfth century BC to protect the lower leg from swords continued to be worn by heavy infantrymen in Greek and Italian armies for about a millennium, but under the Roman Empire came to be restricted to centurions and higher officers. From the second century BC the Parthian heavy-cavalrymen or *cataphracts* — the first fully-armoured warriors in civilized history — wore full leggings of scale, mail, or banded armour that extended also over the feet. They were also the first to wear comparable armoured sleeves covering their arms to the wrist. Roman cataphracts wore similar armour from the second century AD, and transmitted the tradition of armouring arms and legs to the heaviest units of the Byzantine cavalry. By 1410, a fully-articulated, individually tailored, and stylistically uniform *harness* of moulded plate armour covered the whole body of every Latin knight. The gradual discontinuation of armour except for helmets and cuirasses after about 1600 was a result of the perfection of hand-held firearms, whose bullets could penetrate all but the thickest (and heaviest) armour.

JONATHAN BOULTON

Arms serve as our primary connection to people and objects, through our reach and our ability to grasp things: through defensive postures, arms can also prevent connection that might cause us harm. These roles are reflected symbolically both in verbal figurations and in the non-verbal communication that is known as BODY LANGUAGE.

The position of the arms is very important in body language. Arms folded across the chest, in Western cultures, suggest anger, hostility, or defensiveness. Loose-swinging arms suggest ease or confidence; arms clasped behind the back imply gravity or seriousness; arms clasped before the body suggest eagerness. Arms raised above the head convey either submission (especially with palms open and facing the other person) or victory and militancy (especially in conjunction with a fisted hand). In each case the position of the arms relative to the body imitates the EMOTION conveyed through being open or closed.

Relationships between Western people are frequently expressed through the physical connection of arms. Formal relations usually require handshakes, while more familiar relations might permit forearm clasps, shoulder clasps, or even hugs. While different cultures have different standards of personal space, most of them fall within the length of an adult arm. To 'hold someone at arm's length', therefore, is to enforce a somewhat unnatural distance.

Arms have entered the language as symbolic of closeness, connection, or safety. To be 'arm-in-arm', actually or figuratively, is to be in close communication. To 'offer an arm' and 'with open arms' symbolically suggest vulnerability, and so figuratively suggest trust, openness, and willingness. Similarly, the phrases 'within arm's reach' and 'the long arm of the law' both highlight the vulnerability of closeness, especially an inescapable closeness. Finally, to designate someone as one's 'right arm' marks him or her as essential to one's own work, as both connected to oneself and a means of connection elsewhere.

The arms are an important means of defence of our vulnerable points, including the head, chest, and abdomen, as well as of antagonistic connections to others. As such, arms have become our primary metaphor for weaponry, which originally acted to extend the natural capabilities of the arms: reach (spears or swords), throwing or mobility (slings), and blockage (shields). While modern weaponry has far outstripped even the suggested or symbolic capabilities of arms, the connection lives on in our military vocabulary: a soldier was originally a 'man-at-arms'; guns of all sorts are referred to as 'firearms'; to surrender is to 'lay down arms'; to fight or threaten is to be 'up in arms'. The heraldic coat of arms was originally a cover of insignia on shields for fully armoured knights; as nobility became hereditary, the *coat of arms* became an identification of a family.

In anatomical terms, the arm is built around three bones; — the *humerus* in the upper arm, and the *radius* and the *ulna* in the forearm. The

humerus articulates with the *scapula* (shoulder blade) at the SHOULDER, and with the radius and the ulna at the ELBOW. The arm is linked to the trunk by the *shoulder girdle*, formed by the scapula and the *clavicle* (collar bone). The most familiar and obvious muscles of the upper arm, particularly when developed by strength training, are the *deltoid*, *biceps*, and *triceps*. The deltoid muscle fleshes out the curve of the shoulder, and acts to raise the arm, by being attached to the shoulder girdle above and to the humerus below. The biceps muscle on the front and the triceps on the back span the upper arm from the shoulder girdle to below the elbow, so they can flex and extend the elbow respectively. Other, deeper muscles assist elbow flexion. In the forearm, the muscles are mainly those used for movements at the wrist and at the joints in the hand; grasping, and all the finer finger and thumb movements, are achieved by contraction of forearm muscles via the long tendons that span both the front and back of the wrist, assisted by the small muscles within the hand itself. The nerves which serve sensory and motor function in the arm come from the BRACHIAL PLEXUS in the neck, derived through this mainly from the lower cervical segments of the SPINAL CORD. The main arterial channel carrying blood to the arm changes its name from *subclavian*, as it runs behind the collar bone, to *axillary* in the armpit, and to *brachial* in the arm itself, dividing at the elbow into the *radial artery* (familiar for taking the pulse at the wrist) and the *ulna artery*, which both finally supply branches to the hand.   JULIE VEDDER

SHEILA JENNETT

See PLATE 5.

See also BODY LANGUAGE; GESTURES.

Art and the body Since ancient times, artists have visually recreated and re-evaluated the human body. Consequently, it has been used for medical and scientific investigations, as an educational tool and as an allegory for something other than itself. Representations of the body are not merely works of art but can also be read as social documents; paintings and sculptures are direct vehicles of history. To a certain degree all art embodies crystallized history, allowing its cultural values to be portrayed through the iconography of art. For example, cultural attitudes and a society's understanding of sexuality can often be seen through the depictions of the human figure.

The ancient Greeks and the Italian Renaissance artists held the view that the human body should personify 'perfect' forms of balance and symmetry, culminating in equal proportions. Once such a harmony had been understood then the ideal construct of beauty in the form of the body could be achieved. The Renaissance artists were influenced by statements they read at the beginning of the third book *The Planning of Temples* of Marcus Vitruvius' *Vitruvius on Architecture*, which set out rules of the correct human proportions, stating that man's body is a model of proportion because with arms and legs extended it fits into those 'perfect' geometrical forms, the square and the circle. Artists of the Renaissance used this model as a basis for their whole artistic philosophy. Artists were taking an interest in the accurate representation of the human form, and because of this naturalism in art was revived (c. 1450–1550). The Naturalistic movement, combined with access to Greek sources and the revival of learning, produced fundamental changes in the anatomical outlook which found their most natural and forceful expression through artists such as Leonardo da Vinci (1452–1519), Michelangelo (1475–1564), and Raphael (1483–1521). Da Vinci, in particular, treated the human body as an instrument of movement governed by mechanical laws — he thought even the expressions of emotions were controlled in this way. No longer during this period was the body regarded as a sinful instrument which must be hidden or as something sacred that must not be anatomically investigated. Classical ideals were returning and artists were the first heralds of the new age.

In the seventeenth century, distorted, exaggerated poses of the nudes were given the title Mannerism. Painters such as Bronzino, Giambologna, and Correggio produced highly polished and formalized nudes which all had a similar look about them. Mannerism became very popular in France during this period, partly because of its cultivation of the chic female nude in the form of the goddess and in Venus-like postures. Art historian Kenneth Clark states in *The Nude* (1980): 'The goddess of mannerism is the eternal feminine of the fashion-plate.' Mannerist art treated the body as a collection of parts, which could be enlarged and exaggerated at will. Many of the art–anatomy folios also employed this type of visual selecting of anatomical parts. In a drawing by anatomist Govard Bidloo (1649–1713), pinned-back flaps of skin revealed the organs of a female cadaver. However, when the nineteenth-century painter Gustave Courbet later made a similar painting revealing only female genitalia, isolating this part of the anatomy, it prompted a viewer to remark:

> By some inconceivable forgetfulness, the artist, who copied his model from nature, had neglected to represent the feet, the legs, the thighs, the stomach, the hips, the chest, the hands, the arms, the shoulders, the neck, and the head …

Although the Mannerist body was very elegant, with its finely tapered neck, wrists, and ankles, the female shape became far removed from real life. Incorrect proportions of this type were to be challenged in the eighteenth century by the principles of the Enlightenment.

The pursuit of aesthetics for those educated in the eighteenth century did not belong to art academies and paintings alone, but was a way of life. The body increasingly became a visible and tangible medium through which artists could transmit codes of aesthetics that were also interpreted as codes of ethics. Twentieth-century writers interpreted the aesthetics of this period as being politically active in shaping individual taste, knowledge, and moral behaviour, the cultivation of which was considered important to an aesthetic lifestyle. As Eagleton points out in *The Ideology of the Aesthetic* (1990): 'The beautiful is just political order lived out on the body, the way it strikes the eye and stirs the heart'. Cultural ideologies harnessing scientific exactness to artistic beauty were the canons on which paintings and sculptures were produced. Like the reading of text, the reading of art also had its own language and could be deciphered and translated accordingly. In *The Analysis of Beauty* (1753), the artist William Hogarth centres his argument around the 'line of beauty', purporting that figurative art could be regulated by a specific principle which could be expressed by a particular line. The beauty of different physical types is a theme that Hogarth deals with in Chapter XI, entitled 'Of Proportion'. Here he distinguishes between purely formal beauty and the beauty of fitness: the first is governed by the serpentine line; the second arises 'chiefly from a fitness of some design'd purpose of use'. The pictorial distinctions made by Hogarth are an essential part of his language

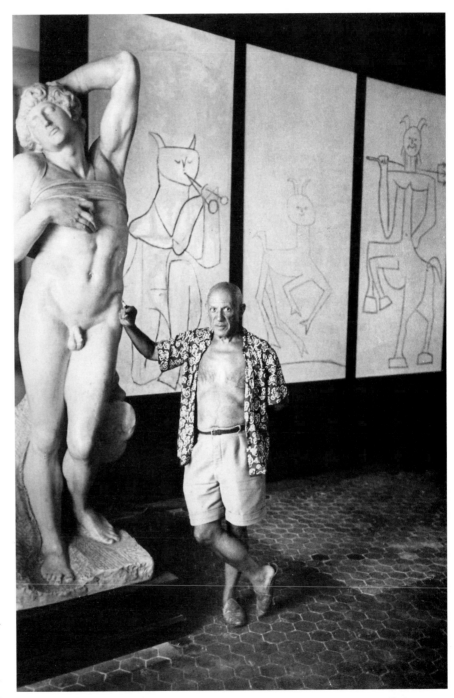

Pablo Picasso in the Grimaldi Museum at Antibes, France in August 1948. Robert Capa/Magnum Photos.

45

as an artist, making his characters and caricatures easily legible.

Sir Joshua Reynolds (1723–92), a renowned artist and socialite, became the first president of the Royal Academy of Arts in 1768. Reynolds, like many of his contemporaries, was a man of the Enlightenment and believed in the harmony of nature, art, science, and medicine, each component relying upon the other. There was very little division for him between art and science. For Reynolds, beauty is not something beyond reach, but tangible and attainable. In one of his lectures to the students and dilettanti, *Discourse III* (1770), he states: 'For perfect beauty in any species must combine all the characters which are beautiful'. The human body was seen by eighteenth-century artists as a tool from which to learn. The body whether real or artificial, dead or alive, took on many guises as a physical being to be scientifically explored and artistically rendered.

While life classes involving a nude female were restricted to married men, there was no shortage of 'anatomized' females adorning the medical folios of this period. Many of the truncated and finely engraved images show female anatomy in all shapes and sizes. The lack of open access to the life class at the Royal Academy of Arts for single men and women artists necessitated their learning anatomy from such folios; consequently, there was a growing medical interest in biological sex and sexual differences, and a growing market for publications of this kind. Anatomical folios used in the teaching of art had a scientific influence on artists in their studies. In addition to the rules of proportion as laid down by the Renaissance architect Vitruvius, classical ideals of beauty, and the slavish adherence to anatomical accuracy, artists were beginning to address new scientific theories concerning female anatomy and biology. Perhaps for the first time, a serious attempt was being made by artists and anatomists to link geometry and the biology of sex together. According to Kenneth Clark:

> 'The fact that we can base our argument either way on this unexpected union of sex and biology is a proof of how deeply the concept of the nude is linked with our most elementary notions of order and design.' (*The Nude*, 1980.)

The study of the nude figure and its physiology was being re-addressed not only by scientists and anatomists but also by artists. Medical inquiry into a woman's biological state began influencing art-anatomy depictions of both her inner and outer physiological structure.

The eighteenth century was culturally redesigning the body, for despite analytical, scientific, and medical mechanization of the human form, art constantly reminds us that we are more than just the sum of our parts. Art–anatomy practices increasingly became multifaceted as both artists and anatomists assimilated a new 'look' and design to the human figure. The shape of the body is both physiologically determined and artificially recreated. This is most noticeable during the Enlightenment,

when fashionable dress, masks and masquerading, corsetry, and the wearing of beauty patches were part of everyday life. Science and art were not alone in measuring the body, for the wearing of stays and the emergence of the fashionable, measured body became part of society's image. William Hogarth's *Line of Beauty*, and Joshua Reynolds' call for harmony, beauty, and proportion, had one thing in common: measurement.

The female body was moulded, measured, masqueraded, and medicalized. Fashion and physique went hand in hand, and consequently anatomists noticed how the slenderness of shoes and the tightness of stays were physically altering the shape of women. Joshua Reynolds urged his students not to disguise the human form or 'disguise nature' by means of 'hair-dressers, and tailors, in their various schools of deformity' (*Discourse III*, 1770). Hogarth, however, encouraged females to change their physical appearance and wear the 'line of beauty', which became a tradename for the corset. The wearing of a corset truncated and fragmented the body, and divided it in two. It covered just enough to reveal parts of the anatomy that were decidedly 'female' — breasts and sexual organs. Thus, the female's anatomy was being reshaped not only by artists but by the means of the fashions that women chose. The process of sectioning, fragmenting, and splitting the female anatomy, therefore, was not peculiar to the realm of man-made art–anatomy images.

The eighteenth-century woman was constantly having something done to her: the man-midwife inspected her, the stay-maker measured her, the scientist demystified her biology, the anatomist dissected her, and finally the artist painted her. Biological and hierarchal divisions between the sexes in terms of their skeletons were explored during the twentieth century by writers such as Londa Schiebinger, whose research found that it was not until 1759 that the 'female skeleton make her debut' (*The Mind Has No Sex*, 1989). Up to this time all depictions of skeletons were of males, even those representing children and females, and it was not until the latter half of the eighteenth century that women were viewed as physiologically different from men. Anatomical understanding of the skeleton, the representation of the human figure and the disfiguring brought about by the wearing of stays had an impact on artistic development. Artists, especially those trained by anatomists at the Royal Academy of Arts, saw dissecting classes as a natural part of art education. Artists and medical men followed iconographic systems resulting in anatomic arithmetic where classical ideals were promoted by using such images as *Apollo* and the *Venus de Medici*.

Cultural iconography of the human figure usually denotes the promise of something 'more'. It can arouse unfulfilled sexual fantasies, commodity–ownership relations or paternal feelings, or question the very existence of 'being' as did the images of life and death during the eighteenth century. Representations of the naked and

the nude portray body images as cultural commodities. For modern writers such as John Berger, Carol Pateman, Dorinda Outram, and Simone de Beauvoir, the body (especially the female) becomes a sign and cultural symbol for external reality, both political and gendered. The 'political culture of the body' that Dorinda Outram speaks of can therefore be seen through images showing types of dress, posture, chosen medium (oil or otherwise), the scale of canvas, and physiology. The body image as a cultural, political, scientific, erotic, and fashionable statement is most evident through visual representation; real, allegorical or symbolic. Part of eighteenth-century understanding of the body was by means of identifying self with images of life and death. The body, in particular, provoked feelings of enquiry and curiosity of self, both external and internal.

By the nineteenth century, the nude and semi-naked female form could be seen as an ever-recurring topic, for, despite the Victorian values of prudity and chastity, the nude survived. French artists such as Ingres, Renoir, Manet, Degas, and Courbet are readily called to mind for their renderings of the body. The British artist William Etty (1787–1849) became wholly absorbed in the study of the nude, and could often be found at the life class housed in the Royal Academy of Art, making copious drawings of his model. The draped and partially-wrapped life models and classical statues located at the Royal Academy, the Government Schools, and the Slade School of Art direct the viewer's attention to the relevant parts of the body by revealing and concealing. Pictorially, the severing of head from body does not always take the form of decapitation and a fine line around the neck, dividing physical space, is sometimes enough. The pearls around the neck of a wax model draw attention to her face; likewise, the black ribbon around the neck of the woman in Edouard Manet's painting *Olympia* (1862–3) draws attention to her social status.

Much discussion has centred around theories of the body, especially since the late nineteenth century. Discourse surrounding the *naked* and the *nude*, Freudian psychoanalysis, the decline of beauty, and the onslaught of feminism have all helped to shape and define what art and the body are, and what they is not. Early twentieth-century artists including Henri Matisse, Auguste Renoir, Pablo Picasso, and George Braque launched new visions of the human figure as each struggled with ideas of form and content. The fragmentation of subject matter, which became the hallmark of Cubism, meant that representations of the body were seen as small fractions of picture-planes, all positioned at irregular angles. Ideas of figurative and abstract art are thought to have been born at this time, especially in the works of Paul Cezanne, a pre-Cubist painter. After 1945, post-war Britain saw artists such as Stanley Spencer, Lucien Freud, Euan Uglow, Allen Jones, Francis Bacon, and Henry Moore extending the boundaries of figurative and abstract renderings of both the male and female body. In America during the 1950s the American Abstract Expressionists also began to reassess the impact of figurative/abstract art, leading Willem de Kooning to paint a series of 'pink nudes', and Pop artist Andy Warhol to make icons of leading Hollywood stars. By the 1960s and 1970s, art was undergoing another metamorphosis, and alternative conventions were being found to re-construct the body in the guise of photo-montage, body-prints, life-size sculpture, concept art, happenings, and performance art. By this time, feminist ideology, the decline of easel painting, and new forms of art were affecting the type of 'body art' made.

Representations of the body have survived the most rigorous tests executed by late twentieth-century artists; interestingly, not unlike in the eighteenth century, art, anatomy, and the body are once again being given centre stage.

ANNE ABICHOU

Further reading

Abichou, A. (1996). *Taught by artists and trained by anatomists: Royal Academy students and art education.* University of London, Institute of Education, London.

Clark, K. (1980). *The nude: a study of ideal art.* Penguin Books Ltd., Harmondsworth.

Eagleton, T. (1990). *The ideology of the aesthetic.* Blackwell, Oxford.

Nead, L. (1994). *The female nude. Art, obscenity and sexuality.* Routledge, London and New York.

See also BODY SHAPE; FEMALE FORM; ICONOGRAPHY; NUDISM.

Artificial feeding

Patients require artificial feeding if they are unable to take adequate food by mouth, or if the small intestine is unable to absorb nutrients from their food. For example, coma or paralysis of the throat muscles can prevent normal swallowing; diseased small intestine may have to be removed by surgical operation which leaves insufficient area to absorb enough nutrients for the patient to survive.

Patients may also require artificial feeding when they have developed major infection or received severe injury such as occurs after a large area of skin is burned. In these situations, patients have a much larger requirement for nutrients and artificial supplements may be required. The aim of artificial feeding is to supply all the nutrients which are essential for the body to survive and, especially in young patients, to allow normal development.

Artificial feeding can be achieved by two different methods. The nutrition can be delivered into the gut whence it can be normally absorbed (*enteral*) or administered directly into the blood stream (*parenteral*).

Enteral feeding is used when a patient has an adequately functioning bowel, but cannot eat sufficient nutrients — such as a patient receiving artificial ventilation in an intensive care unit who is too sedated to be able to eat and drink normally. Enteral feeding can be achieved by passing a fine-bore tube through the patient's nose into the stomach or upper part of the small bowel. If prolonged enteral feeding is anticipated, this *nasogastric tube* is replaced by a *gastrostomy tube*, which passes through a small opening made surgically through the skin of the abdomen into the stomach. Where the patient's upper digestive system has some disease process or has undergone surgery, this can be bypassed by placing a feeding *enterostomy tube* in the lower part of the small bowel.

The major benefit of using enteral feeding is that nutrition is delivered into the small bowel and the normal route is used for nutrient absorption. In addition, enteral feeding may improve the ability of the gut to resist infection, which is extremely important in patients who may already have decreased resistance. This form of artificial feeding minimizes problems of access to a patient's veins, and there is far less chance of infection than parenteral with feeding.

Parenteral feeding

This is used in those circumstances when it is not possible to deliver artificial feeding into the gut. Patients who have disease of the bowel or who have undergone major bowel surgery may then require parenteral nutrition. With this type of artificial feeding, the nutrients are usually delivered directly into the bloodstream. A small tube (*cannula*) is placed into a large vein in the neck or above the collar bone. The insertion of this cannula is a very specialized technique and in some cases may require a surgical operation under general anaesthesia.

This *central venous cannulation* may be associated with several complications, such as blockage of the cannula which then has to be replaced, or infection which may require that the cannula is removed until the infection has been treated successfully. The risk of such complications increases with time, and access to a suitable vein can become increasingly limited as the possible sites for placing the cannula are used. This is especially so in children. Because of these problems the parenteral route for administration of nutrition is reserved usually for patients with high caloric requirements and a non-functioning gut. It may also be used in children who cannot tolerate enteral feeding.

Artificial feeding can improve wound healing and may lead to faster and better recovery after major surgery or other form of severe tissue damage. Even when some food and drink is taken by mouth, it may not be adequate to provide the extra nutrition required for repair.

GAVIN KENNY

See also ALIMENTARY SYSTEM; COMA; EATING; LIFE SUPPORT.

Artificial insemination

The introduction of sperm into the female reproductive tract by means other than a partner's penis. Two categories have been known as *AIH* (using the husband's sperm — now more appropriately AIP) and *AID* (using sperm from a donor). Artificial insemination may be proposed by doctors for the treatment of some types of INFERTILITY, or when there is a strong chance, of an infant having a CONGENITAL ABNORMALITY if fathered by the partner. Social, ethical, and legal issues arise with respect to AID for lesbians and also concerning AIP after the death of a partner, since it is possible to use sperm frozen in advance of anticipated demise. The custom in Aldous Huxley's *Island*, where the semen of great and good men long deceased could be selected from a frozen store is a practical possibility — if a social fantasy.

S.J.

See ASSISTED REPRODUCTION; INFERTILITY.

Artificial ventilation

The body requires a certain volume of air to be inhaled and exhaled to maintain the correct levels of OXYGEN and CARBON DIOXIDE within the tissues. Tissue damage, which leads eventually to death, occurs if the level of oxygen becomes too low or the amount of carbon dioxide becomes too high. The body is therefore critically dependent on breathing to maintain life. When this 'bellows' function of the lungs, moving air in and out, becomes inadequate or stops altogether, the patient must receive artificial ventilation to survive. The 'kiss of life' — mouth-to-mouth breathing — is a well-known 'first-aid' form of artificial ventilation, and is described under RESUSCITATION. Mechanical systems, for more prolonged use, are considered here.

Negative pressure ventilation

The original devices for artificial ventilation developed negative pressure around the patient's chest. One example of these breathing machines was the '*iron lung*' or tank ventilator which was used widely during the poliomyelitis outbreak in the early 1950s, although an early version had been invented long before. The patient was placed inside the tank and a seal completed an airtight fit around the neck. Air was rhythmically sucked out from the tank and blown back in. Thus alternating negative and positive pressure in the tank caused air to flow in and out of the patient's lungs.

Positive pressure ventilation

Since the mid twentieth century the application of drugs such as CURARE (*muscle relaxants*) to cause complete paralysis of the voluntary muscles, including those of breathing, and the development of special rubber tubes which could be placed in the patient's windpipe, has led to the use of a different type of ventilation called *intermittent positive pressure ventilation* (IPPV). This is much more invasive than the negative pressure form of ventilator just described. The patient is first anaesthetized, and given a muscle relaxant which stops the breathing. The *endotracheal tube* is then passed down between the vocal cords and into the patient's windpipe (trachea). A machine then delivers gas in rhythmic bursts at positive pressure which forces gas into the lungs. Each time the positive pressure is withdrawn the

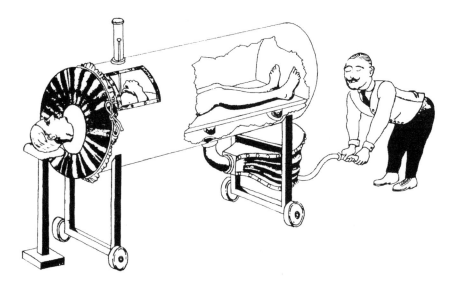

An early tank ventilator.

patient breathes out because of the passive recoil of the lung tissue. This type of artificial ventilation is now the most common type in medical practice. The gas used can be air, or it can be enriched with a higher proportion of oxygen.

Variations on this simple form of artificial ventilation have been introduced which enable the blood to receive higher levels of oxygen, such as applying pressure for a greater part of the breathing cycle (*Positive End Expiratory Pressure* (PEEP)) or which are designed to make it more comfortable for the patient to be gradually taken off the artificial ventilation and to breathe for themselves (types of *supported ventilation*).

Use of artificial ventilation

The most frequent use of IPPV occurs during many types of surgical operations where the anaesthetist administers a drug to paralyze the patient's muscles after inducing anaesthesia. An endotracheal tube is put in place and this is connected to a positive pressure ventilator. The use of the paralyzing drug may be necessary to permit the surgeon to undertake the surgery. An example of this is where the surgeon requires to work inside the abdomen: if paralyzing drugs were not used to relax the abdominal muscles, access to the internal organs would be difficult or impossible. All of the drugs used to produce anaesthesia cause some depression of respiration. Where the surgery is expected to be prolonged, patients may receive artificial ventilation to ensure that they receive adequate delivery of oxygen and removal of carbon dioxide. During the operation, the anaesthetist will monitor the condition of the patient to ensure that the correct volume of air is administered. This is done by analyzing the level of carbon dioxide in the patient's expired air and by measuring the level of oxygen in the blood using a sensor clipped to the finger. At the end of the operation, different drugs are injected by the anaesthetist to reverse the paralysis and the patient then starts to

breathe spontaneously. Once normal breathing has returned, the endotracheal tube is withdrawn, but oxygen monitoring continues until the patient has recovered fully.

IPPV may also be used when patients cannot breathe sufficiently themselves to maintain delivery of oxygen and removal of carbon dioxide from the body. The use of artificial ventilation of this type may be undertaken as a planned procedure — after major heart or brain surgery, for example, when the patient is maintained in a deeply sedated state to permit special treatment to be provided in the period immediately after the surgery. Other examples are in cases of severe brain damage due to head injury or stroke, which interfere with the normal regulation of breathing by the BRAIN STEM, and damage by injury or disease to the parts of the spinal cord involved in breathing movements. When IPPV is required for longer than a week or two, it is usual to establish a *tracheostomy*: a hole made surgically in the front of the trachea, so that a tube for connection with the ventilator can be inserted below the larynx.

Some patients may become unable to breathe sufficiently after severe infection or other disturbance of lung function. In these situations, IPPV must be provided as an emergency. Similar drugs to those used to induce anaesthesia are given and an endotracheal tube is put in place. Patients receiving artificial ventilation are usually looked after in an intensive care unit where specially trained medical and nursing staff monitor the patient continually to ensure that the ventilator functions correctly and that it is set to deliver the correct amount of air with the necessary proportion of oxygen.

While the majority of patients requiring such assistance receive some form of positive pressure ventilation, there is renewed interest in the use of negative pressure ventilation for some who suffer from chronic breathing difficulties, since this form of ventilation does not require paralysis and an

endotracheal tube. This form of respiratory support may only be required overnight and systems have been developed for use in the home.

GAVIN KENNY

See also BRAIN STEM; BREATHING; COMA; CURARE; RESPIRATION; RESUSCITATION.

Asceticism

Asceticism comes from the Greek word '*askesis*', meaning 'exercise' or 'training' — in an athletic sense. It refers to the rigorous and systematic techniques used to alter patterns of life — especially concerning eating, sexual behaviour, and sleep — in order to achieve religious ends. Underlying ascetical practices is the belief that there exists a relationship between such practices and moral development, that is, between the body and the soul or mind. This training or control of the body is seen as the deepest sign of moral transformation. For example, in the early Church it was thought that one could smell sanctity: a virgin would look and smell different, and it was believed that saints' dead bodies, if later exhumed, would be found still intact and would smell sweet. To discipline and train the body is to discipline and train the soul, and thus to purify the soul from its passions in order to love God more perfectly.

Asceticism, in some form or another, is found in most religions, though it is treated with some suspicion in JUDAISM and ISLAM on the grounds that its practices may deny the goodness of God's creation. It has been found amongst certain groups of philosophers, such as the Stoics and Cynics, to indicate practices designed to overcome the vices and develop the virtues.

Asceticism in Christian history

Asceticism developed within early CHRISTIANITY in the context of eschatological beliefs. Early Christians lived in expectation of the second coming of Christ in which all the bodies of those already gathered into Christ's kingdom would share in the glory of His risen body. Living with these eschatological hopes, some began to think that through human control and renunciation of the body — their own ascetical behaviour — they might hasten this second coming of Christ and thus the full redemption of the world. There had been some precedent for this is the community of the Essenes, for example — the community of male Jews living near the Dead Sea in the first century, who had sought to bring Israel back to God by their own disciplined way of life.

Perhaps the first organized Christian ascetics were those who came to be known as Encratites in the second century, some of whom were linked to Gnosticism, or to Ebionite or Docetic groups. They believed that the church should be made up of women and men who were sexually continent and who also abstained from wine and meat. These activities were to be avoided because they linked humans to animals. To engage in a society which relied upon marriage arrangements was to enter into the animal-like cycle of coupling, reproduction, and death. Some of these Encratite communities produced the apocryphal Gospels and

Acts, such as the group in Syria which produced the Acts of Thomas and the Gospel of Thomas. These texts strongly urge abstention from the world: structures of society, such as family, marriage, wealth, and dependents, are all to be rejected. The body is the 'switching-point' where one meets the world and where one must therefore break the connection. All Encratites lived as groups of celibate male and female Christians, not as individual recluses, and they survived and grew by attracting converts.

In the fourth century, with the formation of Christendom after Constantine's conversion, asceticism developed more fully, and celibacy became the ideal for Christians. Historians have often explained this by suggesting that Christians were seeking a form of purity which had been lost with the Christianization of the Empire. Christians ceased to be persecuted and therefore the possibility of the ultimate act of ascetical Christianity — martyrdom — was removed. As Christianity became rich and established, with the building of lavish churches and cathedrals, and the clergy became more powerful and entwined in the state's activities, there seemed to be a new need for a symbolic punishment: the answer, especially for clergy, was to engage in ascetical practices. There is much truth in this explanation — although before the fourth century there were others, as well as the Encratites, who engaged in asceticism.

Asceticism in its 'golden age', within Christianity, took several forms. Some went into the desert, especially the Egyptian desert, to battle their demons — most famously, perhaps, St Antony at the end of the third century. There was a long tradition of people doing this, including Jesus himself: it was seen as a thoroughly biblical activity, a response to a call from scripture. The enormity of the desert represented leaving the 'world' and 'this present age'. Both women and men went into the desert and the sayings of the Desert Mothers and Fathers were collected, as people visited them to seek their wisdom. Their circumstances varied enormously. Some had their libraries with them, while others found a cave or created a cell on the ridge of a mountain where they hoped to survive against the heat, the scarcity of food, and the wild animals. All kept an ascetic regime of vigil and prayer, eating and fasting, and some manual labour. Sexual continence was important but probably not an overriding concern for many, as they struggled to survive both physically and psychically within the vastness of the desert and within the ascetic regime. The greater concern was that the ascetic might lose his or her humanity (what we might call sanity) — break out of the strict regime and approach or even reach mental breakdown. The body was central in all of this activity: these desert ascetics paid great attention to it because they were striving for purity of heart and thereby a future glory for their bodies. Some lived alone while others gathered into groups and in this way, initially in Egypt, monasticism evolved — that is, the organization of monks and nuns into formalized communities. The Egyptian monks, in particular, cultivated a singleness of heart: their practices of self-mortification were designed to reduce the need for food, sleep, and sex, and thereby 'remake' the body, taking it back to its 'natural' or 'pure' state. The fourth-century Life of Antony, traditionally attributed to Athanasius, highlights the ways in which Antony's body did not suffer from being shut up for 20 years, but rather was restored to its natural state.

There were those who wished to lead the ascetic life but could not leave their city. These included women and clergy. Many women, especially élite women, who wished to lead the ascetic life, dedicated their lives as Holy Virgins and created ascetic households: 'the desert in the city'. Girls and women who dedicated themselves to God in this way rejected the calls of society. They tended to be women from the upper orders of society where the primary purpose was to circulate wealth through their marriages and the bearing of male heirs. Ambrose, in his treatise De Virginibus, gave encouragement to those young women who wished to dedicate themselves as Holy Virgins but encountered opposition from their parents. Indeed, Ambrose grew up in such a holy household, for his elder sister, Marcellina, was a consecrated virgin and lived with their widowed mother and companions in their wealthy Italian home. The 'cubiculum', the inner bedroom of consecrated virgins such as Marcellina, was the only 'desert' which Italian Christian men such as Ambrose would have known.

In the Middle Ages, a growing emphasis on the humanity and passion of Christ led to ascetical practices based on an imitation of the physical sufferings of Christ, in particular amongst the mendicant orders. The fifteenth-century Imitation of Christ (most probably written by Thomas à Kempis) instructed the Christian in this sort of ascetic spirituality.

Sixteenth-century Reformation theologies of salvation, which emphasized the depravity of humankind and the worthlessness of any human activities, necessarily undermined the whole rationale for, and practice of, asceticism. Heirs of the Protestant reformation, such as Puritans, well-known for abstaining from the pleasures of the body, cannot be said to have been truly ascetics, for their practices of denial were cast merely in negative terms; asceticism proper is *for* the body and not against it, a view which has continued into the modern period within the Eastern Orthodox tradition.

Asceticism and Buddhism

Buddhist ascetical practices are about releasing a person from desire, suffering, and rebirth as represented by the body, sex, and death. That is, achieving Nirvana, and freeing a person from addictive attachments. But over and against what can often seem a dualistic attitude to mind and body within Buddhism, many Buddhist texts see extreme physical ascetical practices as fruitless. This stems from the Buddha's own experience. In the early stages of his quest for Enlightenment, he embarked on a very extreme form of self-mortification, and he became very thin: his limbs withered, his ribs became gaunt, his scalp shrivelled and his belly clung to his backbone. A sculpture of the Buddha, now in the Lahore Museum, represents him in this state. He found that neither these ascetic practices nor his earlier life of comfort as a prince brought him to any understanding of the questions he had about life, suffering, and death. Thus he developed his 'Middle Way'. His emphasis was on moderation, for he believed both indulgence and denial to be confusing to the mind. In several discourses he was critical of those monks who practised extreme asceticism: those who went naked or wore only rags, those who slept on the ground or on thorns, and those who restricted their food intake very severely. The Buddha allowed 12 optional ascetic practices, all of which emphasized moderation; he resisted attempts to make five of these compulsory for monks.

There is perhaps a tension within Buddhist attitudes about asceticism and the body, as reflected in a set of 13 ascetical practices named the *dhuntangas*. These are: wearing rag robes; using only three robes; begging alms; visiting all houses when begging; eating once a day; eating only from the bowl; not taking second helpings; living in the forest; living at the foot of a tree; living in the open air; living in a cemetery; being satisfied with whatever dwelling one has; sleeping in a sitting position and never lying down. This list is generally not found in canonical texts, and several of the practices have been seen as marginal, and continue to be regarded as marginal today. Indeed contemporary Buddhist monks and nuns, for example in Thailand, have found that physical decorum is important, alongside any of these ascetical practices, in the presentation of their bodies socially. The proper external conduct of the body — such as the wearing of the robe neatly, good deportment, downcast eyes, and observation of good behaviour — is frequently seen as evidence for a state of virtue. This social reality, coupled with an emphasis on moderation in asceticism, contrasts with Buddhist meditations on the body which would seem to present — and sometimes cultivates — a very dualistic notion of mind and body.

Asceticism and other major religions

Sikhs regard asceticism with some caution, for austere practices and penances are seen as irrelevant and unhelpful to spiritual development, though an appropriate self-discipline may involve abstention from alcohol and advocacy of a vegetarian diet. There is an exception in an ascetic order, the Udasis. Islam likewise regards asceticism with suspicion, although fasting during the month of Ramadhan is one of the Five Pillars of Islam, derived from the Koran.

Judaism has generally given little place to asceticism, except in early ascetic groups such as the Essenes, and amongst the Nazirites; Jewish ascetics who vow to abstain from grape products, from cutting hair, and from touching a corpse. A Nazirite is described as 'holy to the Lord' in Leviticus 21: 6. The rabbis expressed varying, sometimes conflicting views about the Nazirites; for example, in one Talmudic passage, one rabbi remarks that the Nazirite is holy because he denies himself wine, and a person who fasts, denying himself all food and drink, is even holier, while another rabbi says the Nazirite is a sinner because he denies himself God's gift of wine, and a person who fasts completely is an even greater sinner.

Rather, in Judaism, the emphasis is always on thanksgiving for daily blessings. For example, fasting in itself is usually seen as displeasing to God and is important only for specific reasons on specific designated occasions, such as Yom Kippur. Nevertheless, a wide variety of views on asceticism are found in the Talmud. In the Jerusalem Talmud it is said, against asceticism, that a person will be obliged to give an account before God for every legitimate pleasure he has denied himself. Medieval Jewish thinkers were often influenced by Greek philosophy, sometimes taking a dualistic attitude to body, with the view that the destruction of the soul occurs in direct proportion to the building up of the body.

JANE SHAW

Further reading
Brown, P. (1988). *The body and society. Men, women and sexual renunciation in early Christianity*. Columbia University Press, New York.

Coakley, S. (ed.) (1997). *Religion and the body*. Cambridge University Press, Cambridge.

See also RELIGION AND THE BODY.

Aspirin or more accurately *acetylsalicylic acid*, is the best known and most commonly used drug after alcohol. Aspirin was originally a trade name, coined by the German company Bayer when the drug was introduced in 1899. The name comes from a combination of *A* for acetyl and *spirin* (from *Spiraea*, the plant family containing salicylates). In 1918 the US Supreme Court ruled that the name 'aspirin' had been so widely advertised that it had become the common name for the drug and the US Patent office cancelled Bayer's rights to the name.

Originally *salicylates* (salts of salicylic acid) were obtained from the bark and leaves of willow and poplar trees; indeed 'salicylate' derives from the title of the willow genus, *Salix*. From early times it was known that salicylates could reduce pain, temperature during fever, and inflammatory swelling (analgesic, antipyretic, and anti-inflammatory actions, respectively).

Instructions for the use of such extracts can be found in Eber's Papyrus (*c.* 1550 BC) and in the writings of Celsus, Pliny the Elder, and Dioscorides in the first century, and of Galen in the second. The four cardinal signs of INFLAMMATION, namely rubor, calor, dolor, and tumor

(redness, heat, pain, and swelling), were described in *De Re Medica* in 30 AD. Celsus described the use of 'boiled vinegar extracts of willow leaves for the relief of pain from prolapse of the uterus and other conditions'. It is possible that this procedure with weak *acetic acid* (vinegar) may have converted naturally occurring salicylate to the acetyl form, that is aspirin itself. The acetyl derivative was thought by Bayer to reduce the nausea and gastrointestinal symptoms associated with salicylic acid itself. In 1980, 97 million kilograms of aspirin were produced in the US alone.

It was to take more than three thousand years after the first descriptions of the therapeutic value of salicylates before their actions were understood. Many of the effects of aspirin are now known to be due to the inhibition of an enzyme in the body, *cyclooxygenase*. This enzyme converts a lipid, *arachidonic acid*, into substances called *endoperoxides*, which are in turn converted to PROSTAGLANDINS I_2, E_1, E_2, D_2, and $F_{2\alpha}$, and to *thromboxanes* A_2 and B_2. Inhibition of formation of prostaglandins and thromboxanes is what prevents many of the symptoms that are relieved by aspirin. The complex biochemical reactions involved in the conversion of arachidonic acid were worked out in Sweden by Bergstrom and Samuelsson, while the effects of prostaglandins and thromboxanes on biological systems were investigated by John Vane and his colleagues in England. All three shared the Nobel Prize for their work in 1982.

Prostaglandins E_1 and E_2 disturb the temperature-regulating centre in the brain, resetting body temperature to a higher level, resulting in fever. By inhibiting the production of prostaglandins, aspirin reduces the temperature in fever; but it has no effect on normal body temperature since no prostaglandins are usually being generated in the temperature-regulating centre. Tissue damage also leads to the production of prostaglandins, which sensitize the endings of the nerve fibres that convey the sensation of pain. Thus aspirin relieves the pain associated with injury or trauma by preventing the formation of prostaglandins. Prostaglandin E_2 and prostaglandin I_2 (*prostacyclin*) are powerful dilators of blood vessels, making injured areas appear reddened. Other agents released in inflammation (e.g. *histamine* and *bradykinin*) increase the permeability of blood vessels. The combination of increased permeability and vasodilation (enlargement of the vessels) allows fluid to escape from the circulation and collect in the damaged tissues, giving rise to swelling — another symptom that is reversed by aspirin.

Considerable interest centres on the recent discovery that low doses of aspirin, taken regularly, reduce the chances of HEART ATTACK and STROKE caused by blood clots. Aggregation of blood platelets is one of the early processes of clot formation and anything that reduces platelet 'stickiness' will help to prevent clots. Platelets synthesize *thromboxane* A_2, which promotes their aggregation, while the cells lining the blood vessel synthesize *prostacyclin*, a powerful anti-

aggregatory agent as well as a vasodilator. Aspirin irreversibly inhibits the cyclooxygenase enzyme in platelets, so the platelets cannot generate thromboxane A_2 until they are replaced (in 7–10 days). What is needed to prevent clot formation is the prevention of thromboxane formation together with the preservation of prostacyclin. This can be achieved with low concentrations of aspirin. Higher concentrations of aspirin inhibit the formation of both agents.

One of the common side effects of aspirin is a feeling of nausea, which may be accompanied by bleeding in the stomach. The stomach lining (*mucosa*) produces prostaglandins, which protect the mucosa itself from attack by gastric acid. Local suppression of prostaglandin formation by aspirin, especially when a tablet lies against the mucosa, can lead to acid attack of the mucosa, even ulceration. The chances of this are greatly reduced by using 'soluble' forms of aspirin which disperse the drug more effectively.

ALAN W. CUTHBERT

See also ANALGESIA; FEVER; PROSTAGLANDINS.

Assisted reproduction Although techniques like *donor insemination* and *induction of ovulation* (stimulation of the ovary to produce eggs) have been used for many years, it was the birth of Louise Brown (the first 'test-tube baby') in 1978 that marked the beginning of new methods of assisted reproduction. The success of *in vitro fertilization* (IVF) showed that eggs and sperm could be manipulated in the laboratory to produce embryos which, when implanted into the uterus, could result in successful pregnancies. The success of IVF opened new horizons in the alleviation of infertility and in the science of embryology. It is now possible to observe the very earliest stages of human development, and with these discoveries came the hope of identifying defects at this very early stage and making it possible to remedy these defects. However, there was unease at the apparent uncontrolled advance of science and the new possibilities for manipulating the early stages of human development. Society was worried.

Because of this concern the UK government set up, in 1982, the *Committee of Inquiry into Human Fertilisation and Embryology* under the chairmanship of Lady Warnock — it is now commonly known as the *Warnock Committee*. This committee considered all aspects of assisted reproduction available at the time and made some 63 recommendations. One of the most important of these was that the government should set up a new statutory licensing authority to regulate both research and those infertility services which the committee recommended should be subject to control. Certain activities were to be made a criminal offence, such as the placing of a human embryo in the uterus of another species. The UK government did not act until 1990 when the Human Fertilisation and Embryology Act was passed. This Act set up the *Human Fertilisation and Embryology Authority*

(HFEA), and the main recommendations of the Warnock Committee were incorporated into the Act, which now regulates the use of assisted reproduction in the UK.

In the period between 1984, when the Warnock Committee reported, and the 1990 Act, the Medical Research Council of Great Britain and the Royal College of Obstetricians and Gynaecologists set up a *Voluntary Licensing Authority* (VLA). This body had no statutory authority but great moral authority and all the centres in the UK using the new techniques were licensed by the Authority after inspection. The VLA set the pattern for the later HFEA, and much of the methodology used by the HFEA derives from the work and experience of the VLA. Unfortunately not all other countries have followed this example. For example, in the USA there is no Federal law relating to embryo research or IVF, and rules tend to be established on a case by case basis. Some other countries have legislated, but what is required is some international agreement to control developments in this area.

IVF was initially instituted to bypass blockage of the Fallopian tubes, but it is now utilized in the treatment of infertility from various causes — male, female, combined or unexplained; also when donor insemination or ovulation induction (see below) have failed.

IVF is carried out in many centres in the UK and elsewhere. The UK centres have all been licensed by the HFEA after inspection by a team from that body. Many centres have evolved specific criteria for inclusion in their programmes. Each couple has to be carefully assessed. Factors like female age and sperm dysfunction affect the success rate considerably. These couples have usually undergone a series of tests before being accepted as suitable for IVF, and this frequently puts a strain on their marriage, so counselling is an important aspect of decision making. IVF treatment should not be used as a panacea for marital or psychosexual disorders but to fulfill the wishes of a well-adjusted couple to have a baby.

In recent years, however, some rather unorthodox requests have been made for IVF. For example a number of lesbian couples have requested IVF using the egg from one of the partners and sperm from a donor. Also, male homosexual couples have requested the use of a donated egg to be fertilized by the sperm from one of them, the resulting embryo to be implanted into the uterus of a woman who would be a surrogate and hand over the baby, when born, to the homosexual male couple. These developments have caused concern to society, as has the use of IVF to enable women past the menopause to have babies. The oldest of such women to date had a successful pregnancy at the age of 63. These new developments require to be reviewed and society must decide what is appropriate and what is not acceptable.

IVF involves the removal of an egg from the ovary and the fertilization of the egg by the partner's sperm in the laboratory. The embryo thus formed is then placed in the woman's uterus, where it will, hopefully, implant resulting in a pregnancy. The incidence of live births resulting from this procedure is on average 20%. Before the egg is removed the ovary is stimulated with drugs (*gonadotropins*). This results in a number of eggs — maybe 10 or more — being available instead of the usual natural single one. All of them are removed and fertilized, and usually 3 are implanted in the uterus at one time. This number is stipulated as a maximum by the HFEA. This gives a higher pregnancy rate than if only one egg is implanted, but if more than 3 eggs are implanted there is obviously a greater risk of triplets or more. Even when only 3 embryos are implanted the multiple births, usually twins, account for 30% of outcomes, so some centres now replace only 2 embryos to try to avoid this situation, as the loss rate with twins is greater than in single pregnancies. The 'spare embryos', as they are called, are frozen and used if the first attempt is not successful. Should a high multiple pregnancy (triplets or above) become evident (and this can be diagnosed early in pregnancy by ultrasound scan) the question of 'fetal reduction' has to be considered. The higher the multiple the greater is the risk of miscarriage or preterm birth of a small baby which may be handicapped. Fetal reduction means the injection, under ultrasound control, of a lethal substance into one or more fetuses to reduce the number from, say, four to two. This gives a much greater chance of survival for the remaining two babies. This method has also caused concern to society but it should be discussed with the couple involved and they should be offered this procedure if they so wish. It follows that with all IVF methods the couple must be well informed of the details of the procedures and the possible outcomes. The message is that, with careful evaluation, persistance in IVF can lead to a successful outcome in a large proportion of cases.

Other techniques which can be used include *GIFT* (gamete intra fallopian transfer) and *ZIFT* (zygote intra fallopian transfer). In GIFT eggs and sperm are transferred to the fallopian tube where fertilization occurs naturally. This seems to be particularly effective in unexplained infertility. In the case of ZIFT the egg is fertilized in the laboratory and then placed in the fallopian tube, where it passes down the tube in the natural way.

A newer technique that is very successful is called *ICSI* (intracellular sperm injection). In this method a single sperm is injected into the egg, which is thus fertilized. The advantage of this method is that the doctor can select and use a single sperm that looks normal and is active. This can be done using sperm from men with very low counts and has therefore greatly improved the results and has given hope to many couples when this is the problem

What are the results for the babies born as a result of these methods? The incidence of preterm delivery is high and there is a 4-fold increase in the number of babies of low birth weight. The reason for this is not clear. The rates of perinatal (around birth) and infant deaths are about twice the national average. This is mainly due to the number of multiple births and the age of the mother — IVF mothers are usually older. There is no greater incidence of congenital abnormalities.

Other forms of assisted reproduction include donor insemination (DI) and ovulation induction. In DI the sperm from a donor is used to inseminate the wife of an infertile man. Provided the husband agrees to his wife being inseminated in this manner he is considered in the UK to be the legal father of the child. However, the birth certificate is false because it says that the husband is the father when he is not. While this is of benefit to the child, ethicists are worried about this falsehood.

Sperm can be frozen and stored and now, to avoid the possible transmission of the AIDS virus, donors have to be tested for the virus at the time of donation and again 180 days later. If the tests are negative on both occasions the sperm which has then been frozen for 180 days can be used. Eggs cannot be frozen at the present time so they have to be fertilized at once, forming embryos which can be frozen and stored. The stored embryos come under the same storage regulations as sperm. The storage of sperm and embryos have sometimes caused difficulties when the partners have separated or one or both has died. Therefore when sperm or embryos are frozen and stored the donors of the gametes now have to record what should happen in such eventualities.

Ovulation induction is a method of assistance for women who are not producing eggs. Drugs (gonadotropins) which stimulate the ovary to produce eggs are used. The dose is carefully monitored by ultrasound scanning of the ovary and the measurement of hormones in the blood.

There are many ethical dilemmas arising out of assisted reproductive methods and the developments therefrom, many of which were not foreseen. Society has to consider which advances are acceptable and which are not. The latest to date is the possibility of 'cloning' human beings by taking cells from a human embryo and forming identical human beings. This has been done with animals and it seems likely that it will be done in the human, probably in a country with no restrictions on such a procedure. Assisted reproduction has enabled many couples to have children who would not otherwise have been able to do so. As long as these methods and the developments from them are kept under control they can be of great benefit to mankind.   MALCOLM MACNAUGHTON

Further reading

Harris, J. and Holm, S. (eds) (1998). *The future of human reproduction*. Clarendon Press, Oxford.

Houghton, D. and Houghton, P. (1994). *Coping with childlessness*. George Allen & Unwin, London.

Bellar, F. K. and Weir, R. F. (eds) (1994). *The beginning of human life*. Kluwer Academic Publishers.

See also INFERTILITY; PREGNANCY.

Astrology took its place in the body of Western knowledge with the spread of astrological lore from Babylon to Greece several centuries before Christ. This transmission began with Berosus, a priest of the temple of Bel, who settled on the island of Cos, the home of Hippocratic medicine, where he established a school of astrology at the end of the fifth century BC. However, the full application of astrology to medicine called *iatromathematica*, was developed subsequently in Hellenistic Egypt.

Both Greek medicine and Greek astrology shared the predominant Aristotelian physics of the day: that everything was composed of the 4 elements of fire, air, water, and earth in varying proportions. The 12 signs of the zodiac were divided into four groups of three, each group or 'triplicity' being associated with one of these elements, whose qualities of heat, cold, dryness, and moisture they symbolized. A particularly Egyptian feature was to give to each zodiac sign signification over certain parts and organs of the body, the first sign, Aries, signifying the head, through to the twelfth sign, Pisces, for the feet. Moreover, the four humours, which Hippocratic medicine held to constitute the human body as the elements composed the physical world as a whole, were assigned planetary significators, along with the organs which contained them: Jupiter ruled the blood, the liver, and the veins; the Moon, phlegm and the brain; Mars, yellow bile and the gall bladder; and Saturn, black bile and the spleen. The Moon in addition represented the humours as a whole, while the Sun denoted the vital spirit of the body, radiating from the heart via the arteries. Venus governed the genitourinary system, while to the seventh planet, Mercury, was given rulership of the mind.

The continuous movement of the planets in their courses, and their mutual interactions, were seen to correlate with the constant changes in the physical world: the cycle of the seasons, its mirroring in the four ages of Man, and the alternations between health and disease in an individual or community. The birth horoscope was used to identify the individual temperament, whether sanguine, choleric, melancholic, phlegmatic, or a combination of these, from which followed advice on the correct diet and lifestyle to maintain health and avoid the diseases to which that particular temperament was liable. The horoscope cast for the time of a person falling ill, called a *decumbiture*, was employed to help identify the nature, origin, and location of the disease, the likely prognosis, the kind of treatment to be given, and the most propitious times for its administration. The critical days in a disease, when an alteration in the condition for better or worse was anticipated, were calculated from the movements of the Moon and Sun for acute and chronic conditions respectively.

Medicine, as systematized by Galen in the second century AD, combined with late Stoic and Hermetic doctrines concerning the influence of the seven planets in the zodiac on terrestrial matters — encapsulated in the notion of a 'cosmic sympathy' and in the phrase '*as above, so below*' — produced a positive science of astrological medicine for medieval men. A more fated attitude took hold among Arab, Jew, and Christian, that everything was 'written in the stars'.

When astrological medicine was transmitted to Western Europe in the later Middle Ages; it required harmonizing with Christian theology. The position came to be accepted that the stars incline but do not compel, keeping intact Man's essential free will. For, although the human body might be subject to alteration and change occasioned by the movements of the planets in the zodiac, Man's immortal soul remained free from such influences so that he could indeed command the stars, insofar as he commanded his passions. This theme, that 'the wise man rules his stars, the fool obeys them', was powerfully developed by Marsilio Ficino, a fifteenth-century Florentine priest and physician steeped in Plato. The notion of a pre-ordained length of life, calculated from the points of life (*apheta* or *hyleg*) and destruction (*anareta*) in the natal horoscope, was overturned by correct physical habit and spiritual development, which nurtured the health of the body and soul, so extending the lifespan. However, the planets were still held accountable for epidemic diseases. The medical establishment in Paris blamed the triple conjunction of Mars, Jupiter, and Saturn for the outbreak of the Black Death in 1348. The spread of syphilis at the end of the fifteenth century was thought to be caused by the conjunction of many planets in Scorpio in 1484, while the very name 'influenza' is testimony of the belief in the celestial origin of that disease.

Nicholas Culpeper, the famous seventeenth-century herbalist and astrologer, was one of the last to practise with integrity the combination of Galenic medicine and astrology, before the celestial art was relegated among the educated to a superstition, along with alchemy, which depended on astrology for its correct operations. Culpeper popularized astrological medicine by issuing inexpensive books in straightforward English on these learned subjects, with the effect of extending people's knowledge beyond the simple rules for seasonal blood-letting, purging, and bathing, and the times for doing so according to the zodiac sign occupied by the Moon, which were common to many popular almanacs of the time.

This astrological medicine, now very much marginalized, was carried on by a small number of enthusiasts. Ebenezer Sibly, an eighteenth-century doctor, believed that Enlightenment learning derived from observation and experiment was improved by a knowledge through astrology of the occult properties of substances. His Solar and Lunar tinctures, for men and women respectively, achieved some efficacy and popularity as medicines, while his edition of

Culpeper's Herbal carried on the iatromathematical tradition. In Victorian England, the astrologer A. J. Pearce, whose career stretched into the 1920s, used to assist his father, a member of the Royal College of Surgeons and a homoeopath, by providing astral diagnoses of his patients. Today, on the fringes of the popular revival of astrology, the iatromathematical tradition continues. GRAEME TOBYN

Further reading
Tester, S. J. (1987). *A history of Western astrology*. Boydell Press.

Athlete Popularly, especially in Britain: participant in track or field athletics. In US and elsewhere, and among sports scientists everywhere: participant in any physically vigorous sport or recreation. A person gifted in and trained for vigorous sport. N.C.S.

See SPORT; SPORTS SCIENCE.

Athletics Original, and still major, British usage: competitive running or walking ('track athletics'), jumping or throwing ('field athletics') — increasingly replaced, especially amongst practitioners, by the phrase 'track and field'. More commonly in US and elsewhere: active sport generally. N.C.S.

Atlas, Charles Charles Atlas was the assumed name of *Angelo Siciliano* (1893–1972), an Italian born in Acri who emigrated to the US with his parents when he was 10 years old. Somewhat small and underdeveloped as a young man, a 97-lb weakling' according to later publicity, he decided to take up body-building and in 1922 won a national contest as 'America's most perfectly developed man'.

Capitalizing on his fame as a strong-man, Atlas produced and marketed, with his business partner Charles Roman, an advertising man, a correspondence course for body-building. He publicized the course in a variety of popular press outlets: comic books were particularly well used. He made frequent reference to his own history, describing the now famous story of having sand kicked in his face on a beach at Coney Island by a life-guard, who then stole his girlfriend. This experience determined him to build up his strength and physique. To do so, he perfected his own methods of 'dynamic tension' — 'secret' exercises that would naturally enhance muscle development and tone. The method used no apparatus or equipment. In addition to these series of isotonic exercises he offered nutritional advice. In his advertising techniques and claims he was following a long tradition of quacks and charlatans, from fairground to the tabloid press, claiming secret knowledge that could lead to an enhanced life, knowledge that could be bought for ready money. There was also a homo-erotic edge to some of his publicity, all those who enrolled in his course being offered 'beautiful photographs of myself in statuary poses'. E. M. TANSEY

See also BODY BUILDING; EXERCISE; ISOMETRICS; ISOTONICS.

Atrophy The word comes from the Greek, meaning 'ill-fed'. In biomedical terms it means *wasting* — loss of mass from a tissue or organ from whatever cause. It is used as a verb: muscles, for example, can *atrophy* with simple disuse; or as a noun (they undergo *disuse atrophy*); or, they become *atrophied* if their nerves are damaged, so that they can no longer be stimulated into action. Another type — closer to 'ill-feeding' — is *ischaemic atrophy* from deprivation of blood supply, such as may happen in parts of the brain after stroke or severe head injury, or in heart muscle in coronary artery disease. Atrophy also happens in the normal course of events to cells or tissues which have fulfilled their useful life (such as umbilical blood vessels after birth or ovaries after the menopause) or as cells die off progressively with age (as in kidneys and brain). SHEILA JENNETT

See also DEMENTIA; MUSCLE WASTING.

Atropine is an alkaloid derived from the solanaceous plants *Atropa belladonna* (deadly nightshade), *Hyoscyamus niger* (black henbane), and *Datura stramonium* (thornapple). These plants contain a mixture of two closely related alkaloids, *hyoscyamine* and *hyoscine*; atropine is a mixture of two isomers of hyoscyamine. In 1867, von Bezold found that atropine blocked the slowing of the heart caused by vagal stimulation. We now know that atropine blocks the action of the neurotransmitter ACETYLCHOLINE at all the nerve endings where the MEMBRANE RECEPTORS are of the so-called *muscarinic* type. This includes those of the parasympathetic nervous system in the heart, glandular tissue, and smooth muscle. Thus atropine causes a rise in heart rate and inhibits secretions (for example of saliva, causing a dry mouth, and of the digestive enzymes). It also relaxes smooth muscle in the gastrointestinal tract, the urinary bladder, and the bronchial trees, by preventing the effects of the normal background discharge of parasympathetic neurons to these organs.

The central nervous system also contains *muscarinic receptors*. Blockade of these by atropine leads to restlessness and mental excitement, and can improve the rigidity and tremor characteristic of Parkinson's disease. Large doses of atropine can cause hallucination.

Long-lasting pupillary dilation results if atropine drops are placed in the eye. The iris has both circular and radial muscles, and the balance between the tonic activities of these two muscle groups controls the pupil diameter. The circular muscle is under parasympathetic control, so when the transmitter, acetylcholine, is blocked with atropine, the pupil will dilate. It is told that Spanish ladies put atropine drops in their eyes for the allure given by large, black pupils: hence the name *belladonna* — 'fine lady'. ALAN W. CUTHBERT

See also AUTONOMIC NERVOUS SYSTEM; NEUROTRANSMITTER; MEMBRANE RECEPTORS.

Aura From the Greek meaning 'breath', the word aura is mostly used in the metaphorical sense of someone having simply 'an aura' about him or, more vividly, one of 'wisdom', 'saintliness', or 'evil'. However, for those suffering MIGRAINE or EPILEPSY, an aura is no longer simply a metaphor relating to their perception of a person in the external world but now a disagreeable perceptual experience heralding an impending attack of their sick headache or CONVULSION (*grand mal*). In the case of migraine the aura is most commonly visual. The images do not relate to previous visual experience but can take the form of scintillating, wavy patterns of bright, silvery light that superimpose on the current visual image — but in contrast to the latter they persist when the eyes are closed.

In epilepsy the simplest form of aura may be an ill-defined feeling of uncertainty or nausea preceding a convulsion. This may be an expression of changes in the cardiovascular and digestive systems induced by the AUTONOMIC NERVOUS SYSTEM as an early aspect of the epileptiform activity within the brain. Undoubtedly the most remarkable 'aura' occurs in the particular type known as 'temporal lobe epilepsy'. At its simplest the aura may take the form of a familiar odour, or more commonly a disagreeable or even disgusting one. At its most complex the aura can be a perceptually complete image of a person with no counterpart in the external world. Such an image is to be distinguished from one summoned voluntarily

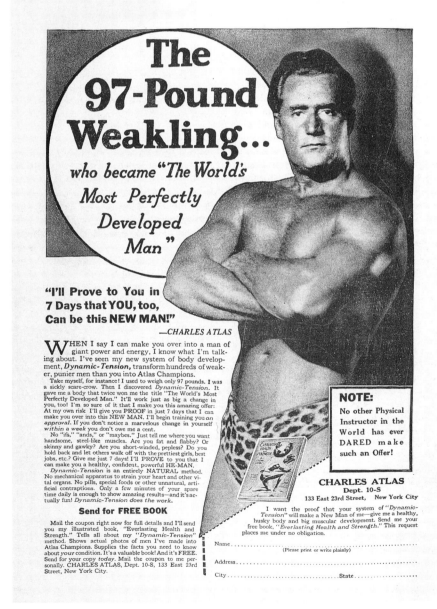

Charles Atlas' body-building programme — advertisement in *Amazing Stories*. Mary Evans Picture Library.

in the mind's eye, or from an illusion due to the brain's interpretation of conflicting visual stimuli from the external world. Instead, that of the aura is a remarkable product of the uncontrollable discharge of neurones associated with an epileptiform focus in the temporal lobe(s) of the brain, demonstrable in the recording of the electrical activity of the brain, and, when the severity of the condition demands, abolished by surgical removal of the offending lobe.   TOM SEARS

See also EPILEPSY; MIGRAINE.

Auscultation is the act of listening to sounds

generated within the body, generally for the purpose of diagnosis of disease. It may be done directly with the unaided ear (*immediate auscultation*) or with a stethoscope (*mediate auscultation*).

Immediate auscultation was practised in ancient times. In both the Hindu and the Greek medical traditions, physicians listened carefully to the sounds which could be heard emanating from within the thorax. The Sanskrit medical texts mention the use of the sense of hearing to determine whether the contents of an abnormal cavity were gaseous. The Hippocratic writings describe the technique of succussion — shaking the patient to ascertain whether splashing noises could be elicited within the chest. Aretaeus the Cappadocian, in the second century AD, described how, in *ascites*, fluid could be heard fluctuating in the abdomen as the patient shifted position, whereas *tympanites* (gas in the abdomen) could be distinguished by the drumlike sound produced if the abdomen was struck with the hand.

In the eighteenth century, the great Italian physician/anatomist, Giovanni Morgagni, valued auscultation, pointing out that attending to the noises made by fluid fluctuating in the abdomen or thorax was useful in the identification of dropsy. The precise location and character of the noises could enable differentiation between the various forms of dropsy. For instance, the otherwise difficult diagnosis of 'dropsy of the pericardium' could be made confidently when the physician could 'distinctly hear the agitation of the water itself in the pericardium'. In 1761, Leonard Auenbrugger, a Viennese physician, published a pioneering account of the related technique of thoracic percussion. The character of the sound elicited when the chest wall was tapped with a finger was indicative of the pathological condition of the underlying tissues.

At the end of the eighteenth century and the beginning of the nineteenth, in a series of developments principally associated with the Paris School, a new approach to internal disease was developed. The holistic, humoral pathology of earlier centuries was gradually replaced by a conception which localized disease in the solid structures of the body. The '*anatomico-clinical*' *perspective* was based, as its name suggests, upon the twin pillars of pathological anatomy, which revealed the structural features of disease after death, and clinical observation, which sought to comprehend the structural features of disease in

the living patient. Within this conceptual framework, techniques of physical examination were revived and their diagnostic potentialities systematically explored. A notable pioneer of the clinical use of the ear was the French physician, Jean-Nicolas Corvisart, whose *Essay on the Diseases of the Heart* contained much that was new in the understanding of cardiac and aortal disorders.

Corvisart's preferred diagnostic technique was percussion, but both he and his Parisian colleague, Gaspard Bayle, experimented with applying the ear directly to the patient's chest. In 1816, Rene Laennec, who had been a student of Corvisart and who knew of Bayle's work, invented the stethoscope, which made examination of the chest much more convenient for both physician and patient. In 1819, Laennec published his great treatise *On Mediate Auscultation*. It has been fairly said that virtually everything that Laennec wrote on auscultation was new at the time, but is now familiar to every medical student. Laennec painstakingly described the normal sounds of the lungs and then identified a large number of abnormal sounds — bronchophony, pectoriloquy, egophony, the metallic tinkling, the cracked pot sound, a variety of 'râles', and so on. The most substantial section of the work is on tuberculosis, which provided him with ideal clinical material upon which to display the utility of auscultation of the lungs. Laennec also investigated the sounds of the heart in health and disease, describing, for the first time, the file, rasp, and bellows sounds, and a variety of murmurs. He showed, among much else, that valvular disease of the heart could be diagnosed by ear in the living patient. Applications for the new instrument were also found in the diagnosis of fractures, of bladder stones, and of liver abscesses. Laennec's investigations with the stethoscope, correlated always with post-mortem findings, laid the foundations of the modern procedures of physical diagnosis.

Laennec's innovation was adopted widely and quickly. The remainder of the nineteenth century saw considerable refinement of stethoscopic technique and design, and improved understanding of the pathological basis of abnormal sounds. Further applications were found for the instrument in the monitoring of pregnancy, of bowel function, and in the measurement of blood pressure. In the twentieth century, however, the ear has been displaced, to some extent, by the eye in physical examination. The invention of radiographic imaging demoted the stethoscope from its place of supreme authority in lung disorders; the ultrasonic scanner threatens the same in disorders of the heart. Blood flow can also now be visualized using Doppler ultrasound. Other imaging modalities provide clear, detailed pictures of all the body's cavities. Yet a trained sense of hearing remains an indispensable aid to the examining physician, and all medical students still have to strive to educate their ears along the lines first set out by Rene Laennec.

MALCOLM NICOLSON

See also DIAGNOSIS; HEART SOUNDS; LUNGS.

Autoimmune disease Every second of our

lifetime, we are exposed to a large variety of MICROORGANISMS in the environment, which are capable of causing fatal diseases. However, normal individuals rarely succumb to such infections and, even if they do, it is usually for a short duration and with limited damage. This is because of an efficient IMMUNE SYSTEM that destroys these organisms and other foreign substances.

An immune response is brought about by two components of the immune system, namely the innate immunity and the acquired or specific immunity, acting in conjunction with each other and with other molecules. Acquired immunity involves the production of *antibodies*, each specifically designed to combat a particular *antigen* — a component of the invading substance or organism. For its normal function of defence, five features of the acquired immune system are essential. These are: (i) specificity for distinct antigens; (ii) diversity; (iii) memory; (iv) self-limitation; and (v) discrimination of self from non-self.

It is the last two features which raise the possibility of Dr Jekyll turning into Mr Hyde. Loss of self-limitation or the failure to maintain self-tolerance can actually turn the immune system from playing a defensive role to causing debilitating diseases. A pathological condition arising from uncontrolled or aberrant immune responses is defined as a *hypersensitivity reaction*, or ALLERGY. Diseases that are caused due to the immune system acting against self-antigens are called 'autoimmune diseases', a situation which has been melodramatically described as '*horror autotoxicus*' by the famous biologist Paul Erlich.

A wide range of diseases have now been classified as having autoimmune causes. At one end of the spectrum of such diseases are conditions like *Hashimoto's thyroiditis*, where the antibodies are directed against one specific organ (in this case the thyroid gland). At the other end of the spectrum are diseases such as *systemic lupus erythematosus* (SLE), where the antibodies are directed against the nucleus of the cells, thereby affecting the whole body; in most instances, specific antibodies can be detected circulating in the blood. In another disease condition, known as *Goodpasture's syndrome*, the autoantibodies bind to components of the membrane that separates air from blood in the alveoli of the lungs and of the glomerular capillaries of kidneys, where filtration occurs. This causes a localized immune reaction and leads to lung haemorrhages and glomerulonephritis. Similarly, in autoimmune *haemolytic anaemia* antibodies are directed against red blood cells, enhancing breakdown and phagocytosis of the cells.

In certain cases, however, the autoantibodies do not cause cell damage, but instead alter the normal physiological functions by mimicking normal signalling molecules. For example, in *Grave's disease* (thyrotoxicosis) autoantibodies bind to the receptors for the thyroid stimulating hormone (TSH) from the pituitary gland and mimic its functions, leading to excessive thyroid hormone production. In another disease, known as *myasthenia gravis*, autoantibodies bind to the receptors on muscle cells for the neurotransmitter, acetylcholine, and thereby inhibit nerve-to-muscle conduction; over a period of time these receptors are endocytosed (taken up inside the cells) and degraded, causing progressive muscle paralysis.

Sometimes, autoimmune diseases may arise because antibodies, which are produced against foreign antigens, cross-react with the body's own proteins ('*self-proteins*'). Thus in acute rheumatic fever, which can develop following a throat infection, antibodies against a cell wall protein of streptococcus bacteria may cross-react with an antigen in the person's own cardiac muscle cells. This leads to myocarditis and damage to the valves of the heart. It is also associated with inflammation of the joints and destruction of the joint cartilage brought about by immune responses.

The immune response involves not only the production of antibodies which circulate in the blood, but also the multiple activities of 'T-cells', the lymphocytes which have been 'programmed' in the thymus gland to recognize specific antigens, and which mediate the 'cellular' component of the immune response. In certain autoimmune diseases, it is the T-cells which become auto-reactive. This occurs in some patients with insulin-dependent DIABETES mellitus. In these patients, activated lymphocytes and macrophages destroy the insulin-producing cells in the pancreas, which leads to the disorders of metabolism characteristic of this condition. Some types of anaemia are thought to be due to antibodies being generated against factors required for absorption from the gut of vitamin B$_{12}$, which is essential for maturation of red blood cells.

Besides the examples described, numerous other pathological conditions have also been classified as autoimmune diseases. Extensive research has been conducted to elucidate the mechanisms by which the immune system discriminates between self and non-self, and the transformation from protector to aggressor in certain pathological conditions of autoimmunity.

One of the cardinal features of immunity is the ability to maintain self-tolerance against self-antigens. Its is an actively acquired process, where self-reactive antibodies are prevented from becoming functionally capable of reacting with self-antigens. A negative selection process plays a major role, whereby immature T-cells, specific for self-antigens, are deleted in the thymus. In certain conditions, the clones may survive but are unable to respond to self-antigens. This is known as clonal ignorance. All these mechanisms lead to the capability of the immune system to discriminate between self and non-self.

Despite these several mechanisms for inducing self-tolerance, autoimmunity remains a significant cause of disease in humans. Multiple factors are implicated in the breakdown of self-tolerance. These factors range from genetic predisposition to microbial infections. Autoimmunity can also arise from abnormalities in lymphocytes following failure of the selection process in the thymus. It is proposed that an individual's 'major histocompatibility' genes, which determine their 'HLA type' (classification based on *human lymphocyte antigens*, used in determining tissue compatibility for organ transplants), influence thymic selection, implying a genetic role in autoimmunity. Studies of a particular strain of mice, which develops an accelerated, severe form of systemic autoimmunity, revealed a genetic predisposition. Indeed, autoimmune diseases are often said to 'run in the family'. HLA typing has shown that some individuals have 90 to 100 times the average predisposition to developing the autoimmune condition called *ankylosing spondylosis*. This may possibly be due to the controlling of T-cell selection and activation by the gene products which determine the HLA type.

Some autoimmune diseases are caused when antibodies or T-cells, stimulated to act against a foreign antigen, recognize a similar molecular component on a self-protein. This '*molecular mimicry*' is often a cause for autoimmunity, as described earlier in the case of rheumatic fever.

A plethora of causal factors are thus implicated in leading to autoimmunity. Recent advances have also been made in elucidating the mechanisms involved in self-tolerance and generation of autoimmunity; these hold promise for development of effective strategies for management of these debilitating conditions.

SHILADITYA SENGUPTA

TAI-PING FAN

See also IMMUNE SYSTEM.

Automata Mythical, manlike monsters permeate the folklore of all cultures, and the dream of building an artificial man has long captured the Western imagination — witness Mary Shelley's *Frankenstein* (1818). Such concerns form part of a wider fascination with mechanical toys and gadgets at large. Automata in general inspire interest by their visual appeal, being intended to induce wonder and astonishment through the magic of their movement; androids in particular are figures in human form designed to walk, talk, play music, write, or draw or perform other distinctive actions.

Few automata constructed before the sixteenth century have survived, but their existence is recorded. Among the earliest was a wooden version of a pigeon, built by Archytas of Tarentum (*fl.* 400–350 BC), a friend of Plato. The bird apparently hung from a pivoted bar, and the complete mechanism rotated by means of a jet of air or steam. Fuller information about similar contraptions is found in the works of Hero of Alexandria (*fl.* first century AD), who recounted devices moved by falling weights, steam, and water.

Reports of Chinese automata date from the Han dynasty (third century BC), when a mechanical orchestra was apparently constructed for the Emperor. By the Sui dynasty (sixth and seventh centuries AD) automata had become familiar. From the T'ang period (seventh to the tenth century AD), there are accounts of flying birds and characters that executed sundry activities, ranging from girls singing to a monk begging. In the Moslem world various inventors were active from the ninth century; best-documented are the water-operated automata — for instance, models of moving peacocks — devised by al-Jazari (thirteenth century).

In Christendom, Roger Bacon and Albertus Magnus have been credited with constructing androids — in Bacon's case, a talking head, and in Albertus', and iron man. In the Renaissance fresh concern was devoted to the making of automata. Sophisticated fountains involving sensational and secret effects became fashionable among the nobility, e.g. the mid-sixteenth-century waterworks and fountains erected in the gardens of the Villa d'Este at Tivoli, near Rome.

The use of coiled, tempered-steel springs made a portable source of motion available from the mid fifteenth century and led to more versatile contraptions. But it was in the late eighteenth and early nineteenth centuries that the most intricate automata made their appearance. Typical are the devices made by the Rochat brothers, who specialized in singing birds. Their mechanical songbirds were designed to materialize suddenly from wide, hinged panels in snuffbox tops, or to operate in cages suspended so that a clock was visible beneath the base. In their magical boxes, a disc engraved with a question would be inserted in a slot in the box, upon which the lilliputian figure of a magician would come to life and point with his wand to a spot where the answer appeared.

Among the more intricate mechanical gadgets popularized in the eighteenth century were *tableaux mécaniques*, or mechanical images — framed, painted landscapes, in which mannikins, windmills, and the like came to life thanks to concealed clockwork. Closely related to the *tableaux mécaniques* were mechanical theatres; the most lavish was put up in the gardens of Hellbrun, near Salzburg, Austria, and involved 113 hydraulically worked figures.

The most acclaimed manufacturer of automata was Jacques de Vaucanson (1709–82), a fertile designer of robotic devices that have proved important for modern industry. In 1738 he constructed an automaton, 'The Flute Player', followed by 'The Tambourine Player' and 'The Duck'; this last imitated not only a live duck's external motions, but also the actions of drinking, eating, and digestion. Nominated Inspector of Silk Manufacture in 1741, Vaucanson managed to automate looms by means of perforated cards that activated hooks coupled to the warp yarns. After Vaucanson's death, his loom was rebuilt and improved by J.-M. Jacquard.

With the exception of a few works by Peter Carl Fabergé (d. 1920), the production of costly artistic automata had virtually ceased by the late nineteenth century. But recent times have brought a rapid development of industrial robots that are increasingly replacing the human workforce in car-assembly plants and similar factories. Such robots are especially beneficial in occupations that would otherwise be dangerous to human health or safety.

The term *robot* stems from the Czech word *rabit* (work). It came into popular use after 1923 to delineate either mechanical contrivances so ingenious as to be almost human, or workers whom repetitive work was reducing to machines. Its prevalent usage is based on the play *R. U. R.* (Rossum's Universal Robots), written by the Czech playwright, Karel Capek, in which the economy is portrayed as depending on mechanical workers called robots, which can perform any kind of mental or physical work and which, when worn out, are trashed and replaced by new ones. In Capek's play the robots evolve intelligence and a temper of revolt, turn upon their bosses, and kill their creators, in a manner perhaps echoing *Frankenstein* on a political plane.

Fantastic machinery has continued to fire the imagination, notably in science fiction. William Heath Robinson (1872–1944), a British cartoonist, book illustrator, and designer of theatrical scenery, won fame for his cartoons featuring fantastic machinery with human overtones. His drawings, collected in *Absurdities* (1934), are particularly notable for the fun he made of machinery. Ludicrously impractical or elaborate machines came to be called 'Heath Robinson contraptions'. ROY PORTER

Further reading

Jennings, H. (1985). *Pandaemonium: the coming of the machine as seen by contemporary observers 1660–1886*, (ed. M.-L. Jennings and C. Madge). The Free Press, New York; André Deutsch, London.

Autonomic nervous system
You wake in the night. A noise? A light? An intruder? Instantly alert, heart pounding, 'butterflies' in your stomach, you are ready to attack, or to run — the classical 'fight or flight' reaction. Or think of a nastier scenario. You are walking in the woods and stumble across a bloody, disfigured human body … you turn away, vomit, and are aware of an ominous urgency of the bowels. You slump in a faint.

How do these extraordinary bodily reactions happen? You certainly have not willed your body to behave in this way. Nor, in more usual circumstances, does one will the heart to vary its rate of beating, or the gut to perform its functions, or the many other continuous internal communications and adjustments that keep the body ticking over. All of these reflect activity of the autonomic nervous system (ANS). The system has two components, *sympathetic* and *parasympathetic*, corresponding to two sets of nerve fibres streaming out from the SPINAL CORD and BRAINSTEM, running towards all the organs they affect.

The autonomy that its name implies is a primary characteristic of the ANS: it is responsible for the body's involuntary reactions to emergencies and for most of our life-support functions except breathing. It also serves as an essential adjunct to conscious voluntary or emotional reactions. For instance, it switches on the digestive system at the time of a meal, and orchestrates the whole subsequent sequence of absorption, storage, or utilization of nutrients according to the body's changing requirements. It also makes sure that waste material is held until the voluntary go-ahead is given to defecate: if control is undeveloped (in babies) or lost (in the incontinent), there is automatic defecation. The ANS regulates the HEART by speeding or slowing the beat and altering the force of its pumping. It regulates the calibre of BLOOD VESSELS to vary the distribution of blood to the organs, whilst also maintaining the correct BLOOD PRESSURE. It adjusts the resistance to airflow in and out of the LUNGS by changing the diameter of the branches of the bronchial tree. It regulates body temperature by varying the blood flow to the skin

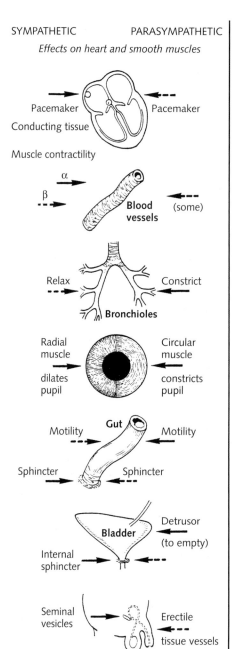

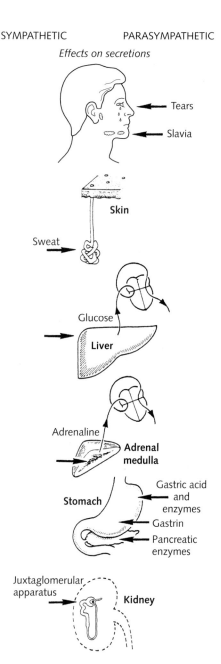

Solid arrows represent stimulation; broken arrows represent inhibition (relaxation)

Arrows to heart indicate release of substance into circulating blood

Actions of autonomic nerves: solid arrows represent stimulation; broken arrows represent inhibition. Left: actions on the heart and on smooth muscle. Right: actions on secretory cells (arrows to heart indicate release of substance into the circulation). After Jennett, S. (1989) *Human Physiology*. Churchill Livingstone, Edinburgh.

and by the control of SWEATING. It varies the size of the pupil and the thickness of the lens of the EYES to adjust for brightness and for distance. It serves reproductive behaviour by controlling ERECTION of the penis and EJACULATION in the male, and engorgement of the nipples and clitoris in the female.

All of these apparently diverse actions and more derive from a fine balance between stimulation and inhibition of the smooth (involuntary) **muscle** (which forms the walls of the several types of tubes in the body), the heart muscle and its PACEMAKER, and the secretion of substances from glandular cells.

The ANS and its relation to the central nervous system

Anatomically, the BRAIN and SPINAL CORD constitute the CENTRAL NERVOUS SYSTEM (CNS) and the nerve pathways outside of the skull and vertebral column are the *peripheral nervous system*. But, on functional grounds, the nervous system is also divided into the *somatic* and *autonomic* systems. Each of these has pathways both within the central nervous system and outside it. The somatic system has (sensory) input from muscles, joints, and body surface, and (motor) output connections to ordinary (skeletal or 'voluntary') muscles. It is responsible for many types of conscious bodily sensation and for the voluntary control of movement — all providing for interaction with the outside world. In contrast, the ANS by traditional definition, has only one-way, outgoing connections. (Its activity is however influenced by a great deal of sensory information, especially that coming in along so-called visceral afferent nerves from the internal organs, signalling such things as the fullness of the stomach or the pressure in the arteries.)

The peripheral nerve fibres (*axons*) of the ANS have their cell bodies in the brain stem and the spinal cord. These nerve cells are influenced by fibres descending within the central nervous system from higher levels, notably from the HYPOTHALAMUS, which contains many of the control centres for HOMEOSTASIS, the process of keeping the internal environment of the body constant.

The axons of the ANS that leave the spinal cord and brain are called 'preganglionic' fibres because they end in ganglia — swellings containing 'postganglionic' nerve cells, with which the preganglionic fibres form synaptic connections. The fibres of these postganglionic cells run out to the final destinations — in the gut, the heart, the blood vessels, and so on — where they make contact with the *effector cells* (smooth muscle, secretory cells, etc.)

The substance ACETYLCHOLINE, first isolated and identified in the late nineteenth century, when injected has many actions on the body similar to those occurring during ANS activity. This is because acetylcholine is the natural chemical NEUROTRANSMITTER released by the endings of preganglionic fibres as a result of nerve impulses (ACTION POTENTIALS) arriving along those axons.

Sympathetic and parasympathetic subdivisions.

The two components of the ANS differ in a number of ways:

(i) *The origin of the preganglionic nerves*: sympathetic from much of the length of the spinal cord, parasympathetic from the brain stem and the lowest part of the spinal cord.

(ii) *The position of the ganglia*: sympathetic ganglia lie close to the spinal cord; parasympathetic ganglia are buried in the final target organ. Hence sympathetic postganglionic fibres tend to be much longer than parasympathetic.

(iii) *The chemical transmitter produced at the terminals of the postganglionic fibres in the effector organ*: mostly acetylcholine for parasympathetic and NORADRENALINE (norepinephrine) for sympathetic.

Sympathetic division Sympathetic preganglionic nerve cell bodies are found in the lateral part of the grey matter of the spinal cord, throughout many segments, from the upper thoracic down to the upper lumbar level. Their axons leave (like all axons that transmit impulses out of the spinal cord) in the anterior (*ventral*) nerve roots that emerge from between the vertebrae. These preganglionic fibres run a short distance from the vertebral column and terminate in a chain of interconnected sympathetic ganglia, behind the *pleura* or the *peritoneum* (the membranes that respectively line the thoracic and abdominal walls). The postganglionic nerve fibres from the cells in these ganglia run out to every part of the body, except the CNS itself (although they do innervate the membranes that surround the brain and spinal cord). Sympathetic nerves run along with all arteries and veins down to their smallest branches, supplying all types of blood vessel except capillaries; from the thoracic ganglia, they supply the eyes and the heart and lungs; in the abdomen, they are distributed in the rays of the SOLAR PLEXUS, to be distributed to the viscera. In the pelvis, they reach the bladder and rectum, and the sphincters that control voiding.

There is one important exception to this plan. Some preganglionic fibres go directly to the medulla of the ADRENAL GLAND, whose cells originate from the same embryonic tissue as those of the sympathetic ganglia. Preganglionic fibres act on adrenal cells (through the production of acetylcholine) just as if those cells were ganglionic nerve cells. But the adrenal cells release hormones (ADRENALINE and noradrenaline, with a little DOPAMINE) into the blood — a process known as *neuroendocrine secretion* — instead of transmitting impulses via a postganglionic nerve fibre.

The best known action of the sympathetic system (and of the adrenaline produced by the adrenal gland) is the dramatic 'fight or flight' reaction. The heart beats faster and more strongly. Blood vessels are constricted and flow reduced in regions, such as the gut, where blood supply is not vital, but not where ample blood supply is needed to deal with the emergency — brain, heart, and muscle. Gut movements are inhibited. Urination and defecation are postponed by relaxation of the appropriate gut muscles; the pupils are dilated and the bronchial tubes are relaxed and widened. However, the 'fight or flight' reaction is only an exaggeration of routine sympathetic nervous activity that is going on all the time, modulating heart rate, setting the diameter of blood vessels to redistribute the blood, and so forth. Adrenaline itself has many effects on the circulation and the METABOLISM, which support any sudden demand for extra energy expenditure.

Parasympathetic division The parasympathetic outflow comes in two parts, from opposite ends of the CNS. The cranial component originates in the brain stem and leaves through the base of the skull in the *vagus* (wandering) nerves. The sacral component has its cell bodies in the lowest part of the spinal cord, with their fibres emerging through perforations in the sacrum — the terminal extension of the SPINAL COLUMN.

The cranial and the sacral components of the parasympathetic system between them distribute themselves around the whole of the head and the trunk. An additional cranial component, which does not leave the skull, supplies the eyes. In the thorax, the influence of the parasympathetic fibres of the vagus nerves on the heart is to slow it down; in the abdomen, their function is to activate the gut and its associated organs. The wandering vagus meets the territory of the parasympathetic outflow from the sacral spinal cord at a point in the colon. In the pelvis, the sacral component innervates the bladder and rectum, where it mediates voiding. In most of the body parasympathetic nerves have no action on blood vessels, but the brain and the penis are major exceptions: parasympathetic stimulation causes their blood vessels to relax, by release of NITRIC OXIDE as neurotransmitter.

In overwhelming circumstances, various actions of parasympathetic nerves slow the heart and lower the blood pressure, depriving the brain of its blood supply — causing FAINTING and thus withdrawing the conscious person from the shocking or frightening experience; stimulation of the gut causes involuntary defecation — 'scared shitless'. In the most extreme conditions the inhibition of the heart can be so severe that it causes death: this is the probable origin of so-called *Voodoo death* and other forms of death without obvious cause.

Although the sympathetic and parasympathetic systems often seem to have opposite actions, for instance in their influences on the heart, they normally work in a complementary fashion, counterbalancing each other and being regulated together to produce fine control of the body's life-support functions.

Historical background: the discovery of chemical transmission

The concept of the ANS is not new. GALEN, in the second century AD, described the sympathetic chain, the *rami communicans* (the bundles of preganglionic fibres coming from the spinal cord), and the path of the vagus nerves. In the seventeenth century the British physician Thomas Willis produced clear descriptions of the component parts of the system; he gave the name 'solar plexus' to the radiating nerve fibres in the abdomen because they reminded him of the sun. Willis and his contemporaries described the '*intercostal*' (sympathetic) and '*wandering*' (vagus) nerves, and he demonstrated that cutting the vagus nerves caused 'trembling' of the heart. By the middle of the eighteenth century similar experiments had revealed that branches of the 'intercostal' system affected the functions of the eye, and that the 'wandering nerve' was associated with the control of involuntary movements of the viscera.

The word 'autonomic' was introduced by the Cambridge physiologist J. N. Langley in the late nineteenth century. It was the work of Langley and his colleague W. H. Gaskell that established our modern understanding of the autonomic nervous system and its integration with the CNS. Langley's observations of the effects of cutting nerves and of applying specific drugs at different points in the ANS led to the realization that there must be specialized sites of action on the cells of end-organs and ganglia, where the autonomic nerves exert their effects. From his experiments, and from the work of Paul Ehrlich in Germany, emerged one of the most powerful concepts in twentieth-century biomedical sciences, the *receptor* theory. Any substance in the vicinity of a cell, however it got there, usually has an action on that cell only if specific receptor molecules, into which that substance 'fits', are present in the cell's membrane. Thus neurotransmitters and hormones are matched to their appropriate targets, and many drugs work by mimicking these natural substances or antagonizing them by blocking the receptors.

This theory has been applied to account for cell–cell and drug–cell interactions in all manner of living tissues. It can explain not only transmission at the ganglia and at the end organs of the ANS, but almost all nerve-to-nerve and nerve-to-tissue communication in the entire nervous system, and all other cell-to-cell signalling mediated by substances released in the immediate neighbourhood, or by hormones circulating in the blood.

Gaskell's studies were predominantly anatomical, and his detailed histological descriptions of the structure and connections of the nerve fibres and ganglia contributed greatly to the unravelling of the component parts of the system, especially his identification of the two major nervous outflows, the *thoracolumbar* (sympathetic) and *craniosacral* (parasympathetic) and the distinction between them. This was a major impetus to the further study of autonomic function, providing the morphological basis for all subsequent studies. A student of Gaskell and Langley in Cambridge in the 1890s was Henry Dale, who was strongly influenced by their work, and spent

much of his own career investigating autonomic mechanisms. One of his early experiments showed that an injection of adrenaline into an anaesthetized animal produced very similar effect (such as increased arterial blood pressure) to those noticed when sympathetic nerves were stimulated. The significance of the observation was not clear at the time, but it intrigued Dale, who gradually elucidated the relationship between the autonomic nervous system and chemical stimulation by discovering that nerves communicate by the release of specific NEUROTRANSMITTER chemicals. It was Dale (later Sir Henry) who showed that acetylcholine can stimulate not only autonomic ganglia, but also the synapses of postganglionic parasympathetic fibres (on smooth muscle, heart muscle, and glands), and even ordinary, skeletal muscle. This implies that all these classes of nerve fibres produce acetylcholine as the transmitter substance at their terminals. On the other hand, the receptors on which the acetylcholine acts vary from one system to another. The acetylcholine receptors in the membranes of cells in the autonomic ganglia and of skeletal muscle are called *nicotinic* because they can be stimulated by the drug *nicotine*. But those in the membranes of the target cells of postganglionic parasympathetic axons are called *muscarinic* since they can be activated by *muscarine* but not by nicotine. The many effects of the drug *atropine*, or Belladonna, are due to the fact that it blocks muscarinic (but not nicotinic) receptors and hence inhibits the parasympathetic system.

The story is different for transmission at postganglionic sympathetic nerve endings. The main hormone produced by the adrenal medulla, adrenaline (or epinephrine, because of the position of the adrenal glands, above the kidneys — Latin *-ren*, Greek, *nephros*) was found to have many effects similar to those resulting from stimulation of the sympathetic system. For some time it was thought that adrenaline was the neurotransmitter released by postganglionic sympathetic fibres, which therefore became known as 'adrenergic' nerves. However, there are important differences. We now know that the principal sympathetic transmitter is the related substance *noradrenaline* (norepinephrine), which is also released as a hormone, along with adrenaline, by the adrenal medulla. The discovery that different drugs can selectively block certain of the actions of adrenaline or noradrenaline led to the view that they act on different receptors in the membranes of the target tissues. Two such types of receptor were distinguished and named *alpha-* and *beta*-adrenoceptors; both types were later subdivided. Adrenaline and noradrenaline both act through these, but disproportionately at different sites. One result of such research has been the well-known beta-blocker drugs, used to treat hypertension and heart disease. They bind with beta-adrenoceptors and hence can prevent some of the constriction of blood vessels and stimulation of the heart by sympathetic nerves and the circulating hormones.

It subsequently emerged that some of the effects of sympathetic nerve stimulation cannot be prevented by drugs that block either type of adrenergic transmission. This is because there are other neurotransmitters, with their own specific receptors, operating at sympathetic nerve endings, either alone or in combination with noradrenaline as 'co-transmitters'.

The work from Dale's laboratory, carried out by physiologists in collaboration with chemists, progressed until his retirement in the late 1930s. Recognition of additional transmitters and of categories of receptors, elucidation of their nature and the consequences of their interaction, are continued by many distinguished contemporary scientists who are unravelling the complexities and diversities of autonomic nervous mechanisms. The powerful techniques of molecular biology are revealing the way in which the GENES produce the ENZYMES that synthesize neurotransmitters and construct the various receptors that they act on.

SHEILA JENNETT

E. M. TANSEY

See also ADRENAL GLANDS; MEMBRANE RECEPTORS; NEUROTRANSMITTERS.

Autopsy In a moment made familiar by television dramas and films, a detective views a dead body, turns to the doctor examining the corpse, and asks for the cause of death. The doctor inevitably remarks, 'Ah, we'll have to wait for the autopsy to be sure.' An autopsy is a standardized biomedical procedure during which trained medical pathologists examine the exterior of the body, dissect the corpse, view the vital organs for any obvious abnormality and weigh them, and collect specimens of tissues and fluids for further analysis. The procedure takes 2–4 hours and ends with the body being prepared either for storage until it can be released, or to go to the undertaker for embalming and burial or cremation. After additional laboratory work on the tissues and fluid specimens to detect the presence of drugs and/or coexisting medical conditions, the pathologist forms an opinion on the cause of death.

A typical autopsy begins with a Y-shaped incision from each shoulder to the lower end of the sternum and in a single incision from there to the pubic bone. The pathologist retracts the skin and superficial muscles from the chest and abdomen, and cuts the cartilages holding the ribs to the sternum, which is then removed. The pathologist removes, weighs and inspects the heart and lungs, often taking a sample of blood from the heart; the abdominal organs are also inspected, removed, and weighed, taking fluid samples as appropriate. The skull is opened by making an incision through the scalp on the back of the head and detaching it from the bone to lie over the face. The skull is then cut through with a bone saw, the bone removed and the brain extracted. Throughout these steps (which can occur in a different order) the pathologist removes sections of tissues to be preserved, with particular attention to those that appear diseased or injured. Photographs may be taken of parts of the body or of organs still in place or after removal. The flaps from the Y-incision are laid back over the thorax and abdomen and loosely sutured; the removed section of skull is replaced and the skin drawn back, which usually means that the face may be viewed during the funeral.

There are two basic kinds of autopsy: the *forensic autopsy* and the *medical autopsy*. A forensic autopsy, as the name implies, is one performed to satisfy the law. In most Western nations, an autopsy must be performed if a person died in suspicious circumstances, was unexpectedly found dead, died without having recently seen a physician who can attest to a cause of natural death, or is suspected of having had a disease that possibly threatens the public's health. In these circumstances, the state requires an autopsy and does not need permission from the deceased's relatives to perform one. If MURDER is suspected, the autopsy is required to establish the cause of death, to determine if the findings support the suspected crime, and to provide as much evidence as possible about how, when, and where such a crime might have occurred.

The medical autopsy has different goals. In these cases, physicians are already satisfied that the person died a natural death. Pathologists then use the autopsy to investigate the details of that natural death. Sometimes they seek additional information about the treatment that the patient had received, such as internal healing after a surgical procedure or evidence of a response to medications, even if these had nothing directly to do with the death. The medical autopsy also serves researchers studying a disease process such as cancer or bone deterioration, and who need specimens from a patient for whom they have a clinical record. Most medical autopsies require the consent of the immediate family, which normally includes permission for the pathologists to take and to preserve organs and specimens of use to medical science.

The word 'autopsy', comes from the Greek terms meaning 'seeing (or seen) for oneself'. The medical and legal use of 'autopsy' to mean anatomical dissection to discover the cause of death carries with it that sense of personal inspection and, when necessary, personal testimony, in court or at a case conference about what the observer saw within the body. '*Post-mortem*' (Latin: 'after death') is often used as a synonym for 'autopsy', but post-mortem examination is actually a general term for inspection of a corpse that does not necessarily include dissection.

History and cultural issues

Most cultures have historically had a strong aversion to mutilating the dead human body or to dissecting it simply to learn normal anatomy. Yet the world's ancient and classical civilizations had equally strong prohibitions against murder. In India, in China, and around the Mediterranean, the ruling orders developed legal systems that defined murder and established procedures in which witnesses testified that external marks on the body, or other visible signs, distinguished suicides, accidental deaths, and natural deaths from murder. In medieval Europe, twelfth-century legal scholars first extended the common practice of viewing the external signs on a body to identify probable cause of death, to examining the *internal* marks of violence or disease. The question of which wound corresponded to the fatal blow, for instance, could be crucial for picking out the murderer from those involved in a group assault. Poison, too, was thought to leave visible marks in the stomach that an expert might identify. Opening the body to serve justice thus outweighed distaste for such procedures. Early autopsies were likely to be quite short and minimally defacing because the inspection was limited to the area of the thorax or abdomen under particular scrutiny. The history of the autopsy in Western Europe and Great Britain is thus closely tied to the evolution of legal systems and court procedures. In English (and later American) law, the development of the duties of the coroner, a lay person, kept the decision to order a medical inspection, whether external or internal, out of the hands of medical experts until the nineteenth century.

Forensic autopsy procedures antedated the introduction of lawful human dissection into medical schools, which first emerged in medieval universities in the early fourteenth century. It is important to distinguish autopsies, where legal officials sought the cause of death, from anatomical dissections, where anatomists and, much later, medical students, learned normal anatomy. The former had a legal purpose; the latter only seemed to satisfy human curiosity. When dissection was introduced into universities and surgical guilds throughout the late medieval and early modern periods, secular rulers only permitted dissections of executed criminals. The continued association of dissection with mutilation and post-mortem punishment helped to maintain cultural aversion to autopsies.

Medical autopsies, where the body is opened simply to determine the cause of a natural death, emerged in Europe only after the rise of the study of normal anatomy in the sixteenth century. Even then, physicians and elite surgeons performed such inspections only sporadically until the eighteenth century, primarily because the dominant theory of the HUMOURS, which explained both health and disease in terms of individualized balances of the body's main fluids, accounted for the visible marks of pathology on organs as being the effects of underlying disease imbalances. Such hidden signs, usually inaccessible to the physician, were not considered particularly useful for understanding or treating disease in the living. In the eighteenth century, however, especially with the publication of Giovanni Battista Morgagni's *De sedibus et causis morborum per anatomen indigatis* (1761), practitioners began to investigate more thoroughly the internal changes associated with diseases, and by the end of the century the study of morbid anatomy was well under way. The early to mid nineteenth century witnessed extensive correlations between the anatomical changes observed at autopsy and the clinical course of diseases in previously living patients, particularly in the bodies of the poor dying in hospitals. With improvements in the microscope, moreover, the enthusiasm for gross pathology shifted to the pathology of tissues and cells, which dominated research in the second half of the nineteenth and well into the twentieth centuries. At the same time, the emergence of biochemistry added chemical investigation of human fluids and tissues to the pathologist's ability to detect both the signs of medical disorders and, eventually, the presence of alcohol and other drugs in a corpse.

Most inhabitants of the industrialized West now see autopsy as a necessary legal and medical protocol. For others, however, an autopsy represents a violation of the spiritual integrity of the recently dead human being. Traditional Hindus prohibit autopsies; Islamic law forbids mutilation of the corpse. While Islamic jurists have long argued that this prohibition does not apply to respectful legal and medical procedures necessary to determine a cause of death, Qur'anic statements about the resurrection of the physical body influence cultural resistance to the procedure. Similarly, modern arguments that humans have ethical obligations to protect life by increasing medical knowledge, and to ensure that justice is done by gathering evidence about crimes, have eased, but not necessarily eliminated, the antagonism towards autopsies held by Orthodox Jews and traditional Christians. As important as autopsies are in the abstract for law and medicine, they will continue to carry important cultural and emotional meanings as humans face the deaths of relatives and friends.

SUSAN LAWRENCE

Further reading

Forbes, T. R. (1985). *Surgeons at the Bailey: English forensic medicine to 1878*. Yale University Press, New Haven.

Encyclopedia of Bioethics (1995). Macmillan, New York.

See also ANATOMY; DEATH; DISSECTION; MURDER.

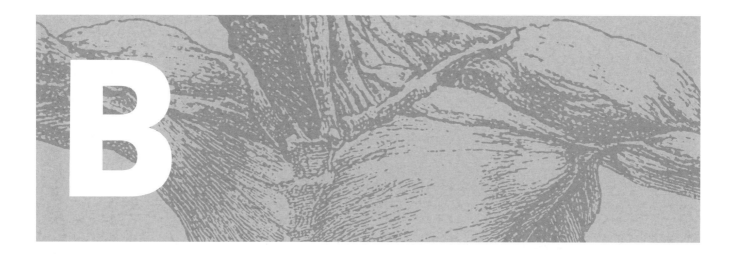

B

Bacchus The Roman god of wine and revelry, Bacchus, seems to have been formed from the hellenisation of the native Italian god Liber, patron of viticulture, to become a Roman version of Dionysos. Like Dionysos (see GREEKS), Bacchus is associated predominantly with female followers (in Greek, these were known as maenads) and is also traditionally accompanied by goat–man satyrs (see CHIMERA) who are in a state of almost perpetual sexual arousal. The secret rites of Bacchus, the Bacchanalia, were introduced to Rome in the third century BC, and were officially banned from Italy in a famous decree of 186 BC, apparently because of fears that the meetings associated with them were being used for political conspiracies; the authority of the leader of a Bacchic cell over those who belonged to it could be seen as threatening the authority of the family and of the patron–client system which linked members of society through vertical ties.

In art, Bacchus is represented as a curly-haired child drinking wine; as a young man, naked apart from a crown of vine leaves and grapes; or heavily drunk, sometimes being put to bed by nymphs and satyrs. HELEN KING

Bacteria From the Greek 'small rod', these are single-celled microscopic organisms found everywhere in the environment and on the human body. They are visible with a light microscope. They are usually harmless, but some are the cause of disease in plants, animals, and humans. They may be broadly split into '*Gram positive*' and '*Gram negative*', depending on their reaction to certain stains (described by Gram, a Danish physician in 1884); or into rod-shaped (*bacilli*) and spherical (*cocci*). They replicate by *fission* (splitting), and most have a complex cell wall structure. A. D.

See MICROORGANISMS.

Balance or equilibrium, is a state in which opposing tendencies are equal. To balance an object means to position it with its centre of gravity above its supports in such a way that

there is no tendency for it to topple over to one side rather than to another. Toppling is not the same as falling. It is the toppling motion that gives rise to the 'sensation of loss of balance' and one feels 'balanced' when such sensations do not occur. We say that someone has a 'good sense of balance' when they appear able to move freely in all sorts of circumstances without obvious signs of accidental toppling. An object topples when the resultant of the stress forces acting on it does not pass through its *centre of gravity* (c of g). Stress forces are the forces of common experience—pushing and pulling—which are always associated with deformation of the molecular architecture of objects in contact. Gravity, on the other hand, is something quite different. It is the force to which Newton attributed the observed accelerations of objects in free fall. It acts at a distance, without contact. It is not gravity that breaks an egg when you drop it, but the stress forces on impact. The egg remains perfectly intact while it is in free fall under the action of gravity. An object can be prevented from falling if it is supported by stress forces exerted at contact with other objects, which are themselves supported in turn on the solid crust of the planet.

An object is said to be in 'stable equilibrium' if any small perturbation generates a force to oppose the displacement. This will be the case if the projection of the c of g falls within an 'area of support', defined as that polygon, with no re-entrant angles, that just encloses the projections of all the available points of support. Balance is maintained by moving the resultant of the supporting forces about in such a way as to resist perturbations. A piece of furniture, such as a table standing on its legs, is stable because, if any attempt is made to tilt it, the support thrusts in the legs alter and their resultant consequently shifts to resist the tilting. If you stand on one leg and pay attention to your standing foot, you will be able to feel changes in the foot as muscular forces alter the position of the thrust exerted between the foot and the ground to compensate for and resist the inevitable swaying arising from movements of the heart and chest.

Role of proprioception

SENSORY RECEPTORS of several kinds are involved in the complex process of maintaining uprightness, as well as in the recognition of the imminence of toppling. There are no 'gravity receptors' as such, in spite of what is generally believed. The parts of the inner ear commonly associated with this function turn out to be accelerometers; i.e. they are detectors of stress gradient, not of gravity. Proprioceptors elsewhere in the body can also act as accelerometers and thus make a contribution to indicating the direction of the resultant support thrust. The actual position of the thrust line is indicated by deformation of the soft tissues of the feet and hands at the areas of contact with the supports. Movements of the head during overbalancing are indicated by the streaming of details in the images of the environment on the peripheral retina.

Stability

Restricting the area of support diminishes the available range through which the support thrust can be moved to resist perturbations, unless the position of the support is itself appropriately moved by the perturbation. When an egg is placed on a hard surface, the area of support is restricted to the very small area of contact. It is, accordingly, very hard to balance an egg on one end, because any accidental tilting produces more movement of the c of g than of the point of support, the centre of curvature of the shell at the ends being below the c of g of the egg. The shift of the thrust line, which necessarily passes through the area of support, is thus not sufficient to correct the tilt. With the egg on its side, however, a brief push in the direction of the long axis of the egg produces temporary rocking, followed by a return to the original position. The centre of curvature in the plane of the long axis is above the c of g, so the shift of the thrust line exceeds that of the c of g. For a sideways perturbation, the centre of curvature is coincident with the c of g, and the egg just rolls away from the perturbation, with the thrust line continuing to pass through the c of g. This is what happens to a wheel: the balance is neither stable nor unstable.

If the body of an animal or of a person is to stay in more or less the same place, any accidental displacement in a particular direction will have to be corrected by a corresponding displacement in the opposite direction. This is achieved by adjusting, by muscular forces, the thrust forces exerted by the limbs against the supports — in magnitude, in direction, in timing, and in point of application.

Anticipatory pre-emptive actions

A number of reflex reactions have been identified that produce the appropriate changes in the musculature, by swaying, hopping, and stepping. In the intact subject, however, many of these reflexes are effectively replaced by 'anticipatory pre-emptive actions'. These are voluntary actions, based on the underlying reflexes, but initiated in response to the detection that the incoming sensory information is changing in a way that might lead to a need for corrective action. Appropriate action is initiated early, before the reflex responses themselves are triggered into action. Frequent rehearsal, from a very early age, leads to these voluntary actions being performed without the subject being aware of what is going on—that is to say, they become habits. Their promptness plays an important role in maintaining smoothness of control, since they are not subject to the delays inevitable in reflex responses.

Overbalancing

The erect posture of man, particularly when standing on one leg, is a condition of precarious equilibrium, because the area of support is small compared with the height of the c of g above the feet. The strategies for avoiding falling over are related to what happens to an egg placed on its side. Small perturbations are met by shifting the centre of pressure at the foot and thus developing an inclined thrust to oppose the perturbation, as in the egg displaced in the direction of its long axis. This strategy will fail when the thrust line reaches the edge of the area of support, because further displacement will cause the body to topple. The imminence of such toppling is detected by the proprioceptive system and a different strategy is brought into play. If another limb is available, it will be thrust out in the direction of the impending fall in a 'rescue reaction' that attempts to find a firm obstacle against which to develop force and thus to extend the effective area of support. This is the basis of stepping. A succession of steps, in locomotion, brings the legs into action in turn, like the spokes of a wheel, so that the body may be moved through an indefinite distance without falling over—like the egg being rolled sideways. The legs do not provide the same continuous support as a wheel because, when one leg is being swung forward in a step, the body topples forward over the stance leg and acquires some downward momentum. This toppling movement has to be corrected when the swing leg eventually touches down, so this leg then at first gives, to absorb the unwanted momentum, and later straightens again to restore

the c of g to its earlier height above the ground. As the body continues to move forward over the new stance foot, that leg extends to provide extra thrust, which propels the body forward into the next step. If this thrust is strong enough, the body can be launched into a free fall phase while the free leg is still swinging. This extends the step length, as in running or jumping.

Uprightness

When an object is at rest on a stationary support, the thrust line is parallel to a radius of the planet, i.e. it lies in the gravitational vertical. Experiments with moving platforms reveal, however, that the direction of the thrust line appropriate to the avoidance of falling over is dependent on the accelerations associated with the movement of the platform. A person standing in a vehicle that is moving in a curved path has to lean inwards, to develop a horizontal component of thrust to accelerate his body into an equally curved path, as well as developing an upward thrust to prevent falling. The best direction for the thrust line is thus not the same as the gravitational vertical.

The thrust developed against the supports, both on moving platforms and on firm ground, is under continuous readjustment by the nervous system to suit the needs of the moment, be it to remain in one place or to move about in locomotion or athletic activity. The successful control of the necessary muscular activity is a matter of skill; the basis of this is first acquired in infancy and it is continually being revised and rehearsed throughout life as different types of activity are undertaken.   T.D.M. ROBERTS

Further reading

Roberts, T. D. M. (1995) *Understanding Balance*, Chapman and Hall, London.

See also POSTURE; PROPRIOCEPTION; SENSORY RECEPTORS; WALKING.

Baldness Over the centuries, male pattern baldness has been a sensitive subject for a great many men. Their desire to restore their crowning glory has led them to try all sorts of supposed remedies, to believe all manner of bizarre theories, and to subject themselves to many methods of attempted restoration which could best be described as torture. One of the earliest over-reactions to the problem concerned biblical prophet Elisha, who summoned forth a bear to kill 42 children who had been mocking him. In an effort to restore their locks, Elisha, and other bald men of the time, turned to rubbing bear grease on their scalps, a treatment that remained popular for many centuries.

What today we sometimes refer to as 'illusion hairstyling' also goes way back in time. Julius Caesar utilized the combed straight forward method to cover his bald area. A second method was to take the hair from one side of the head, letting it grow long, then drawing it all the way over to the other side of the head. Since either method attempted to some extent to defy the law

of gravity, much plastering down of the strands was necessary. Illusion styling remains popular today, especially among politicians. Hippocrates was the first person to describe the pattern male baldness commonly took, but he had no idea what caused the hair loss. He applied sheep's urine to his bald spot, to no avail. Early Romans plastered their scalps with chicken dung. When Napolean and Czar Alexander of Russia (both bald) met to discuss the future of Europe, they got sidetracked into talking about baldness cures.

Wigs and toupees were common at least as far back as the days of the first written medical record — the Ebers Papyrus, *c.* 1500 BC, which contained recipes for baldness remedies. Hair-pieces were desired because baldness was believed to be a sign of servitude or immorality by all ancient nations. After an ancient Greek battle the victor Mausoleus ordered the defeated Lycian males to have their heads shaved, an extremely humiliating punishment. Modern day military organizations of most countries routinely shave the heads of all recruits. Hygiene played some role in the use of this practice earlier in the modern period — it made it easier to control for lice, for example. But it also symbolized the lack of power and passive submission of the recruits. Prisoners and traitors have also had their heads shaved across time and cultures, to declare their worthlessness. Then there was the concept of strength. Caesar worried that his powers might recede with his hair. Another biblical reference was to Samson, whose strength was linked to his hair. When his head was shaved by Delilah his power evaporated, allowing his capture by the Philistines. Only when his hair grew back was he strong enough to tear down the temple. Thus, down through time came images of bald men as weak, impotent, passive, submissive.

Stupidity might have been added to the list if Samuel Johnson had his way, for he thought baldness was due to dryness of the brain and its shrinking from the skull. However, later it became common to declare baldness to be more prevalent among the upper classes. Both of these ideas led to and reinforced theories that lack of hair was caused by mental activity or high intelligence. Desperate for something positive to hold on to, bald men began to popularize the idea that they were more virile, more sexually active than hair-bearing males. With the male hormone testosterone linked somehow to baldness it was easy for the erroneous idea to spread that the more testosterone you produced the more quickly you went bald, and the more completely you went bald. As proof, history had the example of the eunuch. Eunuchs never went bald, and if they were going bald when they became eunuchs the balding process stopped completely. However, lost hair was never restored. The only 100% effective preventive measure against baldness was — and remains — castration.

Widespread acceptance of baldness by the scientific community as heredity-based did not take place until the 1940s. Until then other theories ran wild. The idea for example that hats caused baldness also had ancient roots, with heavy metal helmets blamed for causing hair loss among Roman and Egyptian soldiers. This theory reached its peak of popularity from the late 1800s, lasting into the 1940s or so. What was interesting about hats as a theory was that its proponents had to explain just why it was that hats caused men to go bald but not women — for whom the hat was as necessary and prevalent an item of dress as it was for males. The search for causes often led to strange and convoluted logic. Often the scalp and skull were blamed; there were 'muscle heads', 'fat heads', and the dreaded 'ivory domes'. In one way or another the scalp worked against its owner to somehow reduce or cut off circulation to the scalp, with this loss of blood supply resulting in the death of the hair. This too, led to problems of logic when believers tried to explain hirsute female scalps. Then there was the popular microbe theory, wherein a living microbe or bacillus caused baldness. That is, baldness was contagious. Barbers took a lot of criticism for having unhealthy establishments, which led to the easy spread of those germs. Hair-styling salons for women were somehow much more sanitary: how else to explain the difference? Those microbes were indeed 'isolated' and 'observed' by scientists of the time, with work undertaken to discover a vaccine. One of the more popular preventatives and treatments for hair loss a century ago was blistering of the scalp, by regular application of irritants. One of the more popular irritants was cantharides (crushed insects better known as the reputed aphrodisiac Spanish Fly). Some of the treatments would resurface again and again, over time. The use of electricity to treat baldness had a run in the very early years of the 1900s and reappeared once more in the 1990s.

Of course, quacks had a field day all through the 1900s peddling all sorts of nostrums — tonics such as Lucky Tiger, Herpicide, and Kreml. They grew no hair, stopped no baldness, lightened the buyer's wallet, and sold like crazy. At least most were painless and harmless, but not all. Some of the implant techniques introduced foreign material into the body, with occasionally horrifying results. Implants were first introduced around 1898, only to fall dormant within a few years, then to resurface in the 1970s. Complaints of discomfort, pain, infection, and scarring grew until the US Federal Trade Commission ordered companies to disclose that implants, although cared for like natural hair, require special handling and attention. Equally gruesome was the modern technique called scalp reduction. It seemed to be based on the idea that you didn't have too little hair for your scalp but too much scalp for your hair. Therefore, the answer was to slice out sections of your scalp. The latest rage in baldness nostrums was the drug minoxidil, sold under the label Rogaine.

In recent times many psychological studies have been done on attitudes of people toward bald and hair-bearing men. Generally, bald men have fared poorly, being assessed as less attractive, less confident, less successful, less likeable, and so forth, compared with hirsute men. There were few straws for them to grasp. Perhaps one was the solution to be found on late-night cable television in 1990s America. Those 30 minute 'infomericals' explained it all: for only $40 you just sprayed it on, hair in a can. By 1994 American men spent an estimated $2 billion yearly dealing with hair loss.   KERRY SEGRAVE

Further reading

Segrave, K. (1996). *Baldness; a social history.* McFarland, Jefferson, NC.

See also ALOPECIA; HAIR.

Ballet Imagine your legs rotated, from your hips to the tips of your toes, heels touching, to form an angle of 180 degrees. Every muscle, from the waist down, is contracted. Your buttocks are tight and scooped inwards and under. Your stomach is concave, muscles rippling. You have taken a breath so deep that your waist is floating; your ribs a mile from your hips. Your shoulders press down on your rigid spine. Your head floats on its elongated neck. Gently curved arms flow down to precisely positioned fingers.

Ballet begins here — the head held high, the chest broad, the top half of the body generally quite rigid, with the waist downwards performing whatever skills tradition requires. Every position, from a simple *demi-plié* to the most complex *enchaînement* or *batterie* combination, places exacting, apparently unreal demands on the body. Demands that can, from the best performers, elicit movements of unimaginable agility, virtuosity, and beauty.

Surely, human beings must always have used stylized movement to communicate expression of mood and intent, from ritualistic tribal war ceremonies to dances expressing love or affirming the sense of community. DANCE is a BODY LANGUAGE: one dancer's body is usually in dialogue or in full confrontation (aggressive or friendly) with that of another.

Ballet evolved from the formal *bals* and entertainments held for the pleasure of monarchs and courtiers in the sixteenth- and seventeenth-century courts of Western Europe. The movements articulated in court dances were precise, measured, allowing only the best body lines to be exposed. Thus legs and feet were turned out. The trunk was usually three-quarters crossed (*croisé*) to the partner's body or to the audience, rather than full-face (*en face*) — certainly never side-on, exposing the ugly silhouette of over-prominent buttocks, knock-knees or large stomach. These conventions charted the route to the highly technical forms of classical ballet, as we know it at the start of the twenty-first century.

Louis IV, the Sun King of France (1638–1715), an ardent lover of dance and an enthusiastic dancer himself, established the Académie Royale de Musique. Here the steps and postures that he and his courtiers loved were formalized and refined, and the French terms that had been used well before Louis's reign were consolidated. French ballet terms are now a world-wide language. A classically trained dancer can follow without difficulty a ballet class in New York, Shanghai, Sydney, or Florence.

Over the centuries, ballet skills have become yet more rigorous and exacting. At the same time, poise and ethereal grace must never be lost. Odile's 32 *fouettés* (turning *en pointe*, on one leg, 32 times) in *Swan Lake* must be delivered with effortless finesse. (The audience will think less of the ballerina who does not achieve both the number of turns and the necessary grace associated with the role.)

As with art and music, the nineteenth century witnessed immense changes in ballet, from the aerial romanticism of the ballerinas Taglioni, Elssler, and Cerrito in the first decades to the strict formulaic style of master choreographer Marius Petipa later in the century. Petipa, ballet master and choreographer for the Imperial Russian Ballet in St Petersburg from 1862, sought, above all, sculpted perfection, epitomized in his ballets *The Sleeping Beauty* and *Swan Lake*, to the music of Tchaikovsky. Not only the individual steps but the entire tableaux of *corps de ballet* represent precision itself. As a rebellion against Petipa's formality and rigidity of style came the more expressive works of Russian choreographer Michael Fokine. In the first decade of the twentieth century, after the Russian Revolution, Russian impresario Serge Diaghilev, founder of the Ballets Russes in Paris, extended the boundaries of ballet in experimental, sometimes controversial works, including Stravinsky's *The Firebird*, *Petruschka*, and *The Rite of Spring*. The most enigmatic of Diaghilev's dancers was Vaslav Nijinsky, who interpreted his roles with primitive sensuality and often abandoned classical techniques, such as turnout.

Through the twentieth century, the classical technique and the choreographic masterpieces of the nineteenth century survived, forever preserved, indeed refined in interpretation, especially by the great ballet companies of Europe and North America. But ballet (or modern dance as it became known, to distinguish it from classical ballet) also continued to develop, becoming ever more experimental, improvised, diverging from the rigours of classical ballet. Isadora Duncan, Martha Graham, Merce Cunningham are but a few of the leaders in contemporary dance, in which expression of movement and mood is conveyed through contraction of the torso, flexing of the feet, parallel position of the legs, and many other movements that are out of bounds in classical ballet.

The arduous training pursued by a modern dancer in the search for near-perfect technique results in muscular and anatomical development of the physique — a striking contrast to the first professional ballet dancers of the nineteenth century as we see them depicted in illustrations. Marie Taglioni, who made her début in Paris in 1822, though considered technically brilliant,

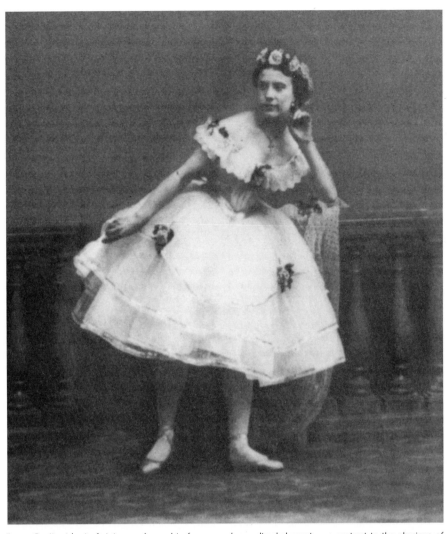

Fanny Cerrito, 'short of stature and round in frame … plump, dimpled arms' — a contrast to the physique of today's ballet dancer. (Photograph by Disdéri: Collection of the International Museum of Photography, George Eastman House.)

was 'stoop-shouldered and skinny with over-long arms'. A famous dancer of the 1840s, Fanny Cerrito, captured in a black and white photograph, appears dumpy and awkward, resembling a mushroom with her legs protruding from a huge knee-length voile skirt. Théophile Gautier, the French poet and sometime dance critic, described her as

> 'short of stature and round in frame … plump, dimpled arms … a delicate ankle and well-rounded leg. Her shoulders, her bosom do not have that scrawniness characteristic of female dancers whose whole weight seems to have descended into their legs.'

Dancers now jump higher, pirouette more times — more than the naked eye can count — spend hours in traction to stretch their limbs and torsos a centimetre or two more. Like modern athletes, their aim is perfection, speed of movement, flexibility of limbs. At the same time, they must retain grace and delicacy. 'Graceful beyond all comparisons, wonderful lightness and absence of all violent effort, or at least the appearance of it,

and a modesty as new as it is delightful to witness,' as Marie Taglioni was described when dancing at the Paris Opéra in the 1820s.

ANDRÉE BLAKEMORE

Further reading

Fonteyn, M. (1980). *The magic of dance.* BBC Books, London

See also BODY LANGUAGE; DANCE; FEMALE FORM.

Baptism is the rite which admits a candidate into the Christian Church, and is considered a sacrament by most denominations. The paradigmatic baptism is that of Jesus himself. As recounted in the Gospels, Jesus was baptised by John the Baptist in the River Jordan; after Jesus emerged from the water, the Holy Spirit descended upon him, in the form of a dove, and the voice of God spoke from heaven, declaring Jesus to be 'my well-beloved son'. Hence the constituent elements of the baptismal rite are water and a Trinitarian formula: candidates are baptised in the name of the Father, Son, and Holy Spirit. According to Matthew's gospel, Jesus commanded his disciples to baptise thus in his post-resurrection appearance to them in Galilee.

The origins of Christian baptism are probably found in the initiation rites of Jewish proselytes and, possibly, those of the mystery religions. Various baptismal rites were developed in the early Church, all designed to bring some or all of the body into contact with the baptismal waters. They generally involved immersion. This usually meant standing in water and having water poured on one's head and upper body. Such rites might involve triple immersion (in the name of the Father, Son, and Holy Spirit) as outlined in the late-first-century practical teaching document, *The Didache*, in which Christians were instructed to baptise the candidate three times in running water or by pouring water over the head three times. The Apostolic Tradition, describing rites and practices in third-century Rome, stated that the baptismal candidates should remove their clothes and enter the waters of the baptistry, where they would be baptised in the name of the Father, Son, and Holy Spirit. Having been anointed with *chrism* (see below), they would put their clothes back on and enter the church to participate in the Eucharist for the first time.

Baptism was quickly seen as necessary for salvation and as the initial moment of redemption; many passages in Acts teach that baptism must be preceded by faith and the confession and renunciation of sins. Paul developed a theology of baptism in which believers, being baptised, come to union with Christ, share in His death and resurrection, are cleansed of their sins, and incorporated into the body of Christ. The believer's sins are metaphorically washed away in the rite. The water is the visible sign of God's grace.

Preparation for baptism in the early Church was serious and lengthy — it could take up to three years. Many public officials in the early Church, and in early Christendom especially, postponed baptism until the end of their lives, knowing that they would be 'sullied' by the activities of their public life. Early creeds developed as simple formulae of Christian belief to be used in the baptismal rite. In the first two centuries, bishops, priests, and deacons (all of whom could be women or men) conferred baptism, but gradually, as the bishop's role was expanded, and women were squeezed out of all of these ministerial positions, it came to be the bishop who baptised. In cases of necessity, baptism could be conferred by anyone — and thus, right through the Middle Ages and into the modern period, it was often the midwife who performed the baptismal rite when a newly-born baby's life was in danger. Easter and Pentecost were the traditional times for baptism, though some churches began to hold baptisms on other feasts, such as Epiphany or Christmas. Baptismal candidates have traditionally had sponsors or godparents to support them in the faith (who, in the case of infants, would accept Christ as the infant's saviour on his or her behalf).

Chrism — holy oil which is a mixture of olive oil and balsam, and consecrated by a bishop — is used in baptismal rites in Eastern Orthodox, Roman Catholic, and Anglican churches. It was used in early baptismal rites. Tradition has it that it is placed on the baptismal candidate's forehead, hands, and feet, to seal the points at which the devil might enter, but there are also understandings of chrism representing — by the richness of the oil and the sweetness of the balsam — the fullness of sacramental grace and the gifts of the Holy Spirit, as well as the sweetness of Christian virtue. John Chrysostom, in the fourth century, wrote of baptismal candidates being anointed with oil from the top of the hairs of the head down to the feet and thereby becoming sharers in the true olive tree, Jesus Christ, and being healed of every trace of sin. An old Roman Catholic baptismal rite involved the offering of blessed salt to the baptismal candidate; this was probably based on the pagan Roman custom of placing a few grains of salt on the lips of an infant, eight days after its birth, to chase away the demons. Salt, because of its preservative quality, represented purity and incorruptibility.

The early Church seems to have baptised both infants and adults (though there is debate amongst historians about this). Gradually, infant baptism came to be the norm in Christendom, especially as a doctrine of original sin developed. Thus baptism became one of the seven sacraments in the Roman Catholic church. At the Reformation, Luther, Zwingli, and Calvin all retained infant baptism, though they interpreted the theology of it differently from the Roman Catholic Church. The Anabaptists rejected infant baptism, advocating believers' baptism, a response of faith by the individual to the gospel.

Today, some Christians — notably Baptists and many Eastern Orthodox — practise full immersion, that is the dipping of the whole body, including the face, into the water. In most Western churches, water is poured or splashed onto the head three times.   JANE SHAW

Barium meal

Some compounds of barium are poisonous, but barium sulphate is a harmless, white, insoluble substance that can be made into a tasteless suspension which is 'radio-opaque'. This can be swallowed as a 'barium meal' to aid diagnosis of disorders of the upper gastrointestinal tract (a '*barium enema*' is a similar suspension that is introduced into the large intestine through the rectum, for the investigation of disorders of the lower tract). The opaqueness of the material allows it to be visualized easily by X-ray as it passes down the oesophagus and through the stomach and upper intestine. The material will fill cavities caused by ulcers, and outline abnormal growths in the tract, thus giving visual information about dysfunction or disease of component parts, such as duodenal ulcer or stomach cancer.

E.M.T.

See IMAGING TECHNIQUES; X-RAYS.

Baroreceptors

are nerves which detect changes in the level of arterial BLOOD PRESSURE, in much the same way as a barometer detects changes in atmospheric pressure. These nerves are found in the walls of certain arteries and are stimulated by the stretch of the artery due to changes in the pressure of the blood. Stretch of the receptors gives rise to nerve impulses, which travel to the brain. They have a *threshold* — the minimum pressure required to cause some stimulation; an *operating range*, where changes in blood pressure cause proportionate changes in the frequency of the nerve impulses: and a *saturation level* — the pressure above which no increase in stimulation can occur. Not all baroreceptors have exactly the same operating ranges, so as blood pressure increases not only is the activity in individual nerves increased, but more receptors become active.

Baroreceptors do not just respond to the static level of blood pressure but they also respond to changes in pressure. These are their *phasic* properties. If blood pressure abruptly increases, baroreceptors initially give rise to a high frequency of nerve impulses, but then this declines to a lower, steady level. When pressure changes in a pulsatile way, as it does in arteries, baroreceptors discharge mainly or entirely during the rising phase of the pulse and are usually silent as pressure falls.

Much of our modern understanding of the ways in which baroreceptors function results from the work of the Belgian physiologist and Nobel Laureate Corneille Heymans and his collaborators. They used elaborate cross-circulation experiments in anaesthetised dogs to investigate in detail the reflex pathways by which the baroreceptors signalled changes in blood pressure.

Baroreceptors provide the input signal for a reflex which controls and stabilizes blood pressure. If pressure rises, baroreceptors are stimulated more and changes are brought about to reduce the pressure. Conversely, decreases in blood pressure are also limited by the baroreceptor reflex.

The best known and most extensively studied baroreceptors are those in the *carotid sinuses*, dilatations of the carotid arteries in the neck. The importance of the carotid baroreceptors is that they are ideally placed to ensure that the brain receives an adequate blood supply. The significance of this region was well known in antiquity, as compression of the carotid arteries could induce drowsiness — indeed, 'carotid' comes from the Greek word for deep sleep. Baroreceptors are also found in other major arteries, including the aortic arch and several of its branches, such as the coronary arteries which supply the heart muscle with blood.

In addition to arterial baroreceptors, *low-pressure baroreceptors* exist and these respond to the degree of stretch of veins and the cardiac atria. The best known of these are *atrial receptors*, which are nerves ending mainly at the junctions of the great veins with the atria. They are stimulated by stretch and can detect heart filling and possibly even blood volume. The reflex responses to their distension are an increase in heart rate, which reduces the filling at each beat, and an increase in urine flow, which reduces blood and extracellular fluid volume.

ROGER HAINSWORTH

E. M. TANSEY

See also BLOOD PRESSURE; BODY FLUIDS; SENSORY RECEPTORS.

Basal ganglia

In classical neuroanatomy this terms refers to the masses of GREY MATTER lying deeply within each cerebral hemisphere, separated from the outer shell of CEREBRAL CORTEX by a wide band of WHITE MATTER. Together these large aggregations of nerve cells or 'nuclei' are described as the 'striate body' (*corpus striatum* — striped because it is partly split by bands of white matter). However as a result of much clinical and animal-based basic research, other structures lower in the brain are now included with the basal ganglia on a functional basis, notably the *subthalamic nuclei* and the *substantia nigra*.

A rich variety of chemical transmitters was identified within the basal ganglia, and sophisticated anatomical tracing techniques employing radioactive or fluorescent 'tracers' to mark out nerve pathways, soon disclosed that they receive information from throughout the frontal lobe cerebral cortex in addition to the motor cortex and frontal eye fields, and also from the substantia nigra in the uppermost part of the BRAINSTEM. Moreover, it was shown that the darkly staining neuronal cell bodies of the substantia nigra, responsible for its name, contained the neurotransmitter DOPAMINE, and that the number of these neurons was severely reduced in the brains of patients who were suffering from Parkinsonism at the time of death. Furthermore, dopamine, and other transmitters such as NORADRENALINE and serotonin, were found to be depleted also in the basal ganglia of these same patients. These observations and the clues they provided to the functional links between these structures led to the remarkable twentieth-century discovery that the substance L-DOPA, the metabolic precursor of dopamine, when given orally in adequate quantities, was very effective in diminishing or abolishing the disabling tremor of what in earlier times was called 'the shaking palsy'. This localisation of the site of the problem promoted more research based on *stereotactic surgery* (three-dimensional positioning of micro-surgical instruments) which, when combined with electrophysiological and imaging procedures, has greatly benefitted patients so severely disabled by tremor that the surgical relief of symptoms has been necessary. Another feature of Parkinson's disease is '*akinesis*' — paucity of movement and slowness in starting or finishing movements. Although initiated by an act of will, most movements are carried out automatically; they are implemented through motor programmes refined by practice throughout life. This is the domain that the basal ganglia appear to be involved in. Crucial to this is the fact that the output from the basal ganglia is not only passed to BRAIN STEM centres and relayed on to the SPINAL

CORD; it also reaches the areas of the THALAMUS that transmit information back to the cerebral cortex, as well as mediating the control of automated movement by the CEREBELLUM. Still more recent research indicates that this system does not simply function by processing the signal flow in a serial mechanism (as suggested by the classical anatomical studies of connectivity between the cortex, basal ganglia, thalamus, and back to motor cortex). Instead, the system consists of multiple segregated pathways, involving the entire frontal cortex, drawing on parallel processing to permit the planning, execution, and co-ordination of eye and limb movements and, by inference, other frontal lobe processes including those of the 'LIMBIC SYSTEM'. TOM SEARS

See also BRAIN; DOPAMINE; GREY MATTER; LIMBIC SYSTEM; MOVEMENT, CONTROL OF.

Basal metabolic rate
The energy output of the body when fasting and completely at rest. All the constituent living cells are continuously metabolizing — releasing energy by the action of ENZYMES on chemical substrates derived ultimately from food. They use that energy for the synthesis or breakdown of vital substances, for maintaining the integrity of the cell by regulating influx and efflux across the membrane which encloses it, and for carrying out their own specialized functions; they release the rest as heat. Some energy is converted into the work of muscle contraction: at rest mainly the heart beat and the breathing muscles. Because the metabolism of the vast majority of body cells requires and consumes oxygen, the BMR can be estimated by measuring the rate at which oxygen is taken up and calculating the energy equivalent. A typical value for a man could be 350 litres of oxygen = 1700 kcal (7000 kJ) per day; or just under 0.25 litre, and just over 1 kcal per minute. Rigorous conditions for basal measurements are difficult to attain; more often the metabolic rate is measured when simply at rest; it varies with BODY WEIGHT and composition, but also between individuals who are similar in these respects. S.J.

See ENERGY BALANCE; METABOLISM; THYROID GLAND.

Bathing
To take a bath is both a pleasure and an act of HYGIENE. It is also an ancient physiological trait shared with other land-mammals who likewise need to groom themselves. When animals bathe, in mud or in water, they are applying a lotion to the skin which eases and moisturises it; they can also cool or heat the body; clear vermin; heal sores and rashes; remove dirt and other adhesions; and, through the external massaging of the skin given by the bath, produce a sense of well-being to the whole organism. So, bathing has a long bio-history, which underlies the social history of its adoption by advanced human societies: when we bathe, we perform a very simple act which reaches back into our own biological past.

The history of bathing in human groups is therefore all about techniques, and access — where and when and how, rather than why. To find a pond and plunge into it is simple enough; to turn it into a regulated, ritualized, custom, made available to large populations 'on tap', is the product of centuries of human endeavour, world-wide. Up until *c.* 3500 BC, when the first urban civilizations appeared, in the valleys of the Lower Tigris and Euphrates, the Indus, and the Yellow River, there is some evidence that the 'natural virtues' of bathing were understood and put to use by tribal human groups as part of their primitive '*techniques du corps*' — their inherited armoury of healing and body care. Several types of 'folk' or tribal cultures of bathing still exist today, while others have been found referred to as past custom: such as 'Finnish' saunas, and the old Irish/Celtic steam huts; the current Nordic and old Teutonic traditions of cold snow and river bathing; Japanese and Turkish mud baths; the use of hot spas everywhere. Archaeological and anthropological evidence provides proof of the additional religious significance which was, at some point, probably in this period, attached to the use of natural springs as the home of gods and spirits.

Bathing for beauty, power, and status was a refinement of bodily care over and above natural 'dipping'. The cosmetic arts of bodily decoration, including bathing for the purposes of both purification and anointing, undoubtedly also formed part of the cultures of tribal societies, as shown today amongst surviving neo-Neolithic groups. But a 'high' cosmetic culture was a major feature of the new-wealth display of the first ancient civilizations of China, India, Mesopotamia, Egypt, and, later, Greece and Rome. The use of bathing in water of all types and temperatures — with all its associated pastes and pomades, perfumes and powders — reached new heights, and the raw ingredients were an important East–West trade. The legendary bathing of Cleopatra in ass' milk is a folk-memory of this period, and such luxurious cosmetic bathing is part of the image of the 'exotic' East. The bathing technologies developed at this stage were those which ultimately spread throughout Western Europe via the Graeco-Roman inheritance.

With the Greeks comes the Western European written 'discourse' on bathing (with which we are mainly concerned — the later Indian or Chinese 'discourses' undoubtedly took a different path). Most crucially, cosmetics were re-classified by new Greek medical science on both moral and professional grounds, as a lowly subdivision of the medical 'art of hygiene'. 'Hygeia' dealt with complete bodily health through the managed regimen of the six bodily 'non-naturals' of air, diet, exercise, sleep, evacuations, and passions of the mind. Bathing was part of exercise, and also assisted the evacuation of the humours. Every part of the regimen was directed by the actions of the four cosmological elements — earth, air, fire, and water — and their correct balance within the body. Thus hot waters heated cold bodily 'conditions'; and cold waters cooled hot conditions. Warm waters were gentlest, the mean between extremes. The wet–dry axis was also important — the body should be carefully wiped, powdered, or dried out after immersion; dry bodily conditions required more or less rich emollients (oils) in the water and afterwards; dry 'frictions' (massage, with a towel) were matched by wet frictions (with loofah or bath brush). Thus bathing was indicated and contra-indicated in various seasons, and at various times of day, as a part of the regimen. The rinsing of the teeth and mouth, and the bathing of the face and hands, was to be performed in the morning; a full body bath was a major operation undertaken before the main meal of the day, with rest and recuperation afterwards, or in the early evening before supper. In classic practice, spring was the time for bathing and blood letting; then the humours rose in the body to be 'evacuated' through pores and veins, and were washed away by the bath. Since spring was also the season for sexual play and courtship, the use of the bath also took on more obvious meanings. The uneasy union between the 'hands on' empiricism of the old school of barber–surgeons, and the philosophic 'mind set' of the new school of physicians is illustrated in Galen's *Hygiene*, the main classical authority on the use of bathing as therapy which describes both the '*logos*' (the reasons) and the '*techne*' (the methods) of bathing, but leaves it to the patient — with or without his professional 'trainer', barber–surgeon, and other body servants — to do the manual labour.

The classical (and Eastern) world used bathing freely. It has always been assumed that there was a hiatus after the retreat of the Roman Empire, and the Roman-built baths and spas did certainly fall into decay, presumably because the lifestyle or bathing culture so dear to Roman imperial administrators disappeared. Moreover, bathing culture was more or less disapproved of by the Church as a bodily vanity; but it was not eradicated. The hot spas were re-colonized locally and developed into communal bathing pools, and used for pleasure and for the purposes for they had always been valued — the healing of skin diseases, the easing of paralysed limbs, a hopeful cure for infertility. For similar reasons small public baths or hot 'stews', in or near barbers' shops, were apparently widespread in European towns and cities *c.* 1100–1550. The barbers' expertise in bathing was protected by the regulations of Guilds of Barbers, while the City Fathers licensed the trade to ensure public order and to protect the public health. When syphilis and the great plagues appeared in Europe after *c.* 1490 the public bathing trade was effectively decimated, and many baths were closed or their activities severely restricted.

Private bathing, however, has a rather different history. At one level, the 'simple waters' (common water without any additives) were available at any water source; and the 'simples', the common ingredients of bathing cosmetics, were available in any coutryside — they were made locally everywhere. In theory, anyone could take a bath. In practice most must have taken the 'strip-wash' in the bowl in front of the kitchen fire, or the shower outside, according to local conditions. In the end, bathing was a question of economics — time and money. Thus, you could not heat water without any fuel, or labour; you could not store, nor take time out for, preparations. Thus the most elaborate arrangements pertained to the royal or courtly bath culture. Ceremonial bathing and ritual bathing for purification (before knighthood, before marriage) were preserved from ancient antecedents; and the cosmetic royal baths were probably always an occasion. To this was apparently later added the outdoor bath-feast, with guests, food, and music — essentially a bath taken in a decorated water tank 'au naturel', in the park or gardens. In the seventeenth-century French aristocratic circles that Georges Vigarello describes, the full *toilette* was impossible without the bath. Domestic plumbing gradually made its way into the upper chambers of the nobility and gentry, where the bathing sets, knapkins, and perfumiery were kept.

The Protestant Reformation in Western Europe brought cold baths, and a renewed interest in the classical philosophy of hygiene. The eighteenth-century Enlightenment spread the message. The classical texts had been gradually exhumed, and their contents and commentaries spread by books. From the 1650s, throughout Europe, natural spas and mineral waters were classified and chemically analysed. By the eighteenth century, spa doctoring was a recognized branch of the medical profession. From Northern Europe came a form of Cold Regimen: cold-water 'hydropathic' bathing, and the development of outdoor spas and coastal resorts. Swimming in the sea became a fashionable hygienic exercise.

During the nineteenth century, bathing moved from being a luxury to being a 'necessity'. *Hydropathy* (the science of bathing) flourished — 'water doctors' developed cold mountain-top 'hydros' or spas, hot Turkish baths, fumigating baths, the shower bath. Philanthropy provided hospital baths, factory baths, and public baths and swimming pools; in England the Public Baths and Washhouses Act was passed in 1846. The Soap Tax — used for laundering and the domestic warm bath — was repealed in 1853. In Europe generally at the beginning of the twentieth century a private bath or shower-room was a luxury; by the end of the century, mass cheap private housing and state health policies had (almost) brought one to every home.

VIRGINIA SMITH

See also HUMOURS; HYGIENE; RELIGION AND THE BODY; SWIMMING.

Beauty In Greek mythology, Paris was called to judge who of three goddesses, Aphrodite, Hera, and Pallas Athene, was the fairest. Eris, the goddess of discord, started the trouble when she appeared at a wedding, and threw a golden apple inscribed 'For the Fairest'. The result was a disrupted wedding and later a war, as Paris abducted Helen to Troy. The gods were unable to make the decision, and Paris' task was not easy. Hera offered him wealth and power, and Athene promised honour and glory, but the ultimate bribe came from Aphrodite: with the promise of Helen, the most beautiful woman on earth, for his wife, Paris ended this beauty contest in favour of Aphrodite.

Like the ancient Greeks, we moderns ascribe high value to beauty and, like them, we have been unable to determine *the* concept of beauty, despite the fact that Miss Universe, Miss World, and a variety of other BEAUTY CONTESTS are staged annually. With the contest still undecided, almost everybody is involved in the pursuit of beauty, and the huge profits of the beauty industry testify to its economic importance. Its significance for the individual can be judged by the time spent in the gym and in front of the mirror, and by the problems that arise from experiencing failure in this pursuit.

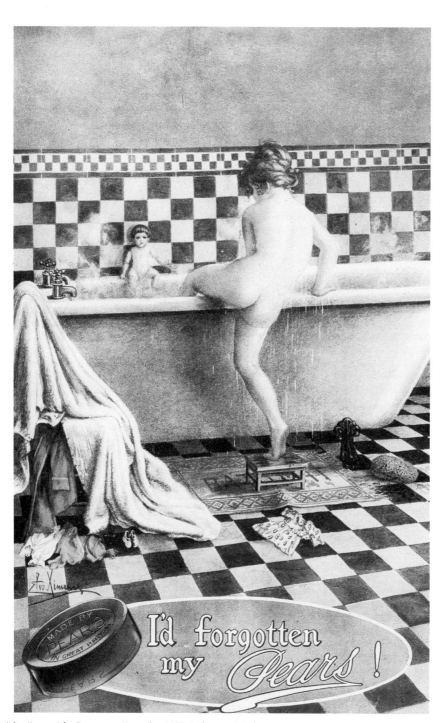

Advertisement for Pears soap, November 1922. Bridgeman Art Library.

Bodily beauty can be defined as the deeply pleasurable experience of someone else's or one's own body. While the beauty of a person might include the person's character, spiritual quality, intelligence, and morals, the beauty of a person's body generally will not. Bodily beauty can be perceived through any of the five senses, and may be concerned with parts of the body, the whole body, or movements. Usually, however, beauty of the body refers to the visual impression of someone's body as a whole.

The origins of interest in bodily beauty were explained by Sigmund Freud, the founder of modern psychology, as being sexual drives: through a transformation, sexual attraction is moved away from the primary sexual characteristics (reproductive organs) and instead to the secondary sexual characteristics (e.g. women's more rounded forms and breasts; men's facial hair and deeper voices).

An anthropological explanation for the human interest in beauty has been offered by Robert Brain: human beings want to set themselves apart from non-humans, and therefore make alterations to the body that animals would not be capable of making. Admiration turns these alterations into marks of beauty. Exactly which alterations are admired depends on cultural preferences. Beautification strategies of one culture might, in another culture, be perceived as mutilations and as marks of ugliness. BODY DECORATIONS can also mark the successful initiation or the identity of a person. But making a difference between humans and non-humans is, according to Brain, basic to those scarifications, tattooings, and colourings of the body that are associated with beauty.

Cultural variations in ideals

Neither the psychological nor the anthropological approaches above can explain the variety over time and between different societies as to what is considered beautiful. All in all, this variation makes a strong case against the idea of some universal components of beauty.

Ideals of beauty vary between and within societies: values, norms, and tastes differ from group to group; the different sexes are used for constituting different genders; and relations of power, e.g. between genders, ethnic groups, and classes, make one ideal of beauty dominant over others. Western cultures have attributed beauty to women to the point where it is difficult to talk of the beauty of men's bodies. The nineteenth-century term for describing a pleasant appearance in a man was neither 'handsome' nor 'good-looking', but 'manly', since beauty was reserved for women, and today 'real men' might be 'handsome' or 'good-looking', but 'beautiful' is considered too effeminate. The ancient Greeks were especially attentive to the beauty of young men's bodies, and the Nuba of Sudan and the Wodaabe men in Niger also have no difficulty in associating men and beauty. Indeed, the latter stage a beauty contest for men, *gerewol*, to express their special birthright

of beauty and their true identity among African people.

The male beauties of the Wodaabe people in Niger challenge any Euro-American attempt to argue for the universality of beauty criteria, and point to the importance of ethnicity. To beautify themselves, the men apply yellow colour to their faces in order to lighten them, draw a line from the forehead to the tip of the nose to make the latter appear longer; blacken their lips; and, at the height of their striving for beauty, squint at the women. Taking the ethnic perspective further, the Nuba of Sudan found little beauty in the appearance of the English anthropologist James Faris; he had a beard, hair on his arms, and white skin. All were appalling features to a people to whom well-groomed hair, a smooth body, and a deep, rich black colour are central ingredients of the body beautiful. Indeed, to the Nuba it was shaving that distinguished humans from animals, and he appropriately got the nickname *wōte* — monkey.

The ethnic component also emerges in the Miss America, Miss World, and Miss Universe contests, which have been strongly hampered by the fact that the finalists and winners are predominantly women with white skin and Caucasian features. Women from other ethnic groups have had little chance of winning these contests, organized by white Euro-Americans, until recently.

Spiritual significance

The importance of bodily beauty has also varied through times and across societies. In Western culture the distinction between the material and the immaterial body, body and soul, and the values that have been attached to them have been central to how beauty was regarded. To the ancient Greeks a beautiful body reflected a beautiful soul and proximity to the gods. To the Gnostics (largely covering the first three to four centuries AD) the divine psychic body was caged in a physical body made by beastly creatures from the underworld. They renounced the material body and sexual drives, and strove for asceticism. In the early Christian era, where a dualism between soul and body prevailed, beauty was considered good if its appeal was spiritual and internal, but evil if its attraction was sexual and carnal. In medieval times the body and the flesh were associated with sin and women, and the immaterial soul with the divine. Thus an ethereal body ideal prevailed for women. Today, Euro-Americans seem to have gone back to an intense interest in beauty, but with a reversal of its significance: work-outs, jogging, and BODY-BUILDING do not any longer reflect a healthy soul, but are assumed to produce one. Further, whereas the ancient Greeks included ethics and cosmological harmony in their beautiful soul, Euro-Americans generally assume the healthy soul to be one that is up to the task of meeting the daily requirements of productive living.

A contrast to Western ideals of beauty and the importance assigned to them can be found in the

study on body ideals for women in Fiji, in the South Pacific, by anthropologist Anne E. Becker. She found that the disparity between what Fijian women themselves identified as the most attractive body shape, and their actual robust appearance, did not pose a problem to them. Most women either thought that they should maintain their present weight, or actually increase it. Anne Becker explains the difference by distinguishing between an ideal of attractiveness, mainly concerned with sexuality and youth, and an ideal based on norms for what women and society ought to be like. In Fiji a robust body indicates a woman, or a man for that matter, who is embedded in a well-functioning network of family and friendship relations. This body, taken to indicate the successful practice of caring and sharing, is more important than the body of attractiveness.

Furthermore, since the Fijian body is primarily seen as constituted through the network of social relations in which the person takes part, beauty is the result of a collective effort and not, as in Western societies, an individual achievement. As a corollary, the body in Fiji was not seen as something that could be worked on and moulded. It is almost unnecessary to mention that no cases of EATING DISORDERS, such as anorexia or bulimia, were found in Fiji.

Changing western concepts

Of course, the slim, firm, and muscular body ideal for women which prevails in the West today, along with the tall thinness of models, are only the latest in the history of Euro-American body ideals. The rise in the sixteenth century of Neoplatonism, which saw concrete forms as expressions of divine ideas, and, as a corollary, saw the body as an expression of the soul, led to higher appreciation of beauty and a change in the ideal. As intelligence and force were divine gifts of the male body, beauty was the divine gift of the female body. Thus female beauty changed from being dangerous to being divine, and the previous ethereal female was succeeded by large, opulent beauties. During the eighteenth century this majestic type was superseded by a more slender and younger ideal for women, while the former, maternal type was denigrated to the status of 'peasant' beauty. This sylph-like early Victorian woman was followed by the voluptuous mid Victorian woman and the Edwardian woman of the late nineteenth century. Where the Victorians stressed a curvaceous hourglass figure, with a full bosom, small waist, and wide hips, the Edwardian woman was taller, weighed more, and had a larger bosom, but somewhat slimmer hips. Thinness was out of vogue and thin women were told to cover their 'angles'.

Shortly before World War I a slender and serpentine type with smaller breasts, slimmer hips, and long legs was fashionable. This 'boyish' and youthful ideal reigned during the 1920s, succeeded by a sensual and voluptuous ideal in the 1930s. The 'boyish' and the 1930s fuller figure persisted throughout the 1950s until the thin look of the 1960s came to dominate. Since then thinness has reigned, with no come-back of the maternal ideal. Changes have taken place within the ideal of thinness, however. Today a woman does not only have to be slim, she has to have a compact, muscular look only achievable through weekly hours of exercise.

The above outline of the changing ideals of women in Europe concentrates on dominant ideology, and suggests a linear succession of different ideals, but the situation is, in reality, more complex. At any given point in time, there will be several competing ideals of beauty. One example, also providing an opportunity to make a small note on the opposite sex, could be mid-nineteenth century North America, where a number of alternative beauty ideals for men coexisted. There was the Byronic man, sensitive and heroic — especially popular amongst young men of the 1830s and 1840s, and modelled after Lord Byron with his leonine head, fair skin, and a body which was regularly subjected to dieting. At the same time, the muscular man of height and physical prowess existed; and a third ideal developed in the 1860s with the portly, rotund man, partner of the voluptuous female beauty, signalling maturity after the dislocating experiences of the Civil War in America and displaying his success in business. By the end of the century, however, the dominant ideal again became youthful, and now associated with the well-trained bodies of sportsmen. Classifying these ideals into the Byronic, the Muscular, and the Solid Man, these models of maleness are also found today.

The changing ideals of both men's and women's beauty is linked to society's perception of appropriate gender roles. The shifts from the maternal, robust body of the mid and late Victorian ages, to the slender ideal of the 1920s, to the compact, slim body of the present reflect changes in the perception of the proper role for women: from mother and caretaker of house and home, through the independent young women of the 1920s, to the active professional and disciplined women of the present.

Beauty, however, does not only relate to the ideal roles ascribed to men and women, but is part of ongoing social identification processes: a person might strive towards a certain ideal to signal man- or motherhood, or independence, but might also be judged differently by others. Furthermore, the interpretation of a body also changes with the context: a woman's thin, muscular body might be seen as representing the disciplined, independent, and professional woman of the 1990s, but seen next to the muscular body of a man she could still represent the fragility and vulnerability of woman.

The ideals of beauty today are defined through different perspectives as the healthy body, the athletic body, the muscular body, the natural body, the aesthetically pleasing body, etc. These ideals do not necessarily overlap. Eating healthy food, getting enough sleep, and having a daily walk might result in a healthy body, but would not produce a muscular body. Doing sports and being fit might result in an athletic body, but would not necessarily produce a healthy or a muscular body. The ideals might even be contradictory, since it is questionable to what extent it is 'natural' to spend hours in the gym to achieve a muscular body, and since the aesthetically pleasing body might be so thin as to threaten health. This is a crucial current issue where 'Even Thinner-ness' has become the ideal.

Bringer of happiness, enchantress, or *femme fatale*? In the intricacies of beauty are promises of happiness and prospects of disruption. Politics of power, gender, ethnicity, and culture are still, millennia away from the Greek gods, part of the indulgence that beauty incites.   CLAUS BOSSEN

Further reading

Banner, L. W. (1983). *American beauty*. Alfred Knopf, New York.

Becker, A. E. (1995). *Body, self, and society. The view from Fiji* University of Pennsylvania Press, Philadelphia.

Brain, R. (1979). *The decorated body*. Hutchinson and Co., London.

Lakoff, R. B. and Scherr, R. L. (1984). *Face value. The politics of beauty*. Routledge and Kegan Paul, Boston.

See also BEAUTY CONTESTS; BODY BUILDING; BODY DECORATION; EATING DISORDERS; FEMALE FORM.

Beauty contests

In its modern form, the beauty contest is an American product. The selection of a woman as a symbol of community solidarity and fertility has a long and continuing history in Europe and North America. In the latter half of the nineteenth century women were frequently displayed in publicly staged events in the US. These rallies and crownings met with little protest as long as the occasion and its organizers were 'respectable', since both American feminists and conservatives regarded women as special guardians of American morality. The public staging of a contest between semi-naked women, however, presupposed the development of modern popular culture, where low and high class values became mixed and bathing beauties could be shown in movies and advertisements. As early as 1854, the American showman P. T. Barnum tried to organize a beauty contest where women were to appear on stage and be judged on their physical beauty. This kind of beauty contest later in the century became widespread at carnivals and other working-class entertainments where physical display was accepted, but P. T. Barnum's 1854 contest was a failure because only women of 'questionable reputation' entered. So he invented the photographic beauty contest, where the appraisal of women was based on the photographs they submitted. The photographic beauty contest, which was acceptable to the dominant values of the middle- and upper classes, quickly spread, and was used by newspapers and city councils for promotional purposes. By the turn of the twentieth century, American Victorian morality was on the wane, and the limits to the appearance of women in public changed: women could be used in advertisements, modelling became a respectable occupation, and film maker Mack Sennett successfully introduced bathing beauties in his movies.

From working class to popular culture

Women's appearance in public in swimsuits did not happen before the early twentieth century. Bathing had long been unpopular in Europe and America, and immersion in seawater did not become an acceptable activity until the early nineteenth century, and then only for health reasons. A bathing beauty contest had been held in Rehoboth Beach, Delaware, US, in 1880, but as this was a working class beach resort, this kind of

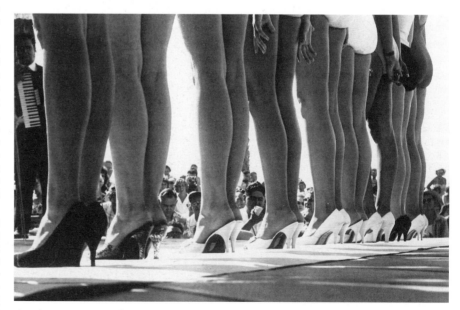

1950s beauty contest. © Robert W. Young/Robert Harding.

contest only became widespread after the turn of the century. The prevalence of Victorian dress codes did not allow for the development of the tight, one-piece bathing suit before the early twentieth century. One of its creators, a professional American swimmer, Annette Kellerman, was arrested when she appeared in public in the swimsuit.

Eventually, all things came together in 1921, when the first Miss America contest was staged in Atlantic City. So as not to offend public morals, the sensual aspects of the contest were obscured by a week-long, elaborate festival with sports events, automobile races, orchestra, and choir competitions. The question of morals led to a rift between the Miss America organization and their main sponsor, a swimsuit company, when Miss America 1951 refused to appear before cameras in a swimsuit after the contest and was supported by the Miss America organizers. In protest, the swimsuit company aligned themselves with Universal Pictures and started the Miss Universe contest the year after, in 1952. The Miss World contest was initiated in Britain the year before.

Previously treated with suspicion, beauty contests proliferated in the 1950s, with civil associations like the Jaycees and Rotary organising them. Through mass media the model of the contest spread all over the world, and today the International Register of Pageants lists more than 3000 pageants worldwide.

Politics of identity and power

Because the contestants represent their group, and the winner the community, beauty contests are often embedded in negotiations of identity and politics of power. In Fiji in 1956 the Jaycees started the Hibiscus Festival, which has been staged annually ever since, and has a Miss Hibiscus Quest at its centre. The aim is to promote tourism and provide a week of entertainment. In its early years, the festival provided the only possibility for the different ethnic groups to participate in a civil celebration together, and the festival became part of the English colonial state's nation-building efforts. However, as usual with beauty contests, the Miss Hibiscus Quest reflected prevailing cultural norms: in the early years, Europeans and part-Europeans predominantly featured as winners, and when the indigenous Fijians came to dominate the state after Independence in 1970, they won most contests. Not before 1979 was there an Indo-Fijian Miss Hibiscus, despite the fact that around 45% of the population is Indo-Fijian.

Similar cases are reported all over the world. In Thailand, the national Miss Universe contest has been used by the state in nation-building efforts since 1934, and is seen as promoting democracy and the nation, and elevating the status of women; in Guatemala, the *Rabìn Ahau*, the 'Indian' Maya Queen, is chosen to represent the indigenous, authentic past, whereas the country's modern national present is embodied by Miss Guatemala, always a Caucasian; and in the Philippines, Muslim gays dramatize through the Miss Gay Super Model conflicts and problems in creating a local identity confronted with globalized media, travel, and consumption.

A notable beauty contest, which is not built on the Western prototype is the *gerewol* staged by the Woodabe of Niger: a three-day celebration is held annually where young men dress up, paint themselves, and dance before a public audience. In the end, three men are selected by three young women as being the most beautiful.

Adapted to local needs, beauty contests take place the world over. Embedded in entertainment signalling 'it's just for fun', they provide a space for the negotiation of standards of beauty, gender roles, identities, and power.

CLAUS BOSSEN

Further reading
Cohen, C. B. Wilk, R., and Stoelthe, B. (1996). *Beauty queens on the global stage. Gender, contests, and power*. Routledge, New York.

Deford, F. (1971). *There she is: the life and times of Miss America*. Viking, New York.

See also BEAUTY.

Beauty spots — not to be confused with BIRTHMARKS or FRECKLES — are associated with a dark spot, usually on the face. Historically they have been seen as a mark of beauty, highlighting and identifying an area on the face such as on the cheek-brow, near to the mouth, or near the chin. The placing, either naturally or artificially, of the beauty spot, is thought to enhance the natural features of the person, making them more attractive, more sexually wanton and, therefore, more beautiful.

The history of FASHION and the wearing of MAKE-UP runs parallel to the evolution of the beauty spot. Originally the beauty spot was artificially worn in the guise of patches and paint. Ovid's manual for lovers, the *Ars Amatoria*, reassured Roman women that: 'No woman need be ugly, for all the remedies can be found in pots and potions.' Whilst freckles were got rid of by scrubbing the skin with mercury, delicate kohl-pencilled beauty spots and other small designs, known as 'patches' were worn on the face, neck, and shoulders. The fashionable Roman woman also pencilled in her eyebrows and wore a patch or two on her cheek or neck, and sometimes on her bare shoulder or arm. The Roman men, like those later in the seventeenth and eighteenth centuries, were also not adverse to the wearing of 'beauty spots' in the form of elaborate patches.

The face patch or beauty spot had two distinct advantages: it enhanced facial features and it concealed battle scars, disfigurement from small pox, and poor complexion. Patches were often

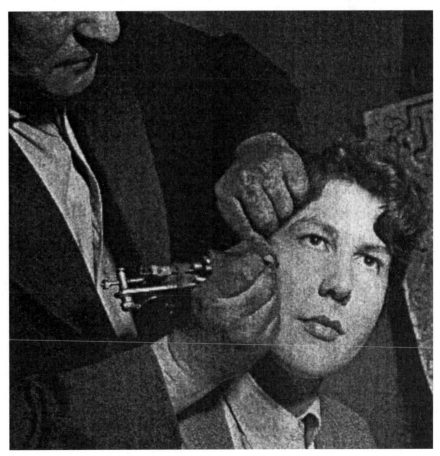

A tattoo artist paints a permanent beauty spot onto the cheek of his client. (Hulton Getty Library.)

made of black taffeta or red Spanish leather and were increasingly worn in larger sizes, in a variety of designs. There developed a 'language of patches', whereby those politically-minded would wear their patch on either side of the cheek depending on political alliance.

By the middle of the eighteenth century the renowned painter, engraver, and satirist, William Hogarth, was creating a furore with his expositions on portraiture and caricature. At the time, essayist William Hazlitt claimed that Hogarth took his painted portraits to the verge of caricature, but never went beyond it. This has been a long-standing debate within the realms of art history: namely, to what extent are Hogarth's faces portraits or caricatures? As David Piper's *The English Face* (1992) reports on Hogarth's portraits:

> [they] carry all the conviction of reality with them, as if we had seen the actual faces for the first time, from the precision, consistency, and good sense with which the whole and every part is made out. They exhibit the most uncommon features, with the most uncommon expressions, but which yet are as familiar and intelligible as possible, because with all the boldness, they have all the truth of nature … *memorable* faces, in their memorable moments. (p. 133)

It is in Hogarth's paintings and prints that we see the beauty spot in use. Though beauty spots and patches are not often found in the history or portrait paintings of the time, Hogarth's use of caricature lends itself to the exaggerated, microscopic view of the face. Thus Hogarth describes in detail, in *The Analysis of Beauty* (1753), the lines and shapes that make a face: 'It is strange that nature hath afforded us so many lines and shapes to indicate the deficiencies and blemishes of the mind, while there are none at all that point out the perfections of it beyond the appearance of common sense and placidity'. An engraving by Hogarth entitled *Morning* (1738), reveals a woman walking to church, holding a fan, with a number of dark spots on her forehead and upper cheek. These are strategically placed for maximum effect, to highlight the physiognomy of the woman.

By the nineteenth century two of the most famous caricaturists, James Gillray and Thomas Rowlandson, chose satire as their form of visual communication, most notably in the tradition of an Italian caricature known as Ghezzi. By emphasizing the physical eccentricities of their subject, they ridicule and shock. Gillray's etching, *Dido in Despair* (1801), shows an elephantine-size female in a night-gown, with dark beauty spots satirically dotted around her face. This is an antithetical depiction of beauty that Gillary offers, reversing the notion of a flawless goddess, ridiculing society for its devotion to such superficial ideals.

By the mid nineteenth century the use of patches and the enhancing of facial beauty was in its decline, and it was not until the 1950s that the beauty spot was to reappear as an aesthetic feature. Post-war Europe and the US looked to beauty and the making of cinematic idols.

Shaking off the drabness of the war years, femininity was back in fashion with Christian Dior's 'new look' tight-waisted dresses, new haircuts, high heels, and the wearing of red lipstick, emphasising the pencilled-on beauty spot. Hollywood icon Marilyn Monroe always wore a beauty spot, strategically placed next to her top lip.   ANNE ABICHOU

Further reading

Piper, D. (1992). *The English Face*. National Portrait Gallery, London.

Pomeroy, S. B. (1975). *Goddesses, whores, wives, and slaves. Women in classical antiquity*. Schoken Books, New York.

Rousseau, G. S. and Porter, R. (ed.) (1987). *Sexual underworlds of the Enlightenment*. Manchester University Press, Manchester.

See also BEAUTY; FASHION; FRECKLES; MAKE-UP.

Belly button The yogi contemplating his navel often figures for Westerners as an object of amusement, being taken as a symptom of indolence or narcissistic self-absorption. In reality nothing could be further from the truth; navel-gazing is, rather, a quest for absorption in realms transcending the individual psyche and even the domain of the human altogether. The navel provides a focus for spiritual concentration.

Beyond its obstetrical and physiological significance, the navel has been an object of great consequence in the light of deep convictions, held in many cultures, about correspondences between the macro- and the microcosm. If the human body is the image and epitome of an orderly and intelligible world, the navel is bound to assume philosophical significance as a key or clue to profound mysteries about the geometry of the universe and perhaps the origins of mankind. An originary myth from Turkey, for instance, relates that on seeing the first man created by Allah, the Devil spat at his stomach. Allah then made a grab at and removed the polluted spot, the resultant scar thus explaining why humans have a belly button. Byzantine mystics for their part thought of their navels as 'circles of the sun', expecting to observe a refraction of the light streaming from sacred Mount Tabor.

Cultures world-wide have striven to locate and distinguish the centre of the universe or at least of the globe. In Greek mythology, Zeus, seeking to discover the precise centre of the earth, arranged for two eagles to fly at the same speed, one from the east and the other from the west. They met at Delphi, and so it was there, in a temple to Apollo, that the Greeks set up an *omphalos* — that is, a holy navel-stone — guarded by two golden eagles. The stones, as revealed by excavations, were in the shape of ornamented half-eggs on squat, quadrangular bases. Apollo, explained Plato, 'has his shrine at the world's centre and navel, to guide mankind.' Further legends state that the omphalos at Delphi stands upon the spot where Apollo killed the serpent Python, or

upon the chasm through which the waters of Deucalion's flood drained away.

The omphalos was regarded as the throne of a deity, notably the Earth Mother. It could serve as a symbol of sacredness, peace, and order. The spinning wheel at which Heracles toiled was an omphalos, as was the shrine where Orestes took sanctuary.

Similar views have been prominent in other cultures too. In India, the *Rig-Veda* depicts the navel of the Uncreated upon which lay the seed of the world, and it was from Vishnu's navel, recumbent upon the primeval ocean, whence arose the Lotus of the universal manifestation. In Hindu thinking, the navel is the 'motionless hub of the wheel'; it may alternatively be viewed as the tree under which the Buddha sat when he achieved illumination at Bodhgaya.

Boundary stones set down as markers in the fields of southern India often resemble the omphalos shape, also being known as 'navel-stones'. The sacred shield of the Jews was likewise given a navel form — reflecting the belief that Jerusalem was the earth's centre. The many 'Bethels' in the Bible (for instance Jacob's sleeping place) are also associated with the navel-stone. In view of their shape, and also since, etymologically, the word 'omphalos' breaks down into *om-phallus* (i.e. penetrating shafts or arrows of enkindling light), navel-stones have been interpreted by folklorists as phallic symbols.

The Suffi people of New Mexico have assorted complicated migration myths which elucidate their search for the navel of the world. Such stories link up with origin myths about their race's appearance from the womb of the earth. Myths amongst some American Indians have held that the navel of the universe is the origin of the four winds. In the sky, the Pole Star, around which the firmament appears to turn, has been styled the 'navel of the Heavens'.

Christian theology and popular traditions have sometimes addressed the troubling question as to whether those not regularly born of woman (and hence lacking an umbilical cord) would possess a navel. Should Adam and Eve be depicted with belly buttons? And, within folklorish speculation, what of naked ghosts? The naturalist and fundamentalist Christian, Philip Gosse (1810–88), wrote a book entitled *Omphalos: An Attempt to Untie the Geological Knot* (John van Voorst, London, 1857), designed to show that suchlike rationalistic speculations (not least, the origin of fossils) were necessarily impious; true religion required faith in the literal word of the Bible, without the posing of such profane questions. It was his answer to the evolutionary controversy.

The belly button has thus provided a major focus for speculations upon the origins both of individuals and of the universe at large. Its shape and nature suggest both links and ruptures.

ROY PORTER

See also UMBILICAL CORD.

Bernard, Claude

Bernard, Claude Claude Bernard (1813–78) was a key figure in French nineteenth-century science, and one of the world's great physiologists. With good reason he has been called the 'father of experimental medicine'.

Bernard was born in St Julien-en-Beaujolais, the son of a winegrower and schoolmaster. The greater part of his education was at the local Jesuit College at Villefranche; at the age of 19 he went to work for M. Millet, a pharmacist in the suburb of Lyons. At this time, Bernard's greatest enthusiasm was for the theatre — he wrote a Vaudeville, *La Rose du Rhône*, and a 5-act drama, *Artur de Bretagne*. M. Millet did not seem to be impressed, and he dispensed with Bernard's services. Bernard found himself, at age 21, in Paris, set on a career as a playwright; but Giraudin, the Professor of Literature who read his work, tactfully suggested a more reliable career.

So in 1834 Bernard became a medical student. He did not seem destined for medical fame, for he came twenty-third out of twenty six in the final examinations for his year. But he greatly admired François Magendie, who was Professor of Medicine at the Collège de France, and the most famous French physiologist of the time. Magendie would break off his ward rounds to test a point with an animal experiment, and Bernard was greatly impressed. In 1841 he became Magendie's assistant ('*préparateur*') and his career as a physiologist began.

His early findings were not striking: thus his MD thesis claimed that the acid in gastric juice was lactic (rather than hydrochloric) acid — a finding from experiments on rabbits, whose gastric juice often contains this acid produced by secondary fermentation. Towards the end of the 1840s, though, he began a series of remarkable discoveries. He began by showing that the PANCREAS, secreting its juice into the duodenum, was capable of digesting foodstuffs. Up to this time the stomach had been thought to be paramount in the process of digestion and the pancreas was believed to be an abdominal salivary gland. Then he demonstrated that both pancreatic juice and BILE were necessary for the absorption of fat from the gut. In 1850 the Académie des Sciences awarded him its prize in Experimental Physiology for his work on the pancreas.

Continuing with his nutritional theme, he proceeded to show that sugar absorbed from the gut was stored in an insoluble form in the liver. Bernard demonstrated that in fasting conditions this insoluble form released its sugar into the blood. He called it '*glycogenic*' (sugar-forming), and subsequently isolated the pure substance, GLYCOGEN, in 1857. Many consider its discovery to be Bernard's greatest achievement. He described the release of glucose from glycogen as 'internal secretion'; unfortunately, when hormones were discovered half a century later, the phrase was also used to describe their entry into the blood — a very different biological process.

Bernard was always intrigued by the role of nerves in controlling the activities of the body, and in 1852 he showed how nerves controlled the diameter of blood vessels, and hence blood flow. His observation was simple enough, but required sound anatomical knowledge: cutting the cervical sympathetic nerve on one side in the neck raised the temperature of the skin on that side of the head. Electrical stimulation of the cut end of the nerve reversed the change, so that Bernard concluded that under normal circumstances the nerve was narrowing the diameter of skin blood vessels: it had a 'vasoconstrictor' function. This 'vasomotor' activity of nerves laid the foundation for the concept of the AUTONOMIC NERVOUS SYSTEM, whose inception had to wait for another forty years or so.

In 1855 Magendie died, and Bernard succeeded him as Professor of Medicine at the Collège de France. His wife felt let down by his lifestyle: she had expected to lead the life of a prosperous physician's wife. Instead Bernard treated no patients, and spent most of his time on animal experiments. Mme Bernard and the daughters disapproved so strongly of his life that they set up a home for stray animals, many of whom, it was said, were subjects of Bernard's experiments. Shortly afterwards he separated from his wife and two daughters. (He had married in 1845.)

His lectures at the Collège de France were published and one of these, in 1859, contained perhaps his most fertile idea. He saw the animal's external environment ('*le milieu extérieur*') as constantly changing: but the composition of the fluids within the body ('*le milieu intérieur*') was kept remarkably constant, so protecting the cells of the body from the vicissitudes of the external environment. This constancy (HOMEOSTASIS) has provided many subsequent scientists with a first step in understanding the body's activities. Many of Bernard's ideas on the internal milieu came from his observations on BLOOD SUGAR.

His health started to deteriorate — though no exact diagnosis of his chronic abdominal pain was made. In 1863 he published nothing and went to live in his house and vineyard in St Julien. During his enforced leisure he tried to provide some sort of rationale to his science, and collected his thoughts in a book, *An introduction to experimental medicine*. This was published in 1865. Bernard believed that there was no 'life-force' (vitalism was a common belief at the time). The only sure way forward in experimental medicine was to design experiments in which every variable was controlled. Furthermore, every experiment should be based on a hypothesis; if the hypothesis were disproved, it should be changed, and the experiment repeated.

The *Introduction* was a great success. The rather disreputable world of the animal experimenter was transformed into an intellectually attractive system of enquiry. It was written with style, and so was read by people who would otherwise have no interest in physiology. Among its admirers was a businessman's wife, Mme Raffalovich, who became Bernard's companion in his last years. The *Introduction* led to Bernard's election to the French Academy in 1868.

His health improved, and he returned to lecturing. But he did little new research, except — in the last year of his life, 1877 — to work on a new theory of alcoholic fermentation. Rather unfortunately, his experimental notes were published after his death, and they were found to contradict some of the findings of his friend Louis Pasteur. In his final days he was diagnosed as having pyelonephritis, a kidney infection, and was nursed by Mme Raffalovich and her daughter, who tactfully withdrew from the room whenever Bernard had a visitor. His death was marked by a ceremonial state funeral: no French scientist had ever been so honoured. His pupil Paul Bert, in a memorable funeral oration, declared 'No one ever made discoveries more simply, more naïvely. He discovered as others breathed.'

JOHN HENDERSON

Further reading
Bernard, C. (1949). *An introduction to the study of experimental medicine*, (trans. H. C. Greene), introduction by L. J. Henderson. Henry Schuman, New York.

Bertillon system

Bertillon system The Bertillon System, invented by French criminologist Alphonse Bertillon in 1879, was a technique for describing individuals on the basis of a catalogue of physical measurements, including standing height, sitting height (length of trunk and head), distance between fingertips with arms outstretched, and size of head, right ear, left foot, digits, and forearm. In addition, distinctive personal features, such as eye colour, scars, and deformities, were noted. The system was used to identify CRIMINALS in the later years of the nineteenth century, but was soon displaced by the more reliable and easily-recorded FINGERPRINTS.

COLIN BLAKEMORE

Bicarbonate

Bicarbonate A salt of carbonic acid, or the dissociated ion HCO_3^-. The extracellular fluids of the body (blood plasma and tissue fluid) contain 20–25 mmol/litre of bicarbonate (about a quarter of the concentration of chloride). Regulation of its concentration (by the KIDNEYS) relative to that of carbon dioxide (altered by changes in BREATHING) is crucial to the function of maintaining ACID–BASE HOMEOSTASIS. Ingestion of bicarbonate is a common remedy for 'INDIGESTION', because it neutralises stomach acid.

S.J.

See ACID–BASE HOMEOSTASIS; BODY FLUIDS.

Biceps

Biceps One of the muscles for bending the ELBOW, and therefore a determinant of strength for lifting — the glass to the lips, or loads a great deal heavier. Being a discrete and visible muscle, especially when well-developed, it is often displayed as the epitomy of BODY-BUILDING. It is so-named because it has two 'heads'; both are attached to the *scapula* (shoulder blade) above the SHOULDER joint. Each 'head' swells into the dual belly of the muscle; this gathers below into a short tendon spanning the front of the elbow joint to be attached on the upper end of the radius.   S.J.

See PLATE 5.

Bile is a greenish-yellow fluid produced by the LIVER, and passing from there into the DUODE-NUM; it has a number of functions, which will be described shortly. But bile also has a remarkable history, for in early medicine bile made up two of the four HUMOURS, which were blood, phlegm, yellow bile, and black bile. For about 2000 years an excess of black bile was thought to make patients melancholic, and an excess of yellow bile to make them choleric.

> But let your friends in verse suppose
> What ne'er shall be allowed in prose,
> Anatomists can make it clear
> The liver minds its own affair;
> And parts and strains the vital juices,
> Still layes some useful bile aside,
> To tinge the chyles insipid tide;
> Else we should want both bile and satire
> And all be burst with pure good nature.

> Matthew Prior, 1664–1721

The belief that bile had such a profound effect on human nature disappeared in the early nineteenth century, when humoral medicine was overtaken by the new scientific rationalism.

Bile is a complex biochemical mixture, made continuously by the liver — 500–1000 ml/day passing down into the duodenum via the bile duct. There is a diversion in this journey: a small 50 ml sac — the gall bladder — fills with bile from the liver, and, by absorbing water across its walls, concentrates bile 5–6-fold. Shortly after a meal the gall bladder contracts and empties, and the concentrated bile is added to the partially digested food ('chyles insipid tide' in Prior's poem above). Bile has two broad functions: it plays a *digestive* role in the breakdown and absorption of fat, and it *excretes* substances from blood which cannot be excreted by the kidneys. These substances are usually fat soluble; they may be produced by the body, or come from outside, like drugs. In composition, bile is 97% *water*; its other major components are *bile salts*, CHOLESTEROL, *phospholipids, bile pigments*, and *electrolytes* (minerals).

Bile acids and bile salts

The function of these remarkable molecules is inextricably involved with cholesterol. The two main bile acids, cholic acid and chenodeoxycholic acid, are both made from cholesterol in the liver and pass into the bile in combination with amino acids, as bile salts. Cholesterol is virtually insoluble in water, and in the words of the 1989 Nobel prizewinners, Brown and Goldstein, 'Cholesterol is a Janus-faced molecule. The very property that makes it useful in the cell membrane, namely its insolubility in water, also makes it lethal.' (The

authors were referring to the crucial part played by cholesterol in the pathological process of atherosclerosis.) So the body has resorted to some remarkable strategies to excrete this difficult substance, and it seems that cholesterol excreted by the liver is partly extracted from the circulation and partly made by the liver itself. The body's main strategy is to use bile salts as detergents: the molecules have a water-soluble (*hydrophilic*) side and a fat-soluble (*hydrophobic*) side. This enables bile salts to make small parcels ('*micelles*') including several different molecules, with cholesterol as contents and bile salts as the wrapping. The hydrophobic aspect of the bile salt faces inwards, and the hydrophilic aspect faces outwards into the aqueous component of bile.

The bile micelles pass into the duodenum, where the detergent action of the bile salts emulsifies fats, which are then broken down by the ENZYME lipase from the PANCREAS. Bile salts also assist the final absorption of the products of fat digestion. Both bile and lipase are necessary for the proper absorption of FATS by the small intestine. Without one or other of these two, there is deficiency of the vital fat-soluble VITA-MINS, A, D, E and K, and malabsorption causes fat to appear in the faeces (*steatorrhoea*).

Bile salts pass down the entire length of the small intestine, but instead of their being degraded or excreted in faeces, a remarkable phenomenon occurs. The bile salts are absorbed as whole molecules at the far end of the small intestine (the terminal ileum) and pass up the portal vein to the liver, whence they are re-secreted into bile. This circuit, known as the *entero-hepatic circulation*, represents extraordinary parsimony, for at any one time only 3–5 g of bile acids are present in the body; this 3–5 g is known as the bile acid pool, and it circulates 6–10 times a day. About 0.5 g of bile acids is lost in the faeces per day, which means that an average bile acid molecule survives in the entero-hepatic circulation for about 3 days, making 18–30 cycles. During this time, it will escort many hydrophobic molecules (such as cholesterol) into the small intestine, and help with the emulsification and absorption of a significant quantity of fat. We have no idea why the body should indulge in this metabolic penny-pinching. If the terminal ileum is diseased, or has to be surgically removed, the bile acids pass into the colon, where they produce watery diarrhoea.

It is of interest that vitamin B_{12} is also absorbed from the terminal ileum, and passes up the portal vein; the liver metabolizes some of it and the products pass into the watery phase of the bile; reabsorption provides an entero-hepatic circulation. Vitamins B_{12} cannot be synthesized in the body, so this is an appropriate device for conservation of a precious molecule. Damage to, or surgical removal of, the terminal ileum produces the syndrome of pernicious ANAEMIA, a consequence of vitamin B_{12} deficiency.

Cholesterol gallstones

The commonest disorder of bile formation is the presence of gallstones, and the commonest type

of gallstone consists of cholesterol, which comes out of solution in the gall bladder. Gallstones cause symptoms by passing out of the gall bladder and obstructing the bile duct; the time-honoured treatment consists of surgically removing the gall bladder. More recently, stones have been treated medically, by increasing the bile acid/cholesterol ratio of bile. This is achieved simply by taking synthetic bile acids by mouth. Unfortunately it may take many months to dissolve existing gallstones, and even if it does have the desired effect, the patient will need to take bile acids indefinitely to prevent the recurrence of stones. Stones can also be disintegrated inside the gall bladder by the ingenious use of high frequency waves ('*lithotrypsy*').

Some races (Finns, Swedes and North American Indian women) have high cholesterol/ bile acid ratios in their bile, and are very prone to gallstones. These races have a high animal fat diet, rich in cholesterol. In races whose diets contain little animal fat (Japanese and Masai for example) the bile contains little cholesterol, and gallstones are rare — but the formation of cholesterol stones is not just a question of diet. It has been found that the cholesterol concentration of bile varies with the time of day, for example, which makes the phenomenon of cholesterol crystallisation much more difficult to analyse.

Bile pigments

The life of red blood cells is about 120 days, and their death is associated with the release of *haemoglobin*, which makes up the greater part of the red cells. *Macrophages* are chiefly responsible for their destruction; the globin protein is reused, while the haem is detached from the iron, which is also reused. Haem is a ring (*tetrapyrrole*) structure and cannot be reused. Within the macrophage the ring is broken, and the four constituent pyrrole groups are arranged in a straight chain — *biliverdin* (green) — and finally *bilirubin* (yellow). The changes in skin seen after bruising represent this conversion, for blood produced by the bruise is taken up by the local macrophages, and the blood in the macrophage undergoes the red to green to yellow conversion.

Under normal circumstances, bilirubin is released by the macrophage into blood. Bilirubin is insoluble in water, and is transported in blood by being attached to very large molecules, *plasma albumin*. When this bound bilirubin reaches the liver it separates from the plasma protein, and enters the liver cell, but, because of its insolubility, some device needs to be employed by the liver to incorporate it into bile. The way that the liver achieves this is not to include it in the centre of a micelle, but to attach, or conjugate, it to *glucuronic acid*, which makes the bilirubin water-soluble. (The yellow-green colour of bile is derived from bilirubin.)

Conjugated bilirubin (or *bilirubin glucuronide*) passes down the bile duct in the bile; unlike bile salts, it has no role in digestion. It passes into the intestine, where bacterial action converts it to *urobilinogen*, which is very water-soluble. Some urobilinogen is absorbed across the gut wall and passes into the blood whence it may be either re-secreted into bile (as an entero-hepatic circulation), or excreted by the kidneys. It is urobilinogen that gives urine its yellow colour. The urobilinogen that is not absorbed from the gut passes down the small intestine to the colon, and its final product, *stercobilin*, gives rise to the brown colour of faeces. Bilirubin is thus a ubiquitous colouring agent.   JOHN HENDERSON

See also ALIMENTARY SYSTEM; JAUNDICE; LIVER.

Biochemistry

The science of biochemistry, nowadays regarded as one of the fundamental pillars upon which the study of medicine rests, is something of a newcomer. It has its origins almost equally in chemistry and physiology, and indeed what we would today call biochemistry was commonly referred to as *physiological chemistry* a hundred years ago. Looking further back we can trace early ideas about the make-up of living things to the birth of organic chemistry, the scope of which seems originally to have been a good deal wider than would be admitted today. In 1806 Berzelius referred to organic chemistry as 'the part of physiology which describes the composition of living bodies, and the chemical processes which occur in them. In the early nineteenth century there was a good deal of debate as to whether the chemical substances found in living things were fundamentally different in character from the 'inorganic' constituents of inanimate matter, and the issue was only resolved (in favour of no difference) with the chemical synthesis of urea by Wöhler in 1828 and by subsequent syntheses of molecules hitherto only associated with living organisms. Thereafter organic chemistry became confined to the study of carbon compounds, and knowledge of the transformations undergone by such compounds in the course of metabolism was left to be re-born as biochemistry decades later. A major influence in that re-birth was the concept of catalysis and the realisation that catalysts must play a vital part in living processes. Here the studies of Pasteur and his contemporaries in the mid nineteenth century played an indispensable part, and led to the broad unifying concept that the nature of life processes must be very similar in disparate organisms, including man, and that catalytic ENZYMES (the word literally means 'in yeast') are responsible for directing and controlling chemical transformations in the living cell.

Given the acceptance of the concept of oxidation, and the demise of the phlogiston theory, thanks to the work of Lavoisier in the late 1700s, it was natural that the early study of METABOLISM should be preoccupied with understanding the processes of respiration, breakdown of sugars, and energy generation. There was also much interest in nutrition and the chemical processes underlying the digestion of food. The identification of enzymes as proteins arose naturally from these efforts and spawned the science of *enzymology*, which remains a major division of biochemistry to the present day. The question of how enzymes work engaged the attention of many of the finest biochemical brains in the 1990s and will continue to do so for the foreseeable future. Moreover, the day is not far away when enzymologists will astonish us all by creating more or less *de novo* enzymes endowed with hitherto-unknown catalytic properties. Already 'catalytic antibodies' have been described, that bind small molecules with exquisite specificity, producing chemical change, and as knowledge of fundamental mechanisms of catalysis emerges from the efforts of physical organic chemists, the practical applications of that knowledge will not be far behind.

It was with the arrival of the twentieth century that biochemistry came of age, so to speak, and made such a major impact on medicine that it was recognised as a formidable science indispensable to the understanding of the human body. Those were the days of VITAMIN and HORMONE research. The pioneering work of Sir Frederick Gowland Hopkins (1861–1947) and his colleagues, which led to the discovery of vitamins, had a lasting influence on generations of biochemists and underpinned the unravelling of intermediary metabolism. The isolation, identification, and eventual production of hormones in sufficient quantity for therapeutic use likewise illuminated some of the most perplexing medical problems, and transformed endocrinology into an important branch of clinical science.

Biochemistry has long boasted of its roots in exact physical sciences and has never been afraid to divert the attentions of practitioners of those sciences to the study of life. By that route some of the most spectacular advances of knowledge in the twentieth century have been achieved, perhaps none more so than the birth of the *enfant terrible*, MOLECULAR BIOLOGY, which nowadays dominates the subject. Molecular biology, rooted in structural studies on proteins and nucleic acids, owes much to the contributions of far-sighted crystallographers and geneticists (aided and abetted by a cohort of physicists and even mathematicians) who built upon the bed-rock of biochemistry to produce a veritable revolution in biology that is still evolving apace. It is sometimes hard to imagine how abstract the concept of a gene was prior to the discovery of the structure of DNA by Watson and Crick in 1953, since nowadays the precise identification of genes and expectations of their manipulation (for good or ill) can be read about in newspapers intended for the man in the street. Biochemistry is no longer the academic tool of medical researchers but, having embraced its sister disciplines in the physical as well as biological sciences, has taken on new meaning as the huge promise of BIOTECHNOLOGY looms before us.

Never has it been more evident how the pace of scientific discovery is driven by technical advances in experimentation, the invention of new techniques, and the application of ideas imported from cognate disciplines. The twin sciences of molecular and cell biology have adapted the foundations laid by the painstaking 'bucket' experiments of the early biochemists to illuminate the marvels and mysteries of molecules and cells in a fashion which can only be described as spectacular. Even philosophers and theologians can no longer ignore the prospects of bio-revolution introduced into our daily lives: genetically engineered foodstuffs; super-athletes; new approaches to treating infertility; eradication of diseases. How many more triumphs (or horrors) attributable to the application of biochemically-based technology await us? And how are we going to cope with them?   M.J. WARING

Biological rhythms

Life has evolved in a rhythmic environment. For example, the daily rising and setting of the sun, and the seasonal variations in day length, temperature, and rainfall are all major factors to which the physiology and behaviour of different species must adapt in order to survive. The most obvious manifestation of human rhythmicity is the cycle of sleeping and waking. Humans are diurnal creatures; that is to say we are active during the light phase of the day and SLEEP at night. Anyone who has kept a pet hamster will know that these and many other species are nocturnal, i.e. active at night. But whilst the sleep–wake rhythm is obvious, virtually all the rest of our functions have their own, less evident rhythms. In fact it would be reasonable to say that everything that happens in our bodies is rhythmic until proved otherwise.

Many different frequencies are present in biological rhythms apart from the sleep wake (a 24-hour rhythm) and seasonal variations. The human pulse rate, at around 72 beats per minute, and the firing of nerve fibres (usually at rates up to hundred per second) are examples of rhythms with high frequencies. Population variations (most evident in sub-human species) are examples of low-frequency rhythms. The MENSTRUAL CYCLE of 28 days has been associated with the lunar cycle, but there is no proof of a definite link.

We know most about our 24-hour rhythms. It would be reasonable to assume that the setting of the sun or the extinction of artificial lights at night, perhaps combined with social conditioning to go to bed in the evening, makes us sleep. These certainly play a role, but the most important factors determining the timing (and structure) of sleep are an internal drive to sleepiness (the biological clock) together with accumulated tiredness since the last sleep. Many years ago, experiments in deep caves and in 'temporal isolation' units showed that, in the complete absence of any known time cues such as changes in the light level and ambient temperature, with no knowledge of clock time, radio, TV, newspapers, telephone, or contact with other people, humans still continue to live on an approximately 24-hour day. This observation is taken as evidence for the existence of an internal rhythm generating system of approximately 24 hours, which has come to be known as the *biological clock*.

Most people in such a time-free environment get up a little later and go to bed a little later each day: their personal in-built periodicity is slightly longer than 24 hours. The average period of the human body clock was thought to be 24.9 hours, but has recently been revised to be about 24.2 hours, on average. This natural rhythm, close to but not exactly 24 hours long, is called a circadian (meaning 'about a day') rhythm. A very few people have a periodicity shorter than 24 hours. Periodicity appears to be an inherited characteristic. Together with the sleep rhythm, many other major body functions exhibit circadian rhythms, including: secretion of HORMONES (e.g. the 'darkness' hormone melatonin, usually high at night, and the STRESS hormone cortisol, usually high in the morning); the production of urine and the variation in deep body temperature (usually low at night); the biochemical composition of the blood; alertness; and the ability to perform cognitive and dextrous tasks. Examples of rhythms that are not internally generated include the salivation and insulin responses to periodic meals.

Endogenous rhythms predict and prepare our bodies for forthcoming events: increased sleepiness in the evening prepares us for sleep, increased deep body temperature in the morning heralds wake-up. Some of the most striking examples of predictive rhythms are seasonal breeding patterns in long-lived animals. Sheep mate in the autumn and give birth in the spring — a time of year most propitious for survival of the lambs. These events are dictated by an endogenous seasonal rhythm of reproductive competence.

Since endogenous rhythms do not have exactly the same periodicity as the corresponding environmental cycle, they have to be reset by external time cues. The most potent of the signals for circadian synchronisation, in the vast majority of species, including humans, is the daily light–dark cycle. The annual change in day length is the primary cue for timing seasonal cycles in most species. An inherent rhythm that is delayed a little each day (such as the natural human circadian clock of some 24.2 hours) must obviously be advanced each day (by 0.2 hours) to stay locked to the outside world. Exposure to bright light in the early morning, shortly after the deep-body temperature reaches its minimum value, will advance the circadian rhythm, while similar exposure to light in the late evening, before the temperature minimum, will delay it. Social interactions, mealtimes, exercise, and knowledge of clock time all help to keep us synchronised.

The major internal rhythm-generating system of mammals is found within the brain, in a pair of tiny structures known as the suprachiasmatic nuclei (SCN). Each SCN is a group of a few thousand nerve cells, sited in the hypothalamus, just above the optic chiasma (the crossing of the optic nerves). Destruction of this small area in rodents abolishes nearly all circadian rhythms, although there is a supplementary 'clock' in the retina itself (at least in hamsters). Amazingly, transplantation of the SCN from one hamster to another in which it has been damaged restores

rhythmicity (of activity–rest) to the host animal, and confers on it the natural periodicity of the donor animal. It is assumed that the same would be true of humans. A small number of nerve fibres branch off from the optic nerve into the SCN. The information they carry enables the mammalian circadian rhythm generated in the SCN to be reset by light.

In most lower vertebrates, both the retina of the eye and the pineal gland in the brain are also capable of generating circadian rhythms. All rhythm-generating tissues (SCN, retina, pineal gland) show circadian rhythms of physiological activity even if they are removed and maintained, alive but isolated, in a cell culture chamber (a *clock in a dish*). Nerve cells of the SCN fire impulses in extremely regular patterns, like metronomes, and the frequency of the pattern varies with the time of day; cells of the retina and the pineal gland secrete the hormone melatonin in amounts that vary with the time of day. Each rhythm-generating cell contains a self-sustaining 'oscillator'. In the case of the retina and the pineal of lower vertebrates, the cells involved are direct photoreceptors. In some non-mammalian vertebrates the pineal gland appears to be the master clock. In the sparrow, *Passer domesticus*, for example, removal of the pineal gland leads to loss of the activity–rest rhythm, and transplantation of a pineal from another bird not only restores rhythmicity but confers the phase of the donor to the host.

The hormone *melatonin* is the main output of the 'clock' of most vertebrates so far investigated. In mammals, where the SCN is the major clock, melatonin is synthesized mostly in the pineal gland under the control of the SCN. It is normally made at night (or during the dark phase). Light serves both to synchronize the rhythm to 24 hours and to regulate the duration of nighttime secretion: in winter (long nights) the secretion profile is longer than in summer (short nights). It is this changing duration of melatonin (the darkness hormone) that acts as a time cue for the organization of seasonal physiology in

photoperiodic mammals (those that depend on daylength to time their seasonal functions). The role of melatonin in circadian organization is very important in those species that use the pineal and/or the retina as a clock. In mammals (humans and rodents) it has only modulatory effects on circadian rhythms. It probably serves to reinforce and elicit physiology and behaviour associated with darkness. And it can also act on the SCN itself, producing 'feedback' resetting of the clock.

The real importance of the biological clock is evident when things go wrong. Disturbed rhythms are found in BLINDNESS, shiftwork, jetlag, certain insomnias, some psychiatric conditions and in some elderly people. Blind people with no conscious (or even unconscious) light perception lack the external light–dark changes that normally reset the body clock each day, and hence many have problems living on a 24-hour day. They manifest their own, endogenous periodicity, which means that, every few days or weeks, when their own clock has drifted out of phase with the world, they go through periods of feeling extremely sleepy and/or napping during the day, and being wide awake at night. Night shift workers are usually unadapted: they are therefore trying to work at the lowest ebb of their alertness and performance rhythms, and have problems sleeping, out of phase, during the day. This is the probable explanation for the increase in accidents on night shifts and for the many health problems of shift workers. A similar problem occurs for people travelling quickly over many time zones (jet lag): the clock adapts only slowly to such abrupt changes of phase. There are moreover a number of other conditions of clock dysfunction, such as delayed and advanced sleep-phase syndrome, and possibly a general lack of robustness of rhythms in some elderly people.

It is reasonable to assume that improper functioning of the circadian system is deleterious to health. Since bright natural light is more effective at synchronizing rhythms than domestic

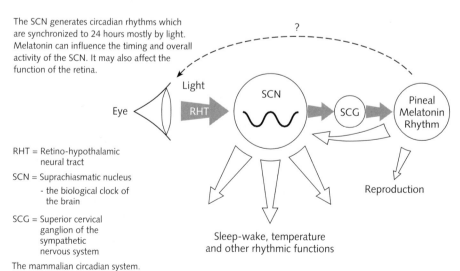

The SCN generates circadian rhythms which are synchronized to 24 hours mostly by light. Melatonin can influence the timing and overall activity of the SCN. It may also affect the function of the retina.

RHT = Retino-hypothalamic neural tract

SCN = Suprachiasmatic nucleus - the biological clock of the brain

SCG = Superior cervical ganglion of the sympathetic nervous system

The mammalian circadian system.

intensity light, urban populations (who generally live in a relatively light-deprived environment) are most at risk. Both bright artificial light and administration of melatonin at night time can be used to reinforce circadian organisation and to hasten adaptation to phase shifts, for instance as a remedy for jet lag. At present there is considerable interest among pharmaceutical companies in the development of artificial analogues of melatonin.   JOSEPHINE ARENDT

Further reading

Arendt J. (1995). *Melatonin and the mammalian pineal gland*. Chapman Hall, London, New York.

Miller, J. D., Morin, I. P., Schwartz, W. J. and Moore, R. Y. (1996). New insights into the mammalian circadian clock. *Sleep* **8** 641–67.

Biological warfare The deliberate spread of agents that cause disease is not just subject matter for thrillers, nor a concern of recent origin. History is replete with examples. The Greeks and Romans provide some of the earliest through their practice of polluting drinking water supplies with corpses. Emulation of this activity occurred in both the American Civil War and the Boer War. Thus cholera and typhoid, both waterborne diseases, may have been two early biological warfare agents.

A more calculated approach, perhaps, was the throwing of the bodies of plague victims over the walls of cities under siege. This stratagem was employed successfully both by the Tartars against the Genoese in the Crimean War of 1346, and in the Russo-Swedish Wars of 1710. Equally scheming was the request of the then British commander-in-chief in North America, Sir Jeffrey Amherst, to encourage the spread of smallpox among 'disaffected tribes of Indians'. Unbeknown to the commander, a subordinate had similar thoughts, handing over, as presents to hostile chiefs, two blankets and a handkerchief from the smallpox hospital. The desired effect followed. In unvaccinated cases some 30% die of the disease within 9–12 days.

More sophisticated methods for spreading bacteria and viruses are now available to the military. The secret lies in ensuring that the organisms are live and viable after dissemination from a grenade, shell, bomb, or missile, or from the spray tank of an aircraft drone. All of these devices have been investigated for their usefulness as delivery vehicles, with some being more effective than others, suitability being as much a feature of the agent being carried as of the battlefield conditions.

Viability both before and after weaponization are equally important for candidate biological warfare agents. Most biological agents have a limited life, with their activity continually declining in storage unless steps are taken to slow the process down. Low-temperature storage or freeze-drying will help retain activity.

Bacteria or viruses would usually be delivered in a finely-dispersed aerosol with liquid droplet sizes ranging from 1 to 5 micrometres — small enough to enable penetration deep into the lungs. Agents unstable in aerosols might be spread in a powder or slurry, efficiency of dispersal being a key requirement.

Candidate biological warfare agents are those that resist environmental degradation through changes in temperature, humidity, or ultraviolet light. Even anthrax, long a favourite biological warfare agent, and renowned for its environmental persistence, will not survive under all circumstances. The wrong temperature, rate of temperature change, or degree of humidity will prevent anthrax bacteria forming spores, the spores being a form of hibernation in which the bacteria can survive more extreme environmental changes, yet retain infectivity.

Anthrax has a considerable biological warfare pedigree. The infectivity of the bacteria was studied on Russian and Chinese detainees, following deliberate contamination by Japanese scientists; some 3000 human subjects in total died as a result of Japanese experimentation, with a range of bacteria and viruses, at Camp 731 in Manchuria during 1938–45. The fruits of this research boosted the US offensive biological warfare programme. Japanese scientists received immunity from prosecution for war crimes by the US in exchange for research results. Less is known about the Soviet programme, but the accidental venting into the air of less than 1 g of anthrax from a military, microbiology laboratory, in Sverdousk in April 1979, led to at least 64 deaths. Thus, it would appear that anthrax was also a part of the Soviet biological warfare programme.

Prior to 1969, the US had an offensive biological weapons programme, with at least eight bacteria and viruses in munitions. A unilateral decision by President Richard Nixon led to their destruction between 1970–1, paving the way for the 1972 *Biological Weapons Convention* (BWC). This prohibits the development, production, stockpiling, transfer, acquisition, or retention of weapons based on bacteria, viruses, or toxins.

The former Soviet Union was a signatory to this Convention, and as such was obliged to disarm. However, as late as 1992, evidence from scientists defecting to the West indicated that an offensive biological warfare programme, run by the State Security Service, the KGB, was still functioning. This programme was stopped by the Russian Federation President, Boris Yeltsin, shortly after it became public knowledge.

No international mechanism exists to police the BWC. Negotiations under the auspices of the UN Conference on Disarmament are continuing to secure a treaty with powers analogous to the *Chemical Weapons Convention* (CWC). Formidable obstacles will need to be overcome before a treaty is ready for signature.

Given the support the CWC received from the chemical industry world-wide, negotiators will be looking to the pharmaceutical industry for equal encouragement to help secure a more robust biological weapons treaty. Culture facilities, such as those employed by the pharmaceutical industry, are required to produce the quantities of agents needed for biological weapons. Attempts were made by Russian scientists, at the Institute of Especially Pure Biopreparations in St Petersburg, to increase the infectivity of plague for use as a biological warfare agent. The plague bacterium under research at this vaccine production facility had developed resistance to sixteen different antibiotics. There is concern that other scientists may be tempted to try to alter the performance characteristics of more candidate biological warfare agents. The expertise and technology necessary to perform this work is becoming more prevalent.

Defences against biological warfare agents will always be limited. Predicting the likely agent(s) that will be used in war is guesswork, and hence vaccination, even if it were possible for a few, can never provide complete protection. Given the continuing interest in biological warfare, and the evidence that Iraq had produced significant quantities of several bacteria, including anthrax, a prescriptive treaty is long overdue. A new treaty will need to ensure that developing countries still have access to technology; that commercial sensitivities are taken into account; and that there are sufficient powers of inspection to detect illicit manufacture. Without a robust treaty, military defence budgets will escalate, but no sum of money will be sufficient to guarantee protection. Only a disarmament regime can provide this security.   ALASTAIR HAY

See also MICROORGANISMS; WAR AND THE BODY.

Bionic man Human life-form integrated with robotic and cybernetic mechanisms. The possibility of a species of bionic men and women has been elaborately imagined in science fiction portrayals of alien races such as 'The Borg' in the Paramount television series *Star Trek The Next Generation*. The scientists responsible for creating a bionic man on Earth in the science fiction television series of the 1970s, *The Six Million-Dollar Man*, claimed that 'We have the technology, we can build him,' but success in transferring fiction into fact has been minimal. While human life has been supported by devices such as heart PACEMAKERS, the development of robotic PROSTHESES for limb and organ replacement remains primitive.

During World War II, American social scientists and physical scientists were mobilised to assist the war effort by developing a range of activities from psychological warfare to breaking intelligence codes and building atomic weapons. Following the war a collection of war-service scientists in the US attempted to explore an interdisciplinary route to developing artificial intelligence that could mimic human behaviour. This group, which included social scientists Lawrence Franck, Margaret Mead, and Gregory Bateson, and mathematicians Norbert Weiner and Jon von Neumann, set up a series of conferences funded by the Josiah Macy Jr Foundation, which met annually between 1946–53 and became known as the 'cybernetics group'. Weiner became a leading figure in post-war cybernetics and the work achieved through the Macy Conferences helped to construct the discipline that now informs the study of both artificial and human intelligence.

Although substantial advances have subsequently been made in the study of robotics, especially in the context of space and military research, the development of either completely artificial or combined artificial and human life-forms remains a distant cybernetic goal. The sophisticated integration of robotic circuitry with organic life-forms, such as that achieved by 'The Borg', may yet have to wait until the twenty-fourth century.   DOROTHY PORTER

Further reading

Heims, S. J. (1991). *Constructing a social science for Postwar America. The Cybernetics Group 1946–1953*. MIT Press, Cambridge, MA.

See also AUTOMATA; CYBERNETICS.

Biopsy

Biopsy A piece of tissue taken from a patient during life to establish a precise diagnosis so that the most appropriate treatment can be initiated. Usually a thin section of the specimen on a glass slide is examined by a pathologist under a microscope, but if the specimen is small and soft it may be more appropriate to make a smear on the slide. On occasion the biopsy may require to be examined biochemically. Biopsies may also be taken, for example, from *chorionic villi* (the projections of fetal tissue around the early embryo after it is embedded in the womb) for chromosomal analysis when a hereditary disorder is suspected.

The technique of biopsy is vital in all branches of medicine. Various methods are used. The simplest is a *scraping* from an accessible site such as the SKIN, or from a mucous membrane, such as in the mouth or the cervix of the womb. One of the commonest is a *needle biopsy* when a small sample is sucked out into some type of syringe through a needle of a calibre appropriate to the consistency of the tissue. This method is applicable to obtaining tissue from the BREAST, KIDNEY, LIVER, BRAIN, or HEART.

In other situations a lesion is biopsied by a surgeon either at an operation undertaken just for that purpose, or in the course of an exploratory procedure. Often only part of the lesion being investigated is taken at operation — an *incisional biopsy*, but if the lesion is small, such as an ulcer, a pigmented spot on the skin, or a lymph node it may be removed in its entirety: an *excision biopsy*. Procedures of this type involve the use of a scalpel. Other instruments may be appropriate: a *curette* is used to take scrapings from the inner lining of the womb (the *endometrium*); small biopsies may be obtained by ENDOSCOPY — from the LUNGS during bronchoscopy, or from the lining of the STOMACH or COLON. Occasionally specially designed instruments are used, in the form of 'punches' or 'brushes'.

One of the commonest reasons for undertaking a biopsy is to establish whether a tumour is malignant or benign. A common example of this is the investigation of a lump in a woman's breast. In such circumstances the pathologist often undertakes an immediate microscopical examination while the patient is still in the operating theatre, the surgeon waiting for the result before deciding how extensive an operation is required. This is also a common procedure during operations for TUMOURS of the brain, or for CANCERS in other sites when lymph nodes need to be examined to establish whether or not they have been invaded by malignant cells.

Apart from the assessment of malignancy, biopsies are taken to examine organs such as the liver or kidneys for evidence of intrinsic disease, or to look for any signs of rejection of a transplanted organ such as a kidney or a heart.

Needle biopsies of SKELETAL MUSCLES are often taken because of the problems frequently encountered in distinguishing clinically among conditions caused by disease in the muscle itself (myositis, muscular dystrophy) and those secondary to an abnormality in its nerve supply.

Healthy individuals are not always exempt — for example they may be recruited as volunteers for muscle biopsy. Enthusiasm for competitive sport and interest in the health-promoting effects of exercise in recent decades have provided an increasing incentive (and funds) for improving knowledge about skeletal muscle and the effects upon it of various training and dietary regimes. Needle biopsy of muscles has become a standard component of investigations in major research laboratories for sport and exercise science.   J. HUME ADAMS

See also CANCER; MUSCLE; NEOPLASM; TRANSPLANTATION.

Biotechnology

Biotechnology is unique amongst the three principal technologies for the twenty-first century — information technology, materials science, and biotechnology — in being a sustainable technology based on renewable biological resources. Such natural resources include animals, plants, yeasts, and microorganisms and have formed mankind's nascent food and beverage industry for several millennia. However, the modern era of scientific biotechnology commenced with the elucidation of the structure of DNA by Watson and Crick in 1953 and the subsequent development of the tools to cleave and resplice genetic material in the early 1970s. Not surprisingly, therefore, the term 'biotechnology' is generally considered synonymous with gene splicing and other forms of genetic engineering. In practice, however, biotechnology refers to a library of advanced scientific tools for the manipulation of biological organisms, systems, or components for the production of goods or services in all sectors of human activity.

The early years of the 'new' biotechnology focused on the technologies required to clone, overexpress, purify, and administer biopharmaceuticals such as INSULIN, GROWTH HORMONE, factor VIII (deficient in haemophilia), and erythropoietin, with some 200 other PROTEINS currently in the pipeline. However, in the future, the most significant breakthroughs in human medicine will result from mapping and understanding the *human genome* — in elucidating the exact sequence of the billions of nucleotides that constitute the estimated 30 000–40 000 genes that are the collective blueprint for human beings and are responsible for some 10 000 genetic disorders. The Human Genome Project was launched in 1990 as a 15-year, $3 billion international effort to map and sequence all human genes. Innovations in sequencing technology have ensured that the project moved ahead of schedule. With less than 5% of all human genes identified at the start of the project, it has become increasingly clear that each new gene discovery proffers new drugs for the diagnosis, treatment, and prevention of human disease. These drugs include therapeutic proteins, diagnostics, gene therapy reagents, and small molecules. A significant proportion of the human genome has been sequenced and many new human disease genes are being characterized. These advances will enable biotechnologists not only to measure disease potential and expand the applications for genomic diagnostics but also to devise fundamental new therapeutic approaches.

Genomics and genetic engineering are also playing a substantial role in the development of *agricultural biotechnology*. This sector is finally moving out from under the shadow of the biopharmaceutical community and is now competing in terms of publicity and investor attention. This is because $1 billion is considered an attractive market in the biopharmaceutical industry, whilst global agricultural markets can readily top $10 billion and the total end-use value of food, fibre, and biomass is estimated to be over $1500 billion. The addressable market on which value can be added and costs cut is at least 6–7 times that of its pharmaceutical counterpart. Two of the factors that have encouraged biotechnologists to enter the genetically engineered food and plant arena are the desire of consumers for better tasting foods and a preference for products grown using fewer pesticides. Calgene was the first company to market a genetically improved tomato which could be ripened on the vine without softening and thereby result in improved taste and texture. Antisense technology was used to inhibit the enzyme polygalacturonase which degrades pectin in the cell wall. Similarly, laurate Canola is the world's first oilseed crop that has been genetically engineered to modify oil composition. Laurate is the key raw material used in the manufacture of soap, detergent, food, oleochemical, and personal care products. Other examples of transgenic agricultural crops include high stearate and myristate oils, low saturate oils, high solids tomatoes and potatoes, sweet minipeppers, modified lignin in paper pulp trees, pesticide-resistant plants, and biodegradeable plastics.

The early goals in the development of *transgenic livestock* were the increase of the meat and of the production characteristics of food animals. However, long research and development timelines and low projected profit margins, especially in developed nations where food is relatively inexpensive, have shifted priorities to the production of protein pharmaceuticals and nutraceuticals in the milk of transgenic animals. Milk has a high natural protein content and is sequestered in a gland where its proteins exert little direct systemic effect. It provides a renewable production system that is capable of complex and specific 'post-translational processing': that is, modifications to the protein that occur after it has been synthesised as a polypeptide (such as conjugation with carbohydrate moieties), which can alter the biological or therapeutic properties of the protein. Such changes cannot easily be accomplished in conventional cell culture systems. As a result, the 'biopharming' focus has shifted to the production of human blood plasma proteins and other therapeutic proteins, in ruminants such as cows, sheep, and goats which are easy to milk.

Marine organisms are also capable of producing a variety of polymers, adhesives, and compounds for cosmetics and food preparation. Bioactive natural products are found in organisms that reside in areas which stretch from easily accessible intertidal zones to depths in excess of 1000 m. Collaborations between marine chemists, molecular pharmacologists, and cell biologists have yielded an impressive library of potentially useful cancer, viral, antibiotic, anti-inflammatory, cardiovascular, and CNS drugs.

The pharmaceutical, agrichemical, and speciality chemical industries are increasingly requiring molecules which have distinct left- or right-handed forms, so-called *chiral compounds*. Whilst chemical and biological techniques for producing single left- or right-handed forms are developing apace, it is apparent that no single approach is likely to dominate. Suppliers and customers alike must continue to draw upon the entire range of chemical, enzymatic, and whole-organism tools that are available to produce chiral compounds. Unfortunately, only 10% of the 25 000 or so ENZYMES found in nature have been identified and characterised, and, of these, only 25 are produced in large quantities. Despite some duplication in activity among enzymes, there is a need to characterise more in order to exploit their unique specificity and activity. However, barriers to enzyme scale-up include product inhibition and a general reluctance on the part of chemists to use water-based reagents in systems which are traditionally non-aqueous. Consequently, enzymes should be made more user-friendly both for bench chemists exploring novel synthetic strategies and for all stages in pharmaceutical scale-up. However, the biologists' toolbox for catalysis is expanding. For decades, there were only two types of catalyst — metals and enzymes — but since 1986 two new

classes of biocatalyst have emerged along with the enzymes, ribozymes, and catalytic antibodies. These novel biocatalysts are prepared both by classical biochemical and immunological methods and by recombinant and phage display technologies. Whilst there are still many catalysts still to be discovered, such biocatalysts will have to exhibit improved performance, stability, turnover numbers, specificity, and product yields.

Biotechnology is also playing a role in *'clean' manufacturing*. Nevertheless, various types of chemical manufacturing, metal plating, wood preserving, and petroleum refining industries currently generate hazardous wastes, comprising volatile organics, chlorinated and petroleum hydrocarbons, solvents, and heavy metals. *Bioremediation* with microbial consortia is being investigated as a means of cleaning up hazardous sites. Methods include *in situ* and *ex situ* treatment of contaminated soil, groundwater, industrial wastewater, sludges, soil slurries, marine oil spills, and vapour-phase effluvia.

Biotechnology is expected to contribute massively to the *global economy*, largely through the introduction of recombinant DNA technology to the production of biopharmaceuticals. In the future, biotechnology will concentrate on the complexity and interrelatedness of biology, with such targets as the human genome project; genetic medicine; gene and cell therapy; tissue engineering; vaccines; factors for transcribing DNA into RNA; signal transduction and the control of gene expression; managing ageing at the level of programmed cell death, and genes that control cell division; neurobiotechnology; agri-industrial biotechnology; drug delivery; cell adhesion and communication; and novel diagnostics. Needless to say, and subject to clarification of certain ethical and public acceptance issues, biotechnology is set to make an indelible contribution to human health and welfare well into the foreseeable future.

C. R. LOWE

Bipedalism When an animal is capable of walking or running on two feet, it is said to be *bipedal* or to show bipedalism. Hence, bipedalism is a style of locomotion. Many animals show bipedalism, some of them habitually (for example, birds and humans) and some sporadically (e.g. some lizards and anthropoid apes). Animals that are capable of bipedal locomotion show anatomical adaptations to this mode of GAIT.

It is instructive to compare a gorilla with a modern human. When a gorilla stands on all fours — its habitual position — its spinal column is at an oblique angle to the ground, not parallel to the ground as in most completely quadrupedal animals. In this position the gorilla's weight-line (or 'centre of gravity' line) falls between the forelimbs and the hind limbs. When the human being stands or walks in the upright position, the axis of the body mass passes from the joint at the base of the cranium, close to the vertebral column, through the hip joints, and

down the lower limbs to meet the ground between the feet.

The conversion of the gorilla's pattern of structure and function to that of humans involves changes of bones, joints, ligaments, and muscles. Adjustments of the SKELETON include alterations at the base of the cranium and of the head–neck alignment: these modifications result in a head which does not hang forward from an oblique spinal column (as in apes), but which is well balanced on an upright column.

Secondly, the SPINAL COLUMN itself develops structural mechanisms for the transmission of body weight down the spinal column to the upper part of the sacrum, and thence through the sacro-iliac joints (the joints between the sacrum and the left and right hip-bones).

Thirdly, substantial differences are seen between the HIP bones of quadrupedal and bipedal primates, involving also the locomotor and postural muscles attached to the hip bones.

Fourthly, there are striking structural differences in the size and form of the head and neck of the femur (thighbone), in the length, curvature, and form of the shaft of this bone; in the structure and function of the KNEE joint; and in the ANKLE, foot, and toes.

There are also other skeletal differences. For instance, there is a restructuring of the upper limb, from shoulder to fingers, as that limb ceases to be employed for locomotion, and becomes an instrument for carrying and for manipulating.

How did bipedal locomotion develop in human evolution? Fortunately, remains of relevant parts of the skeleton from South and East Africa have thrown light on the way in which bipedalism evolved.

The fossils show that elements of the human bipedal complex were developed early in hominisation. However, it would be wrong to imagine that all of the anatomical adaptations to bipedalism appeared at the same time. There is much evidence that many structural and functional complexes evolved piecemeal: some items appeared early, others later; some metamorphosed rapidly, others slowly. We call such patterns of change *mosaic evolution*. The structural complex which makes bipedalism possible is an example. Bipedalism did not arrive on our planet ready-made, but developed in a stepwise manner. For example, the *ilium* (the flared upper part) of the hip bone is distinctive in humans of today, compared with apes. The ilium of ape men of the genus *Australopithecus*, which lived in Africa from four to one million years ago, was much more like that of a modern human than that of an ape; yet it showed features in which it was not perfectly human. The muscles that attached to this bone must have operated in a somewhat different manner from ours. Further changes must have affected the hip bone in later stages, bringing it into line with the structure found in today's human bipeds. Similarly, the foot — an exquisite organ, which permits skilled movements such as ballet dancing and karate —

did not arrive at one giant leap. There is evidence for several stages in the conversion of an ape-like foot to a human-like foot. At least some early African hominids, it seems, possessed feet in which the great toe was separated from the lateral four toes, somewhat as in a chimpanzee's foot. It was a more mobile big toe than in modern humans. Yet such a foot was part of the skeleton of a hominid which was bipedal. The knee joint of *Australopithecus*, too, was in some respects chimpanzee-like and not fully humanised. The shoulder complex of *Australopithecus* showed the persistence of ape-like features, which has given support to the view that the ape men were capable of functioning in the trees or arboreally, for part of the time, while going bipedally on the ground at other times.

The bipedalism practised by modern humans is a *striding gait*. In this form of locomotion a major part is played by the tilting of the pelvis: alternately it tilts downwards to the right, enabling the left limb to clear the ground as it moves forward; and downwards to the left, so that the right limb can stride forwards without the sole of the foot scraping the ground. This tilting of the pelvis is effected by the gluteal muscles, which connect the ilium of the hip bone to the lower limb. If the tilting mechanism is less well developed, as may have been the case in some australopithecines, there is an alternative way in which a lower limb may move forwards without scraping along the ground. In this method, the lower limb that is going forwards is simultaneously *abducted* (swung sideways). This enables it to clear the ground and it is free to move forwards. The process is then repeated for the other limb. This form of bipedal locomotion is a *waddling gait*. It was probably the kind of locomotion used by some or all species of *Australopithecus*, before the striding pattern emerged.

We realise that not only are there different kinds of bipedalism, but also there are differing degrees of adaptation to bipedalism. Moreover, the attainment of bipedalism must have occurred without jeopardy to the other crucial role of the pelvis, as the birth canal.

P. TOBIAS

See also EVOLUTION, HUMAN; JOINTS; PELVIS; SKELETON; WALKING.

Birth Although childbirth is a universal fact of human physiology, where, how, with whom, and even when a woman gives birth are often culturally determined.

Anthropological awareness of the social nature of human birth owes much to the pioneering work of Wenda Trevathan, an evolutionary anthropologist who studied the differences between human and higher primate birth. Because higher primates walk on all fours, their pelvis is wide enough to allow the direct descent of the fetal head, making for easy labours and uncomplicated births. When humans began to walk on two feet, the upright stance they had to adopt made the pelvis narrower, so that the baby

has to rotate as it descends in order to pass through. Non-human primate babies can climb onto their mothers' backs and cling immediately after birth, but the larger brains of human infants made it necessary for them to be born earlier in their developmental cycle, ensuring that human babies would be relatively helpless at birth and require immediate nurturing. These factors encouraged the evolution of birth as a highly social process; women give birth alone and unaided in only a very few societies.

For these reasons, Trevathan postulated that midwifery evolved along with human birth. The presence of other women would have enhanced the success of the birth process as these women acquired skills such as turning the baby *in utero* to ensure the optimal position for birth, assisting rotation of the head and shoulders at birth, massaging the mother's uterus and administering herbs to stop postpartum bleeding, and facilitating breastfeeding. Trevathan suggests that more mothers and babies would have survived in societies that developed midwifery traditions early on, giving such societies a distinct evolutionary advantage.

Both ancient and contemporary figurines and paintings from indigenous cultures all over the world show women giving birth upright: kneeling, sitting on a low stool or chair, or standing with women behind or on either side of them to hold and support them with a midwife kneeling in front with her hands out, waiting to catch the baby. This upright position, with its physiological advantages of facilitating fetal rotation and descent and the mother's ability to push effectively, was pervasive in birth until the advent of Western obstetrics. Its replacement by the flat-on-the-back position common in Western-style hospitals demonstrates the extensive cultural restructuring that has been applied to birth in industrialized countries.

The social nature of birth and its importance for survival ensure that this biological and intensely personal process will carry a heavy cultural overlay. In 1908, Arnold van Gennep noted that cultures ritualize important life transitions — of which birth is a prime example. Anthropologist and childbirth educator Sheila Kitzinger has noted that birth practices point 'as sharply as an arrowhead' to the core values and beliefs of the culture, telling the observer a great deal about the way that culture views the world and women's place in it. Where women's status is high, a rich set of nurturant traditions tends to develop around birth; where it is low, the opposite may occur. For example, in the highly patriarchal Islamic society of Bangladesh, in which the status of women is low, childbirth (like menstruation) has traditionally been regarded as highly polluting. It was believed that women should give birth on dirty linens, attended only by female relatives. An indigenous midwifery tradition never developed, and rates of infant mortality and puerperal infections are high. In contrast, in the matrilineal societies of Polynesia, where the status of women is high, pregnant

women are pampered and nurtured. Skilled midwives administer frequent full-body massages during pregnancy and have a rich repertoire of techniques for assisting women during labour and birth.

Brigitte Jordan's comparative study of birthing systems in Holland, Sweden, the US, and Mexico's Yucatan was the first to demonstrate this wide variation in the definition, the locus, the attendants, and the artifacts of childbirth; it sparked general interest in the anthropology of birth. Jordan's work on American birth was expanded by anthropologists Emily Martin and Robbie Davis-Floyd. They have suggested that American hospital birth, like much of American society, is organized around models of factory production and the technological control of natural processes. In many American hospitals, over 80% of women have their labours artificially speeded up or induced, are routinely hooked up to the electronic fetal monitor, often for long periods, have IVs inserted into their arms to provide the fluids that they are not allowed to drink, and lie flat with their feet in stirrups to give birth. While such technological interventions can sometimes be lifesaving, their routine overuse often generates problems. (The degree of overuse of birth technologies in the US is highlighted by the much lower rates of most such interventions in Great Britain, where a vocal, active, and influential consumer movement arguing for evidence-based care has had a significant impact on obstetrical policies.) Such routine procedures have been interpreted by Davis-Floyd as rituals that symbolically enact and display the core values of the American technocracy, which centre around the supervaluation of technology in many aspects of American life.

The prestige of Western 'high technologies' has induced many developing countries to stamp out viable indigenous midwifery systems and import the Western model even when it is ill-suited to the local situation. Western style hospitals built in the Third World may lack the most basic supplies but are often stocked with several expensive machines that few know how to use or repair. The medically trained personnel who staff these hospitals often have little understanding of or respect for local birth traditions, with the result that local women often avoid such hospitals whenever possible. From Northern India to the Yucatan, indigenous women echo each other's concerns: 'They expose you,' 'they shave you,' 'they cut you,' 'they leave you alone and ignore you, but won't let your family come in'. Ironically, none of the rules and procedures these women find so alarming are essential to good obstetric care; rather, they reflect the importation of the mechanistic Western model and its culturally insensitive imposition on indigenous groups.

In an effort to counteract this trend and build a bridge between technology and tradition, the World Health Organization and UNICEF have been promoting programs to 'upgrade' the skills of traditional midwives. Anthropological studies have shown, however, that because the medically trained personnel in these programmes tend to place a higher value on the Western techomedical approach, they generally fail to take advantage of the knowledge and skills developed by community midwives within the context of their own cultural traditions.

In 1978, Brigitte Jordan called for the 'mutual accommodation' of indigenous and Western birthing systems. In northern Brazil, an obstetrician, Dr Galba Araujo, demonstrated one form this 'mutual accommodation' might take: he oversaw the building of rural community clinics staffed by local midwives (who received culturally sensitive training that honoured their skills while imparting useful biomedical information),

and linked them to one city hospital through a government funded ambulance system. (Lack of transportation to a hospital in emergencies is a significant cause of maternal death in the developing world.)

In the US, obstetricians solidified their control over birth during the first half of the twentieth century and nearly eliminated midwifery by the 1950s. Since then the demands of many women for natural childbirth, coupled with scientific research into the dangers of interventionist hospital birth and the benefits of planned, midwife attended births at home or in freestanding birth centres, have generated a midwifery renaissance. Indeed, in the four countries in which infant perinatal mortality statistics are the lowest in the world — Japan, Holland, Sweden, and Denmark

— over 70% of births are attended by midwives who serve as the woman's primary caregiver.

Deep in the evolutionary past, our ancestors came to understand the benefits of women helping other women to give birth. Today, the most successful birthing systems combine midwifery care with solid scientific research on the physiology of birth. Contemporary midwives work in all settings, from hospital to home, and support women to avoid unnecessary interventions, to give birth in upright positions, to breastfeed, and to enjoy uninterrupted contact with their babies after birth. It has been repeatedly demonstrated that midwifery care results in fewer interventions, less iatrogenic damage to mothers and babies, improved outcomes (both psychological and physical), and lower costs. It is to be hoped that in short order the world will pass through the current phase of high-technology interventions in normal birth and come full spiral, uniting evolutionary understandings with contemporary science through midwives' skilled, nurturant, and woman-centered care.

ROBBIE DAVIS-FLOYD

Further reading

Davis-Floyd, R. E. (1992). *Birth as an American rite of passage*. University of California Press, Berkeley and London

Davis-Floyd, R. E. and Sargent, C. (1997). *Childbirth and authoritative knowledge: cross-cultural perspectives*. University of California Press, Berkeley, California.

Jordan, Brigitte (1993; orig. pub. 1978). *Birth in four cultures: a cross-cultural investigation of childbirth in Yucatan, Holland, Sweden and the United States*, (4th edn) Waveland Press, Prospect Heights, Ohio.

See also LABOUR; PREGNANCY.

Birth defects This term refers broadly to anything that is wrong with an infant at birth, whether it be a true congenital abnormality resulting from maldevelopment of the fetus *in utero* (from either inherent genetic or extraneous causes) or damage to the normally-developed fetus by infection or injury before or during birth. The term may cover both those defects which are evident at the time of birth and also those which reveal themselves later, including inborn errors of metabolism.   S.J.

See ANTENATAL DEVELOPMENT; BIRTHMARK; CLEFT LIP AND PALATE; CONGENITAL ABNORMALITIES.

Birthmark persistent, visible marks on the surface of the body, present from the time of birth, usually a naevus: a local overgrowth of blood vessels, or *haemangioma*.

From ancient times, birthmarks have traditionally been seen as a consequence of a mother's fears, fantasies, or unfulfilled cravings, and this idea acquired a certain doctrinal character during the Enlightenment. Before the eighteenth century the association of maternal passions and emotions with skin blemishes, with certain

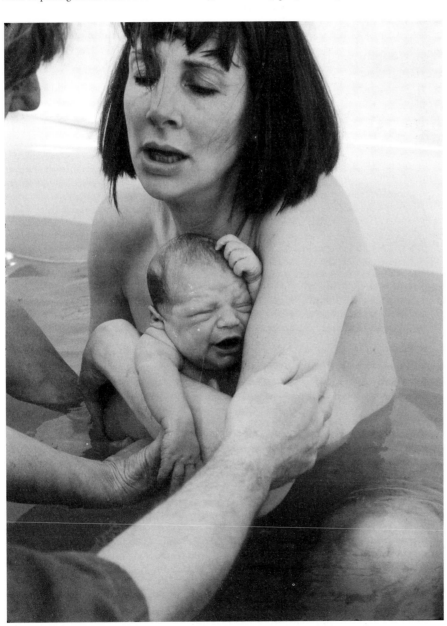

Water birth. A mother holds her new-born baby a few minutes after delivery, which took place in a water pool at home. The father offers a supporting hand. (Hattie Young/Science Photo Library.)

forms of bodily deformities, and, ultimately, with 'monsters' was based on little more than numerous testimonials and anecdotes. Both Aristotle and Hippocrates had cited the maternal imagination to account for birthmarks and abnormalities. It was also in that vein of pathological explanation that the theory survived during the Middle Ages and the Renaissance. Though it was provisionally abandoned by the scientific élite of the seventeenth century, discussion on whether there was any form of correlation between maternal emotions and fetal conformation continued during the eighteenth century and in Romanticism, in popular culture, in folklore, and, to a lesser extent, in scientific and pseudo-scientific literature.

Prior to the first important systematization of the powers of maternal imagination, by the French theologian and philosoper Malebranche in the late seventeenth century, stories about the effects of the mother's thoughts upon the fetus had been on the increase, mainly in compendia and treatises of natural history. These sources show, however, considerable variation in the basic principles: similar causes, the fears and cravings of the mother, did not produce the same effects in all cases, and for the most part, they did not produce any effect whatsoever. On the other hand, even the most fervent upholder of the powers of the imagination on the fetus was willing to call into question the veracity of many of the stories compiled within scholarly or popular traditions. Beginning with the book of Genesis, where Jacob is said to have produced spotted cattle by presenting the animals with lined rods, the alleged powers of the mother's imagination resulted in the most extraordinary fabrications. The French historian Paradin, for example, wrote about the niece of Pope Nicholas III, who gave birth to a child covered with hair, and with bear claws instead of fingers. Another was born with his tripes hanging from his belly because the slaughter of a sheep was contemplated by the mother. And the Dutch scholar Schenkius informs us that a woman from Louvain who conceived on the day of the Epiphany gave birth to three children of three different races.

Despite the lack of evidence traditionally associated with these stories, from 1690 to 1700, communications concerning teratology (the science that deals with fetal malformations) in the *Philosophical Transactions of the Royal Society* London and the *Mémoires* of the French Académie, Paris, frequently debated the possibility of the power of the maternal imagination. Furthermore, after the publication in 1714 of *De morbis cutaneis*, by the English surgeon Daniel Turner, a dispute occurred, first in England and then on the Continent, about the influence of the maternal imagination on the creation of birthmarks and other forms of major or minor abnormalities. The repercussions of this ongoing debate lasted until the late eighteenth century: even after the English surgeon John Hunter had denied the reality of the power of the mother's

imagination in a thoughtful empirical study, the French physician Louis Nicolas Benjamin Bablot wrote opposing treatises on the subject. The French surgeon Jean-Baptista Demangeon did likewise at the beginning of the nineteenth century. Even in the late nineteenth century numerous articles were published in the *Journal of the American Medical Association* which supported the theory. The scholars Gould and Pyle in their famous book *Anomalies and Curiosities of the Medicine*, published in 1896, also supported the belief. And even though most teratologists today would agree that major physical malformations do not result from maternal impressions, some behavioural scientists still consider that certain prenatal events, such as maternal stress, may have an effect on fetal development.

JAVIER MOSCOSO

See also CONGENITAL ABNORMALITIES.

Blackhead is the common name for a type of *comedo(ne)*, the characteristic feature of *acne vulgaris*. They occur mostly on the face, neck, and upper part of the back, because this is where *sebaceous glands* are most thickly distributed. These glands secrete sebum, a fatty lubricant, into the hair follicles. The lining of the follicles, like the skin surface itself, continually sheds and renews its outermost layer, and this debris, along with the sebum, normally escapes onto the surface. When the lining fails to be shed properly the sebum accumulates below it in the hair follicle. The debris of skin cells, pushed outwards by the sebum contains the pigment melanin, and this accounts for the dark plug that closes off the pore. Inflammation may be caused by bacterial action and fatty acids formed in the sebum, resulting in *papules* (lumps) and *pustules* ('boils' or 'plukes'). Male sex hormones enhance the activity of the sebaceous glands along with the stimulation of hair growth, accounting for their exuberant secretion, and hence the likelihood of acne, around the time of puberty, and for the fact that girls suffer less — though they are not entirely exempt. S.J.

See SKIN.

Bladder The bladder is a storage vessel for urine and is lined by a special waterproof skin called *transitional cell epithelium*. There is a similar lining in the *ureters* (the tubes from each kidney to the bladder) and *urethra* (the tube from the bladder to the outside). The bladder is enveloped in a criss-cross of muscle fibres, the *detrusor* muscle. As the bladder fills, these muscle fibres relax in such a way that the pressure within the bladder remains constant at less than 10 cm of water. The normal adult bladder holds approximately 400 ml of urine and when more than this amount has entered the bladder the pressure starts to rise and the desire to void urine is felt. If this cannot be conveniently done and bladder filling continues the feeling becomes very urgent and eventually uncontrollable. Normally, adults

are able to hold on after the first feeling of urgency, but children find this more difficult and in babies the bladder empties automatically. The nerves controlling the bladder belong to the AUTONOMIC NERVOUS SYSTEM and, although such nerves usually function automatically, the bladder is a special situation where voluntary control is superimposed on autonomic. Babies have to learn to control the automatic bladder (POTTY TRAINING) and this is usually achieved by the age of 5 years but may take longer, particularly in boys, and also in some families. Failure to override fully the autonomic nerves to the bladder results in urinary frequency and the need to void urine at night, or bedwetting (*enuresis*). Most children eventually become dry at night but if problems continue beyond the normal age when potty training should be complete then it is important to exclude other problems such as urinary tract infections.

In adults there are two main causes of INCONTINENCE: either *weakness* of the pelvic floor and sphincter muscles (which act normally to prevent passage of urine into the urethra) or *over-activity* of the detrusor muscle, so that the bladder behaves rather like that of a baby (this latter problem is called *instability*). Difficulties in controlling the bladder can also occur in older age, and the number of elderly people with continence problems is a major burden on social services. In this group of people it is important to exclude other causes of incontinence such as cancer, infection, or stones in the bladder. With proper medical, nursing, and physiotherapy measures, many elderly people with problems of incontinence can be helped. TIM HARGREAVE

See Plate 8.

See also AUTONOMIC NERVOUS SYSTEM; INCONTINENCE; KIDNEY; POTTY TRAINING; URINE.

Blindness Surprisingly, blindness rarely means total absence of light perception. Most definitions of blindness are based on measurement of *visual acuity* (the ability to read letters at a certain distance) and assessment of the ability of the person to carry out tasks needing vision. In the UK, the National Assistance Act 1948 states that a person can be certified as blind if they are 'so blind that they cannot do any work for which eyesight is essential'. This rather circular definition refers to 'any work' and not just the person's normal job or one for which he has been specially trained.

Visual acuity is usually tested by asking the patient to read letters of various sizes on a chart viewed from a distance of 6 m or 20 feet (the *Snellen method*). Acuity is expressed as a fraction, the number on top referring to the distance at which a normal person can read a particular size of letter and the lower number the distance at which the subject being tested can read that size of letter. Hence 'normal' visual acuity is 6/6 (European) or 20/20 (American). A person should be certified blind if the visual acuity (while wearing corrective glasses) is 3/60 or below (when a letter that can be recognized from 60 metres by a normal person can be identified only from 3 metres or closer). A person should also be certified blind if their acuity is between 3/60 and 6/60 but they have completely lost the peripheral part of their visual field, hence restricting their vision to the central part of the field. Indeed, if the more useful lower part of the visual field is lost then someone with better than 6/60 acuity can be certified blind.

There is no legal definition of partial sight in the UK, but a person can be certified as partially sighted if they are 'substantially and permanently handicapped by defective vision caused by congenital defect or illness or injury'. All certification must be done by a consultant ophthalmologist. The help from Social Services should be the same for both legally blind and partially sighted groups but Social Security benefits and tax concessions differ.

Definitions of blindness are not the same around the world and the vast majority depend on measured visual acuity with no allowance for any functional deficits. Consequently comparison of the incidence of blindness world-wide is inexact. The World Health Organisation has proposed categories of visual impairment but these have not yet been widely adopted.

The common causes of blindness vary in different countries according to the general levels of economic and physical health. The high rate of blindness in developing countries is mainly due to malnutrition and infectious diseases, coupled with the scarcity of medical care. Moorfields Eye Hospital was founded in London in 1805 to treat the 'Egyptian ophthalmia', a mixture of trachoma and purulent ophthalmitis brought back by British troops from Aboukir after their withdrawal from Egypt in 1803. The disease quickly spread throughout the country when the disbanded soldiers returned to their homes, taking the infection with them. Nowadays the condition is treatable with tetracycline eye ointment and tetracycline taken orally.

Causes of blindness

Lack of vitamin A has a direct effect on the eye, causing clouding and softening of the cornea (*keratomalacia*), but also increases the risk and severity of infections, so that measles can be a blinding or even fatal disease in children who are deficient in vitamin A. Night-blindness due to lack of vitamin A may occur in famines, and cure of this condition by eating liver, which is rich in vitamin A, has been known for over 3000 years.

Another cause of night-blindness is pigmentary degeneration of the retina (*retinitis pigmentosa*) which, combined with partial loss of the visual field, eventually contracting down to 'tunnel vision', can be most disabling. This condition is mainly inherited as an *autosomal recessive condition* (showing itself only when both parents carry the mutant gene), but other forms occur. A high proportion of the population of the Atlantic island Tristan da Cunha was recently discovered to be affected when they were evacuated because

of volcanic activity. The disorder is progressive and untreatable.

Trachoma, an infectious disease, affects some 500 million people world-wide, of whom 7 million are blind and 10 million visually impaired. The infectious agents are bacteria known as Chlamydia.

River blindness (*onchocerciasis*) is the next commonest infection, where microfilarial parasites, spread by black flies, which breed in the tropical, sub-Saharan belt across the whole of Africa and at similar latitudes in Mexico, Brazil, and Ecuador, invade the retina and the supporting, vascularized middle layer of the eyeball, the choroid. Treatment was revolutionized in 1987 when *ivermectin*, already used in veterinary medicine, was registered for human therapy.

From 1976 the total number of people registered blind in Britain has risen, but this rise is limited to those over 75 years old. Fifty per cent of all 75–85-year-olds registered with impaired vision in this country suffer from *age-related macular degeneration* (ARMD). Cataracts are now second as a cause of blindness, at around 40%, but these are essentially treatable by surgery except in those cases where extraction of the cataract reveals underlying, untreatable ARMD.

Damage to the retina caused by *glaucoma* (increased pressure in the eyeball) and by diabetes (*diabetic retinopathy*) make up almost all the remaining causes of blindness. Glaucoma is insidious in onset: acuity in the central visual field is not seriously affected and a diagnosis may not be made until much of the peripheral retina has been destroyed. Diabetic retinopathy is most prevalent and severe in long-standing insulin-dependent diabetes. This emphasises the importance of striving for optimal diabetic control. Routine screening checks for both glaucoma and diabetic retinopathy are essential, but manpower and economic considerations have led to much of this work being transferred to orthoptists and optometrists. *Retinal detachment* (separation of the retina from the pigment epithelium behind it) is a rarer cause of blindness.

There is a long history of visual upsets from *staring directly at the sun*. The high energy optically concentrated at the central part of the retina for only seconds can produce prolonged after-images and even permanent loss of central vision. This is an occupational hazard for astronomers, and for members of the public who sun-gaze in a misguided attempt to strengthen their eyes or when under the influence of hallucinogenic drugs. There is a particular hazard during solar eclipses because the reduced *total* amount of light makes it easier to hold fixation on the sun, but the intensity on the remaining illuminated part of the retina is just as high (and just as damaging) as when there is no eclipse: hence the term '*eclipse blindness*'.

Possibilities for treatment

Given the immense social importance of vision, there is intense effort to develop new treatments for blinding conditions. These are focusing not

only on the conventional approach of developing new vaccines to prevent infection and new drugs to treat specific conditions, but also on more innovative approaches. For instance, attempts have been made to implant an array of electrodes over the surface of the visual cortex, coupled to a video camera or an optical letter reader, in the hope of bypassing the eye and providing visual sensation by direct stimulation of the cortex. Unfortunately, such stimulation produces only the sensation of tiny pin-points of light, which appear to move with movements of the eyes. A more promising approach is the implantation of a thin sheet of light-sensitive electrodes into the retina, to take the place of degenerated receptors and provide direct stimulation to the fibres of the optic nerve.

Cortical blindness

Damage to the visual cortex in the occipital lobe of the cerebral hemispheres can also cause blindness — *cortical blindness*. When fixation is maintained on a point in space, a particular region of the visual field is blind (a '*scotoma*') whether either eye is open, or both (because the cortex receives signals from corresponding regions of the two retinae). Cortical blindness can occur, for example, after a STROKE affecting the posterior cerebral artery, which supplies blood to that part of the brain. If extensive damage occurs in one hemisphere, the opposite side of the visual field becomes blind (*hemianopia*). Often, a small region around the fixation point is spared. This 'macular sparing' is thought to be due to the fact that so much of the visual cortex is devoted to the central part of the retina that some part of this region has a high chance of surviving. Interestingly, even when the occipital visual cortex is bilaterally destroyed, resulting in total blindness with no light perception, the patient does not feel enveloped in darkness: rather, the outside world simply does not exist visually (as for the world behind our heads). This contrasts with blindness resulting from retinal damage (for instance from total bilateral retinal detachment), when the patient complains of being in complete darkness. Indeed, the cortically blind patients are subjectively unaware of their disability — blind to their blindness.

When damage is restricted to the primary visual cortex (not extending into the surrounding cortical areas) some patients are still able to detect certain forms of visual stimulation (especially moving objects and sudden changes in brightness) in the 'blind' part of the visual field. Amazingly, if the stimulus is not very intense or rapidly moving, they are often unaware of their residual visual capacity, but can reliably 'guess' whether, for instance, the stimulus has moved, and even in which direction. This bizarre dissociation of vision from consciousness is known as '*blindsight*'. Recent research even suggests that the facial expression of faces 'seen' in the blind part of the field can be recognized. Blindsight is not magic! Even when the primary visual cortex is damaged, information from the eyes still reaches parts of the midbrain and other visual parts of the cerebral cortex. These secondary pathways presumably mediate the impoverished visual performance.

If a stroke or injury leaves the primary visual cortex intact but destroys visual areas further forward in the occipital lobe of the cerebral hemispheres, remarkable disorders of visual perception, without frank blindness, can occur. These include the inability to see movement, even though stationary objects are quite normally perceived (*akinetopsia*), and a lack of perceived colour, despite normal perception of shape and movement (*achromatopsia*). These observations are entirely compatible with evidence from experiments in animals in which the activity of nerve cells has been recorded with microelectrodes, as well as with studies using positron emission tomography (PET) and functional magnetic resonance imaging (fMRI) to detect activity in the normal human brain caused by different forms of visual stimulation. These experimental approaches have shown that the primary visual cortex is surrounded by a patchwork of other areas in which neurons are devoted to the analysis of one aspect or another of the visual image — motion in some areas, colour in others, etc.

Damage further forward, in the lower part of the temporal lobe, can precipitate even more curious failures of perceptual interpretation, generally known as visual *agnosias* (from the Greek for lack of knowledge). Not uncommon, especially after damage on the right side, is *prosopagnosia* — an inability to recognize faces, sometimes even of family members, although other aspects of object identification (even knowing that a face is a face) are intact. In extreme cases, the poor patient has great difficulty in recognizing a wide variety of everyday objects (until he or she touches them), even though all basic aspects of vision (acuity, colour vision, detection of movement, etc.) are unaffected.

Injury to the rear part of the *corpus callosum* — the great cable of millions of nerve fibres that links the two hemispheres — or to regions at the junction of the occipital and temporal lobes can cause specific disorders of visual integration (*associational disturbances*), such as word blindness (*alexia*).

Provision for the visually disabled

The reaction of the public to handicapped and disabled people remains capricious, and often prejudiced. The deaf have long been figures of fun: they are often ignored and easily retreat into solitude. However, the blind generally receive more sympathy, even admiration. Social Services for the blind unfortunately are not uniformly good throughout the UK. However, some national organizations such as the Royal National Institute for the Blind and Guide Dogs for the Blind give great help and provide funds for research into blindness as well. In 1835 Louis Braille introduced his system of raised writing, where projecting dots represent a letter or number

and are interpreted by touch, but it took 30 years to gain acceptance. In this electronic age there are many devices which can make an enormous difference to the blind person's quality of life. One is a computer that reads out text audibly as it appears on screen. This can be set to speeds as fast as the subject can comprehend the speech. A braille printer and labelling machine help, for example, to identify foodstuffs in the kitchen or deep-freeze, or to catalogue a CD library. Microwave units can respond to and speak instructions and will defrost different foods correctly once they have been weighed. For contact with the outside world there are talking newspapers, which can be sent by compressed e-mail, or put on to the Internet. A CD-ROM of all British daily newspapers is available weekly. Never has so much been available for blind people who can afford it.

PETER FELLS
COLIN BLAKEMORE

Further reading

Cullinon, T. R. (1987). The epidemiology of blindness. In *Clinical ophthalmology*, (ed. S. Miller), p. 571. Wright, Bristol.

Walsh, F. B. and Hoyt, W. F. (1969). *Clinical neuro-ophthalmology*, Vol. 1, (3rd edn), pp. 87–120. Williams and Wilkins, Baltimore.

See also BLIND SPOT; EYE; OPTOMETRY; ORTHOPTICS; VISION.

Blind spot The existence of a small blind region in the normal human EYE was predicted in the seventeenth century by the French scientist Edmé Mariotte. While dissecting a human eye, Mariotte noticed the '*optic disc*' — a hole in the back of the eyeball through which all the nerve fibres that make up the optic nerve leave the eye. He realised that, unlike the rest of the retina that surrounds the hole, this optic disc is devoid of light-sensitive photoreceptors. Applying his knowledge of optics and of the anatomy of the eye, he deduced that every eye should be blind in a corresponding small portion of the visual field. The optic disc lies about 15 degrees to the nasal side of the *fovea* (the part of the retina that we point towards things when we fixate them). Since the image on the retina is inverted by the optics of the eye, the 'blind spot' in the visual field lies to the right of the point of fixation for the right eye and to the left for the left eye.

You can confirm Mariotte's observation and find your own blind spot by viewing Fig. 1. Close your right eye, hold the book about a foot away from your face and look fixedly at the little black dot on the page. Keep looking at the dot as you very slowly move the page towards you. At some critical distance, the round, hatched patch will fall on your blind spot and disappear completely. However, notice that when the patch disappears

you do not experience a black hole or void in its place. You simply see this region as being filled with the same light grey as the background — a phenomenon called 'filling-in' or *perceptual interpolation.*

The Victorian physicist Sir David Brewster was so impressed with this filling-in that he attributed it to God. In 1832 he wrote, 'We should expect, whether we use one eye or both eyes, to see a black or dark spot on every landscape within fifteen degrees of the point which most particularly attracts our notice. The divine artificer, however, has not left his work thus imperfect … the spot, in place of being black, has always the same colour as the ground'. Curiously, Sir David was not troubled by the question of why the 'Divine Artificer' should have created an imperfect eye to begin with.

Since the left eye's blind spot is 15 degrees to the left of fixation and that of the right is 15 degrees to the right, they do not coincide with each other in the visual field. The region of space that falls on the blind area of one eye falls on seeing retina in the other eye. So, if we have both eyes open, we should certainly not expect (as Brewster did) that we should be aware of the blind spot. However, the filling-in of the blind spot that occurs even when the other eye is closed can be explained only by some compensatory process in the brain.

You can explore the limits of the filling-in process by viewing Fig. 2. Notice that when the disc disappears you do not see a gap in the line — you see it as continuous, right through the blind region. It is as if neurons in the visual part of your brain make a statistical estimate: they realise that it is highly unlikely that two separate line segments are precisely lined up on either side of the blind spot simply by chance. So they signal to 'higher' centres in the brain that this is a single continuous line — and that is what you see. On the other hand, if you 'aim' your blind spot at the corner of a line drawing of a square, the corner does get perceptually 'chopped off'. Your visual system does not complete the missing corner. There are clear limits to what you can fill in.

It is unlikely that filling-in is just a quirk of the visual system that has evolved for the sole purpose of dealing with the blind spot. Rather, it appears to be a manifestation of a very general ability to construct surfaces and bridge gaps that might be otherwise distracting in an image — the same ability, in fact, that allows you to see as a complete object anything that is partly hidden from view — for instance, a rabbit behind a picket fence looks like a complete rabbit, not a sliced-up one. In our natural blind spot we have an especially obvious example of filling-in — one that provides us with an experimental opportunity to investigate the 'laws' that govern the process and their underlying physiology.

The physiological organization in the BRAIN corresponding to the blind spot (and possibly to filling-in) has recently been explored in monkeys. In both monkeys and people the retinas of both

Fig. 1

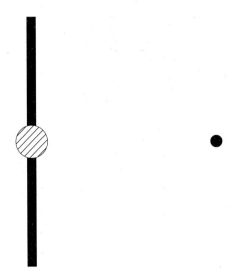

Fig. 2

eyes are mapped systematically on to the primary visual cortex of the cerebral hemispheres (called *area 17* or *striate cortex*). The maps of the visual field seen by the two eyes are in fairly precise registration — an anatomical convergence that provides the basis for *binocular fusion* (singleness of vision) as well as stereoscopic depth perception. But, in each hemisphere (which receives information about the opposite half of the visual world), there is a region of the map corresponding to the blind spot of the opposite eye. Obviously, this region of the visual cortex receives no nerve fibres from the blind region of one eye. So what happens to the map in this region? Does the hole in the map get 'sewn up', or is there a big gap corresponding to the blind spot? The answer is simple. There is indeed a 'gap' in the map in the visual cortex, corresponding to the region that should receive signals from the blind portion of the opposite eye. But this patch of cortex does get signals from the region of the other eye that is looking at the same portion of the visual field. So, in terms of the field, the map in the brain is continuous, even though the input from the opposite eye is missing in the region corresponding to the blind spot.

Intriguingly, within the part of the cortical map that represents the region of visual field that can be seen by only one eye, nerve cells receive input from the region of retina immediately surrounding the blind spot. This aberrant input might help explain the filling-in phenomenon. A cortical nerve cell in this region will fire impulses if a long line straddles the blind spot, or even if two halves of the line are displayed on either side of the blind spot, but not if only half the line alone is displayed. This implies that there is complicated (non-linear) *summation* of signals converging on to the cell from the retina surrounding the blind spot. This process might explain filling-in.

Filling-in can occur for parts of the retina other than the optic disc. For instance, if a part of the *peripheral visual field* (far from the fixation point) is blanked out by an opaque occluder,

lines that run across the occluded region appear complete, just as for the blind spot itself. This suggests that the process that underlies filling-in is not confined to the cortical representation of the blind spot and may play a very general role in the interpolation of contours and surfaces across occluded regions of the visual field.

The blind spot is also important clinically because the optic disc becomes enlarged in certain conditions. An example is *papilloedema* — a swelling of the optic disc that occurs when the pressure inside the skull is increased, for instance because of a brain tumour. Examination of the retina through an ophthalmoscope can reveal such an enlarged disc directly, but it can also be revealed indirectly by mapping out the area of blindness of the blind spot with a device called a *perimeter*, in which tiny spots of light are flashed in various positions across the visual field and the patient is simply asked to say whether they see them.   V.S. RAMACHANDRAN

Further reading

Barlow, H. B., Blakemore, C. and Pettigrew, J. D. (1967). The neural mechanism of binocular depth discrimination. *Journal of Physiology*.

Gatass, R., Fiorani, M., Rosa, M. P. G., Pinon, M. C. F., Sousa, A. P. B. and Soares, J. G. M. (1992). Visual responses outside the classical receptive field, a possible correlate of perceptual completion. In *The visual system from genesis to maturity*, (ed. R. Lent), pp. 233–44. Birkhauser, Boston, MA.

Ramachandran, V. S. (1992). Blind spots. *Scientific American*, **266**, 85–91.

See also EYES; VISION.

Blindness, recovery from

Blindness, recovery from The English philosopher John Locke (1632–1704) received a celebrated letter from his friend William Molyneux, posing the question:

> Suppose a man born blind, and now adult, and taught by his touch to distinguish between a cube and a sphere of the same metal, and nighly of the same bigness, so as to tell, when he felt one and the other, which is the cube, which is the sphere. Suppose then the cube and the sphere placed on a table, and the blind man made to see: query, Whether by his sight, before he touched them, he could now distinguish and tell which is the globe, which the cube? To which the acute and judicious proposer answers: 'Not. For though he has obtained the experience of how a globe, and how a cube, affects his touch; yet he has not yet attained the experience, that what affects his touch so or so, must affect his sight so or so …'

Locke comments (in *Essay Concerning Human Understanding*, 1690) as follows:

> I agree with this thinking gentleman, whom I am proud to call my friend, in his answer to this problem; and am of the opinion that the blind man, at first, would not be able with certainty to say which was the globe, which the cube …

It might seem a simple matter to test this by rearing animals in darkness, to deny them vision, for months or years, then discover what they see when given light. A. H. Reisen found severe

behavioural losses in such experiments; but they might have been due to degeneration of the retina (found to occur in darkness, though less with diffusing goggles) and also to the remarkably passive state of animals, especially monkeys, reared in the dark. It is not acceptable, of course, deliberately to bring up human babies in the dark; but there are cases of adult recovery from blindness. Can these tell us how human perception develops — and answer Molyneux's question?

Some of the reported cases are much as the empiricist philosophers expected; seeing little at first and being unable to name or distinguish between even simple shapes. Sometimes there was a long period of training before the person came to have useful vision, which indeed in many cases was never attained. It is important to note, however, that the reported cases do not all show extreme difficulty or slowness in coming to see. We should also remember that the early surgical operations to restore sight greatly disturbed the optics of the eye, so there could not have been a useful image on the retina until there had been considerable time for the eyes to heal. This was a particular problem in the early cases, in all of which the lens inside the eye was removed, to treat cataract (clouding of the lens). Treatment of the other kind of operable blindness — opacity of the cornea — by corneal transplantation, gives an adequate retinal image far sooner.

The case of SB

Perhaps the best studied case was a person known by his initials, SB, who, following a life of blindness, was given corneal transplants when he was 52. When the bandages were first removed from his eyes, SB heard the voice of the surgeon. He turned to the voice, and saw nothing but a blur. He realised that this must be a face because of the voice, but he could not see it. He did not suddenly see the world of objects as we do when we open our eyes, but within a few days he could use his eyes to surprisingly good effect. He could walk along the hospital corridors without recourse to touch; he could even tell the time from a large wall clock — having all his life carried a pocket watch, with no glass, so that he could feel the time by touching its hands, as he demonstrated with great skill. This was the first

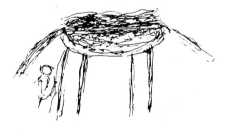

Fig. 1 SB's drawing of an elephant. He drew this before having seen one. Half an hour later we showed him a real elephant, at London Zoo, and he was not at all surprised by it! (Previously published in Gregory, R. L. (1998) *Eye and brain*, (5th edn), Oxford University Press.)

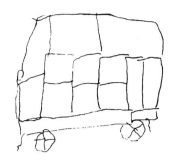
(a)

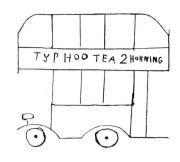
(b)

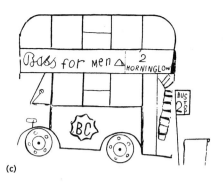
(c)

Fig. 2 (a) SB's first drawing of a bus (48 days after the corneal graft operation giving him sight). All the features included were probably known to him previously through touch. The front of the bus, which would not have been explored by touch, is missing, and he simply could not add it when we asked him to try. **(b)** Six months later. Now he adds writing. The touch-based spokes of the wheels have been rejected, but he still cannot draw the front. **(c)** A year later, the front is still missing. The writing is sophisticated, though he could hardly read. (Previously published in Gregory, R. L. (1998) *Eye and brain*, (5th edn), Oxford University Press.)

intimation that he could use his earlier touch-knowledge for his new-found vision.

When SB left the hospital, we (R. I. Gregory and J. Wallace) took him to London and showed him many things he had not known from touch. At the zoo, to our surprise, he was able to name most of the animals correctly. However, he had stroked pet animals when a boy, and had enquired how other animals differed from the cats and dogs he knew by touch. This use of intelligent inference effectively enhanced his vision. We tried to discover what his visual world was like by asking him questions and giving simple perceptual tests. We found that his perception of distance was peculiar, and this is true of other, earlier cases. He thought he would just be able to touch the ground below his window with his feet if he hung from the sill with his hands; but the distance was at least ten times his height. On the other hand, he could judge horizontal distances quite accurately, presumably by knowledge from walking.

Although his perception was demonstrably peculiar, he seldom expressed surprise. He drew a very odd elephant (Fig. 1) just before we showed him one at the zoo; but then he said it looked much as he expected it would. For one object he did show real surprise — an object he could not have known by touch — the quarter moon. From this common description, and his knowledge that the whole moon is round, he thought it would look like a quarter piece of cake!

SB never learned to read by sight (he read Braille, having been taught it at the blind school) but he could immediately recognise capital letters and numbers by sight. This so surprised us we could hardly believe he had been blind. It turned out, from the school records, that he had been taught upper case though not lower case letters, and numbers, by touch at the blind school. The children were given raised letters on wooden blocks to learn by active touch. The children were not given lower case letters to learn, presumably because they were seldom used for touchable brass plates, and so on. He read upper case letters immediately by sight, but it took him a long time to learn lower case letters, and he never managed to read more than simple words. This finding, that he could immediately read

letters visually, which he had already learned by touch, clearly showed that he was able to use previous touch experience for his new-found vision. This indicates that the brain is not so departmentalised as sometimes thought. There seems to be a general knowledge-base available to all the senses. But this makes these findings of less obvious relevance to the question of how human infants come to see.

SB's use of early touch experience shows in his drawings. The series of drawings of buses (in Fig. 2) illustrate how he was unable to draw things he did not already know by touch. In the first drawing the wheels have spokes. The wheels of buses and other vehicles did indeed have spokes when he was a boy, presumably known to him by exploratory touch. The windows also seem to be represented as he knew them by touch from the inside. Most striking is the complete absence of the front of the bus, which he would not have been able to explore with his hands, and which he was still unable to draw 6 months or indeed a year later. The gradual introduction of writing in the drawings indicates visual learning.

We saw in a dramatic form the difficulty that SB had in trusting and using his vision — when crossing a busy road. Before the operation he was undaunted by traffic; but afterwards, it took two of us holding him on either side to force him across: he was terrified as never before in his life.

Since he was interested in tools, we showed him a simple lathe (a tool he had wished he could use) in a glass case at the Science Museum in London. With the case closed he was quite unable to say anything about it, except that the nearest part might be a handle (which it was), but when he was allowed to touch it, he closed his eyes and placed his hands on it, and immediately said with assurance that it was a handle. He ran his hands eagerly over the rest of the lathe, with his eyes tight shut for a minute or so; then he stood back a little, and opening his eyes and staring at it he said: 'Now that I've felt it I can see.'

Paradoxically, people whose sight has been restored commonly complain of depression. They need very special care. Many of the findings with SB have been confirmed. Alberto Valvo in 1971 described extraordinary operations in Italy

that sound like a Greek myth. The sight of six patients (including a philosopher) was restored by implanting into the eye an acrylic lens, set like a jewel in a piece of tooth (to avoid rejection of the acrylic). Valvo found that earlier experience of letters by touch gave immediate visual recognition of letters. There are new cases of children in Japan, being intensively studied.

It is extremely difficult if not entirely impossible to extrapolate from these cases to the question of what and how babies see. The cases are interesting and dramatic, but they tell us little about the world of the infant, for adults with restored vision are not living fossils of babies. However, the philosophers did not guess there would be transfer of knowledge from touch to new-found vision. So we have learned something surprising and interesting from these rare dramas.

RICHARD L. GREGORY

Further reading

Gregory, R. L. and Wallace, J. (1963). Recovery from early blindness: a case study. *Exp. Soc. Monogr*, 2. Heffers, Cambridge. (Reprinted in: Gregory, R. L. (1974). *Concepts and mechanisms of perception.* Duckworth, London.)

Senden von, M. (1960). *Space and sight*, (trans. P. Heath). Methuen/Free Press, London.

Valvo, A. (1971). *Sight restoration and rehabilitation.* American Foundation for the Blind, New York.

See also BLINDNESS; VISION.

Blister A raised, well circumscribed lesion of the skin, containing a sterile fluid, derived from the serum. Strictly, a blister or *bulla* has a diameter of greater than 5 mm, smaller lesions being called *vesicles*. Commonly they become infected and fill with pus, and are then known as *pustules*. They are caused by trauma (friction, burns, and scalds), allergic contact dermatitis, insect bites, sunburn, etc. In earlier times agents were used to raise vesicles or blisters on the skin to relieve the pain from deeper structures by the process of counter-irritation. A commonly used *vesicant* was a powder derived from the pulverised dried beetles of *Lytta vesicatoria*, containing cantharidin, and commonly known as Spanish Fly or Blistering Beetle.   ALAN W. CUTHBERT

Blood has always held a great fascination, being regarded as a living substance, the very essence of life. The doctrine of the HUMOURS, which dominated Western medical thinking until the Renaissance, held that disease is the consequence of imbalance of the four components of which the human body is composed: blood; phlegm; black bile; and yellow bile. The English physician William HARVEY (1578–1637) wrote that 'blood acts above all the powers of the elements and is endowed with notable values and is also the instrument of the omnipotent creator.' It is, he believed, 'the fountain of life and the seat of the soul'.

Blood is of immense cultural significance. We talk of blood 'being thicker than water' to signify the strength of family loyalty, as also reflected in 'blood brothers'. A massacre is a 'blood bath', the reward for assassination 'blood money'. Blood signifies power, for good or evil; the consumption of blood, metaphorically, lies at the heart of the Christian sacrament, yet many societies produce legends of vampires, whose evil is signified by their taste for human blood. Blood is often equated with strength: the monthly loss of blood through menstrual flow frequently led doctors (mostly male) to assume an inherent weakness in women. But too much blood could also be troublesome: ruddy-faced, plethoric men would make an annual visit to the barber-surgeon each spring (blood's season, according to the doctrine of the humours) to be bled. Barbers and surgeons went their separate ways in the seventeenth and eighteenth centuries, but the red stripe down the barber's pole still commemorates this annual blood-letting ritual.

Knowledge of the structure of blood (such as the notion that it consists of cells suspended in a protein-rich fluid called plasma) slowly accumulated from the seventeenth century onwards. The Dutch microscopist Anton van Leeuwenhoek (1632–1723), examining his own blood under a simple microscope, first described the red corpuscles (cells), and measured their diameter. White corpuscles were first observed by the British physician William Hewson (1739–74), who also discovered the essential features of how blood coagulates, showing that it is due to the clotting of plasma rather than changes in the cellular constituents. In the latter half of the nineteenth century it was found that blood cells are the progeny of more primitive cells in the bone marrow. The modern science of haematology stemmed from the work of the German pharmacologist Paul Ehrlich (1854–1915), who developed a stain that led to a clear distinction between the different types of cells in the blood.

An understanding of the function of blood also evolved over several centuries. William Harvey described its circulation in 1628, and a few years later the English physician Richard Lower (1631–91) observed the change from the dark blue colour of venous to the bright red of arterial blood after its passage through the LUNGS. In 1790 the French chemist Antoine Lavoisier (1743–94) discovered OXYGEN and found that it was the constituent of air that is responsible for the change of the colour of blood. In the mid nineteenth century it was found that OXYGEN combines with a substance in the red cells, which was identified as the protein HAEMOGLOBIN by the German biochemist Felix Hoppe-Seyler (1825–95). By 1900 it was also appreciated that the white cells play a crucial role in defence against infection, an idea first proposed by the Russian zoologist Ilya Metchnikoff (1845–1916).

Blood is the body's major transport system, carrying vital substances to all the tissues and removing their waste products. It delivers oxygen from the lungs and collects CARBON DIOXIDE to be excreted there; it takes up nutrients from the gut, and distributes them for use or storage; and by virtue of its passage through the KIDNEYS it provides an important mechanism for the excretion of toxic waste products of metabolism. The blood also distributes HORMONES from their sites of secretion to their sites of action, and likewise the cells, antibodies, and other substances which combat injury and infection. In performing these functions, the blood continually exchanges substances across the capillary walls with the fluids that bathe all body cells. The total volume of blood, which remains remarkably constant in adults, is approximately 70 ml/kg body weight, or about 5 litres. It consists of a fluid component, plasma, in which are suspended red cells, white cells, and platelets (see figure). In health, the cells comprise about 45% of the total volume of blood: this value is known as the *haematocrit*, and reflects mainly the bulk of the red blood cells.

Red blood cells

The number of circulating red cells in a unit volume of blood — the red cell count — varies at different stages of development. It is relatively high in fetal life and falls quickly after birth, before gradually rising to reach its adult level by the age of 20 (about 5 million/mm^3 of blood). Although it is approximately the same in males and females during childhood, it is higher in males after adolescence. Red cells survive for only about three months in the circulating blood, so production continues throughout life.

The major role of red cells (*erythrocytes*) is to transfer oxygen from the lungs to the tissues. Their rate of production is beautifully adapted to this function. It is regulated by a hormone called *erythropoietin*, produced in the kidney in the adult and in the liver in the fetus. Close to the gene that regulates erythropoietin production are regions of DNA that sense oxygen tension; when this falls, erythropoietin synthesis is stimulated, and more red cells are produced in the bone marrow. When adequate oxygenation of the tissues is achieved, erythropoietin production is reduced. By this biological feedback loop the body is able to respond to varying oxygen demands by modifying the rate of red cell production. In addition to erythropoietin, there is probably some fine tuning of the rate of erythropoiesis by other hormones and protein growth factors.

The site of red cell production changes during development. In the embryo, they are made in the yolk sac, in the fetus in the liver and SPLEEN, and in adult life in the BONE marrow. These sites all contain a primitive, self-renewing population of blood-cell precursors, the haemopoietic stem cells, which are capable of producing all the different cells of the blood. Red cell production (*erythropoiesis*) takes about 7 days. The progeny of stem cells destined to become red cells start out as large, nucleated cells; during their development haemoglobin synthesis begins and, after several divisions, their nucleus is condensed and eventually extruded from the cell. This red cell precursor is now called a reticulocyte. Reticulocytes are released from the marrow into the blood; they undergo fine quality control in the spleen, where unwanted nuclear remnants are removed. (This process is different in birds and amphibians; the nucleus is not removed and is retained throughout the life of the red cell in the peripheral blood.) An adequate dietary supply of iron and of specific VITAMINS is necessary for the synthesis of haemoglobin and the production of normal red cells.

After their release from the bone marrow, red cells spend approximately 120 days in the circulation. During this time they travel over 100 miles, are buffeted at high velocities during their passage through the heart, and have to negotiate tiny capillaries narrower than their own diameter. As they age, subtle structural changes occur which render them identifiable to scavenger cells in the spleen and elsewhere, and they end their days being devoured and digested by these predators.

The red cells of most species are biconcave discs, a shape that offers maximum surface area for exchange of oxygen and carbon dioxide. They consist of a protein and lipid membrane, which encases haemoglobin together with water and a variety of enzymes and salts. Their chemistry is beautifully adapted to their function as an oxygen transporter and to protect them and their haemoglobin from chemical damage.

The oxygen-carrying protein of red cells, haemoglobin, is also closely adapted to its function. In most mammals, adult haemoglobin (haemoglobin A) comprises two unlike pairs of chains of amino acids, or globin chains, called α and β, each of which is folded round one iron-containing haem molecule, to which oxygen can bind. The resulting molecule is designated $\alpha_2\beta_2$. In humans, and some other species, there is a different fetal haemoglobin, haemoglobin F, which has α chains combined with γ chains ($\alpha_2\gamma_2$). In most species adult and fetal haemoglobins are preceded by an embryonic haemoglobin. These different haemoglobins are adapted to particular oxygen requirements at different stages of development. While taking up and giving off oxygen, subtle spatial alterations occur between the globin chains which are responsible for the oxygen dissociation properties of haemoglobin, essential for normal oxygen transport. These functions can be modified by carbon dioxide, pH, and intracellular substances such as 2,3-diphosphoglycerate, the control of which is itself regulated by intracellular pH and oxygen levels. Hence there is an elegant intracellular control network relating oxygen delivery to red cell metabolism which, in turn, reflects the oxygen requirements of the tissues.

White blood cells

The white blood cells, much less abundant than red cells, play a key role in the body's defence against environmental pathogens. They are subdivided — on the basis of their microscopic structure, differences in taking up stains, and functions — into *phagocytic* ('eater') cells (which include *neutrophils, monocytes*, and *eosinophils*), and *non-phagocytic* cells (*lymphocytes* and *basophils*).

Phagocytic white cells derive from precursors in the bone marrow. Their production and maturation is controlled by a family of proteins called haemopoietic growth factors. Following their release into the blood, many of them remain in a so-called storage pool, stuck to the wall of blood vessels. The numbers circulating freely in the blood therefore represent just a fraction of the total body content.

The main function of the neutrophils is to kill MICROORGANISMS. They are attracted to areas of damaged tissue, where they internalise bacteria and other foreign particles, killing any invaders by a complex combination of oxidative and non-oxidative mechanisms. Monocytes have similar properties to neutrophils, and play an important role as part of the macrophage ('big eater') system by presenting foreign proteins (antigens) to T cells (see below). Eosinophils, which are particularly active against parasitic

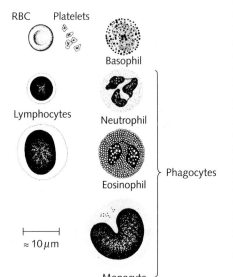

The cells of the blood, drawn to scale—red blood cells (RBC), platelets, and the several types of white blood cells.

infections, exert their action by discharging highly active elements from preformed granules. Basophils, and tissue cells called *mast cells*, to which they are related, also play an important role in combating parasitic infection.

The other important class of white cells is the lymphocytes. These cells play a major role in the body's IMMUNE SYSTEM. They are also derived from haemopoietic stem cells and disseminated in the bloodstream; some migrate to sites known as the '*primary lympho-epithelial organs*', including the thymus gland, where they differentiate further and eventually populate the '*secondary lymphoid tissues*', including the spleen, lymphoid tissue in the alimentary canal, and the lymph nodes. One set of lymphocytes, thymus-derived or *T cells*, migrate to specific areas within these tissues and pass through them into the lymphatic vessels; thus they recirculate from the blood to the lymph, and then back to the blood where the LYMPHATIC SYSTEM drains into it via the thoracic duct. The T cells are responsible for cellular immune responses. The other class of lymphocytes, *B cells*, populate different regions of the lymphatic system. Some of them also recirculate. They are the precursors of antibody-forming cells.

The immune system of a human can differentiate more than one million different foreign proteins, or antigens. T and B cells identify antigen by exposing receptor molecules on their surface: immunoglobulin for B cells, and T cell receptors for T cells. Before their first encounter each lymphocyte can only produce receptors to one particular antigen. When a lymphocyte binds to an antigen, it starts to divide to produce a clone of daughter cells, all with the same specificity — a process known as clonal selection. B cells produce immunoglobulins, or antibodies, in response to particular antigens, while T cells, after being activated by antigen presented to them by macrophages, either kill invading organisms directly, or play more subtle roles in co-ordinating other immune defence mechanisms. The extraordinary specificity and diversity of action of B and T cells is a reflection of a complex series of developmental rearrangements of the genes for immunoglobulins and the T cell receptor.

Platelets and blood clotting

It is vital to have ways to prevent the loss of blood after damage to blood vessels. It is equally important, however, that these processes occur only when they are needed, and do not spread from the site of injury to block off normal healthy vessels. These aims are achieved by the complicated series of cellular and biochemical interactions that constitutes blood clotting. Platelets, the other cellular elements of the blood, play a central role. These small, enucleate cells are produced from large parent cells, the *megakaryocytes*, in the bone marrow.

When a blood vessel ruptures there is immediate reflex constriction, thus narrowing the opening through which blood can escape. Platelets then aggregate at the site of the disruption. The

adhesion of platelets to the exposed tissues beneath the wall of the blood vessel requires the action of a plasma protein called *von Willebrand factor*, which binds to specific receptors on the outer membrane of the platelet. As platelets adhere they release a variety of chemicals that cause further aggregation, leading to the production of a temporary haemostatic plug.

At the same time as platelets are forming aggregates in the damaged vessel wall, a sequence of reactions — the coagulation 'cascade' — is activated. The objective of this complex process is to convert a soluble plasma protein, *fibrinogen*, to an insoluble *fibrin* mesh, or blood clot. This conversion requires the action of the enzyme *thrombin*, which is normally present in the blood in its inactive form, *prothrombin*. Thrombin also stimulates platelets to release several clotting factors and aggregating agents.

The activation of prothrombin results from the action of a remarkable biological amplification system in which circulating, inactive blood clotting factors are converted to catalytically active forms. The properties, and potential dangers, of this system are phenomenal: a sufficient amount of thrombin can be generated from the prothrombin in 2 ml of blood to clot the entire circulating volume. One of the inactive precursors in the clotting cascade is defective in the blood in haemophilia. Four of the factors require vitamin K for their production in the liver. Ionised calcium is one of the necessary factors.

This system is further complicated by the fact that activation of thrombin can occur through the intrinsic coagulation system, that is by the interaction of circulating factors, as well as by an extrinsic system which requires a factor from the tissues to interact with some of the circulating factors.

There is continual minor damage to the lining of blood vessels, so that blood clotting is continually being activated. Therefore mechanisms must exist for terminating the clotting cascade or dealing with the consequences of its activation. These involve either the inactivation of some of the protein co-factors by the enzymatic action of other plasma proteins (such as protein C or antithrombin III), or the digestion of unwanted fibrin (*fibrinolysis*) by the enzyme plasmin, activated from the *plasminogen* which is normally present in the blood.

Haemostasis — the prevention of blood loss — and blood coagulation are thus dynamic processes in which there is continual activation of the complex coagulation pathways, kept in check by inactivation mechanisms together with the removal of unwanted blood clot by the fibrinolytic system.

Plasma

The liquid plasma, in which all the cells of the blood are suspended, contains a variety of substances both in solution and as colloidal particles. There are salts, nutrients from the food (lipids, sugars, and amino acids) and hormones.

A complex mixture of proteins includes *albumin* — the main bulk of the plasma proteins, and of considerable importance in maintaining osmotic homeostasis, as it prevents the accumulation of excess fluid in the body tissues; *globulins* — some acting as 'carriers' for substances such as hormones, and others (gamma-globulins) which are part of the immune system; and also *fibrinogen* and other substances necessary for clotting.

The main functions of plasma are to transport nutrients, waste materials, and hormones; to provide an appropriate environment for different blood cells; to ensure, by exchange of water and solutes across capillary walls, that the chemical composition of the body fluids, both outside and inside cells, remains within normal, physiological concentrations; and — by carrying the coagulation proteins and their antagonists — to ensure that blood loss is prevented promptly after injury.   MARK WEATHERALL

D.J. WEATHERALL

See also ANAEMIA; BLOOD CIRCULATION; BODY FLUIDS; HAEMOGLOBIN; HOMEOSTASIS; IMMUNE SYSTEM; LYMPHATIC SYSTEM; MENSTRUATION; THYMUS.

Blood–brain barrier

Blood–brain barrier The main function of the blood–brain barrier (BBB) is to protect the brain from changes in the levels in the blood of ions, amino acids, peptides, and other substances. The barrier is located at the brain blood capillaries, which are unusual in two ways. Firstly, the cells which make up the walls of these vessels (the ENDOTHELIUM) are sealed together at their edges by tight junctions that form a key component of the barrier. These junctions prevent water-soluble substances in the blood from passing between the cells and therefore from freely entering the fluid environment of the brain cells. Secondly, these capillaries are enclosed by the flattened 'end-feet' of *astrocytic cells* (one type of GLIA), which also act as a partial, active, barrier. Thus the only way for water-soluble substances to cross the BBB is by passing directly through the walls of the cerebral capillaries, and because their CELL MEMBRANES are made up of a lipid/protein bilayer, they also act as a major part of the BBB.

In contrast, fat-soluble molecules, including those of oxygen and carbon dioxide, anaesthetics, and alcohol can pass straight through the lipids in the capillary walls and so gain access to all parts of the brain.

Apart from these passive elements of the BBB there are also enzymes on the lining of the cerebral capillaries that destroy unwanted peptides and other small molecules in the blood as it flows through the brain.

Finally, there is another barrier process that acts against lipid-soluble molecules, which may be toxic and can diffuse straight through capillary walls into the brain. In the capillary wall there are three classes of specialised '*efflux pumps*' which bind to three broad classes of molecules and transport them back into the blood out of the brain.

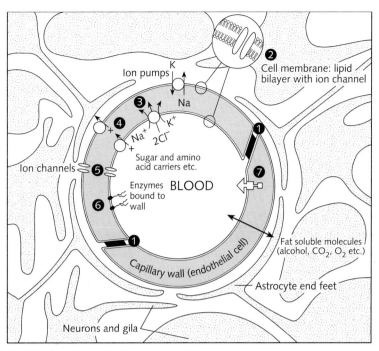

Diagram of a cerebral capillary enclosed in astrocyte end-feet.
Characteristics of the blood-brain barrier are indicated: (1) tight junctions that seal the pathway between the capillary (endothelial) cells; (2) the lipid nature of the cell membranes of the capillary wall which makes it a barrier to water-soluble molecules; (3), (4), and (5) represent some of the carriers and ion channels; (6) the 'enzymatic barrier' that removes molecules from the blood; (7) the efflux pumps which extrude fat-soluble molecules that have crossed into the cells.

However, in order for nourishment to reach the brain, water-soluble compounds must cross the BBB, including the vital glucose for energy production and amino acids for protein synthesis. To achieve this transfer, brain vessels have evolved special *carriers* on both sides of the cells forming the capillary walls, which transport these substances from blood to brain, and also move waste products and other unwanted molecules in the opposite direction.

The successful evolution of a complex brain depends on the development of the BBB. It exists in all vertebrates, and also in insects and the highly intelligent squid and octopus. In man the BBB is fully formed by the third month of gestation, and errors in this process can lead to defects such as spina bifida.

Although the BBB is an obvious advantage in protecting the brain, it also restricts the entry from the blood of water-soluble drugs which are used to treat brain tumours or infections, such as the AIDS virus, which uses the brain as a sanctuary and 'hides' behind the BBB from body defence mechanisms. To overcome these problems drugs are designed to cross the BBB, by making them more fat soluble. But this also means that they might enter most cells in the body and be too toxic. Alternative approaches are to make drug molecules that can 'ride on' the natural transporter proteins in the cerebral capillaries, and so be more focused on the brain, or to use drugs that open the BBB.

Since the brain is contained in a rigid, bony skull, its volume has to be kept constant. The BBB plays a key role in this process, by limiting the freedom of movement of water and salts from the blood into the extracellular fluid of the brain. Whereas in other body tissues extracellular fluid is formed by leakage from capillaries, the BBB in fact secretes brain extracellular fluid at a controlled rate and is thus critical in the maintenance of normal brain volume. If the barrier is made leaky by trauma or infection, water and salts cross into the brain, causing it to swell (*cerebral oedema*), which leads to raised intracranial pressure; this can be fatal.

The blood–brain barrier is thus a key element in the normal functioning of the brain, and isolates it from disturbances in the composition of the fluids in the rest of the body.

MALCOLM SEGAL

See also ACID–BASE HOMEOSTASIS; BODY FLUIDS; CELL MEMBRANE; CEREBROSPINAL FLUID; MENINGES.

Blood circulation

Blood circulation The circulation of blood refers to its continual flow from the HEART, through branching arteries, to reach and traverse the microscopic vessels in all parts of the body, reconverging in the veins and returning to the heart, to flow thence through the LUNGS and back to the heart to start the circuit again. This uninterrupted movement of the blood is necessary to maintain the supply of OXYGEN from the

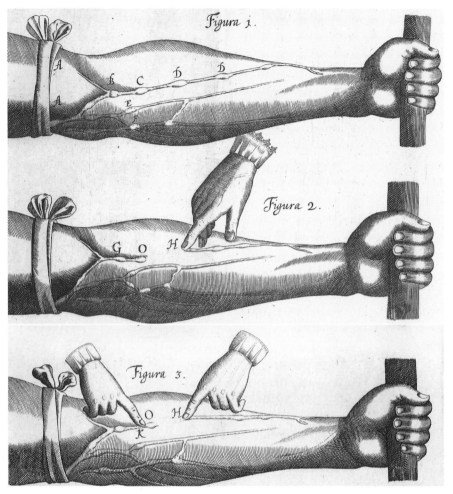

Fig. 1 Illustration from William Harvey: *De motu cordis* (1628). *Figura 1* shows distended veins in the forearm and position of valves. *Figura 2* shows that if a vein has been 'milked' centrally and the peripheral end compressed, it does not fill until the finger is released. *Figura 3* shows that blood cannot be forced in the 'wrong' direction. Wellcome Institute Library, London.

er finger is pressed just above the first and moved along the vein so as to expel the blood towards the heart, then released. Given that there is a valve in the segment of vein which was chosen, as long as the end furthest from the heart remains compressed, the vein remains empty between that point and the valve. It cannot fill from the heart end even when back pressure is applied due to the action of the valves.

The heart is not actually a single pump but, rather, two pumps in series (blood flows in sequence from the first pump round to the second pump and thence back round to the first). The two pumps — the right and left ventricles — are adjacent, sharing the muscular wall which partitions them. The right ventricle pumps blood to the lungs at relatively low pressure (pulmonary circulation). Blood returns from the lungs to the left atrium, enters the left ventricle to be pumped to the rest of the body (systemic circulation) at a much higher pressure, and returns to the right atrium. The various regions of the systemic circulation are perfused with blood through innumerable branching pathways, which are effectively arranged in parallel (Fig. 2).

Because the right and left heart pumps are in series, apart from transient changes their outputs must be identical. Even a minute difference between the outputs, if sustained, would very rapidly empty either the pulmonary or the systemic circulation. In fact, the rates of beating of the two sides of the heart are linked together electrically and the volumes pumped at each contraction are controlled such that each pump ejects at each stroke the volume which it has received, so that the output always matches the input (the *Starling mechanism*).

The importance of venous return

It is axiomatic that the heart, like any other pump, can only pump out the volume of blood that flows into it. If venous inflow is reduced, for example following haemorrhage, no matter how fast and hard the heart beats, it cannot restore flow to normal. When people are resting supine, the return of blood along the veins to the heart is largely a passive process. Sufficient pressure is transmitted from arteries through capillaries to veins to provide an adequate pressure for venous return. However, when we stand, blood distends dependent veins and the return is decreased. Physical exercise, particularly involving the legs, causes an increase in the flow of blood into the leg veins, acting as an auxiliary pump mechanism to enhance the return of blood to the heart.

There are actually two auxiliary pump mechanisms. Veins possess valves and many run deeply in the limbs, surrounded by muscles. Rhythmic movements, as when walking or running, cause alternate muscle tensing and relaxing. During the relaxing phase blood flows into the veins between the muscles, distending them. When the muscle then contracts the veins are compressed, so blood is forced along them. The valves ensure that blood can only move towards the heart.

lungs and nutrients from the gut, as well as for the distribution of HORMONES, many other chemicals, water, and heat, and the delivery of waste for excretion. The 5 litres of blood contained in the blood vessels of a typical adult at rest complete the circuit in about one minute: the blood recirculates 1500 times each day even without any EXERCISE to speed it up.

The beginning of the modern concept of the circulation of blood is attributed in Western society to William HARVEY, who, in a treatise published in 1628, *Exercitatio anatomica de motu cordis et sanguinis*, presented convincing evidence that blood flowed in arteries out from the heart to the tissues and returned back along veins. He did not know how blood passed from arteries to veins, as this was long before Malpighi of Bologna discovered the microscopic capillaries which connect them, but he deduced that some sort of channels must exist. Harvey based his radical conclusions on experiments on a wide range of animals and then demonstrated his results and explanations to his colleagues.

Harvey's contribution was of startling significance. Before his time there had been no serious challenge to the teaching of GALEN in the second century AD. Arguing from gross anatomy, Galen believed that blood passed from the right side to the left side of the heart through invisible pores in the muscular septum which separates the two ventricles. Somewhat paradoxically, Harvey dismissed the existence of these cardiac septum pores' which were widely accepted but had never been seen, whilst simultaneously postulating the existence of components — the capillaries — which he was likewise unable to see.

That blood flows away from the heart in the arteries is clear fom observation following injury, when a high pressure pulsatile jet of blood comes from the heart end of a cut artery and not from the other end. Flow in veins can readily be demonstrated to be only in the direction towards the heart, as illustrated by Harvey (Fig. 1). His experiment is readily repeated. An arm is congested (by letting it hang by the side or squeezing the upper arm) so that the veins stand out; a finger is pressed on a vein and held there; anoth-

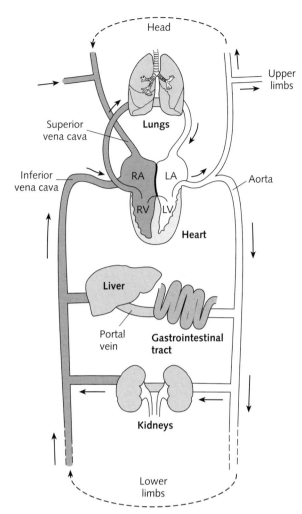

Fig. 2 Simplified diagram of the circulation. Blood enters the right atrium (RA) from the 2 great veins, the *superior and inferior venae cavae* (SVC and IVC). It then enters the right ventricle (RV) to be pumped at low pressure through the lungs. Oxygenated blood from the lungs returns to the left atrium (LA) and is pumped by the left ventricle (LV) at high pressure through the various components of the systemic circulation before returning again to the right heart.

The other auxiliary mechanism is due to breathing. Pressure in the chest is normally negative and that in the abdomen positive. As we breathe in, this pressure difference increases, and the downward movement of the diaphragm compresses the abdominal contents forcing blood into the chest through the inferior vena cava.

Regional circulations

Since the systemic and pulmonary circulations form one continuous circuit, the flow through the lungs is entirely dependent on that through the systemic circulation. Systemic flow is the sum of flow through the many parallel circuits supplying different organs and tissues. Systemic and pulmonary flow must clearly each be the same as the cardiac output — the volume pumped by each ventricle. At rest the cardiac output is typically about 5 litres/min. This can increase during exercise to as much as 25 litres/min in fit young people and 35 litres/min, or briefly even more, in elite endurance athletes. The quantity of blood flowing through each organ or region supplied by the systemic circulation is regulated according to its own particular physiological requirement.

Brain circulation. About 15% of the resting cardiac output supplies the brain. This flow is vital as the brain cannot withstand more than a few seconds of interruption of flow without loss of consciousness, and longer interruptions cause irreversible damage. Overall brain blood flow remains relatively constant, although regional changes occur in response to changes in neuronal activity. For example, shining a light in the eye results in an increase in blood flow to the region of the brain concerned with vision. In the upright position, because of the effects of gravity, the blood pressure in the brain is lower than elsewhere, making it susceptible to low blood pressure. However the brain does show the phenomenon of 'autoregulation', whereby its blood flow is kept relatively stable over a quite wide range of blood pressure. Although the brain blood flow is determined to some extent by nervous control of the diameter of blood vessels, it is more importantly controlled by chemical factors, particularly the level of carbon dioxide which, when it increases, dilates the cerebral vessels and increases flow. Overbreathing lowers the level of carbon dioxide in the body and can cause dizziness due to decreasing brain blood flow.

Muscles. A contracting muscle produces several chemicals which are the end products of its metabolic activity. These 'metabolites' act directly on the resistance vessels (arterioles), dilating them and thus regulating blood flow so that it is appropriate for the level of activity. Although sympathetic nerves do supply muscle blood vessels, they control only the resting blood flow and play no part in the response to exercise. At rest, flow in all muscles comprises only about 1 litre/min out of the cardiac output of 5 litres/min. During exercise, if cardiac output increases to 25 litres/min, 20 litres of this goes to the working muscles.

Heart (coronary) circulation. The flow to the heart muscle via the coronary arteries takes about 5% of cardiac output both at rest and when it increases during exercise. The heart removes nearly all the oxygen from the coronary blood even at rest, so that, when heart work increases, the only way that more oxygen can be supplied is for blood flow to increase. If this cannot happen, as for example if coronary vessels are partially blocked, there is coronary insufficiency and heart pain (angina). Coronary flow is influenced by mechanical factors: left ventricular flow is low or absent during contraction (systole) and maximal during the relaxation phase (diastole). As for skeletal muscle, coronary flow is controlled by metabolites rather than directly by nerves.

Skin. Blood flow to the skin is controlled by the mechanisms of TEMPERATURE REGULATION. If local skin temperature or general body temperature rises, skin vessels, including special arterio–venous shunt vessels, dilate to increase skin blood flow and thereby increase skin temperature and facilitate cooling. Skin flow is controlled partly by nerves and partly by direct local temperature effects (warm hands are red). During very cold conditions blood flow to the entire skin is almost completely cut off. During extreme heat, flow may increase to the extent that most of the output of the heart flows through the skin.

Circulation to the gastrointestinal tract (splanchnic flow). The anatomy of the circulation of the gut (splanchnic circulation) is unusual in that the venous blood does not return directly to the heart, but instead it flows in the portal vein to the liver, and only after this does it reach the hepatic vein and the inferior vena cava. Since the splanchnic circulation is concerned with the digestion and absorption of food, this means that the blood carrying products of digestion passes through the liver before reaching any other part of the body. Splanchnic vessels also serve a 'reservoir' function. Constriction of splanchnic arerioles — the resistance vessels — is under the control of the sympathetic nervous system and makes a major contribution to BLOOD PRESSURE control. The splanchnic veins also constrict in response to stimulation of the sympathetic nerves; this reduces their capacity and increases the flow of blood returning to the heart.

Kidneys. Although the kidneys are relatively small organs they receive about 20% of cardiac output. Most of this blood flow is concerned with the filtration of the plasma and the subsequent concentration of the filtrate to form urine. The blood flow is normally autoregulated and is therefore relatively independent of blood pressure unless this falls to abnormally low levels.

ROGER HAINSWORTH

E.M. TANSEY

Further reading

Vogel, S. (1992). *Vital circuits — on pumps, pipes, and the workings of circulatory systems.* Oxford University Press, New York, Oxford.

See Plate 2.

See also AUTONOMIC NERVOUS SYSTEM; BLOOD PRESSURE; BLOOD VESSELS; HEART.

Blood clotting

Blood which is withdrawn or spilt from the body will separate within minutes into dark red clot and straw-coloured serum. It is normally prevented from clotting (or 'coagulating') in the circulation, but there are substances always present in the blood which will cause clotting when there is a need to plug a damaged vessel. Clotting at a site of injury involves ENZYMES, several specific proteins made in the LIVER, CALCIUM ions, and PLATELETS — all present in the blood — together with substances released from damaged tissue. Their interaction produces fibrin, the stringy framework of a clot. Clots may form inside intact blood vessels where there is an abnormality of the lining, or where blood is unduly static. A clot is also known as a thrombus, and the condition of abnormal clot formation, thrombosis. A tendency to thrombosis can be counteracted by substances which interfere at some stage of the process: e.g. HEPARIN or warfarin, and ASPIRIN is used as a long-term preventative measure. The downside of such anticoagulant treatments is a tendency to bleed more easily.   S.J.

See BLOOD; EMBOLISM.

Blood groups

The giving of blood and its subsequent safe transfusion into a patient is now commonplace. Successful transfusion would not, however, be possible without the realisation that the cells and tissues of individuals are distinct and that introduction of blood of one individual into another may cause an adverse reaction with subsequent destruction of the donated cells. Such reactions come about because there are substances — so-called blood group antigens — on the surface of the cells of the blood, especially on the red cells, or erythrocytes, which may interact with antibodies in another person's blood, leading to red cell destruction. Fortunately, although there are many different antigens on cells, only a small number of them limit transfusion compatibility. These have been designated into major groups, the so-called blood groups. The most well known is the ABO system. If, for example, a donor's cells have the A antigen, that blood cannot be given to a person whose blood contains Anti-A antibodies, because the red cells would be destroyed. Incompatibility of blood groups, usually in this instance of the Rhesus system, is also important in the condition of *haemolytic disease of the new-born* (HDN).

In the ABO system, the surface antigens of the red cells are determined by three genes, *A*, *B*, and *O*. (The genes are referred to by an italicised character, e.g. *A*, whilst the gene product (phenotype) and hence the blood groups are referred to by simple uppercase letter, e.g. group A.) All red cells have on their surface a glycolipid substance called H substance. The *A* gene and the *B* gene convert H substance into substance A and B, giving rise to cells of the A and B groups respectively. The *O* gene has no effect on H substance and thus group O cells have only H substance on their surface. These three genes combine in pairs to give six possible genotypes, *AA*, *AO*, *BB*, *BO*, *AB*, and *OO*. Since *A* and *B* are dominant over *O*, this results in four phenotypes: A, B, AB and O (see table). Eighty per cent of individuals also have A, B, and H substances in secretions such as tears and saliva.

Since, under normal circumstances, individuals do not form antibodies against their own proteins and since all red cells have H substance, no naturally occurring antibodies against H substance are found. Likewise individuals with group A cells (genotypes *AA*, *AO*, or *AB*), do not have antibodies against A substance in their plasma and individuals with group B cells (genotype *BB*, *BO*, or *AB*) do not have antibodies against B substance. However, substances closely related to A and B are widely distributed in nature and absorption of these from the gut, presumably shortly after birth, is thought to give rise to antibodies against A and/or B if that individual does not possess A and/or B antigens on their red cells. Thus, individuals who are group A have antibodies against B substance and those who are group B have antibodies against A substance.

Thus, an individual who is group AB should be able to receive cells of any group, since he would not have antibodies against any blood group substance and the transfused cells would not be destroyed. Likewise, it should be possible to transfuse group O blood into any individual, since the transfused cells will contain neither A nor B substance, but only O, and any antibodies against either A or B substance in the recipient plasma will be without effect. As group O cells do not react with anti-A or anti-B antibodies, people of group O became known as universal donors. But it is not quite as simple as that.

Although the ABO blood group system is the one which is of greatest concern in blood transfusion, approximately 400 blood group antigens have been described and, before blood transfusion is attempted, it is essential that the blood of the recipient and the blood of the donor are directly matched by a laboratory test to avoid incompatibility. The other blood grouping which is a common cause of transfusion incompatibility is the Rhesus system, and occasional reactions are encountered as a result of incompatibility in other systems.

The Rhesus (Rh) system is the usual cause of the so-called haemolytic disease of the newborn, although, rarely, the other grouping systems can be responsible. The Rh system derives its name from the discovery by Landsteiner and Wiener in 1940 that injection of red cells from a Rhesus monkey into a rabbit caused the production of antibodies, and that these antibodies reacted with the red cells of some humans (so-called Rh-positive individuals), but not others (Rh-negative individuals). Similar antibodies were found in the plasma of mothers who had given birth to children with HDN. The development of jaundice and anaemia soon after birth, and the occasional death of such infants was previously a mystery. The definition of the Rh group of an individual depends on the presence of a substance D; those whose cells have the D antigen are Rh positive, and their cells are attacked by D antibodies in blood of a person who is Rh negative. Clinically, only the D antigen and the anti-D antibody are important, although other (C and E) substances also differ between the groups.

Haemolytic disease of the new-born is the result of the passage of antibodies from the maternal circulation across the placenta into the fetal circulation, where they damage the red cells. The condition arises where the mother is Rh-negative but the fetus, and the father, are Rh-positive. At the time of birth in a first pregnancy in these circumstances, there is no damage to the infant, but fetal red cells leak into the maternal circulation, immunising the mother and causing the production of antibodies. These antibodies are small enough in size to cross the placenta and enter the fetal circulation during subsequent pregnancies, causing HDN if the fetus is again Rh-positive. Often this is confined to mild

The ABO system of blood groups.

Genotype	Red cell antigen	Phenotype	Antibodies in blood plasma	Frequency, UK, %
OO	None	O	Anti-A, B	46
AA or *AO*	A	A	Anti-B	42
BB or *BO*	B	B	Anti-A	9
AB	AB	AB	None	3

anaemia, but in more serious cases the baby is severely anaemic and jaundiced because of the accumulation of bilirubin released from damaged red cells. In the 1940s complete 'exchange transfusion' — replacing the whole of the infant's blood via the umbilical cord soon after birth — started to be employed as a life saving measure. Fortunately, the risk of HDN caused by Rhesus incompatibility is now reduced enormously by the administration of an anti-D antibody to the mother at the time of the birth of the first and any subsequent Rh-positive child, thus removing fetal red cells from the maternal circulation before they can stimulate permanent production of antibody. D.E. BOWYER

Blood letting or *phlebotomy*, was one of the most common forms of medical therapy. So pervasive was the practice that the term 'leech', from the use of these animals to suck out a patient's blood, was a synonym for medical practitioner in England from the time of the Anglo-Saxons. *Leeching, cupping* — the use of a horn or a vessel to draw blood to the skin's surface, and *venesection* — the opening of a vein, were in medical use well into the twentieth century and have not entirely disappeared from present-day practice.

Until William HARVEY's discovery of circulation in 1628, blood was thought to be produced continually in the liver and sent around the body by a sort of boiling, fuelled by heat generated from the digestion of food. A normal body nourished itself from this blood, excreting waste material in the form of urine, faeces, sweat, and mucus. Haemorrhoidal and menstrual blood were also considered normal forms of excrement, eliminating from the body the 'dregs' of blood — clotted, dark, and contaminated by black bile or melancholy, one of the four HUMOURS. Certain kinds of 'blood lettings' were thus considered quite normal, and were the body's way of ridding itself of waste products.

Blood letting as a form of medical therapy arose from a belief that fever and inflammation, characterised by redness, swelling, heat, and a quick pulse, were the result of too much blood, which had to be eliminated. The most usual way of accomplishing this was to open a vein, usually the basilic vein at the front of the elbow. Alternatively, blood was drawn to the skin's surface, sometimes by applying suction to an animal's horn with a small hole cut in the tip, or by placing a heated glass cup on the skin. When the air inside the cup cooled, it contracted and drew blood to the skin's surface. This was called dry cupping. Commonly, the bleeder would make small cuts in the skin's surface with a lancet or by using a small box with trigger-loaded knives inside, before applying the cup, which would then fill with blood. Another popular method was to apply leeches, ideally selected with great care for their cleanliness and fitness to the task, which were allowed to drop off after drawing their fill. Three or four were usually recommended, but some nineteenth-century physicians advised 50 at once, a blood letting of nearly vampiric proportions.

One of the purposes of blood letting was to reduce fever, which was indicated by a drop in the pulse after phlebotomy was accomplished. Another was to aid nature, that is to help the body rid itself of 'peccant' or harmful matter that was causing inflammation at a particular site. Medieval Islamic physicians advocated what is generally called 'revulsive' bleeding — blood letting at a place remote from the site of inflammation, in order to draw the peccant matter back into the body where it could be 'digested' normally. Followers of the ancient Greek texts attributed to Hippocrates, like the Frenchman Pierre Brissot (1478–1522) and the Englishman Thomas Sydenham (1624–89), advocated the opposite — a 'derivative' method in which the blood and peccant matter were evacuated close to the site of the inflammation and on the same side of the body. The latter method was in common use after the end of the medieval period.

Medieval medical thinkers often commented on the attraction of the moon both on the tides and on the flow of blood in the body. Many also seem to have associated increased production of blood with the rise of sap in trees during early springtime. Both these beliefs affected the way blood was let. Barbers, surgeons, and the keepers of bath houses, all of whom bled as part of the practice of their trade, were warned not to open veins when the moon caused a high tide, lest too much blood be released. They also typically let blood in the springtime from people who were not ill as a kind of 'spring tonic'.

The discovery of the circulation of the blood only increased the popularity of the practice. By the end of the eighteenth century, blood letting was depicted in novels being performed by lay people as a kind of life-saving 'first aid' to relieve 'congestion' caused by fainting and as the result of accidents. Medical texts before World War II still advocated phlebotomy, either by leeches or by venesection, to 'lower arterial tension' and to 'relieve right side stagnation' of blood in the heart. Nowadays blood letting seems to us a relic of a former age. Its only common use is to reduce the damaging effects of an excess of red blood cells in cases of *polycythaemia vera*. Recently, however, the use of leeches has returned, to remove blood from capillaries after delicate surgery. FAYE GETZ

See also HUMOURS; ISLAMIC MEDICINE; MEDICINE.

Blood pressure In a resting individual the left ventricle of the heart pumps typically 5 litres of blood each minute into the aorta and arteries of the body. Downstream, the small arterioles restrict the outflow of blood from the arteries and are therefore known as the main 'resistance vessels'. The combined effect of the energy generated by the heart and the outflow restriction results in a distending pressure in the arterial system which is referred to as the blood pressure.

The first report of a direct measurement of arterial blood pressure was by Revd Stephen Hales in 1733. He inserted a tube into an abnormally exposed artery of a horse and observed that a column of blood rose in a glass tube to a vertical height of 8 ft 3 in. This represents the force generated by the heart and transmitted to all the major arteries in the body. We do not now express blood pressure as height in feet and inches of blood. However, we sometimes use centimeters of water, so that the horse's blood pressure would be 250 cm of water or blood. Such a column has obvious practical problems for measuring arterial pressure. But for venous pressures which are much lower, a column of saline connected to a major vein is often used clinically to assess the degree of filling of the circulation. Arterial pressure is usually expressed as millimetres of mercury (mm Hg) because mercury is 13.6 times as dense as water and a mercury column of that height is more practicable. Thus the horse's pressure blood would be 185 mm Hg. An alternative unit for expressing blood pressures, which has not been widely adopted in clinical practice, is the SI unit, the pascal or kilopascal (kPa). One kPa is approximately 7.5 mm Hg.

Blood pressure is not normally expressed as a single figure but rather as two, for example 120/80. This means that the pressure in the arteries varies with each heart beat to a peak, called systolic pressure, of 120 mm Hg, and then declines to a minimum value, called diastolic pressure, of 80 mm Hg just before the next beat. These phasic values of blood pressure can be recorded accurately using modern transducers (electronic measuring devices) connected to catheters (fine tubes) inserted into arteries. However, except for research and measurements during complex investigations in patients, blood pressure is not usually determined by direct puncture of an artery. The most common method is to use the device known as a *sphygmomanometer*. This is an inflatable cuff which fits round the upper arm and is connected to a mercury manometer. A stethoscope is applied to listen to the artery below the cuff. The cuff is first inflated with a pressure well above systolic and then slowly deflated. The systolic pressure is taken as the pressure in the cuff when the artery just opens and a sound is first heard. The diastolic pressure is that when the sound either becomes muffled or disappears completely.

Blood pressure, like all biological variables, varies widely in different people and, in the same individual, at different times of the day. Typically a normal value for systolic blood pressure would be 120 mm Hg at age 20, increasing perhaps to 140 mm Hg at 60. Diastolic pressure also increases with age but rather less. Estimates of blood pressure in apparently healthy people show values that can be 20 or even 40 mm Hg higher or lower than the average values. This, and the fact that blood pressure varies considerably during the day, particularly in response to stresses such as visiting a doctor, mean that it is very difficult to decide on the basis of a single measurement whether a patient suffers from HYPERTENSION (high blood pressure). Definitions of hypertension are constantly changing but, generally, if systolic pressure is consistently greater than 160 mm Hg or diastolic more than 95, a person is considered to be hypertensive.

At rest, each time the heart contracts, it ejects typically 70 ml of blood into the arterial system. This causes a steep increase in arterial pressure, the magnitude of which is dependent both on the volume ejected and on the distensibility of the arteries. Older people have less distensible arteries, which explains why their systolic blood pressure is usually higher than in younger subjects. Because the shape of the arterial pressure pulse is roughly triangular, the mean level of pressure is nearer to the diastolic value.

The importance of blood pressure is that it effectively provides a store of energy, generated by the heart, available to cause blood to flow through the working tissues. It is actually the *flow* of blood, providing oxygen and nutrients and removing waste products including carbon dioxide, which is really the important factor, but without pressure there would be no flow. Humans, being upright bipedal animals, have a particular problem in supplying blood to all parts of the body. Due just to gravity, pressure in arteries supplying the head is about 100 mm Hg less than that in arteries in the feet. The fact that the brain must have an adequate arterial pressure places a limitation on the range of effective pressures in the upright person.

Control of blood pressure

Mean blood pressure depends on the flow of blood from the heart (cardiac output) and the resistance to flow in the small arteries and microscopic resistance vessels (arterioles).

$$BP = CO \times PVR$$

where BP is blood pressure, CO is cardiac output, and PVR is the peripheral vascular resistance or the net resistance to blood flow in all the small arteries and microscopic arterioles.

Peripheral vascular resistance is dependent on the radius (r) of the small blood vessels. In fact it turns out to be proportional to $1/r^4$. The equation for blood pressure can now be changed:

$$BP \propto CO/r^4$$

The importance of the degree of constriction of resistance vessels can be seen from this equation because if cardiac output is unchanged a reduction in the average radius of the resistance vessels of only 10% would increase blood pressure by more than 50%. The physiological control of blood pressure is thus effected mainly by regulating the radius of the resistance vessels and, to a smaller extent, the cardiac output. Baroreceptors provide an effective means for detecting changes in blood pressure and bringing about appropriate responses, via the autonomic nervous system. If blood pressure started to fall the baroreceptor stimulation would decrease and the reflex response would cause the small resistance vessels to constrict and the heart to beat faster and harder, by action of the sympathetic nerves. This *negative feedback mechanism* largely

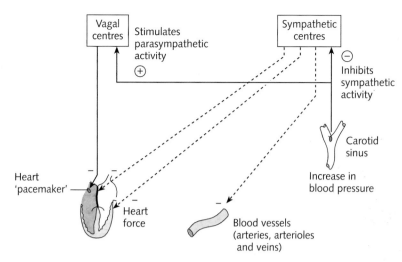

Fig. 1 The baroreceptor reflex. An increase in blood pressure increases the rate of nerve impulses from baroreceptor to brain. Vagal centres are stimulated: increased activity in the vagus nerve to the pacemaker slows the heart. Sympathetic centres are inhibited causing less activity in sympathetic nerves. As these nerves are excitatory, the effect of inhibition is to slow heart rate, weaken force of contraction, and dilate blood vessels. All these changes lower the blood pressure. The opposite effects would be seen in response to a decrease in blood pressure.

restores the blood pressure. Conversely, if blood pressure increases, stimulation of baroreceptors gives rise to nerve impulses which run to the brain and stimulate activity in the parasympathetic pathway in the vagus nerves, which slows the heart; also inhibition of activity in sympathetic nerves decreases both the rate and force of contraction of the heart and dilates of both the resistance and the capacitance vessels (veins) (Fig. 1).

Some factors which affect blood pressure

Baroreceptors are important for minimizing changes in blood pressure: animal studies have shown that blood pressure is much more variable if the influence of baroreceptors is removed. However, they do not prevent all fluctuations from occurring. Continuous 24-hour recordings have been made in healthy volunteers and have shown variations of 30–80 mm Hg in systolic pressure and of 10–80 mm Hg in diastolic pressure. Blood pressure is particularly low during sleep, and high during physical activity or emotional stress.

Physical exercise causes very major effects on the circulation. Due to the enormously increased blood flow through the exercising muscle, the amount of blood pumped by the heart may increase four-fold, or in elite athletes as much as six-fold. The increased volume of blood ejected at each heart beat causes systolic blood pressure to increase, perhaps to 180 mm Hg. However, because blood flows very rapidly out of the arteries, particularly to the working muscle where the resistance vessels are widely dilated, diastolic pressure remains relatively unchanged or may even decrease. Isometric exercise has quite a different effect. Here there is a much smaller effect on the total amount of blood pumped by the heart, but reflexes, particularly those arising from the contracting muscle itself, cause blood

vessels elsewhere to constrict, and consequently both systolic and diastolic blood pressure rise sharply. This response may also be augmented by a straining effect (see below).

Emotional stress can cause quite large increases in blood pressure. Prominent amongst the physiological responses to stress is an increase in activity in the sympathetic nerves. Sympathetic overactivity increases heart rate and force, and constricts resistance blood vessels (Fig. 1). All these effects increase both systolic and diastolic blood pressure and are augmented by increased secretion into the blood of adrenaline and noradrenaline.

Postural changes exert stresses on the cardiovascular system requiring effective reflex responses to constrict arteries and veins and stimulate the heart, to control blood pressure, maintain brain blood flow, and prevent loss of consciousness. The upright position means that blood vessels below the level of the heart are subjected to increased distending pressures due to the effects of gravity. Veins are particularly susceptible to gravitational stress due to their distensibility, and blood 'pools' in dependent veins when we stand. Because of this, less blood flows back to the heart and, were it not for effective reflexes, involving baroreceptors, blood pressure would fall catastrophically, particularly in the brain, resulting in insufficient brain blood flow and consequent loss of consciousness. Blood pressure frequently falls transiently when we stand. This is particularly noticeable if we stand suddenly when warm, for example on getting out of a hot bath, because the resistance blood vessels initially will be dilated. In some people blood pressure control may be inadequate to counter the stress of postural changes and the result is that they faint.

Straining (the Valsalva manoeuvre) induces large and complex variations in blood pressure. The

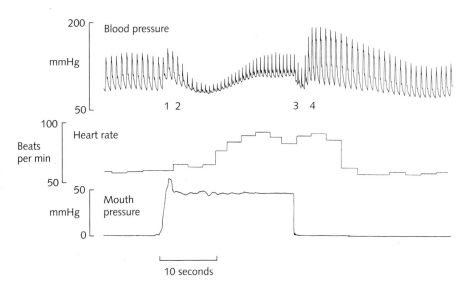

Fig. 2 The Valsalva manoeuvre. The subject blows against a fixed resistance to generate a pressure in the mouth (MP) of 40 mm Hg. This causes 4 phases of blood pressure change. *Phase 1*: blood pressure (BP) rises due to the pressure transmitted to the arteries. *Phase 2*: BP falls and pulse pressure (difference between systolic and diastolic pressures) particularly falls due to the reduced filling, and therefore pumping, of the heart. Pressure subsequently recovers due to the reflex changes. Note also the reflex increase in heart rate. *Phase 3*: BP falls as the pressure is taken off the arteries in the chest and abdomen. *Phase 4*: there is an overshoot as the 'dammed back' blood rushes into the heart and is pumped into a constricted circulation.

sort of stresses that induce these changes include blowing against a resistance, lifting heavy objects, and straining at stool. The effects on the circulation are illustrated in Fig. 2. The primary change is caused by an increase in pressure within the chest (intrathoracic pressure) and within the abdomen. Normally, intrathoracic pressure is lower than atmospheric, due to the tendency of lungs to collapse and their prevention from so doing by the chest wall. This negative intrathoracic pressure aids the flow of blood to the heart from the peripheral veins. Straining causes the pressure in both the chest and the abdomen to become positive. Initially the compression of the heart and large arteries causes an increase in blood pressure. Then, the high pressure in the chest impedes the inflow of blood from peripheral veins (veins in the neck can be seen to distend), so the cardiac output decreases and blood pressure falls. Baroreceptors detect this fall and initiate constriction of blood vessels and an increase in heart rate, so that mean blood pressure is restored. At the end of the strain there is a transient fall in pressure before blood rushes back to the heart, causing an overshoot and often a transient slowing of the heart. In people with some autonomic nerve disorders these responses may be deficient: blood pressure falls continuously, and the overshoot is absent.

ROGER HAINSWORTH

See also AUTONOMIC NERVOUS SYSTEM; BARORECEPTORS; BLOOD CIRCULATION; HEART.

Bloodshot Applied to EYES, this refers to visible blood in or behind the *conjunctiva*. The conjunctiva is supplied by minute blood vessels. Redness is apparent if these are dilated by irritation or infection; actual sub-conjunctival bleeding — a bloodshot eye — may accompany this or more often occurs without infection, from external damage or a surge of blood pressure.　　s.j.

Blood sugar When we refer to 'blood sugar', we actually mean the monosaccharide (simple sugar) glucose dissolved in the blood. Maintaining a stable blood glucose concentration is necessary in order to keep it high enough to ensure normal functioning of the brain, whilst also preventing the harmful consequences which can arise when the concentration is too high. Blood glucose concentration in healthy people, after an overnight fast, will normally be between 3.5 and 5.5 mmol/litre and this is referred to as *euglycaemia*, or normal blood glucose. With more prolonged fasting it can go lower than 3.5, and in some individuals it can exceed 6 mmol/litre. A person would be diagnosed as having diabetes if their blood glucose after an overnight fast exceeded 7.0 mmol/litre: this is *hyperglycaemia*, an abnormally high blood glucose.

When we consume food or drink containing carbohydrates, most of this will be either simple *glucose* (a monosaccharide); *sucrose* (a disaccharide which contains equal amounts of glucose and fructose); or *starch* (which is a polysaccharide — a polymer of glucose). Thus, most of the carbohydrate we consume is available to the body as glucose, and so eating or drinking it will lead, after digestion and absorption, to a rise in blood glucose. The magnitude of this rise is controlled by the release of INSULIN from the PANCREAS. Insulin acts to stimulate the uptake of glucose from the blood into cells such as those of muscle and adipose tissue, its storage as GLYCOGEN (in muscle and liver), and its part in the synthesis of triglycerides, the stored form of fat (mainly in adipose tissue). The relatively slow rate of absorption of dietary carbohydrate (it can take 2–3 hours to absorb the carbohydrate from a normal breakfast), and the effects of insulin, ensure that blood glucose does not usually rise above 8 mmol/litre after meals in non-diabetic people. The figure shows a typical 24-hour profile of blood glucose concentration. The concentration can increase rapidly after consumption of simple sugars, especially glucose itself, either in a drink or in tablet form. This will provide a more rapidly available source of energy than would occur with starchy food.

When blood glucose concentration is normal, the glucose which is filtered from the blood in the KIDNEYS is reabsorbed back into the bloodstream by the kidney tubules, and so none is lost in the URINE. But if blood glucose exceeds about 12 mmol/litre, this causes more glucose to be filtered by the kidneys than they can reabsorb. Glucose is therefore lost in the urine, and, because glucose is a powerful osmotic agent, it draws water with it, causing large volumes of sweet urine to be excreted (characteristic of *diabetes mellitus*). The other undesirable consequence of a persistently elevated blood glucose is that a chemical reaction (glycation or glycosylation) can occur between glucose and proteins, including the important structural proteins in CELL MEMBRANES, and this can damage the membranes, producing harmful effects. Thus the action of insulin to control blood glucose prevents these undesirable effects of hyperglycaemia, and also ensures that glucose is available for use by the body's tissues.

The BRAIN and the rest of the NERVOUS SYSTEM, and also the red blood cells, must receive a constant supply of glucose to function normally. In prolonged starvation it is possible for the brain to satisfy some of its energy requirements by using ketone bodies, which are products of fat breakdown, but under normal circumstances the adult human brain needs approximately 6 g per hour of glucose to function normally. After meals containing carbohydrate this is not a problem, as the absorbed carbohydrate provides a ready supply of glucose. However, if we have a high fat meal, or have an extended period between meals (e.g. fasting overnight), we have to provide glucose from within the body. This is done either by the breakdown of the glycogen stored in the liver, which releases glucose into the blood, or by making glucose from amino acids released from the body protein stores. This synthesis of glucose (known as gluconeogenesis) occurs mainly in the liver, and to a lesser extent in the kidneys. The stimulation of the liver to break down its glycogen store and make glucose from amino acids occurs as a result of the fall in plasma insulin which occurs in fasting, together with an increase in glucagon, which is another hormone released from the pancreas.

In some circumstances the rate of use of blood glucose exceeds the rate at which it is released

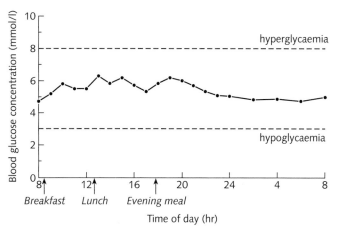

Typical 24-hour profile of blood glucose concentration.

from the liver, and blood glucose concentration falls. When blood glucose falls below 3.5 mmol/litre, the condition of *hypoglycaemia* is beginning to develop. This condition occurs quite commonly in people with diabetes who are treated with insulin injections, but much less so in non-diabetics. However, hypoglycaemia can occur in healthy people if they undertake prolonged periods of quite high intensity exercise, such as ultra-distance running or cycling, without consuming carbohydrate. Another cause of hypoglycaemia in non-diabetic people is the consumption of about 50 g or more of alcohol (about 5–6 units) after either 24–36 hours of starvation or 2–3 hours of exercise to exhaustion. Starvation or exhaustive exercise will have caused liver glycogen to be depleted, so the liver needs to synthesize glucose to maintain the supply to the brain; but alcohol prevents the liver from performing this synthesis, causing blood glucose to fall and hypoglycaemia to develop.

When blood glucose is at hypoglycaemic levels, there are a number of characteristic effects on the brain. Reactions are slowed, the person has difficulty in concentrating and can feel light-headed, vision may be disturbed, and hunger is common. The AUTONOMIC NERVOUS SYSTEM reaction to hypoglycaemia causes sweating and trembling, and the person often becomes aware that their heart is beating more rapidly (they describe having palpitations). With mild degrees of hypoglycaemia (blood glucose between 3.5 and 3.0 mmol/litre) most people would be unaware of anything untoward occurring, although sensitive measurements of brain function would detect a slowing of reactions. As blood glucose falls further, the effects become more noticeable, but provided the symptoms are used to prompt the consumption of carbohydrate, these effects are rapidly reversed. If blood glucose falls to very low levels, unconsciousness can occur, but this is extremely rare, except for people with insulin-treated diabetes.

I.A. MACDONALD

See also INSULIN; METABOLISM; STARVATION; SUGARS.

Blood transfusion

Blood, moved between bodies, has long been thought to rejuvenate its recipient. Though transfusion 'proper' — moving blood directly into a recipient's veins with the intention of healing a variety of afflictions — might have awaited William Harvey's early-seventeenth-century work on blood's circulation, a long and colourful tradition of moving blood preceded it. Homer's Odysseus, for example, fed the blood of sacrificed animals to the shades of Hades to 'substantiate' them, enabling them to communicate with the living. In another blood ritual, the early-sixteenth-century Hungarian countess Elizabeth Bathory became obsessed by the idea that the blood of virgins would preserve her youth and beauty. She enticed local girls to her castle, where she hung them in metal cages and stuffed them into iron maidens, allowing the blood that flowed from their slowly pierced bodies to bathe her.

The perception of blood's movement as regenerative is tied to complex cultural conceptions of blood itself. Blood has long been used as a metaphor for identity: family ('blood is thicker than water'); class ('blue blood'); race ('black blood'); nationality ('red-blooded American'); opposition ('bad blood'). It has also been seen as the intangible carrier of the 'vital spirit' that animates animal bodies. Some Hippocratic physicians dubbed it the highest of the four HUMOURS, the formative substance of body and character. Similarly, blood's movement between bodies has carried and extended these meanings: a sharing of the self and an extension of life. Christians believe communion wine to represent (and, for Roman Catholics, to *be*) Christ's blood. Drinking it prepares the faithful to enter into eternal life and at the same time strengthens the communal Christian identity.

Early history

The first recorded efforts to transfuse blood directly into living veins came in England in 1665, where Richard Lower transfused blood between dogs. In 1667, Jean-Baptiste Denis, of France's Académie des Sciences, successfully transfused lamb's blood into a human. It has been suggested these transfusions were conducted as much to see if science could correct the unhappy consequences of humanity's fall from Grace as to examine the empirical possibilities of blood's circulation. These experiments were cut short after one of Denis' patients died shortly after receiving a transfusion. A subsequent trial exonerated Denis, but banned transfusion without prior approval of the Académie de Médecine. The French Parliament, the Royal Society, and the Catholic Church subsequently issued general prohibitions against transfusion. For 150 years, it fell from orthodox medical practice.

Transfusion was reintroduced by the London physiologist and obstetrician, James Blundell, in 1818. Blundell conducted several transfusions between 1818 and 1834, many of which he considered to have been successful. It is probable that Blundell was inspired to attempt transfusion by his somewhat vitalistic ideas about blood and by a broader cultural interest in reanimation of the 'apparently dead' — evident in scientific movements such as galvanism and resuscitation, and in novels such as Mary Shelley's *Frankenstein* (1818). Blundell came to espouse two main guidelines for transfusion: it was only to be used on women near death from uterine haemorrhage, and only humans could serve as donors. Thus failures were often attributed to the patient being beyond the reach of medical intervention; successes were presented as dramatic resurrections. Further, human donors, unlike their seventeenth century animal predecessors, resisted having their arteries opened for attachment to the recipient's veins. Blundell devised apparatus for 'indirect' transfusion to move venous blood through cups and syringes ('*Impellors*' and '*Gravitators*'), and thence into the patient.

Indirect transfusion inevitably led to another problem: *clots*. Clotted blood gummed up the pipes of instruments and the veins of humans — to the detriment of both. In 1821, J-L. Prévost and J. B. A. Dumas, then working in Geneva, proposed *defibrination* as a solution. Defibrination entailed whipping the blood with a fork or twig so as to collect the fibrin on the whipping object and prevent the blood from coagulating as rapidly. Some, believing fibrin to be a mere waste material, seized upon the procedure, but others opposed it, convinced that fibrin was central to the formation of living tissue. Direct, or 'immediate', transfusion was proposed as a way to circumvent these problems. Suggested independently in London by J. H. Aveling and in Geneva by J. Roussel in 1864, immediate transfusion relied on india-rubber tubes and silver cannulae to carry blood, as it had in the seventeenth century, directly from donor to recipient.

In nineteenth-century Britain, transfusion was primarily the domain of obstetricians, though, from the 1870s, surgeons began to use it as well. By the 1880s, however, physiologists began to question the necessity of using blood to replace blood loss. Guided by blood pressure measurements and histological investigations, they increasingly saw the circulation in material terms: as an enclosed, fluid system that contained cellular parts. From this less vitalistic perspective, lost blood might be replaced by fluids that would refill the circulatory system while avoiding nasty coagulation. By the early twentieth century, blood transfusion had generally been replaced by saline infusion. In Britain, surgery textbooks referred to blood transfusion (once again) as a quaint relic of medical history.

Recognition of blood types

It was at this historical moment, with transfusion distinctly out of medical favour, that the Viennese pathologist, and later Nobel prizewinner, Karl Landsteiner, was conducting his famous studies demonstrating that certain antibodies in human serum were not pathological, but normal. He showed that human blood naturally occurred in three different 'types'. A fourth was discovered in 1902 by his colleagues Decastello and Sturli. These four *blood types* were later given the names by which they are known today: A, B, O, and the fourth type, AB. The discovery demonstrated that the exchange of human blood carried with it the potential danger of haemolysis: if a recipient's blood plasma contained antibodies to the donor's red blood cells, the cells would clump or disintegrate (*haemolyse*), leading to discomfort at best and death at worst. It therefore offered a plausible explanation of transfusion's past failures. Landsteiner's studies did not, however, promptly usher in the modern period of transfusion. Relegated to serological realms, and with medical practitioners generally using saline, blood-typing was virtually ignored by clinicians. Indeed, even after transfusion was again 'rediscovered' a few years later, it was rediscovered in ignorance of Landsteiner's work. '*Typing*' blood for transfusion was not generally regarded as essential until late in World War I; and, even then — given the pressing nature of the circumstances — it was not necessarily conducted. Further, Landsteiner himself abandoned his typing work for decades, only returning to it in the 1920s. In 1939–40, he helped lead the investigations that proved the existence of rhesus types: shedding light upon why even the most careful interwar typing sometimes failed to prevent a haemolytic reaction.

Twentieth century developments

From the turn of the century, the Americans had taken the lead in transfusion. On the basis of experiments on shock, American surgeon and physiologist George Washington Crile became convinced that saline could not, in fact, replace lost blood effectively. In 1905, he began to conduct transfusion experiments on humans. Using a technique pioneered by the French surgeon and future Nobel laureate Alexis Carrel, Crile connected a donor's artery to a recipient's vein, allowing direct transfusion of blood between humans. Americans began practising transfusion with some regularity before the War, even recruiting a growing stream of 'donors' who were paid for their blood.

World War I proved a turning point. Transfusion was imported, first by Canadians, then by US medical officers. Further encouraged by the simplicity of transfusion undertaken with sodium citrate as an anticoagulant — now, blood could be collected in a bottle, moved from room to room, and even held for a while — British and French surgeons at the front increasingly turned to blood to treat soldiers suffering from the collapse they then called 'wound shock'. (The Germans, too, performed transfusions.) Moreover, the British and Americans undertook a special 'anti-shock campaign' from the summer of 1917. 'Resuscitation Wards' were staffed by specially-trained shock teams; in them, collapsed soldiers were given the blood of their lightly-injured brothers-in-arms in an effort to stabilise them for further surgical intervention. It was here that many British sceptics were won over to the benefits of blood transfusion.

Blood donors and blood banks

In the early 1920s, a number of hospitals assembled their own small donor panels: even using the citrate method, donors still had to go to hospital to give blood for each emergency. Initially, they were paid for their blood. Discontented with this adhoc system, some prominent British doctors began calling for a centralised donor service. In 1921, Percy Lane Oliver, master-organiser and Honorary Secretary of the local Camberwell division of the British Red Cross, started just such a system. Moreover — and, more remarkably — his system relied wholly on unpaid donors, at a time when some American hospitals were paying donors up to $100 for a pint. The fledgling voluntary service grew rapidly, being taken up in 1926 by the greater British Red Cross and providing donors to all London's voluntary hospitals by the early 1930s. Under Oliver's firm hand, the new London Blood Transfusion Service also shaped the rights and responsibilities of the modern voluntary blood donor. The London model was quickly adopted throughout Britain and thereafter by national Red Cross and other organisations in a host of other countries. Debate as to the relative merits of paid and voluntary donor systems, and their implied conceptions of blood as commodity or gift, continues to inform the direction of today's donor programmes throughout the world.

Yet, it is difficult to imagine how the current pervasiveness of donor programmes and, indeed, of transfusion itself, could exist without the addition of another innovation: *blood banking*, or, the cold-storage-based exchange of blood. Though initially developed at the Rockefeller Institute in 1916 and applied on a small scale on the French front in 1918, cold storage was virtually ignored until the 1930s, when it was used in Moscow to preserve cadaver blood for later transfusion. The unconventional donors attracted as much attention as did the possibilities of the procedure. Cold storage was given further dramatic introduction to the broader world during the Spanish Civil War, where the international array of doctors

attending to its casualties pooled, cooled, then distributed donated blood to the wounded. Back in the US, Chicago's Cook County Hospital applied the process of cold storage to its own blood exchange system in 1937, creating what is thought to have been the first civilian 'blood bank'. In this odd interplay of war and peace, the place of blood banking (as well as of transfusion more generally) was firmly established in World War II.

Blood products

During the war, the newly-developed procedure of separating the plasma from the blood cells and drying the plasma helped fuel longstanding debates about the best fluids to transfuse in various medical conditions. Dried plasma was indefinitely storable and far more portable than blood. Rehydrated, it appeared to be more effective for example in the treatment of burns than did whole blood. Gradually, a kind of division of labour for blood components was articulated. Today, whole blood is used in relatively few circumstances — for example, to treat severe haemorrhage, and in heart bypass procedures. Red blood cells in suspension are the alternative in operative procedures, and are given to patients with severe anaemia; platelets or white blood cells can be separately extracted and given to those suffering from a lack of them. Whole plasma is transfused to treat fluid and protein loss, and plasma is also used to obtain particular components which are lacking from the blood in certain disorders. The procedure known as plasma 'fractionation', developed in the mid 1930s, has given rise to a host of 'biologicals' for infusion. These include albumin, for treating patients with burns; Factors VIII and IX, which help coagulate the blood of men with haemophilia; and immunoglobulins, to provide specific antibodies to infections such as tetanus or chickenpox, or 'Anti-D' which is given to rhesus-negative mothers to prevent damage to their rhesus-positive babies.

Blood's processing and transportation was facilitated, and the safety of its infusion improved, by the development of plastic '*blood packs*' from the early 1950s. Now a familiar icon of transfusion, these packs were adopted elsewhere, but they did not become the official containers of Britain's blood until 1975, replacing glass bottles.

Despite this medicalisation, blood has in many ways retained its privileged cultural status. Citing Old Testament prohibitions against consuming blood, Jehovah's Witnesses forbid the transfusion of blood into their members. More generally, blood's movement between bodies continues to rest upon donor systems that must grapple with the social meanings of a fluid at once intensely personal, medically essential, and commercially valuable. Indeed, blood's extensive processing has sometimes complicated the task of voluntary donor groups, whose staff must persuade donors that the pharmaceutically-produced powders and potions derived from their blood remain direct 'gifts' to those in dire medical need — not sold at a profit to 'outside' systems.

Current problems

Typing has become more complex, with the recognition of groups within groups, and along with this has come more sophisticated laboratory 'matching'. A hazard that remains, and that requires meticulous screening of donors, is transmission by blood and its products of viral infections, notably hepatitis and HIV. This was tragically brought to public attention in the fate of haemophiliacs in the 1980s. Treated with biologicals derived from large pools of donated blood, many became infected with HIV and later died of complications from AIDS. The medical, ethical, and legal implications of AIDS for blood transfusion are still being determined. While efforts to clone or create synthetic blood continue, transfusion remains bloody — and, as such, intimately linked to its long cultural history.   KIM PELIS

Further reading

Gunson, H. H. and Dodsworth, H. (1996). Fifty years of blood transfusion. *Transfusion Medicine*, 6, supplement 1.

Keynes, G. (1922). *Blood transfusion*. Henry Frowde, London.

Titmuss, R. M. (1970). *The gift relationship: from human blood to social policy*. George Allen and Unwin, London.

See also ANAEMIA; BLOOD; BLOOD GROUPS; HAEMORRHAGE; SURGERY.

Blood vessels are the system of branching and converging tubes which convey blood from the HEART to all the various parts of the body and back again, and from the heart to the LUNGS and back (see BLOOD CIRCULATION). The size of blood vessels varies enormously, from a diameter of about 25 mm (1 inch) in the aorta to only 8 μm in the capillaries. This is a 3000-fold range.

The thickness of blood vessel walls also varies enormously, being largest in the large arteries, much less in veins of comparable diameter, and only a single cell thick in the capillaries. Despite the range of sizes the components of the blood vessel walls have a common pattern. All vessels are lined with a single layer of flattened cells called the endothelium. Except for capillaries, all vessels also contain elastic fibres, stiff COLLAGEN fibres (similar structure to muscle tendons), and SMOOTH MUSCLE fibres which can constrict or dilate in response to chemical and nervous stimuli. The relative proportions of these components vary in different blood vessels in accordance with their functions.

Recently, the endothelium has been recognized to be of importance in the regulation of the state of constriction or dilatation of the vessels themselves. Of particular note in this respect is 'endothelial derived relaxation factor', later shown to be NITRIC OXIDE: when this is released, notably in response to the shearing force of the blood on the vessel, it causes dilatation of the vessel.

Large arteries

The aorta and its main branches are called elastic arteries. Although they also possess fibrous collagen tissue and smooth muscle, about half of their structure is composed of elastic fibres. These give large arteries a characteristic pale yellow colour. Their wide bore means that they offer little resistance to blood flow, so there is little pressure drop throughout the system of major arteries. The physiological significance of the elastic fibres is that they allow the vessels to expand when blood is ejected intermittently into them from the heart and to constrict again as blood flows out of them into the smaller vessels. The combination of a distensible large vessel and a downstream resistance (arterioles) transforms an intermittent cardiac ejection into a continuous capillary flow.

Small arteries and arterioles

These are the resistance vessels of the circulation and are responsible for determining BLOOD PRESSURE. Arterioles are the vessels at the end of the arterial tree and have a diameter of 20 to 30 μm. Their particular significance is that they have very thick walls in relation to their diameters. Furthermore, the main constituent in their walls is smooth muscle, and the degree of contraction of this muscle regulates the diameter of the vessels and consequently the amount of blood flowing through them. Arterioles are responsible for the largest pressure drop in the circulation. Blood pressure in arteries typically varies from 120 to 80 mm Hg, depending on the phase of the cardiac cycle. In capillaries, the pulsatility is lost and pressure is only about 30 mm Hg.

The muscle in the walls of arterioles possesses an inherent tone. That means that they are normally partly contracted, reducing the size of the lumen to less than the widest possible. The degree of contraction is modified by factors external to the vessels. In particular, the chemical products that are formed as tissues use up energy — the 'metabolites' — reach the muscle fibres in the walls of the arterioles and cause them to relax and dilate. This local vasodilatation has the effect of matching local blood flow to tissue energy requirement.

Arterioles can also be regulated by nerves and hormones. These effects tend to be widespread and are concerned mainly with the regulation of arterial blood pressure. Sympathetic nerves have an important role in the control of arterioles. As the frequency of sympathetic nerve impulses increases, more of the transmitter, NORADRENALINE, is released at the nerve endings, and this causes arterioles to constrict. The adrenal glands

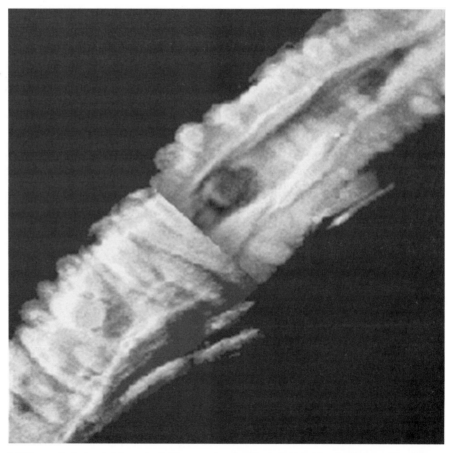

A 3D image of a brain arteriole constructed from a series of confocal microscopy images. An area of the data was 'digitally' removed — effectively slicing open half of the specimen — to reveal inner structures. Although the blood had been washed out, in this case a single red blood cell remains in the lumen, showing the internal diameter to be only 20–25 micrometres. (Courtesy of C. J. Daly, J. C. McGrath, and S. M. Arribas University of Glasgow.)

also release noradrenaline into the blood but their secretion is mainly of adrenaline. ADRENALINE also constricts blood vessels — except those in skeletal muscle, where it dilates them. This diverts blood to the muscle and prepares the body for emergencies as part of the 'fight or flight' response.

Capillaries

These are the 'exchange vessels', allowing passage of substances between blood and the fluids outside them which surround the body cells. They consist of a single layer of endothelial cells, with microscopic spaces between adjacent cells which allow the solutes of the blood, including salts, glucose, and dissolved oxygen, to pass into the tissues, and products of tissue metabolism, including carbon dioxide, to pass into the blood. The number of capillaries is so vast that even though they are microscopic their overall resistance to blood flow is low and blood passes through them slowly. The high density of capillaries means the distance for diffusion by the nutrients and gases is small. The more active tissues tend to have a denser supply of capillaries.

Capillaries are formed as a complex system of branching blood vessels between arterioles and venules (microscopic veins). Those near the arteries are at a higher pressure than those near veins. The gaps between endothelial cells are small enough to be almost impermeable to the protein molecules present in the blood, causing the capillary bed to function as a semipermeable membrane. These molecules exert an osmotic force which tends to draw fluid from the tissue spaces into the capillary. This is opposed by the hydrostatic pressure forcing fluid out. A dynamic equilibrium is established, such that at the higher pressure capillaries fluid leaves the circulation, and at the lower pressure ones it is drawn back in. An additional system of vessels, the lymphatics, are fine tubes which provide an alternative route for tissue fluid, via the lymph nodes and back to the circulation.

Disturbance of the balance of the fluid exchange at capillaries can lead to OEDEMA, which is swelling caused by excess tissue fluid. Major causes of this are: a generalised increase in tissue fluid as in heart failure; obstruction to flow through veins or lymphatic vessels such as by cancer growths; and deficiency of blood PROTEIN, as in liver or kidney disease or malnutrition, which reduces the osmotic reabsorption force.

Veins

Blood returns from the tissues to the heart along veins. Larger veins possess valves which ensure that blood travels in the correct direction and prevents the development of undue back pressure. Sometimes the valves may cease to function, causing veins to distend abnormally and permanently. This is the cause of VARICOSE VEINS.

Veins have another important role in addition to being conduits. Approximately 70% of the entire blood volume is contained within the veins, and these are very distensible. This means that they can readily accommodate quite large changes in their volume, either as a result of a change in the total quantity of blood in the circulation (haemorrhage or transfusion), or because of changes in blood distribution (leg veins distend on standing up, for example). The reason that veins can change their volume with little change in pressure is partly because they collapse when empty, which applies to veins above heart level. When filled, the elastic tissue in their walls is readily distensible, although expansion is eventually limited by the relatively indistensible fibrous tissue (collagen).

There is another, active, way in which the volume of blood in veins can be controlled: some veins have the ability to constrict in response to nerve stimulation. Sympathetic nerves supply smooth muscle in the vein walls, and an increase in sympathetic activity, resulting for example from a decreased stimulus to BARORECEPTORS (falling blood pressure), causes venous volume to decrease. The effect of this is to increase filling of the heart and to enhance its output.

Pulmonary vessels

Although the total flow of blood per minute through the LUNGS is the same as that through the systemic circulation, the pressures are very much lower. Pressure in the pulmonary artery is typically 25/12 mm Hg (systolic/diastolic) compared with 120/80 mm Hg in the aorta and its main branches. The pressure in the lung vessels is lower because they are shorter, wider, have less muscle in their walls, and are very numerous. In particular, there are no muscular resistance vessels like those in the systemic circulation. The pulmonary vessels form a vast low-resistance capillary network which encircles the microscopic air-sacs (alveoli). Gas exchange — of oxygen for carbon dioxide — takes place between blood in the pulmonary capillaries and air in the alveoli.   ROGER HAINSWORTH

See PLATE 2

See also BLOOD CIRCULATION; BLOOD PRESSURE; BODY FLUIDS; LYMPHATIC SYSTEM; MICROSCOPY.

Blushing

Blushing is reddening of the skin of the face and, in some people, the neck, due to an involuntary rush of blood when vessels dilate under the influence of the AUTONOMIC NERVOUS SYSTEM. Blushing usually accompanies embarrassment or self-consciousness. The occurrence of blushing has the effect of revealing feelings of states such as guilt, shame, sexual awareness, or arousal.

One of the acknowledged functions of MAKE-UP, in both men and women, was to conceal the tell-tale blush. However, in the Victorian era cosmetics were generally eschewed. The strict Victorian code of morality emphasized honesty, and the blushing of an open and sincere face became socially acceptable.

In his book *Physiognomische Fragmente* (1775–8), Johann Caspar Lavater, one of the most influential proponents of PHYSIOGNOMY, advocated the division and arrangement of the passions, according to their gradation. Lavater purported that each passion, every emotion of the individual, visually altered the lines and appearance of the face in a particular manner, by co-operation of the nerves, blood vessels, and muscles, and that observers could 'read' the feelings and mental state from the FACE of a subject. The most obvious example of this was blushing. Lavater translated his theories into practical advice for artists. Painters, in particular, were encouraged to understand the inner workings of the human body, including the causes of colouring of the cheeks. Physiognomy advocated that individuals illuminated themselves from inside out, and were reflected in how others saw them.

ANNE ABICHOU

Further reading
Darwin, C. (1872). *Expressions of the emotions in Man and animals.* T. Murray, London.

Piper, D. (1957, 1932), *The English face.* Thames and Hudson, London (1957). Ray Long and Richard R. Smith, Inc., New York (1932).

Bobbitry The name given to the act of cutting off a man's PENIS by a woman, usually an outraged, double-crossed wife. The term derives from a famous case in the US involving John Bobbitt, who successfully had his penis regrafted back in place. Occasional cases of penicide have been reported from China, Japan, and Australia, but in Thailand the practice has reached epidemic proportions, with around 100 cases in a decade, so much so that penis reimplantation has become a surgical speciality.   A.W.C.

Body building Spectacular displays of human strength in modern times were a tradition of the Victorian fun-fair. Systematic methods for building muscular strength were subsequently promoted by highly successful, late nineteenth-century American entrepreneurs such as Eugene Sandow, Bernard Macfadden, and Charles Atlas. Sandow proselytised his muscle-building system as a health philosophy based on the belief that the human body could be made resistant to all disease by keeping all 'cells in perfectly balanced strength … This I contend we can only do by the balanced physical movement of the voluntary muscles.' Macfadden incorporated muscle building into a theory of lifestyle, including sexual, reform. Charles Atlas popularised his fast-track body-building method by humiliating his clients, daring each to turn himself from a 'seven-stone weakling getting sand kicked in his face' into a lion who made all the other animals in the jungle 'sit up and take notice as soon as he lets out a roar'.

Body building as a professional sport flourished after World War II with a newly formed World Body-building Association creating an international competition for the title of Mr Universe, which was judged on muscular bulk and definition. The early systems of Sandow, Macfadden, and Atlas were incorporated into methods for turning muscles into iron — above all by the post-war entrepreneurial giant of the body-building cult, Jo Weider. Weider and his brother funded a separate competition which became the most sought-after world-championship body-building title in the 1980s, 'Mr Olympia', and extended this to provide a female equivalent, 'Ms Olympia'. The Olympia competitions, however, were the tip of a commercial empire including the international supply of gymnasiums and equipment, sports clothes, dietary supplements, and magazine and book publications. Weider, like his predecessors claimed to offer a new lifestyle philosophy along with his methods for increasing muscular size and strength. As a result professional body building has spawned a new EXERCISE and FITNESS cult for the sedentary classes based on the weight-training methods and dietary controls employed by competitive body-building athletes. Weider has given this 'fitness culture' recognition by founding a new competition for the title of 'Ms Fitness', whose chief characteristic is supposed to be the holder's sexual attractiveness defined in terms of weight ratio and body shape.

Another qualification for the Ms Fitness title is that competitors must achieve a developed and defined muscular physique *without* the assistance of anabolic STEROIDS. This criterion differentiates the identity of the 'fit body' because the extravagant bulk of contemporary professional body builders, and all who imitate them, cannot be achieved without the illegal use of SEX HORMONES and/or human GROWTH HORMONE. From the time that Soviet weightlifters, such as Vasily Stepanov, began using anabolic steroids to build strength in the early 1950s, TESTOSTERONE has been a crucial weapon in the cold war in hard flesh. The local gym has become an experimental laboratory investigating the limits to human growth. Professional and amateur body builders have become enthusiastic self-experimenters who exchange a vast quantity of highly specialised knowledge about human health and physique and how to enhance or, indeed, destroy it. The physiological consequences of taking testosterone and human growth hormone are not yet fully known. Apart from distorting normal human muscle proportions, the short-term effects have a number of pathological results ranging from acne to liver damage and the recently identified psychopathology of 'roid-rage'.

The aim of the contemporary body-building cult is not, however, to produce the perfectly healthy human form or even a human form at all. The current criteria for achieving the highly prized Mr Olympia title is body bulk which is also 'cut'. The goals of body building had changed by the end of the twentieth century, taking on a new post-modernist, 'post-human' tonality. As illustrated by one of the currently most popular body-building magazines. *Ironman*, the desire of the contemporary competitive body builder is to look 'alien' — or, in the lingo of the locker-room, to look 'freaky'. As T. C. Louoma, writing in the first edition of the British publication of *Ironman* in 1992, highlights, the competition between body builders is to look 'out of this world'. It is perhaps ironic that the contemporary body-building cult, which can trace its heritage back to the role of the 'freak' strongman in the nineteenth-century fun-fair, chooses to revive this particular Victorian value.   DOROTHY PORTER

Further reading
Berryman, J. W. and Park, R. J. (ed.) (1992). *Sport and exercise science. Essays in the history of sports medicine*. University of Illinois Press, Urbana and Chicago.

Chapman, D. L. (1994). *Sandow the magnificent*. University of Illinois Press, Urbana and Chicago.

See also ATLAS, CHARLES; SPORT; SKELETAL MUSCLE; STRENGTH TRAINING.

Body clock We live in a world that changes its levels of illumination and temperature every day and night of our lives. To make the best of opportunities and to avoid the risks posed by this variability, living things have evolved internal timing mechanisms, called biological clocks, which coordinate their METABOLISM and behaviour with the daily rhythm of the world. The clock mechanism that organizes our cycles of activity and inactivity consists of a number of structures located in the depths of the BRAIN. It sends to the body a variety of nerve and chemical messages that orchestrate our organ systems so that they operate harmoniously with one another as well as with external light and temperature.

The world is full of time-giving signals, particularly the level of light, which could directly rule the patterns of activity of the brain and the body. But remarkably, our body clock (and all other biological clocks) can keep very good time even in the absence of external cues.

The capacity of the human brain clock to maintain its own rhythmic beat was discovered by two German scientists, Jurgen Aschoff and F. Wever, who studied human volunteers, living for many weeks in an underground bunker, isolated from external time cues. Under these conditions, each subject manifested remarkably regular rhythms of body temperature and of SLEEP — wake alternations, with a time-cycle slightly longer than the normal 24 hours. In most cases, the intrinsic cycles of temperature and sleep were locked together in phase, but sometimes they were dissociated (*internal desynchronization*). Because the periodicity of the internal clock approximates to the 24-hour cycle of the natural world, it is called a *circadian rhythm* (*circa-*, about; *dian-*, day); and because it is independent of external signals, it is called a free-running rhythm.

Because the free-running clock is not precisely locked to the 24-hour cycle, it must be reset on a daily basis by signals from the outside world. This apparently inefficient system gives us the ability to deal with the natural variability of the diurnal rhythms of light and temperature. From day to day and from season to season, the times of sunset and sunrise change continuously. If our brain clock could not be reset, we could not deal with these variations, and, over a lifetime, the clock would surely drift out of phase with the rhythm of the world. This dynamic resetting of the body clock is called *entrainment*.

With its artificial lighting and heating systems, the modern world has obscured many of the biologically significant aspects of our body clock. But jet airplane travel reminds us, sometimes painfully, that we are still in the thrall of the primitive and potent timer in our brain. '*Jet lag*' is the discomfort we experience when our brain clock only gradually resets in a new location. After crossing six to twelve of the Earth's time zones in a single flight, we may require 3–5 days to adapt our sleep and temperature rhythms fully to the local conditions of our destination.

Experiments on animals have shown that the body clock system is controlled by a tiny brain region called the *suprachiasmatic nucleus*, lying in the HYPOTHALAMUS on each side of the brain, just above the crossing points (*chiasma*) of the optic nerves, which carry signals from the eyes to the brain. Nerve cells of the suprachiasmatic nucleus generate a continuous train of nerve impulses, with the regularity of a metronome. Even if these nerve cells are isolated from the rest of the brain and maintained for long periods in tissue culture, they still produce a stream of impulses, which gradually shifts in frequency, being faster during the period of the day when the animal would be active (at night for rats) and slower during the period when it would be asleep. This, then, is the heart of the free-running circadian rhythm. A small number of nerve fibres from the optic nerve enter the suprachiasmatic nucleus and provide direct information about the external light level, which somehow modifies the pattern of firing of the nerve cells to reset the clock. The cells of the suprachiasmatic nucleus send signals to other parts of the brain, especially the pineal gland, initiating hormonal and nerve signals that synchronize the body and the brain to the biological clock.   ALLAN HOBSON

See also BIOLOGICAL RHYTHMS; HYPOTHALAMUS; PINEAL GLAND; SLEEP.

Body contact Human beings are unable to survive without body contact. From the moment of birth humans are dependent upon physical contact with others, firstly for the satisfaction of basic needs and secondly for the social support necessary to maintain a personal and fully social identity in the world. The history of human societies can therefore be read as the history of the regulation of body contact. Body contact is essentially an expression of the social classification of human bodies.

Historical and cultural rules of body contact distinguish between physical contact between bodies themselves and contact with body products. In modern Western societies both these sets of rules are closely associated with the separation of social life into public and private areas and the emergence of the self-controlled individual whose rights of privacy include ownership of the body and the right to be free from pollution, physical attack, and sexual interference. There are therefore forms of body contact, for example sexual activity, which are widely regarded as expressive of the private bodily self, and are expected to take place in private spaces. Other forms are regarded as appropriate to the public arena, such as the diplomatic handshake and the sporting embrace.

Contact with body products is similarly subject to distinctions between the public and the private. Excreta, and the menstrual flow, are normally expected to be concealed from public view. The involvement of other people in these bodily functions is only acceptable when an individual is an infant, disabled, or very old. In such cases public handling is permissible in emergencies or when someone cannot function without help; when this occurs, however, the individual in need is usually considered to be excluded from normal adult status.

The rules regulating contact between human bodies and with their products were put into a historical framework by the German sociologist Norbert Elias (1897–1990), in his work on 'the disgust function'. For Elias, personal experiences of disgust over contact with certain kinds of bodies (like the diseased, the dying, and the dead), and with foods that are seen as nauseating (for example the garden dirt that children may put in their mouths), and over bodily functions, are the result of the gradual emergence of good manners and etiquette as techniques for demonstrating social superiority. Superior persons are those who have distanced themselves from their natural functions and whose conduct is correspondingly refined, setting them apart from the 'vulgar' masses. He traces their origin back to early forms of court society where relationships between monarch and courtiers were increasingly regulated by books of manners containing advice on bodily controls (for example belching and breaking wind, or blowing one's nose) and on forms of bodily contact, including the control of interpersonal VIOLENCE.

The direction of historical change as developed in Elias' concept of 'the civilizing process' is the gradual diffusion of codes of good manners from the upper to the middle and eventually the lower classes. The civilized individual is one who experiences disgust over the violation of these rules. Feelings of revulsion over close contact with a sexually inappropriate person, a physically violent individual, a smelly or dirty body, disgusting food, or human excrement (ultimately even the smells of unperfumed bodies, of cooking, and of the closet) come to be experienced as 'natural', a sign of a 'human nature', even though they are essentially historical constructs.

Two forms of contact between bodies exemplify the general issue of regulation. The first is contact between enemies or bodies in potential conflict, and the second is contact between women and men.

In the control of contact between bodies in potential conflict the male handshake reveals that one hand at least does not have a grip on an offensive weapon. A refusal to 'shake hands' is regarded in both public and private life as a rejection of attempts to reduce tension between people and to reconcile conflicting interests. It is a refusal to go through the motions of conciliation or concord, to put up a polite performance and ritually to honour the rules of etiquette. The handshake is only one example of a broader category of ritual gestures involving body contact considered essential for the regulation of good order in complex modern societies. As a highly organized form of contact the handshake exemplifies a high degree of refinement in the expression of self-restraint and agreement about the rules of the encounter. It is an instance of one of the most significant developments in the history of human interaction: the refinement of rules making it possible for individuals to regulate their capacity to inflict violent damage upon one another's bodies and to effect the transition from friend to enemy and back again. As such the handshake is intimately bound up with the expression of the integrity of the self because it is an indication of the trustworthiness of the private self in the public world: 'my word is my bond'; 'let's shake on it'. The handshake therefore belongs also to the important category of body contacts through which the private self goes public; it may function, between men, as a highly restrained expression of deeper positive emotions such as love and devotion.

It is through the rules governing body contact that human emotions are structured and brought to life. The most obvious example is, of course, the regulation of sexual contact between male and female bodies. Contact between men and women is closely monitored according to the beliefs of the day concerning what is sexual and what is sexually neutral. But that boundary is blurred by experimentation with cross-dressing, operations to change the external sexual organs, and the manipulation of male and female self-images. The fact that such experimentation is by no means a recent feature of human history implies that the rules of sexual contact, like all other social rules, are not fixed in tablets of stone but open to negotiation, manipulation, and radical change.

A good example is the Western concept of romantic love. Whilst SEX is clearly a basic biological guarantee of the perpetuation of the human species, its gradual transformation into a vehicle for the expression of the intimate emotional self is the result of specific forms of social organization and culture. As tragedies like the legend of Tristan and Isolde indicate, the romantic notion of 'unrequited love' is made possible by the existence of social barriers preventing the couple from enjoying a sexual relationship. And as many a lover in real life has discovered, the intensity of the emotion is fostered through distance and prohibition. In this cultural context the sexual consummation of the relationship may be less rewarding than was anticipated.

The question of body contact in romantic love raises the broader issue of how the meanings of intimate body contact are constructed and the ways in which they shape personal experience and identity. In love between men and women part of the answer can be found in traditional GENDER distinctions between male and female bodies and the aesthetic beliefs which associate physical beauty (in both sexes) with sexual desirability. The problematic move from looking to touching is exemplified in the Western art of the nude where, until comparatively recently, bodies were sanitized, desexualized, and idealized. This is especially the case in images of the female nude, where the sexual organs are traditionally painted out and the viewer is presented with a safely 'sealed' body with no potential for actual physical sexual relations. Through this device the female body becomes simultaneously desirable and disgusting: desirable in its idealised form yet by implication disgusting in reality. And this complex pattern of associations feeds into the rules of contact between living bodies and the correspondingly ambiguous emotions experienced in everyday life. As the cultural historian Stephen Kern has shown, the move towards more accurate paintings of the bodies of lovers coincides with the demands of women to change the rules of romantic love and to acknowledge the realities of contact with living female bodies. This development provides further evidence of the essential flexibility of the rules of body contact and their close relationship with the social classification of human bodies.

The sealed nude typically encountered, for example, in Victorian art is a reflection of the wider concern over exposing and handling the genitals of the adult human. The problem is that these organs are associated both with the essential and bodily private self and with the close proximity of sex and waste disposal. Having elaborated a social code around the regulation of the 'private parts', society is then faced with the need to dismantle these regulations in order to cope with the potentially embarrassing experience of a medical examination. Research into the social organisation of nursing care and medical examination of the genitals — increasingly common in contemporary society — shows how the associations between sexuality and exposure and contact with the breasts and genitals must be neutralised by doctors and nurses. Techniques of neutralisation are of particular interest because they also involve attempts to depersonalise the 'patient' by fragmenting the body into parts and relegating sexuality to the non-medical sphere, thus implying a significant connection between sexuality and the self. These techniques are also therefore methods of depersonalising body contact by separating the self from the body, a process which is facilitated by the removal of the body from private life into the more public world of the doctor's surgery, clinic, or hospital.

Body contact in close situations involving face-to-face interaction is a feature of everyday life. But as techniques of communication expand there are signs of interpersonal relations becoming increasingly disembodied. Electronic forms of human interaction now make it possible to cultivate a distance from the material bodies of other people. Even intimate sexual contact is being challenged by 'cybersex' on the internet. Violence too is becoming depersonalised in modern warfare as technological innovation enhances the distance between combatants and transforms the destruction of human life into a remote action. Whilst the long-term effects of these changes are uncertain, body contact is beginning to look quite different as technology and science become the culture of the future.

MIKE HEPWORTH

Further reading

Lawler, J. (1991). *Behind the screens: nursing, somology and the problem of the body.* Churchill Livingstone London.

Seymour, W. (1998). *Remarking the body: rehabilitation and change.* Routledge, London.

Body decoration From signs of honour to stigmas, what is drawn on skin or written in flesh is much more than mere body decoration, or a mark of status in the community. The human body and its surface are filled with hieroglyphs telling one of the stories of corporeality in history. The raw material, the 'natural' body itself, seems not to be an anthropological constant, but rather a canvas to be painted or a lump of clay to be moulded: a form and surface to be intentionally elaborated.

The ways in which the body is taught to be used and held and the artifacts supplementing the body have irreversible effects on its constitution and shape, from certain kinds of SHOES to, say, nineteenth-century tight-lacing of women's waists. These techniques can be distinguished from those in which the body itself is an immediate object of elaboration and inscription. The Chinese woman's feet moulded into a form not fit for walking and the spinal deformation caused by high heels are two different things. The one is an intentional irreversible alteration, while the potentially irreversible changes of the other are side-effects of the primary aim of constructing the body image displayed in a social or ritual context.

In moulding and decoration, the body has a double role; as a visual gestalt, which is the raw material to be worked upon, and as the performer of the action. The work may be on one's own body — as in primitive ritual body-painting or in contemporary make-up — or on another's body: this includes compulsion, such as stigmatization or mutilation of slaves and criminals, but unforced forming and marking of the body of the other is often accomplished by a professional, or may be part of an exchange of services.

Intentional body elaboration can have positive or negative value: medals are positive; the Indian caste system is ambivalent; the suppressed or excluded are branded. Then there is the irreversible vs. reversible dimension: the mark of Cain is lasting; changes in hair, nails, and tan recover, and decorations may be removed at any time. Stigmatising branding is irreversible, but alterations such as head shaving may be used as a temporary stigmatising punishment.

The historical roots of stigmatising body-marking are as long as those of more positive forms, and may be traced up until our recent past. In eighteenth-century France criminals were branded, signifying the crimes they had committed, for example 'V' for 'voleur' (thief). At the end of the nineteenth century, the English army still tattooed bad characters 'B.C.', and deserters 'D', and half a century later tattooed number series were used in the concentration camps of the Third Reich.

The modern penal system or, more generally, modern societies in normal circumstances, have in principle given up the use of irreversible body-marking along with traditional corporal punishment. However, even if the techniques have changed, and no longer leave obvious traces, the body is still a locus of intervention, now primarily as an aspect of what Michel Foucault has called the production of 'disciplined bodies'.

Body transformation varies also in extent, from whole to part: from the moulding of the body gestalt to the transformations which do not affect the overall body image or form: from the morphology of the body to the texture of the skin and the textiles covering it.

According to these basic dimensions and distinctions, trends in modern Western body elaboration may be characterized as follows: (i) the emphasis has moved from working on another's body to the elaboration of one's own; (ii) stigmatising body-marking is lessening; this is paralleled by the expanding range of positive body-moulding; (iii) lasting traces are giving way to removable signs; so (iv) transformation of the body gestalt is excluded.

The primitive body

In many traditional and archaic cultures the unformed and unelaborated body is considered imperfect, unfinished, and even ugly. They solve this problem not by covering up, but by moulding and decorating the 'natural' body. Primitive body elaboration consists of a whole range of techniques from permanent body form transformation to temporary painting.

Permanent and temporary body markings have their own specific place. Some markings are inscribed in flesh, giving irreversible changes of status; boys are transformed into men, or unmarried into married. These cumulative body markings are realized in ritual occasions at specific points of the life cycle. They also use non-ritual forms of body marking. The head of the tribe may show off his wealth and superiority by the number of golden rings forged round the necks of his wives; if these neck-stretching rings mould the body gestalt, so much the better.

Reversible decoration, painting, and masking is used primarily in the 'liminal' (threshold) phases of ritual in which the rules of the 'normal state' are annulled and replaced by inverted ones. Medieval carnivals and masquerades are manifestations of this universal phenomenon.

The liminality of the ritual determines the correspondingly limited nature of body-marking: returning to the everyday life of the community after the festivities implies removing the temporal body signs and uncovering the permanent ones. Liminal or exceptional states are not restricted to the festive rituals of a community: they are also manifested in war, in marking the bodies with warpaint.

Permanent body-mouldings and markings vary from culture to culture, and not at random. Colour tattoos have been common, for understandable reasons, among pale-coloured peoples (in Asia, America, and Oceania) and scar ornaments among the dark-skinned Africans. The most elaborate tattoos are found in Japan, where in the seventeenth and eighteenth centuries, after tattoo lost its status-signifying function and before it gained a stigmatising meaning, whole-body tattoos (*irezumi*) developed into an art; an imaginative example is the so called white-tattoo, which becomes visible as the skin blushes — perhaps in a specially captivating way in the realm of erotic pleasures.

Irreversible reshaping or marking of the body manifests the stable and static character of relations in society. It implies neither contempt nor adoration for the 'natural' body image. *Body* is an unfinished piece of art to be completed — to be transformed from nature to culture, by inscribing membership of the community in the flesh. Beyond this, it is an act of artistic creation in a cultural state which does not yet draw boundaries between the ritual, the magic, the erotic, and the aesthetic.

The body painting, decoration, and masking used in the liminal stages and forms of ritual follow an opposite logic to the permanent body marking which transforms the body from nature to culture. The former breaks the coherence of the body image and transforms it into an animal or god figure. This represents a movement beyond the boundaries of the community, towards the natural and the supernatural.

The human body is the origin not only of SCULPTURE and painting but also of jewellery. The body itself is an ornament to be worked upon. In distinction to our 'civilized' trinket-culture, which usually goes no further than ear piercing, in primitive societies, trinkets are often used as tools transforming the body gestalt. Members of the Vietnamese Jörai community use ivory pegs pierced through their ear flaps, to redesign them. The use of rings to stretch the neck (the Chin-women in Padaung, Burma) or plates to stretch the over- or underlip (in Kenya and Tsad) follows the same principle: the material trinket and the body are interacting in a way which makes it impossible to say where the trinket ends and the body begins.

The use of trinkets as removable decoration is equally universal, and not only in liminal rituals. In lighter trinkets — beads, brooches, necklaces — aesthetics and magic unite. Trinkets are not mere decorations to attract fellow men: it is equally important to make oneself favourable to the gods. This is most evident in amulets and talismans, aimed primarily at repelling evil — rather to protect against the evil eye (*mal occhio*) than to draw admiring glances.

The western body

From the Western point of view primitive body art is easily seen as anti-aesthetic deformation. Why? Culturally, this could simply be interpreted as due to differences between aesthetic codes. But there is something else. The Western body image is dominated by a deep-rooted ideal of 'the natural'. This may be traced back to the Greco-Roman body aesthetics on one hand, and the Christian tradition on the other. The Greco–Roman cult of natural, bodily beauty, of both men and women, was — in Foucault's words — part of a whole 'aesthetic of existence', but it allowed decoration and painting of the body only as far as it served 'natural' beauty. Other kinds of body-moulding or permanent marking were disapproved of, and irreversible markings were restricted to stigmatising uses.

The Christian body image and its emphasis on 'the natural' is ambivalent. Man, the image of God, is not allowed to transform or deform his 'sacred' appearance. But on the other hand, man's body is earthly dust — the temporary habitation of the soul and therefore secondary or, as 'FLESH', downright evil. Irreversible moulding or marking of the body is often seen as a profanation of the image of God, and decorating or painting it as shameless articulation of the flesh. The glaringly painted whore is originally a Biblical motif.

In Greco-Roman body aesthetics both sexes were equally represented. In the Christian tradition, as Western art cultivated the eroticism of the female body into an aesthetic norm, the fleshly sins were primarily projected on to the seductive female body. This is highlighted in the English neologism 'nude', appearing at the beginning of the nineteenth century to refer to aesthetically legitimated 'nakedness'. The human body should be 'natural'; untilled and unmarked. The Church banned tattoos officially in the year 787, and with the same prohibition Western man initiated his 'civilizing influence' in the Southern Pacific about a thousand years later.

The body-decoration race went on in the European Courts in spite of the disapproval of the Church, but it left the body form untouched, focussing on removable properties. Ostentation became more and more the occupation of the 'fair sex'. In Puritan England this led to legal measures. In 1649, the year of the execution of Charles I, a Bill was introduced entitled 'The vice of Painting and wearing Black Patches and Immodest Dresses of Women'. Soon after, an Act of Parliament decreed as follows:

> All women, of whatever age, rank, profession or degree whether virgins, maids, widows, that shall from and after such Act, impose upon, seduce, and betray into matrimony, any of his majesty's subjects, by scents, paint, cosmetics, washes, artificial teeth, false hair, Spanish wool, iron stays, hoops, high-heeled shoes and bolstered hips, shall incur the penalty of the law in force against witch-

craft and like misdemeanours and that the marriage, upon conviction, shall stand null and void.

Close to this time, in 1650, John Bulwer's book appeared, analyzing, and moralizing upon, contemporary modes of body decoration. The title of Bulwer's book expresses well the puritanical stance:

> **Anthropometamorphosis.** Men's transform'd or the ARTIFICIAL CHANGELING. Historically Presented in the mad and cruel Gallantry, Foolish Bravery, Ridiculous Beauty, Filthy Fineness, and Loathesome Loveliness of most Nations, Fashioning and altering their Bodies from the mould intended by Nature with Vindication of the Regular Beauty and Honesty of Nature, and an Appendix of the Pedigree of the English Gallant By J. B.

One could suppose that this puritanical flood of words was targeted towards the unnatural body art of the 'natural peoples' rather than against the Western finery which did after all follow the form of the 'natural' body. The peruke still represented real hair and the 'black patch' had its model in the natural mole. Even female body-shaping with the help of the corset, which culminated in the nineteenth century, followed and emphasized the basic 'hour-glass' female BODY SHAPE.

The modern body

In 1863 Charles Baudelaire, the apostle of modernity in Paris, wrote *In Praise of Make-Up* (*Eloge du maquillage*), speaking for the unnatural and artificial character of MAKE-UP. The painted face should not imitate nature, or articulate health and youthfulness, but should be consciously artificial and give an impression of 'supernatural and excessive living'. For Baudelaire, FASHION functions exactly according to this anti-natural principle. Fashion is the sublime deformation of nature, an unceasing and repeated effort to reshape it.

So is the modern a return to the primitive? In a way, yes because in breaking away from imitation and representation of nature, and from the ideal of the 'natural' body, Baudelaire is building a programme of the 'unnatural' which associates with the elements of primitive body art. He even refers to 'savages and babies' who are charmed by garish colours and artificial forms which, according to him, testify to their dislike for reality and also proves, though they do not realise it, 'the immateriality of their art'.

The primitive and the modern are united in anti-naturalism, but this is where the common ground ends. In primitive culture the 'unnatural' body moulding is closely connected to social structure and ritual liminalities. In modern culture, on the contrary, body marking — dressing, masking, and surrounding the body by a repertoire of short-lived signs — functions as the language of the self-expressing 'free' individual.

Fashion, however, is not simply the product of the modern society, it is also part of the system producing it. For Baudelaire fashion was the metaphor of modern life, as it was for the twentieth-century French cultural analysts Barthes

and Baudrillard: 'Modernity is the code and fashion its emblem' (Baudrillard 1993).

The status signs of pre-modern, feudal societies were not any more inscribed in flesh. Tattoos signifying guild or trade ceased to exist, and irreversible body marking became closely associated with stigmatization. Removable signs, especially clothing, still functioned as a restricted code, backed up by rules and sanctions which controlled access to these signs by measures which were not immediately based on money. Dress had to follow the signs of the estate, like a uniform, even if those wearing it could have afforded the clothes of their betters. In feudal society, behind the sign was status, which possessed the right, even the duty, to mark the body with those signs.

The situation is inverted in the dynamics of the modern society where status is increasingly acquired rather than inherited. Now the signs often precede the status, and function as a status-seeking strategy: by surrounding the body with certain signs — clothes, house, interiors, and car — a certain status is reached.

On the one hand the fashion system's sign production broadens the object language surrounding the body into infinity, but, on the other, it also creates a new kind of temporally restricting code: what is in today goes out tomorrow. Fashion is the production of changing sign systems, and thus the production of change within the sign system — in Baudrillard's words, it constitutes 'an aesthetics of repetition'. This transforms material things into 'pure' signifiers which signify each other thus blurring and finally cancelling the difference between function and style — between, say, sport clothes and sporty clothes.

There is a striving towards both the natural and the artificial. The ideal of 'the natural' dominates the body image more than ever — even if it may be cultivated into caricature-like 'unnatural' dimensions (BODY BUILDING) — while the reversible body marks are transformed into 'floating signifiers' overthrowing the whole distinction between natural and artificial. This tendency is not only manifested within the clothes system but also in hair design, which is liberated into new dimensions of expression. The aesthetic code of hair design is moving into the Kantian category of 'free beauty' somewhat in the same manner as the visual compositions of nouvelle cuisine reject the traditional food aesthetics, and turn to the codes derived from abstract and minimalistic painting.

These postmodern tendencies seem to move back towards the realm of irreversible body elaboration. This return of the 'primitive body' does not (yet?) manifest itself in actual body moulding — the plastic surgery still follows the code of the natural body (except for the French performance artist Orlan, whose face-moulding project turns the 'irreversible change' into a continuous metamorphosis) — but rather in smaller scale skin work, especially as real tattoos alongside fake (reversible) ones, and as body-piercing trinkets. The tattoo (and piercing) boom of today is

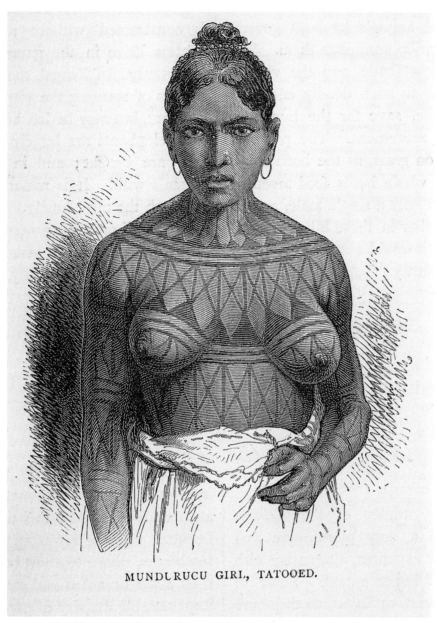

MUNDURUCU GIRL, TATOOED.

A tattooed girl of the Munduruca people, Brazil: engraving by an un-named artist in Brown, *The Races of Mankind*. Mary Evans Picture Library.

Body fluids consist of the water of the body and substances dissolved in it. Water is the main component of the human body, and, in any individual, the body water content stays remarkably constant from day to day. In a 70 kg (154 lbs or 11 stone) man of average build, about 63% of the body weight is water, and hence the total body water (TBW) amounts to 45 litres. In a woman of the same weight, typically only about 54% is water, so the TBW is about 38 litres. The difference is due to the fact that women generally have more FAT (adipose tissue) than men, and there is very little water in the adipose tissues. In both sexes, the proportion of the body weight that is water tends to decrease with increasing age. The functional tissue of the body can be regarded as fat-free, and the percentage of water in the fat-free tissue is very constant in any one individual from day to day, and between individuals. Water accounts for 73% of this 'lean body mass'.

Life as we know it could not have evolved without water. All living things consist of aqueous solutions separated from each other by boundaries such as CELL MEMBRANES. Water has many properties of biological importance. It is a liquid at the ordinary temperatures found on the earth. Compared with other liquids, it has a high specific heat (the amount of heat energy needed to produce a given increase in temperature): this tends to minimize changes in temperature when heat is produced by chemical reactions inside cells. Water has a high latent heat of evaporation (the amount of heat energy given out as a liquid evaporates): this provides the basis for an efficient mechanism for heat loss by SWEATING. Water is a good solvent for ionic compounds, which are essential components of all living systems.

The cells of our tissues and organs could not survive in the outside world. The immediate environment of the cells is the extracellular fluid. This internal environment ('milieu intérieur' — a term first used by the French physiologist, Claude BERNARD) maintains the correct concentrations of oxygen, carbon dioxide, ions, and nutritional materials for the normal functioning of the cells. Maintenance of the constancy of the internal environment, which the American physiologist Walter B. Cannon termed 'HOMEOSTASIS', is achieved by the actions of many body tissues and organs, including the cardiovascular, respiratory, and renal systems, and the liver. These actions are in turn regulated by nerves and HORMONES.

Input, production, and output of water

The body is continually exchanging fluid with the external environment. Water input into the body occurs by drinking (typically 1500 ml/day), by eating (500 ml/day of our water intake is contained in food), and by the metabolism of food (400 ml/day).

The metabolically-derived water comes from the oxidation of food — glucose oxidation for example:

$$C_6H_{12}O_6 + 6O_2 \rightarrow 6CO_2 + 6H_2O$$

glucose   oxygen   carbon dioxide   water

primarily within the younger generations. However, it is hardly a sub- or countercultural phenomenon (with the exception of the body-piercing subcultures related to sexual orientation). There is no 'tribalism' linked to the contemporary tattoo phenomenon. On the contrary, it is clearly a personal issue which is paradoxically both part of the fashion system and its negation: on the one hand it is fashionable to have a (tiny) tattoo, either for public display or for the eyes of the chosen one; on the other hand the tattoo remains irreversible regardless of changes of fashion (provided that it is not tiny enough to be removed) — perhaps as an emblem of coherent and continuous identity in a world of endless change. Luckily Princess Stephanie of Monaco

had a tattoo that was small enough for removal: she had her ex-boyfriend's name cut out of her skin, to give a fresh start to her new chosen one.

PASI FALK

Further reading

Baudrillard, J. (1993). *Symbolic exchange and death*. Sage, London.

Brain, R. (1979). *The decorated body*. Harper and Row, New York.

Seyd, M. (1973). *Introducing beads*. Batsford, London.

Steele, V. (1985). *Fashion and eroticism*. Oxford University Press, New York.

See also BODY MUTILATION AND MARKINGS; MAKE-UP; SCARS; TATTOOING.

The fluid output from the body occurs by several routes: from the lungs (400 ml/day), from the skin (400 ml/day), in the faeces (100 ml/day), and in the urine (1500 ml/day).

The loss from the lungs occurs because as air is breathed in it becomes saturated with water evaporating from the moist linings of the route to the lungs — mainly in the nose or mouth. Some of this water is restored to the same surfaces during exhalation, but much of it is lost. In hot, dry environments, or in sub-zero temperatures (when the air is very dry), the loss of water from the lungs can be considerably greater than 400 ml/day.

The water loss from the skin, termed 'insensible perspiration', is evaporative loss from the skin epithelial cells and occurs at an almost constant rate. It is not sweat. SWEATING, or 'sensible perspiration' represents an additional and adjustable loss, which can exceptionally reach up to 5 litres hour. The fluid lost in faeces, normally 100 ml per day, can be increased to several litres per day by diarrhoea. The loss in urine can vary enormously — between 400 ml/day and 25 litres per day — being adjusted according to the needs of the body relative to intake. Total water loss can never be cut down to less than about 1200 ml per day, so survival without any water intake is possible for only a short time: generally less than one week.

The body fluid compartments

There are two main body fluid compartments; inside and outside the CELLS (intracellular and extracellular). The extracellular compartment is divisible into (a) the plasma, which is extracellular fluid within the BLOOD VESSELS; (b) the interstitial fluid, which is extracellular fluid outside the blood vessels and separated from plasma by the walls of the capillaries; and (c) transcellular fluids, which are fluids with specialised functions. They include synovial fluid (which lubricates joints), CEREBROSPINAL FLUID (which cushions and nurtures the brain), and the aqueous and vitreous humours of the EYES (which maintain the shape of the eyeball and the integrity of structures within it). The transcellular fluids are separated from the plasma by a cellular membrane, which takes part in their formation, in addition to the capillary wall.

The volumes of the body fluid compartments, in a 'typical' 70 kg man, are: 30 litres inside cells and 15 litres outside cells, comprising 3 litres in the plasma, 11 litres in interstitial fluid, and 1 litre in transcellular fluids.

The solutes in the body fluid

The partitions between these compartments (cell membranes between extracellular fluid and intracellular fluid, capillary walls between plasma and interstitial fluid, and cellular layers between interstitial fluid and transcellular fluid) are permeable to water, and hence the osmotic concentrations of the solutes in the different compartments must be essentially identical — otherwise water will move through the barriers until this is the case. However, although the osmotic concentrations (osmolality) in the compartments must be almost identical, the solutes that make up the osmolality are different. The main difference is between intracellular and extracellular fluid.

The major IONS of the extracellular fluid are: sodium (Na$^+$: 142 mmol/litre), chloride (Cl$^-$: 110 mmol/litre), and bicarbonate (HCO$_3^-$: 25 mmol/litre). In the plasma component there is a significant volume of proteins and lipids in colloid suspension, so Na$^+$ concentration is in fact higher.

In intracellular fluid, there is a low Na$^+$ concentration, but a high potassium ion (K$^+$) concentration, and there are large amounts of negatively charged proteins. However, the enclosure of fluids of different compositions in multiple microscopic compartments (organelles) within the cells makes it rather difficult to generalize about intracellular fluid composition.

Exchanges between compartments

A continual exchange of water and solutes takes place between the compartments of the body fluids, which are in dynamic equilibrium with each other. This has an important bearing on the regulation of the body fluids.

Fluid moves between the plasma and the interstitial fluid through the walls of the capillaries, the smallest blood vessels. This movement occurs as a result of two forces, the hydrostatic pressure within the capillaries, pushing water and solutes out, and an osmotic gradient due to the plasma proteins in the capillaries, drawing water into the capillaries. (Since the capillary walls are permeable to other solutes but not to plasma proteins, it is the proteins alone that cause an osmotic pressure difference between plasma and interstitial fluid.) The volume of fluid leaving the capillaries slightly exceeds that re-entering. This excess interstitial fluid is taken up by the lymph vessels and returns to the vascular system at the base of the neck where the main lymph vessel, the thoracic duct, joins the venous system.

Regulation of volume and osmolity

How then is the volume of the body fluids regulated? For intracellular fluid, this is straightforward. Cell membranes are permeable to water, therefore water will cross the membranes if there are differences in solute concentration (osmolality) — and hence differences in osmotic pressure — between the two sides. Individual cells can thus regulate their volume by adjusting their membrane TRANSPORT processes to increase or decrease their solute content; this will lead to corresponding increases or decreases in volume as water osmotically follows the solute.

For extracellular fluid, the regulation of volume is more complicated. Because the extracellular fluid solute concentration (osmolality) is kept constant, the water content will depend on the solute content. For example, if we increase the amount of Na$^+$ in the body by eating salty food, this makes us thirsty so that we drink to bring the Na$^+$ to the correct concentration, and we end up with an increased volume. Because sodium (Na$^+$) and its associated negative ions are the main solutes of the extracellular fluid, the volume is regulated indirectly by controlling the Na+ content of the body. Sensors in circulatory system detect the blood pressure and the amount of blood returning to the heart from the rest of the body. Both of these tend to increase if the extracellular fluid volume increases, and nerve signals from the sensors, relayed to the brain, ultimately lead to changes in the concentrations in the blood of hormones that regulate Na$^+$ excretion by the KIDNEYS. The main hormones are angiotensin II and aldosterone. Both of these act to retain Na+ (and consequently water) so their secretion is inhibited when extracellular fluid volume increases. An increase of volume also has a more direct effect by diminishing secretion of the water-regulating hormone, vasopressin (antidiuretic hormone), the action of which is to promote retention of water in the kidneys.

The regulation of body fluid volume is thus inextricably linked with regulation of the concentration of sodium ions in the extracellular fluid. There are also many other solutes whose concentration in the body fluids are kept within necessary limits by a variety of mechanisms which ultimately adjust their retention or loss, mostly in the kidneys.   CHRISTOPHER LOTE

See also ACID-BASE HOMEOSTASIS; CELL; BLOOD CIRCULATION; HOMEOSTASIS; KIDNEYS; LYMPHATIC SYSTEM; WATER BALANCE.

Body image Towards the beginning of Charles Dickens's *Our Mutual Friend* (first published in 1865), a scene takes place that illuminates the important role played by body image in the formation of our sense of ourselves. The episode, which occurs in a crowded junk shop, features an exchange between Mr Venus, a taxidermist, and Mr Wegg, recent amputee. Wegg has arrived at Venus's shop with the express purpose (now that he has the prospect of regular employment before him) of buying back his own severed leg, which Venus has purchased as part of a 'miscellaneous' lot from a local hospital. Wegg's account of why he wants to complete this transaction is both touching and surreal:

'I have a prospect of getting on in life and elevating myself by my own independent exertions,' says Wegg, feelingly, 'and I shouldn't like I tell you openly I should *not* like — under such circumstances, to be what I call dispersed, a part of me here, and a part of me there, but should wish to collect myself like a genteel person.'

As he makes clear, Wegg is worried that his body may be deficient or vulnerable to attack in its divided state: it is not, he fears, the body of a 'genteel person'. What is at stake in this speech is Wegg's sense of his body: his imaging how his body is and how it appears to others. In fact Wegg has a complicated and multiple sense of how his body exists in the world. First, he knows what it is actually like; it's missing a limb, obviously. Secondly, he has the image of how it might appear to others; ugly, misshapen, perhaps. He is worried about this. Thirdly, he has a sense of how his body could look or perhaps how it should be. This anxious fantasy lies behind his otherwise ponderous sense of his potential gentility. If he can buy back his leg, he reasons, he can begin to restore his belief in his own body image.

The strange case of Wegg's lost leg makes clear what is implicit in all feelings about body image. Our sense of our own bodies emerges from a dialectic between our knowledge of it as a lived experience — its pleasures, its pains; the needs and desires of our physical selves — and a more ambiguous sense of how that body appears to others. In neither case is the knowledge we have, or feel we have, guaranteed to be true. Quite the contrary for most of us; we have no more sense of what we really look like than does Mr Wegg. We might feel we look right or suspect we look wrong; often this will depend on our mood at the time. Despite the potential for misapprehension inherent in our experience of our own body and its appearance, our 'body image', or sense of our physical selves, determines our interaction with the physical world and with other people. A confidence in our body image can reassure us at moments of crisis or indecision. This summary of body image accords with the common experiences of daily life. However, it is possible to codify these sensations, worries, and aspirations in a variety of ways; indeed, body image needs to be specified more closely if we are to appreciate its full significance. There are two ways in which body image has been defined: first, as a medical and psychological term for defining self-perception; second, as a social and cultural phenomenon, which enforces normative expectations. Both of these ideas are, in reality, interconnected — however, it makes sense in the present context to examine them separately.

From the perspective of a medical or psychological practitioner, the term 'body image' describes those PERCEPTIONS of the self that are centred on the individual's sense of their own physical existence, both anatomical and physiological. Paul Schilder defined body image in the 1930s as: 'The picture of our body which we form in our mind, that is to say the way in which our body appears to ourselves'. So defined, body image can be thought from a clinical standpoint to have two main states or modes — the normal and the traumatic. In the first case body image expresses our sense of our body's boundaries and capacities: principally our sense of our height, weight, and physical attractiveness as well as our expectation of the extent of our reach or the length of our stride. It is a normative idea that is held implicitly until we are shocked out of it by some event or remark.

This notion of our physical selves is of course evolving: progressing age, the process of puberty, and the changes of the menopause will cause an individual to update or revise the image of his or her body. However, accidents, surgery, disease, and diet can radically alter body image within a short time. This introduces the problem of a traumatic change in a person's body image. With this crisis in mind, modern nursing requires an under-standing of how a patient's response to changes in their bodily reality will necessarily impact upon their recovery and sense of themselves. Someone who has undergone extensive surgery or who has suffered from a debilitating disease will often require care and support as they form a new image of their body, its shape and capacities. Without such assistance the process can be irreparably damaging to the patient's self esteem.

But why should our self esteem be so affected by our body image? In cultural terms this question can be answered by considering the forces and pressures that cause us to present our bodies — to ourselves and others — in a certain variety of ways. All societies have practices and codes that seek to regulate how the body is permitted to appear. Most often these are a combination of ideas of FITNESS, adornment, FASHION, HYGIENE, size, and DIET. These conceptions provide the basis for how a body is judged, defining the standards to which it is expected to conform. Failure to conform may be condemned, even considered obscene. Contemporary social ills such as anorexia and bulimia are connected, at least in part, with the pressure of these standards. The Western desire for slim figures, for bodies lithe and muscular, rather than rounded or corpulent, produces in some a destructive desire for excessive DIETING, a form of self-denial which, they hope, will realign bodily reality with desired body image.

Women are perhaps particularly exposed to these pressures and are bombarded by more images that seek to privilege one ideal of female form over all others. However, it is not only women in Western cultures who are the recipients of demands upon how their bodies should appear. In other parts of the world, greater stress and more lavish praise is devoted to long necks, small feet, wide girths, and scarification than is generally consistent with European or North American ideals. Despite this apparent divergence, a similar desire to regulate and to judge, as well as to conform, dominates these conceptions of the body. Significantly, the cultural demands placed upon the body are subject to change and revision over time. Nonetheless these codes remain a huge influence on the individual's self esteem and sense of well-being. Our body image in fact is central, if ambiguously so, to our mental and physical well-being.   ROBERT JONES

Further reading

Price, B. (1990). *Body image: nursing concepts and care.* Prentice Hall, New York.

Schilder, P. (1935). *The image and appearance of the human body; studies in the constitutive energies of the psyche.* Kegan Paul, London.

See also EATING DISORDERS; FEMALE FORM; PHANTOM LIMB.

Body language refers to any kind of bodily movement or POSTURE, including FACIAL EXPRESSION, which transmits a message to the observer. Every part of the human body, either in motion or stillness, conveys a meaning which depends upon the physical, social, and cultural context of the action. The message may be deliberately intended, expressed in some sort of accepted code — as when a person points, shakes a fist, or nods the head — or they may be involuntary GESTURES of response, as when someone grimaces or cries aloud in pain.

Body language in history

Specific gestures, such as the 'manual rhetoric' of Roman orators, as well as the general carriage and deportment of the whole body, have been objects of study since Classical times. In the fourth century BC in Greece, upper-class men cultivated an upright, 'firm' stance and an unhurried gait, taking long strides. This distinguished them as persons of leisure, setting them apart from artisans and slaves, who had to hurry to get work done; it also distinguished them from women, who moved in a mincing manner, taking very small steps, while courtesans swayed their hips from side to side while walking. In Classical Rome, strictly moderated and limited gestures were regarded as an indication of a temperate and self-controlled character — requirements of an exemplary Roman aristocrat and orator.

Writings on body language were quite prevalent in Renaissance Europe. Seventeenth-century physiognomists like Giovanni della Porta and Charles Lebrun codified the facial expressions of EMOTION and character; both these investigations, and those of their contemporaries Giovanni Bonifacio and John Bulwer on gestures, were conducted on the assumption of a universal, natural language of expression and gesture which could be assumed and understood by all nations and peoples. In the nineteenth century, the work of Charles Darwin on animal and human 'emotions' tended to support the view that physical expressions might be biologically inherited. In turn, the physical conditions under which people live, and the bodily deportment and habitual actions they perform, have consequences for the structures of their bodies, as discovered by palaeoarchaeologists, who have used the evidence of excavated skeletons to offer generalisations about the body habits of the past. And certain modern ethnologists and zoologists such as Desmond Morris stress the similarities between the bodily movements used by humans and those observed in animals to express hostility, fear, dominance, or territoriality.

Cultural differences

However, most modern studies of body language are based on the assumption that gesture is not a universal or natural language, but the product of social and cultural contexts. The likeness, for example, between the facial gesture used by chimpanzees to express fear and subordination, and the human smile, can serve to underline the differences as well as the similarities between the two species of primates. Among humans, anthropologists such as Marcel Mauss have pointed out that even the most elementary aspects of physical behaviour, such as the ways in which people eat, sleep, walk, or sit, seem to be culturally determined, and vary greatly from society to society. This includes both the deliberate signals used by people to communicate meaning non-verbally, and also seemingly involuntary emotive or physical reactions, such as BLUSHING or WEEPING.

Behaviours which have been represented as spontaneous or instinctive action expressing the emotions are revealed, under closer scrutiny, to be neither spontaneous nor transparent. They are, to a greater or lesser degree, formalised, stylised, and ordered to a specific code of meaning, which may become meaningless or inappropriate in other places or cultures, or in another context. The gesture of greeting displayed by someone who leaps, smiling, to her feet, to throw her arms around another person, may cause discomfort or even offence to a person unfamiliar with this custom; and 'cutting' someone, by passing by with only a distant nod, may fail to have any effect on a person who is not used to expecting displays of affection in public.

Contemporary studies

The study of body language is conducted at present mainly by anthropologists, linguists, and social psychologists, who refer to this science by the name of *kinesics* — the study of non-verbal communication or communicative body movements. These include the study of the ways and frequency with which people touch each other during a conversation, and the distance which they keep from each other during interactions. Linguists have regarded gestures as a form of language, perhaps even the predecessor of all human languages, and have studied the various kinds of kinesic communication used by different cultural and social groups, such as stockbrokers, beggars, and the clergy.

Body language forms an indispensable element in social interaction. Facial expression and bodily movements can amplify, modify, confirm, or subvert verbal utterance, expressing meanings which elude or surpass verbal language. Thus it is a key to the inner psychological and emotional state of the performer: centuries before Freud, early modern writers on decorum discussed the slips or 'leakage' demonstrated by unintentional body language which contradict or undermine the overt declaration or utterance of the speaker.

Gestures also define manners of behaviour sanctioned in collective sensibilities, the general codes and rites which transmit cultural norms. Body language is thus also a key to some of the fundamental values and assumptions, the *mentalité* which underlies any society. It permits the passage from 'nature' (the biological body itself) to 'culture', signified through comportment, demeanour, and the myriad signals and gestures which people employ to express meaning, both deliberate and inadvertent, to each other or even to themselves. And in many formal contexts — liturgical, legal or ceremonial — the speaker's posture and bodily movement may be more important than the words uttered. Body language is extremely important, particularly in non-literate or semi-literate societies, in which commitment is made through ritual gestures, formal spoken words, and symbolic objects. Gestures transmit secular and spiritual power; they make such transmission public, and give political and religious actions a living image.

Social and national distinctions

Additionally, body language is an important ingredient in social differentiation; differences in physical comportment play a significant part in separating social groups from each other, and in fostering feelings of mutual hostility or alienation. For instance, the dignified gravity or refinement esteemed by the elite as signs of superior breeding could be seen as arrogance and affectation by the masses; conversely, the warmth or openness valued by some people could be despised as coarse and heavyhanded by others. This also figures in the creation of cultural differentials between nations. Different languages involve different facial and bodily movements, and there are other, more qualitative judgements and distinctions. As post-Reformation northern Europeans began to employ a more restrained and subtle gestic repertoire, they tended to look with distaste upon the more obvious facial expressions and explicit gestures of southern Europeans. It has been pointed out that the stereotype of the gesticulating Mediterranean fits well into the overall symbolic ordering of the north–south divide, which roughly follows the anatomy of the human body: the south, or the lower parts, are associated with passion, physicality and spontaneity, and the north with the rational faculties, and control of the emotions.

Gender differences

Body language reflects differences of GENDER as well as of class and nationality. Prescriptions for the physical behaviour of women are often different from those of men. Characteristically, women are encouraged to look modestly downward, to walk with small steps, be more restrained in facial expressions than men of their class, and to eat smaller portions of food. Gestures of female assertiveness, like standing with arms akimbo, or legs widely spaced, are regarded, particularly in societies with strong power differentials between the sexes, as unbecoming and aggressive, imitative of male behaviour.

Outward and visible signs

We tend to try to overcome as prejudice what until recently was an oft-stated fact: that the outward appearance of a person is an image of the inward personality and character — dress, gestures, comportment, any motion of the body, are indicative of the inner person. This aesthetic-cum-moral conviction that external bodily behaviour manifested the life of the soul, existed in the Middle Ages and beyond. In medieval Christian Europe, a human being was thought of as double, consisting of a soul and a body, an invisible inside and a visible outside, linked by a dynamic relationship. Gestures figured or embodied the dialectic between inner essence and outer appearance, since they were supposed to express to the viewer the secret movements of the soul within. Thus, bodily control exemplified internal harmony and the superiority of the mind to the body, while inappropriate or excessive gesture was either condemned as clumsy, or disparaged as 'gesticulation'. These 'bad' gestures, transgressive of limits imposed by ethics and social custom, were opposed to virtuous gestures, such as those of charity, penance, and piety, through which salvation could be reached.

Purity and shame

Theories exist as to why variations or changes in bodily behaviour occur: in the 1930s, the sociologist Norbert Elias propounded his very influential argument, based mainly on north European Protestant sources, that, after the relative freedom regarding the body in the Middle Ages, early modern Europe saw an increasing inhibition of bodily impulses. This took the form of a rising threshold of shame or embarrassment surrounding physical functions, and an enhanced concern over the restraint or control of both these and the expression of emotion. Also influential in recent work have been the theories of the anthropologist Mary Douglas, who has argued that, in most societies, the body is a symbol of social relations, and that the control of bodily expression customary in a society is more or less strict according to the degree of group pressure upon the individual.

Cross-cultural surveys demonstrating the variability of bodily gesture and facial expression are supplemented by the experience of travellers to other countries, or even those who see films or listen to music from other parts of the world. It is possible that, given the facilitation of long-distance travel in the later twentieth century, and the globalisation of culture, especially in urban centres which everywhere tend increasingly to be cosmopolitan in their products and attitudes, that certain of these differences have begun to diminish. Cultural homogenisation occurs relatively rapidly in certain aspects (usually confined to the socioeconomic elites) such as fashions in dress, eating of 'luxury' food items, or the importation of foreign words or decorative objects. Yet it tends to take place much more slowly on the level of bodily expression and facial gesture, which entire peoples take rather longer to absorb and alter.

A world of gestures

Body language is both the most basic, fundamental form of expression used by human beings to communicate with one another, and at the same time a part of a highly sophisticated and culturally specific system of coded signals, in which bodily and facial movement play at least as important a part as verbal utterance. It encompasses an infant grimacing in distaste at an unfamiliar or unpleasant sensation; the careful timing and co-ordination of bows between two

Japanese of equal rank; and the complicated series of insulting hand gestures which pass between altercating drivers in Brazil.

NATSU HATTORI

Further reading

Bremmer, J. and Roodenburg, H. (ed.) (1993). *A cultural history of gesture*. Polity Press, Cambridge.

Elias, N. (1939). *The civilizing process*. Blackwell, Oxford.

Mauss, M. (1979). *Sociology and psychology*. Routledge and Kegan Paul, London.

Schechner, R. (1993). *The future of ritual: writings on culture and performance*. Routledge, London.

See also FACIAL EXPRESSION; GESTURE.

Body mutilation and markings

One of the key aspects of human embodiment is the physical frailty of the body in relation to the environment it inhabits. Disease, warfare, and technology not only kill but maim and mutilate. Here, however, we are concerned with the mutilations and markings resulting from social practice. Body painting, scarification, branding, piercing, and tattooing have served as marks of distinction in most societies. Archaeological and textual evidence demonstrates the antiquity of these forms, which were carried out in cultures as diverse as the ancient Egyptians, Celts, Picts, and Germans.

Defining the scope of bodily mutilation and markings is difficult. They encompass a myriad of forms, from genital piercing, to face painting at children's parties. Furthermore, bodily mutilation is culturally relative. Europeans generally interpret female circumcision as an abhorrent mutilation; however, many of those who have suffered the procedure find it an acceptable, even desirable, custom. Accordingly, mutilation can best be defined as any procedure understood by mutilator and mutilated as mutilation. Inclusive within this definition are acts performed for sexual gratification or punishment. Both categories point to the socially transgressive nature of mutilation.

Anthropologists have noted that body markings occur most frequently in pre-literate societies and in repressed or marginalized minorities within the industrial world. Contemporary culture provides illustrations of both. Scarification and tattooing are still practised widely in pre-literate societies. Godna — tattooing using sharp sticks and dyes — remains customary in parts of rural India. In Japan, tattooing was prohibited throughout the Edo period (1600–1868), and was therefore restricted to criminals and prostitutes. Piercing (other than ear piercing) within modern industrial societies is most often associated with 'threatening' or 'deviant' sexual behaviour.

In pre-literate societies, body markings served several purposes. We can extend Gell's view of Polynesian tattooing to encompass most forms of body modification. Gell argues that Polynesian tattooing was deeply embedded in cultural beliefs about personal and social identity. The tattoos acted both as armour and as an expression of the position the individual held within society. Culture is reproduced at the point where the inner individual meets the outer world — the marked skin. Thus, in Papua New Guinea the Kendengei people of the Sepik ritually scarify adolescent men. The patterns produced by multiple incisions over the whole body imitate the scales of crocodiles. Not only is this an induction into manhood, it symbolically reproduces the cosmos of the Kendengei upon the flesh of each male adult, connecting him to the powerful forces of the outer world.

Bodily markings in pre-literate societies were complex. The aesthetic value of the adornments could not be divorced from their social signification. Godna, for example, allows women to conform to their culture's notions of beauty. At the same time, it is bound to religious ritual and social custom. In some places, it is an outward sign of caste. In others, it creates a bond between two people, for example a mother and her daughter, which is said to overcome the separation of death.

Contact between European and non-European societies created new interpretations of, and elaborated, old ideas about bodily markings. In some areas it resulted in systematic attempts by imperial and religious powers to stamp out practices deemed 'barbaric'. The cultural exchange did not, however, flow in one direction. Common mythology insists that the modern European tattoo was adopted as a variant of Polynesian custom. Thus, on Captain Cook's first voyage (1768–71), many of his crew were tattooed in Tahiti. Indeed, the word 'tattoo' is thought to derive from the Tahitian 'tatau' (wound) and the Polynesian root 'ta' (drawing). Whether etymologically accurate or not, it clarifies an important dynamic between Western and other cultures. Bodily markings came to represent the 'exotic', the 'primitive', and the 'savage' — a mark of differentiation between the 'civilized' and 'uncivilized' worlds.

Body modification has traditionally been viewed schizophrenically by Judaeo-Christian societies. The Mark of Cain served as an emblem of sin. Mosaic Law explicitly made body modification taboo (Leviticus 19:28). Tattooing and branding were signs of the outcast and criminal. Mutilation was used throughout medieval and early-modern Europe to inscribe punishment publicly upon the body. Petty crimes met with whipping and branding. Capital punishments were frequently performed with terrifying ferocity accompanied by symbolic mutilation. But while mutilation and marking mostly signified vilification, in other contexts it allowed the expression of piety. ASCETICISM and self-flagellation mortified the flesh. Medieval and early modern pilgrims to shrines in Europe and Palestine were sometimes tattooed as marks of devotion. At the shrine of Virgin Mary in Loreto (Italy), tattooing was linked to the STIGMATA of St Francis. Here, the pain of tattooing was borne in honour of Christ's mortal suffering.

Tattooing, however, appears in Europe to have been exceptional before contact with Polynesia. But as it became more visible, the infliction of punishment became less physical. The two are not unconnected. Scholars have noted that from the eighteenth century, the locus of punishment shifted from the body to the 'soul'. In Britain, for example, branding was statutorily abolished in 1779. During this period the tattoo came to serve a particular function for the penal authorities. Before the advent of fingerprinting and photography a description of a prisoner's tattoos facilitated identification in case of escape. From 1832 identification numbers were even tattooed on French convicts. Tattoos were also transformed into a symptom of criminality. The 'savagery' of Criminal Man, was best indicated by the markings on his body. Cesare Lombroso, the controversial late nineteenth-century criminal anthropologist and author of the celebrated and notorious, *L'Uomo Delinquente* (1876), reasoned that tattooing was so painful that only the racially 'degenerate' or the 'primitive' could endure such mutilation. Thus, he closed the loop between the 'savage' Other, the 'degenerate' criminal, and the 'civilized' European.

But what did the tattoos mean to the nineteenth-century tattooed convict? Fatalism and inherent criminality were the most common motives ascribed to criminal tattooing by contemporary criminologists. For the historian, analysis of nineteenth-century British transportation reveals other traits. Up to 30% of convicts transported to Australia after 1820 were tattooed. Marked upon their bodies were emblems of sentimentality, love, friendship, and the fear of separation encoded in strings of initials separated by hearts, darts, and anchors. Scenes depicting leisure and symbols of devotion appear in abundance. Marks of belonging, to regiment, ship, or nation are also common. Finally, there are records of conviction and a desire to retain control in the face of the state's possession of the convicted body. The culture of the prison hulks combine with that of the urban plebeian, embedded indelibly under the skin. Ironically, the function of the tattoo for the British transportee seems not dissimilar to its function for the Polynesians.

From Lombroso onwards, tattooing remained associated with marginal groups and particular occupations. Exceptions did occur. In late nineteenth-century Britain, tattooing enjoyed a brief vogue amongst royalty and aristocracy, before reverting to its prior associations with the armed forces, merchant seamen, and the twilight world of prostitutes and criminals. It must, nevertheless, be remembered that tattooing was also a commodity with an exchange value. It became increasingly specialised, with professional tattooists appearing at docksides from the 1870s. The influence of Japanese designs, and the invention of electric tattooing machines in the 1890s, transformed the process into a recognisably modern form.

Apart from tattooing and temporary cosmetic markings, other forms of bodily modification a post-industrial phenomenon — the meeting place for the New Primitives is the Internet and MTV.

Older associations remain, however. Tattooing is still mainly carried out in the 'traditional' parlour. And for most, the practices of the New Primitives are, at best, frightening and, at worst, deviant. The outlaw status of the tattooed and pierced remains intact. At the same time, extreme body modification practices, many of which are illegal, are more visible: the work of performance artists like Ron Athey and Stelarc, the content of world wide web sites like the *Body Modification E-zine*, and the prosecution in 1996 of British gay men in 'Operation Spanner' for consensual genital mutilation, raise vitally cogent social and ethical issues about the control and possession of the private body in society.   JAMES BRADLEY

Further reading

Brain, R. (1979). *The decorated body*. Hutchison, London.

Gell, A. (1993). *Wrapping in images. Tattooing in Polynesia*. Clarendon, Oxford.

See also BODY DECORATION; SCARS; TATTOOING.

Body odours The human body produces a wide range of odours, from head to toe. Some of these odours have their source in glandular secretions produced in various parts of the body, such as the scalp, the pubis, and the axillae. Others come from such body products as SALIVA and URINE. Body odours can be influenced by various factors, including age, sex, diet, and state of health. PUBERTY, for example, entails a striking change in body odours as the eccrine, apocrine, and sebaceous glands increase their production of fluids which become odorous through interaction with BACTERIA. Illness, in turn, may alter the olfactory emanations of the body in a distinctive fashion. Thus diabetics have been noted to produce a characteristic sweet scent.

Each individual has a unique blend of body odours. Recent studies have indicated that, even in the relatively deodorized culture of the modern West, most people can recognize the characteristic body odour of close relatives. Parents, for instance, are able, by smell alone, to correctly pick out shirts worn by their children. From a biological standpoint, human body odours probably played an evolutionary role in self and group identification, in regulating reproductive cycles, and in sexual attraction.

Historically, body odours have been a subject of considerable social concern. Among the questions Aristotle pondered in his *Problemata* was 'Why does the armpit have a more unpleasant odour than any other part of the body?' In order to rid their bodies of odours, the peoples of antiquity cleaned themselves regularly with water and/or oil. The public baths of ancient Rome testify to the popularity of frequent BATHING.

The inhabitants of the ancient world further restricted the production of body odours by removing hair (which encourages the growth of

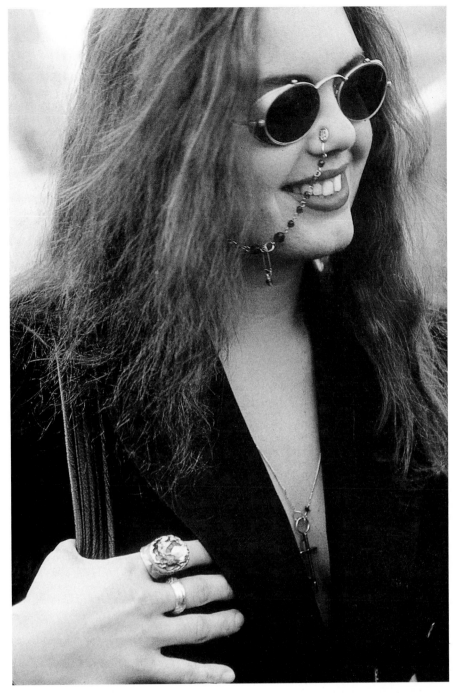
'Fashion victim.' Abbas/Magnum Photos.

remained taboo and, therefore, largely invisible. It is virtually impossible to write a history of piercing. It is said that the genital piercing, the 'Prince Albert', originated at the Victorian court, where it was used to attach the penis discreetly to the inside leg of male courtiers. Other piercings remained uncommented upon, hidden in fantasies retold upon the psychoanalyst's coach or in the murky sado-masochistic demi-monde.

From the 1980s, tattooing and piercing have, to an extent, become desirable commodities bought and sold in hygienically clean high-street shops. In the former, there has been a radical transformation in the nature of the designs: artists have developed a new 'ethnic' style. The latter too has changed: eyebrows, noses, lips, and tongues are now commonplace targets for the piercer's needle; while clothing masks the large increase in genital and nipple piercing. The 'new school' of body modification, termed 'Modern', or 'Urban Primitive', deliberately echoes the customs of pre-literate societies, producing the sense of a shifting, urban tribe locating itself socially and culturally through bodily expression. This is bacteria) from their underarms. Hairy, odorous armpits were considered the mark of an uncouth rustic. The breath, in turn, was made fragrant by chewing on aromatic herbs or perfumed candies. While many people undoubtedly attempted to mask body odours with PERFUME, this practice was widely scorned. Another of the questions raised by Aristotle was: 'Why is it that those who have a rank odour are more unpleasant when they anoint themselves with unguents?'

Body odours, however, were not always considered unpleasant in antiquity. The Roman epigrammatist, Martial, romanticized the fragrance of a kiss as 'the scent of grass which a sheep has just cropped; the odour of myrtle, of the Arab spice-gatherer'.

Significant changes in attitudes towards body cleanliness and odours occurred with the decline and fall of the Roman Empire. The Germanic tribes which invaded the empire tended to eschew baths and perfumes, and therefore — at least according to the Romans — emitted very powerful body odours. The early Christians, in turn, were critical of baths and perfumes due to their association with sensuality and worldliness. A dirty, uncared-for body, by contrast, seemed to many Christians to indicate a preoccupation with matters of the spirit, rather than the FLESH.

According to Christian belief, nonetheless, even a dirty body would exhale a pleasant fragrance if the soul which inhabited it was one of particular holiness. This 'odour of sanctity' was considered to be due to the presence of the divinely fragrant Holy Spirit within the body. In Christian culture, therefore, corporeal fragrance was not, or should not be, an indication of good grooming but of good MORALITY.

The opposite of the odour of sanctity was the stench of sin, a foul odour thought to be exhaled by corrupt, sinful souls. It was said of certain saints that they had the ability to sniff out the virtues and sins of their fellows according to the odours they emitted. As with the odour of sanctity, the stench of sin was believed to be particularly noticeable when the soul left the body at the time of death.

In the Middle Ages bathing was restricted not only due to considerations of morality, but because of a concern that it led to illness. By removing the body's coating of dirt and oil, and by softening the skin, bathing was thought to weaken the body's resistance to disease. Strong body odours, furthermore, were considered to provide a certain protection against illness by warding off pathogenic odours. Thus, even if stale body odours were disliked, it was dangerous to attempt to eliminate them.

Up until the late eighteenth century, washing was usually restricted to the hands and face. Otherwise a scented cloth might be used to cleanse the body of dirt and odour. Hair was similarly cleaned by being rubbed with scented powders. On those rare occasions when the body was bathed, special precautions were deemed necessary to avoid any ill effects from the procedure. For example, the body might first be anointed with oil to prevent water from seeping through the skin.

The peoples of the pre-modern West were preoccupied not only with the odours of the living body, but also with the odours of death. These last were deemed both unpleasant and also potentially harmful, as the odours of decomposition were held to induce illness in the living. The means taken to prevent or disguise such odours included embalming, censing, and perfuming the body. Cemeteries, with their concentration of corpses, were considered particularly dangerous sites of olfactory contagion.

The subject of contagion by body odours — whether of the living or the dead — was of particular concern to the sanitary reformers of the eighteenth and nineteenth centuries. The British physician Hector Gavin, for example, wrote that he found the air in the homes of the poor 'so saturated with putrescent exhalations, that to breathe it was to inhale a dangerous, perhaps fatal, poison'. Previously, 'healthy' body odours had been believed to protect against disease. Now virtually all body odours were suspected of being pathogenic.

In the late nineteenth century this notion was dispelled by a new scientific paradigm which held that germs, rather than odours, caused disease. Nonetheless, the campaign to cleanse the body of dirt and ill odours continued, as these became closely associated both with disease-causing germs and with an 'unclean', immoral lifestyle. According to the new morality, cleanliness, far from being a sign of a sinful preoccupation with the flesh, was next to godliness.

The primary interest which the scientific community of the late nineteenth and early twentieth centuries had in body odours lay in how such odours might constitute a means of differentiating among people, and how they might affect sexual behaviour. Thus attempts were made to chart the characteristic odours of peoples of different ethnicities, and to document instances of an attractive role of body odours in interaction between the sexes. Many of these enquiries were based on anecdotal evidence and coloured by popular prejudices. The customary conclusion was that body odour was stronger among non-Europeans than among Europeans, and played a more important role in sexual behaviour.

Reputed differences in body odour, in fact, had long served to express and enforce social divisions. It was usually the case that all peoples marginalized from mainstream society, whether because of their ethnicity, class, or gender, were associated with ill odours. 'Foreigners', for example, are often typecast as having a 'foreign' — and therefore undesirable — body odour. In the 1930s George Orwell wrote that 'the real secret of class distinctions in the West' consisted in the belief that 'the lower classes smell'. Orwell also pointed out that this belief gave members of the middle and upper classes a sense of actual physical revulsion towards the working class, which helped to maintain class differences.

As regards gender, women have traditionally been considered more odorous than men, either more foul or more fragrant, and sometimes more fragrant due to attempts to perfume their allegedly inherent foulness. The ancient association of women with malodour is due both to their production of odorous menstrual blood and to the (masculine) perception of women as dangerous, corruptive elements in society. The association of women with fragrance, in turn, comes from the characterization of women as attractive (to men) and from romanticized notions of women's sweetness and purity. The customary use of perfumes by women worked to strengthen this association of women with fragrance.

The attitude towards body odours in twentieth-century culture was distinguished by a heightened consciousness about bad body odours or, indeed, *any* body odours, as virtually all odours naturally emanating from the body came to be typified as unpleasant. The term body odour, euphemized as 'BO', refers exclusively to foul body odours in its general usage. This attitude has in large part been shaped by intensive advertising campaigns produced by the marketers of soaps, underarm deodorants and mouthwashes. Such campaigns have played on people's fears of social rejection due to invisible forces of which they are unaware. During the Depression years, for example, soap ads warned people: 'Don't risk *your* job by offending with BO.' While there have been reactions against the stigmatization of all body odours as unpleasant, the naturally odorous body is still the subject of ambivalence and embarrassment.

Relatively little research was undertaken on human body odours in the late twentieth century. This was due to the ambivalence concerning such odours mentioned above and to the low status of the sense of smell in general in modernity. Most of the research which has been undertaken has centred on how human body odours might subliminally affect social behaviour, and on how people might be able to make distinctions of gender, age, and kinship through smelling such odours. Body odours thus remain something of an enigma in contemporary society.

CONSTANCE CLASSEN

Further reading

Classen, C., Howes, D., and Synnott, A. (1994). *Aroma: the cultural history of smell*. Routledge, London.

Schaal, B. and Porter, R. H. (1991). 'Microsmatic humans' revisited: the generation and perception of chemical signals. *Advances in the Study of Behavior*, **20**, 135–99.

See also HALITOSIS; HYGIENE; PHEROMONES; SWEATING.

Body politic The image of the human body and its pervasiveness in both thought and literature attest to Alexander Pope's declaration that the only true study of mankind is man himself. Nowhere is this sentiment more resolutely expressed than in the idea of the body politic. Ostensibly an organicist term for civil society, which enjoyed much currency during the seventeenth century, it nevertheless has a long and interesting genesis. Essentially concerned with organic metaphors for the social order of society, the term has endured into the parlance of the present day, enjoying something of a renaissance, due to the body becoming an object of fashion, and made visible thanks largely to the writing of Michel Foucault.

In classical literature, from Plato to Seneca, the analogy between body and commonwealth is idealised and polemical, rather than literal. Plato, in his *Timaeus* believed the cosmos to be of animate form, literally parallel to the human body. However, the State is not an animate body in a similar vein; moreover, it constitutes an artificial body, necessary for unity and society's evolution. Since Plato's anthropomorphic analogy is largely heuristic, he is more apt to compare the State with the individual man's life than with his body. In the *Republic*, the body plays an important role in Plato's political philosophy, with the three types of guardian, ruled by the tripart head, heart, and belly, each pursuing different goals. Aristotle's conception of the state was more mechanistic than Plato's, which explains Aristotle's use of body analogy in a more specifically corporeal way. This is especially true since the primary quality of Aristotle's association is the perfect integration of many working parts, and is much in evidence at the very beginning of *The Politics*.

Furthermore, the terms can be clarified by recourse to understanding the natural unities among the diversities formed within the human body. The kernel of this corporeal analogy makes an appearance in Shakespeare's *Coriolanus*, with Menenius Agrippa recounting the fable of the belly to pacify the plebeians. This story has its earliest outing in the second book of Livy's *History of Rome*, and has throughout its history followed closely along the lines taken by all the analogies of commonwealth and natural bodies. The belly, corpulent, idle, and seemingly lacking utility, takes in all the nourishment, while the other members, ceaselessly performing their functions, receive nothing for their labours. They rebel, and in some versions actually prevent the belly from receiving nourishment. Soon each member discovers that it is incapable of existence, since the belly not only takes in the food but distributes it accordingly among the other members. The belly therefore stands for some element of society that is perceived as surplus to requirement, the moral of this fable being that not only are tribunes, senators, and clergy indispensable, but also the amputation of any one part of the body politic has serious consequences for all the others. Livy, however, did not go to any great lengths to establish parallels between the body politic and organic analogous equivalents. Anatomical functions were described but not specifically given political equivalents.

The Christian Church has always had recourse to ideas of the body politic. Indeed, the Church regards itself as the embodiment of the mystical body of Christ. The doctrine of the *corpus mysticum* originated in Paul's Epistles. Exceeding Plato, Aristotle, and the Stoics in later influence, yet deriving from them, Paul expanded the analogy in novel ways, to propose theological, sacramental, and ecclesiastical doctrines, totally alien to pre-Christian authors. Paul's new comprehension of the analogy, in 1 *Corinthians* 12.8–31, was essentially a reworking of Seneca's, except an even greater emphasis was placed on the diversity of the body image. However, Paul's later epistles, composed when the danger of schism had somewhat receded, drew from the human body analogy the lesson which emphasized the total dependence of the members upon the head, which was Christ, at the expense of spiritual equality and co-operation between the members. Paul made the analogy more corporeal, by mapping the appetites and functions of the literal body onto the idealised, mystical body of Christ. The body politic, which can be likened to the actual body of Christ, or any other human body, is not merely identical to but actually is the body of Christ. In the mystery of the EUCHARIST lies the doctrine of the sacrament being the body of Christ. Within this framework is a fundamental union of the body politic with the specific, natural body, albeit an idealised one, of Christ. Thus, the Pauline analogy retains some of the flavour of classical rhetoric and idealisation but adds diversity, physicality, and specificity with respect to the body of Christ.

The concepts of *res publica* and *corpus mysticum*, evoked by anthropomorphic analogies, gained currency in the Middle Ages as expressions of the medieval tension between the vision of cosmic unity and the evidence of diversity within the world. This polarity always provided the substance of the microcosmic body image, the analogy of which flourished in medieval thought. However, the unity of the *corpus mysticum* was confounded by the complexity and fragmentation of the medieval world. By the twelfth century, the Church had reaffirmed the actuality of the body and blood in the Eucharist against earlier heresies proposing purely mystical transubstantiation, and in the Church, due to its increasing social importance, the *corpus mysticum* became identified with the body of the faithful.

John of Salisbury in the twelfth century pioneered a full-scale anatomy of the anthropomorphic state. The result, *Policraticus*, detailed the community as a body, fully utilising the lore surrounding the organic theory of the state, with the king as head, administrative officials and soldiers as the hands, and the peasants as the feet. Importantly, anatomical functions within the body politic are understood in precise terms. Nicholas of Cusa ultimately derived his *De Concordiantia Catholica* from Salisbury, although it is a conservative return to the organic and hierarchical vision of Church and State.

The expression of organic theory and of anthropomorphic analogy in Renaissance England, however, the so-called Elizabethan world picture, or the GREAT CHAIN OF BEING, stretching from heaven down to earth, was above all a defence of the hierarchical *status quo*. Probably the ultimate expression of this sentiment is found in ceremony of the Royal Touch, which survived into the eighteenth century. However, Newtonian mechanics and atomistic visions of social order, which appealed to Enlightenment tendencies, replaced organic metaphors with those of a more mechanical kind — 'the ship of state' or 'checks and balances' to name but two.   MARK GOSBEE

Body shape derives from the ceaseless interaction between biological imperatives and historical forces, both cultural and personal. To a large degree the body's size, in terms of height and weight, reach of the arms and length of stride, derives from information in the DNA of the chromosomes, inherited from our parents at conception. The development of muscles, bones, fat, and all that forms the volume and outline of the human body begins in the womb and continues along pathways that take their definition from our genes. This much might be considered demonstrable scientific fact. However, genetic disposition provides only the basis, the foundation, from which the shape of the body proceeds and develops.

Several factors coincide to determine the body's shape at any given time. Of these the most prominent are likely to be: nutrient and dietary circumstances; the intervention of surgery and disease; and the impact of accident and EXERCISE may also play a role. FASHION and custom can also cause a refashioning of the body, whether in line with the latest trend or in honour of the most ancient beliefs. Given the conjunction of these influences (some, if not all, will impact on every human body) it makes sense to acknowledge that body shape emerges from a combination of history and biology. What begins with genetic predisposition (combined with the diet and circumstances of the mother) will ultimately be revised and altered by battles waged against disease, by submissions to fashion, and by the incremental effects of food, habit, and exercise. As a result the shape of the body undergoes constant change. It is perhaps for this reason that the body has given rise to so many cultural anxieties and to many personal crises. Indeed, body shape is something that virtually everyone has winced at or fretted over at some point in their lives.

Nonetheless it is true to say that, in the developed world, the body is now in 'better shape' than ever before. Improved medical knowledge (both diagnostic and surgical) and the increased supply of food enjoyed by most people in Europe and North America have made it possible for many people to imagine a life in which their body shape is not violently altered, or at least not against their will. It is, of course, equally the case that such wealth has brought with it other problems, notably obesity and heart disease. For those who live beyond the luxury of the West, this fact can offer little comfort. Throughout the developing world, common diseases, such as rickets, polio, and post-traumatic infections (gangrene, for example), together with the widespread incidence of malnutrition, continue to ensure that bodies are likely to suffer, if not deformation, then at least stunted or twisted growth. However, despite the unmet promises of Western medicine, some considerable advances have been made.

Previously, if a body suffered major trauma it was inevitable that the marks of that damage would be long-lasting and plainly visible; Melville's frightful Captain Ahab, and Admiral Nelson, are well-known examples of this painful change in body shape. However, surgical advances in the twentieth century ensured that a surprising number of previously disfiguring accidents can now be treated and their worst physical effects ameliorated. Severed limbs have been successfully reconnected and the faces of crash victims restored. It has been one of the aims and greatest achievements of modern Western medicine to succeed in preserving the shape and surface of the body from more and more of the ailments which would otherwise cause it to change or deform.

Despite these advances, Western societies retain an obsessive and sometimes morbid attitude to the body. If greater food provision and vaccination has eradicated the emaciated figure of the nineteenth century, we now worry that we are too fat, too flabby, or too short. The body, now generally fit and well, has risen to even greater prominence in our psychic lives, and a concern with the image and shape of the body seems widely prevalent. Indeed the relationship between body shape and anxiety is an acute one. Often this is the consequence of the ways in which art and advertising, cinema, and television have constructed a dominant ideal of body shape which is young, slim, muscular only as far as it is elegant, smooth, and supple. Given the predominance of these ideals it is not surprising that some people have been led to extreme measures to alter the basic shape of their bodies. COSMETIC SURGERY, to enlarge or reduce breasts, to alter noses, or to reduce waists and thighs, is now relatively commonplace. Pop stars Cher and Michael Jackson are obvious examples of this trend. Cher's well-documented and near-notorious desire to reform and refashion her body has included the removal of ribs (to make her appear slimmer) and the alteration of her nose. More damagingly, the painful experiences of those who have suffered from anorexia or bulimia, or who have sacrificed money, time, and health to pursue a bodily ideal that they could never reasonably hope to achieve, stands as further testimony to both the power of this image and the social consequences of its imposition.

However, the ideal shape of the body has changed though history and remains different between cultures. During the 1920s, the favoured shape for women's bodies was a rather boyish one, with an emphasis placed on straight lines, narrow hips, and flattened breasts. Earlier fashions had encouraged the display of another body

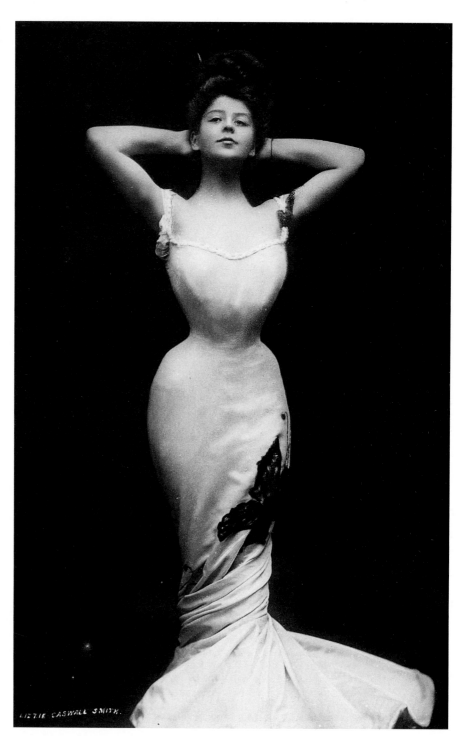

Camille Clifford (1906), actress: 'the girl with the hour-glass figure'. Mary Evans Picture Library.

shape. A more sensuous ('fleshy' to its critics) body shape appears to have dominated conceptions of female form in the Restoration period. Certainly the art produced in that period, notably portraits of court ladies by Sir Peter Lely, depicts women whose bodies might be described as voluptuous or 'full' rather than slim. The male body has also been subjected to regulation and restriction: the eighteenth century saw an emphasis on poise and elegance centred round an image of a slim, restrained body. For upper-class men, the presence of muscle was to be downplayed, as Thomas Gainsborough's work seems to indicate. In earlier times, by contrast, when citizens were more often called to perform military duties, such a slight figure would have been regarded more suspiciously, even derided as 'effeminate'.

It would take a very broad history to take in the whole range of shapes into which the human body has been encouraged to grow. However, it is important to register the variety and changing nature of these requirements. Added to this physical impact made on the body by taste and custom, is the fact that fashion has consistently, through CORSETS, BUSTLES, wigs, and hoops, sought to transform the basic shape of the body. The purpose behind many such designs is to display or to disguise the shape of the body as a signifier of sexual difference and sexual responsiveness.

While the shape of the body can delight, it can also shock. The case of amputees has already been mentioned, but is worth noting again how a real or imagined deficiency in the shape or function of the body arouses some of our deepest fears. During the nineteenth century the reporting of war became more immediate, and photography lent reports immediate impact. The images from Balaclava and Gettysburg of bodies maimed and broken by the increasingly mechanised nature of conflict shocked Victorian newspaper readers and defined, in part, a new anxiety about the body as vulnerable to the might of the industrial age.

It is, however, not only the body of the maimed victim that has the power to shock or disturb. Since antiquity, individuals whose bodies do not obviously conform to dominant images or ideals of the body have been exhibited for curiosity or idle amusement. The sad histories of such 'FREAKS' (John Merrick, the 'ELEPHANT MAN', is a particularly cruel instance) underline the fascination associated with changed or transformed body shape. More recently, the bodies of athletes or near-athletes (such as 'BODY-BUILDERS') have delighted and appalled in roughly equal measure. Such sensitivities indicate that, in most societies, body shape indicates not only personal circumstances and fortune, but also advancing age, sexual difference, and racial and class division. If in our post-modern times these oppositions seems more vulnerable to change or mutation, then this attests more to the power of the body over our imaginations than to any sense that we are free from its limits. ROBERT JONES

Further reading

Felien, M., Nadduff, R., and Tazi, N. (1989). *Fragments for a history of the human body*. Zone Books, London.

See also BODY IMAGE; EATING DISORDERS; FASHION; FEMALE FORM.

Body snatchers
Between the Tudor era and the early nineteenth century, the only legal source of corpses for DISSECTION was the gallows. Not enough bodies were provided to supply the proliferating number of ANATOMY schools and their burgeoning numbers of students. Body snatchers ('grave-robbers' or 'resurrection men') generally obtained fresh corpses from new graves. Their work was crucial to the historical development of anatomical knowledge

and expertise, particularly during their heyday, from the 1780s to 1832. After this the Anatomy Act changed the legal basis of corpse provision.

The earliest grave-robbers were surgeon–anatomists or their pupils. Apprentices' indentures issued by the Edinburgh College of Surgeons in the 1720s forbad trainees to exhume the dead — which suggests that they had been doing so. A contemporary book referred with heavy irony to 'resurrections' by the London Corporation of Corpse Stealers in a number of churchyards. Great museums of medical specimens were being established during this era, and, as with natural history collections, private auctions provided a form of brokerage by which owners could exchange specimens of human origin. Surgical exams at first tacitly, and later openly, recognised that bodies were being procured beyond legal means and dissected in unofficial premises.

Accurate estimates of the demand are difficult to come by. The first period for which figures are available is the early nineteenth century, when 700 medical students were enrolled annually in London alone, each of whom expected to engage in hands-on dissection on three or more corpses.

Until the 1830s, dissection was considered by law a fate worse than death, a 'further Terror and peculiar Mark of Infamy' to public execution itself — to be inflicted upon the worst of murderers. Only beheading; hanging, drawing and quartering; or burning alive exceeded it in severity. There was a widely held belief in some incorporeal association between the fate of the corpse and that of the soul. Dissection mutilated and dismembered the body, and was specifically designed to deny the wrongdoer a grave: in popular belief the spirit denied this repose was doomed to wander, and its future RESURRECTION was in doubt.

The public viewed dissection with terror. Body snatching was greatly feared, and inflicted profound psychological pain upon surviving relatives and friends. Corpses were most desired by the anatomists, and most lucrative to the body snatchers, at their freshest: at the time mourners were experiencing raw grief. Entire communities, on hearing a rumour of body snatchers at work, would repair to the graveyard to dig for their relatives. Severe violence against body snatchers, riots, and even the demolition of anatomy schools could result.

Watchmen, sometimes with guns and dogs, were employed by local inhabitants to protect their dead. Many burial grounds had extra security features. In poor districts, coffins were buried in stacks, reaching almost to the surface, and ordinary folk could do little to protect their dead, other than to make things difficult for the body snatchers. People would delay burial, mix straw with the earth returned to the grave to hinder the body snatchers' shovels, or share stints of watching at the graveside. The rich could purchase better security. Any means by which burial could be made more secure was sure to find a ready market. Better quality coffins were described as 'stout', and extra coffin nails became a status symbol. Double and triple coffins, and

lead coffins, became popular. Ingenious inventors devised and patented special coffin bands, locks, screws, and even cast iron coffins. Yet the wealthy remained vulnerable. Body snatchers were extremely efficient. Sir Astley Cooper, a leading Regency surgeon–anatomist, confidently stated in 1828 that if he was so disposed he could obtain the body of anyone — whoever they were, and of whatever station in life: ready money was always the key.

Prices were affected by market-wide considerations — as when good weather rendered mortality lower than expected — and by local conditions. For example, increased vigilance in one locality could cause greater expense in obtaining corpses from another. Corpses lost value swiftly due to the lack of adequate preservatives: pickling, salting, and other forms of preservation known from food use were used, but neither refrigeration nor formaldehyde had yet been developed, and prices were seasonally variable. An average adult corpse in good condition yielded an average price, one damaged by AUTOPSY or AMPUTATION had considerably lower value. Rising demand, and sometimes severe shortages, caused prices to fluctuate, but the general drift was upwards. In the 1790s, one London gang was said to have been selling adult corpses for 'two guineas and a crown', children's bodies were sold by the inch: 'six shillings for the first foot, and nine [pence] per inch for all it measures more in length'. In the 1820s, when the trade was more difficult, adult corpses cost between ten and twenty guineas apiece.

Collectors paid much greater sums for medical curiosities. In one rare but well-known case in the 1780s, the anatomist John Hunter paid the enormous sum of £500 for the corpse of the 'Irish Giant', whose huge skeleton is still displayed in the Royal College of Surgeons' Museum in Lincoln's Inn Fields, London.

Body snatchers usually worked at night. Daytime reconnaissance informed them of fresh burials, depth, and whether more than one body might be obtained by one spate of digging. Their tools were simple: wooden shovels to lessen noise, a rope with hooks or a crowbar to pull up the coffin lid, and a couple of sacks. A hole would be dug at the head end of a fresh grave; the soft soil would be removed and heaped on sacking. Once visible, the coffin lid would be forced. The weight of earth on the rest of the coffin served as a counter-weight, so when pressure was applied the lid would break across, and the body pulled out. Shrouds or other clothing on the body would be thrown back, and the earth replaced by tipping up the sacking. It was important to leave the grave tidy: if suspicions were aroused future attempts upon the same graveyard could meet with danger. A look-out would be waiting outside with a cart.

In times of dearth, body snatchers would try other sources: country churchyards further afield would be raided if they were on good communications routes — road, canal, or sea. Private vaults were entered secretly, by bribery or force.

Bodies were imported from France and Ireland in casks. Body snatchers posed as grieving relatives at public mortuaries, or stole bodies awaiting inquest.

In law, the body did not constitute property and could therefore neither be bought, sold, or stolen. Body snatchers were convicted, however. A husband and wife, for example, were transported for the theft of grave clothes. Body snatchers generally took the brunt of popular obloquy and judicial punishment for grave-robbery, but the prosecution and conviction of an anatomist in the spring of 1828 — for unlawfully conspiring to obtain and receive a body — effectively incriminated anatomical enquiry, and at last caused Parliamentary action.

The Select Committee on Anatomy recommended the requisition of the bodies of individuals dying in workhouses or hospitals, too poor to pay for their own funerals. Despite opposition, these findings were eventually embodied in the Anatomy Act of 1832. Grave-robbers were rendered redundant by a new breed of body snatcher: the mortuary attendant. Although dissection lost its association with execution for murder, this now adhered to the shame of a death in poverty. It is only in the NHS era that donation has become the major source of corpses for anatomy. 　　　　　RUTH RICHARDSON

See also ANATOMY; BURKE AND HARE; DISSECTION.

Body weight

Weight is probably the most-measured body parameter in Western society — a standard ritual in any medical examination and an obsessive benchmark for those concerned to lose or not to gain it. This is a bizarre reversal: our ancestors were, and multitudes of our contemporaries still are, mainly concerned not to starve — to maintain their weight. The ritual starts at birth — second only to making sure the infant is breathing. (What mother does not know and forever remember the birth weights of her babies?) Birth weight is, of course, quite important, although the normal range is broad even at full term. Body weight in the premature infant is linked to viability; low birth weight at full term can be an ill omen and linked to maternal ill-health or inappropriate indulgence in alcohol or cigarette smoking during PREGNANCY. Weight decreases in the early neonatal days, and then for the first year increases more rapidly than it ever should again. The growth spurts in both weight and height around PUBERTY are common knowledge. Thereafter people generally settle down with their figure until the advent of middle-aged spread, apart from the vagaries which may be associated with pregnancy and its aftermath.

The appropriate ranges for body weight related to sex, age, and height have been derived from healthy population samples, and there are many sources of this information. The '*body mass index*' — defined as weight (kg)/height (m)^2 — gives a 'rule of thumb' guide to OBESITY: 25–30 = overweight and >30 = obesity. Weight gain above the statistical healthy norm is widely acknowledged to be better avoided for both cosmetic and medical reasons, the latter on good grounds since the links between obesity, liability to ill-health, and earlier death are well established, on a statistical if not an individual basis. Unfortunately we are not — or many or most of us are not — endowed with a built-in physiological system which accurately and automatically matches appetite to requirement. So in affluent society a conscious, deliberate balancing act is required, with the aid of the calorie count and the bathroom scales.

But what does our body weight comprise, to add up to the reading on the scales? In the standard average 70 kg man there are over 40 litres of water, so water accounts for nearly 60% of body weight. Small day-to-day fluctuations in weight are often related to varying retention or loss of water, perhaps by excessive sweat loss, or linked to the HORMONES which regulate BODY FLUIDS, including variations in women over the phases of the MENSTRUAL CYCLE. Boxers who are marginally overweight for their class may attempt to achieve their goal by dehydration — although interference with body WATER BALANCE which is rigorous enough to be effective is perhaps unlikely to be good for their general condition.

The solid components can be separated into fat and lean fractions: adipose tissue and fat-free tissue. Body fat can be estimated from measurement of body density. As for inanimate objects, density can be determined by finding the difference between weight in air and weight in water; the fatter you are, the more you tend to float, because fat is less dense than the lean body mass. A person sits on a seat suspended from a weight gauge in a purpose-built water tank, and is briefly submerged, while holding their breath. The amount of air in the lungs has to be measured and allowed for, because this of course affects buoyancy. A formula is then applied which relates density to percentage fat. More practically, body fat is commonly estimated indirectly from *skin-fold thicknesses*: at several specified sites a fold of skin and its underlying fatty layer is lifted and its double thickness measured with graduated calipers. The several measurements are added and the sum used to find total body fat from published tables for different age groups: the tables were constructed by comparing skin-fold measurements in a great many people with the 'gold-standard' from body density estimations. More sophisticated measurements of all the body fat can now be made from scans using the technique known as *DEXA*. The norms for percentage fat are between 20% and 30% of body weight — higher in women than in men.

Weight gain is generally equated with an increase in body fat, although there can be a significant increase in muscle weight during recovery from STARVATION, ILLNESS, or INJURY, or during a rigorous EXERCISE regime. In any state of *positive* ENERGY BALANCE (more caloric intake than output) most of the surplus is converted into fat and stored in the adipose tissues. In *negative energy balance*, it is mostly fat which is used up. When weight loss is deemed desirable, intake has to be cut down and/or output increased. Since an individual's BASAL META-BOLIC RATE accounts for a high proportion of energy output, an extra walk or run each week adds little extra: it may do something for general fitness but makes relatively little difference to fatness.

Body weight can be affected in either direction by different illnesses: some hormonal disorders cause weight gain (e.g. thyroid deficiency, or excess of corticosteroids) and others weight loss (e.g. overactive thyroid, adrenal deficiency). Any injury or acute illness can be accompanied by weight loss, if feeding does not match increased metabolic demands, and weight loss can sometimes be a warning sign of serious disease.

　　　　　SHEILA JENNETT

Further reading
Sumner, M. (1981). *Thought for food.* Oxford University Press.

See also BODY FLUIDS; DEVELOPMENT AND GROWTH; EATING DISORDERS; ENERGY BALANCE; EXERCISE; OBESITY.

Bone

Fairly early in the evolution of multicellular organisms it became an advantage to have a hard body component which could provide protection for soft tissues and a firm base against which contractile elements such as muscle could perform precise movements like those involved in locomotion or grasping. The hard component was often formed from calcium carbonate, as found in shellfish, but other durable defences were provided by *chitin* (a complex carbohydrate), in crustaceans and insects, and even silica, in the glass sponges.

Man and most vertebrates are characterised by an internal rather than an external SKELETON. With the exception of the young animal and the cartilaginous fishes, the hardness is provided by calcium phosphate, laid down as crystalline hydroxyapatite on a template of COLLAGEN (a fibrous protein), forming bone. The collagen confers some elasticity. In man, bone also acts as the major reservoir for several elements such as calcium, phosphorus, magnesium, zinc, and sodium. The storage and release of at least the first three of these into the extracellular space is modified by HORMONES such as parathyroid hormone, calcitonin, and 1,25-dihydroxyvitamin D.

The longest bone is the *femur* (thigh bone), which accounts for a quarter of one's stature; the smallest bone is the stapes — one of the tiny ossicles in the middle ear which transmits the vibrations from the ear drum to the inner ear.

There are over 200 bones in the adult skeleton. They can be divided into two principal types: the long bones such as the femur, tibia, and humerus, which develop principally from within a cartilaginous framework, and the flat bones such as the SKULL, bones of the PELVIS, and scapula, which develop within membranes of fibrous tissue.

Bone development and growth

X-RAYS can detect primary centres of bone formation (*ossification*) in the mid shaft of long bones from the end of the second month of intrauterine life. Secondary centres of ossification appear at the ends of these bones mostly at various times after birth and always earlier in females than males. Some secondary centres, however, such as in the lower end of the femur, occur before birth and this was used in the past as a indication of the maturity of a fetus; this had crucial forensic implications as it could determine whether or not a mother would be charged for concealing the birth of a viable infant.

Towards the ends of the long bones there are specialised discs of CARTILAGE (*epiphyseal plates*) stretching across the entire bone. The cells in this area have a high rate of multiplication, and it is the major site of longitudinal growth in the juvenile bone. The rate of growth is greatest in infancy and around puberty, and growth ceases when the epiphyseal plate itself finally ossifies. It is over 200 years since the anatomist, John Hunter, showed that the mass and width of bone is increased by surface accretion from the *periosteum* — a tough fibrous layer covering the bone — rather than by internal expansion.

The ultimate bone length and mass is largely genetically determined and the average racial differences in bone mass exemplify this, with black people having a higher peak bone mass than white Caucasians and higher still than Asians. However this may be modified by general nutritional status — particularly calcium and protein intake — and by physical load bearing. There is evidence that the impact of such environmental influences may be greatest around the time of PUBERTY, and unfortunately the lifestyle of the average teenager in present day Western society does not favour optimal bone development.

Premature arrest of growth at the epiphyseal plate will result in dwarfism. The cause may be genetic (as in *achondroplasia*), or environmental (as in severe illness or starvation).

Epiphyseal growth is most rapid at the wrists and shoulders in the upper limbs and at the knees in the lower limbs. The increased output of SEX HORMONES at puberty provides a strong stimulus to accelerated bone growth for two or three years and then leads to epiphyseal closure — fusion with the shaft of the bone. Children with precocious puberty end up with stunted growth, whereas in EUNUCHS the epiphyses remain open and they become tall in their later teens. Pituitary GROWTH HORMONE is the other hormone involved in bone growth.

All bone surfaces, with the exception of cartilaginous articular surfaces which form a joint with a neighbouring bone, are invested with the fibrous periosteum, which has *osteogenic* (bone-forming) potential. The flat bones ossify directly from such fibrous tissue rather than from intermediary cartilage. The skull is made up of several bones separated by very irregular interdigitating seams called *sutures*. This arrangement permits the necessary flexibility of the head during the birth process and after ossification is completed the sutures seal up progressively throughout adult life. Examination of the extent of suture union provides a means for assessing the age of an adult skeleton after death, whereas in a child this can be judged by which ossification centres are present and which epiphyses are fused.

Bone structure

About 80% of the skeleton consists of compact or 'cortical' bone which is extremely dense and resistant to trauma, and whose degree of hardness is exceeded in the body only by the enamel of the teeth. Such material forms the thick shafts of the long bones and the surface of all bones. It is perforated by microscopic channels; the *Haversian canals* (described by Havers, an English physician in the seventeenth century). Blood vessels pass through these canals, and bone cells are arranged concentrically around them. These cells, the *osteocytes*, have long extensions which pass down an interlocking network of canaliculi in the bone. This same network also allows nutrients, gases, and solutes to permeate the bone from the Haversian blood vessels.

The other 20% of bone forms a delicate, lacy honeycomb with a high surface-to-volume ratio. Cellular activity in this component (called *trabecular* or *cancellous bone*) is greater than in compact bone, and a variety of metabolic, hormonal, or physical stimuli on the cells renders it more labile. Trabecular bone is found principally in the bodies of the vertebrae, the ribs, the pelvis, and at the ends of the long bones. It contains the red bone marrow where the cellular components of the BLOOD are manufactured. The remainder of the interior of bones — the medullary cavity — contains fat, and the proportion of fat to red marrow increases with age.

Metabolism and remodelling

Live adult bone is not a rigid inorganic framework. If it were, then like other crystalline structures it would be subject to frequent fatigue fractures as a result of the repetitive strains to which it is subjected. At millions of microscopic sites throughout the skeleton, bone is constantly being broken down and then remade in a cellular process first detailed in the mid twentieth century by an American orthopaedic surgeon, Harold Frost, and termed remodelling. At any site and in response to signals which are, as yet, poorly understood, the osteocytes permit access to the underlying bone by *osteoclasts*; these are specialised bone-resorbing cells derived from primitive cells in the marrow which also generate other types of PHAGOCYTES. These large, multinucleated cells dig small pits in the bone over a period of several days and are then replaced by bone-forming cells, the *osteoblasts* — which are derived from precursors of the fibrous-tissue-forming series. Osteoblasts synthesize fibres of the protein collagen and dispose them in a regular pattern determined in part by the direction of local strain forces. They also synthesize matrix mucopolysaccharide and direct the later mineralisation of collagen with crystalline calcium phosphate.

Active metabolites of vitamin D are required to allow adequate provision of both calcium and phosphate at those sites. The osteoblasts are ultimately trapped in the calcified matrix which they themselves have created, and become osteocytes. These cells appear to be able to communicate with each other throughout the bone; their elongated processes form close junctions with each other rather than being joined together.

Whatever the details, one end of a bone can interpret strain and chemical signals from the other. In healthy young adults the remodelling process is in balance, with as much new bone being synthesised as old bone removed. It also permits some adaptation of distribution of bone within a bone (or even within the skeleton) in response to changing physical or biochemical stimuli. Thus the disposition of bony trabeculae or cortical thickness is not haphazard but determined by mechanical and growth signals. Throughout the vertebrates there is a fairly constant ratio between the amount of bone required to cope with the largest forces normally encountered, and that required to deal with average gravitational demands. It is about three to one — for mice through to elephants.

Bone mass and ageing

A minimum regular stress is required simply to maintain your skeletal mass — you either use it or lose it — but the strains required to *increase* your bone mass significantly have to be substantially more than is customary for the individual concerned. Men have more bone than women at all ages because they are larger, but in both sexes bone mass (as measured conveniently by 'dual energy X-ray densitometers') increases into the third decade and plateaus from then till about the end of the fifth decade. It then declines, very slowly in men, but more rapidly in women for some years following the MENOPAUSE. The average woman has lost around 20% of her peak bone mass by the time she is 70 years old (though estimates from different studies vary). This increases her risk of fractures and broken bones. The decline in bone mass in postmenopausal women can be reduced by taking oestrogen, and load-bearing EXERCISE can increase bone mass to a modest extent in both men and women.

Any bone will fracture if it is subjected to sufficient force, but orthopaedic statistics reveal that over the past fifty years in the Western world there has been a striking rise in the incidence of certain fractures in older people, usually associated with only modest trauma. Fractures of the femoral neck (hip fracture), vertebral bodies (spine fracture), and wrist predominate, and appear to relate to populations having less bone at these sites. This condition, where reduced bone mass increases the liability to fracture, is called OSTEOPOROSIS and represents one of our principal medical challenges today. In osteoporosis the remodelling process is not in equilibrium; less new bone is being formed than is being removed. It probably relates to several modern lifestyle changes affecting bone metabolism — notably

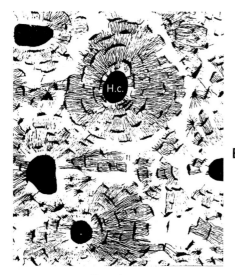

Transverse section of bone from a human femur, × 150 magnification, showing the Haversian canals. The osteocytes lie in the tiny cavities (black) arranged concentrically around the canals. From Le Gros Clark (1971), *The tissues of the body*, Clarendon Press.

diet and physical labour. The fact that Asian populations have smaller skeletons in any event and are adopting many of the same lifestyle features has led to predictions that hip fracture in that part of the world will become one of the greatest health care problems of the twenty-first century.

Several drugs are now available which have powerful actions on bone metabolism: examples are the bisphosphonates and the calcitonins, both of which inhibit bone resorption and can be used in the treatment of osteoporosis. The drug most commonly taken with such an effect is oestrogen, as HORMONE REPLACEMENT THERAPY (HRT). It may also enhance bone formation.

The other common bone pathology is osteomalacia (called '*rickets*' in children). In this disorder the bone is poorly mineralised, permitting softening and deformity such as bow legs. The usual cause is lack of vitamin D in the diet and/or lack of exposure to sunlight, and supplements of vitamin D are the appropriate treatment.

Ancient bones

Of all the body tissues, bone — apart from the teeth — is usually the only one to survive significantly beyond our mortal span. Ignoring palaeological niceties, some 'human' skeletons have been dated at around two million years old and provide us with much of the scanty evidence we have concerning the evolution of our species. Depending on the bones available, careful examination can allow reasonable inference concerning cranial development, height, and nutrition, in addition to the presence of diseases such as tuberculosis and leprosy and the medico-social practice of skull trepanning. The persistence of minute quantities of DNA within ancient bones may, by the application of sophisticated Polymerase Chain Reaction (PCR) augmentation and analysis, permit conclusions on the evolutionary/racial classification of some

prehistoric skeletal remains. Look after your bones — they may tell your story long after you are gone!   IAIN BOYLE

Further reading
Frost, H. M. (1964). *Laws of bone structure*. Thomas Springfield, Illinois.

See also CALCIUM; HORMONE REPLACEMENT THERAPY; JOINTS; PARATHYROID GLANDS; SKELETON.

Bowel This term is more colloquial than strictly anatomical; it may refer to the whole of the gut or intestines, or to any part of them; thus 'inflammation of the bowel', or 'cancer of the bowel' might be anywhere from the small intestine to the rectum; 'small bowel' and 'large bowel' may specify which part. An 'irritable bowel' covers a host of symptoms and an uncertain location, although usually the colon. Bowel movement or *bowels*, plural, (opening of, regularity of, 'any trouble with?') euphemizes defecation. The association of intestines with profound and concealed rumblings has presumably led to usages like 'the bowels of the earth' whereas 'gut-feeling' perpetuates a historical emotional link: compare 'bowels of compassion' or Cromwell's plea 'in the bowels of Christ, think it possible you may be mistaken'. The derivation of the word is from the Latin for sausage.   S.J.

See ALIMENTARY SYSTEM; DEFECATION; TOILET PRACTICES.

Boxing Forget the euphemistic 'noble art of self-defence'; boxing is a human bloodsport in which the intention is to hurt one's opponents by delivering blows to their body and ultimately knocking them unconscious. It sanctions injury in the name of sport.

That said, modern boxing appears almost genteel alongside its prizefighting predecessor in which bareknuckled pugilists fought to exhaustion, with fights often lasting several hours. A round ended only when one combatant was floored; he then had half a minute's respite before placing his toe on a line scratched across the centre of the ring and resuming battle. Not until one fighter failed 'to come up to scratch' was a result declared: no wins on points in those days, just the objective test of an inability to continue. Early rounds were often hard slogging contests but the real physical damage came in the later stages when tiredness slowed defensive reflexes. Imagine too the state of even the winner's hands, protected only by having been soaked in brine.

With their combination of boxing and wrestling moves, early contests were literally 'no holds barred'; grappling, punching, tripping, and throwing all being used to floor an opponent. The widely-adopted Broughton's Rules of 1743 eradicated some of the barbarism by outlawing the hitting of a man when he was down, and the seizing of hair or the body below the waist, but they still permitted butting. Yet it was not the brutality of the prize-ring which brought its demise, but the corruption with which it became associated.

The revival of the sport as boxing in late Victorian Britain saw several changes designed to render it more civilised. Although some of the old practices continued for a while — even the famous Queensbury Rules initially allowed endurance contests — by the turn of the century the general picture was one of boxing in gloves, limited-time rounds, points decisions after a fixed number of rounds had elapsed, and weight divisions, though the latter have accentuated problems of dehydration as fighters struggle to 'make the weight'.

For much of the twentieth century the history of boxing has been one of crumbling resistance to changes intended to protect further the brains and bodies of participants. Between 1984 and 1993 eight boxers had died soon after fights in the UK; bantamweight Bradley Stone was added to the list in 1994. Following a report from a medical working party, which included neurosurgeons, the British Boxing Board of Control subsequently introduced mandatory annual magnetic resonance imaging scans for all boxers to replace the less sophisticated computerised tomography which had been compulsory only for those fighting eight rounds or more. Additionally, any boxer knocked out must wait 45 days (previously 28) before he again enters the ring competitively, and he must also have a hospital check. Ringside doctors may advise referees on a fighter's condition between rounds and may recommend that the contest be stopped. Doctors also examine each boxer at the conclusion of fights and paramedic teams must be on hand at all boxing bills.

The medical profession in several countries has increasingly adopted an anti-boxing stance, citing irreversible brain damage as its major objection to the sport. This is a key point for, in absolute terms of deaths and serious injuries, other sports such as horseracing, mountaineering, rugby, and even cricket appear more dangerous, but in none of them is deliberate and repeated striking of an opponent part of the rules of the game. In contrast a boxer has a licence for physical assault. The evidence is clear that repeated pummelling of the head can cause cumulative damage to the brain: here time is no great healer. Occasionally, acute brain injury can occur during a fight. The greatest danger comes towards the end when a tired man with a loose neck has his head flipped back rapidly by a punch. This can tear a vein outside or inside the brain, which then leaks blood, causing pressure on the brain and eventually leading to a COMA. Only if the clot is removed rapidly can the fighter survive. Fighters now train harder; their bodies are fitter — but their brains are no more resilient than in the past. Some nations, notably Sweden, have already banned boxing on medical grounds.

So far the British government has been reluctant to follow the Swedish lead and since 1981 five private members' anti-boxing Bills proposed in parliament have failed to reach the statute books. Most schools, both state and public, however, have dropped boxing from their physical education curriculum. Yet it should be noted that amateur boxing is exceptionally well regulated: not more than four rounds are fought, headguards are worn, and the referee is allowed to stop a fight to prevent serious injury. However, headguards, whilst absorbing energy from punches, present an even larger target to be hit and thus the number of blows striking home may well increase. Indeed, studies have shown that non-boxing sportsmen outperform even amateur fighters in neurological tests and, notwithstanding the safety precautions, three amateur fighters have suffered serious brain injury in British rings since 1988.

For centuries boxing has been the epitome of overt masculinity, a demonstration of manliness and its embodying characteristics of courage, toleration of pain, and self-discipline. Women were merely ornaments displaying the round cards. This continues, but women have successfully demanded equal rights in the ring. In Britain, girls from the age of 10 are now allowed to spar in amateur boxing gyms, and recently professionalism, too, has been recognised for women — significantly later than its acceptance in the US where fights for women have appeared on the undercard of world championship events.

The moral dilemma of boxing is that it provides an honest opportunity to escape poverty, but it also means for some a legal beating and for all the threat of permanent damage. Hitting below the belt is outlawed to protect the genitals, but surely the brain deserves even more protection, by reducing the concussive power of the boxing glove, developing safer headgear, excluding the head as a target — or by banning the sport altogether. The issue is not how hazardous boxing is but whether the hazards are acceptable.

WRAY VAMPLEW

Further reading

BMA (1993). *The boxing debate*. British Medical Association, London.

Brachial plexus

The nerve fibres that serve SENSATION and motor function in the shoulders, arms, and hands travel to and from the SPINAL CORD in the neck. They are linked to the lowest 4 of the 8 cervical segments of the cord and the uppermost thoracic segment. At each segmental level, on each side, a *dorsal* (sensory) and a *ventral* (motor) nerve 'root' converge to form a spinal nerve that emerges between two adjacent vertebral bones. The major components of these spinal nerves take part in forming the brachial plexus.

The 'plexus' (from Latin for a 'braid') is like a railway junction allowing sensory and motor axons from the different segmental levels of the spinal cord, having exited from the spine, to cross and recross, to travel in the main emerging lines, and eventually, in their branches, to reach their final destinations. The brachial plexus is in the form of a large fissured sheet lying behind skin and muscle in the neck, above the collar bone. It resolves into three main nerve cords, which in turn branch to give rise to the *peripheral nerves* that are distributed via their branches throughout the limb. The three largest are the *radial* nerve, which courses down the outer (thumb) side of the arm; the *ulnar*, down the inner side; and the *median*, in between. These are 'mixed' nerves — they carry both motor and sensory fibres, and give off branches on their way to the hand; some branches also are mixed, some motor, some sensory. The constituent microbundles of nerve fibres (*fascicles*) may change their position within a nerve, thus allowing axons to be directed towards their final target within a tissue (a particular part of muscle, skin, or joint) in the final smallest branches. The longest axons in the median and ulnar nerves, for example, terminate in the sensory branches to the fingertips.

Close to the spine the brachial plexus is joined by fibres from the sympathetic ganglia of the AUTONOMIC NERVOUS SYSTEM; these are distributed to the periphery in the same way, innervating the blood vessels and the glands of the skin. Because of this, damage to any nerve originating from the plexus results in warm, dry skin in the area that it supplies, because the smooth muscle of the BLOOD VESSELS relaxes in the absence of sympathetic tone, and sweating cannot be stimulated.

Whereas lesions of a peripheral nerve give rise to discrete functional disturbance with local weakness, PARALYSIS, and numbness (for example in the case of the median nerve in the 'carpal tunnel syndrome' — or more fashionably a computer-typing-based *repetitive strain injury*), damage to the brachial plexus itself results in widespread loss of both muscle power and sensation throughout the arm and shoulder. Damage may arise from a penetrating missile, from traumatic amputation, or from excessive traction when the constituent spinal nerves are literally torn from their roots, thus causing additional symptoms of spinal cord injury. TOM SEARS

Bradycardia

describes a heart beat which is either habitually slow, or which drops from its usual rate. In health, bradycardia may be the result of athletic training, which reduces the resting heart rate. Persons with HEART BLOCK have persistent or intermittent bradycardia. Sudden bradycardia can result in a dramatic fall in CARDIAC OUTPUT and hence in arterial BLOOD PRESSURE, depriving the brain of blood flow and causing a 'black-out'. FAINTING ('syncope') is one such instance, caused by depression of the heart's PACEMAKER by the parasympathetic (VAGUS) nerves; acute exacerbation of heart block is another. From the Greek for 'slow' and 'heart'   S.J.

See HEART BLOCK; SYNCOPE; FAINTING.

Brain

The brain is a pinkish-grey, wrinkled organ that fills the SKULL — looking, for all the world, like a huge walnut. It is hard to believe, from its appearance, that this ugly lump of jelly contains the mechanisms of thought, PERCEPTION, will, and CONSCIOUSNESS, that it is the seat of our PERSONALITY. Its 100 000 million nerve cells, each with an average of 10 000 connections from other neurons, makes the human brain the most complicated and least understood object in the known universe.

The brain and the SPINAL CORD constitute the CENTRAL NERVOUS SYSTEM. In the human embryo the brain grows from three swellings in the head end of a tube of developing nervous tissue. The frontmost swelling differentiates into the cerebral hemispheres, consisting mainly of the THALAMUS, the HYPOTHALAMUS, the corpus striatum (involved in the control of movement) and the CEREBRAL CORTEX. The two rear swellings form the BRAIN STEM (*midbrain, pons,* and *medulla*) and the CEREBELLUM. When we look at the outside of the human brain we see little more than the cerebral cortex, which is very enlarged in humans compared with other mammals.

The brain is surrounded by protective membranes, the MENINGES, continuous with those covering the spinal cord. The outermost layer, the *dura mater*, is tough and protects the brain physically. Beneath the dura is the *arachnoid mater*, through which cerebral arteries and veins penetrate to reach the brain. The surface of the brain is intimately covered by the innermost layer, the *pia mater*, from which tiny blood vessels plunge into the cortex. A clear fluid, CEREBROSPINAL FLUID (CSF), which is secreted inside cavities called CEREBRAL VENTRICLES, within the brain, circulates in the *subarachnoid space* between the arachnoid and the pia. CSF protects the brain, both physically and chemically. The brain, hungry for oxygen and glucose, receives its blood through a rich system of arteries derived from two major sources, the internal carotid arteries and the vertebral arteries. Sudden blockage or haemorrhage in an artery (a STROKE) can have catastrophic consequences, including almost immediate loss of consciousness or function, and even death.

The adult human brain weights about 1400 g, but there is much individual variation. The side view of the brain is dominated by the highly convoluted cerebral hemispheres, with the brain stem protruding from below, bearing the cerebellum on its back. The axis of each cerebral hemisphere, from the frontal pole, back to the occipital pole, and then down and around to the temporal pole, forms a C-shape — a reminder of the folding process that occurs during embryological development. Each hemisphere is divided into four *lobes*. On the surface of the lobes are variously named convolutions or *gyri*, with fissures, or *sulci*, some of them very deep, separating the gyri (see Fig. 1). The exact pattern of fissures varies enormously from brain to brain, and even between the two hemispheres, but some are very distinctive. The *lateral sulcus*, one of the first to appear in the embryo, divides the *frontal* from the *temporal* lobe. Likewise, the *central sulcus* divides the frontal from the *parietal* lobe. The rearmost of the four lobes is the *occipital* lobe, but there is no sulcus to define its limit

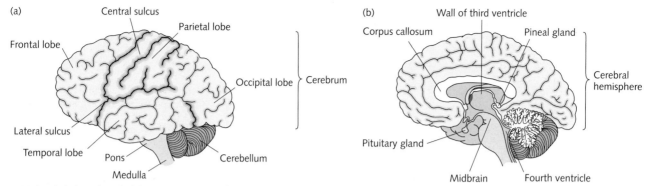

Fig. 1 (a) the whole brain from the left side; (b) a mid-line section.

on the lateral surface. The two hemispheres, roughly mirror-images of each other, are separated by the huge *Sylvian fissure* described in 1660 by Franciscus Sylvius, a physician and anatomist in Leyden (see Fig. 2).

If a cut is made into the depth of the Sylvian fissure, dividing the brain in two, a complex series of structures is revealed on the inner surface of the hemisphere (Fig. 1b). Most apparent is the *corpus callosum* (Latin: 'beam-like body'), a massive tract of nerve fibres (*axons*) connecting the 2 hemispheres. Like the side view of the entire hemisphere, the cut corpus callosum appears as an upside-down C-shape. So too does a smaller longitudinal fibre tract below it called the *fornix* (Latin for 'arch' — Roman prostitutes fornicated beneath the arches!). Just below this is a hole, leading into the cerebral ventricles. This *interventricular foramen* communicates between the *third ventricle* (a midline cavity with the thalamus in its wall) and the *lateral ventricle*, deep within the hemisphere. The third ventricle dips down between the hypothalamus of each side, below which we can see the pituitary gland. The thalamus joins to the brain stem below. The intricate folded pattern of the cerebellum fills most of the space between the bottom of the occipital lobe, above, and the upper surface of the brain stem, below. Beneath the cerebellum the tent-shaped *fourth ventricle* is visible, communicating at this level with the subarachnoid space around the brain. The fourth ventricle communicates with the third ventricle via a narrow tube, the *cerebral aqueduct*, which runs up through the midbrain.

The cerebral hemispheres consist of a thin outer rind of GREY MATTER, containing mainly the bodies of nerve cells (*neurons*), surrounding a core of WHITE MATTER (named after the whitish colour of the axons of the neurons). Deep within the hemispheres are a number of important cell groups (*nuclei*), as well as the ventricular system. Axons arising in the cerebral cortex and those running to it traverse the *internal capsule*, a thick band of white matter in each hemisphere. The largest of the deep nuclei is the *corpus striatum* (named because of its striped appearance when cut), which is of vital importance in integration of muscular action. Another mass of grey matter behind the corpus striatum

is the thalamus, which lies in the walls of the third ventricle. It is a relay station for sensory and motor pathways on their way to the cerebral cortex. Just below the thalamus is the hypothalamus. Although small, it is one of the most important parts of the brain, for it participates in a number of vital activities. It regulates a variety of hormonal functions by direct action on the pituitary gland, and exerts control over the AUTONOMIC NERVOUS SYSTEM, the 'vegetative' part of the NERVOUS SYSTEM, which controls the involuntary activity of, for example, our gastrointestinal tract, heart, and blood vessels.

The hypothalamus is also an integral part of the LIMBIC SYSTEM ('*limbus*' is Latin for a border, and the limbic system forms an almost circular boundary to the inner surface of the cerebral hemisphere). The limbic system is involved in vital cyclical activity — including appetites and sexual cycles, and EMOTIONS such as fear, anger, and aggression — and in all-important short-term memory. It involves not only the hypothalamus but also the thalamus, part of the cerebral cortex called the *hippocampus* (Latin for 'seahorse', because of its shape), and their interconnections. The hippocampus sends its axons backwards in the fornix, which then curves forward, like an arch, to meet the fornix of the other side, ending in the *mamillary bodies* of the hypothalamus. A tract then conveys axons up to the thalamus, which then sends fibres indirectly to the hippocampus again. So the circuit is completed.

The corpus striatum receives information from the cerebral cortex, the thalamus, and a nucleus called the *substantia nigra* ('black substance'), in the midbrain. In Parkinson's disease, the cells in the substantial nigra that project to the corpus striatum degenerate and this leads to problems with motor control and co-ordination (muscle rigidity and tremor).

The cerebral cortex is one of the major features of the mammalian brain, and especially in humans it reaches a very high level of development. It is responsible for the initiation of movements, and for interpreting input from all our sensory systems, as well as for integrating motor and sensory activity necessary for speech and other cognitive functions. It is the seat of our very thoughts, personality, and character.

The cerebellum has on its surface a series of tight folds, called *folia*, similar to, but narrower than, the gyri of the cerebral cortex. The cerebellum consists mainly of two hemispheres that receive their major input from the spinal cord and the cerebral cortex. However, a small, but important, part receives information from the VESTIBULAR SYSTEM, the apparatus in the inner ear that signals information about our position in space and, therefore, helps us balance ourselves. The cerebellum is responsible for unconscious control of motor activity. Although voluntary movement is thought to be initiated in the cerebral cortex, the cerebellum guides such movements. Further, it is involved in learning new skills of movement, often a painfully frustrating business. For instance, when we learn to drive a car, our initial attempts are clumsy and full of errors. We have to learn to co-ordinate movements of hand, eye, and foot in order to turn the key and to control gears, brake lever and accelerator, and clutch and brake peddles so that the vehicle is set in motion and safely stopped again. At first, the whole process demands huge mental effort, as if we were using our cerebral cortex consciously to call up the various movements and muscle groups we need. However, after many attempts, our efforts become smoother and less laborious, and we find that we are achieving the desired results with much less stalling of the motor or threat to the bodywork. Later still, we discover that we can drive around without really thinking about it much, and we are sometimes surprised, if distracted by other preoccupations, to realize that we are on the road and driving safely without clear memories of starting the vehicle and getting under way. We have successfully completed a motor 'apprenticeship', with the cerebellum taking over the routine management of the task from the cerebral cortex. It is as if the cerebellum were a programmable computer controlling the output of the motor system, and its programs have been slowly improved to take more and more change of the operation. Think of learning to play a sport or a musical instrument; but think also of WALKING, talking, and writing. In all these, and many more activities, we can look upon the first, hesitant steps as being essentially cortical, while the final, polished result is more cerebellar.

The brain stem extends between the thalamus and the spinal cord, gradually decreasing in size and in the complexity of its internal structure. It is divided, from top to bottom, into the midbrain, the pons (bridge), and the *medulla oblongata* (usually simply referred to as the medulla). The entire brain stem is largely hidden from view by the highly developed masses of the cerebral and cerebellar hemispheres. The midbrain is attached to the base of the cerebral hemispheres by the *cerebral peduncles*, two massive, flattened bundles of nerve fibres. The longitudinal orientation of the cerebral peduncles is abruptly interrupted by the pons, which gives the impression of a giant ring, slipped on to the brain stem between the peduncles and the medulla. The medulla merges gradually with the spinal cord.

The brain stem contains much white matter, with ascending and descending tracts that can be traced in continuity with those of the spinal cord, including various sensory pathways from the skin and organs, and the *corticospinal* or *pyramidal* tract, conveying motor information from the cerebral cortex down to the spinal cord. There are also various groups of neurons (*nuclei*) within the brain stem. Several of these give rise to the CRANIAL NERVES, through which the brain sends and receives information to and from the head and the organs of the trunk. Other groups of brain stem neurons are vital to the life of the body and to the conscious function of the brain: they generate the rhythmic nerve impulses that maintain breathing, regulate the heart and circulation, and activate the cerebral cortex itself.

Investigation of brain function

Compared with the pulsating heart or blood-filled liver, the brain looks rather unimpressive. No wonder, then, that many ancient cultures chose those other organs as their assumed seat of the mind or soul. Now that we generally accept that the brain is responsible for action, perception, and understanding, one of the greatest scientific challenges is to explain how it works.

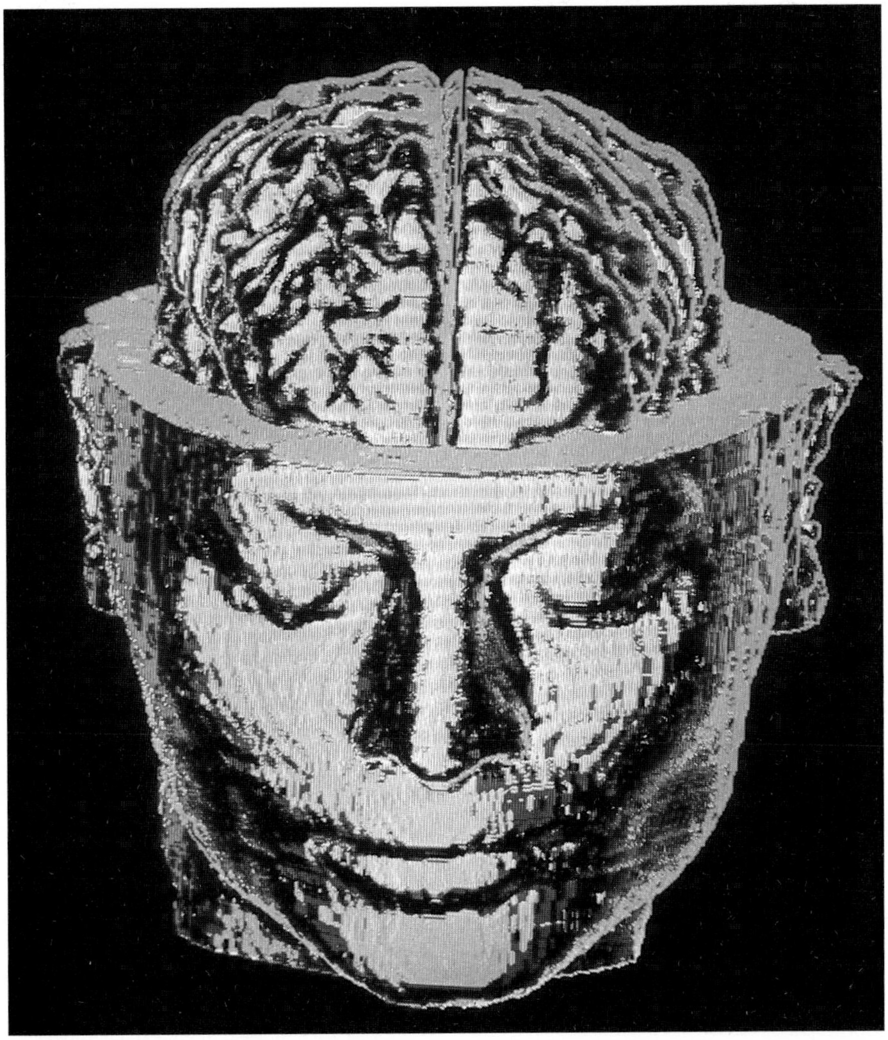

The clues to the functions of the brain were once provided only by 'nature's experiments': the consequences of damage caused by disease or injury. The advent of anaesthesia allowed investigation of the effects in animals of more precisely localized damage and of the responses to electrical stimulation at particular sites. The development of microelectrode techniques made it possible to record the electrical activity of individual neurons in the brains of anaesthetized animals, or in isolated slices of brain tissue. The human brain has been stimulated during neurosurgery under local anaesthetic, and the resulting movements of the body and sensations described by the patient have identified particular regions concerned with motor and sensory function. Electrical activity can also be recorded from the human brain through electrodes on the scalp (ELECTROENCEPHOGRAPHY). Finally, new technologies developed in the twentieth century provided ways of 'mapping', non-invasively, the function of the living human brain. These IMAGING TECHNIQUES can show, for example, the regional distribution of blood flow or metabolic activity, reflecting neuronal activity in the various parts of the brain during different actions or sensations. Thus they are assisting in the understanding of healthy function, as well as in the diagnostic localization of abnormalities.

LAURENCE GAREY

See PLATE 6.

See also BRAIN STEM; CENTRAL NERVOUS SYSTEM; CEREBRAL CORTEX; CEREBRAL VENTRICLES; CEREBROSPINAL FLUID; HYPOTHALAMUS; IMAGING TECHNIQUES; MAGNETIC BRAIN STIMULATION; THALAMUS.

Fig. 2 Three-dimensional computed tomography (CT) scan of a human head, with the skull opened to show the brain. GJLP-CNRI/Science Photo Library.

Brain death applies to the situation when the HEART continues to beat with the BREATHING maintained mechanically after the brain has permanently ceased to function — and it is an unnatural artefact of medical technology.

Under natural conditions when the brain ceases to function breathing immediately stops, and soon after that the heart stops from lack of OXYGEN. If breathing is taken over by a mechanical ventilator, oxygenation is maintained and the heart can continue to beat, for days at least, because the heart muscle acts on its own independently of the brain. That DEATH is a process rather than a sudden event is now well recognised. Most often the process is initiated by the heart stopping, and this is then followed by brain failure due to lack of oxygen. Sometimes it is the breathing that stops first, the lack of oxygen leads to brain failure and later the heart also stops.

The relevant part of the brain for the maintenance of breathing, as well as for the activation of higher cerebral function, is the BRAIN STEM — the lowest part of the brain above its junction with the spinal cord. Because function in this region is crucial for the whole of the brain, cessation of that function, strictly 'brain stem death', is commonly referred to as brain death.

Brain death is the result of unsuccessful RESUSCITATION — the price paid for the many patients whose lives are saved, and who make a good recovery, when a ventilator is used during brain failure which proves to be temporary. When mechanical ventilation was begun it was not known whether or not the brain could recover — only a trial period of ventilation could settle that question.

The problem with waiting for the heart to stop following brain death is that it can go on beating for several days, occasionally for weeks, during which time other organs fail and the extremities may begin to decompose. To continue ARTIFICIAL VENTILATION is therefore regarded as both futile and undignified. In many countries it has been accepted that when the brain is dead the person is dead; in some jurisdictions laws have been enacted to acknowledge this, but in others it has been considered unnecessary.

This matter has, however, been complicated by the development of organ TRANSPLANTATION. Kidney transplantation was well established before the concept of brain death was widely accepted, because it was possible to use organs from donors whose hearts had stopped beating, but the transplantation of hearts, lungs, and livers is possible only from donors whose hearts are still beating, and therefore only from those who are brain dead.

There is clearly need for strict criteria for the diagnosis of brain death, whether or not there is any question of organ donation, because the consequence of this diagnosis will be the withdrawal of artificial ventilation. This is regarded as discontinuing an inappropriate intervention for a person who is already dead, rather than letting that person die. In the UK the medical Royal Colleges agreed criteria for the diagnosis of brain death in 1976. These require satisfying certain pre-conditions and then undertaking tests to confirm that there is no function in the brain stem. The pre-conditions must establish that the patient is in COMA and on a ventilator because breathing has ceased due to irreversible structural brain damage — usually due to severe head injury, brain haemorrhage, or an episode of oxygen starvation of the brain. It is also necessary to exclude reversible causes of failure of brain function, including depressant DRUGS and HYPOTHERMIA. The tests for absence of brain stem function require there to be no reflex responses in the pupils or the muscles of the face, throat, or eyes. The final test is to confirm that there has been no recovery of spontaneous breathing by disconnecting the ventilator temporarily, whilst maintaining a passive flow of oxygen to the lungs. These tests are carried out twice and by two experienced doctors. The time of death, for legal purposes, is when the first set of tests were completed, although death is not declared until after the second test. Additional tests are not required in the UK but are used in some countries. These include demonstrating lack of electrical activity in the brain by ELECTRO-ENCEPHALOGRAPHY (EEG), or lack of blood circulation in the brain using either radioactive isotopes or radio-opaque dyes injected into the bloodstream. BRYAN JENNETT

See also COMA; LIFE SUPPORT; ORGAN DONATION; VEGETATIVE STATE.

Brain stem

The BRAIN within the skull and the SPINAL CORD within the vertebral column constitute the CENTRAL NERVOUS SYSTEM. The cerebral hemispheres (*cerebrum*) of the brain occupy the larger, front part of the cavity of the skull. And at the base of the cerebrum, emerging like the stalk from a mushroom cap, is an elongated structure, the brain stem. With the CEREBELLUM behind and above it, it occupies the smaller, back part of the skull cavity.

The brain stem forms a bridge between cerebrum and spinal cord and also carries the major pathways (*peduncles*) for signals to pass to and from the cerebellum. The brain stem itself consists of three distinct parts. From above down these are the *midbrain*; a bridge-like structure, the *pons*; and the *medulla oblongata*, which merges below with the spinal cord.

From the brain stem emerge pairs of CRANIAL NERVES, analogous to the spinal nerves that innervate the limbs and trunk. These contain motor nerves to SKELETAL MUSCLE fibres that move the eyes, to the facial muscles responsible for the familiar expression or 'set' of a face, and to those controlling the movements of the JAW, the TONGUE, and the LARYNX. Damage to the seventh cranial (*facial*) nerve on one side for example, creates the characteristic asymmetry of the 'set', smile or grimace in 'Bell's Palsy', while motorneuron disease affecting other cranial nerves interferes with SPEECH.

Most of these nerves also carry incoming information: the massive fifth cranial nerve (*trigeminal*) has a rich abundance of sensory fibres contributing to the exquisite tactile sensitivity of the facial skin at the mouth, EYES, cornea and, less agreeably, ones from the dental pulp and gums to cause dental pain. The eighth (*auditory*) cranial nerve carries mainly sensory fibres from two highly specialised structures, the cochlear and vestibular apparatus, concerned respectively with HEARING and BALANCE. The ninth (*glossopharyngeal*) and tenth (*vagus*) nerves also contain the special system of 'parasympathetic' motor fibres of the AUTONOMIC NERVOUS SYSTEM that innervate not only structures around the head and neck (such as the salivary glands) but also, in the case of the vagus nerves, the thoracic and abdominal organs (heart, bronchi, gut). These two nerves also carry important information from receptors in the LUNGS, HEART, and BLOOD VESSELS essential to the reflex regulation of these structures.

By virtue of its nerve connections the brain stem mediates important REFLEXES, including protection of the eyes by closure of the lids, protection of the throat by GAGGING, and elimination of irritant bodies by sneezing and coughing.

The brain stem is very much more than simply a viaduct for the long nerve fibre tracts directly linking brain and spinal cord. It is also a relay for certain categories of MOVEMENT commanded by the motor cortex, as instanced by signals related to hand clenching conveyed in the '*rubrospinal tract*', with its neuronal cell bodies at the upper end of the brain stem. Similarly, signals relating to the sense of touch or limb movement (SOMATIC SENSATION and PROPRIOCEPTION) are relayed in cells within the medulla.

More importantly still, the brain stem is the origin of a multitude of fibre systems, ascending to higher levels as well as those descending into the spinal cord, passing into the cerebellum, or, just as richly, terminating elsewhere within the brain stem.

Networks within the brain stem are at the heart of rhythm generators, for movements such as mastication and the rhythmic EYE MOVEMENTS (NYSTAGMUS) that occur during rotation or when the eye attempts to fixate on a moving object. Most vital of all is the network that generates the rhythm and the command for BREATHING movements and that mediates the central and reflex adjustment of these to match metabolic demands. Closely related networks are responsible for maintaining vascular tone and serve as centres for the reflex regulation of heart rate and blood pressure.

Other networks in the brain stem have been linked to PAIN and its control. Neurons in the '*periaqueductal grey matter*' (PAG), which surrounds the channel (aqueduct) in the midbrain for cerebrospinal fluid, are sites of extensive convergence of sensory information from all over the body. In turn, these signal back to the spinal cord and reduce nerve transmission in ascending pathways carrying signals with the potential of causing pain. This and other systems are engaged when the opiate morphine is used to abolish acute pain and, it is thought, by the body's endogenous production of opioids following severe acute trauma. The PAG also has substantial connections to the cerebrum and activity in these pathways may ultimately form the basis of 'affect'; the emotional adjunct to human behaviour.

Whilst the cerebrum is absolutely essential for sensory perception and conscious, willed behaviour, the brain stem is absolutely essential for life in the absence of artificial life support. Even should the entire brain be destroyed above the midbrain, the brain stem itself, providing the motor pathways to the respiratory motor neurons in the spinal cord are intact, will sustain a living body (though not a 'life' as we normally know it) until death ensues due to starvation, infection, or cardiac arrest. TOM SEARS

See PLATE 6.

See also BRAIN; BRAIN DEATH; BREATHING; LIFE SUPPORT; VEGETATIVE STATE.

Brassière

The word 'brassière' as a description for a woman's undergarment to support and shape the BREASTS was first used in American *Vogue* magazine in 1907. In French the word originally described a small silk or velvet jacket worn under a woman's robe from the late fourteenth century, but the term is rarely used in France to describe the modern brassière. The preferred term has always been *soutien-gorge* (bust support), and this first appeared in 1904. So it looks as if the term 'brassière' was an American invention.

Women had worn CORSETS for centuries prior to this; they were formed and laced to control the shape and dimensions of the breasts, waist, and hips. The fashionable silhouette, at any given date, was moulded by the corset, which was always the principal structural undergarment from c. 1500. However, when the corset gradually shrank in length from c. 1902–8, settling below the line of the breasts, a cover and/or support was needed for them. Essentially, this already existed in various forms such as camisole tops or corset covers in lightweight fabrics, but in 1889 there was a new garment called the 'bust bodice'. This was worn above the corset; it was lightly boned, and laced at the front and back. By 1904 bust bodices were considered essential if only for modesty, and the health-conscious firm of Jaeger produced a 'burst girdle' in that year, possibly one of the earliest brassières. By 1913 it was possible to buy a 'corset cover and brassière combined', and in 1916 it was being reported that 'French and American women all wear them and so must we; a modiste will insist on a brassière to support the figure and give it the proper up-to-date shape'.

These early examples were fairly light, insubstantial pieces of underwear, often just bands of fabric with only the most rudimentary shaping and support, akin to the American Caresse Crosby's two triangles of fabric attached to ribbon straps, which she invented to wear under an evening dress in 1913. She sold the idea to Warner Brothers, the corset firm founded in 1874, for $1500, and later claimed the credit for having invented the brassière. These early examples gave limited support, sizing was inaccurate, and the idea of separating the breasts and having a proper fitting and assessment of correct size came only in the 1930s when Warners devised A to D cup measurements.

Brassières could flatten the breasts, as they did in the 1920s when an androgynous silhouette was fashionable, or they could divide, enhance, and uplift them, as became increasingly common from the 1930s onwards. They were also hybridised, with brassière tops being added to corsets to form the corselette, or attached to petticoats, and so forth. Experiments led to strapless versions for evening wear. Stitching, padding, and underwiring of the cups could rectify apparent deficiencies of nature, just as 'bust improvers' had done in the nineteenth and early twentieth centuries.

Much of the innovative work on the construction and sizing of brassières — or bras, as they tended to be called from the late 1930s — was American. The American film industry quickly recognised the potential of well-endowed actresses with breasts engineered into pointed uplift by padded, whorl-stitched, cone shaped bras, which also produced the required cleavage. The sweater girls of the 1940s and 1950s, such as Jane Russell and Lana Turner, influenced young women around the world and created demand for bras which would emphasise and uplift the breasts. Many surviving bras of this period seem to have a life of their own, with a rigidity of construction which explains the enhancing effect they could create. The reaction against this came in 1965, when Rudi Gernreich designed the 'no-bra bra', a lightweight, minimalist alternative which outlines the natural shape of the breast but no more. Ironically, it was only three years later, in 1968, that Gossard launched the Wonderbra, which fought back courageously for cover-girl curves. Created from twenty-six separate pieces, this was a lightly padded bra that separated and uplifted each breast to offer a décolletage of impressive grandeur with increased comfort for the wearer.

Improvements in manufacture, in the use of man-made fibres such as Lycra, and in marketing a constantly changing range of styles and colours, made underwear a fashion statement in its own right. This occurred against a background of feminist questioning of male exploitation of female SEXUALITY. At the time of the 'bra burning' campaign of the 1970s, groups of young women decided to abandon bras altogether. This liberation of the body, although fine in principle, was less comfortable for larger, fuller-breasted women than for their slim, small-breasted sisters. Stretchy sports bras without hooks which could be pulled on over the head and gave light, natural support became an attractive compromise. More conventional women could select from ever wider ranges of size, style, and colour to suit their bodies and the changes in fashions worn over bras.

By the 1990s there were bras for every figure and circumstance, from pubescent teenagers to the elderly. The combined advertising power of contemporary personalities, such as the American singer Madonna's use of a designer corset and cone-shaped bra as a touring costume in the 1980s, top models promoting structural underwear such as the Wonderbra and the bustier (an elongated strapless bra), and fashions for sheer shirts, have reinvigorated the market for brassières in every size, colour, and construction. Less glamorous but equally important lines include diminisher bras for the overendowed, posture bras to reduce hunched shoulders a variety of styles for full figures which can be worn at night, and so forth. There are sports bras, nursing bras, bras designed to take prosthetic breasts for women who have undergone mastectomies. All this suggests that as an under-garment the brassière has become essential to the majority of the female population in the Western world. Despite this popularity, however, it is known that many women have never undergone a fitting for a bra and few know how to measure correctly in order to ensure that what they wear is the ultimate in comfort and support. VALERIE CUMMING

Further reading

Cartec, A. (1992). *Underwear: the fashion history.* Batsford.

Cunnington, C. W. and P. (1981). *The history of underclothes,* (revised edition). Faber and Faber.

Ewing, E. (1971). *Fashion in underwear.* Batsford.

Probert, C. (1981). *Lingerie in Vogue since 1910.* Condé Nast.

See also CLOTHES; FEMALE FORM.

Breast The human breasts are *mammary glands* — common to all mammals, by definition. There are differences between species in number and in structure, and also in the composition of the milk that they produce for feeding the offspring.

A pair of NIPPLES is of course common to both boys and girls — a relic of the embryological development of the male having been superimposed upon the basic female. As girls approach puberty, female SEX HORMONES produced in the OVARIES circulate in the bloodstream and cause development the rudimentary breast glands, which have been present since before birth. Breast enlargement usually heralds the other changes. Progesterone promotes development of the potentially milk-producing cells, and oestrogens promote the development of the ducts leading to the nipple from the 15–20 'lobes' of glands.

When MENSTRUAL CYCLES begin, the mammary glands also start to undergo cyclical changes: in the second half of the cycle, under the increasing influence of progesterone, the glandular tissue grows, sometimes causing 'lumpiness' and tenderness — one of many preparations for the pregnancy which in most months does not follow.

When conception does occur, the breasts continue to develop. The accompanying increase in blood supply distends the veins under the skin — often the first outward and visible sign of pregnancy. The glandular tissue proliferates, taking the place of connective tissue and fat, and the breasts progressively enlarge. Later in PREGNANCY, the hormones secreted from the fetal tissue of the placenta act on the glandular cells and on the ducts leading to the nipple: thus the fetus itself, along with the hormone, *prolactin*, from the mother's PITUITARY GLAND, prepares the ground for its own later nutrition. This same prolactin would also stimulate the production of milk — but oestrogens from the PLACENTA counteract this, so that milk is not actually made before the time is ripe. After birth of the baby, this suppression stops, so prolactin activity is suddenly uninhibited. Unfortunately for ideal infant feeding, in 'developed' countries nowadays oestrogens are often taken orally, to suppress milk production in those mothers who choose to bottle-feed the baby.

Left to nature, the secretion is initially scanty (*colostrum*) but the volume of milk becomes significant at about the third day after the birth, when the breasts become quite dramatically engorged. The mother's pituitary hormones

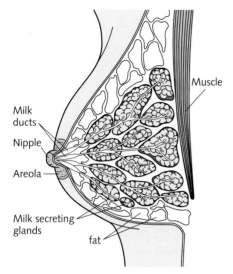

The female breast. After Youngson, *Encyclopedia of family health*.

remain in control of milk synthesis and secretion; under this influence, fats, proteins, and lactose (milk sugar) are made in the gland cells from nutrients taken up from the blood. When the infant sucks, nerve impulses from the nipple reach the HYPOTHALAMUS in the brain; these stimulate nerve cells that have stores of the hormone OXYTOCIN in the ends of their fibres that lie in the posterior part of the pituitary gland. This causes release of the hormone into the circulating blood. Reaching the breasts, oxytocin activates contractile cells, which squeeze milk from its storage sites into the channels that take it to the nipple. This whole 'neuroendocrine reflex' takes about 10 seconds — barely long enough for a hungry infant to show serious signs of frustration.

Lactation will continue for just as long as a baby is regularly sucking away the supply of milk: the more is removed, the more is made. The volume averages about 1 litre per day, but twice that amount can be produced for twins. Weaning of the infant leads automatically to a decrease in the milk supply, and the glandular tissue reverts to the non-pregnant state — until the next time, if any.

The breasts in history and culture

The cultural significance of the breast revolves around its uses as a symbol both of FERTILITY and of sexual pleasure.

Many prehistoric images represent the female body with a high level of body fat and large breasts, the ideals when the food supply was uncertain. Breast milk, as our first and most reliable food, has long been the subject of speculation about its nature and significance. The classical model dominant in Western medicine until the nineteenth century was dependent both on the Greek philosopher Aristotle, who argued that breast milk was a fluid intermediate between menstrual blood and semen in terms of the

degree of 'cooking' it received in the body, and also on the Hippocratic medical writers. It was thought that special channels from the womb to the breasts carried and transformed blood; this meant that, after birth, a child continued to derive nourishment from the same blood that had been its source in the womb.

The medical imperative from such theories was, of course, that a mother should nurse her own child. However, in cases where the natural mother was unable to do this, or as a way of preserving the youthful appearance of the breasts, WET-NURSING could be used. Contracts specifying the duties of a wet nurse, and her fees, survive from Roman Egypt, showing that this form of paid employment was available to women from early times. The second-century AD medical writer, Soranos, offered detailed, and historically influential, advice to Roman men on how to choose a good wet nurse. She should be aged between 20 and 40, have given birth two or three times, and be strong and in good health. Her breasts should be medium-sized, soft, and unwrinkled, with the nipples also of medium size and neither too compact nor too porous. Soranos argued that milk from large women is more nourishing, but regarded very large breasts as a health risk to the infant on two counts: first, they may fall on the nursling, and second, there will be milk left over after each feed, which will lose its freshness and then harm the infant at the next feed. Soranos believed that the wet nurse transmits her own qualities to the child, so an even-tempered woman free from superstition should be found; she should also be Greek-speaking, so that the nursling becomes accustomed to hearing Greek. The wet nurse must abstain from sex and alcohol, both of which could damage the milk. As well as studying the body of the potential employee, a Roman man must taste and smell her milk; after employing her, he should carefully supervise her diet. In the nineteenth century the recognition of the value of colostrum superseded the classical view that, not being 'proper milk', it should be withheld from the baby.

The advice Soranos gives represents both a continuing unease surrounding the use of wet nurses, and a continuing conflict between the nurturing and the erotic breast. Roman writers often accused women of wanting to employ a wet nurse only for the sake of maintaining a sexually desirable figure. Medium breasts on large women may have been good for babies, but classical art suggests that the erotic ideal was the small breasted, boyish woman.

In mid-eighteenth-century Europe when Linnaeus' classification of the natural world put humans among the Mammalia — those with breasts — debate over the use of wet nurses became a state concern. Linnaeus was in favour of mothers nursing their own children; with philosophers, naturalists, moralists, and medical writers, he argued that strong nations were built up from babies fed at the maternal breast. Using the maternal breast was economical, but also

political, part of the good woman's civic duty, and linked to images of the state feeding its children.

When, as a result of Pasteur's discoveries, sterilisation of animal milk for bottle-feeding became possible, even those who could not afford to pay a wet nurse could avoid breastfeeding. A further development was milk substitutes; however, in developing countries there have been considerable problems following the promotion of milk substitutes as an alternative to the real thing, due for example to the formula being made up with non-sterile water or at the wrong strength.

The patron saint of nursing mothers is St Agatha, the legendary martyr who had her breasts cut off, shown in renaissance and baroque art carrying them on a plate. Christian religious art has used the nurturing breast in many ways. In fourteenth-century Tuscan art, during a period of crop failures and plague, the image of the Virgin Mary suckling a greedy Jesus became widespread. Sometimes she is shown directing a stream of milk into Jesus' mouth, or into the mouth of a particularly privileged saint; such images can emphasise the humanity of Jesus, or evoke the analogy of the Christian sucking at the breasts of the church for spiritual nourishment. Images of Charity personified often show a child suckling at each of her breasts.

For Freud, the breast was the first EROGENOUS ZONE, from which a child should move on to the anal and genital stages of its developing SEXUALITY. The baby's complete satisfaction at its mother's breast led to an identification with the mother, after which the baby needed to develop a sense of itself as a separate being. This was achieved by a rejection of the breast, now seen as withholding milk. In adult life, a person therefore longs for the perfect pleasure of the breast which has been taken away. Ideals and representations of the erotic breast show far more variation than the lactating breast. It can be large or small, with a pronounced cleavage or with the breasts entirely separated. The ideal in the Middle Ages was to have firm, white, apple-shaped globes, far from the Hollywood images of Jane Russell or Lana Turner, and even further from the pneumatic breasts of top-shelf magazines. Sixteenth-century kings' mistresses, most notably Agnès Sorel, Diane de Poitiers, and Gabrielle d'Estrées, were painted showing their breasts; Agnès was even represented as the Madonna.

As the size and shape of the ideal breast has varied dramatically over time and space, so fashions have changed to reshape the normal range of breasts to fit the ideal. The breast has been compressed, surgically reduced, padded, enhanced with silicone, pushed up, and armoured by a range of devices including bodices, CORSETS, bras and, most recently, the Wonderbra. Even before the corset or the BRASSIERE, in the Middle Ages pouches sewn in to dresses could give uplift. One of the best-known aspects of the early Women's Liberation Movement was the 'bra burning' of the late 1960s, a form of liberation intended to make men face up to the reality of the breast freed from its fantasy underpinnings.

Breast tissue is more prone than any other in the woman's body to develop CANCER. This accounts for about 1 in 20 deaths of British women, becoming commoner with increasing age. Early detection is assisted by regular X-ray examination (breast screening — *mammography*), and various combinations of surgery, radiotherapy, and chemotherapy can be effective in treatment.

The very high incidence of breast cancer in the Western world has made the breast into an organ associated as much with death as with nurturing life. Fanny Burney's harrowing description of her mastectomy, performed without anaesthetic in 1811, has survived; nowadays 'lumpectomy' may be adequate but mastectomy is sometimes necessary, and women who have had a breast removed may choose to use a prosthesis, or to adjust to a new body shape. The classical myth of the Amazons presents the woman with one breast as powerful, but feared. Currently some women with a family history of breast cancer are offered elective surgery to remove both breasts before disease appears; reactions to those who accept this surgery show that the breast remains a potent symbol of womanhood today.

SHEILA JENNETT
HELEN KING

Further reading
Yalom, M. (1997). *A history of the breast.* Harper Collins.

See also INFANT FEEDING; PUBERTY; SEX HORMONES; WET-NURSING; WITCH'S TIT.

Breath, the air inhaled or exhaled from the body during respiration, is inextricably associated with existence: the first breath marks the beginning of independent life. It is therefore the most commonly held metaphor for life or spirit. The book of *Genesis* states that God formed man from the dust of the earth 'and breathed into his nostrils the breath of life'. By extension, using one's energy to inspire others is referred to, metaphorically, as breathing confidence into them.

Breathlessness is an uncomfortable awareness that arduous respiration is taking place, brought about by the need for increased consumption of oxygen during extended muscular activity. The complete cessation of spontaneous breathing, on the other hand, was for many centuries the prime indicator of DEATH. The common tests for extinction of life were the absence of condensation on a mirror held in front of the mouth (the exit point of the SOUL), or the failure of a feather to flutter in front of the nostrils. But mechanical ventilators have changed all that; and now some relatives will not even accept BRAIN DEATH — which entails the inability to breathe — as the end of life.

For the Greek philosopher Anaximenes (*fl. c.* 550 BC) the breath or *pneuma* was the primeval life force that bound the universe together; inhaling it invigorated the body. Similarly, in Indian yogic philosophy, *prana* is the cosmic energy that fills and maintains the body,

manifesting in living beings as the breath. The fourth step of Patanjali's system of Raja Yoga is *pranayama*, or breath control, practised because the breath is held to influence markedly a person's thoughts and EMOTIONS. In one sense modern medicine concurs in this association, by directly relating HYPERVENTILATION to a disturbed psychological state.

Early advocates of artificial respiration, like the *Society for the Recovery of Drowned Persons*, formed in Amsterdam in 1767, advocated not only mouth-to-mouth respiration to resuscitate the inanimate but also the application a clyster of tobacco smoke blown into the intestines with a tobacco fumigator. Tobacco smoking is man's masterstroke in breath-tainting, which is today sweetened with medicated mouthwash rather than oil-based troches.

Inspired by *Genesis*, literalist advocates of good breathing techniques have pleaded divine sanction for nasal rather than mouth breathing. George Catlin, a nineteenth-century ethnographer of the American Indians (a race little subject, he believed, to fatal diseases of the lungs), insisted, since life was originally breathed into a man's nostrils, 'why should he not *continue* to live by breathing it in the same manner?' The unnatural and addictive habit of breathing through the mouth during sleep, he said, was confined to civilized societies. It allowed impurities into the lungs; affected the voice; caused crooked and protruding teeth; led to nervous agitation; made children into idiots and lunatics, and produced confirmed snorers. In a nutshell, he postulated: 'if I were to endeavour to bequeath to posterity the most important Motto which human language can convey, it should be in three words — *Shut your mouth*.'

FIONA MACDONALD

Further reading
Miller, J. (1978). The breath of life. In *The body in question*. Jonathan Cape, London.

See also ARTIFICIAL VENTILATION; BREATHING; LUNGS; RESPIRATION.

Breathing is the spontaneous taking in and giving out of air from the LUNGS, the product of the visible movements of the ribcage and abdomen. In earlier years breathing was synonymous with life itself, for with the 'last breath' its absence signified DEATH and departure of the soul. However, in the late nineteenth Century, the advent of a scientific understanding of its nature and basis and, later, the development of LIFE SUPPORT measures, meant that this view was no longer tenable, giving rise to new moral and ethical dilemmas as to when life support can be withdrawn.

Breathing is a remarkably robust process compared with other activities involving skeletal (voluntary) muscle. It performs some 400 million or so operational cycles in a sedentary lifetime and, except in disease, does so without fatigue, thus being able to increase in pace with the most strenuous exercise that the heart can support.

Also, breathing continues in SLEEP and in COMA and, fortuitously for patient and surgeon alike, even under ANAESTHESIA that is sufficiently deep to abolish pain. Breathing occurs spontaneously and without conscious attention, notwithstanding its immediate cessation or augmentation in response to volition. Thus it is both the most highly automated of movements, yet, when powering vocalisation during SPEECH and SINGING, the most voluntary.

The neural mechanism responsible for the generation of the basic respiratory rhythm is now attributed to a network of neurons located in the BRAIN STEM. The search for such a rhythm generator, originally conceived as the 'Respiratory Centre', began early in the nineteenth century and notably, perhaps with Madame Guillotine in mind, initiated by the French scientist Le Gallois. In rabbits he successively transected the brain stem and spinal cord at different levels in different sequences. He discovered that if the lower brain stem remains connected to the SPINAL CORD breathing continues, a result in sharp distinction to that following the human experiment by 'Madame,' of sectioning in the neck between the brain stem and spinal cord!

In the fully automatic mode the rate and depth (*tidal volume*) of breathing movements is regulated on the basis of information from sensors in the brain ('central' CHEMORECEPTORS) and a variety of peripheral reflex mechanisms, using sensors detecting the concentrations of oxygen and carbon dioxide in the arterial blood (*peripheral chemoreceptors*) and mechanical events in the heart, lungs and arteries (heart, lung, and arterial *mechanoreceptors*), and also receptors elsewhere in the body. Collectively, these maintain HOMEOSTASIS of the blood gases and pH, thus satisfying tissue metabolic requirements for oxygen uptake and the elimination of carbon dioxide in the face of changing behavioural demands.

The act of breathing can be considered from two points of view: mechanical properties, and the central nervous control mechanism. Insight into the former dictates the problem to be solved by the central nervous system, as through its 'command' signals breathing is maintained and regulated according to the metabolic or behavioural demands of the moment.

Mechanical factors
The lungs are paired, lobed structures which when inflated are in some ways balloon-like: when punctured or surgically removed from the thorax, they collapse under the combined influence of internal elastic forces and surface tension within the terminal air sacs (*alveoli*). As with a balloon they can be inflated through their neck (*trachea*) by air under positive pressure (greater than atmospheric pressure), and the relationship between pressure and volume can be determined experimentally. However, in the living body, the situation is different. For example, at the end of a normal expiration, there is a volume of air in the lungs known as

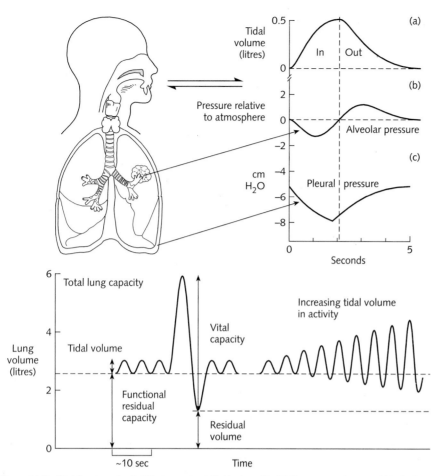

Above: (a) the tidal flow in and out of the lungs at rest that is caused by (b) the pressure changes within the lungs (alveolar), caused in turn by (c) the pressure changes between lungs and chest wall (pleural).

Below: tidal volume at rest, vital capacity, and tidal volume as it increases during muscular activity; the relation of these volume changes to total lung capacity, and to the volume remaining after a normal tidal breath (FRC) or after a full expiration (RV) (see text).

the *Functional Residual Capacity* (FRC); at this point the pressure in the alveoli is atmospheric, there is no airflow, but nevertheless the lungs are held inflated within the chest; this is now by 'suction' from without. Suction exists because the outer surfaces of the lungs are exposed to a pressure less than atmospheric ('negative' pressure) within the thin film of fluid between the two layers of the PLEURA that cover the lungs and line the inside of the chest wall. This pleura fluid both separates the lungs from the chest wall and also links them to it, whilst allowing the lobes to move freely as they inflate and deflate. At FRC this surface pressure, of about −5.0 to −8.0 cm H_2O, is determined by the balance between the elastic recoil forces of the lung pulling inwards and the net elastic recoil of the chest wall pulling outwards. Evidence of the latter is seen during surgery when opening of the chest is accompanied by the collapse of the lungs and the outwards motion of the ribcage. Entry of air into the pleural 'space' due to lung or chest wall puncture constitutes a 'pneumo-thorax'; this is not life-threatening when only one lung collapses, but bilateral collapse is fatal unless artificial ventilation is immediately available.

Even when the breath has been fully expelled by voluntary effort to reach the lungs' minimal volume (*Residual Volume*, RV) the lungs still remain slightly inflated, with pleural pressure still negative at about −2.0 cm H_2O; the expiratory muscular effort to reach RV is needed to overcome the greatly increasing elastic recoil outwards of the chest wall as lung volume becomes low. Similarly, if voluntary effort is used to inflate the lungs to their maximal volume (*Total Lung Capacity*, TLC) the lungs remain intimately applied to the chest wall, held there by a negative pressure of some −25 to −30 cm H_2O; this reflects the increased elastic recoil of the lungs at this higher volume; and the recoil of the chest wall itself is now also a force acting inwards, opposing the voluntary muscular effort to reach TLC. The total volume of air that can be breathed in from residual volume to TLC (or vice versa) is called the *Vital Capacity* (VC), and is in the order of 5.0 litres in the adult. Lung volume, or changes in lung volume, are often expressed as a percentage of vital capacity. The tidal volume during quiet

breathing, about 0.5 litres, therefore represents only 10% VC and is achieved by swings in pleural pressure of −2 to −3 cm H_2O (see figure).

In respiratory mechanics, the term 'chest wall' also includes the abdomen, because a major factor contributing to the balance of elastic forces is that of posture. This is due to the influence of gravity on the large mass of the abdominal organs, which hydraulically generates a negative pressure transmitted across a relaxed DIAPHRAGM to the pleural space at the base of the lungs, so increasing their volume. Thus changing from the supine to the upright posture can increase FRC by some 15–20% of VC (approximately 0.75–1.0 litres). In fact, this major influence of posture can be utilised to achieve artificial ventilation by means of a tilting bed, but the tidal volume achieved is restricted.

The above considerations all refer to the principal 'passive' mechanical properties of the system. In quiet, effortless breathing (*eupnoea*) the resistance to airflow in the lungs and airways is negligible, as also is the viscous resistance to movement of the lungs and surrounding structures, except in disease states. Changes in pleural pressure require appropriate *displacements* of the structures immediately around the lungs — namely the ribcage and diaphragm — and, through hydraulic coupling, the abdominal wall. This would represent a formidable design challenge in engineering, as it would be the equivalent of asking for the hull of a ship or aircraft to change its volume and shape, although the latter is actually achieved in Concorde by articulation of its nose! The articulated ribcage does exactly this, and aided by cartilaginous extensions at the front which flexibly couple each rib pair to the breastbone or sternum, allows the inspiratory rise (inflation) and expiratory fall (deflation) of the chest in 'thoracic' breathing. Similarly, the diaphragm descends relatively freely within the upper abdomen, accommodated by an outward displacement of the abdominal wall — so-called 'abdominal' breathing — until this motion is limited by tension in the abdominal wall. Both expansion of the ribcage and descent of the diaphragm normally cause a decrease in pleural pressure, so either acting alone (as can occur following spinal injury or diaphragmatic paralysis) will cause a paradoxical movement of the other, reducing the change in lung volume. Such paradoxing of the ribcage is seen in the newborn, most markedly in the *respiratory distress syndrome*, when the absence of surfactant which reduces surface tension within the lungs necessitates the development of much greater changes in pleural pressure to achieve an adequate tidal volume. During such inspiratory effort the reduction in pleural pressure due to the diaphragm is greater than the resisting force of the underdeveloped ribcage muscles, so that the chest collapses inwards instead of expanding. Under most circumstances, however, the 2 sets of muscles work in concert and, even when the ribcage may not appear to rise or expand in inspiration, it is stiffened sufficiently to withstand the fall in pleural pressure, enabling the diaphragm to work more efficiently. Similarly, when thoracic breathing is exaggerated the abdomen may move inwards even though the diaphragm is contracting.

The actual elevation and depression of the ribs in quiet breathing is due to the external and internal intercostal muscles, respectively, which bridge each adjacent pair of ribs, aided by other muscles at the front and back, while three layers of abdominal muscle generate active forces for expiratory flow when greater than resting tidal volumes are required. In quiet breathing neither the diaphragm nor all of the chest wall is fully actively engaged in generating the pressures reviewed above. When exercise requires breathing to be increased, the volume and velocity of airflow in and out is greatly accelerated. This is achieved by additional force production involving progressively more of the chest wall and diaphragm; in the athlete this may no longer be fully automatic, but patterned through training to achieve the best performance.

In addition to their role in breathing, the voluntary activation of respiratory muscles is also utilized for generating much higher forces and hence pressures within the system. For example, abdominal pressures in excess of 200 mm Hg help to stabilize the vertebral spine during weight lifting — some 100 times greater than the pressures required for tidal air movement during quiet, effortless breathing. (See Plate 3).

Neural aspects

In order to achieve lung ventilation the central nervous control mechanism has to generate muscular forces, displacements, and hence pressure changes, to oppose the augmenting elastic recoil as lung volume increases. It does this through motor commands issued from the brain stem for a waxing and waning profile of pleural pressure change, with a time course matching the current demand for pulmonary ventilation; in resting breathing this would be approximately 1.0 sec for inspiration, and 2–3 sec for expiration depending on the overall respiratory rate (12–15/min). Inspiration is generated by a progressively increasing co-activation of the diaphragm and external intercostal muscles. This action can either be observed mechanically or more directly visualized by recording the electrical activity of the motor units in the relevant muscles, by *electromyography* (EMG). The EMG shows a strongly augmenting activity pattern paralleling that of the pressure change. At the end of inspiration such activity ceases fairly rapidly, allowing the lungs to deflate due to elastic recoil back to their starting lung volume at FRC. The cycle then repeats. It is generally held that during breathing at rest expiration is a mainly 'passive' process, although some activity in expiratory muscles may maintain the outflow of air.

The inspiratory augmentation in the EMG is due to the progressive recruitment in the number and discharge frequencies (e.g. ranging from 5–25 Hz) of the active motor units in the respective muscles. These discharge patterns correspond to respiratory phased 'trains' of nerve impulses in the motor nerve fibres to the muscles; in turn, their origin lies in the pattern of the electrical activity in the cell bodies of the motor neurons within the spinal cord. Recordings through minute electrodes inserted through the cell membrane of these motor neurons (*intracellular recording*) reveals the presence of rhythmic waxing and waning changes of electrical potential, which are given the name '*central respiratory drive potentials*'. Their time course and amplitude closely mirror a mechanical record of the changes in pleural pressure, and it is during the waxing phase that they generate the augmenting patterns of impulse activity in the motor axons that result in the motor unit activity recorded in the muscles.

The 'central respiratory drive potentials' of respiratory motor neurons, with their slow time course of 2–3 sec duration, reflect the summed synaptic action of impulses in respiratory motor pathways descending from the brain stem, wherein lies the neural network that generates the breathing rhythm. Again, intracellular recording from those 'respiratory' neurones whose axons descend into the spinal cord reveals central respiratory drive potentials, but, in contrast to the motoneurons, their discharge rates are much higher, ranging typically from 50–300/sec within each cycle, depending on the prevailing 'demand' for ventilation. This particular system of neurones corresponds to the 'upper motor neuron system', the corticospinal tract which conveys 'volitional' as well as automated commands for limb and digit movement from the 'motor cortex'. It is these vital pathways which are interrupted following trauma to the highest part of the spinal cord in the neck (cervical spinal cord), leading to total paralysis of the whole body below the neck including both voluntary and automatic breathing movements. Death ensues within minutes unless artificial ventilation is immediately available. A spinal transection at the base of the neck (low cervical region) abolishes thoracic and expiratory-phased abdominal movements, whereas diaphragmatic movements are left intact because their motor neurons are located above the transection.

Much research, of necessity based on studies of anaesthetized animals, is devoted to unravelling the neural connectivity that sustains the respiratory rhythm, and how this is regulated by a variety of reflexes. Such insights should help, for example, to solve the mystery of the *sudden infant death syndrome* (SIDS or 'COT DEATH'), which is usually attributed to an abrupt cessation of breathing — its absence being the first indication of the tragedy to the unsuspecting parents. By recording the electrical activity of a wide range of neurons in the brain stem of anaesthetised animals, several distinctive patterns of neurone activity have been identified, each having different firing patterns within the respiratory cycle and different connectivities one to the other; it is from such information that deductions are made as to how this system could generate the respiratory rhythm. The brain stem emerges as a truly vital structure in the immediate maintenance of

'life' as now understood. Thus following major destruction or inactivation of the cerebral cortex through trauma or deprivation of oxygen, a still viable brain stem can maintain breathing when the former structures are so damaged as not to sustain the conscious state (VEGETATIVE STATE); conversely, if the viability of the brain stem is compromised, breathing ceases; however, although artificial ventilation and other life preserving measures may sustain the metabolic activities of the heart, lungs, and other tissues, the otherwise intact cerebral cortex now lacks the afferent inputs from, and also channelled through, the brain stem that are critical for consciousness itself, a state dependent on a fully-functioning cerebral cortex.　　TOM SEARS

See PLATE 3.

See also LIFE SUPPORT; LUNGS; RESPIRATION.

Breathing during exercise
We breathe OXYGEN into the body from the atmosphere. While this oxygen does not itself contain useable energy, it is the key that unlocks the energy stored in previously-ingested food. As the energy demands of the contracting muscles change during exercise, so must their energy and oxygen provision. But oxygen comprises only 21% of the atmospheric air; one therefore needs to inhale a volume of air each minute which is at least five times the volume of oxygen which is being absorbed out of the LUNGS by the body.

Lung ventilation — the volume breathed in and out per minute — however, is not *five times* that of the rate of oxygen utilization for metabolism, rather, it is *twenty-five times*. This is because most of the oxygen is breathed back into the atmosphere during expiration: only 20% or so of the inspired oxygen is actually taken up by the blood coursing through the lungs *en route* to the cells.

The air taken into the lungs does not all reach the gas-exchange regions (the *alveoli*). Airways that conduct air to the alveoli do not themselves take part in this exchange: only the volume of air that gets beyond this *dead space* into the alveoli contributes to the gas exchange. Consequently the *alveolar ventilation* is less than the total ventilation — and this is the volume which provides the oxygen to be taken up into the body.

The alveolar oxygen concentration, and its equivalent oxygen pressure, is determined by the balance between the supply of oxygen to the alveoli and the demand for its uptake into the blood: the alveolar ventilation per minute and the oxygen consumption per minute. The alveolar oxygen pressure in turn establishes the oxygen pressure in the arterial blood, which is normally maintained at, or close to, a constant level during exercise, the same level as when at rest, despite the body's oxygen consumption increasing more than 10-fold. This can *only* be achieved if the alveolar ventilation increases proportionally. Normally it does so, increasing so that it maintains a ratio of about twenty times the oxygen uptake rate, for moderate exercise, with the ratio for total ventilation being about twenty five.

While this characterizes the ventilation needed to maintain the level of oxygen in the arterial oxygen, it may or may not be appropriate for the other vital breathing requirement during exercise — the defence of blood and tissue acidity.

The exercise-induced challenge to the body's acidity levels has two different origins. Firstly, foodstuffs that serve as energy sources for exercise (CARBOHYDRATES and FATS) are composed entirely of hydrogen, carbon, and oxygen atoms. During the progressive metabolic fragmentation of food molecules, hydrogen atoms are stripped away, to link with oxygen, yielding energy.

For example, for glucose:

$$C_6H_{12}O_6 + 6O_2 \rightarrow 6H_2O + 6CO_2$$

This leaves the carbon and oxygen to be vented into the atmosphere as CARBON DIOXIDE. As the body's carbon dioxide production from this source is normally approximately equal to its oxygen consumption during exercise, the same level of ventilation can serve both purposes: intake and exhaust. However, if ventilation does not increase sufficiently during exercise, the oxygen level will fall in the blood and tissues, and the carbon dioxide level will rise. Such an increase in carbon dioxide would increase blood and tissue acidity.

The body's acidity is determined by the concentration of hydrogen ions $[H^+]$ — the positively-charged protons which form the nuclei of the smallest of all atoms. An increase in carbon dioxide in body fluids increases the concentration of $[H^+]$. For $[H^+]$ to be stabilized in the arterial blood leaving the lungs, the carbon dioxide level needs to be regulated by exhaling the carbon dioxide at a rate equivalent to its production rate.

Normally, for moderate exercise, ventilation does indeed increase in proportion to the increased metabolic rate, thereby maintaining arterial blood levels of both oxygen and carbon dioxide (and hence $[H^+]$) at, or close to, resting levels. This control is mediated through an interaction of neural and blood-borne mechanisms. The neural mechanisms which lead to muscle contraction also simultaneously signal the breathing control centres of the brain; these receive neural information from the contracting muscles as well. If the resulting drive to breathe is not appropriate, then an 'error' in the arterial oxygen, carbon dioxide, and $[H^+]$ levels is sensed by chemoreceptors which 'sample' the blood in the carotid arteries perfusing the brain. This provides the 'fine tuning' of the control system.

The second challenge to arterial $[H^+]$ stability occurs only at higher work rates, where the energy demands cannot be met entirely through aerobic (i.e. oxygen-linked) metabolism. At these work rates the aerobic transfer of energy is supplemented by degradation of carbohydrates to lactic acid — present in the form of a lactate ion $[L^-]$ and $[H^+]$. This component is *anaerobic metabolism* (it utilizes no oxygen). The fitter the subject, the higher the work rate at which it begins to contribute (see figure). The resulting increase in $[H^+]$ has a number of deleterious

effects on exercise tolerance: impaired muscle contraction; perception of limb fatigue; and 'shortness of breath'.

As exercise continues at this high intensity, the body's acidity level can only be maintained (or its increase constrained) if the carbon dioxide-related component of the acidity is reduced. The body therefore 'compensates' by increasing ventilation proportionally more relative to carbon dioxide production. This reduces alveolar and arterial carbon dioxide levels (see figure) as a result of the increased carbon dioxide 'washout'. Clearly, the greater the amount of carbon dioxide 'washed out' under these conditions, the less will be the increase in acidity for any given level of lactic acid production.

The additional drive to breathe which is linked to the increased lactic acid levels is thought to result predominantly from the effects of the $[H^+]$ (and other mediators such as potassium ions released from the active muscles) stimulating the carotid chemoreceptors. Neither hydrogen ions nor potassium ions readily cross the blood–brain barrier, so they do not stimulate the other chemoreceptors on the surface of the brain stem (which in other circumstances also influence ventilation).

The increase in ventilation during exercise could, theoretically, be accomplished by an

infinite variety of depths (tidal volumes) and number (breathing frequency) of breaths per minute. Very deep and slow breathing requires extra effort because the thorax, and the lungs in particular, become very stiff at high volumes. Rapid shallow breathing, on the other hand, mostly ventilates the dead space. The spontaneously-chosen pattern is typically the one which most effectively combines low breathing effort with a high fraction of the breaths reaching the alveoli. Consequently, most people initially increase ventilation predominantly by increasing tidal volume up to a certain optimal maximum; higher ventilatory demands are then achieved predominantly by increasing breathing frequency. In many sporting events, however (e.g. SWIMMING, rowing, and even running), athletes must, or choose to, link the duration of each breath to the cadence of their limb motions.

Physical training or increased fitness does little to improve the lung as a mechanical pump or gas exchanger, unlike the beneficial effects of exercise on skeletal muscles and the heart. Luckily, however, the limits of operation of the lungs normally far exceed the demands placed upon them. For example, at maximum levels of exercise, not only is full blood oxygenation maintained in normal subjects, but also ventilation has not reached a maximum: it can be

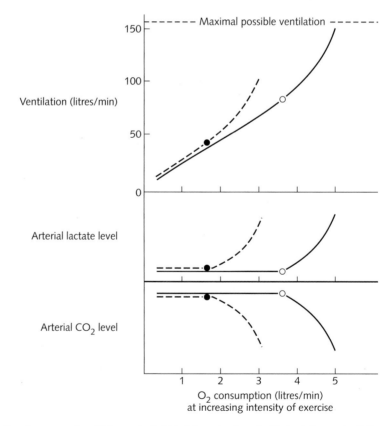

Profiles of response of ventilation and arterial lactate and carbon dioxide levels to exercise that progressively increases to the limit of the subject's tolerance. The dashed line represents a subject of normal fitness, the solid line represents an athlete capable of achieving higher levels of oxygen consumption. The solid circle and the open circle represents the levels at which the subjects begin to increase their lactic acid production. Maximum possible ventilation shows the highest level that can be achieved by these subjects.

increased further by volitional effort (see figure). Elite athletes may be different in this regard. The unusually high metabolic rates they can achieve require unusually high levels of ventilation and of blood flow through the lungs. Those athletes who have not been graced by their genetic make-up to have large lungs with large airways (allowing high levels of airflow), and large capillary volumes (allowing the high cardiac output of rapidly-flowing blood to be exposed to the gas-exchange surface at the alveoli long enough for oxygenation to be completed), can show a component of 'pulmonary limitation' to exercise. This is manifest, only at a very high work rates, by airflow rate reaching a limiting maximum, and by a reduction in arterial oxygenation — but only in those without the appropriate genetically-superior lung structure.

Normal individuals also experience 'shortness of breath' (*dyspnoea*) during exercise. This is quite modest at low work rates — except when the carotid chemoreceptors are sensitized, such as during sojourns at high altitude. At high work rates the dyspnoea is usually more marked and sustained. There is a narrow range of work rates — high but usually sustainable for long periods — for which dyspnoea develops but which then subsides as the exercise continues. This relief of dyspnoea has been-termed *second wind*. This proves difficult to reproduce in the laboratory; consequently its mechanisms are poorly understood. Reduction in the lactic acid-related drive to breathe, as aerobic mechanisms catch up with the high-energy demands, is likely to be contributory.　　　　　BRIAN J. WHIPP

See also ACID-BASE HOMEOSTASIS; BREATHING; EXERCISE; LUNGS; METABOLISM; RESPIRATION.

Bride burning

Bride burning a form of domestic VIOLENCE against women — usually, newly married women. The specific terminology links it to India and to the custom of dowry. It gets its name from kitchen fires or other kinds of fires that are often staged to make the deaths of these women appear to be suicides or accidents. The perpetrators of this form of violence against recently-married women are usually persons belonging to their husbands' families, and often their husbands as well. Though both are derived from the low social value of women, bride burning needs to be distinguished from *sati*, or, widow burning — the practice of widows committing ritual suicide on the funeral pyres of their dead husbands.

The root cause of bride burning, as well as other forms of domestic violence against women, lies in their subordination and their frequent powerlessness within their husbands' family following marriage. Thus, cases of bride burning can and do occur without dowry being the causal factor, although dowry is possibly the single largest cause. Dowry commonly refers to the material gifts given to the bride by her family, usually at the time of the wedding. Scholars, such as M. N. Srinivas, make a distinction between the ancient custom of dowry as *dakshina* or *dana*

(voluntary and often token gifts) and the contemporary practice of dowry. Nowadays dowry refers to material objects demanded (as opposed to voluntarily given) by the bridegroom's family, and often involves significant amounts of cash, property, household objects, and jewellery. In its current form, dowry is regarded, by those who demand it, as a reflection of the social status of the bridegroom's family. Thus, the more eligible the prospective bridegroom (eligibility being perceived as the social standing, the wealth, the educational and career-related achievements, and so forth, of himself and his family) the larger the dowry that his family has the right to demand and receive. M. N. Srinivas, Geraldine Forbes, and other scholars also point out that, in relatively recent times, growing consumerism and the increasing tendency to equate social status with material objects has made it attractive for prospective bridegrooms and their families to use the dowry as a means of enriching themselves at the time of marriage by demanding expensive presents from the parents of the prospective bride. The desire for continuing to benefit materially from the parents of the bride can take the form of pressuring the bride and her family for more dowry even after marriage. The families of prospective brides agree to (or, feel they have no choice but to acquiesce to) the payment of dowry because of the concern that the non-payment of dowry might impair their daughters' chances of marriage. The high social premium still attached to marriage, particularly for women (in the sense that the social status and respectability of women is still largely bound up with their martial status), ensures that families with daughters respond to demands for dowry even when it can ruin them financially. Incidentally, the relatively low social value of girls in Indian society (manifest, for example, in the very recent custom, within some segments of Indian society, of aborting female fetuses) is connected to the financial pressures encountered by their families through the custom of dowry. Dissatisfaction over dowry may find expression through acts of hostility ranging from verbal abuse to actual violence. Bride burning is the most extreme violence against newly married women.

The passage of the Dowry Prohibition Act of 1961 by the government of India formally banned the practice of dowry. The prevalence of the practice, and its link to the perpetration of violence against women, however, continued, and some observers believe that both practices have escalated. Geraldine Forbes points out that the low valuation of women combined with consumerism to bring about a new way of exploiting womens' dependency. Since the 1970s in particular, women activists have made untiring efforts to expose such social ills and to exert pressure on the law courts and on law enforcement agencies to be much more vigilant about reporting and prosecuting such crimes. Their efforts have met with limited success. In 1986, the government of India passed a bill which increased the punishment for accepting dowry and decreed

that in cases where a women died an unnatural death, her property would devolve on her children or be returned to her parents. There have also been criminal prosecutions of those alleged to have been involved in domestic violence against women, including bride burning. Women's organizations, such as Saheli in Delhi (to name one), provide counsel and shelter for endangered women, keep records of women's deaths resulting from suspected domestic violence, and act as a pressure group to demand more thorough investigations by the police. Yet, despite the legislation and the growing efforts of womens' organizations, the problem has not been eradicated. There is, however, greater awareness of the problem, as indicated by its current status as a topic of public discussion in India.

KUMKUM CHATTERJEE

Further reading
Forbes, G. (1996). *Women in modern India. (The new Cambridge history of India IV.2).* Cambridge University Press, Cambridge.

Srinivas, M. N. (1984). *Some reflections on dowry.* Oxford University Press, New Delhi.

Bruise

Bruise Visible bruising is well known to result from a blunt injury to the body surface. It may also follow deeper injuries — sprains or fractures — but this takes longer to show itself. A bruise is due to rupture of BLOOD VESSELS and escape of blood into the interstices among the cells and connective tissue beneath the outermost layer of skin. The red blood cells break down, and their pigment, HAEMOGLOBIN, undergoes chemical changes which account for the sequence of colours in the bruise. The debris is eventually removed by macrophages. A bruise can likewise occur internally on or in any organ or tissue subjected to a blow, squeeze or stretch: contusion is an alternative term.　　　　　　　S.J.

Buddhism and the body

The Buddha and his enlightenment

Guatama Buddha was born between 563 and *c.* 450 BCE in present-day Nepal. Named *Siddhartha*, 'he who has accomplished the goal', after a sage predicted success for him, of either a worldly or spiritual nature, the future Buddha was groomed by his father to take a prominent role in public life. He nevertheless rejected worldly privilege, leaving wife and son to fulfil instead the latter option of the fate predicted at his birth.

The Buddha began his spiritual career during a time of social change, with urban and artisan classes gradually displacing the agrarian order in which the Brahmanic system was entrenched. A mendicant teacher during what was later termed the '*Age of Wanderers*', he travelled, meditated, and followed, only to reject, extreme ASCETICISM. At the age of 35, he sat beneath a tree contemplating the mysteries of death and rebirth through the night, attaining *enlightenment* at dawn.

His insight was that the world, *samsara*, is characterized by suffering; its endless cycle of death and rebirth perpetuated by ignorance. Only *prajna*, wisdom, can overcome ignorance: to this end, the Buddha wandered and taught, bringing into being the *sangha*, community. His teachings were preserved in the oral tradition, and written down as *sutras* within around three centuries of his death. The basic tenets of Buddhism are traditionally ascribed to the first sermon following the Buddha's enlightenment.

The first sermon: the middle way

The Buddhist goal is to realize the true nature of the world, to 'see things as they really are', and to respond with neither repulsion nor attachment, but equanimity. Enlightenment leads to *nirvana*, in which the cycle of death and rebirth (driven by *karma*, an impersonal, universal law of action and reaction) is broken. In his first sermon, the Buddha rejected extremes of sensual indulgence on the one hand, and rigid asceticism on the other, declaring his teaching to be the 'Middle Way'. He also rejected two philosophical extremes: nihilism, with its concept of absolute non-existence; and the opposing concept of *atman*, which posits an essential, continuous self. The Buddha called his philosophy *anatman*, no-self, holding that while there is no absolute non-existence, neither does anything exist which is not subject to change.

The first sermon also contained the teachings of the three *laksanas*, which are descriptive, and the Eightfold Path, or eight *angas*, which are prescriptive. The *laksanas* describe the world as *anitya*, impermanent; *duhka*, painful; and *anatman*, devoid of essence. *Duhka* is the basis for the doctrine of the Four Noble Truths, expressed according to an ancient medical formulation (the Buddha is often likened to a doctor). First, the existence of the disease is stated: the first Noble Truth is the existence of suffering. Next are stated the causes, then the prognosis of the disease. Finally is stated the path to the cure. This last consists of the Eightfold Path, which prescribes: Right Understanding, Right Resolve, Right Speech, Right Action, Right Livelihood, Right Effort, Right Mindfulness, and Right Concentration. Together, the *angas* form a system of psychology, ethics, and mind/body cultivation through meditation.

The spread of Buddhism

Joining the *sangha*, community, at first involved direct contact with the Buddha. This soon became formalized as 'taking refuge' in the Three Jewels: the Buddha as exemplar; the *Dharma*, his teaching; and the *sangha*, the spiritual community, centered around monks and (to a lesser degree) nuns.

The most important new school began around the turn of the first century CE. The *Mahayana* ('greater way') school dubbed previous schools '*Hinayana*' ('lesser way'). Of these, *Theravada* ('the teaching of the elders') survives. Centred in Sri Lanka, it spread to Southeast Asia (except Mahayanist Vietnam) from about the eighth century. Central to *Mahayana* is its aim to attain enlightenment for the benefit of all, rather than as an individualistic goal. *Bodhisattvas* attain full enlightenment, but, motivated by compassion, choose to suffer countless rebirths in the quest to save all sentient beings. *Mahayana* Buddhism spread to China in the first century CE, then to Korea (fourth century), Japan (sixth century), Tibet (seventh century), and Mongolia (sixteenth century).

Buddhism often took on a local stamp as it spread. The arrival of Buddhist missionaries in China sparked off a dialogue between the philosophical traditions of India and China. Chinese philosophy, particularly Taoism, arguably influenced the Ch'an (from Sanskrit *dhyana*, meditation) school. This iconoclastic movement within Chinese Buddhism underwent yet more variation upon its export to Japan, where it came to fruition as Zen. Tibetan Buddhism blends Chinese and Indian schools with elements of indigenous religion.

By the time the Muslim invasions of the twelfth century effectively completed its decline in India, Buddhism had irreversibly altered the religious landscape of its birthplace, and was set on its course to become a world religion. The twentieth century saw the increasing popularity of Buddhism in Euro-America; the politicization on the world stage and survival in exile of Tibetan Buddhism following its repression by the Chinese communist government; and lay revivals in historically Buddhist areas.

Attitudes to the body

Buddhism recognizes neither the mind/body dualism that characterizes much of Western philosophy, nor the concept of an essential self, such as the Hindu *atman*. For the Buddhist, mind and body are both subject to inevitable processes of change. The body is viewed ambivalently: attachment to physical pleasure and repulsion from pain are obstacles to enlightenment; yet enlightenment is of the human realm — even gods must be reborn in human bodies to reach this goal. The discipline of meditation presupposes and aims to enhance mind/body unity. The body can serve spiritual ends. In *Tantra* — an esoteric Indian school which forms a current of Tibetan Buddhism — powerful energy channels in the body are accessed through meditation and yoga. And in Zen, physical gesture is used to cut through discursive thinking and promote the spontaneity characteristic of enlightenment.

KIRSTEN DWIGHT

Further reading

Skilton, A. (1994). *A concise history of Buddhism.* Windhorse, Birmingham, England.

Yuasa, Y. (1987). *The body: toward an Eastern mind–body theory.* State University of New York Press, Albany, New York.

Buildings and the body

The anthropologist Mary Douglas once remarked that, for psychologists and psychoanalysts, everything symbolizes the body; for sociologists, the body symbolizes everything else. In as much as our bodies present a thousand usefully intimate and immediate metaphors, we are all sociologists. The analogy with buildings is, however, a distinctively ancient and durable one, which has been of great rhetorical utility to architects and anatomists, among others.

The 'essence of metaphor is understanding and experiencing one thing in terms of another' (Lakoff and Johnson), and buildings have provided two metaphors essential in the history of Western understandings of the self. The first derives from an even more 'fundamental' one: our conception of our bodies as containers, of our skins as the boundaries between inside and out. We constantly use 'in' and 'out' figuratively in our speech. Because of the form of our bodies, too, we apply metaphorically (think in terms of) 'top' and 'bottom', and this is where buildings are particularly apt containers; Sigmund Freud (1856–1939) noted dream-work's propensity to correlate body-parts with house-parts, including the attic with the mind.

The second metaphor makes reasoning itself a form of construction; we 'build' arguments, and 'demolish' those of others. Again, metaphorical 'constructions' of thinking are not confined to buildings (our ideas can also be 'flowering' plants, for example), but the architectural analogy is one of specific historical importance. Implicit since antiquity — first explicitly addressed by René Descartes (1596–1650) and subsequently institutionalized, notably by Immanuel Kant (1724–1804) — has been philosophy's identification of thinking with building (Wigley). Today the metaphor is of greater instrumental importance than ever, not least to architects surveying the theoretical ground in the wake of 'deconstructivist' philosophy (a term taken from Martin Heidegger's *Abbau*, 1889–1976).

Buildings in minds and bodies

The building–body metaphors of enclosure and construction have given rise to vivid formulations of the workings of the mind. Robert Hooke (1635–1703) — who, as a natural philosopher and architect, was well placed to understand the metaphors — used both in 1680, to describe memory. It is a 'repository of ideas formed partly by the senses, but ... no idea can be really formed or stored up in this repository, without the directive and architectonical power of the soul'; his attribution of architectural power to the soul is a variant of one of the most potent manifestations of the building–body analogy, the conventional praise of God as the architect of creation, and of its microcosmic emblem, the human body. In 1717, Andrew Snape (1675–1742), a divine, preached sympathetically about madness and how the force of the 'labouring imagination' can burst the 'thin partitions and enclosures, that keep ideas separate', resulting in a tragic jumble.

Architectural ruin became a common way of conceptualizing insanity, as real ruins became popular attractions for eighteenth-century tourists playing at melancholy. The fragility of this image, however, belies the comforting sturdiness of that on which it was, ultimately, drawing: God builds, as good architects must, for commodity, firmness, and delight (as the Vitruvian canon was first rendered in English). In *Micrographia* (1665) we can trace Hooke's search for a word to describe, metaphorically, the structures in cork that he saw under the microscope: pores? boxes? He happily hit upon the old architectural term '*cell*', which evoked, not just their uniformity and distinctness, but the evident strength of their slender partition walls. Two centuries earlier, on the other hand, the architect Leone Battista Alberti (1404–72) unreflectingly used the natural architecture of the body in his treatise *On the Art of Building* (1452), as an example of belts-and-braces prudence worth emulating: 'with every type of vault, we should imitate nature throughout, that is, bind together the bones and interweave flesh with nerves running across every possible section: in length, breadth, and depth, and also obliquely across.'

Alberti's verbal description is evocative, but imprecise. Not least of the reasons why the anatomical investigations of the next, sixteenth century were so epochal was the way in which their new, figurative 'construction of an interior body-space' (Sawday) was enabled by new illustrative technologies (including linear perspective) and conventions, which permitted the rendering of three-dimensional forms in two dimensions. In this way, information about the spatial organization of the body's internal volumes was retrievable, without ambiguity, by viewers of the illustration. These innovations were equally transformative for architecture, in a parallel development recognized at the time. The Italian translator of a 1567 edition of the *Ten Books on Architecture* by Marcus Vitruvius, Pollio (act. 46–30 BC), commented on the way that, in preparing a cross-section (in which a building is shown sliced through, to reveal its interior bounded within the outline of external walls), the architect is working as a physician, revealing an ANATOMY. Different kinds of projections (called 'cuts') permitted not just new ways of recording architecture, but a new, formally more integrated kind of architecture, that of the Italian Renaissance. Christian viewers of the new anatomical illustrations were happy to find in them further confirmation of the *beauty* and solidity of God's architecture, now seen in volumetric depth.

To the pictures, in time, could be adduced the verbal descriptions of seventeenth- and eighteenth-century PHYSIOLOGY, which filled the pipes and enclosures with such moving fluids as blood and air. Convinced of the purposefulness of the architecture, physiologists like William HARVEY (1578–1657) could in turn argue from appearances; thus he questioned GALEN's conclusion that the pulmonary veins carried air, because they shared the structure of blood vessels. God's wisdom, wrote the physician Bernard Mandeville (*c.* 1670–1733) in 1729, is nowhere more apparent than in the 'construction' of the

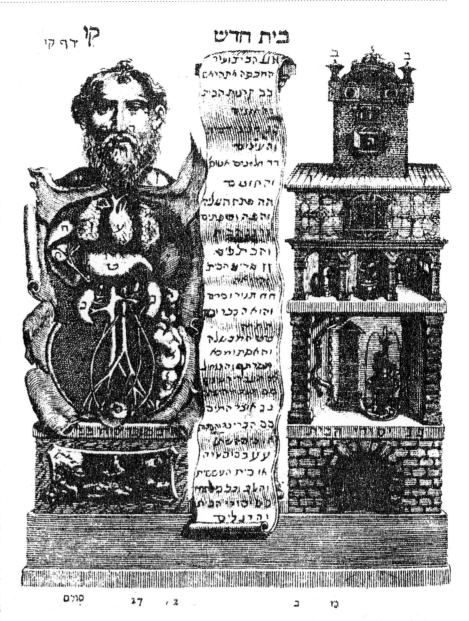

Tobias Cohn's 1708 illustration comparing the cut away torso of a man to the inner workings of a house. From Allen (1984) (see Further reading).

human body, whose every part is 'contrived with stupendous skill, and fitted with the utmost accuracy for different purposes.' Mandeville and others had reached a more machine-like model for the body, but building systems could also be used in explaining dynamism, as by Harvey: 'furnaces … draw away the phlegm, raise the spirit.' No use of the comparison touches that of the physician Tobias *Cohn* (1652–1729), whose Hebrew text *Ma'aseh Tobiyyah* (Venice 1708) illustrated the cut-away torso of a healthy man juxtaposed with a five-storey house: the 'lungs are the upper (ventilated) storey … the kidneys are the water reservoirs, the lower intestines the lavatory, and the feet are the foundation' (Allen) and so forth. This engaging picture (above) must have contributed to the success of the book, last reprinted in 1908.

Bodies in buildings

We still use the building–body metaphor every day in our speech, and anatomists still refer to their subjects' 'architecture'. However, the figurative (and, of course, literal) relation between bodies and buildings has been and continues to be central to architectural thinking in ways more explicit than the one, and more far-reaching than the other. The first and most important treatise about architecture to have survived, Vitruvius' *Ten Books*, virtually single-handedly directed subsequent formulations of the relation.

Vitruvius wrote the book at a time of great political upheaval and, it seemed to many then, architectural chaos in the Roman Empire. Like his contemporaries Horace and Virgil, Vitruvius offered his own version of the admirably old-fashioned, stoic hero. This is the architect who not only works skilfully and dutifully, but who can also explain the reasons underlying his practice: with Vitruvius begins the division between practice and theory. For him, the latter was inextricably bound up with architecture's history, which would redirect it towards its most important goal: to share the immutability, the fixed rules, of *nature*, and in this way to find intellectual coherence. Central to architectural history, or to the myths at least (the difference, which Vitruvius sometimes acknowledged, was, he claimed, not important because myths are made for a reason) had been the human body. A case study: suppose, Vitruvius asked, the architect were to 'set up the marble statues of women in long robes, called caryatids, to take the place of columns … he will give the following explanation to his questioners.' The explanation follows — the women, thus monumentalized, are eternally atoning for the ignobility of Caryae, a Greek state which allied with the Persians, and shared their defeat. Vitruvius went on to explain the origins of the male equivalents, *persics* (Persians). This choice of example, which comes early in his first Book, is significant: it introduces in the most literal way possible an equivalence underpinning an entire theory of architecture. Vitruvius traced the ultimate origins of buildings to bodies. Out of this emerge relationships between the proportions of various types of human body (the man, the maiden, the matron) and the Greek orders; between parts of the body and units of measure (the 'foot'); between the proportioned symmetry of the human frame and that of the temple plan.

Since the fifteenth century authors have emphasized different aspects of the Vitruvian analogy. Alberti used it to develop a critical definition: beauty is that 'reasoned harmony of all the parts within a body, so that nothing may be added, taken away, or altered, but for the worse'. For some, privacy was interesting: the Italian architect Andrea Palladio (1508–80) explained that, 'as the blessed Creator has ordered our members, so that the most beautiful are in places most exposed the view, and the less decent hidden, so too in building.' Sir Henry Wotton (1568–1639) cheerfully gave the image a little dynamism, in 1624 prescribing sewage systems in the well-wrought house:

> 'Art should imitate nature, in those ignoble conveyances; and separate them from sight, … into the most remote, and lowest, and thickest part of the foundation: with secret vents passing up through the walls like a tunnel to the wild air aloft …'

Wotton, and many later English writers, was also interested in sumptuary comparisons; they were perhaps thinking of Alberti's dictum that 'we should erect our building naked, and let it be quite completed before we dress it with ornaments', ornaments which, like *clothes*, should reveal the social status of their owner–occupier. Ornament was thus not superfluous, but the idea of the essential, 'naked' building would, in the eighteenth century, link up with another, privacy-related preoccupation: the status of the build-

ing's façade or '*face*'. Hitherto of fairly casual interest, architectural *physiognomy* became the subject of intense attention in France. Particular preoccupations were the ways in which the façade could exert a direct physical (though perceived as emotional) effect on the viewer; and, concomitantly, its responsibility towards social improvement (fearsome prison façades might deter potential malefactors, for instance). Most far-reaching, perhaps, has been the extension of the building–body analogy to entire towns, and to nations. The figure was sufficiently clichéd by 1685 for the speculative builder Nicholas Barbon (d. 1698) to remark, wearily, that opponents of new urban construction invariably 'use for argument a simile from those that have the rickets, fancying the city to be the head of the nation, and that it will grow too big for the body'; Daniel Defoe (c. 1661–1731) applied the more physiologically-inflected, dynamic form in comparing England's trade to the movement of life's blood around a vast circulation system.

To what extent does the symbolic body in the building live or die with architectural classicism and the Vitruvian tradition? Le Corbusier's (1887–1966) *Modulor* (1951) was a serious attempt to apply the proportions of the male figure to those of building units. In a more abstract way, the concepts of the *objet-type* (the final, mass-producible form of an object as perfected by use) and equivalent *maison-type* with which the same architect was, with others, fascinated after World War I, are themselves metaphors of human *evolution*: 'There are some admirable tools, neat as bones' wrote Paul Valéry (1871–1945). Today, however, architectural Jeremiahs customarily blame a 'modernist sensibility dedicated more to the rational sheltering of the body than to its mathematical inscription or pictorial emulation' (Vidler) — the Vitruvian abstract and mimetic resemblances — for the abandonment of an ancient metaphor and with it ancient satisfactions, for viewers and users alike. This may be to confuse the analogous relations of buildings and the body with other things: architectural style, and quality of design, materials, and workmanship. As Vidler has shown, too, the metaphors do survive, often taking forms explicitly and uncomfortably close to what real bodies are sometimes made to suffer. Images of fracture and dismemberment reoccur in contemporary architectural writing and practice; at their best (and even wittiest) they remind us that the metaphorical relation is inescapable.

CHRISTINE STEVENSON

Further reading

Allen, N. (1984). Illustrations from the Wellcome Institute Library: a Jewish physician in the seventeenth century. *Medical History*, 28, 324–28.

Lakoff, G. and Johnson, M. (1980). *Metaphors we live by.* University of Chicago Press, Chicago and London.

Sawday, J. (1995). *The body emblazoned: dissection and the human body in Renaissance culture.* Routledge, London and New York.

Burke and Hare

These men are universally believed to have been BODY SNATCHERS, but in fact they made a good living in the 1820s supplying an Edinburgh ANATOMY school with dead bodies obtained by MURDER.

William Burke and William Hare never were grave-robbers. They are reputed to have hit upon their calling by accident: an old man died owing rent in Mrs Hare's cheap lodging house, and the men decided to recoup the money by selling the corpse. They were welcomed at Dr Knox's anatomy school, and the £7.10s they were paid amply covered the debt. Burke later confessed that 'that was the only subject they sold that they did not murder, and getting that high price made them try the murdering of subjects.' Soon afterwards, when another lodger fell ill, they helped him on his way with whisky, and smothered him. This first successful murder probably took place in December 1827, and Burke and Hare were paid £10 for the body. The deaths of a further fifteen individuals — twelve women, two handicapped youths, and an old man — followed.

Tales had been circulating prior to the discovery of real events, that children were being stolen and killed for DISSECTION. Such stories had long roots in old tales of abduction of children by gypsies or slavers, but they had a ring of modernity about them too — the corpses were said to be transported to their destinations by the new steamships then being introduced on British sea routes. Medical men may have dismissed these tales as the far-fetched imaginings of popular fantasy, but some of the more reflective individuals among them recognised the possibility that the tales might have some basis. The philosopher Jeremy Bentham — who through his anatomist friend, Dr Thomas Southwood Smith, had inside knowledge of the London anatomy world — had mentioned the dangerous likelihood of murder to the Home Secretary Robert Peel in private correspondence in 1826. In the summer of 1828, while the murders were being committed in Edinburgh, the Select Committee on Anatomy received clear warnings that the high prices then being offered for corpses constituted an incentive to murder. The accuracy of the warnings was proven that autumn.

The murders were discovered not by Dr Knox or the other expert anatomists at his school, but by some of Burke's guests after a party celebrating Halloween in 1828, who became suspicious at the disappearance of an old lady who had been very merry the night before. They discovered her corpse — stripped and ready for packing — in Burke's bedstraw. Mary Docherty had come to Edinburgh from Donegal in search of a long-lost son. She had chanced to beg at a gin-shop where Burke had befriended her. Like all the other victims, she was poor, hungry, and alone. Street folk were not missed immediately as more settled people would have been, and dissection ensured disposal of the evidence.

The mode of death was designed to leave no marks. Since only this last body was available to the authorities nothing could have been proven, despite strong suspicion, had not Hare agreed to give evidence for the prosecution in return for legal immunity. His confederate was hanged on January 28th 1829, an event celebrated with carnival by the Edinburgh populace. His corpse, appropriately enough, was delivered up for public dissection at Surgeons' Hall. Hare left the city incognito, and his fate is unknown.

Burke's execution was witnessed by the novelist Sir Walter Scott, who sympathized with the general opinion that both men's wives had served as accomplices, and that the anatomists had been accessories to the murders. Burke's confessions were published after the execution, and they suggest that this view of the anatomists may not have been altogether misplaced. Burke and Hare were commended by Knox himself on the freshness of a corpse; they were never asked any questions about the derivation of the bodies they delivered to the school, were paid immediately, and were always urged to get more.

A pamphlet, later attributed to a doorkeeper at Knox's school, implicated both the anatomist and his staff in the crimes. According to this witness more than one of the bodies had blood at the mouth, nose, or ears. In at least one instance — that of a well-known Edinburgh beggar, Daft Jamie — identifying features were deliberately obliterated in the dissection room: when it became known that he was missing from the streets, his head and distinctive club feet were severed from his body and dissection was hastened.

Dr Knox was never charged with any crime, nor was he called to give evidence at the trial. He remained silent throughout the furore over the murders. He was burnt in effigy in the streets, ostracised by Edinburgh's medical community, and eventually left the city. He seems to have believed that murder could have been uncovered at any anatomy school, and the fact that it had happened to be his school was simply bad luck. Whether this belief had any objective basis will probably never be known.

The Burke and Hare murders are critically significant to the history of anatomy in Britain. They represent the apotheosis of the market in human flesh. The murders reveal that by the late 1820s, the poor were worth more dead than alive. A further 60 murders (by the 'London Burkers' Bishop and Williams, in 1831) occurred before the Anatomy Act of 1832 provided the anatomists with a free supply of corpses requisitioned from Poor Law workhouses.

RUTH RICHARDSON

Further reading

Richardson, R. (1989). *Death, dissection and the destitute*. Penguin, London.

See also ANATOMY; BODY SNATCHERS; DISSECTION.

Burp A belch, or emission of gas from the mouth. This onomatopoeic word — meant to sound like a belch — was first recorded in American speech in 1932. There are also verbs both intransitive and transitive: 'At the hot springs the mud bubbles and burps,' (*Spectator*) and 'In the USA babies are burped during and at the end of feeds' (*The Lancet*).

Doctors may include burping in the term flatulence, and for a burp may use the old word 'eructation': 'The savour of his meate by eructation ascendeth' (Elyot 1533). Because the burps usually come from the stomach, they often bring with them the smell and taste of partly digested food. This is why carnivores may have very pungent breath, and why cows belch methane.

The gas emitted is mostly air, sometimes swallowed by people eating or drinking nervously, or in a hurry; also by pregnant women, and by others trying to relieve the discomfort of NAUSEA or heartburn. However, burps of other gases can be produced; for example, eating bicarbonate of soda to relieve heartburn causes a chemical reaction with acid in the stomach or oesophagus, and produces burps of CARBON DIOXIDE. Carbonated drinks can generate spectacular carbon dioxide belches. ADAM HART-DAVIS

Bustle The simple dictionary description of a bustle is 'a pad, or wire framework, worn beneath the skirt of a woman's dress, to expand it behind; a dress-improver'. This usage is found in the 1770s and is recorded in a letter to the *Lady's Magazine* of 1786. It is, essentially, a nineteenth-century term, used increasingly from the late 1820s until the disappearance of the bustle from fashionable dress in 1889. However, various aids to change the natural female anatomy at the back of the waist and around the hips had been devised from the fourteenth century onwards. These usually took the form of a padded roll tied around the waist and were depicted in contemporary engravings or caricatures. The practice of emphasising one or more areas of the female anatomy is found throughout the history of fashionable dress and the bustle was only one in a considerable array of undergarments which assisted with this process. It is a wholly impractical structure which distorted the natural curves of the body. Today, examining surviving examples and reading the advertisements of the period, it is impossible not to admire the sheer ingenuity which informed the construction of an item destined not to be seen by anyone other than the wearer and her maid. Lightweight wire, collapsible steel, whalebone, horsehair, and inflatable gutta-percha were used at various times to create or strengthen bustles. They are a tribute to the nineteenth-century delight in new materials and techniques. Undoubtedly they were constricting but they are usually very light in weight and are, in their use of colour, pattern, and imaginative techniques, unintentionally, witty.

The rise and fall of the bustle spans nearly the whole of the nineteenth century. In the early years the high-waisted, fluid dresses only needed a small pad attached to the back of the waist, but this became fuller, and by 1815 it was a separate entity. Gradually, as the waistline reverted to a natural line in the 1820s and 1830s, the crescent-shaped pad became larger and could be layered with one or more additions of diminishing size. Rows of stiffened cotton, like starched frills, were also used or the two types were sometimes combined. By the late 1830s, when dress skirts were widening, a padding was inserted between the dress fabric and the lining to emphasise the area over the hips. This became a rounded, separate bustle once more between 1841 and 1846. By 1849 the discreet euphemism 'dress-improver' was in use, and by 1853 bustles were being made with rolls of crinoline (a mixture of horsehair and linen).

In the late 1860s, as fashions changed, leading to a flattening of the front of women's skirts but compensating by placing emphasis on back fullness, the crinolette (a streamlined, hooped petticoat with back emphasis only) and then the bustle gave support. Initially a few steel or whalebone strips were inserted into a petticoat to support the weight of the ruched-up back of the skirt, but a rounded structure of steel hoops, whalebone, or horsehair quickly became a permanent attachment to the top of the crinolette.

The terminology also changed with the introduction of the French word '*tournure*' as yet another polite word for bustle. This was a structural, full-length petticoat with integral bustle, which emerged between 1870 and 1873. In 1871 it was reported that it rose 'high above the waist and is of vast dimensions.' A brief respite occurred in the mid to late 1870s until the final phase of the bustle began in 1881. It steadily increased in size until it reached its full magnitude in 1885 as an ugly but substantial shelf-like structure. These came in various styles and materials.

Full-length half crinolettes (like aprons but worn at the back and tied at the front) had frills of cloth, horizontal adjustable steels, horsehair padding; half-length versions had collapsible springs and, in line with the health-conscious reform lobby of the 1880s, 'Health Braided Wire Bustles' gained popularity. This American design was marketed as light, strong, pliable, and healthy; it came in several layered and rounded variants and sizes and was intended to support 'the best shapes in the fashionable world'.

By 1890 the bustle had passed from fashion forever and although the term is still used it indicates back interest on a garment, such as bows, loops of fabric, a band of frilled, and layered fabric at the back of the waist — but not a structure under the garment. VALERIE CUMMING

Further reading

Carter, A. (1992). *Underwear: the fashion history*. Batsford, London.

Newton, S. M. (1974). *Health, art and reason: dress reformers of the nineteenth Century*. John Murray, London.

Probert, C. (1981). *Lingerie in Vogue since 1910*. Thames and Hudson, London.

See also CLOTHES; EROGENOUS ZONES; FASHION; FEMALE FORM.

Buttocks Also called the nates, ass, clunes, breech; they are formed by the gluteal muscles which cover the back of each pelvic bone and span the HIP joint to be attached to the thigh bone. These huge muscles are mostly concerned with moving and stabilizing the hip joint. The largest is the *gluteus maximus* ('biggest in the buttock'), which is important in locomotion. (See Plate 5.)

The history of the buttocks has been written either as the history of the physical buttocks or as the history of their symbolic function within cultural systems. Thus Charles Darwin's *The Descent of Man and Selection in Relation to Sex* (building upon the work of earlier anatomists such as Georges Cuvier) assumes the relationship between the 'natural' form of the buttocks and the meaning associated with the human female PELVIS. The pelvis was seen as the most prominent secondary sexual characteristic and the buttocks were read as the pelvis' visible sign. The buttocks became the visual sign of the reproductive system. The BREASTS came to be understood as a sign of the anomalous nature of the human body, as other mammals do not have prominent mammae: only human females do. The breasts came to be perceived as a form which mimicked the buttocks, the 'real sign' of the sexual. The debates about the meaning of the mammae and their defining force in determining the very nature of the 'mammal' has been well documented by Londa Schiebinger in her *Nature's Body: Gender in the Making of Modern Science* (1993).

Buttocks in racism

Beginning with the expansion of European colonial exploration, the form and size of the buttocks became a mode of describing and classifying the races. Thus Darwin's view is a further elaboration on the adaptivity of human form for reproductive purposes. The buttocks become associated with the reproductive organs of the female through the analogy with the form of the pelvis. This is a continuation of the cultural presupposition that 'primitive' races have 'primitive' sexuality, which is represented in their bodies by physical signs of their 'true' nature. Thus Khoikhoi (called the Hottentots by the first Dutch explorers) and San (named Bushman by early Anglophone explorers) women of southwestern Africa were represented from the sixteenth century by their exaggerated buttocks (*steatopygia*) and labia (HOTTENTOT APRON). While these images claimed a greater size for the buttocks, they also claimed that these women (once anatomized) had a smaller pelvic size. The steatopygia was seen as a pronounced, localized accumulation of fat or fatty-fibrous tissue on the upper part of the buttocks. It was understood as rarely manifested prior to puberty, and as an accumulation which enlarged gradually and was a *normal* physical characteristic in women who otherwise may not be obese. As greater pelvic size was understood, in analogy to increased cranial capacity, as a sign of 'progress', the small pelvic size of the 'primitive' was understood as proof of their actual place on the GREAT CHAIN OF BEING. The exaggerated buttocks were understood as an attempt to 'mimic' the higher stages of evolutionary development. Similar representations can be found in the images of the native peoples of South America in early illustrated accounts of European exploration. Here too the breasts and the buttocks are seen as natural signs of the barbarism of the native. After their initial representation as the idealized 'Roman' types, these native inhabitants come to be seen as in need of domestication and conversion. Thus their body forms including their buttocks, come to be represented as grotesque.

Buttocks, gender and gait

In drawing the history of the physicality of the buttocks, works such as Havelock Ellis' multivolume *Studies in the Psychology of Sex* lay stress, following Darwin, on the history of the buttocks as a secondary sexual characteristic which is highly fetishized in European culture. Again Ellis associated the practice of whipping with the overemphasis on the buttocks in British culture. Ellis related this symbolic reading of the buttocks to the primary sexual characteristics (the genitalia) and other secondary sexual characteristics (such as the female breasts). In his case study of 'Florrie' (Volume 7: *Eonism and Other Supplementary Studies*) he showed how 'Florrie' comes to displace the meaning of the buttocks on to other body sites.

Ellis also stressed the function of gait as a manner of measuring the erotic nature of the buttocks. Quoting Virgil, he observed (Volume 4: *Sexual Selection in Man*) that 'the goddess is revealed by her walk.' As Cesare Lombroso and a number of other forensic scientists of the nineteenth century had argued for the relationship between gait and character, the notion that the buttocks could be defined by the appearance and attraction of the carriage is understandable. Thus non-Western women are represented as having a greater 'vibratory movement of the buttocks in their women'. The primitive gait was a further sign of the less civilized (and therefore less self-conscious) sexuality of the 'primitive'.

Buttocks and the Freudian model

Ellis' work on the meaning and the history of the buttocks was paralleled in Austria by Sigmund Freud's discussion of the meaning of the 'anal phase'. First working it out in detail in his *Three Essays on the Theory of Sexuality* (1905), Freud understood the anal phase as the second of three stages of bodily fixation — beginning with the mouth, then moving on to the anus, and then the genitals. 'Normal' development proceeded along this path, but the development could be fixated at the earlier stages. Freud saw anal fixation as the origins of male homosexuality. Again, it is not the anus *per se* which comes to function as the symbolic reference in Freud's system, but rather the buttocks. Here it is not the proximity of the buttocks to the genitalia which is of interest, but rather their adjacent position to the anus. Freud's fascination with the buttocks can be seen in his note to the publication of the anthropologist John Gregory Bourke's *Scatalogic rites of all nations. A dissertation upon the employment of excrementitious remedial agents in religion, therapeutics, divination, witchcraft, love-philters, etc., in all parts of the globe* (1934).

For Freud, too, the question of the symbolic meaning of the buttocks was read in the erotic attraction of the gait. It is in his reading of Wilhelm Jensen's short story *Gradiva* (1903). Introduced to the text by C. G. Jung in the summer of 1906, Freud published his interpretation in 1907, shortly after his work on the stages of human development. It is the first complete study of a work of literature from Freud's pen. In this text the hero recognizes the heroine subliminally by her gait. The classical image, the 'Gradiva', was, according to Freud, a

> sculpture [which] represented a fully-grown girl stepping along, with her flowing dress a little pulled up so as to reveal her sandaled feet. One foot rested squarely on the ground; the other, lifted from the ground in the act of following after, touched it only with the tips of the toes, while the sole and heel rose almost perpendicularly. It was probably the unusual and peculiarly charming gait thus presented that attracted the sculptor's notice and that still, after so many centuries, riveted the eyes of its archaeological admirer.

This description of the act of walking is, of course, also a detailed description of the erotic nature of the gait and therefore a reading of the erotics of the female buttocks in terms of Freud's contemporary discourse. Thus the symbolization of the buttocks as the erotic also has a place within Freud's system of representation.

Consciously building on the Freudian model, the American folklorist's Alan Dundes, in his *Life is like a Chicken Coop Ladder* (1982), stressed the study of the buttocks in terms of their symbolic value as the site of the production of the faeces. Thus anus and faeces become interchangeable. By relating the buttocks to other aspects of the body, Dundes, for example, examined the meaning of scatology in German cultural systems including child raising.

The buttocks are an ever-shifting symbolic site in the body. They are associated with the organs of reproduction, with the aperture of excretion, and with the mechanism of locomotion. Never do they represent themselves. Indeed the very problem of whether they are singular or plural is a sign of their nature as a floating signifier.

SANDER L. GILMAN

Further reading

Gilman, S. L. (1985). *Difference and pathology: stereotypes of sexuality, race, and madness.* Cornell University Press, Ithaca, NY.

Hennig, J. L. (1995). *The rear view: a brief and elegant history of bottoms through the ages*, trans. M. Crosland and E. Powell, Souvenir Press, London.

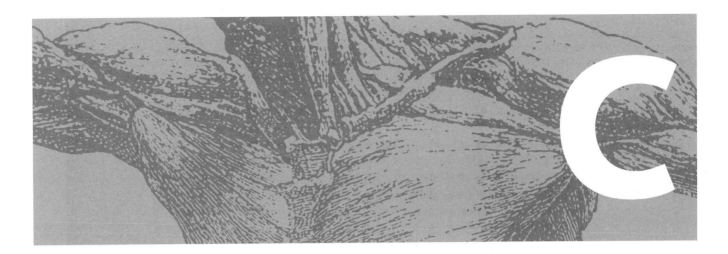

Caesarean section Delivery of a baby by the surgical incision of the mother's abdominal wall and UTERUS has a long history although it is only in the last century that the procedure of Caesarean section has carried any realistic expectation of maternal survival. The origin of the name 'Caesarean' is obscure. Although it is commonly linked to Julius Caesar, his mother is known to have been alive at the time of the invasion of Britain by his Roman army. It is highly unlikely that she would have survived delivery by 'section'. Some have suggested that the term is derived instead from the Latin verb 'to cut', *caedare*.

Many early Caesarean sections were performed post-mortem as attempts to ensure survival of the baby after death of the mother. This may have been the case with MacDuff, who caused the downfall of Shakespeare's Scottish king, Macbeth, and who was 'from his mother's womb, untimely ript'. Caesarean sections were performed sporadically during the seventeenth, eighteenth, and nineteenth centuries as deliberate surgical procedures on living women with obstructed labour, although survival was rare. During the twentieth century, improvements in ANAESTHESIA and the availability of ANTIBIOTICS and BLOOD TRANSFUSION made the operation increasingly less hazardous. It is now commonplace for the mother to be awake during Caesarean section, but pain-free as a result of epidural or spinal anaesthesia.

Caesarean section may be performed as a planned ('*elective*') or an emergency procedure. Reasons for elective operations include breech presentation (a controversial issue), placenta praevia (in which the placenta is below the baby and would bleed during labour), or previous Caesarean sections for recurring complications. Emergency operations are mainly performed for 'fetal distress', or for 'failure to progress' during LABOUR. The main causes of failed progress are poor contractions of the uterus, a baby too large to be accommodated by the mother's pelvis, or an occipito-posterior position (the baby's head facing away from the mother's spine).

Caesarean section is almost always, now, performed as the 'lower segment' operation, which produces a wound in the womb that heals well and which will be strong enough usually to cope with future labours. The formerly favoured 'classical' operation produced a wound that was, in contrast, prone to falling apart in subsequent pregnancies.   J. NEILSON

See also BIRTH; LABOUR; PREGNANCY.

Caffeine is a *methylxanthine* present in tea and coffee, and therefore probably is the most common drug, regularly taken, in the world. Three very similar compounds — all in this same group of alkaloids — are present in common beverages, namely caffeine, *theophylline*, and *theobromine*. The first two are found mainly in tea and coffee, and the third in cocoa. Cola beans, used in the manufacture of well-known soft drinks, also contain caffeine. The three compounds differ very little from each other: simply the number and disposition of methyl groups about the xanthine nucleus is variable. Weight for weight, the caffeine content of coffee beans (0.7–1.5%) and tea leaves (2–3%) is similar, but generally a coffee infusion is stronger than that used for tea. Thus the dose of alkaloid per usual portion of tea or coffee is very similar, namely 50–150 mg, depending on taste.

Infusions made from the leaves of *Camellia sinensis* (i.e. tea) have been consumed in the East for almost two millenia, and the practice reached Europe in the sixteenth century. The demand grew, and plantations were started in the Indian subcontinent. The British remain the most constant tea drinkers, with an average annual consumption of 4.5 kg, equivalent to a daily caffeine intake of 300 mg. In Japan tea is made from powdered green leaves. An elaborate tea ceremony is sometimes performed in which the tea maker performs a series of ritualised procedures in a very precise way. The green tea served at these ceremonies is usually bitter in taste.

Coffee cultivation began in the Yemen in the ninth century, the beans being obtained from a bush, *Coffea arabica*, and they were introduced into Europe alongside tea in the sixteenth century. The major source of coffee is now in the state of Sao Paulo, Brazil. Coffee is supposed to have been discovered by an Ethiopian holy man whose goats had eaten the berries, allowing them to frisk all night long. It was claimed that coffee 'quickens the spirits and makes the heart lightsome' and is 'good against the dropsy', but a distinguished professor of medicine at Cambridge around 1900 claimed coffee caused TREMORS and agitation. Explanations for all these claims can be made, particularly when allowance is made for 'dose'. However, assuming the effects are due to caffeine, tea drinkers as well as coffee drinkers will benefit, or suffer, alike. While lethargy and irritability often result from withdrawal in drinkers, it is doubtful whether true caffeine dependency exists.

The pharmacological effects of caffeine are widespread and various. By inhibition of certain ENZYMES, it allows an increase in the concentration of the 'second messenger', cyclic AMP, within cells, enhancing in turn the systems which this activates. Since caffeine penetrates the BLOOD–BRAIN BARRIER it is assumed that the central stimulant effects, on alertness and counteracting feelings of FATIGUE, are due to this action. Caffeine also acts on the KIDNEYS as a mild diuretic; this combined with its stimulant actions on heart muscle provide good evidence for the claim that it is 'good for the dropsy', both by strengthening the force of the heart beat and by removing accumulated body fluid.

ALAN W. CUTHBERT

Calcium is crucial to all physiological function. It must be obtained from the diet, but since an intake of only about 1 g per day is adequate, shortage is rare; the net daily turnover (the absorption rate into blood, and excretion rate in the urine) is only about one-tenth of that amount again.

The average human body contains just over 1 kg of calcium, more than 99% of it in the SKELETON (and TEETH). Here it is mostly in the form of complex phosphate salts forming the rigid structures that allow bone to fulfil its essential

131

supportive role. Skeletal calcium is not, however, inert. Bone contains cells that lay down new bone and resorb old bone and the regulated activities of these cells, made possible by the extensive blood supply that bone receives, ensure that skeletal calcium actively turns over. Beyond middle age, the rate of bone deposition fails to keep pace with its resorption and the disparity can become severe enough to cause OSTEOPOROSIS, when the bones become fragile and fracture easily. In addition to its structural role, the skeleton serves also as a reservoir from which calcium can be mobilized if necessary.

Calcium absorption from the small intestine and excretion from the KIDNEYS are also regulated to ensure that the concentration of calcium in the plasma is very precisely controlled, probably more tightly than any other component of plasma. The need for such precise calcium HOMEOSTASIS is underscored by the serious consequences that follow deviations from the norm. Excessively low plasma calcium levels (*hypocalcaemia*) are particularly dangerous because they evoke spontaneous activity in both nerves and muscles, causing muscle spasms that can become so severe as to obstruct the airway. Conversely, with too high a plasma calcium level (*hypercalcaemia*), nerves and muscle can become less active, leading to weakness. The longer term consequences of aberrant plasma calcium regulation can include skeletal problems and kidney stones.

Three agents are principally responsible for plasma calcium regulation, acting directly or indirectly at the three sites where the amount entering or leaving the blood can be influenced — bone, kidneys, and intestine.

Parathyroid hormone is a peptide released from the PARATHYROID GLANDS in the neck in direct response to any fall in the plasma calcium concentration. In bone it enhances calcium resorption and transfer into the blood. In the kidneys it both reduces calcium excretion and promotes formation of the active metabolite of vitamin D_3, which in turn enhances intestinal absorption. Thus parathyroid hormone helps to restore plasma calcium levels to normal.

Vitamin D (cholecalciferol) is not only a component of the diet (extra is added to cereals and dairy products) but also is synthesised in the skin in the presence of sunlight. After modification in the liver, vitamin D_3 is further modified to its active form in the kidneys, a step that is stimulated largely via parathyroid hormone, and hence in turn by a fall in the plasma calcium concentration. The active metabolite of vitamin D_3, 1,25-dihydroxycholecalciferol (*calcitriol*) is a hormone that stimulates calcium uptake from the small intestine and mobilization of calcium from bone, both serving to reverse the fall in plasma calcium that triggered formation of the hormone initially. Defects in any of the pathways leading to formation of 1,25-dihydroxycholecalciferol give rise to *rickets*.

Calcitonin is the third, and least important, calcium-regulating hormone. It is released from cells within the THYROID gland in response to an increase in plasma calcium and to several other factors, including GASTRIN, a hormone released during feeding and therefore heralding a potential rise in plasma calcium. Calcitonin serves to reverse any such rise by inhibiting bone resorption.

Clinical disorders of calcium regulation can arise for a variety of reasons, related not only directly to excess or deficiency of the relevant hormones, but also to conditions affecting kidney function and intestinal absorption; there can also be defects in the signalling proteins responsible for mediating the effects of parathyroid hormone on its target tissues. Conditions disturbing ACID–BASE HOMEOSTASIS can alter the concentration of free calcium ions in the blood: alkalinity increases, and acidity decreases their binding to proteins in the plasma.

It is ironic that the insolubility of calcium phosphate that allows it to form so stable a structure in bone was probably also the ultimate cause, in evolutionary terms, of calcium coming to fulfil its other indispensible role as a dynamic regulator of cellular activity. The energy economy of every cell is now dominated by the transfer of phosphate groups, and since calcium phosphate is so insoluble, it is likely that cells have long (in evolutionary terms) been required to actively extrude calcium. Every cell now maintains a very low free calcium ion concentration in its cytoplasm, some 10 000 times or so lower than that in either the plasma or the enclosed calcium stores within the cell. These very steep calcium concentration gradients are maintained by using energy, generated from the metabolism of the cell, to actively export calcium from the cytoplasm, either out of the cell or into the internal stores. There are two benefits of this active calcium transport. Firstly, it allows the energy economy of the cell to operate free of the risk that the key intermediates will be precipitated by calcium. Secondly, it provides steep, ready-made gradients down which calcium can rapidly flow into the cytoplasm when appropriate physiological stimuli cause the opening of calcium ION CHANNELS in either the plasma membrane or the membranes of the intracellular stores. Rigorously controlled leaking of calcium through such channels is ubiquitous in the regulation of cellular activity. The fertilization of an egg, every beat of the heart or contraction of any other muscle, release of transmitters from nerve endings — myriads of physiological responses — all are regulated by transient increases in cytoplasmic calcium ion concentration brought about by appropriate stimuli from outside the cell, that cause calcium channels to open, and allow movement down the gradient into the cell. The ensuing increase in cytoplasmic calcium concentration is detected by specific calcium-binding proteins, the most abundant of which is *calmodulin*. The change in shape of these proteins that follows their binding of calcium allows them to interact specifically with their targets within the cell; these include enzymes, ion channels, and muscle fibres. The intense scrutiny to which calcium channels have been subjected in recent decades has revealed their structures and the stimuli that control their opening (which range from changes in voltage to extracellular and intracellular messenger molecules); it is also beginning to establish the molecular mechanisms underlying their behaviour. Despite the diversity of behaviours, one feature that appears to be shared by all calcium channels is their regulation by cytoplasmic calcium ion concentration itself: each seems to be subject to feedback inhibition by calcium, a mechanism that probably serves to prevent intracellular calcium from rising to levels that could be toxic. This function can fail in sick cells — an excessive influx of calcium is known for example to be destructive to neuronal function when brain cells are damaged by lack of oxygen.

As well as these crucial roles in cellular function and in bone, ionised calcium in the blood plasma is one of several factors necessary for the clotting process: its chemical removal by the addition of citrate solution allows donor blood to be kept fluid for transfusion.   C.W. TAYLOR

See also BLOOD; BODY FLUIDS; CELL; ION CHANNELS; NEUROMUSCULAR JUNCTION; PARATHYROID GLANDS; SYNAPSE.

Callanetics System of exercises, devised by Callan Pinckney in the 1980s, utilising small, exact movements aimed at toning and shaping the body.   N.C.S.

Callisthenics. Programmed, rhythmic, relatively light exercises, performed without weights or other apparatus, and designed to enhance body image, cardiovascular fitness, flexibility and the tone (but not significantly the bulk) of muscles.   N.C.S.

Calorie Calor means heat, and a calorie is defined as the amount of heat which will raise the temperature of one gram of water by 1°C. The Calorie (kilocalorie, kcal) is 1000 calories — a more useful unit and widely used. In a 'calorimeter' a substance can be combusted in the presence of oxygen, to measure the amount of heat generated per gram. From such basic measurements, and by extrapolation to mixtures of different ingredients, the 'calorie count' can be applied as a measure of the energy derivable from a food source. Kcals are also the traditional units for the body's metabolic rate: the energy output or expenditure in kcal/min. Attempts to supplant it by the SI (*Systeme Internationale*) unit, the *kilojoule* (energy defined in electrical terms) have only partially succeeded; the energy content of food is usually quoted in both (1 kcal = 4.2 kJ).

          S.J.

See DIETING; ENERGY BALANCE; METABOLISM.

Cancer The term 'cancer' refers to a diverse group of diseases, characterised by uncontrolled growth of cells, leading to a variety of pathological consequences and frequently death. It is typically a disease of the elderly — the incidence of all forms of cancer increases markedly with age.

However, it also occurs occasionally in children. Often the abnormal cell growth results in the establishment of a macroscopic lump or tumour 'oncos' in Greek, hence the term 'oncology' for the study of cancer), which may grow to a large size and kill the patient by a local effect, e.g. occlusion of vital ducts — even the alimentary tract — or by compromising the functioning of some distant organ. Indeed, the very word 'cancer' derives from the appearance of solid tumours as noted on *post mortem* examination by early physicians, who likened their appearance to that of a crab (*Cancer*) because of the irregular and disorganised appearance of the threads of the tumour radiating from a central body. Some forms of cancer, however, do not grow as coherent lumps but as individual cells diffused through the vascular system; these diseases — leukaemias and lymphomas — are associated with quite a different pathological profile.

Not all tumours of the human body are cancerous, however. Everyone is familiar with the common wart, and probably other skin lesions that result from local proliferation of cells, and which are quite benign. What distinguishes cancerous tumours and renders them seriously life-threatening is the property of *malignancy*, which derives from the capacity of the cells to invade surrounding tissue and to break off from the parent lump, migrate around the body in the blood vessels or the LYMPHATIC SYSTEM, and set up secondary foci of cancerous growth at distant sites. It is the latter phenomenon, metastatic spread of the disease, which most frequently kills cancer patients. The secondary foci — *metastases* — often occur in the brain, lungs, or liver, because these organs have a large blood supply and a well-developed capillary bed of tiny vessels in which single cancer cells or clumps of cells can lodge. By contrast, many common skin cancers (with the singular exception of malignant melanoma) are invasive but not metastatic, so they can be cured by simple excision of the tumour together with a decent margin of surrounding tissue. This emphasizes the seriousness of metastasis in the pathology of cancer. It is also salutary that in many instances cancer patients present with clear evidence of metastatic disease, such as secondary tumours radiologically visible in the lung, but no sign of the primary lump. It may take all the skill of an experienced histopathologist to indicate the probable origin of the diseased cells, knowledge of which is likely to be crucial for any form of clinical management.

Cancer therapy involves four modalities which may be employed singly or in combination: SURGERY, RADIOTHERAPY, CHEMOTHERAPY, or a group of less well-defined treatments, of which immunotherapy is the chief example. It is common practice to employ surgery where applicable (to reduce the tumour burden if a single large mass has been detected e.g. by X-rays or magnetic resonance imaging), followed by localised or whole-body radiotherapy to attack residual disease, and/or chemotherapy to deal with distant metastases. If the disease is advanced,

with obvious metastasis, chemotherapy with a cocktail of three or four powerfully cytotoxic drugs may be the only worthwhile option. Most of these drugs are DNA-reactive chemicals which directly attack the genetic blueprints of the rogue cells. Alternatively a massive dose of whole-body irradiation may be attempted, and the patient rescued from death due to destruction of his bone marrow by subsequent reimplantation of his own marrow cells, collected prior to treatment and 'cleaned up' *in vitro* (*autologous bone marrow transplantation*).

Cancer is increasingly seen as a lifestyle disease, caused at least partly by environmental influences, with important modulation by the genetic inheritance of the individual. Sometimes viral infections may start the process off. In other cases sunlight is to blame, particularly in causing skin cancers among fair-skinned Caucasians living in tropical countries or under the ozone hole of the Southern hemisphere. Sometimes it is diet which seems to trigger disease, especially of the gastrointestinal tract: here fats are held suspect, and a high-fibre diet rich in cereals and vegetables is to be recommended. But far and away the most serious, and preventable, environmental cause of cancer is tobacco smoking, which is inexorably linked to cancer of the lung. On this conclusion the epidemiological evidence is stark — witness the sharp continuing rise in lung cancer among women in the Western world, which correlates precisely with the changes in social attitudes to smoking over the last 50 years.

One of the hottest areas of cancer research by the end of the twentieth century was the identification of genes that impart an inherited susceptibility to cancer of particular organs, or to cancer in general. Early successes have been the discovery of BRCA1 and BRCA2, genes which predispose to breast cancer — still the most common form of malignancy in Western women — and there are more to come. Other cancer-prone individuals carry genes whose products are enzymes known to be intimately associated with the biological phenomena of cell signalling, gene transcription, or DNA repair. A picture is beginning to emerge of cancer development, starting with a single cell exposed to some external influence, which causes a mutation in one of a small number of critical genes, 'initiating' the process of escape from growth control. Other genetic changes, leading to *aneuploidy* (abnormalities in the nature or the number of chromosomes), follow over a period which may be as long as several years, while so-called 'promoter' substances exacerbate the multiplication of the abnormal cells into a small tumour, which begins to invade its surroundings and may start to metastasise. In the later stages of disease the cells enter a 'progression' phase, in which gross re-arrangements of their genetic make-up occur — these, can be seen down the microscope as whole-sale redistribution of chromosomes, involving deletions, translocations, breaks, duplications, and doubtless many more subtle changes. Genetic instability can proceed to a state of chro-

mosomal chaos — a 'point of no return' whereby cells cannot revert to the normal *karyotype* (the characteristics of its chromosomes) and must be killed. At that stage the disease is rampant and only the most aggressive intervention, including treatment with drugs which have dire toxic side-effects, is likely to produce any relief or remission, and cure is most unlikely. Often the side-effects (hair loss, vomiting and diarrhoea, neurological disorders, or bone marrow suppression) are so serious as to be unacceptable to the sick patient, and palliative treatment with powerful opiates is all that can be recommended. The most recent scientific findings emphasize the importance in tumour control of programmed cell death (*apoptosis*) and shortening of the far end, of the 'arms' of chromosomes (the *telomeres*) during replication. Chemotherapeutic and radiotherapeutic strategies induce apoptosis, so escape from programmed death signals is important.

M.J. WARING

See also CHEMOTHERAPY; RADIOTHERAPY.

Cannibalism

Attitudes have changed considerably since the early twentieth century, when Sir James Frazer could blithely ask, of far-flung ethnographic correspondents ensconced among the 'natives', 'Do they eat their enemies or their friends?' The inevitable result of the inquiry was the concept of a universe of customary man-eaters beyond the borders of civilized society eventually enshrined in anthropological texts as 'endo'- or 'exo'-cannibals, depending on the status of the victims, lending a scientific tone to the discussion. Today's post-modern perspective assumes such questions produce 'pre-figured' responses indicating more about those who pose them than about those who have become known as 'The Other' — the exotic objects of discussion. Thus, some believe no objective truth, as opposed to subjective cultural representations, can result from the discourse. In this context considering cannibalism has become a complicated task.

Initially it must be entertained, if not accepted, that travellers' accounts of strange lands with anthropophagic *(man-eating)* inhabitants should be discounted. Famous representatives of this genre, such as Herodotus and Marco Polo, as well as a host of minor peregrinators, never actually encountered the phenomenon in question. (Often they never even encountered the presumed *anthropophagi*.) Instead they relied upon the reports of one exotic people about the peculiar behaviour of others even more distant. Nonetheless, a template had been set for followers, including Columbus and his contemporaries, who subsequently also issued accounts on the fantastical inhabitants of the New World. (In the process they introduced the term 'cannibal', as a perversion of the word 'Carib'). In addition to relying on expectations and unsubstantiated reports, this generation of explorers and Conquistadors had the added impetus to provide a legitimization for their activities, which often had sad consequences for the indigenes.

Subsequent exemplars also inevitably came upon cannibals in Africa, South America, Asia, and the Pacific in the colonization process. In some instances, those who failed to have the encounter merely plagiarized the work of others so as not to be outshone.

In the twentieth century, anthropologists — newly-minted professional interpreters of the exotic — whose self-proclaimed mandate was to de-romanticize the experience by direct observation and objective interpretation of contemporary cultures, continued, despite its absence, to reinforce the cannibalism theme on the authority of previous visitors. The usual explanation for the lacuna was the recent cessation or secret practice of the deed, due to the impact of colonialism and/or missionary activity. The retention of this ethnographic tidbit, as so many others were abandoned, obviously has much to do with the discipline's need for the exotic. This peculiar state of affairs led to the suggestion of a cannibal mythology as a feature of Western cosmology. This does not suggest that those responsible for the vision, including anthropologists, were engaged in a conscious hoax as opposed to maintaining a long-standing cultural projection. (Although their errors are understandable, it could be argued that the discipline had a greater responsibility to be more circumspect in its deliberations on this matter than others.) Nor does the argument imply that cannibalism has never been a feature of some societies; rather that such a conclusion is not supported by evidence. The best way to comprehend the situation in all its complexities invites a consideration of a more recent cannibal belief complex involving a number of academic disciplines, including medicine.

In 1957, while visiting Papua New Guinea, D. Carleton Gajdusek, a medical researcher, learned of an epidemic called *kuru*, savaging the highland area, principally among the Fore people. After arduous initial investigations, his preliminary results allowed for an expanded research team including cultural anthropologists. Of more immediate importance, laboratory results indicated that the disease could be transmitted — via the distillation of human victims' brain tissue — to chimpanzees. A reasonable extrapolation of this fact was that the illness had been transmitted among humans in New Guinea in some unknown fashion. A review of the literature indicates that the pre-figured notion of cannibalism entered into the discussion as the suspected agent of *kuru* transmission, first tentatively, and then with greater authority; the authors, including the anthropologists, began to cite each others' remarks in their publications until cannibalism eventually emerged as a scientific fact. The sensational nature of the claim soon enshrined it in the secondary and popular literature. However, none of the parties intimately involved had ever observed the deed, as opposed to learning of it from previous accounts. The inability to document the activity was explained as usual in terms of the cessation of the practice, or its continued secret occurrence. Thus, a common assertion

about an exotic people was incorporated into an otherwise rational scientific discourse.

The recent concern over the spread of Creutzfeld–Jacob disease (a variant of *kuru*) in Europe provides an instructive example of how the matter is envisioned for 'civilized' populations. The implication of Bovine Spongiform Encephalopathy (BSE) in this instance suggests that the dietary habits of the Fore people, which included the consumption of undercooked pork, including brain tissue, should now be given greater consideration in the transmission of *kuru*. Customary funeral practices, which involved direct contact with the deceased's brain tissue, and institutionalized male homosexuality, also deserve greater appreciation as a disease vector, since they are well-documented activities, as opposed to cannibalism, which was merely assumed.

In sum, it no longer appears reasonable to assume the anthropophagic nature of others in the sense that they have been wholesale consumers of human flesh. This assertion does not deny some cross-cultural variation on the theme. For example, it has been reported on good authority that inhabitants of South America ritually consume the bone-ash of the departed. Yet, similar bodily substances were sold in European and American apothecaries until the beginning of the twentieth century and continue to be used today in some forms for their assumed medicinal qualities. The human use of the human body in all these instances raises interesting questions about the distinction between science and ritual.

W. ARENS

Further reading

Arens, W. (1979). *The man-eating myth*. Oxford University Press, New York.

Gajdusek, D. C. (1977). Unconventional viruses and the origin and disappearance of kuru. *Science*, 197, 943–60.

See also PRIONS.

Carbohydrates

Carbohydrates are one of the major classes of biological molecules, along with PROTEINS, lipids (FATS), and nucleic acids. Carbohydrates range from small molecules — mono-, di-, or tri-saccharides — to large molecules called polysaccharides. As these names imply, carbohydrates are made up of SUGARS.

The most abundant organic compound in the biosphere is a carbohydrate — *cellulose*, a substance which gives strength and integrity to plant cell walls. It consists of linked linear chains of glucose molecules. This configuration allows arrays of long, parallel straight fibrils to form, giving cellulose its characteristic properties. Cellulose is difficult to break down, and only some bacteria, fungi, and protozoa secrete the ENZYMES (*cellulases*) that can do so. So mammals are unable to digest cellulose, except some ruminants that have cellulase-secreting bacteria in their rumens. (If it were not for these bacterial cellulases, the disposal of 10^{15} kg of plant waste per year world-wide would present an enormous

pollution problem.) Nevertheless, in man, cellulose is an important component of the diet as 'roughage'.

GLYCOGEN, another polysaccharide made of linked chains of glucose molecules, is used by mammals as a way of storing energy in the cells of most tissues, but notably in liver cells as a store for the whole body, and in muscles for their own use. Here the type of linkage results in the formation of an open helix, readily broken down by the relevant enzymes (*glycogenases*) when the sudden need for energy arises.

Carbohydrate-rich foods are starchy ones, such as the staples bread, potatoes, and pasta. Large quantities of carbohydrates are ingested as common sugar and in confectionary. Common dietary carbohydrates are sucrose, lactose, and mannose, all *disaccharides* (formed from two simple sugars), which are broken down by digestive processes to monosaccharides and used to derive energy.

The conversion of monosaccharides to energy in the form of ADENOSINE TRIPHOSPHATE (ATP) follows a common pathway — used also for the conversion of fats and, to a lesser extent, proteins into energy — which involves the utilisation of OXYGEN. The end result of this metabolism is that one molecule of glucose generates 38 molecules of ATP. The *respiratory quotient* (RQ) for carbohydrates is 1, where the RQ is the ratio of the number of CO_2 molecules formed to the number of molecules of oxygen consumed in oxidising (burning) one sugar molecule. As carbohydrates have the formula $(CH_2O)_n$, hydrogen and oxygen are in the correct ratio to form water. (When fats are oxidised, extra oxygen is needed to form water, such that the RQ for fats is around 0.7.)

In an ideally balanced diet, about two-thirds of the energy supply should be from carbohydrates. But unlike proteins and fats, which must provide certain essential components, no particular dietary carbohydrates are necessary for health. This may seem paradoxical, in that the brain crucially needs a constant supply of glucose — but this can, if necessary, be made internally from proteins. Excess of dietary carbohydrate, when the glycogen stores are filled, is converted and stored as fat, and this can be released as FATTY ACIDS when needed for energy production. In STARVATION, the mobilisation of fatty acids from body fat results in their uptake by the liver and production from them of *ketone bodies*, an alternative energy source. At this stage acetone can be smelt (like pear drops) on the breath. The same happens when carbohydrate starvation occurs at the cellular level in DIABETES because glucose entry into cells is impaired.

ALAN W. CUTHBERT

See also BLOOD SUGAR; ENERGY BALANCE; METABOLISM; STARVATION; SUGARS.

Carbon dioxide

Carbon dioxide When the body 'burns' food the end products are mainly water and carbon dioxide, together with some nitrogenous chemicals such as urea. The carbon dioxide enters the bloodstream, is carried to the LUNGS, and is excreted in the expired air of BREATHING. The atmospheric air we inhale contains virtually no carbon dioxide, whereas there is about 5% in the air we breathe out.

Carbon dioxide reacts in the blood to form carbonic acid and bicarbonate and, if it were allowed to accumulate, would cause acidosis. This condition is particularly harmful to the cells of the brain. Carbon dioxide diffuses into the liquid in the brain, the CEREBROSPINAL FLUID (CSF); any excess makes it more acid, and this in turn stimulates neural receptors in the BRAIN STEM that increase breathing. The result is that the carbon dioxide is blown off in the lungs and the acidity of the blood and brain are kept close to normal levels. Carbon dioxide is the main chemical stimulus to breathing, which is regulated primarily to keep blood and brain acidity at healthy values. If the carbon dioxide in the lungs increases by only 0.2%, from a normal level of about 5%, then breathing is doubled. Breathholding accumulates carbon dioxide in the body, which leads to an irrepressible desire to breathe (lack of oxygen is also a stimulus, but far weaker than carbon dioxide). Conversely, if we voluntarily hyperventilate, the level of carbon dioxide in the blood will decrease, and breathing may be inhibited until more carbon dioxide accumulates. HYPERVENTILATION can have harmful effects because of the pronounced reduction in blood and CSF acidity. Since decreases in carbon dioxide and acidity constrict BLOOD VESSELS, particularly in the brain, one effect is to reduce the blood supply to the brain.

Carbon dioxide was identified, but not understood chemically, in about 1600 AD by van Helmont, who called it 'gas sylvestre', the gas produced by combustion. He showed that it would not support life. Later Joseph Black, who had a lifelong interest in chemistry and was Professor of Medicine in Glasgow from 1757 to 1766, called it 'fixed acid', because it was absorbed by lime solution, and he showed that it was produced in RESPIRATION. The story goes that in 1764 Black climbed to the ceiling of a church in Glasgow, occupied for 10 hours of religious devotions by a congregation of 1500, and measured the 'fixed acid' that was exhaled by the diligent and sleepy congregation. But it was Lavoisier (1743–94) who definitely established the excretion of carbon dioxide after its formation in metabolism, although he erroneously believed that it was formed in the lungs. Lavoisier was guillotined, and it was said that 'it took but a second to cut off his head; a hundred years will not suffice to produce one like it.' Lavoisier concluded that any series of lectures in an auditorium extending over 3 hours would leave the audience in a soporific state due to the accumulation of carbon dioxide. In theory he was right. Carbon dioxide in excess can act as an anaesthetic and, in animals, major surgery has been performed under its influence alone. Some human lung diseases such as chronic bronchitis may leave the patient drowsy or even comatose because of the build up of carbon dioxide in the

body. It is claimed, probably incorrectly, that in social environments yawning and weariness are due to an accumulation of carbon dioxide. Van Helmont investigated a Grotto del Cane (cave of dogs) in Italy in which it was claimed, rather implausibly, that a tall dog owner would survive while his lowly dog would perish, due to the depressant effect of carbon dioxide, held to the ground because of its greater density than air. Perhaps Black's Glasgow congregation was fortunate.   JOHN WIDDICOMBE

See also ACID–BASE HOMEOSTASIS; BLOOD; RESPIRATION.

Carbon monoxide is a gas which is best

known to us as a product of incomplete combustion. As such, mankind must have been aware of its deadly effect since the discovery and use of fire, and increasingly so as the development of the industrial revolution led to more use of combustion as a source of energy. The important producers of carbon monoxide are industrial processes, heating equipment, accidental fire, cigarettes, and the internal combustion engine. Blast furnace gas contains 25% carbon monoxide, and coal gas, which was used as a fuel in Europe up until North Sea (natural) gas became plentiful, contains 16%. Carbon monoxide POISONING is the most common cause of fatal gassing and is the cause of death in about 90% of fire victims. Domestic gas supplies still lead to carbon monoxide poisoning, but now due to leakage of products of combustion from a damaged flue or poorly maintained equipment, rather than the fuel itself, since natural gas is carbon monoxide free. In the mining industry carbon monoxide contaminates the atmosphere during and after fires or explosions. The 'afterdamp' occurring in such situations is a mixture of carbon dioxide and carbon monoxide.

Carbon monoxide is a colourless, odourless gas which is tasteless and non-irritant. It is somewhat less dense than air and, although it is a product of imperfect combustion, it is inflammable. The gas was first identified by Joseph Priestley in the eighteenth century, but it was Claude BERNARD in 1870 who discovered the affinity between carbon monoxide and HAEMO-GLOBIN which accounts for its deadliness: carboxyhaemoglobin is formed and OXYGEN transport from the lungs to the tissues disrupted. In 1895 J. S. Haldane demonstrated that the formation of carboxyhaemoglobin is an equilibrium reaction which depends upon the relative partial pressures of carbon monoxide and oxygen in inspired gas. Haldane's interest was stimulated by the problems caused by carbon monoxide in British coal mines. By breathing carbon monoxide gas which was passed through a bottle containing a mouse, he was able to determine that man was very much more resistant to the gas. Small animals such as mice and canaries, who are more vulnerable than man due to their high metabolic rate, were used in mines to give an indication of carbon monoxide contamination. Canaries responded to the gas by falling off their perches before workers noticed any ill

effects, and this normally gave ample warning. Occasionally, however, in low concentrations of the order of 0.05% carbon monoxide, the bird adapted to the gas and the workers could collapse while the bird remained well.

Carbon monoxide, like oxygen, has an affinity for iron-containing molecules, but it is about 210 times more effective in binding to iron-containing haemoglobin than oxygen is. Since air contains 21% oxygen this means that only 0.1% carbon monoxide in the air will eventually lead to 50% of the haemoglobin being combined to form carboxyhaemoglobin. Once carboxyhaemoglobin is formed, and after exposure ceases, it takes 4–5 hours for its level in the blood to fall, exponentially, by 50%. The ill effect of the gas can therefore be cumulative, and a person can be poisoned by intermittent exposure during the day.

Because carboxyhaemoglobin does not carry oxygen, a level of 50% means that the oxygen carrying capacity of the blood is reduced by 50% and there is a corresponding reduction in the ability to perform maximum exercise. The body compensates for the blood's reduction in oxygen carrying capacity by increasing cardiac output, and in the early stages of carbon monoxide poisoning the heart beats faster and more strongly. Unfortunately, haemoglobin is not the only molecule affected. Muscle myoglobin also binds carbon monoxide, 60 times more effectively than it binds oxygen. This results in a reduction of heart muscle contractility and a failure of the body's compensatory mechanisms, leading to profound tissue HYPOXIA, which can be fatal. The presence of carboxyhaemoglobin also diminishes the oxygen held by the normal haemoglobin, which further compounds the hypoxic effect. As tissue oxygen level falls, carbon monoxide is able to bind to other iron-containing molecules: notably cytochrome P450, an important drug-metabolising enzyme, and cytochrome A₃, an enzyme in the terminal respiratory chain which can also be poisoned by cyanide.

The scientific history of carbon monoxide is not one of uniform gloom, however. The intense affinity of carbon monoxide for haemoglobin has allowed low concentrations to be used as a marker for measurement of the speed of blood through the lungs and the surface area of the lung available for the transfer of oxygen. This latter remains as one of the standard lung function tests. In 1951 Sjöstrand discovered that Haldane's poison gas is a normal product of the body's metabolism. The enzyme haem oxygenase breaks down the haem from senescent red blood cells, and this reaction produces carbon monoxide and bile salts. The bile salts are excreted by the liver and the carbon monoxide released gives the blood a normal carboxyhaemoglobin level of 0.2–1.0%. This *endogenous* carbon monoxide was thought to be just a waste product, but more recent work by Verma has demonstrated that a type of haem oxygenase is located in specific areas in the brain, and suggested that the carbon monoxide produced acts as a NEUROTRANSMITTER. The carbon monoxide activates the enzyme guanylyl cyclase, as does nitric oxide, regulating the intracellular levels of the second messenger cyclic GMP, which in turn regulates cellular activity. Other workers have demonstrated the haem oxygenase enzyme system in blood vessel walls and demonstrated that the carbon monoxide released causes vasodilation, as does nitric oxide. So far, endogenous carbon monoxide release has been suggested to have a role in the sense of smell, memory, cerebellar function (and hence the body's balance and co-ordination), control of blood hormone levels from the hypothalamus, and control of smooth muscle tone and vasodilatation.

The symptoms of carbon monoxide poisoning depend on the concentration breathed. The victim may pass out without warning, but often the onset of poisoning is slow. Headache, with or without nausea, is common, and this may relate to carbon monoxide's vasodilating effect. Drowsiness and lethargy then occur, along with breathlessness on exertion. At any stage there may be chest pain; this is angina due to cardiac hypoxia. At the stage of lethargy and drowsiness, cerebral function is affected and the person may not be able to think well enough to make an escape effort. Coma follows, and death. Treatment is by removal to an uncontaminated atmosphere and the administration of 100% oxygen. Hyperbaric oxygen speeds up recovery, and there is increasing evidence that it reduces long-term neurological problems.

Endogenous carbon monoxide function is undoubtedly disrupted during poisoning, but at our present state of knowledge it is difficult to say how this contributes to the toxic action of exogenous carbon monoxide. It may well be that our picture of the mechanisms of carbon monoxide poisoning will change as the function of endogenous carbon monoxide becomes clearer. Patients with carbon monoxide poisoning may have very poor balance and yet have good cerebral function. Short-term memory may also be severely disrupted. It is tempting to link these two features with the functions suggested for endogenous carbon monoxide. No doubt time will tell if there is a relationship.

JOHN A.S. ROSS

Further reading

World Health Organisation (1979). *Environmental health criteria 13: carbon monoxide.* WHO, Geneva.

Dawson, T. M. and Snyder, S. H. (1994). Gases as biological messengers: nitric oxide and carbon monoxide in the brain. (Review article.) *Journal of Neuroscience*, 14(9), 5147–59.

Cardiac arrest

Cardiac: pertaining to the heart. Arrest: stop. Cardiac arrest: previously equated with death, but since the advent of modern RESUSCITATION methods, an emergency well known to viewers of hospital soaps. When the heart stops, and the circulating blood therefore comes to a standstill, that part of the brain which allows conscious function has only a few minutes to survive. The heart stops beating if the pacemaker-generated rhythm is halted, or if conduction of the electrical impulses is disrupted, sending the muscle of the ventricles — the heart's pumps — into the irregular and useless twitching state of FIBRILLATION. If the instrument and the expertise are available, electric shocks are administered with a DEFIBRILLATOR, which may or may not restore a normal electrical rhythm and hence a regular beat. When this amenity is not at hand, or access to it is delayed, the first aid measure is *external cardiac massage*, consisting of rhythmic pressure on the chest, at the lower end of the sternum. By squeezing the heart against the spinal column, this can temporarily restore circulation of the blood. Since breathing is likely to have stopped at the same time, or very soon after, the heart beat, attention must be divided between cardiac massage and mouth-to-mouth respiration.

S.J.

See DEFIBRILLATOR; HEART; HEART ATTACK; RESUSCITATION.

Cardiac glycosides

The introduction of the cardiac glycosides into medicine was inextricably linked to William Withering (1741–99), who studied medicine in Edinburgh and then practised in Birmingham. Like many educated people of his time, his interests were wide, and he made significant contributions to chemistry, mineralogy, and particularly botany. In 1776, he published *A botanical Arrangement of all the Vegetables naturally growing in Great Britain*, in two volumes which went through several later editions. His expertise in botany was put to good use when in 1775 his opinion was asked about a family recipe for the cure of dropsy, which had been kept secret by an old woman in Shropshire. He wrote:

'I was informed that the effects produced were violent vomiting and purging . . . This medicine was composed of twenty or more different herbs; but it was not difficult for one conversant in these subjects to perceive that the active herb could be none other than the Foxglove.'

He found that foxglove was a powerful DIURETIC, but he then heard that a colleague in Oxford had cured an accumulation of fluid in the chest with it. This made him undertake a comprehensive study of foxglove, which led to the conclusion that it cured dropsy (the term then used to describe an accumulation of fluid in the tissues) due to cardiac failure, and that it led to a brisk diuresis. He published his findings on 163 cases in *An account of Foxglove and some of its medical uses* in 1785, in which he gave a full account of the botany, preparations, actions, and toxic effects. Of course, the poisonous actions of foxglove were already well known. Leonhard Fuchs had given a good description of the plant in 1542 and noted its action as a diuretic and laxative. However, the focus on the action in HEART FAILURE was entirely due to Withering, and represents the best early account of a rational therapeutic approach.

The main active substance in the purple foxglove *Digitalis purpurea* is *digitoxin*, a steroid (17 lactone with a trisaccharide attached at the 3 position). It is active at nanomolar concentration. Related active substances are found in *D. lanata* (*digoxin*, which is more widely used in current medical practice because of its shorter duration of action), and in *Strophanthus gratus* (*ouabain*), squill, convallaria, hellebore, and many other plants. The main effects on the heart are an increase in contractile force, especially in the failing heart, and a slowing of the rate. The slowing is particularly marked in people with atrial FIBRILLATION, and the heartbeat is also made more regular.

All the active cardiac glycosides are inhibitors of the enzyme Na/K ATPase, present in CELL MEMBRANES, which is responsible for pumping sodium out of the cell and pumping potassium in. It is generally believed that the inhibition of this enzyme is mainly responsible for the strengthening of the contraction of the heart (the resulting rise in intracellular sodium inhibits the sodium/calcium exchanger, which is the main mechanism concerned with extruding CALCIUM from the cell; thus intracellular calcium increases, and this enhances the contractile force of the cardiac muscle). However, the action of the glycosides are complex and involve also the effects of ACETYLCHOLINE and NORADRENALINE released from the cardiac nerves: this may be the main mechanism for reducing the heart rate. Reduction in the rate of beating of the ventricles when there is atrial fibrillation is due to a number of actions: raising of the excitation threshold at the atrio-ventricular node is probably most important (allowing fewer of the disordered waves of atrial activity to be conducted to the ventricles.) The diuretic action is probably due to inhibition of the ATPase in the KIDNEY tubules, resulting in reduced reabsorption of sodium — and therefore also of water — from the tubular fluid, thus increasing the volume of urine.

Toxic effects include anorexia, nausea, vomiting, headache, drowsiness, and visual disturbances, as well as extrasystoles and excessive slowing of the heart rate. The dose range between therapeutic and toxic levels is small: if this were a new drug today, it is very doubtful whether it would receive approval! However, even after 200 years, cardiac glycosides remain of major importance in the treatment of heart failure.

ARNOLD BURGEN

See also CARDIAC MUSCLE; HEART; HEART FAILURE.

Cardiac muscle

Your heart beats about once a second for the whole of your life, and of course has no opportunity to rest. Its output must adjust rapidly to meet the needs of the body, and can increase from about 5 litres of blood/min at rest to more than 25 litres/min in heavy exercise. The special requirements of the heart call for a special type of muscle, *cardiac muscle*, which is not found anywhere else in the body. Cardiac muscle is in some ways similar to SKELETAL and

SMOOTH MUSCLE. For example, all three contract when a rise in CALCIUM inside the muscle cell allows interaction between *actin* and *myosin* filaments. However, cardiac muscle has a unique structure, and differs in the way that contraction is initiated and regulated.

Structure

Under the microscope, cardiac muscle is seen to consist of interlacing bundles of *cardiac myocytes* (muscle cells). Like skeletal muscle it is striated with narrow dark and light bands, due to the parallel arrangement of actin and myosin filaments that extend from end to end of each myocyte. However, cardiac myocytes are narrower and much shorter than skeletal muscle cells, being about 0.02 mm wide and 0.1 mm long, and are more rectangular than smooth muscle cells, which are normally spindle-shaped. They are often branched, and contain one nucleus but many *mitochondria*, which provide the energy required for contraction. A prominent and unique feature of cardiac muscle is the presence of irregularly-spaced dark bands between myocytes. These are known as *intercalated discs*, and are due to areas where the membranes of adjacent myocytes come very close together. The intercalated discs have two important functions: one is to 'glue' the myocytes together so that they do not pull apart when the heart contracts; the other is to allow an electrical connection between the cells, which, as we will see, is vital to the function of the heart as a whole. The electrical connection is made via special junctions (*gap junctions*) between adjoining myocytes, containing pores through which small ions and therefore electrical current can pass. As the myocytes are electrically connected, cardiac muscle is often referred to as a *functional syncytium* (continuous cellular material).

Mechanism of contraction

Cardiac myocytes contract when the voltage across the membrane, the *resting membrane potential*, is reduced sufficiently to initiate an ACTION POTENTIAL. In most parts of the heart this is caused by an action potential in an adjacent myocyte being transmitted through the gap junctions. The action potential starts with a very rapid reduction in voltage toward zero, which is due to sodium ions entering the myocyte. This phase of the action potential is also seen in skeletal muscle and nerves. In cardiac muscle, however, the membrane potential then remains close to zero for about 0.3 sec — the *plateau phase*, which is largely due to entry of calcium ions. It is this entry of calcium that leads to contraction. At the end of the plateau phase the membrane potential returns to resting levels. The plateau means that cardiac muscle action potentials last much longer than those in skeletal muscle or nerves, where calcium does not enter the cell and there is therefore no plateau phase.

When an action potential is initiated in one myocyte, it causes an electrical current to pass through gap junctions in the intercalated discs to its neighbours. This current initiates action potentials in these cells, which in turn stimulate their neighbours. As a result, a wave of activation, and therefore contraction, passes through the heart. This process allows synchronisation of contraction throughout the heart, and is vital for proper function. When it is disrupted, as in some types of heart disease, the myocytes may lose synchronisation. In severe cases, such as ventricular fibrillation, the heart cannot pump at all, and is said to look like a 'bag of (writhing) worms'.

The amount of calcium entering the myocyte during an action potential is not enough to cause contraction. However, its entry causes more calcium to be released from stores in the *sarcoplasmic reticulum*, a membranous structure within the myocyte. This is known as *calcium-induced calcium release*. The amount of calcium released depends on the amount that enters during the action potential, so that contractile force can therefore be regulated by controlling calcium entry. This is increased by ADRENALINE and the AUTONOMIC NERVOUS SYSTEM. At the end of the beat, calcium is rapidly taken back into the sarcoplasmic reticulum, causing relaxation. Excess calcium — the amount that entered during the action potential — is expelled from the myocyte during the interval between beats by pumps in the membrane. If the heart rate increases there is less time to remove this calcium. As a result there is more calcium in the myocyte for the next beat, and so the force developed increases. This *staircase effect* allows the heart to expel blood more rapidly when the heart rate is increased. Drugs that inhibit removal of calcium from the myocyte can similarly increase cardiac muscle force. An example is *digitalis*, which was originally derived from the foxglove and has been used for treating heart disease for centuries.

Special types of cardiac muscle

Some areas of the heart contain myocytes that have specialised functions. One is the *sino-atrial node* or PACEMAKER region in the right atrium,

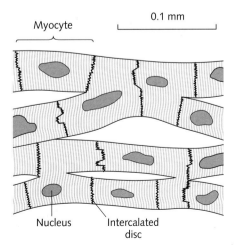

Diagrammatic section of cardiac muscle.

where modified myocytes generate action potentials automatically, and are responsible for initiating the heartbeat. Although nervous activity is not required for the heart to beat, the autonomic nervous system can modulate the activity of the pacemaker, and hence heart rate. The atria and ventricles are separated by a non-conducting band except at the *atrio-ventricular node*. This node consists of small myocytes that do conduct, but delay the impulse from the pacemaker, thus allowing the atria to contract before the ventricles. From here the impulse is distributed rapidly around the ventricles via bundles of specialised large myocytes called *Purkinje fibres*. Defects in any part of this conduction system can lead to a disordered heartbeat.   JEREMY WARD

See also HEART; PACEMAKER.

Cardiac output
The amount of blood per minute pumped out by each of the two ventricles of the heart. A typical value in an adult at rest is 5 litres per minute. The output of each ventricle is the product of the *stroke volume* (about 70 ml) and the *heart rate* (about 70 per minute). The output increases with muscular activity, in work or exercise perhaps to a maximum of 4–5 times the resting rate in an average healthy person, or up to 6–7 times in athletes; heart rate increases by a greater factor than stroke volume.   S.J.

See BLOOD CIRCULATION; EXERCISE; HEART.

Caricature
The caricature is amongst the most prevalent and popular of all 'art' forms. Certainly, comic representations of the rich and famous, the wicked, and the powerful appear prominently in newspapers and magazines the world over. While these images may contain many different aims and agendas, the most striking feature of all caricature is the distortion of the body: the thin are made skeletal, the plump swell to prodigious proportions, noses inevitably lengthen, while eyes either sink or bulge. Distortions of scale are accompanied by exaggerated representations of manner, dress, and temperament. Whether the target is the President of the US, a successful lawyer, or the Queen of England, the caricaturist's intention is to reveal a personality or characteristic through the comic exaggeration of their most visible feature, habit, or trait.

Given its widespread use, the term 'caricature' is often employed rather loosely to describe any form of burlesque, grotesque, or merely ludicrous representation. However, there is more to a caricature than the mere representation of ugliness. A better definition would hold that caricature is an artistic mode, usually in the form of a portraiture, in which the characteristic features of the subject are presented in a way that deforms or exaggerates their shape for comic effect. More precisely, the term 'caricature' (which is taken from the Italian *caricare*) means to overload or to overcharge: as such, caricatures pack meaning and detail onto otherwise simple body shapes.

Works of caricature can therefore be defined as excessive or deformed portraits of known individuals; the purpose of such images is generally satiric.

Given this lurid fascination with the ugly, the representation of comic monstrosity might fairly be said to determine the caricaturist's art. With their gross distortion and exaggerated postures the portraits of men and women provided by caricaturists seem distanced from a real encounter with the human body, its strength and frailties. However, this appearance is deceptive. The study of caricature can reveal a lot about changing attitudes to body shape, diet, and sexual activity. In the seventeenth and eighteenth centuries, caricaturists were much influenced (as were artists in many different genres) by the work of G. B. Della Porter (*De Humana Physiognomia*, 1586); Charles Le Brun (*Expression des Passions*, 1698); and Johann Kaspar Lavater (*Physiognomische Fragmente*, 1775). Le Brun's work described, via a mixture of simple sketches and rather more complicated descriptions, the most striking of facial and bodily attitudes: rage, grief, reverence, and so forth. Le Brun's illustrations provided artists, including caricaturists, with a basic template which they could revise (or distort) for their own purposes.

In the nineteenth century, as research in PHYSIOGNOMY gathered pace, texts such as Charles Darwin's *The Expression of Emotions in Man and Animals* can be seen to have had an influence on contemporary satiric portraits. Certainly anthropomorphic caricature was hugely popular from the middle years of the nineteenth century. As such, caricature provides a record, albeit an oblique one, of changing attitudes to the human body, its form, and its functions. The practice of caricature also has connotations of moral judgement, as well as bodily excess or mere physical form. Writing in 1991, Kenneth Rivers defined caricature as 'the artistic use of deformation for satirical purposes'. Although the intention behind any given caricature can be defined broadly as ridicule or satire, the precise motivation behind a particular piece can be varied. While the work of some caricaturists aims no higher than the exhibition of crude national or sexual stereotypes, many caricatures reveal more subtle ploys, and greater artistic and political aspirations. Indeed, the history of caricature has often been entwined with the history of censorship. The status of the caricaturist's art might fairly be defined as a negotiation between a crude impulse to ridicule and a higher wish for change or reformation.

Although the point will admit of some debate, it is safe to date the emergence of caricature (at least in its pictorial form) to the early sixteenth century. Leonardo da Vinci (1452–1519) is often cited as an early caricaturist. Certainly illustrations in his sketch books depict faces and figures with their features grossly deformed for deliberate comic effect. An equally plausible candidate for the title of first caricaturist is Annibale Carracci

(1560–1609). Carracci's paintings, of which *The Bean Eater* (1583–4) is a good example, blend the conventions of Italian low-life painting with a keen eye for characteristic detail. However, the claim that Carracci was the first caricaturist rests on the knowledge that his works generally represent recognisable individuals, and not anonymous or general types as is the case with da Vinci; witness, for instance his 'portraits' of old men and young girls in his sketch books.

Carracci's foremost achievement was to blend gross distortion with a general likeness, so that while the features of the face were turned and twisted the person portrayed remained easily recognisable. Along with that of his brother Agostino (1557–1602), Carracci's work defined the caricaturist's art as a mode of satiric portrayal which in rejecting the physical reality of the person represented sought to reveal a greater

moral truth through the exhibition of their vices. Unquestionably, it is the work of the Carracci brothers that made caricature both artistically successful and hugely popular, both in the sixteenth century, and arguably beyond. Carracci is even credited with offering the following defence of the caricaturist's art:

> Is not the caricaturist's task exactly the same as the classical artist's? Both see the lasting truth beneath the surface of mere outward appearance. Both try to help nature accomplish its plan. The one may strive to visualise the perfect form and to realise it in his work, the other to grasp perfect deformity, and thus reveal the very essence of a personality. A good caricature, like every work of art, is more true to life than reality itself.

Carracci's statement defends caricature on the grounds of its artistic worth, and its moral seriousness has been used by successive

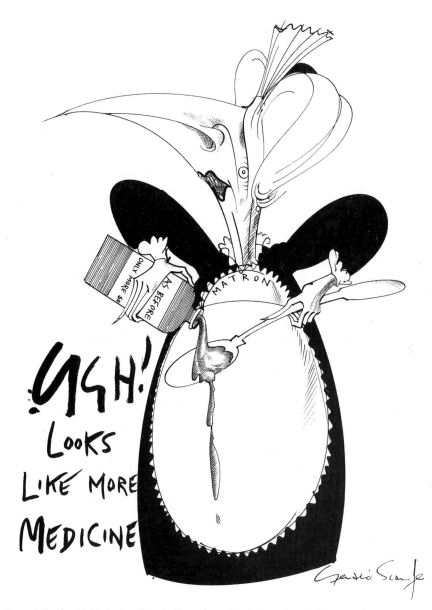

Margaret Thatcher (1983), by Gerald Scarfe. By courtesy of the National Portrait Gallery, London.

generations of practitioners and critics eager to defend caricature.

If Carracci established the worth and value of caricature in the Baroque period in Italy, then the golden age of British caricature was without question the eighteenth century. It was during this period that British art produced arguably some of the more playful, most incisive, and most savage caricatures ever attempted. William Hogarth (1697–1764), Thomas Rowlandson (1756–1827), and James Gilray (1756–1815) all flourished at this time. While Hogarth's graphic satires employ caricature sparingly as part of a more general lambasting of Georgian society, Gilray's cartoons viciously expose the foibles and deformities of his most prestigious contemporaries. Frequent victims of Gilray's pen were politicians such as the Prime Minister Pitt, who is depicted as thin and emaciated as if on the verge of collapse, while his opponent, the more ebullient Charles James Fox, appears fat and swarthy. Like Hogarth, Rowlandson's comedy is broader, but he still uses startling images of personal deformity in order to get his — sometimes cruel — jokes across. With the addition of George Cruikshank (1792–1878), and possibly Sir David Low (1891–1963), Hogarth, Gilray, and Rowlandson represent the finest achievements of British caricature. Today historians regularly cite the social and political satires of Gilray and Rowlandson as valuable evidence of prevailing attitudes and prejudices within eighteenth-century culture.

Undoubtedly influenced by work going on across the channel, French caricature flourished throughout the nineteenth century. In the uncertain political climate that followed the fall of Napoleon Bonaparte in 1815, pictorial satire enjoyed an uneasy existence. Its principal practitioners were Charles Philipon (1800–62) and Honoré Daumier (1808–79). Importantly, Philipon founded the weekly *La Caricature* in 1830, shortly to be followed by the daily *La Charivari*. Both journals provided an outlet for some of the finest caricatures the period produced. Certainly Philipon's representation of the hated Louis-Philippe as an overripe pear on the verge of rotting is a triumph of artistry and political expression. The detested king's flabby features coalesce to form the bulging sides of the fruit, an image which combines, brilliantly, physical ugliness with a distaste for the system of government that Louis-Philippe led. Although quickly repressed, Philipon's and Daumier's work in the 1830s was to have an influence on caricature in France, Europe, and the US for the remainder of the century.

More recently, the twin crises of the early twentieth century — the Great Depression and the rise of Fascism on the continent — have provided caricaturists with fertile if also painful subjects for their comedy. In Germany, George Grosz (1893–1959) used his art to expose the moral bankruptcy of the German state during the Weimar and Nazi periods. Almost entirely self-taught, Grosz drew spare caricatures representing opulent Germans as wholly debauched, their bodies glutted on sexual excess and political corruption. Happily, the twentieth century also saw more pleasurable and prosperous times. In reflecting upon the opulence of the twenties or the wealth of the 1980s, American journals such as *The New Yorker*, and the British comic magazine *Punch*, image an affluent society which they wish to chasten yet also to celebrate. The harsh images of Gilray and Grosz are not present, perhaps, but a canny social commentary remains.

ROBERT JONES

Further reading
Gombrich, E. H. and Ernst, K. (1940). *Caricature*. Penguin Books, Harmondsworth.

Rivers, K. T. (1991). *Transmutations: understanding literary and pictorial caricature*. University Press of America, Lanham, Maryland.

Victoria and Albert Museum (1984). *English caricature 1620 to the present: caricaturists and satirists, their art, their purpose and influence*. Victoria and Albert Museum, London.

See also ART AND THE BODY.

Carnivore One who eats meat; as opposed to a herbivore, who eats plants, or an omnivore who eats anything.   S.J.

See DIETS; FOOD.

Cartilage is a tough, resilient material, found in various sites but especially important in large weight-bearing JOINTS as it lines the articulating BONE ends. Due to its thickness and elasticity it is thought to act as a 'shock-absorber', cushioning the impact of movement. In the knee there is an extra layer of cartilage separating the bone ends (*meniscus*), presumably because of the amount of mechanical stress this joint is subjected to. These can be torn by rotational injuries, particularly in football and rugby players, a condition commonly referred to as 'torn cartilage'. It is sometimes possible to repair the meniscus by 'key-hole surgery' (*arthroscopy*) which avoids having to open the joint; if the damage is too great then the meniscus is removed (*meniscectomy*), usually by arthroscopy. Wear and thinning of articular cartilage in the knee and hip is associated with the development of osteoarthritis. Unlike most tissues in the body, cartilage has no blood vessels within it (it is '*avascular*') and relies on getting its nutrients, essential for the continued well-being of the cells within the cartilage matrix (*chondrocytes*), from the thin film of fluid lining the joint cavity (*synovial fluid*). This fluid is derived from the blood supplying the joint capsule, and its rapid turnover is important for keeping the chondrocytes supplied with oxygen and other essential substances. Cartilage is also found near the ends of long bones (*epiphysis*) in children, where it plays an important role in longitudinal bone growth after birth. New chondrocytes are generated, thickening the epiphysis producing lengthwise growth, whilst the cartilage matrix 'left behind' acquires mineral deposits and forms bone. Cartilage is also found in other sites such as the NOSE, EARS, and LARYNX (externally visible as the 'Adam's apple' in males), where it provides lightweight support or flexibility.   WILLIAM R. FERRELL

See also BONE; CONNECTIVE TISSUE; JOINTS.

Castration means removal of the testicles (TESTES). SPERM (spermatozoa) are made within the seminiferous tubules, which account for most of the volume of the testes. The male hormone, TESTOSTERONE, is made by the 'Leydig cells' (named after a nineteenth-century German microscopist) which lie between the seminiferous tubules.

Because the testicles make spermatozoa and testosterone, their removal results not only in sterility but also in loss of testosterone-dependent characteristics, including sex drive and the more typically male aggressive competitive drive in life. Historically in some societies, these effects were deliberately achieved in the creation of EUNUCHS, who would pose no sexual threat when employed to serve, for example, the women in a Turkish harem or a Chinese palace. Castrated boys retain their unbroken voice, and the history of the 'castrati' is told below. Castrated men tend to put on weight and are more liable to heart attacks.

In medical practice castration is sometimes used in the treatment of prostate cancer. This is because prostate cancer grows in response to testosterone and most of the cancer cells die when deprived of it. The main benefit of castration for an elderly man with PROSTATE cancer is that he does not have to remember to take any medication. Occasionally castration is necessary to treat testicular cancer when it involves both testicles; in this situation male hormone can be replaced by implants or patches and the typical eunuchoid characteristics can be avoided.

The term 'castration' is traditionally applied only to the male, but it is sometimes used also to refer to the removal of the ovaries in the female. The term 'chemical castration' may also be used to describe the hormonal suppression of the function of the testes, which mimics their removal.

Social and historical aspects
Castration was undertaken in earlier times because of the powerful, magical association with the genitalia. Thus the castration of the enemy or the enemy's corpse in some societies was a means of transferring the power of the male warrior to the victor. Slaves in ancient Rome and the Ottoman Empire could be castrated. Their castrated nature reflected their low social status.

Beginning in 1550–60 the practice of castration for musical purposes appears in Ferrara and Rome. In the musical tradition of the early modern period in Europe, the castration of young male singers provided a higher-pitched voice to sing soprano roles. The prohibition against women's voices in the Church had led to the attempt to create male parallels to women's voices. In the secular sphere, these voices became equally central to Italian opera in the seventeenth and eighteenth centuries, indeed the term 'musico' came to be an eighteenth-century euphemism for castrato. From the late seventeenth century the central male operatic role (*primo uomo*) in opera seria was sung by a castrato. The quality of the castrato's voice was unique. Castrati were considered to have 'natural' voices, as opposed to males who sang falsetto (whose studied voices were considered to be artificial). Many, such as the eighteenth-century castrati, Nicolo Grimaldi ('Nicolini') and Carlo Brosche ('Farinelli'), became extraordinarily famous in their own times. Beginning in the eighteenth century (at the height of their fame) there was a concerted attack on the practice and under the rule of the Jacobins in Italy (1796) the practice was banned, albeit temporarily. The last such castrato, Alessandro Moreschi, died in the early twentieth century and an acoustic recording exists of his voice (made in 1902–3).

With the discovery in the 1830s that an implanted testis could produce an internal secretion, a 'scientific' basis for the magical thinking about the relationship of SEXUALITY and power was established. Thus in the course of the nineteenth century ovariectomies were performed as therapy for pathologies such as 'HYSTERIA'. (The analogous procedure was the use of male circumcision as a surgical intervention for 'masturbatory insanity'.) The famed cultural critic Max Nordau wrote his medical dissertation in Paris on the topic of *De la castration de la femme* under the aegis of the neurologist Jean-Martin Charcot in 1882. In the late twentieth century, 'chemical castration' has become discussed as a punishment for sexually oriented crimes such as serial RAPE and PAEDOPHILIA.

In psychoanalysis castration is the fantasy of loss of the penis by the female or the anxiety about actual loss by the male. In the development of this concept of castration and penis envy, there was a powerful association of castration with the origins of anti-Semitism in the act of CIRCUMCISION. In Sigmund Freud's, *An outline of psychoanalysis*, which occupied his final months of life, Freud again returns to the 'meaning' of psychoanalysis in an extended footnote concerning the anxiety which the young boy feels when threatened with castration by his mother, a castration which is to be implemented by the father because of the child's masturbatory activity:

Castration has a place too in the Oedipus legend, for the blinding with which Oedipus punishes himself after the discovery of his crime is, by the evidence of dreams, a symbolic substitute for castration. The possibility cannot be excluded that a phylogenetic memory trace may contribute to the extraordinary terrifying effect of the threat — a memory trace from the pre-history of the primal family, when the jealous father actually robbed his son of his genitals if the latter became troublesome to him as a rival with a woman. The custom of circumcision, another symbolic substitute for castration, can only be understood as an expression of submission to the father's will. (cf. the puberty rites of primitive peoples.) No investigation has yet been made of the form taken by the events described above among peoples and in civilizations which do not suppress masturbation in children. (Standard Edition 23: 190.)

Two factors enter into this discussion: first, again, the theme of the unknown — here the unknown world of an unrepressed sexuality — and second, the universal claims of the phylogenetic model. It is this primary biological model which dominated Freud's biological thinking (as it did most of his contemporaries). Linked to this was the general acceptance of the view that acquired characteristics were inherited (the Lamarckian model). Indeed, Freud's biological model for this was a standard one for most late nineteenth-century biological scientists and physicians. The double model played itself out not only in the realm of the physical development of the genotype, but also in the construction of psychology of the group. It is in the real, phylogenetic experience of earlier generations that the psyche is formed, and it is in such group experience that the psychic development of each of us is mirrored. Employing Freud's theoretical matrix, Arnold Zweig in the 1930s noted that the Jewish prisoners in Rome had very low status because they had been vanquished and because 'they bore the sign of circumcision which was associated in the eyes of the people with castration'. Powerlessness and circumcision are linked because of the involuntary nature of castration in Roman society and because of its association with the status of the slave. This is quoted in the standard German Jewish Encyclopedia of the 1920s. Such a 'Jewish' view echoes those such as Conrad Rieger's that male Jews have a peculiar pathological construction such as a 'loss or absence of the testicles'. Both make the male less than a full-fledged man; a castrated man.

TIM HARGREAVE

SANDER L. GILMAN

Further reading

Barbier, P. (1996). *The world of the castrati: the history of an extraordinary operatic phenomenon*, (trans. Margaret Crosland). Souvenir, London.

Cheney, V. T. (1995). *A brief history of castration*. Crucial Concepts, Ozone Park, NY.

Gilman, S. L. (1993). *The case of Sigmund Freud: medicine and identity at the fin de siècle*. The Johns Hopkins University Press, Baltimore.

See also SEX HORMONES; SPERM; TESTES.

Catecholamines comprise important NEUROTRANSMITTERS and HORMONES, of which the main ones are DOPAMINE, NORADRENALINE (norepinephrine), and ADRENALINE (epinephrine). Other catecholamines occur in trace amounts in the body, and synthetic catecholamines are available; for example *isoprenaline* (isoproterenol) was previously employed for the relief of asthma, while *α-methylDOPA* reduces BLOOD PRESSURE. (They are all *catechols* (3,4-dihydroxyphenyl-) attached to a side-chain which ends in an *amine* group (primary, $-NH_2$, or substituted e.g. $-NHCH_3$).)

Adrenaline is commonly associated with feelings of ANXIETY, STRESS, anger, and excitement ('the adrenaline flowed'). The term 'fight or flight' is well-known in this context. While the overall picture is very complicated, it is clear that the catecholamines produced within the body play important roles in adapting the cardiovascular and other systems to an individual's changing needs in response to physical activity as well as to stressful or threatening events. They have these effects both by means of release as neurotransmitters from nerve endings of the sympathetic division of the AUTONOMIC NERVOUS SYSTEM or within the CENTRAL NERVOUS SYSTEM, and also by discharge into the bloodstream from the adrenal medulla.

The different catecholamines, although closely related structurally, can have widely differing physiological and pharmacological properties; can only be explained if the systems with which they interact have finely evolved ways of distinguishing between them and of coupling them to different cellular events. The differences are not only between the effects of the different substances on similar cells, but between the effects of any one of the catecholamines on different cells, or on the same cells under different conditions.

Adrenaline and noradrenaline

In 1948, in an attempt to provide a framework for explaining the different effects of noradrenaline and adrenaline, Ahlquist proposed the presence of several MEMBRANE RECEPTORS (*adrenoceptors*), coupled to different responses in the various target organs and tissues. His system, refined and extended, has stood the test of time. The two basic types are called α- and β-adrenoceptors, with main subdivisions into α_1 and α_2 and β_1 and β_2 but even further sub-divisions exist. Two major dopamine receptors, D_1 and D_2, have been identified and, again, further receptors and subdivisions have been proposed. All these receptors mediate the actions of catecholamines on target cells by activating intracellular messengers. These trigger the appropriate mechanism controlling the response, which might be contraction or relaxation of SMOOTH MUSCLES (including those of blood vessels, bronchioles, or gut), or stimulation of ENZYME action or of glandular secretion. It follows that the physiological and pharmacological actions of catecholamines can most effectively be described if their relative potencies on the different adrenoceptors, as well as the number and distribution of the adrenoceptors in the various organs and tissues, are known.

With few exceptions, the order of potency on α-adrenoceptors is noradrenaline, adrenaline, isoprenaline, while on the β-adrenoceptor, the order is reversed. Indeed, isoprenaline has virtually no effect on α-adrenoceptors. On the other hand, α-methylnoradrenaline is selective for α_2-adrenoceptors.

α_1-*adrenoceptors* are found on the CELL MEMBRANES of smooth muscle, liver, salivary glands, and sweat glands, and on nerve cells in the central nervous system. When activated, they stimulate a sequence of chemical events of which the end result is mainly the release of CALCIUM ions inside the cell, and this in turn mediates the final action. α_2-adrenoceptors are sited on nerve endings, both in those neurons that use noradrenaline as their neurotransmitter and other neurons that do not. They can also be found on smooth muscle where they mediate contraction. In the CNS, stimulation of α_2-adrenoceptors lowers blood pressure and causes sedation and even unconsciousness. The sequence of events that follows activation of α_2-adrenoceptors results in a reduction in the formation of *cyclic adenosine monophosphate* (cAMP) and this in turn mediates the ultimate effect.

β_1-*adrenoceptors* are the most important adrenoceptors in the HEART, where they mediate increase in heart rate and force. They relax gut smooth muscle, cause breakdown of fat, and cause amylase secretion from salivary glands. On nerve endings, they increase transmitter release. β_2-*adrenoceptors* are on smooth muscle, including blood vessels, bronchioles, uterus, bladder, and the iris, where they mediate relaxation. They cause tremor in skeletal muscle (shivering) and the breakdown of GLYCOGEN in the liver to release glucose into the blood, and decrease histamine release from mast cells.

Dopamine

Dopamine exerts its actions via the D_1 and D_2 receptors, which reside very largely in the CNS. It has much less effect than either noradrenaline or adrenaline on either α- or β-adrenoceptors (because it lacks the β-hydroxyl group which these others have on the side chain). The vast majority of dopaminergic nerves (those which release dopamine as their neurotransmitter, at synapses with other neurons) are restricted to 3 pathways in the CNS, related to movement coordination, to thought, feeling, and behaviour, and to the control of hormone release from the anterior pituitary gland. There are related abnormalities: decrease in dopamine release in the first pathway (or the administration of drugs which block the action of dopamine) leads to disturbances of movement associated with Parkinson's disease; excess dopamine activity in the brain leads to stereotyped behaviours in experimental animals and may account for some of the symptoms of schizophrenia in man; dopamine, and drugs that mimic it, cause nausea and vomiting through an action on a trigger zone in the brain stem. Its action on the pituitary leads to reduced prolactin and increased growth hormone release. It causes vasodilatation of blood vessels in the kidney and mesentery through interaction with dopamine receptors, vasoconstriction elsewhere via α_1-adrenoceptors, and stimulation of the heart via β_1-adrenoceptors.

Endogenous catecholamines are synthesised in neurons and in the *chromaffin* cells of the adrenal medulla, and stored in intracellular vesicles. Dopamine is formed first from the aminoacid, *tyrosine*. Dopamine is the immediate precursor of noradrenaline, which is in turn the precursor of adrenaline. This full sequence takes place only in chromaffin tissue, where all three substances are made, and in a relatively small number of truly 'adrenergic' nerves in the CNS, which release adrenaline as their transmitter. Nearly all so-called 'adrenergic neurons' (comprising most of the final or 'post-ganglionic' sympathetic nerve supply to the various tissues) are, in reality, 'noradrenergic', because they release noradrenaline as their transmitter and are unable to synthesise adrenaline. Likewise, 'dopaminergic' neurons release dopamine and cannot make either noradrenaline or adrenaline.

The actions of catecholamines after their release are terminated by their re-uptake into the sympathetic nerve endings and into certain non-neuronal cells such as smooth muscle. After re-uptake in nerve cells they are broken down by the action of *monoamine oxidase*; this enzyme plays a vital role in controlling the concentrations of catecholamine transmitters while scavenging and destroying unwanted amines. Catecholamines taken up by cells other than neurons are also degraded by enzymes. The combined product of these actions on both noradrenaline and adrenaline is vanilmandelic acid, which appears in normal urine. Raised excretion of vanilmandelic acid can indicate the presence of a catecholamine-secreting tumour.

B.A. CALLINGHAM

See also ADRENAL GLAND; AUTONOMIC NERVOUS SYSTEM; NEUROTRANSMITTERS.

Celibacy

The ideal of celibacy — abstaining from sexual activity for religious or spiritual reasons — exists within several religions. It has been an ideal within Christianity from the earliest times. Jesus spoke of those who are 'eunuchs for the sake of the kingdom of heaven' (Matthew 19: 12), and Paul recommended celibacy as the best way of living, for it enabled a person to be free from distracting 'worldly' concerns, especially the household, children, and sex — and for men, the worldly was particularly represented by the female body — and therefore free to serve Christ. Thus, for many centuries, especially in the West, marriage was regarded as an inferior option for Christians, for those who needed to produce heirs or could not practice self-control because they did not have the 'gift' of celibacy. Only at the Reformation, when Protestant reformers began to privilege and justify marriage, was this view seriously challenged. Even in the post-Reformation period, there have been new Christian groups which have set celibacy as an ideal or rule, most notably the Shakers in nineteenth-century America, who formed communities of celibate men and women to live a simple life together. Roman Catholic, Eastern Orthodox, and Anglican monastic communities retain the ideal of celibacy to this day.

In the early Church celibacy had been an individual vocation, so marriage was not incompatible with holding ecclesiastical office; but beginning with the canons of the Council of Elvira (c. 306), the Church in the West increasingly moved towards clerical celibacy as the norm; married men who were ordained were urged to put aside their wives, go on living with them as sister and brother, or exchange vows of continence with them; their wives might then become deaconesses or join a monastic community. Throughout the later Middle Ages the Roman Catholic Church attempted to enforce clerical celibacy, not always with great success; the second Lateran Council (1139) made clerical marriages invalid. Clerical celibacy remains the rule in the Roman Catholic despite pressures in the late twentieth century to change this. The Church of England allowed clerical marriage in 1549, as did the Protestant churches at the Reformation. The Eastern Orthodox churches have always allowed their priests and deacons to marry before ordination, though not after, and their bishops must be celibate.

Within Buddhism, celibacy is a permanent vocation for monks and nuns. Within Hinduism, celibacy is part of the fourth and final stage — *samnyasa* — for the Hindu who is following the Vedic way. This is the stage of renouncing all ties to family, caste, and property. Within a number of religions, reactions to celibacy are mixed. For Sikhs, it is not an ideal, for the Gurus taught that the married state (*grihastha ashrama*) was the ideal. But there are two Sikh groups that dissent from this: the *Udasis* (meaning 'withdrawn' or 'dejected') are an ascetic order, also forbidden to consume flesh, tobacco, or spirits; they wear salmon-coloured clothing and are clean shaven, though they often have long, matted hair. The *Nirmalas* (meaning 'spotless' or 'pure') are a learned monastic group who live in monasteries called *akharas* (meaning 'wrestling arenas') and wear saffron robes. Islam is generally hostile to celibacy, emphasising the God-given goodness of creation, though *Sufism*, especially in its beginnings, has emphasized the strong control of body and spirit via ascetical practices, including celibacy. Early Sufi leaders saw lust as one of the seven gates to hell, one Sufi leader even going so far as to say that Sufism was founded on celibacy.

Judaism has generally not advocated celibacy, seeing marriage as important for the fulfilment of procreation as commanded in Genesis 1: 28. The High Priest in Temple times had to be married (Leviticus 21: 13) and the unmarried were barred from holding various public offices, though there were two important Jewish first-century Ascetic groups. The *Therapeutae* (Latin, 'healers'), described by Philo, lived in Egypt in solitude, poverty, and (as far as was possible) celibacy, meditating on spiritual writings. Both men and women could be members. Every fiftieth day, they gathered for a meal and sang and danced. The all-male *Essene* community by the Dead Sea (where the Dead Sea Scrolls were found in 1947) sought to bring Israel back to God by their own rigorous and celibate way of life. This relationship between apocalyptic beliefs and the ideal of celibacy forms the backdrop to Jesus' preaching about the coming of the Kingdom of Heaven, which was intimately entwined with his call to follow him and leave behind all family ties. Thus in Christianity, the celibate was seen to anticipate the state of the human being at resurrection — described by some as a state in which the sexes do not exist and there is no place for marriage. The celibate therefore sought to return to his or her original — that is pre-Fall — state. As Genesis records Adam and Eve as having had sexual intercourse only after the Fall, sexual renunciation was a vital component in acquiring this pre-lapsarian 'state'. This meant the transcendence of gender, and while, for some celibates at least, it meant that the body was seen as alien to the true self, many explored the possibilities of that transcendence. Celibacy, and the ascetic way of life in general, were appealing because they allowed any Christian, regardless of gender or social status, to transcend what their body represented in this world; this was particularly appealing for women, especially élite women, whose bodies functioned primarily to produce heirs and thereby circulate wealth in the Roman world. That some writers spoke of Christian women 'becoming male' to indicate their great holiness illustrates the double-edged nature of this ideal of celibacy for women. Suspicion of the female body, and projection onto it of all the male celibate's fears of 'the world' exists within Christianity generally, and has existed particularly within the monastic communities from the fourth century onwards, and is shared by Buddhism and the early Sufis. JANE SHAW

Further reading

Brown, P. (1988). *The body and society, men, women and sexual renunciation in early Christianity.* Columbia University Press, New York.

See also ASCETICISM; CHASTITY ; RELIGION AND THE BODY.

Cell The cell is the fundamental unit of all living things. The simplest forms of life are single-celled organisms; these include both 'prokaryotes' — bacteria, which have a simple internal structure — and the much more complex 'eukaryotes' (*pro*, before or preceding; *eu*, good, normal, and *karyon*, a kernel). Higher organisms, such as man, are sophisticated communities in which groups of eukaryotic cells carry out specialized functions and communicate with each other. Prokaryotes are usually about one thousandth of a millimetre in diameter. Eukaryotic cells are much larger, typically around one to two hundredths of a millimetre. There are about 100 million million cells in the human body. Both prokaryotes and eukaryotes usually multiply by dividing in two, although in multicellular organisms cell division is under strict control.

It was the invention of the microscope, in the seventeenth century, that allowed scientists the first glimpses of individual cells. In particular, the Dutchman, Antoni van Leeuwenhoek described the extraordinary variety of motile single-celled organisms (which he called '*animalcules*') present in pond water. The word 'cell' (from the Latin *cella*, 'a small room') was first coined in 1665, by the English physicist Robert Hooke, to refer to the microscopic structure of cork. Technical improvements in microscopy in the eighteenth and nineteenth centuries allowed more precise observation. It gradually became apparent that cells had a complicated internal structure, and that some features (for example, what we now refer to as the nucleus) were common to most cells, even though the appearance of the cells themselves varied enormously. This in turn hinted that a common basic organization might underlie all living matter.

The first simple distinction had been between nucleus and cytoplasm — the rest of the cellular substance — but by the end of the nineteenth century the principal internal components of cells that we are familiar with today (sub-cellular structures or *organelles*) had been identified. These included the *endoplasmic reticulum* (an extensive network of membranes within the cell), *mitochondria* (cylindrical, membrane-limited structures) and the *Golgi complex* (a stack of flattened membrane sacs, named after the Italian anatomist who described those and other intracellular structures in 1898, and later shared a Nobel prize with Spaniard Ramón y Cajal). The true complexity of the internal structure of cells, however, only became apparent in the 1950s, when cells were examined with the newly-invented electron microscope, which had much greater resolving power than the conventional light microscope — magnifying 20–30 000 times. It was around this time that the field now known as cell biology began to come to prominence, with the goal of understanding how the various organelles acted together to allow the cell to carry out its many functions. As well as simply observing cell structure, cell biologists now began to take cells apart and purify the different organelles using high-speed centrifugation. It was also shown that the purified organelles could be made to work in isolation, which allowed a detailed study of their functions, and the identification of the mechanisms underlying them.

Our current view of the cell is as an organism-in-miniature. The blueprint is contained in the DNA, packaged into chromosomes in the nucleus. Parts of the DNA sequence are replicated into 'messenger' RNA, which exits the nucleus and specifies the sequences of the cell's proteins, which are constructed in the cytoplasm. The power-houses of the cell are the mitochondria, which use nutrients taken up from outside to generate ATP, the energy currency of the cell. (Plant cells have additional organelles, the chloroplasts, which contain chlorophyll, the molecule responsible for capturing the energy of sunlight and initiating the process of photosynthesis. This results in the production of carbon-containing molecules for use by the cell and the generation of oxygen, which is essential for the continuation of life on earth.)

Many cells are responsible for secreting substances which will have external effects. In the pancreas, for instance, some cells secrete enzymes into the gut, where they digest our food,

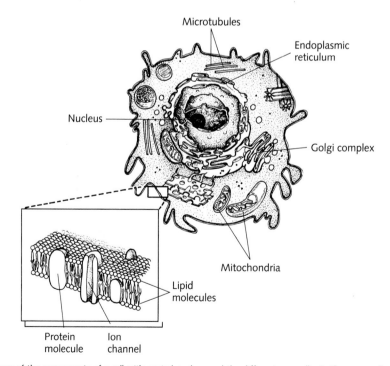

Diagram of the components of a cell with central nucleus and the different organelles in the surrounding cytoplasm; in reality the organelles are very much smaller in relation to the size of the cell and very much more numerous. Inset: enlarged diagram of the cell membrane. The hydrophilic 'heads' of the molecules of the lipid bilayer form both surfaces of the membrane.

whereas other cells secrete insulin into the bloodstream, which instructs cells in the rest of the body to take up glucose. Both the digestive enzymes and the insulin are packaged into the endoplasmic reticulum and are then transported to the surface of the cell via the Golgi apparatus. Thus although each organelle is a discrete structure, there is extensive communication between organelles. This intracellular trafficking system demands that there be strict controls on the movement of proteins between organelles, and that individual proteins be 'tagged' for delivery to particular destinations. Without this control, the organization of the cell would quickly disintegrate.

A single higher organism contains a huge variety of cell types: compare, for example, a neuron with a lymphocyte, or a skeletal muscle cell with a liver cell (hepatocyte). All of these cells were produced from a single fertilized egg, by processes including cell division, migration, differentiation, and death. We are only just beginning to understand how these processes are orchestrated to produce the complete organism. One aspect that is crucial to the development and maintenance of multicellular organisms is communication between cells. Cells are continually signalling to their neighbours through the release of molecules that are detected by specialized receptors on the surface of other cells. In the brain, for example, neurons 'talk' to each other by means of small molecules. These molecules, or 'neurotransmitters', are packaged in small sacs within the neurons, and are released when an electrical impulse passes to the end of its axon. The neurotransmitter then binds to receptors on the neighbouring neurons and changes the electrical properties of these neurons, making them more or less likely to initiate an electrical impulse themselves. In other parts of the body, neurons communicate in similar fashion with muscle cells, causing them to contract, or with glandular cells, causing them to secrete. Many drugs work by blocking or mimicking the action of these neurotransmitters. Again, some cells release molecules which travel in the blood: messengers which communicate with remotely distant cells that have the appropriate receptors on their surface.

Once tissues and organs have been formed it is essential that cell division be strictly controlled in order to maintain normal function. Many proteins are now known which control cell division, often in response to external stimuli. Mutations in these proteins can result in uncontrolled cell division. This can lead eventually to the formation of tumours, which can be life threatening.

We are now familiar with the idea that cells are produced by the division of progenitor cells. This idea, of course, begs the question as to how the first cell was produced. It has been shown that simple organic molecules can form under conditions believed to be similar to those that existed on earth in its early history. How these molecules became assembled into proteins, and more

particularly how the self-replicating 'blueprint' molecules such as DNA came about, are fundamental unanswered questions.

MICHAEL EDWARDSON

See also CELL MEMBRANES; CELL SIGNALLING.

Cell membranes Every cell has a *plasma membrane* that encloses it and maintains differences between the cell contents and the outside environment that are crucial to the function of the cell. All biological membranes consist of assemblies of lipid and PROTEIN molecules. The lipids are rod-shaped molecules arranged in a double layer so that their *hydrophobic* ends, which repel water, point inwards and their *hydrophilic* ends, which attract it, point towards the aqueous environment and the inside of the cell. This *lipid bilayer* provides the basic structure of the membrane, and forms a barrier that is relatively impermeable to most water-soluble molecules. Proteins are embedded in the bilayer; they also have hydrophobic surfaces in contact with the lipids, and hydrophilic surfaces exposed on either side of the membrane. At physiological temperatures, the lipid bilayer is fluid, and so the proteins are able to move about within the plane of the membrane. The two leaflets of the bilayer contain different lipids, and different proteins are exposed on the two faces of the membrane.

The respiratory gases exchange freely across the membrane, because OXYGEN and CARBON DIOXIDE are soluble in lipid. Apart from this it is the proteins that span the membrane which act as pumps and channels for the exchange of materials between the inside and outside of the cell. They allow entry of nutrients into the cell and the exit of waste products. They are also responsible for generating differences in the ionic composition between the inside and the outside of the cell. Finally, proteins act as molecular sensors (MEMBRANE RECEPTORS) allowing the cell to change its behaviour in response to external chemical signals. In addition to the plasma membrane, most cells contain a variety of *organelles* — internal structures that are also surrounded by membranes. These include the nucleus, the endoplasmic reticulum, the Golgi complex, and the mitochondria.

Many membrane proteins are made on *ribosomes* (granules of nucleoprotein) bound to the membrane of the endoplasmic reticulum. Those bound for the plasma membrane are recognised and then inserted into the lipid bilayer locally, before being transported to their final destination by a trafficking system that relies on further signals within the protein. Proteins for the mitochondrial membrane are recognised and then inserted directly from the cytoplasm.

The most fundamental difference between the inside and the outside of a typical cell is in the *ionic composition*. In particular, the inside of the cell has a low concentration of sodium ions and a high concentration of potassium ions; the reverse is true of the fluid outside. This difference in ionic composition is generated by ion 'pumps', which use energy in the form of ATP, produced by

mitochondrial respiration, to drive sodium ions out of the cell and potassium ions in. In addition to this ion-pumping function, most membranes contain ION CHANNELS that let ions diffuse across the membrane passively when they open. The concentration gradients for different ions across the membranes are exploited widely by cells to drive the movement of other molecules across the membrane. For example, glucose enters cells on a carrier protein that carries both sodium and glucose. Furthermore, in specialized cells, such as neurons, the *ion gradients* are also used to generate electrical signals that propagate along their axons and allow neurons to 'talk' to each other through the release of 'neurotransmitter' molecules.

The ability of many proteins to diffuse freely within the plane of the membrane allows them to interact transiently with protein partners, which is often crucial to their function. For instance, many receptor proteins recognize signals outside the cell and then pass the signals on to other proteins that affect cell behaviour. In other cases, though, it is important for the cell to cluster proteins at a particular region of the membrane; this is seen where receptors are localized adjacent to the site of neurotransmitter release at a SYNAPSE. This localization involves the coupling of the membrane proteins to a 'scaffold' within the cell, known as the *cytoskeleton*, via specialized anchoring proteins recruited from the cytoplasm.

Although the many organelles within the cell are enclosed by membranes, they are highly dynamic, and many are in constant communication with each other. Proteins are transported in *membrane vesicles* that bud from one organelle and fuse with the other; for example between the endoplasmic reticulum and the Golgi complex, and between the Golgi complex and the plasma membrane. The *budding process* involves the selection of proteins to be transported and the formation of a protein scaffolding that is able to pinch off a patch of membrane to form a vesicle. The vesicle must then locate and fuse with its target membrane. It is the specificity of these membrane budding-and-fusion events that permits organelles to maintain their integrity despite extensive communication between them.

A particularly good example of the specificity of membrane traffic is found in *epithelial cells*, such as those that form the tubules of the KIDNEY, where the plasma membrane contains two domains that perform different functions and contain different proteins (one facing outwards to the lumen of the tubule where the urine is being formed, and the other facing inwards to the tissue fluid and the blood). The two sets of proteins are synthesized together on the membrane of the endoplasmic reticulum and are later segregated into two populations of vesicles. These vesicles are then able to recognize and fuse with the two separate domains of the plasma membrane. Without this specific targeting of proteins, epithelial polarity would break down, and epithelial secretory and absorptive function would be lost.

Cell membranes are continually in a state of flux. The delivery of new membrane into the plasma membrane is balanced by the removal of membrane by the process of *endocytosis*: inward budding of vesicles. Endocytosis is responsible also for the internalization of important molecules from the outside of the cell, such as CHOLESTEROL in the form of low density lipoprotein, and iron in the form of the protein transferrin. Endocytosis is also used as a route of access into the cell by rogue invaders: certain toxins, such as botulinum toxin, or enveloped viruses, such as the influenza virus.

MICHAEL EDWARDSON

See also CELL; ION CHANNELS; NEUROTRANSMITTERS; TRANSPORT.

Cell signalling

Even the simplest unicellular organisms detect and respond to changes in their environment, but it is in multicellular organisms that signalling mechanisms are most highly developed. The division of labour that allows cells to adopt such diverse and specialised functions as muscle contraction, defending the body from disease, and absorbing and then distributing essential nutrients, is possible only because the activities of all the cells within an organ or tissue are co-ordinated and the activities of every organ and tissue are orchestrated to meet the needs of the body as a whole. Long-distance communication is by means of nerves and circulating hormones; the principal function of many organs, notably the endocrine glands, is to facilitate such communication between organs.

Cells communicate with each other by means of an enormous diversity of signalling molecules. These molecules have traditionally been classified according to the distance over which they act.

Local communication between neighbouring cells is described as *paracrine* signalling. This includes direct physical contact between proteins expressed on the surface of adjacent cells; the release of short-acting messengers, like NITRIC OXIDE, whose ranges of action are limited by their rapid inactivation; and the chemical communication between neurons. This last is provided by synaptic messengers or neurotransmitters (e.g. ACETYLCHOLINE), which are released from the terminal of a neuron into the specialized area of contact that it makes with another neuron or muscle; the SYNAPSE. Such messengers need to diffuse only a few millionths of a centimetre to reach their target and can thereby very specifically address only the tiniest part of the body, perhaps only one of the 100 000 spines on a single neuron from among the 100 000 million neurons in a human BRAIN. *Autocrine* signalling, wherein cells respond to signalling molecules that they have themselves released, is often presented as another category of signalling mechanism, although it too describes local communication, but between similar cells. Another form of local communication is provided by *gap junctions*, which directly link the cytoplasm of certain cells and so allow the exchange both of ions and

of small molecules between them. The co-ordinated contraction of the many individual fibres within a human HEART, for example, depends upon them being linked by gap junctions.

At the opposite extreme are the PHEROMONES released by one person and detected by another. In the middle of the distance range lies *endocrine* signalling, mediated by the hormones (e.g. *insulin*) released from specialised endocrine glands into the bloodstream, which delivers them to their targets. Hormones may thereby exert their effects on many different tissues (in the case of insulin, primarily the liver, muscle, and fat) and so evoke an appropriately co-ordinated physiological response from widely separated organs and tissues.

Receptors are the means by which each of the chemical messengers that mediate intercellular communication are detected and decoded. Some messengers (nitric oxide and the steroid hormones are examples) are sufficiently hydrophobic to pass through the lipid plasma membrane that surrounds every cell and so gain direct access to the intracellular receptor proteins through which they mediate their physiological effects. Most messengers, however, cannot pass directly through the lipid and instead exert their effects by binding to and activating receptors that span the plasma membrane. From both their functional and structural properties, these receptors can be grouped into distinct families. The first comprises those in which the receptor protein forms a *channel* that opens when the receptor binds its messenger and allows specific ions to flow across the plasma membrane. Such receptors are commonly responsible for the fastest forms of chemical communication between cells, and include the nicotinic receptors that mediate the voluntary control of skeletal muscle. A second family includes the many hundreds of receptors that regulate cellular activity by first causing activation of a *G protein*. These G proteins, which themselves comprise a large family of proteins, have an intrinsic timer that allows them to remain active for a period, typically several seconds, after the receptor has caused their activation. A single receptor with its messenger bound is thereby able to sustain the activation of many G proteins and so provide an amplification step in the signalling pathway. Such amplification at both this and later steps in these signalling pathways allows cells to be exquisitely sensitive to very low concentrations of circulating hormones. The active G proteins are responsible for relaying the signal onwards to the ultimate physiological response by regulating either the opening of ion channels or the activities of intracellular enzymes. The latter include the enzymes responsible for both the synthesis and degradation of the intracellular messengers (e.g. cyclic AMP) that serve as the currency for intracellular communication. Earl W. Sutherland, who received the Nobel Prize for Physiology or Medicine in 1971, was the first to recognise that, despite the plethora of extracellular messengers each recognized by a unique receptor, intracellular signalling was

likely to use a far more limited repertoire of signalling molecules or *second messengers*. The idea that specific receptors are the antennae of a cell that are fine-tuned to respond to only very specific signals from the babble of signals to which a cell is exposed, and then direct them to a small range of intracellular messengers, remains the keystone of cell signalling. A third, and very much more diverse, grouping of receptors includes those that are capable of either directly phosphorylating certain tyrosine residues of specific proteins or else activating accessory proteins with that ability. After activation, these receptors (which include the *insulin receptor*) serve as molecular scaffolds around which additional signalling proteins can assemble to generate rather complex webs of intracellular signals, mediated by both small soluble messengers and specific interactions between proteins. These *receptor tyrosine kinases* and their relatives are commonly, though not exclusively, involved in controlling long-term aspects of cellular behaviour, such as cell growth or differentiation.

C. W. TAYLOR

See also CALCIUM; HORMONES; MEMBRANE RECEPTORS; NEUROTRANSMITTERS.

Central nervous system

The central nervous system (CNS) consists of the BRAIN (inside the skull) and SPINAL CORD (inside the vertebral column), which derive from a single, continuous tube of neural tissue that forms at an early stage in the embryo. The head end of the tube develops into the *cerebral hemispheres*, the CEREBELLUM, and the BRAIN STEM. The lowest part of the brain stem, the *medulla oblongata*, merges with the spinal cord at the large hole (*foramen magnum*) in the base of the skull. The spinal cord in an adult human is about 45 cm long, tapering to a cone at its lower end. It has two swellings, the *cervical* and *lumbar enlargements*, which are due to accumulations of nerve cells (*neurons*) responsible for innervating the upper and lower limbs.

Both the brain and the spinal cord are ensheathed by three protective MENINGES (from the Greek for 'membranes'). The outer one, the *dura mater* ('*dura*' because it is relatively hard and strong; '*mater*' because it protects like a mother) lines the skull and the tunnel that runs through the centre of the vertebrae. The delicate, innermost *pia mater* ('*pia*' is Latin for soft) envelops the brain and the spinal cord closely down to the level of the upper lumbar vertebrae. Between the pia and dura is a space, particularly voluminous below where the cord itself ends. The dura is lined by the *arachnoid mater*, which is more fragile than the dura, being likened to a spider's web, the Greek origin of its name. So the space between the pia and dura, which contains CEREBROSPINAL FLUID (*CSF*), is called the *subarachnoid space*.

Twelve pairs of CRANIAL NERVES are attached to the brain, at various levels. Some, such as the olfactory and optic nerves, are purely sensory. Others, such as those supplying the muscles that move the eyeball, are motor. The tenth cranial nerve, called the 'VAGUS' (Latin for wanderer), carries sensory information from some of the viscera and also contains the outflow of *para-sympathetic* fibres (part of the AUTONOMIC NERVOUS SYSTEM) that innervate the heart, the bronchial tree, the smooth muscle of much of the gut, and various glands.

Evolutionarily, the central nervous system is derived from the repetitive, segmented chain of nerve cells found in invertebrates, and this segmental pattern is still clear in the human spinal cord, and even in the lower parts of the brain. It is most evident in the *spinal nerves*, 31 pairs in all, that sprout from the sides of the spinal cord. Strictly, these spinal nerves are part of the peripheral nervous system, but their organization is best understood in relation to the cord itself. For each vertebra, on each side of the cord is a *dorsal root* ('dorsal' means on the top), containing sensory nerve fibres from the periphery of the body, which are destined to end in the cord or the base of the brain. The neuron cell bodies for these fibres are in swellings on the dorsal roots (*dorsal root ganglia*). There is a corresponding pair of *ventral roots* ('ventral' literally meaning on the side nearer the stomach), containing axons from motor neurons in the cord, on their way to skeletal muscles. Additional fibres leave the ventral roots in the middle levels of the cord to innervate smooth muscle (e.g. that of blood vessel walls and the gut), glands, and the heart. These are the *sympathetic* fibres and are also part of the autonomic nervous system. Just outside each vertebra, the dorsal and ventral roots unite to form a spinal nerve on each side.

If you cut a spinal cord transversely, you can see, even with the naked eye, a central, butterfly-shaped core of darker material. If such a section is examined with a microscope it becomes clear that this core consists of GREY MATTER (grey because of a concentration of cell bodies), surrounded by columns of WHITE MATTER (white because it consists largely of nerve fibres — *axons*), running up and down the cord. The dorsal part of the grey matter receives fibres of the dorsal root, relaying information about touch, temperature, pain, and also position sense. The ventral part of the grey matter contains motor neurons that send out their axons in the ventral root to reach the skeletal muscles.

Imagine what happens as nervous impulses arrive at the cord through fibres of the dorsal root. This sensory information is of several types. Firstly, it is either *somatic* (from skin, muscles, and joints) or *visceral* (from the internal organs) in origin. Secondly it may give rise to *conscious* sensation, which presupposes that the information is transmitted from the spinal cord to higher brain centres, and ultimately the CEREBRAL CORTEX. Alternatively it remains *unconscious*, in which case it may be handled by brain centres such as the *cerebellum*, or it may simply feed a pathway within the spinal cord, ultimately resulting in signals passing out to cause muscle reactions (a *spinal reflex*).

Fibres concerned with touch, temperature, and pain end on nerve cell bodies in the dorsal grey matter, which in turn send axons across to the other side of the cord and then up to the brain. Many of them reach the THALAMUS, projecting thence to, amongst other regions, the *somatic sensory cortex* — a strip at the front edge of the parietal lobe of the cerebral hemispheres. Fibres that convey conscious position sense and fine discriminative touch also enter the cord by dorsal roots, but they behave differently in that they immediately turn upward on the same side of the cord and run all the way up through a tract of white matter called the *dorsal columns*, merely sending branches into the dorsal grey matter of the spinal cord along the way. These fibres end on groups of cells in the medulla of the brain stem, whose axons cross to the other side and run up to the thalamus, from where axons run up to the somatic sensory cortex.

The basic function of the central nervous system is to generate appropriate reactions to sensory signals, from inside or outside the body. The simplest form of such a reaction is a '*reflex*' — an involuntary response to a sensory stimulus. The circuit of nerve cells and axons responsible is called a *reflex arc*. The simplest form of reflex arc involves an incoming fibre, which traverses the dorsal grey matter of the spinal cord to terminate at a SYNAPSE on a motor neuron in the ventral grey matter, whose axon runs out to a muscle. Since this circuit contains only one synaptic connection, it is called a *monosynaptic* reflex. The best known example is the '*tendon jerk reflex*': when a muscle is suddenly stretched it reflexly contracts, to oppose the stretching. For instance, when the tendon just below the knee is tapped, stretching the thigh muscles to which this tendon is attached, the same muscles contract, causing the leg to kick. Such tendon jerks are tested as part of a routine neurological examination, to assess the state of synaptic connections. This very simple type of reflex arc is relatively rare, most reflexes being *complex* or *multisynaptic*. This implies that the circuit between incoming sensory fibre and motoneuron includes other nerve cells. As these may innervate several levels of the cord, or even cross to the other side, these reflexes can be much more sophisticated than simple ones. For example, burning the tip of a finger may result in reflex withdrawal of the whole upper limb.

Some reflexes, although involuntary, almost certainly involve connections running through the cerebral cortex, or through the cerebellum, which is particularly involved in the learning and execution of motor skills, especially highly automated ones whose operation does not intrude into consciousness.

As well as major 'ascending' pathways carrying sensory information up to the corresponding regions of the cerebral cortex, the white matter of the brain stem and spinal cord also contains many tracts of fibres running downwards. The largest of these is the *corticospinal*, or *pyramidal*, tract, which originates in large

neurons in motor areas of the cerebral cortex, and descends to the lower brain stem, where most of its axons cross over and enter the spinal cord to end, without interruption, on motoneurons in the grey matter.

This brief account leaves the impression that the central nervous system is little more than a set of cables running up and down, with something akin to a telephone switchboard in between. In reality, the human central nervous system is a monstrous biological computing instrument (although many would contest the analogy with a conventional computer), which is somehow capable of capturing the *meaning* of events in the outside world, representing them in memories and as conscious experiences, and making decisions that go far beyond automatic reactions to immediate events.

LAURENCE GAREY

See PLATE 6.

See also AUTONOMIC NERVOUS SYSTEM; BRAIN; NERVOUS SYSTEM; REFLEXES; SPINAL CORD.

Cerebellum ('little brain'): an intricately corrugated ball of nervous tissue that lies under the rear end of the cerebral hemispheres and is attached to the brain stem by huge bundles of nerve fibres, the cerebellar peduncles, which carry information to and from other parts of the brain.

The cerebellum makes up more than one-tenth of the volume of the human brain. The basic circuitry of nerves within it is essentially similar in all vertebrates and during evolution it has changed much less in size, relative to the body, than have the cerebral hemispheres. These facts suggest that it has some essential, basic function in all vertebrates. Although its exact mechanisms remain unclear, its fundamental role is in the control of MOVEMENT. This was clearly recognised by the seventeenth-century physician Thomas Willis in his book *Cerebri Anatome* (1664) and the idea can be traced back to the observations and interpretations of Galen (*c*. 130–210 AD).

The cerebellum comprises an outer, thin layer of GREY MATTER — the cerebellar cortex — covering a core of WHITE MATTER, within which lie three lumps of grey matter on each side of the midline (the deep cerebellar nuclei). Closest to the midline is the *fastigial nucleus* and furthest from it is the *dentate nucleus*, with the *interpositus nucleus* between.

The surface area of the cortex is greatly augmented by folds that run across from side to side — deep ones that divide the surface into ten *lobules*, and numerous shallower ones cutting each lobule into *folia*. If the cortex were flattened out, it would be a ribbon much longer than it is wide.

The cortex is divided up functionally into longitudinal (i.e. fore-and-aft) strips or zones, each interconnected with a particular deep nucleus. The *vermis*, running down the middle, connects with the right and left fastigial nuclei. This is flanked on each side by a *paravermal cortical zone*

145

related to nucleus interpositus; and most lateral is the pair of large *cerebellar hemispheres*, linked to the dentate nuclei. Since the 1960s studies in animals have shown that each cortical zone comprises many narrower micro-zones, each relating to a particular 'private' portion of the corresponding deep nucleus.

The fine structure of the cortex and the circuits that link it with the deep nuclei vary little from place to place, which suggests that all parts of the cerebellum perform a similar basic 'computation' or operation. If different parts of the cerebellum have different functional roles, this must be due to differences in their input and output connections rather than their internal wiring.

Damage to part or even all of the human cerebellum, on its own, does not lead to clear impairment of intellect, emotion, or vegetative functions (such as the control of the heart and breathing). But there is abundant evidence that the control of movements is markedly disordered. Typically, patients with cerebellar damage are unsteady on their feet, and their hands shake as they try to point or lift objects ('intention tremor'); their eyes swing uncontrollably from side to side (NYSTAGMUS); and even their speech can be jerky ('scanning speech'). These three typical signs, described by the great nineteenth-century French neurologist Charcot, are known as 'Charcot's Triad'.

The movements most affected vary somewhat depending on the location of the damage. No type of movement is completely lost, but movements ranging in complexity from simple reflex actions to walking, speech, and highly skilled manipulations may all be defective in rate, range, force, and timing. Extremely rarely, individuals are born with little or no cerebellum, and although some of its functions may be taken over by other parts of the brain, movements are permanently clumsy and poorly co-ordinated, suggesting that the learning of motor skills is impaired.

The 600 000 nerve cells in the deep nuclei send messages out of the cerebellum along their fibres (or *axons*), which run through the peduncles to a number of nuclei in the brain stem and thalamus. These in turn are connected to the spinal cord and to regions of the cerebral cortex concerned with the control of movement.

Studies of the activity of nerve cells in animals have been the main source of knowledge of how the cerebellum works. Even when movements are not being made, neurons of the deep nuclei are continuously active, producing impulses at rates of 30–50 per second. This continuous background firing arises because the huge number of excitatory nerve fibres that enter the cerebellum, carrying information to the cortex, send side branches into the deep nuclei. In addition, they receive the axons of the 15 million *Purkinje cells*, the largest cells in the cortex. These are all inhibitory, using *gamma-amino-butyric acid* (GABA) as their transmitter. So, the variation of firing of cells in the deep nuclei, which constitutes the output of the cerebellum and hence

modulates movement, is dependent on the relationship between incoming activity and the resulting firing of Purkinje cells.

The incoming nerve fibres, which ultimately control the firing of Purkinje cells, are of two types. The first are the axons of cells in a nucleus in the medulla of the brain stem that glories in the name *inferior olive*, and which receives signals, indirectly, from parts of the cerebral cortex concerned with movement. Each of these axons wraps itself around the huge bush of processes (*dendrites*) of just one Purkinje cell (hence their name, '*climbing fibres*'), ending in around 2000 synapses. As a result, even a single impulse in a climbing fibre will make its Purkinje cell fire an impulse.

The other class of incoming axons are called '*mossy fibres*'. They are the fibres of several different kinds of nuclei in the brain stem and spinal cord. Some 40 million of them arise from cells in a region of the pons called the *pontine nuclei*. Some mossy fibres carry signals from the eyes, inner ears, skin, muscles, and tendons, providing information about the state and POSTURE of the body. Because movements inevitably generate sensory stimulation, these messages must include 'feedback' information regarding current patterns of movement. Other mossy fibres (the majority) carry signals originating in various areas of the cerebral cortex, probably including copies of the current 'commands-to-move' emanating from motor areas of the cortex. They inform the cerebellum about movement intentions even before any motion has begun, enabling it to modify movements before errors have started to occur. This essentially 'predictive' revision is thought to reduce the extent to which the control of movement depends on feedback from sensory receptors about actual, achieved movement. This is very useful because feedback obviously cannot begin until movement has started, and the delay in a control system causes oscillations and other errors, as engineers well know.

The mossy fibres do not contact Purkinje cells directly: they end mainly on the 50 billion tiny *granule cells* in the cortex, whose long *parallel fibres* each form synaptic connections on many Purkinje cells. About 95% of the impulses produced by Purkinje cells result from the stream of signals from granule cells.

But how does it all work? Although we know more about the micro-anatomy of the cerebellum than of any other area of the brain, there is still intense debate about exactly what it does. One of the complicating factors is that the strength of each synapse between any parallel fibre and the large number of Purkinje cells that it contacts can be changed, in ways that are invisible even under the microscope. Technically elegant experiments, involving recording from Purkinje cells in slices of cerebellum, maintained alive *in vitro*, show that when the cell is activated by its climbing fibre, the synapses of any parallel fibres that are simultaneously active are *decreased* in effectiveness, and that this 'long-term depression' lasts a very long time. This implies that the

climbing fibre can, in effect, 'teach' the Purkinje cell to alter its response to any recurrence of the particular pattern of mossy fibre input it was experiencing (representing a particular sensory and motor state of the body) when the climbing fibre was activated. This line of thinking is not universally accepted but has prompted attempts to identify the circumstances (behavioural contexts) in which the climbing fibres increase their activity. At present, the slim available evidence suggests that this occurs when a mismatch develops between the commands-to-move issued to the muscles by the central nervous system and the movements that actually ensue. Climbing fibres may, therefore, function (at least in part) as error-detectors in movement control.

This hypothesis also implies that the cerebellar cortex is the repository of many learned responses or '*motor memories*' that help to ensure the prompt and accurate execution of skilled movements. Whenever these memories prove to be inadequate, either because a novel movement command is required or because they are fading, control errors will be made and the teaching effect of the climbing fibres will automatically come into play, gradually reducing the errors and improving the skill.   DAVID M. ARMSTRONG

See PLATE 6.

See also BRAIN; CEREBRAL CORTEX; MEMORY; MOVEMENT, CONTROL OF.

Cerebral cortex Seen from the outside, the most obvious component of the human brain is the intricately folded cerebral cortex that covers the pair of *cerebral hemispheres*, which conceal most of the rest of the brain. The convolutions, or *gyri*, of the cortex, and the fissures or *sulci* that separate them, vary enormously from brain to brain, and from one hemisphere to the other in each individual. True cerebral cortex is found in the brains of fishes, reptiles, and birds, but is a major feature of the brain in all mammals. In humans it is relatively enormous in size, even compared with our closest relatives, chimpanzees and gorillas. The dominance of the cortex in the human brain led Thomas Willis, the eminent Oxford physician, to propose, in 1664, that it is the seat of 'higher' mental processes, such as PERCEPTION, MEMORY, and will.

The cerebral cortex is the thin outer cloak of GREY MATTER that covers the external surface of the cerebral hemispheres, like the 'bark' of a tree, which is indeed what its Latin root refers to. The total area of cortex in man is estimated at nearly a square meter; it is about 4 mm thick, and it contains 10 000 million or more nerve cells(*neurons*). The number of SYNAPSES (connections between nerve fibres and other neurons) is even more staggering — there are, on average, around 10 000 synapses on every cortical neuron.

When thin sections are viewed under a microscope, with appropriate staining of cell bodies, the cortex is seen to consist of several distinct layers. The almost universally adopted layering scheme is that proposed by the late nineteenth-century

German anatomist Korbinian Brodmann. Most of the cortex, the so-called *neocortex*, has a 6-layered structure, but some areas of the hemisphere are covered with simpler cortex with fewer layers, which is believed to be representative of a relatively primitive stage of brain development.

Cortical neurons and their connections

Cortical neurons are basically classified as *pyramidal* and *non-pyramidal* cells. A pyramidal cell can be recognised by a single, fairly thick process, the *apical dendrite*, which sprouts out of the top of the *cell body* and extends up toward the cortical surface. The other dendrites (branches of the cell body that receive incoming information from the fibres of other neurons), called *basal dendrites*, form a skirt around the lower part of the cell body. All dendrites bear large numbers of *spines*, small excrescences on which incoming nerve fibres terminate to form synapses. Pyramidal cells receive incoming nerve fibres from the THALAMUS and from other areas of cortex, as well as from nearby neurons. The *axon* of a pyramidal cell (the process that conveys impulses away from the neuron to other nerve cells) can extend a long way, for example more than a meter down to the SPINAL CORD, as well as sending branches to other cortical neurons.

The axon of a typical pyramidal cell can make thousands of synapses on other neurons. When the cell fires an impulse it sweeps along all the branches of the axon to reach the synapses at the terminals, where it triggers the release of the excitatory neurotransmitter *glutamate*. This affects receptor molecules in the membrane of the target neuron in such a way that it becomes more permeable to sodium ions, which rush into the cell, making the interior more positively charged. This depolarization increases the probability that the target cell will itself fire off an impulse.

If the target cell of the axon of a pyramidal neuron lies below the cerebral hemispheres, in the BRAIN STEM or spinal cord, it is termed a *projection* axon. If it goes to other cortical areas in the same hemisphere, it is an *association* axon, while if it innervates cells in the cortex of the opposite hemisphere it is called *commissural*.

Other neurons in the cortex are all non-pyramidal cells — a very heterogeneous group. They are called *interneurons* because they have relatively short axons that make local connections and do not leave the cortex itself. Non-pyramidal cells can be either *excitatory* or *inhibitory*. If the latter, they commonly use the important inhibitory substance GABA (*gamma-aminobutyric acid*) as the transmitter at their synapses. Non-pyramidal cells, like pyramidal cells, receive axons from the thalamus, from other cortical areas, and from other local interneurons.

The outermost layer of the neocortex, layer I, consists of a mesh of axons and dendrites with very few cell bodies. The other layers consist of pyramidal and non-pyramidal neurons in varying proportions. Layer IV contains a high proportion of non-pyramidal cells, and receives most of the incoming fibres from the thalamus.

Layers V and VI have particularly large pyramidal cells that project to subcortical centres, such as the spinal cord and thalamus.

Specialized cortical areas

Korbinian Brodmann also recognized that the cortex is divided into a large number of fields or areas, distinguished by slight differences in the appearance of the layers. He suggested that each anatomically distinctive area is specialized for a particular sensory, motor, or associative function.

Each hemisphere is mainly concerned with the control of muscles and with sensory input from the *opposite* side of the body, and also with visual and auditory information from the opposite side of the outside world. Hence damage of one hemisphere tends to affect sensation and movement on the opposite side. The cerebral cortex can be seen as the terminus of all the sensory pathways of the nervous system, in the sense that the cortex seems to be needed for conscious perception. Only when information originating in the eyes, the ears, the skin, or any other sensory organ finally reaches the cortex can it then be felt as a subjective experience. Equally, the cortex is the origin of our intended actions. From the *motor cortex*, axons, especially those from the very large '*Betz cells*' in layer V, project all the way to the spinal cord to contact motor neurons, which relay the signals out to the muscles. But the cortex is also an integrative organ. Large areas of it are *associative* in function, meaning that they bring together activity from different sensory and motor systems to make higher-level functions possible, such as speech, memory, and thought. We know from studies of patients who have suffered damage to various parts of the cortex that some of this association cortex is intimately related to our character or personality.

The visual cortex

An area of the neocortex that has been particularly well studied is the *primary visual cortex* (*area 17* of Brodmann), found at the back of the occipital lobe, mainly on the banks of a deep sulcus. Both EYES send signals, via the THALAMUS, to the visual cortex of both hemispheres, in such a way that each hemisphere receives information about the opposite half of the visual field. Thalamic fibres carrying information from the right eye and the left eye are segregated from each other as they enter the cortex and they form alternating patches of right-eye and left-eye input, about 0.3 mm across, to the cells of layer IV. Since connections between cortical cells mainly run up and down, this has the effect of imposing a pattern of functional 'columns' on the cortex, the neurons below any particular point on the cortical surface tending to be dominated functionally by either the right or the left eye. Such 'columnar' organization is a characteristic feature of the cerebral cortex, reflecting the segregation of different classes of incoming nerve fibres and the arrangement of connections between cortical neurons.

Area 17 is responsible for basic visual feature detection, but there exist dozens of other, interconnected visual areas in the occipital lobe and even in temporal and parietal lobes. Some are concerned with colour discrimination, or complex pattern recognition, certain cells even responding when the eyes view a stimulus as complex as a face. These areas belong to the association cortex, mentioned above, which is a striking feature of the human brain, permitting the integration and further analysis of simple sensory information to form the basis of meaningful, conscious experience, and the accurate control of action.

The primitive cortex

An example of the more 'primitive' cortex described earlier is the *hippocampus* (Latin for 'sea-horse', on account of its appearance in cross-section), which is tucked underneath, on the inner aspect of the temporal lobe. It is unusual in that it has white matter on the outside, and its structure is simple compared with the neocortex, with only three layers. The hippocampus, which receives processed information from much of the association cortex, seems to be involved in short-term conscious memory. It is functionally connected with the HYPOTHALAMUS and the LIMBIC SYSTEM, parts of the brain that control basic life functions such as hormonal systems and basic body rhythms and appetites.

So the cerebral cortex is important for an amazing range of functions, from basic drives for self-preservation to the highest levels of consciousness. LAURENCE GAREY

See PLATE 6.

See also BRAIN; CENTRAL NERVOUS SYSTEM; VISION.

Cerebral palsy denotes 'a disorder of movement and posture resulting from a permanent, non-progressive defect or lesion of the immature brain'. There are a number of causative factors, most of which act before birth, but some can act up until the age of 2 years, to cause a non-progressive disorder of the still-developing brain. The overall incidence of cerebral palsy is about 5 per 2000 infants, although there are quite large variations between countries.

In some cases there are prenatal influences which cause failure of brain development: either definite genetic factors, inadequate supply of oxygenated blood to the fetal brain, rubella in the first trimester of pregnancy, toxoplasmosis transmitted across the placenta, or irradiation.

In about half of all instances cerebral palsy is associated with pre-term delivery and low birthweight. Compared to those at full term and of normal weight, such infants are particularly at risk of developing cerebral palsy if they suffer hypoxia or inadequate blood flow to the brain around the time of birth, or if they suffer brain infection (encephalitis, meningitis) or head injury during early life.

There are many variations in the types of cerebral palsy, and often there is a mixture of neurological abnormalities. The children may have increased muscle tone (spasticity), which most commonly affects all four limbs — the condition of *spastic tetraplegia*; or there may be *spastic paraplegia*, when the arms are apparently unaffected; or the so-called *cerebral diplegia*, often associated with premature birth, when the arms are less affected than the legs. There can also be *hemiplegia*, affecting one half of the body, or *monoplegia*, affecting one limb.

There may also be involuntary movements, such as the writhing (*athetoid*) type and various disturbances of co-ordination, depending on the parts of the brain affected. Less commonly, cerebral palsy takes the form of a *hypotonic tetraplegia*, with no spasticity, when the child has a mobility problem but with floppy muscles.

Children with cerebral palsy frequently have other severe handicaps. About half of them have an IQ less than 70, whilst 25% have an IQ above 90, compared with 3% below 70 and 75% above 90 in the general population. Epileptic seizures are more common than in the population overall. Retarded speech development may parallel the degree of learning disorder, but it is frequently also complicated by the problems of defective muscle control. Different forms of SPEECH defect (*dysarthria*) accompany the different types of movement disorder.

Although the brain abnormality underlying the cerebral palsy is permanent and cannot be corrected, much help can be given to affected children and their families by way of PHYSIOTHERAPY, play and occupational therapy, speech therapy, orthopaedic surgery, and a variety of nutritional, mobility, and educational aids.

FORRESTER COCKBURN

See also MUSCLE TONE; PARALYSIS.

Cerebral ventricles The cerebral ventricles are a series of interconnected chambers deep inside the brain, filled with CEREBROSPINAL FLUID (CSF). The two largest, the *lateral ventricles*, are located symmetrically in each cerebral hemisphere; each has three culs de sac or 'horns', extending into the frontal, temporal and occipital lobes. The lateral ventricles of the two sides are linked by the *interventricular foramen* and they are connected through paired openings (*foramina of Monro*) to the single centrally placed *third ventricle*, for which the *corpus callosum* is the roof and the THALAMUS forms the flanking walls. The third ventricle communicates via a narrow canal (the *aqueduct of Sylvius*) through the centre of the midbrain with the *fourth ventricle* which lies behind the lower part of the BRAIN STEM. The ventricles each contain a *choroid plexus* that secretes cerebrospinal fluid.

The ventricles were observed by the influential Hellenistic physician and anatomist, GALEN of Bergama (129–216 AD) and became known as 'cells'. They were the central feature of a theory of brain function that was endorsed by the medieval philosophers and Fathers of the Christian Church, and which remained dominant until the eighteenth century. The clear fluid within the cells, which was thought to be a distillate of blood and inhaled air, was called 'animal spirit' (from the Latin *anima*: 'mind'), because it was supposed to be the seat of behavioural and mental functions. Information carried by nerves from the sense organs was said to enter the fluid of the *first cell* (the lateral ventricles), where it gave rise to sensations. This cell communicated with the *middle cell* (the third ventricle), which was responsible for 'imagination' and 'estimation', and the fluid then passed into the *final cell* (the fourth ventricle), which was concerned with memory and the control of movement (see figure). Although this hypothesis is, of course, totally discredited, it is interesting that it was essentially mechanistic (rather than mystical) and it incorporated a principle that is clearly established by modern NEUROSCIENCE, namely that the nervous system processes sensory information to provide the basis of thoughts, memories, and actions.

LAURENCE GAREY
COLIN BLAKEMORE

See also BRAIN; CEREBROSPINAL FLUID; HYDROCEPHALUS.

Cerebrospinal fluid The brain floats on a liquid cushion of cerebrospinal fluid (CSF) within the rigid bony skull. The CSF is contained between layers of the MENINGES, the membranes that enclose the brain. It fills the *subarachnoid space* between the delicate *arachnoid mater* that lines the tough fibrous outer covering, the *dura mater*, and the *pia mater* that covers the soft substance of the brain.

ANIMAE SENSITIVAE

Woodcut; anon., 1503. Wellcome Institute Library, London. An early portrayal of the cerebral ventricles.

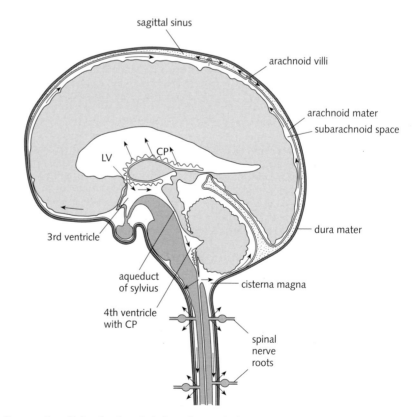

A diagrammatic vertical section through the brain showing the location of the ventricles and the direction of flow of cerebrospinal fluid (CSF). CSF is formed by the choroid plexuses (CP), mainly in the lateral ventricles, and drains into the blood via the arachnoid villi and the spinal nerve roots.

Since the brain floats in CSF, the fluid acts in effect to reduce the weight of the brain from some 1000 g to about 50 g, and also protects the brain from knocks on the head. However, since the brain can move within the CS, it can be damaged on the opposite side by a sudden deceleration such as in a car accident (*contra coup injury*).

The subarachnoid space on the outside of the brain is in continuity with a similar space around the spinal cord and also with the series of interconnected CEREBRAL VENTRICLES within the brain (see figure). Each of the paired lateral ventricles, in the cerebral hemispheres, contains a leaf-like, highly vascular *choroid plexus*. It is from these structures that the bulk of the CSF is secreted. From the lateral ventricles CSF drains into the central *third ventricle*, and thence through the aqueduct in the midbrain into the *fourth ventricle*. Both the third and fourth ventricles contribute to the flow from their own choroidal tissue. From the fourth ventricle, the CSF exits into the subarachnoid space through several openings, and fills the 'basal cisterns' beneath the brain. Thence the flow of CSF is mainly up and over the whole brain surface, whilst some flows down around the spinal cord. Completing the circuit back to the bloodstream, the fluid drains via the valve-like *arachnoid granulations* into the sagittal sinus, the large venous channel lying centrally on the top of the brain; some is also taken up into veins around spinal nerve roots and into the lymphatics of the nose.

The secretion of CSF is an active TRANSPORT process that moves fluid and solutes from the blood plasma into the ventricles, the choroid plexuses being a specialised part of the BLOOD–BRAIN BARRIER. CSF secretion involves the pumping of ions and specialised ION CHANNELS, with the energy coming from glucose and oxygen in the blood. In the adult human CSF is formed at a rate of about 0.5 ml/min; the total volume is about 200 ml, of which 30 ml is in the ventricles and the remainder in the subarachnoid space. The circulation of CSF leads to the fluid being completely replaced about every 4 hours.

CSF is a weak salt solution with similar inorganic ion concentrations to plasma, but with small and significant differences, whereas the protein content is about 100 times less than that of plasma (0.5 g/litre compared to 50–70 g/litre). Abnormalities of the CSF can be important in diagnosis of some medical conditions; the fluid can be sampled by *lumbar puncture* from the extension of the subarachnoid space (the lumbar sac) below the lower end of the spinal cord. CSF is normally a clear, amazingly 'bright' fluid, and if it is cloudy or contains a raised level of protein or traces of blood this is usually an indication of brain infection, some types of brain or spinal cord tumour, or trauma.

The pressure within the brain, the *intracranial pressure* (ICP), is transmitted in the CSF around the spinal cord and down into the lumbar sac. With the body horizontal, it is normally low (about 10 cm H_2O); it is markedly affected by posture, and raised by straining or coughing.

Blockage in the drainage pathways for CSF is one of the causes of a raised ICP, since the CSF is actively 'pumped' into the ventricular system. In an adult this raised pressure can cause expansion of the ventricles, with loss of neural tissue by compression against the rigid skull. In infants, when CSF drainage pathways have failed to develop normally, the raised ICP causes the head to swell because the junctions between the skull bones are not fused, resulting in HYDROCEPHALUS — 'water on the brain'.

A raised intracranial pressure can often be recognised by looking into the eye with an ophthalmoscope, an instrument which shines a beam of light on to the retina at the back of the eye. The beam is focused onto the 'optic disc', where the nerves of the eye converge to pass to the brain. Normally this appears as a clearly-defined, pale concave disc, but if the pressure in the CSF is raised, the disc may bulge forwards into the cavity of the eye. As well as by blockage of CSF circulation, raised pressure can be caused by an expanding tumour or blood clot, or by swelling of a damaged or diseased brain.

The CSF also acts as a drainage route for waste products of brain metabolism, additional to their direct excretion into the capillary blood vessels everywhere in the brain across the blood–brain barrier.　　　MALCOLM SEGAL

See also BLOOD–BRAIN BARRIER; HYDROCEPHALUS; MENINGES.

Cervical smear Cervical CANCER is a disease dreaded by women, but the advent of cervical smear tests has resulted in a significant reduction in the incidence of the disease, to the extent that, in the developed world at least, cervical cancer is justifiably now regarded as being largely preventable.

It was in 1949 that Papanicolaou and Traut published a paper which showed how cells shed from the cervix, popularly known as the 'neck of the womb', could be examined microscopically to diagnose cervical disease. This is known as exfoliative cytology and the name of the pioneer is sometimes retained in the colloquial term a 'Pap smear'. Originally Papanicolaou and Traut intended exfoliative cytology as a test for early cancer, but it then became apparent that precancerous lesions could be detected by this means and treated much more easily and less radically than cancer. Such precancerous lesions, otherwise known as cervical intraepithelial neoplasia (CIN), may or may not become cancer over a number of years. By treating at this stage cancer can be prevented in almost 100% of cases. Programmes were initiated in British Columbia and Finland which proved beyond the doubt of most people that cervical screening saves lives. The key to these exemplary programmes was wide population coverage, the achievement of which is essential for their effectiveness. This has also been clearly demonstrated in the UK, where cervical screening was not sufficiently widespread to have an impact until the late 1980s. At that time the NHS introduced regular, computerised

call and recall for all women between the ages of 20 and 65. As a result over 80% of the population is being regularly screened and there has been an undoubted reduction in deaths, from around 2000 deaths annually at the end of the 1980s to just over 1300 deaths in 1995.

A cervical smear is performed by exposing the part of the CERVIX which protrudes into the upper vagina. This is usually done by either a gynaecologist, a general practitioner, or a nurse practitioner. After exposing the cervix with a speculum, it is then firmly scraped with a wooden or plastic spatula around its entire surface and the exfoliated or surface cells which attach to the spatula are smeared on a glass slide and immediately covered with fixative which preserves the shape of the cells. The slides are then transported to a laboratory where they are stained to enable microscopic assessment.

Some smears are inadequate for examination and as such are labelled as 'unsatisfactory' requiring repeat smears. Five to ten per cent of smears will show some abnormality, but fewer than 1% abnormal smears are associated with cancer. Smears may show a spectrum of abnormality varying from very slight abnormalities, classified as borderline, to cell nuclear changes known as *dyskaryosis* (in the UK) or *squamous epithelial lesion* (in the US). Dyskaryotic changes are graded as mild, moderate, or severe (in the UK), or low grade or high grade (in the US). It must be appreciated that smears do not always accurately reflect underlying change: low grade smear changes *may* be associated with high grade CIN. On the other hand, although abnormal smears *may* suggest underlying precancer, often no significant change is present. Unfortunately many women do not realise this and immediately worry that they have cancer if the smear is not normal.

If the smear is normal, then it is repeated at whatever screening interval is advocated in that country, but it should be at least 5-yearly in the age 20–65. Very young women, even if sexually active, do not require to be screened below the age of 20 because the risk of cancer is extremely remote. Women over 65 who have been regularly screened are also at very low risk indeed of developing abnormal smears.

If the smear is mildly abnormal, a repeat smear in six months may be all that is required, but more severe changes require accurate diagnosis, and for this colposcopy should be performed. This involves looking directly at the cervix with a high magnification instrument; after wiping on acetic acid any abnormal areas become apparent. The area can be biopsied under direct vision and the tiny scrap of cervical tissue is looked at under the microscope by the pathologist. If precancer or cervical intraepithelial neoplasia is found, then the cervix is treated in such a way that the abnormal skin is destroyed or excised using techniques such as laser or diathermy. Fortunately this treatment has been shown not to affect a woman's ability to conceive or to have a normal delivery.

Abnormal smears are thought to be due in large part to infection of the cervix by some of the many types of *human papilloma virus*. Although other types of this virus cause warts, those that infect the cervix do not. The virus is probably transmitted in most cases by sexual intercourse and infection is found in around 5–10% of completely normal women. Scientific endeavour is currently aimed towards development of a vaccine to counter these virus infections.

Inevitably modern technology is beginning to have an impact on how we design our screening programmes. Computerised automated machines have been developed with the aim of reducing the need for cytoscreeners to look at large numbers of normal smears. In this way normal smears might be screened out and cytotechnicians could spend more time examining abnormal smears. These new technologies aimed at making screening more automated have not yet been fully proven, but it may well be that they will establish a role in the future. Another development is cytology in a liquid base to improve the quality of smears.

The absence of screening means that the major burden of cervical cancer is borne by women in impoverished countries, where it is the commonest cancer in women. This is compounded by a relative lack of treatment for the disease. It is to be hoped that improved health education, new technology, and rising affluence will enable many more women around the world to receive protection from cervical cancer by establishment of cervical cytology screening.

HENRY C. KITCHENER

Cervix In full, *cervix uteri*, the 'neck of the womb'. A short thick tube of SMOOTH MUSCLE around a narrow channel leading from the body of the UTERUS to the VAGINA, the first part of the long and hazardous route which SPERM must navigate to reach an ovum, but which, at fertile times, assists them by sperm-friendly modification of the secretions from its lining. In the event of PREGNANCY, the cervix remains a narrow channel until the final weeks: then the muscle of the wall thins out, allowing descent of the infant's head into the PELVIS. During the first stage of LABOUR the opening into the vagina enlarges; when it is 'fully dilated' the second stage begins, heralding descent of the fetus into the vagina. The cervix is one of the common sites for cancer, hence the advisability of regular cervical smears.

S.J.

See CERVICAL SMEAR; LABOUR; PREGNANCY; UTERUS; PLATE 8.

Chastity A confusion of the terms 'chastity' and 'celibacy' has long existed. 'Chastity' — deriving from the Latin '*castitas*', meaning 'cleanliness' or 'purity' — does not necessarily mean the renunciation of all sexual relations, but rather the temperate sexual behaviour of legitimately married spouses, for the purpose of procreation, or the sexual continence of the unmarried. The Greek word for chastity, *sophrosyne*, means moderation, which in the ancient Greek world was the

chief philosophical virtue. This entailed proper self-mastery for men, and the virtue appropriate to a devoted and child-bearing (or potentially child-bearing) wife. For both men and women this meant the avoidance of fornication rather than the avoidance of sex altogether.

The early Church saw a debate between the proponents of chastity and CELIBACY. Paul questioned chastity in favour of celibacy in the first century, as I Corinthians: 7 indicates, for example. This passage was (and has continued to be) variously interpreted. Those in favour of celibacy highlighted Paul's comment that he wished all were like him — that is, celibate — and his urging of those unmarried or widowed to remain so, while those favouring chaste marriage have emphasised Paul's words that it is better to marry than to burn if one cannot practise self-control. A different perspective is seen in 1 Timothy: 3, where a bishop (not, in this period, in charge of anything beyond a local church) is described as a person who must be above reproach, married only once, temperate and sensible, and keeping his children submissive: that is, he must embody the qualities of a chaste, married householder. In the letter to Titus, an elder is described, similarly, as one who must have been married only once, who must be blameless and not rebellious, and whose children are believers.

In the second century, many writers were still advocating chaste marriage. For Clement of Alexandria sexual intercourse should be undertaken in marriage in service of God and for the begetting of children. A well-ordered SEXUALITY was not in itself a problem: sexual relations needed to be ordered just as the rest of Christian life had to be ordered. He was therefore concerned about the continence of unmarried men. He saw marriage and celibacy as equal callings, each having its own and different forms of service and ministry to God. In marriage this entailed the care of one's wife and children (Clement was writing to male householders like himself). The particular readers he had in mind were, perhaps, the members of his own congregation in Alexandria who might be told by the ascetic and celibate encratites who lived in the area that they had accommodated too much to the world in marrying. Clement and others who wrote along these lines were, indeed, trying to accommodate Christian principles within the Roman and Greek household structure.

Tertullian, also in the second century, wrote on the importance of monogamy, the bond between one man and woman, believing marriage to be the lot of most Christians, for VIRGINITY might be splendid and ideal, but it was not for most people. Those who, at this time, privileged celibacy over marriage were sometimes accused of extremism, such as the prophet Montanus, who was said to allow the annulment of marriage.

By the fourth century, however, almost no one was writing of celibacy and marriage as equal Christian callings. Celibacy was seen as decidedly superior. Many people, from Ambrose to Jerome to Gregory of Nyssa, wrote on the importance of

virginity. Only the monk Jovinian denied that virginity was a higher state than marriage, and only Augustine — who himself advocated virginity — wrote anything significant in support of chaste marriage, in his *The Good of Marriage* (*c* 401), in which he outlined the three goods of marriage: offspring, fidelity, and the sacramental bond.

Because chastity in the sense of the continence of the unmarried triumphed (until the sixteenth-century Protestant Reformation) over the chastity of temperate sexual behaviour in marriage, the term chastity essentially came to mean celibacy, though historians debate exactly when this happened. It had happened generally by the sixth century, though as early as the fourth century, '*castitas*' was used in some texts to mean continence rather than non-fornicatory marriage.

JANE SHAW

See also ASCETICISM; CELIBACY; RELIGION AND THE BODY.

Chemical warfare Wilfred Owen, veteran and poet of World War I, understood chemical warfare. *Dulce et decorum est*, Owen's view of gassing by chlorine, sums it up:

> Gas! Gas! Quick, boys — An ecstasy of fumbling
> Fitting the clumsy helmets just in time,
> But someone still was yelling out and stumbling
> And flound'ring like a man in fire or lime . . .

Chemical warfare has evolved since then: from the asphyxiating chlorine; through the irritant, skin penetrating and bone marrow damaging mustard gas; to the acutely toxic skin-and inhalation-hazard nerve POISONS — by-products of research on insecticidal organophosphate chemicals in the late 1930s. *En route*, and since, thousands of chemicals have been screened for their use in war, but the inventory of established chemical warfare agents remains at about twenty.

In parallel with the search for yet more effective agents, research has continued on antidotes and other means of protection. The modern infantryman has protective suits, gas masks, sensitive detectors, and injectable antidotes (but only to nerve poisons). Vehicles with air filtration units, and mobile hospitals with decontamination facilities, offer protection for other service units, the main objective being to avoid contact with the chemical agent.

Antidotes and hospitalisation are no guarantees of a successful recovery following exposure to tabun, sarin, soman, or VX — nerve agents all, and capable at low concentrations of disrupting nerve transmission and the ability to breathe. Nerve agents can kill within minutes after inhalation, and in less than an hour following skin contact. For all chemical warfare agents the degree of injury and subsequent disability depends on the quantity of chemical inhaled or in contact with the skin.

Wilfred Owen captured the terror of chemical warfare, and his fumblers made up a sizeable proportion of the 1.3 million casualties it caused in World War I. Others fell victim because they had either no gas masks, or faulty masks, and latterly, inadequate skin protection when Germany introduced mustard gas in 1917. Some 27 000 servicemen died from the effects of chemical agents in World War I. This ratio of deaths to injuries, lower than with conventional munitions, led some to argue that chemical warfare was a more humane way of fighting.

Civilian casualties, caused by chemical agents being blown beyond the battlefields of northern France and Belgium border villages, numbered roughly 1000. Most civilians survived their ordeal, with some 110–120 deaths being recorded. Approximately 4000 factory workers in Britain, France, and the US were injured during the manufacture of chemical munitions between 1916–18. Iranian and Kurdish victims of Iraq's use of mustard gas and nerve agents in the 1980s were less fortunate. Tens of thousands, largely civilians, were injured, but a high percentage died, some 5000 in the Kurdish city of Halabja alone, according to estimates.

Unlike soldiers, civilians have relatively little protection against chemical warfare agents. The training provided to soldiers equips them, in part, for fighting in a chemical environment. Much of their training is to prevent any fumbling and to overcome the sense of isolation in their protective suits.

Remaining upwind, above ground level, and in a sealed room with an adequate air supply, will provide protection for civilians — if they have time to prepare. Iraq's Kurds had no warning, and the extensive casualties caused by chemical agents caused great panic and led to millions fleeing their homes to seek shelter in neighbouring countries.

The plight of the Kurds galvanized discussions on a chemical disarmament regime. Although most countries are signatories to the 1925 Geneva Protocol, which outlaws (first) use of chemical and biological warfare, this treaty does not forbid retaliation, nor does it have any policing powers. The 1993 Chemical Weapons Convention (CWC) remedies these deficiencies. Following ratification in the parliaments of 65 countries, the convention became international law in April 1997. Well over 120 countries have now ratified the Convention and agree to neither use, make, nor encourage others to produce chemical weapons. As proof of their good intentions all ratifiers have also agreed to inspection, at short notice, of any site, be it military base, chemical manufacturing plant, or area where agents may have been used. Adoption of the Convention requires countries such as the US, with some 30 000 tonnes of chemical agents, and Russia, with some 40 000 tonnes, to destroy all stocks within 10 years. The bill for Russia to comply with these provisions is an estimated $4 billion.

Details about stockpiles, sites, inventories of chemicals, and manufacturing locations are transmitted by governments to the Organisation for the Prohibition of Chemical Weapons (OPCW), based in the Hague. The OPCW oversees the CWC and organizes inspections.

Only two other countries, India and Iraq, are definitely known to have stocks of usable chemical munitions. India has ratified the Chemical Weapons Convention, Iraq has not. Following her defeat in the second Gulf War in 1991, Iraq has agreed to a United Nations Special Commission (UNSCOM) inspecting sites and destroying munitions and chemical and biological warfare manufacturing facilities. UNSCOM never completed this programme. Iraq expelled the UNSCOM team following bombing of the country by the US and the UK in 1999. Negotiations are continuing between Iraq and the UN about a new type of inspection regime.

A number of other countries, including Britain, France, and Italy, have declared that they possess some chemical warfare munitions, many of which were made before 1945. Small stocks of these munitions may be buried on disused military bases, and finding them will probably be more a chance event than the result of a specific investigation. In consequence, countries possessing stocks of these older, largely unusable munitions will have more than 10 years in which to destroy them.

Iraq brought chemical warfare up to date. The most extensive use, prior to this, of chemicals deliberately intended to injure or kill humans occurred between 1915–18. In the intervening years chemical agents have been used in other wars. Italy used mustard gas against Ethiopian forces in 1935–6. Japan is alleged to have used mustard gas against Chinese forces in 1938. In 1967, Britain claimed that an asphyxiating chemical agent had been used by Egypt against Yemeni troops.

Chemical warfare, however, is not only about lethal agents. Many countries adhere to the view that the use of chemical defoliants by the US in the Vietnam War both to remove the forest canopy and to destroy food crops was also chemical warfare. The US disagrees with this interpretation. Defoliants used in Vietnam caused a rapid leaf drop, increasing visibility in large swathes of inland and coastal forests. Destruction of forests and food crops caused considerable hardship in the locality. Regrettably, the concentrations of the chemicals used resulted in the loss of countless trees, and forests being replaced by grassland. The destruction is still evident today.

Riot control agents have also been used in warfare to force combatants to leave entrenched positions, exposing them to enemy fire. Use of riot-control agents in this context also constitutes chemical warfare. The CWC acknowledges this, and the use of riot control agents in war is now forbidden.

A disarmament treaty to prevent chemical warfare is now in place. Negotiations to secure it have taken almost 20 years. More countries are expected to ratify the CWC. Persuading all nations to do so and to follow the new rules is the ultimate goal.   ALASTAIR HAY

See also POISONS; WAR AND THE BODY.

Chemoreceptor Take a deep breath in and hold it. Breath-hold times can range from as little as a few seconds to a much more heroic several minutes — but what limits these times? Certainly a number of factors, including motivation and the volume to which the lung was inflated, are important, but the actual 'breakpoint', defined as the time from the beginning of the breath-hold to the point at which the overwhelming urge to breathe can no longer be resisted, is ultimately determined by the CARBON DIOXIDE (CO_2) and OXYGEN (O_2) levels in arterial blood. These levels are expressed as the partial pressure (P) of each gas with which the blood would be in equilibrium. They rise and fall respectively throughout a breath-hold (as we continue to metabolise foodstuffs for energy) and the break-point is reached when the P_{CO_2} in arterial blood has risen from its normal value of around 40 mmHg (5.3 kPa) to around 50 mmHg (6.7 kPa) and the P_{O_2} has fallen from its normal value of around 95 mmHg (12.6 kPa) to around 70 mmHg (9.3 kPa). Breath-hold times can therefore be increased by prior HYPERVENTILATION (which lowers the initial carbon dioxide) or by breathing pure oxygen instead of air. Combining these two methods will maximally — and dramatically — increase breath-hold times. OK: breathe out, now!

As breath-hold times are ultimately determined by the concentration of gases in the blood, it follows that sensors must exist which can 'taste' the chemical composition of blood. These sensors are known as chemoreceptors, and they play a crucial role in ACID–BASE HOMEOSTASIS and oxygen supply. They help to maintain the appropriate oxygen, carbon dioxide, and pH in the body by initiating a variety of cardiovascular and respiratory reflexes. Such reflexes are required not just during breath-holds but whenever these levels are altered by changes in metabolism, changes in environment, or disease — for example during EXERCISE, at high ALTITUDE, or during respiratory failure caused by lung disease.

Chemoreception occurs both in the brain and in the blood vessels. Sensitivity to brain CO_2 and pH is known to exist in the brain stem — 'tasting' the fluid environment of the neurons where correct pH is crucial to function. Any change in blood carbon dioxide is transmitted to the brain: here, as elsewhere, a rise in carbon dioxide increases acidity; the response of the central chemoreceptor mechanism to such a rise is to stimulate breathing, thus tending to correct the change by the loss of more carbon dioxide. Specific structures mediating these 'central chemoreceptor' responses have not yet however been identified with certainty. In contrast, chemosensitivity to changes in the blood was localised in the 1920s to specialised 'peripheral chemoreceptors'. The most functionally significant group of these receptors is found within the carotid bodies, located bilaterally in the neck close to the carotid artery: there are others in the 'aortic bodies' around the origin of the aorta.

The first descriptions of a small structure, only 5–8 mm long and weighing just a few mg, lying beside the division of the carotid artery in the neck, appeared during the eighteenth century. At first called a 'ganglion', it was later thought to be a gland. It was not until 1927 that Fernando de Castro, an anatomist working in the Cajal Institute in Madrid, recognised the *carotid body* as a sensory organ and postulated its function as a chemoreceptor with afferent nerves to the brain. The sensory function of the carotid (and aortic) chemoreceptors was confirmed by a series of physiological studies performed around the same time by Jean-Frans Heymans and his son, Corneille, in Ghent, Belgium, for which Corneille received the Nobel prize in 1938. By then it had been established that these receptors were stimulated by high carbon dioxide and/or low oxygen in the blood, causing a reflex increase in breathing and in blood pressure. Shortly after these discoveries, a series of studies initiated in Japan and continued in the US described how bilateral division of the afferent nerves from the carotid bodies brought relief in a number of sufferers from asthma. Unfortunately, these results could not be confirmed, and a possible mortality attributable to the surgical intervention led to the banning of the procedure. Studies following such procedures did however provide evidence that people without carotid body function did not show the normal increase in breathing in response to low oxygen.

The carotid body is highly vascular and receives the highest blood flow, relative to its size, of any organ in the body. It is divided into a number of lobules, each containing clusters of two distinct cell types together with arteriolar blood vessels and capillaries, nerve fibres, and a few autonomic ganglion cells. *Type I* cells, of which there are tens of thousands in each carotid body, are believed to be the primary transducer elements. A smaller number of *Type II* cells envelop them and provide a supportive function, like that of GLIA in the nervous system. In the Type I cells there are numerous vesicles containing CATECHOLAMINES; they also store other substances, including ACETYLCHOLINE, certain neuropeptides, and nucleotides as well as the enzymes required to produce the 'messenger' gases, NITRIC OXIDE and CARBON MONOXIDE. Because these features resemble those of the terminal of a nerve fibre, the Type I cell is believed to form the equivalent of a nerve-to-nerve SYNAPSE with the sensory nerve endings close to it, generating ACTION POTENTIALS in them by the graded release of a transmitter. In common with almost all synapses, the release of neurotransmitter is dependent upon an elevation in the concentration of ionic calcium within the Type I cell.

Peripheral chemoreceptors share with central chemoreceptors a responsiveness to acidity and carbon dioxide, but their uniqueness lies in their ability also to sense lowered oxygen (HYPOXIA) in arterial blood. The most likely neurotransmitter released during hypoxia is DOPAMINE, with the other chemicals stored in the Type I cell acting as modulators. (This dopamine-secreting action of Type I cells has led to the recent trial use of surgical autografts of carotid body tissue in the treatment of animal models of Parkinson's disease.) In common with almost all synapses, the release of neurotransmitter is dependent upon an elevation in the concentration of ionic calcium (Ca) within the Type I cell; evidence suggests that Ca ions enter the Type I cell through voltage-gated channels, opened when the cell is depolarised in response to hypoxia or other stimuli. The depolarisation of the cell occurs by the closure of oxygen-sensitive potassium ION CHANNELS in the CELL MEMBRANE. The precise nature of the potassium channel and the mechanism by which it senses the stimulus is not yet known.

At the carotid body, stimuli are thus translated into sensory action potentials that are graded in intensity with the degree of stimulation. Carotid body sensory discharge increases exponentially with increasing hypoxia and linearly with carbon dioxide, and if the two stimuli are applied together the response is greater than the sum of the two responses to each stimulus independently. This means that the receptors are exquisitely sensitive to the combined rise in carbon dioxide and fall in oxygen which occurs in breath-holding, and they act rapidly to cause deeper breaths after even minor interruptions of breathing such as during SPEECH or SINGING. These breath-by-breath adjustments constitute the role of the peripheral chemoreceptors in a normal environment during everyday activity, and they also implement the rapid increase in breathing at the start of exercise. Their responsiveness to hypoxia causes the increase in breathing that is common experience at high altitude, allowing the concentration of oxygen reaching the lungs to be higher than it would be without such a response. In hypoxia also, they initiate vasoconstrictive reflexes which act to maintain the arterial blood pressure. Their response to *acidaemia* — a fall in the pH of the blood — causes increased breathing, and thus tends to correct the acidity by the loss of more carbon dioxide from the lungs.

In summary; the peripheral chemoreceptors perform a vital function in the maintenance of O_2 and CO_2 levels in arterial blood, and of acid–base balance, by translating blood-borne chemical stimuli into electrical activity in afferent nerves, leading to homeostatic respiratory and cardiovascular reflexes.   PREM KUMAR

See also ALTITUDE; BREATHING; HYPOXIA; NEUROTRANSMITTERS.

Chemotherapy

Chemotherapy — broadly speaking, the treatment of disease by chemical means — has had a number of different meanings since Paul Ehrlich (1854–1915) first coined the word in 1907. Then the word referred to the treatment of INFECTIOUS DISEASE by drugs that killed the infective organism, but left the patient unaffected. This led Ehrlich to postulate the concept he called the '*magic bullet*' — a medicine that would knock out a precise target, leaving other tissues unharmed. At the beginning of the twenty-first century 'chemotherapy' is more usually used to refer to treatment of CANCER by powerful chemicals — again based on the original premise of Ehrlich's, that powerful medicinal agents will kill cancerous cells in the body, whilst leaving surrounding cells functioning healthily. In between times, the word gained some currency for the drug treatment of any disease condition.

In the final decades of the nineteenth century, Ehrlich was working on the effects of artificial dyes on living cells, in particular trying to stain PARASITES in animal tissues. In 1891 he discovered that *methylene blue* would selectively stain the malaria parasite, which indicated to him that the dyes had combined with some specific receptor sites on the parasite, which might provide a mechanism for treating the disease. By administering the dye to patients with malaria, he showed that this could indeed be used therapeutically in humans; a few years later he found that the dye *trypan red* showed specific activity against trypanosome infections in mice, although it was not therapeutically effective against trypanosome infections in cattle or humans. From these studies he developed a theory that associated the chemical structure of a synthetic drug with its biological effects. In 1909 he discovered the drug *Salvarsan*, an arsenical compound that was the first effective drug against the organism that causes syphilis, and he used the word 'chemotherapy' to indicate the use of such drugs.

In the early 1930s another chemical agent, *Prontosil Red,* was discovered, which was shown to be an extremely effective treatment against a number of bacterial infections, including erysipelas, streptococcal angina, and puerperal sepsis. Further chemical research on the compound revealed that Prontosil Red was composed of biologically active and inactive parts, the active component being a readily available chemical, a sulphonamide derivative called *sulphanilimide*. This was an important discovery: on the one hand, it encouraged chemists to explore the molecular structures of biologically active chenicals, and in particular opened up the sulphonamide molecule to much chemical modification; on the other hand, sulphanilimide was a simple chemical, easy and cheap to prepare, and free from patent restrictions. Its production and use became widespread, as did the use of its derivatives, and the sulphonamides soon provided effective treatments for a wide range of conditions caused by *Streptococcus* bacteria, including some forms of pneumonia and meningitis. Infections caused by *Staphylococcus* bacteria, however, such as endocarditis and cellulitis, were resistant to sulphonamides.

The discovery of penicillin in 1928 by the bacteriologist Alexander Fleming (1881–1955), and more importantly, its later effective development by a team in Oxford led by the pathologist

Howard Florey (1898–1968) and the chemist Ernst Chain (1906–79), opened up, in the 1940s, a new field of chemotherapy called *anti-biosis*. This was the use of one microorganism, in this case a mould called *Penicillium*, to destroy another, such as a disease-causing bacterium. The successful chemical isolation and preparation of the active agent produced by the mould led to the use of the drug during World War II, especially for the treatment of wounded or VD-infected soldiers. Scientifically, the discovery of penicillin stimulated much chemical research to find similar agents — this involved massive screening programmes of a wide range of MICROORGANISMS, undertaken by institutes and pharmaceutical companies around the world. It also promoted the further investigation of how penicillin killed bacteria, which was by interfering with the manufacture of the bacterial cell wall. This in turn encouraged research work to find other compounds with the same effect. Gradually, synthetic chemicals were manufactured, which did not therefore fit the precise description of 'ANTIBIOTICS', as they were not produced by microorganisms, although the expression 'antibiotics' has continued to be applied to all these medicinal drugs. These antibiotics, whether produced by living organisms, such as mould and fungi, or whether created synthetically in a laboratory, revolutionised the treatment of most infectious diseases. Unfortunately their widespread use has also caused problems, as pathogenic microorganisms are increasingly developing resistance to the powerful drugs designed to kill them. As yet, similar drugs to counteract viral caused diseases have not been produced.

The discovery of the sulphonamide family of drugs in the 1930s coincided with a short period when the word '*chemotherapy*' was often used to indicate the treatment of any disease with a therapeutic chemical. Thus most modern drug therapy can be regarded, in one sense, as 'chemotherapy'. Increasingly, however, the word has come to be used now in association with cancer therapies, cancer chemotherapy having the same connotation as the original usage in infectious conditions — the therapeutic agent will destroy the malignancy without affecting surrounding healthy cells and tissues.

Cytotoxic drugs, which destroy rapidly-proliferating cells such as those found in tumours, started being developed, particularly after World War II, especially in the US. Early trials, on diseases such as childhood leukaemia and Hodgkin's disease, were discouraging, the toxic chemicals used almost invariably proving poisonous not only to the cancerous cells but also to normal, unaffected cells. More advanced developments have produced drugs that are effective against a number of cancers, including some that are effective against cancer cells throughout the body, and so can attack cancerous cells that have spread. Several different types of drugs have been developed — *alkylating agents*, for example, inhibit cell division, whilst *anti-metabolites* interfere with

enzyme systems and block vital processes. These drugs, however, are not readily able to distinguish between healthy and infected cells, and supplementary therapies to protect normal cells and tissues are also given. The concomitant development of drugs to counteract some of the distressing side effects of these powerful medicines, such as nausea and vomiting, hair loss, and fatigue, have also contributed to the success and acceptability of much modern chemotherapy. New fields of research, especially stimulated by developments in understanding the genetic and molecular mechanisms of cancer, have opened up a number of new therapeutic strategies.

E.M. TANSEY

See also CANCER; INFECTIOUS DISEASES.

Chimera In classical myth, the Chimera is one of many creatures combining the identities of human and beast, or merging features of more than one animal. In classical thought, these hybrids are sometimes divine: the god Pan, for example, is represented as part goat. Human–animal hybrids deriving from the Near East or from ancient Greece and with a lasting impact on the Western imagination include the centaur. This was a horse–man combination unable to hold its drink — as witness the centaurs' attempts to rape the wedding guests when they attended the Lapith wedding in northern Greece, depicted on the methopes of the Parthenon. Centaurs represented the violence and sexuality of the world of the beasts and it is

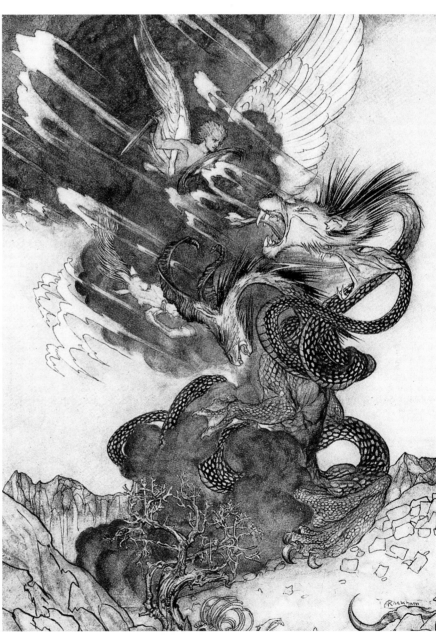

Bellerophon, mounted on Pegasus, attacks the Chimera. Mary Evans Picture Library/Arthur Rackham Collection.

153

significant that some artistic representations show them with two sets of genitalia: a human set at the front and a horse set at the back. Then there were satyrs and silens, goat-men with exaggerated sexuality; sirens and harpies, both bird-women, the sirens being associated with perfume, seductive song, and attractive temptation, the harpies with a foul smell, violent noise, and repulsion; also one-off monsters such as the manticore, a lion–scorpion combination with a human head, the bull-man Minotaur, and the riddling lion-woman Sphinx. Beasts such as these, as well as the MERMAIDS, are encountered by heroes and explorers at the limits of the known world, or in the wild zones between inhabited areas. Frequently associated with boundaries between the forbidden and the permitted, the known and the unknown, or the living and the dead, they are often given the function of guarding a palace or its treasure. But they also provide something for heroes to kill in order to prove their heroism, and they allow myth to explore the boundaries of human identity by asking what counts as civilised behaviour. In medieval art, particularly in illustrated bestiaries, the possible combinations of animals multiplied, as composite beings came to be seen as part of creation, providing evidence of the limitless power of God.

The Chimera herself is the supreme hybrid. She has the head of a lion, the mid-section of a goat and the hindquarters of a dragon. Most versions of her myth say that she is one of many monstrous beings deriving ultimately from the union of Gê (Earth) and Pontos (Sea): from the union of Earth and Heaven the TITANS were born. Among her kin are the harpies, the Sphinx, the snake-haired Gorgons (of whom Medusa is the best known), and the Nemean lion that featured in the labours of Hercules. The members of this bizarre family tree tend towards the repetition of body parts — for example, the many heads of the dog of the underworld, Cerberus. The Chimera has the heads of all three of her component animals, and breathes fire through her goat head. However, Homer refers to her as having been 'kept' by king Amisodarus, which could suggest an alternative tradition in which she was deliberately created as a boundary-guardian or weapon.

Her father was Typhon, half man and half serpent, whose rapid movement makes him the origin of hurricanes and typhoons; he has a hundred hissing snake heads coming from his loins. Her mother, Echidna, also combined human and serpent but, in contrast to her fast-moving, fire-belching husband, she stayed in a cave beneath the earth, only coming out rarely to eat young men. The Chimera was eventually killed by the hero Bellerophon, aided by another hybrid descended from Earth and Sea — the winged horse, Pegasus. Only by rising into the air above the Chimera was it possible to evade destruction by her fire-breathing head.

Because of her triple bodily nature and, in particular, the presence of three different heads, the Chimera is difficult to represent; in art, the lion part often dominates. It has been argued that, because of the uncertainty of her form, the Chimera has become a creature of language, representing the power of the imagination, fantasy, and illusion. It is these associations which lie behind the choice of title for the post-war Florentine literary magazine, La Chimera.

HELEN KING

Chin In modern humans the **mandibular arch** is formed by fusion at the centre of two separate bones, a process complete by two years of age. The thickening of this arch at the centre forms the prominent and distinctive **chin**. The well-defined chin and prominent nose of humans interrupt the generally vertical profile of adult human faces and are said to be distinguishing characteristics separating modern humans from prehuman ancestors and from other primates.

Sitting at the bottom of the FACE, and being the most visible element of the face during speech, the chin plays numerous important physical roles and has acquired several fascinating linguistic associations. The phrase 'to hold up by the chin', and the nursery story's line of escaping 'by the hairs of my chinny-chin-chin' both express the physical prominence of the chin; one conveys the role of the chin as a support that keeps one from sinking while the other marks the chin as a protrusion one must protect. The chin-strap of a hat or helmet secures that accessory to the head, while being 'in it up to your chin' and 'chin deep' — in water or in trouble — both reflect the role of the chin as the lowest point of the face, after which all is lost. To 'keep your chin up' or to 'take it on the chin' signify a measure of psychological or physical courage or fortitude indicated by keeping one's gaze straight ahead and not flinching. Finally, the less common usages of 'chin-wagging' or 'chin-chin' refer to chat or talk, and reflect the fact that the movement of the chin is both highly visible during and a key visual cue of speech.

The chin continues to develop through adolescence and early adulthood as other facial (especially nasal and dental) structures mature. As the size of the face relative to the cranium increases, the angle of the vertical slope from forehead to chin decreases and the chin becomes more protrusive in profile. These changes have been shown to be an important part of the facial cues commonly used to identify the age of individuals. Recent work in experimental psychology suggests that the characteristic differences between adult and infant human faces, and especially the softer, less angular features — including a less prominent chin — of infants play an important role in inhibiting aggression toward infants and stimulating caregiving. As psychologist Leslie Zebrowitz put it recently, 'A baby's face is disarming', an observation confirmed both by experiment and by the everyday experience of adults interacting with infants.

The chin plays a very important part in these experiences, and the presence of an adult chin in an adult face when placed on an infant's body is visually disorienting, as can be observed in portrayals of the Madonna from the late Middle Ages. Cimabue's *Madonna Enthroned* (c. 1280–90), Duccio's *Maestà* (c. 1311), and Giotto's *Madonna* (c. 1310) all portray the Christ child with a baby's body and an adult's face, with adult facial/cranial proportions, eye size and spacing, and nose size and prominence, and also, notably, a very adult chin. Later works, including Parmigianino's *Madonna With the Long Neck* (c. 1535) soften the child's face, showing more features of the 'baby face', including a less prominent chin, and provide a less jarring visual experience.

While a babyish chin and face often elicit caregiving from adults, a 'weak', or relatively undeveloped chin in adults, and especially in adult males, one less angular and elongated than average, often produces less positive reactions from other adults ('Chinless Wonder'). While it is difficult to separate the impact of the several components of a baby face in such responses, some evidence points to a prominent role for the chin. When presented with two similar faces distinguished largely by chin profile and development, the face with a typical adult chin is more likely to be associated with intelligence, physical strength, dominance, and sexual attractiveness, while the face with the more baby-like chin is frequently associated with lower levels of those features and higher levels of warmth, honesty, and agreeability. A quick glance at the profile of the traditional 'leading man' in cinema confirms these reactions; Clark Gable, Kirk Douglas, and other prominent stars display very prominent chins. The undeveloped, receding chin is characteristically a feature of an agreeable if immature or foolish character. In keeping with the association with babyish faces, weak chins are less common in movie villains than in more 'innocent' characters. Such casting and the reactions to it echo the claims of nineteenth- and twentieth-century PHYSIOGNOMY, that intellectual, psychological, and moral fitness can be discerned from facial (and other physical) features. As cited by Zebrowitz, the twentieth-century physiognomist, LeBarr, stated that 'a small deficient chin stands for weakness of will and physical endurance', while the nineteenth-century Swiss physiognomist, J. C. Lavater, categorized chins in men in a similar vein: 'The angular chin is seldom found but in well-disposed, firm men . . . flatness of chin speaks of the cold and dry; smallness, fear; and roundness, with a dimple, benevolence.'

As with most facial features, there are important gender-prototypical differences in the development of the chin. Typical adult females have smaller jaws, noses, and chins, and thus eyes and cheekbones that are more prominent and appear to be larger than in typical males. The less prominent chin in females does not appear to generate the negative reactions it does in men. To judge from the psychological evidence and from experience, conventional assumptions associate attractiveness in female faces with those features most similar to the baby face. Apparently, men but not women (at least in cultures much like our own) are expected to be able to 'take it on the chin', and are deemed more attractive if they can.

JEFFREY M. BARKER

See also FACE; SKULL.

Chiropody

Chiropody as an area of professional practice within health care concerned with the care and treatment of disorders of the FEET, has had both ancient and modern elements in its development. Whilst some health care professions (radiography and occupational therapy amongst others) are products purely of the twentieth century, chiropody, like DENTISTRY, is best understood as an older health-related craft reformed under twentieth-century conditions. The forebears of modern-day chiropodists were the itinerant corn-cutters of past centuries who plied their trade at fairs, markets, and in the streets. Little is known in detail about the history of corn-cutters, but by 1845 Lewis Durlacher, a leading British practitioner, was drawing a distinction between the new professional chiropodist and the humble journeyman cutter.

Durlacher argued that the treatment of foot conditions should become a firmer part of medical practice of his day, and that in particular those with 'the requisite surgical information' after examination should be granted a license to distinguish them from untrained corn-cutters. His attempts to create a trained and recognised new class of practitioner did not come to fruition for nearly half a century, when a 'Pedic Society' was founded in New York, followed in Britain in 1912 by the Society of Chiropodists. Foot care at this time was becoming a major business area, which may have stimulated these professional responses. The Scholl remedial footwear firm had developed in the US, successfully responding to market needs, and had opened its first London branch in 1910. British doctors of the day were generally not interested in this area as part of their practice, and only a dedicated few served as mentors, patrons, and examiners for the new Society of Chiropodists. However, by 1923 its journal, *The Chiropodist*, was presenting the new profession as a collateral branch of medicine in line with Durlacher's earlier ambitions, drawing its scientific principles into a neglected but now crucially important area of health care practice.

The ambitions of the British chiropodists were very much influenced in the 1920s by the general position of dentistry. Dentists were trained, licensed surgical practitioners with a 'body site' of their own, separate commercial premises under their own control, and amicable relationships with other medical practitioners. Although previously licensed by the Royal College of Surgeons, they had attained self regulation in 1921 — but attempts by chiropodists to follow this example with a parliamentary bill in 1928 was strongly resisted by organised, professional medical lobbyists. The British Medical Association's position was to oppose any other class of practitioner outside the formal jurisdiction of the medical profession. Chiropody was modestly defined in the bill as 'the diagnosis and medical, mechanical or surgical treatment of foot ailments such as abnormal nails, bunions, corns, warts and callosities but not the performance of operations for which an anaesthetic is required', but this was not enough to disarm extensive professional rivalries in the inter-war years.

Nevertheless, after further decades of boundary disputes with medicine, chiropody in Britain finally achieved state registration or licensing in 1960, largely within the terms of the above definition. In the meantime, podiatry had developed within chiropody, as a specialised and more surgically ambitious area of bone surgery. The Canadian province of Ontario, for example, now specifically licenses podiatry as 'cutting into osseous tissues of the metatarsals and toes of the foot, including osteotomies and joint surgery' including associated diagnosis. This more advanced type of practice is now internationally common and corresponds with the earlier ambitions of the turn-of-the-century professional modernisers and their vision of a collateral profession. As with other one-time medical auxiliary occupations, chiropody training in recent times has been incorporated into higher education, and now holds a secure place in the broad medical division of labour as one of the preventative and remedial health professions. Students are trained on graduate programmes to offer treatments in the area of biomechanics, sports medicine, and bone surgery under local anaesthesia, in addition to the more traditional concerns with corns, in-growing toenails, veruccas, and local injections. The fully-trained professional group suffers, in its own view, from unfair competition from untrained practitioners, and thus like all professions in such circumstances tries to prohibit their practice, but this claim in Britain at least has not so far been legally successful. Arguably it is more likely that chiropody's next phase of development will lie in even closer links with related medical, surgical, and health professional areas, particularly as health policies try both to contain health care costs and to support increasingly aged populations. Developments in podiatry, however professionally important, may remain a relatively minor part of chiropody's future compared with its wider co-operation with GPs, dieticians, physiotherapists, and others working in primary care services.

GERRY V. LARKIN

Further reading

Larkin, G. V. (1983). *Occupational monopoly and modern medicine*. Tavistock, London and New York.

Chiropractic

Chiropractic is a profession that specialises in the diagnosis, treatment, and overall management of conditions that are due to mechanical dysfunction of the JOINTS and muscles and its effects on the NERVOUS SYSTEM.

The philosophy behind chiropractic is that the body has the capability of healing itself. If factors of accident or lifestyle lead to poor, inadequate, or incorrect function in the spine or the joints, irritation of nerves and muscles can occur, causing direct or referred PAIN or discomfort, or even disease. Chiropractors use their skills and techniques to detect signs of restriction of movement, and to restore normal function and allow self-healing.

The term 'chiropractic' is derived from two Greek words, '*cheir*' and '*praktikos*', denoting treatment by hand, or manipulation. Chiropractic manipulation uses gentle hand movements known as 'adjustments'. The first chiropractic treatment was given by the Canadian Daniel David Palmer in 1895. One hundred years later the chiropractic profession is now established throughout the world, with national associations of chiropractors in over 70 countries.

A chiropractor will always begin a first consultation with a discussion of the patient's symptoms, medical history, lifestyle, and posture. The patient will then be examined, using standard neurological and orthopaedic tests and chiropractic manual tests, before the chiropractor begins treatment. Practitioners use many different techniques to adjust the body, and frequently offer self-help advice and exercise programmes to patients. They may also take X-RAYS when necessary to aid diagnosis. If the examination identifies underlying disease or a condition for which chiropractic is inappropriate they will immediately refer the patient to a general practitioner or consultant. Chiropractors do not prescribe drugs or use surgical procedures.

Restrictions in the movement of joints can often be detected before the onset of pain. For this reason, chiropractors advise people to have regular spinal check-ups, in the same way that they go for dental check-ups, to avoid pain in the future. This is believed to be particularly important for babies and young children, whose constant knocks and tumbles could lead to later joint problems, and for those young people whose developing bodies are liable to imbalance from carrying heavy bags, wearing fashionable footwear, sitting at computers, and an increasingly sedentary lifestyle.

Chiropractic treatment is suitable for people of any age, including babies, pregnant women, and the elderly, and for a wide range of conditions, including back pain; sciatica; tension headaches; migraine; neck, shoulder, and arm pains; sports injuries; repetitive strain injury; and many other joint and muscle disorders.

Treatment consists of rapid, highly specific adjustments to the affected joint, and sometimes soft tissue massage. Although normally painless, treatment may result in a 'popping' noise, which is due to pressure changes within the joint and has no significance. A treatment programme is tailored for each individual, and appropriate techniques are selected to suit that patient's age and overall condition. Manipulation of the spine is aimed at reducing the effects of stress on the particular spinal nerves that are associated with the patient's symptoms; thus, for example, a nerve affected in the cervical part of the vertebral column may be causing headache or neck pain, or in the lumbar part, low back pain. Chiropractors also treat pain in the limbs or the chest.

Manipulation for low back pain has attracted most attention and research. In 1995 the *British Medical Journal* reported on the follow-up of a Medical Research Council trial, which concluded that patients with low back pain treated by chiropractic derive more benefit and long-term satisfaction than those treated in hospital out-patient clinics. In September 1996 the Royal College of General Practitioners issued *Guidelines for the Management of Acute Low Back Pain*; these were reviewed and reissued in 1999, recommending manipulative treatment within the first weeks and confirming that the risks are very low in skilled hands.

Apart from these examples, research into the effectiveness of chiropractic has been relatively sparse. This is due largely to the problems of obtaining finance when drug companies are not involved. However, recent trials have been carried out in the UK, Denmark, Canada, and the Netherlands, with positive results, and an increasing number of UK chiropractors are undertaking comprehensive practice-based research projects.

Patients may also be treated for a range of other conditions such as asthma, indigestion and the irritable bowel syndrome, palpitations, high blood pressure, period pains, infantile colic, and other conditions which may not be directly related to the spine or joints. In cases where these less usual problems are treated, the patient's own doctor is generally contacted and a trial period of treatments agreed upon. Chiropractors believe that if they can reduce, by manipulation, the stress on a spinal nerve within the SPINAL COLUMN, this can affect dysfunctions stemming from the same vertebral level. They regularly report success with such treatment. Researchers world-wide are now investigating such claims. One example is a planned collaborative cardiology–chiropractor study of unexplained chest pain.

In the UK it takes 5 years to become a chiropractor: a full-time, 4-year BSc course, followed by a postgraduate year working in a clinic under supervision. Those who have trained at an accredited college can become members of the British Chiropractic Association; this was established in 1925 and now represents the majority of the 1200 UK practitioners. In North America there is a minimum of 6 years' university-level training: 2 years of qualifying sciences and 4 years of chiropractic college. The practice of chiropractic is licensed by law in all US states and Canadian provinces.

In the UK, the Chiropractors Act received Royal Assent in 1994. The General Chiropractic Council was established in 1997, and its statutory register opened in 1999; it is responsible for setting standards of both education and conduct, and since June 2001 all chiropractors are required to be registered if they are to practise legally in the UK.

Many health insurance companies will now pay for chiropractic treatment, and chiropractors are generally recognised as primary health care professionals by the medical establishment. The Clinical Standards Advisory Group recommended, in 1994, that there should be earlier access to the manipulative therapies and a redistribution of resources within the NHS to make this possible. MANYA MCMAHON

Further reading
Copland-Griffiths, M. (1991). *Dynamic chiropractic today*. Thorsons Publishers Ltd, Wellinborough.

Cholecystokinin (CCK) is a peptide HORMONE that causes contraction of the GALL BLADDER (the meaning of its name) and also release of digestive ENZYMES from the PANCREAS. Originally it was thought that these were the actions of two different hormones, cholecystokinin and pancreozymin, but they were later found to be identical. The hormone originates in endocrine cells in the gut — mainly in the *duodenum, iejunum,* and *ileum.*

This same peptide is found in neurons of the peripheral nervous system, including those in the gut, and in the brain, but little in the spinal cord. The highest concentrations are found in the cerebral cortex, hippocampus, thalamus, amygdala, and hypothalamus. The release of cholecystokinin from the endocrine cells of the gut can be promoted by the presence of digested egg yolk, cream, or olive oil in the duodenum, which also cause the gall bladder to contract. The release of cholecystokinin from neurones can be achieved in experimental studies by depolarisation, like most NEUROTRANSMITTERS, but little is known about its release from nerves under normal conditions.

The functions of cholecystokinin in the gut are clearly related to the need for BILE salts and pancreatic enzymes to digest meals rich in fat and protein, with the partially-digested material acting as the stimulus for release of bile and enzymes into the alkaline gut, once the acid phase of digestion has been completed in the stomach. Cholecystokinin is sometimes injected into patients as a test of gall bladder function.

The neurotransmitter functions in the brain are as yet unclear, although it has been suggested that cholecystokinin is involved in the regulation of hormone secretion, e.g. by promoting release of growth hormone and inhibiting release of thyroid stimulating hormone.

Thus a substance first identified as a blood-borne hormone is apparently widely used in the body to carry 'chemical messages' between cells. ALAN W. CUTHBERT

See also ALIMENTARY SYSTEM; HORMONES; NEUROTRANSMITTERS.

Cholesterol Many people are now aware of their own blood cholesterol level, have it measured regularly and eat diets high in polyunsaturates. This is because they know that high cholesterol levels in the blood, and fat-rich diets, are likely to lead to HEART ATTACKS and STROKES, particularly in later life. Some also know that the narrowing of arteries, particularly the coronary arteries, is due to the deposition of atherosclerotic plaques, made largely of cholesterol, on the walls of the vessels. Narrowing of the arteries reduces the flow rate, especially as flow depends on the fourth power of the radius. Thus, at a given pressure, reducing the radius to one half of normal would reduce the flow rate to one sixteenth of the original value. Adequate flow can then only be maintained by a rise in BLOOD PRESSURE.

The importance of cholesterol in the body can be gauged from the words of Brown and Goldstein in their Nobel Prize Lecture in 1985. They described cholesterol as the 'most decorated' molecule in biology, as no less than 13 Nobel awards had been made to those who spent their lives studying the substance, adding that 'the property that makes it useful in cell membranes, namely its absolute insolubility in water, also makes it lethal'.

Cholesterol was first isolated from gallstones in 1784. It is a neutral lipid, a sterol, and an important constituent of CELL MEMBRANES. Cholesterol is obtained through the diet and synthesised in the body, in the LIVER and the intestine. When the intake is high, synthesis is suppressed. The cholesterol molecule has 27 carbon atoms, yet the synthesis of this complex molecule is from 2-carbon fragments (acetyl CoA) in a very complex biosynthetic process. Cholesterol is the necessary precursor of several *sterol* (steroid) hormones, such as the SEX HORMONES testosterone and oestrogens, and the adrenal steroid hormones, including cortisol. Not surprisingly — remembering that cholesterol was found first in gall stones — cholesterol is used to make bile salts, the constituents of BILE which take an essential part in fat absorption from the gut.

To understand how *atherosclerotic plaques* become deposited in arteries it is necessary to understand how the highly insoluble cholesterol is moved about the body. The agents which transport cholesterol are the lipoproteins — consisting, as their name implies, of a lipid and a protein component. Fats and cholesterol absorbed from the diet are transported as 'chylomicrons' from the intestine to the liver, where the fats are rapidly metabolised, and cholesterol is incorporated into *low density lipoprotein* (LDL) along with phospholipid molecules and one molecule of a huge protein called B-100. LDL is the main cholesterol transporter, transferring it from the liver to all other parts of the body. Since cholesterol is an essential component of all cell membranes it will be needed anywhere new cells are being formed.

The B-100 protein is a key component of LDL, as it is the molecule that is recognised by LDL receptors in the membrane of all cells. After this recognition, the LDL complex is internalised and broken down in the cell, which thus has its vital supply of cholesterol delivered to it. The LDL receptor is recycled back to the membrane to wait for another LDL. When the supply of cholesterol is plentiful the LDL receptors are 'down regulated' (their numbers are reduced), leaving low density lipoprotein circulating in the blood with its potentially lethal cargo of cholesterol. Eventually the cholesterol is deposited in a variety of sites, including the skin, but it is the deposition in blood vessels that leads to the start of atherosclerotic disease.

These processes were worked out in the researches of Brown and Goldstein in the 1970s from studies on patients with *familial hypercholesterolamia* — excessively high blood cholesterol. In this genetic disease, LDL membrane receptors are absent, so the uptake of LDL into cells is prevented. *Heterozygotes* (who have inherited one normal gene and one gene for this disease from their parents) have only half the normal number of LDL receptors. Normal persons have about 175 mg cholesterol per 100 ml of blood plasma, while those with the disease have over 600 mg/100 ml and heterozygotes about 300 mg/100 ml. *Homozygotes* with the disease usually die in infancy of coronary artery occlusion.   ALAN W. CUTHBERT

See also BILE; FATS; GALL BLADDER.

Christianity and the body

Christianity is centred on the life, death, and RESURRECTION of Jesus of Nazareth, yet there is enormous diversity in the interpretation of that life and death, and no agreement about what is meant by resurrection. This multiplicity of interpretation begins with the gospels themselves. Accounts of Jesus' resurrection, for example, range from placing emphasis on the physicality of the resurrected body, which eats boiled fish and honeycomb (Luke 24: 39), to asserting that Jesus could pass through closed doors and was unrecognizable to his disciples (Luke 24: 16–30).

Mirroring claims in the gospels about the resurrection of Jesus Christ, some of the earliest Christian texts understand human salvation in terms of the resurrection of the body. The apostle Paul, for example, uses a number of different metaphors in his letters to express the resurrection of the body, giving rise to the diversity of Christian belief about the nature of the human being in its fallen and saved states. As Caroline Walker Bynum argues, in part because of this emphasis on the resurrection of the body (both of Christ and of the believer), Christianity is the 'world religion' most intent on defending the idea that the body is essential to the self.

The emphasis on MARTYRDOM and ASCETICISM within early and medieval Christianity led many modern commentators, beginning with Enlightenment historians like Edward Gibbon, to claim that Christianity is a world- and body-despising religion. Late twentieth-century historians like Peter Brown and Bynum show that these practices must be seen in relationship to resurrection beliefs and the EUCHARIST.

Although early and medieval Christians sought to transcend the limitations of the body, this occurred through the transformation of the body itself. Martyrologies show Christians joyfully undergoing intense suffering because their bodies have been transformed into Christ's; they possess resurrected bodies that cannot feel the pain inflicted on them. Although early monastic texts are rife with evidence that practitioners fear SEXUALITY, which is associated with the earthly life of the body and its entanglement in society, this asceticism again leads to the transformation of the body. The desert father Anthony (fourth century CE), for example, after years in the desert wrestling with the demons of his own sexuality and other vices, glows; his body is transformed into the spiritual body of the resurrection, attesting to Anthony's victory over vice and his achieved sanctity.

Emphasis on the sanctity of the human body can also be seen in the cult of the martyrs and saints, in which bodily remains are imbued with divine power. For some late medieval saints, often women, the suffering and ascetic body is transformed in life into a source of divine, healing effluvia; manna, sweet-smelling oils, and milk flow from the bodies of many holy women. Even things associated with holy women's bodies become sources of healing sanctity. When Margaret of Ypres' mother (one would have thought wisely) buried the rotting, sweat-drenched cloth that had been bound around the head of the dying holy woman, her confessor unearthed it, demonstrating its miraculous healing powers. Although there is evidence that some medieval holy women rebelled against this association of their bodies with the salvific body of Christ, because of the intense bodily and spiritual suffering it demanded, this is clearly the dominant model of female sanctity throughout the latter Middle Ages.

Arguably, Eastern Christianity is even more bodily in its belief and practices than the West. The Eastern church emphasizes the presence of God through icons, words, and actions. Symbolic actions are crucial to Eastern Christian liturgy and private prayer, most evident in the so-called 'physical method' of prayer taught by the Byzantine Hesychasts. A special position for prayer is advised (sitting on a low stool with the head lowered and chin resting on the knees); breathing is to be regulated in accordance with recitation of the Jesus Prayer; and the practitioner is to seek out his or her 'heart'. The latter seems to refer both to the physical organ and to the spiritual centre of the person, understood as being in some way allied with that physical centre.

Historians are just beginning to turn attention to the place of the body within Protestant and Catholic reformation Christianity, but the complexity of the issues can be discerned in Protestant debates about the nature of the divine presence as body and blood within the Eucharist. Just as sixteenth-century reformers eschewed the cult of the saints and its bodily manifestations, they also began to question

medieval Catholic doctrines of transubstantiation, the real presence of Christ's body and blood in the bread and wine of the Eucharist. Although these debates are far too complex to be summarized here, they began the process of spiritualization that some argue led to a denial of Christ's bodily resurrection and of the bodily resurrection of the believer. When modern philosophy begins to assert a dualistic separation of human mind from human body and the relative autonomy of the former, Protestantism will be in a position to make these claims theologically plausible. This move arguably does not mark a turn away from the body within Western culture, however, but rather its increased objectification and medicalization, as witnessed in the paradigmatic work of the philosopher and scientist René Descartes.

AMY HOLLYWOOD

Further reading
Brown, P. (1988). *The body and society: men, women, and sexual renunciation in early Christianity.* Columbia, New York.

Bynum, C. W. (1995). *The resurrection of the body in Western Christianity, 200–1336.* Columbia, New York.

Coakley, S. ed. (1997). *Religion and the body.* Cambridge University Press, Cambridge.

See also EUCHARIST; HOST; MARTYRDOM; RELIGION AND THE BODY; RESURRECTION; SAINTS.

Chyle

The milky fluid which travels in the lymphatic vessels draining the small intestine. It contains most of the products of digestion of the fat content of a meal, which are absorbed into the microscopic *lacteals* in the *villi* that project from the intestinal lining. Chyle is a particular type of lymph — the general term for fluid drained from body tissues; it flows into progressively larger channels to join lymph from other parts of the body in the *thoracic duct* in the chest, and thence reaches the bloodstream.   S.J.

See PLATE 1.

See ALIMENTARY SYSTEM; LYMPHATIC SYSTEM.

Cinematography and the body

It is difficult today to imagine a world in which we could not record the human image in movement. Yet this was a goal which frustrated many inventors, until in the early 1890s Thomas Edison and others succeeded in devising a practical form of serial photography using strips of celluloid, which could then be viewed and reproduced. The result seemed little short of a miracle. Early reviews of moving picture shows in 1895 spoke of 'bringing the dead back to life', while the experiments that preceded this success solved long-standing questions about, for instance, how horses' legs moved while galloping (Eadweard Muybridge) or how athletes performed intricate actions (Etienne-Jules Marey). By the end of the century, what had started as mainly a scientific quest was already becoming a familiar entertainment, sandwiched between live acts in variety programmes. Soon it became the dominant leisure activity of the twentieth century — watching images of remote humans and animals perform while sitting in a darkened room.

But if lifelike reproduction of movement was the first aim, this was soon overtaken by the realization that cinematography could make the impossible seem credible. Georges Méliès was a French magician turned film-maker who specialized in fantasy from 1898 to 1912, creating images such as his own head appearing to expand like a balloon and explode, and of every kind of grotesque transformation or mutilation of the body. Several basic techniques pioneered by Méliès have remained standard: stop-action permits remarkable transformations; reverse action negates normal causality; overprinted or 'matted' images place the familiar in unrelated settings. The result of these techniques, later reinforced by computer generated images (CGI), has been to create a screen world in which almost any action, however impossible or bizarre, appears convincingly real.

Alongside this largely unforeseen by-product of cinematography, its use as a recording medium contributed to both scientific research and popularization of science from an early stage. The French surgeon Etienne-Louis Doyen had his pioneering operations filmed in 1898, proposing to colleagues that this would teach students more efficiently, but discovered the pitfalls of cinema in 1902 when his film of the separation of Siamese twins was pirated and sold to fairground freak shows. Such occasional scandals did not impede the steady growth of scientific uses of film, which spread to the social sciences as ethnographers became enthusiastic recorders of tribal customs and vanishing ways of life. Explorers also soon realized that film of their exotic adventures could help fund expeditions, as was the case with Captain Scott's tragic Antarctic expedition of 1911–12. Herbert Ponting's record of Scott before he left base camp was actually being shown in London after its subject had died — an eerie reminder of film's 'resurrectionary' quality. Ten years later, Robert Flaherty's portrait of an Inuit hunter and his family, *Nanook of the North*, enjoyed a world-wide success and helped launch the new genre of 'documentary' film.

Much controversy has since arisen from the claim that documentary is or should be truthful. Flaherty did not scruple to teach his subjects how to perform their own forgotten 'traditional' customs, but many other documentarists believe that the camera can either reveal what the unaided human observer would not see (Vertov), or what is provoked by its presence (the Maysles brothers; Rouch). Both of these amount to a claim that film offers a privileged view of human behaviour, although whether this can be regarded as 'objective', given the manipulation of editing, remains highly controversial. What is certain is that much of our information about how 'real' people appear and behave is channelled through the conventions of television news and documentary.

From its beginnings, cinema has also been a powerful source of fictionalized images, of performances intended to entertain, amuse, seduce, and inspire. Erotic display, whether in the form of exotic dances, or a prolonged close-up kiss (which formed the entire action of a 1900 Edison film), or frankly pornographic scenes, were an early source of voyeuristic appeal. This trend arguably helped to shape twentieth-century personal behaviour patterns, replacing national customs with a new international etiquette learned from the screen. Early film stars, such as Asta Nielsen in Europe or Mary Pickford in America, created new ideals of female appearance — essentially slimmer and more athletic — which quickly became global as cinema-going became a universal pastime by the eve of World War I. The male body was also transformed by such popular stars as the dapper Max Linder and Charlie Chaplin's Tramp, both of whom shaped the growth of a balletic slapstick as the main genre of film comedy until the coming of sound in the 1930s.

This period saw the emergence of a genre in fiction cinema that has since become vitally important in popularizing the idea of 'bionic', or mechanically modified, bodies. Although there had been many previous gothic and technological fantasies, the series of 'horror' films produced by Universal in the 1930s launched a new vogue; and in particular the make-up devised for Boris Karloff as the monster in *Frankenstein* (1931) set a pattern which, while often played for laughs, also leads to such conceptually more sophisticated composites as the humanoid 'replicants' of *Blade Runner* (1982), or the eponymous *RoboCop* (1987), or the self-repairing 'cyborgs' of *Terminator 2: Judgement Day* (1991). Through increasingly elaborate special effects, the image of the human body in contemporary cinema can now routinely appear super-human, and can apparently withstand devastating injury. What effect this near-universal entertainment idiom has on our idea of actual bodies, and on attitudes to medical treatment and research, is surely an important, yet under-researched topic. More common is a recurring undercurrent of moral concern about the likelihood of imitative behaviour, often expressed in relation to the portrayal of violence or drug-taking, or the dangerous appeal of extreme thinness, fashionable among film stars, as a role model for young women susceptible to anorexia.

There is, however, renewed research interest in how we perceive and interpret moving images. Historically, four main paradigms in this field can be distinguished. The first, dating from the 1910s, conceived moving pictures broadly as a new form of pictorial language, potentially related to hieroglyphic or ideogrammatic languages, or to primitive sign systems. A second wave of theory challenged this view in the 1920s, inspired by the kinetic editing of Eisenstein, Pudovkin, and other exponents of Soviet Russian 'montage' cinema. Two important influences on this were Ivan Pavlov's study of reflexes and Lev Vygotsky's

investigation of 'inner speech': the spectator's response to a film was conceived in terms of conditioned reflexes to visual stimuli, or as a process of linking seemingly unconnected images by means of pre-cognitive associations such as those involved in metaphor. During the early decades of synchronized-sound cinema, such theories were largely forgotten and most theoretical reflection was based on either the principles of mimesis or generic convention. Thus, it was claimed, we understand film images because they 'model' the world as we ordinarily perceive it; and we grasp the conventions of film narrative because these follow other forms of visual and verbal narrative.

During the 1970s, a new wave of film theory emerged which drew upon semiotics, or the study of sign-systems, and a revisionist psychoanalysis identified with French analyst Jacques Lacan. This identified mainstream cinema as an 'apparatus', which effectively conditions its spectators to believe that they are privileged witnesses of a seamless reality and idealized characters on the screen. But there is also a 'mirroring' effect, similar to that which, according to Lacan, marks a crucial stage in the formation of the individual's sense of self. So, in the cinema we 'recognize' the process of acquiring subjectivity — which is also a misrecognition, an illusion. Through such reasoning, 1970s film theory radically revised traditional theories of 'identification', introducing a sophisticated view of gender relations between viewer and actor, but also encouraging the view that the film 'text' produces its spectator's orientation towards it.

Psychoanalytic spectatorship theory has always been as controversial as psychoanalysis itself, and yet it became something of an orthodoxy in academic film studies during the 1980s and 1990s, and began to influence critical approaches in other media, such as literature and the visual arts. But an opposing paradigm emerged during the 1990s which seems to be gathering strength. Often known loosely as 'cognitivism', this attempts to return to a 'realist' view of what happens when we watch a film. Thus, for example, the philosopher Greg Currie claims that films are actually moving pictures, rather than illusions, that they are realistic, and that they encourage us to imagine the events portrayed taking place — all common sense views, but ones that raise issues of definition. This in turn has led to a considerable amount of philosophical interest in explaining what we mean by such claims and descriptions. It has also prompted some film scholars to turn to experimental physiology and psychology to gain a better understanding of what 'really' happens when we watch and understand films. In this latest, and equally controversial, stage of film theory, the moving image has perhaps returned to its origins, as a by-product of mid-nineteenth-century enthusiasm to explore perceptual phenomena and of technology's ability to exploit them. Meanwhile, the total manipulation of digital image and sound and their use in the simulation of 'virtual reality' promises a new era in which cinema may become a purely historical term.

IAN CHRISTIE

Further reading

Clover, C. (1992). *Men, woman and chain saws: gender in the modern horror film*. Princeton, Princeton NJ.

Hill, J. and Gibson, P. C. (ed.) (1998). *The Oxford guide to film studies*. Oxford University Press. Especially section on 'The film text: theoretical frameworks'.

Williams, L. (ed.) (1995). *Viewing positions: ways of seeing film*. Rutgers University Press, New Brunswick, NJ.

See also PHOTOGRAPHY; SPECTATOR.

Circumcision

Circumcision or *posthetomy*, is the operative removal of all or part of the prepuce of the PENIS. By extension to the female the term is also used for clitoridectomy, which can range from the ritual drawing of blood to infibulation (the removal of the CLITORIS and parts of the LABIA). Male circumcision has been read in the West to be a sign of everything from sexual hygiene, to cosmetic appearance, to tribal identity or a mark of adulthood, to either diminishing or enhancing sexual desire, to increased or decreased fertility, to patriarchal subjugation, to enhanced purity, to the improvement of sexual endurance, to a form of attenuated castration, to menstrual envy, to a substitute for human sacrifice.

In Pharaonic Egypt boys were circumcised between the ages of 6 and 12. The Jews were the group which continued to practise infant male circumcision in Western Europe after the advent of Christianity. Infant male circumcision as practised by the Jews occurs on the eighth day after birth. It represents the covenant of God with Abraham (Genesis 17: 10–14). Even after the Shoah and the increased presence of Muslims, who also ritually circumcise their infants in Europe, circumcision continues to be associated with the image of the Jews.

There are four 'traditional' views of the 'meaning' of circumcision in connection with the Jews. Following the writings of Paul (Acts 15), the first view saw circumcision as inherently symbolic and, therefore, no longer valid after the rise of Christianity. This view was espoused by the Church Fathers, Eusebius and Origen; it continued through the Renaissance (Erasmus) and through the Reformation (Luther). It forms the theological basis for the distinction which Christians were able to make between their bodies and the bodies of the Jews.

The second view saw circumcision as a sign of a political or group identity. The rhetoric in which the accepted science of the late nineteenth century clothed its rejection of circumcision is of importance. It was intense and virulent, and never free from negative value judgments. One central example should suffice. The liberal Italian physician Paolo Mantegazza (1831–1901), one of the standard 'ethnological' sources from the late nineteenth century for the nature of human sexuality, decried the 'mutilation of the genitals' among 'savage tribes' including the Jews.

The third reading of circumcision saw it as a remnant of the early Jewish idol or phallus worship. Thus J. H. F. Autenrieth saw circumcision as but a primitive act practised by culturally inferior peoples such as Jews and African Blacks. Autenrieth, by 1829 the Chancellor of the University of Tübingen, entered the discussion of the meaning of circumcision with a public lecture on its history. For him, as for others, circumcision was a surrogate for human sacrifice. The nineteenth-century British anthropologist John Lubbock saw such rites of sacrifice as a 'stage through which, in any natural process of development, religion must pass'. But the Jews also sacrificed their animals at the Temple as 'symbols of human sacrifice . . . [which] were at one time habitual among the Jews'. Circumcision was a sign of 'the inherent barbarism of this people', a view seconded by a Dr Hacker in a medical journal during 1843. Here again the medical discussion of a social practice becomes contaminated by the racial context into which it is placed. Indeed, this view dominates the discussion of the ethno-psychologists into the late nineteenth and early twentieth centuries about the meaning of circumcision as a semantic sign. The experimental psychologist Wilhelm Wundt sees circumcision as

> of the nature of sacrifice. Along with the offering of hair in the cult of the dead and with the pouring out of blood in connection with deity worship, it belongs to that form of sacrifice in which the sacrificial object gains its unique value by virtue of its being the vehicle of the soul. Thus, the object of sacrifice, in the case of circumcision, may perhaps be interpreted as a substitute for such internal organs as the kidneys or testicles, which are particularly prized as vehicles of the soul but which can either not be offered at all, on the part of the living, or whose sacrifices involves serious difficulties.

For Wundt, politically a liberal in his time, Judaism is '. . . but one of those vanquished cults which struggled for supremacy in the pre-Constantinian period of the Roman World Empire'. And the practice of this substitute for ritual sacrifice is a sign of the barbarism and marginality of the Jew.

The fourth reading of circumcision saw it as a form of medical prophylaxis. This seems to be first claimed in the writing of the Greco-Jewish historian Philo, who was writing in a strongly Hellenistic culture which found any mutilation of the body abhorrent. He claimed that it was a prophylaxis against diseases of the penis, which also promoted the well being of the individual and assured fertility. But the hygienic rationale was also evoked, as we have seen, in the work of Johann David Michaelis, the central German commentator on this practice in the eighteenth century. It is only in the middle of the nineteenth century that the debate about the medical meaning of circumcision impacts upon the Jewish community in Central Europe. Prior to this the discussions concerning the meaning of circumcision in the Christian community remained separate from Jewish concern in Europe. While the image of the circumcised Jew was raised as a central metaphor for Jewish difference in Great Britain with the presentation of the Jewish Naturalization Act in 1753, it only became of importance with the gradual acculturation of the Jewish in Germany and Austria toward the middle of the nineteenth century. The debates within and without the Jewish communities concerning the nature and implication of circumcision surfaced in Germany during the 1840s.

By the end of the nineteenth century, ritual circumcision had grown in disrepute in Germany because of its association with questions of 'race'. However, when Jewish practice was understood as hygienic and could be emulated, circumcision came to be held in higher repute. In a study undertaken by the British surgeon Jonathan Hutchinson in 1854, the incidence of syphilis among London Jews was found to be one-fifteenth of that of the general community. He found that this did not reflect a higher moral stance (as the gonorrhea rate was the same in both groups), but assumed that it was the result of a more general immunity. Hutchinson's views echo the more general assumption of the time, that 'Jews escape the great epidemics more readily than the other races with whom they live'. In the US it came to be associated with the hygiene movement after the Spanish–American war' and was seen as a universal panacea for venereal disease. By the late twentieth century, circumcision for prophylactic reasons had come to be common medical practice in the US, but very uncommon in the UK, and even after the Holocaust it remained a relatively rare medical procedure in Germany.

SANDER L. GILMAN

Further reading

Gilman, S. L. (1993). *Freud, race and gender*. Princeton University Press, Princetown.

Hoffman, L. A. (1996). *Covenant of blood: circumcision and gender in Rabbinic Judaism*. University of Chicago Press, Chicago.

Remondino, P. C. (1891). *History of circumcision: from the earliest times to the present: moral and physical reasons for its performance: history of eunuchism, hermaphrodism, etc. and of the different operations practiced upon the prepuce*. F. A. Davis, Philadelphia and London.

Clairvoyance

Clairvoyance Part of the larger phenomenon know as EXTRA SENSORY PERCEPTION (ESP), clairvoyance is the ability to discern images not readily detected by the five senses. Those with this 'sixth sense' receive messages transmitted over both temporal distances — visions of events occurring in either the past (*retrocognition*) or future (*precognition*) — and geographic distances — events happening simultaneously but in different locations. Other terms for clairvoyance include second sight, shadow sight, prophecy, and spiritual communication. Related abilities include *clairaudience* (hearing inaudible sound), *telekinesis* (moving objects without touching them), and *psychometry* (determining the history of an object or its owner through handling the object). *Parapsychology* is the study of these abilities.

Clairvoyance is based on increased sensitivity and awareness of potential channels for communication. On some level everyone possesses the ability for prophetic sight: an inner voice warns the woman not to get on the elevator with the stranger, a man decides not to board a plane only to learn later that his flight has crashed. Often clairvoyant abilities surface during or following times of heightened stress, such as serious illness or accident, extreme physical danger, or NEAR DEATH EXPERIENCES. A smaller proportion of the population, those traditionally thought of as clairvoyant, appear to have mastered the control of their brainpower, resulting in stronger psychic abilities.

Clairvoyant episodes can occur in a fully conscious state, or while dreaming, fasting, or using hallucinogenic drugs. Messages can also be received while the person is in a suspended state or trance. Often clairvoyants will engage in the practice of scrying; concentrating on the shiny surface of an object such as a mirror, stone, or pool of water to help visions materialize. A common image of such is the fortune-teller with her crystal ball.

While the term 'clairvoyance' first appeared in English in 1840, the phenomenon of second sight itself is much older. Prophetic predictions have been made for thousands of years in cultures and religions all around the globe. Aristotle wrote on prophesying through dreams. Nostradamus offered many predictions for the coming centuries. Other examples include visions by Russian, Scottish, and Japanese seers as well as numerous Australian and North American aboriginal tribal elders. In some cultures, those with second sight are called sages or wise ones. In other cases, such as Europe in the Middle Ages, such abilities bring charges of WITCHCRAFT or heresy.

Often during times of escalated conflict between scientific discovery and religious philosophy a bridge is sought for the gap between the physical and spiritual worlds, and interest in phenomena like clairvoyance, ESP, and the occult rises. Throughout Europe and North America during the second half of the nineteenth century and into the twentieth century, numerous people advertised their services as clairvoyants and spirit mediums. Many subscribed to the belief of spiritualism, and hosting séances became a popular form of social gathering. Following World War II, interest in such activities waned, but with the approach of the new millennium interest in predicting the future increased, and clairvoyance has now gone high-tech with the help of psychic hotlines and the Internet. LYNNE FALLWELL

See also EXTRASENSORY PERCEPTION.

Cleft lip and palate

Cleft lip and palate are congenital deformities of variable severity. The face begins to develop around the fourth week of life in the womb, from five different parts of the developing fetal tissue — a central one and two on each side. These embryonic cellular components normally migrate and fuse to give rise to the nose, the sides and centre of the upper lip, and the palate and the lower jaw. Any failure of fusion of these parts can result in a cleft. The severity may vary from a barely detectable groove or ridge with a gap in the underlying muscles, to a complete cleft on each side of the lip associated with clefts extending back through the gums and the palate. Although genetic factors are implicated, the causes of such deformities are considered to be multi-factorial. Cleft lip and palate (CL/P) and cleft palate alone (CP) are different entities with varying incidence, epidemiology, and genetics.

Clefts of the lip, with or without clefts of the palate, occur in 1 in 750 live births, as compared with 1 in 2000 for clefts of the palate alone. CL/P is commoner in boys and CP alone is commoner in girls. There are racial variations in incidence of CL/P, with a decreasing order of frequency in Orientals, Europeans, and Africans, but there is no heterogeneity in the incidence of CP.

The problems associated with clefts of the lip and palate are both aesthetic and functional.

Aesthetic problems — those related to appearance — are mainly in patients with clefts of the lip. These may be on one side of the central part or on both sides. Clefts of the lip are also associated with deformity of the nose and asymmetry of the underlying facial skeleton which contribute to the problems of abnormal facial appearance.

Functional problems are minor in unrepaired clefts of the lip except in the infant, when there may be difficulty in sucking due to inability to achieve an efficient lip seal, or later, when clarity of speech or whistling may be affected. Unrepaired clefts of the palate, especially the soft palate, cause significant functional problems associated with speech and swallowing. Eustachian tube malfunction in CP patients may result in middle ear infections and hearing loss.

The earliest repairs recorded in history were in China circa 390 AD; in Europe the first report was of surgical repair by a French dentist, le Monier, in 1764. Advances in surgical techniques, and especially anaesthesia, now allow anatomical correction with great precision in restoration of form and function. Traditional repair of the cleft lip is recommended at around the age of 3 months or at a weight of 10 lbs, and of the cleft palate at about 18 months — but various protocols and techniques exist. Current techniques are very successful but there is considerable controversy regarding the effects of surgery and possible adverse influences on facial growth and function. ARUP K. RAY

See also CONGENITAL ABNORMALITIES.

Clitoris

Clitoris Unlike the PENIS, of which it is usually described as the female homologue, the clitoris does not enjoy an array of nicknames, euphemisms or slang terms. There is even some controversy as to its pronunciation, whether this should be clitt-oris or cly-toris; dictionaries vary and some give both as correct (although the *Oxford English Dictionary* prefers 'cly-toris'), but this means that there is still a decision to be made, which may cause hesitation in referring to this organ in speech. The derivation of the word is commonly alleged to derive from the Greek '*Kleis*', meaning 'key', but there is some philological debate about this, as discussed in a 1937 article by Professor Marcel Cohen — reprinted by Thomas Power Lowry in *The Classic Clitoris* (1978).

The anatomy of the clitoris was described in 1559 by Renaldus Columbus of Padua, who claimed that previous anatomists had overlooked the very existence of 'so pretty a thing'. His primacy was, however, contested by another eminent anatomist of Padua, Gabrielo Fallopio. Although they claimed to have discovered this organ, since antiquity there had been a powerful belief that mutual ORGASM was necessary for conception, which suggests that, though unnamed, the clitoris was known to be there. Renaldus had discovered something that had not been named or mapped, but which other people (though not, perhaps, the people he would recognise as colleagues) and other traditions had already known about.

The clitoris is a tiny organ which even the woman to whom it belongs may find difficulty in seeing, except with the aid of a mirror (unless she is very flexible). It may be so concealed as only to come into view when the *labia majora* — the outer lips of the VAGINA — are separated. Located above and in front of the urethral and vaginal openings, it is structurally connected to the *labia minora* (the inner lips of the vagina). The visible *glans* of the clitoris, which is hooded by a prepuce formed by the meeting of the labia minora, is, however, only the outward and visible manifestation of much more extensive erectile tissue, which forms a padding over the pubic bone. These concealed parts are anatomically continuous with and functionally linked to the vagina. The whole structure is densely packed with nerve endings: although there are a similar number to those of the penis, they are much more concentrated and closer together. It may be noted that, although, anatomically speaking, the clitoris is homologous to the penis, the female genitalia are far more differentiated than those of the male: instead of one organ which conveys sperm and urine, and is the source of sexual pleasure, a woman has three different parts for three distinct purposes. When erotically stimulated, the clitoris becomes engorged and erectile; when a high degree of arousal is reached it retracts, with the effect that it appears to have reduced in size. Vaginal lubrication takes place along with the engorgement of the outer part of the vagina. When sexual excitement reaches its peak, orgasm takes place, with rhythmic contractions of the muscles around the clitoris and vagina. Unlike men, women have the capacity for multiple orgasm without an intervening refractory period.

The appearance of the external glans of the clitoris is very various. In some women it may be quite noticeable and an obvious analogue to the penis, in others it may be small and barely visible.

Although these are innate physiological characteristics, the size of the clitoris has been assumed to relate to the sexual activity of the female, and to be excessively developed by masturbation or indulgence in lesbian practices. Successive editions of a standard British textbook of forensic medicine rather gratuitously (since female homosexuality has never been in itself a crime in Britain) included a photograph of a 'tribade's' clitoris well into the middle of the twentieth century.

The role of the clitoris in orgasm has been the subject of very heated controversy. Although for centuries it had been known by medical and religious authorities in Europe that titillating the clitoris had a beneficial effect on conjugal relations, rendering them more pleasant and more likely to be fertile, from the later eighteenth century this information apparently became increasingly hidden. Popular handbooks which went on being reprinted in the nineteenth century underwent expurgation and referred, if at all, much more generally to the necessity of mutual caresses and pleasure between the married couple. However, although the arousing role of the clitoris had been recognised, and even that a woman might bring about an orgasm by self-stimulation if her husband failed to give her an orgasm through intercourse, the assumption was very persistent that if women masturbated, they did so with a dildo in order to mimic penetrative intercourse. (Even today, although vibrators are most often used for clitoral stimulation, the large number of the models available vary in shape from the generally phallic to the hyper-realistically penile.) This supposition extended to the idea of women having sex with one another being thought impossible or else involving this substitution. There are some grounds, however, for believing that there may well have been an oral culture, mainly among women, which, if it could not scientifically name and describe the clitoris, nevertheless knew about its significance. This, however, was increasingly eroded by the rise of a print culture privileging published writings (the vast majority by men) above oral information, and by a variety of social changes including greater privacy and greater separation between social classes.

A new ethos of mutual sexual pleasure in marriage arose during the early twentieth century: though shared pleasure had been an ideal in the Victorian era, suppression and ignorance meant that it had not always been achieved even with the best intentions. Authors of marriage manuals emphasised the important contribution of the clitoris to the sexual arousal and satisfaction of the woman, even going so far as to suggest, in some cases, that the bridegroom should give his wife her first orgasm by manual stimulation before proceeding to defloration. Even so, clitoral stimulation was seen as something ancillary to penetrative heterosexual intercourse, which was defined as the central conjugal act.

The clitoris received, as it were, a setback as a result of the wide acceptance and popularisation of Freudian psychoanalytic ideas. According to this, clitoral stimulation was immature and masculine in its nature (though it may well be doubted that little girls relate this concealed if sensitive spot to the penis, if they have ever seen a penis), and, to be truly women, women needed to abandon clitoral pleasures and effect a transfer to achieving orgasm vaginally. This theory was contested by a developing school of empirical sex research — and it should be noted that marriage advice manuals continued to stress the importance of clitoral stimulation, at least until the wife's sexual responsiveness was 'fully developed' Alfred Kinsey, in his study of the sex life of the American female (published in 1953), noted the vast difference in sensitivity between the vaginal wall and the clitoris and labia minora. (William) Masters and (Virginia) Johnson observed sexual interactions in a laboratory setting, and, on the basis of these observations, which involved various technological devices to measure arousal and orgasm, they concluded that orgasm was always clitoral: even if the clitoris was not being directly stimulated, indirect stimulation was taking place as a result of friction from the pulling on the labia caused by penile thrusting during intercourse. Vaginal contractions were one manifestation of the orgasm produced by the clitoris. These findings came out in 1966, contemporaneously with the enormous social changes which led to the 'second wave' of feminism and the short-lived 'Sexual Revolution'. Women found that this research supplied them with a way of describing experiences which had been neglected or distorted by the masculine assumption that the acme of sexual pleasure consisted of penis-in-vagina thrusting (probably mostly quite uninfluenced by psychoanalytic ideas of the superior maturity of the vaginal over the clitoral orgasm). Works such as Danish author Mette Ejlersen's *I Accuse!* (British edition 1969) and Anne Koedt's 1970 article 'The Myth of the Vaginal Orgasm' made a forceful if anecdotal case for the preceding obliteration of women's actual experience. Shere Hite's more extensive (though methodologically much criticised) survey, published as *The Hite Report* in 1976, to enormous publicity, revealed the importance of clitoral stimulation to women's sexual pleasure. The notion was disseminated in a range of popular publications, handbooks on women's health from a feminist perspective, works of sexual advice, and also in numerous novels taking advantage of a new explicitness.

However, other sex researchers have contested the conclusion that there is only one kind of orgasm, suggesting that, at least from subjective experience, some women do have orgasms, which they describe as 'vaginal' or 'uterine' from penetrative intercourse, and that these are qualitatively distinct from those achieved through specific clitoral stimulation. The connotation of immaturity has been lifted from the clitoral orgasm, and there is some evidence that women who prefer vaginal orgasms tend to be more passive, dependent, and anxious. It can be argued that the focus of attention on the clitoris has perhaps obscured the contribution to sexual pleasure and orgasm of the sensitive erectile tissues of the rest of the vulva.

Although the clitoris is such a small and apparently insignificant organ, there are and have been widespread conceptions that it is dangerous and threatening. There are substantial areas of the world today, in Africa and the Middle East, in which clitoridectomy is still routinely practised on ritual and hygienic grounds — though the number of cultures which practice it are far fewer than those in which some kind of circumcision of the penis is performed on boy children or youths in transition to manhood. The practice is deeply embedded in national and religious cultures, and has proved very difficult to extirpate; attempts to do so have caused crises for colonial powers in Africa. While many of the cultures which practice it are Islamic, clitoridectomy is not coterminous with the Muslim world: it is found among other religious groups in the regions in which it is common, and is not practised in all Islamic nations.

Clitoridectomy takes different forms, from a relatively minor removal of a small amount of flesh from the tip of the clitoris to almost complete extirpation, along with other practices such as infibulation and sewing up of the labia. The effect of this mutilating operation on the subsequent sexual life of the women involved is usually assumed to be deleterious in the extreme, although there is a little, perhaps rather anecdotal, ethnographic evidence that some women who have undergone clitoridectomy are nevertheless capable of experiencing orgasm. This may depend upon how much of the underlying concealed erectile tissue remains. The trauma of the operation, performed normally on young girls around the age of 8, without anaesthetic, by traditional practitioners, must be considerable. Subsequent infection and scarring can have long-term implications for future FERTILITY and safety in childbirth. Such operations are regarded as reprehensible and unethical by Western medicine, although there have been cases of private practitioners performing the operation under surgical conditions in the UK for members of cultures in whom it is regarded as an essential attribute of the marriageable female.

However, there is no reason for an attitude of complacent superiority. During the 1860s the British surgeon Isaac Baker Brown performed an unknown number of clitoridectomies at his London Surgical Home. He believed that female masturbation was widely prevalent and the cause of a number of nervous ailments, including EPILEPSY, a point of view he advanced in his book *On the Curability of Certain Forms of Insanity, Epilepsy, Catalepsy and Hysteria in Females* (1866). The operation was, however, widely regarded as mutilating and shocking (especially given Baker Brown's rather cavalier attitude towards consent), and in 1867 he was expelled from the London Obstetrical Society and the London Surgical Home was closed. Baker Brown subsequently became insane. Clitoridectomy in Britain never recovered from this and did not become part of the medical repertoire, although it went on being practised in the US, to an extent which it is probably impossible to ascertain, well into the twentieth century. While the excesses of the advocates of 'Orificial Surgery', who advocated excising the clitoris as the remedy for a range of ailments, were probably not typical, as late as 1936 Holt's *Diseases of Infancy and Childhood* was not averse to recommending circumcision or cauterisation of the clitoris as a cure for masturbation in girls. These might be extreme options, but there were certainly devices available to prevent girls (and possibly women) gaining access to their clitoris for self-stimulation.

Surgery of the clitoris still takes place. There are, of course, various legitimate medical reasons for operating on this organ, such as various forms of malignancy, but they are fairly rare. These days the clitoris is not, in Western medicine, excised to take away the unruly sexual desires of women, but adjusted to make it more conformable to the demands of penetrative intercourse. It has been observed that, in most coital positions, when the penis is in the vagina, there is rarely direct stimulation of the clitoris as well, without the intervention of hands (or devices such as 'French ticklers'). Operations have been reported endeavouring to relocate the clitoris somewhere where it will be more likely to receive stimulation from simple penile thrusting, nearer the vaginal entrance. The equivalent to circumcision of the penis has also been performed, trimming back the clitoral hood to expose the glans to increase 'sensitivity'. Alleged 'adhesions' have also been removed. The value of these operations is exceedingly dubious. They reflect a mechanistic approach to sexual functioning similar to the use of vaginal dilators for spastic contraction of the vagina: altering or trying to alter the female genitals to make them conform to the cultural norm rather than recognising that the cultural norm has ignored the requirements of the female genitalia.

Perceptions of, and attitudes towards, the clitoris, provide a powerful reflection of wider societal attitudes to female sexuality, whether this is seen as so dangerous that it must be eradicated, or simply needing to be brought into a greater complementarity with male sexual needs.
LESLEY A. HALL

See also COITUS; ORGASM; SEXUALITY.

Cloning is the generation of genetically identical organisms: each group of such organisms is a clone. Ever since Aldous Huxley's *Brave New World*, cloning and clones have been the subject both of science fiction and of serious public concern over their possible biotechnological applications. Before taking a paranoid view, however, it is worth noting that clones occur widely and naturally. Many plant varieties are propagated as clones (for instance by grafting) and the summer aphids preying upon them are asexually produced, genetically identical individuals — clones. Identical TWINS are clones, and the famous Dionne quintuplets born in Canada in 1934 represent a human clone of five people.

Sexual reproduction involves a re-assortment of the genetic material from the two parents and hence the generation of new, genetically distinct individuals. In contrast to this, methods of *asexual* reproduction result in the production of genetically identical individuals. Bacteria, yeast, and the individual cells of multicellular organisms are able to reproduce asexually, and the products of such replication are clones. Thus, for instance, all the cells in a multicellular organism represent one clone derived from the fertilised egg. During the process of development, and indeed at later stages of life, there may be stably inherited restrictions on the use of the genetic material or new mutations which define new clonally-related groups of cells.

The cells of malignant tumours, for instance, usually carry numbers of mutations which were not originally present in the normal cells of the individual; as these cancer cells progress newer mutations may arise so that several discernibly different clones of cells may be found. One question of interest would be whether all the cells arise from one single event — is the tumour a clone? This question may be addressed in individuals where there is already more than one distinguishable clone of cells present. In women, one of the two *X chromosomes* will have been inactivated early in development in a random but stable manner. This results in all the tissues being a mosaic of two alternative types of cell. Tumours typically display a single type, demonstrating their clonal origin from a single precursor cell.

This illustrates another important aspect of cloning: the origin of the clone purifies it from a mixed population. For example, many cultivated plants are deliberately propagated asexually by cuttings or grafting, so that one particular variety may be maintained. In MOLECULAR BIOLOGY, this property — that the isolation of a clone selects, maintains, and propagates as a single pure variant — is used directly for analysis of the genetic material itself; the DNA. Pieces of DNA are inserted into a bacterial or viral host in a form that replicates asexually. One single cell is used to start a colony — a clone — and thus large amounts of a single purified DNA fragment may be isolated.

All the cells of a multicellular organism arising from one fertilised egg are clones and, unless subsequently modified, contain the same genetic information. This was demonstrated in plants by regeneration of a whole plant from a single cell from a carrot root. In animals it was shown possible to transplant the nucleus from a gut cell of a tadpole into a fertilised egg, which had had its own nucleus destroyed, and regenerate a new tadpole which now had the genetics of the donor nucleus. Such cloning was first attempted for mammals using mice, but this did not work with any nuclei other than those from the earliest embryos. In the 1990s, however, Ian Wilmut and a team at the Roslin Research Institute in Edinburgh demonstrated a technique allowing nuclei from cells in tissue culture to be used to clone a sheep. They have now demonstrated that these tissue culture cells can be derived from an adult sheep.

The lamb (named Dolly), who was produced from a nucleus from a cell grown from the breast tissue of an adult sheep, has had major political impact as it is now clear that there is no theoretical reason why this cloning should not be possible not only with sheep but with other mammals, including humans. Cloning people is illegal in Britain, but world-wide legislation is not in place. In some quarters it is argued, however, that the technique *per se* might be useful to regenerate transplant tissues or organs without ever compromising the ethical, legal, and moral susceptibilities that would arise from deliberately generating whole fetuses or people. MARTIN EVANS

See also BIOTECHNOLOGY; STEM CELLS.

Clothes Every human society completes the individual body with a form of dress, which may include painting, TATTOOING, permanent ornaments, and scarification along with the draping, wrapping, and tailoring of fabric into garments. Humans have always believed that the bare adult body is intolerably unfinished; it needs visible modification for acceptance into human society, and thus for self-acceptance. When normal modification consists of clothes that are habitually put on and taken off, absolute nakedness must remain a regular transient state, a nice or dread reminder of bare facts. Clothes themselves may then at times seem to absorb all human wickedness and to be themselves bad, by contrast with the notional purity of the raw organism. On the other hand, clothes may stand for all human effort to transcend brute nature and thus seem inherently good, by contrast with the notional beastliness of the raw organism.

But the true conceptual unity of the body-plus-dress combination is apparent in art that represents human beings, where the dressed form is usually shown as natural and the naked form as a special case, a dressed body with the clothes absent. Artists tend to fashion a nude costume for the naked body, to offer a comforting normative version (complete with orderly variations) of fearfully multiform naked humanity. They will give this nude image the shape and proportions required of normally-clothed bodies, which dress has rendered intelligible.

Animal skins were doubtless the first human clothes in the Northern hemisphere, worn just as they came off the beast, or variously joined together. The skins of trees, in the form of a flexible cloth made by treating strips of the inner bark, were among the earliest sources for human clothes in tropical countries. The earliest woven stuffs were made for use or ornament, before refinements in spinning and weaving permitted textiles malleable enough to clothe the body. Since then, in much of the world, clothing has taken the form of one or more garments made of fabrics that are woven, knitted, or felted in a range of spun fibres (both natural and synthetic), or of treated leather, metal, or synthetic materials. Such garments fall roughly into two categories; cut-and-sewn, or wrapped-and-draped. Schemes of clothing combine these two or use only one of them, employing different methods of stabilizing garments around the body according to whether they are meant to fit closely, to fit more loosely, or to hang free.

Tailored garments made into close-fitting, three-dimensional forms, such as the Renaissance doublet or the modern suit-coat and trousers, must be fitted onto the body with applied attachments such as lacings, hooks or buttons with holes or loops, two-part clasps, or zippers and velcro. Untailored, loose garments sewn into flat forms out of rectilinear pieces, such as the Japanese kimono and the earliest forms of sleeved tunic and trouser, can be held around the trunk and limbs with attached ties or with separate wrapped sashes and belts, or they can hang open and float like the North African djellabah. They, too, may have buttons, hooks or clasps at neck, shoulders or wrists. Untailored garments may also be controlled by drawstrings threaded through flat channels sewn into the cloth, which can gather them close and secure them to the body at wrist or ankle, neck or waist, elbow or knee. Ancient knit garments fitted fairly close without tailoring but usually had fastenings. Synthetic elastic fibres and modern machine knitting have latterly permitted stretchable skin-tight garments that mould to the body without tailoring, fastening, or belting.

Garments made of single woven-to-size and uncut rectangles of cloth were the first fabric clothes, and are still in use. They may be wrapped tightly, and tucked in or tied together around the chest, waist, or hips (e.g. the Tahitian pareo or Javanese sarong); loosely draped around the whole body but anchored with a hidden waistband (e.g. the Hindu sari); or pinned on the shoulders and visibly belted (e.g. the classical Greek peplos). Rectangular, single-piece outer garments may hang down front and back straight from the shoulders, with the arms free and the head through a slit (e.g. the South American poncho); stoles and shawls may be wrapped around the shoulders and held on by the arms. A veil, scarf, or kerchief may be suspended from the head and attached there with a headband or hairpins, or it may variably wrap the head, neck, and shoulders.

Casually fixed on at each wearing, such single-piece garments dress the body in mobile cloth without defining it, so that the body's action creates random play in the cloth, which underscores the body's moving shape and produces the individual aesthetic vitality of the clothes. Taken off, the garment becomes a flat object of which the colour, the woven pattern, and the applied ornament can have separate interest. In wear, if the draped garment randomly exposes the body, as in classical Greece, the acceptable nude costume dresses the unclad and partially clad person, as Greek art amply demonstrates, so that clothes and body remain in aesthetic balance and not opposed.

Ancient Egyptians used modes of regular pleating to control a rectangular garment's behaviour on the body, instead of permitting the random drapery and slippage created by motion. Such pleats, made in stiffly starched white linen that bent and swept around the body, or lay close to it, proposed an aesthetic value for wrapped garments only while they were formally dressing the figure and giving it the required static and abstract look. An idealised nakedness was again necessary to complete the desired effect, as expounded in Egyptian art, since much of the body was deliberately exposed, some of it through transparent fabric. A very different effect was created in China and Japan, with large, untailored silk garments that were so stiffly woven, lined, interlined and disposed around the body as to hide and replace it completely. In such a scheme neither the distinctive shapes nor the articulated movements of the body had any visual authority in the desired clad results, again as expounded in art. Human nakedness was given no added nobility, but unworn noble garments did command separate admiration.

Cutting cloth on a curve was discovered to permit high, round armhole seams and high crotch seams, and to allow for close-fitting, round necklines and for the curved hems that make hanging garments fall evenly around the body with no dropping corners. It was sparingly used to begin with, since precious woven stuff is wasted by this technique, and curved cut edges demand added binding or facing to stop the raw thread-ends from fraying. Leather, on the other hand, has always lent itself well to tailoring — as for SHOES, for example — being non-woven and irregularly shaped in its natural state. Garments of felt may also be edged on a curve without hemming, as for hats and capes.

Modernity, getting under way in late medieval Europe, saw the development of fully-tailored garments that closely covered and modified the body's articulated shape with articulated shapes of their own. These were modelled with subtly curved cutting and seaming helped by stiffening, padding, constriction, and extensions for the clothes of both sexes, including hats, hoods, and shoes. Randomly draped, regularly pleated, or wrapped fabric became only partial elements in the aesthetic scheme for Western clothes, not its main character. European clothes became three-dimensional forms that seemed to compete with the body they covered, even while creating its ideal look; off the body, the three-dimensional garment would look like a ghost inseparable from an individual human soul. Nudity became part of the scheme, too, in despite of climate, with selective exposure requiring the selective idealisation of bodily parts such as the female bosom and the male leg. European nude art shows the amount of variation in the common vision of ideal nakedness that was created by the way clothes shaped the body.

With the complex clothes of the late Middle Ages in Europe came the rise of FASHION. Sophisticated form in dress required a constant shifting of its visual emphasis and stylistic flavour, including erotic, societal, and self-referential flavours. The two sexes were conventionally distinguished by dividing male legs with some form of hose and breeches, and veiling women's legs in flowing or stiff ground-length or shoe-length skirts. Variation was more flexible for the upper body, however, including suggestive similarities as well as vivid differences between the male and female effects that were modish at different periods. For example, fashion might flatten women's breasts and widen men's hips at one time, or enlarge both women's breasts and men's shoulders at another time. Shifts in fashion were first led by powerful and leisured groups at courts and in towns, and realized by their tailors, but fashionable change was eventually promoted among middle and lower class people and their tailors by the increasing dispersal of imagery made possible by the printing-press. Fashion in Western dress more and more became an imaginative sexual, social, and political medium, with the steady help of other media.

Visual art has always been the agent of elegance in dress. For millennia before fashion, sculptors and painters offered stylised versions of clothed persons to public view, so that people could admire, imitate, and feel rightly portrayed by superior visions of accepted clothed appearance. The reproducible graphic arts, however, later helped to hasten the adoption of changes in fashions by emphasising their immediate extremes and priming the public eye for alternatives. By the late eighteenth century, reproduced pictures were affecting general and personal taste through popular journals and magazines, some devoted entirely to fashion in dress. Photojournalism, movies, and television continue to offer stylisations of clothed bodies that guide taste and propel its fluctuations, often in the form of promotion for things other than clothes. Exposure of the body's surface has lately increased among fashions for both sexes, creating a revived need for the stylisation of body parts to go with changing modes in semi-nude costume.

Until the nineteenth century, for all classes of society, clothes were made either at home or by artisans who constructed hand-made garments to individual order. For a very long time, fine spinning and weaving, complex dyeing, and embroidery were the finest arts of clothing, and construction was simple where it existed. This situation still obtains in Japan with respect to the traditional feminine kimono, even though Western clothing has been otherwise universally adopted there. In Europe, during the Renaissance and thereafter, fashionable dress gradually came to demand a similar degree of skill from urban and court tailors and from artisans specializing in headgear, footwear, and gloves, or in lace, braid, and buttons as well as embroidery. Regional clothes were made by local artisans or at home — though not without constant fashionable influence on regional traditions. The very poor in towns and cities could buy second-hand clothes and alter them. Crude work clothes were hand-produced in bulk for labourers, common sailors, slaves, and convicts.

Early in the nineteenth century, the English invention of the tape measure and a new understanding of men's average bodily proportions made it possible for American merchant-tailors to produce many well-tailored coats and trousers at one time, in a range of sizes guaranteed to fit a large number of men. With the development of the sewing machine and later the cutting machine, the ready-to-wear men's clothing enterprise in America expanded to furnish not only the military, but also rural workers, miners, and railroad men with well-made fitted garments — the blue jeans, workshirts and overalls that are still being made and worn. In the twentieth century, although traditional made-to-measure tailoring persisted everywhere at higher social levels, the ready-made suit became the standard public costume of the modern ordinary man. His body was generalized by the suit's smooth, flexible envelope into a useful image of modern male equality. Women's visual equality, among each other and with men, came somewhat later.

Dressmaking had become a women's craft separate from men's tailoring late in the seventeenth century, and thereafter women's clothes more and more outdid men's in visual complexity. Staymaking also became a separate craft, and separate CORSETS became a common part of female fashion, variably modelling the torso under the clothing. At the very end of the nineteenth century, however, fashion began to reduce the expressive shapes and surface embellishments of women's clothes, and they gradually came to match men's in the clarity of line and easy style of bodily fit that had become common for male dress during the previous century. After 1900, everyday skirts were increasingly shortened to allow the shape and action of women's legs to form part of their complete clothed image. By the second decade of the twentieth century, as fashion continued to simplify women's modes of dress, the rules of proportional sizing could be applied to them as well. A large ready-to-wear industry for ordinary women's fashionable garments became possible, spurred by the new needs of working women, whose fashions eventually came to include trousers as well as skirts. Factory-made clothes for both sexes became the staple of mainstream fashion in the industrialized world, and for ordinary clothes everywhere as local artisanal traditions declined.

Just after the middle of the nineteenth century, however, offsetting this incipient trend, the Haute Couture came into existence for women's fashion. This French enterprise specialised in the superior artisanal creation of fashionable feminine clothing, conceived by artist-like designers whose high prices flaunted their distance from both home sewing and mass production, and whose personal fame came to increase the worldwide prestige of their works. Ordinary dressmakers in Europe and America, and eventually clothing factories, therefore copied and modified Haute Couture designs for the general female public.

In the last third of the twentieth century, original creative designers were engaged directly by both the male and female fashionable clothing industries, while the Haute Couture, later including Italian, English, and American designers, came to have a more limited influence on ordinary female dress. The multiple-production aesthetics of industrial design, however, came generally to affect all fashion design for both sexes, as well as for children. With the global clothing markets of the late twentieth century, a certain neutralization has thus occurred in the contemporary look of the clothed human body, which in a great part of the world is commonly clad in the shirts, sweaters, pants, and jackets originally designed as Western masculine gear for work and sport.

Ordinary work and leisure clothes for men, women, and children now look very much alike, and the more traditional fashionable dress that sharply distinguishes sex, age, and social stratum is thought to be special costume for public life, office work, or festal moments. In undeveloped countries, pre-modern woven rectangular shapes still persist, often in combination with tailored factory-made garments; at the same time versions of simple, ancient gear are steadily recurring in tailored, mass-produced Western fashion. It is worth noting that the world's clothing, despite some irreversible changes, has somewhat come full circle, as if returning to the days of wrapped and draped rectangles or T-shaped tunics for every human body. ANNE HOLLANDER

See also FASHION.

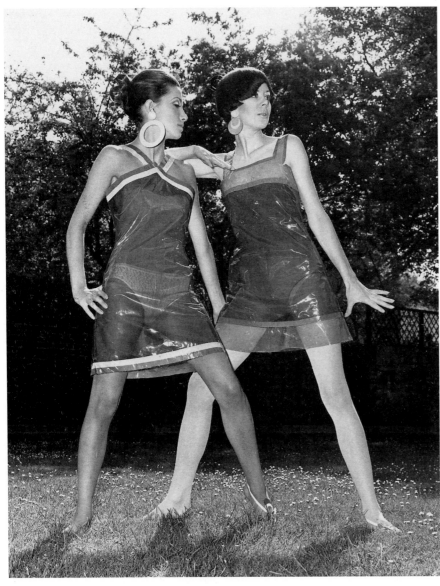

Disposable dresses by Daniel Hechter of Paris, 1966. (Hulton Getty Picture Library).

Clown The word comes from Low German, and originally described the peasant through uncomplimentary association with the soil that he tilled. 'Clown' meant 'clod, clot, lump', with more acerbic overtones of 'clumsy, *loutish*, lumpish fellow' and a female 'hoyden or *lusty* bouncing girl'. A clown was someone with rude manners, *undisciplined physicality*, and an inability to control appetites or impulses. The uncivilized nature of such a rustic stereotype was sometimes symbolized by wild acrobatic dancing, as in Chaucer's *Hous of Fame*:

Tho come ther leapynge in a route
And gunne choppen al aboute
Every man upon the crowne
That al the halle gan to sowne

and in the Scots poem, 'Cocklebie Sow':

Thay movit in thair mad muting . . .
For merrit was thair menstralis . . .
For thay hard speik of men gud
And small thairof vndirstud
Bot hurlit furth vpoun heid

Despite moral disapproval, which until the sixteenth century led to the more common title of 'fool', their energetic antics were popular and the clown was a box-office draw when professional theatres began in 1576. One clown, William Kemp, danced his way, in nine days, from London to Norwich in 1600, probably to rebuild his fame after being sacked from Shakespeare's Company for speaking more than was set down for him. (See *Hamlet* III.ii.45–7.) In Shakespeare's and Jonson's plays, the term 'clown' is often pejorative.

Clowning became more fashionable in the mid seventeenth century when interest in spectacle superceded that for dialogue. Added to the traditional features of clown behaviour — slapstick, rude gestures, and physical distortions — performers vied for success through energetic novelties. The Dutchman, Brederode, mentioned the lusty spring, the spinning, twirling, and turning of English comic dancers. The rope dancer, Jacob Hall, sometimes played straight, turning somersaults on a rope suspended over naked rapiers; as in circuses today the threat that his agility might end in disaster gave vicarious excitement. But sometimes he added an element of clown's satire on his spectators' motives, by suspending the rope over their heads; presumably they rose to the challenge.

After two centuries of being fashionable, physical comedy became respectable in the 1790s through the 'total clowning' of Joseph Grimaldi, which he claimed had resulted in every bone in his body having been broken during his professional life. After his early retirement it was regretted that

Gone is the stride, four steps across the stage
Gone is the light vault o'er a turnpike gate.

Grimaldi astonished his audiences by his ability to make seemingly impossible physical movements. Comic innovation around 1800 also included a satiric reflection of the brutal physicality in the humour of Regency society bucks. Stage directions to Thomas Dibdin's *Harlequin Hoax* read:

To meet Columbine at the street door Harlequin throws himself out of a window and is caught with his head in a lamp iron; the lamplighter pours a gallon of oil down his throat . . . and sticks a lighted wick in his mouth, and a set of drunken bucks, having no better business on earth than to break lamps, knock his nob to shivers.

By a strange coincidence, Tom and Jerry were the names given to two such Regency buffoons in Pierce Egan's *Life in London*.

To a certain extent pantomime curbed the clown's physical expressiveness by pinning him down again with dialogue, but in *silent pictures*, where the only communication was through *action*, various comic techniques emerged. Chaplin reversed the brutalized humour Grimaldi lived with through the success of the little tramp in overcoming bullies with intelligent agility. And in *Modern Times* his athleticism was put to the test inside a machine adversary. But the greatest accolade for ACROBATICS, invention, and physical courage has to go to Harold Lloyd — 'king of daredevil comedy' — with his clownish climb up the skyscraper in *Safety Last*. This did involve a safety platform out of sight of the camera, but far enough below to make the use of it itself a hazard. During one 'take' Lloyd thought he might slip, so chose to fall deliberately so as to be able to aim for the centre and avoid bouncing off into the real void below. Despite the invitation to total trickery which filming allows, *Safety Last* retained a fair proportion of the traditional combination: clowning with risk-taking, particularly in the shots of Lloyd hanging off the clock face.

Circuses which excelled in this in the 1980s and 1990s were Circus Oz and Archaeos. Their acts included sitting and eating upside down on the theatre ceiling, sliding head first down a pole and coming to a halt inches before crashing into the floor, and playing with power machines. As the Circus owner, Signor Truzi, said to Coco the Clown, every clown has first to be an acrobat, then a trapeze artist and a tumbler; he must be able to do everything, and then he can think about being a clown. Such daring is partly in order to be noticed, but the great clown's ability to act out situations which combine comedy with danger are also a way of satirizing the most extreme and ludicrous possibilities thrown up by the society he lives in. The professional's talent in the twentieth century has been to appear incompetent in the face of overwhelming odds but to overcome these by the character's persistence and the performer's physical abilities.

Have we yet to see an astronaut variety?

SANDRA BILLINGTON

Further reading
Baskervill, C. R. (1965). *The Elizabethan Jig.* University of Chicago Press, New York.

Dardis, T. (1983). *Harold Lloyd, the man on the clock.* Viking Penguin, New York.

Findlater, R. (1955). *Grimaldi King of Clowns.* Cambridge University Press, Cambridge.

Club foot is a deformity of which the most common form, known as *talipes equinovarus*, is characterised by the foot being turned upwards and inwards and bent towards the heel. It is frequently congenital, and less severe forms, often believed to be caused by an adverse position in the womb, may be treated with splints, plastercasts, or manipulation: all therapies used since Hippocratic times. Nowadays surgery, to cut restricted tendons and to reposition misplaced bones, may be required for more severe forms. Neurological disorders, such as poliomyelitis and CEREBRAL PALSY, can also cause acquired clubfoot. One of the most famous sufferers was the poet Lord Byron (1788–1824). Contemporary and later accounts differ greatly in their assessment of his lameness, one writer suggesting that he was lame in both legs, the left being severely withered below the knee. However, the consensus opinion seems to be that he had a mild form of talipes in his right foot. He received no treatment until he was ten, when he was put into the charge of a quack called Lavendar who forcibly manipulated and twisted the misshapen foot, and forced it into a vice-like machine. The pain and fruitlessness of these procedures convinced Byron's mother to consult Dr Baillie, a well-known London practitioner, in whose care the boy's foot was straightened to such an extent that he walked thereafter with a slight limp only, although he remained acutely conscious of this small infirmity for the rest of his life.

E.M. TANSEY

Cod liver oil Routine administration of a spoonful of cod liver oil, on a daily basis, to young children, by caring parents, was very common in the 1940s and 50s. Most children were revulsed by the practice because of the unpalatability of the fishy tasting oil, and doubtless extracted a variety of rewards for compliance. As the name implies, cod liver oil is from the liver of the cod (*Gadus callarias*), simply freed from solid fat by filtration at low temperature.

The oil is a rich source of VITAMINS A and D and also contains essential unsaturated FATTY ACIDS. Vitamin A is important for photoreceptor mechanisms in the retina and the integrity of epithelia, so deficiency can lead to night blindness. Vitamin D is essential for the absorption of calcium and phosphorus by the body, a prerequisite for BONE formation. Vitamin D is also formed in the skin by the action of sunlight (*UV radiation*). Children growing up in poor urban areas, with few places to play outside, were commonly the victims of Vitamin D deficiency in the early part of the twentieth century, when rickets was common. Inadequate bone formation leads to bending in weight-bearing bones, giving rise to bow legs and knock knees. Paradoxically, rickets is not uncommon in the tropics because of the swaddling of infants. Vitamin D deficiency in adults leads to *osteomalacia*. There were attempts to make cod liver oil more palatable by forming oil-in-water emulsions with flavoured water, or mixing the oil with malt. It was later discovered that halibut liver oil (from *Hippoglossus hipoglossus*) contains far higher concentrations of both Vitamins A and D so that a daily dose could be accommodated in a small gelatin capsule that was easily swallowed and tasteless.

ALAN W. CUTHBERT

See also VITAMINS.

Codpiece

Codpiece When the early seventeenth-century English playwright John Marston wrote in his *Satires*,

> Nay then, I'll never rail at those
> That wear a codpiece, thereby to disclose
> What sex they are

he pointed to the primary purpose of a codpiece: to emphasise the gender of its wearer. Codpieces appeared in Europe in the early sixteenth century, during a period of economic and territorial expansion, in which the conspicuous display of virility, in public life, sport, warfare, and dress played a major part in a competitive culture of self-presentation, self-aggrandisement, and advertisement. They were designed, along with doublets with massive chests and coats with wide shoulders, to enhance and exaggerate the masculine attributes of the wearer, to 'disclose' rather than conceal or contain, the 'sex they are'.

Codpieces were a distinctive feature of late Renaissance male dress in Italy, Spain, France, and England, reaching their peak of popularity in the mid sixteenth century, before gradually disappearing by the end of the century. They evolved from the pouch-shaped flap which was used to close the front of the close-fitting hose worn by men in the fourteenth and early fifteenth centuries. By the early sixteenth century, the front flap on men's breeches and hose was no longer a flat pouch, but had become a protuberance, often padded and stiffened, to support and accentuate the male genitals. It was essentially a bag made of fabric, usually silk, and was often elaborately embroidered and decorated, either made of the same material as the trunk hose or breeches, or to match the doublet or other upper garments, to which it was fastened by points or lacings. In addition to the padding and ornamentation on the codpiece itself, further attention was drawn to the groin area by the positioning of dagger and sword belts just above it, the dagger often worn with the hilt pointing to or framing the codpiece, creating a visual dialogue between codpiece and dagger, thus amplifying and doubling the phallus.

From its introduction early in the sixteenth century, until its disappearance from fashion in the 1590s, the codpiece served as an emblem for manhood, the part standing for the whole. As Marston's 1598 quote above makes evident, even after its demise, it retained its metaphorical associations with masculine essence. The codpiece, with its sexual connotations, represented the uncontrollable carnal impulses that warred against the rational soul of man. The idea of the sexual organs having a 'will' of their own, independent of their owner's intentions, was a well-established one, dating from St Augustine's laments regarding the 'uprisings' of the flesh. Yet these sexual urges afflict all mankind, and everyone is a victim of his libidinous desires. Hence a character in Shakespeare's *Measure for Measure* condemns judging a man too harshly for a universal weakness: 'For the rebellion of a codpiece, to take away the life of a man?'

During a brief period in the 1570s and 80s in England, around the time that the codpiece was falling into disrepute in male fashion, it became the name for a roughly analogous ornament or appendage, worn by women on the breast. Like the fashion, late in the sixteenth century, of women wearing doublets like those worn by men, the practice of women sporting 'codpieces' on their chests may have exacerbated the anxieties of moralists concerned about the adoption by women of masculine attributes and habits, including those of dress. Pamphlets like *Hic Mulier* (1620) dwelt at length on the insidious dangers presented by a new race of 'mankind women' or female transvestites who usurped male dress and customs such as smoking, swearing, and brawling in public.

NATSU HATTORI

Further reading

Ribeiro, A. and Cumming, V. (1989). *The visual history of costume.* Batsford, London.

Wilcox, R. T. (1958). *The mode in costume: a history of men's and women's clothes and accessories from Egypt 3000 BC to the present.* Charles Scriber & Sons, New York.

Coitus

Coitus is the technical term for sexual conjunction or copulation. It is derived from the Latin 'co', meaning together, and 'ire', a verb form meaning to come or to go. Tracing the etymology of the term, the *Oxford English Dictionary* indicates that during the sixteenth and seventeenth centuries 'coitus' could mean any going or coming together, or a mutual tendency of bodies toward one another. These more general meanings, however, have disappeared from usage. In its narrow medical–anatomical sense, coitus means a specific kind of sexual intercourse: the insertion of the erect penis into the vagina. However, its meaning has been extended to include, for example, axillary coitus, or intercourse with the penis inserted into an armpit; femoral coitus, or intercourse with the penis inserted between the thighs; mammary coitus, or intercourse with the penis inserted between the woman's breasts; and coitus a tergo, or sexual intercourse in which the male enters the woman's vagina from behind.

While coitus, like copulation, is a neutral term, it has in English many vulgar and colloquial synonyms (get it on; do it; fuck; bang, and so forth). Pierre Guiraud's study of the French term 'le coît', which is equivalent to the English 'coitus', lists 1300 words and metaphors culled from French literature that are used to express the concept. These range from the euphemistic *s'abandonner* (to abandon oneself) to the vulgar *foutre* (to fuck), and from the equestrian metaphor, *frémir sous l'éperon* (to shiver under the spurs), to the mythological, '*voyager à Cythère*' (to travel to Cythera, island sacred to Venus). He notes that this list could be infinitely expanded because '*le coît*' theoretically can be described by any action operated by a male subject on a female object. His findings also affirm that '*le coît*' or 'coitus' describes a normative, heterosexual act of intercourse achieved when the active, erect male partner penetrates the passive female. In fact, Guiraud points out that terms suggesting penetration are especially favoured as synonyms for coitus.

Although a natural sexual act, coitus is culturally regulated by legislation, custom, and religious belief. For example, in many societies incest taboos, and statutes forbidding adultery or prostitution, regulate consensual coitus, and forced or nonconsensual coitus is criminalized by laws against RAPE. Many religious beliefs proscribe coitus at certain times (for example, during menstruation), or forbid all coitus except that performed for procreation. Some religious tenets and social conventions ban copulation between unmarried couples or limit coitus to certain postures or positions. The myriad of laws and practices surrounding coitus suggests that this 'natural' act is determined by complicated social and religious conventions which, obeyed or transgressed, are formative of human sexuality.

MARY SHERIFF

Further reading

Guiraud, P. (1978). *Dictionnaire Erotique, La langage de la sexualité*, Vol. 1. Payot, Paris.

See also EJACULATION; ERECTION; REPRODUCTIVE SYSTEM; SEX.

Cold exposure

The body's adjustment

Like other mammals, man normally keeps his body core temperature remarkably constant, so that the temperature of the heart, brain, and other central organs seldom rises more than 2°C above 37°C, or falls more than 2°C below this. The main way that this is achieved in a cold environment is through conscious protective measures, such as putting on warm clothing or entering warm accommodation, when the body's sensory system records exposure to cold. The sensory system itself is a two stage one. Receptors in the skin respond immediately when the body is exposed to cold. If the response to these is insufficient to maintain body core temperature, receptors in the brain record a fall in temperature which induces further sensation of cold.

If the cold exposure continues despite conscious protective measures, the cold receptors trigger internal mechanisms to restore heat balance. The first of these is that sympathetic nerves release NORADRENALINE, to shut down blood flow to the skin. The effect is that blood no longer carries heat from the body core to the surface of the body, and the skin and tissues under it are allowed to cool down. These tissues then provide a layer of insulation between the body core and the surface. An important point is that the thickness of this insulating layer, which is determined in turn by the thickness of the layer of fat under the skin, largely determines the amount of cold stress that the person can undergo without developing HYPOTHERMIA. Hypothermia is defined simply as a fall in body core temperature below 35°C.

The thickness of fat under the skin, described as subcutaneous fat, is particularly important to survival during immersion in cold water, because most of the external clothing is then lost, and internal insulation of the body largely determines the rate of heat loss. When you consider that fat also provides buoyancy to help keep people afloat, and that it provides energy reserves that are needed for many hours of physical exertion, it is obvious why relatively fat people have dramatically better ability than their thinner colleagues to survive in water after shipwreck, and to swim long distances in cold water as in Channel crossings and other long-distance swims.

The exertion of swimming increases heat production, but it also increases heat loss in various ways, and on balance people at risk of hypothermia after shipwreck maintain their body core temperature better by floating still in life jackets than by active swimming. In cold air, physical exertion has a positive effect, helping to maintain heat balance, but it can only be continued for a limited time. It is therefore better for people lost in cold conditions to shelter from the wind than to continue exercise until they are exhausted. Shelter from wind can greatly reduce heat loss, and snow shelters are an important means of achieving this in exposed snow-covered country. If body core temperature drops despite measures of this kind, the cold receptors of the brain trigger shivering, which increases heat production in muscles but without increasing heat loss as much as active movement does. This will normally stabilise heat balance and body temperature, but represents the last defence against cold. If it is insufficient, or if it fails as a result of exhaustion, body temperature will fall progressively and death will eventually occur from hypothermia. The newborn baby has an even more effective method of heat production in the cold by metabolising brown fat, but this is almost entirely replaced by shivering within the first year of life.

Illness in winter

Illness and death from heart attacks, strokes, and respiratory disease increase in winter, even in countries with mild winter climates such as Britain and Greece. Despite some popular perceptions, hypothermia with serious falls in body core temperature from any cause is rare, and is not an important cause of death in urban populations except at times of war or natural disasters when housing is damaged, people are living rough, and food supplies are disrupted.

It has recently become clear that the shutting down of blood flow to the skin, which is the normal first defence against cold, can explain some of the large numbers of deaths that are associated with cold weather. The blood volume has to be reduced to prevent the blood that was displaced from the skin from overloading the circulation; fluid is accordingly lost from the blood to the tissues, which removes the excess volume but leaves the blood more concentrated and therefore more liable to clot. This does no harm to young people with healthy arteries, but increases the chance of a blood clot forming in the arteries of middle-aged or elderly people, resulting in increased heart attacks and strokes.

Respiratory disease is also commoner in winter. The reasons for this are not fully understood, but cross-infection due to crowding in poorly ventilated rooms, and stress hormone responses to cold that reduce immune responses to infection, probably both play a part. The respiratory infections in turn cause changes in blood composition that further increase the risk of blood clots.

Prevention and treatment

Prevention of hypothermia during hill walking, mountaineering, and water sports or shipwreck is a matter for special training and equipment among a special group of people. Although very important in this group, it only relates to around a dozen deaths per year in Britain. With regard to urban illness and death in winter, prevention is directed at around 50 000 excess deaths that still occur annually in Britain in cold weather. Both indoor and outdoor cold exposures seem to play important parts in this mortality; the importance of warm housing has been appreciated for many years, but the realisation that outdoor cold exposure is an important factor in causing illness and death in winter has been more recent. Outdoor activity in which people keep warm by exercise seems to be beneficial, but long waits by elderly people in cold weather with inadequate clothing (for example at bus stops) are not. Official action to improve outdoor facilities such as bus shelters can be important, but much of that kind of cold exposure can best be prevented by action by individuals. Waterproof and windproof clothing when appropriate, as well as sufficient over-clothing, particularly wearing hats, and keeping moving while out, can do much to prevent cold stress outdoors. Keeping enough durable food in the house to prevent the need for shopping excursions in very cold weather, or help by neighbours with shopping, can make outdoor excursions unnecessary for elderly people in the worst weather. Such measures may seem obvious once the awareness of cold hazards is realised, but surveys show that many people in countries with mild winters, such as Britain, do not automatically take the advance measures needed to have suitable clothing and supplies available before a cold spell arrives, or do not use them when it does.

Treatment of people exposed to cold

People who are found confused or unconscious in cold surroundings, particularly in wind and either wet or very cold conditions, may be hypothermic. Many, however, are found to be suffering instead from other illness, or from exhaustion or malnutrition. A mouth temperature above 35°C will exclude hypothermia. A mouth temperature below 35°C does not prove hypothermia as the mouth can be cold when body core temperature is normal, and a rectal temperature below 35°C is then needed to establish whether hypothermia is in fact present.

The first aid treatment for hypothermia is to cover the patient with blankets or other insulation, keep him lying flat, and move him to warm surroundings and to hospital with as little disturbance as possible. This gives minimum risk of precipitating sudden death from ventricular FIBRILLATION, an unco-ordinated contraction of the ventricles of the heart which can result from almost any form of exertion or active interference during hypothermia. The only major situation in which another course is needed is when the victim has cooled so far that the heart has stopped, or has ceased to pump blood because of ventricular fibrillation. In this case, and if a trained person is at hand and establishes that there is no pulse in the carotid artery, external cardiac massage may be useful while the victim is rushed to hospital for specialist treatment. Cardiac massage should never be given if the heart is beating, even slowly, in hypothermia. There is still debate over whether a warm bath (no hotter than is comfortable to your own elbow) is useful for victims who have been rescued from cold water and have suffered rapid body cooling. A warm bath can probably help, but only if given within about 20 minutes of rescue and without great disturbance to the patient, and this is in any case rarely feasible.

Frostbite and immersion injury

Frostbite is the freezing of body tissue. It is obvious in the appearance of hard white areas of skin, developing in air colder than 0°C. Small areas of frostbite, usually on fingers, toes, ears, or face, are best treated by immediate thawing, preferably in lukewarm water. Bending or other injury to the frozen tissue must be avoided. Large areas of frozen tissue, such as whole limbs, must not be thawed rapidly, as potassium ions and other agents can than be released from the thawing tissue into the blood in such quantity as to cause death. Such cases, which are seldom seen except in very cold regions, must be treated by wrapping the frozen area in clothing and transporting the patient as quickly as possible to hospital where limbs can be thawed under full biochemical control.

W. R. KEATINGE

Further reading

Burton, A. C. and Edholm, O. G. (1955). *Man in a cold environment.* Edward Arnold, London.

W. R. Keatinge (1978). *Survival in cold water.* (Reprinted.) Blackwell Scientific Publications.

Neild, P. J., Syndercombe-Court, D., Keatinge, W. R., Donaldson, G. C., Mattock, M., and Caunce, M. (1994). Cold-induced increases in erythrocyte count, plasma cholesterol and plasma fibrinogen of elderly people without comparable rise in protein C or factor X. *Clinical Science*, **86**, 43–8.

See also DIVING; HYPOTHERMIA; SURVIVAL AT SEA; TEMPERATURE REGULATION.

Collagen

The word collagen means 'glue-producing'. Collagen in the body does indeed help to hold it all together, but the notion of glue is not very apt. It strengthens and connects things with a network of tough fibres, rather than sticking them to each other — more like a cat's cradle than an adhesive. Collagen is the PROTEIN which forms the ubiquitous white fibres in all the CONNECTIVE TISSUES of the body, including BONE, TEETH, CARTILAGE, and TENDONS; the SKIN; and all the sheaths, partitions, and supporting frameworks which abound in all organs and tissues. The exception is the CENTRAL NERVOUS SYSTEM, which has its own different variety of internal supporting tissue — the GLIA — though there is collagen in the membranes which cover the brain and spinal cord.

Collagen is one of the 'structural proteins' (the other widespread one is *elastin*), which provide support to the tissues. By crude analogy with string, the principal mechanical property of collagen is its ability to resist distending force (tensile strength), which is vastly greater than its ability to resist compression or twisting (compression and torsion strengths). The tensile strength of collagen is so high as to be comparable, weight for weight, with that of steel. Elastin, by contrast, has a low tensile strength but the important mechanical properties of distensibility and resilience: the capability for relatively long range stretching under load and for returning to the original dimensions when the distending force is removed. Collagen can stretch only by about 2% without damage.

Collagen and elastin fibres often co-exist, notably in tissues which regularly undergo considerable changes in shape, such as skin, LUNGS, and BLOOD VESSELS. The essentially inextensible, high tensile strength collagen is able to exist and function alongside the elastic fibres simply by having considerable slack. This can easily be illustrated if you pinch up the skin on the back of the hand: it returns to its original shape on release by virtue of the elastic fibres (a property progressively impaired in old age due to degeneration of the elastic fibres, with consequent increase in skin wrinkling). Now with the fingertips push the same skin on the back of the hand sideways and note that it slides quite freely until displacement comes to a distinct halt (when the collagen has used its slack and the tough fibres are pulled into alignment, resisting the distending force).

Collagen is synthesized by *fibroblasts*, the living cells present in all connective tissue, so named because they generate fibres — of collagen. There are in fact several types, with minor variations of molecular structure. Like all proteins, collagens are constructed from amino acid units; they are all glycoproteins, meaning that glucose and other simple sugars are attached to the amino acid chains. Each long, thin molecule consists of three chains of over 1000 units; each chain is helical, and the three in turn form a triple helix. A molecule is about 300 nm long — over 3000 end-to-end would measure 1 mm — but in fully-formed collagen they overlap lengthwise, and are also linked side to side, providing longer, wider, and very tough fibres. Again like all proteins in the body, collagen has a finite life span after which it is degraded to the constituent amino acids and replaced by new fibres. The synthesis within the fibroblasts is a complex process; the three chains are separately assembled, and then wound into the triple helix, which is extruded. Once outside the cell, the molecules aggregate and forge links as described.

The complexity of collagen synthesis involves multiple ENZYMES, so that a congenital deficiency of any of these can lead to some disorder of its formation. This accounts for there being a wide variety of clinical syndromes associated with such disorders: there can be fragile bones, with fractures from minimal trauma; fragile blood vessels with widespread bruising; dental defects; readily dislocating joints; a bent or twisted spine; thin, hyperelastic skin; and poor wound healing. Apart from these inborn defects, deprivation of ascorbic acid (vitamin C) at any time of life interferes with a step in collagen synthesis; the resulting bleeding, bruising, and poor healing are part of the picture of *scurvy*.

With ageing, habitually exposed areas of skin in white-skinned people show broken and disordered collagen fibres, related to the effects of UV light. Deficient replacement of collagen also contributes to thinning and wrinkling of the skin, and, together with mineral loss, to OSTEOPOROSIS — decreasing bone mass.

These changes suggest that the continuous production of new fibroblasts, and by them of new collagen, progressively declines. Fibroblasts in culture outside the body divide again and again, but do not continue to replicate indefinitely. When such cultures from different animal species are compared, it is found that the number of cell divisions is related to the lifespan of each species, and is also related inversely to the age of the donor from any one species: a finding of considerable interest in the study of the ageing process.

HUGH ELDER
SHEILA JENNETT

See also AGEING; CONNECTIVE TISSUE.

Colon

Also known as the large intestine, or sometimes the large bowel, because it is wider, although much shorter, than the small intestine, which leads into it via the caecum. There are three components: ascending, from the lower right side of the abdominal cavity; transverse, crossing to the left; and descending, to the lower left where it leads into the rectum. Its main function is the absorption of water, changing the liquid contents received from the ileum into the normally semi-solid faeces. S.J.

See ALIMENTARY SYSTEM; PLATE 1.

Colonic irrigation

is a treatment by ENEMA, practised by naturopaths and designed to clean out the large bowel, which, it is maintained, becomes encrusted with foreign and potentially poisonous material. The enema usually consists of warm water, but sometimes other substances are added to it.

The practice is derived from one of man's oldest treatments — *clysters* — which was especially popular in the seventeenth and eighteenth centuries. These were enemas, which were adjuncts to PURGING. Along with bleeding, emptying the bowels was one of the few active and productive treatments available to physicians in the pre-scientific age. Molière satirized the practice brilliantly in *Le Malade Imaginaire*, describing 'a little insinuative, preparative and emollient clyster to mollify, moisten and refresh his worship's bowels' and 'a good detersive clyster . . . to scour, wash and cleanse his honour's abdomen'.

The popularity of enemas or colonic irrigation did not decline with the development of 'scientific' medicine. On the contrary, they were an obvious form of treatment for 'CONSTIPATION', a subject with which many Victorians were obsessed. In the late nineteenth and early twentieth centuries the theory of *autointoxication* reigned. It was suggested that the bowels should move three times a day but that civilization, unhealthy living, and unhealthy diet had reduced the frequency, allowing foreign matter, poisons, and substances producing 'toxins' to accumulate in the bowel, causing ill-health and many diseases. This theory was widely promulgated by prominent people, including the Nobel-prize-winning chemist, Élie Metchnikoff, the distinguished London surgeon, Arbuthnot Lane, and, in America, John Harvey Kellogg, founder of the Kellogg food empire.

As the twentieth century progressed, orthodox medicine paid less attention to constipation. The idea of 'toxins' and self -poisoning gradually lost its appeal after it was shown that the symptoms of constipation could be produced by cotton wool and were relieved instantly by evacuation. However, many people remained obsessed with the contents of their bowels and continued to believe firmly in their poisonous nature. Some practitioners of alternative medicine have made this the chief feature of the treatment they offer. For many years the London newspaper, *The Times*, carried an advertisement for colonic irrigation on its front page. Even in the 1990s advertisements in the popular press suggested 'A well-balanced diet may not be enough' and announced that a 'colon cleanse' was 'the natural vegetarian food supplement to form a friendlier, health technology'. A colonic therapist announced that she had treated several thousand people and had 'only ever seen one healthy colon'. We were told 'many of us are carrying around between five and twenty pounds of mucus and undischarged debris in our colons'. Mucus in fact is a normal and essential lubricant, produced continually by cells in the lining of the whole of the gut; it is particularly necessary in the colon, where the contents are becoming progressively more solid: the bowel might well become 'encrusted' without it. Excess mucus occurs only in some pathological conditions, and makes its presence known in the stools.

In the last quarter of the twentieth century the fashion for colonic irrigation grew, especially among the rich and idle. As one newspaper put it, 'Where else is there to go anyway, after the facial, the massage, the hairdo and the shops but to a "divine woman I know" who will clean you up and make you feel good on the inside as well?'

The fashion was greatly boosted by royal patronage. When Princess Diana and the Duchess of York took up colonic irrigation, the newspapers became excited. One journalist wrote that it was one of her reader's 'favourite fantasies along with lesbian mud-wrestling. The typical colonic irrigation scheme involved a Stern Matron character clad in five-inch stiletto boots and facemask. I find it quite difficult to picture our future Queen in this situation.' One reporter went to try it and found it delightful: 'For the next half hour you bask in the most satisfying loo-going experience of your life.' She quoted one colonic hydrotherapist from the Well Centre, Chelsea; 'We clean everything else. Why not our insides? It is our encrusted intestines which make us feel lazy and bloated'.   ANN DALLY

See also PURGING; TOILET PRACTICES.

Colour blindness
Some 8% of men exhibit a hereditary deficiency of colour perception, but so imprecise is our common coinage of words about colour that it was not until the eighteenth century that the existence of colour blindness was generally known — and only rather recently was it recognized that there are measurable differences in colour perception between people with 'normal' colour vision.

The novelist Fanny Burney, who became lady-in-waiting to Queen Charlotte, records in her journal an uncomfortable conversation with George III:

> He still, however, kept me in talk, and still upon music. 'To me,' said he, 'it appears quite as strange to meet with people who have no ear for music and cannot distinguish one air from another, as to meet with people who are dumb . . . There are people who have no eye for difference of colour. The Duke of Marlborough actually cannot tell scarlet from green!' He then told me an anecdote of his mistaking one of those colours for another, which was very laughable, but I do not remember it clearly enough to write it. How unfortunate for true virtuosi that such an eye should possess objects worthy of the most discerning — the treasures of Blenheim! 'I do not find, though,' added His Majesty, 'that this defect runs in his family, for lady Di Beauclerk draws very finely.'

In fact, though His Majesty did not know it, most forms of colour blindness do run in families, but in an interesting way. The affected gene is typically on the X chromosome (of which normal females have two and males only one). A woman must carry similar defective genes on both her two X chromosomes if she is to be overtly colour blind; but a man will inescapably be colour blind if his single X chromosome bears the defect. So a woman may inherit an affected chromosome from one or other of her parents and transmit colour blindness to, on average, half her sons. She herself will pass the standard tests of colour vision, but such carriers may reveal themselves in the laboratory by, for example, their judgement of the relative brightness of different colours.

The genes that are affected are usually ones that encode and produce the light-sensitive pigments of the retina. Our daytime vision depends on three types of retinal cell, the 'cones', each type containing a different light-absorbing pigment. One of the pigments has its peak sensitivity in the violet part of the spectrum, a second peaks in the green, and the third peaks in the yellow–green. Our visual system is able to work out the colour by comparing the relative rates at which photons of light are absorbed in the different classes of cone in the area of retina exposed to the light.

In the type of colour blindness called *dichromacy*, one of the three pigments is missing. Typically the cone pigment that is lost is either the type that peaks in the green or the one that peaks in the yellow–green. About 2% of Caucasian men are dichromats of this kind. They are often well content with their residual colour vision, which depends on comparing the light absorbed in the two remaining cone types and allows them to distinguish 'warm' colours from 'cold'. More common, affecting 6% of men, is the milder condition called *anomalous trichromacy*. In such cases, the absorption curve of one of the two pigments in the green–yellow range is shifted in its position in the spectrum so that it lies closer than usual to the other. Anomalous trichromats vary in their ability to discriminate colours: they may be almost as limited as dichromats, or they may be nearly as good as normals, but they always reveal themselves by making anomalous settings in a test called the *Rayleigh match*, where the subject is asked to find the proportion of red to green light in a mixture that will just match a spectral orange. In a lesser — but measurable — way, colour-normal people vary in their Rayleigh matches, and we now know that these differences in our subjective worlds are correlated with small variations in the DNA sequence of our X chromosomes.

In addition to these inherited forms of colour deficiency, there are also forms that arise from eye conditions, such as glaucoma, or systemic conditions, such as diabetes. In these cases, it is often the violet-sensitive cones (or the pathways that carry their signals) that are affected.

In Britain at the beginning of the twenty-first century, coloured lights are still used for signalling on the roads and the railways, and the particular red and green lights employed are easily confused by many colour blind individuals. It is reported that trains are daily driven through red lights and it is a matter of speculation whether any of these incidents arise because colour-deficient drivers slip through testing or monitoring procedures designed to exclude them from such employment. It is clearly critical to screen for colour blindness at entry to professions where coloured signals are used — aviation and navigation, as well as train driving. There are other, less obvious, occupations where colour deficiency is a disadvantage, such as dermatology and market gardening. On the whole, however, colour blindness is a minor handicap in the modern world. And some biologists believe that there must be some compensating advantage that maintains the high incidence of colour blindness in our population. Certainly, one can demonstrate some advantages in the laboratory. For instance, if a screen is filled with an array of small bars randomly coloured red or green, dichromats are more accurate than normals in quickly detecting in which quadrant of the screen there is variation in the size or the orientation of the bars. And so one possibility is that the colour blind person enjoys an advantage in detecting the texture of patterns in the natural world.   J.D. MOLLON

Further reading
Backhaus, W. G., Kliegl, R., and Werner, J. S. (ed.) (1998). *Color vision*. De Gruyter, Berlin.

See also BLINDNESS; EYES; VISION.

Coma
All persons in coma are unconscious, but not all who are unconscious are in coma. SLEEP is a state of unconsciousness from which a person can be roused. The VEGETATIVE state is unconsciousness with the eyes open, the person being awake but not aware. Coma is a state of unrousable, sleep-like (eyes closed) unconsciousness. Although asleep and unaware, only those in the deepest states of coma are unresponsive. Most patients in coma respond reflexly — the pupils react to light and the limbs move in response to a painful stimulus (such as pinching the skin or pressing the nailbed). A person in coma may move restlessly and make sounds, but utters no words.

Different levels of coma, and of impaired consciousness not severe enough to be called coma, are defined by the *Glasgow Coma Scale* or *Score* — often referred to internationally as the GCS. This grades three items of behaviour: eye opening, motor responses (limb movements on command or in response to a painful stimulus), and verbal activity. For each of these there is a score of 1 to 5 according to how good the response is, with higher numbers indicating the more normal responses. At a combined score of 15 the eyes open spontaneously, commands are obeyed, and the patient can say who he is and where he is and when it is. A patient is considered to be in coma if the eyes remain closed, there are no motor responses on command, and no recognisable words are uttered — if all three of these conditions are satisfied, as well as the total score being 8 or less. At the lowest score of 3 the eyes are closed, the limbs show no response even to pain, and no sounds at all are made.

Coma is associated with loss of function in the arousal centre in the BRAIN STEM which is responsible both for eye opening and for activating the CEREBRAL CORTEX, which has to be functioning for a person to be aware of self and surroundings. Some causes of coma temporarily affect the arousal mechanisms alone. These include normal doses of anaesthetic agents, overdoses of sedative drugs or alcohol, and a generalised epileptic seizure. Toxic body chemicals can also cause coma, due to disease in other organs, as a complication of diabetes, or of failure of kidney or liver function. More often coma is a feature of major structural insults in various parts of the brain, such as those resulting from severe head injury, brain haemorrhage, infection, tumour, or oxygen lack (either in part of the brain from a blocked blood vessel (stroke), or in the brain as a whole due to stoppage of the heart or the breathing). In all these conditions the development of coma is a sign that the condition is very serious and that there is much less likelihood of recovery than if coma had not occurred.

The person in coma is at immediate risk of obstruction of the airway, as the normal coughing reflex is depressed. Obstruction may come from the tongue falling back or from inhalation of vomited stomach contents. This complication, which can be fatal, is less likely to occur if as a first-aid measure the person is turned over with the face down — the so-called coma position. Paramedics or doctors will later deal more effectively with this threat by passing a tube through the nose or mouth into the trachea (endotracheal intubation), and artificial ventilation may be set up. Since a person in coma is unable to take food and fluids normally, if coma lasts more than 24 hours artificial feeding will be necessary to ensure survival. This may be by a tube in the stomach (passed through the mouth or nose), or by a infusion into a vein.

Recovery from coma depends on the cause. Chemically-caused coma with no other brain damage or complications can be followed by complete recovery. When there has been a major structural insult the rapidity of recovery and the degree of residual disability will depend on how much permanent brain damage has been caused. How long the coma lasts is often a good indication of how severe this damage is, but a good recovery is still possible when coma has lasted 2 or 3 weeks. On the other hand, severe brain damage can occur without the patient ever being in coma, for example after a severe stroke. In survivors of even the most severe brain damage, however, coma seldom lasts more than 3–4 weeks; the eyes then open and the patient passes into another state of reduced responsiveness such as the vegetative state. Press reports of patients in 'coma' for months or years are therefore misleading.　　BRYAN JENNETT

Further reading

Teasdale, G. and Jennett, B. (1976). Assessment of coma and impaired consciousness. A practical scale. *Lancet*, 1, 1031.

See also BRAIN DEATH; CONSCIOUSNESS; VEGETATIVE STATE.

Companion animals Companion or pet animals are an integral part of many societies. Over the last two decades a body of literature has accumulated highlighting the potential benefits which these animals may bestow on our health.

Pioneering work in this area was conducted by Erika Friedmann and co-workers in the US in 1980. Initially they were interested in the effects of social relationships and personality on the survival of people who had suffered heart attacks, and they included questions about pet ownership. Follow up, one year later, showed that certain aspects of social support, or a lack of it, were found to be important predictors of one-year survival. Unexpectedly, they found that pet owners had a greater chance of being alive one year after a heart attack than non pet owners. This apparent effect of pet ownership was not due to the extra physical exercise which dog owners engaged in, since other kinds of pet owner also seemed to benefit. There were also no pre-existing differences between the personalities of pet owners and non pet owners. The study generated much interest, and led to new studies on the potential health benefits of pet ownership and the mechanisms for these effects. Friedmann also worked on a follow-up study in the 1990s using a much larger number of patients, and again found that pet ownership, and dog ownership in particular, promoted cardiovascular health, independently of social support and the physiological severity of the disease.

A large epidemiological study in Australia provided some evidence that pet ownership may actually reduce the risk factors for developing coronary heart disease. Warrick Anderson, in the early 1990s, examined standard cardiovascular risk factors among 5741 people attending a screening clinic at the Baker Medical Research Institute in Melbourne, Australia. A comparison of pet owners and non pet owners revealed that pet owners had lower systolic blood pressures and blood fat levels (plasma triglycerides) than the non pet owners. When men and women were compared separately, male pet owners had significantly lower systolic blood pressure, cholesterol, and plasma triglyceride levels than non owners. Interestingly, pet owners did not behave in a consistently more healthy manner than non pet owners. They were more physically active and yet they were also more likely to be drinkers, to eat take-away meals, and to consume meat more than 7 times per week. Women over 40 years of age were more likely to have lower systolic blood pressures if they were pet owners than if they were not. Although one could again speculate that dog owners would show the most benefit compared with other pet owners because of having to exercise the animal, in fact no differences could be detected between these two groups in relation to blood pressure, cholesterol, or triglyceride levels.

Apart from there being an interest in the effects pets can have directly on physiological parameters related to coronary heart disease, there has also been interest in the effects these animals have on our general health. James Serpell interviewed 71 adults in Cambridgeshire, UK shortly before they were to acquire a new cat or dog, and then followed them up at 1 and 10 months after acquisition. For comparison purposes, a group of people were included who did not acquire a new pet during the course of the study. In addition to obtaining basic personal and sociodemographic details, the questionnaires filled in by the participants included three self-report measures of physical and psychological health. Not surprisingly, dog owners increased the amount of daily exercise they engaged in. Both cat and dog owners reported significantly fewer minor health problems (e.g. colds, flu, hay fever, indigestion) and fewer emotional concerns during the first month of ownership compared with those who had not acquired a new pet. Only dog owners, however, maintained this over the full 10 months of the study. As with the studies mentioned previously, these benefits for dog owners could not be explained by the increased exercise levels.

A more recent, similar study by Elizabeth Paul and James Serpell in Cambridgeshire considered the effects of new pet dog acquisition on the lives of children and their families. However, unlike the positive effects found in previous studies with adults, dog-owning children were reported to have experienced significant increases in the number of ill health symptoms (e.g. colds, flus, headaches, ear ache, asthma) they suffered in the 12 months after obtaining a new dog. The researchers concluded that possibly for children, if not for adults, a variety of minor zoonoses and/or allergies may be significant consequences of keeping a dog, at least during the first 12 months or so of ownership.

Much interest has also centred on the potential short-term anti-anxiety effects companion animals may have on people. In the early 1980s, Aaron Katcher in the US measured the blood pressures of pet owners while they rested without their pets, interacted with (touched, talked to) their pets, and read aloud in the same room without their pets. The blood pressures rose significantly while reading aloud (this is a common response), however, talking to and handling the pets did not cause an increase in blood pressure.

At about the same time, Erika Friedmann and co-workers in the US studied the effects of an animal's presence only (no contact) on cardiovascular changes occurring during speech. Here they measured children's blood pressures and heart rates while they rested silently and while they read aloud, both with and without an unfamiliar but friendly dog in their presence. The presence of the friendly dogs was found to lessen the blood pressure response to reading aloud.

Mara Baun and co-workers, again in the US, studied the effects of petting one's own dog without talking to it, compared with the effects of petting an unfamiliar dog and with the effects of reading silently. Blood pressures decreased significantly over the assessment period for owners petting their own dogs, but not for those with unfamiliar dogs. These changes in blood pressure paralleled the relaxation effect of quiet reading.

Although interacting with friendly, unfamiliar dogs may not be as good for you as interacting with your own dog, Cindy Wilson in the US showed that they still can reduce the physiological and psychological consequences of stress for dog owners and non owners. She monitored the blood pressures and heart rates of students during three activities: reading aloud, reading quietly, and interacting with (talking to, petting) a friendly but unfamiliar dog. Anxiety was also measured, using a special questionnaire which the person filled out between each activity. All parameters measured (heart rate, blood pressure, anxiety) were found to be significantly higher during the reading aloud period than during the pet interaction period.

While the majority of the research in this area has involved dogs, this does not mean that other animals cannot have the same effects on people. Indeed, watching fish in an aquarium can lead to decreases in both blood pressure and anxiety. Aaron Katcher and co-workers in 1983 found that the blood pressures of normal patients and of those with hypertension decreased significantly while watching fish swim in an aquarium. These reductions were similar to those reported for relaxation therapy or transcendental meditation. Katcher also found that, for dental patients, watching fish swim in an aquarium before dental surgery proved to be an effective means of increasing patient compliance and of decreasing perception of pain during the dental procedure. Additionally, the effect of watching fish was determined to be equivalent to the effect of hypnosis.

However, it is important to note that not all studies have found a positive effect of companion animals on physiological responses to stress. For example, in the late 1980s, John Grossberg and co-workers found that neither blood pressure nor heart rate responses during mental arithmetic and psychological assessment were different for college students accompanied by their own dogs during the experiment than for the dog owners who were unaccompanied.

The ability of companion animals to positively affect our lives is therefore somewhat variable, and this is because there are numerous factors which may influence the way in which we respond to the presence of animals and to touching or talking to them. The type of stress (mental arithmetic, sound of a doorbell, telephone ring), the quality of the human support we have, our personality and relationship with the animal, and the behaviour of the animal can all play a part. Further research is required to determine just what it is about the human–companion animal relationship that can help us both physically and mentally, and under which circumstances.

A.L. PODBERSCEK

Further reading

Wilson, C. C., and Turner, D. C. (ed.) (1988). *Companion animals in human health*. SAGE, London.

Composition of the body By far the largest component of the body is water, accounting for some 60% of the total weight, which in a 70 kg person amounts to about 40 litres. Of the remaining 40% of body weight typical proportions would be 15% protein, 18% fat, and the remaining 7% mineral, largely in the form of bone; but there are large individual variations.

Water is divided into intracellular fluid (that contained within the living cells of the body) and extracellular fluid (that which bathes the cells from the outside). These fluids account respectively for 40% and 20% of the total body mass. The extracellular fluid is further subdivided into the 5% contained within the blood and 15% which is outside the vascular system. The compositions of the intra- and extracellular fluids are very different; further, the blood fluid (plasma) is subtly different to the rest of the extracellular fluid, which is termed interstitial, as it fills the interstices between the cells. Most of the material dissolved within these body fluids consists of charged molecules or ions and clearly there must be the same number of positively-charged molecules (cations) as negatively-charged molecules (anions) to maintain electroneutrality. A major difference between intra- and extracellular fluids is that the main salt in the former is potassium chloride, while outside the cells it is sodium chloride. The body uses a great deal of energy to maintain this difference — the so-called *sodium pump* removing sodium ions which penetrate the cells and bringing in potassium ions at the same time. All cells have sodium pumps in their membranes; these consume energy by hydrolysing *adenosine triphosphate* (ATP).

The differing composition of intra- and extracellular fluids is of vital importance for many bodily processes. For example, the temporary increase in membrane permeability which occurs when nerves are activated allows a flow of sodium ions into, and potassium ions out of the nerve cells. This is the mechanism by which nerve impulses flow along nerve cells, carrying messages from one place to another within the body. After the impulse has passed the sodium pump restores the original resting condition.

The ionic composition of the intracellular, interstitial, and plasma fluids is given below.

Additionally, interstitial fluid and blood plasma contain some non-electrolytes such as glucose. There are many other substances required by the healthy body but their total amounts are generally very small; an exception is iron, which is an essential component of haemoglobin contained in red cells, and hence is essential for the carriage of oxygen from the lungs to the tissues. In addition there are vitamins and trace elements (including cobalt, manganese, copper, zinc, iodine, and bromine).

Disturbances of body composition occur most obviously in dehydration or STARVATION. Estimation of the concentrations of electrolytes and other substances in the plasma is a routine part of many diagnostic investigations, since they can change in characteristic ways in a variety of conditions; in studies of nutritional status and OBESITY, the fat and lean fractions of body mass are measured and compared to standard values for males and females at different ages; estimation of the bone mineral is important in the assessment of OSTEOPOROSIS.

ALAN W. CUTHBERT

See also BLOOD; BODY FLUIDS; BODY WEIGHT; BONE; METALS IN THE BODY; MINERALS; SALT; WATER BALANCE.

The ionic composition of the intracellular, interstitial, and plasma fluids is given below, showing values in milliEquivalents per litre

Intracellular fluid					
Cations	Potassium	157	Anions	Bicarbonate	10
	Sodium	14		Phosphate	113
	Magnesium	26		Protein	74
Interstitial fluid					
Cations	Sodium	143	Anions	Chloride	117
	Potassium	4		Bicarbonate	27
	Calcium	5		Phosphate	2
	Magnesium	3		Sulphate	1
				Organic acid	6
				Protein	2
Plasma					
Cations	Sodium	152	Anions	Chloride	113
	Potassium	5		Bicarbonate	27
	Calcium	5		Protein	16
	Magnesium	3		Phosphate	2
				Sulphate	2
				Organic acid	6

Notice that the total cations are balanced by the total anions in all three fluids. Values in milliEquivalents per litre represent number of molecules x valency, and thus allow assessment of electroneutrality. In other contexts concentrations of substances in the body are more commonly quoted in millimoles per litre.

Conception To conceive usually implies the establishment of a pregnancy — receiving an embryo into the womb for further development, comparable to conceiving an idea in the mind. But conception is essentially defined as the successful entry of sperm into ovum — synonymous with fertilization — even though the fertilized embryo may never attain the privilege of implantation in the uterus and the future which that promises. The point is academic, because the loss of a microscopic fertilized embryo goes unrecognized. When pregnancy is in fact established, conception in the sense of fertilization can be roughly dated, knowing the occasions of coitus, and that the two gametes usually meet as the ovum traverses the Fallopian tube, 7 to 14 days before the next expected period in a 28-day menstrual cycle. s.j.

See PREGNANCY.

Concussion This word originally meant severe shaking, or the shock of an impact, but has come to mean the effect of such violence on the brain. The immediate effect of such an impact — usually when the moving head meets an immovable object, most commonly the ground — is unconsciousness. After a mild injury this lasts only a minute or so and the person is then dazed or confused for a few more minutes before recovering normal consciousness; occasionally recovery may take hours. After more severe impact injury, the patient may remain in COMA for many days and remain confused for many more days thereafter. In either event there will be no memory for the moment of impact, often for a period immediately before this, and always for the period of unconsciousness and confusion: this is known as post-traumatic AMNESIA.

For many years 'concussion' was applied only to mild injuries, when it was assumed that the brief loss of consciousness was due to temporary chemical or electrical events resulting from the mechanical forces acting on the brain. It is now recognised that the effect of the jelly-like brain being distorted by these forces is to stretch or even tear delicate nerve fibres, resulting in some permanent damage. After mild injury this is very limited, but after more severe impact there is more severe and more widespread damage to fibres. There can therefore be both mild and severe concussion and it is misleading to ask 'Was it *only* concussion?'

After only mild concussion there are often symptoms for several days, sometimes weeks — headache, fatigue, dizziness, and poor concentration. In a few patients these post-concussional symptoms give rise to anxiety and other psychological symptoms that can aggravate and prolong the organically-impaired function that the patient suffers. In contact sports there is the risk of repeated concussions, and the small amount of damage sustained each time can be cumulative. Moreover, soon after one concussion the brain may be more susceptible to a second blow, and this is why most sports have rules about

waiting 2–3 weeks before playing again, for example after concussion on the football field or in the boxing ring. The repeated concussions over a period of years that boxers can experience may result in progressive brain damage, evident in altered mental function and control of the limbs — the so-called 'punch-drunk' syndrome. This is now rare, as there are stringent regulations to limit exposure to such a hazard.

BRYAN JENNETT

See also BOXING; COMA.

Conditioning My heart races and my palms sweat during my first attempt to drive again after a traumatic road accident. Alternatively, having discovered that a new joke goes down well at work, I find myself retelling it *ad nauseam*. These two scenarios are examples of different forms of conditioning. The first is an example of *classical conditioning*, and involves learning about the predictive relationship between stimuli. As a result of the car accident, the interior of a car, let alone the touch of steering wheel, has become a signal for a traumatic event and thereby elicits a fear reaction through the activation of my autonomic nervous system. By contrast, my new found humour is an example of '*instrumental*' or '*operant*' *conditioning*. In this case, I have learned about the causal relationship between an action, the telling of the joke, and the apparent attention and interest that it elicits in my friends and colleagues, which only serves to reward this tedious behaviour.

Classical conditioning is often referred to as '*Pavlovian*' because this form of learning was discovered by the renowned Russian physiologist, PAVLOV, in his experiments on the neural control of digestion at the end of the nineteenth century. As is well known, Pavlov signalled the presentation of food to his hungry dogs by turning on a stimulus, such a bell, some seconds before the delivery of each meal. Although the bell initially produced little more than orientation towards its source, after a number of pairings with the food this stimulus began to elicit novel behaviour. As soon as the signal came on, the dogs approached the location of the food and started salivating copiously. The occurrence of the responses depended, or were conditional, upon experience of the predictive relationship between the signal and the food, and thus came to be known as '*conditioned*'. Correspondingly, the signal is called a *conditioned stimulus*, because its property also depends upon learning about the predictive relationship. By contrast, the food is an *unconditioned stimulus*, because the salivation that it elicits, the unconditioned response, does not depend upon the learning experience. Pavlov also referred to the food as a *reinforcer*, as it is the event responsible for strengthening the conditioned response. Although it was originally thought that simple pairings of a conditioned stimulus and a reinforcer are sufficient for conditioning, we now know that only signals that are informative about the occurrence of the reinforcer become conditioned. Moreover, conditioning is not always a

simple, automatic and non-conscious process and, in certain cases, only occurs in humans when they are already aware of the relationship between signal and reinforcer.

The salivation elicited by the signals for food is an *appetitive conditioned response* because the reinforcer, the food, is attractive. By contrast, my hypothetical fear response to the car is an example of *aversive* or *defensive* conditioning, because the reinforcer in this case, the accident, is noxious and distressing. Pavlovian conditioning affects a gamut of response and behaviour systems, from the sexual evaluation of members of the opposite sex to food preference and aversions. Moreover, this form of conditioning also plays a role not only in behavioural responses but also in the regulatory systems of the body. For example, if drinking a fluid with a particular flavour signals an infusion of glucose into the stomach of hungry rats, that flavour will, in future, reduce blood sugar level in anticipation of the glucose load.

The experimental study of '*instrumental*' conditioning also started over 100 years ago, but in this case by an American comparative psychologist, Thorndike, who was interested in comparing the learning capacities of different species of animal. Thorndike studied the rate at which a variety of animals learned to operate a latch in order to escape from a cage to eat some food placed outside. These instrumental tasks were subsequently refined over the succeeding decades, most notably by the behaviourist psychologist, Skinner. As in the case of Pavlovian conditioning, the food acted as a reinforcer to strengthen the conditioned response, the operation of the latch, but in the instrumental case through a positive causal relationship between the response and reinforcer. In contrast to Pavlovian conditioning, however, aversive or noxious stimuli cannot act as instrumental reinforcers through a positive relationship with a response. Indeed, when a response causes an aversive outcome, the behaviour is suppressed or punished. For an aversive event, such as a road accident, to reinforce the appropriate instrumental response (careful and defensive driving) the response has to prevent the event happening and thereby allow us to escape or avoid dangerous and unpleasant situations.

There are two sorts of learning process underlying instrumental conditioning. The first process establishes response habits through the acquisition of a connection between an eliciting stimulus and the response. For example, enhancement of the limb muscle reflexes involved in the movements that the rat must make to reach for the latch can be conditioned by arranging for an appropriate change to be reinforced by the delivery of food to a hungry animal. This simple stimulus–response development clearly plays a role in the acquisition of motor skills. Other learning processes are involved in more complex forms of instrumental conditioning, which support goal-directed actions based upon knowledge of the causal relationship between the action and the outcome that it achieves. This type of instrumental conditioning operates when one explicitly plans a course of action to achieve a specific goal.

In summary, the two forms of conditioning, Pavlovian and instrumental, reflect the processes by which we and other animals learn to adjust our behaviour to the predictive and causal structure of our environment. The fact that, in one form or another, both types of conditioning are to be found throughout the animal kingdom, from relatively simple invertebrates to ourselves, is a testimony to their ubiquitous and important adaptive function.   A. DICKINSON

Further reading

Dworkin, B. R. (1993). *Learning and physiological regulation.* The University of Chicago Press, Chicago.

Mackintosh, N. J. (1983). *Conditioning and associative learning.* Oxford University Press, New York.

See also PAVLOV, IVAN.

Condom

The wearing of penile sheaths made from a diversity of substances — linen, gourds, tortoiseshell, leather, silk, oiled paper — has been known in numerous societies from distant antiquity. But it is less certain that these were employed either as a protection against SEXUALLY TRANS-MITTED DISEASE or for contraceptive purposes, rather than for magical or decorative purposes or modesty. It was the Italian anatomist Gabriello Fallopio (1523–62) who, in a posthumously published work *De morbo gallico* ('on the French disease' — syphilis), recommended as a protection against venereal disease a linen sheath of which he claimed to be the inventor. The manner of fitting it — over the glans but under the foreskin, or inserted into the urethra — sounds neither comfortable nor particularly practicable. A little later, Hercules Saxonia described a larger linen sheath, soaked in a chemical or herbal preparation, which covered the entire penis.

The invention of the sheep-gut sheath has been persistently attributed to a certain Dr Condom, Cundum, or even Quondam, an almost certainly apocryphal figure, during the reign of Charles II. Archaeological evidence, however, suggests that, far from being a product of the licentious Restoration era, gut condoms were already available over 20 years earlier during the height of the English Civil War. Five fragments of shaped animal gut were discovered during the excavation of the garderobe (lavatory) of the keep at Dudley Castle, which had been filled in in 1647. These prototype condoms (*baudruche*, french letters, *capotes anglaises*, etc.), both animal and vegetable, were primarily employed as prophylactics against venereal disease, although there is some literary evidence that their dual purpose as contraceptives was also recognised. There are a number of literary allusions throughout the eighteenth century, most notoriously in the memoirs of Casanova and the diary of James Boswell, to the use of 'armour', or 'implements of safety'. Madame de Sevigné, however, writing of their contraceptive use, considered them 'an armour against enjoyment and a spider-web against danger'. They were manufactured from the caecum or blind gut of sheep, which was soaked, turned inside out, macerated in an alkaline solution, scraped, exposed to brimstone vapour, washed, blown up, dried, cut, and given a ribbon tie. It was necessary to soak them to render them supple enough to put on. The labour-intensive process meant that the products were correspondingly expensive (though reusable) and thus only available to a limited proportion of the population.

The next major technological innovation affecting the condom was the vulcanisation of rubber, enabling the production of cheaper condoms in great quantity. The first rubber condoms had a seam, but around the beginning of the twentieth century a new method of manufacture was introduced, whereby glass moulds were dipped into liquid rubber. Variant forms developed, such as the teat-ended condom and the 'American tip', which covered the glans only. Even these, however, were still beyond the reach of the poorest in the community; moreover they were also coarse and clumsy and perceived as unaesthetic, quite apart from the very pervasive feeling that the condom represented an immoral attempt to interfere with the laws of God and Nature. The device was associated with libertinism, and even the attempts of neo-Malthusian propagandists to promote the social benefits of birth control were tainted by their association with free-thinking secularism.

It is often stated that condoms gained, as it were, a certain currency through being distributed to troops during World War I in an attempt to control the appallingly high rate of venereal diseases. Many approved official prophylactic packs in fact contained antiseptic ointment. With the rise of an articulate birth control movement during the 1920s, condoms became more discussed. They were not the favoured method of most birth control advocates, being seen as unreliable and unaesthetic, and furthermore requiring not merely co-operation but action by the male partner. However, since they did not require expert fitting (as the female pessary did) and could be purchased over the counter and even from slot machines, they were probably the most popular appliance method of birth control until the advent of hormonal contraception in the 1960s.

The technology improved further: the latex process simplified manufacture to the point where it could be automated, making the product cheaper, and created a thinner, more elastic, and more reliable condom. There has been little additional technical innovation, though some brands now include added lubricant or spermicide. Novelty condoms (with no practical value) are produced as sex toys, with a variety of supposedly stimulating excrescences, in different colours, and even flavours.

The reliability of condoms has been a matter of much concern. There was a persistent belief that there was a law requiring one in 10 or 12 to be faulty, or that Catholic workers in rubber-goods factories pricked a certain proportion with a pin. Quality testing, however, gradually made its way into this marginalised industry, in Great Britain stimulated by the possibility of winning the commercially useful accolade of a place on the National Birth Control Association's 'Approved List' of reliable products.

With the advent of the contraceptive pill in the 1960s, the condom lost a good deal of its popularity as a birth control method, while antibiotics meant that venereal disease was no longer perceived as a risk. The condom retained rather louche associations with male promiscuity rather than male responsibility (even though the vast majority were probably used to manifest the latter). The current estimate of its reliability in preventing pregnancy runs from 85–98%, much depending on the user.

The condom has made a comeback, since the advent of the Human Immunodeficiency Virus, as a means of preventing the dangerous exchange of bodily fluids. How extensive condom use actually has become is still moot. The subject is still capable of arousing considerable embarrassment.   LESLEY A. HALL

See also CONTRACEPTION.

Congenital abnormalities

'Congenital' means 'present at birth', but malformations that are obvious at birth represent only a small proportion of the seriously malformed products of gestation. The term 'congenital anomalies' is also used and these are defined as significant, definable, structural and/or developmental abnormalities observed at birth. Some anomalies are produced by adverse environmental agents, such as viral infection of the mother, specific toxins (including hormones), ionising radiations, or inadequate supply of oxygenated blood to developing organs; all these together comprise around 5–6% of the total. Abnormalities associated with a mutant gene account for about 5% and identifiable chromosomal aberrations for a further 10%.

It is estimated that between 60 and 80% of all conceptuses are lost early in gestation. These may be the result of 'bad eggs' (abnormal cleavage, abnormal chromosomes), major early embryonic maldevelopment, or significant embryonic metabolic abnormalities, with early embryonic death and resorption in some cases. Approximately half of all fetuses spontaneously aborted in the first 3 months have significant chromosomal anomalies.

Anomalies of clinical significance are found in 2–5 of every 100 human infants born alive. This does not include infants with hidden defects or those with disorders that only become evident later. For rather more than half of congenital anomalies present at birth no single cause has yet been identified.

The study of congenital malformations is known as *teratology*. Abnormalities evident at birth can arise due to failure of development (for example, absent limb(s), *microcephaly*); failure of parts to unite (CLEFT LIP AND PALATE, spina bifida); failure to divide (*syndactyly* — joined fingers or toes; conjoined twins); failure to canalise (*atresia*: no passage through some part of the gut); failure of tissues to migrate to the proper site (malrotation of bowel, Hirschsprung disease); failure to atrophy — to disappear appropriately in the course of development (branchial clefts, thyroglossal cyst); excess division (*polydactyly* — too many fingers or toes, duplication of kidneys).

Chromosomal and gene mutation abnormalities take effect during all phases of pre- and post-natal life and can cause isolated or multiple congenital anomalies. Regulatory (master) genes code for polypeptides that are active in cell nuclei and modify the array of transcribed genes from the totipotent cells of the 2–8 cell embryo to the specialised cell populations of later organ development, such as that of the brain. Proliferation and differentiation of cells within body organs is largely mediated by growth factors, and by the polypeptides that cause genetic information from the DNA to be transcribed onto messenger RNA in body cells. These *transcription factors*, controlled by regulatory genes, promote a cascade of temporally and spatially organized events that cause the formation of, for example, the neural tube, or the heart. Abnormal transcription regulation can cause profound errors in the forming of the embryo, and a number of genes have been identified that control development of the different segments of the body, from head to tail, and of the organs. The cell replication, programmed cell death (*apoptosis*), induction and intercellular communication, cell migration, and movement of contiguous cell populations are all, in part, determined by regulatory genes and their transcription factors. Nutritional factors, toxic factors, and metabolic disorders present at critical stages of embryogenesis have the potential to interfere with the developmental changes controlled and influenced by the regulatory genes. Maternal infections, physical insults, and metabolic disorders, such as diabetes mellitus or phenylketonuria, increase the risk of congenital anomalies, including brain anomalies; likewise maternal ingestion of some substances (including alcohol and thalidomide), which for this reason are known as *teratogens*.

Mineral and vitamin deficiency states can adversely influence transcriptions through, for example, effects on enzyme systems that depend on particular elements. Notably, severe zinc deprivation during embryonic and fetal development has been shown in animals to have profound effects on virtually all derivatives of the neural tube (the preliminary stage of the central nervous system) and associated structures, including the brain, spinal cord, and eyes. Deficiencies of manganese, copper, iron, selenium, and iodine have all been shown to affect developing organs.

Folic acid is important in, for example, the development of nerve cells, their growth and the myelination of their axons. Normal closure of the neural tube in the human embryo occurs between days 21 and 24. Folate deficiency before and during this stage of development results in neural tube defects (brain and spinal cord abnormalities). A mutation in the genes of some mothers for a certain enzyme (known as MTHFR) is associated with a detectable chemical change in the blood when their dietary folate intake is marginal; this defect has been found in 5–7% of mothers in some European populations. Ensuring adequate maternal dietary intake of folate significantly reduces the incidence of neural tube defects and possibly other central nervous system defects.

Vitamin B$_1$ (thiamine) deficiency is relatively common in the developing world and has been associated with fetal defects; thiamine deficiency may be one of the mechanisms by which chronic maternal alcoholism results in fetal defects. Pyridoxine (Vitamin B$_6$) deficiency, and vitamin A deficiencies and excesses, have also been shown to produce malformations in animals.

Prevalence

The frequency of significant congenital anomalies remained the same or declined slightly overall during the twentieth century in those countries with good registers, despite public apprehension and a number of well-publicised environmental disasters. However, some of the commoner defects have reportedly increased in incidence, according to the birth defects monitoring programme of the Centers for Disease Control in Atlanta. During the 1990s there was a significant increase in ventricular septal defect ('hole in the heart'), patent ductus arteriosus, renal agenesis (failure of kidney development), and hip dislocation, but a decrease in spina bifida.

In the case of some malformations, their manifestations and the likelihood of survival varies among infants who have essentially the same defect, including variation by maternal race, the infant's sex, and birthplace. Neural tube defects are commoner in the UK and Ireland compared with the rest of Europe; this may be partly related to the high prevalence of gene mutations in MTHFR. In Japan, Taiwan, and Singapore there is a high incidence of *anencephaly* (absence of skull and brain) compared with other neural tube defects, and two-thirds of anencephalic infants are female. It may be that anencephalic male embryos are expelled unrecognised from the womb at an early stage.

Whilst about 2% of new-born infants have major malformations, a further 6% have minor ones; also major and minor malformations may co-exist.

Multiple malformations

may be part of

(i) a syndrome in which there is a single cause for the various malformations, e.g. Down's syndrome (extra chromosome 21) and fetal alcohol syndrome (FAS);

(ii) a sequence whereby one malformation has led to other malformations — e.g. failure of kidney development, with lack of fetal urine production, leads to lack of amniotic fluid (*oligohydramnios*), and that in turn to underdevelopment of the lungs (*pulmonary hypoplasia*) because of restriction of fetal breathing movements;

(iii) a condition in which various malformations are statistically associated but there is no known or common cause — e.g. VATER association, which is an acronym for vertebral, anal, tracheal, oesophageal, and renal malformations.

Minor malformations include haemangiomas and naevi (BIRTHMARKS); skin tags; hydrocoeles; webbing of fingers and toes or supernumerary digits; malformed ears; and pigmented skin lesions. Although some of these defects can cause major health problems, malformations considered by convention to be major are those affecting the heart (which may or may not prevent blood from flowing normally through the lungs, and therefore may or may not result in a '*blue baby*': cyanotic or acyanotic *congenital heart disease*); the central nervous system (HYDROCEPHALUS, meningocoele, and encephalocoele); the urinary system (including hydronephrosis and polycystic kidney); the digestive system (various herniae, malrotations, and atresias); cleft lip and/or palate; limb defects (including dislocated hip and club foot); genital disorders (such as undescended testes, *hypospadias* (see PENIS), and ambiguous genitalia); and eye defects (cataract and *microphthalmos* — small eyes). Finally, there may be multiple system defects combining several of these.

Treatment and prevention

There are now medical and surgical therapies available for some malformations detected before birth. Prevention strategies include immunization against rubella; avoidance of alcohol and other potentially embryotoxic chemicals and agents during pregnancy; strict control of metabolic disturbances in the mother; and a balanced nutrient intake from before the time of conception.   FORRESTER COCKBURN

See also ANTENATAL DEVELOPMENT; CLEFT LIP AND PALATE; CLUB FOOT; HYDROCEPHALUS.

Connective tissue

links, separates, supports, embeds, and protects the body's cells, tissues, and organs, and imparts varying degrees of fluidity, elasticity, or rigidity. There are many types. All contain non-cellular fibres together with the living cells which manufacture them and a matrix which ranges from near-liquid to solid. There are fibres of COLLAGEN in all types and also of *elastin* in many. *Loose areolar* tissue is the least solid, with gelatinous material among its fibres. Fatty (*adipose*) tissue has lipid-containing cells in a network of collagenous fibres. Fibrous connective tissue forms a framework among MUSCLE fibres, and among NERVE fibres, as well as sheaths for whole muscles and whole nerves; it also forms membranes such as the thin sheets of *fascia* which separate whole tissue layers from their neighbours, and stronger capsules for individual organs and ligaments which support joints. Elastic fibres in the LUNGS are crucial for the mechanics of breathing, and in the major arteries for their rhythmic expansion and recoil. TENDONS ('sinews') are strong, resilient straps of collagenous and elastic fibres which connect a muscle to a bony attachment. CARTILAGE is a rigid connective tissue; it encircles the windpipe and stiffens the nostrils to keep the airway open, keeps the ears from flapping, and covers the ends of bones in the joints. Finally, BONE is obviously the most rigid in the category, with mineral deposits laid down in a collagen fibre framework.

SHEILA JENNETT

Consciousness The twentieth-century British psychologist Stuart Sutherland once defined consciousness as 'a fascinating but elusive phenomenon: it is impossible to specify what it is, what it does, or why it evolved. Nothing worth reading has been written about it.' Consciousness is indeed hard to define, but most people have an intuitive idea of what it is. It encompasses two different concepts: the notion of a *self*, and the feelings of which the self is aware, especially *qualia* — our raw sensory experiences.

Although some philosophers (*panpsychists*) have believed that all things, including inanimate objects such as chairs and umbrellas, are conscious, most people agree that consciousness is associated with brains (and, some would argue, with inanimate machines that work, in some crucial respect, like brains). Stated simply, then, the problem is how does the activity of nerve cells in the brain give rise to our subjective mental life? Neurons — specks of jelly in the brain, with their electrical impulses and their little squirts of neurotransmitter — seem so utterly different from the redness of red or the flavour of Marmite on toast.

The riddle of qualia is best illustrated with a thought experiment. Imagine a neuroscientist in some future century, who has complete knowledge of the workings of the brain — including the mechanisms of colour vision — but who happens to be colour blind and cannot herself distinguish between red and green. She uses the latest scanning techniques to generate a total description of all the electrical and chemical events in the brain of a normal human as he looks at a red object. The functional account may seem complete, but how could it be so without an explanation of the *nature* of the unique experience of red, which the scientist herself has never had? There is a deep epistemological gulf between descriptions of physical events in the brain and the personal, subjective experiences that we presume to be associated with those events.

Is consciousness a property of the entire brain — does it 'emerge' when the brain reaches a certain level of complexity? Or are only some parts of the brain conscious? (After all, if we argue that only brains and not other organs are conscious, why not imagine that only some parts of the brain are involved?) Indeed, neurological evidence suggests that we are unconscious of most of the activity in our brains — not just the below-stairs business of running the heart, digestion, posture, and so on, but also the pre-perceptual processing of information from the senses, and the complex task of selecting and controlling the individual muscles that carry out actions.

A rare disorder, aptly called 'blindsight', strikingly demonstrates a dissociation between conscious and unconscious visual processing. It results from damage restricted to the primary visual cortex in the cerebral hemispheres, which classically causes 'cortical blindness' in a corresponding part of the visual field. Although the patient denies seeing, say, a small spot of light presented in the blind part of the field, he or she can fairly accurately point towards the spot. Moreover, if a moving spot or a line is shown, the patient can 'guess' the direction of movement or the angle of the line, all the time unaware that it exists! This amazing paradox is explained by the fact that there are two main pathways of interconnected nerve cells from the eyes and through the brain. One goes to the primary visual cortex, and on into the lower parts of the temporal lobe, which is responsible for the identification of objects and the laying down of personal memories. The other projects via the reflex visual centres of the midbrain (which control eye movements) and thence up to the parietal lobes of the cortex, where the information is used to guide hand movements. Since the latter pathway is still intact in the patient with blindsight, he or she can use it for reaching for the object. But the other pathway into the temporal lobe seems to be intimately involved in conscious perception. A more subtle dissociation can occur in patients who have extensive damage to the temporal lobe, which does not interfere with basic visual functions but can cause *agnosia* — an incapacity to distinguish consciously between different objects and shapes. However, such patients can correctly shape their hands to pick up different objects that they cannot perceptually distinguish. It is almost as though there is an unconscious 'zombie' inside the heads of such patients, 'seeing' the world and guiding the hands but not troubling consciousness with what it is doing.

Unconscious vision is not just a neurological anomaly — it occurs even in normal people. If you are driving a car while talking to the person next to you or on a mobile telephone, many parts of your brain are processing enormous amounts of visual information to enable you to negotiate the traffic. Yet little of it reaches consciousness so long as your attention is focused on the conversation. Interestingly, it is hard to imagine the opposite scenario — of having a conversation unconsciously while paying attention to the traffic. At any instant, we seem to be fully aware of only a minute fraction of the things that we could be aware of. As you stand chatting to a friend at a party, you are unaware of the content of the other conversations around you — unless you deliberately eavesdrop out of the 'corner of your ear'.

Equally, our embarrassingly poor ability to recall the detail of a visual scene if the lights are suddenly switched off indicates that we are genuinely aware of only a tiny fraction of the flood of information that pours into our brains from our eyes. Only the focus of current attention seems fully represented in our consciousness, in the sense that it can be remembered. This all suggests that there is a link between consciousness, attention, and MEMORY, and also that we cannot use LANGUAGE creatively without being conscious.

This raises the so-called 'Zombie problem'. If we are able to do so much without being aware of it, what purpose does consciousness serve, and how did it evolve? Imagine an unconscious zombie that looks exactly like a person and does all the things a conscious human does, but without being conscious. There seems to be nothing logically impossible about this. Indeed, we have no way of knowing, for sure, that machines, animals, or even other human beings are truly conscious in the way that we feel ourselves to be. Some philosophers, most notably Gilbert Ryle, have argued that concepts of mind, such as self and intention, are merely 'category mistakes' — muddles that arise from the misuse of language. Such virtuosic philosophical argument reinforces the 'Zombie problem', but is deeply unsatisfactory. We *know* that we are conscious. Indeed, as René Déscartes pointed out, knowing that we are aware is the only thing that we are really sure about — '*cogito, ergo sum*'.

In parallel with Ryle's attempt to explain away the 'Ghost in the Machine', the school of psychology called *behaviourism* also argued that consciousness does not (or need not) exist and that science should confine itself to an attempt to explain externally observable behaviour. To behavioural psychologists, it has indeed been valuable to view the brain objectively, merely seeking accounts of behaviour without the baggage of common-language concepts such as will, intention, and need. However, it is difficult for most people — even brain researchers — to accept the extreme notion of 'eliminative materialism', namely that words such as 'love', 'want', and even 'red' have the same logical status as the once universal but now arcane view that living things have some kind of 'vital essence', which distinguishes them from the inanimate world.

More intriguing is *epiphenomenalism*. Just as the shadow of a running horse appears to run along with it but plays no causal role in the running, consciousness may simply accompany certain brain events but not itself have a function. Can it really be true that when you feel that you are choosing to pick up a cup, it is not the conscious intention that initiates the picking up? In fact, there is growing evidence that our subjective impressions of events in the world and of our intended actions are a kind of post-hoc 'commentary' on things that have already happened. Disturbing though it is, our conscious lives may be a plausible but illusory tale, a translation of the zombie world into the domain of subjectivity.

But why should we have such a self-deluding system in the brain? How did it evolve? What could its value be?

Faced with such philosphical conundrums, many neuroscientists, with Francis Crick as their standard-bearer, have argued that we should simply aim to define the 'neural correlate of consciousness' — the parts of the brain and the nature and activity of nerve cells that implement conscious states. Once we have a clear understanding of the neural activity that is both necessary and sufficient for subjectivity, perhaps many of the philosophic problems will disappear.

The pragmatic advantage of this approach is that it transforms consciousness into an empirical problem that is approachable experimentally. Instead of asking 'What *is* consciousness?', one asks 'What parts of the brain are active, or in what special way are they active, when someone does something consciously?' One experimental approach that is proving fruitful is to monitor the activity of different parts of the CEREBRAL CORTEX (with microelectrodes in animals, or with IMAGING TECHNIQUES in human beings) while the retinal image is unchanging but the content of consciousness changes. For instance, how does activity in the brain change as a person or animal shifts attention from one thing to another? What happens when they view ambiguous visual images that can appear, at one moment, to be one thing, but, at another instant, to be something else?

That other mysterious aspect of subjectivity — the feeling of 'free will' and intention — is more difficult to study. However, fingers of evidence point towards the anterior cingulate cortex, a region on the inner surface of the frontal lobe. Patients with damage here sometimes feel that their own actions occur without being intended — *alien hand syndrome*. Conversely, they may be fully conscious but feel that they don't want to do anything at all — *akinetic mutism*.

The early decades of the twenty-first century will undoubtedly see great advances in our understanding of the neural correlate of consciousness. What is less certain is whether such empirical observations will take us any closer to resolving what philosopher David Chalmers has called the 'Hard Problem', that is, what really is the nature of subjectivity? We may be forced to admit that consciousness, like infinity and the particle-wave concepts in quantum mechanics, is a property that cannot be made intuitively straighforward. Consciousness, like gravity, mass, and charge, may be one of the irreducible properties of the universe for which no further account is possible.

V.S. RAMACHANDRAN

COLIN BLAKEMORE

Further reading

Churchland, P. M. (1996). *The engine of reason, the seat of the soul.* MIT Press, Cambridge MA.

Crick, F. H. C. (1993). *The astonishing hypothesis.* Charles Scribner, New York.

Ramachandran, V. S. (1998). *Phantoms in the brain.* William Morrow, New York.

Searle, J. (1994). *The rediscovery of the mind.* MIT Press, Cambridge MA.

Weizkrantz, L. (1986). *Blindsight.* Oxford University Press.

See also BRAIN; COLOUR BLINDNESS; ILLUSIONS; IMAGING TECHNIQUES; PERCEPTION; VISION.

Constipation

Constipation is a widely used term usually referring to decreased bowel frequency, although it is sometimes used when the stools are hard or when there is pain or difficulty with bowel evacuation. A clear definition of the term is difficult because of the wide range of 'normal' bowel frequency in the general population, which ranges from two or three times a day to less than two per week. Constipation has many causes, the majority of which are not serious and for which there are simple remedies. However, as it may be the presenting feature of a serious condition such as large bowel cancer, in selected circumstances constipation requires further investigation to enable specific treatment to be given. There are a number of important groups of disorders which present as constipation.

Causes of constipation

When the structure of the bowel is apparently normal Most individuals fall into this group, and the most common cause is usually dietary. Low fibre diets result in low faecal residues, which can reduce the frequency of bowel action. In some individuals constipation may be a behavioural problem, possibly related to a life-long suppression of the normal 'signals' to defecate. Other situations like pregnancy and old age and infirmity also slow intestinal transit and can result in constipation. Some patients with irritable bowel syndrome complain of constipation which may alternate with increased bowel frequency.

Structural abnormalities in the colon and rectum Minor anal problems such as 'anal fissure' — a tear in the lining of the anal canal — can result in constipation because of voluntary inhibition of defecation due to the associated pain. Inflammation in the rectum, proctitis, can have the same effect. In addition, there are some important disorders in which there is a developmental or acquired abnormality of the nerves within the bowel wall; examples include Hirschsprung's disease (congenital 'megacolon' described by this Danish physician in 1888) and infection with the parasite *Trypanosoma cruzi*, which causes Chagas' disease (named after the Brazilian physician who noted it in 1909). Abnormalities of colonic muscle produce a myopathy which can also lead to constipation.

Neurological diseases A number of generalised neurological disorders, such as Parkinson's disease and multiple sclerosis, can damage the nerve supply to the colon and rectum and produce constipation. Similar damage to the autonomic nerves can also occur in diabetes mellitus. Colonic function may also be impaired in patients with reduced levels of consciousness and mental retardation.

Endocrine and metabolic causes Reduced activity of the THYROID gland (hypothyroidism) and raised concentrations of CALCIUM in the blood (hypercalcaemia) are the most common disorders in this group.

Psychological disorders Depression and anorexia nervosa are both often associated with constipation.

Adverse drug effects Many drugs can cause constipation, in particular potent painkillers (opiates and opioid ANALGESICS), some antidepressants, and drugs used to reduce high blood pressure.

Investigation and management of constipation

Investigation of constipation which has no simple explanation may require exclusion of a structural problem in the colon; this usually involves a radiological examination (barium enema) or an endoscopic examination using a flexible instrument called a colonoscope. Nerve and muscle disorders sometimes require investigation using methods to measure transit time through the colon, and measurement of pressure within the bowel and electrophysiological tests to study nerve and muscle function.

Simple constipation, in which there is no obvious disease or disorder of the colon, is best remedied by dietary measures such as increasing the fibre content of the diet. Commercially-prepared bulking agents are also available. If bulking agents fail then osmotic laxatives such as magnesium sulphate (Epsom salts) may be required, though there is some evidence that prolonged use can damage the colonic nerves and ultimately make the condition worse.

When constipation is due to colon cancer or an endocrine or metabolic disturbance, then appropriate specific treatment is required. If constipation occurs as an adverse effect of drug therapy for another condition, then it is usually appropriate to try an alternative preparation.

MICHAEL FARTHING

ANNE BALLINGER

See also ALIMENTARY SYSTEM; DEFECATION; TOILET PRACTICES.

Contact lenses

Contact lenses The contact lens provides a good example of the lengths to which some humans will go to overcome deficiencies of the visual system. A contact lens is a foreign body and as such causes irritation and pain. In addition there is an excessive flow of tears to wash out the invading object and a strong urge to rub the eye, with the further risk of causing a corneal abrasion. The contact lens wearer has to be strongly motivated to learn to adapt to this irritant and develop the ocular tolerance necessary for comfortable lens wear. Vanity is a powerful driving force, immortalized by Dorothy Parker's malicious 'Men seldom make passes at girls who wear glasses'. Assuredly there are other advantages with contact lenses in many types of sport, in the rain, and in working in confined and awkward positions, especially if protective goggles are needed as well. An early experiment by Thomas Young in 1801 to eliminate focusing by the cornea involved a convex lens fitted to a short glass socket filled with water which was applied to his eye. He immediately became hypermetropic (long sighted) in that eye, but using his optometer found 'the same inequality in the horizontal and vertical refractions as without the water'. Interestingly, this showed that his astigmatism was not due to his cornea, which is certainly the commonest cause.

The first recorded use of a protective glass for an eye exposed after removal of the eyelid was in 1887. A blown glass contact lens made from a plaster mould of an eye with *keratoconus* (conical cornea) was used for optical treatment in 1888. A year later a ground glass contact lens was made to treat an ophthalmologist's own high myopia (short sight).

Scleral lenses covered more than the area of the eye seen between the eyelids, and ground and moulded glass lenses superseded blown glass until that, in turn, was followed by plastic lenses.

The author was present at a lecture by Wichterle in 1963 at the Institute of Ophthalmology, London when he introduced the soft hydrophilic plastic corneal lens. These cost 1 shilling (5p) each to produce, although Wichterle wryly commented that the cost to the patient would bear no comparison. In fact, having passed through expensive phases, daily wear, disposable soft lenses which are thrown away after use cost only £1 each, nearly 40 years later.

The search for new materials to make contact lenses continues, because a number of important constraints have to be met. The lens must allow OXYGEN and CARBON DIOXIDE easy passage between the air and the aqueous humour, the fluid behind the cornea. It must not interfere with the metabolic pump which maintains corneal transparency. The tear flow must be maintained, but not excessive. Adaptive changes occur in corneal sensitivity, so that the lens is better tolerated, but if sensitivity is blunted too far the risk of abrasions and infections increases. A soft lens is more comfortable because it conforms to the shape of the underlying cornea, but then it may not adequately correct any corneal astigmatism.

The most recent new soft contact lens — silicone–hydrogel — has such high oxygen permeability that up to 30 days of continuous (day and night) wear is advocated. Ophthalmologists always view such claims with scepticism because of the risks of low oxygen flow, drying out of the lens, accumulation of protein debris, and infection. If any contact lens is left in place overnight the further barrier to free oxygen exchange between the eye and the atmosphere imposed by the closed lids may be crucial. Daily wear, disposable soft lenses avoid these difficulties, and because each lens is from a sterile pack the armamentarium of small bottles of sterilizing fluids for reusable, hard lenses is banished.

Contact lens fitting has always been an art, necessitating careful consideration of many factors which allow accurate alignment of the optical centres of contact lens and cornea, with the proper thickness of tear film beneath the lens so that it may move slightly in relation to the globe but re-centres itself naturally. Any long-term effect that a contact lens may have on the underlying cornea shape, and thus its refractive power, must be monitored weekly by the patient checking that his spectacles continue to give optimal vision when worn.

Contact lenses can be used most advantageously to correct myopia, but can also be used for hypermetropia and corneal astigmatism. Any astigmatism not corrected by the contact lens (*residual astigmatism*) is due partly to the patient's own lens within the eye and partly to features of the contact lens itself. Making specially shaped contact lenses to reduce their rotation on the eye can help. Bifocal contact lenses to correct distance and reading vision, so that the obvious bifocal glasses with their ageing implications could be avoided, have not proved successful. Reading glasses for presbyopia still have to be worn over the contact lenses. Another way to overcome this problem is to fit a contact lens for distance viewing to one eye and one focused for reading to the other. There are significant implications for good quality fusion of the images from each eye, in that 3-dimensional vision and depth perception are compromised. This can be important when driving, and spectacles for optimal distance vision should be worn over such contact lenses under these circumstances.

Cosmetic contact lenses fulfil a variety of uses, ranging from different coloured lenses as matching accessories in the fashion industry to films where an opaque scleral lens could be used to simulate a blind or grossly damaged eye.

The new, soft disposable contact lenses can now be used for occasional or social wear, since the long period of adaptation and building up of wearing time with hard contact lenses is no longer necessary.

There are a number of clinical indications for contact lenses, and the irregularly-shaped 'conical cornea' is the principal one. Specially made lenses when held temporarily in contact with the eye assist the opthalmologist to obtain detailed, magnified views of otherwise inaccessible areas of the eye, for example in glaucoma patients. The original scleral contact lenses still have a role in treating severely damaged eyes, now that they are made of a highly permeable polymer allowing good gas exchange but giving essential protection.   PETER FELLS

See also EYES; REFRACTIVE ERRORS; SQUINT; VISION.

Contraception
Many social practices reduce the birth rate — delaying marriage, imposing taboos on the frequency of marital intercourse, and prolonged breastfeeding, for example. Contraception, however, is usually taken to mean deliberate resort to practices to prevent sexual intercourse resulting in the birth of a child, or, more strictly speaking, to preclude conception. Methods can be divided into 'natural' — those not requiring any apparatus — and 'artificial' means. The latter can be subdivided, though not entirely, into barrier and chemical methods locally applied to the genitals; intrauterine; surgical; and the more recent hormonal contraceptives. Magical prescriptions, of dubious efficacy, for the prevention of pregnancy have also proliferated.

Refraining from sexual intercourse may have been an underestimated element in attempts to restrict family size. A modification is indulgence only when the woman is believed to be infertile: however, the relationship between menstruation and ovulation was not reliably established until 1929, and many previous calculations of a 'safe period' were seriously in error — though, due to variation in the cycles of individual women, even an inaccurate idea may have been occasionally effective in delaying if not preventing conception. The independent discoveries of the Japanese K. Ogino and Austrian Hermann Knaus enabled more effective calculations, but nonetheless the 'rhythm method' is widely known as 'Vatican roulette' (as the only method, apart from abstention, approved by the Catholic Church) because of its unreliability. Recently developed devices, however, now enable extremely precise pinpointing of the actual period of fertility through hormonal analysis of the female urine.

Another possibility occurring to the ingenious very early in human history was the practice of coitus interruptus, whereby the man withdraws and ejaculates outside the vagina (cf. Onan — Genesis 38:9). To think of this method means that a connection must be made between emission of semen and conception. Another method requiring no appliances is anal intercourse.

Barrier methods
Barrier methods have a long history. Egyptian papyri describe pessaries and vaginal douches, which could have been effective. The pessaries both formed a barrier, and consisted of substances either spermicidal, or likely to slow SPERM motility, while the douches could have altered the chemical balance of the vagina, rendering conception less likely. Many other societies are recorded as having had similar devices capable of lowering the probability of conception.

The CONDOM, or male sheath, was quite a late development. It became more widely used following the discovery of the vulcanisation of rubber in the 1840s, which also led to the development of various forms of occlusive cap for female use. These required, to be most effective, careful fitting — indeed, the first were custom-made for each individual. The most commonly used type is the 'Dutch cap' or diaphragm, invented by the German physician Wilhelm Mensinga of Flensburg in the 1870s, a domed rubber cap with a metallic spring in the rim, which comes in a range of sizes and is easier to fit than similar devices. Used conscientiously, with spermicide, and left in for several hours following intercourse, it has a success rate of around 95% in preventing pregnancy. The smaller cap, covering only the cervix, has had its advocates. Rubber itself tends to destroy sperm. Using sponges for birth control dates back probably to the eighteenth century, a method particularly efficacious if the sponge is soaked in some spermicidal or sperm-weakening substance, such as vinegar, olive oil, or even soapy water; modern sponges, for a single use only, are permeated with spermicide. The recently-promoted female condom, covering the entire interior surface of the vagina, has a longer history than often realised, and is primarily a protective against sexually transmitted disease.

Spermicides

The nineteenth century also saw the commercial development of chemical contraceptives, usually in the form of pessaries for insertion into the vagina. In theory these contained a spermicidal substance (though some worked because the greasy agents hindered the sperm), but in the unregulated industry of contraceptive manufacture, the unreliability of these products led to the belief (as with condoms) that the law required one 'dud' in every box. In Britain the issue of an 'Approved List' of effective products by the National Birth Control Association (later the Family Planning Association) led to improvement in standards, though spermicidal activity as measured in laboratory circumstances and in practice can still differ widely. Chemical contraceptives currently come as creams and jellies (specifically for use with a barrier method), pessaries, and foam and are recommended to be employed in conjunction with a barrier method.

IUD

As far as can be ascertained, the INTRAUTERINE DEVICE in its modern form dates back to the experiments of Gräfenburg and other German gynaecologists before World War I, although the British obstetrician C. H. F. Routh claimed in the 1870s that women were using uterine pessaries intended for gynaecological conditions for contraceptive purposes. Early IUDs were made of gold or silver; modern ones are made of plastic or copper. They work, it is believed, by irritating the uterus so that implantation of the fertilised ovum does not take place. The method has fallen into some disfavour following the highly damaging effects of the Dalkon Shield, which became apparent during the 1970s.

Sterilization

STERILIZATION may be regarded as a contraceptive method, but unlike other methods it cannot be reversed, or not with any substantial probability of success. In women ligating the Fallopian tubes was originally a relatively major abdominal operation, carried out under general anaesthesia. More recently, sterilizations have been performed using a laparoscope, inserted through a small incision, to locate the tubes so that they can be cauterised; this can be done as an outpatient operation. VASECTOMY is a much less serious operation.

The Pill

The greatest advance in contraceptive technology in the twentieth century was the female contraceptive pill. Ever since the discovery of the SEX HORMONES and STEROIDS there were hopes of a contraceptive which could be taken orally or injected. The earliest combination birth control pill, developed in the late 1950s, contained both oestrogen and progestin, and was taken for 21 days followed by a 5-day break during which menstruation occurred. It caused the suppression of ovulation and the thickening of the cervical mucus, hindering sperm from entering the uterus. The sequential pill (1965) consisted of oestrogen-only pills taken for the first 16 days of the cycle and combination oestrogen-progestin pills for the final five days, inhibiting ovulation but having no effect on the cervical mucus. The minipill, conversely, contains only progestin, is taken without breaks, and works by the constant production of thick cervical mucus which blocks the entry of the sperm. There are a number of other variations, and hormonal contraceptives are also given as implants or injections (e.g. Depo-Provera) with long-term efficacy. Related developments are the 'morning after' pill, a postcoital contraceptive, and the so-far unfulfilled hope of a 'male pill'.

The Pill came into general use in the 1960s. It is an extremely reliable contraceptive method (97–99%) and has the important qualities of being totally detached from the genital organs, not requiring any dexterity to fit, and being unintrusive on the sexual act. This rendered it popular with both doctors and the general public. Side-effects, ranging from mild to extremely serious, and the implications for the dissemination of sexually transmitted disease of a reliable non-barrier method of contraception, have dimmed the initial glowing enthusiasm it generated, but it is still one of the most widely used methods of birth control.

Family limitation and society

Methods of birth control have been known from distant antiquity, but it is less easy to establish to what extent they may have been used. As Angus McLaren pointed out in *A History of Contraception* (1992), the desire of human couples to exercise control over their reproductive capacities may in some epochs veer towards the promotion of conception rather than its prevention. Many factors bear upon the possibility of even imagining that births might be restricted, and upon the putting of such a possibility into efficacious practice. Economic, social, and cultural factors led to increasing debate on the subject during the nineteenth century, particularly associated with the name of the political economist T. R. Malthus and his calculation that the population would always tend to outrun the means of subsistence — though he did not recommend artificial interference with this state of affairs. French peasants were apparently already

limiting their families through coitus interruptus during the eighteenth century, because of their reluctance to let family holdings be divided between several heirs. The cause-and-effect relationship between the decline in infant mortality and the rise of family limitation is not clear: it is often claimed that the increased chances of child survival encouraged parents to reduce family size, but it can also be argued that infants born at wider intervals into smaller families have a better chance of survival through access to more maternal attention, and division of family resources between fewer family members.

In spite of the number of birth control methods available, they are still far from universally employed, due to simple lack of access; economic factors, either local factors encouraging large families, or the inability to afford the means; and in large areas of the world, because of religious objections.

LESLEY A. HALL

Convulsions are movements that result from abnormally synchronous and repetitive activity (*epileptiform activity*) in the brain. Epileptiform activity, as detected by electrical measurements (*electroencephalography* or EEG), refers to persistent abnormal firing patterns in large groups of nerve cells, especially synchronised bursts of nerve impulses. To produce a convulsion such abnormal activity needs to invade regions of the brain that control body muscles. This sequence of events is called a seizure. Prolonged epileptiform activity, whether or not it triggers convulsions, is known as an electrographic seizure. Epileptiform activity leading to convulsions can occur in healthy brains if they are stimulated in particular ways, which implies that it can represent abnormal activity in normal brain circuits.

The factors that can trigger convulsions in people or laboratory animals with apparently normal brains include: administration of convulsant drugs or toxins (e.g. cocaine, certain antibiotics — especially when kidney function is compromised); electrical stimulation (e.g. electroconvulsive shock); the abrupt withdrawal of certain drugs (notably alcohol or barbiturates) after prolonged use; overheating in infants ('febrile' convulsions); and excessive fluid intake (water intoxication).

The term 'convulsion' is also used to describe the muscular spasms (*tetany*) seen when calcium levels in the blood are low (*hypocalcaemia*). This condition can be caused in a variety of ways, including low calcium in the diet, vitamin D deficiency, overbreathing, and prolonged vomiting.

The type of convulsion that results from epileptiform activity depends on the regions of the brain invaded by the seizure and on the pattern of the seizure discharge. The details are difficult to unravel because large parts of the brain can be active simultaneously.

Epilepsy

The most common forms of convulsions are those associated with EPILEPSY (a disorder characterised by recurrent spontaneous seizures). However, just as convulsions do not always indicate epilepsy, neither does epilepsy always cause convulsions. Epilepsy is not normally diagnosed until the patient has experienced more than one seizure without an obvious trigger of the kind listed above. Seizures may result in convulsions (or *motor fits*), but they also can occur without overt motor activity.

It is more accurate to talk of epilepsies, rather than epilepsy, since there is a diverse group of clinical conditions that share the abrupt interruption of brain function, usually with intense, synchronous activity. The classification of these conditions is revised from time to time by the International League Against Epilepsy Commission on Classification. The classification distinguishes between focal epilepsies (those where a site of onset in the brain can be localised, at least to one hemisphere), and primary generalised epilepsies (where a definite site of onset cannot be localised). Focal epilepsies can spread widely and become secondarily generalised. The location of the focus in the brain determines the clinical symptoms.

The primary generalised epilepsies include *tonic clonic seizures*, previously known as *grand mal*, with dramatic convulsions that would be recognised as epilepsy by most lay people. Primary generalised epilepsies also include 'absence seizures', which do not lead to obvious convulsions: these were previously known as *petit mal* and can be mistaken for daydreaming. Other epilepsies in this group are characterised by collapse of posture ('atonic' epilepsy). Focal epilepsies originating in the forebrain area called the *hippocampus*, and associated regions, produce complex, partial convulsions, together with disturbances of consciousness, and often with co-ordinated, if inappropriate, vocalisations.

Mechanisms of epileptiform activity

Animal models of epilepsy have provided detailed theories of how neuronal activity can be organised into epileptic seizure discharges. In the process they have also taught us a great deal about the normal operation of *neuronal networks* in the hippocampus, cerebral cortex, and thalamus.

Experiments, mainly on brain slices maintained *in vitro*, combined with realistic computer simulations, have shown that focal epileptic discharges generally depend on the mutual excitation of pyramidal nerve cells, the main excitatory neurons of the brain, through synapses in which glutamate is the neurotransmitter. The necessary conditions are that there are strong, wide-ranging connections between pyramidal cells, and that the total population of neurons is large. This kind of circuitry, capable of generating epileptic discharges, is present in many cortical areas, but is normally held in check by a variety of mechanisms, including the action of neurons that inhibit the pyramidal cells, using gamma-amino butyric acid (GABA) as their neurotransmitter. When the synapses of these inhibitory neurons are blocked by drugs (such as of picrotoxin or penicillin), the excitatory network can sustain a chain reaction leading to an epileptiform discharge.

This kind of experimental approach has greatly improved our understanding of normal brain function. It has also provided a very convincing account of how brief epileptic discharges, lasting a few tenths of a second, can be induced in experimental animals. These discharges seem to correspond to the abnormal brain activity known as *interictal spikes* that is seen in the EEG between full focal seizures in humans ('interictal' means 'between seizures').

It is more difficult to understand the transition between these 'spikes' and full seizures lasting between tens of seconds and minutes. Indeed, the underlying causes of most clinical epilepsies, both in man and in domestic animals, remain uncertain. In some cases the seizures clearly result from a tumour pressing on the surrounding brain tissue. Head injury can also lead to epilepsy. There can be an inherited disposition to epilepsy, although in many cases, genetics is just one of many risk factors. Focal seizures are often associated with structural abnormalities of the cortex, caused by failures of migration of nerve cells during development or sometimes by adverse conditions around the time of birth.

Anticonvulsant drugs

These work in a variety of ways. Many of them prevent neurons firing rapidly (e.g. carbemazepine, lamotrigine). Others enhance the function of inhibitory synapses (e.g. barbiturates, benzodiazepam, vigabatrin). Some have multiple actions.

JOHN G. R. JEFFERYS
ROGER D. TRAUB

Further reading

Traub, R. D. and Jefferys, J. G. R. (1996). Epilepsy *in vitro*: electrophysiology and computer modeling. In *Epilepsy: a comprehensive textbook*, (ed J. Engel Jr. and T. A. Pedley). Raven Press, New York.

Coronary artery bypass

is a surgical procedure for treating patients with obstructions in their *coronary arteries*. The procedure overcomes the effects of the obstructions, while not directly influencing their underlying causes. The operation was first used in substantial numbers in the late 1960s; it has now become one of the most commonly undertaken surgical operations.

The muscular pumping chambers of the HEART require a copious blood supply, which is conducted by the left and right coronary arteries and their branches. These lie on or near the surface of the heart, giving rise to small vessels which penetrate into the muscle to supply the nutrient capillary networks surrounding individual heart muscle cells.

In many populations, particularly where cigarette SMOKING, diets rich in saturated FATS, low EXERCISE activity, DIABETES, and high BLOOD PRESSURE are prevalent, the coronary arteries are frequently affected by the process known as *atherosclerosis*. This is a degenerative disease of arteries characterised by development of fatty accumulations within the inner portion of the arterial wall, separated from the blood by a fibrous layer or plaque. These lesions predominantly affect the coronary arteries on the surface of the heart, near their origins from the aorta, sparing arteries further downstream (thus fortuitously making bypass surgery feasible).

Atherosclerotic lesions may gradually expand, narrowing the coronary artery, over many years, ultimately restricting blood flow to the heart muscle. This prevents an increase in blood supply to the heart muscle when it is most needed (e.g. during exercise or emotion), and results in an unpleasant, constricting, central chest pain known as *angina*.

Another possibility is rupture of the fibrous plaque with release of the fatty material and clotting of the blood within the coronary artery, abruptly interrupting the blood supply to a portion of the HEART MUSCLE. This is manifested clinically as a heart attack, which may be fatal, may leave part of the heart muscle permanently scarred, or may be followed by near-complete recovery, particularly if the clot breaks up rapidly (spontaneously or in response to *thrombolytic drugs*).

The coronary arteries, and any obstructions, can be demonstrated by the procedure of *coronary angiography*. The passage of a radio-opaque fluid is recorded by cine-radiography, following its injection into the coronary arteries via long catheters introduced through a conveniently placed peripheral artery (e.g. the femoral artery in the groin).

Coronary artery bypass is usually used for treating angina, particularly in those found to have obstructions in multiple coronary arteries, or obstructions at strategic sites. Bypass surgery may be appropriate even when angina is not present, if coronary angiographic study after a 'coronary event' (usually a heart attack) shows severe coronary disease. Coronary artery bypass is only one of the possible treatment options, which include drug therapy and cardiological interventions such as *angioplasty* (inflation of a small balloon at the site of obstruction) and *stenting* (placing a tubular mesh at the expanded site to help keep it open). Surgery is usually reserved for patients with more extensively diseased coronary arteries where angioplasty may be less successful or impractical.

In principle, the operation consists of placing a conduit to conduct blood to the coronary artery beyond the obstruction. The heart is exposed by dividing the sternal bone vertically, and a heart–lung machine is used to maintain the general body circulation while the heart is immobilised to allow work on the coronary arteries. The superficial veins of the legs provide a good source of bypass conduit. The *internal mammary artery*, which lies to the side of the sternum, can be used as a particularly useful conduit for bypassing the anterior descending coronary artery branch. Other arteries, such as the radial artery from the forearm, may also be used as conduits. The coronary artery is opened for a few millimetres at a suitable site beyond the obstruction and the end of the conduit is sewn to the opened artery. The other end of the conduit is sewn to an opening made in the aorta a few centimetres downstream from the natural openings of the coronary arteries, except in the case of the internal mammary artery, when its origin is left undisturbed. Usually several conduits are required, commonly three or four arteries being bypassed. The coronary arteries are typically 1–3 mm in diameter, and magnification is used to enhance surgical precision. If there is extensive coronary obstruction it may be difficult to find a suitable site for insertion of a bypass conduit. In this case it is often possible to open into the diseased artery and extract the atheromatous occlusion from a sufficiently long segment to allow a bypass graft to be inserted (the procedure known as *endarterectomy*).

There is a mortality rate for this operation, usually about 1–3%, and STROKE, bleeding, impaired cardiac function, and chest infections are among the early complications which may occur, depending on age and physical condition.

Bypass of all severe obstructions restores normal blood supply to the heart muscle on exercise. Angina is abolished and normal life can usually be resumed. Over subsequent years there is a gradual return of angina, such that up to 50% of patients have some recurrent symptoms by 10 years after surgery, some even requiring further surgery. Recurrent angina is due either to progression of disease in the coronary arteries to affect new areas, or blocking of conduits (particularly vein conduits) by a process similar to atherosclerosis.

Coronary artery bypass can ameliorate the consequences of subsequent plaque rupture in a bypassed artery. This has been shown to improve the survival prospects of those patients who have multiple major coronary branch obstructions, particularly when there is damage to the heart muscle from previous heart attack.

In attempts to simplify the operation, efforts have been made to undertake coronary bypass without using the heart–lung machine, while the heart is beating, and *video-assisted minimal access* techniques are being developed. These methods are presently feasible only in a small proportion of patients, usually with limited disease. DAVID WEATHERALL

Further reading

Millner, R. and Treasure, T. (1995). *Explaining cardiac surgery: patient assessment and care.* BMJ Publishing Group, London.

Corpse — the body after the moment of death, but prior to the completion of decomposition; also known (particularly in the US) by the Latin term *cadaver*.

In most circumstances, this residue of humanity is regarded as due for disposal. Concern for the future life of the soul or spirit is often reflected in the treatment of the corpse. In all cultures, the corpse is an object of great potency, the focus for a powerful mixture of solicitude and fear: solicitude for the humanity and personality of the dead, embodied in the transformed body of the dead person; horror of death, dread of

bereavement, or terror of the likelihood of further deaths or of haunting.

These lay perceptions have medical parallels. The poet Shelley's corpse was burnt on the beach near Viareggio when it was washed up there after his drowning in 1822, as the Tuscan authorities of the day regarded drowned bodies as a health hazard. In nineteenth-century Britain, corpses were classified as 'nuisances' to public health, and sanitary inspectors were authorized to remove them from the homes of the poor for fear that they might serve as foci for epidemics of scarlet fever, cholera, or smallpox.

Medical solicitude for the corpse derives from its potential value for postmortem diagnosis, DISSECTION, specimen-taking, and TRANSPLANTATION, and depends crucially on its physical condition. Freshness is a key attribute: significant findings at AUTOPSY and the success of transplanted organs and tissues depend upon it, and there is little point in dissecting a body whose structures have badly decomposed prior to preservation, except for forensic or anthropological purposes. Although anatomical dissection may be carried out ultimately on body parts, effective injection and saturation of tissues with preservative requires that corpses be undamaged at the outset. Wholeness is less crucial to transplantation, as organs or tissues from even damaged corpses can be saved for transplant, if saved quickly. For both dissection and transplantation, the cause of death must be known and the corpse ascertainably free from certain transmissible diseases.

Patient organizations such as the Parkinson's Disease Society and the Alzheimer's Disease Society run specialized brain banks, to which sufferers bequeath their remains for research.

The traditional importance of the corpse to medicine is currently being eroded by technological advances. New imaging technologies enable students to explore bodily structures without dissecting, while pathological studies can often be made on tissue located and biopsied in the living patient.

In transplantation, the advantages of using organs from living bodies and the shortage of human 'beating-heart donors' are causing surgeons to seek material from animals. The adequacy, safety, and ethical acceptability of this alternative are as yet uncertain. It seems likely that in time the human corpse will undergo a further process of revaluation. RUTH RICHARDSON

See also ANATOMY; AUTOPSY; BIOPSY; BODY SNATCHERS; BRAIN DEATH; DEATH; DISSECTION; FUNERAL PRACTICES; TRANSPLANTATION.

Corset A close-fitting garment, tightened by laces and reinforced with stays to shape the body from the hips to the breasts. Laced outer garments to shape the body existed from antiquity, but laced undergarments date from the end of the sixteenth century. A 'pair of bodies' was tied at the sides and stiffened at first by paste on linen or cardboard, and later by a removable busk — a flat, tapered strip of wood, ivory, horn, or whale-

bone — inserted down the centre front to keep the body straight. Later, the ideal of a smooth, cylindrical torso, seen in Queen Elizabeth I (1533–1603), was achieved by sewing strips of rigid materials, such horn, ivory, silver, or steel, into the bodies, which became known as stays. Bodies were originally waist-length, but the stays gradually lengthened over the hips, split into tabs and met in a point below the waist. The favourite shaping material of stays was whalebone (*baleen*), cut into thin strips and sewn in a fan pattern to make the torso appear rounder. Though earlier stays did not shape the breasts, by the mid eighteenth century whalebone strips curved around the bosom. Stays dictated very straight posture and necessitated stylized dance movements. As body carriage was essential to good deportment, both girls and boys were dressed in stays at an early age.

The nineteenth-century corset separated the breasts and extended over the hips by the addition of gussets. Some closed in front with metal clips, some laced in back, and some laced in front. Metal eyelets, invented in 1828, allowed for very tight lacing. By the end of the century corsets produced the sinuous body shape of the Gibson girl, with a protruding bust and derrière, and small waist. Despite reports of 18-inch waists, historians have found no Victorian garment with less than a $20\frac{1}{2}$ inch waist.

Tight-lacing generated criticism almost from its inception. Clerics fulminated against the vanity of the fashion as well its sexual nature. Some women viewed corseting as a form of self discipline (an attitude favoured by the Puritans) and the essayist Montaigne recognized how heroically women bore pain to be attractive. Physicians and social critics argued that the corset caused a number of health problems, including spinal deviations, breast cancer, consumption, digestive abnormalities, miscarriages and other obstetrical problems, mental and moral impairment, and even death. During the second half of the nineteenth century, Punch and other humourists satirized the corset.

Tight-lacing has not been limited to women. King Henri III (1551–89) wore stays to accentuate his slim figure. At the end of the eighteenth century, dandies began to wear stays, and the fashion became popular around 1815 with military officers and persisted until the end of the century. Though corsets left the fashion mainstream in the early twentieth century, tight-lacing has been and continues to be part of fetish-dressing for both men and women. Some male cross-dressers wear corsets, and the singer Madonna has appeared on stage in corsets with projectile breast cones.

KRISTEN L. ZACHARIAS

See also CLOTHES; FASHION.

Cosmetic surgery The close of the twentieth century marked the centenary of modern surgical intervention to alter the image of the body. A list of the most common operations which were developed over the past century and are understood as 'cosmetic' procedures today are shown in the table.

Cosmetic operations

Operations on the face

Forehead lift: tightens the forehead and raises the brow

Facelift (rhytidectomy): tightens the jowls and neck

Eyelid tightening (blepharoplasty): tightens the eyelids

Rhinoplasty (nose job): changes the appearance of the nose

Otoplasty (ear pinback): brings the ears closer to the head

Facial implants (chin, cheek): makes the cheek or chin more prominent

Hair transplantation: treats male pattern baldness

Scar revision: improves the appearance of scars

Skin resurfacing (laser, peel, dermabrasion): smoothes the skin

Operations on the body

Breast enlargement: enhances the size of the breast

Breast tightening (mastopexy): tightens the skin of the breast

Breast reduction: reduces the size of the breast

Breast reconstruction: rebuilds the breast after cancer

Abdominoplasty (tummy tuck): tightens skin and removes extra fat

Mini-abdominoplasty: removes the lower abdominal pouching

Liposuction: removes extra fat

Arm lift: tightens the skin of the upper arm

Gynecomastia resection (large breasts in men): reduces breast size

It is, of course, evident that virtually all procedures which could be conceptualized as cosmetic or aesthetic can also have a reconstructive dimension. Breast reconstruction, which used the same type of implant as breast augmentation, was the focus of a major debate within both medical and feminist circles in the US in the 1990s, as to whether it was reconstructive or aesthetic surgery. During the closing decades of the twentieth century these procedures, and also aesthetic orthodontics, came to be a common undertaking. Aesthetic surgery became a focus of interest — being patient-initiated, and non-reimbursable by private or state third-party payers.

While aesthetic surgery is related in many ways to other physical interventions, from hairweaving to TATTOOING and body piercing, it is performed in the quite different context of the institution of medicine. The surgical interventions are understood by doctors and patients alike as aesthetic rather than reconstructive. Even though the term 'aesthetic surgery' was acknowledged only recently, the practice of surgical interventions devoted to making people 'beautiful' rather than to any direct reconstruction of physical anomalies is relatively recent. There is a necessary if rather arbitrary distinc-tion between reconstructive (plastic) surgery and aesthetic (cosmetic) surgery — between not having a nose and having a nose that you dislike. The first represents a functional fault. There is something wrong with the body as well as an unfortunate appearance — a hare lip, a missing jaw, a lost ear — and your desire is to repair the function of the body. Part of that function is, of course, an aesthetic one. Cosmetic surgery, which is part of, and grew from, reconstructive surgery, stresses the latter, subordinate, but essential aspect of the reconstruction. We imagine our bodies as intact and read our intactness as 'beauty'. You may have a functional nose, a jaw, a breast, but it does not represent your self-image of the beautiful nose, jaw, or breast. It inhales, chews, or lactates, but it is not appropriate. The distinction between reconstructive and aesthetic surgery is an arbitrary one. Certain interventions have been labelled as inherently different — such as breast reconstruction vs. breast augmentation, even though the procedures are similar. The former are understood as a means of restoring physical completeness to the body image and therefore of restoring the psyche to a 'happy' state; the latter can be dismissed as 'vogue fashions' (R. V. S. Thompson, Kay-Kilner Prize Essay, 1994). Feminists in the 1990s, such as the American poet Audre Lorde, who underwent a radical mastectomy, argued against breast reconstruction as a refusal to acknowledge the realities of the woman's body. In the Middle Ages, Guy de Chauliac, perhaps the most important surgeon of his time, defined the role of surgery as being threefold: *solvit continuum* (separating the fused), *jungit separatum* (connecting the divided), and *exstirpat superfluum* (removing the extraneous). There is no discussion in his or other texts of that period about the creation of new body parts or their augmentation or reconstruction, although it is evident that virtually all primarily reconstructive surgical procedures also had an aesthetic dimension, even then. As early as the Edwin Smith Surgical Papyrus (3000 BCE), surgeons were concerned about the cosmetic results of their interventions. The Egyptians were careful to suture the edges of facial wounds. Even fractures of the nose-bones were dealt with by forcing them into normal positions by means of 'two plugs of linen, saturated with grease' inserted into the nostrils. The Roman physician Aulus Cornelius Celsus stressed the 'beautiful' suture. This approach can be followed through to the late nineteenth and early twentieth century, with plastic surgeons such as Erich Lexer stressing the cosmetic ends of an operation as 'an always more appreciated requirement of modern surgery'. Such a stress on the neatness and beauty of the closure was part of the image of the return to function following the operation, for the beautiful was a sign of the healthy — but of the healthy body, not the healthy mind.

Yet even as we understand aesthetic surgery as a means of altering our body's 'image' it becomes a means not only of changing our bodies but of shaping our psyches. Aesthetic surgery remains rooted in a presumed relationship between the body and the mind. Sculpting the body comes to be a form of reshaping the psyche.

The central assumption of aesthetic surgery is that if you understand your body as 'bad' you are bound to be 'unhappy'. And in our day and age, being unhappy seems to be identified with being sick. And if you are sick, you should be cured! The idea that you can cure the soul by altering the form of the body became commonplace in the twentieth century. It is the other side of the coin from the argument that to cure specific bodily symptoms you need to 'heal' the psyche.

Elaine Scarry has remarked in her classic work *The Body In Pain* (1985),

> . . . at particular moments when there is within a society a crisis of belief — that is, when some central idea or ideology of cultural construct has ceased to elicit a population's belief either because it is manifestly fictitious or because it has for some reason been divested of ordinary forms of transubstantiation — the sheer material factualness of the human body will be borrowed to lend that cultural construct the aura of "realness" and "certainty".

It is this realness and certainty ascribed to an imagined as well as the real body which is operated upon by the aesthetic surgeon.

During a period of revolutionary change in science, from the mid nineteenth to the early twentieth centuries, two major developments took place which enabled surgeons to introduce aesthetic changes, and patients to overcome their anxiety and undertake such procedures. Antisepsis and ANAESTHESIA became central to the practice of surgery, following the discovery of

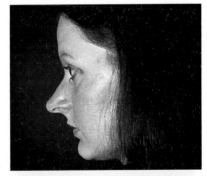

(a)

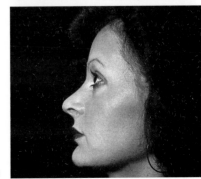

(b)

Nose-reducing surgery, (a) before and (b) after. Alex Bartel/Science Photo Library.

ether anaesthesia in 1846 and the development by the 1880s of local anaesthesia. The movement toward antisepsis paralleled the development of anaesthesia: the model for antisepsis provided by Joseph Lister in 1867 became generally accepted by the end of the century. Aesthetic surgery became a context in which the ideology of the medical alteration of the body (and its state) was accepted by both the patient and the physician. All of these concerns can be understood as concerns of 'HYGIENE' in the broadest nineteenth-century sense, a hygiene of the state of both the body and the psyche. This set the stage for the development of the procedures used today. Take the case of Jacques Joseph, a young German-Jewish surgeon practising in *fin-de-siècle* Berlin. In 1896 Joseph undertook a corrective procedure on a child with protruding ears (*otoplasty*), which, although successful, caused Joseph to be dismissed from the staff of the orthopaedic clinic at the Berlin Charité. One simply did not undertake surgical procedures for vanity's sake, he was told upon his dismissal. The child was not suffering from any physical ailment which could be cured through surgery. Yet, according to the child's mother, he had suffered from humiliation in school because of his protruding ears. It was the unhappiness of the child that Joseph was correcting. The significance of protruding ears was clear to Jacques Joseph and his contemporaries at that time. There is an old trope in European culture about the Jew's ears that can be found throughout the anti-Semitic literature of the *fin de siècle*, and it is also a major sub-theme of one of the great works of world literature, Heinrich Mann's *Man of Straw* (1918). In that novel, Mann's self-serving convert, Jadassohn (Judas's son?) 'looked so Jewish' because of his 'huge, red, prominent ears' which he eventually went to Paris to have cosmetically reduced; his ears signified his poor character. Jacques Joseph went on to pioneer the intranasal procedure for the reduction of the size of the nose and came to be known among the Jewish community in Berlin as 'Nose-Joseph'.

The social and psychological significance of the introduction of aesthetic surgery is relevant to other external markers of difference, from ageing (*face lifts*), to sexuality (*transsexual surgery*), to notions of beauty of face (*orthodontics*) and of body (*liposuction*). The norms of the acceptable change with time, but the desire to become invisible, to become a member of a class or group to which one does not naturally belong, maintains itself over the entire history of aesthetic surgery.

SANDER L. GILMAN

Further reading

Gilman, S. L. (2000) *Making the body beautiful: a cultural history of aesthetic surgery.* Princeton University Press, Princeton.

Maltz, M. (1946). *Evolution of plastic surgery.* Froben Press, New York.

Wallace, A. F. (1982). *The progress of plastic surgery: an introductory history.* Willem A. Meeuws, Oxford.

Cot death Sudden unexpected death, with no cause identified after post-mortem examination, accounts for between one-third and one-half of deaths occurring in babies between the ages of 1 month and 1 year in developed countries.

In 1855, Thomas Wakely, the founder editor of the *Lancet*, wrote about 'Infants found dead in bed'. At that time infanticide was common and accounted for over 80% of all coroner's reports of murder in England and Wales. Disraeli said that infanticide was 'hardly less prevalent in England than on the banks of the Ganges'. Deaths from unintended smothering were also common, perhaps because of overcrowding in bed and the prevalence of drunkenness.

There was a period during the first half of the twentieth century when cot deaths were mistakenly attributed to the enlargement of the thymus gland (part of the IMMUNE SYSTEM, found in the upper chest and lower neck). Pathologists, inexperienced in childhood post-mortems, would attribute the death of these infants to a disease, which they called *status thymo-lymphaticus*. Surgical removal of the thymus as a prophylactic measure became quite fashionable. Thymus enlargement is now known to be normal in this age group, and the erroneous theory, like many postulated before and after this time, gradually fell into disrepute.

During the 1940s the concept of 'cot death' became more clearly defined, but it was not until 1969, at the second conference on causes of Sudden Deaths in Infants, that cot death was defined as 'any sudden death of an infant or young child, which is unexpected by history and for which a thorough post-mortem examination fails to demonstrate an adequate cause of death'. Most forensic post-mortems in the UK are now performed by experienced paediatric pathologists and more accurate records of the prevalence of what is now know as *Sudden Infant Death Syndrome* (SIDS) have been available in the UK during the past 25 years. The rate of cot deaths during this time has reduced from about 2.3 to 1.3 per thousand live births — that is about 10 deaths per week. This improvement may have been due to changes in behaviour in response to four identified risk factors for babies: (i) being placed face down to sleep; (ii) having a mother who smokes cigarettes; (iii) not being breastfed; and (iv) sharing the bed with parents.

Because of remaining uncertainty as to the cause of SIDS, many other theories have been put forward. *Hyperthermia* (over-heating), due to an excessively heated bedroom or too many bed coverings, may be involved. *Unidentified infections* remain an unproven cause, and they might also contribute to hyperthermia. Another suggested cause is exposure to *noxious chemicals*. For a time there was a theory that fungi attacked the coverings of cot mattresses, releasing trace amounts of toxins such as arsenic and antimony, but this idea has now been discredited. It is likely that, as further information is acquired, a number of different contributory factors will be identified.

The sudden loss of an apparently healthy baby causes enormous anguish in parents and results in inevitable feelings of guilt and fear about the outcome of future pregnancies. Groups of affected families have established support organizations and have raised funds to sponsor research.

ANN DALLY
FORRESTER COCKBURN

Cough is an onomatopoeic word in most languages (e.g. *kuchen, tosse, tossa, toux*). It has been called the 'watchdog of the lungs'. When it barks it warns you that there may be an intruder (inhalation of an irritant), there may be something wrong in the house (lung disease), or perhaps the dog is asking for attention (communication). Cough always requires interpretation.

A cough is a deep inspiration, followed by a powerful expiratory effort while the LARYNX (voicebox) is reflexly closed by bringing together the vocal cords; then the larynx suddenly opens, allowing a rapid flow of air from the lungs which will repel the intruder or expel the material in the airways that needs to be coughed up. Cough is the most violent of respiratory acts. Put your hands on your abdomen and cough and you will see. Expiratory pressures in the chest may be three times that of blood pressure (and occasionally coughing can break blood vessels), and the airflow velocity in the larynx may approach supersonic levels. During coughing the airways in the chest are squeezed, and the expiratory blast forces *mucus secretions* through these narrow passages out into the open air. The associated cough sound is part of the definition of cough. The sound varies, from a simple single or double pattern of 'dry' cough, due, for example, to laryngitis, to the bubbling, rumbling cough sound of disease with much mucus in the airways.

Cough is the commonest and sometimes the most distressing symptom of lung disease, far more so than breathlessness or pain, and can be caused by over 100 chest and lung diseases. Probably the most frequent cause of coughing is cigarette SMOKING, but this has never been assessed because smokers do not complain to the doctor; they would be told to stop smoking, which is not what they want to hear. Although only the first breaths of cigarette smoke cause cough, and the smoker rapidly becomes acclimatized, smoking causes mucus secretion in the bronchi, and this produces the typical early morning smokers' cough. Later, and unfortunately, the smoker may develop *chronic bronchitis*, characterised by chronic cough and PHLEGM production.

The commonest disease to cause cough is upper airway infection (due to influenza, sinusitis, etc.), but there are some bizarre causes, such as an earwig in the external ear (which is supplied by the same nerve as the lungs). Cough can be psychological, as Sigmund Freud recognized when some of his patients presented with 'hysterical cough', including the first historical case of psychoanalysis, Anna O. Unlike sneezing, hiccough, and yawn, cough can be voluntarily produced with its complete pattern, and we may use it as a form of communication. The speaker may cough (clear his throat) to attract the attention of his audience, and the audience may get its revenge by 'coughing him down'. Voluntary or not, coughing can 'drown the parson's saw' (Macbeth).

It seems common experience in concert halls and theatres that we cannot suppress a cough, although the cougher and his neighbours may disagree about this. However, cough due to upper airway infection can be suppressed for quite long (5–20 min) periods, so perhaps the old adage that 'love and cough cannot be hid' is wrong in both respects.   JOHN WIDDICOMBE

Cramp Muscle cramps are one of the most common clinical problems suffered by athletes in endurance events. A third to a half of marathon runners and two-thirds of triathletes have been reported to experience *exercise-associated muscle cramping* (EAMC) at some time in their lives. Other forms of cramp affecting healthy people include nocturnal foot and calf muscle cramps, those arising from certain occupations (such as hand cramps in pianists and typists) and those associated with PREGNANCY. Cramps can also occur in a variety of relatively rare medical conditions, congenital or acquired, including metabolic or neuromuscular disorders, POISONINGS, and drug effects. This article will focus principally on EAMC — a spasmodic, painful involuntary contraction of SKELETAL MUSCLE that occurs during or immediately after muscular EXERCISE — since it is the most studied of the common forms, and has recently become better (though still not completely) understood.

The interest in skeletal muscle cramping associated with exercise was first stimulated at the turn of the century by reports that it occurred during physical work in hot, humid environments, including steam ships and mines. In these early studies the proposed explanation was a disturbance of body fluid and salt balance. The early observations led to the 'serum electrolyte depletion' and 'dehydration' theories for the cause of the cramps. Such theories are consonant with the fact that widespread cramping is one of the symptoms of severe *hyponatraemia* (salt deficiency). Thus they are still accepted by some clinicians and applied in practice by many athletes who believe adequate salt and water intake to be important cramp-preventatives.

Recent evidence, however, challenges the salt-and-water view. More than one careful study has shown that most runners with acute EAMC are not salt-deficient, dehydrated, or overheated. Also, cramp among sports people can occur in cold conditions (such as cold water, for swimmers). Factors actually associated with EAMC have been identified using three research approaches: epidemiological investigations; studies on spinal reflex activity during muscle FATIGUE in animals; and recording of muscle electrical activity (electromyography, EMG) in human volunteers

during EAMC. The latter technique demonstrates intense electrical activity, at exceptional frequencies (up to 300 Hz), in both EAMC and occupationally cramped muscles, and indeed in the cramps associated with a number of medical conditions, though not quite all. Critical analysis of these factors has led to the development, by Scwellnus and colleagues, of a novel hypothesis for the cause of EAMC.

It seems that most forms of exercise-associated cramp result from an abnormally sustained activity of the nerve cells in the SPINAL CORD which control skeletal muscle, the *alpha* MOTOR NEURONS. Fatigue appears to be the central factor in EAMC. Fatigue enhances the input to the alpha motor neurons from the main receptors in the muscles (*muscle spindles*) and inhibits the input from the receptors in their tendons (*Golgi tendon organs*) that signal tension. As the spindle signals excite alpha motor neurons, while those from tendon organs are inhibitory, these fatigue effects can combine to promote uncontrolled activity in the relevant regions of the spinal cord. It is a common experience that cramp may be precipitated by contraction of the muscle from an already shortened position, and this of course is when the tension signal from its tendon is weakest.

In a recent epidemiological study of over 1300 marathon runners, risk factors for EAMC were identified. Cramps were more likely with older age, a longer history of running, a higher body mass index, shorter daily stretching time or irregular stretching habits, and if there was a family history of cramping.

In addition, runners themselves identified specific conditions that were associated with EAMC: high-intensity running (racing), long duration of running (most cramps occur after 30 km in a standard marathon), hill running, subjective muscle fatigue, and poor performance in the race.

The two most important observations from these data are that cramp is associated with running conditions that can lead to premature muscle fatigue, and that poor stretching habits appear to increase the risk.

The muscles most prone to cramping are those that span two joints (for example, the *gastrocnemius* spanning knee and ankle). These muscles are typically activated when shortened — as in swimming, when the gastrocnemius contracts while the toes are already pointed. In runners, the situation is less clear-cut, but activation is common when only one of the two joints is extended. As the foot strikes the ground, the toes are pointed — the ankle is extended by contraction of the gastrocnemius — whilst the knee is also extended. Then in the load-bearing phase of the stride the foot has flexed, which would stretch the gastrocnemius — but now the knee is bent. The gastrocnemius is then activated again in this relatively shortened position. Such contractions are presumed to produce significantly less tension in the tendons than contractions starting near full extension, resulting in less inhibiting effect on motor neuron activity of the sort described above.

In localized cramp, confined to one or 2 muscle groups, the typical scenario is as follows: there is distressing pain in the muscle that develops gradually over a few minutes during intense or prolonged exercise. The muscle is contracted and hard, and an observer can see *fasciculation* — small twitchings — over its surface. The onset of the cramp is usually preceded by muscle fatigue and more immediately by a feeling of twitching in the muscle ('cramp prone state'). This is followed by spasmodic spontaneous contractions and frank cramping if the activity is continued. Relief from the 'cramp prone state' occurs if the activity ceases or, temporarily, if the muscle is passively stretched. Once activity stops, there may be alternating periods of cramping and relief.

The athlete who has generalized severe cramping, extending to non-exercising muscle groups, or who is also confused or comatose, presents an emergency. This condition is not typical EAMC as a result of fatigued muscle, but a whole body, usually metabolic, disturbance requiring immediate hospitalization and full investigation.

The immediate treatment for acute EAMC occurring in a sports event, or for cramp experienced in bed, should consist of passive stretching of the affected muscle groups, holding the muscle in stretched position until return to normal muscle length does not lead to recurrence of cramp. General supportive treatment includes maintaining a comfortable temperature and providing fluids if required.

The key to the prevention of acute EAMC is to protect the muscle from developing premature fatigue during exercise. The following advice to athletes is recommended: be well conditioned for the activity; perform regular stretching exercises for the muscle groups that are prone to cramping; and have adequate nutritional intake (carbohydrate and fluid) to prevent premature muscle fatigue during exercise. However, athletes who continue to be prone to EAMC must face the need to perform their activity at a lower intensity or a shorter duration.   MARTIN SCHWELLNUS

Further reading

McGee, S. R. (1990). Muscle cramps. *Archives of Internal Medicine*, **150**, 511–8.

Maughan, R. J. (1986). Exercise-induced muscle cramp: a prospective biochemical study in marathon runners. *Journal of Sports Sciences*, **4**, 31–4.

Schwellnus M. P. (1999). Skeletal muscle cramps during exercise. *Physician and Sportsmedicine*, **27**(12), 109–15.

Schwellnus, M. P., Derman, E. W., and Noakes, T. D. (1997). Aetiology of skeletal muscle cramps during exercise: a novel hypothesis. *Journal of Sports Science*, **15**(3), 277–85.

See also FATIGUE; REFLEXES.

Cranial nerves are those that carry information directly to and from the BRAIN, entering or emerging through openings in the cranium (SKULL). There are twelve pairs, known by Roman numerals according to the sequence in

The 12 pairs of cranial nerves

I	**Olfactory**

Special sensory, for smell. Consists of small bundles of fibres passing from the nerve endings in the olfactory epithelium, through perforated bone at the top of the nose, to enter the olfactory bulb, underneath the frontal lobe.

II	**Optic**

Special sensory, for vision. Made up of fibres that converge from the whole of the retina. Pass backwards to the base of the brain from the back of the eyeballs.

III	**Oculomotor**

Mainly motor to small muscles that move the eyeball. Also carry autonomic (*parasympathetic*) nerve fibres that constrict the pupil.

IV	**Trochlear**

Mainly motor to the muscle that turns the eyeball downwards and outwards.

V	**Trigeminal**

The largest of the cranial nerves, with 3 main divisions: ophthalmic, maxillary, and mandibular. Mainly sensory, from most of the tissues of the head, face, and mouth; motor to the muscles that move the lower jaw.

VI	**Abducens**

Motor to the muscle that moves the eyeball outwards.

VII	**Facial**

Motor to the facial muscles; sensory, for taste, from the front part of the tongue; also parasympathetic nerve fibres to salivary glands.

VIII	**Auditory (vestibulo-cochlear)**

Mainly sensory, for hearing and balance; enter the brain from the inner ear (vestibulocochlear) (cochlea and vestibule).

IX	**Glossopharyngeal**

Sensory and motor, for the mouth, neck, including pharynx, larynx, and tongue (taste from the back part); also transmit sensory information concerning blood gases and blood pressure from the neck arteries; parasympathetic fibres to salivary glands.

X	**Vagus**

Carry visceral sensory information from thoracic and abdominal organs; motor to the larynx (speech) and oesophagus (swallowing); parasympathetic to heart, lungs, and to muscle and glands of the alimentary tract as far as the middle of the colon.

XI	**Accessory**

Shares the functions of X, and joins with uppermost spinal nerves to innervate muscles that move the head and shoulders.

XII	**Hypoglossal**

Motor to the tongue muscles.

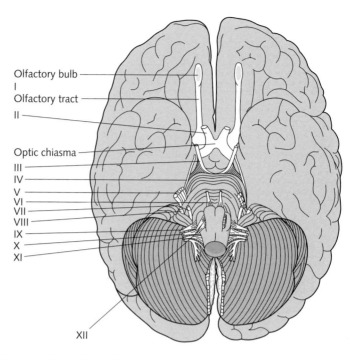

The human brain viewed from below to show the cranial nerves.

which they are attached to the brain. Those that serve the special senses of smell and vision are purely sensory, and differ from the rest in being essentially extensions of the brain itself. The others are part motor, part sensory; for these, the relevant MOTOR NEURONS (analogous to those in the spinal cord) are in collections of cells (nuclei) in the BRAIN STEM, and the cell bodies of the sensory neurons are in ganglia outside the brain stem (analogous to those in the dorsal roots of spinal nerves). Also, nerve fibres belonging to the cranial component of the parasympathetic division of the AUTONOMIC NERVOUS SYSTEM arise from neurons in the brain stem and form a part of some of the cranial nerves.

SHEILA JENNETT

Craniometry is the study of the shape and form of the human head or SKULL, sometimes known also as craniology (the difference lies largely in that the former implies precise measurement, the latter less so). As it is such an obvious observation that people vary considerably in the size and shape of their heads and faces, it is hardly surprising that attempts to put this to scientific and other uses stretch well back in time. The modern and quantitative study of craniology derives essentially from the nineteenth century, when it became widely accepted that evolutionary ideas could be explored through detailed comparisons of skulls. In effect it is a specialized branch of ANTHROPOMETRY, the quantitative study of the human body.

The practice of craniometry consists of taking precise measurements using 'landmarks' on the skull (see figure). The skull is not a single bone, but is made up of several interlocked plates, such as the two parietal bones at the sides and the central frontal bone. Where these bones meet can be easily identified, and these places form many of the major landmarks of the skull — for example, the 'bregma', where the two parietals and the frontal meet, which is in effect the highest part of the skull. The distances between the various points can be measured, and thus form the basis of craniometry. In this way, a structural model of the skull, consisting of the angles and lengths between the landmarks, can be formed, and thus it is possible to compare one skull with another, and to make statistical comparisons between populations. Measurements are made most easily on skulls, but some can also be taken from the heads of living people as part of more general anthropometric studies.

The development of craniometry owes much to many pioneers of the nineteenth and twentieth centuries, of whom perhaps the most important was Rudolf Martin, professor of ANTHROPOLOGY at the University of Zurich (1864–1925). He provided the systematic basis for craniology, much of which is used today. Another important contributor is W. W. Howells, emeritus professor of ANTHROPOLOGY at Harvard University, who developed a more practicable set of measurements, and greatly enhanced the statistical treatment of such data. Although often confused with PHRENOLOGY, the study of variation in the size and shape of the human skull within the biological sciences owes more to classic medical and comparative anatomy than to this discredited and largely subjective approach.

The study of the human skull has been one of the most fertile, important, controversial and abused branches of anthropology. Comparisons of human skulls with those of fossil hominids that have been unearthed have been the main source of information and inference about the pattern of HUMAN EVOLUTION, and the relationships between humans and other primates. Differences in shape reflect evolutionary history and relationships. Furthermore, data on cranial variation was used extensively in discussions in the earlier part

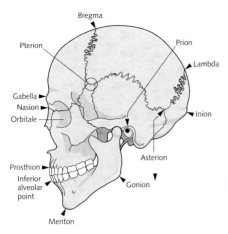

Craniometry: major landmarks used for measurements of the skull, from *Gray's Anatomy* (Longman).

of this century, following the rediscovery of Mendel's work, in debates concerning the continuous or otherwise nature of evolutionary change.

Comparisons can also be made between human populations. Externally we can see that people from different parts of the world look different, and this is reflected in their cranial anatomy. The patterns of measurements can be used to explore relationships between populations, and the history of human diversification. For example, modern European skulls are characterized by large FACES and NOSES, and relatively long skulls; modern East Asians are lightly built, with very short, flat faces. Craniometry allows these similarities and differences to be treated not as racial types, but as patterns of biological variation, and to be understood in terms of history and adaptation.

However, although modern craniometry eschews the use of head shape to classify people into races, this has not been the case in the past, and craniology has a blacker history. Cranial shape was assumed by many to be a direct measure of racial affinity, such races being seen as fixed biological units. In Nazi Germany such measures as the *cephalic index* (how broad a skull is) and nose shape were used to categorize people, and to define the Jewish population and degrees of Jewish admixture. Similar but less extreme programmes occurred in other countries, either as part of attempts to introduce EUGENICS programmes or through attempts to define CRIMINAL types.

The scars left after World War II by these atrocious programmes of research meant that the study of human skull shape and size fell into disrepute. Human variation, the core subject of anthropology, was increasingly explored through genetics and other biological markers, and became functional and adaptive in orientation rather than a search for racial affinities. In recent years, however, the introduction of new computer-based techniques of measurement, and the greatly enhanced power of statistical analysis, has meant that there has been a resurgence of interest in this subject, and, stripped of its non-Darwinian

and racist past, the study of the human head remains a topic of major importance.

ROBERT FOLEY

Further reading

Lahr, M. M. (1996). *The evolution of modern human diversity: a study of cranial variation.* Cambridge University Press.

Spencer, F. (ed.) (1982). *A history of American physical anthropology.* Academic Press, New York.

See also ANTHROPOLOGY; ANTHROPOMETRY; EVOLUTION, HUMAN; HEREDITY; SKULL.

Craniotomy By derivation, this word covers any surgical opening into the SKULL, but it is now usually used only to describe the fashioning of a hinged flap of bone which allows the intracranial cavity to be reached. Opening the skull (*trepanning*) in the belief that this would let out evil spirits is one of the oldest operations in the history of SURGERY, as evidenced by the finding of man-made holes in skulls from very early periods. In these cases, pointed flints were probably used to bore out the hole, and some skulls show evidence of subsequent healing with new bone formation — indicating that people survived such procedures. Until the middle of the twentieth century, skull openings were still being made by some tribes in Kenya. Indications probably included mental illness, EPILEPSY, and perhaps severe, recurrent headache such as

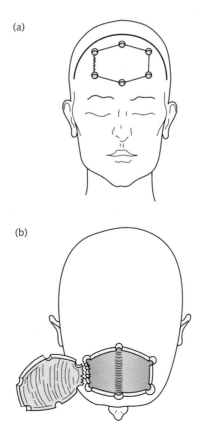

(a)

(b)

Diagram of frontal craniotomy: (a) burrholes; (b) the hinged flap.

MIGRAINE. Recently an eccentric small group have advocated do-it-yourself drilling of the skull, supposedly to restore the alleged benefit of allowing a pressure outlet similar to that in infancy before the fontanelle closes. Technical instructions for this bizarre procedures have even appeared on the Internet.

By the seventeenth century the 'trephine' was an instrument in the surgical armamentarium for opening the skull. This was a circular crown saw with a central pin, which would cut out a disc or button of bone. It could vary in diameter from 1 cm or so up to 8 cm; sometimes more than one disc was cut to give adequate access. The larger discs would be put back in place, but smaller holes were left as permanent defects. A further development was to use a brace and bit to ream out (as bone dust) burr holes about 1 cm in diameter. Through trephine or burr holes, blood clots that were threatening life by compression of the brain could be let out, and lives were saved. Burr holes are still used today for releasing surface clots and also to allow probes to be passed into deeper parts of the brain. These may be for measuring the pressure in, or draining fluid from, the CEREBRAL VENTRICLES; for obtaining BIOPSY specimens of brain for microscopic examination; to record electrically from the deeper parts of the brain; or to produce controlled damage in parts of the brain for the correction of abnormal functioning (e.g. epilepsy or tremor). The limited access provided by a burr hole may be increased by nibbling away more bone with forceps, the resulting procedure being termed *craniectomy*. This leaves a permanent defect in the skull, with the brain covered only by the skin and other soft tissues.

The Gigli saw, invented by this Florentine obstetrician in 1894 to enlarge the pelvic outlet in obstructed labour, made the craniotomy flap possible. This saw is a serrated wire that can be passed under the bone from one burr hole to the next one and used to saw the bone in between. This is done along the lines joining each pair of burr holes, except the line which underlies the fold of skin and other tissues that has been turned back. This base section of unsawn bone is then cracked as the bone flap is raised. The bone flap remains hinged on the soft tissues attached to it, preserving its blood supply (see figure). This allows major intracranial surgery to be performed, such as the removal of a tumour, and when this has been completed the bone flap can be turned back into place and the soft tissues and skin also replaced. The use of a brace and bit and Gigli saw has recently been replaced by power driven drills and saws.

An unusual use of the term 'craniotomy' is in obstetrics. This is when a dead baby with an abnormally large head has caused obstructed labour, and the obstetrician has to reduce the size of the head by perforating it in order to allow delivery.

BRYAN JENNETT

Crash impact Along with the increasing speeds of transport and fighting machines in the twentieth century have come the study and

185

implementation of methods of limiting human damage in the event of a crash. Body restraint has been a crucial consideration in aircraft since the beginning of aviation, and the high incidence of head injuries occurring in accidents in military jet aircraft led in the 1950s to the introduction of protective helmets for military aircrew. The use of seat belts in the front seats of cars has been required by law in the UK since 1983, and motor cyclists have been required to wear helmets since 1974. Since the late 1980s many pedal cyclists wear helmets by common consent or institutional requirement. All these measures, enforced by law or adopted by choice, reduce the risk of serious injury from crash impact.

An abrupt acceleration, imposed upon the human body by a collision between a person in motion and a stationary object, or by an object striking a stationary individual, can cause injury which may be fatal. The sudden change of velocity which occurs, whether it be produced by a fall from height onto solid ground or by the vehicle in which a person is travelling hitting a stationary object, is the cause of the injury. The degree of injury is related to the magnitude, duration, and direction of application of the accelerative forces. The inertial force which results from the application of an acceleration and which causes displacement of organs within the body is equal and *opposite* to the applied acceleration. The effects of short duration acceleration (less than 0.5 sec) are related principally to the structural strength of the part of the body upon which they act, the peak acceleration (measured in G, i.e. multiples of the acceleration due to gravity) (see G AND G-SUITS), and the duration of the acceleration.

The direction in which the accelerative force is applied to the body is a major factor in determining the body's tolerance to an impact and the risk of injury. The other major factors are the support to and restraint of the body, and the possibility of a flailing head or limb impacting with a solid structure. The levels of acceleration which occur on the crash of a road vehicle or an aircraft can vary from a few G to a peak acceleration of 150–200 G, acting for 0.2 to 0.4 sec.

Human tolerance

The effects of short duration accelerations are usually categorised as tolerable, injurious, or fatal. Tolerable forces may produce bruises and abrasions but do not incapacitate. Injurious forces result in moderate to severe trauma, including fractures and injuries to internal organs such as liver, spleen, and brain, which may or may not incapacitate. The limits of human tolerance — for the seated adult subject, well supported by a seat, and effectively restrained by a harness which prevents impact with other structures — have been estimated for different directions of acceleration, from experiments using whole or parts of human cadavers, non-human primates, anthropomorphic dummies, and human subjects. The lowest tolerance (around 11–12 G for 0.1 sec) is for sideways accelerations

and the highest (greater than 45 G for 0.1 sec) is for forwards acceleration. The limit of tolerance for headwards acceleration (25 G for 0.1 sec) is an important factor in defining the performance of ejection seats in high-performance military aircraft and of attenuating devices designed to reduce the risk of injury on a vertical impact with the ground. The limit of tolerance of backwards acceleration is important in relation to provision of crash protection in motor vehicles and aircraft with conventional forward-facing seats.

Restraint systems

The more effectively the occupant is restrained in a seat, the higher is their tolerance of an impact acceleration. The seat in turn must be adequately secured to the structure of the vehicle. There has been, for example, a progressive increase in the strengths of aircraft seats and their attachments to the aircraft floor, which in the past were woefully inadequate. The familiar restraint *harness* comprises one or more straps which are secured across the trunk of the seated individual by means of a quick-release buckle. The simplest type is the lap strap, which, whilst easy to use, does not restrain the upper trunk, leaving it free to jack-knife on impact with backwards or sideways accelerations, which may well result in serious injury, especially if the head hits the vehicle structure. The addition of a diagonal strap running from the origin of one of the lap straps, up over the front of the trunk and the top of the opposite shoulder, to be secured to the seat or vehicle structure — the 'three point' harness as fitted to the front seats of cars — provides very good restraint provided that it is well designed and adjusted. Most modern fighter aircraft are fitted with a 'five point' harness, which comprises two lap and two shoulder straps, and a strap from the seat structure between the legs to the quick-release box. This harness gives excellent restraint both during aerobatic manoeuvres and on crash impact and ejection.

Another method of enhancing tolerance of impact accelerations in use is the *air bag*, which is located in front of the seat occupant and inflates automatically in response to deceleration to prevent the occupant moving forward and striking the vehicle structure. An air bag typically inflates in less than 0.1 sec and then deflates slowly over the next few seconds.

Head injury and protection

Head injury is common in all forms of crash impact. One third to a half of car crash fatalities are due to injury to the head. Blows to the head may cause fracture of the bones of the skull, tearing of the membranes lining the inside of the skull — causing bleeding which may raise the pressure within the skull — and local damage to the brain itself where it underlies a fracture. But the brain is often damaged within the intact skull by the linear and angular acceleration of the head induced by the blow; the brain moves within the skull, and layers of its substance move relative to other layers, causing

distortion or at worst disruption of connections between neurons. A relatively minor blow to the head can give rise to CONCUSSION — a transient paralysis of cerebral function, with loss of consciousness, which is followed by complete recovery. The concussed individual may, however, be unable to escape other consequences of the crash such as fire. Whilst the factors responsible for the concussion are complex, it is generally accepted that the human brain can withstand crash impact forces of 300–400 G without either concussion or skull fracture, provided that there is no local deformation of the skull to inflict direct injury.

Prevention of injury to the heads of the occupants of a vehicle on crash impact depends upon adequate restraint of the trunk, the presence of an adequate space free of rigid structures around the head, and making sure that any surface with which the head may come in contact is made of a material which deforms when hit, allowing a measure of energy absorption. Frequently, however, especially where the risk of head impact is increased, the most satisfactory solution is to provide personal head protection. A well-designed protective helmet comprises an outer semi-rigid shell and a suspension system either of a strap harness or a layer of crushable foam beneath the shell. The shell distributes the impact over a larger area and provides some attenuation by partial disintegration, whilst the gap (18–25 mm) between the shell and the head reduces the average acceleration applied to the head to 1/6–1/8 of that applied to the surface of the helmet. Such protective helmets have done much to reduce the toll of fatalities and serious head injuries in motor cyclists and in military aircrew.   JOHN ERNSTING

Further reading
Ernsting, J. and King, P. (1988). *Aviation medicine*, (2nd edn). Butterworth-Heinemann, Oxford.

Glaister, D. H. (1978). Human tolerance to impact acceleration. *Injury*, **9**, 191–8.

See also CONCUSSION; FLYING; G AND G-SUIT; INJURY.

Creation myths
The essential metaphysical question that creation myths seek to answer is that of origins, or where things come from. The emergence of day from night, the growth of plants from seeds, the provenance of weather and the seasons, the birth of living things, all provoke questions regarding the source of these phenomena. Creation myths serve, in most societies, to give an account of such origins.

The central bodily image in most recorded myths of creation is that of human birth. This leads to a widespread anthropomorphization of the original principles or powers of creation as being primeval parents, male and female. In the classical Greek myth of Hesiod, the Earth Mother, Gaia, is impregnated by the Sky Father, Uranos, and gives birth to Kronos, who later kills his father and unites with his mother to produce a race of giants, the first mortal living beings in the world. The genders of earth and sky are reversed in an Egyptian creation myth, which depicts the cow-goddess Nut with long hair and hanging breasts, overarching the earth-god Geb, her spouse, as his sky-protectress.

In patriarchal cosmogonies the 'normal' imageries of divine motherhood are taken over by the father, as in the Christian myth of creation by the Word spoken by a male creator, who calls things into existence by naming them: 'Let there be light'. Alternately, in the Hindu story of the world's beginnings, Lotus, which grows from the navel of the reclining god, Vishnu, and is a symbol associated with the female powers of reproduction, is transmuted into an image of creation springing from the male. For, since the lotus is associated primarily with the goddess, Padma, whose body itself is the universe, the long stem from Vishnu's navel to the lotus should properly connote an umbilical cord through which the flow of energy would run from the goddess to the god, mother to child.

The image of Athena springing, fully grown, from Zeus' head, is an example of the appropriation of birth and its transference away from the lower regions of the body, to the higher faculties. As the mother gives birth from the womb, so the father gives birth from the mind, through the faculty of speech: in this latter transformation, the mouth, with its tongue (in Western cultures sometimes regarded as the alternative male member) produces that precious child of civilisation, the word.

The *Brihardaranyaka Upanishad* (c. 700 BC) tells of how, in the beginning, the universe was nothing but the Self in the form of a male. 'It is I!' he shouted, whence the concept I arose. Feeling lonely, however, he split himself in half, and his other half was in the form of a woman, whom he embraced. To escape him, she transformed herself into a cow, then a goat, then a sheep, and all the female animals that exist, while he followed, transforming himself into the male of these animals in order to embrace with her, and thus all pairing things were formed. Seeing the proliferation of living beings from his own and his mate's inventive metamorphoses, the male Self congratulated himself, saying, 'I, actually, am creation; for I have poured forth all this', rather overlooking the fact that it was his other half's reluctance to embrace him, and desire to escape him, that produced this animal abundance.

Procreative desire may give rise to land as well as the animals that inhabit it. The emergence from the sea of the volcanic islands of Japan is explained in terms of childbirth, the islands being the offspring of two heavenly spirits, Izanagi and Izanami. The first children of the pair, however, were abortions, caused by the fact that, when their parents first joined together, it was the woman who had first exclaimed at the man's beauty. The second time round, the order of precedence was corrected, the man spoke first, and the births were successful, forming the eight islands of Japan, and all their forests, mountains, rivers, and valleys. While sexual desire serves as the explanatory model for these myths of creation, there exist other myths that purport to explain the origin of sexual desire itself.

Several creation myths tell of one primeval body, out of which all the parts of the world were made: in a Norse myth, when the frozen wastes of the north met the fiery realm of the south, the melting ice transformed into the shape of the sleeping giant, Ymir. From his flesh was formed the soil, his bones became mountains and stones, his hair became vegetation, and his blood the sea. More frequently this primeval body is female, as in the Mayan myth of the great female Earth Monster, who was torn in half by the gods Quetzalcoatl and Tezcatlipoca: her lower half ascended to form the heavens, and her upper half descended to form the earth. In a Mayan myth describing the origin of plants, the corpse of a god provided the basis for a thousand varieties of fruits and grain. From his hair grew cotton; from his ears, seed-bearing plants; from his nostrils, healing herbs; from his fingers, the sweet potato; from his fingernails, maize.

Creation myths in many cultures ascribe different parts of the cosmos to different parts of the body of a divine being, or give alternative origins for the sexes. In Babylonian myth, Marduk slaughters the serpent Tiamat and makes the sky and the earth from her divided body. In Norse myth the three creator gods kill the bisexual giant Ymir, making the earth from his body, the sea from his blood, and the sky from his skull. The giant Purusha's body is the basis of the universe in Vedic myth.

The notion of the many growing out of the one is counterposed in mythology by the idea of two opposing principles of existence, the struggles and foment of which provide the seeds of creation. In the Zoroastrian myth of creation, the world is made and maintained by two contrary powers; Ahura Mazda, the Lord of Life, and Angra Mainyu, the Demon of the Lie who, when the world had been made by Ahura Mazda, corrupted every particle of its being. Yet it was Angra Mainyu who, by shattering the fixed order of the stars, caused celestial motion to being, and by dessicating the first created plants, and spreading their powder over the world, covered it in vegetation; and by destroying the sole created being, a primaeval ox, made all living things arise from its seed, from the birds of the air to the fish in the waters and beasts on land. A parallel story of the world created through the dynamic tension between opposing forces is found in the Huron creation myth, which tells of how the world was made by the twinned offspring of the Woman Fallen from the Sky. The evil twin, Taweskare, kicked his way through his mother's armpit, and killed her, while the good twin, Tsentsa, was born in the usual manner. So when Tsentsa created fertile plains and valleys, Taweskare heaved up parts of them to create barren mountains, and cleft others to make swamps and chasms; the first made flowers and fruit trees, and his brother put thorns on the stems and made the fruit small and gritty; the good twin made fish and other animals to eat, and the bad twin gave them sharp teeth, and scales, and horns.

Creation myths thus have a dual relationship with the body, in that they seek both to mimic, as well as explain, bodily processes such as birth and growth. The functions and qualities of the human body, or microcosm, are seen to mirror those of the external world, or macrocosm. Body and earth become one in these myths, and human origins, geological formations, plant life, and animal life, are all explicated by means of metaphors and images related to human reproduction and development. Similarly, the observable oppositions and dichotomies in the world are accounted for as the competing expressions of two siblings, whose rivalry drives the diversity of creation.
NATSU HATTORI

Further reading

Campbell, J. (1960–5). *The masks of God*, Vols 1–3. Secker and Warburg, London.

Graves, R. (1961). *The White Goddess*. Faber and Faber, London.

Taube, K.A. (1993). *Aztec and Maya myths*. British Museum Press, London.

See also GREEKS; METAMORPHOSIS; MYTHIC THOUGHT; MYTHOLOGY AND THE BODY; REPRODUCTION MYTHS.

Criminals An important figure in the early history of scientific criminology was the Italian Cesare Lombroso (1835–1909). Notoriously, Lombroso suggested that some (although not all) offenders are 'born criminals', characterised physically by a variety of morphological features reminiscent of lower primates, and therefore are atavistic throwbacks to an earlier stage in evolution. In the century since the publication of Lombroso's work, there has been a regular succession of 'disclosures' about links between crime and biology, many of which, like the atavism hypothesis, have been subsequently falsified. For example, in the late 1960s and early 1970s, suggestions were made that the small minority of males with an extra Y chromosome (in addition to the normal, single X and Y sex chromosomes) frequently exhibit extreme aggressive antisocial tendencies. More recent research fails to support these suggestions, though there is some evidence that the XYY anomaly is associated with factors (such as low IQ) that indirectly increase the likelihood of more minor antisocial acts.

Given this unfortunate intellectual history, it is hardly surprising that many sociologically-oriented criminologists have, in the past, denied, and some continue to deny, any link between biology and crime. Viewed dispassionately, the empirical evidence does not support such a position. However, the best evidence now suggests that links between biological characteristics and crime work in a probabilistic rather than a deterministic fashion, and that the extent of any genetic or other biological influence is, in general, only modest to moderate. Contrary to earlier speculations, there is no 'criminal gene' — nor indeed could there easily be, given that the concept of 'crime' is not a natural behavioural category, but a socially constructed concept, which varies between different societies, and in the same society over time.

How then might biology–crime links work? An example might be helpful. Research on criminal careers in several countries has consistently demonstrated, using both officially-recorded indices of crime and self-report studies, that a small minority of male persistent offenders is responsible for a very disproportionate percentage of all criminal acts. Longitudinal studies show that certain factors, identifiable at age 7–10, or earlier, can reliably differentiate subsequent persistent offenders, occasional offenders, and non-offenders. Among these identifiable factors are some that are unambiguously environmental, such as poor parenting. It is also clear, however, that pervasive, early-onset hyperactivity/inattention/impulsivity is associated with a greatly increased risk of criminal behaviour in adolescence and adulthood; and there is some evidence to link these traits with abnormalities of certain NEUROTRANSMITTER systems in the BRAIN. It is not hard to see that a trait of persisting impulsivity might be causally linked to later *property crime* (giving instant rather than delayed gratification) and VIOLENCE (impulsive aggression). Yet, despite such links, we also know that hyperactive children reared in supportive and prosocial environments often do not become delinquent. For these and other reasons, predictive studies based on individual factors observable at age 7–10, while reliably predicting group differences, usually over-predict the incidence of subsequent persistent criminality.

This line of evidence and theorisation strongly suggests that biological associations with criminality, while they certainly exist, can be understood properly only within a firm biosocial framework. To date, however, the specialisation of academic disciplines, together with the unfortunate history of the search for a rigid link between biological characteristics and crime, has militated against much real progress in developing adequately detailed, interactive, bio-social explanations of crime.

An example illustrates the potential scope for such interactive explanations. Sociologists have observed that, in all modern societies, both official criminality and self-reported serious or persistent criminality is consistently associated with four variables: *sex* (males more criminal than females); *age* (peak age of criminality in adolescence); *social class* (lower class more likely to commit 'street crimes', such as burglary or robbery); and *urban–rural differences* (urban areas more criminal, even when other relevant variables are controlled for).

The standard research methods for attempting to infer possible genetic influences on criminality are studies of TWINS (looking for differences between genetically identical, monozygotic twins and non-identical, dizygotic pairs), and of adoptees (looking for similarities between the behaviour of the biological parents and their children, adopted and reared separately). Twin and adoptee studies have shown that inferred

genetic effects seem consistently *greater* among samples of female offenders, adult offenders, higher-class offenders, and rural offenders. In other words, apparent genetic influences on criminality are proportionately greater within social contexts in which crime is generally low, and genetic factors diminish in influence as the group crime rate rises. The increased crime in general populations (disproportionately associated with urban, lower-class young men) is, then, largely produced by social factors.

There has been a significant renewal of serious scholarly interest in the field of biology and crime in the last decade. Given this, and the present underdeveloped state of interactive, biosocial explanations, significant intellectual progress might be expected in the fairly near future. In such research, the real interest will lie not in the quantification of the genetic or other biological components, 'but rather in understanding *how* the risk is mediated and *how* [biological] factors combine with environmental influences to predispose to antisocial behaviour' (Sir Michael Rutter).   A. BOTTOMS

Further reading

Brennan, P. A., Mednick, S. A., and Volavka, J. (1995). Biomedical factors in crime. In *Crime* (ed. J. Q. Wilson and J. Petersilia).Institute for Contemporary Studies Press, San Francisco.

Ciba Foundation (1996). *Genetics of criminal and antisocial behaviour.* John Wiley and Sons, Chichester.

Raine, A., Brennan, P. A., Farrington, D. P., and Mednick, S. A. (ed.) (1997). *Biosocial bases of violence.* Plenum Press, New York.

See also DEGENERATION.

Cults and the body
Everybody knows what a cult is. But few realize that the word 'cult' has both a common and a technical meaning, and that these meanings are significantly different. What most people seem to mean by the word is a social group whose members adhere to a strange, unorthodox, and even dangerous set of religious beliefs and practices. Cults vary in beliefs and scope of activities, and range from zealous and satanic groups at one extreme to New Age religions and HEALING circles at the other. The more famous cults are often organized around a charismatic leader, like Vernon Howel, a.k.a. David Koresh, of the Branch Davidians, an offshoot of the Seventh Day Adventists, or science-fiction-writer-turned-guru, L. Ron Hubbard of the Church of Scientology, or Elizabeth Clair Prophet of the Church Universal and Triumphant. People are beginning to realize that Hitler's Nazi movement in Germany was also a kind of mystical cult.

Cults pop up all over the world, and have done throughout human history. Hinduism has spawned cults of this sort, as with the groups centred around such charismatic teachers as Bhagwan Shree Rajneesh, and Maharishi Mahesh Yogi, the founder of the Transcendental Meditation (TM) movement. Such religious groups may

advocate beliefs and carry out practices that sometimes lead them into trouble with authorities, and may, in certain extreme situations, lead members to bodily injury and even death, as with the tragic Jonestown cult. Groups of this sort may or may not be loose-knit in their organization, and may or may not endure much beyond the death of their leaders.

Social scientists who study religion use the word 'cult' in a more technical sense. For scientific purposes, a cult is simply *a set of institutionalized beliefs and ritual practices pertaining to cosmological, spiritual, and religious knowledge.* Used in this sense, all societies on earth, as well as all religious institutions in our own Euro-American societies, have their cult aspects. The Roman Catholic Church has its set of standardized beliefs and ritual practices, such as the Mass, 'doing the rosary', marriage ceremonies, and BAPTISM services. Buddhists have the teachings of the Buddha pertaining to awakening and the cessation of suffering, and carry out pujas and other kinds of devotional and meditative rituals. It is important to understand that all the world religions began as 'cults' in the more common sense of the term. They began as small, localized organizations led by charismatic leaders like Jesus, Mohammed, and the Buddha. But instead of falling apart after the death of their leaders, these 'cults' endured, continued to attract adherents, and grew into vast, worldwide organizations.

The body in cultic systems
In religious terms, the human body is simultaneously a symbol, an agent, and a problem. The human body is often a profoundly meaningful cult symbol. Most cultic systems place the human form at the very centre of the cosmos as they understand it. The body is viewed as a microcosm which reflects within its nature the organic principles that motivate the greater universe. Thus, in the cosmology of the Navajo people of the American Southwest, the body is symbolically positioned within the *hogan*, or traditional house, and the *hogan* is positioned in proper relation to the four cardinal directions within Navajoland (which is defined by four sacred mountains), and Navajoland is positioned at the centre of the world. The human body is sacred to the Navajo precisely because of its relationship to everything in the world. When they wish to heal someone of a disease, this relationship between body, house, land, and world is enacted in a ceremonial way to bring all the proper relations back into alignment.

Parts of the body may have particular significance relative to a cult's belief system. For example, the sexual organs (phallus or vagina) may signify the generative or fertility principle operating in the universe. Dismemberment of the body may be symbolic of a stage in the development of one who has become wise in the ways of the cult. Footprints along a path may symbolize the many way-points in the process by which a novice becomes an adept.

Most cultures on the planet alter the form of the body of their members in symbolically meaningful ways. Very few, if any, cultures leave the body unchanged through life, and these changes often have sacred significance. As many writers have noted, our English words *cosmos* and *cosmetics* derive from the same ancient Greek root for universe and ornamentation. The hair is styled or a wig donned, the skin is pierced, tattooed, painted, the body is adorned with often elaborately patterned raiments and ornaments, and the face is covered with paint or a mask. Alteration of the body may be severe and even brutal, as among those cults that require scarification and cicatrization of the face and body, physically injurious ordeals that leave SCARS, elongation of the neck, deformation of the head (usually done in infancy), CIRCUMCISION, or clitoridectomy.

Put in a word, our body is a symbol to ourselves — a symbol of our gender, our group membership, our status, our role in life, our aspirations, and, in many cultic systems, our place in the universe. Our body is not merely an object to ourselves. If we are a cult member, it may be a symbol of our sacred relations to the divine principle operating in the universe. We may wear a costume (robes, cassock, prayer shawl, etc.) that signals both to others and to ourselves that we are practicing members of a cult. All these transformations of the body are meaningful within the cultic system of beliefs and practices that gives rise to the changes. Stages of entry into the cult may be marked by transformations of the body or its adornment. Buddhist monks everywhere shave their heads and wear distinctive robes. Tibetan Buddhist monks in addition signal the status of the religious hierarchy by even more elaborate robes and headgear.

Moreover, the movements of the human body may also be meaningful, particularly when they are used to communicate. Formal postures and GESTURES often go hand in hand with dress and ornamentation in signalling important information about the beliefs of the cult to members and to others outside the organization. The signalling aspect of the body may become quite elaborate, as in the case of Balinese sacred dance, where costume, posture, movement, and gesture are all highly choreographed for the purposes of religious performance.

As the signalling function of human actions suggests, the body is the central agent of cult activities. No religious system is ever comprised solely of beliefs, but rather of beliefs and their actualization through behaviour. It is insufficient merely to believe; one must act in accordance with belief. And cultic actions are at least partially ritualized. *Ritual* by definition is a set of appropriate formal acts established by custom and directed toward some socially appropriate goal or purpose.

For most people, the body also presents a profound existential problem. The body is universally recognized as the locus of both HEALTH and DISEASE, both life and DEATH. People everywhere experience those around them getting sick and sometimes dying. Disease and death pose a

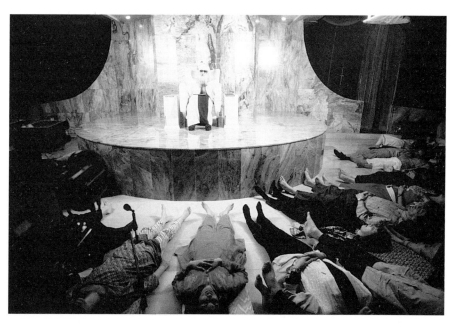

Bhagwan Shree Rajneesh at his nightly sermon, seated on the marble throne dais. Rene Burril/Magnum Photos.

dilemma for people everywhere, for they must ask themselves, 'If my body gets sick or grows old and dies, what happens to my spirit?' Such questions are what Paul Tillich in his book *Systematic Theology* called 'matters of ultimate concern' for people in all cultures. As a consequence, cults and religions always provide some kind of account of disease and death in their belief system, as well as some means for alleviating suffering and for facilitating the dying process. This is why all religions incorporate some form of healing system and such systems almost always involve rituals.

Dualism and cultic systems

Moreover, virtually all cult systems develop some view of what happens to the human spirit or psyche after death. As Ernest Becker noted in his book *The Denial of Death*, it is as though people cannot fully come to terms with the implications of their 'creatureliness' — with the implications of being a physical being with an embodied CONSCIOUSNESS — without the notion of some form of an afterlife. Again, the problem is an existential one. People everywhere perceive that the physical body dies and decomposes, and at the same time there seems to be a need to view the psyche, or some inner spiritual essence, as passing on to another form of existence, be that a new world, another plane of existence, or reincarnation back into this earthly realm. For this reason, all cultures show to at least a minimal degree a mind–body dualism. Cultic systems everywhere hold that, at least to some extent, the mind is separate or separable from the body. There is usually a soul or some spiritual essence that does not depend upon the body for its existence and that survives the dying process to pass on to some kind of continued existence.

The ritual control of experience

Whether we consider cults from the popular or the technical point of view, we find that rituals are the single most common and effective means of controlling and transforming the mental state of cult members. This is because, embedded within many rituals, there are activities and stimuli that directly act upon the body in such a way as to alter the state of consciousness of practitioners. A very common cross-cultural example is the use of ritual among the Umbanda cult, a tradition of healing that arose in the 1920s and that continues to the present day in Brazil. In Umbanda rituals, trained practitioners lead patients into a trance state in which the patient identifies with and acts out the role of the spirits. It is by contact with the power of the spirits that the healing is accomplished. This identification with spirits is in no sense a 'brain-washing' exercise, but appears to have distinct therapeutic effects on the subsequent well-being of the patient.

The components of rituals that alter states of consciousness are called *drivers*, because they activate various combinations of body functions, and particularly those of the nervous system. It is by way of drivers that ritual activities actually penetrate into and evoke the physiological processes that underlie mental processes. A useful way to think of drivers is to distinguish between those that are extrinsic and those that are intrinsic to the body. *Extrinsic drivers* are elements such as drumming or concentration upon an icon — they depend upon stimuli external to the body. *Intrinsic drivers*, such as fasting or breathing techniques, are staged within the body. The table overleaf lists some examples of both types of drivers.

Intense concentration upon a cult's core symbolism may result in profound transformation of the state of mind and body — as is the case in the

Types of drivers used in ritual production of experience

Intrinsic drivers	Examples
breathing exercises	Buddhist meditation
auto-rhythms: chanting	Hindu and Buddhist mantra

visualization
  vision quest
  dream incubation
	Plains Indian vision quests
	Tsimshian shamanism

fever	Iroquois Handsome Lake movement, Tsimshian shamanism
circadian rhythms	
fasting	
physical exertion	long-distance running, Tibetan trance-running
fatigue	vision quest
concentration	Navajo stargazing, Zen koan meditation
directed intention	Jungian active imagination
seclusion	Tsimshian shamans
sensory deprivation	Kogi mamas (with seclusion)

Extrinsic drivers	Examples

rhythm:
  dancing
  drumming
  group chanting
  flickering light
	Bushman trance dancing
	Tsimshian healing
	Tsimshian healing

psychotropic drugs	Southwest US datura complex

imagery:
  art
  skrying
  Meditation symbol
  mnemonics
	Navajo sandpainting
	shaman's mirror
	Buddhist basic 10
	meditations
	Tsimshian power songs

ordeal:
  scary task
 	
  pain
	firewalking, snake
	handling, drinking
	poison
	plains vision quest, burial in
	ant hill

heat	Plains Indian Sundance, sweat lodge
performance	Tibetan cham dances
bloodletting	Maya ritual bloodletting

trance induction techniques of the Umbanda practitioners. A core symbol may be presented to a practitioner as a meditation, or the practitioner may imagine the symbol before the mind's eye (as in visualization practices). This would be driving the mind and body 'from the top down', so to speak. On the other hand, fasting (intrinsic driving) or ingesting psychotropic substances (extrinsic driving) may result in significant alteration of sensory and cognitive activity of the nervous system and thus alter the state of consciousness 'from the bottom up'. Much of a cult's ritual activity may be directed toward significantly altering the state of consciousness of its

members, which in turn may produce radical changes in the members' sense of identity, their value orientation, and their cultural affiliation. Possibly it is the power of ritual to alter states of consciousness that is the source of the fear people feel about cults. They perhaps become concerned that the cult is 'brain-washing' its members. While it is not true that a person can be literally 'brain-washed', in the sense of erasing their identity and previous cultural conditioning, ritual procedures do have the power to alter these in profound ways, in part by driving the body and its processes into alternative states. But most of the social science evidence on cultic ritual practices suggests that, in the case of most cults, the effect of these rituals is harmless and even therapeutic.

In conclusion, cults, whether in the popular or the technical sense, are concerned with the body as symbol, the body as agent, and the body as a source of existential dilemma. The body, its parts, and its transformations often provide a symbolic reference point upon which to ground and centre cultic beliefs. The body is also the principal agent for the realization of the cult's belief system. The belief system is enacted through ritual practices that frequently alter the state of consciousness of cult members. And because the body is perceived to sicken, age and die, cults everywhere must account for how the consciousness or spirit of the being may transcend the death of the body.

CHARLES D. LAUGHLIN

Further reading
Lewis, I. M. (1996). *Religion in context: cults and charisma*, (2nd edn). Cambridge University Press, Cambridge.

Rambo, L. R. (1993). *Understanding religious conversion*. Yale University Press, New Haven, CT.

Wallace, A. F. C. (1966). *Religion: an anthropological view*. Random House, New York.

See also BODY MUTILATION AND MARKINGS; RELIGION AND THE BODY.

Curare is the name of a crude drug, existing in the form of a dark brown, sticky, plant extract, and characterised by containing considerable amounts of poisonous alkaloids. Curare was prepared by the South American Indian tribes living in the valleys of the Amazon and the Orinoco. The extracts were used as arrow POISONS, for hunting, in a way which demonstrates a profound understanding of mechanisms. The flesh of animals killed by a poisoned arrow could be eaten with impunity, showing that the poison was lethal when injected, but not absorbed when taken orally. History does not tell us just how many attempts to develop arrow poisons had less fortunate outcomes. When Westerners turned their attention to the nature of South American arrow poisons there were considerable problems in discovering the active principles. Individual samples from the same region were often variable in composition. In some samples several

hundred constituents could be detected, mainly of plant origin, but often including animal material, such as excreta, and sometimes soil. Attention eventually focussed on extracts of plants from the families *Menispermaceae*, particularly *Chondrodendron* species, and *Loganiaceae*. Curare became available in three major forms with different regional origins: packed into bamboo tubes (*tube-curare*); in gourds (*calabash-curare*) containing material from Strychnos species; and in earthenware pots (*pot-curare*). In 1935 Harold King, a chemist working for the Medical Research Council in London, extracted, from a sample of tube-curare from the British Museum, a crystalline alkaloid which he called *tubocurarine*. This was to have a major impact in medicine.

Tubocurarine blocks the effects of the neurotransmitter acetylcholine in sites where it acts on the type of post-synaptic membrane receptors which are known as *nicotinic*. Quite the most important sites of these receptors are the junctions between motor nerves and voluntary skeletal muscle. When injected — and this includes injection by poisoned arrow — control of voluntary muscles is lost and flight or escape is not possible. Long before King had investigated the structure of tubocurarine, Claude Bernard had shown in 1856 that curare blocked neuromuscular transmission, without affecting conduction in the nerve or the contractility of the muscle. We now know that curare competes with acetylcholine for combination with the receptors on the muscle membrane — causing *neuromuscular block*.

In surgery, access to body cavities is hampered by tension in the voluntary muscles. These can be relaxed using anaesthetics, but only if dangerous dosage levels are used. Another, rather awkward solution is for assistants to hold open the incision with retractor. Motor paralysis by tubocurarine offered a surer and less cumbersome alternative. Use of such *muscle relaxants* became widespread for major surgery from the mid twentieth century. Not all voluntary muscles are equally sensitive to tubocurarine, and fortunately the respiratory muscles are the most spared. Thus by careful control of the dosage respiration can be maintained, although it is usual for anaesthetists to control the ventilation of the lungs mechanically.

For many years the commercial supply of tubocurarine was by extraction from crude curare extracts. New synthetic drugs, such as *atracurium*, have now largely replaced tubocurarine in medical practice. Nevertheless, for a while, surgery owed a debt to the experimentation of primitive peoples with their need for an arrow poison.

ALAN W. CUTHBERT

Further reading
Sneader, W. (1985). *Drug discovery — the evolution of modern medicines*. Wiley, Chichester.

See also ACETYLCHOLINE; ANAESTHESIA, GENERAL; NEUROMUSCULAR JUNCTION; PARALYSIS; MEMBRANE RECEPTORS.

Curse A term sometimes used colloquially for the menstrual period. It has been in use for centuries, because menstruating women were believed to produce many horrifying effects. They were considered unclean, unfit for coitus and capable of spoiling food, drink, and crops. Early Hebrews, for example, punished women who had intercourse during menstruation and in medieval times menstruating women were prevented from going to church or even entering a wine cellar in case they spoiled the wine!

S.A.W.

See MENSTRUATION.

Cyanosis this, like any word with the prefix *cyan*, derives from the Greek for dark blue. It refers to a blue tinge seen on the surface of the whole or part of the body, due to lack of OXYGEN in the blood. The apparent colour of the skin depends on the state of oxygenation of the blood in the microscopic vessels below the surface. Blood in the arteries is normally bright red, the colour of red blood cells when the HAEMOGLOBIN they contain is carrying its full quota of oxygen. In conditions of HYPOXIA due to ALTITUDE, lung disease, heart defects, or HEART FAILURE, the blood leaves the lungs without being fully oxygenated, and the arterial blood is less red. The degree of desaturation of haemoglobin at which such 'central cyanosis' is detectable varies between observers as well as between patients. Detection also depends on the superficial blood vessels being well-filled; if they are largely 'shut down' the skin is simply pale whatever the colour of the blood. Undoubtedly, however, if blueness is evident, there is significant hypoxia.

When arterial oxygen saturation is normal, the extent to which the blood becomes desaturated as it flows through the skin depends on the rate of blood flow. If blood flow is sluggish, a larger fraction of the oxygen is removed than if it is florid. Thus when cheeks are flushed, increased blood flow brings bright red blood near the surface; the oxygen supply is far in excess of need, with very little being removed. But when hands and feet are cold, the reflex constriction of blood vessels — to conserve heat as part of body TEMPERATURE REGULATION — reduces the flow, so a higher proportion of the oxygen is removed to supply the skin tissue, and the blood becomes bluer before it moves on. Hence we can become 'blue with cold' — but only superficially. The arterial blood itself remains bright red, if everything else is normal. For similar reasons of diminished blood flow, cyanosis is seen locally in a part of the body — say a leg or a big toe —

when the circulation in that part is compromised by arterial disease. SHEILA JENNETT

See also BREATHING; HAEMOGLOBIN; HYPOXIA; LUNGS; OXYGEN.

Cybernetics is the science of control. Its name, appropriately suggested by the mathematician Norbert Wiener (1894–1964), is derived from the Greek for 'steersman', pointing to the essence of cybernetics as the study and design of devices for maintaining stability, or for homing in on a goal or target. Its central concept is *feedback*. Since the 'devices' may be living or man-made, cybernetics bridges biology and engineering.

Stability of the human body is achieved by its static geometry and, very differently, by its dynamic control. A statue of a human being has to have a large base or it topples over. It falls when the centre of mass is vertically outside the base of the feet. Living people make continuous corrections to maintain themselves standing. Small deviations of POSTURE are signalled by sensory signals (PROPRIOCEPTION) from nerve fibres in the muscles and around the joint capsules of the ankles and legs, and by the *otoliths* (the organs of BALANCE in the inner ear). Corrections of posture are the result of dynamic feedback from these senses, to maintain dynamic stability. When walking towards a target, such as the door of a room, deviations from the path are noted, mainly visually, and corrected from time to time during the movement, until the goal is reached. The key to this process is continuous correction of the output system by signals representing detected errors of the output, known as 'negative feedback'. The same principle, often called *servo-control*, is used in engineering, in order to maintain the stability of machinery and to seek and find goals, with many applications such as guided missiles and autopilots.

The principles of feedback apply to the body's regulation of temperature, BLOOD PRESSURE, and so on. Though the principles are essentially the same as in engineering, for living organisms dynamic stability by feedback is often called 'HOMEOSTASIS', following W. B. Cannon's pioneering book *The wisdom of the body* (1932). In the history of engineering, there are hints of the principle back to ancient Greek devices, such as self-regulating oil lamps. From the Middle Ages the tail vane of windmills, continuously steering the sails into the veering wind, are well-known early examples of guidance by feedback. A more sophisticated system reduced the weight of the upper grinding stone when the wind fell, to keep

the mill operating optimally in changing conditions. Servo-systems using feedback can make machines remarkably life-like. The first feedback device to be mathematically described was the rotary governor, used by James Watt to keep the rate of steam engines constant with varying loads.

Servo-systems suffer characteristic oscillations when the output overshoots the target, as occurs when the feedback is too slow or too weak to correct the output. Changing the 'loop gain' (i.e. the magnitude of correction resulting from a particular feedback signal) increases tremor for machines and organisms. It is tempting to believe that 'intention tremor' of patients who have suffered damage to the CEREBELLUM is caused by a change in the characteristics of servo control.

Dynamic control requires the transmission of information. Concepts of information are included in cybernetics, especially following Claud Shannon's important mathematical analysis in 1949. It does not, however, cover digital computing. Cybernetic systems are usually analogue, and computing is described with very different concepts. Early Artificial Intelligence (AI) was analogue-based (reaching mental goals by correcting abstract errors) and there has recently been a return to analogue computing systems, with self-organising 'neural nets'.

A principal pioneer of cybernetic concepts of brain function was the Cambridge psychologist Kenneth Craik, who described thinking in terms of physical models analogous to physiological processes. Craik pointed to engineering examples, such as Kelvin's tide predictor, which predicted tides with a system of pulleys and levers. The essential cybernetic philosophy of neurophysiology is that the brain functions by such principles as feedback and information, represented by electro-chemical, physical activity in the nervous system. It is assumed that this creates mind: so, in principle, and no doubt in practice, machines can be fully mindful.

RICHARD L. GREGORY

Further reading

Cannon, W. B. (1932). *The wisdom of the body*. New York.

Craik, K. J. W. (1943). *The nature of explanation*. Cambridge.

Mayr, O. (1970). *The origins of feedback control*. Cambridge, M.A.

Shannon, C. E. and Weaver, W. (1949). *The mathematical theory of information*. Urbana.

Weiner, N. (1948). *Cybernetics*. New York.

See also BALANCE; HOMEOSTASIS; PROPRIOCEPTION; VESTIBULAR SYSTEM.

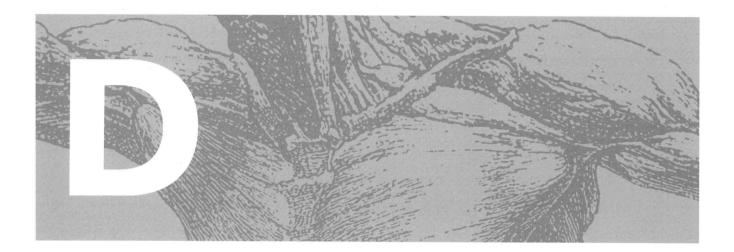

D

Dance Like 'body', dance's meanings and functions have been constituted differently at distinct moments in history. Louis XIV, for example, asserted that dance provides the ideal bodily preparation for the warrior, imparting the agility and adeptness necessary for effective combat. The British sexologist Havelock Ellis identified dance as the consummate elaboration of the sexual impulse, evident in the behaviour of a wide variety of species. The American choreographer Martha Graham described dance as the truthful expression of the psyche's deepest feelings, revealing through the body's movement the innermost impulses of the human soul. The dance anthropologist Joann Kealiinohomoku, having noted the marked differences in dictionary definitions of dance during the twentieth century, offered the following definition:

> Dance is a transient mode of expression, performed in a given form and style by the human body moving in space. Dance occurs through purposefully selected and controlled rhythmic movements; the resulting phenomenon is recognized as dance both by the performer and the observing members of a given group.

If dance has been construed as fulfilling a variety of expressive and social functions, histories of dance have likewise been structured around distinctive conceptions of dance, reflecting in both their organization and choice of subject matter specific notions of dance's meaning. Dance, they assert, has evolved from sacred to profane, or from ritual to spectacle, or from communal play to individual discovery. What seems clear at the beginning of the twenty-first century is the historical and cultural specificity of each of these claims. The following comments, therefore, reflect this author's and this moment's assessment of dance's significance. For who can say how the meaning of dance might change for those who pass their time absorbed in the virtual technologies that the future promises to offer us?

Dance provides a rare opportunity to experience body as both functional and symbolic. While dancing, the individual is embroiled in body as the creative producer of 'ideas', as a medium for communicating ideas, and as the disciplined executant of those ideas. Ideas generated by the dancing body can include images of physical identity, such as a body's characteristic postures, stances, or gestures, or they might include physical representations of thoughts, feelings, moods, intuitions, or impulses. Ideas issuing from the dancing body also consist in pronouncements about its nature — its shapes, its differentiation of body parts or regions, its rhythms, and its tensile qualities of motion — as it negotiates its surroundings and the force of gravity, and as it encounters other bodies. Through the articulation of these ideas, dance both reproduces and generates key cultural values.

Bodies engaged in dancing typically learn a dance — the orchestrated movement patterns known as the choreography — and they also learn to perform the dance, according to the criteria of proper performance of the movement patterns. Both the dance's choreography and performance resonate strongly with more general cultural concerns. BALLET, as practised in Europe and the US, emphasizes the abstract geometry of bodily form exploring the heights and extensions the body can achieve both on the floor and in the air. It constructs unique roles for male and female performers who work together to create a unified whole. Ballet recognizes a hierarchy of skills and physical prowess, and commemorates that hierarchy in the arrangements of soloists and corps de ballet. At the same time, the dancers are asked to mask the extraordinary labour entailed by their bodily elevations, and to make their jumps, balances, and turns appear effortless. In contrast, the West African dance repertoire elaborates a vital connection to earth. Its dances display the capacity of the body to engage in multiple rhythmic patterns simultaneously and to move among different rhythmic structures. It also offers opportunities for improvised dialogue between dancers and musicians. The large number of dances in this tradition, performed at a range of social and religious occasions, provide numerous opportunities for non-professional dancers to participate. In each of these cultural contexts, dance works to illuminate attitudes toward the body and to exemplify patterns of physicalized sociability through which all bodies relate.

Many dance forms require extensive bodily training in order to attain competence at performance. Pedagogies of dance training typically engage the body in extended repetition of movement sequences. These exercises may be taken directly from specific dances or they may consist of sequences that are especially designed to enhance flexibility, strength, endurance, coordination, dexterity, or other physical attributes deemed necessary for successful performance. Each of these training programmes produces a body with distinct capacities and limitations. In ballet, exercises develop the musculature so as to construct ideal lines for arms, legs, and torso, which the choreography then displays. In West African dance, practice is required to learn rhythmic acuity and to extend the body's endurance and its capacity to articulate complex rhythms. For Tongan choreography, dancers work to acquire an articulateness of hands and arms, and a cordial relationship between gesturing appendages and central body, in keeping with the overall aesthetic demands of that form. Bodily competence in each of these forms is highly distinctive, and only rarely can a dancer adapt the training from one tradition for use in a different form.

Through the process of learning to dance, the body is made over into the kind of medium of expression required for a given dance form. The dancer extends and alters the body's physical capacities, and, also, the dancer develops a new symbolic conception of body, of what and how it means. The early modern dancer Isadora Duncan established the diaphragm as the central source of bodily movement and as the place that connected body with soul. In contrast, the Argentine tango locates bodily centre and the source of movement in the constantly changing interplay between male and female partners. The eighteenth-century ballet theorist Jean Georges

Noerre asserted that the face provided a window onto the soul, but that the bottom of the foot offered the key to balance and postural alignment. Dance training inculcates the symbolic interpretation of body as well as the patterned movement responses required by a given form. As these examples demonstrate, there are as many distinct conceptions of body and mappings of bodily meaning as there are dance forms.

Dance provides a vision of what it is to be a body for those who watch it, and an experience of being a body for those who do it. Dance connects this corporeal identity to subjectivity and sociality, so that the dancing body achieves a locatedness in relation to self and others. Dance's transcendent power stems, in part, from just this ability to synthesize physicality with individual, gendered, ethnic, and social identities. At the same time, dance places this experience of identity in motion so that the dancing body comprehends the transitoriness of each moment and its changing relation to the flux of the world.

SUSAN FOSTER

See also BALLET; MUSIC AND THE BODY.

Dance notation

Dance notation approaches the body and its movement in an analytic, abstract, and systematic way, using specific symbols for documenting movement. Not every written documentation of movement can be called dance notation, just as not every movement necessarily constitutes dance. Systematic notation of dance differs from the arbitrary and unsystematic usage of stick figures, verbal descriptions, and floor patterns which can be observed transculturally and transhistorically. During the history of Euro-American dance since the Renaissance, more than fifty different systems of notation have been developed. The high number of systems emphasizes the fact that dance lacks the achievement of European music, where one system of notation has been used since the sixteenth century.

Up until the beginning of the twentieth century, notation was used primarily to record the formalized movements of theatrical dance, mainly ballet, and to a certain extent also of social and folk dances. It is possible to identify several categories in the variety of notational approaches that developed within Europe between 1500 and 1900. The first two categories, 'letter codes' and 'floor plans', used primarily in the sixteenth to eighteenth centuries, concentrate on the execution of dance steps as the primary element of dancing. Body movements beyond those of the feet are either neglected or described in only rudimentary terms. 'Letter codes' are featured for the first time in Thoinot Arbeau's 1588 *Orchesographie*. This book presents a fictional dialogue between a dancing master and his student, in which dance steps are described in the text, and reduced to their initial letters and presented in temporal order in the so-called 'tabulations', which are connected with the musical notes. Arbeau complements these descriptions with drawings showing the whole body in certain steps and postures.

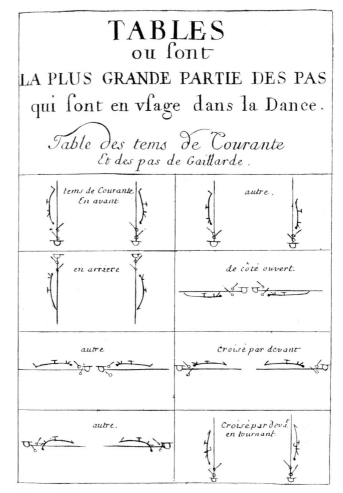

Feuillet system of dance notation.

Notation, featuring 'floor plans', appeared in *Chorégraphie* — a system invented by Pierre Beauchamps and published by Raoul Auger Feuillet in 1700 in Paris. This very influental 'Feuillet System' represents the spatial execution of the steps as seen from a bird's eye view, thus establishing the 'floor plans'. Feuillet's procedure was analytical; he broke up the steps into their mechanical parts, invented symbols for each of those parts, and organized them temporally by bars on the progression line. These bars reflect the temporal sequence of the steps according to the musical score.

In the nineteenth century, two categories of notation systems became prevalent, namely 'stick figure' notations and systems using 'musical notes'. The characteristic feature of both approaches was the isolation of specific movement elements. Notation was no longer limited to the documentation of dance steps alone, but sought to capture the complexity of the whole body movement. The focus shifts from a bird's eye view to a frontal view: the inventors of 'stick figure' systems place themselves in front of or behind the dancers. In his *Stenochorégraphie*, published in Paris and St Petersburg in 1852, Arthur Saint-Léon used a scheme consisting of five horizontal lines for the movements of the legs and one additional line for the actions of the upper body. The figurative notation signs appear directly above the musical score, relating them approximately to the musical values. 'Stick figures' have continued in use as, for example, in *An Introduction to Benesh Notation*, published in 1956, or in the 1973 *Sutton Movement Shorthand*.

Yet another innovate approach to dance notation in the nineteenth century used 'musical notes' to record movement on bars and staffs. Thus, procedures of sound notation are transferred to movement notation: addition (a movement is, just like a musical sound, the sum of several elements) and duration (the temporal value of a movement is indicated by the time value of the note). In his *Alphabet du Corps Humain*, published in 1892 in Paris, Vladimir Stepanov described the human body within a scheme consisting of nine lines, divided into three parts. The top two lines are used for the movements of the head and torso, the three middle lines indicate the actions of the arms, and the bottom four lines the movements of the legs. The position of the tail of a note indicates whether the movement concerns the left or the right body part: for the left parts, the tail is directed upwards, for the right parts, it is directed downwards. The notation system developed by Vaclav Nijinsky in the early 1910s is quite similar: like Stepanov, he used a system of lines consisting of three sections; in contrast, however, he assigned five lines to each of them, thus shifting the focus of movement analysis from the legs toward the torso.

In the twentieth century, dance began to be recorded in 'abstract signs'. This new approach creates a dynamic relationship between notation, the spatial/temporal occurrences and corporeality. Rudolf von Laban's early attempts at notating (his) dance are based upon the concept of 'natural' movement, which for Laban meant emotional and visionary dancing as well as notating. His experiments in the 1920s with notation not only have practical consequences for documenting movement, but also manifest a strong theoretical concern; they relate to his concepts of *Eukinetics* and *Choreutics* — terms describing the patterns of expression he found in the temporal and spatial dynamics of the movement. The original continental *Kinetography Laban* of the late 20s and early 30s as well as the *Labanotation*, a slightly different American version of the 40s, are both still used today — *Kinetography* in continental Europe, *Labanotation*, to a greater extent, in the Anglo-Saxon countries. Both versions go far beyond Laban's initial experiments by shifting their focus from the 'natural' view to the phenomenological aspects of dance. Laban, *Kinetography*, and *Labanotation* use geometrical shapes as symbols that indicate not only directions, but also specific levels and duration. Direction symbols modify the basic rectangular shape and show the directions forwards/backwards and left/right as well as the diagonal directions in between; the shading of the shape indicates the direction upwards/downwards, and its length shows duration. The body is represented within a vertical system from behind that is to be read from the bottom of the paper towards the top: following the central line, the right side of the dancer is also the right side of notation. The central line represents the vertical centre line of the body, and also the progression of the movement. Next to this line, on both sides, there are the columns for all movements transferring weight. The body parts themselves are identified by particular symbols. Their various movements are observed and notated separately and then synchronized in the notation score.

Like *Kinetography* and *Labanotation*, the *Eshkol/Wachmann Notation* of 1958 also conceives movement in its complexity. It consists of various components that can be identified with a finite alphabet of abstract symbols within a system of coordinates. *Eshkol/Wachmann* lists the body parts along the vertical axis; temporal information is given along the horizontal one. The movements themselves are digitalized by using the mechanical potential of the joints: their physical structure forces each movement either into a circular or into a conical shape, and this shape can be identified by evaluating its vertical and horizontal coordinates.

Eshkol/Wachmann Notation shifts the focus of movement analysis from phenomenology toward mechanics. This approach is neutral and abstract, featuring movement observation and composition, but not necessarily dance documentation; it allows to describe movement beyond historical or stylistic definition of dance. Thus, it establishes a new strategy that enables notation to react to contemporary dance concepts: both declare any movement to be able to operate as dance movement, and shape up dance sequences that decidedly transgress traditional and conventional choreography.

CLAUDIA JESCHKE

Further reading

Davies, M. (1972). *Understanding body movement. An annotated bibliography*. Arno Press, New York.

Hutchinson-Guest, A. (1984). *Dance notation*. Dance Books, London.

Hutchinson-Guest, A. (1989). *Choreo-graphics*. Gordon and Breach, New York.

See also BALLET; DANCE.

Deafness For most of us, the term 'deafness' conjures up a frightening image. Becoming deaf in the prime of life must be akin to becoming hard-of-hearing in old age, only infinitely more traumatic. We imagine ourselves turning desperately for help to an *audiologist* (a specialist in the assessment of HEARING), or to a clinician specialised in the diagnosis and treatment of disorders of the ear (an *otologist*). Music, bird song, the warning sound of an approaching car: all of these, plus, most importantly, the possibility of engaging in spoken interaction with our fellows, are lost to us. Yet being deaf has always been much more than this. Throughout much of European history it meant to be an outcast: cut off not only from human society but, far worse, from the word of God.

Recently, a new 'cultural construction of deafness' has emerged. According to this view, to be 'deaf' is to identify with a community in which the dominant medium of communication is sign language, and with its own history, social institutions, and cultural forms. The medical understanding of deafness as hearing loss and the cultural understanding of deafness as social and linguistic difference coexist uneasily in modern societies.

Because of differences in the degree and nature of hearing loss, the overall incidence of deafness is difficult to estimate. However, it is likely that around 15% of the population have impaired hearing, which, in many cases, is accompanied by TINNITUS (ringing in the ears) and BALANCE problems. Deafness is associated with many hereditary and non-hereditary diseases and may also result from pre- or post-natal exposure to a variety of toxins and traumas. The degree of hearing loss can vary greatly, from a very slight impairment in one ear to total deafness in both ears.

Causes of deafness

Although tumours and other disorders may impair the function of the auditory nerve or of those areas of the brain that are responsible for our perception and recognition of sounds, most causes of deafness involve a defect in the ear and may be divided into two types. A *conductive hearing loss* results from conditions that interfere with the transmission of airborne sound through the EXTERNAL EAR and the middle ear. These structures normally conduct sounds efficiently to the sensory apparatus within the cochlea of the inner ear. As sound waves pass through the external ear to the eardrum, their amplitude is increased as a result of the resonant properties of the outer ear and of the ear canal. Vibrations of the eardrum are then coupled by the middle ear ossicles, the three smallest bones in the body, to the fluid-filled cochlea. Conditions that impair sound transmission to the inner ear will therefore attenuate the incoming sound. Conductive hearing loss does not involve damage to the receptor cells or any other nerve cells in the auditory pathway.

The second major type of deafness to originate from abnormalities of the ear is known as a *sensorineural hearing loss*, which is sometimes referred to, albeit usually inaccurately, as 'nerve deafness'. Sensorineural hearing loss most often arises from defects in the cochlea itself, but also describes the hearing deficit that results from damage to the auditory nerve.

Hearing sensitivity varies with sound frequency (or pitch) in a very characteristic way. Decreases in sensitivity at particular frequencies can provide valuable clues as to the nature of the hearing loss. Moreover, although sounds are most effectively conducted to the cochlea by the external and middle ear, they can also reach the cochlea by bone conduction if a vibrating object, such as a tuning fork, is applied to the skull. When airborne sounds are attenuated by disorders of the external ear or the middle ear, hearing by bone conduction should remain normal. On the other hand, sounds transmitted to the cochlea by bone conduction will be heard less well in cases of sensorineural deafness.

Abnormalities of the external ear that result in conductive hearing loss include obstruction of the ear canal, most commonly by wax, and inflammation of the skin surrounding the canal. The eardrum can be ruptured as a result of injury or middle ear disease. Build up of viscous fluid within the normally air-filled middle ear cavity can impede the mobility of the drum and the ossicles. This condition characterises *otitis media* with effusion (glue ear) and is particularly prevalent in infants and young children. Damage to the middle ear ossicles may follow head injury. And in *otosclerosis*, bone growth between the third of these bones — the stapes or stirrup — and the membranous oval window that provides the entrance to the cochlea will immobilize the ossicles and reduce the amount of sound energy that is transmitted. Most forms of conductive hearing loss are characterised by more or less the

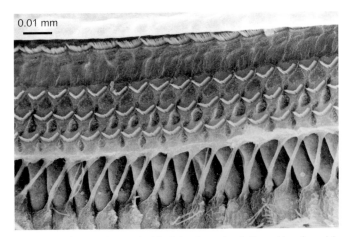

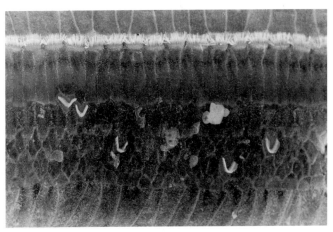

(a) Scanning electron micrograph of the hair cell receptors in the cochlea of a gerbil. The cylindrical structures in the lower part of the picture are outer hair cells, which are arranged in 3 rows. Each outer hair cell has a W-shaped bundle of fine hairs projecting from its apical surface. A single row of inner hair cells bearing hair bundles that are arranged in an approximately straight line can be seen at the top. Mechanical vibrations within the cochlea will deflect the hairs, leading to the generation of electrical currents within the hair cells, which give rise to the sensation of hearing. The scale bar represents one hundredth of a millimetre.

(b) The hair cells in a guinea pig that had been treated with the antibiotic gentamicin for 10 days. Most of the outer hair cells have been lost and replaced by an expansion of supporting cells. The inner hair cells appear to be intact. Damage to outer hair cells can produce hearing losses of up to 50 dB. Kindly supplied by Dr Andrew Forge of the Institute of Laryngology and Otology, University College, London.

same degree of deafness across all sound frequencies. In general, the causes of conductive hearing loss can be remedied by drugs or by surgery. Otherwise, hearing aids provide an effective means of amplifying the sound so that normal hearing can be restored.

In humans, each ear contains about 15 000 sensory hair cells, so named because of the bundle of fine hairs, the *stereocilia*, that project from their apical surfaces. These hair cells convert sound energy into electrical signals, which are conducted to the brain by the fibres of the auditory nerve. In birds, hair cell regeneration occurs following injury. However, if mammalian hair cells die, they are not replaced and so a permanent sensorineural hearing loss results. A variety of factors can cause the hair cells to die. One of these is ageing, and it is a sobering thought that one hair cell dies, without being replaced, approximately every two weeks. This condition, which is called *presbyacusis*, first affects those hair cells that are responsible for high frequency hearing, so the upper frequency limit of hearing progressively declines over a period of years. This leads to difficulties in distinguishing consonants, making it harder for the listener to understand what is being said.

Hair cells can also die as a result of certain infections and as a consequence of exposure to drugs, including therapeutic compounds with 'ototoxic' side-effects, such as the aminoglycoside antibiotics (see figure). However, the commonest cause of acquired sensorineural deafness is excessively loud noise. This used to be referred to as 'boilermaker's disease' because of the incidence of hearing loss among workers subjected, often without ear protectors, to intense industrial sounds. Noise-induced deafness affects all ages and may result from a history of exposure to gunfire, extensive wearing of personal stereos, or

attending too many discos or rock concerts. As with ototoxic drugs, noise trauma involves damage to the stereocilia and, in more severe cases, destruction of the hair cells. High frequencies again tend to be affected first and the hearing loss may be restricted to frequencies around 4 kHz.

In addition to reduced or lost hearing over particular frequency ranges, people with sensorineural deafness often have problems understanding speech in noisy environments and experience an unusually rapid growth in loudness as sound intensity rises. In contrast to conductive hearing losses, surgery rarely helps in the treatment of sensorineural deafness. Hearing aids are therefore used to boost residual hearing, and in cases of total or near total deafness, a new technology, *cochlear implantation*, has been used successfully to bypass the damaged hair cells and to stimulate electrically what remains of the auditory nerve.

The deaf in society

The rehabilitation of the deaf is by no means restricted to attempts to restore or improve hearing, but also includes the utilisation of non-verbal modes of communication. When speech seemed the single most important quality distinguishing man from beast, the question of how the 'deaf and dumb' were to be humanized loomed large. Many eighteenth-century texts contain examples of cures for deafness, of 'deaf mutes' spontaneously bursting into speech, of highly secret techniques for teaching speech to the deaf. In France, however, matters took a different turn. In 1760 the Abbé L'Epée, inspired by ideas taken from the *philosophes* and from John Locke, founded a school based on quite different assumptions. L'Epée distinguished speech from language, concluding that it was the minds, not the tongues, of deaf people that had to be united.

To this end he studied the gestural form of communication that he found among the deaf, and used it to develop a sign-based form of education. Diderot, making a similar distinction between language and its oral expression, developed related ideas in more abstract form, particularly in his *Lettre sur les sourds et muets à l'usage de ceux qui entendent et qui parlent*. Inspired by this work, in the nineteenth century sign-based education spread rapidly, though more easily in some countries than in others.

Towards the end of the nineteenth century the tide turned. A leading figure in the re-establishment of speech-based education was Alexander Graham Bell, best known for his invention of the telephone. Bell had a deaf mother, worked initially as a teacher of the deaf, and subsequently married a deaf woman. Bell feared that the high rate of intermarriage among the deaf would ultimately lead to the 'formation of a deaf variety of the human race'. He argued that both institutions and language (sign language) that facilitate formation of social relationships among the deaf should be banned by law. It did not go so far. But after the Congress of Milan on deaf education (1880) oralist approaches gradually became universal. Sign language and signing teachers were banished from schools for the deaf.

The turn of the nineteenth century saw the emergence of organized deaf clubs and national associations for the protection of the interests of the 'deaf and dumb'. Today, older deaf people tell stories of their schooling: dominated by speech lessons, forced to sit on their hands, punished for signing. Few received any education worth the name, though some found their way into technical trades.

In 1960, and despite widespread scepticism, an American linguist, William Stokoe, embarked on a study of communication among deaf people. It gradually became clear that what was involved was no system of primitive gestures but true language, with all the properties of natural languages. The deaf need no longer be seen as a collection of deprived individuals handicapped by lack of (reflexive) communication. Research on sign language paved the way for sociological investigation of the deaf community and for historical research on the social life of deaf people. The fruits of these researches were to be an important resource: gradually, deaf people began to press for the recognition of sign languages and of their own minority status. Sign language gradually re-entered the schools. In 1980 an important milestone passed. The Swedish government recognized Swedish sign language as an official minority language, with deaf children now having the right to education in their 'own' language. Few countries have as yet followed suit, and in most countries oral and sign-based education are both to be found (together with a mixed form, Total Communication). Nevertheless, where older deaf people are frequently ashamed to use sign language in the presence of hearing people, younger ones sign proudly. Productions in sign language are to be found on television and on the stage.

What does it mean to be deaf today? Few people deafened in middle age become proficient in sign language or identify strongly with deaf culture. What of the child born deaf? Ninety per cent are born to hearing parents. Do those parents try to rear their child to be as like them as possible, as indistinguishable as possible from its hearing peers? Or do they set out to master sign language as best they can, and help their child realize its identity as a culturally Deaf person? Some do one, some the other. Much depends on the advice they receive in those first months of fearsome uncertainty. There is no answer to the question of what it means to grow up deaf. All depends on the choices made by the family, on the child's own personality and attainments, on the educational, social, and cultural environment in which he or she grows up. But growing up deaf is still marked by conflict and uncertainty, for there is little sign of reconciliation between medical and cultural understandings of deafness or those who espouse them. STUART BLUME
ANDREW J. KING

Further reading

Ballantyne, J. and Martin, J. A. M. (1984). *Deafness*, (4th edn) Churchill Livingstone, Edinburgh.

Pickles, J. O. (1988). *An introduction to the physiology of hearing*, (2nd edn). Academic Press, London.

Sataloff, R. T. and Sataloff, J. (1993). *Hearing loss*, (3rd edn) Marcel Dekker, New York.

See also EAR, EXTERNAL; EUSTACHIAN TUBE; HEARING; HEARING AID; TINNITUS.

Death Reports of the first human heart transplants in 1967 made controversy over the definition of death seem as unprecedented as heart transplantation itself — a radically new issue produced by a radically new technology.

But disagreements over the meaning of death long predated the 1960s, and such debates never were simply products of new technical knowledge. From the intense fear in the eighteenth and nineteenth centuries that people were being mistakenly buried alive, to current controversies over BRAIN DEATH, death has long been a contested and changing construct, shaped by scientific discoveries in RESUSCITATION and vivisection, the changing social powers of the medical profession, and changing cultural values. If death means the end of *life*, defining death implies defining life — a long-contentious issue indeed.

1740–1880

For much of the eighteenth and nineteenth centuries, an intense fear of 'premature burial' haunted Western culture, from the tales of Edgar Allen Poe to European laws that imposed long waiting periods before interment. This concern was neither an isolated curiosity nor an outbreak of mass hysteria. Rather, it reflected major changes in the concept of death itself, prompted in large part by new scientific discoveries in resuscitation and experimental vivisection. For example, beginning in the 1740s a series of widely-publicized cases demonstrated that BREATHING and heartbeats could be restarted after they had stopped. To make sense of such resuscitations, London physician John Fothergill proposed that suspended animation was a curable form of death. Like a machine, life could be turned off and on; reanimation was a form of resurrection. However Fothergill's view was rejected by such vitalists as Scottish medical theorist William Cullen (1710–90). Cullen redefined death, not as the actual cessation of heart and lung functions, but as the loss of the potential for muscle and nerve activity ('irritability' and 'sensibility'). His approach reconciled resuscitation with the belief that death was by definition irreversible. However, it offered no way of diagnosing when this vital potential had been lost, and thus no way of knowing for certain when resuscitation efforts should be ended. Others rejected both these new definitions of death, denying that 'suspended animation' was real. They postulated that undetectable levels of heart and lung activity must by definitions have been continuously present in all cases of successful resuscitation.

The mid seventeenth-century discovery that the heart and lungs could be maintained alive in an animal that had been decapitated also challenged concepts of death, by dramatizing the distinction between the death of an organism and the death of its component parts. The guillotine, invented by a doctor to make execution swifter and more humane, also seemed to demonstrate that human heads and bodies could show signs of separate life. Based on such observations, many eighteenth-century medical writers concluded that death was not a single event but a long process taking place at a succession of physiological levels, and that death could not be diagnosed with certainty until the process had concluded with decomposition of body tissues. Such

doctors' doubts about their own ability to diagnose or define death played a key role in triggering the cultural concern that people were being buried alive.

However, the specific fear of premature burial was not simply a product of medical uncertainty. To make sure that their bodies would be dead before burial, some people requested that they be cremated or embalmed. Their terror of being buried alive was more than simply a fear of being mistaken for dead. Romantic fascination with the claustrophobia of isolated helpless confinement, anti-Semitic opposition to traditional Jewish rapid interments, and post-Enlightenment doubts about the afterlife helped shape medical uncertainty about death into the specific horror of being buried too soon.

1880–1960

While the fear of premature burial was triggered by the discoveries of eighteenth-century scientists and physicians, late nineteenth-century doctors generally concluded that new technologies, from the STETHOSCOPE to X-RAYS had solved the problem of diagnosing death. These new instruments did not resolve any of the underlying conceptual controversies over the meaning of death, but an unprecedented faith in technology, from the 1880s through the first half of the twentieth century, led both the medical profession and much of the lay public to stop expressing concern over the persisting philosophical uncertainties. The fear of premature burial never disappeared, but it was largely relegated to such marginal organizations as the *Association for the Prevention of Premature Burial*, an international group of vitalists, anti-vivisectionists, and antibacteriologists, united by their opposition to the growing philosophical materialism and social power of twentieth-century medicine. Women also were disproportionately active in this movement. Some opposed the new technological medicine for undermining nineteenth-century women's efforts to integrate moral and physical healing. Others worried that women were particularly at risk of premature burial, because women were believed to be especially susceptible to FAINTING spells, catatonic fits, and spiritual trances that mimicked death.

Dramatic new discoveries, including recoveries from prolonged HYPOTHERMIA and successful animal head transplants, continued to complicate the era's concepts of death. The resulting uncertainties were widely debated by scientists and the public. Many physiologists agreed with Boston embryologist Charles Minot that organisms were illusory, and that life and death could be defined only at the cellular level. Alternatively, neurologists like Charles Sherrington redefined the life of an organism as the nerve-mediated capacity to integrate organ and tissue functions. Mass culture, from journalism to science fiction, avidly reported these discoveries and disputes. However, unlike in prior centuries, when such scientific developments sparked public panic, in the first half of the twentieth century they were represented as wonderful marvels of modern science, possibly leading to RESURRECTION or immortality. Also, while physiologists, philosophers, and the public continued to ponder the meaning of death, few of this era's practitioners of clinical medicine joined the discussion.

Since 1960

The brain death debates that began in the late 1960s thus did not constitute an unprecedented change in the meaning of death. But the 1960s did mark two new developments: a revival of interest in the issue on the part of clinicians, and a change from optimism to renewed concern on the part of the public. In the late 1960s, several medical leaders such as Harvard University anesthesiologist Henry K. Beecher proposed that patients be declared dead if their brains had irreversibly lost all functioning, even if their other vital functions were being maintained by mechanical ventilators. At first, 'brain death' was explained primarily as a means of defending organ TRANSPLANTATION, and of protecting medicine against the era's renewed social criticism of professional authority. But in the early 1980s, this representation of the issue was dramatically reversed. Brain death now was promoted, not as a defence of medical technology against public criticism, but as a defence of the public against that technology's invasive indignities. Redefining death was understood as logically distinct from EUTHANASIA, but each provided a different way to answer the same clinical question: when should a physician stop treating a patient? Growing public support for a 'right to die' and 'death with dignity' proved crucial to the rapid adoption in the US of the brain death legislation advocated in the 1981 report of the President's Commission on bioethics. To diagnose brain death, the commission specified that the patient must have suffered permanent loss of all brain functions, both 'higher-brain' based activities, such as CONSCIOUSNESS, and basic BRAIN STEM reflexes, such as gagging and pupil constriction. Great Britain adopted slightly different criteria, promoted by Christopher Pallis, under which the permanent loss of brain stem functions was considered sufficient to diagnose brain death.

Despite the success of brain death legislation, the fear of being treated too long was added to, not substituted for, the fear of being abandoned too soon. Mass culture continued to link brain death with organ-stealing doctors, as in the 1977 book and subsequent motion picture *Coma*. Orthodox Jews, traditionalist Japanese, and 'right to life' supporters are all deeply divided over whether to accept any brain-based definition of death. Some African Americans expressed concern that brain death was being used to take organs prematurely from blacks for transplantation to whites.

On the other hand, many philosophers, such as pioneer bioethicist Robert Veatch, attacked 'whole brain' legislation as failing to resolve crucial conceptual ambiguities. They promoted various 'higher-brain' alternatives that define human death as the permanent loss of consciousness and personal identity — as in the persistent VEGETATIVE STATE.

Thus, while the whole-brain definition of death has won wide acceptance, death remains a controversial and contingent concept, as it has been for centuries, at the intersection of changes in physiological research, medical practice, social structure, and cultural values.

MARTIN PERNICK

Further reading

Pernick, M. S. (1988). Back from the grave: recurring controversies over defining and diagnosing death in history. In *Death: beyond whole-brain criteria*, (ed. R. M. Zaner), pp. 17–74. Kluwer Academic Publishers, Dordrecht and Boston.

Pernick, M. S. (1999). Brain death in a cultural context: the reconstruction of death 1967–1981. pp 3–33 In *The definition of death*, (ed. S. Younger, R. Arnold, and R. Schapiro). Johns Hopkins University Press, Baltimore.

President's Commission for the Study of Ethical Problems in Medicine and Biomedical and Behavioral Research (1981). *Defining Death*. US Government Printing Office, Washington, DC.

See also BRAIN DEATH; COMA; CORPSE; EUTHANASIA; FUNERAL PRACTICES; LIFE SUPPORT; ORGAN DONATION; RESURRECTION; RESUSCITATION; TRANSPLANTATION; VEGETATIVE STATE; ZOMBIE.

Death rattle the gurgling sound produced by air passing through mucus or fluid in the lungs of a dying person. It is said to indicate approaching death, or sometimes to be the sign of the arrival of death itself; the last sound a dying person makes.

Gustave Flaubert described Emma Bovary's death rattle in vivid terms:

> At once her breast began to heave rapidly. Her tongue hung at full length from her mouth; her rolling eyes grew dim like the globes of two lamps about to go out; and one might have thought her dead already but for the terrifying, ever-faster movement of her ribs, which were shaken by furious gasps, as though her soul were straining violently to break its fetters.

SARAH GOODFELLOW

Death's head The figure of the death's head has been a prominent symbol of human mortality and the vanity of life in Western culture. Whether it appears in the hands of Shakespeare's Hamlet or as an emblem for a 1980's heavy metal band, the human SKULL brings DEATH to mind; as a well-known and popular image, its primary purpose is to draw attention to the end of life. Although the death's head has roots in more macabre images of the *transi*, or rotting, worm-infested CORPSE, the meanings of the death's head, and the animated SKELETON in general, have multiplied over the last several centuries.

The skull is the most recognizably human element of the entire skeletal frame; it is also a strange, disconcerting object to reflect on because the fleshless face, hollow eyes, and bared teeth anticipate the future state of all who contemplate it. When the skull is detached from the rest of the skeleton and inserted into a particular context, it communicates a general message about the human condition. This message can be related to inevitable change and dissolution, Christian conversion, or simply existential horror; the supporting iconographic field of images usually determines the symbolic valences of the death's head.

As historian Philippe Ariès argues, the appearance of the skull in a variety of artistic expressions and everyday objects, beginning in the sixteenth century, was linked to a new sensibility about life known as the *vanities*. The sentiments associated with the vanities expressed a range of rather sombre, melancholy notions, including the swift passage of time, the fragility of human life, and the centrality of death in all human affairs. Whereas the earlier expressions of the macabre often imagined death as a supernatural threat existing outside of human nature, the vanities reconsiders the power of death as an integral condition of life itself. The ideas tied to these sentiments related both to distinctly religious strategies for conversion, and to more secular musings about the brute facts of physical death and the transitory nature of this world. Indeed, after the sixteenth century the death's head becomes one of the most popular versions of the *memento mori* theme: 'Remember, you must die!'

The range of possible meanings identified with the death's head depends very much on cultural setting. In Puritan New England, for example, this symbol had specific religious value to the community understanding of death. Cotton Mather captured the common religious assumptions associated with contemplating the death's head when he wrote: 'That man is like to die comfortably, who is every Day minding himself, that he is to die shortly. Let us look upon every thing as a sort of Death's-Head set before us, with a Memento mortis written upon it.' In the ICONOGRAPHY of early New England cemeteries, the death's head was combined with an array of images, including scythes, crowns, hourglasses, and wings, to represent both the swiftness of time and the possibilities of spiritual regeneration.

In more recent times, the symbolism of the death's head has less to do with the vanities theme and more to do with modern fears and anxieties about violence and death. Although it has retained its function as a *memento mori*, the death's head does not always lead to melancholy contemplation of the shortness of life and inevitable decay. It can often bring to mind the presence of evil in the world and, in many cases, it serves as a general symbol alerting individuals to impending mortal danger.

GARY LADERMAN

Further reading

Ariès, P. (1991). *The hour of our death*. Oxford University Press, New York.

See also DEATH; SKULL.

Debauchery A formula for debauchery may be reduced to the single-minded pursuit of flagons, feasts, and fornication. Traditionally one who over-indulgences in the sensual appetites, particularly EATING and drinking, the debauchee is laid bare in Thomas Warton the Elder's poem *The Glutton* (1747):

> Fat, pamper'd *Porus*, eating for Renown,
> In Soups and Sauces melts his Manors down;
> Regardless of his Heirs, with mortgag'd Lands,
> Buys hecatombs of Fish, and Ortolans;
> True Judge of Merit, most disdainful looks
> On Chiefs and Patriots when compar'd to Cooks;
> With what Delight Pigs whipt to Death he crams
> On fattn'd Frogs, or Essences of Hams;
> For fifty thousand Tongues of Peacocks sighs
> Mix'd with the Brains of Birds of Paradise;
> Loud ring the Glasses, powder'd Footmen run,
> He eats, drinks, surfeits, still eats, is undone!
> See the swoln Glutton in terrific State,
> Behind his chair what dire Diseases wait?

Warton goes on to make explicit the relationship between gluttony and morbidity, by indicating what diseases lurk behind the piled high plates of food. To his catalogue of illness, which includes GOUT, Asthma, and APOPLEXY, may be added OBESITY and heart disease. Gluttony is a slave to a passion which turns feasts into orgies of immoral excess. A table-fellow of the glutton is invariably the gourmet, whose debaucheries tend to be more qualitative than quantitative.

Connoisseurs of food become debauched once eating becomes an act of immorality. Aside from obvious examples such as gratuitous CANNIBALISM or the eating of live animals, the debauched gourmet offends cultural codes by going beyond the limits of good taste. Such transgressions may include the preparation of a domestic pet or the creation of a tasty fricassée out of certain taboo animals. Nowadays, there is even greater condemnation of 'delicacies' involving ingredients containing endangered species — like the ancient Chinese speciality, Panda Paw Casserole, the recipe for which was given to M. Urbain Dubois, chef to the Prussian monarchy during the nineteenth century.

The Renaissance French author, François Rabelais, was caricatured as a drunken buffoon, whose most enduring legacy was his comic fiction *Gargantua* (1534–5). The eponymous giant–hero and his creator have become synonymous with images of engorgement, as in the proverbial gargantuan appetite and Rabelasian excesses.

No better example of the latter can be found, albeit anachronistically, than in the Roman banquet, whose corollary was the aptly named *vomitarium*. The most famous account is that of Trimalchio's feast narrated by Petronius in his *Satyricon* (*c.* 65AD). Here guests had wine poured over their hands before being presented with sows' udders, plump fowls, and a hare with wings fastened to its back to look like Pegasus. The centre-piece was an enormous platter carried into the dining room on which lay a wild boar with a basket of Syrian dates and one of Theban dates

hanging from its tusks. A slave drew a hunting knife and stabbed the wild boar in the belly. Out of the gash flew live thrushes, which were caught and distributed to guests. An enormous pig was served up on the table, whose stomach was slashed open, a cornucopia of black puddings and sausages pouring out of it.

Nostalgia for a more extreme example of the dissipations of ancient Rome is expressed by the Comte de Gernande, who, mercifully, is only a fictional character in the Marquise de Sade's *La Nouvelle Justine* (1797):

> I admit that I have often wanted to imitate the debauchery of Apicius, that most famous of Roman gourmets. He had slaves thrown live into his fish ponds so that the flesh of his fish would achieve a greater delicacy. I am cruel in my lusts and would be even more so when it came to such acts of debauchery. I would sacrifice a thousand if necessary, just to eat a dish which was more tempting or recherché

The conflation between cruelty and food was not confined to the Roman Empire. The lunch and dinner of Tz'u-hsi, the Chinese Dragon Empress, who reigned between 1861 and 1908, consisted of hundreds of dishes from which she always picked her favourites. Aware of this, her chefs did not replace most other dishes for up to ten days, with the result that they would be crawling with weevils. A favoured lady-in-waiting, at the Empress's possibly sadistic invitation, would be forced to sample, with a smile, one of those rotting dishes. Imperial decadence can be seen here in wasting food on a gargantuan scale in an inversion of satiation. Whoever was unfortunate enough to have to entertain the Emperor Charles V for lunch, was expected to serve up no less than 400 dishes. De Sade's Comte de Gernande's more modest fare was in evidence during the feast he had hosted, which consisted of 89 dishes. During the meal, however, he drank 12 bottles of wine followed by a Tokay, a Paphos, a Madeira, and a Falernian with the fruit. His night-cap consisted of two bottles of *liqueurs des îles*, two bowls of punch, a pint of rum, and 10 cups of coffee.

The libertine used such banquets to stimulate lust, particularly as the ability to eat a huge meal has been seen as a signifier of sexual prowess. Descriptions of food are often used in novels to sublimate sexual desire. The Marquise de Sade's notorious sweet tooth provided him with yet another tool of debauchery, as when he secretly fed some prostitutes, the aphrodisiac Spanish Fly, disguised in chocolate, making them severely ill. Sexual practices that have been regarded as the height of debauchery are the kind of sadistic bedroom activities to which the Marquise gave his name. As John Henry Meibomius points out in *A Treatise of the Use of Flogging in Venereal Affairs* (1718): 'there are Persons who are stimulated to *Venery by Strokes of Rods, and worked up into a Flame of Lust by Blows*, and that the Part, which distinguishes us to be Men, should be raised by the Charm of invigorating Lashes.'

Far more benign was the pseudo-Aristotelian, anonymously written sex manual, *Aristotle's Master-piece* — even though it was described as 'an hoary old debauchee as acknowledged by no-one' by D'Arcy Power, the twentieth-century surgeon. Ironically this mine of medical misinformation about SEXUALITY was intended to exalt the state of matrimony. To see *Aristotle's Master-piece* as debauched in its dissemination of sexual advice, over the course of three centuries, is a legacy of Victorian prurience. The mark of true debauchees is, surely, when individuals have become so consumed by the excesses of their own sensual desires and carnal appetites that they can no longer function as whole and integral human beings. MARIE MULVEY-ROBERTS

Decompression sickness may be defined as the illness associated with the formation, following a reduction in ambient pressure, of bubbles from gases dissolved in the body.

The clinical syndrome of decompression sickness was recognised in divers and compressed air workers in the middle of the nineteenth century, but the first description of the similar condition induced by exposure to ALTITUDE was not made until 1930, and altitude decompression sickness was not widely acknowledged until the late 1930s.

Bubble formation

Man's tissues at sea level have dissolved gas tensions in equilibrium with the atmosphere. At a raised environmental pressure, there is further uptake of gases from the lungs into solution by the blood and tissues until equilibrium is achieved with the new raised partial pressures of the respiratory gases — quickly by some tissues, and more slowly by others such as cartilage. On decompression these dissolved gases are excreted through the lungs until a new equilibrium is achieved at the new pressure. When the rate of decompression exceeds that at which the excess gases dissolved in the tissues can be excreted, gas may come out of solution and form bubbles.

In DIVING, therefore, the longer the exposure, and the higher the pressure, the more slowly a diver must return to the surface, to avoid decompression illness, which includes also the consequences of barotrauma — damage by expansion of gases in body cavities.

Those combinations of depth and duration of dive that allow the diver a direct return to atmospheric pressure without incurring the overt manifestations of decompression illness form the '*no-stop curve*'. Very approximately, he may surface directly after unlimited time at slightly less than 10 m, 60 min at 18 m, and 20 min at 30 m; at the extreme, experience from submarine escape suggests a safe duration of only about 30 sec at around 180 m. Increasing depths and durations beyond this fuzzy curve represent an increasing risk of decompression illness and require the use of a slow decompression profile to minimise bubble formation and its consequences. For many years the presence of bubbles in the bloodstream was thought to be synonymous with acute decompression sickness, until bubbles were detected by the use of ultrasound in divers who developed no subsequent manifestations. Thus another aspect in the causation of decompression sickness is the response of the individual to the presence of bubbles and their effects.

The causes of decompression *sickness*, the dissolved-gas variety of decompression *illness*, include omission of the accepted decompression stops, the use of decompression tables or of a personal diving computer based on inappropriate mathematical models — and, perhaps most commonly, individual variation. Many factors affect individual susceptibility, such as dehydration, adaptation to decompression, in-water exercise, and water temperature.

Decompression illness can occur even in those who have followed all the rules meticulously. The causes of its most severe form, neurological decompression illness from *gas embolism*, are the same as those of *pulmonary barotrauma*, but this neurological condition can arise with no evidence of lung injury. Thus the diagnosis of the underlying cause of a case of decompression illness can be difficult but, as the treatment procedures are virtually the same, a general diagnosis of decompression illness is all that is needed in this emergency.

Decompression sickness can be a hazard also when ascending to altitude in an aircraft. Some of the nitrogen normally dissolved at ground level is excreted in the expired gas, but the rate at which it can be excreted through the lungs is slow relative to the rate at which the environmental pressure is reduced in flight; some tissues therefore eventually become supersaturated with nitrogen. Under certain circumstances this supersaturation gives rise to the formation of bubbles of gas within the tissues and blood. The bubbles are carried in the blood to the right side of the heart and thence to the lungs. Bubbles can be detected in the chambers of the right side of the heart after exposure for several hours to altitudes of the order of 15 000–18 000 feet, but symptoms of decompression sickness do not occur until the altitude exceeds 18 000 feet. The incidence and intensity of the symptoms increase with the altitude and the duration of the exposure. The incidence of severe symptoms necessitating immediate descent varies from 0.7% after 1 hour at 28 000 feet to 45% after 4 hours' exposure to 35 000 feet.

Symptoms and signs

The commonest symptom of decompression sickness is a 'bend', which is a deep seated pain in or near a limb joint, probably caused by bubbles in the ligaments around the joint. Itching, tingling, and 'formication' (sensation as of crawling insects) are also common symptoms due to bubbles forming in the skin. Much less common but more serious are respiratory disturbances, 'the chokes', comprising a tightness in the chest, an inspiratory 'snatch,' and coughing. These symptoms are believed to be due to bubbles being carried from the periphery to the lungs. Other serious symptoms of decompression sickness include visual disturbances and severe headaches, and sensory disturbances. Less frequently, weakness or paralysis of a limb or limbs, or unconsciousness, may occur. Decompression sickness can give rise to circulatory collapse. Very rarely, recovery does not occur and death supervenes.

Prevention

For divers and compressed air workers, prevention is based upon adherence to a slow decompression procedure designed to permit the safe excretion of dissolved gases. The printed Decompression Tables available and the online personal decompression computers used by some divers are all derived from the concepts of Professor J. S. Haldane nearly a century ago. These predictions, although validated by the experience of large populations, do not always hold for every dive. Illness still occurs even when everything appears to have been done correctly.

For aircrew, there are three ways of avoiding or preventing decompression sickness at altitude. The most satisfactory way is to avoid exposure to altitudes at which it occurs. Provided that an individual has not been exposed to breathing air at pressures greater than one atmosphere in the 24 hours prior to the ascent, decompression sickness does not occur at altitudes below 18 000 feet. Since the susceptibility to decompression sickness varies considerably from one person to another it is possible to select for high-altitude flights those who are relatively resistant to the condition. This approach was widely used during World War II. The third method of prevention is to remove the nitrogen from the tissues of the body by breathing 100% oxygen prior to the ascent — a procedure known as pre-oxygenation or denitrogenation. Complete protection requires that 100% oxygen is breathed for at least 4 hours before ascent, but even 30 min pre-oxygenation is effective for ascents up to 45 000 feet provided that the duration of exposure at more than 18 000 feet does not exceed about 20 min.   JOHN ERNSTING
DAVID ELLIOTT

Further reading

Bennett, P. B. and Elliott, D. H. (1993). *The physiology and medicine of diving*, (4th edn). Saunders, London.

Ernsting, J. and King, P. (1988). *Aviation medicine*, (2nd edn). Butterworth-Heinemann, Oxford.

See also DIVING; GASES IN THE BODY; HYPERBARIC CHAMBER; NITROGEN; OXYGEN.

Decongestant: a drug used to relieve congestion caused by swelling in the mucous membranes of the nose and sinuses. This condition is brought about by an allergic response (as in hay fever), or by an infection with *rhinoviruses* (as in the common cold) or influenza viruses: local inflammation occurs in which the blood vessels are dilated and mucus secretion increases. Decongestants contain agents which cause *vasoconstriction* when applied locally to the nose — usually ones which act on α-adrenoceptors (see MEMBRANE RECEPTORS). Ephedrine and phenylephrine are common examples. While decongestants bring speedy relief, it is often short-lived, and may be followed by a rebound congestion. Prolonged vasoconstriction of the blood vessels of the nasal mucous membrane can lead to chronic *rhinitis* (Greek: *rhis*, nose; *itis*, inflammation).   A.W.C.

Defecation is the process by which FAECES (stools) are ejected from the rectum. This is a co-ordinated neuromuscular process involving relaxation of the muscles that normally maintain continence at other times.

When sufficient faecal material has entered the rectum, the 'call to stool' is evoked. Distension of the rectum by inflating a balloon can reproduce this sensation and invoke the relaxation of the sphincters which allow defecation to proceed. Providing the continence mechanisms are intact the relaxation can be voluntarily overridden—the 'call to stool' can be delayed until it is socially convenient to defecate.

The most common physiological stimulus to defecation is eating. This initiates the 'gastro–colonic reflex' which results in increased motor activity in the colon and the passage of faeces from the colon into the rectum. Sitting or squatting straightens the angle between the rectum and the short anal canal, and contractions in the colon force additional stool into the rectum to initiate a defecation reflex and sphincter relaxation. Although many individuals 'strain' (perform a Valsalva manoeuvre: see BLOOD PRESSURE), which increases intra-abdominal pressure and facilitates movement of faeces into the rectum, this is not strictly necessary since the process will proceed automatically.

There are two major — and opposite — disorders of defecation, namely faecal incontinence and obstructed defecation.

Faecal incontinence results when the anal sphincter is no longer competent to prevent the unscheduled evacuation of faeces. This may occur as a result of injury to the local nerves serving the sphincters or as a result of disease of the CENTRAL NERVOUS SYSTEM, notably DEMENTIA, mental retardation, STROKE, brain tumours, and spinal cord lesions. Local nerves may be affected as part of widespread nerve damage (*polyneuropathy*) in conditions such as as DIABETES mellitus, although perhaps the most common situation is that of sacral nerve damage associated with PREGNANCY and delivery. Incontinence may also occur as a result of primary muscle disorders or as a result of direct sphincter damage following surgery, radiation, or inflammatory disorders. Incontinence can also occur in the irritable bowel syndrome and in situations of extreme anxiety.

Obstructed defecation. Recently it has become apparent that some individuals with constipation have a problem with co-ordination of the process of defecation, and a failure to relax pelvic and sphincter muscles to allow the evacuation of faeces. This may be part of the spectrum of sacral nerve damage, although there is also evidence that there may be a psychological component in addition.

Management of defecation disorders

Degenerative neuromuscular disorders which affect the defecatory process are extremely difficult to treat and in some instances a *colostomy* is the only socially acceptable intervention. However, when there is evidence of traumatic damage to the anal sphincter, surgical repair is a possibility. In individuals with only partially impaired sphincter function, continence can be maintained for some time with the use of simple anti-diarrhoeal drugs and possibly bulking agents. There is no universally accepted treatment for obstructed defecation, although psychotherapy and behaviour therapy, particularly using biofeedback techniques, have been successful.

MICHAEL FARTHING
ANNE BALLINGER

See also ALIMENTARY SYSTEM; AUTONOMIC NERVOUS SYSTEM; CONSTIPATION; FAECES; TOILET PRACTICES.

Defibrillator
This is a device used in the treatment of life-threatening disturbances of the rhythm of the heart beat which may occur as the result of a HEART ATTACK or a variety of serious injuries or illnesses. Its effect is to 'reset' the electrical activity of the HEART in the hope that the natural PACEMAKER cells can then regain control of the rhythm. Defibrillation using direct current, in the form of an unsynchronised countershock, is usually the only way to halt ventricular fibrillation. The countershock from the defibrillator produces a sustained simultaneous excitation (and hence contraction) of all cardiac muscle fibres, which can terminate ventricular fibrillation and other abnormal rhythms. The countershock is administered by pressing a button on each of two defibrillator 'paddles' placed on the chest wall. Firm pressure is applied to these paddles to ensure good electrical contact with the skin; this also forces air out of the lungs to bring the chest wall in closer contact with the heart. While the shock is discharged, the patient often 'jumps' because motor nerves and SKELETAL MUSCLES are simultaneously, unavoidably stimulated.

DAVID J. MILLER
NIALL MACFARLANE

See also CARDIAC ARREST; ELECTROCARDIOGRAM; HEART; HEART ATTACK.

Degeneration
The idea that a nation, a 'race', or even human civilisation is on a path of inevitable decay and decline has appeared in different guises throughout history. But from the later nineteenth through the early twentieth centuries, such theories gained unprecedentedly wide circulation in European science and culture, as observers perceived alarming increases in criminality, morbidity, and mental pathology. Indeed, as Daniel Pick has shown in his thorough study of the concept, ideas of medical decline — or degeneration — were deeply intertwined with the political and scientific developments of this period, becoming the central focus of numerous social and biological investigations.

The French physician Bénédict-Augustin Morel (1809–73), traditionally seen as the first theorist of degeneration, expressed these ideas in an influential treatise entitled *Traité de dégénérescence*, which appeared in the same year (1857) as Baudelaire's *Fleurs du mal*, a volume of poetry concerned, in a sense, with similar themes. Having devoted himself to the study of '*cretinism*', an allegedly incurable, heritable mental and moral disorder, Morel viewed the so-called cretin as a symbol of humanity's racial degeneration, which manifested itself in deteriorating physical, mental, and even cultural conditions. Though rather controversial at the time of their publication, Morel's ideas attained increasing influence in the aftermath of France's disastrous military performance in the Franco-Prussian war of 1870, and critically informed a growing body of medical studies on crime, prostitution, and insanity toward the end of the century.

These ideas had perhaps their greatest impact on the emerging sciences of *psychiatry, anthropology*, and *criminology*, and deeply influenced such thinkers as the Italian–Jewish criminologist Cesare Lombroso (1835–1909). Lombroso's theory of *atavism* posited the existence of an unevolved 'criminal type', a biological anachronism, which harkened back to a primitive stage of development and was detectable through morphological and physiognomic stigmata. In contrast to French thinkers, who tended to focus on the invisible, 'internal' signs of degeneration, Lombroso concentrated on these outward, visible characteristics, which are well encapsulated in the following litany:

> … enormous jaws, high cheek bones, prominent superciliary arches, solitary lines in the palms, extreme size of the orbits, handle-shaped ears found in criminals, savages and apes, insensibility to pain, extremely acute sight, tattooing, excessive idleness, love of orgies

Another key theorist of degeneration was Max Nordau (1849–1923), a Hungarian-born physician and journalist, who eventually became a major Zionist leader. Nordau lamented increasing rates of hysteria and mental disorder — and their reflection in 'degenerate' cultural forms — in a widely read and controversial 1892 book entitled simply *Degeneration* (Entartung). For Nordau and numerous contemporaries, nineteenth-century technologies had exerted a deleterious effect on the mind and body, leading to a fatigue-induced HYSTERIA, which was then passed on through the generations.

More mainstream medical figures, such as the American physician George M. Beard (1839–83), the French neurologist Jean-Martin Charcot (1825–93), and the British alienist Henry Maudsley (1835–1918), also saw causal connections between degeneration and nervous disease. Even Charles Darwin (1809–82) subscribed to theories of degeneration, viewing madness as closer to a primitive, animal-like state than to human civilisation.

The idea that, due to centuries of 'inbreeding', Jews were disproportionately degenerate, or most susceptible to mental illness, was popular among many of these thinkers; such claims were most famously made by Charcot and the German psychiatrist Emil Kraepelin (1856–1926), but were assumed by Nordau and other Jewish writers as well. Meanwhile, anthropologists and biologists applied these theories to non-white 'races', alternately viewing entire peoples as degenerate, and seeing particular individuals as having decayed (or fallen) from the true properties of their racial type through exposure to foreign cultures and climates. Similarly, turn-of-the-century sexologists and psychiatrists raced to document degenerate sexual types and the alleged degeneracy of Hottentot or African sexuality. A reaction to scientific concern with sexual degeneracy took the form of the '*Decadence*' a cultural moment most associated with Oscar Wilde, which celebrated subversive sexual styles and challenged normative GENDER roles.

Thus in these late nineteenth-century formulations, degeneration connoted a kind of collective genetic decay variously plaguing a specific nationality or the entire human species, and allegedly manifested in a series of medical, moral, and cultural crises. Influenced by these ideas — and the widely bemoaned therapeutic inefficacy of psychiatric medicine against the allegedly growing incidence of mental illness — various scientists sought collective, eugenic solutions which aimed to root out genetic impurities by directly intervening in reproductive choices and processes. So-called *negative eugenics* — first applied in the sterilisation laws of several American states — became integral to the biologistic vision of Nazi Germany and helped motivate the brutal murder of tens of thousands of psychiatric patients. Indeed, the Nazi period saw the return of degeneration in both its cultural and medical forms; the concept facilitated the simultaneous condemnation of the physical condition and the artistic expressions of Jews and other targeted groups, such as homosexuals, gypsies, and the mentally ill. To radical right-wing ideologues, modern, avantgarde art, like the degenerate body, represented an evolutionary failure, causing the pathological persistence of the primitive in the midst of the healthy and new.

PAUL LERNER

Further reading
Gilman, S. L. and Chamberlin, J. E. (1985). *Degeneration: the dark side of progress*. Columbia University Press, New York.

Pick, D. (1989). *Faces of degeneration: a European disorder*. Cambridge University Press.

See also EUGENICS; CRIMINALS; RACISM.

Delirium
is a widely-used diagnostic category used to denote a confused and excited state. It has been recognized ever since antiquity. Plato

stated that there were four kinds of delirium; that of the prophets sent by Apollo, that of the 'initiated' sent by Dionysus, that of the poets due to the Muses, and that of lovers caused by Aphrodite and Eros.

The core symptoms are disturbances of CONSCIOUSNESS accompanied by a change in cognition. The disturbance develops over a period of hours or days, and tends to fluctuate. A patient may be coherent and co-operative in the morning but at night insist on leaving hospital and going home to long-dead parents. Maniacal excitement often sets in, sometimes accompanied by violence. Other physical manifestations include muscular tremors and sweats.

The disturbance in consciousness is marked by a muddled awareness. Attention is impaired, and a delirious person is difficult to engage in conversation and easily distracted by irrelevant stimuli. There is an accompanying change in cognition — MEMORY impairment, disorientation, or LANGUAGE disturbance — and sometimes the emergence of perceptual disturbance, usually manifested in disorientation with respect to time or place. In some cases, speech is rambling or incoherent. Language disturbance may be evident, as in *dysnomia* (impaired ability to name objects) or *dysgraphia* (reduced ability to write). Perceptual disturbances are common. A banging door may be mistaken for a gunshot (*misinterpretation*); bedclothes may turn into terrifying animals (*illusion*); or the person may 'see' enemies when no one is actually there (*hallucination*).

The debates over delirium as a diagnostic label concern its relationship to mental disease and, hence, more broadly, to the MIND-BODY PROBLEM. Until the nineteenth century, disorientation with memory loss, and loss of the sense of time and place, was routinely considered a sign of mental disease. Since then, it has become accepted that many types of mental disorder occur without delirium (*manie sans délire* in the formulation developed by Pinel and Esquirol in France). There has, by consequence, been a growing tendency to stress the organic aetiology of delirium.

In modern medical thinking it is axiomatic that delirium is primarily an organic condition. From the patient's history, physical examination, or laboratory tests it will be apparent whether it arises as a physiological consequence of some medical condition (e.g. fever), or through injury to the head, or through substance intoxication or withdrawal, or through use of a medication (for instance, bromides or barbiturates), or by exposure to POISON.

Substance-induced delirium has achieved considerable prominence nowadays. This includes the diagnosis of *delirium tremens* — a state of confusion, agitation, and tremulousness, associated with alcohol or its withdrawal, first identified as a separate clinical entity in 1813 by Thomas Sutton, who coined the term. Alcoholic delirium is a product not merely of excessive alcohol consumption but of accompanying exhaustion, lack of food, and dehydration. The patient has usually been deteriorating physically because of vomiting and restlessness. Vitamin B deficiency is also implicated.   ROY PORTER

Further reading
Berrios, G. E. (1996). *The history of mental symptoms: descriptive psychopathology since the nineteenth century.* Cambridge University Press.

See also MIND-BODY PROBLEM; PSYCHOLOGICAL DISORDERS.

Dementia

… Last scene of all,
That ends this strange eventful history,
Is second childishness, and mere oblivion,
Sans teeth, sans eyes, sans taste, sans everything

[Shakespeare, *As You Like It*]

We all fear disintegration of the mind, and rightly so; it robs us of our dignity. Bereft of reason we cannot contribute to society, vote, write a will, nor with time care for our basic needs. The disintegration of the mind, or dementia, is a familiar occurrence in the elderly but can occur at any age and result from a vast array of diseases. The loss of acquired intellectual skills — the characteristic feature of dementia — is distinct from developmental failure, which results in learning difficulties of variable severity. We may also be robbed of our senses by SLEEP or inebriation, and so the term 'dementia' is restricted to individuals who are awake and alert. Similarly, patients with a restricted cognitive deficit such as impairment of LANGUAGE following a STROKE may have a very different prognosis, with preservation of other intellectual functions, when compared with the widespread disintegration commonly seen with the dementing diseases. A definition of dementia has thus emerged to describe an individual who is alert but who suffers impairment in more than one cognitive domain, of sufficient severity to impair social function. A difficulty in applying the definition is to decide what is a specific cognitive domain. Impairment of MEMORY is considered essential, or more specifically impairment of event memory: that which allows us to recall day-to-day events and maintains our sense of continuity; impairment of memory is a salient feature of *Alzheimer's disease*, the commonest cause of dementia. Other cognitive domains may include language; visuospatial and visuoperceptual functions, which allow interpretation of our visual world; and so-called 'frontal executive skills', which allow us to plan and select appropriate responses to our environment.

It is important to emphasise that dementia is a syndrome and not a disease. The challenge to the clinician is to identify the underlying cause, of which there are many. Alzheimer's disease is the commonest, particularly in the elderly; it is thus the main cause of 'senile dementia', a term that is becoming obsolete. It was described in 1906 by Alois Alzheimer, and was considered a rarity occurring in relatively young people ('*presenile dementia*'), until the 1960s, when it was recognized that the microscopic abnormalities described by Alzheimer were also found in the demented elderly. This led to an apparent epidemic as patients were reassigned from the categories of 'just old age' or 'senile dementia' to Alzheimer's disease.

Alzheimer had exploited the newly-discovered silver staining method for microscopic examination of nerve tissue, to visualize abnormal cellular changes in the brain. He studied the brain of a 51-year-old patient, Auguste D., whom he had seen whilst working in Frankfurt and who died at the age of 54 years with severe dementia. He reported the hallmark features: 'neurofibrillary tangles' and 'senile plaques'. Recent research has shown that the neurofibrillary tangle results from a collapse of the 'internal skeleton' of brain cells (the *neuronal cytoskeleton*). Senile plaques consist of disrupted neuronal connections, axons, and dendrites, around a core of abnormal deposits of a protein called *beta amyloid*. This protein undergoes a change in shape that renders it harmful to the cell; exactly how and why these changes occur is the subject of intense research aimed at finding effective treatments.

Alzheimer's disease is the prototypic dementia, characteristically starting with mild forgetfulness and a tendency to repetition in conversation: memory failure worsens, with appointments and recent events forgotten. Losing their way, at first in unfamiliar and then in familiar surroundings, patients become increasingly bemused and testy. Failure of language follows, with increasing difficulty in making sense of the world around them. Dressing, feeding, and toileting all require help before the final stage 'sans everything'.

A variety of other degenerative diseases have been, and are being, identified as causes of dementia, including *Creutzfeldt Jakob disease* and *Pick's disease*. The latter was described as long ago as 1894. Arnold Pick, a neurologist from Prague, reported a patient with loss of language who was found to have circumscribed shrinkage or atrophy of the temporal lobe, the area of the brain involved with language function. Pick reported the case to disprove the prevailing dogma that all senile atrophies inevitably involved the whole brain. It was Alzheimer's subsequent analysis of such cases that identified silver-stained 'Pick bodies' as distinct from the neurofibrillary tangles of his own eponymous disease. Pick's disease is rare and cannot be reliably diagnosed without examination of brain tissue after death, and so is generally swept up in the wider diagnostic category of the fronto-temporal degenerations. Reflecting the areas of the brain affected, such patients present with impairment of language or of social behaviour; whilst at first the symptoms may be confined to one cognitive domain, other functions decline and the clinical picture becomes that of a dementia.

Before the demonstration that the changes of Alzheimer's disease were the common accompaniment of dementia in old age, it used to be thought that such cases were due to a failure of the blood supply, starving the brain of oxygen. There is no evidence that this is so, but multiple strokes can result in dementia, as can multiple haemorrhages into the brain. These are subsumed within the broad category of *vascular dementia*, which represents the second commonest cause of cognitive impairment, according to some reports.

The 'use it or lose it' school of thought argues that education may in part protect us from Alzheimer's disease. But no one is exempt. Scholars, scientists, artists, and statesmen have all succumbed. The publicity surrounding Ronald Reagan's diagnosis of Alzheimer's disease has done much to focus research funding, whereas the same diagnosis in Finland's President may have affected his ability to govern in the last few years of office in the early 1980s.

A small minority of dementias are eminently treatable, and vascular dementia is anticipated to become less common with better management of risk factors such as heart disease, hypertension, and SMOKING. The major challenge is Alzheimer's disease, and the challenge is a global one, with a predicted 34 million affected individuals by the year 2025. Most will be in the emerging nations, where life expectancy is increasing. In China this is combined with a policy of one child per family, such that the future work force will have to provide for a disproportionate dependent population; the solution will owe as much to politics as to medicine.

The conceptual shift in our understanding of dementia has been profound; no longer is it seen as an inevitable concomitant of old age. Instead we can view Alzheimer's disease, the major cause of late life dementia, as a disease with distinct physical changes, which should be amenable to treatment. However, we should not confuse this with the inevitable changes of ageing. We cannot run as fast at 90 as at 20, nor can we think as fast. We can, though, anticipate the preservation of wisdom and knowledge; to exploit the latter is a challenge for society, to preserve them and avoid dementia is a challenge for medicine.

MARTIN ROSSOR

See also AGEING; MEMORY; PSYCHOLOGICAL DISORDERS; SENILITY.

Dentistry is the art or science of treating diseases of the teeth and of the gums around them. As with medicine, dentistry is subdivided into a number of specialities. *Oral surgery* includes tooth extractions and operations on the jaw bones and the soft tissues of the mouth. *Oral medicine* deals with the treatment of local or systemic diseases affecting the mouth. *Restorative dentistry* involves replacement of parts of teeth or missing teeth. Fillings may be made from 'plastic' materials, such as amalgams or tooth-coloured composite resins, or pre-cast inlays; larger restorations may require metal or ceramic crowns. Restorative dentistry also includes *endodontics* (treating the pulps or root canals of teeth) and *prosthodontics*. In prosthodontics, missing teeth are replaced either with fixed bridges (using crowns placed on healthy teeth to support the 'pontic' that replaces the missing tooth or teeth) or removable dentures (false teeth) that may be partial or complete, depending on whether some or all of the natural teeth have been lost. *Periodontics* covers treatment of diseases of the gums (*gingivitis*) and other tissues around the teeth (*periodontitis*). *Orthodontics* is the correction of misalignment of teeth using appliances ('braces'), which may be held by brackets glued to the teeth (*fixed appliances*) or retained with wire clasps (*removable appliances*). *Paedodontics* covers all aspects of dentistry in children.

The earliest references to teeth and dental diseases are inscriptions written on clay tablets around 5000 years ago in Mesopotamia. The first known dentist was Hesi-Re. He lived in Egypt around 3000 years ago, and was described as 'the greatest of the physicians who treat teeth'. In ancient times, dental 'treatment' consisted mainly of tooth cleaning and perhaps some tooth extractions. *Dentures* (false teeth) first appeared in Sidon (Lebanon) and Tuscany around 630 BCE. Here, gold bands and wires were used to attach false teeth (usually carved from ivory) to adjacent healthy teeth. The Romans were very oral hygiene-conscious. They washed their teeth and cleaned them with tooth powders (*dentifrices*). In ancient Greece and Rome, as in Egypt, dentistry was performed by general physicians. Practitioners were skilled in restoring carious teeth with gold and replacing missing teeth with false ones. These false teeth were ridiculed by the poet Martial, who wrote in the first century AD:

> Lucania has white teeth; Thaïs brown. How comes it? One has false teeth, one her own.

During the Dark and Middle Ages in Europe (approximately from 500–1500 AD), progress in medicine halted and there were no real advances for nearly 1000 years. However, during this period knowledge was sustained by Islamic scholars such as Albucasis, who wrote extensively on teeth and tooth cleaning. The importance of oral hygiene was widely recognised in the Orient. During this period Hindus and the Chinese developed various dental treatments and complex surgical procedures. In Europe, by the fifteenth century 'dentistry' was undertaken by barber–surgeons, physicians or apothecaries, blacksmiths, and other 'tooth-drawers'. Herbal concoctions were the main 'remedies' for toothache and 'treatment' was confined mainly to extractions. The upper classes cleaned their teeth with cloth or sponges, and some even had gold or silver toothpicks. These were often hung round the owner's neck as an item of jewellery.

Knowledge blossomed in the Renaissance. Many of the new anatomical texts, such as Andreas VESALIUS' great work *De humani corporis fabrica*, contained sections on teeth. Some purely dental texts were published in the sixteenth and seventeenth centuries, but the foundations of modern dental practice were laid in Pierre Fauchard's *Le Chirurgien Dentiste* (1728).

Fauchard's book was a comprehensive discourse on a wide range of treatments. He described techniques for scraping out caries and filling the cavities with soft metals such as tin, lead, or gold. His book also gave rise to the modern term 'dentist' or 'dental surgeon'.

Prior to 1844, there were no anaesthetics to abolish the pain of surgery. However, opium and laudanum (tincture of opium) were freely available 'over the counter'. Dorothy Wordsworth (sister of the poet William) wrote: '*I had toothache in the night. Took laudanum*.' In 1844, an American dentist, Horace Wells, was the first person to experience tooth extraction under nitrous oxide analgesia. Two years later, William Morton extracted a tooth under ether anaesthesia. In 1884, a Dr Nash was the first person to fill a tooth using cocaine injected as a local anaesthetic. In 1905, cocaine was replaced by the synthetic drug *novocaine* (procaine). This in turn was replaced by *lignocaine* (lidocaine), which is in use today.

In the eighteenth century, dentures were hand-carved from materials such as ivory, and so did not fit well. Springs were sometimes used to help improve the stability of these loose dentures. However, dentures did not improve until the invention (by Nelson Goodyear) of a hardened rubber ('Vulcanite') which allowed closely-fitting denture bases to be constructed on casts made from impressions of the patient's mouth. As well as fitting better, vulcanite dentures were cheaper to make.

Other developments in the nineteenth century included the reclining dental chair, amalgam fillings (which were controversial even in the 1850s), and the treadle engine for driving the dental drill. The first electric-powered dental drill was invented in 1868. Many of the technical aspects and skills of dentistry were established by the end of the nineteenth century and some have remained more or less unaltered to the present day. The principles of cavity cutting, formulated by G. V. Black in the 1880s, have been supplanted only recently with the advent of adhesive filling materials. Developments in the twentieth century included improvements in dental materials, the introduction of the 'high-speed' drills (powered by compressed air), and greater emphasis on instrument sterility and cross infection control.

The modern dentist is part of a team, which includes a dental nurse (dental assistant), a technician, and ancillary operators such as dental hygienists, dental therapists, and dental radiographers. Dentistry is changing from being a pain-relief and patch-up service to a profession which places emphasis on prevention of tooth decay (dental caries) and gum disease (gingivitis and periodontitis). These diseases are largely preventable with good diet and effective oral hygiene. Their effects can be minimised by early diagnosis and treatment. Fluoride can help prevent caries, by making the enamel more resistant to attack by plaque acids, but it can also cause staining or mottling of the teeth (*fluorosis*). Artificial fluoridation of water supplies would reduce the incidence of caries, especially amongst people with poor standards of oral hygiene. However, fluoridation of public water supplies is a controversial political issue. The recent improvements in dental health can be illustrated by data from Great Britain. In 1968, 37% of adults in England and Wales had no natural teeth. In Scotland in 1972, 44% of adults had lost all their teeth. By 1988, these figures had fallen to 20% in England and Wales and 26% in Scotland. These improvements were due mainly to the better dental health in people under 35 years of age.

In spite of these improvements in dental health, teeth are still extracted because of decay. General anaesthesia (GA) was widely used for tooth extraction in young children and in some adults with a fear of injections. In the UK, the use of GA for dental procedures has been restricted. This is intended to eliminate the small numbers of deaths each year associated with dental GA. Since 1998, GA can be administered only by suitably qualified anaesthetists in clinics where proper emergency facilities and staff are available. One alternative to GA is *conscious sedation*. Here, the patient is awake and can respond to verbal commands, but is 'relaxed'. Sedation is produced using drugs such as a nitrous oxide–oxygen mixture, or tranquillisers such as *diazepam* (*Valium*), and is normally used along with appropriate local anaesthesia.

What of the future? The improvements in dental health must be sustained. A major priority is to find effective alternatives for injected local anaesthetics and replacements for the dental drill. One interesting area of development is the use of chemicals to remove caries without the need for drilling. The decay is dissolved by acids and the softened debris is scooped out. Laser technology, too, is developing and in time may replace the drill in restorative dentistry. The advent of adhesive, tooth-coloured fillings has revolutionised restorative dentistry. It is no longer necessary to cut large cavities for amalgam fillings. Instead, fillings can be placed with the minimum loss of healthy tooth substance. In prosthodontics, metal posts implanted in the jaw bones can be used to improve the support and efficiency of dentures. Nowadays, people live longer and can expect to have their natural teeth when they die. The science of dental gerontology has emerged to meet the dental needs of elderly people. Cosmetic dentistry, too, is a growth industry. Thin veneers can be used to correct defects on the outer surfaces of anterior teeth. The current trend of body adornment has extended to teeth, and small gems or gold shapes ('Twinkles') can be glued to the tooth surface. But cosmetic dentistry is not new. Many societies in Africa and America file the teeth for decorative and ceremonial purposes. In the ninth century the Mayans placed decorative inlays in anterior teeth. These inlays of semi-precious stones were fixed into cavities cut with a simple bow drill. Such skills were not introduced to Europe until many centuries later.   ROBIN ORCHARDSON

Further reading

Hillam, C. (1990). *The roots of dentistry*. British Dental Association, London.

Ring, M. E. (1993). *Dentistry: an illustrated history.* H. N. Abrams Inc., New York.

See also TEETH.

Depilation or the removal of body hair, is an extraordinarily ancient and widespread practice. As with the removal of teeth, foreskin, and other bodily substances, hair removal is usually performed in accordance with prevailing social customs. In ancient Greece, for instance, Athenian women reduced and shaped their pubic hair in order to increase their sexual attractiveness. In modern-day Turkey, where beards and moustaches are signs of political and religious sympathies, depilation often serves to identify villagers with particular fundamentalist, Marxist, or nationalist interests. Depending on the particular culture and historical period, depilation might be used to distinguish individuals by military rank, religious belief, political affiliation, occupation, ethnic or racial identity, sexuality, age, health, or economic standing. Hair removal is a relatively simple way to assert social distinctions.

Because such social distinctions have long been matters of intense preoccupation, different cultures have developed many ways to remove hair. Unwanted hair has been singed off through close contact with heat; scraped from the skin with abrasives such as pumice stone or with sharp implements such as razors; poisoned with depilatories made from sulphides, thallium acetate, or other chemicals; ripped out using string, tweezers, waxes, resins, or mechanical coils; and destroyed with electric needles, radium, or X-ray radiation. Significant effort continues to find the 'one best way' to remove human hair painlessly and permanently. In the United States, liposome-based gene therapies are under investigation as the next big step in depilation technology.

Depilation may be a universal human activity, yet modern Western societies have exhibited a particular fascination with 'excessive' body hair. Hair has a long history of connotations in the West, ranging from wolf-men and witches to 'dog-faced' boys and bearded ladies. Beginning in the mid-nineteenth century, however, a series of cultural, economic, and political transformations revised these conventional images of human hairiness. In the wake of Darwinism, body hair became more deeply invested with evolutionary and racial significance. As popular and scientific writings on hair began to emphasize the importance of 'hereditary' characteristics in determining the growth of body hair, excessive hair was reconceived as an indication of racial and ethnic difference. Shifting patterns of immigration further established the role of hair in comparative racial PHYSIOGNOMY. At the same time, body hair became a critical sign of sexual dimorphism. As greater numbers of white middle- and upper-class women entered public spheres traditionally reserved for men, 'masculine hair growths' among young white women provoked increasing public dismay. One typical beauty manual reported in 1874 that unwelcome hairiness in girls was brought on by 'high living among middle-class people'.

By the last quarter of the nineteenth century, dermatologists had created a new medical term for the condition of excessive hairiness: 'hypertrichosis'. Physicians defined hypertrichosis as 'an unnatural growth of hair', and diagnosed the disease when hair was determined abnormal in location, quantity, or quality. Abundant body hair, newly attached to fears of evolutionary atavism, transgressed sexual roles, and individual pathology, was suddenly perceived as a threat to public health. Beauty specialists, physicians, and 'afflicted' patients all began to seek new ways to 'remedy the evil' of unwanted body hair.

Anxiety over human hairiness still affects life in the West, where depilation products and services are now a massive and lucrative industry. Ironically, the history of hair removal in Western cultures has closely paralleled a rise in concern over hair *loss*. Technologies designed to 'cure' baldness are now nearly as widespread as those designed to remove 'superfluous' hair. The transformation of hair, 'the human body's most versatile raw material', continues to captivate.

REBECCA HERZIG

Further reading

Hope, C. (1982). Caucasian female body hair and American culture. *Journal of American Culture*, 5, 93–99.

Niemoeller, A. F. (1938). *Superfluous hair and its removal.* Harvest House, New York.

See also HAIR.

Deportment consists in how one carries and moves one's body. The term 'deportment' came into English usage around 1600, and is allied with the earlier ideas of *chivalry* and *courtesy*, and the later ideas of *etiquette* and *good manners* — in short, with conduct according to the rules of behaviour accepted by polite society. These rules helped to provide social stability in changing times, and people clung to them to maintain the appearance of stability. Such ceremonial rules contrast with the more substantive rules of *morality* and *law*.

Europe

Since antiquity, rules for deportment have guided the behaviour of the more privileged classes and those who served them. Throughout the Middle Ages a person's position within the social hierarchy of the nobility determined proper deportment. By the thirteenth century, however, the disciplined restraint dominating the visible conduct of nuns became a model for the laity, and eloquent poems and texts on courtesy began to appear in Italy. A somewhat problematic causal relationship between chivalry and the development of courtesy exists. From the ninth through the eleventh centuries, codes governing knights' behaviour reflected crude and practical military exigencies. Later on, however, as economic and political developments during the twelfth century enabled knights to settle, the focus of chivalry moved away from the military and towards the social realm of ritual and ceremony. A romanticized notion of chivalry, with an elaborate code of conduct, began to emerge.

Thirteenth-century prescriptions for women's deportment focused on the manner of WALK-ING, the method of riding a horse, modesty of glance, and proper management of the gown. Men received admonitions against poor table manners, and knights received advice on the proper way to approach a woman in the open. Deportment was informed by the persistent notion that the inner character revealed itself through outward bodily movement.

Economic and social changes in the early modern period enabled people to rise in social standing by learning proper deportment in the service of the nobility as knights, squires, pages and ladies-in-waiting. For example, a fifteenth-century page learned how to display a proper demeanour, to defer to superiors, to effect the proper stances for serving and conversing, and to become skilled in aristocratic amusements such as riding, singing, dancing, and playing musical instruments. Noblemen's houses thus functioned as finishing schools for the young.

The control of the features in laughing, eating, and talking, and the control of larger movements in walking, sitting, standing, and greeting someone, formed the subjects of careful instruction. The bow and curtsy, very similar in the Middle Ages, diverged by the seventeenth century. Sliding the left foot backward, while bending the knee, gave rise to the expression 'bow and scrape'. When greeting a superior, a gentleman doffed his hat, making certain that he executed this courtesy with the proper arm and body movements. A lady slid back her hood. Dancing schools acquired a particular importance, for DANCE involves gracious movement.

As many of the conventions of good deportment in Europe involved the wearing and handing of voluminous CLOTHES, which reflected high social status, the rules did not readily apply to the peasantry. SHOES governed the manner of walking. For example, out-of-doors, well-to-do Elizabethans wore two pairs of shoes, an inner slipper and the outer shoe (pantofle), which required some practice to keep on while walking. The pantofle was removed indoors, particularly while dancing, so that one could 'trip light-footed'. In some countries in the seventeenth-century, outer shoes had very thick cork soles, which resulted in a careful, slow manner of walking. When sitting or walking, women had to manage farthingales, trains, hoop skirts, or BUSTLES, covered with voluminous petticoats and skirts, as fashion changed, all the while constrained by the wooden Elizabethan bodice (which led to wooden movements) or its successor, the CORSET. Men had to learn how to move elegantly in stiff, padded Elizabethan doublets, with swords at their sides —

though their clothing became less restrictive as time passed. No one hurried; women walked in dainty steps and men in moderated strides. In standing, the whole leg was turned outward, a stance still seen in classical ballet.

The rules for deportment reached a zenith of artificiality at the end of the seventeenth century. Body carriage relaxed during the eighteenth century, but the fashionable set still made sure that their children received training in deportment, mainly at the hands of the dancemaster. In the nineteenth century, rules for standing, walking, and sitting were simplified. Though the corset remained in style, the erect posture of women in sitting and walking relaxed somewhat, while men's fashions achieved a modern appearance. Some were quite critical of the new ease that some men affected.

After World War I the earlier focus on gracious manners yielded to an emphasis on the rules necessary to avoid being snubbed. Jane Wildeblood, a historian of deportment, has attributed this change to a contemporary emphasis on efficiency.

United States
Etiquette in the US developed along different lines, as most of the colonists came from the peasant or working classes and brought no tradition of polite behaviour. Legislation and education brought some civility to the colonies, and during the eighteenth century certain groups looked to the English for higher codes of conduct. In the 1820s a steady stream of American etiquette books appeared, divided into two philosophies: one was the idea that manners are 'character in action', the other was an adaptation of Lord Chesterfield's views that manners are a set of rules to be learned. With their egalitarian origins, the Americans generally scorned European pomp, until a new wealthy class arose after the Civil War. A cult of elegance, borrowing heavily from the hereditary leisure classes of England, and especially of France, developed, and ended only with World War I.

KRISTEN L. ZACHARIAS

Further reading
Aresty, E. B. (1970). *The best behavior*. Simon and Schuster, New York.
Wildewood, J. (1973). *The polite world. A guide to the deportment of the English in former times*. Davis-Poynter, London.

Development and growth: birth and infancy
The Latin word *infans* means 'not speaking' and by convention the word infancy has come to mean the first year of childhood. There are very great differences between mammalian species in the degree of maturity of their newborn young. Deer, cattle, sheep, and guinea pigs are described as *precocial* for they are born with a protective covering of hair and are able to stand and walk almost immediately after birth. In contrast mice, rabbits, and humans — born naked, helpless, and vulnerable — are described as non-precocial or *altricial* (from the Latin for

nurses or feeders). The human infant is known as *neonatal* for the first month after birth.

Comparison of the gestation period in man (266 days from the date of conception, or 280 days from the last menstrual period, to delivery) with that of other animals shows that whilst a number of species have longer periods of gestation they are all born in a state of greater functional maturity. The human is unusual in having a long gestation period without obtaining great size or maturity at the time of birth. Another peculiarity is the size of the brain which already weighs about 350 g at birth or 10% of the average total body weight of about 3.5 kg.

Adaptation from complete dependence upon the maternal uterine environment and placenta to the extra-uterine environment requires major changes in the infant body organs. Within a minute of cessation of placental blood supply and delivery from a watery to a gaseous environment, the infant lungs, heart, skin, and the alimentary, renal, and nervous systems undergo a series of dramatic functional changes.

By means of the exchange of substances between their respective bloodstreams, the fetus has depended on the mother for obtaining OXY-GEN and nutrients, and for excretion of CARBON DIOXIDE, heat, and other metabolic waste products. Now it must fend for itself. More blood flow must be directed through the lungs for gas exchange, to the gut for nutrient absorption, to the kidneys for urine formation. But first and foremost, BREATHING must begin.

Breathing
Fetal breathing movements are necessary for normal lung development in the womb. The patterns of these movements are related to the 'sleep' and 'awake' states of the fetus but can be affected by extrinsic factors such as maternal SMOKING. Fetal lung produces a fluid which is normally swallowed although some may be expelled into the amniotic fluid. Nearer to the time of delivery this lung fluid contains SURFACTANT which at delivery is critically important for the stability of the alveolar air spaces once they are cleared of fluid and filled with air sucked into the chest by the first breath. Lack of this surfactant material is one of the major causes of breathing difficulty in infants born prematurely.

Normal vaginally-delivered infants make their first breathing movements within 20 to 30 sec from the emergence of the nose. Within 90 sec of complete delivery most infants have started to breathe rhythmically. The strong initial inspiratory efforts and subsequent rhythmic activities of respiratory muscles are largely dependent upon neurones in the BRAIN STEM, in turn stimulated by the carbon dioxide and hydrogen ion concentration in the blood and in the cerebrospinal fluid. Breathing is also stimulated by a low level of oxygen in the blood, acting on CHEMORECEPTORS in the carotid bodies; this hypoxic drive may assume great importance if the brainstem centres have been depressed by the infant becoming hypoxic during delivery or by anaesthesic and analgesic drugs given to the mother.

Circulation

At birth the CIRCULATION OF THE BLOOD is drastically re-routed. In the fetus there was relatively little blood flow through the lungs. Oxygenated blood reached the fetus from the placenta in the umbilical vein and joined the blood entering the right side of the heart. Most of this blood bypassed the lungs — shunted through to the left side through a hole between the right and left atria of the heart (*foramen ovale*), and through a channel from the pulmonary artery to the aorta (*ductus arteriosus*); thence to the rest of the body and the umbilical arteries. Now, after birth, the right ventricle must pump all the blood it receives through the lungs. This change is assisted by the onset of breathing itself. The expansion of the lungs with air reduces the resistance to flow in their blood vessels. Flow through the foramen ovale stops mainly as a result of altered pressures. Constriction of the ductus arteriosus and dilation of the lung vessels is mediated by the increased oxygen content of the blood in them, and by locally released substances that act on the muscle in the vessel walls. Anatomical closure of the fetal channels ensues. Closure of the umbilical vessels is accompanied by increased blood flow to the abdominal organs.

Nutrition and metabolism

Newborn polar bears weigh about 550 g, which is 0.3% of the mother's weight, whereas a newborn lesser horseshoe bat weighs 2 g, 30% of its mother's weight. The human lies between these extremes at 5–6%. In spite of these great species differences in prenatal vs. postnatal growth there is in all mammals a continuum of nutrient supply by the mother from conception until after complete weaning. Even after weaning in most human societies and other mammalian species, the mother is primarily responsible for helping the immature offspring to obtain adequate nutrition. The importance of optimal nutrition in human fetal and neonatal life has been highlighted by Barker and his colleagues in Southampton who have noted the association of disordered growth in early life with an increased incidence of HYPERTENSION, STROKES, DIABETES, and coronary artery disease in later life.

Energy The human infant born at term (37–42 week's gestation) has relatively large stores of lipid, carbohydrate, and important nutrient elements such as iron. After birth, fat and lactose supplied in the mother's milk are the major sources of energy, whereas before birth glucose supplied by the placenta provided the energy for fetal growth. This abrupt transition in nutrient supply causes major challenges to the digestive, absorptive, and metabolic processes of the infant. Until lactation is established stores of GLYCOGEN in the liver and muscles, and triglyceride fat from adipose tissue, help to maintain the infant body temperature, metabolic activity, and tissue growth. Release of these energy stores is mediated through signals from the HYPOTHALAMUS which change the ratio of glucagon to INSULIN released from the PANCREAS. When the infant blood reaching the hypothalamus is low in glucose a higher ratio of glucagon to INSULIN stimulates the release of more glucose from the glycogen stores and of triglycerides from subcutaneous fat stores.

Temperature If the infant's temperature falls, neural thermostats stimulate the sympathetic nervous system to release heat and FATTY ACIDS from *brown fat*. Brown fat looks brown because its cells are full of mitochondria, which are cellular power-houses for the release of energy from fat; it is located mainly between the shoulder blades in the newborn infant and there is relatively little in later life. (Animals which hibernate retain brown fat stores in adult life and it is from these stores, replenished in the summer months, that they maintain their body temperatures during winter.) Maternal body heat, and covering the head and body of the infant with clothing to reduce heat and fluid loss, greatly reduce the energy and fluid needs of the newborn. Throughout life the skin is an important organ for TEMPERATURE REGULATION by means of heat and fluid loss or retention, and the relatively high surface-to-volume ratio of the infant enhances its importance. Temperature receptors in the hypothalamus acting through the sympathetic nervous system regulate blood flow to the skin and thus help to control heat and water loss, but the infant at first lacks the additional mechanisms of SWEATING and SHIVERING.

Colostrum and milk Once the immediate needs for an adequate supply of oxygen have been met the infant normally within minutes begins to 'seek' a supply of water and nutrients at the mother's breast. During the first few days the mother supplies *colostrum*, which is specifically designed for her own infant in that it contains antibodies, cells, and other protective substances which will safeguard her infant from virtually all of the infections to which she has been previously exposed. Thereafter, the volume of milk produced by the mother increases to meet the demands of the infant. It may take 4–6 weeks to achieve a complete balance of maternal milk output and a satisfied infant. To meet the demand of one infant the mother will produce 700–750 ml/day, but she can easily double this volume to meet the needs of twins. The same levels of protection from infections, particularly of the gastrointestinal tract and upper airways, that were provided in the first few days by colostrum, are provided by these larger volumes of milk.

There are a series of brainstem-mediated reflexes which together with help from a supportive mother ensure that the infant finds, attaches, and obtains nutrition from her BREASTS. Rooting reflexes are initiated usually by contact of the infant's cheek with the mother's NIPPLE. They are mediated by the trigeminal nerve (which carries sensory nerves from the face and activates the jaw muscles) and they ensure that the infant's head turns towards the stimulus and the mouth opens to accept the nipple. If the infant is hungry these reflexes are enhanced so that a stimulus applied anywhere on the face will elicit the rooting responses. Once the infant has located the nipple it is drawn well into the mouth so that outer margin of the nipple (*areola*) lies at the level of the infant's gums. By closing the gums (fixing) and with rolling movements of the tongue, milk is squeezed from areolar milk ducts into the PHARYNX where a series of reflexly co-ordinated muscle actions stop the infant breathing while milk is directed down the OESOPHAGUS and into the STOMACH. The gums and tongue are relaxed whilst the infant breathes through the nose, the milk ducts refill and a further cycle commences. Newborn infants are obligatory nose breathers which is why nasal obstructions can interfere with normal feeding. Suckling is the major stimulus to further milk production in the glandular tissue of the breasts, mediated by a reduction in the maternal hormone oestrogen and increase in prolactin. Muscle sphincters at the nipple prevent leakage of milk between feeds. Reflex propulsion of milk from the alveoli and relaxation of the nipple sphincters is mediated by maternal OXYTOCIN release from the posterior PITUITARY GLAND. The main stimulus for this so-called 'draught' reflex is suckling by the infant but it can be initiated even by the cry of the hungry infant. Once the draught reflex has been initiated milk may continue to flow from both breasts even when the infant is not suckling. This reflex greatly helps the infant obtain milk. If the mother cannot relax during feeding the draught reflex may be delayed and the infant becomes frustrated. These early feeding interactions between mother and infant are important determinants for the subsequent behaviour, communication, and language development of the infant.

Digestion Over 90% of the fat present in human milk can be digested and absorbed by the infant intestine even though the activity of the pancreatic fat-digesting enzyme (lipase) is low relative to adult values, and bile salt production (which helps absorption of fats) is also low. Fat digestion is possible because lipases are present in the milk, and are also released from glands in the infant tongue. These enzymes remain active in the environment of the stomach.

Lactose, the sugar present in milk, is split in the small intestine by the enzyme lactase into its constituent glucose and galactose molecules, allowing absorption of the glucose. Absence of this enzyme, from an inherited defect, or through damage to the intestinal mucous membrane from viral or bacterial infection, can result in intractable DIARRHOEA.

There are no digestive enzymes for protein in human milk or (unlike the adult) in the infant's stomach and duodenum. This is significant because there are important proteins in the milk — immunoglobulins and growth factors — which might otherwise be damaged before they can be absorbed from the intestine.

Weaning is the process of expanding the diet to include foods and drinks other than breast milk or infant formula. A Department of Health working group in 1994 recommended that most infants should not be given solid foods before the age of 4 months and that a mixed diet should be offered by the age of 6 months. Cow's milk is not recommended as a main drink during infancy but during the second year it can make an important contribution to the intakes of several different nutrients and energy. By the end of the first year the child should be able to drink from a cup with help and have been introduced to most of the range of foods eaten by the family, with the exception of highly spiced foods.

Growth

If comparison is made between the *Madonna and Child Enthroned* of Cimabue (1240–1302) and the Castelfranco painting of the same subject by Giorgione (1477–1510), the change from the conception that the human infant is a diminutive adult to the reality of early infant body proportions is very obvious. The change in relative size of head, body, and limbs, constructed from photographs in which height has been standardised, is shown on page 209.

Factors which influence growth are genetic, nutritional, endocrine, and psychosocial. Diseases of essential organs or generalised disease will also have secondary effects on growth. On average, girls are slightly smaller than boys at birth and there remains a slight average difference in height and weight throughout childhood. In general, when both parents are above average height and come from tall families the children are likely to be tall, and the converse is also true. Undernutrition, specific nutritional deficiencies, and disease can prevent children achieving their genetic growth potential. In all countries in which the standards of living have improved during this century there has been a progressive increase in the average heights and weights of the children.

Growth in length is most rapid during the first 6 months of postnatal life and gradually decelerates during the pre-school years. By convention, body 'length' is measured up to the age of 2 years and 'height' thereafter. Measurements of height and weight of individual children are of most value when carried out at regular intervals and when compared with data obtained from large groups of children with similar age and development. Since children may be small or large depending on their inheritance and prenatal growth much greater importance should be attached to their growth increments than to their actual size. No individual child should be expected to conform to the mean childhood population growth data throughout the whole growth period.

Neuroendocrine function

Neural inputs or stimuli from eyes, ears, nose, skin, muscles, tendons, joints, and from most body organs through various types of SENSORY RECEPTORS enter the brain stem and higher

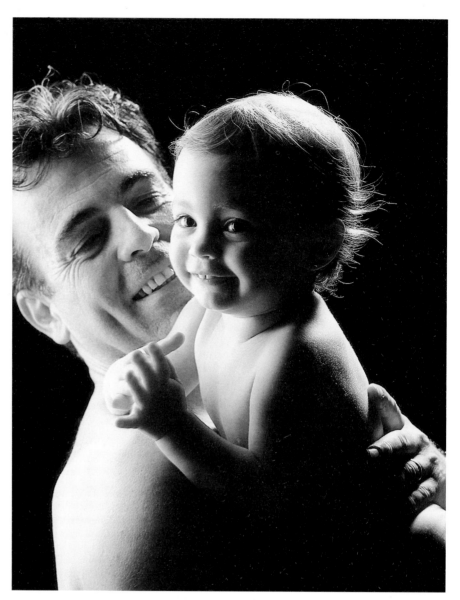

Father and baby. Oscar Burriel/Science Photo Library.

centres of the infant brain where they are integrated, interpreted, and responded to. Chemical messengers pass signals between nerve cells and between nerves and other tissues such as muscles. Nerves of the sympathetic and parasympathetic systems link with blood vessels, muscles, intestine, the CENTRAL NERVOUS SYSTEM, and endocrine glands to regulate the many automatic functions of the infant body. The brain also links with endocrine gland chemical messengers through the HYPOTHALAMUS and pituitary gland.

At birth much of the underlying brain and neuroendocrine system development is equipped to integrate newborn infant body functions, but it is becoming evident that if there is failure during the first year of life to use and develop a good pattern of response to a given stimulus from the environment, then there may be significant impairment in the ability to respond in later life to stresses both physical and emotional.　　　　FORRESTER COCKBURN

Further reading

Rennie, J. M. and Roberton, N. R. C. (ed.) (1999). *Textbook of neonatology*, (3rd edn). Churchill Livingstone, Edinburgh,

Department of Health (1994). *Wearing and the wearing diet*. Health and social subjects No. 45. HMSO.

See also ANTENATAL DEVELOPMENT; INFANT FEEDING.

Development and growth: early childhood

The transformation that occurs in the first five years of life is extraordinary. William Blake speaks of the baby at the time of birth:

> My mother groan'd: My father wept
> Into the dangerous world I leapt:
> Helpless, naked, piping loud:

Like a fiend hid in a cloud.
Struggling in my father's hands:
Striving against my swaddling bands,
Bound and weary I thought best
To sulk upon my mother's breast.

Arnold Gessell who worked in the Yale Clinic of Child Development described the 5-year-old as a 'self-assuming conforming citizen of his small world'. During these five years, the child builds up a store of knowledge about the environment, masters motor skills, and learns to look after itself. Language with which to communicate and think, and socially acceptable patterns of behaviour, are built on the confidence gathered within a secure relationship with parents or other carers. Thus they learn how to relate to and behave appropriately with others. This mental growth or development is dependent on maturation of the NERVOUS SYSTEM and on experience. Piaget, a psychologist working in Geneva in the first half of the twentieth century, stated that 'maturation of the central nervous system only opens up the possibility for new responses and functional development but does not result in actualisation of any given response unless the appropriate environmental circumstances are available.'

Learning and development

During the first year the BRAIN of the infant increases in weight by about 750 g to reach 1100 g. Much of this increase is membrane phospholipid — CELL MEMBRANE material — which forms the many new dendritic processes, developing multiple links among the nerve cells which were themselves already established during fetal life. As many as 10 000 or more 'boutons' or dendritic connections may form on each neuron. At the same time there is an increase in the brain cells — the *glial cells* — which are not neurons, but which support the functioning of the neurons by providing nutrients and regulating the chemical environment. Neuroglial cells cover with a MYELIN sheath the long processes (*axons*) of the neurons which transmit messages over long distances (e.g. head to toe). The process of myelination of the axons speeds the rate at which messages are transmitted.

There is evidence that the chemical composition of brain phospholipids can be affected by the type of dietary fats fed to the infant in the first year of life and it is thought that these differences in chemical composition might affect learning processes and longer-term functioning of the brain cell membranes. It is the phospholipid membrane and different NEUROTRANSMITTER receptors installed in the membrane which subserve the processes of learning and MEMORY. These developing interconnections between cells result in patterns of behaviour which determine the general similarities and basic trends of child development. However, the acquisition of knowledge and the refinement of skills depend on the child's opportunity to observe, copy, and experiment. Children actively construct their understanding of the world by interactions with it, thus developing schemes and strategies that can be applied to a wide variety of situations. Intelligence reflects the child's capacity to initiate and assimilate new experiences and to profit by past experience.

Language and communication

There are no innate ideas or memories in the brain of a newborn infant. They must all be acquired. Many of the normal infant cyclical activities, such as breathing, feeding, sleeping are controlled at lower BRAINSTEM level. Interactive imitative behaviours between mother and infant, e.g. smiling at 6 weeks, are processed at higher cerebral cortical levels and are learned behaviours. These interactions promote the development of pathways of communication between the retina of the eye of the infant, the occipital region of the brain and the motor cortex which controls the facial muscles to produce a smile, and also begin to build a memory bank which gives the associated 'pleasant' feeling which goes with smiling and happiness. Similar patterns of behaviour are mediated and built up for aural signals. Mothers quickly learn to distinguish a cry of hunger from one of discomfort or frustration and respond appropriately.

Babies are born with a preference for looking at the human face and responding to the human voice. Within a few days they are able to distinguish their mother's face, voice, and smell. When babies are awake in their parents' arms, they will spend a lot of time staring at their faces. Trevarthen from the Department of Psychology in Edinburgh University has videotaped such interactions and has shown that babies only a few weeks old will copy a parent's facial expressions. However, the baby is not for long a passive recipient and by 3 months is shaping the interaction by smiling, scowling, turning away, vocalising, and so forth. This intricate human dialogue (reciprocity), which gives enormous pleasure and delight, is immensely important for the child in learning about social interaction and in forming a trusting bond with one or more adults. This secure bond allows children to broaden their horizons and explore the world with confidence. Failure to develop appropriate learned patterns in early life can cause permanent disruption to the child's later emotional responses.

Re-learning or restructuring of these learned processes is possible but difficult to achieve in later life. The establishment of the interneural connections associated with this learning requires the provision of an adequate supply of nutrients for brain growth as well as the environmental stimuli from the parents. Evolutionary processes in the mammal over the last 100 million years and in modern man over the last 0.5 million have resulted in the development of a milk specifically adapted to the needs of the human infant and its complex brain. Maternal–infant interactions during breast feeding are important determinants of early acquisition of language and behaviour in later childhood.

From 5–6 months, the infant starts to look at objects in the wider environment. Parents follow the infant's gaze, will bring or take them to the object, name it, and let them handle it. This coincides with the time that the child is able to produce an increasing variety of sounds and thus will slowly start to approximate the sounds made to the words heard — allowing the realisation that objects have names. Children will often use one word for a wide range of similar objects, only slowly refining its use (e.g. 'dog' for all animals). Parents' responses of delight, and their willingness to interpret and elaborate the child's first SPEECH sounds, enhance not only language development but also communication and social skills such as taking turns.

Children clearly do not learn their early language just by copying. The sentences they use in the third year of life are telegraphic; they select the important words and make an attempt at correct grammatical order; they eliminate small words and sometimes word endings; they can create combinations they have never heard, e.g. 'light bye bye' (when a candle is blown out). Children can create sentences to convey their experience from whatever vocabulary they have.

Motor development

Children's motor development depends not only on improved control of body and limbs resulting from maturation of the brain but also on the child building up a mental scheme of the environment and of their own body; they learn where their arms and legs are from VISION, from touch, and from PROPRIOCEPTION, sensing stretch and position in muscles and joints. The child has to learn through experience to judge the depth of a step, the speed and trajectory of a ball, and the weight of an object, and that MUSCLE TONE and body POSTURE can be automatically adjusted to perform the task. If we pick up what we think is a full teapot but it is empty, we use too much muscle effort and it will shoot up into the air — but the brain also learns to make very rapid adjustments on the basis of sensory feedback.

Hand function matures from crude swiping movements, through whole-hand palmar grasp, to the accurately controlled reach and pincer grasp of a one-year-old child. This allows the child to use tools such as a spoon or a pencil. During the fourth year the child learns to cut with scissors and to thread beads, develops a mature pencil grasp, and learns to draw. By 3 years the child is capable of drawing circles, lines, and crosses and uses these to draw the sun, and people with increasing numbers of body parts. The ability to draw a square for a car is acquired at age 4–5 years.

Social development

When children learn to crawl and walk, they are physically able to move away from their parents but initially they will be continuously checking and will get very anxious if their parent disappears. A child who is securely emotionally attached to parents will become increasingly confident in exploring and being separated. In this way they develop a sense of self which can lead to stubborn negative behaviour — the 'terrible twos' or toddler omnipotence. At this age, children become much more aware of other children and will watch them intently, but will play in parallel, talking to themselves and not expecting an answer. By 3 years the child will begin to play with others and get involved with complex social interchange and is ready for nursery experience. Gessell described the 3-year-old as ready to come out of the home but almost completely ignorant of the wide world.

During the nursery years motor and self help skills improve so that with some prompting children are able to look after themselves in school. Language becomes increasingly complex so that by 5 years they are able to converse with adults and other children with only minor errors of grammar and pronunciation. They move away from being able to think not only of the here and now but also about things which have been or might be. This is associated with a love of imaginative stories, but there may be confusion over what is real and what is not; this can lead to fears and fantasies. Children of this age constantly ask questions and clearly are beginning to consider and solve problems. They require time and patience from adults who are able to put themselves in the child's shoes and explain and explore the world with them. There is a fundamental urge to make sense of the world and young children will behave in ways which produce results with no rewards except success. The child needs to be encouraged to see the options, to solve incongruities, and to risk errors rather than avoiding them. What children work out for themselves will be far more meaningful than anything they are told.

Growth

Meanwhile during all these developments, the body has been steadily growing and its proportions changing (see figures). Growth decelerates in the early years — it is never again as rapid as in the first year of life — but between 3 and 5 it is still as fast as it will be again later in the pre-pubertal 'growth spurt'. Given good health and an adequate diet, final stature will be genetically determined, but undernutrition or severe illness can slow down growth towards that potential at any stage. On recovery there is an acceleration until the child has caught up with the predicted growth curve, although severe malnutrition or disease can cause permanent growth restriction. Increasing height implies lengthening of the leg BONES. This growth occurs at the *epiphyses*, where the main shaft of a bone joins the parts which are shaped to fit a joint at each end. Solid fusion does not occur here until growth is completed. All the bones of the skeleton, including the spine, are also continually enlarged and remodelled. Many HORMONES are involved and necessary for normal growth throughout the body, notably GROWTH HORMONE from the PITUITARY.

What progress has been made in the first five years?

> At first, the infant
> Mewling and puking in the nurse's arms
> And then the whining schoolboy, with his satchel
> And shining morning face, creeping like snail
> Unwillingly to school.

Shakespeare. *As you like it*

RUTH DAY

FORRESTER COCKBURN

Further reading

Donaldson, M. (1978). *Children's minds*. Fontana, London.

Gessell, A. (1950). *The first five years of life*. Methuen, London.

Sylvia, K. and Lunt, I. (1983). *Child development — a first course*. Blackwell, Oxford.

Development and growth: school age and adolescence
Growth is a complex biological phenomenon and is a vital part of a child's development. The rapid growth of childhood depends on increases both in the number of cells and in the size of individual cells. PUBERTY is the unique stage of growth and development associated with the social and psychological changes referred to as adolescence.

The nervous and endocrine (hormone) systems are the principal mediators of growth. The hypothalamus, at the base of the brain, contains nerve cells which produce a family of regulatory hormones whose effect is to stop and start the production of further hormones from the PITUITARY GLAND. The latter, weighing only 0.5 g, has been termed the 'conductor of the endocrine orchestra', as its hormones exert effects on many aspects of growth, metabolism, and reproductive development.

Growth and puberty

From 4 years of age until the onset of rapid growth in puberty (the adolescent growth spurt) the average rate of growth for boys and girls is about 5–6 cm/year. During this time the 'typical' boy is slightly taller than the 'typical' girl. This situation is temporarily reversed when girls reach their adolescent growth spurt at around 11 years old, some two years earlier than boys. At age 14 years, boys are near the peak of their growth spurt and overtake girls, whose growth spurt has nearly finished. The difference in magnitude of these growth spurts largely explains the difference in final heights attained by boys compared with girls. Weight velocity is almost constant from age 3 to puberty (rising from an average of 2.0 to about 2.7 kg/year), since the increase in fat velocity balances the drop in velocity of muscular and skeletal dimensions. Body shape continues to change, since the rate of growth of some parts, such as the legs and arms, is greater than the rate of growth of others, such as the trunk. The change is a steady one, a smoothly continuous development to the final prepubescent physique, rather than any passage through a series of separate stages.

At puberty, a very considerable change in growth rate occurs. There is a swift increase in body size, a change in shape and body composition, and a rapid development of the OVARIES and TESTES, the reproductive organs, and the characters signalling sexual maturity. Some of these changes are common to both sexes, but most are sex-specific. Some children grow slightly more slowly than others and reach puberty later than average. They do, in the end, reach a normal height, though children who have short parents tend to be short themselves. At puberty, boys have a great increase in muscle size and strength, together with a series of physiological changes making them more capable than girls of doing heavy physical work, and running faster and longer. The changes specifically adapt the male to his primitive primate role of hunting, fighting, and foraging. Such adolescent changes

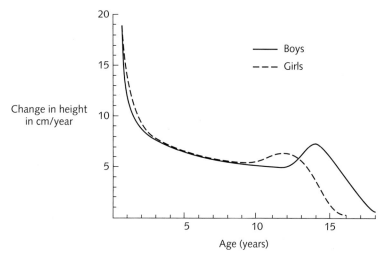

Rate of growth with age. Note that growth is fastest during the first 2 years of life and that the growth spurt occurs sooner in girls than in boys

occur generally in primates, but are more marked in some species than in others. Man lies at about the middle of the primate range, in terms of both adolescent size increase and degree of sexual differentiation. During the adolescent growth spurt, for a year or more, the velocity of height increase approximately doubles; a boy is likely to be growing again at the rate he first experienced about age 2.

Practically all skeletal and muscular dimensions take part in the spurt, though not to an equal degree. Most of the spurt in height is due to acceleration of trunk length rather than length of legs. There is a fairly regular order in which the dimensions accelerate: leg length as a rule reaches its peak first, followed by trunk length and the body breadths, with shoulder width last amongst them. The earliest dimensions to reach their adult size are the head, hands, and feet. At adolescence, children, particularly girls, sometimes complain of having large hands and feet. They can be reassured that by the time they are fully grown their hands and feet will be a little smaller in proportion to their arms and legs, and considerably smaller in proportion to their trunk (Fig. 2).

The adolescent growth spurt in skeletal and muscular dimension is closely related to the rapid development of the reproductive system, which takes place at this time.

In boys the first sign of puberty is usually an increase in the size of the testes and scrotum, with reddening and wrinkling of the scrotal skin. Slight growth of pubic hair may begin about the same time, but is usually a little later. The spurts in height and penile growth begin on average about a year after the first testicular acceleration. Axillary hair appears on average some two years after the beginning of pubic hair growth. In boys, facial hair begins to grow at about the same as the axillary hair appears. Breaking of the voice occurs relatively late in adolescence, and is often a gradual process and so not suitable as a criterion of puberty.

In girls the appearance of the 'breast buds' is as a rule the first sign of puberty, though the appearance of pubic hair sometimes precedes it. The UTERUS and VAGINA develop simultaneously with the BREASTS. MENARCHE, the first menstrual period, is a late event in the sequence. It almost invariably occurs after the peak of the height spurt has been passed. Though it marks a definitive and probably mature stage of uterine development, it does not usually signify the attainment of full reproductive function. Early menstrual cycles may be more irregular than later ones, and often there is no ovulation. There is therefore frequently a period of adolescent sterility lasting a year to 18 months after menarche, but this cannot be relied upon in an individual case.

Nutrition

Adolescent growth proceeds at an astonishing pace — average weight increment during the adolescent growth spurt is 16 g/day for females and 19 g/day for males. It is also during adolescence

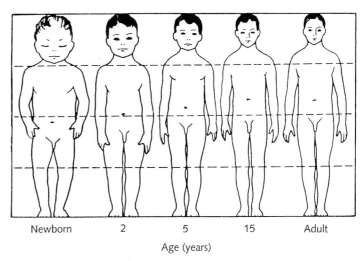

The changing proportions of the growing body.

Newborn 2 5 15 Adult

Age (years)

and young adulthood that BONES complete their maturation.

Overweight and obese conditions occurring at this age show persistent health effects decades later. Atherosclerosis (blood vessel narrowing) begins to accelerate at this age. The peak incidence of anorexia nervosa and bulimia nervosa is in adolescence. Food habits which develop as adolescents enjoy increasing independence and responsibility for their own dietary intake are believed to persist into adulthood, making this a critical time for preventive health interventions.

Dietary guidelines consist of principles based on scientific and practical knowledge about nutrient requirements, which are translated into terms that can be taught to each adolescent. Adolescents must be most aware of foods and cooking practices that result in an adequate intake of all nutrients. The basic principles of good nutrition are:

Eat a variety of foods The best defence against nutrient deficiencies and excesses is to vary the intake among diverse groups of good foods.

Maintain a healthy weight by balancing energy intake with output. This is the most difficult nutritional task for adolescents. OBESITY is increasing at an alarming rate among adolescents. Malnutrition secondary to chronic disease is also significant world-wide. Over the past four decades, habitual physical activity has declined for adolescents and children, while energy intake has not changed, resulting in increased overweight and obesity. Restriction of intake must be accomplished carefully to assure adequate nutrient intake. Encouragement of more physical activity is critical in maintaining good body weight and composition.

Choose a diet low in fat, saturated fat, and cholesterol This is important for prevention of chronic disease in adulthood as well as of overweight in adolescents. Arteriosclerosis is the major cause of death in adults in industrialised countries. Its antecedents are clearly in early life and must be dealt with early.

Eat plenty of fruit, vegetables and whole grains, avoiding high-fat foods and ensuring good bowel habits.

The 'food pyramid' is a straightforward way of teaching good dietary practices. It classifies foods into groups and recommends the numbers of each that should served daily to achieve the principals outlined above. The guide is this:

bread, cereals, and pasta: 6–11 servings

vegetables: 3–5 servings;

fruits: 2–4 servings;

dairy products: 2–3 servings;

meat, poultry, fish, and legumes: 2–3 servings;

and, at the top of the pyramid, fats, oils, and sweets, to be used sparingly.

Impaired growth is an invariable feature of children who are undernourished, whatever the cause of the malnutrition. In developed countries, the provision of inadequate amounts of food is less common but does occur, and may be the main reason for the poor growth of deprived children. Inadequate intake also occurs as a result of chronic illness, especially renal disease, infection, and psychological disturbances such as anorexia nervosa and depression. Chronic bowel disease may lead to malnutrition and poor growth.

Motor development

In its simplest terms motor development refers to movements. It includes the waddling, clumping, ungainly movement of the toddler, the fine skills of the dancer, and the enormously intricate, delicate touch of the watchmaker.

An example of fine motor skills, extending to an older age range, is that of handwriting. Up to 5 years, copying is frequent. At 5–6 years, children learn to write their own name with large writing and some reversals. At 6–7 years, the alphabet can be printed on request but there is still some reversing. From 7–8 years most children can now write and most attempt to make their letters smaller. There is some evidence of consciousness of design. At 8–9 years, some, but not all, letters are joined. This can lead to untidiness and an apparent deterioration in ability, made worse if the child is also mastering skills of punctuation and spelling. By 9–11 years, writing is now well established, with each child's individuality beginning to show. It is essential that teachers allow for individuality; for example, if a child writes naturally without joining letters this should be accepted. From 11 years upwards individual styles flourish and should be encouraged.

Understanding, learning, and behaviour

Early human understanding involves elementary forms of SPEECH, development of the use of symbols, and consideration mostly of one's self. Thinking is limited by the difficulty the child has in taking into account more than one feature of an object at a time. Thus a red chair cannot at the same time be thought of as wooden as well as red.

Once children start school, number concepts develop quickly. At the same time comes the ability to use number-related words: 'more', 'less', 'four', 'several', and so on. Time concepts are developed more or less uniformly, at least in Western cultures. At first comes the ability to locate one event in terms of another; breakfast comes before dinner. Other concepts follow; the child's own age (approximate age 3 years) morning or afternoon (4), the day of the week (5), the approximate time (7), the month (7), the year (8), the day of the month (8). Telling the time also follows a fairly consistent pattern; at first children tell time by the hour, then by the half hour, and then quarters, and they usually develop reasonable accuracy by the age of six or seven.

From 7 to about 12 years, children learn about size, weight, and number. They begin to think logically about things they have experienced. They realise that the number of objects in a set remains constant even if the pattern is changed. They can also think backwards and forwards in time. In mathematics, this is the same as realising that if 2 plus 2 equals 4, then 4 minus 2 must equal 2. Underlying this development is an increase in 'flexible' thought, being able to see things from someone else's point of view.

From about 12 years to adulthood the main characteristic is the ability to formulate general laws and principles. The thinking of this period is, in essence, the sophisticated, flexible, symbolic thought of the adult. Children become able to reason in an abstract way about matters that they have never themselves experienced. But not everyone reaches this stage, even in adulthood.

Socially, for the first two or three years the family remains the paramount influence, but from then on there is competition from peer groups and from significant adults outside the family. The first day at school is a major event in childhood and the child's first teacher is a key figure in subsequent development. From 6 years to adolescence, the more or less formal group, created by children themselves and sometimes referred to as a gang, becomes increasingly important. It offers a relief from adult supervision and meets needs not adequately catered for in an adult-orientated society. Its function has much in common with the formal groups like Brownies or Scouts but is not identical. Gangs vary in size and activity. Some devote themselves almost entirely to antisocial behaviour; others are entirely benign. What they all do is offer members opportunities to measure themselves against others, to learn co-operation between peers, and to develop a sense of 'belonging'. This progress in socialisation may be seen as a gradual transition from dependence, via interdependence, to independence.

Adolescence is recognised as a period of risk-taking behaviour, including experimentation with smoking, alcohol, drug-taking, and sexual activity. One form of risk-taking activity may lead to another, for example the association of alcohol and substance abuse with sexual initiation. At this stage, behaviour may be in turn impulsive, exploratory, excitable, disorderly, and distractible.

DONALD C. BROWN
CHRISTOPHER KELNAR

See also PUBERTY.

Dexterity It is intriguing that, although this word derives from the Latin *dexter*, meaning 'on the right', its definition in *The Shorter Oxford English Dictionary* lists 'right-handedness' as only the fourth meaning, and describes that usage as 'rare'. The more common meanings are:

1. Manual skill, neat-handedness; hence, address in the use of the limbs and in bodily movements
2. Mental adroitness or skill; cleverness, address, ready tact. In a bad sense: Sharpness.
3. Handiness, conveniency.

Dexterity has clearly expanded its meaning to incorporate attributes that have generally been associated with right-handedness. The positive value of these attributes reflects the fact that the great majority of people are right-handed, and are more proficient at using the right hand than the left. This is especially evident in fine motor skills like writing, as well as in some skills, like throwing, which involve the whole arm. This gives rise to the first of the above definitions of dexterity as manual skill and neat-handedness. It is further generalised to *mental* qualities in the second definition.

About 10 percent of the population are left-handed, and are therefore more 'dexterous' with the left hand, while a few are approximately equally skilled with either hand, and are therefore termed 'ambidextrous.' Although HANDEDNESS is probably innate, and possibly influenced genetically, it is possible for right-handers to acquire considerable dexterity (in the generalised sense) with the *left* hand, as in those who play musical instruments, such as the piano and violin, that require skilled action by both hands.

Other terms linked to handedness have acquired even more metaphorical significance. *Sinister*, the Latin for 'left', has taken on the meaning of evil-suggesting, or malignant. The term *adroit*, meaning dexterous or skilful, comes from the French *à droit* ('according to the right'), while *gauche*, the French for 'left', has taken on the meaning of socially awkward, or tactless. The German word for 'left' is *link*, and the word *linkisch* has taken on the general meaning of awkward, while *recht* for 'right' means just or true, as does the word *right* in English. In Italian, the left hand is termed either the *stanca*, meaning tired, or the *manca*, meaning defective. These and countless examples from other languages testify to the universal preponderance of right-handers across all human cultures, and the linguistic prejudice directed against left-handers.

Although right-handers are indeed clumsy when using the left hand, there is no reason to suppose that left-handers themselves are especially awkward, except when using implements, like scissors, that are specifically designed for the right hand. In the Old Testament, Judges 20: 16, we read that out of 26 000 soldiers, 700 were left-handers who could 'sling stones at an hair breadth, and not miss'. Dexterity, then, is not confined to the right-handed.

MICHAEL CORBALLIS

See also HANDEDNESS.

Diabetes usually refers to the condition known in full as *diabetes mellitus*. '*Diabetes*' can be translated, from its Greek derivation, as 'going through' — describing the characteristic copious production of urine. '*Mellitus*' comes from the Latin for honey. There is an excess of sugar (*glucose*) in the blood and this 'spills over' into the urine, bringing an excess of water with it. The cause is either a deficiency of production of the hormone INSULIN by the PANCREAS, or defective response of body cells to the action of this hormone, which normally enables glucose and other nutrients to be taken up from the circulating blood. The derangement of metabolism leads to extensive complications. The type of diabetes due to lack of insulin production was fatal before the early 1920s, when treatment with an extract from animal pancreatic tissue was shown to be effective.

The illness with 'the passing of too much urine' was known in 1500 BC to the Egyptians; Aretaeus wrote of it in the second century AD as 'diabetes … a melting down of the flesh and limbs into urine'; Paracelsus described it in the sixteenth century; but it was the English physician Thomas Willis who first reported in 1679 that the urine was 'so wonderfully sweet'.

A much rarer condition, *diabetes insipidus* (with copious urine which is not 'sweet'), is caused by deficiency of *antidiuretic hormone* (*ADH*) (also known as *vasopressin*) from the PITUITARY GLAND. ADH normally acts in the kidneys to prevent any greater escape of water in the urine than is necessary to maintain constancy of the salt concentration and volume of the BODY FLUIDS. When ADH is lacking, due to disease or injury in or near the pituitary gland, the daily output of dilute urine can be 25–30 litres, with extreme thirst to match.   S.J.

See BLOOD SUGAR; BODY FLUIDS; INSULIN; PANCREAS; PITUITARY GLAND.

Diagnosis, systems of

Medical diagnosis is concerned with the determination of the nature of a diseased condition; a process usually undertaken by a doctor. It requires the identification of the disease by careful investigation of its symptoms and history.

First we must define what is meant by the term 'disease'. To many a broken leg may not be regarded as a disease, whilst unquestionably cancer of the lung or diabetes would be so described. For the purpose of this article, the definition of disease will follow that of the *Oxford English Dictionary*: 'a condition of the body, or of some part or organ of the body, in which its functions are disturbed or deranged'. It may also be defined as a departure from the state of health, especially when caused by structural change.

The process of diagnosis in medicine now often requires a team of doctors, nurses, and technicians. It involves: (i) the careful assessment of the history of the *symptoms* of the disorder; (ii) clinical examination to determine whether there are any *signs* of abnormalities of the body; (iii) investigation of the blood or other body fluids to reveal any abnormalities indicative of the nature of the disorder; (iv) the use of special techniques for visualisation, such as radiological examination or ENDOSCOPY.

The history is obtained by first asking the patient to tell the story — to give an outline of the symptoms of their condition — without asking leading questions. Thereafter the doctor may ask specific questions in order to clarify the sequence of events and to elicit any features which might be diagnostic; for example, has there been any blood in the stools or urine, any breathlessness? In some illnesses, for example MIGRAINE or EPILEPSY, the diagnosis may be evident from the history alone. The clinical history is always vitally important, since it often suggests the direction in which further investigations should be pursued; on the other hand the patient's account may not always be relevant to the diseased state. All alert doctors are aware of the patient who gives a long history of headaches, or tiredness, or of something else and then, when leaving, turns back from the door to say 'And by the way, doctor …' Only then may the significant symptoms emerge. Often, the symptoms presented by the patient may cover up the real nature of their disorder, particularly in the case of psychiatric problems, or when the main difficulty may lie in family relationships. Experienced doctors know that the clinical history more often than not provides the main clues to diagnosis.

After the clinical history has been recorded, the doctor turns to physical examination. This involves four steps: observation, palpation, percussion, and AUSCULTATION. Careful observation detects whether there are any abnormalities such as pallor of the skin (indicating ANAEMIA), JAUNDICE (indicating possible LIVER disease), or the bluish-purple colour of cyanosis (indicating HYPOXIA from lung or heart conditions). Where a clinical history of breathlessness has been elicited and cardiac disease suspected, any abnormal pulsations or distension of the veins in the neck will be looked for. Any unusual lumps or moles which may have been enlarging are noted. There might be visible evidence of THYROID disease, as indicated by tremor and staring eyes (*thyrotoxicosis*) or sluggishness of demeanour (thyroid underactivity or *myxoedema*). The PULSE is examined to detect any abnormality of cardiac rhythm, and the BLOOD PRESSURE measured to establish whether there is hypertension.

The 'systems' of the body are then examined — first usually the HEART and LUNGS, then the abdomen, where palpation may be of great importance in revealing tumours or other palpable masses. Percussion is helpful in detecting fluid in the chest, and is equally important in examining the abdomen: the tapping finger detects resonance where there is air in the lungs or gas in the guts, but dullness where there is an abnormal collection of fluid.

Examination of the NERVOUS SYSTEM takes a little more time. Power and sensation are tested in the limbs, and the tendon REFLEXES are examined. After a STROKE, for example, there may be loss of power in one side of the body and the reflexes will be unusually brisk. The *optic fundi* (the retina and optic nerves in the EYES) are then examined with an ophthalmoscope: they provide a window not only on the brain but also on the state of the body's blood vessels: brain damage can be reflected in swelling, and conditions such as hypertension and diabetes also show characteristic changes.

At the first interview certain simple tests may have been carried out already. The urine is examined for the presence of sugar (indicating diabetes), albumin (indicating kidney disease), or bile pigment (indicating liver or gall bladder disease). The next stage involves the various pathology laboratories. In the *haematology* laboratory the BLOOD is examined: the numbers of the white and red blood cells are measured, using an automatic cell counter. Diseases such as anaemia due to iron deficiency, pernicious anaemia, and leukaemia are diagnosed in this way. In patients with a history of bleeding, studies of blood clotting may be indicated. The *microbiology* laboratory is extremely important in cases of fever, sepsis, DIARRHOEA, pneumonia, or SEXUALLY TRANSMITTED DISEASE. Isolating a specific MICROORGANISM from, for example, stool, urine, or blood, and determining its susceptibility to different antibiotics, often not only provides the diagnosis but also indicates the correct treatment. In the *clinical chemistry* laboratory, the blood electrolyte levels (concentrations of the different IONS) are measured; measurement of chemical substances related to liver function is also usually carried out as a routine. The measurement of the blood glucose level is important in the diagnosis and management of diabetes. The levels of immune globulins and of certain antibodies in the blood may indicate a problem in the IMMUNE SYSTEM. Some tests may be useful in screening for disorders which have not yet produced symptoms. The finding of a raised *prostate specific antigen* (PSA) may indicate cancer of the prostate, often permitting treatment in the early stages when the condition is most likely to be amenable to treatment.

In many disease conditions the final achievement of an accurate diagnosis lies with the *histopathologist*. In disorders of the female reproductive tract, for example, where screening techniques offer the hope of early diagnosis, it is the pathologist or trained technician who will make the diagnosis, on the basis of microscopic examination of a sample of tissue in a CERVICAL SMEAR. There are a number of BIOPSY techniques (taking a sample of living tissue) which are often vital in clinching a diagnosis suggested by the clinician. Liver or kidney biopsies, taken by a needle through the skin, provide the pathologist with material that is often diagnostic. Jejunal biopsy — obtaining a small knuckle of the lining membrane of the intestine — provides material from which the pathologist may make an almost instant diagnosis.

The pathologist is also of vital importance in establishing the diagnosis in conditions such as cancer of the BREAST, when the surgeon operates to obtain tissue for immediate histological examination before deciding on what operation to carry out.

In the modern era, IMAGING TECHNIQUES have virtually made the human body transparent, from the first use of X-RAYS at the end of the nineteenth century, to the various imaging techniques now available. Ultrasound has been particularly helpful in pelvic disorders. The use of radioactive tracers makes it possible to outline a wide range of conditions, the take-up of the tracer being detected by a radioactive scanner. Whilst conventional radiological examinations are still an important part of diagnosis, particularly for example in injuries involving fractures of limbs, scanning techniques using computerised axial tomography (*CT scanning*) have greatly increased the accuracy of diagnosis, particularly in the detection of tumours or of abnormalities of the different organs of the body. In such instances, however, it is often necessary to obtain tissue either by needle biopsy or at surgery before the diagnosis can be certain.

Abnormalities of the heart and blood vessels are best shown by the introduction of a contrast medium (*radio-opaque substance*) via the bloodstream into the relevant area, followed by X-ray examination (*angiography*), a technique now routinely used in the diagnosis of the common condition of coronary heart disease. Ultrasonic techniques are also valuable in cardiac diagnosis.

A more recent development has been the introduction of *magnetic resonance imaging* (MRI), a remarkable scanning technique which has made it possible to diagnose abnormalities of the skeletal system and within the central nervous system with great accuracy. The earliest abnormalities in the brain in multiple sclerosis may be revealed in this way. MRI is also being exploited for the determination of brain and liver function, as well as providing evidence of metabolic disorders.

These and other contemporary body imaging techniques have made it possible to reveal not only structural defects but also disordered function.

Likewise in the modern era, the practice of ENDOSCOPY has revolutionised diagnosis, particularly in common conditions such as stomach ulcer or cancer of the colon. Endoscopy has made it possible to obtain specimens from stomach or colon, or from the bronchial tree in the lungs, which can be examined by histological techniques, allowing an accurate diagnosis to be made.

The number of techniques that may be used in the investigation of human disease has increased enormously in recent years. Many of these tests are extremely costly, so that the expense of obtaining a precise diagnosis has to be balanced against how precise the diagnosis needs to be for effective decision-making and treatment. Neither are they all entirely free of risk to the patient's well-being, whether by causing some physical complication, or through the mental stress of a 'false-positive' finding which proves to be a false alarm.

In the utilisation of medical diagnostic technologies, nothing can replace the importance of the clinical history and physical examination, since these determine the diagnostic pathway that should be followed. Doctors, aware of the risk of litigation should the diagnostic process not prove accurate, tend to carry out too many investigations; the patient then becomes locked in to a series of complicated and expensive procedures that may be neither necessary nor in their best interest. As in all things in medicine, medical diagnosis requires prudence, and more than a modicum of common sense. CHRISTOPHER BOOTH

See also BIOPSY; ENDOSCOPY; IMAGING TECHNIQUES; RADIOLOGY; X-RAYS.

Dialysis
Failure of the KIDNEYS, whether acute (rapid onset) or chronic (gradual onset), is life-threatening, since waste products accumulate in the body and there are disturbances of body fluid volume and composition. There are two possible treatment: dialysis, or kidney TRANSPLANTATION. A period of dialysis may enable the kidneys of a patient with acute renal failure to recover. In patients with chronic renal failure, dialysis is generally used until a suitable donor kidney becomes available for transplantation. However, many kidney patients have been maintained for over 20 years, with a reasonable quality of life, by dialysis.

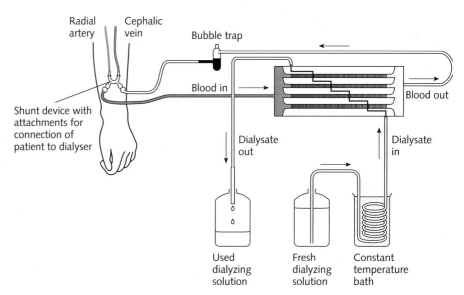

Fig. 1 Haemodialysis.

Dialysis is a way of removing toxic substances from the blood, and restoring the body fluid volume and composition to close to normal. Two kinds of dialysis are now common, though both types have long histories. *Haemodialysis*, using dialysers which are sometimes called *artificial kidneys*, was pioneered by the Dutch physician Willem Kolff, initially at Gronigen University Hospital, and then at Kampen Hospital. Kolff treated his first patient with an experimental haemodialyser in 1943, and in 1956 introduced the first practical haemodialysis machine.

Peritoneal dialysis has a longer history but a shorter period of practical application. The first peritoneal dialysis of a patient was performed in 1923, but the procedure did not become accepted until 1959, when developments in tubing and catheters had made the technique safer.

Neither peritoneal dialysis nor haemodialysis bear much resemblance to the way the kidneys normally work. The kidneys have a *filtration* process which is essentially non-selective: with the exception of the proteins, all the constituents of the blood plasma are filtered, whether or not the body needs to excrete them or retain them. The selectivity comes after the filtration process, when the *nephrons* (kidney tubules) reabsorb some substances into the blood, secrete others, or simply allow the filtered substances to continue along the nephron to escape in the urine. No artificial kidney works like this.

Haemodialysis
The principle of haemodialysis is that blood from the patient passes over a 'dialysis membrane' of very large surface area, on the other side of which is a dialysing fluid. Hollow fibres are often used instead of a flat membrane. Molecules pass from the blood into the dialysis fluid (and vice versa) by *diffusion*. The dialysis membrane is permeable (porous) to all the plasma constituents, with the exception of plasma proteins. If the concentration of a substance (such as urea) is greater in the patient's blood plasma than in the dialysis fluid, there will be net transfer of the substance to the dialysis fluid. Conversely, it is possible to raise the concentration of substances in the patient's blood plasma by having a higher concentration of substances (e.g. glucose or bicarbonate) in the dialysis fluid.

The rate of movement of any individual solute across the dialysis membrane depends on four factors: (i) the permeability of the membrane to the solute; (ii) the surface area of the membrane; (iii) the concentration gradient for the solute across the membrane (the difference in concentration between plasma and dialysing fluid); (iv) the length of time that the plasma and dialysing fluid remain in contact with the membrane.

The maximum rate of solute transfer will occur when the concentration difference is greatest. For urea, for example, this will be when the dialysis is begun, because the patient's plasma concentration is high, but the difference becomes smaller as the solute moves from blood plasma to dialysis fluid. This dissipation of the concentration gradient can be minimised by having high flow rates for blood and/or dialysis fluid.

In modern dialysers, the dialysis membrane or hollow fibre has significant permeability to water, so that water (and solute) can be removed from the blood by ultrafiltration (also called bulk flow). The process of carrying solute across a membrane by bulk flow of solvent (water) is *convection*. The rate of ultrafiltration will depend on the four factors listed above, and on the hydrostatic pressure difference between the blood compartment and the dialysing fluid compartment of the apparatus. Some artificial kidneys do not use dialysing fluid, and rely on ultrafiltration and bulk flow to remove water and solute across a membrane. This process is termed *haemofiltration*.

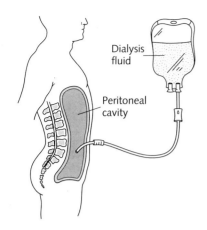

Fig. 2 Peritoneal dialysis.

For both haemodialysis and haemofiltration, easy access to the patient's blood supply is essential, and since access may be required every few days over a period of many years, special arrangements are necessary. In general this involves a '*shunt*' — an artificial connection from an artery to a vein, usually in an arm or leg. One such shunt is shown in Fig. 1. It is then a simple matter to connect the 'artificial kidney' to the patient's blood supply.

The total volume of blood in the artificial kidney at any moment is small (about 500 ml), with a flow rate of about 300 ml/min, and a total dialyser membrane area of 1–3 m; this means that the equivalent of the whole blood volume of about 5 litres in an adult circulates through the dialyser every 15–20 min.

Peritoneal dialysis

This is commonly termed CAPD — *continuous ambulatory peritoneal dialysis* — since most patients undergo the procedure while going about many of their normal activities. The principle of the method is that the peritoneal membrane, which lines the peritoneal cavity in the abdomen, is used as the dialysis membrane.

The patient has a tube (*catheter*) inserted through the abdominal wall into the peritoneal cavity, and this remains in place on a semi-permanent basis. Dialysis fluid (0.5–3 litres) is allowed to flow into the peritoneal cavity via the catheter, left in typically for several hours or overnight and then drained and replaced with fresh fluid. Movement of fluid and solute occurs across the peritoneal membrane by diffusion and *solvent drag* (convection), as described above.

The high urea content of the blood in renal failure creates an osmotic attraction across the peritoneal membrane, so that water would tend to move from the peritoneal cavity into the patient. To prevent this, and ensure that water moves from the patient's blood to the dialysis fluid, an osmotically active substance is incorporated in the dialysis fluid. This is usually dextrose, but amino acids and glucose polymers can also be used.   CHRIS LOTE

Further reading

Gabriel, R. (1990). *A patient's guide to dialysis and transplantation*, (4th edn). Kluwer Academic.

See also KIDNEYS; ORGAN DONATION.

Diaphragm The term has come to be applied to any thin partition, either in a man-made instrument or in biology. But the original meaning from the Greek referred more to hedging around or fencing in; that meaning is well fitted by the contraceptive diaphragm: a thin rubber cup which fences in the neck of the womb against invasion by sperm.

The human anatomical diaphragm is a part muscle, part tendinous sheet, convex upwards, that separates the thorax from the abdomen. It is described as doubly 'domed', accommodating below it the LIVER on the right and the STOMACH and SPLEEN on the left. It is attached to the inside of the lower margin of the 'rib cage': from the sternum (breast bone) in front, the cartilages interposed between this and the lower ribs around the sides, to reach the vertebral column behind. It is a complete partition except for openings to allow passage between thorax and abdomen: for the OESOPHAGUS to join the stomach, for the main artery (aorta) and for the main vein (inferior vena cava) that carry blood to and from the lower body, and for nerves and lymphatics vessels.

When the muscle of the diaphragm contracts, its convexity is flattened. This, together with other mechanical factors and muscular actions, causes an increase in the capacity of the thorax, which in turn draws air into the lungs. The motor nerve supply to the diaphragm comes to its upper surface in the *phrenic nerves* from each side of the neck. These carry the rhythmic bursts of impulses, relayed from the BRAIN STEM via the phrenic MOTOR NEURONS in the SPINAL CORD, which cause regular inspiration. Each time these stop, the diaphragm relaxes and rises, and air leaves the lungs. Although this cyclical control of the diaphragm and other breathing muscles occurs automatically, it is of course possible to control them voluntarily — to stop, start, or deepen breathing. The extent to which the diaphragm is used relative to the muscles of the thorax can also come under voluntary control, by selecting 'abdominal' breathing rather than chest expansion.   SHEILA JENNETT

See PLATE 3.

See also BREATHING.

Diarrhoea is a world-wide health problem. It ranges from a trivial nuisance for travellers to a fatal illness, particularly among children in underdeveloped countries. Infection is the commonest but not the only cause of diarrhoea. The several causes will be reviewed, but first it is necessary to be clear about the meaning of the term itself.

Diarrhoea is commonly defined as a change in bowel habit resulting in an increase in stool frequency or fluidity or both. Since stool frequency and consistency varies widely in the normal population it is the change from what is usual that is important. Stool frequency alone is not a good indicator of 'true diarrhoea' since stool frequency can increase in 'irritable bowel syndrome', but the total amount of stool passed each day may be unchanged and within normal limits. It is for this reason that diarrhoea is best defined by stool weight, which for an individual in the Western world is usually less than 200 g/day. In the developing world, stool weight is higher in the normal population (250–400 g/day). Diarrhoea may be acute — an illness of abrupt onset lasting 3–7 days — or chronic (persistent), which is usually defined as lasting more than 14 days.

Mechanisms and causes of diarrhoea

Normally, during a 24-hour period, about 9 litres of fluid enter the small intestine. About 2 litres come from the diet, and the remaining 7 litres from secretions into the alimentary tract which carry the ENZYMES and other substances necessary for the digestion and absorption of food: saliva, gastric juice, biliary, and pancreatic secretions, and additional fluid secreted by the small intestine itself. Of these 9 litres only 1–2 litres pass on into the colon, so under normal circumstances the small intestine reabsorbs 7 litres of fluid into the bloodstream. The colon also retrieves the major part of the fluid with which it is presented, so that only about 100 ml finally leave the body in faeces. Diarrhoea results when these absorptive mechanisms fail to retrieve the large volume of fluid entering the small intestine, or when there is excessive secretion of fluid into either the small or large intestine. In some circumstances both decreased absorption and increased secretion are combined.

Acute or chronic diarrhoea may be due to a variety of pathophysiological mechanisms and is often categorised into four major groups as follows:

Osmotic diarrhoea Failure of the intestine to absorb certain solutes results in an increase in the osmolality of intestinal contents which draws an excess of water into the gut from the body fluids down the osmotic gradient. This occurs in conditions that involve carbohydrate malabsorption (monosaccharide intolerance, lactase and sucrase deficiency) or ingestion of non-absorbed saccharides, such as sorbitol, which is used as a sweetener in sugar-free confectionery, and the laxative, lactulose. Magnesium sulphate (Epsom salts) is effective as a laxative because of its osmotic effects. Other conditions which produce malabsorption syndromes, such as coeliac disease, also produce diarrhoea because of the presence of non-absorbed solute in the intestine.

Secretory diarrhoea Cholera toxin is an example of a bacterial product which produces high-volume watery diarrhoea by promoting massive secretion from the lining of the small intestine. The non-osmotic laxatives, phenolphthalein and senna, partly act by stimulating secretory mechanisms in the intestine. Bile salts, which aid in the process of digestion and absorption of nutrients, are normally absorbed in the last part of the small intestine (*terminal ileum*). Surgical removal or disease of this part of the bowel causes bile acids to move on into the colon where they interfere with water absorption, causing diarrhoea.

Exudative diarrhoea occurs usually as a result of damage to the lining of the gut, which leads to impaired absorption or increased losses of body fluids into the lumen. Common causes include intestinal infections, inflammatory bowel diseases (*Crohn's disease* and *ulcerative colitis*), other forms of colitis including those due to irradiation and ischaemia, and coeliac disease.

Increased motility Rapid transit through the intestine can result in true diarrhoea due to the reduced time available for intestinal absorption. This mechanism is thought to be important in some forms of laxative abuse, diabetic diarrhoea, and thyrotoxicosis. Certain functional disorders, such as irritable bowel syndrome, are also associated with more rapid intestinal transit, although in these conditions the change in bowel habit is often regarded as 'pseudodiarrhoea' because the increase in bowel frequency is not accompanied by an increase in stool weight.

Acute diarrhoea

Patients with acute watery diarrhoea generally have an intestinal infection. In infants and young children this is most commonly due to a virus infection (rotavirus or adenovirus). There are reported to be no less than 130 million cases annually worldwide, of which about 1 in 150 are fatal.

In adult travellers a frequent cause is a type of *E. coli* bacterium, which thrives in hot countries and forms toxins that disturb the function of the gut lining. In the indigenous population of industrialised countries, the commonest organisms are bacteria of the *Salmonella, Campylobacter,* or *Clostridium* families. The last is particularly common in the elderly and in immunocompromised patients undergoing anti-cancer chemotherapy. Acute diarrhoea accompanied by blood (dysentery) usually indicates infection with an invasive enteropathogen (an organism that attacks the cells of the lining of the gut) such as a member of the genus *Shigella* (causing bacillary dysentery), an invasive strain of *E. coli*, or amoebiasis (amoebic dysentery).

Organisms cause acute diarrhoea either by multiplying in a food source, and surviving to be ingested if it is not fully cooked (e.g. *Salmonella* in chickens), or through living in the gut of people or animals, whose faeces contaminate food or water by reason of defective personal or social hygiene (e.g. *E. coli* and *Shigella* from humans; *Campylobacter* from farm animals, birds, or pets).

In many instances the presence of infection can be determined by microscopic examination of the stool for evidence of parasites and microbiological culture for bacteria.

When acute diarrhoea is due to infection it is usually self-limiting and will remit without specific therapy. When the illness is more severe, oral rehydration therapy with glucose–electrolyte solutions is the mainstay of therapy to correct dehydration and acidosis. There is no need to modify food intake during episodes of diarrhoea, although secondary deficiency of lactase absorption can occur and it sometimes wise to restrict milk and milk products. Breast feeding of infants should continue despite diarrhoea.

Anti-diarrhoeal agents, such as loperamide, are sometimes helpful to reduce bowel frequency but should be avoided in children. Antibiotics are not routinely used for the treatment of acute infective diarrhoea although it is well established that a short course can reduce the severity and duration of symptoms. Some infections, however, do require antibiotic therapy, particularly the invasive organisms that cause dysentery such as severe *Shigella* and *Salmonella* infections and amoebiasis.

Persistent diarrhoea

When diarrhoea is persistent, measurement of stool weight over a 3-day period may be needed to confirm whether this is true diarrhoea or 'pseudo-diarrhoea'. Laxative abuse may be revealed by urine testing. Chronic parasitic infection can be sought and excluded by microscopic examination of the stools. Inflammatory bowel disease usually requires an examination of the colon by endoscopy and possibly a small bowel radiological examination using barium by mouth — a barium 'follow-through' examination. If a small bowel disorder such as coeliac disease is considered likely then a small intestinal mucosal biopsy may be required to confirm the diagnosis.

The treatment of chronic diarrhoea depends entirely on the causes. Chronic infections due to certain parasites such as *Giardia lamblia* and *Entamoeba histolytica* require anti-microbial chemotherapy. Chronic diarrhoea due to inflammatory bowel disease usually requires treatment with anti-inflammatory drugs such as corticosteroids or 5-aminosalicylic acid. Dietary therapy is sometimes required when the problem is a food sensitivity, such as coeliac disease when a GLUTEN-free diet is appropriate.

MICHAEL FARTHING

ANNE BALLINGER

See also BACTERIA; INFECTIOUS DISEASE; PARASITES; VOMITING.

Dieting While one can diet to gain weight, or for specific physiological needs such as allergies or diabetes management, 'dieting' tends to refer to the process of manipulating food intake and energy output in order to reduce BODY WEIGHT for health or aesthetic reasons. To reduce weight, fewer calories than the body needs are ingested, forcing the body to obtain its energy from fat stores. To lose 1 lb per week, about 3500 kcal, (the weight of 1 lb of fat tissue) must be subtracted from the diet.

But the Latin root *diaeta*, 'a way of life', more accurately describes the daily realities of contemporary dieters. Fostered by Western medical and beauty standards, which prize slenderness, a 30 billion dollar diet industry has produced a wealth of diet plans ranging from hazardous fad diets to the nutritionally healthful. Recent research has emphasized the efficacy of drug therapies such as amphetamines and leptin, but the potential side-effects continue to pose serious problems. Since the majority of people who lose weight via dieting eventually gain it back, dieting has become a constant way of life for large numbers of Western people.

Dieting, particularly in order to achieve a thin ideal, only makes sense in the midst of affluence. Where food shortages endure, dieting (versus FASTING for religious or cultural reasons) holds little value. On the other hand, affluent Western societies admire successful dieters for their self-discipline and willpower, as well as for their slim bodies.

Diet regimens, including those for weight loss, have existed for centuries, but modern dieting gained popularity in the late nineteenth and early twentieth centuries. Scientists who turned their attention to nutrition in the nineteenth century began to argue against overeating. Researchers such as Wilbur Atwater and Ellen Swallows 'discovered' VITAMINS, MINERALS, and calories as well as an understanding of how the body converted fat into energy. From this knowledge, the 'new nutritionists' laid the groundwork for modern dieting. They advocated lower body weights and smaller meals, and encouraged people to make dietary decisions based on the chemical composition of food (its nutritional value) versus taste or appearance. They encouraged everyone to count calories. Though invisible to the naked eye, excess calories would pile on very visible fat.

At the same time, a new, slender ideal of beauty, especially for women, gained cultural prominence. As historian Lois Banner has pointed out, in the late nineteenth century several popular ideals of female beauty, including robust and curvaceous images, competed for public attention, but by the 1920s, the slim-hipped, small-breasted, straight-lined flapper became the popular ideal. Though the exact dimension and shape of beauty ideals have shifted, the thin standard has never waned.   MARGARET A. LOWE

Further reading

Banner, L. (1983). *American beauty*. Knopf, New York.

Schwartz, H. (1987) *Never satisfied: a cultural history of diets, fantasies, and fat.* Collier–Macmillan, London.

See also DIETS; ENERGY BALANCE; OBESITY.

Diets A diet is a pattern of FOOD consumption which is followed by a population or an individual. The diets of populations are affected by local factors including geography, climate, food availability, culture, and religion, whereas the diets of individuals within populations are further influenced by factors such as socio–economic status, personal preference, and health considerations. To maintain life, all diets must supply the essential amounts of energy, PROTEIN, essential FATTY ACIDS, VITAMINS, and MINERALS, but these needs can be met by a wide variety of diets, each of which will be sufficient for growth, survival, and reproduction but may also have obvious or subtle effects on the long-term state of health.

Traditional diets

The traditional diets of populations around the world vary greatly. The diet of Inuit hunters in the Arctic is composed almost entirely of meat and fish, but most hunter-gatherers in other parts of the world obtain more food from gathering plants than from hunting animals. Pastoralists keep different animals according to where they live, varying from reindeer in the north to camels in hot arid areas, but they always have a diet rich in animal foods such as milk, meat, and blood. Peasant agriculturalists grow different staple crops according to local conditions, but usually have diets composed largely of plant foods with only small amounts of animal foods.

The traditional diets of populations have been followed for hundreds or thousands of years and, except in times of severe food shortage, are certainly compatible with the maintenance of health sufficient for the survival and growth of infants and children, and for successful reproduction. However, traditional diets are sometimes far from optimal and may be accompanied by serious nutritional disorders, from which the people may have suffered for many generations. For example, approximately one-fifth of the population of the world is at significant risk for developing iodine deficiency disorders; pellagra was formerly common in populations subsisting largely on maize due to deficiency in the vitamin niacin and the amino acid tryptophan; and high BLOOD PRESSURE and STROKE are common in populations with a diet high in SALT.

'Western' diets

The diets of affluent Western populations changed very rapidly during the twentieth century. In comparison with the diets of peasant agriculturalists, Western diets are usually much higher in animal protein and fat and much lower in starch and dietary fibre, and ample food is available throughout the year. It is well known that Westernization of the diet is usually associated with increases in the rates of some diseases, such as ischaemic heart disease, large bowel CANCER, and OBESITY, but it should also be appreciated that Westernization is generally accompanied by an increase in overall life expectancy and by decreases in the rates of some diet-related diseases such as stomach cancer, as well as decreases in the incidence of most infectious diseases.

Diets for health

Within Western populations, the word 'diet' is commonly used to refer to patterns of food consumption which are followed for reasons of health or for ethical or religious reasons (VEGETARIAN and VEGAN diets are discussed in separate entries). A good diet is of profound importance for the maintenance of good health; nutritional deficiencies severe enough to cause obvious diseases such as scurvy and pellagra are now very rare in Western societies, but diet is a major determinant of the risk for developing many of the commonest fatal diseases, including ischaemic heart disease, stroke, and cancers of the large bowel and stomach.

The commonest type of diet followed for health reasons is one intended to cause weight loss in the treatment of overweight, and the term DIETING is often assumed to refer to a weight-reduction diet. Numerous types of weight-reducing diets have been marketed. Most will cause some initial weight loss, but this is difficult to maintain because obesity is associated with the typical Western lifestyle of low physical activity and constant availability of highly palatable, energy-dense foods.

After obesity, the most common reason for requiring dietary changes is a high blood cholesterol concentration and associated ischaemic heart disease. The blood CHOLESTEROL concentration is increased by diets high in saturated fat and cholesterol. Reducing the intake of these factors causes a reduction in blood cholesterol, but most individuals find it difficult to change their diet sufficiently to have more than a small effect. Other diets followed for health reasons include low salt diets for the reduction of raised blood pressure and GLUTEN-free diets for individuals with coeliac disease.

High-fibre diets have become popular since the work of Denis Burkitt and others in the early 1970s. Fibre is now defined as non-starch polysaccharides, and is supplied by unrefined cereals, vegetables, and fruits. Fibre has several benefits, including the prevention of CONSTIPATION and probably reducing the risk for coronary heart disease and cancer of the large bowel.

The topic of diet and health is covered extensively by the media and many people are confused as to what constitutes a healthy diet. Government bodies in many countries now make dietary recommendations. In Britain, the Committee on Medical Aspects of Food Policy (COMA) reviews various aspects of the relationship of diet with health. In their recent report on nutritional aspects of cardiovascular disease, COMA made several recommendations for adults, including that total fat and saturated fat should provide no more than 35% and 10% respectively of food energy, that average salt intake should be reduced to 6 g per day, and that the consumption of vegetables, fruit, potatoes, and bread should be increased by at least 50%. These recommendations reflect a growing consensus that a healthy diet should be based on starch-rich foods such as cereals and should include generous quantities of fruit and vegetables. This type of diet is also rich in dietary fibre and many vitamins, and the emphasis is on supplying these nutrients from ordinary foods rather than from special high-fibre foods or vitamin supplements.

Future needs — more science in the choice of diets for populations and individuals

Traditional diets have evolved out of necessity, to be sufficient for life, but are often far short of ideal. Western diets have come from traditional roots but have been radically changed by affluence, developments in agriculture and food processing, advertising, fashion, etc. Most people now eat a diet determined by a mixture of tradition, availability, convenience, taste, and peer pressure. The health effects of the resulting mix are themselves mixed, with some diet-related health problems decreasing and others increasing. We already have sufficient knowledge to do much better than this, and need to introduce more science into all the components of society which affect food consumption, including agricultural policy and the education of children, caterers, and politicians. Evidence from sound scientific studies should be continually fed into society with the aim of producing improvements in the health of the population and in the optimal use of land and other resources.

TIM KEY

Further reading

Report of the Cardiovascular Review Group Committee on Medical Aspects of Food Policy (1994). *Nutritional aspects of cardiovascular disease.* HMSO, London.

See also DIETING; FOOD; HEALTH FOODS; VEGAN; VEGETARIAN; ENTRIES ON THE SEPARATE DIETARY CONSTITUENTS.

Diffusion The name applied to a physical process by which individual particles move randomly, within a fluid, from areas of high concentration to lower concentration until the particles are evenly distributed throughout the space. The particles referred to can be molecules or ions and the fluid can be either gaseous or liquid. For example, a person wearing perfume can be noticed on entering a room because molecules of the odiferous substances contained within the perfume diffuse in the air and are detected by the nose. Similarly, a drop of dye dropped into a glass of water will eventually colour the whole volume as the molecules of dye diffuse evenly throughout the volume. Because of thermal motion and vibration, a molecule, ion, or small particle undergoes 10 to 10 collisions per second with molecules of the fluid. The particle is said to undergo a *random walk*, in which the result of a particular collision is independent of the effects of previous collisions. The statistical consequence of this is that the displacement of a particle from its original position will depend on the elapsed time. Where the diffusing particles are at high concentration, many collisions will be between the diffusing species, so that they will move away from each other, thus creating a flux from high concentration to low until the concentration is even throughout the volume. Diffusion is influenced by many factors, such as viscosity and electric charge. Thus diffusion in treacle will be slower than diffusion in water, and particles carrying the same charge will exert mutual repulsion.

Diffusion is an important process for bodily function. Important substances, such as OXYGEN and CARBON DIOXIDE, not only need to diffuse within a particular fluid volume but need to diffuse from one bodily compartment to another across barriers, where generally diffusion will be slower than within a fluid. Consider the position in the LUNGS; oxygen from the air has to diffuse across the walls of the alveoli and of the capillaries within the lungs to reach the blood, and then across the walls of the red cells to reach the HAEMOGLOBIN. Fortunately it combines with the haemoglobin to form oxyhaemoglobin, thus maintaining a steep concentration gradient. At the same time carbon dioxide, released from the venous blood, needs to diffuse in the opposite direction, down its concentration gradient, into the lungs, in order to be exhaled. As the transit time of blood in the lungs is just a few seconds, the diffusive process needs to be rapid. (If, for example, the lungs are filled with thick, viscid mucus, as in bronchiectasis or cystic fibrosis, then the diffusive process is impaired and full oxygenation will not occur). Conversely, when oxygenated blood arrives at the tissues the conditions are such that oxygen is released and needs to diffuse into the cells to maintain tissue respiration, whilst carbon dioxide, a product of tissue respiration, needs to be loaded into the blood for conveyance back to the lungs.

Diffusion is similarly important in the absorptive processes in the gut. The purpose of digestion is to break down complex molecules into simple ones such as SUGARS, FATS, and PEPTIDES. The lining of the gut wall has many specialised transporters to take the breakdown products into the cells and to transfer them to the blood, for delivery to tissues where they can be used as a source of energy, stored, or used for growth and repair. However, to arrive at the transporters the products of digestion need to diffuse from the gut contents, through the aqueous stationary layer closest to the lining of the gut, to reach the transporters. Diffusion therefore is a universally important process affecting every aspect of living tissue. A single living cell is a hive of activity. Substances produced within the cell which are important for its normal functioning may be produced at one site but then interact with another part of the cell, which they reach by diffusion, moving from high concentration to low by way of thermal motion, an inherent physical property.

ALAN W. CUTHBERT

Digestion The process whereby the constituents of food are broken down into simpler organic chemicals that can be absorbed through the lining of the gut. Mastication in the mouth and churning in the stomach assist mixing with the secreted juices which contain the necessary ENZYMES to catalyse the chemical processes. The linings of the mouth, stomach, and small intestine, together with the pancreas, contribute three main types of enzyme: amylases for carbohydrates, lipases for

fats, and proteases for proteins. The end products are simple sugars, lipids, peptides and amino acids.

SHEILA JENNETT

See ALIMENTARY SYSTEM; EATING; ENZYMES.

Dimples Small indentations in the surface of the SKIN, usually, though not always, on the FACE. The primary use of 'dimple' is in reference to small hollows formed by the cheeks when smiling or to a small dent in the surface of the chin. Dimples can be permanent or transient, and can occur in any part of the body with sufficient flexibility of skin and plumpness to allow their formation, including shoulders (especially in children), legs, and buttocks.

The origin of the term 'dimple' is obscure and, unlike most other English words describing facial features, use of the word is in evidence only relatively recently, from about the fifteenth or sixteenth century onward. Shakespeare mentions dimples in *The Winter's Tale* (1610–11): 'The pretty dimples of his chin, and cheek' (II.iii.101). Occurrences of the use of the term increase after this period.

Some anatomical uses of the term lack the pleasant connotations commonly associated with a pretty chin or cheek. Certain genetic disorders produce conditions referred to as 'dimples'. For example, occlusions of the gastrointestinal tract can be caused by the failure to form a true anus; instead, those with this defect are born with a dent or 'dimple' that must be corrected by surgery.

Dimples and dimpling extend well beyond references to the body. One possible (though historically unsupported) origin of the term, the Middle High German *tümpfel* and modern German *tümpel* — pond, pool, or puddle — conveys the sense of 'dimple' as used to refer to depressions or dips in a geographic surface, including the dip in surrounding land made by the surface of a pond or a 'dimple' caused by a low spot in a meadow or hill.

Dimples are generally considered attractive features when located on the cheeks or chin. SMILING tends to enhance social interactions and life in general, and has been shown in recent studies to increase perceptions of attractiveness over neutral expressions. Dimples tend to accentuate a smile and thus may increase perceptions of attractiveness and sociability. Dimples, especially on the chin, also increase the angularity and definition of the male face, creating the impression of a strong visage. It is probably not coincidental that many of Hollywood's leading men of the 'Golden Age' of movies, identified with competence, strength, and fortitude, had well-defined chins or lively smiles notable for their dimples.

JEFFREY BARKER

See also BEAUTY; FACE.

Disability Which one of us is not disabled or 'challenged' in some aspect of our physical or mental capacity? The spectrum of human ability is wide, and it is on their capabilities that people with a disability would like society to focus.

Definitions

There is no single commonly-accepted, straightforward definition of disability. The subject is complex and controversial. Three of the main sources for definitions of disability are the medical, social, and legal models. The medical model uses the World Health Organisation (WHO) definition. The WHO (1980) outlines the relationships between impairment, disability, and handicap. The simplified working definition is called the International Classification of Impairments, Disabilities, and Handicaps (ICIDH). It uses these terms to describe the inter-relationship, aiming to achieve consistency in the meaning and use of the labels. The focus is on functional difficulties.

> A disease, disorder or injury produces an impairment causing a change to ordinary functioning. Impairment refers to failure at the level of organs or systems of the body. This means loss or abnormality of psychological, physiological or anatomical structure or function. A disability refers to the resulting reduction or loss of ability to perform an activity in the manner considered normal for a human being e.g. climbing stairs or manipulating a keyboard. A handicap is a social disadvantage resulting from an impairment or disability which limits or prevents the fulfillment of a normal role.

This medical model demonstrates an interplay of factors acknowledging that grey areas requiring interpretation are acceptable within the definition. For purposes of assessment, quite often what matters is not the medical condition but the accompanying decrease or loss of function resulting from a disability.

The social model separates a person's specific impairment from his or her disability. In this approach, 'a person with an impairment becomes 'disabled' when the organisation of the society in which they live excludes them from mainstream activities' (Employers' Forum on Disability). The Royal College of Physicians stresses the need to consider disability in the context of 'a disabled person's encounter with daily living, the environment and society, not only in specific circumstances, but in the whole of that experience'. This then can meet the needs of individual differences and concentrate on the external, reversible factors. Clarifying 'barrier-free' policies for everyone rather than 'special case' policies for people with labels creates a more dynamic approach.

The third model incorporates the legal aspect and includes the rights of the individual. The current UK Disability Discrimination Act (DDA), 1995, was introduced to progress individuals beyond the limitations of the 1944 register for disabled people and the quota system. The Act states that a person has a disability for the purposes of this Act if he has: 'a physical or mental impairment which has a substantial and long term adverse effect on his ability to carry out normal day to day activities.' The purpose of this legislation is to protect individuals with a disability which makes it difficult for them to carry out ordinary, routine, day to day activities. The disability can cover physical, sensory, or mental faculties. It must be substantial and last or be expected to last for at least one year. The Act requires employers with 15 employees or more to make 'reasonable provision' for disabled workers.

Interpretation

The definitions above utilise the words 'normal' and 'reasonable' which are of course wide open to interpretation, escalating to contentious and litigious argument whenever the financial stakes are high. This frequently results in queries around settlement of legal, industrial, discriminatory, or insurance claims, assessment for medical aid, supply of high-tech equipment, provision of expensive prostheses, and access to special facilities, including education. Allocation of these increasingly expensive, sophisticated, and necessarily limited resources always hinges on the assessment of the degree of disability. Thus, whatever the formal definition, it is crucial to relate the disability to the level of purposeful functioning. For example, a short-sighted person might meet one test for disability, whilst with corrective lenses few would regard his myopia as a disability. Yet, if the myopia was severe or seriously progressive, no one would argue that this visual problem or partial sight did not constitute a disability, a handicap, and an impairment. A significant disability like blindness does not prevent a senior politician from performing a leading role, although he has to find creative ways and support to overcome the functional handicaps of his impairment. A relatively minor impairment, the loss of a finger to a violinist or of a thumb to a labourer, would be both a major disability and an occupational handicap — although not so to a majority of lecturers or teachers. Many people manage life well with asthma, but for a plasterer this would signal a major life and job change.

The definitions given generally refer both to physical disabilities and to mental health problems. Care is needed with respect to the latter, since many people appear 'normal' and also cope well much of the time, although in practice their day to day functioning can be seriously affected. Mental illness is therefore at risk of going undetected, with the individual consequently deprived of the necessary support until significant inappropriate behaviour is displayed. The reasons are a combination of the invisible nature of the disability, the not infrequent lack of a formal diagnosis, and the poor level of awareness of mental health issues amongst the healthy population.

Disabled people do not form a static or easily-identified group distinct from the rest of society. Some impairments improve with time while others are exacerbated. There are disabilities that are invisible, like diabetes, dyslexia, hearing loss, and mental illness. People not born with impairments can acquire them through accident or illness, and others born with them may gradually deteriorate.

What becomes important is not the label, though in some cases like dyslexia (specific learning difficulties) the label is important in gaining access to resources, but the assessment of loss of function in the context of employment and of day to day living.

Assessment

When it comes to assessment for resources and state benefits, few of the disabled person's rights depend on what the condition is called. Rather, the allocation of the benefit or service depends on the effect of the disability on day to day life. Someone with a severe facial disfigurement, not deliberately acquired, may not have a named disability but can suffer severe embarrassment and social stigma to such an extent that there is a long-term adverse effect and considerable handicap. They would be defined as a disabled person under the DDA.

Within health assessments, it is common to distinguish between two levels of activities of daily living (ADL): basic ADL are those that are essential for all aspects of self care; instrumental ADL are those activities such as shopping, housekeeping, and using private or public transport that are necessary for someone to maintain a level of independent living, especially in the absence of a carer.

The purpose for which the results are to be used is a necessary prerequisite in making an assessment. If, for example, the information is for inclusion in a survey this would necessarily be less stringent than for access to a facility or resource.

Objective assessments attempt to measure disability in a standardized form to provide information for individual health care, educational access, job requirements, and legal rights. Health professionals may use a variety of structured approaches from screening questionnaires to diagnostic tools involving physical tests. Psychometric tests can also be used for assessments. They have to be reliable and valid and can be used to measure ability, aptitude, reasoning, and aspects of personality.

It is appropriate to allow for self- as well as observer-based assessments. The person most likely to know the constraints and possibilities of their condition is the individual, who may also be one of the best sources for describing creative solutions to get around the difficulties. Self-assessment together with objectivity from health or support workers is likely to provide a realistic picture of limitations and potential.

In general, assessment gives an indication of need, can help with prediction of problems, and can give measures of outcome and output. Any system of assessment needs to be reliable, valid, sensitive to change, acceptable, relevant, realistic, and practical to use.

Perceptions

There is a strong need to combat bias and to dispel preconceptions in any review of disability. The disabled want the focus of their social relationships and medical interventions to be on their capabilities as far as that is reasonably possible. They wish to be accepted within society on an equal footing with equal rights. Typical situations include the doctor who addresses the carer rather than the individual, implying a perceived inability to communicate. Or, an employer may assume that disability will be an insuperable burden, dismissing the potential and commitment of the individual, in ignorance of the practical experience that disabled workers are frequently highly motivated, effective workers with good attendance records. Disabilities obviously can impose restrictions; but the goal many want as a right is unprejudiced, unfettered, and equal opportunity to demonstrate their creativity and their capability to function in day to day life and work.

Information

For the newly injured or diagnosed access to good information is crucial to dealing successfully with the trauma. The obvious sources are the institutional ones (hospitals, social services, and relevant government bodies). At the next level are the organisations usually related to particular conditions or lobby groups. Frequently, informal support groups have developed precisely because there may be limited practical support and information available. These can usually be accessed via helplines or the media. Other sources include:

(i) the *Disability Rights Handbook*, updated annually, published by Disability Alliance Education and Research Association;

(ii) the Internet;

(iii) the local library;

(iv) special Olympics and sporting organisations;

(v) the DDA information line;

(vi) *Ability*, 'The computer magazine about disability issues';

(vii) The Employers' Forum on Disability.

MARIAN BORDE

See also BLINDNESS; DEAFNESS; PARALYSIS.

Disease can be broadly defined as any ILLNESS or sickness that impairs or disrupts the normal functioning of the human body. Definitions of disease, however, have varied over time and place, and diagnostic categories vary. We will be concerned here with concepts of disease in the Western medical tradition. MEDICINE itself can be defined as 'the science and art concerned with the cure, alleviation, and prevention of disease, and with the restoration and preservation of health'. Thus the definition, treatment, and prevention, of disease is intimately associated with the development of medicine itself, and several specialist areas of medicine are specifically concerned with broad aspects of disease. For example *nosology*, the classification of diseases, was for many centuries the cornerstone of medicine; *therapeutics* is the treatment of disease; DIAGNOSIS is the art the physician uses to determine from the patients' signs and symptoms what the underlying causative mechanism may be; *epidemiology* is the study of disease in populations.

The Hippocratic tradition maintained that diseases were physiological, arising from an imbalance between the four HUMOURS, the correct balance of which maintained health. Each individual had a unique humoral balance which could be easily disrupted by conditions such as cold, biting winds, poor air, or injudicious eating. It was Paracelsus (*c.* 1492–1541) who provided an alternative to such classical ideas by suggesting that disease was the product of active agents independent of the human patient. The English Hippocrates, Thomas Sydenham (1624–89), also believed that diseases were specific entities, which might be manifest in variable ways in individual patients, but which could be recognised by observant clinicians. Sydenham also advocated that specific remedies could be applied to each such disease, his favourite example being the prescription of Peruvian bark for intermittent fever or ague. It was during the eighteenth century that the classification of diseases became a dominant part of medicine, such taxonomies often being based on the presenting symptoms. Increasing attention to pathology and cellular mechanisms during the nineteenth century provided additional criteria whereby diseases could be described, recognised, and treated.

An increasing array of diagnostic techniques have become available during the twentieth century, and these have made it possible for even more diseases, syndromes, and conditions to be classified, and the International Classification of Disease goes some way to providing international standardisation in the categorisation of modern disease.

Disease categories

One broad classification divides diseases into two principle categories, defining disease as primarily *congenital* (present at birth) or *acquired* subsequently. The acquired category can be further subdivided to include infectious, neoplastic, traumatic, and degenerative diseases, which are not necessarily mutually exclusive. Modern concepts and definitions have obscured many of these classificatory boundaries, and occupational, nutritional and deficiency, autoimmune and allergic, and psychiatric diseases can now be included in contemporary nosologies. As the molecular mechanisms of diseases and their causations are increasingly understood, so classifications are increasingly becoming blurred and overlapping, and many diseases are now recognised as being multi-causal. The following sections will give brief overviews of some broad classes of disease.

Genetics and diseases

Hereditary diseases may be passed down from generation to generation, but are not necessarily genetic disorders unless determined by one or more genes. The experiments on peas by Gregor Mendel (1822–84), on the transfer of characteristics from generation to generation, established the basic principles of HEREDITY. Mendel and his successors determined a number of factors to define genetic inheritance, including its occurrence in known proportions amongst relatives, but not in unrelated individuals, such as in-laws. Applied to human conditions, some diseases were now identified as hereditary, including haemophilia and sickle-cell anaemia — although it had been recognised for centuries that some diseases 'ran in the family'.

CONGENITAL ABNORMALITIES are present at birth, though some do not immediately become apparent. They are not necessarily inherited, many in fact being environmentally determined during intrauterine life. It is now known that many common diseases, including heart disease, insulin dependent diabetes, some forms of psychiatric illnesses, and autoimmune diseases, have a genetic component. But these susceptibilities are often triggered by some environmental influence, and represent a complex interaction between *nature* (genetic makeup) and *nurture* (external influences). Some forms of CANCER are increasingly recognised as having a major genetic component. The genetics of some diseases, such as cystic fibrosis, beta-thalassaemia, and Duchenne's muscular dystrophy, are now well known, and it is possible to screen parents, and unborn fetuses, to detect genetic abnormalities, and to offer termination of an affected fetus. The development of *in utero* GENE THERAPY offers the hope of treatment, whilst modern medicine can do a great deal to maintain individuals who, in earlier periods, would have died because of their genetic constitution.

Infectious diseases

INFECTIOUS DISEASES caused by microorganisms or parasites have been powerful forces in shaping human history. As early humans formed hunter–gatherer societies in about 3000 BC and began to contain and domesticate wild animals, so they became susceptible to the infections carried by the animals with which they now shared their living space. Smallpox, distemper, and measles are amongst the diseases known to have entered human populations at this time. The devastating effects of these diseases gradually became ameliorated as immunity built up in communities — major EPIDEMICS (and PANDEMICS) were often caused by the movement of communities where such diseases were endemic into non-immune populations. Urbanisation provided fresh opportunities for infectious diseases to flourish and to decimate populations — close living conditions encouraged the transfer of infections; migration into the cities from rural communities, and the dependency of urban populations on the countryside for food, provided fresh avenues for infection. Until almost the end of the nineteenth century, sustaining cities was a constant problem, and the large metropolitan areas of Western civilization were known to be centres of disease, malnutrition and starvation, and ultimately death. Diseases such as smallpox, syphilis, typhoid fever, and whooping cough were all endemic and accounted for a high infant mortality — estimates have suggested for example that the mortality rate for children under 5 was as high as 50% for much of the nineteenth century in the English city of Manchester. By the latter half of that century, the experiments of Robert Koch (1843–1910) in Germany and Louis Pasteur (1822–95) in France, amongst others, increasingly provided evidence that microorganisms were the cause of several infectious diseases. Efforts were made to utilise this knowledge in the manufacture of *vaccines*, preparations of modified or killed bacteria that could be administered to produce a mild form of the disease and to confer immunity. Although the precise mechanisms of how such immunity was created were unknown, a number of therapeutic substances were developed, the biggest breakthrough coming at the end of the nineteenth century with the appearance of serum anti-toxins. Since then, increasing understanding of the underlying cellular mechanisms of immunity and of the biology of microorganisms; the growth and development of the pharmaceutical industry, especially the discovery of antibiotics; and the development of public health measures to prevent and treat infectious diseases, have led to a notable decline in mortality and morbidity from such diseases in the Western world. The same cannot be said for the developing world, and concerns grew at the end of the twentieth century about resistance to antibiotics, the appearance of new infectious killers such as HIV (which causes AIDS), and the re-emergence of drug-resistant forms of diseases such as TB.

Autoimmune diseases

AUTOIMMUNE DISEASES occur when elements of the immune system, normally responsible for recognising and attacking 'non-self' cells — such as the microorganisms that cause infectious diseases — fail to distinguish between 'self' and 'non-self'. Such cellular attacks on healthy constituent parts of the body can contribute to a variety of disorders, including myasthenia gravis, some thyroid disorders, and rheumatoid arthritis. There is growing evidence that conditions such as diabetes and multiple sclerosis also have an autoimmune component.

Diseases associated with food: deficiencies, excesses, and intolerances

Deficiency (nutritional) diseases arise from lack of one or more essential nutritional component, such as a VITAMIN or MINERAL, in the diet, or because of the body's inability to digest, absorb, or utilize particular nutrients. A nutritional deficiency can also occur if the body's metabolism is abnormal or if essential elements are excessively excreted. Historically, deficiency diseases have arisen in populations forced, by war or famine, to abandon their traditional diets, or by the adoption, perhaps for religious reasons, of a restrictive diet. Expeditions into new territories have always been vulnerable to dietary diseases because of the difficulty of carrying adequate supplies. The most notable example was that of *scurvy*, and the development of its treatment by eating citrus fruits, which occurred long before the rationale was understood — namely that this corrected a vitamin C deficiency due to lack of fresh fruit and vegetables. Subtle changes to farming or cooking methods can also lead to unexpected deficiencies. One of the best known examples is the use of white (huskless) rice instead of brown (husked) rice. This can lead to *beri-beri*, particularly prevalent in the Far East, which is characterised by ascending weakness in the legs and accompanying muscle tenderness, and can lead to widespread nerve irritability and congestive heart failure. This is due to a lack of thiamine, a vitamin that is essential for the mechanisms by which energy is released from foodstuffs.

Excess consumption of certain kinds of foods has been shown to be associated with the onset of conditions such as heart disease or diabetes — often exacerbating a genetic predisposition, and thus once more blurring the distinctions between different disease categories. Over consumption of alcohol, cigarette SMOKING, and taking other damaging drugs can all lead to disease conditions that can be classified as 'self-inflicted' (a category that can also include SEXUALLY TRANSMITTED DISEASES contracted during unprotected sex).

Food intolerances have been increasingly recognised in the latter part of the twentieth century, as some individuals show anaphylactic responses to particular allergens, such as nuts or dairy products.

Occupational diseases and the effects of pollution

Concern about the workplace as a source of disease has grown, particularly since World War II, as have the specialities of public and occupational health. Safety procedures, including the use of PROTECTIVE CLOTHING, have been proposed to limit workers' exposure to dangerous chemicals or to hazardous practices. Working conditions, such as those for office workers using video display equipment, have received attention, and exposure to noise, bad ventilation, and poorly designed furniture have increasingly been recognised as playing a role in STRESS. Stress in turn is recognised as contributing to high blood pressure, heart disease, and STROKE.

These concerns are not, however, entirely new. Lead POISONING amongst miners was recognised by Hippocrates (*c.* 450 BCE), but it was really the impact of the Industrial Revolution that focused the attention of reformers and some physicians on the impact of working conditions on health. A Leeds physician, Charles Thackrah, wrote *The effects of arts, trades and professions on health and longevity* (1832), which described the occupational hazards attached to numerous trades, including flock dressers, maltsters, coffee grinders, and corn-sillers. The effects of adverse and dangerous conditions on the ordinary working man became an issue for the growing number of trade or labour unions, and reform movements throughout the twentieth century campaigned for safer working conditions and adequate health care and compensation for those injured in the workplace.

Increasingly, however, environmental dangers have been recognised as having wider impact than just at the workplace. There can be pollution from accidental contamination and from large-scale industrial accidents. Disease and disasters can arise from cynical exploitation by manufacturers who ignore concerns for the welfare not only of their own workforce, but also of those living in the vicinity of their production facilities, such as the workers in the asbestos industry or the victims of the Bhopal explosion in India that killed 2000 people. Dispersal of pollutants, by air as after the Chernobyl disaster in Ukraine, or by river systems, can cause disease at vast distances from the original site of contamination.

Psychiatric diseases

Mental illness can refer to disorders in perception, understanding, emotion, and behaviour, and can range from the milder PSYCHOLOGICAL DISORDERS and PSYCHOSOMATIC ILLNESS to the severe PSYCHOSIS. Psychiatric disorders have not always been seen to be the province of the medical profession: theories about demonic possession, for example, have led to religious remedies or persecution. For many centuries doctors had little to do with those classed as 'insane'. The insane were incarcerated and contained, rather than treated. In the twentieth century increasing acknowledgement of the interplay of social, psychological, and physical factors in the causation of many psychiatric disorders, and the development of specific pharmacological therapies, led to improved care. Here again, the categories of disease classifications have become blurred, as faulty chemical processes in the brain and genetic defects have been shown to account for some manifestations of mental disease.

Degenerative diseases

Ironically, as infectious diseases were increasingly conquered during the twentieth century, degenerative diseases emerged in the Western world, primarily affecting the elderly. Degenerative processes can strike in particular organs or tissues, resulting in damaged JOINTS, such as hips and knees; in weakened bones, as a result of OSTEOPOROSIS; or as degeneration of the brain, causing severe mental deficits, such as DEMENTIA. It has been argued, most notably by the epidemiologist, Thomas McKeown (1912–88), that the main risks to life and good health have occurred in 3 distinct historical phases: accidents and injuries; infections; and finally degenerative diseases of longevity, which can include diseases such as Alzheimer's disease, Parkinson's diseases and some cancers.

One of the best known degenerative diseases is Alzheimer's, first described in 1906 by Alois Alzheimer, but then recognised as only a very rare brain disorder associated with cognitive dysfunction. This type of dementia is now the most common acquired progressive brain syndrome, although its cause remains unknown. Recent figures from the US have shown that Alzheimer's affects more than 4% of the over-60s population, whilst prevalence grows to 20% of the over-80s age group. The impact of chronic degenerative disease is felt not only by individuals and families, but also by social welfare and health care systems.

Cancer

Cancer is caused by a breakdown in the normal processes of cell division and multiplication, resulting in uncontrolled cell growth producing a tumour. In the industrialized world, at the beginning of the twenty-first century, it is estimated that one-third of the population will develop cancer, with the probability currently increasing. This is partly because it is predominantly a disease of middle and old age, and as life expectancy has increased, so too has the incidence of cancer. Several cancers are known to have a genetic basis, and also the environmental impact of some pollutants, known as carcinogens, is becoming increasingly well understood.

Iatrogenic diseases

These diseases arise from medical treatment for another condition. Sometimes the problem may be due to recognised undesirable side-effects of therapeutic drugs, or to an unusual, idiosyncratic reaction to a medicament. A scheme of reporting adverse drug reactions, the so-called 'yellow card scheme' was introduced in Britain in the early 1970s, in an attempt to identify such reactions. Surgical procedures, when mishaps or infections result, can also inadvertently cause further disease.   E.M. TANSEY

Further reading
Kiple, K. F. (ed.) (1993). *The Cambridge world history of human disease.* Cambridge University Press.

McKeown, T. (1979). *The role of medicine: dream, mirage or nemesis.* Oxford University Press.

McKeown, T. (1988). *The origins of human disease.* Oxford University Press.

See also ALLERGY; DRUG ABUSE; ENVIRONMENTAL TOXICOLOGY; GENETICS, HUMAN; ISLAMIC MEDICINE; MEDICINE; MIND–BODY INTERACTION; WORK AND THE BODY.

Dissection of the human body is the act or art of cutting open the body in order to display and study the topographical ANATOMY and structure of its parts. It has its origins in antiquity. The evolution of the practice of dissection is a curious history of heroic academic endeavour, ingenuity, artistic idealism, romance, and iniquity. Claude BERNARD, the French physiologist, rightly described anatomy as the basis of all physiology. Without a proper understanding of both there could never have been a scientific approach to the study and practice of medicine.

The story of the systematic dissection (anatomizing) of human corpses really begins in Alexandria (*c.* 300–250 BC). It was here that anatomy first became a recognized discipline and that a proper systematized description of the structure of the human body was made. This was largely due to the work of Herophilus and Erasistratus. Herophilus is universally acknowledged as the 'father of anatomy' and is believed to be the first person to have performed a public dissection of the human body. He is thought to have performed approximately 600 dissections during his career, and it is alleged that some of these were vivisections (dissections of live persons) of condemned criminals. His contemporary, Erasistratus, also performed dissections. Together they made significant contributions to the study of abdominal and pelvic viscera, vascular anatomy, and neuroanatomy. Following the decline of Alexandrian science, the seat of serious anatomical study shifted to Rome. Here, GALEN of Pergamum (129–216 AD) was the pre-eminent anatomist. Galen based his anatomical observations solely on animal dissections, and made the serious misjudgement of inferring that human anatomical features were identical to those in animals. Galen's authoritarian teaching held powerful sway throughout his lifetime and for a considerable period thereafter, resulting in the propagation of many erroneous concepts. For over a thousand years following Galen's death, there was a virtual cessation of any form of original anatomical inquiry. The practice of dissection had stopped altogether, chiefly due to contemporaneous religious proscriptions. This period of general intellectual stagnation is termed the Dark Ages. The resumption of the exploration of human anatomy by dissection, and the scientific impulse to verify or challenge Galenic doctrine, were part of the general intellectual reawakening (the Renaissance) that commenced in Italy during the thirteenth and fourteenth centuries and spread rapidly through the rest of Europe. The proliferation of this intellectual activity owed much to the many universities which were established in Italy and elsewhere in Europe, notably those in Salerno, Bologna, Padua, Florence, Louvain, Paris, and Montpelier. There is evidence that human post-mortem examinations were conducted in Bologna towards the end of the thirteenth century. These, however, were done not primarily for anatomical study, but to ascertain the cause of death. The first comprehensive human dissection to be done in post-Alexandrian times was performed in Bologna, in 1315 AD, by Mondino de Luzzi, a professor of medicine at the university in Bologna. In the following year he published his treatise, *Anathomia*, which reads remarkably like a practical dissection manual. Mondino's dissections were public events. He performed these in person and was largely responsible for restoring to anatomy its original respectability and status as a recognized discipline. None of Mondino's successors in Bologna made any significant contribution to anatomical knowledge.

The next milestone in the history of dissection occurred in 1543, when Andreas VESALIUS, a young professor of anatomy in Padua, published his masterpiece *De Humani Corporis Fabrica*

Libris Septem ('the seven books on the fabric of the human body'). This was an exhaustive and systematically classified compendium of anatomical observations, sumptuously illustrated with accurate depictions of dissections based on Vesalius' vast personal experience, and laying to rest all Galenic misconceptions. Vesalius was largely responsible for inspiring the modern scientific study of topographical anatomy based upon direct observation at dissection, as opposed to the traditional ecclesiastical method of interpreting the written word. Realdus Columbus, Gabriel Fallopius, and Heironymus Fabricius continued the Vesalian anatomical tradition in Padua. Between the thirteenth and seventeenth centuries, Bologna and Padua (principally the latter) were the leading centres of anatomical study in the world.

It is generally acknowledged that Joannes Caius, a colleague of Vesalius, was the first to popularize the study of practical anatomy by dissection in England. Caius taught anatomy in Cambridge. However, neither Caius nor any of his immediate successors made any original contributions, and anatomical study in England was generally barren until the advent of William HARVEY. Harvey's great intellectual triumph, *De moto cordis et sanguinis*, was published in 1628, and proved conclusively the circulation of blood. He reached his findings 'by reason and experiment' based on observations made in the course of dissecting several bodies, including those of his own father and sister (post-mortem) — a most unusual manifestation of clinical detachment.

During the fifteenth century, in the wake of the revival of anatomical dissection, there appeared a movement in Western art toward accurate representation of the human form. Prime among the exponents of this new school of naturalism in art were LEONARDO DA VINCI, Michelangelo Buanorroti, Albrecht Durer, Andrea Mantegna, and Andrea Verrocchio. Such was their obsession for scrupulous anatomical accuracy in their artistic depictions that they took to performing elaborate dissections (often in collaboration with eminent anatomists of the day) to enhance their understanding of the structure of the human body.

Availability and procurement of cadavers

Until the eighteenth century, the only lawful source of cadavers for dissection was the gallows. In Italy, papal consent was necessary before the corpse of an executed criminal could be dissected. In Scotland and in England royal assent was required in order to dissect the bodies of hanged felons. These legitimate dissections were intended as nominated public events and were conducted in large halls or amphitheatres. From the early eighteenth century onwards, anatomical theatres, specifically designed for dissection, were built in many of the major centres of anatomical study in Europe, including Leyden, Dublin, Edinburgh, London, Paris, and Louvain. These theatres were the forerunners of the

modern-day dissection halls in medical schools. Towards the end of the eighteenth century, France repealed the law allowing dissection of executed criminals. Other European nations, including Britain, soon followed.

Thereafter only unclaimed bodies of persons dying in civil hospitals, prisons, and poor-houses could legitimately be used for dissection. However, the limited availability of legally-obtainable cadavers during the early days of dissection led to the unsavoury practice of 'grave-robbing' or 'BODY SNATCHING' — the illegal exhumation and theft of freshly interred bodies for dissection. The scandal of 'BURKE AND HARE' who committed murder to supply corpses to anatomists, led to the very first act of legislation regulating the acquisition and use of cadavers for dissection in Great Britain, the Anatomy Act of 1832. In the present day, laws in different countries ensure that only such bodies as are legally bequeathed to medical institutions are used for dissection.

Preservation of cadavers

From the very earliest days of human dissection until relatively recently, a problem for anatomists was that there was no satisfactory method of preserving cadavers that would allow dissection to be carried out in an unhurried manner. The natural decomposition of the body, a rapid process, dictated the need for the dissection to be accomplished quickly and efficiently (in a matter of 3–4 days at most) before the unbearable stench of the putrefying cadaver made it impossible for the dissector to continue his task. In conditions of excessive humidity and warmth the problem was worse still, for which reason anatomists preferred to perform dissections during the winter months.

Robert Boyle's observation in the 1650s that decomposition of animal and human tissues could be prevented by immersing them in spirits of wine was a notable advance. This remained the principal method of cadaveric preservation until the latter half of the nineteenth century, when the antiseptic and preservative properties of formaldehyde were discovered. In the present day, preservation of cadavers (embalming) is usually accomplished by inserting tubes into a large artery and vein (usually the femoral artery and vein), washing out the blood, and then infusing a mixture of formalin (a 40% solution of formaldehyde), industrial alcohol, phenol, and glycerin. This mixture ensures that the body is both sterilized and preserved, and the glycerin prevents the tissues from becoming excessively hardened, thereby facilitating the process of dissection. As a result of these preservation techniques, there are several museums of human anatomy today containing permanent displays of beautifully dissected specimens. Among the finest and most comprehensive of these is the Wellcome museum of anatomy at the Royal College of Surgeons of England in London.

The study of human anatomy by dissection remains, today, an integral part of the basic undergraduate curriculum in medical schools the world over. A relatively recent innovation is the establishment of centres where experienced surgeons can revise and refine their anatomical knowledge of a particular surgical operation by cadaveric dissection, using precision instruments for incising tissues, operating microscopes for better visualization of structures, high-power drills for cutting bone, and endoscopes for viewing internal anatomy.   VISHI MAHADEVAN

See also ANATOMY; BODY SNATCHES; BURKE AND HARE.

Diuretics
Diuresis is increased URINE flow, and diuretics are substances which elicit diuresis. Strictly speaking, by this definition, water is a diuretic, because ingestion of excess water increases urine flow. In medicine and pharmacology, however, the term 'diuretic' has come to have a more specific meaning. Diuretics are therapeutic agents which act on the KIDNEYS. They are used to reduce the extracellular fluid volume (see BODY FLUIDS), and they also reduce the effective circulating blood volume. They are widely used in patients with hypertension and with congestive HEART FAILURE. In the latter group, diuretics are used to reduce OEDEMA (tissue swelling due to excess fluid). They have also been used as an aid to slimming, though this is not medically approved.

In the first 20 years of the twentieth century, the diuretics used were *theophylline* (found in dandelions) and *caffeine* (in tea and coffee). In 1919, mercurial drugs came into use, followed in the 1950s by thiazides. Details follow of diuretics still widely used.

In the kidneys, water and dissolved substances are filtered from the circulating blood into the microscopic nephrons; most of this water is normally reabsorbed into the blood, whilst the solutes are variously dealt with — retained or rejected according to need.

Water reabsorption from the fluid in the tubules of the nephrons is dependent primarily on reabsorption of sodium ions — the more sodium ions are retrieved, the more water accompanies them back into the blood. The term 'diuretic' therefore generally refers to agents which inhibit tubular sodium reabsorption, which occurs to the greatest extent in the first (*proximal*) part of the tubules through which the fluid flows. With the exception of osmotic diuretics (see below), most diuretics are organic acids, and as such are secreted from the blood into the fluid in the proximal tubules, whence they exert their effects. There are a number of different chemical types of diuretic, and several sites of action within the nephron.

Osmotic diuretics
A straightforward cause of diuresis is the filtration of large amounts of any substance which cannot be reabsorbed by the nephrons. In diabetes mellitus, for example, the plasma glucose concentration (BLOOD SUGAR) is increased, and the amount of glucose filtered overwhelms the nephrons' reabsorptive mechanism, so that glucose is excreted in the urine, and there is an increased volume of urine. The glucose is acting as an osmotic diuretic. Likewise, a completely non-reabsorbable sugar, mannitol, is often used as an osmotic diuretic agent. So, how do osmotic diuretics work?

When the proximal tubule reabsorbs sodium ions, water normally follows by osmosis, causing the concentration of non-reabsorbable solutes in the tubular fluid to increase. This limits water reabsorption. If there is additional solute in the fluid (as in the glucose example above) less water than normal follows the sodium ions. This discrepancy results in a lowering of sodium ion concentration in the tubular fluid, and in turn a diminished rate of sodium ion reabsorption. Hence there is increased excretion of both sodium ions and water.

Loop diuretics
Most of the diuretics introduced in recent years are 'loop' diuretics — their primary sites of action in the kidneys are the *loops of Henle*, which the fluid reaches after leaving the proximal tubule. Here sodium ions are normally 'pumped' out of this fluid and into the fluid which surrounds the loops and the next channels, the *collecting ducts*, helping to establish an osmotic gradient which will draw more water out of the incoming fluid. Ethacrynic acid, bumetanide, piretanide, and frusemide are loop diuretics. They act by blocking this movement of sodium, so both sodium and water reabsorption are impaired, and more remains to reach the urine. Loop diuretics also increase potassium loss in the urine, so they are often combined with a dietary potassium supplement.

Other diuretics
Spironolactone competes with the hormone aldosterone for receptor sites in the cells of the distal tubules of the nephrons, which the fluid reaches from the loops of Henle. Since aldosterone promotes absorption of sodium from the tubular fluid, and secretion of potassium into it, spironolactone opposes these actions, enhancing excretion of sodium in the urine — and of water along with it — and decreasing potassium excretion. The diuretics *triamterene* and *amiloride* have similar overall effects, though by different molecular mechanisms.   CHRIS LOTE

See also KIDNEYS; URINE; WATER BALANCE.

Diving
As divers descend below the surface of the sea, they are affected by the increased pressure on their bodies which occurs because water is heavy (just consider the weight of one bucketful). At the relatively shallow depth of 10 m of seawater the environmental pressure is 200 kPa, twice that at the surface. Because the body is composed predominantly of incompressible fluid, the effects of increased pressure may not be evident to the diver, except as applied to the gas-containing spaces — notably the lungs. As Robert Boyle observed in 1670, when pressure is doubled, gas volume is halved.

The effects of increased environmental pressure upon the body can be considered as: (i) effects on the gas-containing spaces; (ii) effects of the increased partial pressure of the respiratory gases; (iii) direct effects on cells and molecular mechanisms; (iv) consequences of the uptake by the blood and tissues of dissolved respiratory gases.

As well as the effects of pressure itself, there are other complications at great depths, such as thermal imbalance. There are also some long term effects of diving, of which the precise causes are less certain.

Early diving
The breath-hold diver was certainly the first to venture below the surface, and divers who have no external source of gas to breathe underwater are at work today around the world, mostly gathering shellfish. During descent they hold their breath and at the same time must equalise the pressure in their middle ears via the EUSTACHIAN TUBES to avoid rupture of the ear-drum.

The compression of the air within the chest means also that, for a diver with full lungs who is just buoyant at the surface, descent reduces chest volume and makes his buoyancy progressively negative: he will not spontaneously float to the surface.

Similar effects are experienced by recreational breath-hold divers; they may also use a snorkel to allow breathing when on the surface. The duration of a breath-hold dive is determined by the rise of carbon dioxide in the lungs and blood, and hence the need and the stimulus to return to the surface for a breath of fresh air. Thus a diver may be tempted to prolong underwater duration by prior hyperventilation in order to wash out as much carbon dioxide as possible. This poses an additional hazard because hyperventilation reduces the carbon dioxide, but does not increase the oxygen, in the blood. The dive is prolonged because the carbon dioxide level remains tolerable for longer, but towards the end the oxygen has diminished significantly. A diminished blood content of oxygen at depth is at increased pressure and so may be sufficient to sustain consciousness but, during the inevitable return to the surface, the partial pressure of that oxygen diminishes and the breath-holder may lapse into unconsciousness — a potentially lethal situation.

The first attempts to remain underwater longer than breath holding allows may have included the use of hollow reeds as breathing tubes for concealment in battle, but many of the early drawings of submerged men breathing through long tubes to the surface are physically impossible because of the compression which would be imposed upon the chest by hydrostatic pressure.

The invention of the diving bell reputedly allowed Alexander the Great to descend to depth, but duration would have been limited by build up of carbon dioxide in the trapped air within. The bell used in the river Thames in 1691 by Edmund Halley, the Astronomer Royal, was replenished by barrels of air lowered down to it.

When a reliable force pump was invented in 1788, those who ventured underwater could for the first time get sufficient compressed air, with the result that entirely new medical and physiological problems emerged. These were noticed first among men in new industrial applications: tunnelling below water and working in caissons.

Development of compressed air diving

Simply pumping air down a hose may seem a crude technique, but it is still used today by many native fishermen. They hold the open end of a hose between the teeth and wear simple goggles. Such fisherman have a high incidence of crippling decompression illness (see below), but this is due not so much to the equipment as to lack of knowledge and training, since it occurs even when they are provided with modern underwater breathing apparatus.

A hose leading into a bucket inverted over the head, with a window, provides the simplest example of an early diving helmet and is similar to equipment being used today by attendants in large marine aquaria. One advantage is that gas is supplied for breathing at exactly the pressure of the depth of the helmet. The development in the early nineteenth century of the copper helmet attached to a closed dry suit made this system commercially viable.

Prolonged durations became practical but brought with them a greater risk of bubble formation in the tissues on return to atmospheric pressure. Joint pains after surfacing were considered by compressed air workers to be just routine. During the salvage of the Royal George off Spithead in 1843 the first case of neurological decompression illness in a diver was reported.

Problems associated with the exchange of respiratory gases at depth also became apparent and the work of John Haldane and others in the early twentieth century showed the importance of avoiding a build up of carbon dioxide. The greater the depth, the greater the volume of air that had to be pumped to the diver: at record depths of greater than 90 m, teams of 12 or more attendants were needed to man the pumps.

There was concern that divers at such depths sometimes behaved irresponsibly; it was not until 1934 that Al Behnke showed that this was due to the increased partial pressure of nitrogen. The so-called inert gas was acting like alcohol, an anaesthetic, or any narcotic.

The substitution of oxy-helium for compressed air was first demonstrated to be practical by Max Nohl in 1938, with a dive in the Great Lakes of the US. In the 1960s it was recognised that, due to the direct cellular effects of pressure during rapid compression to depths greater than 100 m, a number of manifestations occurred which became known collectively as the High Pressure Nervous Syndrome (HPNS) (see later).

Breathing apparatus

The design and use of underwater breathing apparatus (uba) presents its own problems. A complex closed-circuit rebreather apparatus was designed by Henry Fleuss in 1878. The diver breathed from a bag of pure oxygen (a 'counterlung'), which he topped up with more oxygen 'as required'. His exhaled air was returned to the bag through a 'scrubber' which chemically removed the carbon dioxide. This is a hazardous procedure but nevertheless the apparatus was used successfully for the salvage of the flooded Severn Railway Tunnel. Because no bubbles emerge it was further developed for use in clandestine military operations in World War II — leading to recognition of the problems of acute oxygen neurotoxicity. Within strict depth limits it has also been useful for photographers and biologists.

Semi-closed-circuit uba is similar but uses an oxygen-nitrogen mixture rather than pure oxygen, enabling a greater depth to be achieved than with closed-circuit uba; the gas is supplied at a constant mass flow rate, which means that some bubbles emerge. This type of apparatus was developed as acoustically safe for those highly trained men whose underwater task was the clearance of enemy mines, but has recently been adopted by recreational divers. They require special training to minimise the risks from hazards peculiar to such apparatus: 'dilution hypoxia', 'shallow water blackout', and 'soda-lime cocktail'.

Enjoyment of recreational diving depends on a sense of freedom in the water and, in particular, freedom from the encumbrance of helmets and hoses. This was made available to the world in the mid twentieth century by the development by Cousteau and Gagnan of a 'demand regulator'. This allows just the right volume of gas, at the correct pressure for the diver's depth at that moment, to be delivered to the diver's mouthpiece from a tank of compressed air which he carries. Though not the first demand valve to be invented, it was the first to be adopted almost universally, and it is used widely for air and mixed gas diving by recreational and professional divers. Other types of uba with lower resistance have been developed to reduce the work of breathing at greater depths as gas density increases.

In the 1970s the need to exploit offshore oil and gas reserves led to the adoption of 'saturation diving' which had been pioneered by George Bond of the US Navy. The commercial diver avoids daily and prolonged decompressions from great depths by living at the surface in a chamber with an internal pressure similar to that of the worksite, until the task has been completed. Each day he descends by means of a pressurised diving bell to his work and, at the end of an in-water shift of several hours, returns to the deck chamber in the closed bell.

The gas-containing spaces and barotrauma

Aural barotrauma Unless additional gas can be admitted through the eustachian tube into the middle ear cavity during descent, to compensate for the reduction of gas volume there, the developing pressure differential may lead to injury — 'barotrauma'. At depths as shallow as 3 m transudation and possible haemorrhage into the middle ear cavity, and ultimately an implosion of the ear-drum, can occur. The sudden influx of cold water into the middle ear is an abnormal stimulus to the labyrinth of the inner ear, and can cause total disorientation. Most divers avoid such trouble by learning to 'clear their ears' from the moment they leave the surface by using a simple swallowing technique. Even lesser degrees of aural barotrauma, perhaps if only one ear is 'sticky', can lead to underwater disorientation; this can become a hazard, especially as immersion also reduces sensations from limbs and joints, and as visibility may be impaired.

There is a risk of infection to a middle ear exposed by barotrauma. Even worse, attempts to 'clear' the ears by forcing gas through the eustachian tube too vigorously can raise the cerebrospinal fluid pressure enough to rupture a membrane which separates the middle from the inner ear, causing permanent damage to hearing and balance.

Pulmonary barotrauma In contrast to the middle ear, which is damaged predominantly during the compression phase, the lungs are at risk during ascent: when the diver has inhaled gas at a pressure greater than atmospheric, this gas will expand progressively as he approaches the surface, and failure to breathe out the expanding gases can lead to pulmonary barotrauma — probably the commonest cause of death among sports divers. (The breath-hold diver should not be affected by this, since during ascent his lungs are merely re-expanding to their original volume.) Clearly the risk of lung damage is greatest if the diver holds his breath during ascent — yet lung rupture *can* occur even when he has exhaled continuously and even when it is known that he has no abnormality in his chest which might impede the venting of gas; rapid expiration may itself tend to collapse the small airways, trapping gas in the lungs.

Rupture allows gas to escape from the lungs into the pleural cavities (*pneumothorax*) or into the lung blood vessels (*gas* EMBOLISM) — a serious form of 'decompression illness'.

Barotrauma due to equipment can arise when there is a gas-containing space which becomes rapidly smaller with increasing pressure, if there is no adequate inflow to maintain the volume. An unanticipated rapid fall through the water by a traditional helmeted diver whose helmet pressure is controlled at the surface can lead to a fatal 'chest squeeze'. A squeeze of the half mask of a scuba diver, if not equalised by small exhalations through the nose during descent, can damage the eyes by conjunctival oedema and haemorrhage. Even a dry suit, worn for thermal protection, can lead to painful pinches of the skin if compression of the air within it is uncompensated.

Increased partial pressure of respiratory gases

When the total pressure is increased, the partial pressure of each component gas in the inspired air (or other mixture) is increased proportionately;

these increased pressures in the lungs equilibrate with the blood, resulting in greater 'tensions' of the gases in solution in body fluids.

Oxygen neurotoxicity Oxygen can cause an epileptiform fit, but only when breathed at pressures greater than that of pure oxygen at normal atmospheric pressure (~100 kPa). A partial pressure of 150 kPa in oxy-nitrogen mixtures is an acceptable upper limit for short-term use, but military divers rebreathing pure oxygen for swimming use a limit of 176 kPa which occurs at 7.6 m. The threshold for oxygen toxicity varies greatly between and even within individuals and

from day to day, and is influenced by the amount of physical work being done. For a diver at rest, requiring oxygen treatment, up to 280 kPa is commonly used. Intermittent oxygen breathing, with 5 min air breaks every 20 min or so, reduces the risk of oxygen toxicity.

Characteristically the diver has no warning of an impending fit. Occasionally there is an impression of hearing the sound of an engine within the head, but this comes too late for the diver to avoid a CONVULSION. If this occurs in the water, especially when wearing some kinds of uba, it is likely to be fatal; those using a helmet or with some other guaranteed airway are less likely to drown.

Oxygen pulmonary toxicity In contrast to neurotoxicity the ill-effects of prolonged oxygen breathing on the lung are relatively slow in onset. Characteristic first signs are a dry cough with chest pain; vital capacity shows a progressive impairment which at first is reversible. Later there may be pulmonary oedema which can become irreversible. These effects can usually be avoided by estimating and controlling the cumulative oxygen dose. With more prolonged exposures at lesser partial pressures (~30 kPa), there can be a slow diminution in the ability to transfer oxygen to the blood.

Nitrogen narcosis Like all 'inert' gases, NITROGEN has actions on nerve cells like those of alcohol and some anaesthetics. At increasing nitrogen partial pressure (proportional to depth when breathing air) the diver becomes incapable of behaving responsibly and this can have disastrous effects upon in-water safety. For this reason amateur divers are recommended to stay shallower than 30 m and commercial divers are restricted to 50 m when breathing compressed air. Some amateur divers practise '*extreme air diving*' and a number of potential record breakers have achieved 90 m — but not all have returned to the surface. Extreme air diving is really rather stupid.

Carbon dioxide may build up in some types of breathing apparatus and create breathlessness and headaches. A number of divers have been shown to tolerate raised carbon dioxide: they do not respond to it, as normal persons, by increasing their breathing. While one might expect this to be a potentially useful adaptation, in fact the synergism of carbon dioxide with nitrogen and with raised partial pressures of oxygen is thought to be a cause of otherwise unexplained loss of consciousness. '*Carbon dioxide retainers*' may therefore be at a greater risk of an underwater accident than others.

The direct effects of pressure

The High Pressure Nervous Syndrome (HPNS) begins in the compression phase of deep diving when oxy-helium is used to avoid nitrogen narcosis. It is worse with rapid compression rates and increases with depth. The neurological manifestations include tremors, nausea, and vomiting, and there are changes in the ELECTROENCEPHALOGRAM. Helium itself has

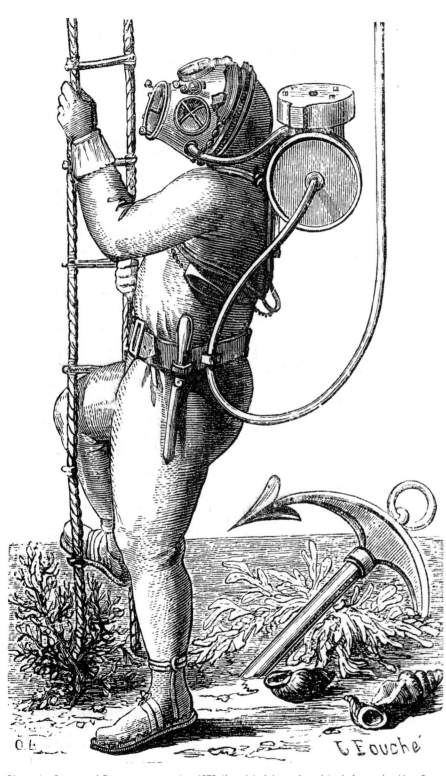

Diver using Rouquayrol–Denayrouze apparatus, 1872, the original demand regulator before scuba. Mary Evans Picture Library.

no significant narcotic effects at depths to around 600 m and it has been shown that the HPNS is not a gas effect. It is thought to be due to the direct effects of pressure upon transmission of nerve impulses. Paradoxically the HPNS can be ameliorated by the addition of a narcotising agent, and 5% nitrogen is the one most readily available for oxy-helium divers. Such 'trimix' dives have been shown to be an effective solution for very deep diving, but are not used commercially for reasons of expense related to the difficulties of gas recovery and purification; rather, a very slow staged compression rate is used to avoid HPNS in oxy-helium diving, developed over years of experience.

Uptake of gases into solution in the body

Nitrogen accounts for 80% of air breathed into the lungs, so is at 80% of the total gas pressure, but it is relatively insoluble in the blood so that body tissues at sea level contain very little. At depth, breathing air, progressively more nitrogen slowly dissolves in blood and in all body tissues. The amount that accumulates depends on both the depth and the duration of the dive. Then, when rising to the surface, nitrogen is released, and can cause decompression sickness (including 'the bends') if the rise is too rapid.

Long-term health effects

The only known long term hazard of diving is aseptic necrosis of bone (*dysbaric osteonecrosis*), a disintegration in the substance of the head, neck, and shaft of the long bones, where it causes problems very rarely, or under the cartilage in the shoulder and hip joints, where it can be painful and crippling. It can occur even after only a single exposure to raised environmental pressure and has a latency of months or years before symptoms arise. Cases among sports and European commercial divers are rare, but the condition is prevalent in shell-fishing divers who tend to be unaware of safe decompression procedures.

Much has been said about the possible long-term damage to the central nervous system caused by diving, but when sequelae from known episodes of neurological decompression illness are excluded, the evidence is not dramatic. There may be some pathological changes but there is little or no evidence that these are harmful.

In conclusion

Those who dive must be mentally, medically, and physically fit to do so. Some obvious contraindications are EPILEPSY and cardiac inadequacies, while those who are diabetic or paraplegic should dive only under the careful restrictions of an appropriate organisation. Lung and other diseases require assessment of fitness to dive by a doctor experienced in this environment. Assessment is not easy but is justified not only by the subsequent avoidance of unnecessary diving accidents but also for the safety of those who otherwise might suddenly become rescuers.

Those who wish to dive should do so only after rigorous training and each must recognise that the most important feature of every subsequent dive plan is to include the recognition, assessment, and control of risk. Diving is hazardous and the sea is an unforgiving environment.

DAVID ELLIOTT

Further reading

Bennett, P. B. and Elliott, D. H. (1993). *The physiology and medicine of diving*, (4th edn) Saunders, London.

Bove, A. A. (1997). *Bove and Davis diving medicine*, (3rd edn). Saunders, Philadelphia.

Edmonds, C., Lowry, C., and Pennefather, J. (1994). *Diving and subaquatic medicine*, (3rd edn). Butterworth-Heinemann, London.

Undersea Medical Society (1983). *Key documents of the biomedical aspects of deep-sea diving selected from the world's literature, 1608–1982*. Undersea Medical Society Bethesda, Maryland.

See also DECOMPRESSION SICKNESS; GASES IN THE BODY; HYPERBARIC CHAMBER; NITROGEN; OXYGEN.

Dizziness The term 'dizziness' is used to describe both 'lightheadedness' and vertigo. Lightheadedness may consist of a clouding of consciousness, a difficulty in focusing rational thought, or a difficulty in concentrating. Vertigo is the illusion of movement either of oneself or of the surroundings.

The illusion of movement, when the neighbouring train departs the station, or the feeling of being drawn toward the ground or the sea when standing on a high point, are recognized by many. The feeling of falling is a part of our dreams. We enjoy the illusion of movement in 3-D and circular surround cinemas. Children enjoy the vertigo they can trigger by spinning on the spot. All these are perceptions we have in the absence of illness, but many people experience dizziness as part of an illness, which can ruin their quality of life and lead to a loss of independence. Lightheadedness and vertigo can lead to a final common pathway of ANXIETY and HYPERVENTILATION, resulting in a spiral of deteriorating lightheadedness. This overlap of symptoms and the final common pathway justify the acceptance of the term 'dizziness'.

Balance information is processed within the *vestibular nuclei* of the BRAIN STEM. Inputs include the sensory organs of the ears and eyes, proprioceptive and tactile sense, and higher centres in the brain. There is no single area of the CEREBRAL CORTEX involved with balance information alone. On the contrary, PET scanning (positron emission tomography, which 'maps' relative activity in the different regions of the brain) reveals that balance-related inputs influence many large areas of the cerebral cortex. Therefore, dizziness can lead to a myriad of symptoms, depending on which areas of the brain are involved. The extent of these complex connections is highlighted by the effect of stimulating the balance organs of the left ear, by

running cold water into the left ear canal, in patients with left-sided sensory 'hemi-neglect' due to a right cerebral hemisphere STROKE. For several minutes after the irrigation of the water into the left ear, during the dizziness which this causes, function may be improved in the previously numb and poorly-used left side of the body. This complex neuronal networking is also crucial to our ability to suppress dizziness with training or rehabilitation, as pilots, gymnasts, and dancers demonstrate.

Any factors that can alter the function of the many parts of the brain dealing with balance function can lead to dizziness and a variable cluster of symptoms. These include any cause of inadequate blood flow (and therefore of OXYGEN and glucose supply) to the brain — as for example at the onset of FAINTING, or in illnesses causing heart failure or obstruction of the blood vessels — or impaired nutrient supply due to decrease in BLOOD SUGAR (hypoglycaemia). Inadequate brain blood flow may result from overbreathing (HYPERVENTILATION) — from whatever cause, including PAIN. Dizziness may also be the result of environmental agents, such as carbon monoxide poisoning from faulty domestic appliances or car exhaust fumes, which again impair the brain's oxygen supply. Likewise with other causes of oxygen shortage (HYPOXIA) such as high altitude or lung disease.

Damage to the balance organs themselves, as a result of trauma, infection, or other disease affecting the inner ears, may result in dizziness, though the brain has a remarkable capacity to compensate fully for such pathology. For reasons that are currently being investigated, some patients become over-reliant on visual clues for stability, and they become dizzy when they are exposed to excessive visual clues, such as in shopping malls, even when there is no definable structural pathology.

Dizziness can therefore be a manifestation of illness anywhere in the body; to determine the cause, a careful evaluation of the patient and their circumstances is essential.

PETER SAVUNDRA

See also BALANCE; FAINTING; PROPRIOCEPTION; VESTIBULAR SYSTEM.

DNA The abbreviation stands for *deoxyribonucleic acid*, a double-stranded nucleic acid, in which the two strands twist together to form a helix. The strands consist of sugar and phosphate groups, the sugars being attached to a base — *adenine, thymine, guanine,* or *cytosine*. In DNA the bases pair to form a ladder-like structure, with adenine paired with thymine and guanine with cytosine. DNA forms the basis of inheritance in all organisms, except VIRUSES, the DNA code being sufficient to build and control the organism. DNA is located in the nucleus of all cells; it is the substance of the *chromosomes* that separate out from the nucleus when cells divide, and it carries the GENES, each of which is a segment of a DNA molecule. A small fraction of total DNA is present in mitochondria that codes for a few mitochondrial proteins. This DNA is passed down the female line from the mitochondria contained in the ovum. A.W.C.

Further reading

Watson, J. D. (1968). *The double helix*. Weidenfeld and Nicolson, London.

See CELL; GENETICS, HUMAN.

DNA fingerprinting

DNA fingerprinting also known as DNA typing or genetic fingerprinting, is a method for identifying individuals by the particular structure of their DNA. It gained its name because the structure of the DNA of each person is different, and hence, just as each of us is unique with respect to the pattern of our fingerprints, so we can be identified from our DNA.

As well as containing the 100 000 or so GENES that encode the structure of the thousands of PROTEINS from which human beings are constructed, there are large regions of our DNA that do not consist of genes and appear to serve no useful purpose. Part of this functionless, 'junk' DNA is made up of long stretches of repeated sequences of the four nucleotide building blocks from which DNA is constructed. There is, however, some order in these repeats. For example, they may form what are called *hypervariable regions*, also known as mini-satellite DNA, which consist of blocks of tandem repeats of a short 'core' sequence. Nearly 100 of these hypervariable regions have been found in the human genome, many but not all of which are close to genes that encode different proteins. The number of copies in these different families of repeats varies widely between unrelated people and thus constitutes a unique genetic profile, or fingerprint. They are of particular value because they are apparently dispersed randomly throughout the genome and therefore are inherited independently of each other.

To produce a DNA fingerprint, DNA from a cell sample is digested with enzymes that cut it up into many different sized pieces and the mixture is placed in a gel. This is then exposed to an electric field and the fragments migrate to different positions by virtue of their size. In this way a pattern is obtained that reflects different numbers of repeats in different individuals; the length of a particular DNA fragment is a function of the number of repeats present.

After the separation of the fragments is complete, the DNA is transferred to a nitrocellulose filter, on which it is immobilised. The position of the fragments containing the repeats is identified by the use of a radioactively labelled DNA probe designed to bind to the core repeat sequences. The fingerprint is visualised by placing an X-ray plate over the filter and developing the film. Since mini-satellite DNA has a relatively high mutation rate, and this varies between different hypervariable regions, in practice it is important to ensure that the rates of mutation of the mini-satellites used for testing are not too great, so as to avoid false exclusions.

DNA fingerprinting is used for many purposes, particularly paternity testing and for forensic work. Of particular concern to the criminal fraternity is that DNA for fingerprinting can be obtained from whole blood, semen, vaginal fluid, hair roots, almost any tissue, and even from bones that have been buried for a long time. The probability that two unrelated individuals show exactly the same pattern varies depending on the particular hypervariable regions that are chosen. In one commonly used system the region analysed yields up to 36 different sized DNA bands, or alleles, for each individual. A band-sharing statistic is estimated at 0.25; that is, the probability of two unrelated individuals sharing the same pattern is 0.25^{36} or one in 5000 billion billion!

Because of its extreme sensitivity, and because appropriate hypervariable regions can be amplified from minute traces of DNA to produce diagnostic patterns, this technique has revolutionised forensic medicine over recent years.

D.J. WEATHERALL

Further reading

Gill, P. (1994). DNA typing. In *The enclycopaedia of molecular biology*, pp. 286–8. Blackwell Science, Oxford.

Jeffreys, A. J. *et al.* (1986). DNA fingerprinting and segregation analysis of multiple markers in human pedigrees. *American Journal of Human Genetics*, **39**, 11–24.

See also GENETICS, HUMAN.

Dolls

Dolls As miniatures of human bodies, dolls have had many meanings. Across cultures, dolls have served as religious or magical icons for adults, thought to contain the power and personality of a god, an ancestor, or even a personal enemy. Because they were often made of perishable materials, few children's dolls have survived from earlier than 3000 BCE, but these figures abound in ancient civilizations, presumably used to act out adult roles and to learn skills. Archaeologists sometimes find it difficult to distinguish an icon from a children's doll, and in some societies, like ancient Japan, adults passed religious dolls down to children as toys after their ritual use. Similarly, fashion dolls, used by adults from the fourteenth century to display the latest style, were gradually transformed into girls' playthings. Miniature silver soldiers and self-animated figures were first made for medieval aristocrats and entered boys' playworlds in the eighteenth and nineteenth centuries as lead soldiers and wind-up toys. Replicas of the male body had many descendents — the rubber and plastic toy soldier from the 1930s; the dress-up military doll (GI Joe or Action Man) from 1964; the action figure popularized by *Star Wars* in 1978. But the term 'doll' has been associated primarily with the female form. Despite secularization and the separation of children's from adults' culture, dolls still retain associations with powerful personalities and are closely linked to the imaginations of adults.

In the twentieth century, innovations in the doll's body and face reflected changes in the culture of childhood. Late Victorian dolls assumed the proportions of adult women and were used to imitate women's household and society roles. Others were plain cloth figures used as manniquins to help teach girls the essential art of sewing. From about 1900, dolls were increasingly portrayed in the bodily proportions of children (chunky torso and short legs) and with sweet and impish faces (Campbell Kids and Kewpie dolls). They fostered a positive image of childhood, increasingly favoured by parents encouraging girls to be affectionate and to retreat into a playful world with their companion dolls. Baby dolls also appeared in large numbers from 1900, encouraging maternal feelings at a time of popular concern about decreasing fertility.

The Barbie doll of Ruth Handler's Mattel Toys (1959) marked another major change. Barbie's distinctive grown-up face and exaggerated shape (long legs and pronounced breasts) invited the girl to anticipate the freedom of young womanhood. Despite adults' dislike for this disturbingly sexual image of the female body and threat to the play patterns of the old companion and baby dolls, girls embraced Barbie. Mattel exploited the little girl's association of the woman's shape with entry into a wider world of adults. Barbie's body and face has remained relatively unchanging, symbolizing growing up to the little girl. Yet Barbie's clothing, playsets, and friends (siblings, boyfriend, and playmates) change yearly, reflecting a modern childhood of fashion and an ephemeral consumer culture. GARY CROSS

See also MANIKINS AND MANNEQUINS.

Dopamine

Dopamine is a CATECHOLAMINE, from which other important catecholamines (ADRENALINE and NORADRENALINE) are derived, but it is also an important NEUROTRANSMITTER in its own right, especially in the BRAIN. Of particular importance are central nervous pathways involved with the co-ordination of MOVEMENT and with behaviour and EMOTION. As with the other catecholamines, dopamine is released from nerve endings where it acts upon receptors on other nerve cells to produce its effects. There are two sorts of receptors for dopamine, namely D_1 and D_2, of which the second are of greater importance. After release the dopamine is rapidly destroyed or taken up back into the nerve fibres for reuse. A number of medical conditions are associated with underactivity or over-activity of dopamine pathways in the brain. The rigidity and tremor, together with the *hypokinesia* (relative lack of voluntary movement), of Parkinson's disease are associated with lack of dopaminergic function in the nigrostriatal pathway in the brain. One form of treatment for this disease is to give large amounts of L-DOPA, the precurser of dopamine, so that some reaches the brain, is converted to dopamine, and restores some lost functions. Another approach is to transplant fetal dopamine-secreting cells into the relevant brain nuclei to take over the function of the diseased nerve cells. Over-activity of dopaminergic nerves, especially in the LIMBIC system, is associated with schizophrenia. It has also been claimed that individuals with mutations affecting the dopamine D_2 receptors show enhanced risk-taking behaviour. Some drugs, like the amphetamines, release dopamine from nerve endings in the brain, leading to hyperactivity and manic behaviour. Dopamine pathways are also associated with the vomiting centre in the brain, so drugs which block the dopamine receptors, such as the phenothiazines, have a calming effect on schizophrenics and are also useful anti-emetic drugs. There are a few dopamine pathways in other parts of the body, for example the kidney, where activation causes vasodilation. Dopamine increases the force of contraction of the heart and an infusion is sometimes used to treat shock resulting from blood loss.　　　　　　ALAN W. CUTHBERT

See also BASAL GANGLIA; DRUG ABUSE.

Doppelganger

The coinage of the term *Doppelgänger* (commonly Anglicized as 'doppelganger') is not certain, but it was a sufficiently unfamiliar term for the writer Jean Paul Richter to have to gloss it in a footnote to his novel, *Siebenkäs*, of 1796. According to this founding definition *Doppelgänger* (literally 'doublegoer', by contrast with the German *Einzelgänger*, or loner) is the name given to 'people who see themselves'. It seems, then, that there is uncertainty from the start as to whether the apparently original self or its alter ego is the double in question. This indicates the fundamental level at which the phenomenon challenges conventions of identity, by making the self see itself double (or, more precisely, see itself going double, as a duplicate body which may go its own way).

Seeing is the primary category here; the *Doppelgänger*, as it appears and reappears in literary and other cultures, is above all a thing of visual fascination and terror. It corresponds in this sense to the clinical condition of autoscopy: the relatively rare cases of psychological bilocation where individuals see themselves in another body. But the *Doppelgänger* challenges the location of the self in a coherent and singular body in other ways as well. Thus, it specialises in ventriloquism, appropriating the voice as sound-image of a bodily identity (more akin in this to the clinical shape of schizophrenia). In most cases of the *Doppelgänger*, sound and image work together to ensure potentially successful imposture.

Classic literary cases like R. L. Stevenson's *Strange Case of Dr Jekyll and Mr Hyde* show how the *Doppelgänger* may appropriate the body in particular in order to commit excesses of violence and sex. In the case of Jekyll and Hyde, this appropriation works through metamorphosis, a violent changing of bodily shape, rather than the purloining of a body's original appearance, its mirror-image, its portrait, or its shadow (as in the many variations on the myth of the Schlemihl figure who sold his shadow to the devil). Thus notions of doubling involve not only replications of identity, but also transformations in identity, where the self appears to be in the wrong body. A case which combines the two possibilities would be Oscar Wilde's *Picture of Dorian Gray*.

At its extreme, transformation into an other self can challenge perhaps the most primary of bodily identifications: that of gender. The *Doppelgänger* as a cultural construct has been largely the preserve of men, representing the Faustian prerogative to be split between two souls or identities. In the canonical versions of the *Doppelgänger* story any cases of female doubling tend to be a symptom of objectification for the schismatic desires of a male subject rather than exploring the possibility of constitutional splits in female subjectivity. The eponymous protagonist of Robert Musil's *Man without Qualities* is doubled by his twin sister, but, given that the female form — *Doppelgängerin* — has no proper currency in German, the transgender double can only be framed here as the '*Doppelgänger* in the other sex'. If the *Doppelgänger* is indeed gendered male, then it frequently embodies gender trouble for the masculine subject.

As a cultural figure or figment, the *Doppelgänger* has a special relationship to theories grounded in the psychosomatic. It recurrently operates against the context of scientific or pseudo-scientific theories of psychological schism, and especially of the constituent splitting of bodily and psychic identities. It is supplied variously by mystical theories of the astral body, by the conjecture of ANIMAL MAGNETISM, and by the subsequent cults of hypnosis and somnambulism. And it sees a resurgence in the early twentieth century as a corollary of psychoanalytic theories of the split ego. Indeed, in the culture of Modernism, it can be seen as figuring the ambivalent fascination which Freudian psychoanalysis held for contemporary literature and film. Early cinema in the style of *The Cabinet of Dr Caligari* offered a particularly apt medium for the projection of double identities, for case-histories on release from the cabinets of Drs Freud and company. For Freud, the *Doppelgänger* is the archetypal figure of the uncanny, embodying the return of the repressed, of all that 'should have remained hidden but has emerged' to haunt the security of the psychic household.

While it has been conventional to follow Tzvetan Todorov in seeing the extensive theorization of the split self in psychoanalysis as producing the endgame of the *Doppelgänger* as cultural construct, this now seems premature. The post-Freudian age yields no shortage of material for a reactivation of the Gothic bogey-man. Feminism helps enable the bogey-man to become a bogey-woman, a *Doppelgängerin* proper (such as in Emma Tennant's reworking of Stevenson's strange case as that of Ms Jekyll and Mrs Hyde in her *Two Women of London*). The troubling of corporeal and psychological identity in the age of computer and genetic science, and the projections of alternative identities afforded by film and other media, also open up new dimensions for the *Doppelgänger*. The likes of David Cronenberg's *Dead Ringers* or Kryzstof Kieslowski's *Double Life of Veronique* would suggest that the late twentieth-century cultural psyche was not simply at home in, and at one with, its body.　　ALAN W. CUTHBERT

See also HALLUCINATION; PSYCHOLOGICAL DISORDERS; PSYCHOSOMATIC ILLNESS.

Double-jointed

Some individuals are referred to as being 'double-joined'. In reality these individuals do not have 'double' joints, but have a greater than average range of joint mobility — the joints are hypermobile. This can have career advantages (e.g. for contortionists) but can sometimes result in painful joints even though there is no clinical evidence of joint disease (*hypermobility syndrome*).　　W.R.F.

See JOINTS.

Douche

A douche is a stream of water or other liquid directed at the body or into one of its orifices; in French it is simply a shower. Douching in English usage usually refers to washing out the VAGINA, both for hygienic purposes, especially when there is an infection, and after sexual intercourse, although the procedure has little contraceptive effect. The use of chemical substances such as deodorants or detergents can cause local irritation, and the use of excessive pressure can force liquid, contaminated with vaginal organisms, into the UTERUS and Fallopian tubes and hence into the peritoneal cavity, where damage and infection can result. Excessive douching, which removes the vagina's normal, beneficial microorganisms, can also be dangerous.

The term has also been applied to washing out the rectum or colon — by ENEMA or COLONIC IRRIGATION.　　E.M. TANSEY

Dreaming

is a mental state associated with sleep whose characteristics have important implications for theories of normal CONSCIOUSNESS as well as for its extreme derangement in major mental illness. The advent of modern sleep laboratory science has provided an objective aspect to the study of dreams and has opened the way to a brain-based theory of dreaming. Recent excitement about the prospects of this agenda stems from the application of brain IMAGING TECHNIQUES that allow dream activity in humans to be correlated with the selective activation and deactivation of various BRAIN regions. The modern scientific study of dreaming thus provides an avenue of access to the MIND–BODY PROBLEM, one of the most obdurate philosophic conundrums of human history.

While dreaming can be broadly defined as any kind of mental activity occurring in sleep, most people and most brain scientists are interested in a more specific state of mind that is normally unique to sleep. When we say 'I had the craziest dream last night' we refer to a conscious experience during sleep marked by visual imagery, delusional misidentification of our state as waking, difficulties with thought processes, emotional intensification, and very significant recent memory loss. It is important to emphasize this particular definition of dreaming for two reasons. The first reason is that this kind of dreaming is so highly correlated with the physiology of the stage of sleep known as paradoxical or REM (*rapid eye movement*) sleep as to invite an integration of dream psychology with the specific brain processes of REM. The second is that this kind of dreaming shows many of the formal features of such major dysfunctional states as schizophrenia, manic depression, and organic PSYCHOSES. But even these intense dreams are not restricted to REM sleep. Furthermore, many other cataclysmic states of mind, like the night terrors of normal children and the horrifying replay of experiences in people who have been brutalized or traumatized, occur almost exclusively in other, non-REM stages of sleep (*NREM*).

Until recently, the traditional approach to understanding dreaming has emphasized its narrative or scenario-like character and attempted to elaborate an interpretive scheme that could bring order to the emotional and cognitive chaos of dreaming. The most famous approach of this type is the psychoanalytic theory of Sigmund Freud, who abandoned his early hopes for a brain-based approach because the necessary neurophysiological data were then non-existent. Freud was therefore obliged to account for all of the formal properties of dreaming in psychological terms, a heavy burden, which caused his ingenious speculations to become Byzantine in their complexity and comical in their interpretive oversimplification.

For Freud, every dream was caused by unconscious wishes that were released in sleep. These forbidden impulses threatened to invade consciousness and to cause an awakening if their unacceptable meaning was not censored and disguised by symbolic transformation. The hallucinatory character of dreams, the bizarreness of dream perception, the defective cognition, and even the memory loss were all ascribed to psychological defence mechanisms whose function was to protect sleep. For Freud, the common existence of strong negative emotion in dreams was a factor that his theory could not explain.

The discovery of the biphasic cycle of NREM and REM sleep and the possibility of waking people up at particular stages of sleep in the laboratory, immediately provided an alternative approach. The flood of data quickly overthrew many age-old assumptions about dreaming, as well as challenging Freud's ideas. For example, it was soon clear that everyone dreams, every night, and that dreaming of the vivid kind emphasized here occupies finite amounts of time — up to one and a half or even two hours of sleep. Unless we awaken spontaneously, or are awakened by an external stimulus (such as an experimenter), we may recall nothing. More interestingly, the most vivid and sustained dreaming occurs in association with REM sleep. Moreover, dreaming intensifies the intermittent bursts of eye movement that punctuate that sleep phase. These discoveries showed that the subjective experience had been not only grossly inadequate but also downright misleading in suggesting, for example, that dreams are rare, colourless, evanescent events that occur in the instant before awakening. Furthermore, Freud's speculative hypotheses about the instigation of dreams by unconscious wishes, and about censorship and repression moulding the content of dreams, were called into question.

To develop the detailed brain-based theory of dreaming that Freud himself yearned for, it was also important to utilize information from animal experiments that identified the specific brain cells and molecules involved in REM sleep generation in all mammals, including man. For example, the electrical activity of the brain (recorded by electroencephalography) and the movements of the eyes are very similar in the awake state and during REM sleep. However, in REM, the activated brain is operating without those NEUROTRANSMITTER chemicals known to be necessary to order attention, perception, thought, and MEMORY. No wonder dreaming is so chaotic, bizarre, unfocused, and unremembered. No need to postulate psychological defences, symbolic transformations, or any other Freudian fantasy to understand what is going on.

This is not to say that dream narratives are without interest or without meaning. The interpretive stance taken by modern dream science is that the emotionally salient aspects of dreams mean exactly what they appear to mean, while the meaningless nonsense is simply a by-product of the brain's physiological handicap. In other words, dream psychology is of interest precisely because it so directly and undefensively reveals the dreamer's psychological concerns. On this view, dream meaning is transparent, not disguised, and is synthesized as the dreamer tries to make sense of the activation of his emotional and perceptual brain without the aid of the organizing and directive powers available to it during waking.

Neuropsychological evidence

The capacity to deduce regional activation patterns in the human brain during natural sleep is afforded by imaging techniques, such as *positron emission tomography* (PET) and *functional magnetic resonance imaging* (fMRI), which measure differences in local blood flow and thus infer the increases in nerve cell activity that call for more oxygen. For the first time in history scientists are able to study the depths of the human brain in action and to correlate the differences between, say, waking and REM sleep with the psychology typical of these states.

Recent PET data affirm the importance of the brain stem in REM sleep dream generation, that was suggested by animal studies, but they also emphasize the importance of emotion centres in the limbic system. The integration of the emotions and internally-generated perceptions of dreams is facilitated by selective activation of a specific cortical zone at the junction of the parietal, temporal, and occipital lobes, whose damage typically results in disintegration of these functions, and to a loss of dreaming. Dreaming is also lost when strokes damage the deep basal forebrain area thought to mediate emotional and motivational drive, a finding that would have thrilled Sigmund Freud in 1895 when he was still struggling to produce a brain-based theory of the mind.

But the most significant finding of all may be the discovery that the brain region responsible for working memory, critical evaluation of behavioural options, and decision-making is selectively deactivated in REM sleep. How, and why, this critical area of the frontal cortex escapes the activation process that is otherwise at least as prominent in REM as in waking is as yet unknown, but it is irresistibly attractive to speculate that it may be related to the regional differences in chemical modulation of the brain that have been discovered in animal studies.

Whatever the answer to detailed questions such as these, it can safely be concluded that no one interested in dreaming, including the most die-hard psychoanalyst, can any longer afford to be either ignorant of or indifferent to the findings of modern brain research.

J. ALLAN HOBSON

See also BRAIN STEM; CONSCIOUSNESS; EMOTION, BIOLOGICAL BASIS OF; LIMBIC SYSTEM; MIND–BODY PROBLEM; SLEEP; SLEEP DISORDERS.

Drowning

Drowning has always enjoyed mythic power. The Deluge, the sinking of the Titanic, and the drowning of Virginie in J. St Pierre's eighteenth-century bestseller *Paul et Virginie* (1788), are just some of the memorable drownings that carry with them arresting images of mankind's relation with nature, death, God, and itself. But as a theme in the history of the body, drowning's significance lies not among myths, but in its critical role in the discovery of resuscitation. The possibility of reversing the effects of drowning excited in the late eighteenth century new systematic inquiries into the physiological states and processes of life and death. The implementation of resuscitation, informed by these fresh accounts of the way the body worked, entailed new practices surrounding drowned bodies that in turn required a shift in the way the body carried commonsensical and religious meanings.

The idea that drowning could be 'cured' enjoyed little currency in medical literature before the 1760s. However, in late eighteenth-century Europe, with the advent of the Humane Movement, drowning for the first time enjoyed widespread attention as a reversible and preventable accidental death. Before the emergence of medico–philanthropic societies that embodied this movement, rescue and recovery of the drowned was practised, but in a haphazard and limited way characterized by ignorance and fatalism. As champions of the Enlightenment's optimism in science, reason, and progress, the founders of these societies sought more effective and reliable methods. Beginning in Amsterdam in 1767, and spreading in the next 30 years throughout Europe and on to America and the Indian Subcontinent, these organizations publicized methods of recovery from all states of accidental and sudden apparent death, including drowning, strangulation, narcotics, and lightning.

It was drowning that most intrigued those who wanted to explore the latent powers of recovery in a near-dead body. This was for three main reasons. First, it began to be believed that drowning led to a brief suspension of the vital powers, rather than an immediate extinction. In this the drowned body appeared to epitomize a state of 'apparent death', a notion that had gained a high profile in Europe following the publication of J.-J. Bruhier's *L'incertritude des signes de la mort* (Paris, 1742). In this book Bruhier argued that the body could display the signs of death yet spontaneously recover. This argument shed doubt upon the possibility of knowing the moment of death with any precision, and hence made the idea of a 'suspension' of life intelligible. Second, because drowning happened to healthy bodies, and did not necessarily involve internal destruction of the organs, or extensive lesions, its reversibility seemed more likely. Third, on the busy European rivers, where drowning was both conspicuous and plentiful, resuscitation could be tested in practice.

The desire to perfect a therapy for drowning led medical men back to the body. The patronage of the Royal Humane Society of London (RHS), founded in 1774, ensured the publication of experimental works, such as Edmund Goodwyn's *The Connexion of Life with Respiration* (1788), that investigated the effects of drowning on animal bodies. These explorations sought reliable knowledge of the signs of life and death, as well as the mechanical and chemical processes of vitality. Because drowning in humans was impossible to reconstruct experimentally, these researches entailed extensive dissection of freshly drowned puppies and kittens. Here drowning figured as an experimental method and analytical device, which generated new data on respiration and circulation, and provided greater conceptual and empirical clarity about the relationship between states of life and death. This work represented the cutting edge of physiology, but was later eclipsed by the subsequent influence of French morbid anatomist Xavier Bichat, whose definition, in 1800, of life as 'the totality of functions which resist death' replaced the Aristotelian notion of death as the absence of life used by Goodwyn.

The new knowledge had to be translated into action if deaths by drowning were actually to be averted. The act of translation was a frictional process for, in exhorting people to change their behaviour towards drowning bodies, the RHS required alterations in popular accounts of the body itself, and these cut across beliefs about how the world was and ought to be. First, to discourage witnesses of drowning from believing that the moment of death had already passed and that further activity was useless, the RHS had to overcome existing assumptions about the signs of death and replace them with the counterintuitive idea of apparent death. Second, the RHS had to override popular reluctance to interfere with the CORPSE, either for fear of obstructing the law, or for fear that the corpse might bring about bad luck. (Local fishermen in Germany, for example,

would not rescue drowning persons for fear of eliciting the wrath of the river spirits.) Third, the RHS had to challenge those ideas about Providence which sat uneasily with the concept of an 'accidental' death, and which saw resuscitation as an impious and hubristic activity that, Prometheus-like, mimicked the animating power of God. Clergymen supporting the RHS attacked such charges of impiety, and reinterpreted scriptural accounts of body–soul activity at death to make way for the idea of apparent death. In other words, in order to fashion a cultural ambience favourable to the rescue and revival of a drowning/drowned body, which we take for granted, men and women of the eighteenth century had to unlearn their assumptions about these cosmic, practical, and ethical fundamentals that were mediated by the drowned body.

Interest in resuscitation no longer grips the imagination as it did between 1770 and 1830, when it unleashed a more general interest in reanimation that brought about anaesthesia, blood transfusion, and Mary Shelley's *Frankenstein* (1818). Consequently, drowning no longer constitutes such a generative locus for new knowledge of, and practices surrounding, the body.

LUKE DAVIDSON

See also NEAR-DROWNING.

Drowning: clinical aspects

When victims of immersion die, it is not usually because of inhaling water. Rather, most have swallowed copious amounts of water, which exacerbates the effects of immersion hypothermia. Only when they become unconscious as a result of HYPO-THERMIA does water rush into their lungs.

The witness at the water side may believe the victim to be dead from drowning, but should not be discouraged from starting RESUSCITATION, because ultimate revival may be possible. A victim who is not breathing should not be assumed to be dead: a hypothermic person does not need to breathe very much. The action to be taken is first to clear the airway and start artificial respiration (mouth-to-mouth or mouth-to-nose), then to take wet things off and wrap the victim in whatever dry warm coverings are available. If there seems to be no circulation — no pulse — the advisability of starting external cardiac massage is somewhat dubious, since it may convert an imperceptible, weak, slow, but regular heart rhythm into ineffectual ventricular FIBRILLATION. Once started, the rhythmic cardiac compression would have to be maintained until professional help and hospital treatment became available.

Once started, cardio-pulmonary resuscitation should be continued until body core temperature has risen to near normal. Only then, if there is still no spontaneous heart activity, can the victim be said to have drowned. Up to that time they were suffering a NEAR-DROWNING event.

G.R. GREY

Drug

The term 'drug' has become something of a misnomer. Strictly, a drug is a chemical substance used to treat disease in animals,

including man. Today, a drug is a pure chemical substance whose structure is known and is formulated, by mixing it with other materials, into a preparation suitable for administration. This results in the familiar tablets, pills, injections, liquid mixtures, emulsions, and syrups; ointments, creams, and salves; infusions and tinctures; drops for eyes, ears, and noses; sprays for inhalation, gases delivered by machine, supositories, and the like. In earlier times drugs were not always pure, single substances, but mixtures of substances together with many unknown constituents, and were derived from medicinal plants. Here the dried leaves, roots, stems, bark, or rhizomes of plants were ground into powders or used to prepare infusions, tinctures, syrups etc. For example, malaria was treated with infusions made from cinchona bark, and constipation by extracts of casacara sagrada bark. Today, the same diseases might be treated with tablets containing quinine or emodins, respectively.

Approved drugs are those which have passed all the stringent tests for safety and efficacy granted by organisations such as the Committee on the Safety of Drugs (in the UK) and the Federal Drugs Administration (FDA) (in the US). Approved drugs then become listed in National Formularies and pharmacopoeias of various countries. The designation BP, USP, or EP after the name of a drug implies it conforms to the standards described in the British, US, or European Pharmacopoeias. Even crude drugs, made from medicinal plants, were standardised during preparation to give *galenicals* having the same potency from batch to batch and as given in the pharmacopoeias.

With the advances in science and medicine it became appropriate to extract and purify drugs of plant origin, separating them from other plant constituents so that they could be formulated as with pure drugs. As the chemical structures of drugs were discovered it became clear that it could be economically sound to synthesise the compound chemically, rather than to rely on its synthesis by plants, together with all the attendant problems of extraction and purification. The commonly-held view that drugs produced naturally are good while synthetics are bad is a myth. The same substance produced by nature or by chemical synthesis is identical in its actions. The idea of vital force, believed to be locked away in molecules of natural origin, was destroyed in 1828 when Wohler produced the naturally-occuring substance urea from inorganic starting materials.

Open any newspaper or listen to any news broadcast and you are likely to read or hear about drugs — drug problems, DRUG ABUSE, drug culture, drug barons, drug smuggling. While it is true that Harry Lime smuggled penicillin in the *Third Man*, the film portraying racketeering in post World War II Europe, today's references refer almost exclusively to drugs of abuse which lead to addiction. It is entirely possible for a drug to be a useful therapeutic agent as well as a drug of abuse. Properly used, morphine and its derivative heroin are excellent ANALGESICS, which can be used without causing addiction. In former times cocaine was the local anaesthetic used by most dentists, and currently cannabinoids (from marajhuana) are being examined for their usefulness in multiple sclerosis.

Chemical modification of a drug can be made without necessarily affecting either its biological effects or its potency. In this way a new substance is produced which is not covered by any legislation. So-called designer drugs produced from drugs used for their abuse potential thus enter the illicit marketplace. In these situations rapid actions are necessary to prevent the rapid spread of their use.

The potential of chemical substances to modify biological function in disease states is still a largely untapped area. The appearance of new diseases (e.g. HIV, BSE) creates urgent demands for drug discovery. The cloning of the human genome, and identification of genes and their functions, combined with high throughput screening methods and combinatorial chemistry, will lead to a revolution in drug discovery programmes. The control of drug abuse is likely to be a more intractable problem.

ALAN W. CUTHBERT

See also ADDICTION; DRUG ABUSE; DRUG ADMINISTRATION.

Drug abuse
Mechanisms of addiction

Drug abuse is an increasing problem in our affluent societies and carries great social and economic costs through its impacts on crime and health. Official policy in the Western world for the past 50 years has been to treat addicts as criminals and to punish them, but this has manifestly failed to prevent the increase in drug abuse. Nor have campaigns to educate people about the dangers of drugs, tobacco, and alcohol had anything other than relatively minor effects. From the neuroscientist's point of view addiction is increasingly seen as an organic disorder of brain function; if this could be better understood we might be able to offer more effective treatments to addicts.

The definition of addiction has changed in recent years. The term was previously applied only to such 'hard' drugs as HEROIN, where there are obvious signs of tolerance and physical dependence in regular users, and a painful or even life-threatening physical withdrawal syndrome when drug use is stopped. Psychiatrists now use the term '*substance dependence*' to include both psychological dependence (where there may be no obvious withdrawal syndrome or tolerance) and physical dependence. The cigarette smoker who cannot stop SMOKING or the cannabis smoker whose drug habit has come to dominate their life is no less addicted than the chronic heroin user, even though they may suffer only mild withdrawal signs when drug use is stopped.

Great progress has been made in understanding the mechanisms by which the various classes of addictive substances act in the brain. These include the '*psychostimulants*' — a large group of drugs encompassing COCAINE and various amphetamines. These drugs all act in the brain to stimulate receptors that recognise the chemical messenger substance DOPAMINE. Cocaine works by blocking the inactivation of dopamine after its release from nerve terminals in the brain — a process that involves recapture of the released chemical into the nerve endings. Blocking this process makes more dopamine available to stimulate brain receptors. The amphetamines work by displacing dopamine from nerve terminals. The 'rave dance' drug, *ecstasy*, is an amphetamine derivative that combines psychostimulant (dopamine) properties with a mild hallucinogenic effect — thought to be due to stimulation of receptors for another brain chemical messenger, SEROTONIN. The OPIATES (for example heroin), cannabis, and NICOTINE all act on specific receptors that are present in the brain and which recognise these different drugs. When the drug binds to the receptor it triggers activity in nerve cells. One might wonder why the brain should contain such receptors, since the drugs themselves are plant products that do not exist naturally in the brain. The answer is that in each case there are naturally-occurring brain chemicals which activate these receptors, and the drug molecules hijack these normal brain mechanisms. Precisely how alcohol works remains unclear, but it is increasingly thought to act by modifying the responsiveness of the brain to the principal 'on' and 'off' chemical signals, glutamic acid and GABA — thus lowering neuronal excitability.

Knowing how these drugs act, however, does not explain why they are addictive. Furthermore, there seem to be a bewildering number of different brain mechanisms activated by the different classes of drugs. Consequently, great excitement has been generated in recent years by the first glimmers of some common themes of understanding in this area. One important series of research findings points to a common brain mechanism that is triggered by all known drugs of addiction — namely, the activation of dopamine mechanisms in a region of the forebrain known as the *nucleus accumbens*. This is a small dopamine-rich brain region underlying the larger dopamine-rich movement control centres, the caudate nucleus and putamen. The nucleus accumbens is part of the limbic forebrain, a brain region known to be important in emotional behaviour and in PAIN and PLEASURE. By direct measurements of dopamine release from animal brains, using tiny probes inserted into the nucleus accumbens, it has been found that cocaine, amphetamines, alcohol, nicotine, and cannabis all share the ability to cause increased levels of dopamine. When low doses of the drugs are used, the nucleus accumbens is the only brain region that shows such increased levels of dopamine. Furthermore, rats

in which the dopamine-containing nerve terminals in the nucleus accumbens are selectively destroyed (by means of the selective chemical neurotoxin, 6-hydroxydopamine) no longer self-administer amphetamines or cocaine. Could it be that dopamine release in the nucleus accumbens is the common mechanism underlying the pleasurable actions of these drugs? According to this view the drugs simply subvert a normal brain mechanism in which pleasurable or 'reinforcing' stimuli assist the animal in learning to repeat a behaviour. Addiction can be viewed as an 'aberrant form of learning' — the drugs recruit brain mechanisms that have a normal place in cognitive and emotional behaviour and cause these to malfunction, so the addict 'learns' to continue using the drug.

Historical perspective

There have been remarkable changes in attitudes to psychoactive drugs in Western society over the years. What was considered safe and beneficial in one era often comes to be seen as an evil scourge to a later generation. Nowhere is this more obvious than in the place that opium has played in British history. Imported as an important trade commodity from Turkey and India, opium was widely used in all strata of British society in the eighteenth and nineteenth centuries. The poor sought solace from the miseries of their daily lives, working mothers used opium-containing 'cordials' to calm their children while they went out to work, middle-class housewives took *laudanum* (an alcoholic extract of opium) to calm their nerves, and artists sought inspiration from it. The literary movement in Europe known as the Romantic Revival relied extensively on opium to free the users to flights of fantasy and imagination, and included such figures as Schlegel, Madame de Staël, and Pushkin, in continental Europe, and Coleridge, Wordsworth, Scott, Shelley, Keats, and Byron in Britain. Thomas de Quincey's famous autobiographical *Confessions of an Opium Eater* (1821), was the first literary account of the powerful addiction that opium can cause.

In mid-nineteenth-century France, cannabis was introduced from Egypt, following the Napoleonic campaign, and became fashionable among many in the literary world who frequented the 'Club des Hashischins' in Paris. The work of Alexander Dumas, Gerard de Nerval, and Victor Hugo was much influenced by the drug, and Charles Baudelaire wrote a classic description of the cannabis (hashish) experience in *Les Paradis Artificiels* published in Paris in 1860. It was not until the latter half of the nineteenth century that restrictions were placed on the use of opium in Britain. Even as late as 1895, the Royal Commission appointed to report on the use of opium in India concluded that the drug had no harmful effects on the local population. A similar conclusion had been reached a year earlier by the Indian Hemp Products Commission, which reviewed the widespread use of cannabis in India.

In much the same way, when cocaine was first discovered a century ago as the active component in coca leaves, many experts extolled its virtues, and it rapidly gained a short-lived medical acceptance for a multitude of uses. Ironically, one of its popular uses was in the treatment of opium addiction! Sigmund Freud experimented with this and other uses of cocaine and took the drug himself for many years. By the turn of the century, however, the party was over; it had become clear that cocaine was a dangerous drug of addiction.

A more recent example of changing attitudes is the way we view tobacco smoking. Cigarette smoking grew rapidly in the Western world in the first part of the twentieth century. In the US by 1945 half of all adult men were smokers — consuming an average of 20 cigarettes per day. Smoking was glamourised by Hollywood movies and even advertised as having medical benefits. Things began to change, though, after the discovery of the link between cigarette smoking and lung cancer, and the growing recognition that nicotine is a drug of addiction. Today cigarette smokers have become pariahs, no longer permitted to indulge their habit in many public places or on aeroplanes, and tobacco companies are seen as 'evil empires'.

The historical perspective perhaps teaches us that during the late twentieth century we may have moved towards over-emphasising the damaging effects that psychoactive drug consumption has on society. While the regulation of such dangerous drugs as heroin and cocaine may be necessary to protect citizens from them, the use of the criminal law to prohibit the use of drugs such as cannabis and ecstasy, which are less likely to cause damage, is less rational. It may have to do with our demonisation of drug use as almost a modern equivalent of heresy in the Middle Ages — a crime to be punished by penalties that are more severe than the crime itself.

The way forward

Despite the importance of scientific research in this area for improving future treatment strategies, there is lamentably little effort or resource devoted to it at the moment. In thinking of treatments that might help to wean addicts from their drug habit we need to think of a range of different goals aiming to reduce craving for the drug, assist in overcoming the withdrawal signs 'both psychological and physical', and help the reformed addict not to relapse. We are not very close to achieving any of these at the moment. The most effective strategy we have currently is to treat addicts with a safer form of the drug itself — the heroin addict with methadone, the cigarette smoker with nicotine patches or gum. We must learn approaches that are both more sophisticated and more effective if we are to make any real impact on the problem.

LESLEY L. IVERSEN

Further reading

Berridge, V. (1999). *Opium and the people. Opiate use and drug control policy in nineteenth century and early twentieth century England*. Free Association Press, London.

Musto, D. F. (1999). *The American disease. Origins of narcotic control*. Oxford University Press, New York.

Robbins, T. W. and Everitt, B. J. (1999). Drug addiction: bad habits add up. *Nature*, **398**, 567–70.

See also ADDICTION; DRUGS; MEMBRANE RECEPTORS; OPIATES AND OPIOID DRUGS.

Drug administration

Medicines and other chemicals, for both diagnostic and therapeutic reasons, and for purposes such as IMMUNIZATION or ANAESTHESIA, can be administered in a wide variety of ways. The administration of drugs concerned the very earliest physicians. The ancient Babylonians (*c.* 3000 BCE) compounded laxatives — mixed vegetable and animal components with oils and honey for oral administration — and volatile oils were prepared using the newly-discovered technique of distillation. Ancient Egyptian papyri (*c.* 1900–1100 BCE) also mention many medicines prepared as potions, made up in water, milk or alcohol, or mixed into pills with dough or honey. There were ointments and vapours, and also suppositories and purgatives. These basic methods of administering drugs to patients have remained in use, improved by refinements of preparatory technique — especially with the advent of machinery to compound medicines — and the preparation of purer, unadulterated ingredients. To these have been added techniques for delivery by other routes — most notably that of injecting substances into the body.

The aim of therapeutic administration is for the active components of the medicine to reach the target site where it is intended to be effective. The technique and route used, such as an injection into a muscle, application of a cream to the skin, or ingestion of a pill, are influenced by both the formulation of the compound and the desired site and rapidity of action. An additional constraint is that medicines that could be degraded by natural digestive processes, or which would not be absorbed from the gut, cannot be given by mouth.

Injection and infusion

Injection is the act of introducing a substance into a body by means of some impulsive force, usually employing a syringe. The substance so injected is usually in a liquid form, and is employed to have a therapeutic effect either at the site of application (local actions including cooling, heating, antibiotic, and anti-inflammatory) or elsewhere in the body. Injected drugs usually act faster than those taken by mouth — and some substances, such as INSULIN, need to be injected, because they would be destroyed in the gut.

Injections can be made into practically any tissue, or cavity of the body, hence for example *intradermal* (into the skin), *subcutaneous* (just under the skin), *intramuscular* (deep into a muscle), or, less commonly, *intra-peritoneal* (into the peritoneal cavity), or *intra-pleural*. The site used depends on the purpose and the nature of the injection. Injection directly into the bloodstream (*intravenous*) has the most rapid effect — within minutes or even seconds — and so is suited to urgent treatment, such as reviving, by glucose injection, a diabetic person who has had an overdose of insulin. Substances given by intramuscular injection take longer to be absorbed into the circulation. The subcutaneous route has the slowest effect, and by comparison with the intramuscular route does not allow as large a volume to be injected without discomfort.

Infusion usually into a vein, but also sometimes into a body cavity, differs from injection in being a continuous, slow introduction of material, usually under pressure of gravity (as in a blood or saline infusion, or transfusion), and sometimes by a slow, mechanically-driven syringe (as in some methods of delivering post-operative ANALGESIA). Materials to aid diagnosis, such as radioactive chemicals, or radioopaque dyes which show up on X-ray, are injected or infused, most commonly into veins or arteries.

One of the earliest attempts at intravenous injection was made in 1656 by the young Christopher Wren (1632–1723). Although best remembered for his architectural work, Wren was also a poet, a mathematician, and a keen experimentalist in the natural sciences, who was strongly influenced by William Harvey's views on the circulation of the blood. With colleagues in Oxford he experimented on introducing a slender quill into a dog's veins, and is recorded in the historical records of the Royal Society as '… the first Author of the Noble Anatomical Experiment of Injecting Liquid into the Veins of Animals'. This technique did not find immediate therapeutic application. Early attempts at inoculation did sometimes open a vein with a needle or scalpel, but the insertion of infective matter into a person's arm was usually accomplished by scratching an area of skin, a technique which continued for vaccination against smallpox until its eradication in the 1970s.

It was not until 1853 that the *hypodermic syringe* was invented by Charles Pravaz (1791–1853). Its first purpose was to inject iron perchloride into the veins to induce clotting, which he was using as an experimental treatment for aneurysms. In the same year, an Edinburgh doctor, Alexander Wood (1817–84), first thought of using a hollow needle to introduce medicinal agents through and under the skin. Originally thinking the technique could be used to remove birthmarks by injection directly into the blemish, he rapidly extended its application, by using a mixture of morphine dissolved in sherry to produce pain relief in a patient suffering from chronic neuralgia. Despite the fact that his patient fell into a deep sleep, Wood seemed to believe that the drug only acted locally, at the site of injection, rather than passing into the bloodstream and acting on the central nervous system. His views were of some importance, as many practitioners were not therefore alerted to the addictive nature of narcotic substances. Wood and others continued to develop injection techniques, principally for pain relief, despite practical problems such as the development of abscesses at the site of injection — this was before the recognition of bacterial infection and of the concomitant importance of antisepsis. A great variety of substances were injected into hapless patients: whisky and coffee to overcome opium poisoning, ammonia for snakebite, potassium permanganate for diphtheria.

It was the use of morphine injections that moved the technique of hypodermic drug administration from the realm of medical practice, into the underworld. The increasing availability of mass-produced syringes and uncontrolled access to narcotics, whose addictive properties were not known, not only led to many respectable people becoming inadvertent morphine addicts, but also facilitated illegal recreational use. Literature from the late nineteenth and early twentieth centuries frequently portrays morphine addicts, including the fictional detective Sherlock Holmes, created by the Edinburgh-trained doctor [Sir] Arthur Conan Doyle. Modern concerns about infection, especially by AIDS sufferers, amongst intravenous drug-users has led to schemes of syringe and needle exchanges, offered by charities and local authorities, to encourage the hygienic use and disposal of equipment used by addicts.

Despite advances in hypodermic administration, at the turn of the twentieth century intravenous injection was still regarded in practice as a surgical procedure — the skin would be cut, a vein exposed, and a cannula tied into it. Increasing demand and practice, especially by anaesthetists; the production of improved needles and syringes; and the advent of sterilization of needles and aseptic procedures, all contributed to increasing confidence in the technique. Similarly, enhanced methods of drug preparation, especially to produce sterile material, and improved formulations, enabled further refinements. For example, enclosing the active medicinal agents in an inert vehicle, such as an oil, will delay its absorption and prolong its activity; these are called depot injections, and a range of preparations, including contraceptive drugs, can be administered in this form. Very powerful drugs, such as those used in CHEMOTHERAPY, which could damage healthy tissues, are given by slow intravenous injection, so that they have an affect at their target site and are then rapidly diluted and removed by the circulation.

Oral medication

Drugs to be given by mouth are produced in a wide array of formulations, including tablets, pills, and liquids. ASPIRIN, and also alcohol, are absorbed in the stomach, but most oral medications are designed to be absorbed in the small intestine, where nutrients are normally absorbed, and they are coated with a protective material so that they pass through the stomach intact.

Fluid mixtures and elixirs have been used for centuries, and provided a convenient method by which a measured dose could be administered to a patient. Pills 'balls cut from a solid mass and hand-rolled' and lozenges 'shaped pieces also cut from a solid mass' have been known since ancient times. Various coatings were devised to disguise any bitter or unpleasant taste, gold and silver being particularly valued. There is some evidence that the Romans devised ridged stones on which the pill mass could be easily cut into equal portions. But it was not until the eighteenth century that 'pill tiles' were introduced into England from Delft. They had graduated grooves into which the pill mass, formed into a tube, was placed before being cut. These all depended on hand cutting and rolling of the pills, usually done by the druggist who dispensed the medicine. Later, mechanical mixing, rolling, and cutting instruments were devised, which greatly increased the production of pills, and heralded the advent of commercial manufacture.

During the 1830s a French pharmacist devised a mechanism for making soft-gelatin capsules which could then be filled — usually with unpalatable, oily, or semi-solid medicaments that could not easily be made into pills. In the following decade came a great breakthrough, the invention by William Brockedon in England of a hand-punch machine to make compressed medicines. Taken up by some English and American manufacturers, the products became known as '*tablets*' because of the usage of that word by the pharmaceutical firm of Burroughs Wellcome and Co. In 1884 the company registered the word 'Tabloid' as their tradename for such medicines. The advantages of these compressed medicines were that they were convenient to carry, did not deteriorate in extremes of temperature, and were easier than other methods for the preparation of a standardized dose. One problem that remained, however, was that of ensuring that the tablet would disintegrate in the intestine. This was solved by the discovery that adding starch to the coating facilitated the absorption of water, and the consequent break up of the tablet.

Other routes

Some drugs are best absorbed through MUCOUS MEMBRANES — such as the lining of the mouth, especially under the tongue — one of the best known being nitroglycerine for angina. Other sites for absorption can include the rectum, vagina, urethra, or nasal cavity, although these are more often used so that the drug can act locally, as in the case of anti-allergic nasal sprays, vaginal pessaries in the treatment of local infections, and spermicide preparations in contraception. Rectal suppositories are usually bullet shaped, and moulded from a substance that will slowly dissolve at body temperature, such as glycerine, and may be used to carry drugs for absorption as well as the commoner local lubricant function. Some drugs which would normally be given orally may have to be administered through the rectum, in cases where, for example, a patient is vomiting

excessively, or is unconscious and unable to swallow. Approximately 50% of a drug can be absorbed through the rectal mucosa, although irritation often occurs. For a period in the nineteenth century the rectal route was also used to induce anaesthesia, being especially favoured by Russian military surgeons for the administration of ether.

Ointments are preparations of a fatty or oily consistency, for the application of medicines to the skin or mucous membranes, and are intended either to exert a local effect — such as warming, cooling, pain relief, anti-infection; or to provide a protective barrier — or to be absorbed and spread through the body to have more widespread effects.

Few drugs penetrate readily through the layers of the SKIN. Absorption is determined by both the surface area over which an ointment is spread, and the solubility of the ointment. Some chemicals, such as toxic substances in organic solvents, can be absorbed rapidly through the skin and cause poisoning. Absorption through skin patches can provide low-maintenance levels of drugs, such as oestrogen replacement therapy (a form of HORMONE REPLACEMENT THERAPY) for post menopausal women, or a patch worn to release anti-MOTION SICKNESS drugs whilst travelling. Absorption is enhanced through skin damaged by burns, wound, or abrasion, and particular care must be taken when applying medicaments to such injuries. Ointments are also prepared for application to the EYES, principally for their local effects, usually from absorption through the conjunctiva, often for infections or trauma. More recently, ocular inserts have been developed to provide continuous delivery of low levels of drugs, somewhat analogous to skin patches.

Some drugs can be delivered by *inhalation*, in the form of vapours or aerosols. They can be absorbed rapidly into the circulation through the pulmonary epithelium — the lining of the LUNGS. This route is used particularly for the treatment of respiratory diseases, such as asthma, and for the administration of volatile anaesthetics. Absorption is rapid because of the large surface area of the lungs. The main disadvantages to this route are the difficulties of regulating the dose, and the fact that many of the gases used in this way also act as irritants. During the twentieth century the main advances were to improve anaesthetic apparatus so as to control and monitor the dose received by the patient, and to minimise that accidentally received by the anaesthetist and other operating theatre staff. This can also be the route for inadvertent absorption of toxic chemicals in the environment, and substances used in CHEMICAL WARFARE, such as mustard gas.   E.M. TANSEY

Duodenum The first and shortest segment of the small intestine. For up to 3 or 4 hours after a meal it receives spurts of partly digested food (*chyme*) from the stomach. Juices pour into it at this appropriate time from the PANCREAS and from the GALL BLADDER, both close by, stimulated to do so by HORMONES secreted from the duodenum itself in response to the chyme's arrival. Because the juices are alkaline, stomach acid is normally neutralized here, but excessive acidity has been linked to the duodenum's propensity to develop ulcers.   S.J.

See ALIMENTARY SYSTEM; PLATE 1.

Dwarf is a general term given to animals, plants, and other things which are significantly smaller than would ordinarily be expected. The term 'dwarf' has historically been attributed to people of profoundly short stature, especially those whose bodily proportions are notably different from those of average people. By contrast, the term 'midget' has generally been reserved for people of profound short stature whose bodily proportions are consistent with those of average height. Activists of very short stature prefer to call themselves 'little people' because of the negative connotations 'dwarf' and especially 'midget' have accrued, and because, while not all little people fit strict medical definitions of 'dwarfism', all little people face the same sorts of social hardships, regardless of the exact cause of their short statures. 'Little people' usually refers to people whose height will not exceed 4 feet 10 inches over the course of their lifetimes.

The causes of short stature are very numerous, and not all well understood. In several historically-isolated groups, 'short' stature is actually the norm. For example, some peoples indigenous to Africa and the Malay Peninsula rarely grow over five feet tall. (Europeans have tended to lump these peoples together under the single name 'Pygmy'.) Among 'average' sized peoples, short stature can result if children are given inadequate nutrition or inadequate emotional nurturing. Medical researchers believe that the latter kind of phenomenon, known as 'psychological dwarfism', occurs when emotional stress in childhood leads to a growth-hormone deficiency and consequent cessation of growth. Major illnesses in childhood, such as kidney failure, can also contribute to stunting. Children whose growth rates appear slower than normal should therefore be examined carefully so that dangerous metabolic diseases can be ruled out.

Medical professionals use the term 'dwarfism' to refer to a host of metabolic conditions which result in profound short stature. In the US, about 1 in 10 000 births is of a child with dwarfism, although diagnosis may not occur for several years. The most common form of dwarfism is *achondroplasia*. The heads and trunks of achondroplastic dwarfs are average, but their limbs are relatively short and thick. Achondroplastic dwarfs are typically healthy and enjoy the same range of intellect as average-sized people. (As adults they may suffer back and limb pain from the hazards of living in a world designed for much larger people.) In a different syndrome, the bodies of hypopituitary dwarfs — while proportioned in the way typical for 'average'-height people — produce less than the average amount of GROWTH HORMONE, and so, unless they take regular injections of growth hormone, they will remain small. In contrast to achondroplastic dwarfs, hypopituitary dwarfs often suffer from underlying metabolic health problems. Other conditions, too numerous to mention here, can also result in dwarfism.

Joan Ablon, a medical anthropologist who has studied the lives of little people and their families, has noted that categorizing dwarfism as a disability is inappropriate for at least two reasons. First, 'although dwarfism is a dramatic, physically distinctive, and immediately identifiable condition, dwarfs are usually not physically disabled or handicapped in the general sense of these terms …'. As one parent of a dwarf child said, 'Their bodies are just packaged a little differently.' Short stature is not a disease, nor does short stature necessarily signal an underlying disease state (if we define disease to mean a metabolically dangerous or physically painful condition).

Secondly, as Ablon writes, 'in our cultural tradition dwarfs belong to the mythic world, not the mundane world of our daily experience or reality. Dwarfs carry with them the historical and cultural baggage of special and even magical status much more than do persons with various other physical differences.' In centuries past, dwarfs were commonly displayed, held as captive entertainment, and even given as gifts. Still today, adult dwarfs often find themselves the subjects of unwanted attention. Many report encountering strangers who, without permission, insist on picking them up and treating them like children or dolls. For many dwarfs, acting is the only career available to them — employers are reluctant to hire dwarfs, and on the job many suffer harassment — but even then, dwarfs are typically assigned only to play elves or other charmed or 'cute' people.

Our culture rewards tall stature and denigrates small stature. (At least for men, income is positively correlated with height, and tall men are more likely than shorter counterparts to be married or elected to office.) For this reason, some parents of short-stature children have sought treatments to increase the ultimate height of their children. (The available treatments do not work well after puberty, and so they are not an option for adults.) These treatments are extremely expensive and are still considered experimental. One involves the cutting and progressive stretching of the bones of the limbs. A more common approach is the regular injection, throughout childhood, of growth hormone supplements. Until 1984, growth hormone supplements were typically derived from cadavers, but the discovery that some recipients thereby developed Creutzfeldt-Jakob disease ended that practice. Since 1985, clinicians have instead employed synthetic growth hormone developed from recombinant DNA technology.

Because injections of growth hormone might make any child grow taller than she or he would otherwise (note that this is not proven), the possibility has arisen that these treatments could be used on any child, regardless of her/his condition. Indeed, some parents of children who are short, but not growth hormone-deficient, have sought these treatments. This raises many ethical issues, touching on the right of parents to take risks on behalf of a child who has a cosmetically-challenging body, distributive justice, the rights of people with atypical anatomies, and so on. These questions about 'designing' or 'engineering' children have also been raised by the recent discovery, in 1995, of the genetic basis for achondroplasia. Parents are now able to screen fetuses for achondroplasia and selectively abort them. At the same time, given the hardships of raising a child who quickly grows bigger than oneself, some achondroplastic dwarfs have apparently even considered selectively aborting fetuses who, via the genetic screening, are shown *not* to be achondroplastic.   ALICE DREGER

Further reading

Ablon, J. (1988). *Living with difference: families with dwarf children*. Praeger, New York.

Berreby, D. (1996) Up with people: dwarves meet identity politics. *The New Republic*, 214(18), 14–9.

Dyspepsia A set of symptoms attributed to a disorder of digestion and usually focused upon the STOMACH — upper abdominal pain or discomfort, nausea, flatulence, 'heartburn'. Such problems may indeed be due to disordered function in the stomach itself, but also or alternatively in the OESOPHAGUS, LIVER, GALL BLADDER, DUODENUM, or PANCREAS.   S.J.

See ALIMENTARY SYSTEM; INDIGESTION.

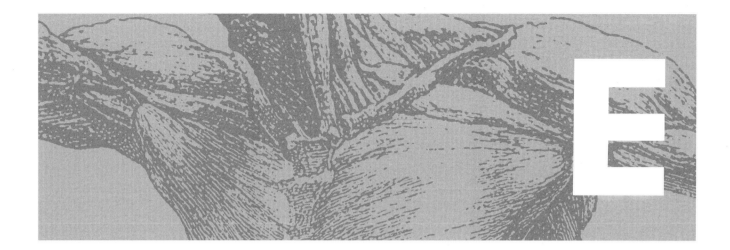

Ear, external The ear of a mammal is divided into three regions: the external or outer ear, the middle ear, and the inner ear. The external ear is the only part that is visible from the outside and is what people are usually referring to when they talk about their ears. It consists of a skin-covered flap known as the *pinna* or *auricle*, which leads like a funnel into the *ear canal* (external auditory meatus). Apart from the soft earlobe, the pinna possesses a framework of CARTILAGE moulded to form several ridges and depressions, the most important being a cavity known as the *concha*, which lies just behind the opening to the ear canal.

The ear canal, which is also lined by skin, is a tubular structure, about 25 mm long, with a cartilaginous outer region and a bony inner region. Fine hairs and glands (which secrete wax) are found in the outer part. The ear canal terminates at the *eardrum* (tympanic membrane), which forms the boundary between the external ear and the middle ear. The external ear is responsible for collecting airborne sounds and for protecting the delicate eardrum from mechanical damage.

Although experiments carried out in the late nineteenth century provided insights into the role of the external ear in HEARING, many textbooks give scant attention to it and even state, quite erroneously, that it is a vestigial structure in human beings, having little function compared with the larger, more erect, and often moveable ears of other mammals. This is largely due to the fact that research on hearing in the twentieth century mainly involved the delivery of sound by headphones, which cover and therefore remove the influence of the pinnae. However, beginning 30 years ago, acoustical measurements using tiny microphones inserted into the ear canals of either real or artificial pinnae have shown how incoming sound waves are modified by the different components of the external ear in ways that aid our ability to detect and localize sounds in the environment.

The external ear has two key functions. Firstly, the resonances of the external ear, particularly of the concha and ear canal, increase the sound pressure at the eardrum for some frequencies of sound by as much as 20 dB. In adult humans, this gain in amplitude is greatest at sound frequencies from 2 to 7 kHz. Consequently, sounds in this frequency range are transmitted by the external ear most efficiently, which, in turn, contributes to an improvement in the listener's hearing sensitivity. (It may be significant that the sound of human speech is largely concentrated in this frequency band.)

Secondly, interaction of sound waves with the external ear provides information that helps in judging the *location* of sound sources. The primary cues for sound localization result from the fact that we have two ears, one on each side of the head. Sounds that lie to one side of the straight-ahead direction differ in their time of arrival and in the amplitude of the sound at the two ears. These differences can be detected by neurons in the brain, which underlie our ability to determine the direction of a sound source. However, studies in humans and other animals have shown that the external ear, by differentially filtering sounds from different directions in space, provides additional information. Therefore, filling the cavities of the pinna or inserting tubes into the ear canals to bypass the pinnae altogether leads to errors in localization of sounds, particularly in the vertical direction, and to a decreased ability to discriminate sounds in front from those behind. Although two ears are definitely better than one for recognizing the positions of sounds, the filtering of sounds in the external ear can enable us to localize sounds under circumstances where the so-called binaural cues are ambiguous or missing. Such monaural listening conditions occur not only in people who are deaf in one ear, but when a sound on one side is too quiet to reach one of the ears, because of the shadowing effect of the head.

The convolutions of the external ear, particularly the concha, act to increase or decrease the amplitude of different frequency components of a sound as it passes from the free field to the eardrum. These filtering effects are dependent on the location of the sound, giving rise to spectral patterns — characteristic variations in amplitude with frequency — that vary with both the horizontal and vertical angle of the sound source. These spectral cues are most useful when the sound contains energy over a wide range of high frequencies. Eliminating the influence of the pinna by wearing headphones — for example, when listening to music on a personal stereo — gives rise to the impression that the sound is located inside the head. However, if sounds in the free field are first recorded with microphones placed in the ear canal, hence spectrally transformed by the pinna, and then played back over headphones, the listener experiences the vivid illusion of a sound originating from a particular direction outside the head. Generating virtual space sounds in this way not only helps in the scientific study of sound localization: computer-generated virtual environments are also used in training simulators and are found in many amusement arcades.

Because no two ears are exactly the same, we might imagine that each person has to learn to use the spectral cues generated by the particular dimensions of his or her own ears. Thus, listeners usually localize less well when listening to sounds as filtered by another person's external ears.

Some mammals, such as cats and bats, can precisely and independently alter the shape and orientation of their pinnae. Dogs tend to 'prick up their ears', i.e. raise their pinnae. Cats readily direct their ears toward the source of environmental sounds, usually in concert with movements of the eyes and head. These movements of the pinna appear to optimize sound reception by placing it at the position where the increase in sound pressure provided by the external ear is maximal, and may also help in sound localization. In bats, pinna movements are additionally thought to play an important role in echolocation.

As well as their auditory function, the external ears can help in the regulation of an animal's body temperature, via control of their extensive blood supply; and they may contribute to the threatening gestures made in encounters with other animals.
                                        ANDREW J. KING

Further reading

Carlile S. and King, A. J. (1993). From outer ear to virtual space. *Current Biology*, 3, 446–8.

Pickles, J. O. (1988). *An introduction to the physiology of hearing*, (2nd edn). Academic Press, London.

See also HEARING.

Eating

To survive, humans must ingest FOOD — must eat ideally from an abundant, varied diet, several times per day. Perhaps due to this fact — the basic necessity of eating to human survival — the rituals and habits surrounding it have flourished across cultures and throughout history. Why do individuals, societies and particular classes or ethnic groups eat specific foods? Why do eating rituals develop and change over time? Historians, economists, and anthropologists debate the relative importance of various influences, but tend to agree that a combination of factors motivate eating habits. It is neither strictly cultural influences nor economic conditions that determine eating behaviour but the interplay of both. Variables such as survival strategies, agricultural patterns, industrial development, gender, and familial structures, and the symbolic perceptions of particular foods and foodways, interact to determine eating patterns. Though it is clearly a physiological function linked to vitality, cultural and social expectations have had a profound influence upon the act of eating. As Roland Barthes has stated, 'food is but a system of communication, a body of images, a protocol of usages, situations and behaviors'.

Social meanings

In subsistence or peasant societies, economic realities may severely constrain food types and amounts, often leading to malnutrition and disease. In pre-industrial Europe, for example, while the upper classes enjoyed a varied diet including substantial amounts of meat, the masses ate an undiversified diet, primarily of cereals. Lacking meat (most consumed only about 2 oz per week), they suffered from diseases associated with a lack of protein. Similar conditions persist in Third World countries as well as among the poor in the most affluent of societies. Yet even where material circumstances limit dietary intake, food and eating customs contain social meaning. The great feasts of medieval Europe, while infrequent occurrences, settled status conflicts in feudal society, while gender relations were clearly marked by female responsibility for preparing food in African–American slave communities.

In regard to the symbolic meanings given to food and eating, folk and religious customs, class stratification, gender definitions, and ideas about health have had the most significant impact. In most cultures, religious beliefs have included specifications about food and eating. Prehistoric peoples, faced with erratic food supplies, devised elaborate ceremonies hoping to sway the Gods to provide bountiful foodstuffs. All of the major religious faiths contain food regulations. For example, Hindus, guided by their belief in reincarnation, avoid killing animals and thus do not eat meat. Class stratification is also at work as those in the highest castes follow the strictest vegetarian diet. Principles of 'right action' also encourage Buddhists to avoid killing animals, while Islam and Judaism both proscribe pork or blood. Moslems also undertake the mandatory fast of Ramadam. Christian practices vary by faith and denomination. Catholicism includes a prohibition of meat on Fridays as well as abstaining from meat, fish, and dairy products on certain fast days. Seventh-Day Adventists follow a vegetarian diet, while Mormons are expected to avoid tobacco, alcohol, and hot drinks.

Eating rituals have acted to differentiate the classes from one another. In what people eat as well as when and how, their class status emerges. Since prosperity permits the most elaborate food purchases as well as the furnishings of meal times (crockery, china, silver, linen, decorations, etc.), minute differentiations can signal economic and social standing. In the economic uncertainties of nineteenth-century America, the newly-middle class proved their status by acquiring the coveted accoutrements of a fine dining room and then entertaining, while in the early twentieth century, slenderness and its attendant dieting distanced middle-class women from their 'robust' working-class sisters. In the twentieth century, food knowledge as well as dining out at the finest restaurants demonstrated social status.

Eating the right thing in the right manner has also served to define masculinity and femininity. In modern Western cultures, prior to the late twentieth century, that has tended to mean dainty or polite eating for women and hearty eating for men. Once fat became disdained for both sexes, correct, healthful food choices came to dominate.

History

Ideas about healthy nourishment, particularly with the development of food science in the nineteenth century, spawned new eating behaviours. In the last 100 years, 'healthful' eating has meant a turning away from heavy, simple, protein-rich diets to ones dominated by fruits, vegetables, and complex carbohydrates. At the same time, Westerners tend to consume more and more 'unhealthy' but commercially viable, 'fast' foods. As a result, a constant tension exists between what one wants to eat and what one 'should eat'.

Though eating patterns have differed widely by region and culture, some broad historical patterns can be outlined. Until about 12 000 years ago, humans sustained their diet by food gathering which included hunting. Small, isolated populations moved from place to place, foraging for plants, animals, and eventually fish. Though they had little control over their food supply, anthropological evidence suggests that they practised food sharing. Food production emerged in different sites between 9000 and 12 000 years ago as humans began to control their food supply through animal husbandry and domestication of plants. Some argue that this marked the 'rise of civilization'. Malnutrition decreased and populations increased, resulting in more sedentary living and leisure, the rise of cities, complex political organization, and more aggressive societies.

The four major early civilizations (Mesopotamia, Egypt, the Indus Valley, and the Huang He Valley) intensified animal husbandry, tool and weapon development, and pastoralism. Ancient Greece (2000 BC), considered the birthplace of modern civilization, actually emerged with food habits about 1000 years behind those of earlier civilizations. Until about the fifth century BC, the Greek diet consisted of cereals, breads, olives, fish, root vegetables, some fruit, and wine. In the Hellenistic period, food rituals began to signify class difference. The wealthy enjoyed a wide variety of imported foods, while the poor existed on a simple, bland diet. The same can be said for Ancient Rome during the Republic (509 BC–27 BC). The upper classes imbibed wine (diluted to reduce salt content) and dined on plentiful meat, fish, figs, and fruits, while the poor ate porridge, bread, olive oil, and water. The Roman Empire (27 BC–AD 476), with its vast territory, produced or imported almost every type of food we know today. Wealthy Romans were known for their opulent dinner parties and gargantuan appetites. With so many food pleasures to chose from, it was as though they could not be satiated. Though the Romans emulated all things Greek, it is said that 'they became gluttons, rather than gourmets'.

During the Middle Ages — known as the Years of Famine — food and eating, like most other activities, became severely restricted due to crop failures, disease, and war. Still, eating habits reflected the strict hierarchy of the feudal system. Serfs produced their own wine, ate wild game, raised pigs and chickens, and eked out seasonal vegetables. In contrast, feudal lords enjoyed plentiful meat and a wide variety of imported foods, including spices from the Mid-east. The Renaissance brought more trade and exploration and — again, for the most affluent — an increasingly abundant diet.

The economic and cultural contact ushered in by the fifteenth- and sixteenth-century travels and immigration to the 'New World' highlighted the different values held by those in the East and West with regard to land, food production, and eating. Amidst much death, war, and disease, there was also sharing of skills and resources, especially in the mid-Atlantic region.

By the eighteenth century, people's relationship to food was increasingly infused with moral meaning. Embedded in religious language of self-control, eating behaviour began to signify one's moral standing. In the nineteenth century, the new science of dietetics began to elaborate basic nutritional standards. Much of the research, conducted on soldiers and workers in order to determine the minimum nourishment necessary to maintain health, emphasized models of efficiency. The body became just one more machine. To keep running smoothly, it needed the right balance of food, which acted as 'fuel'.

MARGARET A. LOWE

Further reading

McIntosh, E. N. (1995). *American food habits in historical perspective.* Praeger, Connecticut.

Minnell, S. (1985). *All manners of food.* Blackwell, New York.

See also FOOD.

Eating disorders

The modern term that covers all forms of the conditions known as *anorexia nervosa* and *bulimia nervosa*. It also sometimes includes OBESITY. The recorded prevalence of all three has increased during the past 40 years.

Anorexia nervosa, a form of food refusal, is mostly found in young girls, though 1 in 20 cases is a boy. Sometimes it improves spontaneously and sometimes it continues throughout life. The sufferers are usually intelligent high achievers and are often ambitious, and come from families who have ample food. Some have markedly 'hysterical' personalities, tending to be dramatic, to overreact, and to manipulate those in their environment. Others are more obsessional, ruminate constantly about food, and develop rituals connected with it. Anorexia means a lack of appetite, but the condition is misnamed because sufferers control rather than lose their appetite. It has been called 'the relentless pursuit of thinness'. Sufferers rigorously suppress their desire for food in order to be thinner, avoiding all food that they think contains more than the minimum of calories. They often tell lies about the food they do or do not eat, perhaps hiding it or disposing of it secretly to give the impression that it has been eaten. They think about food constantly, weigh themselves several times a day, and have distorted ideas about their bodies, believing that they look fat when they are actually dangerously thin. They tend to wear many layers of loose clothes, partly to hide their condition and partly because they suffer from the cold. Many exercise obsessively and constantly in an attempt to lose further weight. Some, like sufferers from bulimia, have episodes of binge-eating, after which they make themselves vomit to get rid of the food. The most severe cases are medical emergencies and require the most skilled care of a physician in hospital to avoid death. The underlying condition, and the full care of less severe cases, is usually managed by psychiatrists.

Bulimics, who are usually of normal weight, gorge food, but then induce VOMITING, sometimes several times a day. They deliberately vomit, at least initially, in order to become thinner. However, it frequently becomes a habit that is hard to break and their whole lives may be concentrated on bingeing and vomiting. Frequent vomiting leads to unpleasant mouth odour and can promote tooth decay, so sufferers tend to be secretive, to avoid close contact with other people, and to clean their teeth several times during the day. Famous bulimics have included Princess Diana and Audrey Hepburn.

Anorexia nervosa and bulimia nervosa are sometimes regarded clinically as different forms of the same illness.

A number of 'causes' are believed to underlie these conditions. Those most discussed are disturbed family relationships and social pressures to be thin. Some sufferers also use their obsession with food as a means of controlling their families, perhaps by creating parental anxiety or by insisting that they do all the family cooking and preventing their parents going away because they are doing this. Some have very dominant mothers and feel that the only way in which they can gain power themselves is by controlling their intake of food.

A theory has arisen that anorexia and bulimia are 'caused' by sexual abuse in childhood. Sometimes there is an association between the two. However, therapists of doubtful training and repute have suggested that those with eating disorders have invariably been abused in childhood. In pursuit of this belief they may have used persuasive techniques to elicit many apparent 'memories' of sexual abuse of which the patient was previously unaware. This has given rise to what has been labelled 'false memory syndrome', which has disrupted many otherwise intact families. The current view among most psychiatrists is that true memories of sexual abuse in childhood are seldom if ever repressed and that 'memories' which emerge for the first time during treatment, especially with a therapist who believes that they *must* be there, should be treated with great caution.

Anorexia nervosa was identified by William Gull in the nineteenth century. It has certainly existed for much longer, perhaps throughout the history of civilization, wherever there was ample food. It used to be regarded as a rare condition, partly because doctors tended to believe what their patients told them, and to look for physical disease. Many cases in the past were probably misdiagnosed as TUBERCULOSIS, endocrine disease (such as Simmond's disease, a failure of the PITUITARY GLAND), or loss of weight from unknown cause. The secretiveness and deceptiveness of the patients made the diagnosis difficult for those who were unaware of this tendency. Since then doctors have realized that anorexia nervosa is usually not difficult to identify and that bulimia is much more common than was supposed.

The recorded incidence of anorexia nervosa increased greatly during the 1950s and 1960s, and it became a worrisome epidemic, especially in girls' boarding schools. This rise was undoubtedly partly due to the increasing recognition of the condition by doctors, but partly because of the fashion for thinness, which became popular and was accompanied by hostility to plumpness and fear of gaining weight. Those responsible for the care of young girls have shown hostility towards the FASHION trade's flaunting of skeletal models to display and advertise clothes, but the custom persists, as does the epidemic of anorexia, which is found at ever younger ages, even as young as 6 or 7. Some of the youngest sufferers are the children of anorexics and bulimics, many of whom raise their families with bizarre attitudes towards food. Doctors have expressed anxiety about the threat to health in children who are fed on skimmed milk and high fibre food, virtually free of SUGAR and FAT. Such a diet is unsuitable for growing bodies and can cause long-term damage. The fact that eating disorders tend to run in families may not be entirely due to parental feeding practices: it seems likely that there is a genuine genetic factor in their causation.

The 'epidemic' of anorexia may now have peaked as the incidence seems no longer to be rising. According to figures from the Eating Disorders Unit in the University of London, during 1988–93 the incidence of anorexia remained stable at about 20 cases per 100 000 of the population, whereas the incidence of bulimia rose from 15 to 50 cases per 100 000. This apparent dramatic rise in bulimia can be at least partly explained by the fact that the disease was first described in 1979: doctors and the public have only gradually become aware of it. Probably it was common before it was identified. Since the sufferer usually looks normal, the condition is unlikely to be diagnosed unless the sufferer admits to having the problem or their behaviour is noticed by others.

Some people with these conditions recover spontaneously but many need help, which they are often reluctant to seek. Various treatments have been tried, including incarceration with 'rewards' (such as having visitors) for weight gain, sedatives (to suppress activity), and various forms of psychotherapy. Antidepressant drugs are often quite effective and many clinicians believe that there is considerable overlap between eating disorders and depression.

Obesity represents the other end of the eating disorders spectrum. Classically, it is a problem of middle age, but its incidence has been rising, even among young children, especially in the developed world. It affects women more than men and lower social classes more than upper. It is associated with higher than average morbidity and mortality. Heart disease, high blood pressure, diabetes, and even accidents are much more common in overweight people than in those of normal weight. Obesity is commonest where food is ample but protein is expensive and it is particularly likely to develop in people whose diet is high in processed foods, since these often contain many 'hidden' calories in the form of fat and sugar. The recent increase in obesity is thought to be related to the sedentary and labour-saving characteristics of modern life in the developed world. People drive cars rather than walk, guide the vacuum cleaner rather than scrub the floor, and spend much time watching television. A sedentary lifestyle makes it difficult to lose weight. Many people control any tendency to gain weight by deliberately taking EXERCISE, perhaps joining a gym or playing an energetic game regularly, but others dislike taking exercise. It is often harder to persuade a patient to take exercise than to keep to a slimming diet.   ANN DALLY

See also DIETING; DEVELOPMENT AND GROWTH; OBESITY.

Echocardiography is the clinical technique, developed with related ULTRASOUND techniques in the 1960s, of producing images of the functioning HEART by reflecting pulses of ultrasound from the structures of the heart and then recording the reflected ('echoed') sound signals. It is a close relative of the methods used to produce live images of the fetus developing in the womb. With this technique, physicians have a further powerful 'non-invasive' method to aid both diagnosis and treatment of many heart complaints. The 'echo' images can reveal the size of the heart's chambers, the width of the major veins and arteries entering and leaving it, and the status of the valves that define the direction of blood flow into and out of the chambers. Powerful computing techniques mean that the echocardiography can be done in 'real time', with the patient fully conscious, enabling the dynamic features of heart function to be observed over the course of many heartbeats.

The method involves two basic elements, a transmitter and a receiver. The transmitter emits an electrical signal to a *piezo-electric crystal* each time an oscillation is required. The electrical signal is converted by the crystal to an ultrasound wave. The ultrasound beam is directed through the chest and the sound wave is transmitted and reflected as internal structures of the chest are encountered. The reflected waves are collected by the receiver. Currently, most echocardiographers use *sector scanners* to produce images of the heart. With these instruments the ultrasound beam is swept in an arc across the heart from a single point on the chest wall. The solid parts of the heart walls and even the very thin valves produce strong reflections, whereas blood-filled spaces produce little reflection and so are reported as 'empty' by ultrasound. The received pattern of sound waves is often displayed in a video format, but a permanent record can be produced by using photography or chart recorder technology. Since the time between the emission and reception of an ultrasound signal can be accurately measured, it is possible to display the depth at which a structure lies within the chest using a simple formula: $D = V \times T$ or, distance = (velocity of the ultrasound signal) × (time between emission and reception of the signal). In this way, an image of a 'section' of the heart can be built up over a number of cycles. Cross-sectional images can be produced by electronic sector scanners which have small multi-element transducers cut from the same piezo-electric crystals.

The narrowing (*stenosis*) of heart valves is a typical clinical problem that can be studied by echocardiography. In association with valve narrowing, the speed of blood flow and chamber dimensions are increased. By applying the Bernoulli principle it is possible to estimate the pressure differences across a damaged valve. CARDIAC OUTPUT can be assessed by measuring the velocity of blood flow leaving the heart and multiplying this by the echocardiographically-derived cross-sectional area of the aorta.

Doppler imaging, usually performed at the same time as echocardiography, utilizes the principal of the Doppler shift of ultrasound to measure velocity of blood flow in the chambers of the heart and in the aorta. In the 'continuous wave Doppler' technique, two piezo-electric crystals are utilized; one continually sends and another continually receives the ultrasound wave. Information is thus received from the entire length of the beam and range resolution is not possible. Its great advantage, however, is that high maximal velocities of blood flow, such as occur when blood is being ejected from the ventricles, can be reliably measured. In the pulsed Doppler system, the transmitter is turned off after sending the pulse to the crystal, while the receiver is immediately turned on. The receiver waits for the pressure wave-front to return to the crystal and amplifies it to allow frequency analysis. This technique is useful for localizing high velocity flow, as commonly associated with defective ventricular exit (aortic and pulmonary) valves, rather than for measuring an absolute velocity.

The current uses of cross-sectional and Doppler echocardiography are to record the dimensions of heart structures, cardiac output, jet velocities, and flow disturbances. Abnormal flow patterns can also be recorded and used, for example, to map jets of blood leaking from damaged valves. Recent technology has allowed colour coding of blood flow direction using a combination of cross-sectional and Doppler echocardiography.

DAVID J. MILLER

NIALL G. MACFARLANE

See also HEART; IMAGING TECHNIQUES.

Ectopic pregnancy

Ectopic pregnancy 'Ectopic', from the Greek, means out of place. Fertilization usually occurs in one of the Fallopian tubes, and the embryo proceeds to be implanted in the uterus. Occasionally it becomes lodged in the tube, and may continue to grow there, with consequences which are fatal to the pregnancy and may be hazardous for the mother because of internal bleeding. Much more rarely, an ovum can lose its way between the ovary and the receiving end of the tube, wandering into the peritoneal cavity, and ascending sperm can even find and fertilize it there — again a hopeless future for the embryo. The signs and symptoms of ectopic pregnancy are usually evident as early as, or even before, the first missed menstrual period, so prompt diagnosis and operative treatment can prevent major trouble. The inevitable loss of one of the tubes reduces the chances of subsequent conception.

SHEILA JENNETT

See PLATE 8.

Ectoplasm

Ectoplasm Spiritualism began in the mid nineteenth century and spread rapidly, until by the 1890s spiritualist seances were being held in major cities all across America and Europe. In the most dramatic seances, mediums not only transmitted messages from the dead, but generated 'physical phenomena' such as levitating tables, speech through trumpets, direct voices from the dead (i.e. without any trumpet or other instrument), and even full-body materialization of spirit forms.

The question then arose of how the dead could influence the physical world, and one answer was that they used a substance called ectoplasm. Ectoplasm was produced only by the most accomplished mediums, and was said to depend on their special physiological make-up. This white or grey fluid substance could sometimes be seen emerging from a medium's mouth, although it was said to come from other orifices as well. Usually ectoplasm was described as cold to the touch and rubbery or leathery, but sometimes it was said to be fluid and slimy, or gauzy and wet. Often it began by flowing out of the body and later hardened into a solid.

There are several photographs of well-known mediums producing ectoplasm. For example, in the 1930s, photographs of Jack Webber show him producing long ribbons of a white material that seem to grip on to tables or trumpets and lift them physically in the air, while he is seen bound to the arms of a chair on which he is seated. Eva C. was photographed with a strange gauzy substance stretched across her naked chest, and Helen Duncan with a mass of white cloth-like ectoplasm pouring from her mouth. Perhaps the oddest experiments were conducted by a Dr Crawford in the 1910s. The medium, Kathleen Goligher, apparently produced 'psychic structures' made of ectoplasm, which emerged from the several orifices of her body and were strong enough to lift tables, register on weighing scales, and make impressions on specially positioned trays of sand. She was searched and provided with clean underwear before experiments, and special dye was used to trace the route of the ectoplasm back into her body.

Ectoplasm normally appeared only in total darkness. Light was said to damage the delicate substance, and even harm the mediums who were producing it. So, although it was occasionally photographed by flash, investigators wanting proof were usually disappointed. In the archives of the Society for Psychical Research in London, there is still a piece of Helen Duncan's ectoplasm. This looks very much like a large piece of fine muslin and even has stitching around the edges. Although, like most other mediums, she was regularly searched before seances, many believe she swallowed and later regurgitated the material.

Ectoplasm has rarely been reported since the 1930s. Indeed, the advent of infrared photography, and of other methods of recording in the dark, seems to have coincided with the end of the truly dramatic physical phenomena of spiritualism, including the once popular ectoplasm.

SUSAN BLACKMORE

Effigies

Effigies An effigy is a likeness or image, usually sculpted, and usually of a person, which is distinguished by its capacity to substitute for the individual it represents. Effigies commonly have a

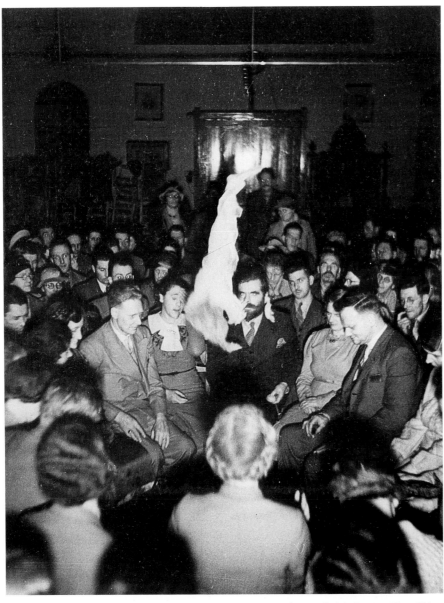

Medium Colin Evans producing ectoplasm at Rochester Square Spiritualist Temple (1938). Mary Evans Picture Library/ *Psychic News*.

Westminster Abbey. It was cut from stone imported from Tournai, a dark limestone, commonly called black marble.

Throughout Europe, effigial sculpture showed a gradual evolution, where low relief carving gave way to increasingly higher relief, and rigid poses to greater naturalism and more realistic detail. This was particularly the case in England, where effigial sculpture was to attain its highest stage of development. Representative examples are the effigies of thirteenth-century ecclesiastical figures in Ely Cathedral; the effigy of Eleanor of Aquitaine, Queen of England, shown holding a devotional book, in the church of Fontevrault Abbey; and the mail-clad, crossed-legged knights entombed in cathedrals, abbeys, and parish churches throughout England. The stones used were the black 'marble' of Tournai, the dark brown or gray 'marble' of domestic Purbeck, and, in the case of the queen's effigy, a pale limestone, which, because it could be quarried in blocks rather than slabs, gave masons a freer hand in creating projecting surfaces.

Effigies carved from true marble were a French innovation. The earliest known example is that of Isabella of Aragon, the first queen of Philip III of France, who died in 1271 and was buried in Saint Denis Abbey. Her effigy was completed in 1275, a decade or so after Louis IX commissioned the carving of effigies of all the rulers who had preceded him, going back to the seventh century, to be kept in the abbey. Since their likenesses had not been preserved, the effigies were symbolic. By the mid fourteenth century, French monarchs and others, as concerned about their image as any modern politician, had their effigies fashioned while they were alive.

Bronze effigies were cast, and brass effigies were engraved or cut, and while commoners' effigies often served as church pavement, those of people of higher station were lifted up onto tomb covers. Subsequently, the tombs themselves were raised — mounted on the backs of carved lions, for example, and, later, on short columns. The elevation of the effigy created problems. Comparatively flat figures were barely visible from below. In Italy, where wall tombs predominated, effigies were tilted to enhance visibility — an unsatisfactory solution that left the images in a seemingly precarious position. In Italy, as elsewhere, the problem was solved as the comparatively flat figure evolved into one that was three-dimensional. The figure, freed from the slab, took on the dimensions of sculpture. In the fourteenth century, by which time churches were becoming cluttered with tombs, recumbent effigies were often made to stand up and commence a new life, as statues. In Bamberg Cathedral, to cite one example, the effigy of Pope Clement II, carved around 1240, was separated from the tomb lid and set up, vertically, against a pier. A number of later tomb effigies appear to have been specifically designed for vertical attachment.

As effigial art rounded out in form and swelled in ostentation, it began to assume a homilitic

symbolic resonance, as in the case of Uncle Sam or Guy Fawkes; they do not necessarily differ from portraits in how they are produced, or even how they appear, but in their function and use. While the term 'effigy' (from Latin: *effingere*, to fashion) may, broadly speaking, refer to any likeness, it has come to be applied most consistently to likenesses produced in connection with death — whether carved tomb sculptures or painted representations of the deceased.

The effigies of antiquity were created to perpetuate the memory of the deceased as he or she looked while alive. The earliest known tomb effigy is that of King Djoser (*c.* 2686–13 BCE), found in the worship chamber of an Egyptian pyramid. Such Egyptian portraits were intended to house the soul after death, and to identify it as it travelled through the realm of the dead. The

most lifelike effigies of the ancient world were those fashioned by the Etruscans of the sixth and fifth centuries BCE; their mortuary art features full-scale effigies of the deceased — sometimes an individual, sometimes a married couple — taking their ease, recumbent on a casket cover. Neither the Greeks nor the Romans memorialized their dead in the form of full-scale recumbent effigies. This form of mortuary art reappeared in the eleventh century, in Germany, in bronze grave slabs. Among the oldest of these is a grave slab at Merseburg Cathedral, which dates to 1080. At the wealthy Quedlinburg monastery, grave slabs dating to the mid twelfth century preserve the appearance and costume of three abesses. The oldest recumbent effigy in England is thought to be that of Abbot Crispin, who died in 1117 and was buried in the cloisters at

237

function: below the effigy of the living person, shown in his or her splendid attire, lay the same body, now shown in a state of decomposition or reduced to a skeleton. An early example is the mid-fifteenth-century tomb of John Fitzalan, in which Fitzalan is shown, his head on a pillow, his hands folded in prayer, lying above a Gothic cage containing his cadaver. A curious, latter-day French example dating to the second half of the sixteenth century depicts an aristocratic woman, Valentine Balbiani, reclining, reading, her cheek resting on her hand and a lapdog at her side, above a low-relief of her corpse, whose skull rests on the same pillows on which her effigy rests its elbow. Following the Council of Trent (1545–63), Catholic reformers began to inveigh against grandiose effigies, with a resultant hiatus in their production. The recess did not last long. Many tombs of the seventeenth and eighteenth centuries exhibit hyperactive effigies, such as Louis–Francois Roubiliac's monument — completed in 1761 — in Westminster Abbey, showing Joseph Nightingale trying to shield his wife from a dart about to be flung by Death. More dramatic yet is the tomb of General William Hargrave, also in Westminster Abbey, by Louis–Francois Roubiliac, in which the deceased is shown breaking free of his cerements, apparently already confident of his salvation.

Effigies, of course, had a life outside the church. Those crafted of straw of other materials were thrashed or burned to vent public fury, as when a guilty party managed to escape from his captors, or, famously, to celebrate the foiling of the Gunpowder Plot. Effigies of Guy Fawkes, a conspirator in a plot to blow up Parliament and King James I on November 5, 1604, are still burned in England on November 5. In the latter half of the twentieth century, effigies representing Uncle Sam have been burned at various times in various countries, providing not only a means of venting emotions, but good film footage as well. It is the capacity of the effigy to substitute for the individual it represents that accounts for its long history of use in a funereal context as well as in the more popular contexts of Guy Fawkes Day, for example, or in the practices of the *vodun* religion.   CLAUDIA SWAN

See also FUNERAL PRACTICES; IDOLS; RELIGION AND THE BODY; SCULPTURE.

Ego In the history of philosophy and pre-Freudian psychology, the word 'ego' (Latin for 'I') has usually meant the 'self': the rational, autonomous subject of CONSCIOUSNESS, which, at the same time, is the object of the individual's self-consciousness. At least since the end of the Renaissance, the notion of the self has been fundamental to human identity. Whereas Man had previously been represented as an entity connected with and dependent upon a divinely ordered cosmos, the meaning of humanity came, by the Enlightenment, to be located increasingly in the interior of individual human beings, characterized by reason and by autonomy from the outer cosmos.

Immanuel Kant emphasized that morality was inseparable from true autonomy: the autonomous human agent *chose* to submit himself to the moral law. This law was not imposed by external authorities but by what Kant called the *noumenal ego*, a part of one's own self that could be shown by philosophical argument to exist beyond doubt but was wholly imperceptible and inaccessible to empirical investigation. Unlike the *phenomenal ego*, which was perceptible to self as well as others, and roughly synonymous with the personality, the noumenal ego was the inviolate and inviolable source of human reason and morality — and, therefore, of human autonomy.

The Kantian concept of the ego contrasted sharply with that of David Hume, who believed, scandalously, that there was nothing called the self — human beings were mere bundles of sensations. In the late nineteenth century, a similar idea was argued with great force by the Austrian physicist Ernst Mach. A thoroughgoing phenomenalist — Mach also rejected the concept of the atom — he argued that human individuality was simply due to different ways in which the Humean bundles of sensations were configured in different individuals. 'The ego', Mach proclaimed in 1886, 'is beyond salvage' (*Das Ich ist unrettbar*). As it happened, the ego was salvaged over the next few decades by one of Mach's own compatriots, Sigmund Freud — but the Freudian ego was a puny caricature of the heroic Enlightenment conception that Mach was attacking.

His early experience with hysterics had shown Freud that the self was not necessarily unitary: one part of the self could remain rational, intelligent, and moral, while another went completely crazy. His study of dreams had convinced him that there were regions of the mind seething with activity but inaccessible to the waking consciousness. Freud's first model of the mind was laid out topographically like a feuding empire (rather like the tottering Habsburg Empire at the turn of the century, of which Freud was a citizen) in which individual regions battled for supremacy with each other. Soon, Freud replaced this scheme with the more sophisticated structural model, using a new vocabulary of different psychic *agencies*, not of different *regions*. The mind, he now felt, was a system but not a closed system. The agency of the mind that was directly open to the external world, Freud called simply the 'I' (*das Ich*) but his English translators turned it into the 'ego'. The Freudian ego represented rationality and common sense, ensured safety and self-preservation, translated thoughts into action, and repressed unacceptable impulses. Consciousness was attached to the ego but not all of the ego was conscious: whatever consciousness it possessed was largely due to its links with the perceptual system, with the body. The ego was intimately related to another agency of the psyche, the *id*, which was fully unconscious, completely irrational, understood only immediate satisfaction, and was the ultimate source of the passions driving human beings. The 'power of the id', Freud asserted,

'expresses the true purpose of the individual organism's life. This consists in the satisfaction of its innate needs.' Instead of being a totally rational being, the individual human was merely 'a psychical id, unknown and unconscious, upon whose surface rests the ego'.

What, however, of morality? It had no necessary link with consciousness, Freud argued — locating it almost casually in a third agency of the mind: the *super-ego*, which developed out of the ego and was an unconscious mental representative of one's parents and parent-surrogates such as teachers. The major reason for its development was the fear of castration: consequently, Freud asserted, the female super-ego never attained the strength and implacability of the male. The super-ego was punitive, of course, and often irrationally so, but it was not merely the conscience. It was also the vehicle of the ego-ideal, the standard by which the self judged itself, the ideal it tried to emulate, and whose demands for ever greater perfection it strove to fulfil.

The Freudian self as a whole, then, was, at best, a consortium of potentially conflicting members. The conscious ego maintained psychic unity by mediating between external reality, the demands of the id, and the strictures of the super-ego. 'We are warned by a proverb against serving two masters at the same time,' Freud wrote. 'The poor ego has things even worse: it serves three severe masters and does what it can to bring their claims and demands into harmony with one another . . . No wonder that the ego so often fails in its task.' In such a messy situation, psychological problems were to be expected, and the task of the psychoanalyst was to strengthen the ego: to make it as independent of the super-ego as possible, to widen its field of perception, and to enlarge it so that it could take over fresh portions of the id. 'Where id was, there ego shall be' was how Freud summed up the therapeutic endeavour of psychoanalysis. The ego, that valiant warrior of the Enlightenment, had been cut down to twentieth-century size: robbed of its sovereignty and unassailable might, it now needed a therapist's help to conquer unreason!

    CHANDAK SENGOOPTA

Further reading

Freud, S. (1961). The Ego and the Id (1923). In *The standard edition of the complete psychological works of Sigmund Freud*, Vol. 19, (ed. J. Strachey et al.). Hogarth Press, London.

Porter, R. (ed.) (1997). *Rewriting the self: histories from the Renaissance to the present*. Routledge, London.

Taylor, C. (1989). *Sources of the self: the making of the modern identity*. Harvard University Press, Cambridge, MA.

See also CONSCIOUSNESS; PERSONALITY.

Ejaculation of SEMEN is the final outcome of a complex series of reflexes induced by sexual arousal and stimulation. The reflexes involve both the sympathetic and the parasympathetic branches of the AUTONOMIC NERVOUS SYSTEM, as well as spinal motor nerves and descending nerves from the BRAIN. Three phases of the ejaculatory response can be defined — ERECTION, *emission*, and *ejaculation* itself.

Erection is caused by changes in blood flow to the PENIS that can be induced by tactile stimulation of the genital region, particularly the glans penis, which has a high density of tactile-pressure receptors. This sensory information is relayed by sensory nerves to the lower SPINAL CORD which, via parasympathetic nerves, causes dilation of arterioles in the penis. As a result blood inflow to the spongy sinuses increases dramatically and they become engorged. Because these erectile regions are surrounded by a strong fibrous coat, the penis becomes enlarged and rigid. Also, as the erectile tissue expands the venous outflow from the penis is compressed, so while inflow of blood increases, through flow does not, and erection results. Simultaneously, parasympathetic nerves stimulate the bulbo-urethral glands to produce a mucoid substance to aid lubrication. Erection can also occur in the absence of any tactile stimulation, when thoughts, visual cues, or emotions stimulate descending nerve pathways from the brain. These, in turn, activate the same nerves as those reflexly stimulated by sensory stimulation of the genital region.

During the second phase of the response (*emission*), contractions of the smooth muscle in the walls of the vasa deferentia, and the ejaculatory duct formed by their junction, push sperm into the upper part of the urethra. At the same time the seminal vesicles and PROSTATE gland contract and release seminal fluid into the urethra. (See PLATE 8)

In the third phase, ejaculation proper, which occurs at ORGASM, the SEMEN (sperm plus seminal fluid) is expelled from the posterior urethra by contractions of the muscles which surround it. During COITUS ejaculation is also associated with involuntary rhythmic thrusting of the pelvis. The role of the sympathetic branch of the autonomic nervous system at this point is to contract the sphincter round the neck of the BLADDER, so that ejaculation cannot backfire in that direction.

A feeling of intense pleasure usually accompanies ejaculation, and the whole event is known as orgasm. After this there is the *resolution phase* in which all the physiological changes which have occurred are reversed and a man becomes refractory to any further sexual stimulation for a while. This period can last from a few minutes to several hours.

Any interference with the relevant spinal reflexes can cause IMPOTENCE and other sexual dysfunction, although libido will be unaffected. The central nervous system plays an important role in regulating the sexual response, not only in normal individuals but also in cases of disordered sexual function. Whilst sexual arousal can be stimulated or enhanced by visual or other inputs of a sexual nature in the absence of tactile genital stimulation, conversely the sexual response may be suppressed by the central nervous system,

either consciously or subconsciously. This can lead to impotence, loss of sexual interest, premature ejaculation, ejaculatory failure, or a loss of the usual generalized accompaniments of orgasm. These are all common defects of this complex reflex response and may have a psychogenic basis in some patients. They are often amenable to behavioural therapy.

SAFFRON WHITEHEAD

See also COITUS; ORGASM; PENIS; SEMEN.

Elbow

Elbow An example of a hinge joint (uniaxial) with movement essentially limited to flexion and extension. The *condyles* at the lower end of the *humerus* in the upper arm articulate with the heads of both the *radius* and the *ulna* in the lower arm. Twisting movements of the lower arm (*pronation* and *supination*) are possible because the top end (the head) of the radius can rotate against the lower end of the humerus. Flexion of the elbow is achieved by action of the BICEPS muscle, which shortens and bulges, a muscle often shown to advantage in the classic pose of the body builder. Extension involves the triceps muscle, and when fully extended the arm should be in a straight line — the elbow angle at 180 degrees. This joint can also hyperextend; this is much more common in females than in males. Another difference in females is that the lower arms tend to be bent slightly more outwards when extended at the elbow (valgus carrying angle), thus clearing the hips, which are broader than in men. The most common problems associated with the elbow are colloquially described as 'tennis elbow' or 'golfer's elbow'. However, these are not really a dysfunction of the elbow joint itself, but arise from over-indulgence in the named activity, or some equivalent muscular

effort. Over-activity, particularly if the sport is not practised regularly, can result in small tears of the fibres in the TENDONS of muscles which are anchored at the lower end of the humerus (at the *epicondyles*), resulting in inflammation in this region (*epicondylitis*). Characteristically there is pain at this site which is aggravated by gripping or twisting movements. Treatment may involve a local injection of anti-inflammatory agents (STEROIDS). WILLIAM R. FERRELL

See also JOINTS; SKELETON.

Electrocardiogram

Electrocardiogram This means of studying the activity of the HEART from electrical signals detectable from the body surface stemmed directly, early in the twentieth century, from the invention of the *string galvanometer* by the Dutch physiologist, Einthoven. Electrocardiography was demonstrated to the Royal Society in London in 1909.

The 'ECG' (or sometimes still 'EKG' in the US, from the German spelling) has become an icon representing the heart's activity. The waveform is the most familiar 'high tech' sign of the electrical behaviour of the heart. In various versions, its characteristic shape (see figure) reporting a healthy rhythm, or the flat line suggesting the patient's demise, is familiar to any viewer of television medical soap operas. A clever variation on the theme forms the distinctive logo for the British Heart Foundation, the largest UK charity dedicated to funding cardiovascular research.

The electrocardiogram (as a paper trace or a TV monitor display) shows the changes in the voltage, detectable during the time course of the heart beat, between pairs of electrodes placed at certain points on the skin. The basis of the ECG is that the heart, like other muscles, is triggered to contract by electrical activity. The heart is a

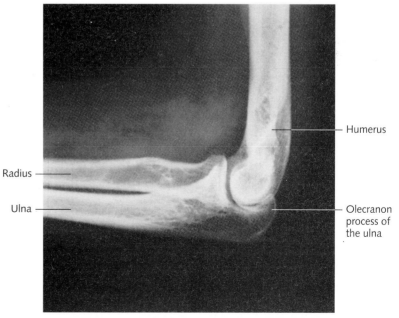

Radius

Ulna

Humerus

Olecranon process of the ulna

X-ray of adult elbow joint. Reproduced, with permission, from *Cunningham's textbook of anatomy*, (12th edn), OUP.

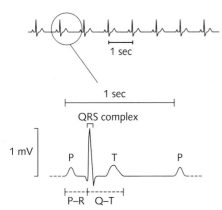

Characteristic ECG pattern of a healthy heart beating at 60/minute.

relatively large piece of tissue, so the flow of electrical current associated with (and immediately preceding) contraction produces detectable voltages (typically a few millivolts) on the surface of the body. Electrode pairs can be placed at various positions on the body to yield information about the status of the heart. The classic '*limb leads*' are attached to one leg and two arms; other pairings are placed at defined positions on the chest itself. Even more detail can be obtained with leads inserted in the *oesophagus* (the gullet) or even from within the heart itself (with the electrode introduced via a vein). Abnormal enlargement (*hypertrophy*) of the heart's various chambers produces characteristic distortions of the 'ideal' ECG form which are readily interpreted by experienced users.

The spread of the electrical wave across the heart varies in speed (see HEART). Simple physics dictates that where a change in potential of a large fraction of the heart occurs in a relatively brief time, the resulting ECG wave is large too. When most of the heart is at a similar potential, no voltage *difference* will appear at the surface. Thus, prominent waves in the ECG indicate the synchronized start (or finish) of activity in significant fractions of the heart.

These potentials amount to one or two *millivolts*. The impulse of electrical activity causing the heart to contract in a co-ordinated manner progresses through the heart in a complex three-dimensional pattern. The appearance of the electrocardiogram, therefore, varies from person to person as heart shape and position can be significantly different even in entirely normal individuals. Any person's pattern further alters with the location of the recording electrodes. Nevertheless, there are significant, consistently observed deflections and intervals in a typical electrocardiogram; the main 'peaks' are labelled as P, QRS, and T (see figure).

The most basic feature of the ECG is that the time from any one such 'peak' to the same one in the next cycle indicates precisely how long the heart cycle is taking. At slow rates, the timing of the waves can be easily correlated to the HEART SOUNDS heard with the stethoscope. But far more precise information can be gleaned once

the relationship of the waves to the phases of the cycle is understood:

The *P-wave* indicates the electrical activity associated with contraction of the cardiac atria, the heart's upper chambers.

The *P–R interval* is the delay between the beginning of activity in the atria and the ventricles (atrio–ventricular conduction time). In adults, normal P–R intervals range between 120 and 200 milliseconds, occasionally being shorter in children and slightly longer in the aged. The P–R interval shortens at high heart rates (e.g. due to exercise or to fever) and increases at lower heart rates (e.g. during sleep).

The *QRS complex* indicates the onset of contraction of the ventricles. The shape of the QRS complex may be modified by a number of physiological factors (e.g. body position and breathing pattern). In normal adults, the duration of the QRS complex varies between 60 and 100 milliseconds; in children it tends to be shorter.

The *Q–T interval* is measured from the beginning of the QRS complex to the end of the T-wave and represents the time between activation of electrical activity in the ventricles and their return to the resting state. Like the P–R interval, the Q–T interval shortens at high heart rates and increases at lower rates.

The *T-wave* indicates when the electrical activity associated with the cells in the cardiac ventricle returns to the resting state after electrical activation. Thus, it signals the start of relaxation of

the ventricle walls. It tends to be longer lasting than QRS because the onset of relaxation across the ventricle is less tightly synchronized than that of contraction.

Some stark deviations from this classical sequence can occur, including the chaotic waves associated with *ventricular fibrillation*. This is the uncoordinated, apparently random electrical activity (and thus contraction) of the ventricles that can readily prove fatal without defibrillation. HEART BLOCK is a condition readily identified by ECG analysis.

There are characteristic changes in the wave pattern of the ECG in *myocardial ischaemia* (inadequate blood supply to the heart), which may be evident at first during exercise in sufferers from *angina*, and which may confirm or exclude an ischaemic episode or *myocardial infarction* in instances of unexplained chest pain.

DAVID J. MILLER
NIALL G. MACFARLANE

See also HEART; HEART ATTACK.

Electroencephalogram (EEG) Recording of electrical activity from the brains of animals was first reported by the British physiologist Caton in 1875. Berger, a German psychiatrist, described the human EEG in 1929, but it was only after a further description of 'the Berger rhythm', by Adrian and Matthews in Cambridge five years later, that it began to be used in research and diagnosis.

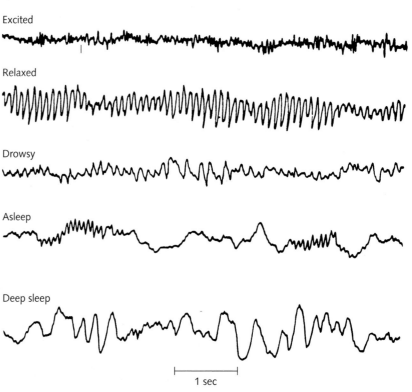

An early EEG. Effect of general excitatory states. Normal electrograms as varied by conditions of generalized excitation, relaxation, drowsiness, light sleep, and deep sleep. (From W. Penfield and T. C. Erickson (1941), *Epilepsy and cerebral localization*, Charles C. Thomas, Baltimore.)

Electroencephalography records, from electrodes placed on the scalp, the weak electrical activity generated by the BRAIN, its voltage ten times smaller than that from the heart displayed by an ELECTROCARDIOGRAM (ECG). This makes the EEG very sensitive to interference from muscle activity in the scalp or from electronic equipment in the vicinity. Moreover, whereas in the heart the origin of the activity is very well understood, the EEG records the collective activity of large populations of neurons in the CEREBRAL CORTEX. For all the sophistication of modern recording equipment and computerized analysis of the records, it has to be accepted that the EEG remains a relatively crude measuring device, although it enables recognition of the different phases of normal SLEEP, and is of diagnostic value in some abnormal conditions.

A number of electrodes (typically about 20) are positioned on the scalp and connected in pairs, yielding 8–16 channels, each recording the potential between two electrodes. Each electrode receives signals from an area of cortex of 2–3 cm diameter. But a third of the cortex is inaccessible, in the depths of the indentations (the *sulci*), on the basal surface, or hidden within the larger folds of the brain. Some 10–15 min of recording results in 20–30 pages of paper that can be bound and read like a book — and often also analyzed by computer.

Information lies in the frequency and amplitude (voltage) of the waves recorded in different channels. At rest, relaxed and with the eyes closed, the frequency of these waves is 8–12 Hz (cycles/sec). This 'alpha' activity is believed to reflect the brain in 'idling' mode, because if the person then either opens the eyes, or does mental arithmetic with the eyes closed, these waves disappear, to be replaced by irregular patterns (so-called *desynchronized activity*). In normal sleep there is characteristic higher voltage activity, in patterns which vary according to the level of sleep.

When there is severe diffuse brain abnormality, such as encephalitis or conditions causing COMA, there will be usually be no alpha activity, whilst in the vegetative state there may be alpha activity that fails to desynchronize on eye opening. Faster frequencies (*beta*, at >13 Hz) or slower (*theta*, at 4–8 Hz) can be normal in infancy and childhood. Even slower 'delta' waves (<4 Hz) can be normal in sleep and in infancy, but in awake adults indicate severe abnormality. When localized they may indicate pathology such as a tumour or abscess in the brain, causing the adjacent cortex to produce abnormal rhythms; however, modern IMAGING TECHNIQUES have replaced EEG as a means of detecting and locating such lesions.

It is in the investigation of EPILEPSY that EEG has proved most useful — both in diagnosing epilepsy as the cause of abnormal behaviours and in localizing the site in the brain from which abnormalities are originating. During an epileptic seizure there are bursts of high voltage activity in the region of the brain affected. The problem is the low probability of a patient having an attack during routine recording. However, the record in a person with epilepsy is often abnormal between attacks, and these abnormalities are more likely to be found if the patient hyperventilates (producing temporary alkalosis in the brain), or is fasting (with temporary mild HYPOGLYCAEMIA). But some patients who never have a clinical seizure may show such abnormalities on EEG, whilst a third of patients who do have seizures have a normal record at times between attacks. To increase the chance of securing a recording during an attack patients may be fitted with electrodes that transmit by radio to a receiver. Such telemetry allows 24-hour recording during normal activities — which may also be monitored on video in order to visualize any seizure that occurs.

When patients with epilepsy are being investigated with a view to possible surgery the location of the seizure-producing lesion may be identified by using electrodes placed to cover areas not available to those placed on the scalp. Electrodes introduced through the cheek to the base of the skull can detect activity from the under surface of the brain, whilst those inserted through a burr hole (a small opening in the skull) on to the surface of deeper parts of the brain, or even into the substance of the brain, bring other areas under surveillance.

A visual, auditory, or somatic stimulus will normally evoke an altered wave form from the appropriate area of the cortex (for example the occipital region for a visual input). It is therefore possible with the EEG to explore the integrity of sensory pathways by means of these *evoked potentials*. This method is also used during operative procedures to help surgeons to identify such sensory pathways by observing the effects of electrical stimulation on the EEG, so as to avoid damaging them.

An occasional use of the EEG is in confirming the diagnosis of BRAIN DEATH, when an *isoelectric* (flat) record may be obtained, but technical difficulties can lead to equivocal results. In some places, but not in the UK, EEG is mandatory after clinical tests have been completed.

BRYAN JENNETT

See also CONVULSIONS; EPILEPSY.

Elephant man The life of Leicester-born Joseph Carey Merrick (1862–90), 'the Elephant Man', has become surrounded by myth, entering popular culture as a symbol of gross deformity and noble spirit. Attention has focused not on his body, but on the man beneath the skin, with his story becoming one of physical and personal metamorphosis. Merrick's life, portrayed in print, on stage, and on film, has been made into a moral tale.

At birth Merrick showed no obvious signs of his later deformities, which began to emerge only after eighteen months. Disfiguring industrial diseases at that time produced a wide range of deformities, and this perhaps made Merrick's adolescent condition more acceptable. Certainly he was not so deformed as to prevent him from attending school until he was twelve. After that he worked for two years rolling cigars. However, the gradual deterioration of his right arm forced him to seek employment peddling goods from his father's haberdashery shop. Here his progressive abnormality worked against him, and Merrick entered Leicester workhouse 'demonstrating his deformities' to escape unemployment and his harsh stepmother. It was Merrick who decided to exhibit himself as a 'freak', turning his disorder to his advantage. The decision brought him to London and to the attention of the surgeon (later Sir) Frederick Treves, at the London Hospital; of the medical community; and of fashionable society.

Treves discovered Merrick in 1884 at a private view opposite the London Hospital. Appalled by the 'most disgusting specimen of humanity', Treves arranged to examine Merrick and presented his case to the London Pathological Society. Continuity was maintained: where Merrick had been exhibited to the public, now he was presented to the medical community by an ambitious Treves. The *British Medical Journal* felt Merrick was 'a man who presented an extraordinary appearance, owing to a series of deformities'. His body was difficult to define (see figure). In his *Reminiscences*, Treves described Merrick as below average height with a limp caused by a childhood hip disease. He recorded an 'enormous and misshapen head' where a huge bony mass 'like a loaf projected from the brow' and 'fungus-looking skin' comparable to 'brown cauliflower'. From the chest and buttocks 'hung a bag of the same repulsive flesh'. Merrick's mouth was so deformed, with a jaw protruding 'like a pink stump', that he was unable to speak clearly. A trunklike growth had been removed while he was in the workhouse. The right arm was large, with the hand shaped liked a paddle and a thumb like a 'radish'. Only his left arm and genitals were unaffected. In his early descriptions of Merrick, Treves was inclined to refer to him as 'repellant', 'loathsome', and 'horrible'. From his appearance, Treves assumed Merrick was an imbecile, but later discovered that he was intelligent and sensitive. Treves did not at that time rescue Merrick, who, with his self-exhibition hounded by the police, was bought by an Austrian who took him to Brussels. But he was too repugnant for continental tastes. Robbed of his savings, Merrick was abandoned to return to London, where he was admitted to the London Hospital in 1886 through Treves' intervention. A charitable appeal was made to pay for Merrick's care, and a room, known by some as the 'Elephant House', was provided in a quiet part of the hospital.

At the London, Merrick became a celebrity, an object of curiosity, visited by fashionable society women and royalty. Treves encouraged these visits to help normalize Merrick and arranged a trip to the theatre and a country holiday. In one sense, Merrick's time at the London can be seen as reflecting Victorian concerns to domesticize the savage. With cure out of the question, efforts were made to make Merrick comfortable. Daily baths removed the foul smell that had previously surrounded him.

In 1890 Merrick was found dead 'lying across the bed', with no signs of a struggle. His head had grown so large that he had to sleep in a 'crouching position' and at the time it was suggested that during an afternoon nap his head had fallen forwards onto his windpipe, suffocating him. Others, including Treves, argued that Merrick's head fell backwards, dislocating his neck when he attempted to sleep lying down: Merrick's urge to conform makes this probable.

Merrick was first described as a case of 'congenital deformity'. In 1884 some speculations were made that he suffered from 'dermatolysis', a pendulous condition of the skin, combined with 'pachydermatocele', or tumours arising from an overgrowth of the skin, but no definite diagnosis was reached. It was not until 1909 that Parkes Weber retrospectively 'diagnosed' *neurofibromatosis*, a genetic disorder where a failure of cellular control results in tumours of fibrous and nervous tissue. The disorder had been identified by von Recklinghausen in 1882, but in 1884 this was overlooked. Usually, however, neurofibromatosis produces relatively few visible signs. The diagnosis made Merrick extraordinary in degree but not in kind. Weber's view became widely accepted until 1986, when Tibbles and Cohen offered a different diagnosis. They suggested that Merrick exhibited signs of the 'Proteus syndrome', a term derived from Greek mythology and first used in 1983 to identify a disorder with varying and shifting manifestations. Tibbles and Cohen supported their diagnosis by explaining that there was no family history of neurofibromatosis, and argued that when Merrick was examined in 1885 there were no '*café au lait* spots' — the patches of unusual skin pigmentation that are the clearest indication of neurofibromatosis, present in 99% of cases. For them it was evident that Merrick's condition was more grotesque than that associated with neurofibromatosis, while he had many features of Proteus syndrome; these include thickened skin and subcutaneous tissue; hypertrophy of long bones; and overgrowth of the skull. To press their diagnosis, a second case was described who was Merrick's double. The rediagnosis led to a remythologizing of Merrick, although those suffering from neurofibromatosis continued to be confronted with the stigma of the Elephant Man's disease.

Merrick was the Victorian ideal of a deserving cause: a man bowed down by a condition no fault of his own, willing to work and repay those kind to him with handmade gifts. He also challenged basic nineteenth-century assumptions about humanity and the divisions between man and animal. In the twentieth century his deformity came to symbolise something different, showing that it is mind that matters more than appearance.   K. WADDINGTON

Embolism When fragments, usually of blood clot, are let loose in the bloodstream, they lodge in and obstruct the first vessels they encounter which are too narrow for them to pass. Such a fragment is known as an *embolus* (plural *emboli*) and the event as embolism. Pieces may break off from a clot (*thrombus*) which has formed, usually during prolonged immobility, in the deep veins of the legs or pelvis (*deep vein thrombosis — DVT*). The clots travel to the HEART through progressively larger veins, thence from the right side of the heart to the LUNGS; there they obstruct branches of the pulmonary artery, where the severity of their effects depends on their size and number. Large *pulmonary emboli* can be fatal; very small ones lodge in microscopic vessels causing some impairment of oxygen intake. Thrombi which form on damaged lining of the left heart valves or of major arteries can release fragments which reach the BRAIN (*cerebral embolism*) causing a type of STROKE. There can also be *fat embolism*, when particles enter

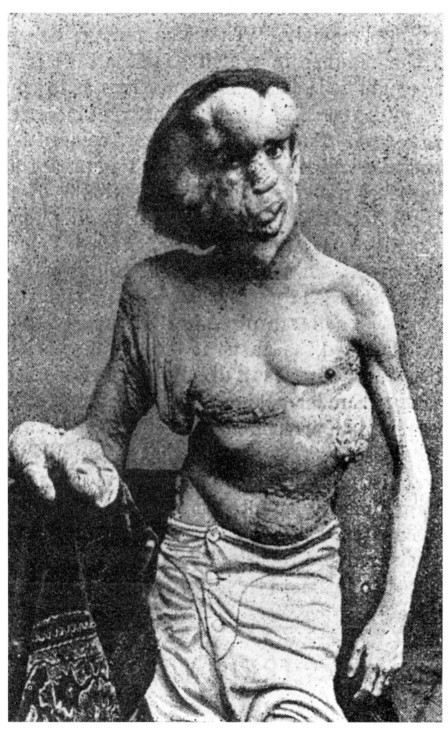

Joseph Carey Merrick, the 'Elephant man' in 1889. Wellcome Institute Library, London.

veins from the marrow of fractured bones, or *air embolism* if air is injected or sucked into an open vein.   SHEILA JENNETT

Embryo An organism in its early stages of development. The developing human is known as an embryo for about its first two months in the womb. Conventions differ in defining when the name first applies — whether it is immediately after FERTILIZATION or after IMPLANTATION of the fertilized ovum in the UTERUS a week or so later.   S.J.

See ANTENTAL DEVELOPMENT.

Emotion has usually, in the European–American tradition, been seen as the opposite of reason; the definitions provided in the *Oxford English Dictionary* emphasize emotion as agitation, perturbation, and 'feeling' or 'affection' — as distinguished from cognitive or volitional states of consciousness. Philosophically this split became entrenched through the thought of Rene Descartes, with his famous 'I think, therefore I am'. Emotion has thus come to be associated with the body the way reason has been associated with the mind.

The European–American tradition often values reason over emotion, except in specifically defined events such as funerals, weddings, or births. Some cultures, notably that of Japan, are even more reserved, wanting to avoid negative emotional expression altogether. Other cultures, especially those of South and Latin America, and some south-east Asian cultures, see emotional expression as essential to living life, and value a wide range of emotional experience.

Emotion's connection to the body is frequently reinforced through our metaphoric description of emotion; it is frequently described as a visceral event. Disappointment means a sinking heart; nervousness, butterflies in the stomach; depression, weight in the chest area; joy, lightness and freedom of movement; excitement, racing heart and blood and tingling nerves. Emotions are conveyed to others through bodily configurations, including FACIAL EXPRESSIONS, POSTURE, muscle tension, voice tone, and GESTURES.

While emotions and their physical expression are culturally specific (especially gestures), studies have suggested that facial expressions are remarkably similar across cultures, with the biggest differences or confusions occurring for anger or surprise. We learn to identify and reproduce facial expressions as infants, where we study the expressions on adult faces and learn to associate them with emotions. Western cultures have long attributed special emotional intelligence and capability to women, who have traditionally borne the largest burden of emotional work in the culture.

Emotion frequently plays an important role in religious ritual. Many Christian sects revere emotional ecstasy as a direct encounter with the Holy Spirit and an expression of our oneness with God. Buddhism, on the other hand, rejects both self-denial and self-indulgence in a quest to extinguish the craving for physical or material pleasures. Religious emotion is often balanced through paired rituals; Catholic cultures often have a festival period preceding the asceticism of Lent.   JULIE VEDDER

Emotion, scientific aspects Emotions are subjective states produced by rewards and punishments. Rewards are things for which an animal (including humans) will work, and punishments (technically called 'punishers') are stimuli that an animal will work to escape from or avoid. Rewards and punishers are called 'reinforcers' because they strengthen the probability of certain sorts of behaviour. Some emotion-producing stimuli (such as the taste of food to a hungry animal, or PAIN) are unlearned or 'primary' reinforcers. Other, initially neutral stimuli produce emotions because they have been associated with such primary reinforcers, thereby becoming 'secondary' reinforcers. For example, you may experience the emotional state of fear if you hear the voice (the conditioned stimulus) of someone who has previously caused you pain (a primary reinforcer).

The wide variety of different emotions that we feel depend not only on whether the stimulus is rewarding or punishing, and how strong it is, but also on present and past associations surrounding the experience. Even the type of response that is possible can alter the emotional state. Denial of an expected reward, which might normally produce an outburst of anger, will trigger only silent sadness or grief, if the situation forbids an active response.

The functions of emotion

Emotions seem irrational and maladaptive, occupying the body and the mind with apparently irrelevant thoughts and actions. However, they can result in a variety of adaptive functions:

1. Emotions can trigger useful responses of the AUTONOMIC NERVOUS SYSTEM (e.g. a change in heart rate) and the release of hormones, such as ADRENALINE, which prepare the body for action.

2. Emotions act as a simple and flexible 'interface' between sensory inputs and motor outputs. The kinds of stimuli that act as primary (unlearned) rewards and punishers may somehow be directly specified in our brains by genetic information, and these stimuli define 'goals' for actions. For example, genes may specify that strong stimulation of the skin or deep tissues produces a state of pain, which animals (including humans) are built to avoid or escape. The state produced by the painful stimulus is an emotional state, which has the adaptive function of identifying and maintaining the goal for an action. This is an efficient design, for the genes involved need only specify the goals, and not the actions themselves, so that the actions can be selected flexibly to meet the goals.

3. Emotion is motivating. For example, fear provides the motivation for actions performed to avoid painful stimuli.

4. Emotions may aid communication, as emphasized by Charles Darwin. For example, monkeys may communicate their emotional state to others by making an open-mouth threat, thus indicating the extent to which they are willing to compete for resources, and this may influence the behaviour of other animals.

5. Emotions enhance social bonding, for instance between parents and their young.

6. The state of mood may help in the continuous interpretation of the reinforcing value of events in the environment.

7. Emotion may facilitate the storage of memories, particularly so-called 'episodic' memories of particular events in life. Vivid memory of the circumstances surrounding a powerful reward or punishment may help to guide behaviour in the future.

8. Emotion may also help to trigger the recall of memories.

9. By enduring for minutes or longer after a reinforcing stimulus has occurred, emotion may help to produce persistent and continuing motivation and direction of behaviour, to help achieve a long-term goal.

Brain mechanisms of emotion

Animals are built with nervous systems that enable them to evaluate which environmental stimuli, whether learned or not, are rewarding and punishing, i.e. produce emotions that will be worked for or avoided. Sensory stimuli are normally processed in the brain to produce a 'neutral' representation of the object or event, before its emotional significance is decoded. For example, in monkeys, signals from the taste buds of the tongue are relayed to a region of the CEREBRAL CORTEX, the 'primary taste cortex', in which nerve cells respond selectively to different tastes, regardless of their reward values to the animal. Then, signals are passed to the 'secondary taste cortex', in a region of the frontal lobe called the *orbitofrontal cortex* where neurons respond to the taste stimulus only if the monkey is hungry. Similarly, visual stimuli, which frequently carry information about potential reward or punishment in the environment, are initially processed in the visual parts of cerebral cortex, leading to the lower part of the temporal lobe, where objects are represented, independent of their emotional significance. Then, in structures such as the orbitofrontal cortex and the *amygdala* (part of the LIMBIC SYSTEM), which receive fibres from the inferior temporal visual cortex, associations are learned between the objects and the primary reinforcers associated with them.

Emotional states are thus represented in the orbitofrontal cortex and amygdala. Consistent with this, electrical stimulation of the orbitofrontal cortex or amygdala is rewarding (even in humans it produces a sensation of pleasure), while damage to these structures affects emotional behaviour, leading to inappropriate reactions to emotive stimuli.

The behavioural selection system must deal with many competing rewards, goals, and priorities. This selection process must be capable of responding to many different types of reward, which are decoded in different brain systems that have evolved at different times, even including the use in humans of LANGUAGE to enable long-term plans to be made. These many different brain systems, some involving implicit assessment of rewards, and others explicit, verbal, conscious evaluation and planned long-term goals, must all enter into the mechanism for the selection of behaviour. Although poorly understood, the issue of emotional feelings is part of the much larger problem of CONSCIOUSNESS.   E. T. ROLLS

Further reading

Darwin, C. (1872). *The expression of the emotions in man and animals*, (3rd edn). University of Chicago Press.

Oatley, K. and Jenkins, J.M. (1996). *Understanding emotions*. Blackwell, Oxford.

Rolls, E. T. (1999). *The brain and emotion*. Oxford University Press.

See also CEREBRAL CORTEX; CONDITIONING; CONSCIOUSNESS; LIMBIC SYSTEM; PAIN; PLEASURE; TASTE; VISION.

Endocrine

Endocrine Internal or hormonal secretion. Endocrine GLANDS are discrete organs (e.g. pituitary, thyroid, adrenal) which discharge HORMONES into the circulating blood; they are sometimes known as 'ductless glands', in contrast to EXOCRINE glands, which pass their secretions through ducts to an external or internal body surface. There are also cells with endocrine function scattered among other types of tissue (e.g. G-cells, secreting GASTRIN, in the stomach lining) or grouped within an organ which has other functions as well (e.g. insulin-secreting 'islets' in the pancreas; sex hormone-secreting cells in the gonads).   S.J.

See HORMONES; PLATE 7.

Endorphins

Endorphins During the 1960s and early 1970s, it became apparent that opioid drugs such as morphine and heroin produced their profound actions in the body by interacting with specific receptors on the outer membrane of nerve cells. This raised the intriguing question of why the body goes to the trouble of synthesizing such receptor proteins. Surely it was not just on the off chance that a drug such as morphine might be administered. In 1975 the group in Aberdeen, Scotland led by Hans Kosterlitz and John Hughes, isolated from the pig brain two related molecules, the *enkephalins*, which bind to and activate opioid receptors. These enkephalins are short peptides, each comprising five amino acids. Although at first glance the enkephalins did not look similar in chemical composition to morphine, they proved to have a crucial component in common. We now know that the brain contains as many as thirteen such *endogenous*

(internally generated) opioid peptides, which have come to be referred to collectively as 'endorphins'.

There are three classically defined opioid receptor types, named the μ, δ, and κ receptors, and each of the endorphins shows a different spectrum of activation (*agonist* action) at these different receptors. The endorphins function as inhibitory NEUROTRANSMITTERS and neurohormones: they are released from nerve cells to act on other cells that bear opioid receptors and thus dampen the activity of those cells.

To probe the physiological functions of the endogenous opioid systems, either antagonist drugs can be administered or transgenic mice lacking one or more of the receptors can be developed. From such studies it is evident that the endorphins play little part in our normal routine daily functions. If, in ordinary circumstances, one were to be given an opioid antagonist such as naloxone, little change would be observed. It is when the body is stressed that the endorphins are important. Then they are released to activate their receptors and help to protect the body. Thus endorphins interacting with the μ and δ receptors have been implicated in the inability of some accident victims to sense the severe PAIN that their injuries should be causing and also in the 'high' that is experienced following EXERCISE. Endogenous opioids may also be responsible for part of the ANALGESIA experienced during ACUPUNCTURE therapy.

Recently a new, endogenous neuropeptide system, very closely associated with the endogenous opioid system, has been discovered. Unfortunately, at present the terminology used to label the receptor and its endogenous peptide agonist is still quite clumsy. The receptor is referred to as the *ORL1 receptor*, and the endogenous peptide that is an agonist at the receptor is called either *nociceptin* or *orphanin FQ*. The term 'nociceptin' derives from the initial belief that this peptide acts in the opposite direction to the endorphins in that, rather than being pain relieving, it actually enhances pain (cf. noxious, from the Latin *noceo*, to injure). It is becoming apparent that this is an oversimplification and that this peptide in some circumstances inhibits the action of morphine and the endorphins but in other circumstances can also itself suppress pain.

What is very exciting is that this new system appears to be involved in other important brain functions apart from the sensation of pain. The discovery that it may be involved in MEMORY, anxiety, and appetite control make it an exciting new area for drug development. Several major pharmaceutical companies are currently developing non-peptide molecules (more stable and brain-penetrating than the peptides) that will act as agonists and antagonists at the ORL1 receptor, to advance our knowledge of the physiological and pathophysiological functions of this receptor. Hopefully this will result in the discovery of novel therapeutic agents.   G. HENDERSON

See also ANALGESIA; OPIATES AND OPIOID DRUGS; MEMBRANE RECEPTORS; PEPTIDES.

Endoscopy

Endoscopy is the process whereby an optical instrument is introduced into one or other of the body tubes or cavities so that the organs of the body may be directly inspected. The instruments of endoscopy are most usually inserted through existing orifices, such as the mouth and rectum, but in certain cases an incision may be made so that otherwise inaccessible body cavities may be examined. The word is derived from the Greek *endon* 'within' and *scopeo* 'examine'.

The earliest endoscopic examinations, introduced in the mid nineteenth century, were of the throat and LARYNX. Using mirrors placed carefully at the back of the throat it became possible to examine the vocal cords directly. The key technological advance was the ability to develop a light source which could be directed at the organ or tissues to be examined. *Laryngoscopy* became the technique which encouraged the development of ear, nose, and throat surgery.

Gradually, other endoscopic techniques were introduced. Examination of the rectum and colon were made possible by the development of *colonoscopes*, but in the early days the rigidity of the instruments available limited examination to the lower colon and rectum. Similarly, at the upper end of the alimentary tract, rigid instruments were used for the examination of the oesophagus (*oesophagoscopy*) and for the stomach, the earliest *gastroscopes* were introduced in Germany during the 1930s. During the next two decades, *bronchoscopy* (introducing an instrument into the bronchial tree via the locally anaesthetized throat, larynx, and trachea) became a significant technique because of the increasing incidence of cancer of the LUNG, for which this was for some time the most important tool in diagnosis. At the same time, urologists were using comparable instruments to examine the BLADDER, a technique of great importance in the diagnosis of cancer or of prostatic disease. Since there was no direct access to the thoracic or abdominal cavities, instruments were inserted through incisions made in the chest wall or abdomen, enabling operators to examine the lungs directly and to carry our surgical procedures (*thoracoscopy*), or to examine the liver and other abdominal organs (*peritoneoscopy*: looking within the peritoneal cavity). Peritoneoscopy also became an important technique which enabled the gynaecologist to examine the pelvic organs of women. By the 1950s there were therefore a wide range of endoscopic techniques available which greatly improved the methods of diagnosis of a variety of illnesses. The rigidity of the instruments, however, limited their use for the doctor and were in many instances particularly unpleasant for the patient, the passage of a rigid or semi-rigid gastroscope requiring the skills of a sword-swallower. Nevertheless, a whole generation of gastroenterologists became proficient in the technique, which was widely used for the diagnosis of peptic ulcer or cancer of the stomach.

A revolution in endoscopic techniques, however, followed the discovery of fibre optic instruments, since their flexibility permitted a far wider application than hitherto. Such techniques were to be of particular value in gastroenterology. It was at a social meeting in London that a physician, Hugh Gainsborough, met the physicist Harold Hopkins. He was pretty well appalled at the use of the rigid instruments in use for gastroscopy at that time and wondered whether Hopkins, already the discoverer of the zoom lens, could make an instrument that was flexible and therefore much more tolerable for the patient. Hopkins, then working at Imperial College in London, recruited a young research student (N. S. Kapany), and together they were able to develop a flexible fibreoptic bundle of glass fibres through which it was possible to examine an object. The significance of their invention was at once apparent to a distinguished British gastroenterologist, Sir Francis Avery Jones, who encouraged a young South African research worker, Dr Basil Hirschowitz, to try to explore the technique for clinical studies. It was not, however, possible to obtain the help of British industrial firms in this venture, and Hirschowitz later went to work in the US. There, he successfully pioneered the use of a fibreoptic bundle which could be introduced with relative ease into the stomach and, for the first time, beyond that into the duodenum, enabling duodenal ulcers to be directly examined. His work was at once followed up by Japanese workers in association with companies such as Olympus. It was they who introduced the new range of gastrointestinal endoscopes that have enabled clinicians directly to examine virtually the entire alimentary tract, as well as making it possible to visualize, with associated radiological techniques, organs such as the PANCREAS, which had until then been examined only by a major operation involving the opening of the alimentary tract. In addition, skilled operators were able to remove gallstones from the bile ducts. Flexible colonoscopy in particular brought the entire colon within view, as well as making it feasible to remove lesions such as polyps, considered to be premalignant, through the endoscope.

The use of fibreoptic endoscopy has been extended to other organs since its introduction, initially for the alimentary tract, so that it is now possible, for example, to introduce such instruments into the JOINTS or major BLOOD VESSELS to carry out surgical procedures.

There is little doubt that, in the history of endoscopy, the invention of the fibreoptic bundle by Hopkins and Kapany was a technological achievement that has transformed the practice of medicine in the modern era. Endoscopic 'keyhole' surgery continues to advance.

CHRISTOPHER BOOTH

Further reading

Hirschowitz, B. I. (1961). Endoscopic examination of the stomach and duodenal cap with a fiberscope. *Lancet*, i. 1074–8.

Hopkins, H. H. and Kapany, N. S. (1956). A flexible fibrescope using static scanning. *Nature*, 173, 39–41.

See also ALIMENTARY SYSTEM; SURGERY.

Enema The introduction of fluid into the rectum. Warm saline or oil may be used for the purpose of clearing the faeces when there is serious constipation. Also popular, from time to time, among those who believe that washing out the bowel is a healthy thing to do, even in the absence of constipation. By derivation from the Greek, the word means 'sending in', rather than washing out, so is appropriately applied also to the administration of drugs by this route, and to the diagnostic use of barium sulphate to visualize the colon and rectum by X-RAY.   S.J.

See COLONIC IRRIGATION; CONSTIPATION.

Energy balance It is important for the human body to regulate the total amount of energy which it receives in the FOOD eaten so that this will balance the total amount of energy which is expended. The sources of energy available to the body come from solid food plus fluids (such as milk, juices, or alcohol). There are several ways in which the body expends energy: most importantly: (i) as the basal metabolic rate (BMR); (ii) in the processes of digestion and absorption of foodstuffs; and (iii) in physical activity.

(i) The BMR is the total amount of energy expended when the body is apparently at rest: that is, it refers to the work of breathing, contraction of the heart, circulation of the blood, kidney function, and so on, including the metabolism of all the body's living cells. These are all essential functions and closely represent the minimal total metabolism of the body, though it may be further reduced during sleep. The BMR for an adult woman of average body size would be about 1400 kcal/day and for an average man about 1700 kcal/day. These amounts account for roughly 60–70% of the total daily energy expenditure.

There is considerable variability in BMR among individuals who are superficially similar, and since BMR accounts for a large portion of total energy metabolism, the extent of this variation can have important implications. For instance, two people who might appear to be physically similar in BODY WEIGHT and in body composition (with respect to the relative proportions of fat and lean) might differ in BMR by 300–400 kcal/day, meaning that one of them could eat food with an energy content of 300–400 kcal/day more than the other with the same end result for energy balance. In our present day Western lifestyle, this would impose a penalty on the biologically more efficient individual, whose BMR is comparatively low and who will therefore be somewhat unfairly constrained to a life of partial self-denial if OBESITY is to be avoided. The low BMR means that the total energy requirement of such a person will also be relatively low, compared with others with a similar pattern of physical activity, and will therefore be satisfied by a smaller total food intake — which may not be to that person's particular liking. The compensation for these people is a somewhat inadequate one in a privileged

society; faced with a famine situation, they could expect to survive better and longer than those with average BMR.

(ii) After a meal, the processes of *digestion and absorption* are initiated and continue for some hours. This involves an expenditure of some energy, equivalent to roughly 10% of the total calorie content of energy of the food and drink taken. The more food you eat, the more energy is used up in processing it.

(iii) *Physical activity* obviously affects energy expenditure. Its influence on energy balance can go in either direction. With increased physical activity the extent of the greater energy expenditure will obviously depend on the intensity and duration of the exercise. If the energy expended is sufficiently large, this leads to a state of negative energy balance and part of the energy which would normally be supplied by the food will be obtained from the breakdown of energy stores (mostly from FAT). The consequence is a reduction of body weight, and increased physical activity is indeed often prescribed as a treatment for obesity — albeit not always with marked success.

On the other hand, if physical activity is reduced, the requirement for energy is also diminished, and less food needs to be eaten — which often causes dissatisfaction. Because the situation is basically disheartening, the end result is often a gradual increase in fatness and body weight.

So far, this seems straightforward, but the effect of physical activity on energy balance is a source of some confusion. For example, if we know that Joe Bloggs regularly goes jogging for half an hour three times a week, we look on him as an active person expending much more daily energy than the average non-active person. However, the actual amount of extra energy used up at this level of exercise would amount to perhaps 200–300 kcal in the half hour; 600–900 kcal over the week or an average of about 90–130 kcal/day Out of a total daily energy expenditure of about 2700 kcals this is a relatively small quantity (equivalent, say, to the energy content of a pint of beer, or a small packet of hula hoops). It could influence energy balance only on a long-term basis. Other forms of activity which may be of considerable severity, but of short duration, may have a similar and surprisingly small effect.

One of the difficulties associated with maintaining energy balance in the kind of lifestyle of most people in our industrialized society is that obligatory physical activity, necessitated by the occupation, has become progressively diminished over the past few decades. Indeed, a great deal of time and ingenuity has gone into removing or minimizing any physical effort which would previously have been an essential part of the working day. The amount of physical activity indulged in by most people is therefore dependent on a voluntary decision, which, unhappily for a majority of people, requires a considerable mental effort.

Obviously, there are still a variety of jobs which involve whole body movement — working as a waiter or waitress, or in a shop, nursing, some types of construction work (as a joiner, bricklayer), and so on. The changing pattern of work over the years is interestingly illustrated by comparing present-day values with the rates of energy expenditure for various occupations given in a table in a book entitled '*Energy, work and leisure*', published in 1967. People with jobs which at that time were regarded as requiring appreciable expenditure of energy — such as colliery clerks, factory workers, steel workers, farmers, coal miners — have no present-day equivalents because of the altered patterns of work: housework, which used to involve quite strenuous tasks, is reduced to minimal levels because of the development of household appliances.

All of these tendencies contribute to a situation where total energy expenditure is reduced and where therefore it becomes increasingly difficult to limit our intake of food to avoid the development of a positive energy balance, giving rise to overweight and, eventually, obesity.

Energy balance and age

Children At varying stages of the life cycle, physiological changes occur which may affect energy balance. In infancy and up to early adulthood, growth is a factor which would commonly be believed to have some influence. Mothers particularly would account for the 'healthy appetite' of their offspring as resulting from growth: 'He's a growing boy', they might say. Yet the actual amount of energy needed for normal growth is comparatively small. A 2-year-old child would normally expend daily a total of about 1200 kcal, of which only 30 kcal or so would satisfy the growth requirement. At the age of five, the total expenditure might be 1500 kcal/day with only 35 kcal for growth. Even at adolescence, when growth is occurring at its maximum rate, this is satisfied by no more than 50 kcal/day. The energy requirement for growth *per se* is therefore of little consequence for energy balance.

Of much greater import is the amount of energy that is required by the normal activity of children now, compared with previous years. There is considerable indirect evidence which seems to show, particularly in adolescents, a progressive reduction in energy expenditure: 13–15-year-olds expend several hundred kcal/day less than 13–15-year-olds did 50 years ago. Perhaps this diminution in total daily activity is not surprising when one considers the alteration in lifestyle during this period, with the considerable amount of time spent nowadays watching TV and using public and private transport instead of walking.

The elderly At the other end of the age range, from about 50 onwards, additional factors may affect energy balance. One of these is an apparent progressive reduction in BMR resulting from a diminishing quantity of active body tissue. However, there is some doubt about whether this lowering of overall energy metabolism is a normal AGEING process, because of decreased metabolism of most of the body tissues, or whether it is dependent on an alteration in body composition due to relative physical inactivity. Where only comparatively small changes have taken place, as in the case of elderly individuals who have remained physically active throughout their whole life span and have retained good muscular and cardiovascular development, BMR does not change appreciably until advanced age — perhaps up to 70. A physically active existence is of great importance for the elderly. However, whether or not there is much diminution in the total energy expended by elderly people is something which can obviously be affected by health and mobility. Gross arthritic changes will inhibit activity to an extent where total energy expenditure becomes very low and even a moderate diet may produce a positive energy balance and the possible development of obesity. It may seem incongruous that obesity is a potential hazard in a situation where food intake is low and appetite is poor. It is nevertheless a real hazard and there may also be an inadequate intake of several nutrients, such as PROTEIN and some of the MINERALS and VITAMINS. Increasing physical activity has a two-fold benefit: the greater expenditure of energy necessitates a larger intake of food, making nutritional deficiencies less likely, and the improved MUSCLE TONE enhances the feeling of well-being and the capabilities of the elderly person.

The energy involved in gaining and losing weight

If there is a positive energy balance, with intake greater than expenditure, there will be a gain in body weight. Conversely, when energy expenditure is in excess of energy intake, body weight will become less. It is interesting to examine the actual amounts of energy represented by these weight changes. The weight which is added to or lost from the body does not consist only of fat itself but is mostly adipose tissue which is a complex mixture of fat (lipid), connective tissue, and fluid. One kilogram of lipid has an energy equivalent of about 9000 kcal. The energy content of the connective tissue and fluid is comparatively low, but these form 10–30% of the total mass of adipose tissue, which therefore has a lower energy equivalent than pure lipid: about 7000 kcal/kg. When the body is losing weight, each kilogram of adipose tissue which is being consumed has therefore provided 7000 kcal of energy. In the opposite circumstance, when the body is gaining weight, each kilogram of added adipose tissue increases the body energy stores by about 7000 kcal. However, the positive energy balance needed to effect this change is more than 7000 kcal/kg, because depositing adipose tissue is a chemical process which is metabolically rather inefficient, and adding an extra kilogram of adipose tissue to the body requires something like 10 000 extra kcal.

There are some interesting extrapolations which can be made from these data. Some slimming regimes advertise a loss of 10 lb (a little more than 4 kg) during a week of their therapy. Four kilograms of lost weight represents the equivalent of 28 000 kcal. If this amount of energy is lost during 7 days, this means a negative balance of 4000 kcal/day. Of course, any food which is eaten during this period will negate part of the energy deficit so that the negative balance of 4000 kcal/day will only be applicable if there is absolute starvation. An intake of, say, 1500 kcal/day will require an energy deficit of 5500 kcal/day. To increase the normal energy expenditure by this amount is virtually impossible for almost everyone (equivalent to continuous hill-climbing, say, at about 550 kcal/hour for 10 hours/day) and, in any case, could be continued for only extremely brief periods. A weight loss of 10 lb per week is therefore a gross distortion of what would actually happen. A more realistic possibility capable of being continued for many weeks would be to reduce energy intake by about 1000 kcal/day, thus producing an energy deficit of 7000 kcal per week, which is the energy equivalent of 1 kg of adipose tissue.

Extended effects of exercise on energy metabolism

It has been suggested that the increase in energy expenditure caused by physical activity continues for some time after the activity has stopped. This has not been convincingly demonstrated except in the case of severe and prolonged exercise which may have a limited effect over some hours.

Energy balance and pregnancy

Theoretically, PREGNANCY would normally be expected to increase energy requirements. There is no doubt the development of the FETUS, the PLACENTA, the increase in BREAST and uterine tissue as well as in energy reserves, all need extra supplies of energy, and indeed it is possible to calculate with a fair degree of precision what the actual amounts should be. For a healthy mother leading the sort of lifestyle common in an industrialized country, the amount would be about 80 000 kcal. One would therefore expect an increase in energy intake of about this amount in order to maintain energy balance. Far from it! In many instances there is no increase whatever over the pre-pregnant level. There are no indications of any improved metabolic efficiencies: BMR remains at pre-pregnant levels and muscular efficiency stays the same. Although it is difficult to measure, it appears most likely that physical activity is subtly reduced, with an energy saving equivalent to the extra energy needs.

J. V. G. A. DURNIN

Further reading

Cottrell, R. (ed.) (1995). *Weight control: the current perspective*. Chapman and Hall, London.

Garrow, J. S. (1978). *Energy balance and obesity in man*, (2nd edn). Elsevier, Holland.

See also DIETING; EXERCISE; METABOLISM; OBESITY.

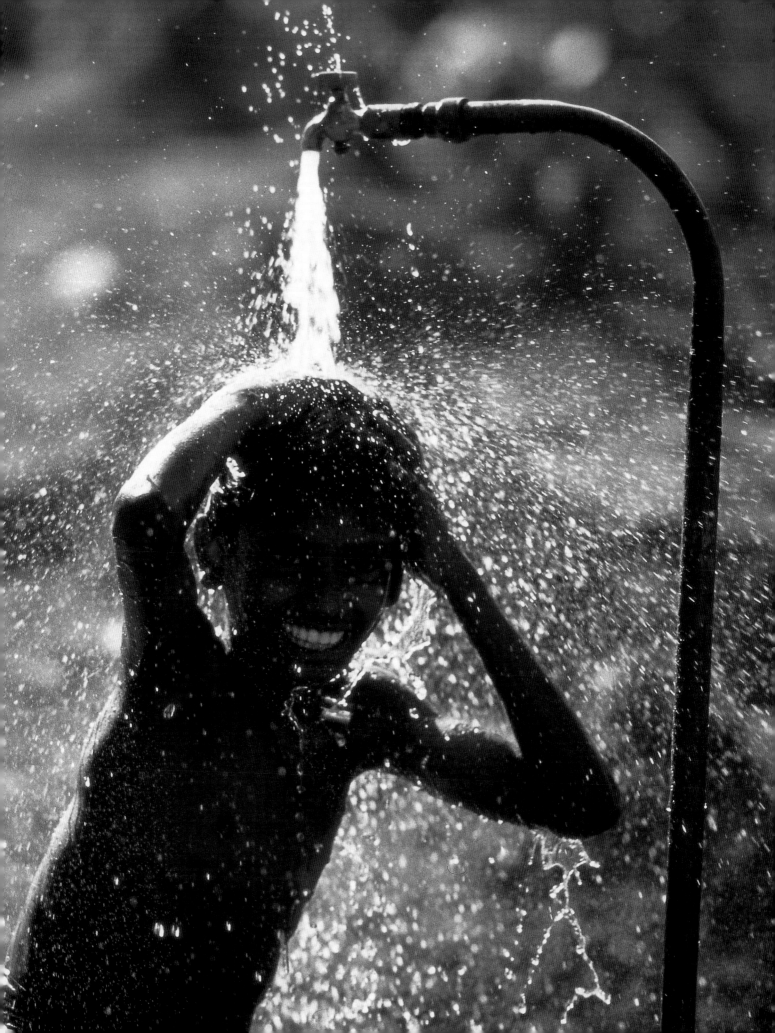

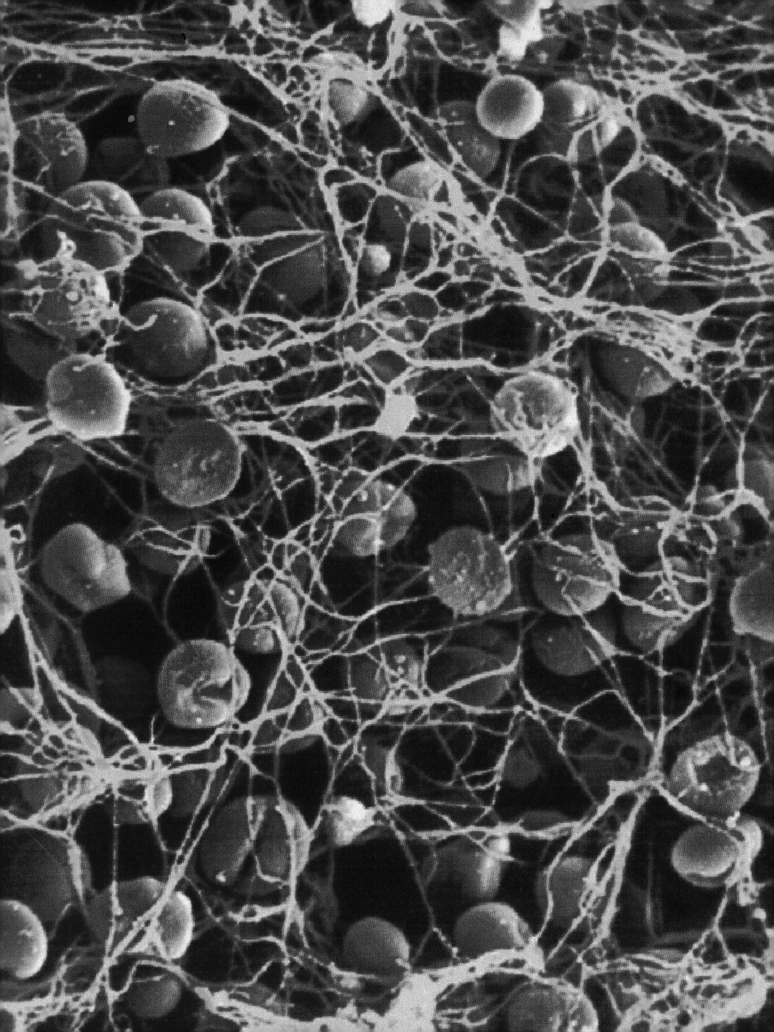

Environmental toxicology Most toxic agents in the environment are present at very low levels. In exceptional cases, however, the levels of environmental pollutants become so high that the effects on health are readily apparent, and severe enough to precipitate remedial action. The persistent London fog of 1952 led to so many cases of death due to respiratory problems that within a few years an Act of Parliament was passed which laid down limits on urban air pollution. Most large conurbations around the world have experienced episodes of dramatic increases in pollution that have led to legally enforced changes in lifestyle, such as the introduction of restrictions in the use of private cars in Athens on days when air pollution rises above a certain level.

Contamination of the atmosphere by the products of combustion has been a problem ever since the beneficial effects of fire were discovered. The blackened roofs of caves known to have been inhabited in prehistoric times are a silent reminder that environmental pollution is by no means a modern phenomenon. Any combustion in the atmosphere inevitably leads to the production of oxides of nitrogen (nitrogen makes up 80% of the atmosphere) and oxides of sulphur and carbon (by combustion of organic matter). The nitrogen oxides are potent pulmonary irritants and concentrations as low as 0.5 parts per million can lead to respiratory problems. Incomplete combustion of complex organic molecules leads to the formation of *polyaromatic hydrocarbons* (PAHs), which are known to be potent carcinogens. The interaction between nitrogen oxides and PAHs leads to formation of *nitrated PAHs*, which are in turn even more potent carcinogens. However, ascribing increased risk of certain chronic diseases, such as lung cancer, to atmospheric pollution in general, or to individual components in particular, has proved rather difficult. For example, levels of many atmospheric pollutants are so low that active or passive exposure to cigarette smoke is the major contributor to exposure. Indoor air pollution is a particular case where exposures can be high simply because of the confined space and slow rates of exchange of air with the outside. Most combustion processes also lead to the production of particulate matter of such small dimensions (less than 10 microns in diameter) that they penetrate deeply into the lungs, where they lodge in the bronchioles or in the alveoli and cause local inflammation. Automobile emissions share many of these properties of all combustion processes, but can also contain particular toxic agents such as lead, benzene, and 1,3-butadiene.

Water is, in principle, the easiest of the environmental matrices to obtain in a pure state. Even the most contaminated water supply is likely to be greater than 99% H_2O. However, our requirement for drinkable water of 1–2 litres per day lays quite stringent limits on the levels of contaminants which are compatible with a healthy lifestyle. The provision of clean water supplies has been, and continues to be for many parts of the world, one of the greatest contributions to improved public health. Contamination of water by industrial processes can contribute to episodes of human POISONING either directly or indirectly, for example through the food chain. Perhaps one of the most dramatic examples of the latter in recent times was an incident of mercury poisoning caused by consumption of contaminated fish by families in a fishing community in Minimata, Japan. A proper balance has to be found between various risks from various toxic agents in the environment. For example, chlorination of public water supplies has been found to lead to the production of low levels of organochlorine compounds via the reaction of chlorine with natural humic acids; as with many organochlorine compounds there have been concerns about possible toxicity from these substances. However, the hazards of not chlorinating water supplies were highlighted most recently by epidemics of cholera in Peru, when flooding led to contamination of water supplies and public health officials were hesitant about the use of chlorine.

Environmental pollutants can also be found in foods through contamination of soil. Metals (such as mercury, cadmium, and arsenic) and organohalogen compounds (containing chlorine and bromine) are examples of the kinds of toxic compounds that are absorbed through roots or leaves of plants.

Much attention has been focused on the effects of environmental toxins on non-human species (*ecotoxicology*). A high incidence of tumours in the livers of bottom feeding fish, such as flounder in Boston Harbour, has been attributed to the effects of carcinogenic constituents of heavy marine motor oils. Toxic effects in species which share our environment can sometimes act as an early warning of effects in humans in an analogous manner to the miner's canary, which at one time acted as a marker of poisonous gases in coalmines. In 1962 Rachel Carson published a highly influential book, *Silent spring*, which graphically described the deleterious consequences of the pollution of our environment by manmade chemicals, particularly pesticides. The widespread use, in the postwar years, of organochlorine and organophosphate pesticides for the eradication of agricultural pests and control of health hazards such as malaria began to be seen as a mitigated success. The persistence of some pesticides in the environment led to unforeseen side-effects, such as the thinning of eggshells resulting in the dramatic reduction of bird populations in agricultural areas. However, it is perhaps as a consequence of the heightened public awareness of environmental toxicology as a result of *Silent spring*, that the dramatic 'Fable for Tomorrow', describing the widespread loss of wildlife due to contamination with pesticides, which opens the book, has not (yet) come to pass.

DAVID SHUKER

Further reading

Carson, R. (1962). *Silent spring*. Penguin, London.

Klassen, C. D. (1996). *Casarett and Doull's toxicology: the basic science of poisons*. McGraw Hill, New York.

See also POISONS.

Enzymes are most familiarly associated with digestion, as substances in the alimentary tract that are necessary for the breakdown of food into simpler stuffs that can be absorbed into the body proper. These are indeed important, but they are in a small minority among the vast population of the body's enzymes. They also differ from the majority in acting outside rather than inside the cells that make them.

All living cells are teeming with enzymes. The name comes from the Greek meaning 'in leaven' or yeast. They are PROTEINS, synthesized in cells, which act as catalysts, causing all the body's chemical processes to advance with the necessary rapidity and completeness. Enzymes are ubiquitous in body cells and fluids, and they are specific — each enzyme is responsible for catalyzing one particular chemical process. Their existence and their function came to be recognized during the nineteenth century; understanding advanced with burgeoning twentieth-century BIOCHEMISTRY; and molecular biologists continue to elucidate their ultimate structure and mode of action, and the GENES that make them.

The names and nature of enzymes

The naming of enzymes in most cases reveals their function; '-ase' is added to the name either of the substance (the *substrate*) on which they act (like *peptidase* for those acting on peptides), or of the type of reaction induced (such as *hydrolase*, for those causing hydrolysis, the splitting of a substance with addition of water, or *transferase*, for those moving some chemical group from one molecule to another). Some of the first enzymes to be discovered have unique names, such as *pepsin* in the stomach, and *trypsin* from the pancreas, which are both *proteinases*.

So what sort of proteins are they, and how do they function? With molecular masses of 10 000 to 1 000 000, enzymes are themselves large molecules, but some also exist in larger complexes that facilitate a sequence of changes. An enzyme molecule is a 'globular' protein that has an area on its surface to which can be bound only the specific substrate that the enzyme is designed to accept. This binding leads to changes in both molecules that result in the formation of the required product, and restoration of the enzyme molecule to its original state, ready to take on another substrate molecule. With progressively higher concentrations of substrate the rate of product yield increases, but the increment in rate diminishes as it approaches a maximum at a certain substrate concentration; beyond this point only an increase in the concentration of the enzyme itself can accelerate the process. This behaviour is consistent with progressive occupation of binding sites on all available enzymes, until they are all functioning at a maximal turnover rate.

Range and sites of enzyme function

Enzymes operate at every stage of life. Even the head of the sperm releases an enzyme that dissolves its path through the outer covering of the ovum to reach and penetrate it. Cell division in the embryo and throughout life involves replication of the DNA that carries the genetic information. A series of specific enzymes is needed for this, to unwind the double helix, to replicate it by the synthesis of new strands, and to put it and the new pairs back together again — whilst other enzymes meanwhile supply energy by the breakdown of ADENOSINE TRIPHOSPHATE (ATP). Yet others are involved in the formation of messenger RNA and in all subsequent synthesis of proteins in a cell that results from the genetic coding.

Enzymes implement every event in the internal life of every cell in the body, and in its interaction with its environment. Each enzyme, or chain of enzymes acting in rapid sequence, has a specific function. There are those that are necessary for RESPIRATION and energy production; for transport mechanisms across the CELL MEMBRANE and between internal components; for modifications of cellular metabolism in response to hormones; and for any specialized activity, including secretion by glandular cells, contraction by MUSCLE cells, synthesis, release, and reuptake of NEUROTRANSMITTERS by nerve cells. The continual potential damage to tissues by the generation of free radicals is crucially limited by the body's antioxidant enzymes.

All cells have enzymes in their membrane, in the cytoplasm, and in the organelles within them. Those at the heart of cellular metabolism are the complex sequence of respiratory enzymes in the mitochondria that make possible the utilization of oxygen for the conversion of nutrient substrates to carbon dioxide and water, synthesis of ATP, and its breakdown for release of energy.

Cell membranes are furnished with 'sodium pumps' — protein molecules spanning the cell membrane that pump sodium ions out and potassium ions in. Facing inwards is an enzyme site that binds and breaks down ATP to supply the energy for pumping. Other enzyme molecules in the cell membrane may have, in addition to a site for substrate-binding, another that acts as receptor for a 'messenger' that activates the catalytic process: for example, the insulin receptor spans the cell membrane of muscle or fat cells; its outer site binds insulin, and its inner site handles the first of a series of enzyme-catalyzed reactions inside the cell that result in the several effects of insulin.

At SYNAPSES between nerves, and at NEUROMUSCULAR JUNCTIONS, enzymes are present that break down redundant neurotransmitters, preventing persistence of their effects. An example is acetylcholinesterase, found in the synaptic clefts on motor end plates in SKELETAL MUSCLE, which hydrolyses excess ACETYLCHOLINE, the neurotransmitter released by the motor nerve terminals.

Within skeletal muscle fibres, the enzymes vary according to their type of metabolism: whether it is predominantly aerobic (utilizing oxygen: 'slow' or 'red' muscle) or anaerobic ('fast' or 'pale' muscle). The sequence of events leading from activation of a muscle fibre by neurotrans-

mitter, to contraction by means of interaction between myosin and actin filaments, depends on enzymes at every stage.

Enzymes in the blood

In the circulating BLOOD there are enzymes both inside the blood cells, and outside in the plasma. Blood cells, in common with all cells, have the necessary enzymes for membrane transport and energy production. White blood cells have respiratory enzymes for aerobic metabolism, and others suited to their particular functions. Red blood cells are without mitochondria and respire anaerobically, so have enzymes appropriate to anaerobic glycolysis. Important for their function in whole-body respiratory gas exchange, they contain *carbonic anhydrase*, which promotes the uptake from the tissues of carbon dioxide and its carriage in the blood as bicarbonate, by catalyzing its combination with water to form carbonic acid, and its release in the lungs by this reaction in reverse.

Some enzymes exist as *pro-enzymes* or *zymogens*; they require some molecular change to be triggered into their active forms. These include proteins in the plasma that are involved in blood clotting: *prothrombin* is synthesized in the liver, and becomes *thrombin* when clotting is activated, and *plasminogen* can come into action as *plasmin*, a clot-dissolving enzyme. In the stomach, *pepsinogen* is secreted, and activated into *pepsin* by the acid that is secreted at the same site.

Enzymes that are normally secreted only into the gut or inside cells may, in pathological conditions, appear in significant quantities in the plasma, so that their measurement may be clinically useful. Examples are digestive enzymes that leak into the blood in acute pancreatitis, and *creatine kinase*, an enzyme from muscle tissue, that can appear in skeletal muscle disorders or, along with other intracellular enzymes, after a coronary thrombosis resulting in breakdown of some of the CARDIAC MUSCLE.

Conditions for enzyme activity

All enzymes need the right environment for effective function, notably an optimal acidity, which differs in accordance with the site at which a particular enzyme acts (for example, more acidic inside cells than outside, and, for digestive enzymes, acidic in the stomach and alkaline in the duodenum). Like any chemical reactions, the rate of those that are catalyzed by enzymes varies with temperature. Local heat generation, for example in exercising muscle, enhances all such reactions within it. Likewise, whole-body metabolic rate increases in fever and decreases in hypothermia, because of the effect on all enzyme-catalyzed reactions. Extremes of pH or temperature irreversibly abolish enzyme activity, and so also do some substances that bind to the active sites of particular enzymes. These include an organophosphate 'nerve gas' that blocks acetylcholinesterase (causing persistent accumulation of acetylcholine at neuromuscular junctions, and thus uncontrollable muscle contraction). Poisoning by cyanide is due to blocking an

essential enzyme in mitochondria and so fatally preventing all tissue respiration.

Medical applications

It is possible to inhibit the action of an enzyme without destroying it, and this has important therapeutic implications. There are substances that compete with the natural substrate for binding to an enzyme by having a similar structure, and others that act on other components of the enzyme molecule, preventing its ability to catalyze. Acetylcholinesterase inhibition is again an example — though in this context useful and reversible — in the treatment of the condition of *myasthenia gravis*, when the receptors on muscles cells for acetylcholine are deficient; the similar molecular structure of *neostigmine* allows it to bind to the enzyme, preventing binding and breakdown of acetylcholine; this can then accumulate sufficiently to enhance neuromuscular transmission. Drugs are used similarly to reverse the neuromuscular blockade deliberately induced during general anaesthesia. A different and important medical application of enzyme inhibition is in the use of antibiotics that block enzymes in microorganisms that are essential for their life or growth.

There are also many necessary *co-enzymes*, or co-factors for enzymes — organic non-protein molecules, smaller than the enzymes themselves, which either enhance or are necessary for the enzyme's activity. These again are widespread throughout the body, and are of many different molecular structures. Some require for their synthesis small amounts of essential substances from the diet. This is the basis of the need for the vitamins of the B group — they provide components for co-enzymes which could not otherwise be made in the body. Ions of several metals are also essential as co-factors, as well as for incorporation in some enzyme molecules themselves.

SHEILA JENNETT

See also ALIMENTARY SYSTEM; CELL; CELL MEMBRANE; METABOLISM; RESPIRATION; TRANSPORT.

Epicanthic fold In human anatomy, this is the fold of skin covering the inner corner (*canthus*) of the EYE, normally from the top of the eye downward in a semilunar form. The epicanthic (or epicanthal) fold is a normal feature of fetuses of all races but is present in a pronounced form and in high concentrations in humans of certain geographic races and subraces. The epicanthic fold is sometimes referred to as the 'Mongolian eye fold', because of its high incidence in and historical association with the Mongoloid (Asian) geographic race. The presence or absence of the epicanthus, which helps produce in Asians a distinctive eye shape and facial appearance, has helped fuel controversies in physical anthropology and evolutionary theory, including historical attempts to establish racial hierarchies based on evolutionary fitness and disputes concerning the nature of evolutionary adaptation. In addition, epicanthic folds in individuals of groups without a high normal incidence of its presence is often phenotypic of genetic or congenital disorders. In some recent debates, the alleged absence of the fold in some depictions and descriptions of humans from Chinese and Indian history has led some Afrocentric historians to claim an African origin of at least some aspects of Indian and Shang dynasty Chinese culture.

In addition to Asians and eastern subarctic and arctic Eurasians, some native American peoples (especially those of Middle America and some populations in South American lowland areas), the Capoid local race of southern Africa, and some of the composite racial groups of Pacific island peoples have high incidence of developed epicanthic folds. The fold occurs less frequently in Southeast Asian populations and in North American Indian groups but occurs occasionally in some European groups, for example in some Scandinavians and Poles.

While epicanthic folds occur more frequently in Asiatic groups and those peoples genetically linked to Asia, its presence is not universal in these peoples and it occurs less frequently in other groups. The incidence of epicanthic folds varies widely among the nine major geographic races and their local races. Attempts to define racial groups by the presence or absence of such features, by phenotype, rather than by genotype and specific inherited traits, are historically problematic and scientifically unreliable. There is substantial variation in phenotype within geographic races and subraces produced by the gene flow inevitable in an aggressively mobile species such as our own, by environmental conditions, and simply by individual variation due to a number of causes, including genetic mutation and the 'small-sample' effects of isolated population groups. Modern genetics rejects the notion of a 'pure' race; while the historical origins of some geographic groups are obscure, contemporary racial groups are mixtures of the gene pools of many geographic races. Thus, the presence or absence of a developed epicanthic fold, while an indication of one of a number of genetic origins and an important diagnostic feature of certain genetic disorders, cannot bear the cultural freight often bequeathed to it by history, pseudo-science, and prejudice.

The association of the epicanthic fold with Mongolians and Asians more generally served to reinforce notions of racial and cultural supremacy in nineteenth and early-to-mid twentieth century European physical ANTHROPOLOGY, PHYSIOGNOMY, and racial theory. Humans with the genetic anomaly now known as Down's syndrome, caused by having three copies (trisomy) of chromosome 21, have limited physical growth and mental retardation of varying severity, and an increased risk of other serious physical problems. Down's syndrome is one of the more common chromosomal defects, occurring on average in 1 in 900 live births. The Down's syndrome infant is quickly recognized by both facial and more general cranial characteristics, including a rounded head, short neck, thin and usually fine hair, flat nose, small mouth, and, especially, slanting eyes with pronounced epicanthic folds.

John Langdon Haydon Down first described this syndrome in 1866 and termed it 'mongolism' because of the eyefold and other facial features that Down believed linked the European children he observed to geographic races with a high incidence of such features, including the Asian geographic race (of which the Mongolian people constitute a local race). Down's report on this condition is an important example of the influence of cultural assumptions both on reading facial features and on the construction of anthropological theories designed to categorize and judge peoples: his comparison of European children born with a chromosomal disorder with the normal features of many Mongolians was both scientifically inaccurate as an analysis of the condition and a patronizing mischaracterization of Mongolians. Down argued that these children represented a degeneration of the superior (European) human type, stating that 'A very large number of congenital idiots are typical Mongols.' The racial theories used by Down and others have been decisively rejected by modern science, but it is only recently that the descriptions of Down's syndrome as 'mongolism' or 'mongolian idiocy' and persons with Down's syndrome as 'mongols' or 'mongolian idiots' have begun to fade from view.

In addition to Down's syndrome, epicanthic folds occur in other, less common genetic disorders, including Trigonocephaly 'C' syndrome and two types of 'Blepharophimosis, Ptosis, Epicanthus Inversus Syndrome' (BPES). In the latter condition, the epicanthic fold is inverted, extending from the lower eyelid up the side of the nose. Folds also occur in certain congenital conditions, including fetal alcohol syndrome. While the facial anomalies of infants with fetal alcohol syndrome are usually less pronounced than those of a Down's syndrome child, some of the same features occur, including a flat nose and nasal bridge, and developed epicanthic folds.

JEFFREY H. BARKER

Epidemic

Epidemics come with wings and slowly limp away
(from a French proverb).

The word 'epidemic' has an emotional ring to it. This is probably the reason why it is often used wrongly when, strictly speaking, other epidemiological terms such as *pandemics* or *outbreaks* should be employed to enumerate disease. An epidemic (from the Greek: *epi* upon; *demos*, people) is usually defined as a large-scale, temporary increase in the occurrence of a disease in a community or region which is clearly in excess of normal expectancy, whereas a *pandemic* (*pan*, all) is the occurrence of a disease which is clearly in excess of normal expectancy and is spread over a whole geographical area, usually crossing national boundaries.

At the other end of the scale are *outbreaks* and *sporadic cases*. An outbreak may be a *household* or a *general* outbreak. A household outbreak involves two or more persons resident in the same household whose illness is associated in time but not apparently connected with any other case or outbreak. A general outbreak involves two or more persons who are not confined to one household but are associated in time and location. A sporadic case refers to a person whose illness is not apparently connected with similar illnesses in any other persons.

A disease or infectious agent is said to be *endemic* when it is constantly present within a given location or population group.

Although the term 'epidemic' is used widely to describe clusters of disease in general, and even in a non-medical sense (e.g. an epidemic of road rage), it has traditionally been used when infection strikes a population. This often occurs when there is crowding together of humans (or, for that matter, animals, fish, or birds), as this provides the necessary conditions to allow microorganisms to multiply and spread. When humans led nomadic lives there was often less chance for epidemics to occur; the main opportunities came when large numbers gathered for such things as pilgrimages or wars — and when subsequently the group dispersed the chances of carrying the infection elsewhere were multiplied.

The threat of epidemics in overcrowded and difficult conditions is particularly well illustrated in military history; on many occasions the germ has been as important as the sword or gun in determining the outcome of a campaign. The Spanish conquest of Mexico owes much of its success to an epidemic of smallpox that destroyed about half of the Aztec population. The typhoid bacillus caused severe effects during both the American Civil War (1861–5) and the Boer War (1899–1902). The use of typhoid vaccine in the latter years of World War I meant that the main impact of typhoid in this war subsided after 1916. Similarly, typhus was rife in the Civil War in Britain (1642–9), when both the Parliamentary and Royalist armies were affected.

There are three main patterns of epidemic, determined by the mode of transmission of the microorganism.

Firstly, the *explosive epidemic*. This is characterized by the occurrence of many cases in a relatively short period; there is a sharp rise and fall in the number of infected persons, since the usual cause of such an event is a common source of infection. This type of epidemic is thus also frequently termed a *common source epidemic* or a *point source epidemic*. This pattern of infection often occurs when water or food becomes contaminated, although other vehicles of infection can also be responsible.

Secondly, *person-to-person spread*. These epidemics usually have a more protracted course, taking longer than explosive epidemics to build up and subside. An infective agent may be passed from person to person by a variety of routes (e.g. respiratory or gastrointestinal). Diseases such as influenza or chickenpox often follow this pattern.

Thirdly — a combination of the two — an explosive epidemic with subsequent person-to-person spread. This pattern is apparent when there is contamination of a common water or food source and the initial cases then infect their contacts. Although this type of epidemic starts in the same way as an explosive incident, there is a slower decline.

The importance of keen observation and recording of epidemics in order to deduce the likely cause has been demonstrated on many occasions, and may be considerably in advance of microbiological proof. In 1849, 34 years before the identification of *Vibrio cholerae* by Robert Koch (1843–1910), John Snow (1813–58), a London physician, proved by epidemiological observation that cholera is mainly spread by drinking infected water, rather than through the air in the form of a miasma as was commonly thought at the time. Similarly, William Budd (1811–80), a general practitioner in Devon, showed in 1873 how typhoid was caused, even though it was not until 1885 that *Salmonella typhi* was first isolated in the laboratory. More recently, William Pickles (1885–1969), a general practitioner in Wensleydale, Yorkshire, was able to elucidate many of the epidemiological characteristics of viral hepatitis well before microbiological advances were to confirm his observations. DANIEL REID

Further reading

Pickles W. N. (1939). *Epidemiology in country practice.* Wright, Bristol. (Re-issued in 1972 by the Devonshire Press, Torquay.)

Tyrrel, D. A. J. (1982). *The abolition of infection. Hope or illusion?* Rock Carling Fellowship Lecture. Nuffield Provincial Hospitals Trust, London.

See also INFECTIOUS DISEASES; PANDEMICS.

Epidural Epidural strictly means 'on the dura'. In anatomical usage it means outside or around the *dura mater*, which is the outermost of the membranes (MENINGES) that ensheath the BRAIN and SPINAL CORD. In the vertebral canal there is a narrow space between the dura mater and the lining (*periosteum*) of the bones; local anaesthetic injected into this space abolishes sensation from those parts of the body served by nerves that enter the spinal cord below the level of injection. In the skull, the dura has two layers, and the outermost is itself the lining of the bone and firmly adherent to it. Head injury that involves fracture in the region of the temple where there are particularly vulnerable blood vessels, can lead to an epidural ('*extradural*') collection of blood, stripping the dura from the bone, and requiring drainage by trephining to alleviate compression of the brain. S.J.

See ANAESTHESIA, LOCAL; ANALGESIA; LABOUR; MENINGES; SURGERY.

Epiglottis A leaf-shaped piece of cartilage covered by mucous membrane, sited vertically against the back of the root of the tongue and in front of the *glottis* — the opening into the larynx.

The upper part of the epiglottis is free to bend back and down; also the arrangement of nearby folds of tissue and bands of muscle allows the rim of the glottis to be drawn against a thickening on the back surface of the epiglottis. These mechanisms provide for closure of the glottis during swallowing, preventing food and drink from entering the larynx and trachea (windpipe) and directing it further back into the opening of the oesophagus (gullet). S.J.

See SWALLOWING; PLATE 1.

Epilepsy may well be one of mankind's oldest diseases. Hippocrates (*c.* 450–377 BCE) wrote *On the sacred disease*, which is usually interpreted as being epilepsy, arguing that it could be treated by regular attention to a healthy way of life, especially by the proper and moderate use of food and drink, which would correct the causative physiological blockages. That is, the Hippocratic tradition regarded epilepsy as a disease as natural as any other, and not due to supernatural influences, whilst prior to the Hippocratic corpus a range of disturbed gods had been invoked to account for epilepsy's signs and symptoms.

Further, Hippocrates argued that the disease was inherited and was caused by a disturbance in the BRAIN, and thus firmly fixed epilepsy as a natural disease, treatable by doctors and not by priests, an important development for both market and medical practices. This view was long held by learned doctors: the influential physician Alexander of Tralles (525–605), however, recommended treatments that included making the nail of a wrecked ship into a bracelet, which was to be decorated with 'the bone of a stag's heart taken from its body whilst alive', adding that this should be worn on the left arm, for 'astonishing results'. Somewhat earlier, the Roman physician Pliny (*c.* 23–79) had also reported that epileptic patients could be cured by drinking blood, especially of gladiators. Throughout the Middle Ages, the view that epilepsy was a medical problem continued to coexist with causative theories of demonic POSSESSION and spiritual imbalances. Treatments including Christian prayer (St Christopher was drafted in as a patron saint with special responsibility), pagan ritual, and humoral medicine all emerged. A prominent medieval surgeon, Guy de Chauliac (1298–1368), prescribed magic and prayer for epileptics — they were to write the names of the Three Wise Men in their own blood on parchment, and daily recite three Pater Nosters and Ave Marias for three months. It was at this time that mistletoe acquired a special association with epilepsy — mistletoe was hung around children's necks in Central Europe as a protective against seizures, and in Scandinavia knife handles were cut from oak mistletoe, for the same purpose. By the sixteenth century epileptics could be branded as WITCHES, and little medical progress had been made. In the middle of the seventeenth century, Robert Boyle, a founder member of the Royal Society of London, was still advocating crushed

mistletoe to be taken during the days of a full moon.

Gradually however, some effort was made to classify the different types of seizures, and by the beginning of the nineteenth century epileptics were often hospitalized. One advance occurred in 1838, when epileptic children in Paris were provided with education, rather than being completely hospitalized, although often epileptics were separated from the insane because of the growing belief that epilepsy was infectious. Thus epileptics were increasingly confined in separate wards, and soon in separate institutions.

By 1860 special hospitals for epileptics had been founded in Germany, France, and Britain. One of these was the Hospital for Epilepsy and Paralysis in Queen Square, London (later the National Hospital for Nervous Diseases). This meant that epileptics were increasingly seen and treated by physicians attached to such institutions, who became particularly experienced in the diagnosis and treatment of the disease. This led in particular to a more detailed differentiation and classification of epilepsy, including terms still in use today, such as *grand mal*, PETIT MAL, absence seizures, and *status epilepticus*. By the latter part of the nineteenth century, the theories of the British neurologist, John Hughlings Jackson (1835–1911), and his French counterpart Jean Charcot (1825–93) began to define the neurological basis of the disease and its complex symptomatology. W.R. Gowers (1845–1915) authoritatively described the 'aura' that preceded a *grand mal* attack (although Hippocrates had not been ignorant of it).

In terms of treatment, *bromides* were the first successful medicine for epilepsy, from the 1850s onwards, abolishing attacks in some, and diminishing them in number or violence in most others; they started to be displaced only after the introduction of *phenobarbital*, first prescribed in 1912. Barbiturates continue to be one of the effective treatments, although further understanding of the underlying mechanisms have led to the development of alternative modern anticonvulsant drugs: those that potentiate or imitate the inhibitory NEUROTRANSMITTER GABA, or stabilize the neuronal cell membrane, and thus prevent excessive firing.

It may seem obvious in the present day that the origin of the CONVULSIONS that characterize epilepsy lies in the brain — but this was not in fact established until the latter half of the nineteenth century. Indeed, there had been at that time a belief that they originated as abnormal REFLEXES from the SPINAL CORD. This, together with the notion that there was not any localization of function in the CEREBRAL CORTEX, was based on faulty interpretation of experimental studies. Broca initiated the concept of localization in the 1860s, with his description of the part of the left hemisphere responsible for SPEECH function, followed by Hughlings Jackson's conclusion from his studies that convulsions on one side of the body are due to discharge from certain convolutions of the cortex on the opposite side of the brain. (Hippocrates had noted this association somewhat earlier in his writings on injuries to the head, but the knowledge had been submerged.) Studies on electrical stimulation of the brain of animals in the 1870s supported Hughling Jackson's suppositions. Anaesthesia and antisepsis followed by asepsis allowed the beginnings of modern brain surgery, and another historic event was in 1886, when Victor Horsley in London operated on the brain and cured a young man's fits by removing scarring resulting from a head injury in childhood.

The next landmark in the history of epilepsy was the ELECTROENCEPHALOGRAM (EEG) — the first demonstration in the late 1920s that the electrical activity of the brain could be recorded through the intact skull, and that abnormal patterns appeared during an epileptic attack. In subsequent decades, electroencephalography advanced the diagnosis of epilepsy, and the localization of its site of origin in the brain. Meanwhile, exploration of the effects of electrical stimulation of the human brain, with relevance to the site of onset of focal seizures, culminated in the detailed mapping of functional localization of the parts of the body in the motor and sensory regions of the cortex, by the Canadian neurosurgeon Wilder Penfield and his colleagues in the 1930s.

Deliberate induction of epileptic seizures was used during the twentieth century in attempts to treat mental illness. Camphor, which had been observed to precipitate attacks in epileptic patients, was introduced to induce shocks, but it produced such violent convulsions that bones were broken, and symptoms remained unaffected. INSULIN shock therapy inducing seizures by the lowering of BLOOD SUGAR was used with some success in schizophrenics. Electroconvulsive therapy (ECT), first applied in the late 1930s, and nowadays performed under anaesthesia, remains in use and is effective in the treatment of depressive illness.

Epilepsy would now be defined as a paroxysmal and transitory disturbance of the functions of the brain, involving repetitive discharges in large groups of brain cells, and commonly causing convulsions. The disturbance develops suddenly, ceases spontaneously, and is subject to recurrence. The current understanding of epileptiform activity in the brain, its types, nature, and mechanisms, is described under 'CONVULSIONS'.   E.M. TANSEY
SHEILA JENNETT

See also CONVULSIONS; CRANIOTOMY; EEG; MAGNETIC BRAIN STIMULATION.

Episiotomy Once memorably described as 'the unkindest cut of all', episiotomy is a surgical cut in the perineum that is effected by knife or scissors shortly before delivery of a baby. The procedure has undoubted merit when there are signs of distress in the baby, or a need for forceps delivery, or where there is a risk of serious and extensive tearing of tissues. However, episiotomy has been applied, in some countries, to an extent

that is almost routine; thus hence the controversial nature of this procedure. The wound is stitched immediately after delivery.   J. NEILSON

See also BIRTH; LABOUR.

Epithelium Epithelia are tissues lining the outer surface of the body (SKIN), or the inner surface of organs which have a direct connection to one of the body's orifices. The latter group includes tissues lining the airways; the alimentary canal and its associated organs and glands; and the genito-urinary system. In some organs the epithelium consists of a simple layer of cuboidal or columnar cells — as in the alimentary canal, gall bladder, and airways — while in others there are multiple layers of cells arising from a *germinal epithelium*, with many dead cells in the outermost layers — as in the skin. In man, the skin forms an impervious and protective layer. Important absorptive and secretory functions are carried out by epithelia lining the body organs. After eating, products of digestion are absorbed from the stomach and small intestine, and glands secrete fluid and enzymes to help the digestive processes. In internal organs the cells are continually sloughed off and replaced by new cells. The life time of an epithelial cell in the gut is just a few days; for cells lining the airways it is about 40 days. To perform their secretory and absorptive functions, epithelial cells are equipped with a variety of ION CHANNELS, ion pumps, ion exchangers, and solute carriers, which enable TRANSPORT of substances across the CELL MEMBRANE. These are distributed asymmetrically in the cells: some are present exclusively in the face of the cell exposed to the lumen (cavity) of the organ or tube, while others are found on the opposite face. This arrangement of the transporters allows movement from one side of the epithelium to the other. Some epithelia are specialized for absorptive functions, moving substances from the lumen into the body fluids; others only secrete substances by transport into the lumen, and still others can have both functions.   ALAN W. CUTHBERT

See also GLANDS; MUCOUS MEMBRANE; SKIN.

Erection Turgidity in a tissue brought about by distension with blood: usually referring to the enlargement and stiffening of the penis in a state of sexual arousal; also applicable to the clitoris. Given the appropriate stimulus, the arterial blood vessels dilate, blood floods into specialised 'spongy' tissue, and the engorgement itself blocks outflow through the compressible veins.
S.J.

See COITUS; EJACULATION; IMPOTENCE; PLATE 8.

Ergonomics Why is the video recorder one of the most frustrating domestic items to operate? Why do some car seats leave you aching after a long journey? Why do some computer workstations confer eye strain and muscle FATIGUE? Such human irritations and inconveniences are not inevitable — ergonomics is an approach

which puts human needs and capabilities at the focus of designing technological systems. The aim is to ensure that humans and technology work in complete harmony, with the equipment and tasks aligned to human characteristics.

Ergonomics has wide application to everyday domestic situations, but there are even more significant implications for efficiency, productivity, safety, and health in work settings. For example:

(i) Designing equipment and systems, including computers, so that they are easier to use and less likely to lead to errors in operation — particularly important in high STRESS and safety-critical operations such as control rooms.

(ii) Designing tasks and jobs so that they are effective and take account of human needs such as rest breaks and sensible shift patterns, as well as other factors such as the intrinsic rewards of work itself.

(iii) Designing equipment and work arrangements to improve working posture and ease the load on the body, thus reducing instances of Repetitive Strain Injury/Work Related Upper Limb Disorder.

(iv) Information design, to make the interpretation and use of handbooks, signs, and displays easier and less error-prone.

(v) Design of training arrangements to cover all significant aspects of the job concerned and to take account of human learning requirements.

(vi) The design of military and space equipment and systems — an extreme case of demands on the human being.

(vii) Designing working environments, including lighting and heating, to suit the needs of the users and the tasks performed. Where necessary, design of personal protective equipment for work in hostile environments.

(viii) In developing countries, the acceptability and effectiveness of even fairly basic technology can be significantly enhanced.

The multi-disciplinary nature of ergonomics (sometimes called 'Human Factors') is immediately obvious. The ergonomist works in teams which may involve a variety of other professions: design engineers, production engineers, industrial designers, computer specialists, industrial physicians, health and safety practitioners, and specialists in human resources. The overall aim is to ensure that our knowledge of human characteristics is brought to bear on practical problems of people at work and in leisure. We know that, in many cases, humans *can* adapt to unsuitable conditions, but such adaptation leads often to inefficiency, errors, unacceptable stress, and physical or mental cost.

The components of ergonomics

Ergonomics deals with the interaction of technological and work situations with the human being. The basic human sciences involved are *anatomy*, *physiology*, and *psychology*. These sciences are applied by the ergonomist towards two objectives: the most productive use of human capabilities, and the maintenance of human

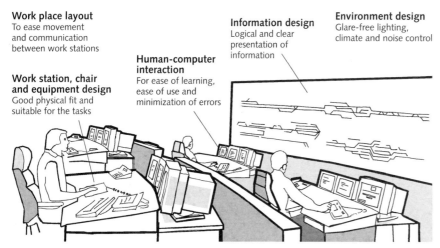

Work place layout
To ease movement and communication between work stations

Work station, chair and equipment design
Good physical fit and suitable for the tasks

Human-computer interaction
For ease of learning, ease of use and minimization of errors

Information design
Logical and clear presentation of information

Environment design
Glare-free lighting, climate and noise control

Office ergonomics. Davis Associates.

health and well-being. In a phrase, 'the job must fit the person' in all respects, and the work situation should not compromise human capabilities and limitations.

The contribution of basic *anatomy* lies in improving the physical 'fit' between people and the things they use, ranging from hand tools to aircraft cockpit design. Achieving good physical fit is no mean feat when one considers the range in human body sizes across the population. The science of anthropometrics provides data on dimensions of the human body, in various postures. Biomechanics considers the operation of the muscles and limbs, and ensures that working postures are beneficial, and that excessive forces are avoided.

Our knowledge of human *physiology* supports two main technical areas. Work physiology addresses the energy requirements of the body, and sets standards for acceptable physical work-rate and workload, and for nutrition requirements. Environmental physiology analyses the impact of physical working conditions — thermal, noise and vibration, and lighting — and sets the optimum requirements for these.

Psychology is concerned with human information processing and decision-making capabilities. In simple terms, this can be seen as aiding the cognitive 'fit' between people and the things they use. Relevant topics are sensory processes, perception, long- and short-term memory, decision making, and action. There is also a strong thread of organizational psychology.

The importance of the psychological dimension of ergonomics should not be underestimated in today's 'high-tech' world — remember the video recorder example at the beginning. The ergonomist advises on the design of interfaces between people and computers (Human Computer Interaction or HCI), information displays for industrial processes, the planning of training materials, and the design of human tasks and jobs. The concept of 'information overload' is familiar in many current jobs. Paradoxically, increasing automation, while dispensing with human involvement in routine operations, frequently increases the mental demands in terms of monitoring, supervision, and maintenance.

The ergonomics approach — understanding tasks ... and the users

Underlying all ergonomics work is careful analysis of human activity. The ergonomist must understand all of the demands being made on the person, and the likely effects of any changes to these — the techniques which enable him to do this come under the portmanteau label of 'job and task analysis'.

The second key ingredient is to understand the users. For example, 'consumer ergonomics' covers applications to the wider contexts of the home and leisure. In these non-work situations the need to allow for human variability is at its greatest — the people involved have a very wide range of capabilities and limitations (including the disabled and elderly), and seldom have any selection or training for the tasks which face them.

This commitment to 'human-centred design' is an essential 'humanizing' influence on contemporary rapid developments in technology, in contexts ranging from the domestic to all types of industry.

DAVID WHITFIELD
JOE LANGFORD

Further reading

Kroemer, K. (1997). *Fitting the task to the human*, (5th edn). Taylor and Francis, London.

Norman, D. A. (1988). *The psychology of everyday things*. Basic Books Inc., New York. (Reprinted in paperback as *The design of everyday things*. Doubleday, New York, 1990.)

Erogenous zones are those areas of the body that arouse sexual desire. Erogenous has two general meanings. The first refers to the genitals or breasts, which when stimulated produce pleasurable sensations in their owner. The phrase 'erogenous zones' was coined near the end of the nineteenth century and used in the early twentieth century by some psychologists to describe how simple pressure to these parts of the body could arouse complete orgasm in what were defined as 'hysterical persons' (generally understood to be women). The second general meaning of the phrase, to be dealt with at some length here, refers to a visual phenomenon associated with clothing and body adornment. For cultural anthropologists, erogenous zones are those areas of the female body which men find sexually arousing and which women alter or adorn to attract the male eye.

Erogenous zones vary from culture to culture and over time. Asian men prize the nape of the neck while Europeans are unique in their fixation on the waist. In defiance of common sense, the genitals rarely become erogenous zones. Suggestion is more arousing than exposure so male desire is displaced from the vulva to parts of the body like the mouth or the foot which symbolize or resemble it. Humans then increase this likeness through body painting, cosmetics, mutilation, or other procedures. Western women paint their lips bright red, enhancing the resemblance to the labia. Aristocratic Chinese women bound their feet so that these tiny, curled appendages more closely resembled the vulva. All societies alter erogenous zones to make them more 'beautiful' or prominent. Polynesians tattooed the thighs and buttocks of nubile girls; Africans scarred them. Both procedures were designed to exaggerate the secondary sexual characteristics, thereby helping the girl attract a mate. Westerners have not escaped this tendency to 'perfect' nature. In the nineteenth century, tight-laced CORSETS produced bulging hips and buttocks that made women more 'feminine' — that is, erotic.

When not laced, bound, stretched, pierced, or tattooed, erogenous zones are usually concealed or only partially exposed. In his influential study, *The Psychology of Clothes* (1930), psychoanalyst J. C. Flugel observed that bare flesh is boring. Male curiosity is sustained by veiling the erotic site, by covering and exhibiting it at the same time. In Africa and Polynesia, scarring and tattooing performed this function: erogenous zones appeared covered but were naked on a second glance. In the West, CLOTHES perform this function, for they conceal while drawing attention to the erotic site. For example, heavy skirts concealed European women's legs for centuries, while colourful or decorated petticoats directed the eye to the feet and ankles. This ploy was so successful that Victorian men became faint-hearted at the sight of a well-turned ankle. Then legs lost their sexual allure when hemlines rose after World War I. Female legs were exposed for the first time in centuries and the erogenous zone moved elsewhere, to the back in the 1930s and the breasts in the 1950s.

Erogenous zones should be distinguished from sexual fetishes. According to Freud, a *fetish* is an inappropriate object (a shoe for example) that is substituted for a woman and used for sexual gratification. An erogenous zone is a body part (a foot, for instance) that arouses sexual curiosity and draws a man's attention to the whole female body. FETISHISM is an individual personality disorder, while erogenous zones are sexual preferences shared by most men at a given time or place. Fetishes belong to the science of psychopathology while erogenous zones belong to the social world of costume and FASHION.

It was in fact a dress historian, James Laver, who first discussed 'shifting erogenous zones' in the 1930s. He used this concept to explain fashion or rapid changes in female dress. Influenced by psychoanalyst Flugel, Laver argued that women are born exhibitionists whose social subordination forces them to acquire male protection. Consequently, women dress mainly to attract men, and in order to do so they emphasize their erogenous zones by means of their attire. Male sexual curiosity is, however, highly unstable. Men quickly tire of a given erogenous zone and move on to other feminine body parts. Women must follow and adopt a new form of dress. The instability of male sexual curiosity means that women's dress is in a constant state of flux. This change of fashion and its dictates are directly related to shifting erogenous zones.

Unlike women, modern men have escaped the tyranny of fashion. In medieval and early modern times, male dress was opulent and highly erotic, as the Renaissance codpiece attests. Around 1800 male dress changed: men forswore exhibitionism and renounced brightly coloured, erotic attire. This 'Great Male Renunciation', as Flugel called it, produced the sober, undemonstrative suit, which two hundred years later men still wear. Male attire is impervious to fashion because it is indifferent to sexual display or allure: it need not follow shifting erogenous zones.

For fifty years, historians accepted this version of costume history and believed that shifting erogenous zones fuelled fashion. Then in the 1980s a new generation of costume scholars (most of them women) challenged the old theory. Art historians insisted that costume was a part of a broader visual culture and obeyed the same laws as painting or architecture. Feminists pointed to the sexism that underlay Flugel and Laver's theories and argued that women dressed to please themselves as much as to please men. Costume historians observed that fashion always produces its opposite anti-fashion and menswear, appearances notwithstanding, conveys subtle but strong erotic messages. All these scholars agreed that SEXUALITY was not the primary motive for dress. People dress, the young scholars insisted, to express themselves, to project their ideal self image, to display their political views, to signal their racial and national identity, and to assert their social position. In the new costume history, sexuality still shapes costume; dress is too close to the skin to avoid it. But the erogenous zone no longer dictates fashion nor serves as the only explanation for the human compulsion to decorate, ornament, and alter the body.

KATE NORBERG

Further reading
Steele, V (1985). *Fashion and eroticism: ideals of feminine beauty from the Victorian era to the Jazz Age.* Oxford University Press, New York.

Wilson, E. (1985). *Adorned in dreams.* Virago, London.

See also BODY DECORATION; BODY MUTILATION AND MARKING; BUTTOCKS; FASHION; FETISHISM; SCARS; TATTOO.

Eroticism is a curious word — there even seems to be some confusion over whether it should be 'eroticism' or 'erotism'. The earliest example given for the related term 'eroticise' — defined as to make erotic or to stimulate erotically — dates from as late as 1914, citing Geddes and Thomson's handbook *Sex*, which deals with the 'eroticisation of the brain' that takes place during adolescence. The term as used conflates various rather different meanings, and this indeterminacy may be indicative of both the haziness of the concept and of a particular elusive quality characteristic of eroticism.

There is a specific psychoanalytic meaning for 'eroticism', which is seen as an inherent quality not originally attached to the genitals at all. Freud, in *Three Essays on Sexuality* (1905) outlined his theory of infantile sexuality and the development of various manifestations of eroticism around different erotogenic zones of the body. The key phenomenon for him was thumb-sucking: this was sensual, characterized by rhythmicity; it bore no relation to the primary purpose of obtaining nourishment (though was initially associated with this need for self-preservation), and involved a complete absorption in the process, leading to sleep or even to something resembling orgasm. Freud noted that the early erotic manifestations he delineated were additionally characterized by being auto-erotic; directed towards the attainment of satisfaction from the individual's own body rather than being directed towards other people.

He generalized from this instance to define certain common features in zones which became imbued with erotic interest. They were MUCOUS MEMBRANES, or parts of the SKIN, which evoked feelings of pleasure of a particular quality when stimulated in a certain way. A rhythmic character seemed to be an important component of why these stimuli were significant (Freud found the analogy of TICKLING 'forced' upon him). But any part of the body might become an erotogenic zone. However, there were certain areas which were particularly liable to do so, and for Freud the oral eroticism of sucking was the model. The development of erotic attachment to anal activity, and the stimulating effects of the faecal mass on a sensitive portion of mucous membrane, was a later manifestation. Genital stimulation was a still later development: Freud concluded that it was not 'the vehicle of the oldest sexual impulses'. Its earliest arousal was often brought about in connection with urination, but general hygienic activities (such as washing) or accidental stimulation (e.g. by threadworm infestation) could direct the child's attention towards this area.

This concept of eroticism relates to the wider meanings and connotations of the term, in that it

clearly situates eroticism as a form of pleasure drawing on sexual sources but detached not only from the primary reproductive purpose of sex but from its more socialized functions such as creating relationships. Eroticism implies a conscious and deliberate concern with the subsidiary aspects of the sexual drive, and thus it is strongly associated with ideas of TABOO and the transgressive. The French theoretician of eroticism, Georges Bataille, in *L'érotisme* (1957: UK publication 1962) argued that it performs a function of dissolving boundaries. It is something disruptive and disorderly.

Eroticism should be distinguished from sensuality. The latter tends to denote a certain wallowing in pleasures of the senses: eroticism, however, is concerned to heighten these pleasures. The means of doing so are various, but often involve strategies by which final gratification is delayed, and which intensify the period of yearning desire. This ties in with the counter-natural quality of eroticism; it is not about proceeding to satisfaction by the most direct route possible, but about finding means of making the satisfaction greater and even transcendental when it is attained.

MARRIAGE is often seen as the deathbed of eroticism, since it is a public and institutionalized relationship forming the basis of societal ties. Moreover, the husband and wife have largely unrestricted sexual access to one another (the maximum of temptation with the maximum of opportunity, as George Bernard Shaw put it), which is something antipathetic to the idea of eroticism, for which barriers impeding the consummation which is striven towards are a necessity. Sexual intercourse within marriage tends to become habitual and routine. This problem exercised early-twentieth-century writers who were endeavouring to import an erotic quality into marriage, in order to cancel out the threats to national and individual health posed by forbidden pleasures, by integrating these into the licit and conjugal. Authors such as Havelock Ellis and Marie Stopes put the case for periodic abstinence within marriage to make the pleasures of union sweeter. All writers of sex advice warned couples, and particularly the husband, to avoid falling into a banal routine of marital relations and to make each union a unique experience, a point of view which had already been advanced by the French novelist Honoré de Balzac in his work *The Physiology of Marriage* (1826).

How far eroticism, as an experience both transcendental and transgressive, can be incorporated into an approved state such as marriage is problematic. However hard a couple may try to import eroticism into the marriage, particularly in these days of sexual liberation, there is very little which can be done by two consenting adults which has the *frisson* of the forbidden. This may lead us to re-evaluate the erotic potential of the marriages of earlier epochs, such as the Victorian, when so much was (at least in public rhetoric) forbidden or disapproved of, that a sense of the transgressive might be readily achieved by quite small matters, such as mutual nakedness, or slight alterations of coital position such as placing the woman on top. The doctrine of conjugal continence also placed restrictions upon the frequency of marital intercourse and thus may have made the occasions when it did occur much more intense. Changes in sexual morality during the 1960s and 70s may provide part of the explanation for the rise of 'swinging' or partner-swapping parties during the 1970s: not so much an expression of sexual liberation as a reaction to the idea that 'anything goes' by finding some form of sexual activity that could still generate a sense of the transgressive. The recommendations in *The Joy of Sex* (1974) for the use of bondage to heighten the sexual experience may also be seen as a way to achieve an erotic transcendance which cheerful, guiltfree, 'straight' sexual romps could not provide.

Anything can become eroticized. Different parts of the body signify the erotic in different cultures: the example usually cited is that of the bound foot which exercised such a strong influence over the erotic preferences of the Chinese for many centuries. Fashion both follows and creates new areas of erotic interest. Clothes or habits which were associated with prostitution became themselves erotic signifiers — for example, make-up, bright lipstick. The actual allusion to sexual activity may be exceedingly distantly displaced. There is no obvious reason, apart from social coding, why an earring in one ear or the other should advertise particular sexual preferences, and in fact there is some doubt as to whether (outside limited circles) it does this rather than being merely a choice in individual decoration. Ankle-chains worn by women may make some distant reference to bondage.

Because of its mutable, unstable, and floating quality, eroticism often turns up in places where it might be assumed to have been completely eradicated. It has often been pointed out how close a connection exists between eroticism and religion, though this is seldom so explicit as in the famous erotic temple carvings of India, or the rituals of Tantric Buddhism. The metaphors of yearning, of desire, of satisfaction withheld and then overwhelmingly achieved, which have obvious erotic connotations constantly crop up in religious contexts. The lush and poetic eroticism of the *Song of Songs* in the Old Testament has been read as an allegory of the union between God and his people. St Theresa of Avila's writings of her mystical ecstasies seem to the modern reader unmistakably sexual, and this eroticism is made quite explicit in the famous statue of her by Bernini, swooning in ecstasy when pierced by an angel with a sword. Hymns can express a desire for a passionate consummation.

Given Freud's derivation of eroticism from a primary oral source, it may be suggested that all eroticism, with its promise of an exquisite culmination, hearkens back to the infant sucking on its mother's breast. He himself noted that the

blissful satiation of the flushed baby after feeding was the 'prototype of the expression of sexual satisfaction in later life'. This may explain why, although enacted through sexuality, eroticism has the persistent quality of being contrary to, even detached from, the usual ends of sexual activity, both personal and social.

LESLEY A. HALL

Erythema From the Greek for 'flush' — redness of the skin, due to persistent engorgement of microscopic blood vessels. A descriptive term; not in itself a diagnosis. Sunburn, or sitting too close to an open fire, causes erythema; it surrounds a nettle or insect sting, or an inflamed wound. A rash, whether due to INFECTIOUS DISEASE, to ALLERGY, or to drug reactions for example, is described as *erythematous* if blotches of redness are a feature. It is characteristic of such blotches that they can be emptied of their colour by pressure; this distinguishes them from actual bleeding into the skin. S.J.

See SKIN; SUN AND THE BODY.

Eucharist The Eucharist — also known variously as the Mass, Holy Communion, the Lord's Supper, according to doctrinal position — is a central act of worship in Christianity which commemorates or 'follows' the Last Supper as recorded in Matthew 26: 26–8, Mark 14: 22–4 and Luke 22:17–20, in the eating and drinking of bread and wine, thought either to be or to represent Christ's body and blood. From the Greek, meaning 'thanksgiving', there is evidence of the earliest Christians participating in this liturgy, believed to have been instituted by Christ in his celebration of the Passover meal on the night before he died and during which he 'gave thanks'. Both Acts and the Epistles of Paul show early Christians participating in this service; Paul emphasized participation in the Eucharist as a Christian duty because it signified the unity of Christians in one body — the body of Christ. Early Christian art, including wall paintings in the catacombs, illustrates Christians eating and drinking bread and wine together, and several written texts provide evidence of the different ways in which the Eucharist was celebrated by the early Christians. For example, the first Christian handbook, the *Didache,* documents a ritual which is part proper meal and part sacramental, introduced by a confession of sins, and expressed as a foretaste of the future coming of Jesus.

The early Church and the patristic period saw variety of practice in the ritual, but general acceptance of the idea that the eucharistic elements of the bread and wine were the body and blood of Christ. The notion that the bread and wine were transformed into Christ's body and blood during the eucharistic service became a matter of debate in the West in the Middle Ages, by which time the Eucharist was firmly established as one of the seven sacraments in the Roman Catholic church. This debate led to a

more precise formulation of transubstantiation of the Fifth Lateran Council (1215) and by Thomas Aquinas, who used Aristotelian physics to explain the process by which, during the act of consecration by the priest, the substance of the bread and wine changed into the body and blood of Christ (that is, changed their essence) while remaining in the accidental forms of bread and wine. The later Middle Ages saw great eucharistic devotion, especially amongst religious women who imitated and shared Christ's suffering by eating nothing but the host — that is, Christ's body — so that they might become so united with the body of Christ that their own bodies would be no longer ordinary human bodies, but a body like Christ's. The institution of Corpus Christi ('Body of Christ') as a feast day in 1264 indicated a more popular, widespread (and less extreme) eucharistic piety.

The Protestant Reformation saw much dispute about the meaning of the Eucharist, and it was the issue on which the mainstream German and Swiss Protestant reformers broke with each other, at the Colloquy of Marburg in 1529. The dispute turned on the extent to which Christ was thought to be present in the bread and wine, with Zwingli holding the extreme position that the Eucharist was a mere memorial of the Last Supper and there was no change in the bread and wine at all (thus the Eucharist is simply the Lord's Supper), and Luther adhering to the doctrine of 'consubstantiation' in which, during the Eucharist, both the bread and wine and Christ's body and blood co-existed. Their disagreement was expressed particularly in their interpretation of Jesus' words at the Last Supper — 'this is my body' and 'this is my blood', with Zwingli insisting that 'is' means 'signifies'. Behind Zwingli's position lies his belief that 'the body and spirit are such essentially different things that whichever one you take it cannot be the other' (*Commentary on True and False Religion*, 1525). The Roman Catholic Church, in its sixteenth-century reforming Council of Trent, reaffirmed its belief in transubstantiation.

Debate also began in the late Middle Ages, developed in the Reformation, and continues to this day on the extent to which the Eucharist is a sacrifice. In part this debate is about the nature of priestly and lay power, for the notion of sacrifice in the Eucharist suggests that the priest is exercising a particular kind of spiritual power and authority in the re-enactment of the events of the Passion, in which the body of Christ is broken and his blood shed, and in effecting the transformation of the elements from bread and wine to the body and blood of Christ. This spiritual authority is often signified by the bodily gestures of the priest while he or she is consecrating the elements while presiding at the Eucharist. On the whole Protestants have rejected this notion of sacrifice in the Eucharist, partly because it might be seen to detract from Christ's once-and-for-all act of self-giving on the Cross (in which singular act they believe he redeemed humanity from sin), by suggesting that humans constantly have to petition God to act for our salvation, and partly because of their understanding of the priesthood of all believers by which the authority of their ministers lies in their proclamation of the Word and leading of congregations rather than in any form of sacramental ministry. In the West, Roman Catholics and 'high' Anglicans have continued to debate the notion of sacrifice in the Eucharist, while the Liturgical movement of the twentieth century emphasized the importance of the Eucharist for the corporate life of the Church, thereby reaffirming the notion of the Church as the body of Christ and the active participation of the laity in the Eucharist. Vatican II also stressed these points. JANE SHAW

See also CHRISTIANITY AND THE BODY.

Eugenics

Eugenics The founder of eugenics, Francis Galton, identified it as 'the study of agencies under social control that may improve or impair the racial qualities of future generations either physically or mentally'. Galton was Charles Darwin's cousin and believed that human EVOLUTION could be consciously directed, by using *biometry* to explain the mechanisms of inheritance that would prescribe new rules for human reproduction. Eugenics, therefore, was both a theoretical system and a social cause, which aimed to bring about social and biological improvement of the human race through the application of the study of HEREDITY to human affairs.

Galton developed probabilistic statistics by inventing the correlation coefficient to analyse heredity — his main interest in the 1870s to 1890s. The idea that heredity could be understood through statistical analysis alone, however, was challenged when the works of the Austrian monk, Gregor Mendel, were discovered at the end of the nineteenth century. In the 1860s Mendel had outlined the 'law' of biological inheritance of positive and recessive characteristics. Something of an intellectual rift subsequently developed between biometric and Mendelian research into heredity, symbolized above all by the hostility of Galton's disciple, Karl Pearson, to Mendelianism. Pearson, who held the first Galtonian Chair of Biometry at University College London, refused to join the Eugenics Education Society, founded in Britain in 1907 (and later known as the Eugenics Society), because he believed that they remained too sympathetic to Mendelian research into heredity. In fact the Eugenics Society tried to turn Galton's creed of human racial improvement into a reality by supporting both Mendelian and biometric research into heredity and helping others to develop a method which synthesized both theories, 'pedigree analysis' — and it was renamed the Galton Society after World War II.

Following the establishment of the Eugenics Education Society, enthusiasm for eugenics crossed national boundaries and it promoted an international discourse on the relationship between the quality and quantity of population.

Eugenists believed that modern economies encouraged undesirable — '*dysgenic*' — differential birth rates by facilitating the survival of 'unfit' mental and moral defectives, the chronic sick, residual idlers, recidivist CRIMINALS, and the unemployable. The productive had to bear ever greater tax burdens in order to support the growing numbers of degenerates, and higher fiscal exactions naturally persuaded the prudent middle classes to go in for practices of family limitation. Declining fertility amongst the professional and middle classes, rising birth rates amongst the working classes, and massive reproductive surges amongst the '*lumpenproletariat*' — the unemployed and unemployable — had to be corrected in order to avoid race suicide.

The self-appointed mission of eugenics was to protect 'the unborn' through a programme of selective breeding. Positive eugenics aimed to achieve racial improvement by encouraging the fit to breed, while the goal of negative eugenics was to prevent breeding amongst the unfit. In Britain, Europe, and the US, eugenic reformers advocated MARRIAGE regulation, sequestration of the mentally deficient, and STERILIZATION — voluntary or compulsory — of the unfit. Methods for controlling human reproduction and directing demographic change were applied, however, in different ways in different national contexts.

Before World War I eugenists in Britain concentrated on obtaining the sequestration of the 'feebleminded', which included the mentally retarded, alcoholics, and women who had more than one illegitimate pregnancy. British eugenists also advocated voluntary and compulsory sterilization for various social categories, and some flirted with the idea of the 'lethal chamber' for ridding society of its unwanted; this idea had its most profound expression in Germany in the inter-war period. In Germany and elsewhere, however, negative eugenics can be seen to have accommodated rather than invented a set of political goals whose origins had a much broader cultural base.

Eugenism combined with other ideological cults in Germany during the 1930s and 40s to produce a murderous science which legitimated the '*final solution*' implemented under the Third Reich. When Hitler held a meeting, on August 20 1942, to appoint Otto–Georg Thierack as Reich Justice Minister and Roland Freisler as President of the 'People's Court', he raged about the need to reconstruct the criminal justice system. He vented a tirade about the dysgenic effects of war which left only the poorest stock to breed for the future. The justice system had to be used to rebalance the equation by killing off the 'negative' elements of the population. Punishment was subsequently used to cleanse the 'body of the race' of its undesirable members. Criminals — who, according to the Führer, included the frivolous and the irritable — were not, of course, the only undesirables who were being referred to. Cleansing meant targeting Jews, Gypsies, the mentally ill, and political dissenters for elimination. The relationship between eugenics, social

Darwinism, racial hygiene, and the Nazi policies of elimination is highly complex and fiercely debated by historians. Nazi population policy could be seen as a mixture of science and pseudo-science which informed but did not solely determine the murderous ideology of Fascism. However, although eugenics may not have led directly to the construction of the Final Solution, it played a significant role in providing it with a rationalist authority. It provided similar legitimate authority to the debate about population quality elsewhere.

Eugenics won enthusiastic disciples during the Progressive Era in the US, appealing to both the conservationist and the technocratic ideas of the movement. Eugenics was embraced by a number of reform movements, which espoused the ideas of Progressivism. Sex educationalists in the social hygiene movement believed that 'eugenics will destroy that sentimentalism which leads a woman deliberately to marry a man who is absolutely unworthy of her and can only bring disease, degradation and death.' Margaret Sanger supported her leadership of the birth control movement with eugenic arguments about stemming the tide of the reproduction of the unfit. In the US and elsewhere, however, other eugenists were extremely cautious about the question of birth control. Some were concerned that those whom they wanted to breed actually used CONTRACEPTION most — the middle class and the economically prudent. In Britain the Eugenics Education Society were hostile to the activities of the Neo-Malthusian League because they feared that the widespread availability of contraception would simply enhance the decline of the middle-class birth rate, which was already fearfully low.

In the US eugenics successfully influenced three other policy areas: marriage regulation, sterilization of the unfit, and immigration restriction. By 1914 thirty states passed laws preventing marriage of the mentally handicapped and the insane, together with laws restricting marriage between people suffering a venereal disease, or between those from various categories of 'feebleminded'. The first state sterilization law was passed in Indiana in 1907, and by 1917 fifteen other states had followed suit. Sterilization was legal for habitual criminals plus various categories of the insane, mentally handicapped, and epileptic. Eugenics in the US also provided ideological justifications for immigration restriction and the development of IQ testing.

By the inter-war years eugenics in Britain focused on the declining birth rate, the changing demographic structure of the population, family allowances and family tax relief, voluntary sterilization, popularizing the idea of the eugenic marriage, and raising a eugenic consciousness throughout society. The British biologist, Julian Huxley, and the long-serving secretary of the Eugenics Education Society in the 1920s and 30s, C. P. Blacker, suggested that eugenics should become a form of social consciousness, which elevated the needs of the community above those of the individual, thereby facilitating the creation of a planned Utopian society.

'Reform' eugenics in Britain and Europe in the inter-war period claimed that social systems and philosophies based upon individualism, such as capitalism and nationalism, were dysgenic because rigid social stratification failed to maximize the reproduction of hereditary talents, which were distributed throughout all social divisions. Capitalism, for example, failed to provide favourable conditions for the most able amongst the labouring classes to rise to higher social and economic status and reproduce their hereditary endowments. Equally, the least able in all classes were not prevented from reproducing their inadequacies in their offspring. In place of the class system, a eugenic utopia would provide an equalized environment maximizing the possibility for the expression of desirable genetic qualities. Improvement of the social environment was crucial if a eugenically sound society was to be achieved.

While concern over the differential birth rate remained central amongst eugenic thinkers, the demographic debate broadened to include discussions of the changing age structure of the population. The transformation of the demographic structure of modern industrial societies, with smaller productive populations supporting expanding numbers of ageing, chronically sick, and unproductive dependants, led eugenists in Britain and Europe to advocate the introduction of family allowances and tax relief to encourage large families amongst both the working and the middle classes in order to check these trends. The broadening of the demographic debate was accompanied by the modernization of discussions about sterilization. The eugenic campaign for voluntary sterilization in Britain and elsewhere in Europe now suggested that the people most likely to be enthusiastic about legal voluntary sterilization would be working-class mothers with no other access to reliable birth control.

Eugenism in this period became a loose synthesis of widely divergent ideologies. The *Eugenics Review* reflected the broad cross-section of eugenic interpretations of demography and degeneration. British eugenists were enthusiastic about the first sterilization laws set up in Germany in 1933, admired the Nazi policy of family allowance and tax relief, which assisted 'Aryan' early marriage and large families, and approved of the courage of the new regime in introducing compulsory sterilization of the mentally defective. However, British eugenists were at pains to point out the differences between German and British proposals for legal sterilization. The British Eugenics Society wanted a law based on consent, with legal protection for the 'liberty of the individual'. Blacker, in particular, perceived the need, early on, publicly to separate the identity of British from German eugenics, although he was privately aware of the members of the Society who wholeheartedly approved of the German measures.

In Britain, Europe, and the US, the popular appeal and intellectual legitimacy of eugenics declined after World War II following revelations of the mass murder perpetrated by the Third Reich. Nevertheless, eugenic ideology did continue to influence post-war ideas about the social applications of medicine. Enthusiastic supporters of social medicine, for example, believed that a form of whole-person clinical practice should mix prevention and cure by synthesizing an understanding of the effects of environment and endowment upon physiological variability. In this context doctors could use knowledge of susceptibilities to advise a pattern of life and a policy of reproduction for their patients which would prevent the onset of disease either in themselves or their offspring. Such ideas eventually provided a blueprint for genetic counselling.

The development of MOLECULAR BIOLOGY and embryology since World War II have greatly enhanced the possibilities of genetically engineering future populations. While genetic counselling has currently been limited to providing prospective parents with advice about known hereditary diseases, such as Huntington's Chorea and Cystic Fibrosis, there has been popular speculation about the possibility of 'designing' the babies of the future. Tests for fetal gender have already resulted in controversial ABORTION practices amongst communities throughout the world who place a higher cultural value on a male than a female life.

For the first three decades after World War II, genetics limited its investigations largely to the hereditary nature of physiological diseases and characteristics. By contrast, contemporary molecular biology is once again beginning to cross into the social and psychological realm by claiming to be able to identify the genetic source of various forms of behaviour. The determinants of human behaviour, however, continue to be highly disputed amongst social, psychological, and biological scientists, and what has been identified in the Western media as the 'New Eugenics' is once again at the forefront of public debate. Some public commentators from both the scientific and lay communities have speculated that this debate is likely to become one of the most urgent in the post-industrial societies of the twenty-first century.

DOROTHY PORTER

Further reading

Evans, R. (1997). In Search of Social Darwinism. The histiography of the concept. In *Medicine and modernity. Public health and medical care in nineteenth and twentieth century Germany*, (ed. M. Berg and G. Cocks). Cambridge University Press.

Kevles, D. (1985). *In the name of Eugenics. Genetics and the uses of human heredity.* Knopf, New York.

Mazumdar, P. M. H. (1992). *Eugenics, genetics and human failings.* Routledge, London.

Soloway, R. (1990). *Demography and degeneration.* The University of North Carolina Press, Chapel Hill.

See also GENOCIDE; HEREDITY; STERILIZATION.

Eunuchs From the Greek 'eunouchos', meaning 'eunê' (bed) and 'echein' (to have charge of), the word eunuch literally means 'chamberlain'. As the traditional sense of the word seems to imply, not every person referred to as a eunuch was necessarily castrated. In ancient and oriental history not every favourite minister of the king who was given the name eunuch had necessarily 'suffered the cut'. It was rather the humility and loyalty of these chamberlains, along with other behaviourial characteristics traditionally associated with eunuchs, which gave them their name. There were three different types of eunuch identifiable by the three different methods of CASTRATION. The slaves whose PENIS and TESTES had both been severed were called *castrati* by the Romans and *sandali* or *es-sendelle* by the Arabs. *Spadones* was the word used to describe those eunuchs whose testicles had been literally torn from their bodies, but not cut off. By far the most common method of emasculation was to detach the testicles by a single cut, and these eunuchs, who were called *thlibias* or *semivir*, retained their penis.

From a physiological point of view, two different types of eunuchs can be distinguished depending on whether castration has taken place before or after PUBERTY. In the latter case, eunuchs retain, in some instances, the capacity to achieve ERECTION, and the penis, if still present, maintains its normal size. In the case of emasculation before puberty many features of childhood are prolonged. The voice, for example, stays high-pitched, the body develops a rounded contour, and the loss of HORMONES produces an unusual tallness and also prevents the skin from tanning.

From the point of view of mythological beliefs, many ancient sources seem to point to Semiramis, a mythical Persian queen, as the initiator of this cruel practice. The French erudite Ancillon, who anonymously published a book on the subject at the beginning of the eighteenth century, refers to Poliphar as the first eunuch mentioned in the Bible. Apart from those who were castrated as a result of their defeat in warfare — a practice very well documented throughout the course of history — eunuchs constituted political or religious institutions in Assyria, Persia, Greece, Egypt, Ethiopia, Russia, Italy, and China. In China, the existence of eunuchs can be traced to the eighth century BC. In many of these cases, eunuchs were subject socially to a mixture of respect and repulsion. According to the English historian Gibbon, they constituted a moral plague in the court of the Roman emperors Gordiano III, Constancio Honorio, and Arcadius.

Eunuchs are also found in religious rites. The cult of Artemisa, in the sanctuary of Ephesus, was hosted by virgins and eunuchs, and the priests of the goddess Cybele shared the same condition. Furthermore, the spring festivals of this latter goddess, who, according to the legend, had fallen in love with Attis, who was either castrated while he slept or emasculated himself, seemed to have favoured self-mutilation among their followers. This practice, usually connected with the attempt to avoid the sin of fornication, has continued until relatively recent times among certain Russian religious sects.

Historically, the most famous eunuchs have been the Muslim slaves who were in charge of the seraglio. The life of these eunuchs was described by the French philosopher Montesquieu in his *Letters persanes*, published in 1721. Equally famous were the singers of Italian baroque music, the most renowned among them being the Italian castrato Carlo Broschi Farinelli (1705–82).   J. MOSCOSO

See also CASTRATION.

Euphoria The French novelist, Michel Tournier, believed that euphoria carried within its etymology the key to a fundamental transformation in the Western conception of the self. The word, which is now interpreted as little more than a feeling of light-headedness or a general sensation of well-being, originally occupied a much more moral position. Its Greek root of *eu*, meaning goodness, happiness, or contentment, and *phoria*, signifying the act of carrying, reveal a more effort-bound situation in which the individual supports happiness or bears themself with joy. The etymology suggests that contentment and joy are states demanding a persistent and active engagement. Tournier draws a parallel with the coterminous etymology of Christopher, from the martyred giant who achieved his sainthood by carrying Christ.

This idea of euphoria as a state achieved through effort and activity has now largely disappeared. With the advent of Christianity and the rise of Calvinism, in particular, a more passive view of the self and its EMOTIONS has emerged. Euphoria is now regarded as a state which overwhelms the personality. In medical terms euphoria is defined as a form of mood elevation inappropriate to circumstances, brought on by diseases of the NERVOUS SYSTEM such as syphilis or multiple sclerosis. In religious terms it connotes the epiphanies and awakenings of passive soul. The American psychologist, William James, described the state as one 'in which the will to assert ourselves and hold our own has been displaced by a willingness to hold our mouths and be as nothing in the floods and waterspouts of God.' James offered his own explanation for this connection between euphoria and passivity, arguing that the emotion emerged only when the self gave up its struggle with the world and instead surrendered to the uprushes of the subconscious life.

In recent years, a middle way has emerged between the active and passive models of euphoria. The growing use of euphoriant drugs such as MDMA ('ecstasy') and MDEA ('eve') has encouraged a new perspective in which the emotional life is seen as the passive product of the brain's biochemistry whilst the self maintains the familiar control and discrimination of the modern consumer.

In medical terms, as well as its association with such drugs, euphoria, defined as mood elevation inappropriate to the circumstances, may accompany mental illness and diseases affecting the nervous system, such as syphilis and multiple sclerosis.   RHODRI HAYWARD

See also EMOTION; PLEASURE.

Eurhythmics was the name given by Emile Jaques-Dalcroze (1865–1950), a Swiss composer and teacher of music, to his system of training that linked musical rhythm with movements of the body. He gave instruction in his method in Dresden before World War I, and later, in 1915, he founded his own Institute in Geneva. Marie Rambert was one of his notable disciples: she learnt the method from him, passed it on to the Diaghilev BALLET and later applied it in her own company. 'Eurhythmy', or 'eurhythmic', from the Greek meaning good proportion or rhythm, had been used earlier in several contexts including architectural harmony, postural grace, and regular pulse.   S.J.

See BALLET; MUSIC AND THE BODY.

Eustachian tube Lying beyond the eardrum is the *middle ear*, a tiny air-filled cavity in the *temporal bone* of the skull, which is connected to the back of the throat by the eustachian tube. In adult humans, the eustachian tube, which was first described by Bartholomeo Eustachio in the sixteenth century, is just less than 4 cm long and lies at an angle of 45° relative to the horizontal plane. The bottom end of the eustachian tube, which opens into the *nasopharynx*, is composed of membrane and CARTILAGE and is normally closed. However, it is essential for proper sound conduction through the ear that the eustachian tube opens periodically, so that the air pressure within each middle ear can be matched to that of the surrounding atmosphere. This occurs as a result of the contraction of the muscles that surround the eustachian tube during sneezing, forceful nose blowing, yawning, and SWALLOWING (both when eating or drinking and throughout the day and night as build up of saliva and mucus stimulates the swallowing reflex). Opening of the eustachian tube also serves to drain any fluid that builds up in the middle ear into the nasopharynx.

The discomfort in the ears that sometimes follows marked changes in atmospheric pressure — caused, for example, by rapid descent in an aircraft or compression in a DIVING suit — is due to differences in pressure on either side of the eardrum. The unpleasant feeling can usually be overcome by yawning or some other means of opening the eustachian tubes. This is why scuba divers are taught to hold their noses and blow as they descend, and the same technique helps when an aircraft is landing.

The middle ear cavity, eustachian tube, and upper respiratory tract are lined by a continuous layer of MUCOUS MEMBRANE. It is therefore not surprising that infections of the nasopharynx — including the common cold — readily reach the

middle ear via the eustachian tube. Infants and young children are particularly susceptible to such acute infections, which usually cause ear pain and fever, possibly because the eustachian tube is wider, shorter, and more horizontal than it is in adults. This can lead to a build up of fluid in the middle ear in a condition known as *otitis media* with effusion or 'glue ear'.

Accumulation of mucus in the eustachian tube, associated with inflammation of the middle ear, impedes the flow of air along the tube and results in negative pressure within the middle ear cavity. This causes the eardrum to be pushed inwards by the greater pressure of the atmosphere. Occlusion of the eustachian tube produces a sense of fullness in the affected ear and a mild conductive HEARING LOSS, which may be increased if there is fluid in the middle ear. The sensation of popping in the ears that results when the nose is blown vigorously during a cold is due to air being forced up a blocked eustachian tube. Because of the increased difficulty in equalizing middle ear pressure, people with upper respiratory tract infections are more likely to suffer from ear discomfort when flying.   ANDREW J. KING

Further reading

Bluestone, C. D. and Klein, J. O. (1995). *Otitis media in infants and children*, (2nd edn). W. B. Saunders, Philadelphia.

See also DIVING; FLYING; HEARING; SWALLOWING.

Euthanasia The ideals of bodily incorruptibility and immortality have been envisaged in many cultures and religions: Christianity, for instance, holds that, had man not sinned and been expelled from Paradise, there would have been no disease and death. In truth, mortality has been the great, omnipresent mystery — beyond man's powers and in the hands of the gods or fate. Hence man has tried to tame death.

On the one hand, there have been efforts to prolong life with a view to creating quasi-eternal existence on earth. With the alchemy of the Middle Ages, partly borrowed from the Arabs, an ambitious quest for the prolongation of life entered Western culture. The thirteenth-century cleric Roger Bacon claimed that Christian medicine would surpass pagan science by the conquest of senescence. Francis Bacon and the later philosophers of the Enlightenment expressed confidence that the advancement of science would produce the indefinite prolongation of life.

On the other hand, there has been the ambition of mastering death, not by preventing it, but by controlling its timing, means, and manner. Within traditional Christian culture, a good death (as prescribed by the *ars moriendi* — the art of dying well) was a Christian death; departing in a state of grace, denouncing Satan, praying to God, repenting one's sins, and (for Roman Catholics) receiving the sacraments.

Increasingly, from the eighteenth century, the good death became a rather more secularized concept, and within that framework euthanasia assumed relevance. In its original meaning, however, 'euthanasia' referred to any means for securing an 'easy' death; for example, by leading a temperate life or by cultivating an acceptance of mortality. The *Discorsi della vita sobria* (*Discourses on the Temperate Life*) of Luigi Cornaro (*c.* 1463–1566!), written in his eighties and frequently consulted into the eighteenth century, featured both an easy (or holy) terminus in advanced years and the prospect of longer life — up to 120 years — through the pursuit of moderation in food, drink, and lifestyle.

Francis Bacon praised prolongevity as the 'most noble' purpose of medicine. He also argued that relief of suffering was a desideratum in terminal care, and that the physician may sometimes hasten death. The Enlightenment brought intense interest in prolongevity. Benjamin Franklin boldly declared senescence to be not a natural process but a 'disease' to be cured, and he predicted that longevity might stretch to a thousand years or more. The Marquis Condorcet and William Godwin speculated about virtually immortal life.

But 'euthanasia' increasingly came to connote measures taken by the physician, including the possibility of hastening death to prevent pain or suffering. At the same time, the idea of dying well was secularized. The traditional good death scenario — calling upon God and renouncing Satan — gave way to an emphasis upon a quiet and peaceful death. Tranquil death, it was argued, should be like sleep. A peaceful death betokened a serene conscience, a life well lived. It squared with Romantic notions of the beauty of death, particularly in those who died young. Thus, in the new idea of euthanasia emerging in the nineteenth century, it was the duty of the doctor to ensure a peaceful death, by careful management, and judicious application of opiates to dull pain and induce coma. At the wishes of family or patient, the family doctor was doubtless the frequent agent of informal (and illegal) euthanasia in the nineteenth and twentieth century.

Any trend there had been towards the informal acceptance of euthanasia was rendered more problematic in recent times. The Nazis introduced legal euthanasia, approved by doctors, for selected people such as the severely mentally disabled, on the grounds that they had a life which was not worth living. The later extension to persons considered simply undesirable — Jews, Gypsies, and homosexuals — perverted euthanasia to supremely evil purposes. The Nazi 'final solution' has created suspicion that any broader acceptance, practice, or legalization of euthanasia would be the thin end of the wedge that in due course would lead to (possibly compulsory) public euthanasia programmes for problematic or costly people, especially the very old, the poor, and the demented.

In addition, death now increasingly occurs in public institutions, notably hospitals and hospices. This may make humane euthanasia more difficult, as physicians and nursing staff involved in such practices may be justifiably afraid that they thereby risk exposure and legal prosecution.

Those liable to promote such exposure are established religious groups, including Roman Catholics, Orthodox Jews and pressure groups such as 'Life'. They fundamentally disapprove of mercy killing on religious grounds, and may believe that suffering is God's will and that God alone should determine when life ends.

Yet the conditions of modern death and recent developments in medicine are also increasing advocacy and desire for euthanasia. Life-saving and life-supporting technologies now make it possible to interrupt and extend the natural dying process. RESUSCITATION or ANTIBIOTICS may defer death, and life may be sustained by ventilators or tube feeding when there is no prospect of recovery. It has become widely accepted that withholding or withdrawing treatment in such circumstances — for example for those with advanced CANCER or PARALYSIS, or in a permanent VEGETATIVE STATE — is good medical practice and also legal. At the same time developments in palliative care aim to ease the pain and distress of the conscious dying person by the judicious use of drugs. Such drugs may hasten death, but provided the intention is to control symptoms this is accepted morally and legally by the doctrine of double effect. Whilst these humane approaches — non-treatment decisions, and drugs for symptom control — are generally accepted, there remains acute controversy about the deliberate administration of lethal doses of drugs or other measures to ensure death, whether as active euthanasia, or 'physician-assisted suicide'.

Euthanasia may be squared with the professional ethics of the physician and with normal morality through the argument that, while it is the doctor's duty to save life, that duty does not run so far as to prolong life through artificial means in all circumstances.

Changes in opinion, public policy, and medical practice have been most marked in the Netherlands, where since 1984 the national medical association has accepted medical euthanasia, under strictly controlled circumstances. Although this remained unlawful until 2001, there were no prosecutions provided that doctors abided by strict guidelines based on a patient's valid request. By 1995 a survey suggested that active euthanasia (a physician humanely intervening to end a terminally-ill patient's life at the request of that patient) was taking place in around 1.8% of all deaths. (In some 87% of such cases, the patient was expected to be able to live, or to be kept alive, only for a further month.) Public acceptance of this practice had been facilitated by the development of 'living wills'. Since 1994 in the Netherlands, physicians have been legally obliged to honour 'living wills' — a measure welcomed by the medical profession as it absolves them of legal problems. Acceptance of euthanasia seems equally widespread amongst religious and non-religious Dutch people, though members of the Dutch Reformed (Calvinist) Church still tend to be distrustful of the practice. Such practices have met with a

much more divided reception elsewhere. In Britain, where euthanasia remains illegal, the pressure group Exit has been subject to prosecution, as has the controversial American pathologist, Dr Jack Kevorkian, who has advocated and participated in doctor-assisted suicide at the patient's request.

The advance of modern medicine presents deep dilemmas. If a patient is in a permanent coma, should LIFE SUPPORT measures be employed? And should a patient near death from both painful cancer and debilitating heart disease be resuscitated? No easy answers are available to any such questions, which set the sanctity of human life against the question of personal autonomy, and raise fundamental legal and moral questions as to the ownership of the body.

ROY PORTER
BRYAN JENNETT

Further reading

Baruch, A. B. (ed.) (1989). *Suicide and euthanasia: historical and contemporary themes.* Kluwer, Dordrecht.

British Medical Association (2001). *Withholding and withdrawing life-prolonging medical treatment: guidance for decision making.* 2nd ed BMJ Books, London.

See also DEATH; EUGENICS; SUICIDE; VEGETATIVE STATE.

Evil eye Belief in the evil eye — that a human being can cause injury or death through a malevolent glance or stare — is a very widespread one, found in ancient Greek and Roman literature, in the Jewish, Christian, Bhuddist, Islamic, and Hindi traditions and, more generally, in the culture of most pre-literate societies. The exact nature of the damage which the evil eye is supposed to cause varies between cultures, but children and animals have often been thought to be most vulnerable, while already problematic experiences such as marriage or childbirth were also considered to be occasions when the evil eye could act especially effectively. Very often, the harm inflicted by the evil eye was linked to the envy of the person doing the harming, and the possession of an evil eye was often thought to reside in persons who displayed more general anti-social tendencies, such as meanness, selfishness, and envy. Accordingly, in many cultures (for example, pre-World War II central European Jewry) people were at pains not to advertise their wealth, talents, or achievements, lest this should bring down retribution from the malevolent and envious, while new-born babies, prominent men, and beautiful women were thought especially likely to attract the evil eye. Most cultures also recommended means of protection against the evil eye. Most often this was by amulets or charms, but sometimes by more immediate action such as spitting in the presence of, or making obscene gestures at, the person thought to possess the evil eye.

Although ethnographers and folklorists have noted the frequency with which belief in the evil eye has existed, they have been less forthcoming on the most important concern for the historian of the body: where the power to do harm in this way is thought to come from and how it is exercised. Again, ideas on this matter vary between cultures, but a few general points seem clear. Many religions believe in the existence of an all-seeing deity, which links the power of VISION, and hence the eye, very clearly to wider considerations of power and knowledge. These wider considerations led to such conceptualizations as that current in Christian Europe by the late Middle Ages, that the eye is not just the window of the soul, or a visible portrait of the invisible soul, but also a visible centre from which rays of sight emanate. There was proverbial wisdom in England around 1600 that the eyes were the window of the heart or the mind, for joy or anger could be seen through them.

A demonstration of how various ideas on the evil eye might run together at about that date is provided by Reginald Scot, an English gentleman who in 1584 published *The Discoverie of Witchcraft*, a sceptical tract which denied the existence of witches. Scot devoted a chapter of his book to 'inchanting or bewitching eies'. Here he cited such classical authors as Virgil, Theocritus, Cicero, Plutarch, and Philarchus. Some people, according to these writers, had two eyeballs, one of which was the seat of evil power which could be used to hurt young lambs or young children. Other people, it was held

'reteine such venome in their eies, and send it foorth by beames and streames so violentlie, and therewith they annoie not onlie them with whom they are conversant continuallie; but also all other, whose companie they frequent, of what age, strength or complexion so ever they be'.

Scot wrote of more general beliefs, which held that spirits emerging from the eye could infect the hearts of those against whom they were directed. He also noted that occult powers were ascribed to the gaze of

'old women, in whome the ordinarie course of nature faileth in the office of purging their naturall monethlie humors'.

Froth would therefore be left on mirrors which post-menopausal women had looked at.

These sorts of belief were clearly widespread, as was another set of beliefs, those in sympathetic magic or occult forces more generally. Thus it was easy to accept that malicious power could be transmitted through the eye, the window into the soul of the malevolent person. Some traditions gave a more elaborate explanation: post-Talmudic Jewish literature held variously that the evil eye contained the element of fire, and hence spread destruction, or that the glance of an angry man called into being an angry angel who took vengeance on the object of wrath. Belief in the evil eye also connected with a broader folklore about the eye. One very relevant belief, again seemingly widespread, was that meeting a person with a squint might lead to misfortune or loss. Here the connection is clear enough: an obvious physical deformity is linked with a supposed

inner deformity, the willingness to do harm. But, at the very least, this widespread belief in the power of the evil eye demonstrates how one of the human senses, and the organ connected with it, could be seen as a channel for spreading harm, and also provides an interesting way of exploring some aspects of the folklore of the human body.

J. A. SHARPE

See also WITCHCRAFT.

Evolution The theory of evolution is the view that species change over time. Before Charles Darwin (1809–82), most people in the West followed Aristotle in thinking of species as immutable. Dogs could only ever give birth to dogs, and so one species could never 'transmutate' into another. This view was increasingly challenged during the eighteenth century, but it was not until Darwin published the *Origin of Species* in 1859 that the theory of evolution became widely accepted. Darwin's originality lay in proposing a mechanism by which evolution could occur — natural selection.

For a species to evolve by natural selection, three conditions must hold: (i) the members of the species must differ with respect to their chances of surviving and having offspring; (ii) these differences must be capable of being passed on to offspring; (iii) there must be occasional mutations that cause offspring to differ from their parents in ways that affect the survival chances of the offspring.

Once these conditions are in place, the species will evolve, and may in time become so different as to warrant being described as a different species.

Before Darwin, the few people who did subscribe to the theory of evolution tended to believe that the gradual change of one species into another was guided by some kind of purpose or plan. On this view, the theory of evolution was not a great threat to the idea of a divine creator. The idea that evolution occurs by means of natural selection changed all that because it assumes that the mutations which are the ultimate source of all evolutionary change are essentially random. This introduces an irreducible element of contingency into the evolutionary process, which is antithetical to any idea of a divine plan. In Darwin's theory, human beings and all other living things on this planet are, in an important sense, just accidents.

The idea that mutations are random does not mean that they are not caused. It simply means that mutations occur without any consideration for the future direction of evolution. Mutations are, so to speak, 'blind'. Most mutations are deleterious, because for any complex organism there are far more ways of making it less effective than of improving it. These deleterious mutations are selected against. The bulk of the work of natural selection thus consists of winnowing out the bad mutations. Only occasionally does a good mutation come along, but these are retained by natural selection and over time they accumulate to produce adaptations.

Adaptations are features of organisms that show complex design and that serve (or once served) some vital function. For example, the eye is an adaptation for seeing; its complex, camera-like design is suited for that function and not any other. Before Darwin, many people argued that such complex designed features were proof of the existence of a designer, i.e. God. By showing how complex designs could emerge without the aid of a supernatural designer, Darwin demolished this argument for the existence of God.

Though Darwin's theory of evolution by natural selection was rapidly accepted by many biologists after the publication of the *Origin of Species*, its explanatory power was weakened by the fact that there was no satisfactory theory of HEREDITY until the rediscovery in 1900 of a seminal paper written in 1866 by Gregor Mendel (1822–84). From Mendel's work came the idea of hereditary particles (now called 'GENES') that were transmitted from parents to offspring and that caused the development of particular traits. This idea paved the way for the crucial distinction between genotype (the set of genes possessed by an organism) and phenotype (the physical and behavioural traits of the organism, which develop as a result of the genes interacting with the environment).

The distinction between genotype and phenotype allowed certain refinements to be made to Darwin's theory of evolution by natural selection. In the modern theory, information passes in only one direction — from the genotype to the phenotype. This is why mutations are random with respect to the direction of evolution, because the genes have no way of 'knowing' how best to mutate. This contrasts with the view put forward by Jean Baptiste de Lamarck (1744–1829), which Darwin himself accepted, according to which organisms could pass on to their offspring characteristics that they had acquired during their lifetime. In Lamarck's famous illustration, ancestral giraffes strenuously extended their necks to reach the leaves at the top of the trees, and their necks grew as a result of this effort. Their offspring were then born with longer necks. For this to occur, information would have to flow back from the phenotype of the adult giraffe and change the genes in some way so that the offspring would inherit genes for a longer neck. The mutations would not then be random with respect to the direction of evolution.

Twentieth-century developments in the science of genetics showed Lamarck to have been wrong. The 'central dogma' of modern genetics supports the view that information can only flow from the genotype to the phenotype, and not vice versa. In fact, the development of genetics was crucial to Darwinism in many other ways too. For example, the theory of population genetics, developed by Ronald Fisher (1890–1962), J. B. S. Haldane (1892–1964); and Sewall Wright (1889–1988), in the first few decades of the twentieth century, allowed evolutionary problems to be tested quantitatively. The principle achievement of these theorists was to

259

integrate Darwinian theory and genetics into a single body of theory which is now known as 'neo-Darwinism', or the 'modern synthesis', after the title of a book by Julian Huxley, *Evolution: The Modern Synthesis* (1942).

In population genetics, evolution is now defined as change from one generation to the next in gene frequency. Suppose we take all the organisms in a particular population and look to see what genes are present at a given locus in the genome. On the one hand, all the organisms might have exactly the same kind of gene at that locus: in that case, there is no variation in the population at that locus, so there can be no evolution at that locus. On the other hand, we might find that half the organisms have one variant of the gene at that locus, while the other half have another variant (in technical terms, the two groups are said to have different 'alleles'). If we then looked at the population a generation later, and found that the frequencies of the two variants had changed — for example, if only 25% of the population had the first variant, while the second variant was now found in 75% of the organisms — then and only then could evolution be said to have occurred. In fact, it would still be a case of evolution even if the change in gene frequency had no observable phenotypic effect (that is, no detectable difference between individuals with the different variants).

Natural selection is not the only means by which evolution occurs. Gene frequency can change from one generation to another as a result of other forces, such as random drift, mutation, and migration. However, unlike natural selection, these other forces cannot produce adaptations. One of the debates in contemporary evolutionary theory concerns the relative importance of natural selection *vis-à-vis* the other forces, such as random drift. On one side, thinkers such as George Williams and Richard Dawkins have emphasized the role of natural selection, because they are primarily interested in studying adaptations. On the other side, writers such as Stephen Jay Gould have emphasized the role of non-adaptive forces, like random drift.   DYLAN EVANS

Further reading
Darwin, C. (1859). *The origin of species*. Penguin, Harmondsworth (1968).

Dennett, D. (1995). *Darwin's dangerous idea: evolution and the meanings of life*. Penguin, Harmondsworth.

Evolution, human The human body is the end product of a long period of evolution, stretching back millions of years. In the case of some aspects of our body, the ancestry goes back not just a few million years, but hundreds of millions. The basic layout of the human body, for example, is that of the vertebrates (being bilaterally symmetrical, organized around the backbone) and of the reptiles and amphibians (in having a pair of hind limbs and forelimbs, each with five digits — fingers or toes — at the end of

them). But like every species, humans have a shape that is unique to themselves. Among primates, our closest evolutionary relatives, humans have three features that stand out — upright POSTURE and WALKING, a relatively large BRAIN, and relative hairlessness.

Most primates live in trees, and they do so like all mammals by using all four limbs (or in the case of spider monkeys, five — their tails are also prehensile and can grasp things). Their HANDS and FEET can both be used for grasping. In this sense, all non-human primates are quadrupedal. In the case of something like an orang utan, LEGS and ARMS, hands and feet are equally mobile and dextrous, and in a way all act more like arms than legs — for holding and grasping, rather than support. With baboons the forelimbs and hindlimbs are both rather leg-like, and support the animal as it moves quadrupedally over the ground, rather like a dog. For the gibbon, the only truly arm-swinging primate, the arms are long and flexible, and the legs, short and reduced — basically to get them out of the way as the owner brachiates through the trees.

Everything about the human body is either a retention of these basic characteristics, or else has been modified by evolution. The grasping hand, the relatively mobile shoulder, the eyes that look forward with stereoscopic VISION, are all part of the human being's ancient primate heritage. Each evolved for some reason in our past, long before any movement towards the human condition, but has remained useful and has been built upon. The close-set eyes that look directly forward, with overlapping fields of vision, evolved among the earlier primates, to allow them to judge distances in three-dimensional space — an essential part of leaping perilously from one tree branch to another. The ability to co-ordinate this vision with dextrous hand movements is an old evolutionary heritage, but one that is used every time we catch a ball or calculate whether it is safe to overtake a car at 100 km per hour.

While our body is a cumulative and often messy mix of this ancient past, it is also the product of a unique evolutionary history shared with no other living primate. It is often said that humans are the most generalized of species, lacking all the specializations that characterize other animals such as giraffes, with their long necks, or elephants, with their trunks. In actual fact, as primates we are very specialized in one way — BIPEDALISM. Unlike virtually all other primates, we are highly dedicated ground-dwellers, and indeed are fairly poor at climbing and clambering in trees. Our ability to walk upright habitually and easily is our most distinctive and in many ways most divergent characteristic. It has also shaped virtually all aspects of our body, from head to toe. Our foot is effectively a highly sprung platform, with arches in two directions to take the endless pounding of hitting the ground, and to push off into the next stride. It is heavily built compared with the feet of monkeys and apes, and has lost any ability to grasp. The knee is

also built to take pressure, being large, and heavily constrained in sideways movement. The leg as a whole is very long, to ensure a large stride. The PELVIS is perhaps the most modified part of the body, being turned from a long baton for connecting upper and lower parts of the body, to a large bowl to take all the weight of the upper body, which is now resting entirely on two legs. The vertebral column is also robust. Unlike the back of a quadruped, which is built with a single arch like a cantilevered bridge, the human spine is S-shaped. The head is also modified, being perched more vertically on the spine.

The overall impression of a human from an evolutionary perspective is a tall, cylindrical shape, a linear design. There has been considerable debate as to the evolutionary pressures that have shaped the human body, and it looks as if there are two main factors involved. The first is that bipedalism is an energy-saving way of moving on the ground: since our ancestors had to cope with the disappearance of forests, and search widely for food in dry African environments, it was the most evolutionarily effective way, turning an arm-swinging, tree-dwelling ape into a terrestrial specialist. The other factor is temperature. The open savannas where the earliest bipeds evolved were hot, with little shade, and the effect of the sun would have been severe. One of the effects of an upright posture is to reduce the area of the body that receives direct sunlight, and to remove more of it away from the reflected heat of the ground. The human body, then, was forged by selection in the heat of the more open plains of Africa.

Evolution is the process of change over time, over thousands and millions of years. The fossil record has shown that the basics of bipedalism go right back to the roots of our evolutionary history, back to over four million years ago, soon (in evolutionary terms) after our ancestors diverged from the ancestors of the living chimpanzees, our closest relatives. The modern form of bipedalism, with the cylindrical, linear pattern, is probably about two million years old. With bipedalism would have come other changes. The hand, no longer needed to support the body in movement, became the highly dextrous and finely-tuned structure that we use today for so many activities.

The upright stance is such a universal and uniform human characteristic that it is taken totally for granted: it is the essence of humanity. Around the world, though, the human body comes in enormous variety — tall, short, fat, thin, hairy, smooth, dark, and light. Unlike the basic upright body plan, these variations are not millions of years old, but just a few tens of thousands or even less. But they are still the product of evolution. Once again the environment has played a major part. Although humans vary in the amount of hair cover they have, they are, by comparison with apes, largely hairless. This is again a response to heat. Humans have evolved a copious SWEATING system — we use the evaporation of moisture from the skin to cool our body, and this built; people in the tropics are small, linear, and lean.

While the human body has evolved to suit the environment, especially the temperature, it has been affected by one other major factor — sex. Evolution is driven by selection — the survival of those best suited to the environment — but Darwin pointed out that there were two elements to this; natural selection and sexual selection. Most of the characteristics described so far have been the product of natural selection, but much of the human body is probably the result of how males and females have chosen their mates, and how well they are able to reproduce. Out of this has arisen the differences between the sexes. Some of these differences have a direct function — women have wider hips than men, compensating for the narrower birth outlet forced by bipedalism. Others are probably related to the preferences of men or women — larger breasts and curvaceous hips in women, for example. These secondary sexual characteristics may have their basis in some function, but are as much a signal and a symbol, and selected as such — in this case, a signal of FERTILITY. Men also give signals with their bodies — simple ones related to strength and size, but also more subtle ones, such as grey hair or BALDNESS as a sign of having lived a long time — and therefore being a successful male. Most characteristics, though, are a mixture of the sexual and functional. Men often prefer women who are more curvaceous, which is often related to fat deposition — women lay down fat more easily than men. This fat is also necessary for ensuring that a woman is well-nourished, and thus better able to withstand the costs of pregnancy and lactation. Women may prefer large, strong men, but such men may also be better at other things, such as hunting or fighting, and thus better adapted.

In the end, the evolution of the human body is a seamless mix of sex, reproduction, activity, and environment; it is also a mix of the very old and the very new, and over evolutionary time has changed and shifted. In some ways it is a sleek and efficient machine; in others, it is full of flaws. In this sense it is like any other evolutionary product, a compromise between all the demands placed on it during the course of the many different lives that humans have to live, have lived in the past, and will live in the future.

ROBERT FOLEY

Further reading

Aiello, L. and Dean, M.C. (1990) *An introduction to Human Evolutionary Anatomy.* Academic Press, London.

See also BIPEDALISM; EVOLUTION; HEREDITY, LANGUAGE AND THE BRAIN.

Excretion is the transfer of substances out of a living organism into its environment. At its simplest, for single-cell forms of life, this involves extrusion across the cell membrane of the unwanted or potentially toxic by-products of respiration and metabolism. This is also what is

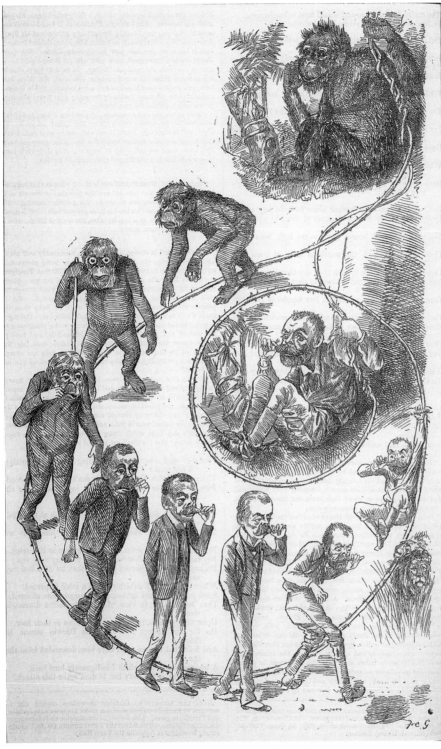

The ascent from ape to man: a Victorian representation. Mary Evans Picture Library.

works more effectively where the air can move freely over the skin — that is, where there is no hair. As a whole, therefore, the species is 'naked' — not actually hairless, but with a miniaturized hair cover. And those people who have a long history of living in the hotter parts of the world are the most hairless. SKIN COLOUR follows this pattern, with darker skins, produced by higher levels of MELANIN, acting as a compensatory mechanism to reduce the effect of high levels of solar radiation on the skin. Body shape is also affected by the environment — larger, shorter-limbed bodies are better at keeping in heat, where thin, long-limbed individuals are better at dissipating heat. As a result, people who live at higher latitude have shorter limbs, and are often robustly happening continually in the individual CELLS of the animal body, but from their immediate environment substances must move into the BLOOD to be carried away to the site of their ultimate disposal. In the animal body there is also another type of excretion: expulsion of the residue of substances which have not been absorbed into the body proper from the gut (which can be considered a tunnel through the body of the external world).

In human terms 'excreta' normally refers only to URINE and FAECES, whereas the definition of excretion would also include both carbon dioxide and heat, and these will be considered first.

Carbon dioxide

CARBON DIOXIDE (CO_2), along with water, is the end-product in cells which use oxygen to release their energy supply from food sources, and those cells are in the vast majority. If this CO_2 were to accumulate the cells would become too acidic for their internal chemistry to proceed. Continual generation of CO_2 maintains a concentration gradient from inside to outside so that it moves by DIFFUSION out of the cells into the surrounding fluid, and thence into the blood in the nearby capillaries. So the blood picks up CO_2 as it circulates, until it converges from the whole body into the right side of the heart, carrying an amount of CO_2 which varies with the total rate of energy release by body cells. This venous blood, low in oxygen and high in CO_2, is pumped through the lungs, where CO_2 is excreted by the reverse process to that of its uptake from cells — it diffuses out down a gradient, because breathing keeps the concentration lower in the gas in the lungs than it is in the incoming blood.

Heat

Heat is continually generated by resting metabolic activity, and to a much greater extent by working muscles. Unless conservation of body heat is required in cold conditions to maintain body temperature, it is 'excreted' from the surface of the body when there is a temperature gradient from the skin to the environment. This gradient, and therefore heat loss, is regulated by the mechanisms for TEMPERATURE REGULATION: dilation of skin blood vessels brings heat to the surface and increases the gradient; when this mechanism is inadequate, sweating comes into play as well.

Excretion in the urine

The KIDNEYS are responsible for filtering off a continual sample of the watery component of the blood plasma, with its solutes, at a rate equivalent to the whole of the plasma volume about every twenty minutes. The further processes within the kidneys could be likened to 'quality control' and correction. Not only the filtered water, but also many dissolved substances, are largely reabsorbed, but the reabsorption is fine-tuned according to any need for correction of the blood composition; nitrogenous waste (mainly urea) from protein breakdown is allowed to escape, and waste acid (H^+) and other substances present in excess are actively secreted into the urine. The end result is production of urine at a variable rate depending on fluid intake, but on average less than one-hundredth the rate of filtration of fluid from the blood, and containing all that needs to be excreted minute by minute.

Excretion from the bowel

That which is voided consists of the residue that remains after digestion and absorption of food breakdown products in the stomach and small intestine, and after absorption of most of the remaining water in the large intestine. This is also the route for voiding of cholesterol, excreted by the liver into the bile. The colour of the faeces is derived from bile pigments: although these are recycled to a large extent, the remainder becomes *stercobilin* and leaves by this route.

SHEILA JENNETT

See also FAECES; URINE.

Execution Capital punishment has, historically, been a mainstay of most systems of judicial punishment, although it is only recently that systematic work has been carried out by historians either on the incidence of the use of the death penalty, or on its broader cultural significance. If we confine ourselves to Europe in the late medieval and early modern periods, we find that at least initial studies have been completed on England, France, Amsterdam, and parts of Germany. The English and German evidence in particular suggests that levels of capital punishment rose in the late sixteenth and seventeenth centuries, and dropped in the later seventeenth and eighteenth, although both levels of execution and methods of killing varied enormously between individual territories. Perhaps more interestingly for the history of the body, it is possible to trace changes in the ceremonial of execution. The continental European evidence is perhaps more relevant here than the English: in England, condemned CRIMINALS were usually hanged, whereas in many continental states what were considered more atrocious crimes were followed by aggravated punishments. Perhaps the best documented of these is breaking on the wheel, where the condemned was tied by the arms and legs to a large wheel, the limbs being subsequently broken. Other refinements (rarely administered) were the tearing of the flesh of the condemned with red-hot pincers, the cutting off of hands, and the cutting out of tongues.

Obviously, study of both the actual practice of execution (public in most European states and in North America before the nineteenth century) and the symbolism and rituals attached to the phenomenon is of considerable interest to historians of the human body. Unfortunately, direct comment on this matter was rarely made by contemporaries, and the historian of such matters has usually to work by inference. It is therefore interesting to consider the remarkable commentary that the English judge and legal writer Sir Edward Coke (1552–1634) made on the punishment in England for male common-ers convicted of High Treason, namely hanging, drawing, and quartering. Here the various elements of the punishment are directly related to contemporary ideas surrounding various parts of the human body.

The convicted person was dragged to the place of execution on a hurdle, and since 'God hath made the head of man the highest and most supreme part, as being the chief grace and ornament', Coke wrote that 'he must be drawn with the head declining downward, and lying so near the ground as may be, being thought unfit to take the benefit of the common air'. The convicted man would then be hanged by the neck, but only briefly, before he could die, and was then 'to have his privy parts cut off and burnt before his face as being unworthily begotten, and unfit to leave any generation after him'. After this, 'his bowels and inlay'd parts' were to be 'taken out and burnt, who inwardly had conceived and harboured in his heart such horrible treason' (it should be noted that every effort would be made to keep the convicted man alive and sensible up to this point). The traitor's head, 'which had imagined the mischief', would then be cut off, and, finally, his body would be quartered, 'and the quarters set up in some high and eminent place, to the view and detestation of men, to become a prey for the fowls of the air'. It is instructive that Coke followed through this discussion of punishment in terms of the symbolism of body parts with a medical analogy: 'and this is a reward due to traitors, whose hearts be hardened: for that it is a physic of state and government, to let out the corrupt blood from the heart'.

In England the usual means of capital punishment was hanging, which left the body more or less intact, and hence in good condition for the fate which awaited the bodies of many condemned criminals: DISSECTION in the medical schools. Elizabethan legislation had allowed for a limited supply of such corpses to be made available for dissection, but the rising professional standards of the eighteenth-century physician made the legal supply insufficient, and a brisk trade developed in the bodies of the hanged until, in 1752, an act was passed making it easier for the bodies of executed murderers to be sent to the ANATOMY classes. Interestingly, fear that such a fate should attend the corpse of a convicted criminal frequently provoked crowd action, led by the relatives or friends of the deceased, who attempted to rescue the corpse in hopes of keeping it intact and giving it a decent burial. Here we see popular ideas about the body coming into direct conflict with official ones. It should also be remembered that the corpses of executed criminals were thought to have therapeutic powers, and that a touch from their hands was considered efficacious in curing illness or injuries. Moreover, the practice of gibbeting, that is leaving the corpses of especially heinous criminals to rot in public places (normally the location where the crime had been committed), was another way in which the body of the convicted would enter the domain of the general consciousness.

The folklore which surrounded executions was rendered redundant when, in the nineteenth century, most states began to carry out death sentences in private, while a few abolished the death penalty altogether. The causes and significance of this shift have given rise to considerable theorizing among historians, social scientists, philosophers, and commentators on penal policy. One of its central themes, however, has been that of changing attitudes to the human body, and, more particularly, changing sensibilities about the infliction of pain and suffering. But whether displayed on a public scaffold in the eighteenth century, or the result of a scientific killing within the confines of a modern prison, the body of the executed criminal remains a vivid and striking symbol of the power of the law.

J. A. SHARPE

See also KILLING.

Exercise

Muscle activity

Exercise is muscular activity. When the word is used, there is almost always the additional implication of the activity being extended over time, but for how long is up to the user. More commonly explicit are the adjectives of intensity (mild, moderate, strenuous/high) and body region (leg, upper body/arm). An important distinction, from the point of view of physiological response, is between exercise predominantly involving movement (dynamic exercise) and that in which the muscles brace against each other or an unmoving outside load (static exercise). Static exercise is also known as 'isometric' because the muscles stay at (approximately) constant length.

All exercise, then, starts with the activation of voluntary muscle. Whether there is significant movement depends on whether the force the muscle is producing exceeds, matches, or falls short of the load against which it is acting. The first situation produces dynamic exercise of the form we usually think of; technically, the muscles, successfully shortening, are said to be contracting 'concentrically'. However, the last situation is dynamic too; here the muscles, extending under the greater external force, are active 'eccentrically' (often pronounced 'ee-centrically'). Only in the middle case, where muscle force equals that against which it is acting, will the exercise be static. Finally, it must be made clear that the muscles need not be working flat out in any of these situations. That will depend on their degree of activation by the NERVOUS SYSTEM; full activation is uncommon in daily life.

The chemical demands of the muscles underlie most of the other phenomena of exercise. In particular, ample supplies of oxygenated blood must be supplied to every active muscle. Both the HEART and the circulation, and the respiratory system, respond accordingly. Scientific understanding of these responses, however, depends on our ability to measure both muscular performance and the metabolic energy input upon which it is based.

Measuring muscular performance and metabolic input

It is a fairly simple matter to measure isometric force production. All that is required is a spring balance or, better, an electronic strain gauge, against which the body-part of interest exerts force through a virtually inextensible wire or rigid lever system. Grip strength, bite force, elbow flexion, or knee extension are easily measured by 'dynamometers' (force measurers) of this broad type.

In dynamic exercise, measuring force as such is not often sufficient for the physiologist, though transducers placed in bicycle cranks, or in 'force plates' let into a rigid laboratory floor, are examples of instruments which can provide this information. The overall demand of dynamic exercise is, however, most completely indicated by the power output achieved by the body, for power embodies both the force and the rate of movement. Power output is assessed by 'ergometers' (work measurers), and can be most readily measured for rhythmic movements against external load, such as in cycling or rowing.

The input of energy from metabolism can be estimated with reasonable precision when the exercise lasts long enough at a steady rate for breathing to come into balance with the muscles' demands ('aerobic' exercise). Then the effort may be considered to be entirely founded upon the 'burning' of fuel molecules in OXYGEN. As all the body's fuels (CARBOHYDRATE, FAT, and — normally used to a much lesser extent — PROTEIN) release rather similar amounts of energy when reacted with the same volume of oxygen, measurements of the volume of oxygen consumed per minute ($\dot{V}O_2$) are the basis of the energy–input calculations. Such measurements are made by collecting the air breathed out by an exercising subject, assaying the percentage of oxygen left in that air, and subtracting that from the percentage of oxygen which would have been in the same volume of air when it was breathed in. The result gives the 'aerobic power' of the subject performing that exercise. The maximum aerobic power a subject can achieve ($\dot{V}O_2max$) is a fundamental indicator of exercise potential.

Changes in heart and circulation

Considering the heart first, its rate of beating rises appreciably even as we stand up and walk gently through the house. In the highest intensity exercise, the pulse rises to its maximum. This varies with the age of the individual, but negligibly with gender and, more surprisingly, only a little with FITNESS. The thumb rule is that maximum heart rate (HR) (in beats per minute) = 220 − (age in years). People who are trained to sustain high intensity dynamic exercise for periods of many minutes at a time ('aerobic' athletes) actually have maximum HRs 10–15 beats per minute *lower* than would be calculated by that formula. This seeming paradox makes more sense when it is considered that the amount of blood pumped by their hearts in every beat (their 'stroke volume', SV) is greater in any given state of rest or exercise

than that of an untrained person; thus the aerobic athlete's resting pulse will be slower than the average person's by at least as much as the shortfall at maximum HR, and so allows a greater percentage increase from rest to maximum exercise.

During the responses to increasing exercise intensity there is some increase of SV as well as of HR in everybody, so that in an untrained but healthy young adult, of 70 kg body weight (the standard textbook figure), pulse might rise about threefold, from say 70 beats per minute at rest to 200, SV by about 1.7 times, and thus total CARDIAC OUTPUT (CO) from 5 to 25 litres/min. Equivalent figures for the internationally elite aerobic athlete might be from 45 to 185 beats per minute (HR) and 5 to 40 litres/min (CO), implying a near doubling of the already large SV. Notice, however, that the resting CO is the same for both, as the metabolic demands of sitting still are much the same for everybody of a given weight.

Nevertheless, even the élite athlete's eight-fold increase in CO is far from sufficient by itself to explain the total blood flow through each of the muscles that is working flat out. Modern indications are that muscle blood flow can increase by the order of 100-fold from the resting level. Great increases of flow through the active muscles are achieved by dilatation of BLOOD VESSELS running through them, assisted to some extent by constriction of the vessels supplying organs, such as the gut and kidneys, which do jobs that can take second place during the exercise. (How vessels constrict and dilate is discussed under 'Blood vessels'.) Finally, the active muscles' METABOLISM is enabled to increase by yet one more factor — enhanced extraction of oxygen and nutrients from each ml of blood flowing through them. In the case of oxygen, this increase is typically about three-fold.

The limit to maximum power output

Pursuing our figures, if muscle blood flow rose 100-fold and oxygen extraction/ml of blood rose threefold, 300 times as much oxygen would have to be extracted from the air each minute for all muscles in the body to be maximally active at once. Actually, this cannot happen: it has been calculated that the heart can only supply 30–40% of the total musculature, fully active, simultaneously. This puts a significant limitation on running and cycling, and an even more substantial one on activities demanding direct propulsive power from all four limbs — such as cross-country skiing and swimming. Tellingly we find that, if any one of the measures of whole-body effort (such as maximum CO, maximum power output, or maximum oxygen consumption — $\dot{V}O_2 max$) is considered, its values over all these exercises are within about 10% of each other — strongly indicating that the chief limitation on them all is a central function upon which each depends. One expression of this central limitation is the ceiling, just noted, on cardiac output.

Changes in breathing

The limit shows itself in respiratory function, too. However, it is not in the obvious feature, ventilation (the volume of air breathed in and out each minute); this increases several times more than CO — namely 15–35-fold, according to aerobic fitness. (Typical patterns of the increase of ventilation during the first few minutes of both moderate and strenuous exercise are described under BREATHING DURING EXERCISE.) That the maximum ventilatory rate is more than sufficient to meet requirements is indicated by the fact that oxygen extraction from each litre of air goes slightly *down*, not up, at high exercise intensities. At such intensities the time available for oxygen to diffuse from the air in the lungs into the blood as it races past, begins to become a limiting factor. In normally healthy people near sea level the limitation is barely, if at all, detectable; but in top athletes racing at sea level the arterial blood, fresh from the lungs, falls clearly short of full saturation with oxygen — comparable to its condition in a resting person at the altitude of an Alpine ski resort.

Anaerobic exercise

A distinction which has been avoided until this point must now be confronted. The discussion has focused on exercise continued long enough (say 4 min or more) that it must be performed in balance with oxygen uptake. Any track race longer than 1500 metres is of this kind once the athlete's body has adjusted fully to the pace. Briefer activities (like a 400 metre race) can be more intense, but only on the basis of the extra power, greater than the aerobic maximum, being supplied via anaerobic metabolic pathways. Such very intensive, short-term exercise is termed 'anaerobic'; but note that, while aerobic exercise, when we have settled into it, is totally aerobic, even the briefest high-intensity exercise is never wholly anaerobic.

Upper body exercise

Before leaving dynamic exercise, we should note that exercise using only the arms provides less power at a given HR than exercise predominantly using the legs. Among the reasons for this is that external (and therefore measurable) work done by the arms usually requires the trunk to be braced by muscular effort which needs energy but does not move the load.

Static versus dynamic

Bracing actions of the trunk muscles are in fact examples of static exercise. Other instances are the guardsman's posture at attention, the weightlifter's few seconds of triumph with the bar above his head, and the dinghy crew's efforts to hold the body horizontal over the water, balancing the boat. In all these situations HR is raised (in the latter two instances, very considerably), yet compared with dynamic exercise giving the same HR — especially leg exercise — two things are markedly different:

   (i) oxygen consumption is much lower;
   (ii) BLOOD PRESSURE is higher, especially during diastole.

The first point is explicable chiefly by the fact that isometrically contracting muscles require substantially less oxygen than the same muscles cyclically shortening and lengthening. The second arises because, in dynamic exercise, blood flows through the active muscles during the *periods of relaxation* which alternate with their contractions; during the contraction phases it is impeded. There being no relaxation periods during a static exercise, blood pressure must be raised if any flow at all is to be forced through the tensed muscles. This rise is brought about by reflex mechanisms originating in the muscles themselves.

Hormonal adjustments

In addition to the cardiovascular and respiratory adjustments which the body makes in the face of exercise, substantial hormonal adjustments also occur. ADRENALINE flow is elevated, especially in anticipation of vigorous exercise; and as exercise proceeds, cortisol and (particularly in really protracted efforts, such as marathon races) GROWTH HORMONE concentrations are both substantially raised, and may not return to basal levels for some hours afterwards. All these promote mobilisation of both carbohydrate and lipid fuels, and growth hormone also promotes tissue adaptation and repair when the activity is over. INSULIN flow, however, is *reduced* during exercise. This at first seems a paradox, for the function of insulin is to promote glucose entry into tissues such as muscle, and exercising muscle surely needs its glucose? It is now clear that increased availability of glucose transporter molecules in the membranes of exercising muscle fibres enables them to take in glucose with less insulin than usual. Suitably controlled exercise therefore has special benefits for diabetics.

Fuel sources

In short bursts of intensive exercise, carbohydrates are the main fuels used. At lower intensities, fats contribute more and, as endurance efforts proceed, they become the major energy source. Four-fifths of carbohydrate storage is as 'glycogen' (animal starch) within the muscle fibres themselves. The rest is as glycogen in the liver, from which it can be released as glucose (BLOOD SUGAR) when circulating levels fall. However, the brain, which uses no other fuel, makes priority demands, so blood-borne glucose does not contribute a major fraction of the energy used by the muscles in a long event unless its concentration is kept topped up by glucose drinks or carbohydrate food.

Fat is stored both within some muscle fibres and in fat cells. The balance, however, is the converse of that for carbohydrate: most activities seem to draw more upon the fat cells than the intramuscular stores.

Health benefits

Clearly, all exercise constitutes a degree of training for the muscles which it uses. All exercise also enhances cardiovascular and respiratory health

to some extent, though aerobic exercise benefits these systems most. The hormonal and metabolic consequences of any but the most severe exercise are almost always advantageous too. Of these benefits, the cardiovascular ones are normally emphasized. Sustained aerobic exercise trains the heart, lowers blood pressure, tends to reduce body fat, and promotes a switch from 'bad' to 'good' lipids — from low to high density serum lipoprotein — thereby reducing the risk of atheromatous plaques.

How much exercise is necessary, and of what form, has naturally been much researched. Recent work indicates that the most marked gains, relative to a sedentary lifestyle, are achieved by a mere 30 min of moderate exercise (such as brisk walking), on each of 3 days a week. The more exercise is taken, within a normal lifestyle, the greater the health benefit; yet a law of diminishing returns applies.

As to the form of exercise, it is clearly undesirable for an unfit person to leap straight into short-term, high-intensity activity. Worse still, isometric exercise will always, in the short term, raise the blood pressure. So exercise for health, in those who have been sedentary, should be dynamic and essentially aerobic. Such exercise will not build up much muscle. Effort against high resistance, in the weights room or equivalent, is the way to achieve that; but such 'resistance exercises' are best not embarked upon by people who have not already achieved a fairly good aerobic fitness base.

Exercise in different cultures

Finally, it may be salutary to recall how rare, and for the most part recent, in human societies is the disposition to take exercise when it could have been avoided. Exercise has been toil, for the great majority of mankind, at least until an industrial revolution was well advanced in the society concerned. Wealth and status thus meant indolence and often corpulence, whether in medieval Europe or over a similar period in China. Yet in such civilizations as that of Sparta and Rome, and in sectors of Japanese society over many centuries, exercise was cultivated in the expectation of war. Perhaps it is ancient Athens that, in its attitudes to exercise as in so many other ways, most closely anticipated our own outlook: exercise for sport, for health, and to maintain/improve the body image were all recognized by the contemporaries of Plato, as they are once more by us. It is to be hoped, however, that our physiological understanding is at least a little better.
      NEIL SPURWAY

Further reading

Bursztyn, P. (1990). *Physiology for sportspeople: a serious user's guide to the body*. Manchester University Press.

Noakes, T. (1991). *Lore of running*. Human Kinetics, Champaign, Illinois.

Wilmore, J. H. and Costill, D. L. (2000). *Physiology of sport and exercise*. 2nd ed. Human Kinetics, Champaign, Illinois.

See also BREATHING DURING EXERCISE;
FATIGUE; FITNESS; SPORT.

Exocrine refers to glands, or to secretions, where the discharge of the secretion is onto a body surface. This may be either onto the skin or onto one of the lining surfaces within the body: of the alimentary tract from the mouth to the anus; the respiratory tract from the nose down to the alveoli of the lungs; the urinary tract (urethra, bladder, ureters, and tubules of the kidneys); or the genital tract (vulva, vagina, uterus, and Fallopian tubes, or vasa deferentia and tubules of the testis). These tubes or cavities are all in continuity with the outside world, and exocrine secretions all deal in some way with the external environment, or with exchanges between it and the body. Thus secretions onto the skin (e.g. from *sweat glands, sebaceous glands*) deal with heat loss and surface protection; those into the gut (e.g. *digestive enzymes, bile*) deal with food; those into the respiratory passages (e.g. *mucus, surfactant*) with the filtering of inhaled air and facilitation of gas exchange in the lungs; those into the urogenital system with excretion and reproduction (e.g. *substances in the urine, seminal fluid, cervical mucus*). By contrast, *endocrine* refers to glands, or to secretions, where the discharge is internal, into the bloodstream.   S.J.

See EPITHELIUM; GLAND.

Extrasensory perception The twentieth century witnessed the rise of *parapsychology*, which set out to prove the reality of extrasensory perception (ESP). Historically, widespread credence has been given to such phenomena in most if not all cultures, and this holds true today for large sectors of the West. Debates about ESP have been dominated by the question of its existence. Writers about the subject usually take sides, denigrating it as a figment of the imagination, or valorizing it as one of the most fundamental propensities of our being. The history of these debates indicates the changing interconnections between religion, popular belief, conceptions of psychology, and the role of science in demarcating and producing the real.

At the end of the nineteenth century, an increasing number of investigators, including leading psychologists, physiologists, and philosophers, took up the study of psychical phenomena. Many were attempting to find something with which to refute materialism and provide a basis for religious belief, and so to enable a transformation of society. Thus the very definition of *telepathy* (previously termed 'thought-transference'), in 1882, by the English psychical researcher Frederic Myers, as 'the communication of impressions of any kind from one mind to another, independently of the recognized channels of sense' presents itself as part of a polemical argument, which has framed how the phenomena have subsequently been approached, or dismissed. The interest was not in the phenomena *per se*, but in whether their existence

could give some evidence of a mechanism which would be able to render intelligible how the dead could communicate with the living, and hence establish the *post mortem* survival of the soul.

All sorts of invisible forces — either physical or purely psychical — were invoked to explain telepathy, and variations along these lines continue till this day. In 1896 the chemist William Crookes speculated that telepathy was like radiation. By contrast, Myers claimed that the telepathic impression was registered in subconscious or subliminal aspects of one's being. In so doing, telepathy played a crucial role in the creation of the unconscious as a non-material interiority in which past and future, self and other intermingled. Following this, Myers and the French philosopher and psychologist, Henri Bergson, speculated that, beneath the manifest occurrences of telepathy, such processes were taking place all the time. Telepathy thus became the hidden substrate of the social bond, its intimate communion. It was only the restriction characteristic of consciousness that hid this awareness.

Psychical researchers attempted to provide evidence for telepathy by the experimental pursuit of the 'guessing game', which was then a popular pastime, and through the collection of firsthand testimonials, presented in *Phantasms of the Living* (1886). Having convinced themselves of the reality of the phenomena, their subsequent investigations of mediums were dominated by the problem of how to establish that a telepathic message came from a defunct, rather than living source: that phantasms of the dead were not simply phantasms of the living.

It is important to note that concern with such phenomena lay at the forefront of the psychological agenda at the end of the nineteenth century. In commenting on the first congress of physiological psychology in Paris in 1889, William James noted that the most striking feature of the discussions was their 'tendency to slope off to some one or other of those shady horizons with which the name of "psychic research" is now associated.' Consequently, a vast census of hallucinations was set up, in which the question of the telepathy was paramount. For James, and for other subliminal psychologists such as Théodore Flournoy, the task confronting psychology was that of providing a differential account of all human phenomena — including supernormal phenomena — and studying their interrelation. It was through a process of limitation and exclusion that the agenda of mainstream psychology was established, and with this, its conceptions of the PERSONALITY and of sensory perception.

By and large, psychical researchers failed to convince the majority of the scientific and academic worlds of the existence of telepathy. Subsequent investigators attempted to set right this situation; rather than locate themselves in private societies, they attempted to gain a foothold in the universities, usually through large endowments. Taking on the regnant experimental methodology in psychology, they attempted to

show that the phenomena could be taken out of the seance and reproduced in laboratory settings. To mark these changes, the field was redubbed 'parapsychology', and 'telepathy' and CLAIRVOYANCE' became 'extrasensory perception'. It was J. B. Rhine at Duke University who was responsible for the latter term, and he gave such research its modern cast with his *Extra-sensory perception* (1934). No longer content to posit the existence of yet-unrecognized senses, Rhine reformulated Myers' definition to read: 'perception in a mode that is just not sensory'. Rhine subjected individuals to rigorously controlled experiments. So-called Zener cards bearing a cross, circle, rectangle, star, or three parallel wavy lines were placed in sealed envelopes, and subjects had to guess their shapes in prolonged trials which were statistically analysed.

For Rhine, no less than his forebears, the prime interest in ESP was its use as an argument against physicalism. He claimed that the proof for the existence of ESP had repudiated the view that the mind was just a physical brain function, and had proved the existence of a 'minimal concept of the soul', which he dubbed the 'psychological soul'. Salvation for religious belief had apparently been found in the shape of undergraduate card guessers in laboratories. Rhine was not markedly more successful in promoting belief in ESP than earlier investigators. As William James had noted, it seems as if there is sufficient evidence to persuade those who have the requisite 'will to believe', and insufficient to sway those who do not.

At the same time, theories of perception and extrasensory perception continue to be wedded. Conceptions of extrasensory perception presuppose conceptions of what constitutes perception itself. Perception has generally been linked to particular sense organs. An exception to this was the psychologist J.J. Gibson's ecological theory of perception. According to this, all perception could be said to be 'extra-sensory'.

SONU SHAMDASANI

Further reading
Gurney, E., Myers, F. W. H., and Podmore, F. (1886). *Phantasms of the living*, Vols 1 and 2 Trübner and Co., London.
Rhine, J. B. (1934). *Extra-sensory perception*. Boston Society for Psychical Research, Boston.

See also CLAIRVOYANCE.

Eyes are both windows and beacons for the mind. They provide VISION — our most precious sense. But they also transmit signals to others — signals of anger, lust, fear, compassion, happiness. Eyes can desire ('A lover's eyes will gaze an eagle blind'; Shakespeare, *Love's Labours Lost* 1595); but also violate ('They rape us with their eyes'; Marilyn French, *The Women's Room* 1977); and eyes can reflect our innermost thoughts ('Her eyes are homes of silent prayer'; Alfred, Lord Tennyson, *In Memoriam A.H.H.* canto 32, 1850). GAZE is arguably the most powerful component of BODY LANGUAGE.

An eye is a part of the body specialized for catching light and translating it into nerve impulses. Defined in such basic terms, eyes have been around for a very long time. The fossils of primitive arthropods (ancestors of insects, crustaceans and spiders), 530 million years old, show clear signs of eyes, and the first eye-like organs probably date back to the very beginning of multicellular life, 600 million years ago.

In the depths of the ocean, in underground rivers, inside the bodies of other animals, there are creatures without eyes. And organisms such as corals and sea anemones, which simply stay still and grow, have no need of eyes. But wherever there is light and a reason to move around, animals have eyes.

Scrutiny of the fossil record, and of the diversity of extant animals, suggests that eyes have been 'invented' by natural selection at least 40 times during the EVOLUTION of life on earth. 'Re-invented' might be more accurate, because there is genetic evidence that there may have been a single origin for all eyes. A gene called Pax-6, which has a very similar, 'conserved' DNA sequence in a vast range of animals, from fruit flies to human beings, appears to determine when and where eyes form during development.

Light, the diet of eyes, constitutes a tiny part of the entire spectrum of electromagnetic radiation. The various forms of such radiation (ranging from that associated with mains electricity through to X-rays and gamma rays) differ in the frequency at which their electrical and magnetic fields oscillate, and therefore the distance travelled during one complete cycle of oscillation — the wavelength.

The sun is a powerful source of electromagnetic energy. The sun's rays that reach the surface of the earth belong mainly to the so-called optical band. This extends from about 1 mm to 100 nanometres in wavelength (a nanometre is one billionth of a metre). The longer wavelengths constitute infrared radiation, which we feel as warmth, and the shortest are ultraviolet, which can be damaging to the skin and to the eyes. Visible radiation — true light — lies in the middle of the range, extending from about 400 to 750 nanometres. All our visual experience rests on the detection of this narrow band of wavelengths.

Sources of light (the sun and other visible stars, lamps, camera flashbulbs, etc.) appear bright because the radiation that they emit enters the eye directly. But most of the light that reaches our eyes has been reflected from the surfaces of objects around us: that is how we see those objects. The brightness and colours of surfaces are determined by the amount of light they reflect and the wavelength composition of that reflected light.

These facts now seem self-evident, but the whole process was deeply mysterious to the ancient Greeks. Plato imagined that some sort of 'spirit' streamed out from the eyes to palpate the world. Aristotle, ever contrary, suggested that light flowed into the eyes. Isaac Newton's famous

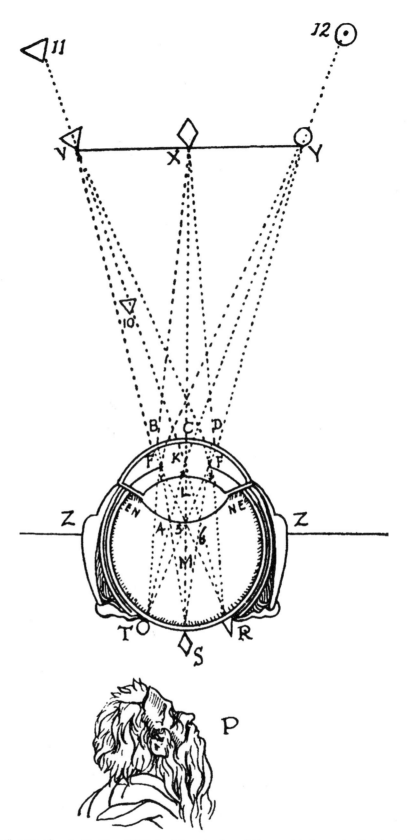

In this illustration from *La Dioptrique* (1637), René Descartes shows fairly accurately the way in which the optics of the eye form an inverted image in the plane of the retina (seen here through a window cut in the back of an ox eye). The Jesuit astronomer Christopher Scheiner (1573–1650) was the first to observe the image in this way, although Johannes Kepler (1571–1630) had already geometrically deduced its likely organization. Before this time, most philosophers had imagined the lens to be the point of focus of light.

experiments with prisms demonstrated that white sunlight is composed of a rainbow of different sorts of light, appearing to be of different colours, from violet, through blue, green and yellow to red. Newton concluded that these forms of light vibrate at different frequencies. Light of short wavelength appears blue, the longest visible wavelengths appear red.

The most essential feature of a true eye is a mechanism for catching the energy of light and using it to trigger a chemical reaction. This is achieved in all eyes by substances called photopigments. Every photopigment consists of a derivative of vitamin A (*retinal*) linked to a protein molecule called an opsin. Here again is evidence of the antiquity of seeing: *opsins* are similar in structure and are encoded by very similar, conserved genes throughout the animal world. Even certain bacteria have photopigments in their membranes. The capacity to catch light was one of the first tricks discovered in the story of life.

In a famous passage in *The Origin of Species*, Charles Darwin played Devil's (or perhaps God's?) Advocate:

> To suppose that the eye, with all its inimitable contrivances … could have been formed by natural selection, seems, I freely confess, absurd in the highest degree.

But he went on to argue:

> Reason tells me, that if numerous gradations from a simple and imperfect eye to one complex and perfect can be shown to exist, each grade being useful to its possessor … then the difficulty of believing that a perfect and complex eye could be formed by natural selection … should not be considered as subversive of the theory.

There is indeed evidence for numerous, useful gradations of eye. The earliest eye-like organs, still found in present-day limpets, probably consisted of depressions lined with cells containing photopigment, which were connected to the nervous system. Such photosensitive pit organs can detect the presence of light and even give crude information about its direction (enabling the organism to turn towards or away from the light — *phototropism*). But proper eyes have something more — a system to focus the light to form an image on the array of photoreceptive cells. Like telescopes, microscopes and cameras, almost all eyes form images with lenses or mirrors. Humans, indeed all seeing vertebrates, have so-called *simple* eyes: they have a single lens system, focusing light to form one, continuous image of the outside world. But all sighted insects have *compound* eyes, consisting of a mosaic of tube-shaped optical lens systems, with photoreceptors at the base of each tube. Scallops have eyes that form images with reflective mirrors. And the primitive mollusc *Nautilus* has an eye with only a pinhole at the front, forming a crude image on the array of photoreceptors inside.

The eyes of cephalopods (squid and octopus) are uncannily like human eyes. They too are simple eyes, with muscles to make them move, and a pigmented *iris*. They have an internal lens and they form an image on a light-sensitive retina. But there the similarity ends. There are differences so fundamental in the anatomy of the retina that it is generally believed that cephalopod eyes arose independently of vertebrate eyes. The striking similarity of these unrelated organs is a dramatic example of convergent evolution — the separate emergence of similar structures to solve the same problem.

The adult human eye is roughly spherical, about 24 mm in diameter, with a transparent bulge — the *cornea* — at the front, around which the white of the eye — the *sclera* — is visible. The cornea has no blood supply; hence transplanted corneas (replacing damaged, opaque originals) are rarely rejected. The cornea provides two-thirds of the focusing power of the eye. Much of that power is lost, hence causing blurred vision, when the eye is immersed in water. Immediately behind the cornea is the *anterior chamber*, filled with fluid called *aqueous humour*. The continuous production of this fluid by epithelial cells generates a hydrostatic pressure inside the eye (normally about 15 mm of mercury). The fluid percolates out of the eye through an epithelial meshwork inside the rim of the cornea, enters the Canal of Schlemm, which runs beneath the surface of the eye, around the edge of the cornea, and drains into the veins of the eye. The potentially blinding condition of *glaucoma*, which is an elevation of intraocular pressure above about 25 mm of mercury, is usually caused by structural defects in the anterior chamber associated with extreme short-sight, or degenerative changes in old age.

Visible through the cornea of the eye is the pigmented epithelium of the iris (which gives the eye its characteristic, genetically determined, colour). Contraction of smooth muscle within the iris changes the diameter of the hole in the middle — the *pupil*. When the circular muscle around the edge of the aperture of the iris contracts, the pupil constricts. This muscle is controlled by *parasympathetic* nerves, coming from the midbrain. There are also *radial* muscle fibres in the iris, innervated by *sympathetic* nerves, which make the pupil enlarge or dilate.

The main function of the pupil is to optimise the quality of the retinal image and the retinal illumination. The eye is not a perfect optical system. It has many sources of error, which can reduce the sharpness of the image. The effects of spherical and chromatic aberration increase as the pupil expands. The blurring effects of diffraction (due to interaction of the wavefront of light with the pupil) become worse as the aperture decreases, as in all lens systems. In bright light, the pupil is usually just over 2 mm in diameter — providing an optimal compromise between diffraction and the aberrations. However, in very dim conditions, the pupil dilates, sacrificing image quality in order to catch enough light to sustain vision.

The pupil also serves as a signal to others. Generalised activation of the sympathetic system (the 'fight or flight' reaction) causes the pupil to dilate — a clear sign of anger or fear. Activation of the sympathetic nerves to the pupil also occurs in sexual arousal, and the sight of dilated pupils can itself be arousing. If people are asked to rank the attractiveness of photographs of the opposite sex with small pupils or large, they generally prefer the latter. Indeed, Belladonna ('beautiful woman'), an extract of deadly nightshade containing the drug ATROPINE, which blocks the action of parasympathetic nerves and hence dilates the pupil, used to be applied to the eyes as a cosmetic.

Immediately behind the pupil is the *crystalline lens* — a transparent protein gel in an elastic sac, which provides the additional optical power needed to bring light to a focus at the back of the eye. The part of the eyeball behind the lens is filled with a jelly called *vitreous humour*. The margin of the lens is attached to the *ciliary body*, which, like the iris, contains a circular muscle innervated by parasympathetic nerves. When this muscle contracts, the tension on the lens decreases and it becomes more

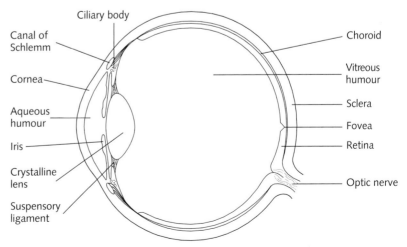

The structure of the human eye.

spherical, and hence more optically powerful, focusing the eye on closer objects — a process called ACCOMMODATION.

An 'ideal' (emmetropic) eye is exactly focused on the extreme distance when its ciliary muscle is completely relaxed, so that the entire range of additional power provided by accommodation is available to focus closer objects. During the first few years of life, the growth of the eyeball is normally regulated, in some uncertain way, according to the quality of the retinal image, so as to tend to make the eye emmetropic. Eyes that are not optimised in this way are said to have REFRACTIVE ERRORS (long sight or short sight).

The thin shell of the eyeball is made up of three layers or tunics: the outer sclera, consisting of strong protein fibres; the *choroid*, a spongy layer filled with blood vessels; and the *retina* or nervous layer. The retina forms as an outgrowth of the embryonic brain, and is strictly part of the central nervous system. It consists of alternating layers of nerve cell bodies and their processes and connections. The photoreceptors lie at the back of the retina, so light has to pass through all the other layers of transparent neurons to reach the *outer segments* of the receptors, containing membranous discs, packed with photopigment. The tips of the receptors are in contact with the *pigment epithelium*, which contains enzymes that regenerate photopigment that has been 'bleached' by light. Retinal detachment occurs when a gap opens between receptors and pigment epithelium.

There are two kinds of photoreceptor. The 120 million, thin *rods*, which operate in dim conditions, contain a photopigment called *rhodopsin*, which is most sensitive to short wavelength (blue) light. Each of the 6 million or so *cones*, which are more conical in shape, contains one of three pigments, absorbing maximally in the blue, yellow-green and red parts of the spectrum. The perceived colour of a light (whether a pure, monochromatic light or a mixture of wavelengths) depends on the relative stimulation of these three classes of cone receptor. There is a very dense concentration of slender cones in a dimple, called the *fovea*, in the centre of the retina. Shifting gaze towards something involves rotating the eyeball to bring the image of the object of interest on to this special region. It has very high visual acuity (the capacity to resolve fine patterns of light and dark, as in reading) and excellent colour vision.

The electrical potential inside an individual rod changes detectably when one of its millions of rhodopsin molecules absorbs a single photon or quantum of light (the smallest, indivisible unit of energy). This exquisite sensitivity is achieved by a 'cascade' of four chemical reactions, 'amplifying' the response. The final step is the constriction of ION CHANNELS that normally allow positive sodium ions to leak into the cell. Hence, light makes the voltage inside the photoreceptor more negative, which reduces the release of transmitter substance at synaptic connections at the foot of the receptor. Photoreceptors cannot produce

nerve impulses: indeed, out of the five basic types of nerve cells in the retina, only those in the innermost layer, the ganglion cells, reliably produce full-blown impulses. The roughly 1.5 million *ganglion cells* have long axons, which run across the inner surface of the retina towards a round patch called the *optic disc*. Here the fibres form a bundle and plunge back through a hole in the sclera to form the optic nerve. This nerve connects the eye to the BRAIN, which learns of the world through the chatter of impulses reaching it from the eyes.

The retina is not merely a passive device, like the film in a camera. Its complex network of nerve cells compresses the information flooding into the eye, and detects important features in the visual image. Most of our knowledge of retinal function has come from the study of anaesthetized animals, in which electrical responses can be recorded from individual nerve cells, while images are presented to the eye. Most ganglion cells (in cats and monkeys) do not respond well to overall illumination of the retina, but to a local difference in brightness (i.e. *contrast*) between their particular region of the retina and the surrounding area. Half respond to local brightening, half to local darkening. In monkeys, many of the ganglion cells are also 'colour-selective', responding best to one colour of light.

The eyes rest snugly in slippery cups of fat, inside the *orbits* — cavities in the skull on each side of the nose. Six thin, flat muscles, stretching from the back of the orbit to various parts of the eyeball, enable it to rotate extremely quickly (up to hundreds of degrees per second) around any axis perpendicular to the direction of gaze. Some torsional rotation around the axis of gaze is also possible. The precious front surface of the eye is well protected against blows and flying objects, by the bony brow ridges, the hairs of the eyebrows, the eyelids and their lashes. A delicate translucent epithelium — the *conjunctiva* — covers the visible part of the sclera, folds back under the lids and attaches all around the inner margins, thus sealing off the contents of the orbit.

Lacrimal glands, embedded in the upper eyelids and controlled by parasympathetic nerves, secrete watery tear fluid, which flows through tiny ducts on to the surface of the cornea. The fluid is distributed over the cornea by *blinking* — rapid closing of the eyelids, combined with upward rotation of the eyeball, which normally occurs spontaneously about 10 times a minute. This continuous bathing maintains the smoothness and transparency of the cornea, which are essential to its function. When the process is compromised, the painful condition of *dry eye* occurs. Tear fluid normally collects in the inner corner of the eye and drains down into the nose through a tube called the *nasolacrimal duct*, but can tumble over the lower lid and run down the cheeks when secretion increases, e.g. in windy conditions, or when the eye is irritated. Crying or weeping occurs as a result of excessive secretion of tears.

Is it not remarkable that such mundane, though essential, physiological functions as lubrication of the cornea, enlargement of the pupil, fluttering of the eyelids, and movement of gaze have been 'captured' as potent, normally unconscious, social signals of extreme emotion. Metaphorically, eyes can dance, twinkle, drink (to me only!), even kill, as well as beginning the remarkable process of vision.

COLIN BLAKEMORE

Further reading:

Oyster, C. W. (1999). The Human Eye: Structure and Function.: Sinauer Associates, Sunderland, Mass.

Gregory, R. L. (1998). Eye and Brain: the Psychology of Seeing, 5th edition. Oxford University Press, Oxford.

See also ACCOMMODATION; AUTONOMIC NERVOUS SYSTEM; BLINDNESS; BLIND SPOT; COLOUR BLINDNESS; EYE MOVEMENTS; GAZE; NYSTAGMUS; RADIATION, NON-IONIZING; REFRACTIVE ERRORS; SENSORY RECEPTORS; SQUINT; VISION; WEEPING.

Eye movements

We move our eyes for a variety of reasons. We may look upward as a surreptitious signal that we do not believe what someone else is saying, or avert our gaze out of embarrassment or modesty. But even when we are not sending or responding to social signals, our eyes are often on the move for a quite different reason — to satisfy the needs of VISION. One might think that animals move their eyes in order to look from place to place, but oddly enough the oldest (in evolutionary terms) and commonest function of eye movements is to keep the image of the world stationary on the retina. The eyes sit in a mobile container (the head), itself attached to an often mobile body: if the eyes did not move to compensate for movements of the head, the image of the world would slither around on the retina and so be more difficult for the brain to analyse.

Some privileged animals, especially humans and other primates, can actively move their eyes to shift the image around on the retina. We do this because the central part of the retina, the fovea, is specialized for acute vision. When you try to recognize something, such as the printed letters on an optometrist's chart, you point your fovea directly at it and can then resolve gaps in the letters as small as 1 mm at a distance of 6 m (the usual distance for an optometrist's chart). If you were to look at the chart 'out of the corner of your eye' (with your far peripheral retina), the letters would have to be 100 times larger to be recognized. Because the fovea is so small, it is necessary to move the eyes in order to explore the scene at high resolution. To convince yourself how quickly visual resolution falls off in the peripheral retina, try to read the words at the edges of the page of a book while holding your eye fixedly on the middle of the page. Whatever the merits of 'speed reading', there is no possibility, as some claim, that every word can be recognized if the line of sight is simply moved down the middle of the page.

(a)

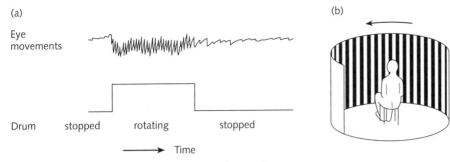

Fig. 1 The optokinetic response to rotation of the visual surround.

A proper classification of human eye movements, still valid, was provided by the American psychologist Raymond Dodge, at the beginning of the twentieth century. He distinguished two types of compensatory movements: the *vestibulo-ocular reflex* (VOR) and the *optokinetic response* (OKR), both of which compensate for head movement. And he described three types of active, exploratory movement: (i) *saccades* — rapid shifts in the line of sight that are used to look at new targets; (ii) *smooth pursuit* — smooth movements of the eyes to follow a moving target; and (iii) *vergence* — alteration of the angle between the lines of sight of each eye, either increasing the angle (*convergence*) to look at close objects, or decreasing it (*divergence*), so as to look at things far away.

Stabilization movements

The most common cause of instability of the retinal image is one's own movement. If this is slow, then the whole image begins to slip across the retina; this overall movement is detected by the brain, which initiates a reflex, compensatory optokinetic eye movement. But when the head moves quickly, signals from the retina itself are too slow to drive useful compensatory movements: it takes 1/20 sec or so for visual signals to leave the retina, let alone travel through the various brain pathways to control eye movements. On the other hand, the organ of BALANCE (the vestibular apparatus) in the inner ear, which detects both rapid rotations and linear motion of the head, has negligible internal delays. Its signals cause vestibulo-ocular reflex movements of the eyes, which compensate quite precisely for the head movement, even in complete darkness. Of course, if the head were to continue to rotate through a very large angle, uninterrupted counter-rotation of the eyes would carry them to the limit of travel in their sockets. In fact this does not happen because the smooth movement is frequently interrupted by rapid jerks of the eyes in the opposite direction, tending to re-centre the eyes in the orbits. This fast-slow-fast-slow, back and forth movement of the eyes is called *nystagmus*.

The VOR operates for rotations about all axes, even around the direction in which the eye is looking. Get someone to sit on an office chair that can turn, looking directly upward along the axis of the spindle of the chair. If the chair is rotated gently, a torsional VOR occurs: the eyes counter-rotate around the line of sight, flicking back from time to time.

While the VOR is remarkably accurate for fast head movements, even a small error will cause the image to slither across he retina during head movement. Such image movement activates a second stabilization response: the OKR. This visually-driven response may be demonstrated by placing a volunteer inside a rotating drum, the internal walls of which are covered with stripes, to create uniform motion of virtually the entire visual field, as shown in Fig. 1(b). The eye movements so elicited are called 'optokinetic nystagmus' (OKN): the eyes move smoothly in the direction of drum motion (*slow phases*) and intermittently flick rapidly back in the opposite direction (*fast phases*). (See Fig. 1(a).) Another interesting effect of sitting in such a rotating drum is that, after a few seconds, most observers feel that the drum has slowed down and even stopped, and that their body is rotating in the opposite direction. This is a sort of rotational analogue of the common experience, when sitting in a stationary train at the railway station, of mistaking the adjacent train pulling out for the departure of one's own. The rotation illusion is called *circular vection* and was studied by the nineteenth-century physicist Ernst Mach.

Exploratory movements

When you wish to scrutinize an object in the visual field, it is important to place its image on the fovea, where visual acuity is highest. Rapid saccadic eye movements do this. Even when you try your best to shift your gaze slowly and smoothly, for instance when reading, the eyes actually move in a series of small saccades (see Fig. 2). Saccades have fairly stereotyped time-courses, and the movements themselves last between only 1/40 sec, for the smallest saccades, and about a tenth of a second, for the largest. They are thus some of the fastest movements the body can produce.

Saccades are *conjugate* (i.e. matched in size in the two eyes) when gaze is transferred between two objects at the same distance from the viewer, but are *disconjugate* (different in size in the two eyes) when shifting gaze between two objects at different distances as well as in different directions in the field. If you are looking at something and another object of interest appears unexpectedly in your visual field, there is a delay of about quarter of a second before you make a saccade to look at the new object. But if the current target is suddenly removed before the second one appears, the delay in making the saccade to a new target can be as short as one tenth of a second. This suggests that the normal long delay is not entirely due to the time taken to process information about the new object in the brain; part of the delay is the time needed to disengage attention from what one was previously looking at.

Smooth pursuit eye movements are used to follow a moving target that one is looking at directly. For predictable target movements of

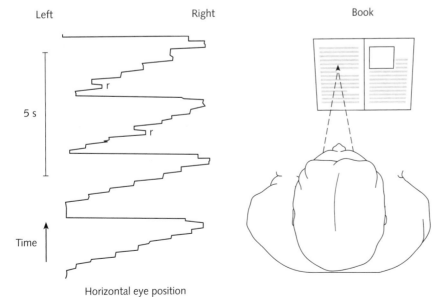

Fig. 2 Eye movements in reading.

modest velocity, eye velocity comes close to matching target velocity. Unlike saccades, smooth pursuit cannot easily be initiated voluntarily without a moving target to follow. When a target first starts to move, it shifts off the fovea before the smooth eye movement can start (because there is a delay of about one eighth of a second). Therefore there is often an initial 'catch-up saccade' mixed with the beginning of the smooth pursuit.

Dodge noticed and objectively documented the curious fact that patients in an asylum for the mentally ill (suffering from what we would now call schizophrenia) had imperfect smooth pursuit, in that they followed a swinging pendulum bob with a chain of tiny, rapid, saccadic eye movements rather than by continuous motion. Dodge's methods of recording eye movements were cumbersome and probably somewhat painful, but, contrary to what one might have expected, he found subjects in the asylum generally very co-operative — perhaps because they were otherwise so bored!

Vergence eye movements are the disconjugate movements made when shifting gaze from one distance to another. The 'cross-eyed' movement needed to look at close objects (for instance, at the end of your nose) is called *convergence*. The reverse movement is called *divergence*. Pure vergence movements, uncontaminated by saccades, occur when changing gaze between two targets, both lying straight ahead, but at different distances. These vergence movements are smooth, and approximately five times slower than conjugate saccades of a similar size. Convergence is normally closely associated with *accommodation* (focusing) of the eyes and constriction of the pupil, forming together the so-called 'near response' (because they all prepare the eye for looking at a near object).

Even when one does one's best to fixate a small object, tiny eye movements occur involuntarily. One of the most remarkable of all findings in this field is that the minute instability caused by these miniature eye movements is actually essential for vision. If the retinal image is artificially *completely* stabilized (for instance by monitoring eye position and using a feedback system to move the visual scene so as to exactly compensate for all eye movements), then vision fades out completely after a few seconds.

Eye muscles

Each eye is rotated by six extraocular muscles, which can achieve rotation about any axis, centred on a point approximately 13 mm behind the cornea. Rotations have awkward mathematical properties — e.g. one rotation followed by another about a different axis does not generally have the same effect as the two rotations applied in the opposite order. A complete description of eye movement needs advanced mathematics. In general the effect of contraction of any one eye muscle depends on the degree of contraction of all the others. This is just one of the complications that the brain must deal with as it programmes eye movements.

Why don't we see the world move when we move our eyes?

We have remarkably little awareness of our eye movements, which is perhaps just as well considering that we make several hundred saccades each minute! One issue that has attracted a great deal of attention is how a stable impression of the world is achieved from a series of 'snapshots' of information gained during each saccade. Passive displacement of the retinal image (by tapping the side of the eyeball gently, for example) produces a dramatic sense of movement of the visual environment, whereas the same retinal image displacement brought about by a voluntary saccade has no such consequence: the visual world is stable. It seems likely that the brain makes some sort of comparison between signals from the retina and internal messages from the eye movement control system, and 'assumes' that the world is stationary unless there is blatant contradiction between the two.

Very little is seen during saccadic movements themselves. This is mainly because the very rapid slipping of the image smears the detail. However, there is also a genuine decrease in sensitivity to light during a saccade — called *saccadic suppression*. This can be demonstrated by testing how bright a flash of light must be in order for it to be seen, either when the eye is still or during a saccade. (The flash must be so brief that it is not blurred by the movement.) The loss of sensitivity is very small, and this makes it unlikely that (as some argue) saccadic suppression is actively programmed to help to block signals to the brain during saccades. In any case, the resolution of this issue will not greatly advance the understanding of how the world comes to be perceived as stable, because no amount of alteration of visual sensitivity during saccades can alter the fact that before a saccade the retinal image is in one place and after it is in another.   STUART J. JUDGE

See also ACCOMMODATION; EYE; GAZE; VESTIBULAR SYSTEM; VISION.

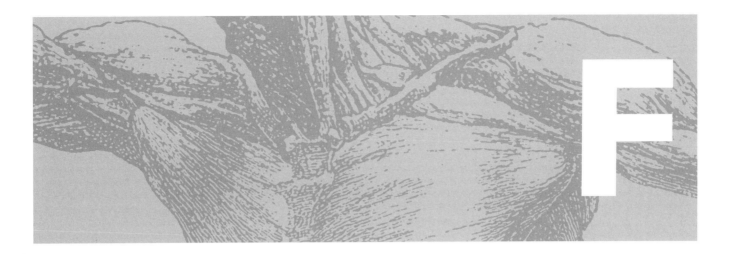

Face The face is the most complex-surface structure of human and other vertebrate anatomy — in humans containing a total of 14 bones and 32 teeth: it includes the frontal bone supporting the forehead; a cartilaginous nasal cavity; prominent cheeks supported by malar bones; circular muscles around the mouth and each eye; other musculature radiating from the circular muscles; a fixed upper jaw (maxilla) and movable lower jaw (mandible); and sensory apparatus for VISION, HEARING, TASTE and SMELL.

The human face is commonly seen as the key to identifying individuals and comprehending their emotional states and intentions. Its characteristic structures and expressions have been the focus of much of culture, both East and West, making the face perhaps the most important anatomical subject of mythology, religion, art, and literature. When Marlowe had Faustus ask of Helen,

‘Was this the face that launched a thousand ships
And burnt the topless towers of Ilium?’,

he echoed the elders of Troy, whom Homer had murmur,

‘Terrible is the likeness of her face to immortal goddesses.’

The terrible beauty of the human face, its potential to reveal and to conceal, its alleged power to disclose essential features of the individual, the race, or the species, its ability to inspire love and motivate acts of utter unreason, together with its capacity for pretence and deception, mark it as a subject of unending interest and complexity.

Physiological and evolutionary development

The human face begins in fetal development as a forehead protrusion above an incipient mouth at approximately four weeks gestational age. At seven months the face has achieved much of its early development — though the proportion of facial surface to cranium; the growth of nasal structures; the eruption of teeth; the fusion of facial skeletal sutures; and the relative facial dimensions in depth, height, and width continue to develop, some well into adolescence.

While it is possible to find evolutionary traces of the modern human face at each stage from early vertebrates to *Homo sapiens*, facial structures are important boundaries between humans and our prehuman ancestors. The *Australopithecenes* and other prehumans had relatively large faces in proportion to the size of their heads, whereas modern humans have proportionally smaller faces and larger braincases filled with larger brains. Jaw and tooth structure are less complex and smaller in modern humans, resulting in less protrusive jaws and a more vertical profile. Prominent and distinctive in this profile are the nose and the well-defined chin separating modern humans both from prehuman ancestors and from other, contemporary primates.

Evolutionary variation in facial features has helped physiognomy and physical anthropology attempt to define racial categories. While certain features are more prominent in one geographic racial group than in another, such categorization is not definitive or entirely reliable. Attempts to make such judgments have had profound social consequences, however.

The face in the mirror

The idea that the face both reveals and conceals or masks identity is a very ancient one. In classical drama, great literature, and bank robbery alike, masks obscure or conceal facial features and thus conceal identity. Facial recognition is an early and primary skill; very young infants have been shown to prefer the sight of the human face to other images.

Facial cues have been shown to be vital in several areas of recognition, including age, sex, ethnicity and race, emotional state, honesty and deception, and personal identity. The most important aspect of recognition is that of individual identity. While individual features of a face are important in recognizing other aspects of a person, identifying an individual flows largely from identifying their face as a whole. The ability to pick out one's adult friend from a group photograph taken in his youth seems an unremarkable task and yet requires remarkable powers of discernment. Family resemblance marks faces as of a type, allowing identification of siblings and different generations, but recognizing individuals requires more than specific features. This ability is strongest when one identifies individuals within one's own racial group; research has shown that cross-racial and perhaps cross-ethnic recognition is more difficult than identification within one's own race or ethnicity. Psychologist Leslie Zebrowitz hypothesizes that facial recognition is much like language acquisition, and that early immersion in another racial group may be necessary to facilitate cross-racial identification.

Facial recognition of personal identity appears to have a specific location within the brain. *Prosopagnosia*, a disorder in which there is a deficit of facial recognition, is caused by lesions in a specific part of the visual system of the brain. Prosopagnosics are often able to identify aspects of faces, but they are unable to recognize persons — sometimes even themselves — by using facial cues. In such cases, identity reverts to other cues, including voice.

Reading faces

Children are usually taught ‘not to judge a book by its cover’, and most adults recognize the ability of a façade — architectural or otherwise — to misrepresent in Potemkin-village fashion what it seeks to conceal. LEONARDO DA VINCI's *Mona Lisa* is a commonly-cited example of both the centrality of reading faces for the meaning they represent and the difficulty of doing so. Despite this, psychological research and the clear evidence of artistic and literary experience demonstrate that our judgments of physical, mental, and moral health often proceed from the first glance of facial appearance.

A remark to a friend that she doesn't ‘look’ well is usually an elliptical reference to the friend's facial appearance. Traditional Japanese and Chinese medicine use facial appearance as a key diagnostic indicator. In contemporary Western medicine, the term 'facies' is used to describe the general facial appearance of a patient, especially useful in the diagnosis of disorders marked by phenotypic facial characteristics. Some of these conditions (for example, Down's syndrome and Patau syndrome), are caused by genetic anomalies and produce serious physical and mental abnormalities, while others (fetal alcohol syndrome, for example) are congenital in nature, and still others (syphilis and measles, for example) are caused by infectious agents.

Genetically-linked and congenital disorders are often associated not only with specific facial anomalies but also with a general tendency toward facial asymmetry. Many INFECTIOUS DISEASES produce distinctive facial appearances that are helpful and sometimes central to diagnosis. Parents know that, at first (facial) glance, the indication of a child's common cold or fever is found in changes in facial appearance. Beyond changes in appearance caused by diseases or disorders, correlations have been suggested between specific facial structural types and certain diseases, including polio and some types of ulcer. Some evolutionary theorists have gone beyond these results in asserting a correlation between facial asymmetry and an increased susceptibility to infectious and genetically-linked disease. The experimental evidence for this claim is inconclusive.

The evidence linking specific facial appearances both with underlying causal disorders and increased vulnerability to specific conditions is slightly better, however, especially where the facial characteristics and expressions are indicative of living patterns and personality types. The veined, red nose associated with chronic alcoholism and the frequent scowls, raising of upper eyelids, and tensing of eyes of a 'Type A' personality can help diagnose their immediate causes. Even here, however, one must be careful, since these same facial characteristics can be caused by other conditions: the red nose of the 'alcoholic' could indicate instead the skin disease rosacea, or even something as simple as a bad cold or allergies. Likewise, the scowls and other features of the 'Type A' may indicate specific neurological damage or, if one is observing a single instance, simply a bad case of indignation or even indigestion.

Ordinary experience and results in experimental psychology demonstrate that many people judge the mental or moral health of others by their facial structures and expressions. Classical Greek medicine attributed many mental (especially emotional) disorders to an imbalance of the four HUMOURS (blood, yellow bile, phlegm, and black bile) and, in a forerunner of the contemporary use of 'facies', diagnosed mental and physical disorders in part by the surface expressions of the imbalance of colour or physical shape in the face. The development of PHYSIOGNOMY as an explanatory framework for describing and predicting psychological (and later social and moral) conditions on the basis of facial and other physical conformation provides a more

subtle if no less flawed understanding than the theory of the four humours. A work attributed to Aristotle (*Physiognomonica*) gives the first recorded systematic treatment of physiognomic principles, with both a description of the diagnostic method and a catalogue of results. Aristotle's treatment of the topic relies on analogies to the facial characteristics of animals, a practice nearly universal in human culture. Greek mythology and art, astrological traditions, medieval bestiaries and heraldry, children's fables, personal naming practices in Native American and other cultures, and many colloquial expressions ('a face like a dumb ox') all make use of such analogies. Classical references attempt to describe the systematic correlation between face and mind, while medieval efforts joined description to prediction.

By the eighteenth century, physiognomy had assimilated many modern advances in biology, especially improvements in anatomical knowledge. By the end of that century and throughout the nineteenth century, physiognomists developed a theory of mental, moral, and especially evolutionary fitness that could be determined in large part by facial characteristics. Swiss physiognomist J. C. Lavater's 1772 work on reading faces was very influential. (Charles Darwin relates the story of how he was nearly denied passage on HMS *Beagle* because the captain, influenced by Lavater's views, was convinced that the shape of Darwin's nose indicated insufficient 'energy' and 'determination' for the voyage.) Textbooks in psychiatry and criminology regularly assumed the truth of these theories. In one recently cited example, Krafft–Ebing's 1879 textbook on insanity claimed that 'every psychopathic state, like the physiologic states of emotion, has its own peculiar facial expression and general manner of movement which, for the experienced, on superficial observation, makes a probable diagnosis possible.' Illustrations in such texts provided carefully categorized examples of such correspondences.

Reading faces as a way of detecting criminality and moral or social degeneracy is an important aspect of nineteenth- and early twentieth-century physiognomy. The Italian physician and criminologist Cesare Lombroso saw criminality (for the most part) as an atavism, with the natural criminal one who 'reproduces in his person the ferocious instincts of primitive humanity and the inferior animals.' The marks, the *stigmata* — as Lombroso revealingly termed them — of the criminal type once again reflect the analogy with animal types. Lombroso found the stigmata concentrated both in 'primitive' non-European races and in Europeans from the lowest socio-economic classes. While the stigmata include features of the feet, arms, hair type, etc., the most significant are facial or facially-related. The frontispiece to his work *Criminal Man* is a veritable rogue's gallery of facial types, arranged by the type of crime to which their anatomical destiny condemned them. Stephen Jay Gould's critique of Lombroso lists the facial stigmata of the criminal

man, including large jaw size, high face-to-cranium proportions, pronounced wrinkles, a less prominent forehead, large ears, and darker skin. This last feature reveals the assumptions colouring much of Lombroso's pseudo-science and by extension much of criminal anthropology and physiognomy: natural criminality and natural superiority coincided very nicely with then-existing assumptions about natural hierarchies in intellectual, social, political, and economic life. One's face, together with other salient physical features, truly was one's destiny, and while the natural criminal is not to be blamed in any ultimate sense, neither could he be changed. 'We see in the criminal man,' Lombroso wrote, 'a savage man and, at the same time, a sick man.' These 'sick men' were 'true savages in the midst of our brilliant European civilization'. Such biological determinism was very influential at the end of the nineteenth century and helped pave the way for the early-to-mid twentieth-century EUGENICS movement that marked the naturally (physiologically, culturally, morally, racially) defective for passive elimination by controlled breeding or, as in the hands of Nazi racial theorists, for active elimination in the gas chambers of Auschwitz.

While the theory of the humours is a quaint antiquity and the sometimes pernicious theories of physiognomy have been dismissed by modern science, it is clear that many continue to read physical, mental, and moral health in faces. The long and deeply held view that the face reveals essential aspects of the self, that facial cues tell us more than science is willing to admit, remains. Schopenhauer's comment on the subject, that 'as a rule a man's face . . . is the monogram of all his thoughts and aspirations' is more reflective of how we actually live than many of us care to acknowledge.

A smooth impostor or the motions of the mind?

The face has been exploited in its essential ambiguity in culture generally, and in art and literature in particular. Portraiture no less than caricature draws upon generalizations about human nature and character to depict the face as concealer and revealer, and Western literature has used the set of a face to paint the intellectual, emotional, and moral scenes of its dramas. To be faceless is to be without identity and thus without weight, and yet artistic and literary portrayals of the face often fail to deliver on the promise of portraying a clear and unambiguous identity. Da Vinci's characterization of his portraits as depicting 'the motions of the mind' sits face-to-face with Pierre Corneille's remark that:

> The face is often only
> A smooth impostor.

In addition to the attempt to describe through portrayal the emotional reality of the subject, the art of the face has been put to other purposes. Idealized political types, psychological traits, and moral principles have been conveyed through artistic representations of the face since ancient times, serving political, religious, and commercial ideals. From the distorted Paleolithic faces on the cave walls at Les Trois Frères in southern France, which may have had a magical function; to ancient Egyptian and Mesopotamian use of the face in art, serving in large part religious and political purposes; to classical Greek depictions of an aesthetic ideal; to iconography and religious art in the Christian world; to nineteenth- and twentieth-century 'faces' of liberty and revolution; to the modern use of well-scrubbed young faces in commercial advertising, the human face has been a vehicle for both artist and society, giving form to their ideals.

In some contemporary philosophy the face has taken on a new and important role, though one that echoes earlier humanisms. In the twilight of postmodernism, some philosophers in the European continental tradition are looking to the human face as a, if not the, mark of the ethical. Emmanuel Levinas has stated that

'the other becomes my neighbor precisely through the way the face summons me, calls for me, begs for me, and so doing recalls my responsibility, and calls me into question.'

Levinas points to the twentieth century's remarkable accomplishments in defacing or effacing individuals, both in body and in spirit, and points out that ethical individuality is accomplished — if it is accomplished — only in the gaze of the other, of the 'epiphany of the face as a face'. Perhaps the terrible beauty of the face can find its ethical reflection in the mirror of the other. It is sure to retain its ambiguity, its complexity, and its centrality in human life. JEFFREY H. BARKER

Further reading

Davies, G., et al. (1981). Perceiving and remembering faces. Academic Press, London.

Ekman, P. (1973). Darwin and facial expression. Academic Press, New York.

Gould, S. J. (1981). The mismeasure of man. W. W. Norton and Company, New York.

Zebrowitz, L. A. (1997). Reading faces. Westview Press, Boulder, Colorado.

See also PHYSIOGNOMY; SKULL.

Facial expression Can we trust our interpretation of a foreigner's facial expressions; do we need an expression translator? Are expressions, like gestures and words, socially learned and therefore culture-specific in their meaning? Or are our expressions the product of our evolution and therefore universal? Why do the eyebrows go up in surprise rather than down? Do other animals have facial expressions, and if so do they have the same meaning as they do in humans? Can we use our expressions to lie about how we are feeling, or are they more reliable than words?

The great evolutionary theorist Charles Darwin wrote a book about facial expression. *The Expression of the Emotions in Man and Animals*, in which he considered these questions (except the one about lying). Remarkably, many of his observations, first published in 1872, have recently been proven to be largely correct. As Darwin suggested, the facial expressions of a number of EMOTIONS are universal, not culture-specific. The muscles that contract to produce the facial expressions of anger, fear, sadness, disgust,

and enjoyment are the same the world over, regardless of sex or culture. Three kinds of research have established this. When people from various cultures have been asked to identify the emotions represented by photographs of different expressions, they have, by and large, given the same answers. In one set of studies the people studied were from an isolated, Stone Age culture in New Guinea, who, at the time, could not have learned how to make or interpret expressions from outsiders or the media. A second type of research asked people to use their faces to imitate different emotions, and found members of different cultures produced the same expressions. The figure shows people from the isolated New Guinea culture posing three of the emotions. The last type of research measured spontaneous expressions when people in different cultures were subject to the same emotional conditions, and found that the same expressions were shown under the same circumstances.

There may also be universal expressions for surprise, contempt, and embarrassment as it is for anger, fear, sadness, disgust and enjoyment, but the evidence is not as complete. Love and hate — which probably don't have unique facial expressions — involve strong feelings, but those feelings endure much longer than the emotions, which can last only seconds or at most minutes. Love and hate may be better thought of as affective attitudes rather than momentary emotions. There may be facial expressions for other emotions such as shame or awe, but these have yet to be identified.

Not everything about facial expressions of emotion is universal. All people learn, in the

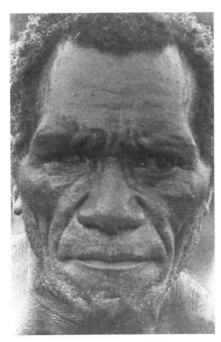

(a) show me what your face would look like if you were about to fight.

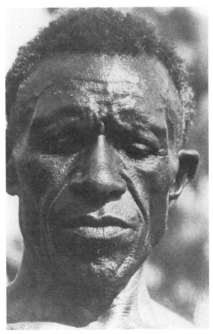

(b) show me what your face would look like if you learned your child had died.

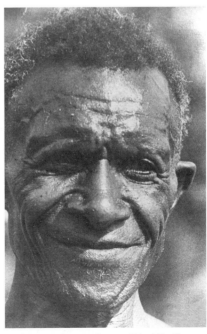

(c) show me what your face would look like if you met friends.

Photographs from Ekman, P. (1980). *Face of Man: universal expression in a New Guinea village*. Garland, New York.

course of growing up, to manage their facial expressions. Polite and proper behaviour requires that we employ what have been termed *display rules* that dictate who can show which emotions to whom, and when. For example, in many societies, people who lose in a public contest try to inhibit any sign of their disappointment. Although we know what we should do, that does not always mean that a display rule is actually followed. There are cultural differences in display rules. For example, in one experiment, when a person in authority was present, Japanese masked with a polite smile the sign of any negative emotions more than did Americans. When there was no one present, then American and Japanese subjects showed the same emotional expression when watching different emotional scenes. Misunderstandings in cross-cultural communication occur when people do not realize that it is a difference of display rule that makes for a different expression, not the underlying emotion.

Darwin also tried to explain why we make the particular expressions that we do for particular emotions. Why do the eyebrows go up rather than down in surprise? Building on Darwin's ideas, contemporary theorists believe that these expressions originated in movements that were of functional value — raising the brows might let in more light, raising the upper lip exposes the teeth, and so forth. Over the course of our evolutionary history these movements have been ritualized, to communicate intentions to others. The most difficult expression to explain is the smile.

Darwin claimed that emotions and their expressions are not unique to humans but shared with other animals. Nearly all of our facial muscles can be found in other primates. Chimpanzees, for example, show some expressions that bear a resemblance to human expressions. But do they actually feel the same emotions? Without the capacity for words they probably cannot think about or make plans about their emotions as easily as we do. But they do show similar expressions to ours when they are playing, threatened by harm, about to attack, or when their young offspring are removed. When we look at animals with less developed brains, we find that vocalizations play a more important role than facial expressions. In humans, both the face and the voice signal emotions.

Facial expressions of emotion are involuntary and are produced almost immediately when an emotion occurs. Yet we can, to a large extent, interrupt or suppress expressions if we concentrate on doing so. We can also deliberately put on expressions of certain emotions when we do not feel them. This is hard to do for fear and sadness, because most people do not have voluntary control over the specific facial muscles that are deployed in those expressions. False expressions of enjoyment, anger, disgust, and surprise are easy to make, although careful measurement of the speed, symmetry, and specific muscular activity suggests that it is possible to distinguish

the spontaneous from the false expressions of even these emotions.

Different areas of the brain are involved in the recognition of emotion (what does that person feel?) and the recognition of identity (who is that person?). Patients with damage (from STROKE or accident) to one brain area may not know who other people are, but they do know how they feel, while those with damage to another brain area know who people are but not how they feel. Recent research has found that the perception of different facial expressions of emotion activates different brain areas, suggesting that not only are we highly sensitive to facial expression, but very specialized mechanisms have evolved to process this information.   PAUL EKMAN

See also EMOTION; FACE.

Faeces
Adults in Western societies excrete approximately 200 g of faeces each day. Faeces consist of unabsorbed water, undigested fibre, short chain fatty acids (which are a major product of fermentation), relatively low concentrations of salts, and an extremely large number of bacteria including anaerobes, lactobacilli, yeasts, and coliforms. Faeces are normally 'formed' rather than fluid; this is advantageous as it indicates effective retrieval of fluid and electrolytes, and is a component of the continence mechanism. The colour of faeces relates predominantly to the presence of bile 'pigments; in obstructive jaundice, when bile pigments are unable to enter the intestine, the faeces become pale and sometimes almost white.

Faeces may change consistency in pathological states (see DIARRHOEA and CONSTIPATION). Faeces become offensive in malabsorption states, particularly when increased quantities of fat enter the colon and are then available for bacterial degradation. This also results in increased quantities of gas being present in faeces, which accounts for the fact that faeces float when there is fat malabsorption. Faeces become hard and more difficult to pass when the diet is low in dietary fibre. Other conditions which result in slow intestinal transit also tend to produce hard faeces.

Faeces act as a vehicle for many intestinal infections when the organism can exist in its natural state or in the form of a cyst which enables the infective agent (usually a parasite) to exist outside its host in the environment. Careful disposal of faeces and clear separation between sewers and domestic water supplies has been one of the most important primary public health interventions to prevent the spread of infectious gastrointestinal diseases.

MICHAEL FARTHING
ANNE BALLINGER

See also ALIMENTARY SYSTEM; CONSTIPATION; DEFECATION; DIARRHOEA; TOILET PRACTICES.

Fainting
is a transient, reversible loss of CONSCIOUSNESS due to an acute reduction in blood supply to the brain. Lack of cerebral perfusion for 2–3 sec can cause premonitory symptoms (such as light-headedness, DIZZINESS); after

10 sec fainting results. Fainting is synonymous with *syncope* (from the Greek 'to strike' or 'cut off'). Slumping in a chair or falling to the ground characteristically occurs because of loss of postural MUSCLE TONE, although occasionally there may be jerky movements, muscle spasms, or urinary incontinence as a result of transient 'decerebration'. Fainting usually occurs when the subject is upright, and falling results in recovery of cerebral blood flow and spontaneous recovery.

Fainting does not cause damage to the nervous system, unless there is injury from the fall, but it can cause concern, embarrassment, and loss of confidence. However some of the conditions associated with fainting are potentially serious or even potentially fatal. It has been said that 'the only difference between fainting and sudden death is that in one you wake up' (Engel, 1978).

Maintenance of blood flow to the brain is dependent on an adequate BLOOD PRESSURE and on patent and responsive cerebral blood vessels. These vessels dilate to maintain flow when blood pressure falls within its normal range of variation, but a major or rapid fall can defeat this compensation. Thus, there are numerous causes of fainting.

Low blood pressure (*hypotension*) may occur with postural (*orthostatic*) change, on moving from the horizontal to the upright position such as when rising after sleep. The sympathetic nervous system normally responds to gravitational change and prevents pooling of blood in the lower limbs by an increase in its activity, which causes constriction of blood vessels. The majority of the population do not faint, as adaptive mechanisms to standing erect are well developed. However, in certain situations even the fittest can faint (such as guardsmen standing still at attention on a hot day), and there are some disease conditions, and some drugs, which impair the reflex response. Fainting caused by postural hypotension classically occurs on assumption of the head-up posture, with relief by lying flat.

Intermittent abnormal activity of the AUTONOMIC NERVOUS SYTEM (*neurally-mediated syncope*) also may occur. During these episodes increased parasympathetic activity slows the heart rate whilst diminished sympathetic activity allows blood vessels to dilate, lowering blood pressure. The most common form is known as *vasovagal syncope* — the 'emotional' or 'common' fainting. This is often of teenage onset, in females, and with a family history.

A variety of factors, such as fear of needles, sight of blood, or pain, can precipitate this type of fainting. There is often prompt recovery on attaining the horizontal position. In the elderly, similar autonomic effects on the heart and circulation may occur, when there is hypersensitivity of the BARORECEPTORS in the carotid sinus in the neck; tightening the collar, or moving the head whilst shaving, stimulates nerves that normally signal a rise in blood pressure. The result is a 'correction' of this false signal — a fall in heart rate and blood pressure. This can be a potentially serious condition, with severe injury from falls, and may require treatment with a cardiac PACE-MAKER and drugs that maintain blood pressure.

There are other, rarer, causes of fainting mediated by the nervous system, precipitated by a range of factors such as urination, coughing, or swallowing.

Another cause of fainting is a change in cardiac rhythm, when the heart beats too fast or too slowly, resulting in a poor cardiac output and inadequate blood flow to the brain. The best known is the *Stokes–Adams attack*, when the ventricles of the heart fail to beat because of HEART BLOCK.

There are also more direct — mechanical or hydraulic — causes of low blood pressure; these include depletion of the circulating blood volume due to HAEMORRHAGE or plasma loss, and inadequate fluid intake or excessive fluid loss due to VOMITING or DIARRHOEA, or from the kidneys in some abnormal conditions. Excessive dilatation of blood vessels, due to drugs (such as glyceryl trinitrate used in angina, or from excessive alcohol ingestion), circulating vasodilator substances, or venous disorders (extensive varicose veins), may be contributory.

Finally, constriction of the cerebral blood vessels may contribute to fainting. For example, during HYPERVENTILATION, even in healthy people, low carbon dioxide in the blood causes constriction of the blood vessels. Or when a major vessel supplying the brain is partly or severely occluded in *carotid artery stenosis*, even small decreases in blood pressure or changes in cardiac rhythm threaten the blood supply.

In summary, fainting may occur in any individual, from the young (*vasovagal syncope*), to the elderly (*carotid sinus hypersensitivity*). It is estimated to occur at some time in 3% of the adult population, and sometimes in extremely healthy and fit people (oarsmen, athletes, and in particular weightlifters). There may be an occupational hazard — as in trumpet players. Fainting is usually involuntary, but it may be deliberately induced, as in the so-called 'fainting lark': a combination of squatting, overbreathing, forceful expiration, and standing up suddenly. The 'Mess trick' is a variation of this.

Fainting can sometimes be ominous, especially in those with an untreated cardiac rhythm disorder, consistent with ancient observations that 'those who suffer from frequent and severe fainting without cause often die suddenly' (Hippocrates, *Aphorisms* 2.41). But in many other conditions, such as vasovagal syncope, the prognosis is excellent.   C. J. MATHIAS

See also AUTONOMIC NERVOUS SYSTEM; BLOOD PRESSURE.

Fallopian tubes
Fallopio was an outstanding sixteenth-century Italian anatomist (a pupil of VESALIUS, who challenged the teaching of GALEN); in 1561 he published a description of these tubes, which are also known as oviducts. Each of the two symmetrical tubes has a fringed open end close to an OVARY, and leads into the

cavity of the UTERUS. One of the tubes 'catches' the ovum discharged from an ovary at the monthly ovulation. The wall is muscular and the lining is covered in cilia — fine fronds whose movement waves the ovum along the tube. If sperm are ascending at the crucial time, fertilization takes place usually in mid-tube, and the embryo is conducted onwards to the uterus.

s.j.

See MENSTRUAL CYCLE; PREGNANCY; PLATE 8.

Farting
or 'breaking wind', is releasing gas from the anus. The English word 'fart' has been around for a long time; in 1386, Chaucer wrote: 'This Nicholas anon let flee a fart.'

The medical word for a fart is *flatus* (rhymes with hiatus); farting is flatulence — which is sometimes used to mean belching as well. 'Pease and beans are flatulent meat' (Blount, 1674) — and there are flatulently, flatulentness, flatuosity, and flatuous — 'If a man eat them [mulberries] alone . . . they swell in the stomack and be very flatuous' (Holland's translation of Pliny, 1601). However, there seems to be no verb 'to flatulate'.

Some old people claim that they fart more with increasing age. Doctors do not regard flatulence as a problem in the absence of other serious symptoms.

Farting has always been viewed as vulgar and comical. In the opening scene of Aristophanes's comic play *The Frogs*, the slave Xanthias, trying to raise a laugh from his master (and the audience), says:

μηδ' ὅτι τοσοῦτον ἄχθος ἐπ' ἐμαυτῷ φέρων,

εἰ μὴ καθαιρήσει τις, ἀποπαρδήσομαι;

which means, roughly, 'Well, how about this: If nobody will take away my pack, I'll let a fart and blow it off my back!'

Noise
The Roman Emperor Claudius felt strongly that people should have no inhibitions about farting, even at parties, and issued an edict to that effect. In the 1530s, Erasmus wrote that to hold back wind is dangerous, but that one should hide the sound with a cough, for 'the sound of farting, especially of those who stand on elevated ground, is horrible.' Today most people try to hide the sounds of farts in public places, and smart public lavatories in Japan are equipped with wall-mounted gadgets that make a loud flushing noise when a button is pressed, thus covering the noise of a fart the occupant feels is coming.

However, one man made his living from the sounds of his farts. Joseph Pujol, who called himself *Le Petomane*, found he could inhale air through his anus, and developed amazing control of the farting sounds he made. He appeared on stage at the Moulin Rouge in Paris, wearing a red tail-coat and black satin breeches, and delivered a long repertoire that ranged from the sound of a young girl farting to that of a strip of calico tearing. He blew out candles, and, through a tube, played *Au claire de la lune* on a little flute,

and smoked a cigarette. During the 1890s he could earn 20 000 francs in one day at the box office, while Sarah Bernhardt earned only 8000.

Chemistry
Farts are actually gas bubbles produced in the colon by the action of bacteria on food. The idea that farts are bubbles of swallowed air that have been passed right through the digestive tract has been disproved by American research: the gases in farts are mainly carbon dioxide (up to 50%), hydrogen (up to 40%), nitrogen (about 20%), and methane. One person in three produces about 15% methane; the rest of us produce none. This probably arises because we all have hundreds of types of bacteria in the gut, and they vary widely from person to person.

Hydrogen and methane are highly flammable, which has led to some tragic accidents on the operating table. In April 1978, for example, at the University Hospital in Nancy in France, surgeons were trying to remove a polyp from the colon of a 69-year-old man, using an electrically heated wire loop. When they switched on the power to the loop there was a loud explosion inside the colon, and despite emergency surgery the patient died within minutes. Their conclusion was that even though his bowels had been thoroughly cleared and seemed to be completely clean, an explosive mixture of air and hydrogen or methane must have collected. After this incident the official policy was changed, and such patients were insufflated with carbon dioxide before and during surgery.

There have been rumours that cases claimed to be SPONTANEOUS HUMAN COMBUSTION were in fact caused by farts being ignited by electrostatic sparks from synthetic fibres in underwear.

A vet in Holland was smoking a cigarette while working on a cow. It farted, and after the subsequent explosion the barn burned to the ground. Cows and other ruminants produce methane and other gases from both ends. In 1799 these gases were thought to have possible medical benefits, and were tried out on the patients at Dr Beddoes' Pneumatic Institution in Bristol, under the supervision of the medical superintendent, the 19-year-old Humphry Davy.

Today the farts from cows are asserted by some to yield enough methane to cause a greenhouse effect in the upper atmosphere, thus contributing seriously to global warming.

Beans
Almost all people fart, typically once an hour, producing between 200 ml and 2 litres a day, although both rate and quantity can be enormously increased by stress, and by eating particular foods — notably cabbage, onions, and beans.

Foods are broken up by the acid in the stomach to produce sugars and various other fragments. The sugars reach the small intestine in the form of oligosaccharides — a few sugar molecules stuck together. We digest most of these oligosaccharides by hydrolysing them with the aid of enzymes to form simple monosaccharides, which in turn are absorbed into the bloodstream.

However, there are three rogue oligosaccharides — raffinose, stachyose, and verbascose — which we cannot digest. Hydrolysis (breakdown) of these requires the enzyme α-D-galactopyranosidase, which does not exist in the human gut. So they pass through into the large intestine, where bacteria digest them anaerobically to make carbon dioxide and hydrogen.

The flatulent effects can be reduced, some people claim, by soaking dried beans for at least 5 hours, then draining, rinsing, boiling for at least 10 minutes in fresh water, and draining and rinsing again before the final cooking.

Alternatively, proprietary medicines are available containing the missing enzyme, and the manufacturers claim that if you take these (drops or pills) when you eat beans you will be able to digest the rogue sugars, and you will not fart. Indeed, the American manufacturers go further, and sell a similar product for pets, to curtail the farting of cats and dogs!

Smell

The smell of farts can be memorable. Sir Thomas More, Chancellor to Henry VIII, was famed for his witty Latin epigrams, some of which were quite fruity:

> Sectile ne tetros porrum tibi spiret odores;
>   Protinus a porro fac mihi cepe vores;
> Denuo foetorem si vis depellere cepe:
>   Hoc facile efficient allia mansa tibi;
> Spiritus at si post etiam gravis, allia restat;
>   Aut nihil, aut tantum, tollere merda potest.

Sir John Harington, incorporating his own puns, translated this as follows:

> If leeks you leeke, but do their smell disleeke,
>   Eat onions, and you shall not smell the leeke:
> If you of onions would the sent expell,
>   Eat garlick, that shal drown the onions smell;
> But against garlikes savour, [if you smart],
>   I know but one receipt. Whats that? [A fart].

Martin Luther boasted he could 'drive away the evil spirit with a single fart.' In 1825 Thurlow asserted 'There are five or six different species of farts' — a fact known to every schoolchild.

The smell was for many decades thought to be due to the traces of indole and scatole the gas bubbles pick up from the faeces, but recent research suggests that at such concentrations these compounds smell only of mothballs. The smell of farts has been shown to come mainly from sulphur compounds; hydrogen sulphide and organic sulphides. In general, vegetarians fart more than meat-eaters, but their farts are less smelly. However, some vegetarians are said to have more sulphur-producing bacteria in their guts, and so produce much smellier farts.

When a fart is suppressed the gas may be absorbed by the gut. Most of the hydrogen and other gases eventually escape in the breath, but luckily the smell does not get through.

ADAM HART-DAVIS

Fashion In a fairly literal translation from its French and Latin origins, the word fashion describes the make or cut of an item, the forming of its shape. However, over the centuries, the word has acquired a specific association with the design, making, and wearing of clothing. Fashion now implies an awareness of and a desire to be at the forefront of changes in styles of dress and personal appearance. It can be used to suggest an extravagance and frivolity far removed from the mere functional need to clothe the body for reasons of modesty or to offer protection.

Origins

There is general agreement amongst costume historians that the origins of what we understand as fashion are to be found in the late fourteenth century. The flowing, unemphatic full-length lines which had characterized the dress of both sexes since late antiquity were gradually abandoned. Men's dress changed faster than women's, with the adoption of short tunics and closely-fitted garments. This coincided with the newly formed guilds of tailors developing skills in cutting and fitting fabric to the figure, thus allowing a much wider repertoire of stylistic effects to be achieved, with fabric and padding emphasizing or exaggerating the contours of the body. Better trading links with the Near and Middle East had introduced wider ranges of fabric, new techniques for their manufacture, and fresh ideas about colour and decoration. Inevitably, fashion, even in this early phase, was the prerogative of the wealthy who could afford the rich silks and fine linens which supplemented the staple Western European woollen fabrics. Over the next two centuries the emergence of a wealthy merchant class with international interests in trade and banking widened demand for luxurious possessions. Sumptuary laws were introduced, prohibiting the wearing of certain fabrics and colours, and meting out punishment to those who dared to presume that mere wealth could ensure equality of choice with the ruling class. This reinforcement of the notion that fashion was the prerogative of the few recurred throughout the succeeding centuries.

Fashion changed relatively slowly in the period c. 1500 to 1700, and the finest clothing was a valuable commodity, finding its way into inventories and wills, being remade and, not infrequently, stolen. The limited terminology of dress began to expand from the late seventeenth century onwards, with a proliferation of new terms indicating an increased rate of change in fashionable dress. This acceleration was underpinned by a more sophisticated process of manufacture and further improved skills but, of course, the speed of change also maintained the status quo. To be dressed in the height of fashion meant being rich or heavily in debt.

Fashion was both national and international with, in succession, Burgundian, French, and Spanish styles in the ascendant with some Italian, German, Dutch, and English elements in the mix. Curiosity about the fashions of others found expression in the costume books which began appearing in the late sixteenth century and, by the late seventeenth century, when Europe began to be dominated by all aspects of French culture, the production of exquisite engravings — precursors of the fashion plate — depicted what the most stylish French courtiers were wearing. This French hegemony was supported by the production of superb silks, delicate lace, and an ingenious array of accessories, and by a centralized court at which all the fine and applied arts from painting to dress were accorded equal attention. It is hardly surprising that the first dressmaker of international renown was Rose Bertin, who made clothes for Marie Antoinette at the French court in the 1780s; she and other dressmakers despatched fashion dolls dressed in the latest styles throughout Europe to add miniature, three-dimensional verisimilitude to supplement the available fashion illustrations.

Design and production

By the late seventeenth century a division had occurred between the provision of male and female clothing. Tailors continued to produce men's tailored garments, but female dressmakers undertook the making of women's clothing, with the exception of riding habits and CORSETS. A limited democratization of fashion occurred in the eighteenth century as some ready-made and partly made clothing allowed the less wealthy to keep in step with the growing pace of changes in fashion. The principle of exclusivity was reasserted by the continued use of the finest tailors and dressmakers by those able to afford their services and the expensive fabrics they recommended. By the nineteenth century the rise of the couturier whose name and clientele implied the height of fashion reinforced such distinctions. The idea of men being equally as interested in fashion as women declined sharply in the nineteenth century. The beaus, macaronis, and dandies of the eighteenth and early nineteenth centuries, who were caricatured and ridiculed for their dedication to the more outré details of personal appearance, were replaced by dour, dark-suited men of business.

Fashion, from the period of the Englishman Charles Worth's rise to dominance over the design of women's dress, during the Second Empire in France (when he became the first great couturier as understood today), until the 1950s, was, in the main, about women's clothing. The origins of the late twentieth century's multibillion pound fashion industry can be traced back to Worth and his two sons. He created new designs to show to his clients rather than deferring to their ideas, a notable change from previous practice. These garments were displayed on human models for his clientele of royalties, aristocrats, and the rich bourgeoisie. His clothes were bought by foreign buyers, and became available in the capitals of Europe and the US, and he was treated like an artist rather than as a tradesman by his clients, although he always thought of himself as the latter. He also reinvented the idea that a man can understand and design for women as well, if not better, than another woman. This dichotomy has been preserved; there have been inventive, even great female couturiers — Chanel, Vionnet, Schiaparelli, Grès — but the male dominance of female fashion in France, in Italy, in America, and in Great Britain has been a feature of the last 150 years.

During this period there were important technical changes which influenced the creation and marketing of fashionable clothing. The introduction of the sewing machine in the 1840s, of aniline dyes in the 1860s, and of artificial fibres from the 1890s onwards offered important improvements to the process of production. Fashion also benefited from the growing sophistication of the media: specialist magazines, dedicated newspaper articles, photographic images, and the advertising opportunities offered by film, radio, and television all contributed to an international awareness, at many levels in society, of the latest fashion trends and ideas. Increased demand for novelty in all matters to do with dress caused misery amongst the employees of many dressmakers; cramped conditions, long hours, and pitiful pay combined to create sweat shops. Unfortunately, despite legislation, this problem is still found today, and not just in the so-called Third World.

Fashion designers, especially in the period from the 1920s onwards, diversified into ranges of ready-to-wear garments, scent, and cosmetics. Specialist suppliers of accessories became equally aware of the possibilities inherent in designer footwear, jewellery, luggage, and much more. Ultimately, as both compliment and curse, talented copyists ignored patent law to produce cheap facsimiles of the most luxurious labels, and, within the law, chain stores 'imitated' the latest suit, dress, shoe, or scarf, to offer affordable fashion to mass markets.

Even in the area of alternative fashion in the post 1945 period, the world of Teddy boys, mods and rockers, hippies, punks, new Romantics, and so on, the driving force has been a masculine one. And, to a degree, alternative fashion is about men reasserting their right to attention through the adoption of unusual, exotic, or bizarre forms of dress. Ironically, these so-called street fashions have in turn, influenced the expensive, handmade creations of the powerful fashion designers.

Today, so we are led to believe, we can create our own fashion statements by buying across the spectrum from charity shops to couture houses. Fashion is fun, it is adventurous, it defines us and our approach to life. In fact, the majority prefer to conform to the dress codes of their social group, accepting or rejecting the dictates of fashion according to their circumstances and means.

Theories about dress

No overview of fashion, however basic, can ignore the corpus of criticism and theoretical analysis that has surrounded it across the centuries. The Judaeo-Christian tradition laid considerable emphasis on modesty and simplicity in all matters concerning personal adornment. As a consequence both clerical and secular moralists felt able to criticize fashion on the grounds of the supposed morality or immorality of clothing and personal adornment. Any excessive display could be construed as the sin of pride and any unnecessary revealing or emphasizing of the body could be deemed a provocation to immoral behaviour. Women's fashions were a favourite target for such moral condemnation; undoubtedly this criticism expressed real or imagined concerns about loss of CHASTITY or adultery.

Caricature and ridicule had also partnered the vagaries and absurdities of fashionable dress throughout the centuries. Artists disapproved of fashions that distorted and unbalanced their portrayal of sitters and, from the seventeenth century onwards, a number used so-called 'timeless' draperies to replace the fashions they disliked. In the nineteenth century, medical opinion was enlisted in order to question the effects on health that distorting the anatomy in quest of a fashionable silhouette might provoke. More idealistically, there was an interesting conjunction between groups of artists, doctors, and political thinkers which produced theories about aesthetic dress, dress reform, and universal suffrage which, if followed, would release women from their slavery to fashion.

Towards the end of the nineteenth century criticism was overtaken by a more analytical approach to fashion. Exponents of this approach were interested in applying their knowledge of anthropology, economic and social theory, sociology, and psychology to the reasons for the creation and popularity of certain fashions. A detailed consideration of these theories can be found in Valerie Steele's *Fashion and eroticism* (OUP, 1985). A few influential examples will indicate the range of their analysis. For instance, the American economist Thorstein Veblen, in his book *The Theory of the Leisure Class*, criticized fashionable dress as a symbol of conspicuous consumption, conspicuous leisure, and conspicuous waste. In contrast, the German historian of dress and manners, Max von Boehn, promoted the appealingly simple idea that fashion is 'a visible manifestation of the Zeitgeist' in his book *Modespiegel* (1919). The sexual significance of dress was discussed by the psychologist J. C. Flügel in *The Psychology of Clothes* (1930), a work which popularized the theory of 'shifting erogenous zones'; an idea he had extracted from the earlier work of Havelock Ellis. Flügel suggested that all clothing is charged with sexual symbolism. This was not a wholly new approach, for Richard von Krafft–Ebing had discussed 'erotic fetishism' and its place in the interpretation of dress in the *Psychopathia Sexualis*, published in 1886.

There have been many subsequent studies, some descriptive, some analytical, all of them drawing upon a wide range of source material. A recently launched quarterly publication — *Fashion Theory; The Journal of Dress, Body and Culture* — has chosen to begin its examination of fashion from the viewpoint that it is 'the cultural construction of the embodied identity'. This offers a late-twentieth-century, multi-disciplinary approach to the subject by broadening and democratizing the term across the boundaries of gender, multi-culturalism, and sexual preference. This merging of body decoration, clothing, and fashion into one subject area for critical analysis suggests that the ephemeral nature of clothing the human form will continue to be debated for the indefinite future. VALERIE CUMMING

Further reading

Newton, S. M. (1974). *Health, art and reason: dress reformers of the nineteenth century*. John Murray, London.

Ribeiro, A. and Cumming, V. (1989). *The visual history of costume*. Batsford, London.

Ribeiro, A. (1986). *Dress and Morality*. Batsford, London.

See also CLOTHES; MODELLING, FASHION.

Fasting In fasting, individuals or whole communities abstain from food and drink, usually for a specific reason and a specific amount of time. Fasting differs from DIETING or avoidance of certain foods, in that it implies complete abstinence from food, with only small modifications such as time limits or subsistence liquids. Documented in a wide array of cultures and throughout history, the motivations for fasting are many. Religious tenets have most commonly instigated fasts, but so have RITES OF PASSAGE, special occasions, political beliefs, and health ideals.

All of the major religions have called for some form of fasting. Though many factors motivate religious fasts, successful fasting demonstrates one's ability to subsume physical needs to spiritual desires, and has been thought to bring the faster closer to the divine. According to Islamic precepts, Moslems undertake Ramadan, a month-long fast (no food until after sundown), as well as other lesser fasts, such as Ashura. Buddhism requires ascetic behaviour, including fasting, by its monks, but not from other followers. HINDUISM encourages fasting on the eleventh day after a new moon, after the full moon, and every Monday in November.

JUDAISM also calls for regular fasting as a part of its doctrine. The major fast, Yom Kippur (Fast of Atonement), the holiest Jewish holiday, falls on the tenth day of the Hebrew month of Tishri. The Old Testament specifies at least six other minor fasts. During all of these except Yom Kippur, which demands abstinence from sunset to sunset, faithful Jews fast from sunrise until the first night stars.

Most sects within CHRISTIANITY have also advocated periods of fasting. The early Church called for voluntary fasts, but by the fourth century specific fasting practices were enumerated. In the past, the Roman Catholic Church required numerous fasts, including all Sundays during Lent, Easter week, and all Fridays except from Christmas to Epiphany and from Easter to

Ascension. Today, the Church recommends only a few fasts. Adults (those over 21) and youths (those over 14) are expected to conduct limited fasts on Ash Wednesday and Good Friday, as well as a one hour fast before communion. The Greek Orthodox Church lists over 250 fast days, including the 40 days before Christmas and Easter. The Eastern Orthodox Church proscribes meat during the first week of Lent and then precludes other foods, including fish, cheese, oil, butter, and milk, for the duration.

In all faiths, religious ascetics, especially saints and holy figures, have undertaken extreme fasts as a path to spiritual perfection. Hindu Yogis, Greek priests, and Christian martyrs all fasted. Recently, historians have taken great interest in the fasting practices of medieval women. Rudolph Bell suggests that the fasting rituals of such figures as Catherine of Sienna mirror present-day anorexic behaviour. Others suggest that though the behaviours may appear similar, their meanings, deeply rooted in each era's specific prescriptions about women, food, religion, and the body, make them distinct phenomena. Medieval saints fasted to receive God and to offer service to others, while modern anorexics fast for a complicated set of more individualistic reasons, including a desire for self-control and slenderness.

Many cultures have marked rites of passage and special occasions with fasting. Puberty is often accompanied by fasting, as for example among Sioux boys and some Africans, while Orthodox Jews fast before the marriage ceremony. Initiation in the cults of the ancient Isis and Mithra required fasting, and fasting has commonly accompanied grieving and mourning customs. Certain special occasions, such as celebratory feasts or, on the other hand, crises, provoke fasting — often in order to appease the gods.

Political activists have used fasting or 'hunger strikes' to gain attention, dramatize their cause, or force the hand of their opponents. The modern hunger strikers in Ireland protesting against British rule in Northern Ireland were preceded by the tradition of 'fasting on' someone to force them to make legal restitution. Mahatma Ghandi made effective use of political fasts, as did the British suffragists, who brought hunger strikes to the American suffrage movement.

Fasting to 'purify' health has long historical roots, especially among utopian societies. A number of such nineteenth-century American communities, led by such figures as Sylvester Graham and John Harvey Kellogg, recommended various dietary restrictions, including fasting. The health movement of the 1960s and 1970s, combined with the 'cult of slenderness' spawned new fasting fads (juice, liquid formulas, fruit only, etc.), including Alan Cott's *Fasting as a Way of Life.*

While dieting or abstaining from particular 'fattening' foods differs from strict fasting rituals, many who want to lose weight undertake fasts. It is this type of fast that is perhaps most common in modern Western cultures, where, even among the faithful, religious fasts are commonly evaded.

Many fast intermittently for aesthetic reasons (to slim the body to fit beauty ideals) without incident, but such rigid weight-loss regimens have also contributed to the increase in EATING DISORDERS among young females.

MARGARET A. LOWE

Further reading

Brumberg, J. (1988). *Fasting girls: the emergence of anorexia nervosa as a modern disease.* Harvard University Press, Cambridge, MA.

Bynam, C. W. (1987). *Holy feast and holy fast: the religious significance of food to medieval women.* University of California Press, Berkeley.

See also DIETING; EATING DISORDERS; RELIGION AND THE BODY; STARVATION.

Fatigue

Not a simple topic

'Fatigue is multifactorial' — it has diverse causes and many components, and expresses itself in varied ways. Even if we postpone discussion of mental fatigue, the purely physical dimensions of the word will prove more flexible than the first-time enquirer probably suspects. A hockey or rugby winger, after sprinting 60 metres, has to stop; but the fatigue experienced is of a palpably different kind from that at the end of a day's hill walking, yet alone a marathon race. Another sprint down the wing is possible within 1–2 minutes; another marathon is not possible that day. We will take these two extremes of sports fatigue, and related experiences, in that order. The entry on SKELETAL MUSCLE should, however, be read first, and that on EXERCISE may also be helpful.

'Sprint' fatigue

Very intensive exercise, such as that involved in sprinting, is powered predominantly by anaerobic metabolism. This form of metabolism produces lactic acid, and it is normally considered to be the acidity of this which stops muscles working. No form of fatigue has a single cause, but very intensive dynamic exercise probably comes nearer to being brought to an end by one mechanism than any other form of activity.

Degrees of acidity are expressed scientifically in terms of pH units, lower values indicating greater acidity. The pH within resting muscle cells is about 7.2. If it falls to around 6.4, which can happen after about a minute of really intensive activity in mammals and humans, the great majority of experiments indicate that both force-generation and further metabolism will be severely inhibited. (The musculature of salmon, after 30 seconds' swimming flat-out up a salmon ladder or striving to jump a weir, has been reported to touch pH 6.0; warm-blooded animals cannot tolerate this value.) Recovery from the major part of the fatigue is almost as rapid as onset. One of the few anomalies in the account is that the recovery of pH within the cells is not as quick. Also the inhibition of force-production by acidity is much more marked in experiments done on isolated

muscles at the salmon's body temperature than at our own. So the mechanisms involved may be less direct than has long been thought, but the association between acidity and fatigue remains very strong.

Decline of speed and power

It is never more obvious than towards the end of a burst of sprinting that fatigue consists not only in loss of the force that muscles can produce but in impairment of their shortening speed. Since many actions in life depend not on either force or speed alone, but on *power*, which involves both, the effect of fatigue is redoubled. Power is the essence of such varied actions as a high jump, a javelin throw, a tennis serve, an axe-stroke, or work with a saw.

Isometric fatigue

Intensive isometric (static) exercise produces no power at all, since it causes no movement. Nevertheless, isometric fatigue has about the same time-scale as that of intense dynamic exercise, and near-complete recovery is also comparably fast. Build-up of acidity is part of the mechanism here, too, but there are other factors. Muscles exerting more than about a third of their maximum static force squeeze the intramuscular blood vessels so hard that they cut off their own blood supply: effectively they operate under a self-imposed tourniquet. This produces a more profound loss of force than sprinting. Our fit hockey winger, if she slowed down by 20–30% after her 60 metre dash, could go on running for many minutes. A maximal isometric contraction falls to half or less in the first minute, and starting at 70–80% maximum force retards the subsequent decline only a little. (Try applying your utmost effort to undoing a recalcitrant jar-top; maintaining it for more than 3–5 seconds is impossible.) Only when force has fallen to 10–15% of the original maximum does a steady state ensue which can be maintained for long periods, because only then has the muscle's self-tourniquet been fully released. Fortunately it is this level of force which muscles involved in posture need to maintain, when a guardsman stands to attention for long periods.

During self-tourniquet, muscles trap within themselves many products of contractile effort in addition to lactic acid. Perhaps the most important other product is potassium. Potassium ions come out of all electrically-active cells, including muscle fibres, in the second half of each electrical impulse ('ACTION POTENTIAL'). Outside the muscle cells they probably contribute to fatigue in at least three ways. Firstly, they may lead to failures of impulse transmission down the finer motor nerve branches within the muscle, so fewer muscle fibres receive the instructions to go on contracting. Secondly, by accumulating particularly in the narrow 'transverse tubules', which have the function of conveying activation from the surface to the depth of each muscle fibre, they can block propagation of further impulses at that

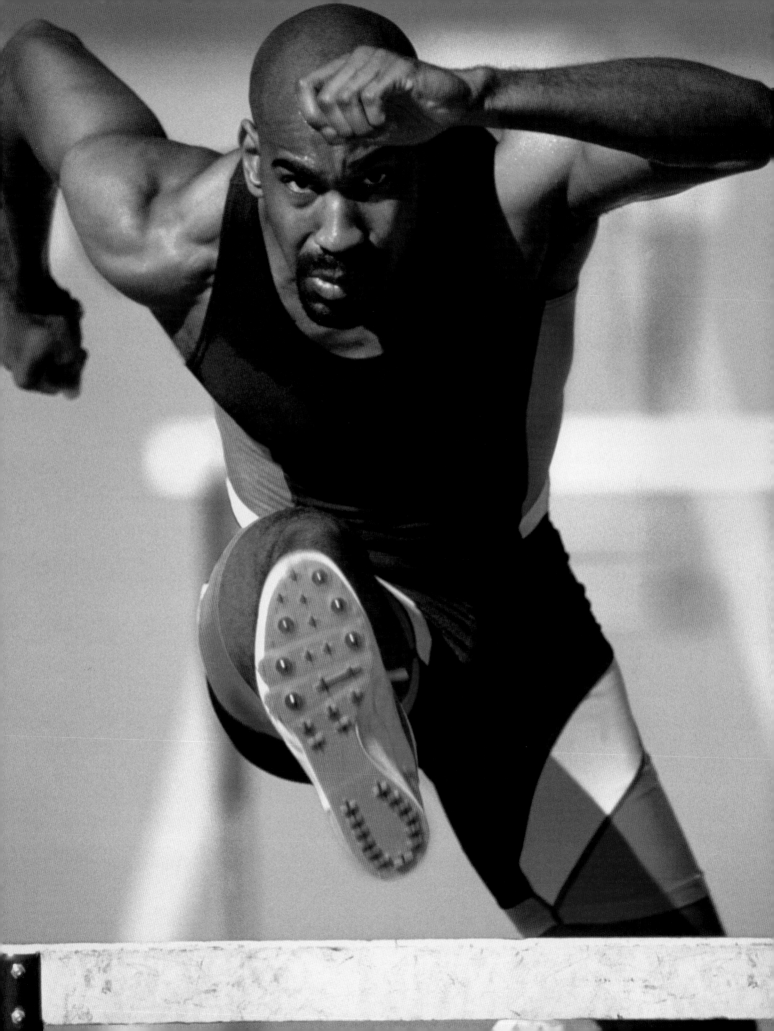

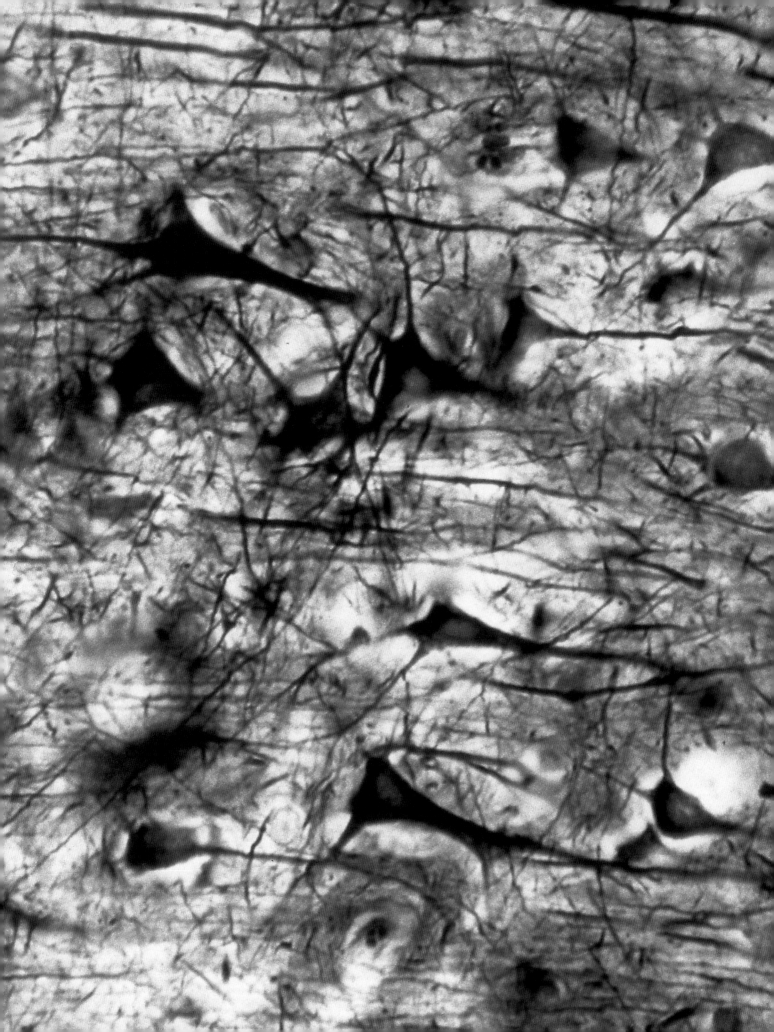

point; consequently the centre of the fibre may cease to produce force, even when the surface is still doing so. Thirdly, by depolarising sensory nerve endings embedded in the interstitial spaces between muscle fibres, potassium ions are thought to contribute to the pain of sustained contraction, and to a number of other effects such as increased respiration and elevated blood pressure. An organic product of metabolism, adenosine, also probably contributes to the pain, and contrary to a common assumption it is almost certainly more significant in this than lactic acid.

Long-lasting activity

At the end of a day in the hills, or even a marathon race, muscle pH is not significantly lowered; the metabolism has been aerobic not anaerobic, so negligible lactic acid has been produced. The main causes of fatigue in these 'endurance activities' appear to be microscopic muscle damage, and simply running out of fuel.

The fuel concerned is GLYCOGEN, the animal body's stored carbohydrate. Untrained people have only enough glycogen for perhaps 6–10 km at a racing pace; athletes who are highly trained, and have loaded themselves with carbohydrate food for the last few days before a race, will normally reach the finish with just a little left. Without glycogen one is not immobile, but maximum speed drops severely. The explanation for this hinges on the fact that muscles are composed of different types of fibre. The fastest fibres can utilize only carbohydrate, and many others — perhaps, in human beings, all others — can work faster on carbohydrate than on their alternative fuel, fat. Ultramarathons, channel swims, and other competitive events lasting many hours have traditionally been performed almost entirely on fat. However, technology can alter this situation to some extent, and cyclists on such events as the Tour de France (who can carry drinking bottles easier than runners) take high-carbohydrate drinks throughout the day to ward off total depletion of their carbohydrate stores as long as possible; the drink keeps blood glucose concentration high, and the muscles can use the glucose direct or turn it into glycogen.

As to the micro-damage, this is often marked enough to see in electron micrographs of endurance runners' leg muscles, and might prove even more severe after strenuous climbs. However, a form of damage on a yet smaller scale probably affects the internal activating mechanism of every fibre in a profoundly fatigued muscle. Experimentalists have called this 'low frequency fatigue', for it shows as substantially subnormal force when the muscle is artificially stimulated at fairly low frequencies (mimicking gentle voluntary activation). High-frequency stimulation overcomes the shortfall, and voluntary 'superhuman effort' has the equivalent effect: presumably high rates of natural or artificial stimulation release, even from a somewhat damaged system, enough of the required agent, calcium ions, to activate the contraction fully.

Intermediate intensities

In running races from 1500 to 10 000 metres and cycling, swimming, or rowing events of similar duration, many of the mechanisms described thus far probably mingle. Lactic acid builds up, but more slowly than in a sprint; glycogen depletion may be significant in some of the fastest fibres, though not generally; calcium release is probably impaired in more than one way; and so on. One additional mechanism, however, may have its greatest importance in activities lasting from a few minutes to half an hour. The key biological energy-molecule, ADENOSINE TRIPHOSPHATE (ATP), is broken down to adenosine diphosphate (ADP), hydrogen ions, and phosphate ions in the process of force-generation and then must be reconstituted by metabolism. Reconstitution seems to lag increasingly behind breakdown as exercise proceeds; significant concentrations of the breakdown products thus build up in intensively working muscle. In the events we are now considering this is especially true of phosphate ions. Hydrogen ions, when not also being released at great rate by the additional mechanism of anaerobic metabolism, are better 'buffered'. The effects the two ions can have are discussed in the next section.

Action of ATP breakdown products

If two water tanks are linked at the bottom by a pipe, and one starts empty while the other is full, water at first flows into it rapidly; gradually, however, the build-up of water in the receiving tank slows down further flow between them. In rather the same way the build-up of the products of any chemical reaction weakens its forward drive. This is a key mechanism by which both hydrogen ions (acidity) and phosphate ions are generally thought to contribute to muscle fatigue. No doubt ADP would do so too, did not metabolism ensure that ADP concentration never rises far.

Muscle contraction is brought about by the concerted action of submicroscopic structures called 'cross bridges'. Their power-generating strokes are weakened, and may also be individually slowed, when hydrogen and phosphate ions accumulate. In addition, in the majority of experimental conditions, hydrogen ions inhibit the amount of calcium released from intracellular stores by electrical excitation — which has the consequence that fewer cross-bridges are even active.

Notice that 'running out of ATP' does *not* appear among the mechanisms inducing fatigue. ATP concentrations are maintained quite close to resting value by muscle metabolism; evolution has ensured this, since to let them fall far could be fatal. The fatality would not be due to weakened contractions but to a single over-strong one: not fatigue but 'rigor mortis', the rigidity of death, is what sets in when ATP concentrations fall seriously low! So muscle fatigue is not due to an energy crisis in a direct, simple way, though some of the fatigue mechanisms we have discussed could be said to represent energy crises in broader senses.

Systemic fatigue

So far, all the mechanisms discussed have been of 'muscle fatigue', but the body can tire of prolonged work in other ways. Fluid loss, notably in sweat, is a major factor. Even 2–3% loss (1–2 litres, according to one's size) impairs performance. Thus sportspeople competing in hotter countries than their own should check themselves each morning for weight loss, which is likely to occur even without their being active. Heat in fact presents a double challenge, for blood is diverted from muscles to skin, so that it may be cooled there by evaporating sweat; when there is less fluid circulating, due to SWEATING, circulation in both regions is compromised. Furthermore if core temperature rises more than about 3°C, bodily and mental functions are seriously impaired, and heat stroke may set in. Thus the importance of maintaining fluid intake during prolonged activity, even in temperate climates and more so in hot ones, cannot be overstated; and it is unfortunate that thirst is an insufficient guide — in these circumstances we always need more fluid than the thirst mechanism indicates.

At the other extreme, cold is (in a purely arithmetical sense) even more dangerous than heat, for in many people core temperature need only fall 2°C to produce the severe impairments of physical and mental function characterizing HYPOTHERMIA. This is a thermal risk associated with exercise in exposed conditions, though not due to it, and involving fatigue-like symptoms rather than fatigue itself. Furthermore, the best preventive on land, however wet the conditions, is to maintain activity; so hypothermia in these circumstances becomes not a cause but a consequence of fatigue. (In cold water, however, attempts to swim are counterproductive, for stirred water extracts body heat faster than muscle activity can generate it).

Irrespective of temperature, though more challenged by cold than heat, blood glucose must be maintained. If it is not, the organ that suffers worst is the brain, which can only operate on glucose fuel. About one fifth of the glycogen in a rested body is stored in the liver, not the muscles, and it is from there, as exercise goes on, that it is released into the blood as glucose. When this mechanism fails and blood glucose ('BLOOD SUGAR') falls below about half its resting value, mental functions become seriously impaired.

The heart is a muscle, and both it and the muscles of breathing can in principle be subject to fatigue. When healthy people exercise at ordinary altitudes, however, neither of these categories of muscle fatigues sufficiently to impair the body's performance — though either heart or lung disease can alter this situation profoundly.

Central nervous fatigue

This may be regarded as the physiologist's name for what others would term 'mental fatigue'; however, it carries the specific implication that a physical mechanism can be identified, which is not (or not yet?) the case in all mental fatigue.

A particularly interesting mechanism has recently been proposed, which would make central nervous fatigue a direct consequence of prolonged muscle activity. Muscles running short of carbohydrate fuel instead take up increased amounts of certain amino acids, notably the branched chain amino acids (BCAA) such as valine. Consequently, after a while, less of these remain in the blood than were present when the exercise began. Now, there is a transport mechanism across the walls of brain capillaries which normally shares out its services between BCAA and other large, uncharged amino acids — the most prominent being tryptophan. As muscle demands continue, less BCAA and instead more tryptophan is taken into the brain. The neurotransmitter substance serotonin ('5-HT') is made from tryptophan, so the consequence of the shift in uptake is that more serotonin is synthesized. The crux underlying all this is that increased brain concentrations of serotonin appear to promote the symptoms and sensation of fatigue.

Inverting the direction of brain–muscle interaction, every sports coach knows that psychology has profound effects on the most physical of performances; even shouts of encouragement can be crucial. Fatigue, however, occurs in more situations than those involving muscular effort. Can anything be said about the others? We all know that, when tired, we perform less well at both motor and mental tasks — indeed, the mental ones are often impaired earlier and more severely, so that physical exercise can be a fruitful way of throwing off mental fatigue. That there are physical aspects even to mental fatigue is strongly suggested when we recall that hunger or severe thirst, extremes of cold or heat, oxygen lack, alcohol, and other drugs can all increase fatigue — while drugs with the opposite effect, such as CAFFEINE or amphetamines, can help ward it off. Altered levels of brain transmitters, particularly in regions of the brain stem — increased SEROTONIN and ACETYLCHOLINE, decreased NORADRENALINE — have been demonstrated in certain experimental studies of fatigue. But it is probably fair to say that scientific investigation is still only scratching the surface of the problem, as the most universal and ultimately irresistible cause of mental fatigue is lack of sleep. Despite the best efforts of committed researchers, we do not yet really understand sleep. Until we do, there seems little hope of comprehending what happens when we have had too little.
NEIL SPURWAY

Further reading

Gandevia, S. C. *et al.* (1996). *Fatigue: neural and muscular mechanisms.* Plenum, New York.

Newsholme, E. A., Blomstrand, E., and Ekblom, B. (1992). Physical and mental fatigue: metabolic mechanisms and importance of plasma amino acids. *British Medical Bulletin*, **48**, 477–95.

Wilmore, J. H. and Costill, D. L. (2000). *Physiology of sport and exercise.* 2nd ed. Human Kinetics, Champaign, Illinois.

See also COLD EXPOSURE; EXERCISE; HEAT EXPOSURE; SKELETAL MUSCLE.

Fats or, more technically, lipids, together with CARBOHYDRATES and PROTEINS, are one of the three staples of the diet. As the seventeenth-century nursery rhyme relates, 'Jack Sprat he ate no fat/His wife she ate no lean'. This does not mean, however, that Jack Sprat could not get fat, because excess carbohydrates and proteins can be broken down in the body and the fragments synthesized into fat. But had he eaten no fat whatsoever he would have been deprived of certain essential FATTY ACIDS, and of the fat-soluble VITAMINS. Fats serve many purposes: they not only provide thermal insulation and a source of energy, with stores in reserve, but also are involved in important functions, providing for example the materials for components of CELL MEMBRANES, of the MYELIN sheaths that electrically insulate nerve fibres.

Chemically, fats are *esters* — that is, formed by combination of an alcohol with an acid. In this case the alcohol is *glycerol*, which has three alcohol groups, allowing it to combine with three acidic groups. The acids are *fatty acids*: long chains of carbon atoms linked to a carboxyl (acidic) group. Three fatty acids therefore combine with one glycerol molecule to form a *triglyceride* or neutral fat molecule.

Triglycerides are the main fats in the diet. After breakdown and absorption in the ALIMENTARY SYSTEM, they are resynthesized and stored in special cells in which fat globules coalesce to form a large droplet, almost filling the cell. Aggregations of fat cells form *adipose tissue* (as in the white fat of uncooked meat). White fat can be deposited in a variety of tissues, especially beneath the skin and in muscles — but a great deal of human endeavour is today devoted to getting rid of adipose tissue collected around the waist, even to the extent of having liposuction. Fat acts as a rich fuel reservoir that can be utilized during STARVATION. Oxidation of fat yields about twice the energy that can be derived from equal amounts of carbohydrate or protein. However, white fat is not easily got rid of physiologically, since it is poorly perfused with blood. Hence hormones that mobilize fat do not reach the target in high concentration, nor is there a high flow rate to carry the energy-giving molecules in the blood to the tissues, such as MUSCLES, where they can be burned.

There is a second type of fat deposit, namely *brown fat*, found at the base of the neck and between the shoulder blades. This tissue is specialized for *thermogenesis*, i.e. the rapid mobilization of fat to generate heat. The cells contain many small lipid droplets, a pigment, and many mitochondria, the latter essential for breaking down the lipids into simple two carbon fragments from which energy can be rapidly generated. Furthermore the tissue is well perfused with blood and has a rich innervation by nerves liberating NORADRENALINE, one of the hormones that can rapidly mobilize the breakdown of fats. Brown fat is important for heat production in infants, and is retained variably into later life. Those who retain the most brown fat into adulthood find it easier to avoid putting on weight. Hibernating animals lay down large amounts of brown fat to see them through the dormant period.

Many different fatty acids are found among the lipids. They vary in the number of carbon atoms in the chain, which in some cases are branched, and also in the number of double bonds they contain, if any. Those with double bonds are known as *unsaturated*, and those without as *saturated*. For example palmitic acid and palmitoleic acid both have 16 carbon atoms, but the latter has one double bond (*mono-unsaturated*). Oleic, linoleic, and arachidonic acid have respectively 16, 18, and 20 carbon atoms in the chain and 1, 2, and 4 double bonds. Oleic and linoleic acids are essential fatty acids, that is they cannot be synthesized in the body and are therefore essential dietary constituents. Readers will be familiar with the term 'rich in polyunsaturates' applied to many supermarket products like margarines, sunflower oils, etc. There is evidence that diets rich in polyunsaturated fats are less likely to cause atherosclerosis than ones rich in animal fats, with their predominance of saturated fats.

Fatty acids are essential constituents of *phospholipids* and *glycolipids*. In phospholipids the glycerol moeity is combined with only two fatty acids, the remaining alcohol group being combined with a phosphate group linked to an alcohol (e.g. to serine, choline, or inositol, to give the phospholipids phosphatidylserine, phosphatidylcholine, and phophatidylinositol). These compounds are 'amphipathic', that is, they have a polar head group, which is compatible with an aqueous environment, and a non-polar tail, which is not. Such molecules can form films (as does oil spread on the surface of water) in which the hydrophobic tails interact with each other, projecting out of the aqueous surface, while the polar head groups remain in the water. Now imagine such films are brought together so that the hydrophobic tails of one film are opposed to those of the second. This is a very close approximation to the structure of all cell membranes, where the polar head of one lipid layer contacts the extracellular environment, while the head groups of the other layer contact the aqueous environment within the cell. These structures, so-called *lipid bilayers*, form flexible membranes, which are very impermeable to the movement of substances across them, whilst particular permeability properties are provided by the inclusion of protein molecules in the membrane. Some membrane fatty acids can be mobilized as *autacoids* (released to affect other cells) and as intracellular messengers. For example, arachidonic acid gives rise to PROSTAGLANDINS in cell membranes, and phosphatidylinositol is the source of the important 'second messenger' inositol triphosphate, implementing an internal response to a chemical message from outside the cell.
ALAN W. CUTHBERT

See also BODY WEIGHT; CELL MEMBRANE; METABOLISM; OBESITY.

Fatty acids are a constituent of dietary fat and important components of the body's *phospholipids* and *glycolipids* (e.g. in CELL MEMBRANES, lung SURFACTANT, the NERVOUS SYSTEM). They consist of long carbon chains, each with a carboxyl group at one end. If the chain contains double bonds the fatty acids are said to be polyunsaturated; when no double bonds are present the fatty acid is saturated. Examples of saturated and unsaturated fatty acids are palmitic acid and linoleic acid, with 16 carbons and no double bonds, and 18 carbons with three double bonds, respectively. Fatty acids form esters with alcohols, and the common esters are glycerides, because the alcohol involved is glycerol. As glycerol has three alcoholic groups, most fats are triglycerides, and this is the major form of energy storage.

Fatty acids are absorbed from the gut as products of fat digestion, or made in the body from the other forms in which fats are absorbed. They are a major fuel for energy production at any time, except after a carohydrate-rich meal, and they are the main nutrient mobilised from fat stores in prolonged EXERCISE. There are several essential polyunsaturated fatty acids which must be obtained from the diet for the synthesis of vital substances.   ALAN W. CUTHBERT

See CELL MEMBRANE; EXERCISE; FATS; METABOLISM.

Feet BIPEDALISM, emerging about 3 million years ago, is considered to have been a crucial step in evolution, especially as it allowed the hand to develop into a distinct and specialized appendage. Not simply a primitive hand, the human foot is adapted to a form of bipedalism distinctive for the efficacy of its stride. *Australopithecus africanus*, for instance, had a fully 'modern' foot 2–5 million years ago, and probably walked with a stride. Unlike other primates, the human foot is not prehensile — that is, not able to grasp objects with the aid of an opposed first digit like the thumb. Though the toes of the human foot are generally not capable of independent or precise movement, the flexor muscles of the big toe are vital to our GAIT. The human foot is stable, yet adaptable to WALKING and running on rough and sloping ground. Like FINGERPRINTS, footprints are unique to each individual; thus, the footprints of infants are often recorded as part of birth records in hospitals.

Structure and movement
The feet have two distinct functions: to support the body when standing, and to act as levers when walking. For support, they need to be as rigidly flat on the ground as possible, but the bones and joints which form the skeleton of the foot have an arched form, both from front to back and from side to side, which requires strong support from fibrous ligaments and from muscular contraction to withstand the stress when it is performing as a lever.

The bones, from heel to toe, are the tarsal and metatarsal bones and the phalanges. One of the

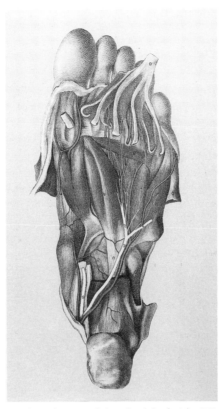

Muscles and nerves of the sole of the foot by G.H. Ford, from dissection by G. V. Ellis of University College (1864). The tendons from the muscles of the calf have been turned back to reveal the intrinsic muscles of the foot. Mary Evans Picture Library.

tarsal bones takes part in the ankle joint. Under this is the largest bone (calcaneum), which is cushioned by soft tissue below to form the heel; attached to it is the exceptionally thick and strong tendon of the calf muscles, which spans the back of the ANKLE, allowing contraction of the muscles to lift the heel. This tendon can sometimes be torn — a painful condition which seriously interferes with walking — and it is known as the ACHILLES TENDON, from the 'heel' of mythological vulnerability. In front of the ankle, a prominent tendon from the shin muscles stands out when the foot is pointed upwards. Other leg muscles can tilt the foot inwards or outwards.

Movement of the whole foot at the ankle is achieved mainly by contraction of muscles in the lower leg, and the same is true of some other foot movements. Within the leg are the muscles which *extend* (point up) the toes — via their long tendons, which cross the front of the ankle (held close to it by fibrous bands), and reach to the small bones (*phalanges*) of the toes. Muscles which *flex* (curl down) the toes (including a separate important one for flexing the big toe) lie deep in the calf, and their tendons run behind the bony knob (*malleolus*) on the inner side of the ankle, and thence across the sole to reach their insertions. Behind the malleolus on the outer side, tendons from other leg muscles run in

the sole to the metatarsals, such that their contraction plants the foot firmly on the ground. Attachments of tendons of leg muscles from both sides to the underside of the foot bones is important for retaining the 'arches'. Each of these long tendons has a lubricated *synovial sheath*, which can become inflamed and painful in the condition of *tenosynovitis*.

There is also a complex set of small muscles within the foot itself, mainly in the sole, arranged in no less than four layers and protected by a very strong fibrous sheet reaching from heel to toes. These muscles can flex the toes, splay the big toe and the little toe outwards, or pull in the sides of the foot; they actively modify the foot's shape, and maintain its strength and flexibility in the face of the continually changing strains and pressures of walking and running. The foot muscles themselves assist in retaining the arches, but it is mainly a failure of the leg muscles which leads to 'fallen arches' or 'flat feet'. In unusual circumstances, the remarkable achievements of some foot-painting artists show the extent to which the movements of feet and toes can sometimes be trained into hand-like precision.

The foot as a measure
The foot has been used as a standard linear measurement in various cultures. The English foot, still in use today in the US, was defined in 1959 as being 30.48 cm. The foot is also a unit of measure in poetry, indicating the smallest unit; a foot is usually defined as one stressed and one or two unstressed syllables, as in the word 'poet'. The number of feet per line determines the metre of a poem: if a single line contains one foot, it is called monometer, two feet is diameter, three is trimeter, etc.

Religions and the feet
The washing of another's feet has long been performed as a gesture of humility in Western culture. An act of hospitality in ancient Palestine, servants or the wife of the host might wash a guest's feet. Jesus is said to have washed the feet of his disciples at the Last Supper (John 13: 1–15), and the early Christian Church introduced foot washing as a ritual (*pedilavium*) imitating the humility and selfless love of Jesus. Foot washing on Maundy Thursday, the Thursday before Easter, appeared as a rite in the Roman Catholic Church during the seventh century. In some European countries, the social elite would wash the feet of the poor and give them gifts on this day, a practice which continued in England until the mid eighteenth century. Many Episcopal and some other Protestant churches, for instance the Mennonites, still practice foot washing today.

The *Buddha's footprints* play an important role in Buddhist iconography. Emphasizing the transiency of all things, for several centuries after his death in the fifth century BC, the Buddha was represented only by his footprints. For instance, his footprints in stone can be seen at the base of the tree where he is said to have attained enlightenment.

Historian Sander Gilman has analyzed the cultural meaning of the Jewish foot, which he claims has been associated in Christian societies with the cloven hoof of the devil. During the nineteenth century, the 'weak' feet of the Jewish male were perceived as a sign of his unfittedness for military service, and hence his inability to participate fully in the European nation state. The Jew's feet were partially responsible for his or her allegedly idiosyncratic and heavy-footed gait. Flat-footedness in particular was believed to be a racial characteristic of Jews, and also blacks, throughout the Nazi period. Interestingly, while a sign of atavism, flat-footedness was also considered a result of 'modern', urban living and its unhealthy and disabling influences.

Foot-binding

Like the Jew's feet, the tiny bound feet of Chinese women have served as a complex social signifier. Though a less severe form of *foot-binding* is also practised by the Kutchin Indians of Alaska, the most well-known form of foot-binding first became popular among Chinese women under the T'ang dynasty in the seventh century, and continued to be practised well into the twentieth century. The goal was to achieve the look of tiny, delicate, 'golden lily' feet; this was accomplished by tightly binding the feet, stunting their growth and breaking the bones. Beginning as early as the age of five, cultural critic Mary Daly (1978) discusses foot-binding as a form of painful and crippling mutilation imposed on women by a deeply patriarchal society. The process is indeed extremely painful and can last for over 10 years, until the feet have stopped growing and have adopted the desired shape; Chinese women continue to bind their feet throughout their lives in order to maintain and improve their form. A sign of status and desirability in marriage, foot-binding was practiced on all levels of Chinese society, including among the working class. A girl's bound feet were an indication not only of her sexual desirability, but also of her self-discipline, her ability for self-sacrifice, and the care with which she had been raised by her mother. The psychological implications of such torment being inflicted upon a young girl by her mother has been the subject of much speculation. There is a Chinese adage that a mother cannot love both her daughter and her daughter's feet at the same time. As a sex-segregated ritual, men were excluded, in theory, from knowing anything about the process or pain involved. This taboo in some ways reconciled the practice with Confusion teachings which clearly forbade self-mutilation. C. Fred Blake argues that the female mystique of foot-binding helped to exempt men from direct responsibility for dominating and degrading women.

Blake has re-examined the relationship between foot-binding and women's labour in China, and revised the traditional interpretation that foot-binding was a way in which women made themselves useless as a sign of the wealth and status of the men on whom they depended. Blake argues that foot-bound women perform all sorts of manual and menial labour, including agricultural field work and domestic service. What foot-binding does is to make women's labour less visible; the foot-bound woman only appeared 'useless' and helpless, while in fact her labour, both economic and reproductive, made vital contributions to the family economy and to society in general.

An imperial edict prohibiting foot-binding was issued in 1644 and remained in effect until 1911, but the practice lingered until the Great Leap Forward in 1958–60. Part of the problem was that these were political movements, propagated by men and medical professionals, while foot-binding continued to be a traditional female practice. Interestingly, in traditional Chinese culture, two types of women had natural-sized feet: uncivilized, clumsy, and crude women, and extraordinarily powerful women, like legendary female warriors, goddesses, and Guan Yin, the Buddhist redeemer of humanity.

The bound foot was highly eroticized, often compared to a 'golden lotus', a central symbol in Buddhism. It was not unusual for a man to have a pet name for his wife's feet. The suggestion that foot-binding was part of sexual maturity, a prelude to the trials of marriage and childbirth, is indicative of an association between the foot and the womb in Chinese culture. Sigmund Freud proposed that by maiming their own feet, Chinese women allayed the castration anxieties of men.

The Chinese are not the only culture to eroticize the foot. Ancient Egyptians decorated feet with henna, and toe rings are common in many cultures. Pedicures and all manner of products to beautify and eroticize the feet, including nail polish and various forms of foot jewellery, are widely available throughout the world today. Foot and shoe fetishes are well-known forms of 'perversion' in European and Asian cultures as well. Stressing that it is often not possible to trace the origins of subconscious connections, Freud mentions the foot as an age-old sexual symbol, and a frequent locus for the displacement of desire. The shoe or slipper, he notes, often operates as a symbol of the female genitalia.

SARAH GOODFELLOW
SHEILA JENNETT

Further reading

C. Fred Blake, (1994). Foot-binding in Neo-Confucian China and the appropriation of female labor. *Signs*, **19**(3), 676–712.

Sander Gilman, S. (1991). *The Jewish Foot. The Jew's Body*. Routledge, New York.

See also ANKLE; SKELETON; WALKING.

Female form In many respects, images of the female body serve to define some of the most important discourses of Western culture — the appreciation of Fine Art (beauty, and the tradition of the nude); the application of the law (the prosecution of obscenity and the licensing of pornography); and religious worship (the Virgin Mary and the goddesses of ancient religions — images still prevalent in art). To this list might be added, in certain respects, the practice of medicine (principally obstetrics and gynaecology) as an investigation into the form and interior of the female body. Each of these practices regard the image of the naked woman as the object alternately of fascination and suspicion. Alongside these privileged discourses, the ubiquity of images of women's bodies in both advertising and art, make the female form one of the most familiar, if also most contested, images in newspapers, on cinema screens, and along any public street.

In each case a question of legitimacy arises. How are these images to be judged? Which are acceptable? Which are, by contrast, obscene? The latter question is crucial. Indeed, one way to begin to think about 'female form' and its cultural significance is to think of representations of the female body as less of a static object and more as a limit point or set of exclusions, for while an image of the body of a woman can represent all that is pure or worthwhile, it can also embody that which is thought to be the most contaminated and disgusting. The history of art, and indeed that of medicine and the law, is replete with campaigns designed to contain or to repackage the materiality of the female body within the reassuring assumptions of aesthetics. Let us consider some of the ways in which that demand for order has shaped discourses about female form historically.

The most conspicuous example of this social regulation comes from within the languages of aesthetics and art history. Within the tradition of Western aesthetics, female form has been defined and judged on the basis of the plasticity of its parts, the smoothness and fullness of its shape, and its capacity for completeness. Although the judgement of female form has retained a sense (inherited from Aristotle) of the value of order, symmetry, and definiteness, most aesthetic accounts of female form add an appreciation of the sensual and tactile qualities imagined to be defined in the female body. The imagined refinement and poise of the female figure led, by the eighteenth century, to the assumption that an ideal female form was the logical antithesis of the body defined by physical labour or warfare. Unlike the male body, which disclosed the signs of labour through muscular development, the female body was thought to remain whole, and undisrupted by apparent effort. Above all, the female body was assumed to be moulded, enclosed: all openings sealed, all passage denied. In many cultures the assumption of the perfectibility and completeness of the female form has also led to its endorsement as a national or cultural symbol: witness Britannia, Marianne, and the Statue of Liberty, amongst others.

Examples of such reverence for the female form are not hard to find. One of the more notorious is Edmund Burke's, *A Philosophical Enquiry into the Origin of Our Ideas of the Sublime and Beautiful* (first published in 1757). Throughout the *Enquiry*, Burke describes female form in a way that stresses both its formal resolution and the continuity of its surfaces. Burke writes:

'Observe that part of a beautiful woman where she is perhaps the most beautiful, about the neck and breasts; the smoothness; the softness; the easy and insensible swell; the variety of the surface, which is never for the smallest space the same.'

Despite the air of sexual excitement, Burke's description succeeds in laying its emphasis on the harmonies and varieties of a completely closed and completed form. Female form for Burke represents the perfection of beauty because it embodies no excesses or disunities that might shock his roving eye. Burke is a useful example, as his opinions were to codify aesthetic opinions about the beauties of the female form for over a century after their publication.

This tradition continued into the twentieth century, most notably in the work of the art historian Kenneth Clark. Clark's 1956 study *The Nude* remains a landmark (albeit an increasingly controversial one) in the description of the female body as art form. Indeed, for Clark the female nude represents the triumph of art: the ultimate transformation of matter into form. In these terms the image of the female nude is a pure form, one that, rather than provoking action, encourages contemplation, even reverence. To make his point Clark differentiates between the celestial and the earthly Venus. The former represents a perfection of the female form, so abstracted from sexual pleasure that it can sanction the male gaze and turns the female body into a work of art. The earthly Venus, by contrast, is warmly sensual, its wanton form always on the brink of immodesty. As such it is taken to be a less deserving object. Clark's statement is a classic example of the ways in which art criticism has sought to regulate the female form.

The opinions of men such as Burke and Clark — they are but two examples from a long tradition — image the female form as potential perfection. It is doubtless for this reason that the nude study has retained its high prestige within

art practice and teaching. In order to achieve such prominence and such apparent respectability, the female body is assumed to require transformation and realignment. It is commonplace within the tradition of aesthetics to argue that while mere flesh is pornographic, art requires the contemplation of purified form: the body's orifices are either passed over or discreetly sealed. The exclusivity of such a position should be made evident: the bodies of women which do not fit this profile are imagined not to count as art or imagined to be deficient, excessive, or disgusting. This might include: bodies of aged, disfigured, or impoverished women; the body during parturition or menstruation; the pornographic image; the apparently savage or bestial. In each case the rejected form is taken to embody that which is beyond the bounds or transgresses the limits of, variously, decency, acceptability, or good taste. Of this latter category the nineteenth-century interest in the 'HOTTENTOT VENUS' will serve as a good example. During the 1860s, the protruding buttocks and pendulous BREASTS of Hottentot (Khoikhoi) women provided Victorian society with an object of both anthropological inquiry and almost pornographic curiosity. Certainly the differences between African and white women were both examined and exaggerated as part of the spectacle of imperialism. Most importantly, the physical form of other peoples was imagined to define the greater perfection of Europeans.

Since the 1970s, feminist art practitioners have sought to challenge and to overturn the restrictive and complacent assumptions of this dominant tradition. From the late sixties onwards there was a growing sense within the Women's Movement that such discourses had a profound and detrimental effect not only on women's self esteem, but more forcefully on women's health. Seeking to break the stranglehold of a tradition that upholds only one image

of the female body, artists have sought to emphasize the divergence and difference of the female form. In place of the insistence upon the pure form of the feminine body, artists such as Judy Chicago, Cindy Sherman, and Jo Spence represent their own bodies as both different and distinctive, and in so doing reject the dominant aesthetic tradition represented by Burke and Clark. In so doing, many artists, most controversially performance artists, have rejected the assumption that the female body is best presented by the stasis of its exterior surfaces, and have represented the female body as potentially difficult, open, or inclusive. Such a movement is both utopian and critical in its insistence on the multiplicity of women and the diversity of female form. The success of such a project would transform the language of aesthetics irrecoverably.   ROBERT W. JONES

Further reading

Clark, K. (1956). *The nude: a study of ideal art.* John Murray, London.

Nead, L. (1992). *The female nude: art, obscenity and sexuality.* Routledge, London.

See also ART AND THE BODY; BEAUTY.

Feminism

Feminism and woman's nature

> The most far-reaching social development of modern times is the revolt of women against sexual servitude (Margaret Sanger, 1920).

While feminism takes many forms and cannot be characterized in any seamless way, it nonetheless encompasses the struggles of women to secure their economic and political agency. From the Women's Suffrage Movements of the late nineteenth and early twentieth centuries to the Women's Liberation Movement of the 1960s and 1970s, feminism is typically associated with particular historical moments when a coalition of women succeeds in bringing issues of gender equality, sexual oppression, and sex discrimination into the public arena. Whether it takes the form of an explicit demand for the vote (as did the Suffrage Movements) or a more generalized demand for women's freedom (as did the Women's Liberation Movement), feminism is invariably engaged in resistance to prevailing notions of women's 'nature'.

In the nineteenth century, the ideological ascendancy of science and medicine joined the spread of industrialization to promote the 'sexual division of labour' based on the assumption that 'biology is destiny'. Women's fixed role as caregivers was ideologically determined by their biological capacity to bear children. Associated with that biological capacity was a host of psychological attributes — passivity, dependence, moodiness — which further reinforced a growing emphasis on the gendered separation of the domestic and the public spheres. The qualities requisite to economic or political success were linked to biologically based notions of masculinity and femininity, according to which men's

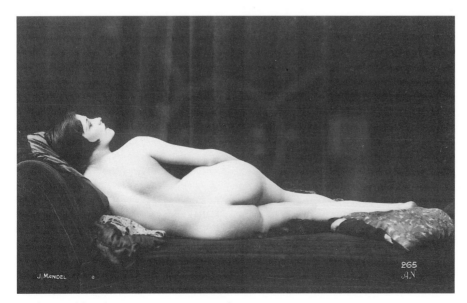

French postcard from the 1920s. Mary Evans Picture Library.

bodies and minds are naturally suited to positions of power and women's are naturally suited to positions of subordination. While the resistance to this view of sexual difference varies historically and culturally, it is against this backdrop that modern and contemporary feminism must be understood.

Feminism and political activism

Not surprisingly, feminism often consolidates into a political movement as a result of women's participation in other radical, reformist, or revolutionary activities. For example, women were active in the anti-slavery movements of the nineteenth century. Yet, at a World Anti-Slavery Convention held in London in 1840, Lucretia Mott and Elizabeth Cady Stanton were forced to sit in the gallery because the convention's organizers had determined that women could not be delegates. Eight years later, Mott and Stanton convened the Seneca Falls Women's Rights Convention, which adopted a platform explicitly revising the US Declaration of Independence to accord women the same guarantees that it granted to men. ('We hold these truths to be self-evident: that all men and *women* are created equal . . .') In addition, it specified a set of grievances regarding the usurping by men of women's political, legal, and economic autonomy. It would not be the last time that the hypocrisy of demanding rights for some while denying them to others would initiate a women's movement. Women's experience as coffee-makers, typists, and sexual attendants to men in the anti-war and civil rights movements of the 1960s similarly activated both the demand for women's full participation in the public sphere and denunciation of masculine sexual prerogatives.

The Women's Liberation Movement of the 1960s and 1970s, the backdrop to contemporary feminism, is characterized by two intersecting trajectories. On the one hand, in spite of the liberalization of non-marital sex (occasioned in part by the wide distribution of the birth control pill), women remained men's sexual subordinates. Feminists challenged 'sexist' images of women in popular culture and in the pornography industry in relation to a growing understanding of women's 'political subordination under patriarchy'. Women's bodies, then, became the ground on which the struggle for liberation was waged. On the other hand, a connection was made between women's 'consciousness' and their sexual subordination. While feminists like Margaret Sanger had long before identified women's complicity in perpetuating their own subordination, the concept of 'consciousness raising' as an instrument of liberation emerged only in this later period. Consciousness raising, a collective activity of mutual support and critique, encouraged individual women to see the ways in which their habits of thought conformed to a particular set of ideological presuppositions about women's nature and women's roles — why am I supposed to wash the dishes, change the diapers, watch soap commercials, stay within the budget, and worry about cellulite, while he earns the money, fattens happily, determines when we will have sex, and metes out judicious punishment to the children when he returns from his important work in the real world?

Though this characterization of consciousness raising might appear a parody of the concerns of middle-class married women, the fact that such women were drawn into the movement in large numbers was crucial to the widespread recognition that women were no longer content to sit on the sidelines of political/public life. The slogan 'the personal is political' captured the Movement's insistence that what goes on behind the closed doors of the domestic sphere has everything to do with what goes on outside it. On this basis, despite serious differences among feminists as to whether the goal was equality with men or freedom from them, a broad agenda for change could be articulated. The women's health movement demanded everything from an increase in the number of women doctors, to access to abortion and contraception, to freedom from sterilization abuse, to a full understanding and celebration of women's bodies in feminist terms. (*Our Bodies/Ourselves*, still the principal women's health handbook, was first published in 1971.) More generally, women demanded ready access to the political arena, to economic self-sufficiency, to childcare, to freedom from male violence, to divorce, and to workplaces free from sexual harassment.

Understanding power and oppression

While feminism must be seen as an activist demand for political and economic reform, it has always been informed by serious reflection on the nature of sexual difference and the mechanisms by means of which sexual difference is enmeshed in, even created out of, relations of power and oppression. Mary Wollstonecraft (*A Vindication of the Rights of Woman*, 1792), John Stuart Mill (*The Subjection of Women*, 1869), Margaret Sanger (*Women and the New Race*, 1920), Simone de Beauvoir (*The Second Sex*, 1949), Betty Friedan (*The Feminine Mystique*, 1974), and bell hooks (*Ain't I a Woman? Black Women and Feminism*, 1981) are among the many feminists who have endeavoured to understand the causes and forms of women's oppression, and to reconceptualize sexual difference. Contemporary feminism has achieved more systematic interventions into the arenas that authorize representations of sexual difference, in large part because feminists have secured a greater presence in academia (and in elite domains of business, politics, medicine, science, and the mass media). For example, feminist historians have unmasked the assumption that history is determined by great wars and great men, and have succeeded in drawing attention to the ways in which women's work has significantly affected historical developments. Feminist scholars have demonstrated the extent to which male bias has determined the normative assumptions of the social, natural, and behavioural sciences. In the arts, literary and artistic canons are no longer restricted to the work of men.

Though feminism's relation to other struggles for political liberation has always been an element of its self-understanding, this has become particularly salient in recent years as feminism is increasingly exposed as beholden to a pernicious set of assumptions about class, race, sexuality, ethnicity, and nationality. Feminism has been challenged to re-think the centrality of a unified and singular *woman's* identity to its political aspirations, since that identity too often comes at the expense of other, equally significant forms of identification. For example, African–American women's identity is constructed in relation to the history of slavery in which white women were complicit. The institutionalized racism that persists in spite of legal reforms continues to ensure white women's relatively greater access to those who uphold multiple systems of domination and subordination, namely, white men. Adding class as a factor further complicates the feminist agenda, for upper-class white women have considerable economic and social power over lower-class men and women, irrespective of race or ethnicity.

The feminist programme has been unsettled as well by the claim that, however unwittingly, it privileges heterosexuality as a normative feature of women's identity. According to this view, for example, the focus on abortion and contraception as the principal items on the feminist reproductive freedom agenda has too often ignored the realities of lesbian (and gay male) sexuality. Lesbian and gay procreation face challenges very different but, it is argued, equally compelling as those faced by women who wish to resist the heterosexual reproductive paradigm.

Whatever its fragmentation, within those arenas where it has a relatively secure footing, feminism can be credited with effecting profound changes in the ideological construction of womanhood, not only in the US and Europe, but more globally. The issue of women's autonomy in relation to reproduction and to work, and the issue of women's health more generally, have found themselves on the global political stage. Feminism continues in its struggle to establish itself as the ground for women's political, economic, and cultural ascendancy in the face of its own internal debates about the significance of differences among women.

MEREDITH W. MICHAELS

Further reading

Jaggar, A. and Rothenberg, P. (1993). *Feminist frameworks*. McGraw–Hill, New York.

Schneir, M. (1994). *Feminism: the essential historical writings*. Vintage, New York.

Fertility The French word '*fertilité*' entered the English language in 1490 to characterize the richness of the soil. By the seventeenth century, writers adapted 'fertility' to describe creative imaginations. In the course of the nineteenth century, the term 'fertility' came to account for the number of children a woman bore. In this period, too, fertility and another French term, 'fécundité', were used to refer to female procreative abilities. In 1866 J. M. Duncan differentiated fecundity from fertility with this explanation: '. . . by fecundity I mean the demonstrated capability to bear children . . . fertility implies fecundity, and also introduces the idea of number of progeny' (*The Oxford English Dictionary*, 1989, 2nd edn). After 1866, especially among demographers, fertility increasingly came to refer to the number of live children a woman delivered.

Technically, fertility simply denotes successful production of offspring. This requires the development in the potential parents of mature eggs (OVA) and SPERM, sexual intercourse, the opportune encounter between sperm and egg in the woman's body, FERTILIZATION, IMPLANTATION of the embryo in the uterus, successful ANTENATAL DEVELOPMENT, and a safe BIRTH. In the human female, the opportunity for fertilization lasts only a day or two following ovulation (the release of an ovum), which occurs about every 28 days, in the middle of the menstrual cycle. Sperm are present in vast numbers in the semen, so that, despite many hazards along the way, some survive the necessary journey to the egg. Given the typical frequency of COITUS between habitual partners of reproductive age, the odds are in favour of PREGNANCY occurring within a few months of the first encounter, in the absence of CONTRACEPTION or any specific physical cause for infertility.

Fertility, however, is not simply the expression of a woman's bodily capacity to procreate (fecundity). Recent anthropological and feminist theory advocates understanding fertility as the product of individual actions situated within a particular historical and cultural context. Women and men, responding to local and global changes in the political economy and available resources (e.g. social networks, abortifacients, and contraceptives), act as individuals to produce the family arrangement they prefer (Greenhalgh 1995).

Women and men promote or control their fertility to meet particular needs and concerns at different moments in their life cycle, and these needs and concerns alter depending upon their sexual partner and the changing circumstances of their lives. A woman might attempt, for example, to limit her fertility with an extramarital partner, but not her spouse. Or a widow might attempt to control her fertility after her husband's death in her attempt to retain a particular social standing in her community or limit the economic strains on her household.

People negotiate the circumstances of their fertility differently according to their social position and their personal needs, interests, and concerns. In many societies, bearing a child grants a woman adult status in her community, provides her with a legitimate place in the adult community, and garners her political power in her household and sometimes in her community. The desire to have a child has led many women who wish to conceive to seek the assistance of herbalists, ritual experts, and clinics. The efficacy of fertility treatments depends not only on the male and female partners' reproductive capacities, but also on their financial ability to pay for the treatment and the quality of the drug or procedure. Places where women and men can have their fecundity tested and treated abound throughout the world.

The desire to limit fertility exists in concert with the wish to procreate, and many women experience both desires in their lifetimes. Women in countries around the world seek contraceptives and ABORTIONS to limit their fertility, with or without the consent of their partners. A recent study by Bledsoe and colleagues in West Africa, for example, found that some women who have just had a miscarriage elect to use contraceptives for a period to give their bodies a chance to recuperate before they choose to become pregnant again.

Beyond individual preferences, however, fertility responds to a number of factors. Chief among them are health, nutrition and environmental factors. A woman's nutritional status, age, and experience of disease contribute to the probability of subfecundity (reduced capacity to conceive), miscarriages, and stillbirths. The tragedy experienced by residents of the Love Canal, New York State, where unsuspecting families lived on toxic waste dumps, provides an example of how environmental hazards have increased the incidence of miscarriage.

Cultural and religious values relating to the onset and duration of sexual relationships, use of contraceptives, and frequency of coitus (with a fecund male), determine a woman's exposure to the possibility of pregnancy. Obviously, women who begin their reproductive careers immediately after the onset of puberty have a greater window of opportunity to experience pregnancy than women who delay childbearing. Additionally, women in societies that condone the sexual relationships of women before, between, and after marriages could feel more comfortable being pregnant during more of their childbearing years than women living in less open communities. However, the ease with which a women can contract sexual liaisons does not directly translate into a socially sanctioned pregnancy and birth. Experiences of miscarriages and the duration of breastfeeding are also factors in the time during which a woman can get pregnant. The longer the breastfeeding period, the longer the possibility of lactational amenorrhoea — the time when a women is unlikely to be ovulating and therefore to get pregnant. Referred to as the 'proximate determinants of fertility' by demographers, myriad factors impinge on a woman's reproductive experiences.

Governmental programmes and policies that attempt to limit or promote women's fertility also affect the number of children a woman bears. For example, China's urban policy of one child per family sends a strong message to the community about the importance of controlling fertility. In contrast, when a country limits women's access to contraceptives or abortion, as some states in the US do, some women are forced to bear children they are not able to raise.

Women's fertility outcomes are also a response to international pressures. The economic crises of the 1980s and 1990s that plagued many African countries forced many Africans into extreme poverty. The recognition that poverty limits a woman's or couple's ability to care for many children leads women and men to limit the number of children they have. In Kenya, for example, where an unstable government is unable to pay international debts and secure internal peace, demographic studies conducted during the 1990s linked the decline of women's fertility to the current economic crisis. Kenyan women and men faced with growing uncertainty in their everyday lives are electing to limit their fertility.

SHERYL A. MCCURDY

Further reading

Bledsoe, C., Bahja, F., Hill, A.G. (1998) Reproductive mishaps and Western contraception: an African challenge to fertility theory. *Population and development review.* **24** (1), 15–59.

Greenhalgh, S. (ed) (1995). *Situating fertility: anthropology and demographic inquiry.* Cambridge University Press.

King, M. (1990). All in the family? The incompatibility and reconciliation of family demography and family history. *Historical Methods*, 23 (1), 32.

Levine, D. (1987). *Reproducing families: the political economy of England's population history.* Cambridge University Press. Cambridge, New York.

See also CONCEPTION; CONTRACEPTION; FERTILITY RITES; INFERTILITY; PREGNANCY.

Fertility rites

Fertility rites The promotion of the generative powers of earth, water, and human, animal, and fish populations is a common concern of major religions and small-scale cults the world over. In this general sense Christian farmers praying for a bountiful harvest, Muslim prayer leaders seeking to hasten the rains, and 'magicians' of the Trobriand Islands, chanting harvest charms to enrich 'the belly of the garden', pursue similar objectives despite varied ritual styles. These types of performances have existed in human cultures for thousands of years. Palaeolithic societies of hunter-gatherers from the Pyrenees to the shores of the Black Sea fashioned figurines and cave images dedicated to feminine and masculine, human and animal powers of fertility. In the third and fourth millennia BCE, small scale societies of farmers in forested Europe and on central Mediterranean islands, as well as the complex palace societies on Crete, active participants in maritime commercial networks, created order from ceremonies dedicated to deified powers of procreation and renewal. Further archaeological evidence from the Italian peninsula and Sicily in roughly the same period reveals the existence of elaborate

285

fertility cults centred in caves. These employed symbols of a ceremonial hunt to promote the fertility of domestic animals, plants, and humans in everyday life, and linked to notions of an after-life in another world, perhaps itself subter-ranean. In the Roman world, the festival of Saturnalia marked the death and propelled the rebirth of the sun, the seasons, the fertile powers of fields and bodies, and indeed the social order itself, as slaves and servants temporarily assumed positions of power in a festive season of controlled misrule. Many aspects of this festival were assimilated in Christian celebrations of Christmas, in particular the ritual disorder overseen by lords of misrule, and became a significant source of conflict after the Reforma-tion. Yet on the Rogation days of the Easter cycle, down to the modern period, many Christian priests, Protestant and Catholic, led local proces-sions around the boundaries of parishes praying for absolution of sins and for divine blessings on local fields and harvests — a variation of ancient festivals known as Terminalia, dedicated to the guardians of boundaries and fields.

Several important debates in the social sciences resulted from efforts to understand this historical interrelationship among religious sys-tems. In the late nineteenth and early twentieth centuries, a search for the origins of culture and social order led to the isolation of fertility cults and rituals as the most primitive human efforts to make sense of the world and the cosmos. The British anthropologist and folklorist (Sir) James Frazer (1854–1941) interpreted early human societies as using fertility cults and their magical power in efforts to renew the generative powers of the natural world. Frazer labelled these sys-tems 'magic' — as 'nothing but a mistaken appli-cation of the very simplest and most elementary processes of the mind' — and differentiated them from religion, which he saw as a later stage of cultural development. Frazer and many con-temporaries viewed the notion of personal agents, characteristic of religion, as more com-plex than the 'simple' observations of magic: observations perceived as closer in principle if inferior in practice to the modern natural sci-ences. More recent scholars prefer to examine how the terms 'religion' and 'magic' have been used politically in the past to differentiate legiti-mate and illegitimate uses of claims to super-natural power. This approach has been especially fruitful in the study of European witchcraft, now seen in part as an assault on the ritual inheritance of the ancient past in the Christian culture of early modern Europe.

As applied to the human body, fertility rites tend to open the system to the influence of pow-erful external forces and to situate the reproduc-tive and recuperative powers of the body in a hierarchic relation to the unseen forces of the cosmos that are understood to surround it and to influence its functions. Among the Kasena of northern Ghana, male elders present wives newly arrived in the family compound before the altar of the ancestors and sacrifice chickens in exchange for the power of the ancestors to give children. A similar use of ancestral power has been observed in Chinese patrilineages, despite a distinctive symbolism and ritual. In Cantonese funerals, daughters-in-law cover their abdomens in cloths of green — the color of spring, growth, and fertility — and rub their bodies against the coffins, exposing themselves to the pollution of death to attract the procreative power of the deceased. In this context, as in many others, the ends of fertility are interrelated with the rites of death. The Christian churches of early modern Europe sanctioned prayer as the primary means to marshal spiritual power for reproductive ends, although Catholic communicants were also encouraged to believe that their participation in the Eucharist could, among its other miraculous powers, ease a pregnancy or end barrenness. In addition, early modern Europeans could have recourse to a variety of unsanctioned or 'magical' techniques to promote or restrict fertility. A vari-ety of plants, such as coriander, saffron, and satyrion, stimulated erection or — to use the terms of humoral physiology and cosmology that defined the potency of these remedies — supplied heat to cold semen and thus increased male virility; according to the same principles, a woman's powers of conception might be enhanced by drinking potions of powdered hare's womb, sparrow's brain, or wolf's penis, by wearing amulets of lodestone or quail's heart, or by walking in the shadow of a 'lusty' woman; on the other hand, if children were not desired, liga-tures, amulets, and charms, such as the teeth or fingers of a dead child or the testicles of a weasel, might be used in sexual intercourse to inhibit procreation.

These substances harnessed the invisible forces of the cosmos in order to secure a desired out-come amid the myriad uncertainties and dangers of sexual relations. Knowledge of the principles and the use of the techniques of this process sometimes but not invariably belong to a class of specialists. Bronislaw Malinowski observed in the taytu gardens of the Trobriand Islands that the performance of fertility rites — if not the knowl-edge of their operations — belonged to an official class of 'garden magicians'. In early modern Europe, by way of contrast, a rudimentary knowl-edge of 'magical' means to address issues of health and fertility ranked among conventional domes-tic arts, dominated though not monopolized by women. Particular neighbours might acquire reputations for superior skill in such arts and accumulate a local clientele — perhaps inspiring fears of witchcraft in the process — but this expertise did not amount to office.

Many forms of fertility rite use simple forms of association to build a complex metaphysics of generation. These associations have been classified as the two laws of sympathy: (i) the *law of similarity* ensures that 'like acts on like', 'opposites act on opposites'. Accordingly, a liga-ture or knotted cord will produce impotence or inhibit procreation, and water will overwhelm dryness to produce rainfall; and (ii) the *law of contact* dictates that objects once joined share a special sympathetic relationship, even when separated. Consequently, the middle finger of an aborted child will retain a power to limit fer-tility, and the shadow of a 'lusty' woman will communicate her fertility to the barren. Recent scholars have used these 'laws', which modern science would reject, to explain why preindus-trial societies experienced high fertility even though they practised sometimes elaborate forms of fertility control.   DAN BEAVER

Further reading

Ginzburg, C. (1966). *The night battles*, (trans. J. and A. Tedeschi). Penguin Books, New York.

Malinowski, B. (1935). *Coral gardens and their magic*, 2 vols. Allen and Unwin, London.

McLaren, A. (1984) *Reproductive rituals: the perception of fertility in England from the sixteenth century to the nineteenth century*. Methuen, London, New York.

See also FERTILITY; INFERTILITY; REPRODUCTION MYTHS.

Fertilization Union of a male and female *gamete*: an ovum and a SPERM (*spermatozoon*). If COITUS has occurred within a few days of dis-charge of a ovum from an OVARY (normally around the middle of the MENSTRUAL CYCLE or about two weeks from the start of the last peri-od), one among the sperm which have survived the hazards of the journey to the Fallopian tube meets the ovum there, and enters it. This event instantly triggers changes in cellular chemistry and physics in ways which, among other things, prevent access of any rival sperm. A new unique individual is formatted from the conjunction of genetic material, and cell division begins.   S.J.

See OVA; PREGNANCY; SPERM.

Fetishism The concept of erotic fetishism originated with the French psychologist Alfred Binet (better known for his work on intelligence testing) in an article published in 1887 in the *Revue Philosophique*, and was given further currency by the Italian criminologist Cesare Lombroso. However, the idea was put into wider circulation by the great collator of sexually diverse practices, Richard von Krafft–Ebing, in many editions and translations of his *Psycho-pathia Sexualis*, up to his death in 1902. He defined erotic fetishism (differing somewhat from earlier writers) as associating strong emo-tions of sexual pleasure with physical or mental qualities of, or even objects used by, a beloved person, and considered this part of normal sex-ual attraction. However, he also suggested that a predisposition to be sexually aroused by particu-lar characteristics could be the motive for falling in love with or becoming infatuated with a specific individual associated one way or another with those characteristics, rather than an indi-vidual leading to an obsession with characteris-tics connected with them.

Krafft–Ebing made a distinction between what he called '*physiological fetishism*', or a preference for certain particular physical characteristics in persons of the opposite sex, and what he defined as '*pathological, erotic fetishism*'. This was not merely directed to particular portions of the body, but extended to inanimate objects, usually articles of female apparel, or towards particular materials such as furs or velvet. But there was no hard and fast dividing line. The fetishist of the body part was stimulated by something which would normally arouse the sexual instinct, but his sexual interests were restricted to that particular part. There were also fetishists attached to some bodily part with no obvious connection to sex, and those interested in particular kinds of bodies, e.g. those exhibiting some kind of deformity. In the case of object fetishism, Krafft-Ebing noted transitional states, from 'mere physiological preferences' in which intercourse with the fetish was more pleasurable, through coitus feeling less satisfactory if the fetish were not present, to complete impotence if it were absent.

Krafft-Ebing attributed the development of fetishism to some event whereby erotic feelings became associated with some particular body part or object; this is still today usually considered to play a significant part in its aetiology. While invoking environmental circumstances, he also suggested that individuals who formed these bizarre associations were predisposed to psychopathic states and excessive sexual desire, in keeping with his theories about the role of degenerate heredity and neuropathy in the aetiology of sexual disorders. Recent writers on the subject, e.g. John Bancroft in *Human Sexuality and its Problems* (1989), cite experimental demonstration that the male erectile response is capable of being conditioned to react to unusual stimuli. The reason why the conditioned response to particular stimuli which results in the formation of a fetish is so much more prevalent in the male may be, Bancroft suggests, because of the obviousness of penile erection. This sets up an unmissable visual and sensory link between the object of the stimulus and sexual arousal. Women may be less likely to identify pleasurable feelings invoked by certain objects or textures as specifically sexual in nature (experimental evidence demonstrating women's physiological signs of arousal, even though they denied erotic response, to sexually stimulating visual materials tends to corroborate this possibility).

The questions remain why some particular stimulus becomes the focus of erotic sensation, and why some are more likely to be conditioned than others. Fetishes are seldom completely random objects or attributes, although Bancroft points out that the particular object chosen by an individual may well have purely personal significance. There continue to be various definite areas of fetishistic interest, which, however, change over time. Krafft-Ebing considered hand-fetishism common, but Bancroft reports this as now being extremely infrequent. Feet, however, and shoes, remain an area of considerable interest. Rubber is not mentioned by Krafft–Ebing as of particular interest alongside furs,

velvet, and silk, but the twentieth century saw the rise of a definite sub-group of rubber fetishists. This may be connected with the more widespread use of various rubber items for child care (sheets for changing the baby, waterproof pants, etc.). Leather and PVC also have their subcultures of devotees. This suggests that fetishes are not only psychologically determined but subject to various social influences.

The designation of particular bodily parts as sexually stimulating by particular societies could be considered as a culturally-produced form of fetishism. Certain attributes — large breasts, bound feet, a glimpse of ankle — may be preferences so deeply encoded into a particular culture's sensibility as to appear 'natural' and not in need of any explanation. Therefore, a man (and fetishists are almost exclusively male) whose sexual response is very specifically tied to some such apparently universal stimulus is unlikely to consider himself as a fetishist even if interest in the stimulus greatly outweighs that towards the person whose breasts or feet they may be. If, however, he is aroused by some other body part or some unusual quality in the approved attribute (small rather than large breasts, for example), he may at least be aware of something that distinguishes him from the multitude, without describing himself as a 'fetishist'.

The strict Freudian psychoanalytic interpretation of the fetish is that it represents the penis, and operates as either a protection against the fetishist's fear of castration, or a denial of the penis-less state of the woman. It seems certainly to be the case that the fetish operates as a defence against IMPOTENCE if it is employed in a coital situation: it may do this by acting as a reliable stimulus to arousal and erection, or possibly more magically by its association with sexual arousal.

Not all fetishes are capable of being deployed within a reciprocal sexual relationship. Men may feel hesitant about revealing their particular quirk to a partner, or may eschew employing the fetish within marital life, going instead to prostitutes. The fetish may be associated with other minority sexual practices: in descriptions of the pleasures of rubber it is not always clear whether it is the sensation of rubber against the skin or the sense of being tightly bound in this clinging substance which is the main component of the sexual kick. Fetishism may be overtly combined with sadomasochist rituals: Maurice North, in his study of rubber fetishism, *The Outer Fringe of Sex* (1970) notes the pervasive elements of domination in fantasies written for the rubber market, and that rubber fetishism is but one component in a 'syndrome' including boots, leather, PVC, and sadomasochistic tendencies.

While many of the statistically less common forms of sexual behaviour can be shown to have been practised by individuals throughout the course of human history, even if they were not conceptualized as sexual perversions, fetishism is not so readily detected before its identification by late-nineteenth-century sexologists. It is merely conjectural that it was the 'liquefaction' of Julia's

silks rather than Julia which allured Robert Herrick, that the abundant and curling tresses celebrated by poets were the real focus of attraction. Impotence occurring when the fetish was not present occasionally brought fetishism to medical attention, but in many cases its significance was probably not recognized. It has seldom figured in divorce proceedings. Krafft– Ebing noted that it did, however, have forensic implications in cases of fetishists compelled to steal the items of their desire — but, again, the erotic motivation may not have been recognized before he pointed it out. North, in his study, was writing at the time of the 'Permissive Society', when a certain degree of 'kinkiness' was fashionable and designers incorporated themes (such as high boots) from the sexual underworld, but he found nevertheless that rubber fetishism was largely a hidden deviance, kept deeply secret by its practitioners because of their own shame: this may also apply to other fetishes. For example, while men may readily reveal a 'normal' predilection for legs, breasts, or bottoms, it is less likely that a fondness for feet would be admitted.

While North found publications circulating among individuals sharing this obsession, there was no subculture comparable to that of homosexuals or even sadomasochists. At the time he wrote (and it is doubtful whether this has changed radically) most rubber fetishists wanted a relationship involving rubber items with a consenting female, but extremely few women were interested: and these were either prostitutes catering to a niche market, or wives or partners introduced to rubber sex by their male partners. Thus there was very little motivation to join a community which would include few potential partners, but competitors for any possible partners available. Most of the rubber fetishists investigated by North contented themselves with fantasy and MASTURBATION, sometimes with the aid of fetish products and special-interest publications. As a very private vice, it did not have the visibility or social implications of other transgressive sexual behaviours. The incorporation of fetish motifs into mainstream fashion, and the appearance of a few fashionable fetish clubs in major urban centres, is not necessarily any indicator of a wider acceptance of fetishism.

LESLEY A. HALL

See also EROGENEOUS ZONES; EROTICISM.

Fetus The term used for the developing individual in the womb, by convention when it ceases to be called an EMBRYO after about the first two months. The adjective 'fetal' is however often applied from an earlier stage to the cellular elements of the embryo during and after IMPLANTATION in the womb, when distinguishing them from the 'maternal' tissue. Again by convention, the baby remains a fetus until BIRTH, when it becomes an infant (or, for a month, a neonate). 'Foetus' was the traditional British spelling until recent years.

S.J.

See ANTENATAL DEVELOPMENT.

Fever a term derived from the Latin *febris*, refers to an elevation of body temperature due to disease or injury. Man is a *homeotherm*, meaning that body temperature is kept within narrow limits by complex control mechanisms. This is distinct from *poikilotherms*, such as reptiles and amphibians, whose body temperature is just above the ambient temperature, and varies with it. Measured in the mouth, body temperature is close to 37°C (98.6°F), and does not usually vary by more than 1.5°C, although a rise up to 40°C can occur transiently in strenuous muscular exercise. In excessive HEAT EXPOSURE, normal TEMPERATURE REGULATION is defeated, resulting in *heat stroke*. In other circumstances any deviation from the norm in an upward direction constitutes fever. Fever, or *pyrexia*, refers to a rise of up to 40.5°C and *hyperpyrexia* to a greater rise. Above about 41.5°C a person loses orientation and may become unconscious.

In some diseases the word 'fever' is incorporated into the common names, such as in puerperal, scarlet, typhoid, and yellow fevers, indicating that a rise in termperature is associated with the condition. Before the advent of mass vaccination programmes those with infectious fevers were taken in to isolation hospitals, often called fever hospitals. The word 'fever' is sometimes used in other contexts, such as 'fever pitch', when an individual, group, or crowd (such as a football crowd) becomes over-excited or agitated.

The body has a complex mechanism for controlling temperature that balances heat production against heat loss. Heat is continually produced by metabolism of all body cells, to an extent that varies with the activity of glands and organs, and of the muscles (SHIVERING is an effective way to increase heat production). Heat is lost by radiation and convection, particularly from exposed parts such as the face and hands, and by evaporation of sweat. The control of the balance between heat production and heat loss is centred in the brain, in the HYPOTHALAMUS, which acts basically as a thermostat. Input signals from heat- and cold-sensitive receptors in the skin relay information to the hypothalamus (these receptors are extremely sensitive: the heat receptors are able to detect a rapid rise in temperature of 0.007°C, while the cold receptors can detect a rapid fall of 0.012°C) and the 'thermostat' also senses the temperature of the blood passing through. While the discomfort of the experience of hot and cold environments resides in the skin, it is the body's 'core' temperature that matters, as many processes within the body are disrupted if the core temperature changes. Thus if the blood temperature rises, then the output signals from the thermostat lead to vasodilation of blood vessels in the skin and to SWEATING, thus increasing heat loss. Or, if body temperature falls, then heat loss is curtailed by vasoconstriction of surface blood vessels, and heat production may be increased by shivering.

In fever the hypothalamic thermostat becomes set at a higher temperature. The normal blood temperature is therefore sensed as being too low, and temperature-raising mechanisms come into action, accounting for initial pallor and shivering. Conversely, when fever is abating the set temperature is lowered, and the warm skin and sweating represent heat loss mechanisms.

The commonest cause of fever is infection by VIRUSES, BACTERIA, yeasts, or PARASITES. Substances are released by these organisms which are collectively called *pyrogens* (substances causing a rise in temperature — pyrexia). The pyrogens act upon white blood cells to produce further, endogenous, pyrogens; these latter can also be released from tumours, from the brain after INJURY or STROKE, from blood clots, or in AUTOIMMUNE DISEASE. The endogenous pyrogens interact in the brain with *prostaglandin synthetase*, the enzyme necessary for synthesis of PROSTAGLANDINS, which in turn are the main agents that alter the setting of the 'thermostat'. This explains why taking ASPIRIN can abolish fever, since it inhibits prostaglandin synthetase; it also explains why, in the absence of fever, aspirin has no effect on body temperature.

In general, it is the practice to use drugs to reduce fever, but this may reduce the effectiveness of MACROPHAGES (white cells) to engulf and destroy bacteria. Experimental evidence indicates that prevention of pyrexia is detrimental to survival in infected animals. It is equivocal whether or not fever can be universally regarded as a body defence mechanism, particularly as its usefulness or otherwise where there is no infection is obscure.

ALAN W. CUTHBERT

See also HEAT EXPOSURE; INJURY; PROSTAGLANDINS; TEMPERATURE REGULATION.

Fibrillation

Fibrillation Non-rhythmic and mechanically ineffective contractile activity in the heart muscle, associated with disordered electrical activity. *Atrial fibrillation* is not uncommon, and not in itself a serious threat: the heart can function without effective contraction of the atria, because the main pumps (ventricles) continue to beat effectively (though not regularly). But *ventricular fibrillation* stops the pump and is fatal, unless it can be promptly reversed. S.J.

See DEFIBRILLATOR; HEART; PACEMAKER.

Fingerprints

Fingerprints In the minds of many people, fingerprints are significant only for the identification of CRIMINALS. But the skin corrugations that produce fingerprints are a functionally important part of the structure of the finger pads, not only in human beings, but also in a number of other mammals, especially primates, which use prehensile HANDS (and FEET) for active exploration of surfaces and for the fine manipulation of objects.

Fingerprints form naturally during the development of the human fetus, starting about 13 weeks after conception. The inner surfaces of the fingers and the palms of the hands, which are covered with hairless (*glabrous*) SKIN, develop tiny 'pods', which are the precursors of the pores of sweat glands. These pods, or ridge units, expand and coalesce with neighbouring pods, producing roughly linear ridges, with the sweat pores distributed along their crests, raised above the surface of the surrounding skin. These form the familiar parallel and swirling ridges and intervening furrows, the exact pattern of which is determined by complex, irregular stresses in the skin. They can be seen not only on the pads of the fingers and thumb, but over much of the glabrous skin on the undersurface of fingers and toes, and on the palms and soles of the hands and feet. (A little talcum powder dusted over the surface of the skin makes the pattern more easily visible.)

The ducts of the sweat glands open through the pores on the crests of the ridges. The moistening of the ridges, combined with the texture of the corrugations, increases friction when in contact with objects and hence improves grip. The regions of glabrous skin that have these epidermal ridges are especially richly supplied with cutaneous sensory nerves. These include large fibres that terminate in specialized endings that are sensitive to mechanical stimulation, in particular structures called *Merkel's discs* and *Meissner's corpuscles*, which are acutely sensitive to touch and to low-frequency vibration of the skin, respectively. The individual nerve fibres innervating the finger pads branch over areas of skin that are tiny compared with similar classes of fibres in other parts of the body surface. Thus the *receptive field* of each such fibre in the finger pads (the area of skin over which the application of an appropriate stimulus will cause an individual nerve fibre to respond) can be smaller than 1 mm². The skin of the fingertips therefore excels in its capacity to detect and discriminate the texture and three-dimensional shapes of surfaces. As the fingertips are moved over a non-smooth surface (when a blind person reads embossed Braille characters, for example), the resulting pattern of impulses generated in these nerve fibres and transmitted up to the brain provides remarkably acute tactile perception.

Serendipitously, the sweat secreted onto the skin ridges leaves an oily image of the pattern of corrugations on any surface that is touched. Since the exact forms of the corrugations are unique to each individual, and do not alter from birth to death (unless the skin is badly injured), fingerprints provide an infallible method of identification.

History

The discovery of the uniqueness of fingerprints is very ancient: the Chinese and Assyrians used them on legal documents more than 2000 years ago. The great Czech anatomist, Jan Evangelista Purkinje (who gave his name to the main class of nerve cells in the CEREBELLUM), studied the pattern of skin ridges and, in 1823, suggested a method of classification. The first Police Fingerprint Bureau was established in Argentina early in the 1890s by a Croatian immigrant, Juan Vucetich, whose system of classification is still used in South America. But the best-known system was devised a few years later by a police official, Khan Bahudur Azizul Haque, of the Bengal police, under the direction of Edward (later Sir Edward) Henry. When Henry was appointed Assistant Commissioner of Police for the Metropolis in London at the turn of the twentieth century, he established the first British Fingerprint Bureau at New Scotland Yard. The Henry System, based on prints of all the fingers, spread throughout the world. It quickly replaced the BERTILLON SYSTEM for identification, devised in 1879 by the French criminologist Alphonse Bertillon, which involved anthropometric measurement of parts of the body and detailed records of personal features, such as SCARS and eye colour.

The appearance of fingerprints

A record of an individual's fingerprints is made by inking the pads of the fingers and thumb and pressing or rolling them onto paper or some other suitable material. The most distinctive overall fingerprint patterns (arches, loops, and whorls) occur on the pads of the fingers, thumbs, and toes. The one illustrated is a magnified image of a 'loop', the commonest such pattern, which almost everyone has at some point on their skin. The sweat pores appear as little white dots at intervals along the ridges. Within such overall patterns are individual features known as 'ridge characteristics', 'ridge detail', or 'minutiae'. In places, the parallel ridges split into two (a fork or bifurcation), stop dead (a ridge ending), or divide into two and then join up again (a lake or enclosure). These features were studied and named by the British anthropologist and founder of the science of EUGENICS, Sir Francis Galton. It is such features (marked in the figure) and their proximity to one another that define the unique individuality of fingerprints. The prints of each finger pad typically contain about 100 such minutiae.

In many people, the overall macro-patterns on corresponding fingers of the left and right hands are roughly mirror images of each other. But it is possible to have a different feature pattern on every digit. Although the gross patterns (arches, loops, and whorls) may be passed on through family lineage, the individual ridge details are not. Since these minutiae are presumably not directly genetically determined, they differ between identical twins, and presumably would not be the same even in the clone of an individual.

Minor cuts and abrasions, and some skin diseases (e.g. psoriasis and eczema), may temporarily disturb the ridged skin features, but after healing the structure is exactly the same as before. More serious injuries or burns, involving the deeper layer of the skin (the dermis), can damage the cells that are responsible for regeneration of the skin, and leave a scar within which the ridge pattern is lost or changed. However, identity can still be established from surviving features outside the area of damage. A notorious American criminal, Roscoe Pitts, eliminated the prints of his fingertips by having them sewn into incisions in his chest until new skin grew over the ridge pattern. But he was later identified from prints of his palm, left at the scene of a crime!

Use in crime detection

When a surface is touched by a human hand, oily sweat is deposited from the skin ridges. This 'latent print' is often invisible to the naked eye, but can be revealed by a light dusting of powder, using a fine brush. Nowadays, aluminium flake powder is usually applied with a fibreglass brush, but a whole battery of physical and chemical processes is also available to develop prints on almost any surface.

Fingerprints collected at the scene of a crime are then matched against those taken from previously convicted criminals (now held as graphics files on computer databases), or from suspects. Although there have been encouraging developments in automated, 'expert system' computerized methods for the matching process, identifications are still made exclusively by experienced Fingerprint Officers.

Fingerprints are not the only means of identifying individuals. Voiceprints, lip prints, ear prints, glove prints, and DNA profiling provide additional or alternative methods for recognition.

S. E. HAYLOCK

See also DNA FINGERPRINTING; SKIN; VOICEPRINT.

Fitness

Fitness for what?

When we speak, perhaps with a hint of envy, of a 'fit' young man or woman — and even more when we refer, with undisguised admiration, to a 'fit' old person — there is little ambiguity as to our meaning: we are referring to fitness to cope with life in general, not only with SPORT, and certainly not a particular sport. Furthermore the international athlete, in peak of condition, is 'fit' for only a limited number of very similar events: the sprinter could not possibly run a marathon, the power lifter could compete with neither kind

of runner at their events. The fitness of the racing driver is radically different from that of the dinghy sailor, the gymnast from that of the mountaineer and, perhaps most radically of all, the oarsman from that of the pistol shooter. Furthermore, many highly trained athletes, particularly those conditioned for endurance events, display greater, not less, vulnerability than the average person to many forms of illness.

Clearly then, we must distinguish 'fitness for life' from 'fitness for sport'; and, when considering the latter, must specify which sport.

Fitness for life

This is a condition which we almost all desire, but few of us pursue with vigour. To attain and maintain it requires adequate and balanced nourishment, adequate and varied EXERCISE, adequate but not excessive SLEEP, avoidance of excess in using social DRUGS, plentiful stimulation without excessive STRESS, and psychosocial well-being. The Aristotelian precept, 'moderation in all things', remains as good a guide as any to the balances which must be struck. Fitness for work, for LEISURE and recreational exercise, for family life and parenthood, and even for childbearing itself, and fitness to cope with emergencies — all are optimized in these broad ways. The influences of genetics and of environment are inescapable, so the fitness attained by one person will be very different from that attained by another, but all will approach their individual optima by personal application of the same balanced principles. Even Western and Eastern, secular and religious wisdoms (disregarding the most extreme of the latter) have much more in common than divergence in their guidelines for 'fitness', whether or not they would recognize that term; and modern science, while adding a few details on matters like trace nutrients, takes little issue with them about the broader picture.

Endurance fitness

If there is one aspect of specialist, sports-oriented fitness which embodies the greatest part of the lay ideal, it is probably endurance fitness — the ability to continue a demanding physical activity many times longer than the untrained person can. Whether the challenge is a London–Brighton cycle race, an ascent of the Matterhorn, or a Channel swim, the fundamentals of this category of fitness are the same. Each of these activities is trained for in essentially the same way — namely, by covering large mileages several days a week for many months, with few if any periods of exertion that are flat out, either in strength or speed. Each activity is, in turn, necessarily aerobic — an activity performed in balance with oxygen intake — and consequently requires that the HEART can pump blood to the working muscles at several times its resting rate throughout the long duration of the exercise; also that the LUNGS can adequately oxygenate this enhanced blood flow as long as the exercise continues. 'Cardio-respiratory fitness' is thus a common feature of all endurance events, though they

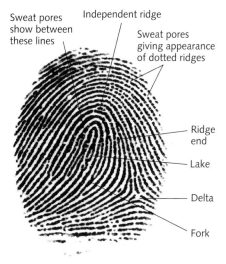

Magnified ink fingerprint from the pad of a left forefinger.

Sweat pores show between these lines

Independent ridge

Sweat pores giving appearance of dotted ridges

Ridge end

Lake

Delta

Fork

differ in the SKELETAL MUSCLES used, and the movement patterns these muscles perform.

When muscles have been endurance-trained they are typically only a little larger than before the training began, months or years before. They become furnished, however, with a much more copious system of blood capillaries. Within the muscle fibres, mitochondria, the organelles involved in oxidative energy provision, may be 2–3 times more numerous than in untrained or differently trained fibres. CONNECTIVE TISSUES within the muscle as well as the associated tendons and ligaments are stronger too. The NERVOUS SYSTEM must also participate in the training, for patterns of movement in the exercise concerned are usually measurably more economical than before the regime began.

Other forms of training

Pure STRENGTH TRAINING contrasts most markedly with the low-force, multiple-repetition work just described. Though increasing the bulk of the muscles and the maximum loads which they can handle, it adds little or nothing to their endurance. However the more commonly undertaken 'weight training', in which less extreme loads are worked against, with several times as many repetitions during the course of each gymnasium session, imparts 'strength endurance', a balance between the two extremes which arguably develops the most useful form of fitness for everyday life. Speed training, 'plyometric' (resilience) training, and flexibility training are other forms in which it is possible to specialize: in particular, yoga places a degree of emphasis upon flexibility which most other schools of physical educators would consider disproportionate. Nevertheless a programme of muscle stretching and joint flexibility should be part of the regime of every sportsperson seeking to improve not only performance but resistance to injury. Finally, between speed and endurance comes 'anaerobic endurance' — the ability to maintain a power output only a few per cent below flat out for several tens of seconds (as in 400 metre running) or to repeat short bursts many times in a period of about 90 min (as in hockey, soccer, and other 'multiple sprint' sports).

Specific versus general fitness

It would be widely agreed that the broader-based forms of fitness are of greater value in daily life than the extreme forms, such as pure endurance, pure strength, pure flexibility, or pure speed. Older literature embodied the ideal of breadth in the term 'general fitness'. However, it is now appreciated that the dominating principle underlying the response of the body to training is its 'specificity'. A particular exercise elicits the adaptive responses we call 'training' only from the specific muscles and other tissues exercised, and enhances only the specific property (endurance, strength, speed, or extensibility) which the exercise challenges. At best only very modest improvements of other properties or at other muscle sites ('cross-training') are ever

reported, and they cannot be counted upon. A sport requiring many forms of fitness must thus have a training programme including many elements. There is probably only one sense in which 'general fitness' can be enhanced by most individual forms of exercise, pursued in isolation: since it is impossible to undertake any exercise without raising both pulse rate and ventilation, every form of exercise provides some cardio-respiratory training, and hence some degree of 'general fitness' in respect of these central organs. More thorough-going general fitness can only be attained by an exercise programme which is itself broad-based.

A broad-based programme can, of course, be achieved by regular visits to a well-conducted gymnasium; however, such a clinically purposeful regime is not the only way. Someone who, in a typical 2-week period, goes for a 40-minute run, plays a game of squash, spends an active 30 minutes in the swimming pool, does a couple of hours' heavy gardening, polishes the car energetically, chops wood, vacuum cleans the stairs twice, and scrubs the steps, especially if (s)he precedes at least the first three of these activities with 5–7 minutes of stretching and flexing exercises, will be as fit for life as a neighbour who visits the local gym three times a week. Any difference between them which is non-genetic may well be determined by which of them gets more sleep, or eats less fat.

Women, children, and the elderly

In modern, Western societies, women, children, and the elderly are particularly prone to take insufficient exercise. The Allied Dunbar National Fitness Survey found that, in England during 1990, only one woman in ten, whether aged 20 or 50, took the amount of exercise really recommended for health whereas, among the men, 30% of 20-year-olds and 20% of 50-year-olds did so. Dunbar's standards were admittedly high — among the 20-year-olds, for instance, it hoped to see three games of squash, or equivalent, per week. More recent research has shown that statistically demonstrable improvements in cardiovascular fitness, compared with the effects of taking no exercise at all, can be had from only three 20–30 minute periods per week of moderately vigorous walking. Nevertheless, about a quarter of women in the working age-groups do not even achieve this, which is a much more modest goal than the vibrant fitness sought by Dunbar.

Modern children are distracted by television and computer games and are more likely to be transported to and from school, so that they almost certainly take less exercise than their predecessors before the 1939–45 war (although incontrovertible figures for the past are hard to establish). They should be urged to the maximum amount of physical activity of which they seem capable. No damage will accrue, provided they wear well-fitting trainers, are provided with shock-absorbing landing mats for gymnastics, and don't spend more than 90 minutes, 3 days a week, with specialist, competitive coaches.

Amongst the elderly, a 'disuse–disability spiral' operates. Well-meaning younger carers can be the old person's worst enemies. If daily activities fail to maintain independence — the bottle top, the heavy kettle, and worst of all independence at the toilet, being critical markers of diminished capacity — exercise regimes can be of enormous benefit. Often this benefit is proportionately greater than in younger adults, because, through disuse, the elderly have declined further below their genetic capability. Instances of elderly people running marathons are well known, but strength training is at least as effective in the very old as endurance training, and may be even more beneficial.

NEIL SPURWAY

Further reading

Morris, J., et al. (1992). *Allied Dunbar National Fitness Survey*. The Sports Council, London.

Sharkey, B. J. (1990). *Physiology of fitness*, (3rd edn). Human Kinetics, Champaign, Illinois.

Wilmore, J. H. and Costill, D. L. (2000). *Physiology of sport and exercise*. 2nd ed. Human Kinetics, Champaign, Illinois.

See also EXERCISE; HEALTH; SPORT.

Flagellation

During the Middle Ages, various ascetic sects within the Mediterranean and Hibernian world adopted the practice of flagellation; ritual scourging of the flesh with a whip for the purpose of cleansing the soul of sin. Among Christian religious communities, where flagellation was most systematically integrated into devotional life, flagellation was performed as a memorial to an act of sacrifice that occurred centuries in the past, the suffering and martyrdom of Jesus Christ. Personal acts of self-immolation by monks, nuns, and other holy people imitated biblical descriptions of Christ's journey to Calvary for crucifixion, the primordial moment of Christian sacrifice, when life beyond the grave was supposed to have been achieved. Mimetic flagellation was done in the belief that bodily suffering atoned for offenses against God and satisfied divine justice.

Penitential obligations imposed by the church hierarchy over the lay population extended the practice of remunerative suffering in the high Middle Ages. Flagellation of a voluntary nature was appropriated soon thereafter by lay members of society in Italy, Greece, Germany, and Poland. During the fourteenth century, public processions of ritual scourging were formed with the intention of appeasing God's wrath in order to secure communal health against the bubonic plague. At a slightly later date, towards the end of the fifteenth century, voluntary scourging became public in Spain, where it took on its most elaborate and ceremonial forms. Young men who called themselves *disciplinantes*, the flagellators, organized into religious brotherhoods for the specific purpose of scourging the flesh 'in payment for all the sins of the Christian people'. These collective orders of storytellers reproduced during Holy Week the mournful scriptural saga of redemption by inscribing on their backs the blood that was thought once to have been shed by Christ. The men who chose to participate in the annual performances of penitence initially met together in private in parish churches and local monasteries, to contemplate Christ's suffering and share in evening meals. They extended to one another signs of affection and goodwill and offered apologies for past offences. Wedded in a state of grace and freed of animosity, they silently journeyed out on to dirt and cobblestone streets, walking barefoot through narrow corridors of urban and rural thoroughfares for distances of some two to five leagues. On the way they scourged themselves, flailing long, knotted and wax-tipped ropes across their backs until blood drenched their linen tunics and spilled over on to darkened pavements. As much as a pound of coagulated blood was noted to have been shed by individual flagellants during these paschal ceremonies. It was because of the physical strength and endurance required to perform in front of the public with unwavering resolve that corporate legislation required that flagellation only be performed by men under the age of fifty in good health.

The flagellants' re-enactment of Christ's sacrifice, in processions that riddled the surface of public streets with the blood of inhabitants, exposes for us a dual meaning to bodily ritual in the religious observances of traditional communities. Ritual is a means first and foremost, as Mircea Eliade has demonstrated forcefully in *The Sacred and the Profane*, of spanning the chronological distance between present and past and perpetuating memories of a people's supernatural origins. The theological message of ritual scourging was made clear to spectators in formal pronouncements. As young men solemnly raised lashes over their heads, public oracles announced that

'this is done in honor and reverence of the shedding of His precious blood, and in honor of the five thousand lashes that they gave Him in order to redeem and save us'.

Along with this commemorative function, a second, more immediate and personal meaning was expressed in these ceremonial acts. Suffering and affliction experienced by all who followed Christ, it was collectively articulated, had the continued power to cleanse, to heal, and to restore moral order. This was why Holy Week exercises did not merely recall, in an abstract manner, an act of sanctifying pain that had occurred once already in the past, but actively *emulated* this sanctification process in the present.

Through the experience of genuine pain, penitents were laying claim to their immediate sense of control over morality and collective justice. Flagellants were rehearsing a past that continued to live on in their emotional appreciation of the world, causing their own blood to mingle with that of Christ's memory to bring down upon the community divine grace.   M. FLYNN

See also BODY MUTILATION AND MARKINGS; CHRISTIANITY AND THE BODY; STIGMATA.

Flesh

An anecdote from the material culture of the late twentieth century may serve to introduce the layers of meaning associated with flesh; its epistemological, moral, and biological implications.

From the 1960s the manufacturers of Crayola crayons included in their colour range a tone called 'flesh', a salmon-pink which was intended to approximate the skin tone of Caucasians. In recent years, the heightened sensitivity, particularly in North America, to politically incorrect designations of race and colour, has caused Crayola to withdraw its 'flesh' tone, replacing it with a separately packaged selection of oranges and browns, appropriately named 'Skin Tones of the World'.

The action of Crayola crayon manufacturers in removing the offensive 'flesh' from their colour palate is an illustration, albeit a very historically specific one, of the problematic connotations associated with the flesh in the West. But 'flesh' refers usually to that which lies under the skin, or on the bones — fat and muscle — rather than to the skin itself. In the current affluent West, where surfeit is a far more common phenomenon than famine, excess flesh and lack of bodily 'FITNESS' is interpreted as a sign of laxity, overindulgence and weak will. Anorexia nervosa, the medical condition in which food is deliberately avoided, results from a loathing of the flesh and a desire to discipline bodily appetites. Unlike medieval Christian ASCETICISM or other religious movements which seek to discipline the body to strengthen or elevate the spirit, anorexia victims have as their principal aim the attainment of a less fleshly, and therefore to their mind a better, body.

'The flesh' has long carried overtones of transgression, rebellion, and disgust, particularly strong in Christian cultures. This is due largely to a number of commentaries on the Old and New Testaments by early Church Fathers such as St Augustine and St Jerome. By elaborating on the opposition and struggles for supremacy between the spiritual and physical parts in a human being, they denigrated the desires and promptings of the body, or 'the flesh', as emblematic of original sin and of man's fallen state.

The first reference to flesh in the Bible is neither a negative nor a condemnatory one. It appears in Genesis 2, when God removes a rib from Adam while he is sleeping, and from it creates Eve to be his companion and helpmate. On waking, Adam declares,

'This is now bone of my bones, and flesh of my flesh: she shall be called Woman, because she was taken out of Man. Therefore shall a man leave his father and mother, and shall cleave unto his wife; and they shall be one flesh' (21–5).

Flesh and bone, or, as in the later idiom, flesh and blood, thus epitomizes kinship, the tangible bonds between family members. The physical union between man and wife is symbolized and ritually celebrated, by their becoming 'one flesh', or one body.

This description of the state of matrimony before the Fall was tendentiously placed by Jerome, as occurring *after* Adam and Eve had sinned, thus tainting all fleshly union with evil. Jerome further points out that Jesus himself remained 'a virgin in the flesh and a monogamist in the spirit', faithful to his only bride, the church. The passage to which Jerome alludes is that in Romans (7:24–5), in which Paul says,

'O wretched man that I am! who shall deliver me from the body of this death? . . . with the mind I myself serve the law of God; but with the flesh the law of sin.'

The response to Paul's desperate call is, of course, Jesus Christ, whose law of the spirit will free mankind from the law of sin and death: 'For if ye live after the flesh, ye shall die: but if ye through the Spirit do mortify the deeds of the body, ye shall live' (8:13).

In the *Confessions*, Augustine identifies the question of self-government with the rational control of sexual impulses. He recalls how, 'in the sixteenth year of the age of my flesh . . . the madness of raging lust exercised its supreme dominion over me.' The first government in Creation was the rule, within Adam, of the rational soul over the body. This hierarchy reflected the obedience and subjection of all Creation to the Creator, an order which was first overturned by Adam's transgression and rebellion against God's rule. Augustine points out the aptness of the punishment for this uprising, which was none other than disobedience within Adam's own self:

'After Adam and Eve disobeyed . . . they felt for the first time a movement of disobedience in their flesh, as punishment in kind for their own disobedience to God . . . The soul, which had taken a perverse delight in its own liberty and disdained to serve God, was now deprived of its original mastery over the body.'

In the beginning, Augustine insists, Adam and Eve enjoyed mental mastery over the procreative process: the sexual members, like the other parts of the body, enacted the work of procreation by a deliberate act of will, 'like a handshake.' Ever since Eden, however, spontaneous sexual desire is, Augustine contends, the clearest evidence of original sin. What epitomizes our rebellion against God, is the 'rebellion in the flesh — the spontaneous uprising in our 'disobedient members'.

The battle specifically for CHASTITY, or freedom from sexual urges of the flesh, is discussed by Cassian, the first-century ascetic, in his *Institutiones*, and in several of his *Conferences*. Within the deadly sins, fornication is coupled with greed: like greed it is rooted in the body; they are 'natural' vices and hence difficult to cure. While sins like anger or despair can be fought only in the mind, fornication cannot be eradicated without chastising the body. There must therefore be severe mortification which still permits us to 'depart from this flesh while living in the body', to gain deliverance from the corruption and moral vicissitudes of the flesh.

The passage in Romans quoted above inspired legions of physically punitive practices of worship in Christianity, in which the filth of the world was combatted by the discipline of the self, the voluntary annihilation, self-torture, and deformation, of the foul and bestial flesh. Self-flagellation and mutilation, prolonged fasting or the eating of distasteful or rotten food, sleep deprivation through night vigils, continuous kneeling in prayer upon stones or nails, the wearing of vermin-infested clothes, exposure to extreme cold and heat, degrading and back-breaking labour, were expressions of the desire to subdue, castigate, and mortify the sinful body in order to liberate the soul imprisoned by its needs and desires. 'Let us kill this flesh,' cried the first-century monk, John Climacus, as he ascended the *Santa Scala*, the holy ladder to monastic perfection, 'let us kill it just as it has killed us with the moral blow of sin.' St Bernard of Clairvaux in the 12th century wrote in his *Meditationes* that

'This flesh . . . is no better than filthy Rags . . . froth and bubble, clothed with a gay, but frail and decayed beauty; and time will shortly come, when all its boasted charms shall sink into a rotten Carcass.' Man, concluded Bernard, is nothing but stinking sperm, a sack of dung, and food for worms.

The feelings of disgust and horror invoked by the body and the flesh in the Christian ascetic tradition find a distant parallel in the many and varied customs of flesh food avoidance found around the world. The use of living creatures for food is everywhere influenced by rules, prejudices, and conventions. The feelings associated with unacceptable foods of animal origin are much stronger than those associated with foods of plant origin, as animals are forceful vehicles for highly emotionally charged ideas.

Ideas of contact or contagion suggest that, by ingesting flesh, one can take on the undesirable qualities of the animal or part of the animal one eats. These reveal concerns over purity and pollution, and the disgust at different flesh foods derives from a dread of being contaminated or debased. This fear of defilement is generated principally by waste products of human or animal bodies, which in a broad sense may extend to anything coming from the body. As St Bernard says, 'Consider a little those constant evacuations, the discharges of thy mouth, and nose, and other passages . . . and ask thy self how much this differs from a Common Shore [sewer] . . .' The dietary purity of the animal may enhance its status as flesh food: hence herbivores, especially those pastured or which graze in the wild, are considered 'clean' compared with carnivores, the disgusting qualities of whose flesh are enhanced by the disgusting things they may consume. Most unclean of all are those animals who are fed on refuse scraps, human or animal excrement, or who scavenge dead animals: omnivores such as pigs, dogs, or carrion crows.   NATSU HATTORI

Further reading

Camporesi, P. (1988). *The incorruptible flesh: bodily mutation and mortification in religion and folklore*, (trans. Tania Croft-Murray). Cambridge University Press, Cambridge.

Pagels, E. (1988). *Adam, Eve and the Serpent*. Wiedenfeld and Nicolson, London.

Simoons, F. J. (1994). *Eat not this flesh. Food avoidances from prehistory to the present*. University of Wisconsin Press, Madison.

See also ASCETICISM.

Flying Transport by air became a very common activity during the second half of the twentieth century. It provides a rapid means of transport over long distances, in relative comfort. Commercial air travel is amongst the safest forms of transportation. Military aircraft have played a very major role in war since the late 1930s. The modern fighter-bomber is a very formidable weapon.

The environment in which aircraft operate differs markedly from that on the ground. The fall in the pressure and temperature of the air which occur with ascent to ALTITUDE have major effects upon the body, including expansion of gas in gas-containing cavities, HYPOXIA (oxygen lack) due to the fall in the partial pressure of the OXYGEN (PO_2) in the air, DECOMPRESSION SICKNESS due to the formation of bubbles of gas in the tissues, cold injury, and HYPOTHERMIA. The ability of aircraft to execute turns at high speed exposes the occupants to far greater accelerations than are normally encountered in terrestrial life. These accelerative forces produce profound effects upon the cardiovascular and musculo–skeletal systems (see G AND G-SUIT). The additional freedom of motion and abnormal accelerative forces which occur in flight can give rise to misinterpretation of the information provided by the senses, giving rise to *spatial disorientation*, with potentially dangerous consequences.

Gas expansion

The pressure of the atmosphere falls in an approximately exponential manner with increasing altitude, but the proportions of the major components of the atmosphere — oxygen (20.9%), nitrogen (78.1%), and the rare gases (1%) — however, remain constant up to 300 000 feet. The fall in pressure which occurs on ascent to altitude is transmitted throughout the tissues and gas-containing cavities of the body, namely the middle ear, the sinuses, the lungs, and the gut. The gases in these cavities expand as the pressure falls. If the escape of gas to the atmosphere is hindered, then the cavity will be stretched, and discomfort, pain, and tissue damage may ensue. With normal rates of ascent, the only site in which failure of venting may occur is the intestines, especially if the altitude exceeds 25 000 feet, when it can cause abdominal pain. If the fall of pressure occurs very rapidly the gas in the LUNGS may not be able to escape and the lungs may be damaged by over-expansion, and gas may enter the circulating blood (gas

EMBOLISM) with potentially fatal results. On descent from altitude, gas must enter the middle ear and sinuses. The valve-like function of the tube which connects the middle ear cavity to the back of the nose (the pharyngo–tympanic, or EUSTACHIAN TUBE) may prevent air re-entering the middle ear cavity on descent, causing pain in the ear and DEAFNESS, and, on occasion, rupture of the ear-drum. Voluntary actions, such as SWALLOWING, open the tube in about 50% of healthy individuals. Others find that they must raise the pressure in the mouth and nose in order to force gas into the middle ear. A head cold may make inflation of the middle ear much more difficult.

Hypoxia

The fall in the partial pressure of oxygen (PO_2) in the air which occurs on ascent to altitude reduces the PO_2 in the tissues — the condition termed 'hypoxia'. Normal cellular function is impaired when the local PO_2 falls below a critical value. The effects of hypoxia are seen first in the central nervous system, especially the higher centres. Thus the time taken to learn a new task is increased at an altitude as low as 5000 feet. Impairment of the performance of well-practised tasks does not occur until the altitude exceeds 10 000–12 000 feet. Subjects seated at rest exhibit virtually no symptoms of hypoxia at altitudes below 15 000 feet. Moderate physical exercise will, however, induce breathlessness at altitudes above 10 000 feet. Breathing air at altitudes between 15 000 and 18 000 feet rapidly produces impaired mental performance, lack of insight, and loss of judgement and self-criticism, leading to euphoria and neuro-muscular uncoordination. The increase in pulmonary ventilation stimulated by the hypoxia removes an excessive amount of CARBON DIOXIDE from the body. This *hypocapnia* causes light-headedness, apprehension, tingling sensations, and muscle spasm in the face and limbs. Acute exposure to altitudes above 18 000–20 000 feet causes gross impairment of mental function and leads in a matter of a few minutes to unconsciousness and CONVULSIONS. Prolonged exposure to these or higher altitudes is fatal. The time which elapses between a sudden exposure to breathing air and serious impairment of consciousness falls from 3 to 5 min at 25 000 feet to 40 sec at 35 000 feet and to 15 sec at 45 000 feet.

Two methods of preventing the hypoxia induced by ascent to altitude are employed in aviation. The first is to maintain the PO_2 in the inspired gas by increasing the concentration of oxygen in the gas breathed, which requires the individual to wear a mask. The second method is to limit the fall of environmental pressure to which the individual is exposed by raising the pressure in the crew and passenger compartments of the aircraft above that of the external environment.

The pressure cabin

The cabins of all modern civil transport and military combat aircraft are pressurized with air supplied by the engines. The flow of air through the cabin is determined principally by the requirements for ventilation (removal of carbon dioxide and body odours) and thermal comfort. The differential pressure between the pressure cabin and the environment is controlled by the cabin air outlet valves. In passenger-carrying aircraft, the degree of pressurization of the cabin is determined by the requirements to prevent significant hypoxia at altitude and damage to the middle ear on descent. Present international requirements allow the pressure in the cabins of these aircraft to be reduced to the equivalent of 8 000 feet. Breathing air at this altitude, however, impairs the ability of aircrew to respond to a new task, which may be significant in an emergency situation. There is also evidence which suggests that this degree of hypoxia when combined with sitting for several hours can produce deterioration of the condition of individuals suffering from certain cardio–respiratory diseases. In practice, therefore, the cabin altitudes of many passenger-carrying aircraft do not exceed 6000 feet.

The pressure cabins of military aircraft normally employ a smaller pressure difference between inside and outside ('low differential pressure') in order to minimize the weight of the cabin and to reduce the consequences of a failure of its structure. The crew of these aircraft breathe oxygen-enriched gas throughout the flight. The maximum cabin altitude in a combat aircraft is determined by considerations of the time available in the event of a failure of the oxygen supply and reversion to breathing air, and the incidence of decompression sickness. Typical maximum cabin altitudes lie between 18 000 and 22 500 feet.

Pressurization of the cabin introduces the possibility of decompression of the cabin in flight due to a failure of the structure, of the air supply to the cabin, or of the air outlet valves. A major structural failure may well be associated with break-up of the aircraft. The fall of pressure produced by a more limited failure, such as the loss of a window or door, may be less catastrophic, although individuals close to the defect may be blown out of the aircraft. The major hazard is hypoxia. It is likely that only a small proportion of passengers would succeed in using the drop-down oxygen masks. The life-saving measure in the event of a decompression is immediate rapid descent of the aircraft to low altitude. It is essential, therefore, to prevent hypoxia in the flight deck crew, by the correct use of efficient oxygen delivery equipment.

Pressure breathing

Breathing 100% oxygen at an altitude of 40 000 feet produces a PO_2 in the lung gas equal to that produced by breathing air at 10 000 feet. The PO_2 in the lung gas can be maintained at this value at higher altitudes by breathing 100% oxygen at a raised pressure — a procedure termed *positive pressure breathing*. Breathing oxygen at pressures above 30 mm Hg requires a counterbalancing pressure to be applied to the external surface of the trunk to aid breathing and prevent over-distension of the lungs. At higher breathing pressures (above 50 mm Hg) counter-pressure must also be applied to the lower limbs to minimize the circulatory disturbances induced by the high pressure in the chest. Several types of partial pressure suits based upon these principles are used to provide emergency short-duration protection against hypoxia at altitudes between 40 000 and 80 000 feet. Longer duration protection against the effects of exposure to altitudes above 40 000 feet requires the use of a full pressure suit: this is essentially a personal pressure cabin which applies counter-pressure to the whole body and can thus protect against both hypoxia and DECOMPRESSION SICKNESS.

Spatial disorientation

Nearly all aircrew experience illusory sensations of the attitude or motion of their aircraft, or fail to detect changes in the orientation of the aircraft, at some time during their careers. These incidents are due principally to the limitations of the sensory mechanisms of the body. False perceptions of orientation may give rise to errors in the control of an aircraft which can, in turn, cause an accident. Disorientation has been implicated in about 10% of all civil airline accidents and in about 20% of military fixed wing aircraft accidents. The principal sources of information which provide the perception of the spatial orientation of the body are the EYES, the VESTIBULAR SYSTEM of the inner ear, and sensory endings in the skin, joints, muscles, and ligaments. Vision is of prime importance to spatial orientation both on the ground and in flight. The vestibular apparatus of the inner ear, and the SENSORY RECEPTORS in skin muscle and joints, provide information which ensures balance and spatial orientation on the surface of the earth even when the eyes are closed. The vestibular apparatus frequently provides erroneous information in flight because the magnitude and time course of the motions to which the pilot is exposed are atypical and outside the normal dynamic range of this system.

There are two important classes of illusion which can arise from the vestibular organs in flight. The first is the perception of linear acceleration, which is sensed by the *otolith organs* of the vestibular apparatus, which signal the position of the head relative to the gravitational vertical. They also respond to linear accelerations of the head so that when an aircraft accelerates, the pilot has the sensation that the aircraft is rotating nose-up. This 'somatogravic' illusion may be so strong, especially in the absence of visual cues in fog or at night, that the pilot pushes the control column forward in an attempt to regain level flight, which may well increase the strength of the illusion. The pilot may then push the control column further forward and rotate the aircraft into a dangerous position — a pattern which has occurred in crashes associated with overshoot from an abandoned approach in poor visibility.

The second class of vestibular illusions is concerned with angular accelerations which are sensed by the fluid-filled *semicircular canals* of the vestibular apparatus. The commonest form of spatial disorientation is a false sensation of roll attitude. It occurs typically on recovery from a co-ordinated turn to level flight. The pilot enters the turns gradually and smoothly so that the angular velocity in roll is well below the level of detection by the semicircular canals and the pilot feels that the wings of his aircraft are level. If recovery from the turn is made relatively abruptly so that the semicircular canals are stimulated, the pilot now feels that the aircraft is flying one wing low when in fact the wings are level. This false sensation of bank, the *leans*, can persist for many minutes. In situations where the aircraft performs a prolonged spin the pilot will at first experience a sensation of spinning in the direction of the rotation. This sensation, however, ceases after 7–10 sec. When the spin ceases the pilot feels that he has entered a spin in the opposite direction and this somatogyral illusion may cause him to re-enter the original spin in an attempt to counter the apparent new one. These sensations are very disorientating, and the powerful control which the vestibular system has over the movements of the eyes can also seriously impair vision at the beginning of a spin and on recovery from a spin.

Pilots are taught to recognize conditions (e.g. poor visibility, landing and take off, and particular manoeuvres) which may lead to disorientation, to reject bodily sensations as unreliable, and to rely upon the visual information of aircraft behaviour and orientation provided by flight instruments.

Long-duration flight

Long-distance flight can cause fatigue in aircrew due to excessively long periods of duty, disturbances of sleep, and transmeridian travel. A critical factor in ensuring that excessive fatigue and disturbances of sleep do not occur in long-distance operations is to limit the total duty hours in a given period. Thus aircrew operating worldwide routes are considered able to cope with a total of 50–55 hours in the first 7 days and a total of 75 hours by the end of 14 days. Performance of the flying task by a pilot who is well rested typically increases over the first 5 hours of the duty period, but then falls precipitously over the next few hours, levelling out after 16 hours. Time of day also exerts a marked effect on performance (*circadian rhythm*). Performance rises during the day and falls during the late evening and overnight, reaching its nadir at about 05.00 in the morning. Very low levels of performance will occur if the fall in performance produced by a long period of duty coincides with the fall of performance produced by circadian rhythmicity early in the morning. Flight schedules for aircrew are designed to avoid such a gross impairment of performance.

Transmeridian flight through a number of time zones introduces the additional complication of the changes in the circadian rhythm, the magnitude of which depend upon the number of time zones crossed, and the speed of adaptation to the new time zone, which varies with the direction of travel. The adaptation phase is associated with disturbances of sleep, appetite, and bowel function, general discomfort, and reduced mental performance ('jet lag'). The circadian rhythms of the body adapt to a new time zone more rapidly on westbound travel than when travelling towards the east. Typically a flight through 6 time zones in an eastward direction produces disturbed sleep for 3–4 days, with the greatest disturbance occurring on the second night in the new time zone. Worldwide, aircrew flight schedules take account of these disturbances. They are designed to ensure that the aircrew obtain adequate sleep between duty periods. In military operations it may be impossible to ensure that adequate sleep can be taken at the appropriate time of day and it has been shown that the induction of sleep by the controlled use of hypnotic drugs can greatly enhance the maintenance of intense and sustained air operations.

JOHN ERNSTING

Further reading

Ernsting, J. Nicolson, A.N., and Rainford, D. J. (1999). *Aviation medicine*, 3rd edn. Butterworth-Heinemann, Oxford.

See also ALTITUDE; BALANCE; BODY CLOCK; DECOMPRESSION SICKNESS; HYPOXIA; VESTIBULAR SYSTEM.

Fontanelle A soft place in the scalp over a gap between four bones of the skull (the *frontal* and *parietal* bones on each side) which is normally present in the newborn infant. It gradually closes during the first 12–18 months of life, as bone formation extends until the edges come together at the *sutures*. The fontanelle reveals changes in pressure inside the skull: it tends to bulge when the baby cries, and to become sunken in a state of dehydration. The pulsations of the underlying brain with the heart beat can be felt at this site through the scalp.   S.J.

See SKULL.

Food What is food? Looked at in biological terms, it would appear that food is merely a source of the energy and nutrients essential for life. However, viewed from an anthropological perspective, it becomes evident that food has played a central role in human history. While the everyday quest for food shaped the life of prehistoric man, the onset of the production of a reliable and sufficient supply of food is likely to have led to the rise of civilizations, and to human population expansion. Furthermore, the ability of man to colonize almost every part of the world is at least in part due to his adaptability with regard to food. Not only are humans omnivorous, they have also shown remarkable ingenuity in identifying and preparing nutritious foods out of unpromising materials. For example, bitter cassava (*Manihot esculenta*), a root crop that contains toxic levels of cyanide-producing compounds, comprises, after thorough processing,

the major food item in the diet of millions of people worldwide.

Food for prehistoric man

The evidence used to determine which foods were eaten by prehistoric man is scarce and can be very difficult to interpret. The majority of clues about food usage come from the study of collections of animal bones, sea-food shell mounds, plant food remnants, and faecal remains, at or close to sites of human habitation. Studies of these food leftovers provide some hints as to what foods were available to and used by prehistoric man.

Until 10–12 000 years before the present (BP), humans relied on hunting and gathering for their food. They hunted wild animals such as gazelle, antelope, and deer, as well as fish, crabs, and migratory waterfowl, and gathered foods including shell-fish, root vegetables, grains, pulses, nuts, and fruit. The period between roughly 11 000 and 6000 years BP, which has been termed the Neolithic, was a time of crucial and widespread agricultural revolution. Wild crops such as wheat and barley began to be cultivated, and wild animals such as sheep and goats were tamed and then domesticated.

This shift from hunting and gathering to domestication and cultivation was very gradual and by no means universal (indeed some small isolated populations continue today to practise hunting and gathering as a mode of subsistence). However, the nature of the diet was altered considerably by the advent of farming. Pre-Neolithic man may well have consumed a large proportion of his diet in the form of animal products, with a lesser contribution coming from plant items. In contrast, the advent of plant cultivation led to certain crops, such as grains and root vegetables, becoming the main, or staple, part of human diets. As a consequence, the diet of Neolithic man was likely to have been dominated by these staple crops, with animal products making a considerably reduced contribution.

Food acquisition by hunting and gathering was time consuming and unpredictable. With the advent of farming, Neolithic man was, for the first time in human history, able to provide himself with a reliable and sufficient source of food. A major consequence of this was that as humans were no longer merely struggling from day to day to find sufficient food to survive; they could devote time to other matters. Most importantly, the availability of sufficient food led to a massive and unprecedented growth in the human population.

Food for modern man

Over the past 2000 years there have been substantial increases not only in the quantity but also in the quality of the food available to man. Early inventions such as new forms of plough enabled the cultivation of virgin lands, and practices such as crop rotation, which allowed soil to become reinvigorated between plantings, significantly increased food production. The mechanization of seed planting, harvesting, and threshing during the Industrial Revolution made agricultural production even more efficient.

However, this enhanced production led to a new set of problems, as it demanded innovative storage techniques and improved transport capabilities to avoid the produce spoiling before it was consumed. Salting and smoking had long been known as methods for preserving foods over extended periods of time. Canning was perfected in the early 1800s and quickly became popular as a convenient, cheap, and safe method of conserving pre-cooked food. Chilling or freezing was originally only available as a method of food preservation to those with a ready supply of ice. However, with the invention of ice-making machines in the 1830s, ice became widely available, and fresh fruit, meat, and fish could be conserved. Finally, the advent of fast and refrigerated transportation enabled fresh foods to be delivered in their original form to consumers around the world.

In order to ensure that the food supplied to the public is of adequate quality, many countries have set up agencies to monitor food safety. These agencies are designed to protect the consumer and improve the health of the public in relation to food by providing advice and information on food consumption. Furthermore, such agencies develop policies relating to food safety, and, by carrying out their own research, monitor relevant developments in science, technology, and other fields of knowledge related to food.

As a result of the slow but continual development of production, preservation, and safety technology, contemporary humans in developed countries have access to an astonishing quantity and diversity of foods. In the past, only locally-produced, in-season foods were available to consumers, but modern technology has now made it possible to supply consumers with foods produced in countries from around the world throughout the year.

Food for thought

The question of whether there is sufficient food to feed the world's ever-increasing population has exercised the minds of philosophers, economists, agronomists, and demographers for many centuries. In 1798, Thomas Malthus, an English political economist, wrote a paper entitled *An essay on the principle of population*, which still provokes heated debate. Malthus suggested that the world's population, growing at a geometric rate, was increasing at a much faster rate than the world's food production, which only increased arithmetically. Malthus argued that if a balance between population and food was not maintained, and the world's population grew to a size that was not sustainable by contemporary food production practices, then the consequence would be widespread famine.

The opposing viewpoint to that of Malthus suggests that increased population size is both a sign and a cause of prosperity, and that flexible and efficient markets can overcome any problems associated with an imbalance between population size and food production. This argument assumes that improving technology via scientific and agricultural innovation will ensure a steady and continual increase in food production. To support this assumption, anti-Malthusians suggest that increased population size will lead to a larger number of farmers tending ever-larger amounts of land, and that this will in turn precipitate innovation in land use and agricultural techniques.

There is good evidence that food production and crop yields have indeed increased sufficiently to cope with the increase in population size, but there are worrying signs that the rate of increase of crop yields is declining. This slowdown is no doubt due to a combination of causes: farmers may well be approaching the absolute maximum possible crop yields, and the cumulative effects of environmental degradation, partly caused by agriculture itself, may also be responsible. Considerable evidence suggests that, at least in some of the world's poorest countries, years of intensive agriculture, often coupled with long periods of drought, have led to the nutrient-exhaustion and desiccation of farming land. Such land is significantly less fertile and quickly becomes unable to support an ever-increasing population. Areas where this has occurred have been labelled *demographically entrapped*, as their projected population exceeds that which can be fed by local food production capabilities. In the absence of international food aid programmes, these countries, which typically lack trade and migratory safety valves, are thought to be facing uncertain futures of STARVATION, disease, and internal conflict.

Since Neolithic times, humans have carefully selected and bred plant and animal organisms that have demonstrated favourable traits. These selectively-enhanced descendants, with characteristics such as greater yield or improved flavour, often show little resemblance to the wild varieties. This ancient technology was further exploited between 1960 and 1980, during which laboratory-bred, high-yield cereal grains fed much of the world's expanding human population: the so-called 'Green Revolution'. However, these increases in yield may have led to environmental degradation through the exhaustion of ecological capital such as topsoil and groundwater. In response to the need for more productive and more environmentally friendly crops, modern advances in BIOTECHNOLOGY have produced genetically-modified or GM crops. GM crops typically contain gene alterations which confer agronomic benefits such as resistance to pests or to herbicides. These traits can reduce costs to the farmer and can also be beneficial to the environment, as they theoretically decrease the amount of insecticides and herbicides required. However, while such advances may be extremely useful in balancing world food production with population, there has been considerable public concern about this new technology and much more long-term research is still required.

Ironically, while the health of people in developed countries suffers from an excess of food leading to OBESITY, many developing countries face a stark future. Recent estimates have suggested that almost one-tenth of the world's population is malnourished in ways that impair health, and that the absolute number of malnourished persons, especially children, continues to grow. It is clear that food will continue to play a crucial role in human history for the foreseeable future.   ALAN DANGOUR

Further reading
Dyson, T. (1996). *Population and food: global trends and future prospects.* Routledge, London.

Tannahill, R. (1988). *Food in history.* Penguin Books, London.

See also ALIMENTARY SYSTEM; DIETS; EATING; ENERGY BALANCE.

Forehead The forehead, or brow, has been seen, literally and figuratively, as a place of expression. As Lord Byron remarked, 'Thy calm clear brow, Wherein is glass'd serenity of soul . . .' Ancient Egyptian women traced designs in henna on their temples. A furrowed brow marks distress or concern; being beetle-browed means one is of bad temper and surly, and a modest or meek person is 'tender-foreheaded'.

The form of the forehead is also believed to reflect the character of a person. A high brow, or being 'high-brow (ed)', indicates a superior intellect and sophistication; a low brow or prominent ridge above the eyes, on the other hand, is associated with primitive species of humanity, like the Neanderthal, and hence is a sign of primitivism and ignorance.

The forehead or brow is also a significant location in Christianity. Being cast from the Garden of Eden, Adam was to earn his living 'by the sweat of his brow'. Baptism, one of the sacraments of the Christian Church, may involve either total submersion, or simply the pouring of baptismal water over the forehead. In early Christianity, grievous sinners wore sackcloths and were covered with ashes during Lent as a sign of their penitence; around the ninth century, faithful Christians in general began to put ashes on their foreheads on the first day of Lent, Ash Wednesday, as a reminder of their need for penitence. These ashes came from the burned palm leaves from the previous Palm Sunday. Today, Roman Catholics receive the mark of a cross of their foreheads on Ash Wednesday.

The forehead is a site of spirituality in other religions, too. The centre of the forehead in Hindu tradition is the location of a third eye, a location of spiritual insight. Hindu gods are also frequently represented with a third eye in the middle of their foreheads, representing their divinity. Muslims touch their foreheads to the floor when bowing toward Mecca, and some Tibetan meditation practices focus on the centre of the forehead.

Anatomically, the forehead is formed by part of the frontal bone of the SKULL, whose shape is likened by Gray's Anatomy to that of a cockleshell — rounded rim above; below, a central projection forming the bony basis of the root of the nose, and low arches at each side over the eyes; the smooth convexity accommodating the frontal lobes of the underlying brain. The bone of the forehead is covered by a continuation of the layers of the scalp: a sheet of muscle under the forehead skin is joined above to a fibrous sheet which covers the skull and is in turn connected to muscle at the back of the head. Thus the scalp can be shifted back and forth, the brow furrowed, the eyebrows raised and lowered — contributing to a whole range of FACIAL EXPRESSION. The paired frontal sinuses are cavities in the frontal bone which drain down into the NOSE, and draw unwelcome attention to one's forehead if afflicted by sinusitis.

SARAH GOODFELLOW
SHEILA JENNETT

See also FACE; SKULL.

Frankenstein The clanking, bolted Boris Karloff, whose latest incarnation is the parodic Herman Munster, has become the popular image of the Frankenstein monster — in defiance of the illustration — accompanying the 1831 edition of Mary Shelley's novel, *Frankenstein,* which depicts the creature as a far more human and personable-looking being. The monstrous brood of her creation is a hideous progeny that has found its way into cinema, popular fiction, and critical theory by taking literally the injunction in her introduction to the 1831 edition to 'go forth and prosper'. The proliferation of the monstrous body is the anxiety that afflicts the mad scientist hero, Victor Frankenstein. His experimentation allegorizes not only the way in which science is not always in control of its metaphors, but also how men can lose control of the monsters they themselves create.

In preparation for his monstrous experiment Victor scours charnel houses, places for vivisection, and graveyards, for parts from which to assemble his New Adam or Modern Prometheus, which is the novel's subtitle. BODY SNATCHING was rendered obsolete a year after the third revised edition of *Frankenstein* by the 1832 Anatomy Act, which made available for DISSECTION the bodies of unclaimed paupers. For this reason, the blasphemy of Victor's nefarious activities has impacted less on the modern reader than on Shelley's contemporaries. The monstrosity of his creation is predicated upon the dilemma that, despite his having selected the most beautiful parts, only God can harmonize the whole. The product of Victor's labours is a creature that is eight foot tall with yellow skin and straight black lips, from which he recoils in horror. Victor's reaction, in regard to SKIN COLOUR, is replete with racist overtones. His creation is a mirror-image of colonization since, in wanting to reshape the world anew, he plunders the old. His aversion to his 'hideous progeny' can also be seen as a post-natal rejection of a newly-born infant by its mother. Some feminist critics have interpreted *Frankenstein* as an allegory of childbirth which, in this case, is the product of solitary male propagation, being the proverbial scientist's brain child.

Mary Wollstonecraft, Mary Shelley's mother, wrote about the importance of a maternal and nurturing presence in the upbringing of a child. Despite having mastered language and the range of human emotions, abandonment and the withdrawal of affection has warped Frankenstein's creation into the actuality of a monstrous self. Taking revenge on Victor, the creature murders his young brother William and pins the blame on a young family servant, Justine, who is eventually wrongly executed for the crime. Later he kills Victor's best friend Henry Clerval and his fiancé Elizabeth Lavenza. At the end of the novel, we are left to assume that he takes his own life in the Arctic wastes following the final confrontation between creator and created — which is foreshadowed by John Milton's *Paradise Lost* (1667) from which the epigraph of the novel is taken. The trail of destruction and waste has been interpreted as a warning of the potential dangers of modern science. Had Victor not abandoned his original mentors, necromancers like Paracelsus, Cornelius Agrippa, and Albertus Magnus, he might have created a harmless homunculus instead of the creature, who exacts revenge upon him.

The monster has been seen by Marxist critics as representing the new social order of the industrial proletariat, the destruction of the body politic by the mob in the Reign of Terror during the French Revolution, and a Malthusian dystopia born of a monstrous growth in population (see Thomas Malthus, *An Essay on the Principle of Population*, 1798). The fear of breeding a race of monsters leads Victor to destroy the female mate he has created for his creature by dismembering 'the thing' he had put together. The perception of both creature and mate as subalterns, who are subhuman, is integral to the process of colonization and the concept of 'thingification' whereby the colonizer assumes a position of power and superiority over the colonized. Once it was known that the author was a woman, the novel become a trope for the monstrosities produced by the female imagination as a source of patriarchal anxiety. For this reason, Mary Shelley may have felt it to be incumbent upon herself to explain in her later introduction, 'How I, then a young girl, came to think of, and to dilate upon, so very hideous an idea?' (1831).

The impetus for completing the novel is thought by critics such as Marilyn Butler to have arisen from the interest of Mary and her husband Percy Bysshe Shelley in current debates between the schools of vitalism and materialism as to the creation of life, experiments in galvanism on executed criminals, and a general vogue for automata. The genesis of the novel, which was first published in 1818, is explained in the preface to the revised 1831 edition, where Mary Shelley describes her participation in the ghost-story competition at the Villa Diodati in 1816. After a nocturnal conversation about Erasmus Darwin's apparent animation of a piece of vermicelli, she has a terrifying waking dream that gives her the idea for the creature.

The real nightmare described in the book, however, is the predicament of a being trapped in a monstrous body, who is sickened by his own image and shunned by human society. The text encourages the modern reader to reconsider the responsibilities of science, particularly in relation to such controversial areas as genetic engineering, CLONING, and reproductive technologies. Victor's teratological experiment may even be read as a parable for the dangers of male science, which have escalated subsequently into the nuclear arms race. By questioning our received notions of aesthetics, particularly the way in which the creature is rejected by society on account of his appearance, the novel invites us to consider afresh the relationship we have with our own body and its interaction with the outside world.　　　MARIE MULVEY-ROBERTS

See also MONSTERS.

Freaks The word 'freaks' generally refers to individuals or animals with physical anomalies or to sideshow entertainers able to perform acts which would be impossible or gruesomely painful for most people. For each of these groups, the title 'freak' is short for '*freak of nature*'. This terminology stems from a long-standing cultural belief that the usual processes of nature have set standards of normalcy for human form and ability. Freaks with physical anomalies are often called monstrosities because their deformities are congenital. Self-made freaks, on the other hand, define themselves according to their skills. These contortionists, sword-swallowers, glass-eaters, human-pincushions, geeks (those who eat live animals and raw meat), fully-tattooed men and women, and others who can safely hammer nails up their noses, refer to themselves as novelty act performers. Few exhibiting themselves as freaks before the early twentieth century found the term 'freak' denigrating. To a large degree, the current stigma associated with 'freaks' stems from the modern affiliation of physical deformity with illness.

In the historical record on freaks, from Aristotle to the twentieth century, several physical anomalies have consistently captured human interest. The most commonly cited types include cyclopes, giants, dwarves, joined twins, hermaphrodites, hirsuits and bearded women, individuals with severe skin disorders, living skeletons, the obese, and animals and humans born either without arms or legs or with extra pairs. Proclaimed animal–human mixes were also popular. Foreigners constituted another group of freaks. Sometimes freakish foreigners were purely mythical, like the reported races of men with tails. In other instances, the foreigners' freak status relied on Western European and North American fantasies of imperial and racial hierarchies. For example, nineteenth- and twentieth-century sideshow managers, doctors, and anthropologists alike described 'freaks' from Africa, South and Central America, the South Pacific, and Australia as the missing links in evolution, the last of the Aztecs, or savage cannibals. Known for her large buttocks and genitals, Saartjie Baartman (the Hottentot Venus) was the most famous 'exotic savage' in nineteenth-century Europe. Finally, there were the artificial freaks, the prime example of which was mermaids. P. T. Barnum's 'Fejee' Mermaid was apparently created by sewing the shaved head and torso of a red monkey onto the body of a fish.

The specific causes of many physical anomalies still remain a mystery, but present day doctors assert that most extreme cases result from genetic and chemical influences during the embryonic period, the first seven weeks of development. Dwarfism is one imperfection that doctors now trace to genetics. The thalidomide disaster of the late 1950s and early 1960s underscored the significance of toxic substances in reproduction. In this case, the thalidomide that pregnant women took to decrease nausea created a myriad of fetal deformities, including limb reduction. Doctors have also argued that maternal diabetes and multiple fertilizations increase the risk of birth defects.

Many other explanations for physical anomalies preceded today's. In ancient Greece and Rome, it was widely believed that monstrous births were caused by astrological forces or capricious gods. Interpreting deformities as portents or signs of divine displeasure continued well into the sixteenth century. As Ambroise Paré's treatise of 1537 shows, however, the Renaissance community also attributed unsightly births to the quantity and quality of seminal fluid, the size of the womb, maternal posture, heredity, accidental illness, bestiality, and maternal injury, as well as to divine or demonic influences. Since ancient times, communities have also asserted that maternal imagination and experiences could cause anomalies. Joseph Carey Merrick (the ELEPHANT MAN, *b*. 1862) revealed the persistence of this belief as he traced his deformity to the fact that his pregnant mother was nearly trampled by an elephant.

In 1981 the historians Katharine Park and Lorraine J. Daston observed that the Reformation heralded a shift away from the explanation of freaks as divine punishments. Instead, seventeenth-century communities saw freaks as relatively innocuous curiosities that revealed nature's power. By the late seventeenth century, the educated community believed in a nascent form of the embryological theory of reproduction. In addition, theories that deformities were caused by damage *in utero* gained momentum against the belief that anomalies were preordained and present within the seeds of life. Although philosophers and medical men continued to argue over the influence of God in human reproduction well into the nineteenth century, conceptualizing the body as a faulty biological system helped to justify the medical study of freaks. Isidore Geoffroy Saint-Hilaire's 1832 publication of *Histoire général . . . des anomalies* also marks a significant shift toward the modern study of physical anomalies. Rejecting the notion that freaks were sports of nature, Saint–Hilaire argued that *teratology* (the medical study of congenital monstrosity) should link normal and abnormal development.

Representations of human and animal freaks in culture are numerous. In *The Odyssey*, Polyphemous is one of a race of giant cyclopes. Goliath and Og, king of Bashan, are the star giants of the Bible. Japanese prints from the Edo period (1615–1867) depict a variety of freaks including a king of freaks and demonic cyclopes. In the *Tempest*, Shakespeare's Trinculo suggests that if he painted Caliban, he might make a good fortune exhibiting this savage to the curious. Swift's *Gulliver's Travels* addresses Gulliver's own exhibition as a freak. Velásquez's painting *Las Meninas* reflects the popularity of dwarves in seventeenth-century Spanish courts. Sixteenth- and seventeenth-century European handbills and similarly illustrated wonderbooks depict both freaks known to have lived and others that could only have been mythical. Expressing the optimism of Baconian science and hoping to record all the wonders of the natural universe, seventeenth-century elite gentlemen formed academic and philosophical societies to discuss nature's oddities. They also collected specimens of human and animal freaks in private curiosity cabinets. Others took notes on the freaks they witnessed at local fairs. Well into the nineteenth century, doctors also avidly collected freak specimens in medical college museums, exhibited these specimens and living freaks in their medical lectures, and described them in the major medical journals. Freaks also featured in twentieth-century movies such as Todd Browning's *Freaks* (1932) and David Lynch's *The Elephant Man* (1980). In 1972, Diane Arbus' photographs of freaks were published posthumously in *Diane Arbus: An Aperture Monograph*.

The most notorious venue for freaks has been the travelling raree or sideshow. Cities like London and Paris were the focus markets, but showmen also travelled around the European countryside. Particularly in the seventeenth and eighteenth centuries, freak shows could be quite casual, set up both inside and outside taverns. They were also common at the great fairs, the most reputed of which was the Bartholomew Fair, held at Smithfield for two weeks each year from the Middle Ages until 1855. By this time, several managers including P. T. Barnum, Uffner, Johnson, and Watson had already begun to consolidate the trade. They offered multi-starred spectacles in great rented halls, the most popular of which was the Egyptian Hall, Piccadilly. Although freak shows still continue today, their age of glory ended in the 1940s. Their decline resulted from the combined effects of competition from new kinds of entertainment, the disability rights movement, and the redefinition of physical abnormality in relation to medical disease.

Within the sideshows, the balance of power between manager and freak varied. Some freaks handled their own display entirely, but most relied on business partners to advertise and schedule shows and to create the essential aura of mystery that drew audiences. Certainly some exploitation existed — freaks were kidnapped, and their corpses were sold without their permission. Nevertheless, and despite long work days, most entertainment freaks appear to have been content in their careers and to have lived in relative comfort. A few, for example the midget Charles S. Stratton (Tom Thumb), amassed great fortunes. In addition to profits from admission and from the sale of illustrated pamphlets, which recounted their life stories, skills, and physical features, exhibition freaks sometimes received gifts from private audiences. Queen Victoria was quite generous in this respect.

Audiences for the shows came from all classes, as entry fees varied according to one's class status or the time of the viewing. Most freak shows admitted women and children as well as men, although with some 'delicate' subjects women and children were barred. In nineteenth-century France several freak shows were banned for fear that the shocking spectacles would cause women to bear monstrous children.

Some of the more famous freaks in Western culture include the (mythical) Bird Boy of Ravenna illustrated by Paré and the two-headed Bengali boy whose joined skulls are in the Hunterian Museum of the Royal College of Surgeons. Claude Ambroise Seurat (*b*. 1798) was the most famous 'living skeleton' and Patrick Cotter 'O'Brien' (*b*. 1760) and Chang Wow Gow (*b*. 1845–6) were well-known giants. The midgets 'Tom Thumb' (*b*. 1832) and his wife Lavinia Warren (*b*. 1841) are still the most celebrated little people. Since the exhibition of Chang and Eng Bunker (*b*. 1811), joined twins have also been called 'Siamese twins'. Matthew Buchinger (*b*. 1674) was a skilled draftsman who had neither hands nor legs. In the tradition of armless freaks, Charles Tripp (*b*. 1855) performed tasks with his toes.

HEATHER MCHOLD

Further reading

Bogdan, R. (1988). *Freak Show: presenting human oddities for amusement and profit*. University of Chicago Press, Chicago.

Daston, L. and Park, K. (1998). Wonders and the Order of Nature, 1150–1750. Zone Books, New York.

Gould, G. M. and Pyle, W. L. (1896, 1956). *Anomalies and curiosities of medicine*. Julian Press, New York.

Wilson, D. (1993). *Signs and portents: monstrous births from the Middle Ages to the Enlightenment*. Routledge, London.

See also DWARF; ELEPHANT MAN; GIANTS; MONSTERS.

Freckles (or *ephelides*) are small, usually yellow or brown spots on the skin, often seen on the face but capable of occurring in freckled individuals on any part of the body that has been exposed to sunlight. Freckles are produced by the action of ultraviolet radiation on the level of MELANIN in the melanocytes (pigment cells). In individuals of a certain genetic makeup and usually having red or blonde hair, the level of melanin increases to form freckles that contrast with the otherwise fair skin that such individuals possess. Freckles are found most frequently in older children and young adults and sometimes become less distinctive in older adults, in part because facial skin — where freckles are most noticeable — tends to darken and become coarser, more wrinkled, and more blemished with age. While the use of make-up can conceal freckles, there is no way for those disposed to freckling to avoid them other than by avoiding exposing their skin to sunlight.

Freckles can appear similar to and are sometimes confused with pigmented (or melanocytic) naevi, BIRTHMARKS, or moles. A pigmented naevus is quite distinct from a freckle, however, being a congenital anomaly produced by any of a number of abnormalities in the structure of the skin. While freckles are harmless, some naevi are pre-cancerous or are associated with a higher level of risk for cancer or other diseases.

While not freckling in the usual sense of the word, the rare genetic condition *xeroderma pigmentosum* resembles freckling in some ways. In affected individuals there is little natural resistance to ultraviolet radiation, producing large numbers of pigmented spots on the skin after exposure to the ultraviolet radiation in sunlight. Unlike freckles, these spots often become cancerous.

There are wider uses of 'freckle' than the primary reference to spots produced by increased melanin in some of the fair-skinned. Various types of mottling or spotting of bodily surfaces are sometimes called freckling, including spotting caused by several diseases. The presence of brown 'freckles' on the lips can indicate *Peutz-Jegher's syndrome*, which is characterized by intestinal polyps, while chronic liver disease can produce 'spider naevi' on the skin surface.

The use of 'freckle' extends beyond references to the skin, covering descriptions of a range of small spots. In Shakespeare's *A Midsummer Night's Dream*, a fairy tells of service to the Fairy Queen:

> The cowslips tall her pensioner's be
> In their gold coats, spots you see
> Those be rubies, fairy favors
> In those freckles live their savors. (II.i.13)

'Freckle' also acts as verb, and in less common usages refers to a wide range of coverings-up with small spots or discolorations.

While some adults consider mild freckling an attractive feature of youth, aesthetic appreciation of freckles has been absent from much of literature, art, and popular culture. Samuel Pepys wrote in his diary of his sister Pall, 'a pretty, good-bodied woman and not over thick, as I thought she would have been, but full of freckles and not handsome in the face.' In a subtle line that none the less invokes the image of a horse, John Cheever describes a character in *The*

Hartleys: 'There was a saddle of freckles across her nose.' Freckles are sometimes seen as a mark of immaturity, and children in contemporary societies are often teased about their freckles — and just as often about the red hair that can accompany freckles. Styles and preferences change, however: while many fair-skinned people prone to freckling continue to avoid the sun, a recent work on makeup and skin care, *Woman's Face*, advises the freckled to avoid attempts to conceal freckles with heavy makeup: 'Instead, rejoice in your freckles.' JEFFREY H. BARKER

See also SUN AND THE BODY.

Free radicals A free radical is any chemical species which contains one or more unpaired electrons and which is capable of an independent existence. An unpaired electron is one that can alone occupy an atomic or molecular orbital, conventionally denoted by a superscript dot: $X^{\bullet}$.

The biologically important free radicals are the oxygen species, superoxide $O_2^{\bullet-}$, the hydroxyl radical $OH^{\bullet}$, and the reactive nitrogen species $NO^{\bullet}$; each may play a significant physiological or pathophysiological role in the body. E. K. M.

See AGEING; NITRIC OXIDE; OXYGEN.

Freemartins The freemartin, an occasional anomalous development in domestic cattle, has long been recognized. It was observed at least as long ago as the Roman Empire that when a cow bore male and female twins the apparent female did not develop as a cow should, could not be bred from, and did not give milk — there was a Latin term '*taura*' (female form of *taurus*, a bull), meaning a barren cow, and a similar expression in Greek. In many other ways the freemartin resembled a bull, or a spayed heifer, more than a normal cow, and was also readier to mount other heifers when they came into oestrus. The term 'freemartin' (and its variants) in English, for this anomaly, can be traced back to the seventeenth century. It is often suggested that the term derives from the butchering of cattle around Martinmas (11 November) to preserve for the winter: these particular cattle, unsuitable for breeding or dairy production, would be prime candidates for not keeping throughout the lean months. This may, however, be purely coincidental, given that the word 'martin', a generic term for cattle, can be traced in variant forms back to the thirteenth century, and that 'ferry', 'farrow', and related words are found in both English and Scottish dialects to mean a barren or dry cow.

Although the external genitalia of the freemartin may appear normal, the internal organs are abnormal in greater or lesser degrees. In a few cases, one in ten or twelve, a heifer born as twin to a bull calf will be normally fertile, but these odds are such that stockbreeders discourage breeding for the trait of mixed-sex twins. The condition occurs as a result of the placentas of the two embryos uniting during pregnancy, allowing the two embryonic circulations to combine. A hormonal substance which organizes the development of the reproductive system of the

male enters the bloodstream of the female. This inhibits the development of the ovaries and causes abnormal development of the heifer's reproductive tract, affecting the oviducts, uterus, cervix, and parts of the vagina. The degree to which the reproductive system of the heifer is affected relates to the stage at which the placentas join: the earlier, the more extensive the masculinization which occurs. Other abnormalities — two cervixes, absence of one uterine horn, or blockage of the oviducts — have also been reported as a result of this uterine exposure to male hormones. Stockbreeders are advised to have a veterinarian examine suspected freemartin heifers by rectal palpation to ascertain whether the reproductive organs are present and functional. If they are not, culling of the heifer for beef is usually recommended — although freemartins were sometimes used as draught animals in the past, this is no longer relevant to modern agriculture. Freemartins are sometimes employed as oestrous detectors, being readier than normal females to mount other cows when these become ready for breeding.

Freemartins became an object of particular interest to anatomists in the seventeenth century, and were the subject of correspondence between A. M. Malsalva and G. Baglivi, pupils of the great Italian anatomist, Malphigi, in 1692. In 1779 John Hunter reported to the Royal Society of London on his dissection of three freemartins. The specimens, which were retained in the internationally-renowned anatomical collections of Hunter and his brother William, excited the interest of another Italian anatomist, Antonio Scarpa of Modena. Scarpa acquired a freemartin to dissect on his own behalf, and generated a considerable stir in Italian scientific circles. However, the major advances in the elucidation of this fascinating but mysterious condition did not take place until the twentieth century and the early investigations into the SEX HORMONES. Following morphological investigation by Tandler and Keller of Vienna, F. R. Lillie of Chicago established that the freemartin was a genetically female embryo which had been affected by the circulation of the male hormones of its twin via the joined placenta, and he published this conclusion in a paper in the *Journal of Experimental Zoology* in 1917. This conclusively overturned the arguments of some contemporary scientists that freemartins were in fact defective genetic males, and had far-reaching implications for the development of embryology and in particular for the relationship between the gonadal hormones and sexual differentiation. The exact nature of the hormonal influence remains a little obscure, since attempting to replicate the condition experimentally by injecting testosterone into pregnant cows does not produce the same effect. A similar effect in rodents, however, does seem to be due to transfer of testosterone or oestradiol. Freemartin births have sometimes been reported in other mammals, e.g. sheep. This phenomenon of one normal and one sterile twin may possibly be responsible for

the superstition that, in human twins, only one will be capable of childbearing, but as this is said to apply to identical twin females, perhaps not.

Freemartin cattle (and their male twins) played an important role in the work by P. B. Medawar and his colleagues on skin grafting. He had assumed that grafts between heterozygous twins (which mixed-sex twins are) would be rejected whereas those between monozygotic (identical) twins would not (transplantation between identical twins having already been proved to be possible). In fact, it turned out that skin and other tissue could be transplanted between such a twin pair of cattle at any stage in their lives, since they were tolerant of each other's tissues as a result of exposure to one another's tissue antigens as embryos. This demonstrated a state of acquired tolerance. Two papers describing this unexpected result and its implications were published in *Heredity* (Billington, Lampkin, Medawar, and Williams, 1951; Anderson, Billingham, Lampkin, and Medawar, 1952). Equivalent tolerances were subsequently induced in new-born mice: given skin or bone marrow transplants from unrelated animals, they became permanently tolerant of the new tissue. This work led to the award of the Nobel Prize to Medawar in 1960 and heralded the dawn of a new era in immunology with wide-ranging implications for the prevention and treatment of diseases in humans and animals.

LESLEY A. HALL

Frostbite The effect of severe cold on the body's most exposed parts, most commonly affecting feet, hands, ears, nose. Tissues freeze, and the damage depends on the scale and duration of the exposure. In mild cases, if thawing is not long delayed, only the superficial layers freeze; injured skin is shed and replaced by new growth. Deeper tissues — muscle, bone, and tendon — may suffer in more severe frostbite, and cell damage may be irreversible. Damage to nerves may cause permanent sensory loss. Damage to blood vessels makes them leaky so that restoration of the circulation during thawing leads to escape of fluid into the tissues, hence OEDEMA and viscosity of the blood, and obstruction of the local circulation, sometimes leading to gangrene and loss of the affected part.

S.J.

See COLD EXPOSURE.

Frown Produced primarily by the action of the *corrugator* muscle, which lowers the brows and pulls them together. In adolescents and adults, a vertical wrinkle often appears on the brow, and there may also be a horizontal wrinkle across the bridge of the nose.

Charles Darwin in his book *The Expression of Emotion in Man and Animals* called the corrugator the 'muscle of difficulty'. Darwin was quite correct: frowning occurs with many kinds of difficulty, mental or physical. People who lift something very heavy will frown when doing so, as will people who are having a difficult time remembering something or figuring out the answer to a difficult mental task. Frowning is shown during concentration, perplexity, and determination to accomplish a difficult task. Darwin noted that lowering the brow provides a natural sunshade, and indeed people do frown when they are in bright sunlight without sunglasses.

When people frown, they are often perceived by others to be feeling unpleasant, resentful, or angry, although this is often not the case. This interpretation may occur because the frown is part of the anger expression, which also typically involves glaring eyes and tense lips.

PAUL EKMAN

See also FACIAL EXPRESSION.

Funeral practices: British customs

Funerary practices are observed in every culture when a dead body is to be disposed of. In times of exigency such as war, disaster, pestilence, or in cases of violent death where the imperatives of pathology and judicial rules take precedence over family wishes for the care of the body, norms of funerary behaviour are often breached, adding to the trauma of events.

Corpse care

In Britain, funerary practices begin with the lay or official declaration of death, and consist of small attentions to the body itself, such as closing the eyes and covering the face. The 'laying-out' of the body — or 'rendering the last offices' was in the past a job traditionally done by women, often the local midwife. It involved undressing and washing the body, plugging its orifices, if necessary placing coins (traditionally pennies) on the eyelids, and a bandage under the chin, to hold these parts closed, dressing the body in its grave clothes, and holding limbs straight (with bandages or ribbons around the body at the elbows, wrists, and ankles, and sometimes a thread around the big toes) ready for placing in the coffin. Today the female tradition is continued to some extent inasmuch as most hospital, hospice, and district nurses who do the job are women. However, in cases of death at home undertakers are now generally swiftly called to remove the body, and the process of laying-out is done by available staff — male or female — away from the location of death or mourning.

Multipotent custom

In the past, each aspect of lay funerary ritual had multiple levels of practical justification and traditional meaning. The eyelids are generally the first part of the body to set in RIGOR MORTIS, just before the jaw, hours after death. A corpse whose eyes refused to close was traditionally believed to presage further deaths, so closing the eyes was imperative to forestall the omen, and to prevent survivors' unease.

Funerary practices altered a great deal in the twentieth century, and the meanings which attached to them in past ages have become attenuated. Yet even at the beginning of the twenty-first century, relatives of victims of murder or

accident — including drowning at sea — continue to do all they can to retrieve lost bodies in order to give them decent disposal.

The dead body is an object of great potency, with a powerful presence of its own. Part of this effect derives from its embodiment of the power of death, part from the strangeness death works upon it. While the CORPSE retains identity, personality is absent. British funeral practices reveal that there existed a conception, said by anthropologists also to operate in many other societies, of a transitional period between death and burial in which the body was regarded as 'neither alive nor fully dead'.

In a physical sense, of course, we are all familiar with this notion — in the currently continuing difficulty in defining the *precise moment* of death, the possibility of RESUSCITATION, and in the phenomenon of organs, which, though extracted from corpses, are yet sufficiently alive to support life again in the body of another. Old British customs and beliefs — such as the belief that a signature taken while the corpse is still warm had the same status as in life, that a corpse could indicate displeasure if a will read before it was false, or that it would bleed if a murderer came into its vicinity — seem to attribute sentience to the dead body.

The corpse also had ambiguous spiritual status: the care it received was thought somehow to influence the future life of the soul. Washing cleansed not only the sweat of death, but the sins of the earthly life, a sort of lay absolution. A woman interviewed in 1980 in a Suffolk village told me 'the washing is so that you're spotless to meet the Lamb of God'. The emblematic whiteness of grave-clothes dates back at least to the Jacobean period, when the epigraph to John Donne's poem *Death's Duell* stated: 'just as the body is shrouded in white linen, [so] may be the soul'. Although the traditional desirability of linen has long since waned, most mass-produced 'coffin-sets' (matching shrouds and coffin linings) currently provided by undertakers are nevertheless white. Several traditional funerary practices — such as the customs of viewing the dead, kissing or touching the body, placing refreshments beside the body, watching the body during the period between death and burial, waking (celebrating the funeral with food and drink), placing personal objects in the coffin, and tending graves — possessed a multipotent character: practical for mourners, respectful to the dead, and solicitous towards the soul.

Mortuaries

Modern changes in funerary practice are particularly noticeable in key areas: the location of the dead between death and disposal, the rise of cremation, and the declining significance of the funeral. The undertaker's 'private chapel' or 'chapel of rest' was a late Victorian development. There had been a move to open public mortuaries in the mid nineteenth century, but they foundered on the rock of parochial parsimony — lacking facilities for mourners to care for or

watch over their dead, they were often attached to the local workhouse and partook of that institution's terrible stigma. If no one arrived to claim a body from a public mortuary within a certain period, the dead could legally be requisitioned for dissection. Public mortuaries were places associated with sudden death, death by crime, death in the public highway, suicide, and the deaths of the unknown, and were bitterly unpopular among the poor.

A change in attitude towards the corpse had begun to develop towards the end of the nineteenth century — probably as a result of the public health reformers' activities (see CORPSE) — whereby the older attitude of solicitude towards the dead was supplemented, even superseded, by a growing perception that dead bodies were unhygienic. This attitude emphasized the need to segregate the dead away from the living. For extra payment, undertakers began to offer wealthier people new facilities without the taint of the public mortuary to store their dead away from home.

One undertaker has estimated that when he began working in 1936, 90% of bodies would be kept at home between death and burial; today the figure is only about 5–10%. This significant change in customary behaviour reveals something of a revolution in attitudes towards the corpse: a new squeamishness which means that many people accept the physical removal of the dead with relief; indeed, seem to require it for their own psychological survival.

Location of death

The transformation of corpse storage parallels changes in the location of death consequent upon the institutionalization of the elderly and greater access to hospitals and hospices in casualty and terminal illness. These developments have precipitated the decline of some long-standing funerary practices — such as viewing, touching and kissing the dead, and a number of domestic observances which derived from having the dead at home, such as darkening windows, stopping clocks, and covering mirrors.

The twentieth century also saw a significant transformation in the disposal of the dead. Although cremation was available as a mode of disposal in 1900, less than 1% of bodies were cremated; today the figure is over 70%.

Funeral feasts

In 1800 it was customary to have a meal, or a 'funeral feast', after the funeral. Usually this was a cold meal for mourners returning to the house of the deceased. In 1900 such a meal was still customary, even among the wealthy, and considered highly important among the working class. Stock phrases are used to describe these events, which indicate both the key ingredient, 'we buried him with ham' and the nature of the occasion; 'a real spread', 'the best feed we'd 'ad for ages'.

Today the gathering is still common among the traditionally minded, although after World War II it dropped from favour in many circles, and cold ham is no longer seen as crucial. In addition to the generally older observers of the custom, there is a newer, more self-consciously celebratory readoption of the idea of a post-funeral party among younger people. The old idea of the feast is having a comeback as more people recognize the value of such events for family and social cohesion, and as understanding develops of the dangers of incomplete mourning.

Fading taboo

Whilst several of the older customs appear to be undergoing long-term decline, especially those associated with exposure to the dead body itself, the re-emergence of the funeral feast may not be an isolated development, but part of a more general change. The last twenty years or so have seen a growing willingness to talk about death, dying, and funerals in the press and on radio and television, and among the public generally. The hospice movement for the care of the dying has developed apace in the UK, and the 'palliative care' developed in the hospices to control deathbed pain is being increasingly adopted by doctors all over the country. Charitable fundraising for these institutions ensures that the dying are a higher priority than they were twenty years ago. The same is true of mourning — there is now a much wider acceptance that grieving is a natural process, and a greater understanding of the need for appropriate rites of passage in its resolution.

In addition, new funerary customs are emerging. The old custom of marking the site of an accident or a sudden death has developed considerably since the mid 1980s — as the sites of national and local disasters, accidents, murders, and so on become transformed into wayside shrines, smothered in flowers laid by many hands. The public response to the death of Princess Diana was quite in keeping with a long-term process already well underway at the time of the tragic accident which killed her.

Funerals in general and the cremation ceremony in particular are widely perceived as unsatisfactory. During the last two decades people have been taking custom and ceremony into their own hands, and they can be very inventive. News stories cover burials at sea, and sprinkling of cremated ashes from aircraft, or in fireworks. Princess Diana's funeral, with its de-emphasis on the liturgy and open acceptance of non-religious elements, was a manifestation of this change, and evidence of its acceptance by the Church. The Booker prize was awarded in 1996 to a fine novel *Last Orders*, detailing the last journey of a Londoner's ashes, a theme previously unheard of in fiction. Press stories often feature individuals who have already purchased their own coffins, or who have prearranged their own disposal. 'Green' developments, such as recyclable coffins, woodland burials, and memorial trees in place of conventional gravestones, are frequently in the news. Virtual memorial gardens can be accessed on the internet, where 'tombstones' display exposition of a person's biography unlimited by churchyard regulations or the costs of carving on stone.

Memorial gatherings

Another noticeable change is the process of separation which seems to be developing between the physical disposal of the corpse — whether by burial or cremation — and the celebration of the dead person's life. The ceremony at the disposal — the funeral itself — seems to be diminishing in importance. Memorial gatherings, typically occurring some time later and so entirely detached from the presence of the dead body, have noticeably increased not only in number but in significance. These memorial events are designed to celebrate the life of the dead person in a more positive way than is generally possible at a funeral. The corpse is increasingly perceived as merely a repository of identity, whereas personality resides in the nature of the life lived, and in the memory of survivors. Once again, many people are formulating bespoke events appropriate for their own dead, for themselves in advance, and for those who are left behind.

Funerary practices are therefore perhaps becoming more elaborate: not in the nineteenth-century sense of florid trappings in mourning wear or funerary panoply, but in the development of informal, celebratory secondary ceremonies and convivial gatherings for survivors. Rather than dwellings, as the nineteenth century did, on the bleakness and sorrow inflicted by death, the emphasis is increasingly positive — in the expression of thankfulness for life.

RUTH RICHARDSON

See also DEATH.

Funeral practices: cultural variation

Quite when humans began ritually disposing of their dead, rather than just leaving corpses lying there for animals, birds, and insects to consume, as is the way of other mammals, is not entirely clear. The desire for ritual disposal, however, certainly goes back to pre-history, and is deep rooted in humans as we now know them.

This is clearly shown by those occasions when a funeral is deliberately denied. Denying the corpse a socially approved ritual disposal is one of the most potent ways in which disrespect can be shown to a person. The Holocaust, desecration of graves, eating your enemies, or chopping up and displaying the body parts of a traitor on the city wall, are all ways of publicly stating that this person, these people, either had no part in your society or belonged to another group, entirely unworthy of respect. We give a person a funeral, we pay ritual respect to the corpse, as a mark that this person was one of us, and therefore deserving of respect. In liberal democracies, in which there is some identification not just with the group but with all human beings, to be denied a funeral is to be deemed sub-human. Hence the not uncommon wish to deny proper funeral rites to war criminals and mass murderers.

There are a number of ways in which humans ritually dispose of their dead.

(i) Nearest to the natural process are the Parsees (Zoroastrians residing in India), who leave their dead in towers of silence, where they are eaten by vultures, and certain Buddhists in the Himalayas who chop up the corpse and leave it on a rock for the birds to consume.

(ii) A number of ancient peoples ritually placed their dead in a cave (as was the case with Jesus) or in a long barrow (as with some European Neolithic peoples). This practice finds an echo in modern Italy, Spain, and the US, where the coffin is often placed in a niche within a mausoleum — a building constructed for the purpose of housing human remains.

(iii) Burial in the ground is also common worldwide. The degree of contact of the corpse with the earth can vary. Muslims bury in a shroud, as was also typical at certain times in Christian Europe; the insects of the earth can get to work straight away. The British place a simple coffin directly into the earth. North Americans are first embalmed, and then placed in a strong casket, possibly made of steel, which is placed in a concrete-lined grave, so that the body never comes into the contact with the soil. The process of decomposition is therefore more akin to that in an above-ground mausoleum than in a Muslim burial.

(iv) Burial at sea is less common, usually occurring when someone dies on the high seas and return of the corpse to land is not feasible. With motorized ships and refrigeration, burial at sea is now uncommon. A small number of Americans, Britons, and others who die on land but who have sentimental attachments to the sea choose to be buried at sea.

(v) Cremation, followed by ritual disposition of the cremated remains, is very common, globally. The product of cremation is not ashes in the sense of a powder, but fragments of bone, whose size is determined by the temperature of the cremator or pyre. In some Western countries, the remains are mechanically pulverized to produce 6 pounds or so of 'ashes'. The remains may be ritually thrown on to running water, as in Hinduism, so that they eventually mingle with the vastness of the ocean; or they may be placed in a pot and buried in a family grave for cremated remains, as in Japan or Hong Kong; or they may be placed in a container that is buried individually, as is often now done in English churchyards; or they may be interred in an existing ordinary family grave, as in Finland; or they may be scattered over land, as is often the case in Britain and the US; or scattered over the ocean, as is frequently done in California. Mourners may actively participate in the cremation. In India, relatives circle the pyre and one crushes the partly burned skull in order to release the spirit; in Japan relatives use large chopsticks to pick up the cremated bones and place them into the burial pot. In contrast, many Westerners choose cremation precisely because they take no part in the body's destruction; the cremation is carried out invisibly and by nameless operatives. Clean and hygienic, such cremations remove from the mourner's consciousness the physical reality of death, so evident in burial or in Indian or Japanese cremation.

Today, earth burial, cremation, and placement in a mausoleum are the most common forms of disposal. Cremation is the norm in Hinduism and Sikhism, which teach reincarnation, and common in Buddhism, which teaches rebirth, though it is only in the past century and a half that cremation has become standard in Buddhist Thailand or Japan. Burial is historically common in Islam, Judaism, and Christianity, all of which teach resurrection of the body. In medieval Christianity, numerous altar paintings and cathedral portals depicted the dead getting out of their graves on the Last Day, to be judged on their way to either heaven or hell. Even today, Catholics, when asked why they prefer burial to cremation, often answer 'because of the resurrection'. In medieval Europe and still today in Islam, following gruesome deaths in war, in which body parts might be missing, great concern can be expressed if the whole body cannot be buried, as this might impede resurrection.

Cremation has increased markedly in some Western countries. In most European societies there were experiments in cremation in the late nineteenth century and the earliest Western crematoria date from that time. Cremation prospered in secular and Protestant areas; only in 1965 did the Pope allow cremation, and the Catholic church still does not encourage it; Orthodox Christians do not cremate. The popular mythology that the most crowded countries cremate the most is not born out by the facts. In the West, cremation is highest in secularized Protestant countries, and lowest in religious, Catholic, and especially Orthodox societies. Great Britain (72%), Denmark (71%), and Sweden (63%) contrast markedly with Eire (4%) and Italy (3%) (all figures for 1997). The US has a curiously low cremation rate at 24%. The American cremation rate is extremely low in the deep religious South; and lower than the national average in areas of high immigration, where permanent burial in the American soil is a symbol, if not of having achieved the American dream, at least of having arrived.

In most societies two funerals are conducted. The first is the 'wet' funeral, the initial disposal of the fresh corpse. The second is a subsequent relocation of the dry remains. In the case of cremation, this may follow quite soon, with the ritual interring or scattering of the products of cremation. In the case of burial, the secondary ritual is typically years later once the flesh has decomposed; the bones are removed, as in medieval Europe or in Greece today, to an ossuary, or disposed of in some other way. Following the studies of Robert Hertz and Arnold van Gennep in the early twentieth century, anthropologists have noted that this in-between period, in which the corruption of the body is being cleansed, may parallel both the period in which the soul is thought of as being prepared for its next existence and the period in which mourners have to reorganize their lives. In this period, body, soul, and mourners are all 'in limbo', and the end of the limbo period needs to be marked by the final funeral. Many Western funerals, however, have only one ritual, or a number of rituals (cremation, church service, refreshments) all on the same day.

The funeral then usually has three main participants: corpse, soul, and mourners. In the US, the embalmed and cosmeticized corpse plays a central role. With the high levels of religious belief in the US, the soul is also of considerable concern. In Britain, however, there is a trend toward minimizing the presence of the corpse, while secularization reduces the importance of the soul. This leaves the mourners as the sole participants. Reflecting this, a number of recent commentators see the funeral's purpose as having little to do with the deceased's body or soul and being simply to ease the grief of mourners (though this is largely an article of faith, since little research has been conducted into the circumstances in which funerals might help or hinder grief). Such funerals focus more on memories of the deceased, which may form a secular equivalent of the soul.

Socially, the funeral is an occasion in which the family, explicitly or implicitly, displays its status and resources. Gordon Childe has argued that, if that status is uncertain, there is an incentive to produce a more elaborate funeral in which a claim to status can be staked out. Hence the scale of funerals does not always reflect income *per se*, but the need to display income. This may account for the relative cheapness of the typical twentieth-century funeral in Britain, a society in which most people knew their place, compared with both nineteenth-century Britain and twentieth-century US — both societies with high rates of migration from, respectively, the countryside and around the world. Migrants are unsure of where they fit, and the funeral becomes a way to demonstrate respectability in the new society. In the US, cremation, equated there with cheapness, is primarily chosen by those whose ancestors migrated to the US some generations ago; they have proved themselves in life, and have nothing more to prove in death.

The economics of the funeral is a matter of some concern in a number of countries. On the one hand, people are prepared to pay funeral directors a lot of money to handle the corpse, which they themselves are frightened of. On the other hand, mourners are vulnerable, needing to know they are doing the right thing for the deceased in the eyes of God or their neighbours. They have therefore always been open to economic exploitation by priests or funeral directors. The implication is that, if you don't pay up, the dead, or your social standing, or your psychological health, or all three, will be harmed. Jessica Mitford, a Briton criticizing the American way of death, wrote a best-selling exposé of this kind of exploitation.

At the beginning of the twenty-first century, a few very large American funeral companies are buying up funeral homes, crematoria, and cemeteries in other countries. The biggest, Texan-based Service Corporation International (SCI), now has a major presence in Europe, Australia, and the Far East. Its basic strategy is to retain local funeral directing outlets but to centralize most operations, including embalming, thus reducing costs (but not prices). The dearly beloved corpse is therefore carted to-and-fro

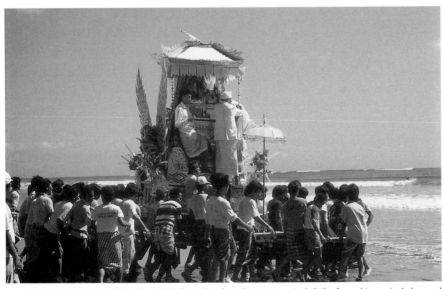

In many societies, mourners help dispatch body and soul on their journey. In Bali the funeral tower is shaken and run around in circles to disorientate the deceased's spirit so that it cannot find its way home. Michael Macintyre/Hutchinson Library.

around town in unmarked vans, in the care of total strangers, while the family mistakenly presumes it is all the while in the care of the nice gentleman with whom they arranged things in their local funeral parlour. The extent to which the funeral market can be globalized, however, is still an open question, and SCI has experienced some difficulty acculturating to the funeral habits of its new European customers. In the global village, in which Coca-Cola or Japanese cars may be found even in the remotest jungle or desert, there is still remarkable variation in funeral customs between one country and another.   TONY WALTER

Further reading

Davies, D. (1997). *Death, ritual and belief*. Cassell, London.

Mitford J. (1999). *The American way of death revisited*. Virago, London.

See also CORPSE; DEATH.

Funny bone

Funny bone Usually applied to the projection, the *olecranon*, at the back of the elbow, which is the upper end of the *ulna*, one of the two forearm bones. On the inner side of this is a smaller protuberance, the *medial epicondyle* of the *humerus* — the bone of the upper arm. The *ulnar nerve* runs in a groove on the back of the epicondyle, between this and the olecranon. The nerve can be felt and rolled under the fingers, most easily when the elbow is at a right angle, and because it is near the surface it can be painfully tweaked if the inner side of the elbow hits a hard surface. The sensation is funny only in the sense of peculiar. (Tempting though it be, there is apparently no pun intended to link it to the humerus — whose name is Latin for shoulder, referring to its upper end.)   S.J.

See ELBOW; SKELETON.

Furniture and the body

Furniture and the body Furniture is both the body's surrogate, and its slave. Terms for chair parts reveal the surrogacy very clearly, from 'rounded shoulder' to 'arm', 'back', 'knee', cabriole 'leg', and 'foot'. ('Seat' seems to have migrated in the other direction — first used to indicate the place where sitting occurs, only later did it refer to the body part involved.) Slavishness can be inferred from the iconography of the decorative motifs we impose, from a vanquished enemy or beast carved crouching under the seat of an African throne to the ubiquitous ball-and-claw foot of rococo chairs, signalling the captive poise of a raptor, or an orientalizing dragon's taloned grasp. In the modern period, signification has moved away from such applied motifs; the form and its materials themselves situate the user in a particular ideological scheme. The blatant anthropomorphism and zoomorphism of earlier ages have given way almost entirely, with technological materials and computer modelling now used to provide floating ergonomic platforms to support bodies trained to work in relative stillness for long periods of time.

Seats of power

Furniture was initially a perquisite of the ruler, never of the ruled. Graceful, slim beds and elegant stools were interred with Egyptian pharaohs as signs of their divinity, and guarantors of their comfort in the afterlife. In these Pharaonic objects, the various animal-headed gods (cow-headed Hathor, falcon-headed Horus) occasionally make appearances as finials behind thrones or on bedposts; the only allusions to bodies are in the legs of thrones, which can appear with muscled thighs, calves, and paw-like feet. As for the non-royal Egyptians, even well-born scribes and functionaries are shown kneeling or sitting cross-legged, in the non-propped positions still used by the majority of peoples around the world.

Access to furniture was more widespread among the ancient Greeks, whose patrician classes demanded a refined type of chair called the *klismos*. Less interested in the upright regality and animal symbolism that preoccupied the Egyptians, the Greeks provided their chairs with a low back support and a seat shaped to the lounging human body, anchored on splayed legs that remained stable whatever the sitter's position. Judging from sarcophagi that portray scenes from everyday life, the chair seems to have become truly common in well-born households only during the Roman empire, when the increasing height of the chair back began its long life as a signifier of nobility and power. Ancient pharaohs needed only an armchair and a crown to place their heads above their squatting attendants, but when even lowly potters and tradesmen sat on stools, the Romans were forced to enlarge the vertical back of the armchair to amplify its authority.

This trajectory reached a kind of apogee with the medieval chair, a stiff-backed, excessively vertical affair that originated in the monastic orders and was reserved for the clerical elite. The laity sat in aptly named *misericordia*, bench-like pews, with decorated backs and undersides that presented the distracted worshipper seated behind them with scenes of hellfire and worldly suffering. Medieval bench, chair, and stool were austere combinations of vertical and horizontal planes that trained the body in appropriate disciplinary modes. The ecclesiastic model governed domestic interiors as well: the armchair, symbol of moral and spiritual authority, was reserved for the higher orders, and most medieval diners and dwellers sat on long, backless benches, if they sat at all. *Where* they sat at the long, plank-like dinner table (above or below the salt) was all that mattered — there was no concept of comfort or beauty to be found in the table itself. In contrast to the sumptuous tapestries and cushions that adorned it, furniture was a prop for bare bones, made to be dismantled and ported around by a restless nobility. The Latinate words for furniture (*mobiliers* in French and *mobilia* in Italian) reflect this acknowledgement of the object's (and the body's) 'movability' and unimportant worldly status.

Domestic props

There is little place for furniture in nomadic, shepherding societies, nor in subsistence agricultural ones. Sleeping with the cows made good sense in an unheated peasant household in Northern Europe, and the North African nomad's tents and metal cookware were enough to carry without lugging around cumbersome objects to prop up the body. Cultural historians relate how the notion of the 'domestic', tied intimately to the development of furniture, only emerges with force in settled bourgeois societies of urban merchants, such as those in the seventeenth-century Dutch 'golden age', or perhaps a bit earlier in pre-Renaissance Tuscany. In the growth of capitalistic urbanity that began in the Renaissance, there was a shift from the medieval bed, built to hold up to ten people, to a more modest two-person model, fitted with curtains that could be pulled by the chambermaid to enclose the married couple for the night. Concepts of privacy, and models of the learned, pious scholar, were articulated in new built forms — the bookshelf, the enclosed study, the reading stand (constructed at the height of a standing reader — used primarily by elites. The reading body finally achieved its apotheosis in the professorial 'chair' (roofed, with a built-in lectern and reading stand for a seated reader), a term since conflated to the person of the endowed academic or the ruling business leader (the 'chair-man').

Surging, twisting, dynamic compositions, engaging as many senses as possible, emerged in art after the Renaissance, pioneered by the sculptor Gianlorenzo Bernini and epitomized in his 'furniture' for the Catholic cathedral, St Peter's, in Rome; the twisted, black-and-gold Solomonic columns called the *Baldacchino* (1624–33). The opulent and effusive schemes of the Italian Baroque were brought to France and harnessed for the glory of the *roi soleil*, Louis XIV. Furniture at Versailles incorporated the contradictions of the 'Sun King'; the oxymoronic play of sunlight and absolutism. Mirrors multiplied the glories of the king's body, yet their reflections were manifestly contained by gilded plaster festoons. The royal bed was the veritable *omphalos* of power — yet, when curtains were drawn around the sleeping king, by implication, darkness reigned. Again, the 'Louis quatorze' chair is held to instantiate the values of the court elite, and to echo the ornament employed for the king's body: shapely tapered legs and slender frames, painted in colours and encrusted with gilt, decorated with the court emblems of fleurs-de-lys, feathers of exotic birds, and, of course, the centred rays of the sun. Royal chairs were built to be so lightweight that they could easily be moved to the side for the more important choreography of courtiers and king.

The taste for pomp diminished after Louis XIV's death, and as Paris resumed its dominance of French life a more playful style of ornament ensued among the aristocracy, named after, its central motif, the *rocaille* (rock-work) — hence,

'Rococo'. The rococo piece of furniture presumed a body lost in pleasures: lounging *en déshabillé*, listening to music, or engaged in the serious pursuit of culinary marvels. Built of solid mahogany, adorned by gilding, and upholstered with cut velvet or damask, the chair, couch, or *chaise-longue* was further laden with cushions and draped with exotic cloths. It signalled the opulence of a culture importing stuffs from around the world, and the intimacy of those who would indulge their deepest desires for literature and romantic intrigue. The front legs of rococo chairs were undulating symphonies of curves and counter-curves. Still following the anthropomorphic echo of a mammalian leg, the thigh surged forward, often capped with a decorative shell, a curving bit of foliage, or even a Sphinx-like torso; occasionally this retreating thigh shape was paved with the scales of a fish. The knee swooped down and back, relatively unremarked in decorative terms, only to come forward again into the foot, which resolved itself into the talon and ball marking the tenacious terminus of the body that was the chair.

The Revolutionary condemnation of the sybaritic aristocratic body was expressed in its furniture, which, like every aspect of visual culture, conformed to the new rigours of a self-consciously 'Republican' neo-classical taste. Once again, prevalent verticals intersecting stable horizontals became points on a moral compass. Geometry replaced surprise and delight, sobriety reigned in the choice of striped satins over the earlier velvets and brocades. The age-old association of furniture parts with anthropomorphic or animal forms was broken in favour of architectural motifs. Now legs were slim classical columns, tapering toward a minimized, possibly Doric-looking foot. Leaves, rocks, shells, fish scales, all vanished in favour of a few urn-like finials, a hint of metope or columnar fluting, or the suggestion of a pediment. The bodies invited into such furniture possessed an egalitarian decorum in keeping with the Enlightenment ideals of the age.

Modern living

The burst of industrial and imperial energies that culminated in Victorian England produced a furniture suited for the various bodies of divergent classes, occupations, and pocketbooks. Market differentiation combined with eclectic and exotic tastes to produce a dizzying array of objects to fill the crowded Victorian home, citadel of domestic virtue and fortress of the regimented body. The domestic was now woven into the urban fabric with networks of gas, water, and, soon, electricity; in this industrialized context, symbols of the private and individual became more and more important. Rooms proliferated along with furniture functions, many differentiated along class, age, and gender lines. The anthropomorphic identity of furniture's parts returned, and with it a Victorian anxiety over nakedness that resulted in the 'skirting' of legs on everything from pianos to armchairs to bathtubs. The severe lines of William Morris' 'Arts and Crafts' style, which found many American adherents, was an antidote to most Victorian overstuffed profiles, while providing yet another correction to the perceived excesses of an earlier age. Furniture was believed to educate both mind and body in nineteenth-century moral behaviour.

The birth of *art nouveau* (called *jugendstil* in German-speaking countries) was a self-conscious effort to address the new century and determine its modernist pulse. Bodies were being reconfigured dramatically, particularly female ones — the corset and chignon were abandoned for the unconstructed sack dress and bobbed hair of the *femme nouvelle*. As art nouveau evolved into 'deco' (shorthand for '*l'art decoratif*'), furniture participated in a dramatic redesigning of interiors to house the new modern figure — sinuous, asymmetric curves echoed the baroque and rococo periods, but the heavy-handed symbolism of earlier centuries (with their putti, shells, and claws) was recast into simplified, abstracted shapes and lines. The flapper silhouette of deco would glorify a pre-pubescent female figure, just as the forms of art nouveau evoked tender spring buds and swaying reeds rather than fleshy, full-grown acanthus leaves. Much of these vegetal forms were cast in iron or blown into glass moulds on an industrial scale.

Modernist architects and designers entered the fray with a dramatic rejection of such artifice. 'Ornament is crime,' opined Adolf Loos in 1908, and in 1927 Le Corbusier echoed, 'A house is a machine for living in . . . an armchair a machine for sitting in and so on.' The new 'machines' drew explicitly on other technologies of the body — bicycles, for example, whose tubing served as the inspiration for the famous (and mostly uncomfortable) seats manufactured by the famous German art and design academy, the Bauhaus. Techniques of steaming and bending wood allowed this grained organic material to assume the same linear, undecorated form as the chrome-plated steel and leather chairs of Bauhaus fame. Connections to the body were now instrumental, not mimetic — and the bentwood technologies developed by Charles and Ray Eames for their 1946 chair were first worked out in moulding 150 000 leg splints for soldiers wounded in the battles of World War II.

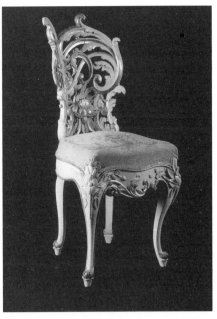

Art nouveau painted and gilded chair decorated with flowers from art nouveau Quinta Gameros Chihuahua Mexico. Designed by LaTorre 1907–10. The Art Archive/ Nicolas Sapieha.

Never again could designers turn a slim-ankled cabriole leg without indulging in a 'period' style. But the bodies destined for the twentieth-century's 'machines for sitting in' were not yet adapted to the new spatial hygiene of modernity. Bodies need motility, and furniture needs to support a shifting variety of poses in which the long-sitting human frame can refresh itself. Adjustable office furniture, and the efforts of efficiency experts, came together to address the new need for 'ERGONOMICS' — equipment and objects designed with the human body in mind. Plastics, and the almost endlessly inventive forms they encouraged, finally released furniture from the need for legs, arms, and even an obvious seat. But while cantilevers and knee-supports may have decoupled chairs from their traditional representational functions, bodies still have visual appetites for the comfortable, overstuffed look of the surrogate/slave.   CAROLINE A. JONES

Further reading

Aries, P. and Duby, C. (ed.) (1987–90). *A history of private life*, Vols I–IV. Harvard.

Rybczynski, W. (1986) *Home: a short history of an idea*. Penguin, London.

See also BUILDINGS AND THE BODY; ERGONOMICS.

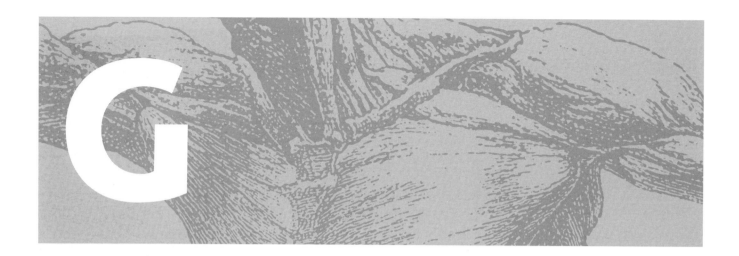

G

G and G-suit Life on earth has evolved in the accelerative force of *gravity*, which attracts all material towards the centre of the earth and gives a mass of material the characteristic which we term weight. Changes in the speed or direction of travel of a vehicle such as a car or an aircraft generate accelerative forces which may be many times the accelerative force of gravity. For a given mass the force generated is directly proportional to the acceleration of the mass (Newton's Second Law of Motion). It is convenient to state the latter in multiples of the acceleration due to gravity, the gravitational constant (9.81 m/sec^2). The ratio of the acceleration of a body to the gravitational constant is the 'G'. Thus a body which has a weight of 1 kg at 1 G will weigh 5 kg when exposed to an accelerative force of 5 G.

The ranges of accelerative forces to which the occupants of aircraft and space vehicles may be exposed in flight and the durations for which these forces may operate are extremely large. Thus the passengers of a wide-bodied jet aircraft will be exposed to accelerations of 1.2 to 1.3 G sustained for several seconds during take off, landing, or a tight turn. The pilots of modern combat aircraft are exposed to accelerative forces up to 9–10 G for many seconds, whilst the crew of a space vehicle which is in orbit around the earth or which has attained escape velocity will be exposed to *microgravity* — 1×10^{-4} to 1×10^{-5} G. (See SPACE TRAVEL). Finally, aircraft and spacecraft may crash on landing, exposing the occupants to accelerative forces of the order of 50 G or greater (see CRASH IMPACT.)

The effect of an accelerative force upon the body depends upon the magnitude of the force, its duration of action, and the direction in which it is applied. It is useful to classify accelerations into short duration (where the force acts for less than 1.0 sec), when the main determinant of the effect is the structural strength of the body; and long duration, where the force acts for several seconds or longer and the effects are due to the sustained distortion of tissues and organs, and alterations in the distribution of blood within the body. The direction in which an accelerative

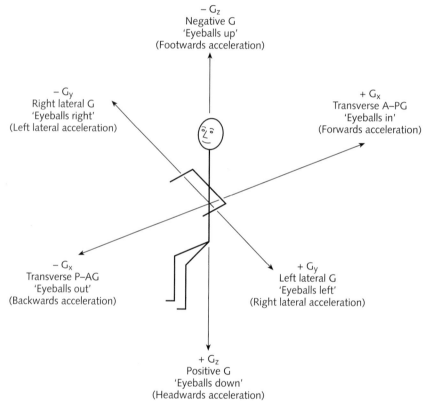

The standard Advisory Group for Aeromedical Research and Development (AGARD) aeromedical terminology for describing the direction of acceleration and inertial forces. The vertical G$_z$ axis is parallel to the long axis of the body, the G$_x$ axis runs from the anterior to the posterior surfaces of the body, and the G$_y$ axis runs from one side of the body to the other. The vector arrows indicate the direction of the resultant inertial forces. A-PG is antero-posterior acceleration and P-AG is postero-anterior acceleration.

force acts is described by the use of a three axis co-ordinate system (X, Y, and Z) in which the vertical axis (Z) is parallel to the long axis of the body (see figure).

Common aircraft manoeuvres such as co-ordinated turns or pulling out of a dive apply an accelerative force parallel to the long axis of the seated pilot which tends to displace tissues towards the feet (+G$_z$). The increase of the weight of the tissues and organs of the body

produces sagging of the soft tissues of the face at +2 G$_z$; makes it impossible to stand up from the seated position at +3 G$_z$; makes upward movement of the upper limbs very difficult at +5 G, and impossible above +7 to 8 G$_z$; and makes it very difficult to raise the head at +5 G$_z$, once the neck has flexed, and impossible at +6 to 8 G$_z$. Accurate movements of the fingers can be performed, however, at +9 G$_z$, provided that the hand and forearm are well supported.

Of even greater significance on exposure to $+G_z$ is the increase in the weight of the blood. The pressure of blood in the vessels above the level of the heart is decreased whilst the pressure below the heart is increased, and the blood moves from the upper to the lower parts of the body. At about $+4.5\ G_z$ the pressure in the arteries supplying the retina of the eye falls below the pressure within the eyeball (20 mm Hg), blood flow to the retina ceases, and loss of vision, termed *blackout*, follows in about 5 sec. At $+5–6\ G_z$ the blood flow to the brain of a seated, relaxed individual ceases, and unconsciousness supervenes in about 5 sec.

Several procedures are employed by fighter pilots to maintain the BLOOD PRESSURE at head level, and hence consciousness and vision, on exposure to high $+G_z$. Raising the feet, a technique used in the Battle of Britain, will raise tolerance by about 0.5 G. Reducing the amount of blood which pools in the lower limbs and abdomen by applying counter-pressure to these regions by a *G-suit* will increase tolerance by 1–3 G, depending upon the area of the lower body covered by the G-suit. Raising the pressure in the chest, either actively by performing a hard expiratory effort against a closed glottis, or passively by means of *positive pressure breathing*, can greatly increase tolerance of $+G_z$ by raising the arterial blood pressure. When active expiratory effort is employed it must be interrupted by taking a rapid breath once every 3–4 seconds, to allow blood to flow back into the chest to the heart and to maintain respiratory gas exchange. The pilot also tenses the muscles of the trunk and limbs while performing this manoeuvre, which is termed the *Anti-G Straining Manoeuvre (AGSM)*. The AGSM together with a G-suit will increase the tolerance to 8–9 G. It is, however, very fatiguing. Positive pressure breathing combined with a G-suit which fully covers the lower limbs and abdomen will maintain performance at 9 G for many seconds.

Much less common in flight is for a pilot to be exposed to $-G_z$ which forces the blood towards the head. $-G_z$ is produced by simple inverted flight and outside loops and spins. Tolerance of $-G_z$ is much lower than tolerance for $+G_z$ acceleration. Thus exposure to $-2\ G_z$ causes severe discomfort in the head, and is followed usually by a severe headache which persists for several hours. Exposure to -2.5 G for only a few seconds causes rupture of blood vessels in the skin of the head and neck and on the surface of the eye. It frequently causes bleeding from the nose. The increased pressure in the arteries of the neck acting through the carotid sinus BARORECEPTORS causes very marked slowing of the heart and often produces loss of consciousness.

JOHN ERNSTING

Further reading

Ernsting, J. Nicolson, A. N. and Rainford, D. J. (1999). *Aviation medicine*, (3rd edn). Butterworth–Heinemann, Oxford.

See also CRASH IMPACT; FLYING; SPACE TRAVEL.

Gagging (gag reflex) When a food bolus is transported towards the back of the TONGUE, its presence usually elicits an automatic series of muscle contractions designed to propel the bolus further onwards through the PHARYNX and OESOPHAGUS all of which comprise the swallow. The stimulus eliciting this process is primarily a mechanical one.

If a mechanical stimulus is applied to the back part of the tongue or to the soft PALATE and the resultant motor response is unsuccessful in moving the food bolus or is unsuccessful in dislodging the source of the stimulus, then a gag response is elicited. Efforts at removal first increase, and then the movements are converted to those of expulsion. The soft palate is elevated (closing off the nasal airway), the jaw lowered, and the back of the tongue lifted followed by a forward sweep of the lifted part. If there is a continued failure to remove the source of the stimulus, retching and finally VOMITING can be triggered.

Gagging is a term that tends to be used somewhat differently by neurologists and by dentists. Neurologists are interested in the competence of the reflex for diagnostic purposes; they may use the term to mean simply that a mechanical stimulus to the back of the mouth elicits one element of the complex pattern described above: reflex elevation of the soft palate; this confirms the integrity of the reflex pathway, via CRANIAL NERVES and the BRAIN STEM. Dentists tend to use the term to refer to the response of those individuals in whom the threshold for the whole complex pattern is so very low that even a simple dental examination can provoke violent rejection movements followed rapidly by retching and vomiting.

ALLAN THEXTON

Gait is a general term covering a series of modes of forward progression. In humans, it encompasses the only two familiar types: WALKING and running. However, other bipeds like kangaroos have radically different mechanisms of gait, and quadrupeds such as the horse have a much fuller repertoire of gaits including walking, trotting, cantering, and galloping, that involve quite different patterns of movement. Human walking and running varies only in speed.

The general principle is that increases in speed are associated with lifting each foot earlier in the stride cycle and placing it so that stride length is increased.

The choice of gait is largely determined by the energy cost of progression. In each case the most economical gait is selected, although the mechanism by which the CENTRAL NERVOUS SYSTEM makes the selection remains unknown.

The power requirement for gait increases linearly with speed in each mode of gait. However, the efficiency with which this power is converted into forward motion varies. In general, each limb is used like a pendulum, swinging forward passively at low speeds and accelerated forward at higher speeds of progression. The increased flexion of the limb at the knee as humans change from walking to running can be regarded as a attempt to shorten the length of the pendulum, so allowing faster swings forward. This pendulum action is supplemented by storage of energy in the elastic components of the limb, with its subsequent release in the next phase of movement. This is obvious in the 'spring in the step' of youngsters, that allows smooth storage and release of energy during gait. It also allows a low energy cost of movement. (This reaches its most sophisticated form in the bouncing gait of the kangaroo and, as a consequence, kangaroos have the most energy-efficient gait in the animal kingdom.)

The management of energy transfer between its kinetic and potential forms requires complex control within the central nervous system. The limbs have to be folded to allow swing phases and stiffened to allow stance in precisely co-ordinated ways. In addition, muscle contraction can be used to stiffen the natural springiness of TENDONS, so allowing more energy storage.

Many neurological conditions, such as Parkinson's disease and STROKE, affect the timings of the muscle activity. This severely affects the efficiency of movement and imposes a large additional demand for muscle activity, which is obvious in slowed gait and reduced endurance.
R. H. BAXENDALE

See also WALKING.

Galen of Pergamum (AD 129–216), the most influential and prolific of all the physicians of antiquity, produced a philosophically sophisticated synthesis of earlier medical theories of the body that was dominant until the seventeenth century. The son of a rich architect, he began his medical career in AD 145–6; due to his family's wealth, he was able to train in his home town of Pergamum, and then at Smyrna and Alexandria for the unusually long period of ten years. From AD 157 he worked as physician to the gladiators in Pergamum, where he claims to have significantly reduced the death rate, before moving to Rome in AD 162. He left Rome in AD 165, alleging that other physicians in Rome were jealous of his success. His abrupt departure is, however, more likely to have been due to an attempt to avoid the smallpox epidemic which hit Rome soon after. On his return in AD 169 he became doctor to the emperor Marcus Aurelius and his family, although he managed to avoid accompanying the imperial household on a dangerous campaign in Germany by claiming that he could not go on religious grounds.

His work claimed to continue the tradition of Hippocrates, the fifth-century (BC) doctor to whom a large and disparate corpus of ancient Greek medical texts was attributed. Galen attacked other doctors of the time for failing to understand what Hippocrates really meant, but this is merely rhetoric; the 'Hippocrates' Galen gives us is one created in the image of Galen. Galen's very personal judgements of which treatises in the Hippocratic corpus were the 'genuine works' of Hippocrates have influenced all subsequent work on that corpus.

Galen's model of the body combined ideas from Hippocratic medicine, Plato, and Aristotle. The scientific logic is Aristotelian. The notion of three body systems – governed by the HEART, the BRAIN, and the LIVER respectively — comes from Plato, the fourth-century (BC) Athenian philosopher whose dialogue, the *Republic*, divides the soul into three parts, namely reason, 'spirit' or emotion, and desire. From some Hippocratic texts, Galen adopted the idea of four HUMOURS, or body fluids, the balance between which is necessary for health, and used these as the basis of a more far-reaching system in which each humour can be tied to a quality, a season, and a period of life. Blood, the warm and moist fluid, is associated with spring and predominates in childhood; yellow bile is warm and dry, and is associated with summer and youth; black bile, thought to be cold and dry, is associated with autumn and adulthood; phlegm, cold and moist, is the humour of winter and of old age. Healing for Galen involved the application of general principles to specific, individual cases. The maintenance of the correct balance amongst the four humours in any individual body constitutes health, while imbalances can be corrected by attention to air, food and drink, exercise, sleep, repletion and evacuation, and emotion.

In the Galenic body, heat plays a central role: the three 'faculties' of the body are, in ascending order of importance, the nutritive, the vital, and the logical faculties. In the nutritive sphere, food is partially cooked by the stomach, and then moved in the form of chyle to the liver where it is heated further. The portal vein then carries chyle to the liver, where further heat refines it into blood and adds the 'natural spirit'. The liver draws in the chyle by 'attraction', and other parts of the body then attract to themselves for nourishment most of the 'venous blood' which the liver makes. Some fluid, however, travels on, by way of the vena cava, to the heart, where in a further stage of cooking it takes in 'vital spirit' to become lighter and thinner, as 'arterial blood'. This transmits to other parts of the body the vital faculty, which gives warmth and the power of growth and can be measured through the pulse. The brain gives the blood psychic *pneuma*, which is distributed through the body by means of the nerves; with the brain is associated the logical faculty — the power of thought, will, and choice. In the Galenic body, veins, arteries, and nerves are thus separate systems with different functions. Veins originate in the liver, and carry food to nourish the body, while arteries proceed from the heart and carry vital spirit, although they also contain some blood.

Galen believed that medicine required both practical and theoretical elements. He claimed that he dissected every day, sometimes in public, even asking members of the audience to nominate the part to be dissected; his experiments on the spinal cord, in which he demonstrated that muscles are controlled by nerves, are still famous. However, these experiments were performed on animals, particularly pigs and apes, rather than on humans. Some parts of the Galenic body, which were questioned — and their existence eventually disproved — in the Renaissance, derive from incorrect analogies between animals and humans. The '*rete mirabile*' at the base of the skull is one example. Other errors, such as the 'invisible pores' which Galen insisted must be present in the interventricular septum of the heart, were logically necessary to his model of the body.

Galen was a highly prolific writer, whose works included not only philosophically and logically argued treatises on the body but also texts on the practical side of being a doctor in the Roman world. He insisted that his enemies spread malicious rumours about him, including the slander that his extraordinary success in prognosis was due to magical rather than medical skills. On one famous occasion, described in his treatise *On Prognosis*, he detected that a woman's pulse rate increased when the name of the man she loved was mentioned. Galen himself attributed his prognostic skills to following Hippocratic principles based on reading bodily signs and being aware of all relevant features of the patient's life.   HELEN KING

Gall bladder

The gall bladder receives BILE from the LIVER, stores and concentrates it, and delivers it to the intestine as required. It is a slate-blue sac, partly sunken in a groove on the under surface of the right lobe of the liver. It is 7–10 cm long, 3 cm in maximum breadth and, under usual circumstances, has a 30–50 ml capacity. Bile acids and other constituents of bile produced in the liver are carried to the gall bladder via the hepatic and cystic ducts. A 10-fold concentration effect is achieved by the transport of water from the bile to the bloodstream within the gall bladder wall. When fatty food passes from the stomach into the intestine, the gall bladder is stimulated to contract by CHOLECYS-TOKININ, a hormone released from the lining of the intestine. Concentrated bile is then released into the intestine via the cystic and common bile ducts. The high concentration of bile acids turns fat in the diet into an emulsion which is easily digested by the action of the enzyme lipase from the pancreas, and absorbed across the intestinal wall. The efficiency of this system is enhanced by the reabsorption of bile acids from the intestine, minimizing the quantity lost in the FAECES. Reabsorbed bile acids are then carried by the bloodstream back to the liver, where they are available for further recycling into the bile. If the gall bladder has to be removed, unconcentrated bile drains directly into the intestine from the liver, but in most people digestion of fatty food can still occur quite adequately.

The formation of gallstones within the gall bladder represents the most common cause of gall bladder disease. Gallstones were first described by Gentile da Foligno in Padua in 1341, who noted many stones within the post-mortem gall bladder of a woman whose viscera had been removed so that the body could be embalmed. Gallstones occur commonly in people of all races and at all ages (even in the teens). Although their prevalence varies, there is some truth in the well-known aphorism that the typical patient with gallstones is a fat, fair, fertile woman in her forties.

Bernard Naunyn's classic monograph published in 1892 is credited as containing the first discussion of the chemical composition of gallstones. It is now common to speak of three types of gallstone: pigment, cholesterol, and mixed. Patients with excessive breakdown of their red blood cells, resulting in increased production of bilirubin, are at increased risk of the formation of pigment gallstones, which are predominantly composed of calcium bilirubinate, carbonate, phosphate, and palmitate. Conversely, supersaturation of bile with insoluble cholesterol, as a result of metabolic defects, promotes the formation of cholesterol gallstones.

Autopsy series suggest that gallstones are formed in at least 15% of the adult population, the majority of whom have never experienced symptoms. Indeed, it has been estimated that only about 1% of people with gallstones will develop complications of them each year. These occur when gallstones obstruct either the cystic or the common bile ducts. The most common symptom is abdominal pain, which may be due to inflammation of the gall bladder (*cholecystitis*), bile duct obstruction (biliary colic), or inflammation of the pancreas (*pancreatitis*). Partial obstruction of the common bile duct by a gallstone is the commonest cause of *cholangitis* (inflammation of the bile ducts), marked by the appearance of '*Charcot's triad*' of abdominal pain, fever, and jaundice (named after the Parisian professor who described 'biliary fever' in 1876, although he was mainly famed as a neurologist).

'Acalculous' cholecystitis, in which gall bladder inflammation occurs in the absence of gallstones, accounts for about 10% of all cases of acute cholecystitis and also a proportion of those with chronic gall bladder inflammation. Gall bladder inflammation may occur during the course of typhoid fever. In a minority of cases, the responsible bacterium, *Salmonella typhi*, even persists in the gall bladder after the acute illness has resolved, and is intermittently excreted in the faeces. After a year, about 2–5% of individuals still excrete this organism and some, mostly females, continue to do so indefinitely. These 'chronic carriers' may spread the infection to others if their personal hygiene is careless, by the faecal–oral route. The most notorious carrier was 'typhoid Mary' who, in her capacity as cook to many households and institutions in the early 1900s, left a trail of typhoid victims across the US and Canada.   STEPHEN M. RIORDAN
ROGER WILLIAMS

See PLATE 1.

See also ALIMENTARY SYSTEM; BILE; JAUNDICE; LIVER.

Gargoyles A gargoyle is a waterspout designed to throw rainwater away from the walls of a building. The German term is *wasserspeier* (water spitter). The English word 'gargoyle' derives from the French *gargouille* and in turn from the Latin for throat, *gargula*. Gargoyles usually take the form of humans, animals, or grotesque combination of the two. They are found on the exterior of gothic buildings often in combination with other grotesque and marginal sculpture on corbels and parapets, which are sometimes also mistakenly called gargoyles.

Lion-head water spouts were used in classical architecture. The earliest medieval examples date from the twelfth century. Squat and few in number to begin with, by the thirteenth century gargoyles became more numerous and had developed the projecting form characteristic of gothic cathedrals. Because of their exposed position gargoyles are vulnerable to erosion, consequently most are reproductions or inventions of the restorer.

The profanity of medieval gargoyles contrast with sacred images decorating doorways and the interior of churches, though grotesque imagery on a smaller scale is found here too. This opposition is partly explicable in terms of purpose and location. Gargoyles are placed high up on buildings disgorging water, that flows along concealed channels through gaping mouths. Occasionally other orifices are employed, as at Autun Cathedral where a man appears to defecate on unwary passers-by.

Human figures usually adopt either abusive or fearful attitudes. Figures shouting or pulling their mouths open with their fingers are common. Other characters are found clinging to buildings in apparent fear, or there can be depictions of individuals who imagine they support the entire edifice. Gargoyles combining a number of figures are not uncommon. At Heckington (Lincolnshire, England) a winged devil carries off a woman. Others, derived from antiquity, pour water from large jars (e.g. St Mark's, Venice).

Until recently scholars have largely ignored or declined to interpret such images. Emile Mâle (1913) considered them meaningless. Some nineteenth-century antiquarians thought of them as pagan survivals. Recent scholarship has interpreted such sculptures as images of sin and folly or references to vernacular culture: Michael Camille calls them the opposite of angels, 'all body and no soul — a pure projector of filth'.

Literary references include Hardy's *Far from the Madding Crowd*, where a gargoyle, 'too human to be called like a dragon, too impish to be like a man, too animal to be like a fiend, and not enough like a bird to be called a griffin', vomited a stream of water 'into the midst of Fanny Robin's grave' scattering the repentant Troy's flowers. In Victor Hugo's *Notre–Dame de Paris*, Quasimodo is a living gargoyle.

With the Gothic revival the gargoyle, made redundant by the drainpipe, acquired a picturesque role. In France, Viollet–le–Duc was responsible for more gargoyles than any medieval mason, whilst Ruskin mentions them only once in more than 40 volumes, delighting in their fantastic outline, 'when they had no work to do but open their mouths and pant in the sunshine'.   BRIAN O' CALLAGHAN

Further reading
Camille, M. (1992). *Image on the edge: the margins of medieval art*. Reaktion Books, London.

Gases in the body Man evolved from animals living in water, but occupies an OXYGEN-containing gaseous environment. The body uses food as fuel for what can be loosely termed a combustion reaction, in which the fuel combines with oxygen and is oxidized, producing CARBON DIOXIDE, water, and energy. The necessary oxygen is taken into the body by breathing air into the LUNGS, where it is absorbed into the blood which is then pumped round the body by the HEART. The same blood then transports the carbon dioxide formed in the tissues back to the lungs, where it diffuses into the alveoli and is breathed out.

Air is only about 21% oxygen; its other components are nitrogen (about 78%), argon (about 0.9%), carbon dioxide (about 0.03%), and other rarer gases, including CARBON MONOXIDE, neon, helium, krypton, hydrogen, xenon, and radon, which together generally form about 0.03%. Of course human activities can markedly alter the concentration of some of these agents in air, and carbon monoxide and carbon dioxide levels can be locally much higher.

Whatever is breathed into the lungs dissolves to some extent into the blood and passes via the blood to the tissues — so the body contains all the same gases as the surrounding air. Some gases are more soluble than others and some, notably oxygen, combine chemically with blood. Gases can also be absorbed into the body, to a limited extent, across the SKIN and MUCOUS MEMBRANES. This latter route allows gases formed in the gut, such as methane, also to be present in blood and body tissues.

The effect that a gas has on the body depends on the number of gas molecules that are available to act on receptor molecules in the body. The number of molecules in a given volume of gas at a fixed pressure and temperature is the same no matter what the gas is (Avogadro's principle). Since body temperature is more or less constant, the number of molecules of a gas is dependent only on its partial pressure. This is calculated from Dalton's law, which states that the pressure exerted by a mixture of gases is the sum of the pressures exerted by the individual gases occupying the same volume alone. So air, approximately 79% nitrogen and 21% oxygen, has a partial pressure of these gases of 79% and 21% of the prevailing atmospheric pressure. Atmospheric pressure varies but, at sea level, it can be taken to measure approximately 1 bar, 1,000 millibar or 100 kiloPascals (kPa). The partial pressures of nitrogen and oxygen in air at atmospheric pressure at sea level are therefore 79 kPa and 21 kPa respectively. As atmospheric pressure is reduced, for example with increased ALTITUDE, then, although the percentage composition of air remains the same, the partial pressure of the gases falls. The main effect of this is to cause oxygen lack — HYPOXIA. If atmospheric pressure is increased, for instance during DIVING, the partial pressure of oxygen and nitrogen rise. The most obvious effect of this is that nitrogen is breathed in sufficient quantities to cause partial anaesthesia or intoxication. The partial pressure of oxygen in the body can be raised easily at atmospheric pressure by adding it to the inhaled air. This technique is used to reverse the hypoxia of altitude in aviators and climbers, and of course is of great benefit in diseases that lower blood oxygen levels. Abnormally high partial pressures of oxygen in the blood, however, are toxic.

The amount or mass of a gas contained in the body depends directly on its partial pressure in the gas breathed, its solubility in the blood and various tissues, and whether it combines chemically with other substances. The solubility of a gas in another substance is expressed as the volume of gas which dissolves in the substance under stated conditions of temperature and pressure. Since the temperature of the body is more or less constant this factor does not normally influence gas uptake. The mass of gas dissolving is directly related to its partial pressure so if this is doubled the amount of gas dissolving is also doubled. This is important in conditions where decompression occurs (divers returning to the surface and astronauts during space walks, for example), since time must be allowed for excess gas to be cleared from the tissues and blood without the formation of bubbles of gas leading to decompression illness.

In addition to being simply dissolved in blood and tissues, some gases actually also form chemical compounds. For example, carbon dioxide forms bicarbonate and also combines with haemoglobin in the blood. Carbon monoxide combines with haemoglobin in the blood and many other iron-containing compounds in the tissues. Chemical combination allows very much larger amounts of gas to be held in the body than by simple solution. The amount of nitrogen gas, which is held only in solution in the body, is about 1 litre for someone weighing about 70 kg, while chemical combination allows the same person to contain about 35 litres of carbon dioxide.

Gases are not only taken up into the blood and tissues of the body but may also be contained, as gases, in body cavities. The lungs and upper and lower airways, of course, contain gas but so too do the bony sinuses of the skull and the middle ear. All these compartments are open to the atmosphere. The Eustachian tube connects the middle ear to the nasal cavity, and all the skull sinuses also open into the nasal cavity. This ensures that the pressure in these spaces remains at atmospheric pressure. If for some reason these connections become blocked, most commonly by a upper respiratory tract infection, and atmospheric pressure changes (for instance during flying or diving) then the tissues around the gas spaces can become damaged due to barotrauma (pressure-induced tissue damage); this is usually associated with a great deal of pain. Small pockets of gas may also exist under improperly maintained dental fillings and, if there is no connection to atmosphere, the expansion or contraction induced by changing pressure can cause toothache — *barodontalgia*. Extreme effects in teeth can cause the gas pocket to rupture or explode (dontopraxia). Free gas can also be present in the joints; this is commoner with increasing age and is of unknown significance. There is, however, some suggestion that such gas spaces are important in the causation of decompression illness. Free gas also exists in the intestinal tract but, since this is highly distensible and open to atmosphere (at both ends!), changes in atmospheric pressure rarely cause problems except under the most severe instances of sudden or explosive decompression. However, if the gut wall becomes perforated, such as occasionally happens due to a perforated ulcer, the appearance or free gas under the diaphragm on an X-ray picture is typical.

Some metabolic processes actually produce gases. NITRIC OXIDE is formed in the lining of blood vessels; it regulates their diameter and is very important in controlling blood pressure. Nitric oxide is also formed in the brain and is an important neuromodulating agent. CARBON MONOXIDE is formed from the metabolism of the haem in haemoglobin. This gas is also a vasodilator — like nitric oxide, but less potent. Recently carbon monoxide has been identified, like nitric oxide, as a possible neurotransmitter in the brain.

JOHN A. S. ROSS

See also CARBON DIOXIDE; OXYGEN; NITROGEN.

Gasp

Life may begin with a gasp and end with a gasp, but the causes and results are quite different.

A gasp is a deep, near maximal inspiration through an open mouth, followed by breathing out which, unlike that of COUGH and sneeze, is not particularly forcible and is through an open larynx and mouth.

At birth the newborn emerges into a world suddenly filled with sensations, including possibly a slap on the bottom. The baby is blue and somewhat asphyxiated, the latter signalling to the brain to start the breathing process. The LUNGS, full of liquid, and collapsed by the squeezing confines of the birth canal, also send nerve signals to the brain to initiate the first gasping breath. As a result of these stimuli the first breath is exceptionally powerful, as it has to be, to overcome the strong resistance to airflow entering the liquid-filled lungs. Once air is in the lungs breathing becomes less forceful.

Gasping breaths continue to be taken throughout life, for much the same reasons as for the baby. In quiet breathing occasional deep breaths are always taken, usually every 5–20 min,

as a kind of restrained gasp. These are called *augmented breaths*. The main cause is that in quiet breathing the lungs slowly and progressively deflate. Nerve endings in the lungs become sensitized to the deflation and, when their activity is great enough, their signals to the brain become strong enough to stimulate a deep, gasping breath. This large inflation of the lungs reverses the deflation and inhibits the sensory nerves, so the process is switched off until the lungs have slowly deflated again. The augmented breaths are not conspicuous when breathing is vigorous, as in EXERCISE, and although colloquially we may talk of gasping from exertion this usually occurs after the effort. Augmented breaths are more frequent in some diseases where there is lung collapse or when the lung sensory nerves are activated, possibly in asthma, for example.

Other sensory inputs cause a gasp. Step under a cold shower or receive a painful stimulus, and an irrepressible gasp is almost inevitable. One can argue that this deep breath prepares the lungs and breathing for a rapid escape from the assault. The deep, gasping breath also reflexly stimulates heart rate, so the circulation is simultaneously brought to a state of readiness.

We gasp with EMOTION, as every romantic novelist knows too well. Again this may be a preparation for avoiding or other action, but it can also be a form of *communication*, so that observers see the strength of our reaction. We may 'gasp out' words in an urgent attempt at speech, but this is a physiological misuse of the term. Lie detectors rely in part on a deep, gasping breath when the subject is asked a question that activates his guilt.

In unconsciousness after a traumatic accident, the patient sometimes shows repetitive gasping instead of normal breathing, and this is an ominous sign, implying damage to the brain stem where breathing is controlled. The 'last gasp' in a dying patient is probably also an indication of brain stem malfunction, and is traditionally regarded as the last sign of impending death. But an ill or dying patient may have many 'last' gasps, and at death breathing usually fades quietly away.

JOHN WIDDICOMBE

See also BREATHING.

Gastrin

is a HORMONE produced in the stomach which stimulates gastric acid secretion after a meal. It was discovered in 1905 by John Sydney Edkins (1863–1940), working in St Bartholomew's Hospital, London. Edkins reasoned that gastric acid secretion might be regulated by a mechanism analogous to the control of pancreatic secretion by the intestinal hormone secretin which had been discovered by W. M. Bayliss and E. H. Starling three years earlier. He then showed that when extracts of the lowest part of the stomach were injected into the jugular vein they stimulated gastric acid secretion, and he called the active factor 'gastrin'. Gastrin is a polypeptide. It occurs in several different molecular forms, the most important of which are molecules of 17 and 34 amino acid residues.

In 1919 the Russian physiologist L. Popielski showed that histamine was a powerful stimulant of gastric acid secretion and for some years thereafter it was widely thought that Edkins' 'gastrin' was in fact histamine. The issue was clarified by S. A. Komarov, who established that histamine-free extracts of gastric mucosa stimulated acid secretion when injected into the blood. However, the low concentrations of gastrin in stomach tissue frustrated early attempts to obtain the hormone in a pure form. Success was finally achieved by Rod Gregory and Hilda Tracy at the University of Liverpool, who in the early 1960s purified from pig stomach the 17 amino acid form of the hormone. Their work required the routine processing of many hundreds of pig stomachs obtained each week from a local abattoir. Together with their colleague, the chemist George Kenner, they established the structure of gastrin and noted that a sequence of 4 amino acid residues was sufficient to produce the full range of actions of the molecule they had purified. A synthetic compound based on this sequence, pentagastrin, is used clinically for tests of gastric acid secretion. A closely related sequence occurs in the brain–gut peptide CHOLECYSTOKININ, and a similar peptide is also found in high concentrations in skin glands of certain amphibians, for example the South African clawed toad, *Xenopus leavis*.

Gastrin is released from specialised cells in the mucosa of the final part of the stomach. Secretion into the bloodstream is increased by the presence of food, particularly protein, in the stomach, and is also stimulated by neural reflexes. Gastrin is then carried by the blood throughout the body, but it exerts its action by virtue of specific receptors on cells of the acid-secreting (middle and upper) part of the stomach. Gastric acid, in turn, passes to the lower part of the stomach and there inhibits the release of gastrin, providing a mechanism to limit acid secretion during digestion. In the absence of acid due either to loss of the parietal cells that secrete it (pernicious anaemia) or to administration of drugs that block the proton pump in parietal cells, e.g. omeprazole, the concentration of gastrin in the blood becomes elevated. It also becomes elevated in the blood of patients with the rare condition of Zollinger–Ellison syndrome, due to a gastrin-producing tumour typically sited in the PANCREAS.

Gastrin increases acid secretion both by direct stimulation of the acid-producing parietal cells, and by increasing the release of histamine from specialized cells, known as enterochromaffin-like cells, in the mucosa adjacent to parietal cells. Histamine then diffuses through the mucosa to parietal cells, acting as a local regulator. Gastrin is also a stimulant of the growth of the gastric mucosa, and in particular of the enterochromaffin-like cells. In extreme cases, elevated concentrations of gastrin in blood may be associated with the development of nodules of enterochromaffin-like cells, known as gastric carcinoid tumours.

The actions of gastrin are mediated by receptors on the surface of parietal and enterochromaffin-like cells, activation of which leads to increased intracellular calcium. The same receptor responds to cholecystokinin, and is known as the gastrin/cholecystokinin-B receptor. Cholecystokinin is normally present in blood in concentrations about ten times lower than those of gastrin and so its actions on these receptors in the stomach are relatively unimportant. Cholecystokinin also acts at a different type of receptor (the cholecystokinin-A receptor) which responds weakly to gastrin. Actions at cholecystokinin-A receptors account for the capacity of gastrin to stimulate pancreatic enzyme secretion and gall bladder contraction when given in high doses. The gastrin/cholecystokinin-B receptor is abundant in the central nervous system. Gastrin is not normally present in the brain and does not normally penetrate from the circulation; however, cholecystokinin does occur in the brain and so is the natural stimulant of this receptor in the central nervous system.   G. J. DOCKRAY

See also ALIMENTARY SYSTEM.

Gaze It is unsettling to be gazed at. Staring is a threat for monkeys and apes, and perhaps humans share some trace of this response. On the other hand, good 'eye contact' is recognized in most cultures as important for effective interpersonal communication, especially during dialogue. So it may be the combination of looking intently and protractedly without verbal communication that is particularly unsettling or threatening. There was a time when, in the Southern States of the US, it was a sexual offence, punishable by law, for a black man to look overly long at a white woman.

Mutual gaze is, however, one of the delights of lovers; as Shakespeare writes (Sonnet 24):

Mine eyes have drawn thy shape, and thine for me
Are windows to my breast, where-through the sun
Delights to peep, to gaze therein on thee.

Francis Bacon went so far as to describe the appropriate pattern of gaze for courtship — 'sudden glances and darting of the eye', but not a fixed stare.

The lover's gaze may be accompanied by enlargement of the pupil (a 'wide-eyed' look) — a sign of activation of the sympathetic nervous system. Experimental psychologists have shown that if male subjects are shown two copies of a photograph of a girl, one modified to enlarge the pupils and the other to make them smaller, the subjects will describe the girl with the larger pupils as more attractive, even if unaware of the size of the pupils. Presumably the involuntary enlargement of the pupil acts as a signal of sexual arousal. Indeed, Southern European women are said to have put extracts of the plant Deadly Nightshade (containing the drug belladonna or atropine) into their eyes to enlarge their pupils, in order to make themselves more attractive to the opposite sex.

When we gaze directly at an object, we hold our eyes in such a position that the image of the object falls on the central, specialized region of the retina — the *fovea* or *macula* — where visual acuity and colour vision are best. If we look around a scene, thinking that our eyes are roaming smoothly, they are, in fact, making a series of step-like shifts of gaze. The line of sight or direction of gaze rests briefly on one object, before jumping to the next, as often as three or four times a second. Even when we try to fixate — to look fixedly in one direction — tiny shifts of gaze still occur. This pattern, in which the line of sight is either briefly fixed or rapidly jumping to another position (rather than slithering around), is characteristic of any situation in which the visual surroundings are stationary. This is true even if the head is moving, because as the head rotates, signals from the organ of balance (the vestibular system) trigger the powerful *vestibulo-ocular reflex*, which automatically causes the eyes to rotate through the same angle, in the opposite direction. So, remarkably, movement of the head does not cause a change in gaze. Only an active shift of the eye in the orbit alters the line of sight.

Perhaps because the fixity of the line of sight is so nicely maintained when the head is moving, 'gaze' has come to have a technical meaning for scientists who study eye and head movements. It means the 'position of the line of sight *in space*', rather than its direction relative to the head.

Even though our eyes are constantly shifting from place to place, visual perception occurs almost exclusively during the brief pauses. Very little is seen during a shift of gaze. The ability to maintain gaze can be profoundly disturbed by damage to the brain stem or hindbrain.

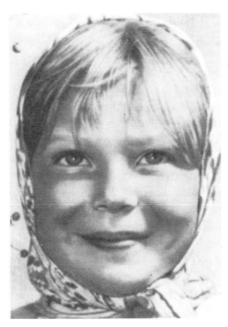

How eyes search a picture. Such records show what the brain thinks it needs. This depends on what it is seeing and the current task. Movements when driving a car are very different from reading, or looking at pictures such as this. For portraits, eyes and noses are specially selected. (From Yarbus 1967.)

Another, now rare, cause of difficulty in maintaining gaze is damage to the hair cells of the inner ear by high doses of particular antibiotics. Not only is hearing affected but so too is the sense of balance, because hair cells in the organ of balance in the inner ear are also destroyed. These hair cells normally detect head rotation, so the vestibulo-ocular reflex is affected and gaze becomes unstable. There is a well known account by a patient (who happened to be a physician) who suffered from this condition, which described how difficult it was to read because even small head movements shifted the line of sight unexpectedly.

STUART J. JUDGE

Further reading

Argyle, M. and Cook, M. (1976). *Gaze and mutual gaze.* Cambridge University, Press.

See also AUTONOMIC NERVOUS SYSTEM; EYE; EYE MOVEMENTS.

Gaze in medical perception
Michel Foucault's book *La Naissance de la Clinique*, first published in France in 1963, reached an English-speaking audience in 1973. The opening sentence read: 'This book is about space, about language, and about death; it is about the act of seeing, the gaze.' This was the first reference to a new concept underpinning much subsequent understanding of Western clinical practice and the body. Ironically, for a term that has achieved such widespread recognition as a key component of Foucault's analysis of Western medicine, it was the choice of his translator, A. M. Sheridan Smith. Indeed, in a translator's note he referred to the problem of translating the French noun, *le regard*. As Foucault made clear in his opening sentence, he was not referring to a passive visual process, but to something more active, an 'act of seeing'. Accordingly Sheridan Smith felt that the term, 'the gaze', though unusual, was a useful way of registering the breadth of Foucault's concept, and this is the word used throughout the book except in the subtitle (*An Archaeology of Medical Perception*), which was a 'concession' to the unprepared reader by Sheridan Smith.

Foucault went on to describe an eighteenth-century report of a medical treatment that was said to have resulted in a patient discarding her insides in her urine. He then compared this strange account to a nineteenth-century description of the meningeal layers of the brain. Between these two ways of describing the clinical world, Foucault argued, lay a transformation in '...the relationship between the visible and the invisible', a process in which knowledge and clinical practice were radically changed as medicine began to 'see' by means of this novel gaze into the depths of the body.

In earlier models of ILLNESS, disease was mobile, a sum of the trail of symptoms that marked its passage through the inside and outside of the body. In contrast, the new pathological medicine construed illness as a specific anatomical lesion located in the analyzable three-dimensional structure of the body. The gaze was the literal ability to see through the density of the corporal tissues to the hidden lesion that was bringing about the patient's distress. The gaze therefore encompassed both a system of knowledge that equated illness to the underlying pathological lesion and a new method of clinical practice. The post-mortem that could finally reveal the truth of the pathological lesion, the techniques of the clinical examination that enabled the three-dimensional volume of the body to be explored, and the neutral space of the hospital in which these practices could occur, all were both consequences and manifestations of the new clinical gaze. Thus, perception and cognition, seeing and knowing, were brought together within an overall framework of clinical practice.

The new clinical gaze underpinned the development of medicine in Western countries throughout the nineteenth and twentieth centuries' as increasingly sophisticated searches were devised to penetrate and 'read' the patient's body. And yet, despite this intensification of the gaze into the body, it was also accompanied by a widening of its field to other objects during the latter half of the twentieth century as medicine increasingly explored the patient's mind and social context. This extension represents further evidence that the gaze is an active process: the gaze does not simply see what is there but constructs the conditions of possibility, to use a Foucauldian term, for the emergence of certain (medical) objects that in their turn are brought to the senses. The notion of the gaze therefore stands opposed to a conventional account of medical progress that would claim that two centuries ago a means was found of sweeping away the veils of ignorance and revealing things as they really were. Modern Western medicine is only one version — historically and culturally located — of how illness and the body relate together: according to Foucault, this order of the solid visible body was only one way 'in all likelihood neither the first nor the most fundamental in which one spatialises disease. There have been and will be, other distributions of illness.'

DAVID ARMSTRONG

Gender Apart from its narrow application in languages that assign masculine/feminine/neuter status to linguistic terms, gender is a category used to differentiate women and men, boys and girls, male and female, masculinity and femininity. Increased attention to gender as a category of analysis, particularly in the social and behavioural sciences, has coincided with the rise of academic feminism. The category itself has undergone many revisions over time, but is typically employed to distinguish sex from gender in the following way: there are clear biological differences (sex differences) between men and women, and those biological differences serve as the basis for the social construction of different roles for men and women (gender differences), though these may vary from one culture to the next.

Although biological difference does not necessitate the roles assigned to men and women, it enables differential social relations which are then often (mis)understood to be 'naturally' determined by biology. Recently, this formulation of the relation between sex and gender has been challenged as endorsing 'gender essentialism' (see below).

Gender as sex

That men and women have different natures is an ancient idea, but in the nineteenth century it gained the epistemological authority of medicine and science as the idea became an object of formal investigation. Victorian science placed particular emphasis on what it identified as the weaker constitution of women, and fluctuated between assigning to them either through-going sexual passivity (attributed to bourgeois women) or rampant promiscuity (attributed to lower-class women and women of colour). However it was characterized in medical or biological terms, and women's nature was said to be decidedly inferior to that of men. The emergence of the science of psychology seemed to confirm women's inferiority by locating female pathology in a psychosomatic nexus. Freud is an exemplar of the view that female 'hysteria', characterized by a complex interweaving of physical and mental disorders, results from somatizing unfulfilled sexual fantasies. While Freud was certainly ready to admit that both men and women suffer from mental disorders, his overall approach was that the 'anatomical differences between the sexes' determine gender-typed psychopathologies. The rigid adherence to the biological model enforced the belief that homosexuality was pathological, as well. Sexual desire for the 'opposite' sex was thought to be a *sine qua non* of normal gender identification. The 'mannish woman' or the 'effeminate man' could only be understood as forms of deviance.

In the early twentieth century, Margaret Mead was among the first explicitly to forge a distinction between sex understood as a biological category, and sex or gender *roles* understood as a social category. Mead's ethnographic study, *Sex and Temperament in Three Societies* (1935), argued that, 'many, if not all, of the personality traits which we have called masculine or feminine are as lightly linked to sex as are the clothing, the manners, and the form of head-dress that a society at a given period assigns to either sex.' This prying apart of sex and gender forms the basis for feminist efforts to displace biologically based assumptions about women's inferiority and/or the 'naturalness' of the maternal role. For feminism, gender becomes a *critical* category by means of which women's degraded status can be understood and transcended.

Feminism and gender

Early (1970s) feminist sociology and anthropology sought to identify how those with female bodies are solicited into particular gender roles that are then seen as stereotypical. An explosion of research proposed both that (i) gender

stereotyping occurs at all levels of social and cultural organization; and that (ii) the analytical tools by means of which different disciplines organize knowledge are themselves permeated by gender bias. Sherry Ortner (1972), for example, argued that because women's reproductive functions are associated with nature, and because nature is subordinated to culture (which is associated with men), it follows that women are assigned a status subordinate to that of men. Carol Gilligan (1982) argued that cognitive–developmental categories employed by the dominant research on moral development assumed the superiority of categorical over relational thinking. Since men are more likely to reason categorically, and women rationally, it follows that women's moral reasoning will be deemed deficient in relation to that of men. This would explain why moral authority is granted to men in both the public and the private spheres, as both the Judge and the Father. Gilligan attempted to develop an analytical framework that re-evaluated the development of women's moral reasoning in light of the particular contexts of women's experience. Thus, she juxtaposed women's 'ethic of care' to men's 'ethic of justice', and argued that the former is just as structurally complex as the latter.

Feminists made analogous claims concerning the gendered nature of the subject matters and the methodologies of other fields. Evelyn Fox Keller (1978) argued that the very terms of scientific investigation — objectivity, disinterestedness, rationality — are themselves highly invested in a masculinist regime of domination and control over nature (including women). According to Keller, the relatively small number of women scientists reinforces the genderization of science by excluding women's ways of knowing from its arena. Feminist literary theorists scrutinized the literary canon for its exclusion of women writers, and for its masculine preoccupations (the pursuit of power, women, and whales). By analyzing representations of women in literature, and by unveiling the work of women writers, feminist scholarship revealed both the gendered nature of literature and our gendered ways of reading it. These approaches to the study of gender, sometimes called 'gender standpoint theory', assume that women's 'identity' can be defined and demarcated, and that the world is constituted in unique ways by women's 'subjectivity'.

Gender essentialism and beyond

Apart from a general conservative backlash against the disruption to business as usual, feminist critics themselves offered counterexamples to the presuppositions that seem to underlie gender standpoint theory, that is, that women are universally subordinated to men, that men and women are always differentially associated with culture and nature respectively, that nature and culture are universally distinct categories, that male and female are universally distinct categories, and finally, that the category of woman is a stable category in and of itself. Cross-cultural evidence, for example, has been marshalled to show that there are widespread differences in the ways that reproductive labour is apportioned between men and women. Other critics have demonstrated that race, class, sexuality, and ethnicity must be interposed with gender in order to account for the cultural and historical variability of social relations and subjectivities. Given the effects of racism on the distribution of material and symbolic resources, the category of *woman* cannot be applied univocally to white women and to women of colour. Similarly, 'queer theory' has challenged the assumption that gender provides a singular axis of sexual orientation. Along these lines, Monique Wittig (1991) argues that, understood in relation to the categories of sexual difference, lesbians are not women. How many genders might there then be?

Thus, revisionist accounts of gender attempt to displace 'gender essentialism', the view that women's experience and embodiment can be distilled into a unified form of subjectivity. Some theorists replace gender essentialism with the idea that subjectivity is not fixed by intersecting social categories (gender, race, etc.) but is 'positional', 'provisional', and 'performative'. According to this view, the initial feminist impulse to distinguish sex and gender must be resisted because, though it attempts to break the ideological tie between the 'natural' and the 'social', it in fact reproduces the categories of *man* and *woman* at the level of the sexed body. Judith Butler (1990) argues that sex construed as a biological category is as heavily socially constructed as gender, and that biological sex itself is a gendered category. According to Butler, while feminist analysis successfully identified the social practices that produce gender as a category of identification, they have failed to see that sex itself is produced as a category that precedes gender. Butler's postmodern conception of gender draws on the assumption that nothing exists prior to systems of representation, thus it is wrong to think that gender identity is inscribed on a pre-existing sexed body. According to this view, the meanings attached to the female body as an object of scientific scrutiny are determined not just by the practices of science, but in conjunction with other cultural and economic formations, for example, global capitalism, the mass media, institutional racism, or homophobia. Gender, as such, is best seen as a heuristic category, a means of investigating the variability and contingency of our understanding of sexual diference.

MEREDITH W. MICHAELS

Further reading

Fausto-Sterling, A. (1985). *Myths of gender: biological theories about men and women*. Basic Books, New York.

Rosaldo, M. Z. (1980). The use and abuse of anthropology: reflections on feminism and cross-cultural understanding. *Signs: A Journal of Women in Culture and Society*, 5(3).

See also FEMINISM; SEX DETERMINATION; SEXUAL ORIENTATION; SEXUALITY.

Gene A gene is part of a DNA molecule within the nucleus of all cells. Each gene codes for a particular PROTEIN. Thus a gene is a unit of the inheritable characteristics of the organism. Humans have tens of thousands of different genes; these determine the PHENOTYPE of the individual.   A. W. C.

See CELL; GENE THERAPY; GENETIC TESTING; GENETICS, HUMAN.

Gene therapy is the treatment of human disease by gene transfer. Many, or maybe most, diseases have a genetic component — asthma, cancer, Alzheimer's disease, for example. However, most diseases are *polygenic*, i.e. a subtle interplay of many genes determines the likelihood of developing a disease condition, whereas, so far, gene therapy can only be contemplated for *monogenic* diseases, in which there is a single gene defect. Even in these cases only treatment of recessive diseases can be considered, where the correct gene is added in the continued presence of the faulty one. Dominant mutations cannot be approached in this way, as it would be necessary to knock out the existing faulty genes in the cells where they are expressed (i.e. where their presence shows an effect), as well as adding the correct genetic information.

Gene therapy for recessive monogenic diseases involves introducing correct genetic material into the patient. This can be approached in two different ways. Cells can be taken from the patient, modified in the laboratory ('in vitro'), and then re-introduced, or a carrier ('vector') of the correct genetic material can be delivered directly into the patient. Examples are adenosine deaminase (ADA) deficiency and cystic fibrosis, respectively.

ADA deficiency is a lethal monogenic disease in which *adenosine* is not normally metabolised, leading to high levels of $2'$-deoxyadenosine, which is selectively toxic to cells of the immune system (T and B cells) and leads to immunodeficiency. The gene therapy for this disease is to isolate T cells from patients and treat these cells *in vitro* with a retroviral vector — a virus, normally capable of causing disease, which has been modified to carry the required genetic information. Cells that have incorporated the new genetic information into their genomes are selected and reinfused back into the patient, allowing the appropriate metabolism of adenosine to occur.

Cystic fibrosis (CF) is also a lethal disease resulting from a single gene mutation. It disables normal cell membrane function. The gene codes for a protein, the cystic fibrosis 'transmembrane conductance regulator' (CFTR), which acts as a chloride ION CHANNEL in the EPITHELIA of the airways, alimentary canal, and numerous other hollow organs. The correct genetic sequence can be incorporated into a type of virus which ordinarily can infect the respiratory tract (*adenoviruses*), or into genetic particles (plasmids) linked to lipids to form *lipocomplexes*. Either of these can be delivered directly into the patient's lungs.

Both the examples given must still be regarded as at the experimental stage. In ADA deficiency the transformed T cells persist for only 6 months, while in CF the new genetic material is not incorporated into the genome and is expressed outside of it (*episomally*) for only a few weeks. The major problems with gene therapy relate to the delivery of new genetic instructions to the appropriate body targets. Ideally, delivery should be to stem cells — the progenitor cells which give rise to replacement cells as adult, mature cells die. Furthermore, the material should be incorporated into the genome so that all future generations of cells carry the correct instructions. *Retroviral vectors* (viruses carrying the genetic material) are incorporated in the genome, but this can only be used in the *in vitro* type of procedure, when the treated cells are outside the body. Incorporation of the new material into an inappropriate position may switch on an *oncogene* which can lead to tumour formation. Thus it is very necessary to be sure that cells transformed *in vitro* behave normally before reintroducing them to the patient. These problems do not occur with *adenoviral vectors*, but expression persists for only a short time, thus requiring repeated administration, leading to immune reactions. Use of lipoplexes avoids this latter problem, but the efficiency of gene delivery by this route is very low.

Gene therapy will undoubtedly have much to offer for the future. Unlike many conventional therapies, it aims to cure disease rather than simply treat the symptoms. The principles of gene therapy are established, but technical problems, primarily related to efficient and safe ways of delivery, have still to be overcome.

ALAN W. CUTHBERT

See also GENETICS, HUMAN; IMMUNE SYSTEM.

Genetic testing is now possible, as both the structure of DNA is known and methods to determine the sequence have been developed. Genetic testing brings with it benefits of diagnosis and treatment, but raises many other issues, both sociological and ethical. It is known that a great number of diseases have a genetic input; in some instances, such as single gene diseases, the genetic mutation is the sole cause of the disease. In polygenic diseases there are a number of mutations in different genes, none of which individually may have any measurable effect, but which in combination one with another may increase the likelihood that a complex disease condition, such as high blood pressure, will result.

What is genetic testing, what does it involve, and how is it done? We all have 22 pairs of chromosomes, one of each pair from each parent plus an X and Y chromosome in the male and two X chromosomes in the female. Paired genes are arrayed along the length of each pair of chromosome. Thus we all have two copies of each gene, one from each parent, plus either an X and a Y or two X chromosomes. Suppose the particular gene on a particular chromosome carries a defect responsible for a disease, while the other gene on the paired chromosome is normal, yet the person has the disease. Then the mutant gene is said to be *dominant*. If no disease is present then the gene is *recessive*; the person is a carrier, but may pass on the defective gene to the offspring. It is important to know in genetic testing whether an individual has two normal genes or one normal and one abnormal gene. Some genetic diseases are associated with X and Y chromosomes and are described as *sex-linked*, while genetic diseases due to gene defects on the non-sex chromosomes are called *autosomal*; i.e. these can affect males and females alike. Genetic testing therefore consists of looking for the gene mutation, together with the normal gene in a DNA sample, from a patient. Providing a sample is very easy; for example, simply lightly brushing the inside of the mouth yields enough cells to examine the DNA. Techniques are available to *amplify* (copy) the DNA in the sample, and, since the sequence of the gene involved is known, probes are used to look for the presence of normal and mutant genes. If only one type of gene is found then the sample is from a *homozygous* individual, who may have two normal or two abnormal genes. If both types of gene are found then the individual is *heterozygous*, that is they have one normal and one abnormal gene. Given this information, the consequences for the offspring follow clearly defined genetic rules. Examples of dominant inherited disorders are *Huntington's chorea* and *retinoblastoma*; of recessive disorders are *cystic fibrosis* (CF), *sickle cell anaemia*, and *thalassaemia*; and of sex-linked inherited disorders are *haemophilia* and *muscular dystrophy*.

Consider an example. A perfectly healthy pregnant female is offered a genetic test and discovers that she is a carrier of CF. It is most important that confidentiality is maintained and that the patient is not made to feel somehow responsible. If the father is also a carrier then the chances are 1 in 4 that the child will have CF. The chances that the child will also be a carrier, like the parents, is 50%, and the chance that the child inherits a normal gene from both parents is again 1 in 4. Testing the father involves some delay and, of course, concern for the parents. In some instances the father will be unknown or parentage of the child may be in doubt, raising further embarrassments for those involved. If the father cannot be found or refuses to take part it is possible to test the fetus by *amniocentesis*. In this procedure a small volume of fluid is drawn from around the foetus. This contains sufficient fetal cells to collect the DNA. If, when all the tests are done, the unborn child is found to have CF, then termination may be offered, again an ethical problem which the originally unsuspecting parents had never envisaged. Counselling is very important at this stage.

Looking to the future, it is possible that babies will be genotyped at birth and that this may allow prediction of diseases that might arise in later life. In this way prophylactic measures taken early may be able to prevent the disease appearing, or delay its onset. Furthermore, if the disease does develop, knowledge of the genetic profile will allow the most appropriate drug regimens to be prescribed. This sort of benefit will be most useful for polygenic diseases, such as high blood pressure, various forms of cancer, and asthma. It must be remembered, however, that complex diseases of this type have causes that are due both to nature and nurture. Clearly, much disease prevention can be achieved by appropriate attention to nurture — lifestyle, diet, and the like.

ALAN W. CUTHBERT

Genetics, human Surely, people must always have been curious about how physical traits and aspects of character are passed down from generation to generation. But, until the middle of the nineteenth century, thoughts about heredity were extremely confused. Indeed, throughout the medieval period in Europe, all organisms were thought to grow from replicas created by God at the beginning of the universe. In these terms, Eve literally contained within her ovaries the whole of the rest of the human race, generation after generation of miniatures packed one inside the other, each waiting for an act of fertilization. Even after the discovery of sperm this 'pre-formation hypothesis' was not discarded, and some held that an individual was pre-formed in the sperm, and simply nurtured by the mother. Towards the end of the nineteenth century, anatomists found that they could see thread-like objects, which could be stained with coloured dyes, inside dividing cells. They called these structures chromosomes, and later suggested that they might carry heritable information from cell to cell. At about the same time, based on a series of breeding experiments on ornamental plants, Gregor Mendel formulated the concept that later became known as the gene — a unit of heredity, passed from generation to generation in a way that follows simple mathematical laws. These disparate observations were finally unified during the middle of the twentieth century with the discovery that genetic information carried by chromosomes resides in the double helix of *deoxyribonucleic acid* (DNA), first described by Francis Crick and James Watson. DNA has the remarkable property of self-replication — it copies itself faithfully each time a cell divides. It was soon clear that genes consist of lengths of DNA, and that their major function is to direct the synthesis of proteins, ensuring that the structure of proteins is always the same and that they are made in the right amount in the right place at the right time.

Proteins are made up of 20 different amino acids, and the extensive differences in their structures — from the fluid haemoglobin of our blood to the tough keratin of our skin — reflect differences in the number and order of amino acids in their constituent peptide chains. The information responsible for selecting and arranging the amino acids in these peptide chains is encoded by the order of the four bases that make up each strand of the DNA helix — adenine (A), guanine (G), cytosine (C), and thymine (T). Each individual amino acid is represented by a unique three-letter 'word', spelled out by a particular sequence of three bases in the gene. Even more remarkable, the code is the same throughout almost all of the animal kingdom.

In recent years it has been feasible to isolate human DNA, cut it into pieces, and insert these into bacterial cells, where they grow and multiply. In this way, it has been possible to prepare 'libraries' containing most of a person's genes (the '*genome*'), to isolate individual genes, and to examine their structure and function.

The human genome

Normal human cells (except eggs and sperm) have 46 chromosomes, arranged in pairs, one member of each pair coming from each parent. Twenty-two pairs are called autosomes and the other pair are the sex chromosomes, designated X and Y. Females have two X chromosomes (one from the mother, the other from the father) while males have one maternal X and one paternal Y sex chromosome. '*Germ cells*' (sperm and eggs) are unusual in having only 23 unpaired chromosomes, each of which is created by a process in which maternal and paternal chromosome pairs become closely wound round each other in the germinal cells that give rise to the eggs and sperm. The closer together a pair of genes are on the same chromosome the less chance they will have to cross over from one to another. Hence the number of crossovers is a measure of the distance between genes. Indeed, many years ago it was realized that if two different genes are on the same chromosome, and particularly if they are close together, they will tend to be inherited together. They are then said to be linked.

Through studies of individual families, and later by generating genetic markers by analysing DNA itself, geneticists have been able to obtain a 'linkage map' of the human chromosomes, assigning many different genes to particular chromosomes. In essence, this looks like a road map in which the towns (genes) are clearly marked, although it tells us nothing about the state of the roads (DNA) in between. Early in the new millennium, as part of the Human Genome Project, this work will be extended, and the complete sequence of all the bases that make up the 30–40 000 genes of the human genome will be worked out.

Mutations and human diversity

Occasionally, during cell division, when new strands of DNA are synthesised, a different base is inserted, by mistake, into a gene. This is called a mutation. Without this slight imperfection in the mechanism of DNA replication we would still be swimming round in the primeval soup. For, while many mutations, or *polymorphisms*, are neutral (that is, the slight changes in the proteins produced have no effect on the function of the organism), others may be beneficial.

Although it is still a topic of some controversy, there is general agreement that this is the way in which Darwinian evolution has occurred; the occurrence of mutations occasionally leads to changes in organisms that enable them to adapt better to their current environments, or to new ones. While this may not be the only mechanisms for the gradual emergence of different species there is compelling evidence that it has been a major force behind human evolution. The existence of polymorphisms, and our new-found ability to analyse DNA with ease, are providing major insights into the origins of human beings, the ways in which different races have evolved, and, indeed, the whole basis of human diversity. As well as the DNA that resides in the nuclei of our cells, our mitochondria, the chemical dynamos that energize the cell, have their own DNA. Since mitochondrial DNA is all derived from our mothers, it is of particular value in tracing our evolutionary past in a direct line.

Harmful mutations

Unfortunately, not all mutations are simply neutral or even beneficial; occasionally they cause disease, because they affect some vital process in the body. Inherited diseases due to single defective genes usually follow Mendelian patterns of inheritance. Some are said to be '*dominant*' because they occur with the inheritance of a single defective gene on only one of the pair of chromosomes. Others are '*recessive*' — it is necessary to inherit the mutant gene from both parents to have the disease. '*Carriers*', or '*heterozygotes*', are individuals who have a recessive disease gene on only one of the pair of chromosomes, and who therefore are not affected by the disease but can pass it on their children if they mate with a partner who is also a carrier. Yet other diseases are sex-linked; that is, they are carried on the X chromosome and, if recessive, are not expressed in females (who have two X chromosomes) but may be transmitted to a son to whom the mother passes down an X chromosome bearing the mutant gene.

Although there are over 4000 single-gene (*monogenic*) disorders, most are very rare because they produce such severe disorders that they usually prevent reproduction, and therefore cannot disseminate within a population. However, a few monogenic diseases — the inherited anaemias, sickle cell anaemia and thalassaemia, for example — are extremely common. This is because carriers are made more resistant to malaria by the presence of the mutation in their cells. Therefore they tend to survive slightly longer than non-affected individuals in malarious countries, and hence have more children. In this way, the frequency of the disease increases until it reaches an equilibrium, at which it is balanced by the loss from the community of severely affected *homozygotes* (those who have received the defective gene from both parents). This kind of interaction may explain why cystic fibrosis, a disease that affects the lung and bowel, is so common in European populations: the mutation may have made carriers resistant to one or more

of the severe infections that swept through Europe in the past, possibly cholera.

Many of the common diseases of Western society — heart attacks, stroke, diabetes, and dementia, for example — are the result of complex interactions between our genetic make-up and the environment. These diseases do not run predictably through families like single-gene disorders, but there may be a familial tendency, which probably reflects the action of several different genes combined with the effects of lifestyle. Other common diseases, cancer in particular, also reflect interactions between our genes and environments.

Many cancers result from the acquisition of mutations in a family of genes called oncogenes, which normally serve important housekeeping functions for our cells. They tell the cells how and when to divide, identify those with damaged DNA and either ensure that it is repaired or programme the potentially harmful cells to die, and regulate how they interact with their fellow cells. Cancer appears to be due to the acquisition of mutations in these genes; the frequency with which this occurs may be related both to exposure to environmental mutagens such as tobacco smoke, and to chemical agents that are by-products of our metabolism.

Other genetic defects are responsible for congenital malformation and for mental retardation. Sometimes these conditions result from major chromosomal abnormalities, involving either their numbers or structure. However, many malformations of this type can be traced to the action of single mutant genes — an observation that is providing clues about the mechanisms that control human development.

Manipulating the human genome

Our new-found ability to analyse human DNA, which has led to the discovery of the mutations that cause many monogenic diseases, means that they can be identified in carriers and appropriate counselling and advice can be given. It is also now possible to diagnose most of these diseases prenatally by *chorionic villus sampling* — removing and genetically analysing a tiny amount of tissue from round the fetus between 9 and 13 weeks of pregnancy. This allows prenatal diagnosis, and gives the mother the option of termination of a pregnancy if the fetus has a particularly severe condition. Soon it may be feasible to correct genetic disease or alter the genetic machinery of cells in a way that may be used to treat cancer or other acquired diseases. The treatment of single-gene disorders can, in principle, be approached by either *germ-cell gene therapy* (in which a 'good' gene is injected into a fertilised egg and therefore distributes among all the cells of the body, including future germ cells) or *somatic-cell therapy* (in which the gene is inserted into a particular cell population in the body of one individual — the stem cells of the bone marrow for example). Although germ cell gene therapy offers the prospect of eliminating disease from a family for all future generations, it is

currently not permitted because of the possible risk of making damaging errors to the genes. On the other hand, somatic-cell gene therapy poses no major ethical problems beyond those of any form of tissue or organ transplantation. Human genes can also be inserted into cultured cells or whole animals (a process called *transgenesis*) in order for the recipient cells or animals to produce molecules of therapeutic value — insulin to treat diabetes, or clotting factors to treat haemophilia, for example.

Biological determinism and the future

The remarkable developments in human genetics over the last half of the twentieth century led to the notion that most of people's mental achievements, personality traits, and behaviour can be explained by their genetic make-up, shaped in the past by Darwinian evolution. Much of this thinking ignores the important role of the environment in making us what we are. But because it carries such conviction, and because it is assumed that we will gradually learn how to manipulate our genetic make-up, this view is causing considerable concern about the possible resurgence of the *eugenics* movement — a philosophy for the 'betterment' of mankind by selective breeding, which stimulated the study of human genetics at the end of the nineteenth century. Although it will be a long time before we know the relative role of nature and nurture in shaping human beings, there is little doubt that our ability to modify the human genome will increase dramatically during the new millennium, and society will be faced with the dilemma of deciding how far it wishes to shape its destiny in this way.   D. J. WEATHERALL

Further reading
Bodmer, W. and McKie, R. (1994). *The book of man.* Little, Brown and Co, London.
Bowdler, P. J. (1989). *The Mendelian revolution.* Johns Hopkins University Press, Baltimore.
Jones, S. (1993). *The language of the genes.* Harper Collins, London.
Lewin, B. (1997). *Genes VI.* Oxford University Press, Oxford.
Raskó, I. and Downes, C. S. (1995). *Genes in medicine.* Chapman and Hall, London.

See also EVOLUTION, HUMAN; GENE THERAPY; HEREDITY.

Genitalia The genitalia are the organs of reproduction which characterize the male or the female. In common usage, 'the genitals' applies only to the *external genitalia* — the LABIA and the CLITORIS, forming the VULVA, in the female, and the PENIS and SCROTUM in the male. The female *internal genitalia* are the OVARIES, FALLOPIAN TUBES, UTERUS and VAGINA. In the male, although the TESTES in fetal life are internal, they become externalised by descent into the scrotum; the vasa deferentia link the external components to the internal — the seminal vesicles and the PROSTATE gland.

In an early fetus there are rudimentary precursors of the future genital organs which are not distinguishable as male or female: sex glands, which will become either ovaries or testes, and two pairs of blind-ended ducts opening into the *cloaca*, in common with the gut. It is only after about the sixth week that male–female developments diverge. Of the two pairs of ducts, one is destined to mature into the female apparatus, or the other pair into the male, whilst the undeveloped pair in either case normally shrivels away, apart from small anatomical vestiges. The primordial female genital ducts were described by Müller, a distinguished German anatomist and physiologist, in 1825, and hence are known as Müllerian ducts. The innermost parts of these ducts remain separate, and become the Fallopian tubes, or oviducts; the lower parts fuse, and develop into the uterus and vagina. The primordial male genital ducts are known as Wolffian, after the description in 1759 by Wolff, a German anatomist and physiologist (regarded as the founder of the scientific study of embryology). These remain separate on the two sides: the innermost parts develop branches of multiple coiled tubules, which link up with the developing testes, forming the *epididymis*; the rest of each duct forms a vas deferens (opening into the urethra) and a seminal vesicle. Each testis at first lies in the back of the abdomen but gradually descends to the groin, and usually at about seven months of gestation travels through the *inguinal canal* — a channel between attachments of abdominal muscles and ligaments — to reach the scrotum.

The rudimentary external genitalia are similarly common to male and female in the early weeks of fetal life. A midline 'genital tubercle' appears and enlarges into a primitive *phallus*, destined to become either a clitoris or a penis; two *labioscrotal swellings* grow on either side and later fuse into a scrotum in the male, or remain apart as the labia in the female.

A fetus with male chromosomes starts to produce testosterone in its gonads in the second month. It is this which causes the primitive ducts to develop in the male direction. In the absence of such influence, development will be female.

The appearance of the external genitalia at birth is of course the acknowledged diagnostic criterion of sex. But it is occasionally misleading. Some rare individuals who are genetically male may have apparently female genitalia, and vice versa. From the above embryological account it is not difficult to imagine, for example, that a failure at one stage of development could leave the potential scrotum unfused: combined with nondescent of the testes, the infant would appear more female than male.   SHEILA JENNETT

See PLATE 8.

See also ANTENATAL DEVELOPMENT; GENDER; SEX DETERMINATION; SEX HORMONES.

Genius The notion of 'genius' has been used, primarily since the Renaissance, as a way of describing and explaining individuals of surpassing intellectual or artistic brilliance — it may

thus be seen as a secular analogue to the religious idea of holiness. Like that sacred attribute, genius is mainly marked by qualities that are moral, mental, and spiritual; but in certain traditions genius has also been supposed to be indicated by certain physical traits, and even perhaps caused by essentially somatic factors.

For 2000 years a body image bequeathed by Greek philosophy held sway amongst doctors and the educated, known as the 'humoral model'. The body's state was broadly grasped in terms of natural rhythms of development and change, determined by the major fluids constrained within the skin envelope, their balance producing health, their upset causing illness. Classically, these crucial juices sustaining vitality were blood, choler (or yellow bile), phlegm, and melancholy (or black bile). Excess of black bile would produce pathological conditions that would lead to depression. Aretaeus (*c.* AD 150–200), in his *De Causis et Signis Morborum*, thus described the condition:

> The patients are dull or stern: dejected or unreasonably torpid, without any manifest cause: such is the commencement of melancholy, and they also become peevish, dispirited, sleepless, and start up from a disturbed sleep. Unreasonable fears also seize them …They are prone to change their mind readily, to become base, mean-spirited, liberal.

But in a parallel tradition attributed to Aristotle, that self-same black fluid (melancholy) was also said to be the humour of genius. A combination of fundamental physical attributes (dark hair, a swarthy complexion, black eyes) and personality traits (sudden and erratic movements, rapid mood swings from lethargy to excitability, indifference to hunger and other bodily needs and wants) were supposed to distinguish gifted and creative individuals. Melancholy malcontents like Prince Hamlet, dressed all in black, were difficult, disdainful, dangerous. Yet, for Hamlet' or for Jaques in *As You Like It*, there was also something bittersweet to be savoured in a contemplative sorrow; Jacques spoke of sucking 'melancholy out of a stone'. Melancholy thus was seen as the midwife of poetry and philosophy, as was exhaustively discussed in Robert Burton's *Anatomy of Melancholy* (1621).

A newly eligible mode of melancholy emerged in the age of sensibility and in the Romantic era. Amongst social and artistic élites, it became rather fashionable to parade as a hypersensitive soul, one whose personality was too delicate, whose nerves were too highly strung, to cope with a high-pressure urban milieu. For a fashionable man-about-town like James Boswell (1740–95), who wrote a magazine column under the penname 'The Hypochondriack', it became the done thing to be depressed, or to put on a show of depression, because torment and suffering were hallmarks of a beautiful soul, proofs of superior sensibility.

Fashionable melancholy had an exquisite future ahead of it. On both sides of the Atlantic, eminent Victorians revelled in hypochondria (mainly a male condition), hysteria (strictly for

the ladies), and the 'blue devils' (a form of dyspepsia, validating invalidism).

In particular, élite depression underwent a gender switch, becomely closely associated with women — and with 'effeminate' males. Traditional images of creative depression had been man centred. The traditional genius, poet, or artist was male. From the eighteenth century, however, and especially with the foregrounding of the image of the hysteric, melancholy genius became feminized. The novels of Mary Wollstonecraft (1759–97) popularized the image of a heroine becoming victimized and crazed through being too sensitive to survive in a heartless world. Depressive, hysterical, suicidal, and self-destructive behaviour among unstable artists have become deeply associated, since early-Victorian times, with images of womanhood; in the psychiatric profession, in the public mind, and amongst women themselves. The old links between writing, genius, and melancholy were traditionally fixed upon male intellectuals like John Milton, author of *Il Penseroso* (1632), or Matthew Green, author of *The Spleen* (1737). During the last 150 years, they have undergone a sex-change, clustering around female writers like Emily Dickinson, Virginia Woolf, Sylvia Plath, Anne Sexton, and Janet Frame. The explanation was said to lie in female physiology — above all in creative gynaecological disturbance or more sensitive nervous physiology.

In modern times, the linking of melancholy with genius has assumed two further twists. The Romantic movement renewed the interest in the mad genius that had been cultivated by Renaissance Platonism but dampened by the age of reason. From Blake, through Hölderlin, to Schumann, poets and composers either gloried in their transcendental visions or believed that madness was the inevitable price of creativity.

Then, in the last third of the nineteenth century, *degenerationist psychiatry* turned the tables. Leading clinical spokesmen for the 'degenerationist' position, notably the Italian Cesare Lombroso, or, in Britain, Theo Hyslop, began to contend that the 'madness' of artists and writers (including their Bohemian disregard for conventional respectabilities) revealed them as sociopaths, moral cripples, and, generally, undesirables. Lombroso summed up and added to a long tradition that held that geniuses (and their cousins, degenerates) were visibly distinctive through physical and physiognomical marks as well as by personality traits. Amongst the main physical signs, he believed, were large ears, irregular teeth, asymmetry of the face and head, left handedness, stammering, a tubercular disposition, and a tendency towards sterility. Lombroso was also convinced that geniuses were commonly short of stature — he cited by way of evidence Aristotle, Linnaeus, Gibbon, Beethoven, Heine, and both the Brownings. Such traditions lingered into the twentieth century; Havelock Ellis believed that a statistically significant proportion of geniuses suffered from gout.

The close of the nineteenth century brought a further extraordinarily fruitful development. A new possibility opened up for the hordes of neuropaths, neurasthenics, hysterics, and hypochondriacs who had emerged in Biedermeier and Victorian bourgeois society and filled the clinics and health spas of affluent Europe and America: *Freudian psychoanalysis*. Since the eighteenth century, the depressed person had been depicted as attention-seeking. From the time of Freud (1856–1939), neurosis offered the possibility of being infinitely fascinating — but its stress on the unconscious threatened to severe the ties long linking genius to the body. ROY PORTER

Further reading

Murray, P. (ed.) (1989). *Genius: the history of an idea*. Blackwell, Oxford.

See also HUMOURS; HYPOCHONDRIA; INTELLIGENCE; NERVOUSNESS.

Genocide

The term 'genocide' was introduced in 1944 by Raphael Lemkin, who had escaped from German-occupied Poland to the US. As a child in the new Polish state Lemkin sensed the vulnerability of Jews, as an ethnic minority, to coercive states; his expertise in international law prompted him to develop the term to describe the systematic annihilation of an ethnic group, religion, or culture. To Lemkin's dismay, the Nuremberg Medical Trial did not recognise genocide as a crime, although medical experiments were defined as a crime against humanity. Lemkin drafted the International Convention on the Prevention and Punishment of the Crime of Genocide, which was adopted by the United Nations General Assembly in Paris on 9 December 1948. It was only in 1988 that the US ratified the Convention.

Although medicine at its best is antithetical to genocide, at its worst it has facilitated genocidal atrocities. The biomedical sciences (broadly conceived) have supplied rationales for defining degenerate races. Anthropologists collecting specimens accelerated the demise of the Tasmanians, who at the turn of the century were regarded as one of the most primitive races. Physiological sciences assisted in racial classification, for example with the use of blood groups, which were linked to racial types. This reached a culmination with the Nazi measures of racial screening and genocide in the occupied East. Josef Mengele had doctorates in anthropology and medicine, and other racial experts attempted to identify residual Germanic elements among the Slavs. Not only Jews, but also gypsies were defined by the Nazis as meriting total eradication, and numerous other 'races', such as the Slaves, were subjected to atrocities. Medical expertise was essential to maintain the fitness of higher races by eliminating the mentally ill and the severely disabled, and preventing reproduction of carriers of inherited diseases.

Medical expertise has provided techniques of extermination. The development of the Zyklon gas chamber was transferred from sanitary practices of delousing. Instead of killing the insect vectors of diseases, the Nazis tried to kill the human hosts of the pathogens. Each of the Nazi crematoria at Auschwitz could kill and dispose of a thousand bodies each day. This represented a highly medicalised form of genocide, using techniques and ideas of hygiene.

Genocidal measures provided an opportunity for advancing medical knowledge by the performance of human experiments, and the collection of specimens of the killed. Again, this is well illustrated by Nazi medicine. Anatomical collections included the skeletons, brains, organs, and tissue samples of persons deemed racially inferior. These collections often remained in German medical institutes until the 1990s. The anatomical atlas of Pernkopf, long a standard work, contained material from children killed in a Viennese hospital, and he also used corpses of executed persons for teaching purposes. German concentration camp experiments were conducted to determine the point that death sets in under extreme conditions of cold or immersion in seawater. Other experimental victims were used to test new vaccines and drugs after deliberate infection.

Despite Lemkin's efforts to prevent repetition of Nazi atrocities, the crime of genocide can all easily occur. '*Ethnic cleansing*' in the former Yugoslavia had a number of disturbing features, not least the prominence of physicians among the Bosnian Serb leadership. Large-scale massacres do not necessarily require medical expertise: the Turkish killing of the Armenians during World War I or the tragic massacres in Rwanda in 1995 show that all that might be necessary for such measures is to set in motion death marches — when persons would die from exhaustion — or to wield a simple machete. Genocide seems likely to remain one of the most horrific forms of pathological human behaviour.

P. J. WEINDLING

Further reading

Kuper, L. (1977). *The pity of it all*. Gerald Duckworth, London.

Horowitz, I. (1976). *Genocide: state power and mass murder*. Transaction Books, New Brunswick.

Weindling, P. J. (1989). *Health, race and german politics between national unification and Nazism*. Cambridge University Press.

See also EUGENICS; KILLING; RACISM; WAR.

Genome

The total DNA sequence that characterizes a species, including man. The Human Genome Project, aimed at sequencing the DNA in human chromosomes, was completed at the end of the millennium. A.W.C.

Genotype

The total set of *alleles* possessed by an organism. (Alleles are genes, which may be different or identical, that occupy matching sites on each of a pair of chromosomes.) Expression of these is responsible for the PHENOTYPE of the individual, which can be modified by environmental pressures. A.W.C.

See GENETICS, HUMAN; PHENOTYPE.

Germ cells

(germinal cells) Cells which will eventually mature into SPERM or OVA, which are also known as gametes. In the early embryo germ cells migrate from the yolk sac into a group of cells known as the *gonad primordia*. The primordia develop into either a TESTIS or an OVARY. In the testis the germ cells become *spermatogonia*, which will divide and eventually become spermatozoa. In the ovary the germ cells become *oogonia*, are enclosed in a follicle, and are then capable of maturing into ova. S.A.W.

See OVA; SPERM.

Gestures

According to the *Concise Oxford Dictionary*, 'gesture' refers to 'a significant movement of limb or body' or the 'use of such movements as expression of feeling or rhetorical device'. This is a broad definition, encompassing essentially the whole carriage and deportment of the body. Though this was the original meaning of the term, today it is generally limited to indicating a movement of the head (including FACIAL EXPRESSION) or of the arms and hands. A gesture may be inadvertent (BLUSHING, fumbling with one's clothes, etc.) or deliberate (nodding, making the V-sign, etc.). Most scholars agree that a degree of volition should be implied. They also acknowledge that there are no watertight divisions between posture and gesture, or between voluntary (or 'conventional') and involuntary (or 'natural') gestures; indeed, these divisions have a history of their own.

Many gestures function independently of the spoken word. A lucid survey of such 'autonomous' gestures may be found in *Gestures: Their Origin and Distributions* (1979; revised as *Bodytalk: A World Guide to Gesture* in 1994) by the ethologist Desmond Morris. Particular types of autonomous gesture are the sign languages of the deaf and dumb and of various tribal and monastic communities.

Since the 1970s most studies undertaken by anthropologists, sociolinguists, and social psychologists have focused on gestures that accompany SPEECH ('gesticulation'). Using video and other audio-visual techniques it was shown that speech and gesticulation are produced together, as though they are two aspects of a single underlying process. Many studies have been devoted to the nature of this matching, to the question of how phrases of speech production are related to phrases of gesticulation. In addition, older classifications of speech-related gesture were qualified and new ones introduced. A well-known classification is that of 'beats', 'pointers', 'ideographs', and 'pictorial gestures'. Beats (or 'batons') beat time to the rhythm of the words. Pointers (or 'indexical gestures') point to the object of the words (either a concrete referent in the immediate environment or an abstract referent, such as a point of view brought forward by the speaker). Ideographs only refer to abstract referents; they diagram the logical structure of what is said. In contrast, pictorial gestures, essentially the gestures of the mime artist, refer to concrete objects and activities.

315

Gesture has been studied (and practised) from many perspectives. Since antiquity, speech-related gesture has been part of rhetoric. For example, both Cicero (106–43 BC) and Quintilian (c. AD 35–100) wrote extensively on delivery (Greek *hupokrisis*; Latin *actio* or *pronuntiatio*), deeming it no less important than the other four departments of oratory: *inventio*, *dispositio*, *elocutio*, and *memoria*. Quintilian was the first to explicitly distinguish delivery into *vox* (voice) and *gestus* (i.e. the general carriage of the body). Interestingly, Cicero was already using notions such as 'body language' (*sermo corporis*) or the 'eloquence of the body' (*eloquentia corporis*).

Both Cicero's and Quintilian's writings were crucial to the flowering of rhetoric in the Renaissance. Delivery, however, had a modest impact. It is true that classical 'contrapposto' was more or less 'reconquered' by Leon Battista Alberti (1404–72) (and by later authors such as Leonardo da Vinci, Michelangelo, Georgio Vasari, and Giovanni Paolo Lomazzo) on the basis of a passage from Quintilian. However, it is significant that the text in question was not on delivery. It merely referred to the Discobolos of Myron (c. 450 BC), one of the finest examples of classical contrapposto, as an illustration to *elocutio*. Just as this statue in abandoning the straight line suggests movement and grace, the speaker too should favour an ornate style and introduce grace and variety. Even when, at the beginning of the fifteenth century, the complete text of Quintilian's *Institution oratoria* and Cicero's rhetorical works became available, scholars kept complaining about the impracticability of classical delivery. They found it hardly conducive to contemporary oratory and some, including the German rhetorician Philippus Melanchton (1497–1560), disposed of classical *pronuntiatio* altogether.

The tradition of the 'civilization of manners' is another perspective in which the study and practice of gesture has been prominent (and still is!). The sixteenth century experienced an explosion of such texts, though many of these display a disinterest in classical *actio* or *pronuntiatio* similar to that in the contemporary texts on rhetoric. One can hardly say, as did Jacob Burckhardt and so many later historians, including Norbert Elias, that the rules propounded in these manuals originated in the classical or courtly tradition. As was shown by the English historian Dilwyn Knox, many of these texts derive from the *disciplina corporis*, from the monastic and clerical precepts of comportment which from the thirteenth century on had been communicated to the laity. For example, it was this tradition — reaching back to the *De institutione novitiorum*, possibly composed by the canon regular Hugh of St Victor (d. 1142) — that provided the framework for Erasmus' idea of *civilitas*, set forth in his *De civilitate morum puerilium* (1530), and for all the texts based on it, including other manuals on proper comportment, the numerous Latin school curricula, and the regulations of the new Catholic orders, including the Jesuits.

The second half of the sixteenth century witnessed a new interest in gesture. At this time notions of civility were adopted in most European countries, both by the court and by the urban elite. Generally, this development followed a course of restraint, compared with the excess of gesture attributed to the peasant population, the inhabitants of southern Europe (in particular, from the seventeenth century onwards, the Italians), and many of the newly-discovered peoples in the East and West. At the same time, the concept was set off against the mere appearance of manners and all exaggerated civility. The background to all of this was the late medieval aesthetic-cum-moral conviction already implied in the monastic and clerical codes of comportment of a close correspondence between physical expression and inner disposition.

It was also in this emphasis on the moral, or universal, rather than the conventional nature of gesture, that civility and the study of PHYSIOGNOMY came together. An informative example is *De humana physiognomonia*, published in 1586 by the Neapolitan dramatist Giambattista della Porta (1535–1615). Later studies related physiognomy to the passions, as in the *Conférence sur l'expression* (1698) by the French court painter Charles Lebrun (1619–90), or to the so-called 'moral sentiments', as in the *Ideen zu einer Mimik* by the German scholar Johann Jakob Engel (1742–1802). As these studies reveal, gesture was now also studied and practiced from the perspective of contemporary painting and stagecraft.

The late sixteenth and seventeenth centuries also witnessed a philosophical interest in gesture. In 1572, for example, the Spanish scholar Arias Montanus published his *Liber Ieremiae, sive de actione* (also dealing with dress!), in which he argued for the universality of gesture. Similarly, Giovanni Bonifacio's *L'arte de' cenni* (1616) and John Bulwer's *Chirologia: or the Naturall Language of the Hand* (1644) were conceived as manuals of rhetorical delivery. However, both authors professed their belief in a natural, universal language of gesture, opining that its often noted diversity could be reduced to a few general principles, thus facilitating the conduct of trade, not only in Europe, but also in the recently discovered New World and Far East. In the process, classical delivery was revalued, as 'natural' gesture — in contrast to merely 'conventional' gesture — became increasingly identified with the Graeco–Roman tradition. Eventually this philosophical interest inspired the late seventeenth- and eighteenth-century discussions on universal language schemes.

A quite different, strongly antiquarian, approach to classical gesture was offered by the Neapolitan scholar Andrea de Jorio in his *La mimica degli antichi investigata nel gestire Napoletano* (1832). Based on the idea that the lively gestures of his poorer fellow townsmen, the *volgo*, were a direct legacy of the Romans, he interpreted them as a key for understanding the mimic codes on antique vases, murals, and reliefs. Offering an extensive survey of all the gestures he witnessed in

the streets of Naples, de Jorio's study is still highly original. At the same time, he was very much a nineteenth-century scholar in his selection of a contemporary phenomenon among the lower classes, not for its concrete significance to these individuals, but as a 'relic' or 'survival' of the past. In the same decades the romantic folklorists, in particular Jacob Grimm, professed a similar approach aimed at the Germanic past, just as later in the century well-known evolutionists, including E. B. Tylor or Wilhelm Wundt, took an interest in gesture, not for its role within their own contemporary culture, but for the entry it was supposed to afford to the origins of language. Remarkably, both evolutionists were careful not to associate the more lively gesticulation of Italians (and southern Frenchmen) with a 'lack of civilization' or with any 'primitivism'.

In a famous essay, called *Les techniques du corps* (1935), the French anthropologist Marcel Mauss discussed gesture independently of any evolutionary schemes. Defined as 'the ways in which from society to society men know how to use their bodies', his 'techniques' included a wide range of phenomena: from sitting, standing, walking, dancing, swimming, and sleeping to table manners and matters of hygiene. At the same time his comparative approach ranged from the gait of American nurses (Mauss spent some time in a New York hospital), to the delicate balancing of the hips displayed by Maori women in New Zealand. Anticipating the writings of American anthropologists, in particular those of Ruth Benedict and Mary Douglas, Mauss was greatly interested in the ways physiology, psychology, and sociology converged in his techniques, and he emphasized the role of education, adopting (well before Pierre Bourdieu) the notion of *habitus* in its Aristotelian and Thomist sense of *hexis* or 'acquired ability'.

Mauss' essay is one source of inspiration for current research, another is David Efron's *Gesture, Race and Culture* (1972; first published in 1941, under the title *Gesture and Environment*), actually the first systematic study of cultural difference in gesture. Encouraged by the anthropologist Franz Boas, for two years Efron studied the use of gesture of two ethnic groups in New York City: Jewish Yiddish-speaking immigrants, and immigrants from southern Italy. Using drawings, photography, and film, Efron and his colleagues found some significant differences. The Italians, for example, used both arms, generally needed more space for their gesticulation, and stood mostly apart from one another. In contrast, the Jewish immigrants gestured mostly in front of their faces or chests, stood together in small groups, and touched one another frequently. Similarly, the Italian immigrants displayed a range of 'symbolic' gestures (many corresponding to de Jorio's inventory), while the Jews displayed a preference for 'beats' and 'ideographs'. Arguing against theories that regarded gesture as racially determined, Efron could also show that the various differences were already less conspicuous in the second generation of the two groups, as they absorbed much of the American mimic code they saw around them. Efron's study was also one of the first to focus on speech-related gesture.

In the 1950s, a group of anthropologists, sociolinguists, and social psychologists turned to the study of non-verbal communication. The anthropologist Ray Birdwhistell coined the notion of 'kinesics' (the study of communicative body movements), just as his colleague, Edward T. Hall, and others introduced such terms as 'proxemics' (the study of the distance people keep from each other when talking), 'haptics' (the study of the way they touch each other during the conversation), and 'social space'. In the following decades many of these insights were included in the fast-growing fields of studies on face-to-face interaction and semiotics. In the 1970s, art historians, such as Michael Baxandall and Moshe Barasch, turned to the study of gesture in Italian painting of the fourteenth and the fifteenth centuries, followed in the 1980s by a much broader interest in gesture (and also in posture and comportment) on the part of intellectual historians — literary historians; historians of rhetoric, the stage, and dance; and a wide range of historians of everyday life, including Jean–Claude Schmitt and Peter Burke. Only recently, however, have attempts been made to develop an interdisciplinary approach: to integrate more fully the insights of anthropologists and sociolinguists with a historical approach, and also to follow the history of gestures as encoded in everyday life and in their 'recoded' quality in painting, sculpture, stagecraft, literature, and so on.   HERMAN ROODENBURG

See also BODY LANGUAGE.

Ghost When asked if he believed in ghosts, Coleridge replied that he had seen too many to put any trust in their reality. Verifying their existence does not, according to psychics, always depend upon believing the evidence of one's eyes or ears. Freud attributes a belief in ghosts to our sense of 'the Uncanny', whereas the Society for Psychical Research, who first met in 1882, attune themselves to empirical manifestations, as in monitoring changes in atmosphere such as unaccountable drops in temperature.

The moot point is whether ghosts are real or whether they belong in the eye or sixth sense of the beholder. Aside from such epistemological questions regarding the nature of reality, even the question of belief in the ghostly is fraught with ambivalence. For example, while denying that she believed in ghosts, Madame du Deffand admitted to being afraid of them. The reality of such fears is borne out by the evidence of tombstones testifying to those who died of fright after seeing a ghost. Those foolhardy enough to spend the night at London's most famous haunted house at 50 Berkeley Square, for instance, did not always live to tell the tale.

Traditionally being a deceased person who appears to the living, a ghost can also appear as a reanimated corpse or even be a supernatural spirit of a non-human variety or animal spirit phantom, as in Edgar Allan Poe's *The Black Cat* (1843). Associated often with a particular building, ghosts can be the restless spirits of suicides, those denied a resting place, or those who have met a violent death; hence the grisly apparitions of mutilated or dismembered bodies, like Matthew 'Monk' Lewis' Bleeding Nun, or the headless woman, whose image graces many a public house sign across Britain.

Women have been regarded as being particularly sensitive to psychic phenomena. Spiritualism was in vogue for the Victorians, especially since the mechanics of spirit possession involving the female medium, who was overwhelmed by a greater force, reinforced the normative feminine ideal of passive surrender. The empowerment this entailed for women, both mentally and physically, once in the spirit mode was a subversion of the restrictions of femininity. The potential for transgressive behaviour when 'out of the body' could manifest itself through blasphemous and obscene language that would drive sitters away from the seance table. Not only could the medium be unruly, but so too could be the spirit or apparition, especially if it turned into a poltergeist which specialized in creating physical disturbances. In Noel Coward's play *Blithe Spirit* (1941), the troublesome ghost of Elvira appears after a table-rapping session to meddle in her ex-husband's new marriage.

Control over the spirit world through necromancy or the raising of the dead has traversed history from the biblical Witch of Endor, who raises the prophet Samuel's spirit (1 Samuel 28: 11–19) to Aleister Crowley's invocation of the Great God Pan, the result of which allegedly drove him mad. The ghosts of those who died insane or incarcerated against their will have 'lived on' to torment their captors and ancestors. Jenny Spinner, after being imprisoned in the East Wing of Knebworth House in Hertfordshire, supposedly worked so hard at her spinning wheel that she went mad. One version of her 'autobiography' describes how she faked suicide to effect her escape by impersonating her own ghost. That her ghost was reputed to have haunted the East Wing until it was demolished in 1811 is an irony she had not foreseen. Spinner's story probably inspired a later owner of Knebworth House, Edward Bluwer–Lytton, who wrote the short story *The Haunted and the Haunters* (1857). At his ancestral home, Bulwer–Lytton entertained Charles Dickens and Wilkie Collins, fellow ghost story writers, who picnicked at midnight in the tower bedroom, which is reputed to be still haunted.

The origin of the term 'ghost' is shrouded in cobweb-like uncertainty, which dates back to pre-Teutonic origins. Like the wailing banshee who is a harbinger of death, the ghost cries out for a narrative context, since even the most disembodied ghost needs to be fleshed out with a ghost story. Apparitions and spectres are the cast of a story-line replayed through time, like the lonely sentinel who haunts Chester's Roman ruins or the hungry ghosts of famine-stricken Ireland. Such phantom theatre is captured best by a narrator reciting a spine-chilling tale in a haunted setting to a receptive audience. Ghosts need ghost stories in order to preserve for themselves their most tangible and enduring after-death existence.

Whether ghosts emanate from some mysterious ECTOPLASM, or are the product of psychical projection emanating from electromagnetic fields glavanized by certain individuals and generated by certain locations, or are psychosomatic HALLUCINATIONS, is still unknown. Do the ghost and ancestral spirit stories of so many cultures represent a subconscious challenge to a collective fear of death, or do they express the uncertainty surrounding our individual corporeality? Having survived the advent of the electric light bulb, ghosts appear to be here to stay. Neither do they fear to tread beyond the traditional boundaries of the ivy-covered Gothic ruin. Nowadays psychic investigators and exorcists are invited to hauntings that take place on recently built housing estates. Like Oscar Wilde's eponymous hero in *The Canterville Ghost* (1887), for whom clanking chains and a creaking suit of armour were *passé*, the modern ghost is moving into new territory, such as the world of the computer, where its ghostly presence ventures to compete with the virtual realities of cyberspace.

MARIE MULVEY-ROBERTS

See also ECTOPLASM.

Giants Stories of men of great stature are found everywhere in legends and traditions of almost every culture in the history of mankind. The presence of these beings of extraordinary height, usually called giants, was traditionally associated with feelings of terror and impotence, their enormous size being closely related to the fear or wonder that they produced. In the West, we find early examples of such stories in the mythology of the classical world and in the Bible. The Titans, for instance, were described as beings of astounding stature and even greater strength who dared to rebel against the Olympian gods. The most clear representative of physical strength, however, has always been associated with the figure of HERCULES, whose height was said to be about 7 feet. In the sacred texts, many other allusions can also be found to peoples and races of extraordinary height. The Nephilim were the first people to be referred to by the name of giants in the book of Genesis. Equally interesting, but perhaps more famous, are the cases of Og, king of Basham — whose story is related in the book of Joshua — and Goliath, in the second book of Samuel, who was said to have measured about 10 feet.

Legends like these, and many others, survived in both Eastern and Western traditions. They were compiled in medieval encyclopedias and books of wonders, and extended by the accounts provided by new chronicles or traveller's reports. Apart from being the subject of mythological legends and fairy tales, this phenomenon of

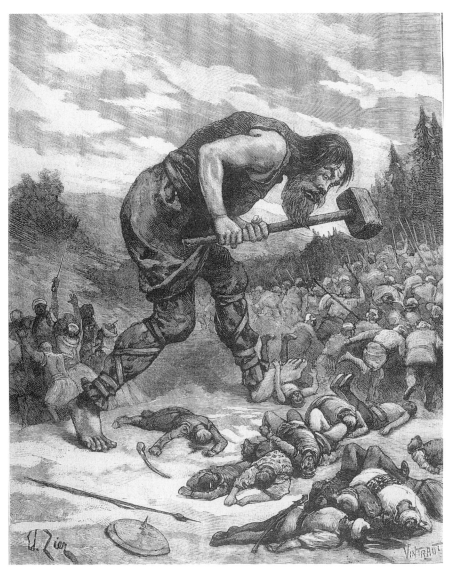

When the Saracens invaded southern France, a giant is said to have driven them back with his hammer, near Castelsarrasin (near Albi) as illustrated in *Journal des Voyages*, January 1897. Mary Evans Picture Library.

sixteenth century onwards, many giants attracted the attention of kings and served as janitors, as porters, or as members of their private bodyguard. Specially famous was Oliver Cromwell's giant porter, named Daniel, whose height — of approximately 7 feet 6 inches — is marked by a big 'O' in the walls of Windsor Castle. Equally notorious was the army of giants that the king of Prussia, Federick I, stationed in Postdam at the beginning of the eighteenth century, and that became so famous throughout Europe that even the philosopher Voltaire occasionally made reference to it. One of the most celebrated cases of the eighteenth century was that of Charles Byrne, 'the Irish giant', who was 8 feet 4 inches tall, and whose skeleton ended up in the Royal College of Surgeons, very likely stolen by the famous anatomist and surgeon John Hunter. At the beginning of the eighteenth century, the Abbé Henrion, a member of the French Academy, taught that, as a consequence of original sin, there had been a progressive reduction of the height of men from the time of Adam until the arrival of Christ. Following his own calculations, Henrion stated that Adam had been 125 feet high, Eve 118, Noah 100, Abraham 28, Moses 13, Alexandre 6, and Julius Caesar 5. Though this idea never gained credibility among the scientific community, it remained quite popular within the Republic of Letters.

During the nineteenth and twentieth centuries, unusually tall persons were exhibited for profit in circuses and freak shows. Given the social and physical barriers they had to encounter during their lives, many of these 'giants' were forced to make a career as human oddities. Specially notorious was the case of the American Robert Wadlow who, despite his height of 8 feet 11 inches, tried desperately until the moment of this death in 1940 to be considered neither a freak nor a medical case. He sued the American Medical Association for having cast him as a 'preacromegalic giant'. Though he lost the case on technicalities, he may legitimately be credited with having been the last 'giant' of the twentieth century.　　　　J. MOSCOSO

Further reading

Bonheim, H. (1994). The giant in literature and in medical practice. *Literature and Medicine*, 13, 243–54.

See also GROWTH HORMONE; PITUITARY GLAND.

inordinate bodily growth has been a clinical problem since the condition of '*acromegaly*' was first described, and related to enlargement of the PITUITARY GLAND, in the nineteenth century. '*Pituitary gigantism*' is now known to be caused by excessive secretion of GROWTH HORMONE, starting before the length of the long bones is irrevocably fixed after adolescence. Abnormal growth elsewhere in the body, whether in such rare 'giants' or in those who (more commonly) develop the pituitary problem in their maturity, constitutes the condition of acromegaly. The symptoms of this illness are legion, including widespread abnormal growth of tissues and organs, with swelling of the lips and ears, pain in the joints, and impaired vision. As the scholar Helmut Bonheim has shown, many of these symptoms are also found in mythological figures and explain part of the lore of giants in myth and literature. For example, Polyphemus, the cyclops described by Homer, and who was depicted as

being of extraordinary stature, could have gained his reputation of being one-eyed as a result of an abnormal growth of his pituitary gland, which, pressing on the optical nerves, may have diminished vision in both eyes or produced blindness in one of them. Bonheim also argues that perhaps the same condition of the giant's sight could have been advantageous to David in defeating Goliath, as some illustrations of this biblical scene seem to confirm. Many other features traditionally associated with giants, like their extraordinary appetite or their bodily deformities, may be explained in terms of the symptoms associated with acromegaly.

From a mere historical point of view, one of the first giants we have an account of was John Middleton, who lived at the end of the sixteenth century and reached a height of 9 feet 3 inches. As in many other similar cases, 'the childe of Hale' attracted so much notoriety that he was given audience by King James I. Indeed, from the

Gland A group of cells with a communal secretory function. EXOCRINE *glands* incorporate a duct, or a system of ducts like tributaries leading to a river, which open onto an external or internal body surface. Some are simple or spiral pits (such as sweat glands in the SKIN or those which secrete acid and enzymes into the STOMACH) with a few secreting cells in their depths; others vary in size and complexity from the small *salivary glands* to the *mammary glands* (BREASTS). ENDOCRINE *glands* by contrast are ductless, and secrete hormones directly into the bloodstream. The activity of all glands is regulated by chemical or nervous signals, or both. Molecules in the local environment, or brought by the blood, or released from nerve endings of the AUTONOMIC NERVOUS SYSTEM bind to cell MEMBRANE RECEPTORS, starting a sequence of signals within the cells which results in an increase (or decrease) in extrusion of their own particular secretion.

The nodular enlargements which can be felt under the skin in association with an infection (such as those in the neck with a sore throat) are commonly called swollen 'lymph glands', but they are not secretory and are more correctly called *lymph nodes*.   S.J.

See ADRENAL GLANDS; ALIMENTARY SYSTEM; BREASTS; HORMONES; PANCREAS; PARATHYROID GLANDS; PITUITARY GLAND; SWEATING; THYROID.

Glia

(or glial cells) and *neurons* (nerve cells) are the two major types of cells in the NERVOUS SYSTEM. While neurons are excitable — generating electrical impulses that transmit information throughout the CENTRAL NERVOUS SYSTEM (CNS) and the peripheral nervous system (PNS) — glia are non-excitable cells that serve a wide range of essential functions in support of neurons.

The term 'glia' was coined by Virchow in 1846 and can be translated as 'glue' or 'putty'. The classical view of glia is that they form the packing material within which nerve cells are embedded, similar to the CONNECTIVE TISSUE of peripheral organs. Indeed, a major function of glia, recognized a century ago by the great Spanish anatomist Ramón y Cajal, is to provide structural and physical support for neurons. However, glial cells account for half the bulk of the CNS and outnumber neurons 10 to 1: a window with 10 parts putty to 1 part glass would not be very enlightening! In fact, glia are dynamic elements of the nervous system, performing a variety of other essential functions. The different types of glial cells can collectively be considered as supporting and protecting neurons in the healthy brain and also defending it in all forms of pathological insult.

The main kinds of glia are *Schwann cells* in the PNS; *astrocytes* and *oligodendrocytes* in the CNS; and *ependymal* cells, forming the lining of the ventricles of the brain. In common with neurons, all these glia are produced by cell division in the *embryonic neuroectoderm* (indeed, early in development some of the dividing stem cells produce both neurons and glia among their 'daughter' cells). Unlike neurons, glia can undergo cell division in the adult and are capable of self-renewal and regeneration.

Oligodendrocytes and Schwann cells have, as their main role, the production of the fatty MYELIN sheaths that insulate many of the fibres or axons of nerve cells, throughout the nervous system. Myelination increases substantially the speed of conduction of nerve impulses (ACTION POTENTIALS). Destruction of the myelinating glial cells leads to *demyelination*, which causes slowing and eventual block of impulse conduction and hence loss of function (both sensation and the control of movement). The results can be devastating, as in the human demyelinating diseases Multiple Sclerosis (MS) and infectious polyneuritis, which respectively affect the CNS and the PNS.

There are many Schwann cells in the PNS and oligodendrocytes in the grey matter of the CNS that do not form myelin, and little is known about their function. In the developing PNS, and following injury and degeneration of peripheral nerve fibres, Schwann cells have an important 'trophic' role — meaning that they produce substances (called 'trophins') that promote regrowth of the axons. Conversely, for reasons that remain somewhat mysterious, damaged axons in the adult CNS do not spontaneously regenerate (at least not over long distances) and this is partly due to the fact that oligodendrocytes actually produce proteins that inhibit axon growth. It is noteworthy that transplantation of Schwann cells from peripheral nerves into the CNS can promote regeneration of damaged CNS axons in animals, and this procedure is being pursued in the hope of developing new treatments for damage to the human spinal cord and brain.

Astrocytes are star-shaped (stellate) cells with long, radiating extensions or processes (rather like the dendrites of neurons). During development, the primitive nervous system first appears as a tube (the neural tube) running along the back of the embryo. The first astrocytes extend their processes to span the walls of this tube (some of these are called 'radial glia'). The stem cells that give rise to neurons (*neuroblasts*) attach themselves to these glia, and the immature nerve cells that they produce migrate along the glial processes to take up their final positions (for instance forming the layers of the cerebral cortex at the head end of the neural tube).

Astrocytes in the developing, and in the injured, nervous system release trophins that encourage proliferation and maturation of other glial cells. In the adult CNS, the processes of astrocytes stretch out to wrap around cerebral blood vessels and induce their cells to stick tightly together, thus playing an important role in maintaining the BLOOD-BRAIN BARRIER. Astrocytes are also the true 'glue' of the brain. Their ramifying processes contain fine, strong filaments, giving the brain its physical framework. They also stretch to the boundaries of the CNS, forming a delicate meshwork, the *pia mater*, which covers the entire surface, helping to maintain the shape of the brain.

Besides providing structural support, the processes of many astrocytes wrap themselves around the dendrites, cell bodies, and axons of neurons and play an essential role in HOMEOSTASIS or stabilization of the chemical environment around them. They absorb potassium, which is released by active neurons, and which would, if allowed to build up, depolarize neurons, first causing *hyperexcitability* — a state of affairs akin to epilepsy — and eventually *inexcitability*. Astrocytes near SYNAPSES also mop up the neurotransmitter *glutamate*, which, in excess, is also highly toxic to nerve cells. The build-up of glutamate that occurs when blood flow to an area of brain is inadequate (ischemia) or is cut off (stroke) can cause widespread death of neurons in surrounding areas of the brain. Astrocytes absorb other NEUROTRANSMITTERS, including the inhibitory transmitter, gamma-aminobutyric acid (GABA). This helps to terminate the action of a neurotransmitter when it has taken effect at the appropriate synapse, and to ensure that it does not spread and act inappropriately on neighbouring synapses. Astrocytes also synthesize and release NITRIC OXIDE (NO), which has a variety of actions on blood vessels and on neurons (possibly even involved in the strengthening of synapses that underlies memory).

Astrocytes are involved in brain metabolism, because they are capable of *glycogenesis* (conversion of glucose into GLYCOGEN for storage) in response to various hormones and to potassium and glutamate. They can produce lactate, which neurons can metabolize. Astrocytes are extensively coupled to each other via areas of leaky membrane. These 'gap junctions' allow the passage of calcium, from cell to cell, which spreads in waves, over long distances. These calcium waves can be initiated in response to a variety of physiological and pathological stimuli and in turn regulate many functions of astrocytes, including their response to injury.

Ramón y Cajal noted that astrocytes form scar tissue in damaged brains and nowadays we know that this is due to an increase in the production of the protein (GFAP) that makes up their filaments. The glial scar isolates undamaged brain areas from the site of injury and has a protective role, but it is also believed to inhibit regeneration of axons.

Finally, there is a class of small glial cells, called *microglia*, uniformly distributed throughout the CNS, which are not 'born' in the nervous system but are formed by transformation of certain white blood cells called MACROPHAGES or their precursors, monocytes. Microglia are now thought to be part of the IMMUNE SYSTEM, defending the brain against infection and injury. Like the macrophages from which they develop, they act as scavenging cells or phagocytes — removing debris in the developing or injured CNS. Again like macrophages, they can 'digest' foreign proteins (parts of viruses or bacteria, for example) and display fragments of them on the outer surface of their membranes (called *antigen presentation*). These antigen fragments then stimulate certain white blood cells to produce antibodies to the foreign protein. Microglia also, on activation, secrete various ENZYMES and other molecules that can attack foreign material (proteases, cytokines, reactive oxygen species, and nitric oxide) in the brain. The presumed function of this reaction is to protect the CNS from immunological insult, but it can be damaging. It might, for example, be a factor in killing oligodendrocytes, and hence triggering demyelination in Multiple Sclerosis, an autoimmune disorder.   ARTHUR M. BUTT

Further reading
Ransom, B. R. and Kettenmann, H. (1995). *Neuroglia*. Oxford University Press.

See also BRAIN; CENTRAL NERVOUS SYSTEM; MYELIN.

Glucose is an important source of fuel for the body, especially for the BRAIN and for red blood cells, which use no other fuel. Chemically glucose is a *hexose sugar* or *monosaccharide* — that is, a sugar with 6 carbon atoms and the formula $C_6H_{12}O_6$. Most glucose in the body is derived from the digestion of *polysaccharides* and other sugars: starch, for example, is *polyglucose*; common sugar, or sucrose, a *disaccharide*, is one molecule of glucose combined with one of fructose. In blood the level of glucose is around 90 mg per 100 ml. Glucose is stored in the body in the form of GLYCOGEN in body cells, especially in the liver and muscle, and is metabolised in tissues to generate the ADENOSINE TRIPHOSHATE (ATP) which provides energy.   A. W. C.

See BLOOD SUGAR; METABOLISM.

Gluten The term 'gluten' comes from the Latin word for glue. The use of the word gluten to describe a sticky proteinatious component of dough was established by the middle of the nineteenth century. Mrs Beeton in her famous *Book of household management* observed that when flour and water were mixed and kneaded, an elastic dough was produced which was best using wheat flour, less satisfactory with rye flour, and inadequate with barley, maize (corn), oats, or rice. This sticky elastic substance, or gluten, is essential for making satisfactory leavened bread. Bubbles of carbon dioxide released from fermenting yeast are trapped by the visco–elastic protein, ensuring a light honeycombed texture for the dough. The elastic nature of gluten also holds particles of the dough together, preventing crumbling during rolling and shaping.

Wheat gluten can be extracted from wheat flour by adding sufficient water to make a kneadable dough which is then washed with a stream of cold water. The water-soluble protein and starch granules are thus flushed away, leaving a sticky mass high in structural plant protein. About 70% of the mass is water and 30% is protein. With drying, a pale, yellow-grey powder is produced. Gluten is poorly soluble in water, but the fraction known as 'gliadin' is soluble in aqueous alcohol. Two thirds of gluten protein is in the form of glutenins, which are insoluble in ethyl alcohol but soluble in a mixture of ethanoic acid, urea, and cetrimide. There are more than 40 different gliadin proteins, which traditionally have been separated by starch gel electrophoresis. The fraction with the fastest mobility is known as alpha gliadin, with progressively slower mobility groups classified as beta, gamma, and omega. These proteins have molecular weights between 30 000 and 40 000. The glutenin proteins are much larger units, mostly around 2 000 000 molecular weight. The glutenin protein chains form a three-dimensional net when hydrated (mixed with water) and this gives the elastic properties to gluten.

Not all sticky plant cereals in our diet contain gluten. A type of rice grown in the Far East known as glutinous or sticky rice contains no proteinatious gluten and owes its sticky nature to a waxy carbohydrate.

The sticky nature of gluten has been utilized as a paper and fabric glue, as in making papier-mâché and wallpaper paste. Wheat gluten has also been used as a cattle feed and as a starting point for the manufacture of the food flavour enhancer, monosodium glutamate.

Although the presence of gluten in wheat flour has been utilised to create a variety of pasta shapes, such as noodles, spaghetti, and tagliatelle, gluten is not an essential human nutrient. There is however, some experimental work to suggest that dietary gluten may be protective against some toxic substances. For example, gluten in the diet of rats reduces the liver toxicity of a known toxic chemical, D-galactosamine.

Gluten and coeliac disease
The importance of gluten in the human diet however, relates to the fact that 1 in 200–300 of the European Caucasian population are intolerant to wheat, barley, and rye gluten.

The lining cells of the small intestine become damaged and the patients develop a condition known as *coeliac disease* or permanent gluten-induced enteropathy. The classical presentation was of a pre-school child with DIARRHOEA and weight loss. Possibly due to nutritional campaigns to delay the introduction of gluten to infant diets, an insidious onset later in childhood, with ANAEMIA and poor growth in height, is now more frequently seen. Onset in adult life may occur, with anaemia, INFERTILITY, and vitamin D deficient bone disease amongst the possible presenting features, although gastrointestinal symptoms and weight loss may, as in children, be the main complaints.

Although this medical condition was described in the first century AD by Aretaeus and accurately, clinically, delineated by a London physician, Dr Samuel Gee, in the late nineteenth century, its cause and cure were not discovered until the 1940s. Dr W. K. Dicke, an astute Dutch physician, noticed that in Holland children with coeliac disease were temporarily cured and improved in health during the World War II famine created by Nazi occupation. He then observed the relapse in their condition when wheat flour was flown in by the Swedish authorities. Subsequent work by Dicke and colleagues and later investigators identified the toxic factor to be an oligopeptide in alpha gliadin.

The practice of cereal cultivation by man started first in the Middle East around 8000 years BC. There was subsequently a gradual spread north and westward. Cereal cultivation arrived late in southwest Ireland, at around 3000 years BC, and wheat was not a staple food until after the potato famine of 1847. The majority of patients suffering from gluten-induced enteropathy (coeliac disease) are of tissue type HLA B8. The incidence of coeliac disease in southwest Ireland, particularly Galway, is amongst the highest in Europe, and there is correspondingly a high prevalence of HLA B8 tissue type. It has been suggested that when populations consume large quantities of gluten from wheat cereals the susceptible HLA B8 individuals develop disease and are at a reproductive disadvantage compared with those not genetically predisposed to the disease, leading to a reduced proportion of B8 individuals in subsequent generations.

Many commercially-prepared foods in Europe contain gluten. Wheat flour is added as a bulking agent in many items of confectionery, as thickeners in sauces, to give bulk and to reduce the cost of meat products, such as sausage meat, and even in some pharmaceutical preparations. It is therefore difficult without a detailed knowledge of the constituents of manufactured foods for an individual to adhere strictly to a gluten free diet. Some food labels indicate the product is gluten free, either in words or as a symbol — an ear of wheat with a cross through it. 'Gluten free' flour and bread are available and usually contain starch from maize (corn) or rice, with some of the elastic properties of gluten being provided by guar gum or similar substances.   T. J. EVANS

See also ALIMENTARY SYSTEM; DIETS.

Glycogen In the 1840s and 50s, Claude Bernard was applying his great scientific mind to the problem of 'sugars' in the body, in particular how the LIVER could apparently make sugars and 'squirt them into the blood … in a regulated manner' when he had fed an animal only on protein. In 1855 he coined the term 'matière glycogene' — sugar-making material. He removed a liver, washed it out with water, and found that there was still sugar in a subsequent wash-out. He concluded that the sugar-forming substance was stored in the liver, and was not water soluble. Eventually he succeeded in isolating the 'emulsive material of the liver', found it to be similar to starch, and listed its properties in an account so complete as to be valid to this day. It was to be over 70 years before the medical significance of glycogen storage came to light, when defective storage in liver, kidney, and heart became recognized. Another 70 years on, and the several associated diseases are well understood, mainly as enzyme deficiencies, whilst deliberate boosting of glycogen storage in muscle before a marathon run is common knowledge.

Glycogen is the form in which CARBOHYDRATE is stored in the body. Each molecule of glycogen is formed by the linkage in branching chains of many thousands of glucose molecules. Thus, glycogen is a natural polymer, a *polysaccharide*, which has a similar structure to the starch which is found in plants.

Most tissues of the body are able to store small amounts of glycogen, but the main sites of glycogen storage are the liver and SKELETAL MUSCLES. In both cases, glycogen is made from glucose within the cells in which it is stored, and the synthetic process is stimulated by the hormone INSULIN. When glycogen is stored within muscle and liver cells, it retains water along with it (approximately 3 g of water for each gram of glycogen), so changes in glycogen content can cause quite noticeable changes in total body weight. For example, in the first few days of STARVATION, glycogen is used by the liver to maintain BLOOD SUGAR and by muscle metabolism, and the associated water is excreted from the body in the urine, accounting for a major part of 1–2 kg loss of weight.

There are important differences between the major functions of liver and muscle glycogen. The main role of liver glycogen is to provide a reserve supply of glucose in order that blood glucose concentration can be kept at an adequate level to supply the brain (which does not use other fuels) during periods of fasting, or when glucose use is increased during physical work and exercise. Thus, after meals some of the carbohydrate consumed is stored as liver glycogen, and during fasting (even just overnight) this glycogen is broken down and the glucose is released into the blood. In a healthy adult, the liver glycogen store is usually between 50 and 100 g, containing enough glucose to satisfy the brain's requirements for up to 24 hours.

The main role of muscle glycogen is to provide fuel for the muscle's own contraction during EXERCISE. In fact muscle glycogen cannot be broken down to glucose and so cannot be used to raise blood glucose concentration directly. However, in some circumstances, when their metabolism is partly *anaerobic*, skeletal muscles produce lactic acid from glycogen. When this lactic acid passes into the blood it is taken up by the liver, where it is converted into glucose; thus it can be used indirectly to raise blood glucose. The major stimulus causing the breakdown of muscle glycogen is contraction of the muscles. Thus, the onset of exercise is accompanied by the initiation of glycogen breakdown. The extent to which the muscles continue to use their glycogen store depends on the intensity of the exercise. With low intensity exercise (such as slow walking, cycling, or swimming) the muscles do not use much glycogen as they are able to take up fat from the blood as a source of energy for contraction. However, with higher intensity exercise (jogging, brisk uphill walking, running) the muscles need to use glycogen or glucose from the blood to support the higher rate of energy expenditure. (See figure). A well-nourished person will have enough glycogen in their muscle to enable them to exercise for 1–2 hours at approximately two-thirds of their maximum capacity for aerobic exercise. However if people consume a very high carbohydrate diet, especially for at least three days after first depleting their muscle glycogen levels, it is possible to double this normal glycogen content, ensuring that a longer period of exercise can

be sustained before it is used up. This is known as *carbohydrate loading*, or glycogen supercompensation, and is often used by distance — especially marathon — runners before an important race.

I. A. MACDONALD

See also BLOOD SUGAR; EXERCISE; METABOLISM; MUSCLE.

Glycolysis The first stage in the production of energy by breakdown of glucose in body cells; a chain of chemical events requiring a specific set of ENZYMES, and resulting in formation of ATP (ADENOSINE TRIPHOSPHATE). In aerobic METABOLISM subsequent sequences produce several times more ATP, thereby providing a greater quantity of energy per molecule of glucose, utilizing oxygen, and producing carbon dioxide and water — comparable to burning organic fuels in air. In anaerobic metabolism (metabolism which does not use oxygen) glycolysis is the only means of energy production from glucose, and lactate is the end-product. This occurs in cells which cannot utilize oxygen (red blood cells), predominately in some components of SKELETAL MUSCLE (fast, 'white' fibres), and probably to some extent in all cells when there is a shortage of oxygen. However, it also occurs in the first 1–3 minutes after a sudden increase of demand in cells which will subsequently make all the necessary ATP aerobically, because the glycolytic system can respond within seconds whereas both the biochemical pathways of aerobic metabolism and the systems for supplying them with oxygen take time to adjust; the

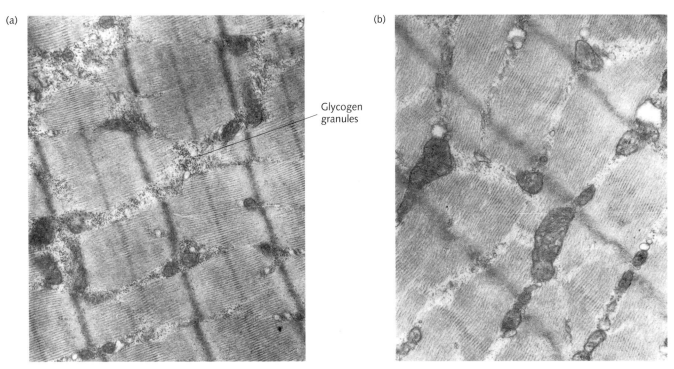

(a)

(b)

Glycogen granules

A subject exercised *one* leg only to exhaustion. Specimens of the quadriceps muscle were taken from *both* legs immediately after the exercise (by 'needle biopsy'). The figure shows the microscopic appearance of the muscle, magnified × about 25 000; (a) from the leg which was *not* exercised; normal glycogen content is seen as granules (black dots) between the muscle fibres; (b) from the leg which *was* exercised; the glycogen granules are depleted. Reproduced with permission from E. Hultman.

start of vigorous EXERCISE, even in a trained athlete with large numbers of 'red' muscle fibres, is the most obvious example. SHEILA JENNETT

Goitre is defined as an enlargement of the THYROID GLAND which can be seen as a swelling in the front of the neck. There are several types of goitre which are features of different thyroid disorders.

Endemic goitre

On a worldwide basis, this is the most notable class of goitre. It arises because of insufficient iodine in the diet. This occurs in regions of the world where the iodine content of the normal diet or drinking water falls below the minimum requirement of about 25 μg/day. At least 1 billion people worldwide are at risk of iodine deficiency. Whereas most of these live in mountainous areas of developing countries, even in Europe 50–100 million people (15–30%) inhabit areas of at least moderate deficiency. In Britain the best recognized region is the Peak District and this is the reason why this goitrous condition is known colloquially as '*Derbyshire neck*': but iodination of table salt has now made it rare.

The thyroid is unique in its ability to extract iodine from the blood and utilize it for the biosynthesis of HORMONES. The thyroid gland itself is positively regulated by a hormone from the PITUITARY GLAND named 'thyroid stimulating hormone', (TSH). The relationship between the pituitary and the thyroid is a classic example of *negative feedback*: the secretion of thyroid hormones influences TSH secretion from the pituitary; excessive secretion from the thyroid gland raises the concentration of thyroid hormones in the blood, which switches off TSH secretion by the pituitary. Conversely, if the rate of thyroid hormone secretion is inappropriately low, TSH from the pituitary increases.

It is this negative feedback regulation which results in the endemic goitres found in iodine-deficient regions. Iodine is an essential component of both thyroid hormones (T3 and T4). When there is insufficient iodine in the diet the thyroid is unable to synthesize and secrete sufficient quantities of T4 or, in the most restrictive conditions, of T3. As a consequence, pituitary secretion of TSH increases. This 'trophic' hormone stimulates both the function and the growth of the thyroid gland, so that it enlarges, eventually forming a goitre. In stimulating growth, TSH acts in conjunction with other growth factors, produced locally within the thyroid gland itself. Endemic goitres are however limited in size, and it is now thought that one of the local growth factors acts as a negative regulator.

Iodine deficiency is prevented by its addition to staple foods such as household salt, bread, and cheese. Iodine can also be effective when given by injection as an intramuscular depot of a slowly resorbable iodized oil. On a long-term basis this leads to the disappearance of goitres, but a more rapid resolution may be obtained surgically.

The correct level of iodine supplementation for household salt was first determined in the

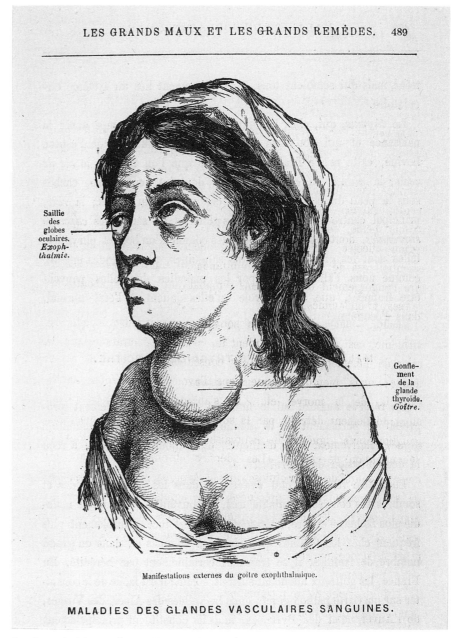

Saillie des globes oculaires. *Exophthalmie.*

Gonflement de la glande thyroïde. *Goître.*

Manifestations externes du goitre exophthalmique.

MALADIES DES GLANDES VASCULAIRES SANGUINES.

From Rengarde, J. *Les grands maux*. Mary Evans Picture Library

1930s by Purves, in the University of Otago, New Zealand. He showed that when the salt was appropriately supplemented, the levels of iodine excreted in the urine of nurse volunteers in the city of Dunedin increased to equate with those excreted by a control group selected from the inhabitants of an iodine-replete Pacific island. When the suitably iodized salt was subsequently used prophylactically throughout Otago, there was a dramatic decline in the incidence of goitre in the populace of this province.

Goitres in iodine-abundant environments

A variety of goitrous conditions occur which are not due to iodine deficiency in the diet. These range from non-toxic, so-called 'sporadic',

goitres to those associated with autoimmune hyper- and hypothyroidism. In addition there are rare inborn errors of thyroid hormone biosynthesis which usually cause congenital HYPOTHYROIDISM, high TSH, and a goitre. Thus a goitre *per se* does not reveal the thyroid status of the person, as it may be associated with either under- or overactivity of the gland or may be present in a 'euthyroid' individual — one with normal hormone levels.

There is a range of techniques for investigating the nature of a goitre, from manual examination by a skilled thyroidologist (needle aspiration BIOPSY), to IMAGING TECHNIQUES such as radiology, ultrasound, radionuclide scanning, computed tomography, and, more recently, magnetic resonance imaging. These are useful both in discriminating the goitre type and also in observing changes such as shrinking of thyroid volume following treatment. Conventional radiology provides information on the effects of goitre growth on surrounding tissues; for example it identifies goitres which are pressing on the windpipe, causing breathing difficulties, and require prompt surgical intervention.

A large proportion of patients who have either an over- or an underactive thyroid suffer from autoimmune conditions and their thyroids exhibit varying degrees of infiltration by lymphocytes. In the HYPERTHYROIDISM of *Grave's disease* we have a unique example of antibodies (known as thyroid stimulating antibodies) which mimic the action of a pituitary trophic hormone, namely TSH. This leads to persistent and unregulated stimulation of the thyroid. A diffuse and symmetrical goitre is often present. Conversely in the hypothyroidism of *Hashimoto's disease* there is autoimmune destruction of thyroid follicular cells, leading to underproduction of the hormones and eventually to thyroid failure. Large multinodular goitres are characteristic of this condition; there is extensive lymphocytic infiltration and with the passage of time mere remnants of thyroid follicles.

Aberrant growth within the thyroid may produce solitary nodules. These can be 'hot', when they avidly accumulate orally administered radioactive isotopes of iodine and usually suppress the activity of the surrounding thyroid tissue. Alternatively they may be non-functional — 'cold' — when iodine uptake is abnormally low. About 10% of these 'cold' nodules are malignant; however the overall incidence of thyroid cancer is very low, with only about 750 newly diagnosed cases reported annually in all of England and Wales.

Thus goitres occur in several different forms, due to a variety of widely differing causes, some of which are at present only poorly understood. It is likely that advances in our knowledge of local regulators of thyroid growth, including some subtle effects of iodine which have recently come to light, will lead to improved understanding and management.

Goitres are long-recognized clinical and cosmetic problems: they influenced even male fashions in the Regency period when high collars were adopted to alleviate the embarrassment of the Prince Regent who suffered from an unsightly goitre. Indeed his search for a cure, by daily drinking several pints of sea water, presumably influenced his choice of Brighton for the location of his Pavilion. Conversely, small goitres, particularly in women, have been considered marks of beauty. Examples are seen in some of Lely's portraits of ladies of the seventeenth century Dutch court.　　　　N. J. MARSHALL

See also HORMONES; HYPERTHYROIDISM; HYPOTHYROIDISM; THYROID.

Gout is a metabolic disorder characterized by excessive concentration of uric acid in the blood occasioning the deposition of sodium urate in the JOINTS — particularly the extremities, and notoriously the great toe. Joints become swollen and very painful ('like walking on my eyeballs', remarked the Revd Sydney Smith, himself a sufferer). Chalky deposits called *tophi* (routinely likened to crab's eyes) often form around the joints and under the skin, especially of the ear. Thomas Sydenham, the illustrious clinician and another sufferer, gave the classical description of gout in the 1670s. The parts affected, according to Sydenham, became 'so exquisitely painful as not to endure the weight of the clothes nor the shaking of the room from a person's walking briskly therein'. By the eighteenth century different kinds of gout were distinguished. The classic swelling of the toes, heels, ankles, and wrists was labelled '*regular gout*'. Then there was '*irregular gout*' (also called 'visceral', 'metastatic', or 'repelled gout') — gout which, failing to be expelled in the standard way, allegedly rebounded from the extremities to the vital organs — head, brain, liver, heart — where it was judged more ominous. A third type was '*flying gout*', where the pain flitted, apparently randomly, around the body.

Greek medicine had understood gout as a humoral disease, and the Hippocratic aphorisms *inter alia* noted that eunuchs do not get gout; nor women, unless their menses be stopped; nor even youths, till they indulged in coitus. Gout, in other words, was a disorder of mature, sexually-active males.

The sixteenth-century iconoclastic Swiss physician Paracelsus repudiated humoral thinking and sought a chemical explanation. Later developments supported Paracelsus' general outlook. In 1776, the Swedish chemist, Karl Scheele, isolated uric acid, and in *A Treatise upon Gravel and Gout* (1793), Murray Forbes speculated that gout was attended by an excess of uric acid. Four years later, William Hyde Wollaston obtained uric acid from a gouty tophus. And the victory of the theory was assured when, in 1859, Alfred Garrod tendered his classic analysis. In a normal healthy person, he argued, uric acid is excreted in the urine; if that process be interrupted, deposition of uric acid occurs in the form of urate of soda. Not least, Garrod devised an effective clinical test — the thread test — for uric acid. His *The Nature and Treatment of Gout and Rheumatic Gout* (1859) proved a milestone in the scientific understanding of the disorder.

Gout became one of those body-disfiguring diseases that acquired a distinctive personality, so much so that it could even be regarded as a desirable acquisition. It was widely viewed as exclusive to the upper classes, and therefore a mark of a good breeding, wealth, social status, and cultural superiority. 'Gout is the distemper of a gentleman', insisted Lord Chesterfield in the mid eighteenth century, 'whereas the rheumatism is the distemper of a hackney coachman.' 'Gout loves ancestors and genealogy,' declared Sydney Smith, 'it needs five or six generations of gentlemen or noblemen to give it its full vigour'. Hence, like melancholy in the Renaissance or tuberculosis in the Romantic era, gout achieved a social cachet.

More singularly, perhaps, gout assumed an identity, amongst doctors and sufferers alike, as a 'healthy' disease which protected sufferers against the depredations of worse diseases. 'I have so good an opinion of the gout', remarked the long-suffering Horace Walpole, 'that when I am told of an infallible cure I laugh the proposal to scorn and declare that I do not desire to be cured … I am serious … I believe the gout a remedy and not a disease.' For that reason, the apparent incurability of gout paradoxically caused no problems. If gout was indeed truly protective, then a cure might be worse than the disease.

The theory underlying such views was that gout was a healthy response through which a strongly constituted body attempted to divest itself of morbid matter by expelling it to the extremities, like the big toe, where it could do no harm. Hence, though a chronic disease, it was at bottom a symptom of basic good health. The poet William Cowper congratulated a friend on becoming gouty, 'because it seems to promise us that we shall keep you long.'

Gout thus affords a good instance of what Susan Sontag has called 'disease as metaphor', one laden with meanings that transcend strict medico-scientific bounds.

Gout is still with us, but rarely in its florid form: an excess of uric acid in the blood can be recognized and controlled by drugs which diminish its excessive formation or enhance its deficient excretion — either of which may account for the excess. The link with affluence has some foundation, since a high protein diet can be a factor; uric acid is a breakdown product of *purines*, which are essential body constituents — for example of DNA. Purines are abundant in a protein-rich diet, and both ingested and internally synthesized purines contribute to the turnover which produces uric acid; so a high intake combined with subnormal ability of the kidneys to handle the load can cause excess in the blood.　　　　ROY PORTER

Further reading

Copeman, W. S. (1964). *A short history of the gout and the rheumatic diseases.* University of California Press, Berkeley, CA.

Sontag, S. (1978). *Illness as metaphor.* Farrar, Straus and Giroux, New York.

Gray, Henry Henry Gray (1827–61) was a London surgeon, who, in 1858, published the first edition of a medical text book entitled *Anatomy: descriptive and surgical.* In later years — first informally, and, after 1938, formally — the book became known as *Gray's Anatomy.* It is one of the few medical texts known by name to the general public.

Henry Gray was born in Windsor Castle, but lived in Belgravia for most of his life. The family had moved to be closer to Buckingham Palace on the accession of William IV, to whom Gray's father, William, was Deputy Treasurer. Aged 18 Henry entered St George's Hospital at Hyde Park Corner in Central London, and he qualified as a Member of the Royal College of Surgeons in

1848, the same year in which he won one of the College's triennial essay prizes for an account of the nerves of the human eye. As a student he was known for his diligent attention, especially in anatomical studies, and in particular for performing numerous DISSECTIONS himself. Gray remained at St George's in House Surgeon positions, and continued his anatomical work, publishing several of his anatomical observations in papers in the *Philosophical Transactions* of the Royal Society. In 1852 he was elected a Fellow of the Royal Society. From that time on he devoted himself to anatomy, serving St George's as a demonstrator, later as Lecturer on Anatomy, and as Curator of the Museum.

The appearance of his book was timely. Medical education in Britain was being professionalised and formalised — in that same year, 1858, the Medical Act was passed in Britain, creating the General Medical Council (GMC), the regulatory and licensing authority of the medical profession. This epitomized the growing professional status of medicine in Britain, with regulated access and recognized training procedures and courses taking place in properly accredited institutions. Simultaneously, new scientific approaches to medicine were developing, which were being incorporated into the medical curricula. Gray's book was not the first anatomy textbook — especially since the passing of the Anatomy Act of 1832 (which provided legitimate sources of bodies for dissection), guides and manuals had been produced for medical and surgical students. What distinguished Gray's book was the number and quality of illustrations, and his emphasis on anatomy as the practical basis of surgery. The premier medical journals of the time, *The Lancet* and *The British Medical Journal*, praised its style and content, and the latter's review prophesied that it would become *the* manual of anatomy. A year after its appearance in Britain, an American edition was produced, and a second edition was produced in London in 1860 — just before the death of its young author, at the age of 34, from smallpox contracted after nursing a nephew. Gray's loss to anatomy was mourned by many colleagues; one of them, Timothy Holmes, who was a fellow surgeon from St George's, continued to produce new editions of Gray's book up to 1880 (the 9th edition). He in turn was succeeded by another practising surgeon, T. Pickering Pick, and it was not until 1901 (the 15th edition) that a professional anatomist — one who earned his living by teaching and studying anatomy, rather than from surgery — was appointed as editor.

In 1995 the 38th edition appeared. Continuing the tradition of generous illustrations begun by its eponymous founder, *Gray's Anatomy* now provides a coherent account of the structure of the human body from the ultra-microscopical to the population level — and anatomy is now presented as a central discipline in the natural sciences, not merely of relevance to the practising surgeon. E. M. TANSEY

See also ANATOMY.

Great chain of being

A holistic worldview which linked all of nature's wonders together into a continuous chain: the inorganic was connected to the organic, the natural world to its omnipotent Creator. The idea was related to ancient concepts of nature's plenitude and continuity — that the universe is filled with all possible forms arranged according to degrees of perfection — but flourished under its familiar name in the eighteenth century. All natural objects were considered 'chained' together in a hierarchy according to increasing physical complexity and mental sophistication, from stone pebbles through higher primates and finally God.

Unlike modern evolutionary thought, this was principally a static view of nature. All 'beings' were created in what was pictured as a linear, continuous series, and all always remained in their relative position on the chain. However, providing empirical proofs for fine gradations was challenging. Far from seeing smooth continuity in a collection of natural objects, specimens placed next to each other all too frequently revealed 'gaps' in the chain, which frustrated naturalists who wanted to find convincing proof of God's perfectly ordered universe.

The search for structures of increasing complexity in nature often led to complications in determining the 'natural' hierarchy of specimens. From Aristotle onwards, constructing classification systems had always been predicated on arbitrary judgements, many of which formed the basis of naturalists' debates, and which led some natural philosophers to declare that only individuals, not species, exist in nature. But even looking at individual specimens led to problems in establishing patterns in nature, and many naturalists alternated between thinking of nature as a continuous chain and assuming particular criteria to demarcate groups of species.

For a long time, *zoophytes* (primitive marine creatures) and shell-carrying molluscs were classic examples of the continuity between minerals, plants, and simple animals. Similarly, certain amphibians could be used as links between sea and terrestrial creatures. Frequently, however, it was difficult to determine where in the natural hierarchy a creature should be placed. The eighteenth-century Swiss naturalist and popularizer of the chain of being, Charles Bonnet, for example, had troubles determining where in the continuum between fish and birds he should place sea lions or flying fish. Further complications in classifying nature's wonders were created by imaginary sightings of monsters and sea creatures such as mermaids, a myth which flourished in the eighteenth century as a result of increased voyages of exploration, and sailors anxious to tell tales of their heroic travels.

While some imagined that creatures might be found to fill gaps between species, others were beginning to find new reasons to suppose discontinuities between animal forms. The early nineteenth-century, influential French comparative anatomist, Georges Cuvier, reconstructed animals based on palaeontological remains, and

not only proposed that species were created separately and at different times, but claimed proof from his interpretation of the fossil record that species went extinct. This could not only be taken as a contradiction to the chain of being, according to which no gaps were supposed to exist in nature, but also as offensive to religious belief in a rational and benevolent Creator who would not allow species to die out. In short, the strength of the chain of being was not to be threatened by a weak link.

Perhaps more embarrassing or problematic to the legitimacy of the chain of being was the placement of humans in the scale. A chain that linked all natural objects together by subtle degrees of difference tended to humble humans' estimate of their unique and special position in the world. Humans were generally regarded as residing in the middle of the Great Chain, with angels, spirits, and 'intellect' among the 'links' to God. While many figured that the upward space between humans and God was infinite, the close proximity of man to beast could be disturbing to theologians. The matter was confounded when, after the 'discovery' of African apes, anatomists revealed the similarities between human and animal bodies and brains. Such close ties were exemplified during the eighteenth century in the famous classification system of Carl Linnaeus, who grouped humans with apes in the same order (*primates*) and even the same genus (*homo*) as orang-utans. Linnaeus' designation of humans in the species *sapiens*, meaning 'wise,' was a gesture toward making man essentially different from animals, and a degree closer to the intelligent beings higher up in the chain.

Even human varieties could be reduced to fine degrees of difference, with a particular person's position in the chain corresponding to a social position. The chain of being could be used as a model to conceptualize different human 'types', or races, savages. This led to an apparently 'natural' social hierarchy that could then be used to legitimate the development of such programmes as social medicine, evangelical philanthropy, or even colonialism. BRIAN DOLAN

Greeks

In ancient Greek culture, the body was the object of display and the subject of debate. For example, athletic competition was a central part of the life of the Greek city, and young men were expected to train in the public space of the gymnasium: but, while poets praised victorious athletes, medical writers warned of the dangers of body-building, claiming that excessive development of the body was unnatural. The ideal of a glorious death (the *kalos thanatos*) was for a young man in his prime to die for his city in another form of competitive display of the body, namely war.

From the sixth century BC onwards, medical and philosophical writers debated the constituents of the body, often drawing parallels with the wider cosmos. Some saw the body as dominated by one element, such as air or fire, but the need to explain different illnesses, combined with observation of body fluids meant that, by the fourth century, most people thought that the body was composed of several different substances needing to be kept in balance in order to ensure health. These could be bile and phlegm; bile, phlegm, water, and blood; or, in the version which was to become GALEN's theory of the 'four HUMOURS', yellow bile, black bile, phlegm, and blood. All of these alternative versions of the interior of the body meant that one was expected to take responsibility for one's own health through individual control of regimen: diet, exercise, environment, and appetites. As for bodily organs: the heart, the liver, or the brain were seen as dominant. The female body was seen as inherently unstable; the womb was thought to be able to move around the body, while homologies existed between the top and the bottom of the body so that lips, a mouth, and a neck were present at both ends. This is reflected in our Latinate medical terminology, since 'cervix' means 'neck' and labia are 'lips', but was taken rather further in the ancient world; for example, it was thought that one could detect from a deepening of her voice whether a girl had lost her VIRGINITY.

The body was seen as something which needed to be controlled: just as POSTURE and GESTURES were used consciously to convey meaning, particularly in the public context of the oratory so important to Athenian democracy, so one's body needed to avoid revealing unintentional messages which could be read by hostile others. PHYSIOGNOMY was a recognized science, claiming to interpret all human activity.

The images of the body which are found in Greek art include open display of human sexuality; costumes worn in Greek plays included exaggerated sexual organs, enormous models of the penis were carried in religious processions, and vase paintings include sexually explicit scenes of intercourse with multiple partners. The images which have had most impact on our perception of 'Greek art' are, however, the statues. In constructions of the classical Greek past, in particular in the Victorian period, people have chosen to see these images as pure, white, and serene, part of 'the glory that was Greece' — but all stone statues would originally have been painted in bright colours, the eyes inlaid with glass or coloured stone, and metal hair, jewellery, and weapons added. Only faint traces of paint and the holes for the attachment of metal pieces now remain, but even these are sufficient to sully the vision of purity. In the mid fifth century BC, statues start to indicate more emotion, but it is not until the Hellenistic period that sculptors depict pain and grief in their subjects. This was also the period when old age, drunkenness, and deformity were shown, and sculpted bodies were represented with swelling muscles and with attempts to capture violent motion. We are far from the idealized serenity of the classical body, and it is significant that Hellenistic art has subsequently been labelled by art historians as 'debased'.

Although the male body is usually shown naked in Greek art, to demonstrate musculature and strength, the female body is usually clothed, although the diaphanous drapery may reveal as much as it conceals. Exceptions, such as statues of the goddess Aphrodite, often involve the creation of some sort of narrative to account for their nudity; hence Aphrodite is often shown preparing for, or completing, her bath. Nudity usually indicated vulnerability, but could be used in initiation rituals to represent the removal of one social identity before the assumption of a new one.

In its reception of the classical tradition, Western civilization has chosen to identify two competing attitudes to the body in ancient Greece, identifying each of these with a different Greek god and labelling them the 'Dionysiac' and the 'Apollonian' approach.

Dionysos was the son of the mortal Semele and Zeus, the main god of the Greek pantheon. Twice-born, he was taken from his dying mother and placed in Zeus' thigh as an incubator. Although he appears to have been a thoroughly Greek god, known in ancient Mycenae, the Greeks told stories of his 'foreign' origin as part of their perception of him as representing the 'Other'. He transgressed many boundaries designated as being socially important: at his festivals, for example, men and boys dressed in women's clothes, while he himself could be represented as an effeminate youth. His violent behaviour was associated with his discovery of the process of making wine, while myths told how his followers — in particular the women, known as maenads — engaged in ritual murder and cannibalism. Dionyosis is also associated with the theatre, where masks covering the identity of the person not only permitted individuals to take on another persona, but also allowed men to act the roles of women. Myths of Dionysos stress his fluidity and powers of transformation.

Nietzsche, widely followed by nineteenth-century scholars, opposed 'Dionysianism' to 'Apollonianism', claiming that Greek tragedy was the result of Apollo controlling Dionysos. To reach this binary opposition, he stressed the otherness and irrationality of Dionysos, contrasting these with the apparently rational characteristics associated with the god Apollo. Apollo, another son of Zeus, but with a different mortal mother, Leto, has been seen as the most Greek of Greek gods, because of his connection with qualities which scholars have preferred to associate with the Greeks in their role as our cultural ancestors. Apollo is associated with healing — although he also fires the arrows which bring plague — purification, prophetic knowledge, poetry and the music of the lyre, education, and the sun. He is represented with a bow, and is linked to the laurel tree, the leaves of which were used by his priestess at the oracle of Delphi. The calm, orderly image of Apollo has historically been opposed to the rampant disorder of Dionysos. However, the opposition is our own construct, buttressed by the Greeks' own deliberately erroneous insistence that Dionysos was a foreign import. In fact both deities are equally 'Greek',

Dionysos representing an attempt to control the darker side of Greek culture.   HELEN KING

Further reading
Cartledge, P. (1995). *The Greeks*. Oxford University Press.

See also ART AND THE BODY; SCULPTURE; VENUS.

Grey matter comprises those regions in the BRAIN and SPINAL cord that consist predominantly of the 'cell bodies' of nerve cells (*neurons*).

The NERVOUS SYSTEM is composed of many types of body tissue, but the most important is nervous tissue itself. The component cells are nerve cells or neurons. Just like cells elsewhere in the body, each neuron has a cell body, with a nucleus (containing the chromosomes with the genetic programs) and cytoplasm for metabolism and the production of proteins. But neurons also have several rather special features, in particular two types of processes extending out from the cell body. Typically, there is a nerve fibre or *axon*, which can be a metre or more in length, along which impulses travel to convey information to other neurons, or to muscles or glands. In addition, there are several dendrites (from the Greek for 'wood' or 'tree'), up to 2 mm long, on which the axons of other neurons terminate, forming SYNAPSES.

In the CENTRAL NERVOUS SYSTEM (CNS) — made up of the brain and spinal cord — nerve cell bodies are usually found closely packed together in characteristic regions. Such a concentration of cell bodies, together with their dendrites, but with a relatively small proportion of axons, appears grey in a fresh cut through the brain or cord and is called 'grey matter'. It forms a relatively thin surface layer, called 'cortex' over the cerebral hemispheres and the cerebellum. The spinal cord has a central core of grey matter, which has the shape of a butterfly when cut across. Elsewhere, there are clumps of grey matter called 'nuclei', making up such structures as the hypothalamus, the thalamus, and the basal ganglia.

Where mainly axons are concentrated, in most of the rest of the brain and around the outside of the grey matter of the spinal cord, the predominant colour when cut is whitish, because many of the axons are surrounded by a pale, fatty sheath, consisting of MYELIN. This forms the WHITE MATTER.

The brain, and particularly the cerebral cortex, has for long been associated with 'intellect'. The use of the expression 'grey matter' has, therefore, appeared in common parlance to mean intelligence, but there is little evidence to suggest that this quality is directly connected to the size of an individual brain.   LAURENCE GAREY

See PLATE 6.

See also CENTRAL NERVOUS SYSTEM; NERVES.

Growing pains After headache, growing pains appear to be the most frequent form of pain in otherwise healthy schoolchildren. They have been found to affect around one in every six children aged 6–11 years, more girls than boys, and affect many fewer children over the age of 13. However, the pains usually described as 'growing pains' probably have little to do with growth other than that they usually do not persist after a child reaches his or her final height. The process of growth in a child is so slow at any given time (at a daily rate only perceptible to the most highly accurate precision measuring devices) that the process of growth alone would be unlikely to cause pain. This is supported by the fact that many millions of normally-growing children do not develop such pains. Nor do the pains increase or 'grow' as the child increases in size.

The child usually complains of intermittent and frequently quite incapacitating pain localised deeply in the arms and/or legs. The pain is not situated at or near any of the joints (ankles, knees, hips, elbows) and if it is, should mean that the child is seen by a doctor to rule out more serious causes of such pain. Growing pains are sometimes accompanied by feelings of restlessness in the arms or legs, but if there is tenderness, redness or swelling, the pain will again need to be assessed and perhaps treated medically. The pain in the legs should not be made worse by walking and the way the child walks should be normal, without any limp.

The vague, nebulous discomfort of 'growing pains', for which no cause can be found, ranges from a mild ache, sometimes associated with tiredness, to severe pain that may even waken the child from sleeping. The pain or ache is commonly situated in the front of the thighs, in the calves, and behind the knees. The groin is sometimes affected. The pain is usually felt on both sides may come on suddenly or gradually, and does not usually occur every day. The pains typically occur late in the day and in the evening. When the child wakes up in the morning, the pain has usually disappeared.

These pains most commonly occur in children and young adolescents, but they may commence in early infancy and disappear once the child reaches maturity. In older children, the pain may resemble what adults more accurately describe as CRAMPS in the legs, creeping sensations, or restless legs. Growing pains may be made worse by running during the day. In contrast to growing pains, the pain of fatigue, which may occur with or without excessive physical activity, disappears after rest.

It was once said that emotional growth can be painful but physical growth is not. Perhaps it is simply best to admit ignorance about the cause(s) of such pains and recognize that (except in the uncommon situations described above) they are harmless and self-limiting.

DONALD C. BROWN
CHRISTOPHER J. H. KELNAR

See also DEVELOPMENT AND GROWTH.

Growth hormone also called SOMATO-TROPHIN, is secreted from the anterior part of the PITUITARY GLAND. It is a major product of the gland, which contains 5 mg of the hormone (about 10% of its dry weight). As the name implies, growth hormone is important in controlling linear growth and, together with the thyroid hormones and the sex hormones, is important in determining the final height and development of an individual. It also has a role in controlling metabolism of foodstuffs, so that lack of the hormone in children results in short stature with the whole body in proportion, whereas deficiency in the adult results in weakness and depression.

Growth stops when the epiphyses (ends) of the BONES fuse to the main shaft between them. Oversecretion before this occurs results in *gigantism*, whereas oversecretion afterwards results in *acromegaly*, a condition characterized by coarsening of the facial features and enlargement of the hands and feet. Interest in dwarfism, gigantism, and acromegaly has spanned the centuries; literature, especially for children, is filled with stories about dwarfs and giants, while Old Testament writings have several descriptions of giants. A study of paintings can also reveal subjects with disturbances of growth hormone secretion. A portrait from about 1365 BC of Tutankhamun's father-in-law illustrates some of the chacterisitics of acromegaly, but it was not until the late eighteenth century that Saucerette, a French surgeon, described a subject with features suggestive of this condition. During the nineteenth century a number of reports appeared and the term 'acromegaly' was coined in 1886 by Pierre Marie. In the following year, Minkowski (who also performed some of the early experiments important in the discovery of insulin) noted that acromegaly was associated with a pituitary tumour. Such tumours are now known to be the cause of gigantism and acromegaly. Once this was established, surgical treatment of the condition began to be attempted in the 1890s. In 1912 Cushing, a famous American neurosurgeon who also made major contributions to endocrinology, pioneered the technique of operating on pituitary tumours via the nasal route.

The nasal approach to the pituitary is possible because the gland itself lies in the midline at the base of the brain. Part of the visual pathway, the 'optic chiasma', lies in front of the pituitary, so a spreading tumour may lead to visual defects. This could explain why Goliath of Gath failed to see the pebble launched by David.

Growth hormone is a large PEPTIDE of 191 amino acids and is relatively species-specific, so only primate growth hormone is effective in man. This meant that until 1985, when it became possible to synthesize it, treatment of short stature employed growth hormone extracted from human pituitaries. As with some preparations of human gonadotrophins previously used in fertility treatment, some of the preparations were contaminated, leading to 1 in 1000 patients developing Creuzfeld Jacob disease, resulting in dementia and death. Currently biosynthetic growth hormone is employed.

Growth hormone is always detectable in the plasma of healthy individuals throughout life; it is not secreted continuously over the 24 hours, but in bursts. The most marked increase follows the onset of SLEEP, so there may be a basis for the old wives' tale that you will not grow if you do not get a good night's sleep. The hormone is present in the fetus, but does not appear to be necessary for growth until soon after birth. Its release is increased in PUBERTY, at an earlier stage in girls than in boys. Secretion of growth hormone is controlled by the HYPOTHALAMUS, a region of the brain which is important in regulating many functions including a major role in the response to STRESS: growth hormone is released in response to a number of stresses such as EXERCISE, anaesthesia, and surgery. Prolonged stress may however suppress growth hormone release, so that children with marked emotional deprivation can show secondary growth failure. One such case is said to be Sir James Barrie who was short of stature and may have had some affinity with his creation, Peter Pan.

Release is stimulated in response to a rapid fall in blood glucose, which can be produced by an injection of insulin in a clinical test for growth hormone secretion. The hypothalamus controls growth hormone secretion by means of its own secretion of two peptides; *somatostatin*, which inhibits secretion, and *growth hormone releasing hormone*, which is stimulatory; these hormones reach the nearby anterior pituitary through local blood vessels.

Growth hormone stimulates the growth of the long bones, not directly but through the action of *somatomedins*, which are insulin-like growth factors made in the liver, and which also inhibit release of the hormone. It has a direct effect on metabolic processes throughout the body, supporting growth through enhanced formation of protein and nucleic acids (anabolic action) and of other constituents of lean body mass. By contrast its effects promote breakdown of carbohydrate and fat, with the energy released supporting growth. Because of the anabolic effects and because detection is difficult, growth hormone has been used by athletes to improve performance, although studies have shown it to be of little value.

MARY L. FORSLING

See also DEVELOPMENT AND GROWTH; HYPOTHALAMUS; PEPTIDES; PITUITARY GLAND.

Gut In developmental and evolutionary terms, the gut is simply a 'tube' from head end to tail end, extending the outside environment into the shelter of the body, allowing the processing and absorption of nutrients from an internal surface: an advance upon absorption from only the external surface in the simplest organisms. In human terms, although the 'tube' runs from mouth to anus, the term 'gut' usually refers to the stomach and intestines; gut sensations and functions have strong psychosomatic links involving the AUTONOMIC NERVOUS SYSTEM — a physical basis for the traditional association with unreasoned responses and EMOTIONS: 'gut reactions' and 'gut feelings'.

S.J.

See ALIMENTARY SYSTEM.

Gymnastics is the practice of athletic exercises for the development of the body, especially those exercises performed with apparatus such as rings, pommel horse, bars, and balance beam. Although gymnastics was likely practised in ancient Egyptian and Chinese cultures, its roots for Western culture lie in ancient Greece, hence the derivation from the Greek word *gymnazein*, which literally means 'to train naked' (*gymnos*: naked). The early Greeks practised gymnastics in preparation for war, as jumping, running, discus throwing, wrestling, and BOXING helped produce the strong, supple muscles necessary for hand-to-hand combat. Because military training was necessary for the production of Greek citizens, and because the Greeks viewed the training both of the body and the mind as inextricably linked, gymnastics became a central component of ancient education. Gymnasia, the buildings with open-air courts where such training took place, evolved into schools where youths learned gymnastics, rhetoric, music, and mathematics. Gymnastics also provided a way to train for the athletic festivals around Greece, the most famous of which was the Olympic Games, held every four years from 776 BCE until 393 CE.

With the end of the Olympic Games, Greek-style gymnastics training declined, not to be revived until the eighteenth and nineteenth centuries in Western Europe. With this revival came a concomitant revival of the corporeal values associated with gymnastics: upper body strength, musculature, elasticity, litheness, flexibility, poise, and equilibrium. Underpinning the re-emergence of gymnastic training is the same assumption held by the Greeks, that a healthy body and a healthy mind are intimately connected.

In the mid 1800s Friedrich Jahn did much to re-introduce gymnastics into German education and became known as the 'father of gymnastics'. Jahn introduced the horizontal bar, parallel bars, side horse with pommels, balance beam, ladder, and vaulting bucks. His gymnastics program was promoted in Turner societies, clubs established to develop self discipline and physical strength in the name of national unity. In Sweden, Pehr Henrik Ling followed closely behind Jahn, systematizing Swedish pedagogic gymnastics with a strong emphasis on the medical benefits.

In the early nineteenth century, educators in the US imported German and Swedish gymnastics training programs. With the American integration of gymnastics into the general education curriculum, its connections to nationalism

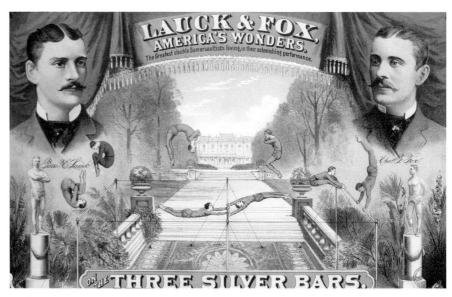

Lauck & Fox, America's wonders on the 3 Silver Bars, American poster late 19th–early 20th century. The Art Archives/Bibliothèque des Arts Décoratifs Paris/Dagli Orti.

and military training re-emerged stronger than ever. By the early twentieth century, the armed services published drill manuals featuring all manner of gymnastic exercises, drills which, according to the US Army *Manual of Physical Drill* (1910), provided proper instruction for 'a body of young and active men' and were thus 'all important'. The US Navy's *Gymnastics and Tumbling*, published in 1944, asserts that 'Gymnastics and tumbling contribute in large measure to the demands of a democracy at war.' Nonetheless, as military activity moved away from hand-to-hand combat and toward fighter planes and contemporary computer-controlled weapons, gymnastics training as the mind/body connection, so important for the Greek, German, and Swedish educational traditions, began to lose force. As a result, physical and intellectual training in schools are now almost completely separate; although in Germany the term 'gymnasium' still persists as the term for a place of secondary education, the gymnasium is more commonly cordoned off for physical training, while the privileged intellectual education takes place in traditional classrooms. The mind/body split is more pervasive than ever.

The nineteenth and twentieth centuries saw the powerful emergence of a strand of gymnastics,

similar in form to gymnastic training for educational and military purposes, but practised for different ends. The first Modern Olympic games in 1896 featured competitive gymnastic events for men, which have been included in every Olympics since. Men's gymnastics events are scored on an individual and team basis, and presently include the floor exercise, horizontal bar, parallel bars, rings, side horse (also called pommel horse), vaulting, and combined exercises (the all-around), which combines the scores of the other six events. Combined exercises for women were first held in 1928, and the 1952 Olympics featured the first full regime of events for women. Women's gymnastic events include balance beam, uneven parallel bars, combined exercises, floor exercises, vaulting, and rhythmic sportive gymnastics. Olga Korbut, Nadia Comaneci, and Mary Lou Retton have helped popularize women's competitive gymnastics, making it one of the most watched Olympic events as they performed difficult manœuvres on some of the very apparatus developed for bodily training by Friedrich Jahn in the eighteenth century.

DEBRA HAWHEE

See also ACROBATICS; EXERCISE; SPORT.

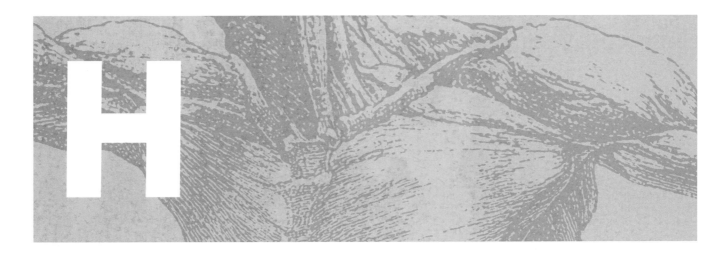

H

Habituation You are sitting quietly, reading a book. Suddenly, a tap on the window startles you. Your heart rate rises momentarily and you glance at the window to see if someone is there. But you see that the wind has strengthened and the branch of a tree has touched the glass. As your interest returns to the book, repeated taps of the branch on the window evoke progressively smaller reactions, until they hardly intrude into your reading at all.

The gradual reduction of existing responses to repeated presentations of a stimulus is 'habituation'. At first sight, it might seem that habituation is nothing more than some sort of fatigue process in the relevant sensory or motor neural pathways. But habituation has several key characteristics that identify it as an active process that is biologically useful. For example, once the response to a familiar stimulus has habituated, another intense stimulus can cause the response to the familiar stimulus to return immediately, by a process of *dishabituation*. Furthermore, habituation is relatively stimulus-specific, so that responses to the repeated stimulus are reduced but responses to different, novel stimuli are not. Neither of these characteristics is consistent with a fatigue mechanism for habituation. Instead, they indicate an active, stimulus-specific form of learning. More complex forms of learning, such as CONDITIONING, involve an association between two or more stimuli or events. Habituation does not, so it is regarded as a non-associative form of learning.

Habituation is ubiquitous in the animal kingdom. It has been observed in the gill-withdrawal reflex of marine molluscs, in limb-withdrawal reflexes mediated by the spinal cord of mammals, and in the auditory startle response discussed above. Just like more complex forms of memory, habituation initially depends upon short-term mechanisms that last between minutes and hours. With more stimulus presentations occurring over hours or days, long-term mechanisms take over and these can support habituated responses over much longer periods.

Habituation is present from an early stage of development and can be seen in infants as young as two months, who like to fixate and inspect novel visual stimuli. When presented with pairs of pictures that always include both a familiar and a new scene, the infants will fixate the new picture — indicating a habituation of the fixation response to the familiar scene. Habituation to previously presented stimulus maximizes input from the new stimulus. Other novel stimuli may be of great significance because they may signal danger. Reflex responses to such stimuli provide appropriate defensive behaviours. But if the stimuli are not intense and no damage is done, then repeated presentation leads to habituation.

Habituation allows the nervous system to optimize sensory–motor processing by eliminating unnecessary responses. It allows us to adapt to the familiar in order to preserve our ability to react rapidly and appropriately to the new.

CHRISTOPHER YEO

Haematoma A discrete internal collection of blood which has leaked from damaged blood vessels. At some sites blood can seep away between layers of tissue, but where there are tighter compartments it remains a circumscribed mass which can cause problems by putting pressure on its surroundings. A small one, for example, appears under a fingernail which has been hit with a hammer. At the other extreme a life-threatening one can occur on the surface of the brain (*subdural haematoma*) following a head injury.   S.J.

See BRUISE; HAEMORRHAGE.

Haemoglobin Both the red badge of courage and the blue blood of the aristocrat are due to haemoglobin, the pigment that gives blood its colour. Take it away, by removing the blood cells, and the resulting plasma is a very pale yellow. Haemoglobin combines with OXYGEN, enabling blood to carry 70 times more than if the oxygen were simply dissolved. Animals that are physically active and larger than a pea could scarcely survive without it. 'But for haemoglobin's existence, man might never have attained any activity which the lobster does not possess, or had he done so, it would have been with a body as minute as the fly's' (J. Barcoft).

Haemoglobin, contained in the red cells of the blood and constituting the main site of iron in the body, is present in all vertebrate species. In the human adult it is synthesized in the developing red cells in the bone marrow. Many worms have haemoglobin, but others and also most molluscs have different and more primitive oxygen-carrying pigments, which have not survived into higher forms of evolution.

Haemoglobin not only distributes oxygen as it is required by the tissues but is also an important store of the gas. Healthy humans have about 15 g of haemoglobin per litre of blood, and this can bind with 200 ml of oxygen per litre. With the body at rest the tissues only remove about one-quarter of the available oxygen reaching them in arterial blood, the other three-quarters remaining in the venous blood returning to the lungs. This constitutes an important reserve of oxygen supply which can be called on in conditions of work and exercise. In a typical total blood volume of 5 litres, even though more than half is in the veins, we thus have about 0.75 litre of oxygen combined with haemoglobin in the blood, and we have about the same amount as gas in the lungs. If we stop breathing, for example by holding our breath, these stores will maintain the functions of the brain for at the most a few minutes — but without them brain function would cease almost immediately.

The amount of oxygen free in solution in the blood plays no important role in carriage of oxygen to the tissues. The amount depends on the pressure of the gas in the lungs (see figure). If we breathe pure oxygen the amount in solution rises almost seven-fold and it can become a significant contribution to the body. If we were to breathe pure oxygen in a chamber at a pressure of three atmospheres, all the oxygen we need could be carried in solution and we would not need haemoglobin. This treatment is used for some conditions when haemoglobin is seriously deficient, but there are significant hazards of breathing high-pressure oxygen.

Each haemoglobin molecule consists of four iron-containing parts (*haems*) and four protein chains (*globins*). The fact that blood contained iron was discovered in 1747 by Menghini, who showed that if blood was burnt to an ash, iron-like particles could be extracted by a magnet. Chemical analysis of haemoglobin began in the mid nineteenth century and culminated in one of the great early triumphs of molecular biology, when in the 1960s the full chemical structure of haemoglobin was worked out.

Each haemoglobin molecule can combine with four oxygen molecules, but with no more. The complete combination is called *oxygen saturation*. The degree of combination depends on the pressure of the gas; in healthy humans the pressure in the alveoli of the lungs is above that needed for saturation. If the alveolar oxygen pressure is increased, for example by breathing more deeply or by inhaling pure oxygen, the haemoglobin in the blood will not take up any additional oxygen (see figure). However in patients with arterial blood not saturated with oxygen, for example with lung or heart disease, stimulation of breathing or administration of oxygen should increase the oxygen carriage in the blood and be beneficial or life-saving.

The combination of oxygen with haemoglobin is not related linearly to the oxygen pressure, and this is crucially important in its function. As oxygen pressure reduces below that required for full saturation, haemoglobin is relatively little desaturated until and unless the oxygen pressure reaches about the level which blood normally encounters in the oxygen-using tissues: it then parts with it readily. Thus in breath-holding, or in disease, or at ALTITUDE, alveolar oxygen pressure can approach half its normal value before haemoglobin saturation declines steeply in the blood leaving the lungs; and saturation is not itself halved until the oxygen pressure is reduced by almost two-thirds. Thus the properties of haemoglobin defend the oxygen supply against interruptions of breathing or shortage of oxygen in the atmosphere, whilst promoting its off-loading around the body.

The combination of haemoglobin and oxygen is weak, and oxygen can be pulled from the blood if the surrounding pressure of oxygen is low; indeed a vacuum will extract all the oxygen from a sample of blood. When blood flows through the capillaries of tissues which are using oxygen for metabolism, the low oxygen pressure in the tissue cells draws oxygen from its combination with haemoglobin and the gas flows into the cells. The resulting venous blood contains less than its full oxygen saturation, and the haemoglobin is partly 'deoxygenated'. Such haemoglobin does not have the bright red colour of saturated haemoglobin, but is more blue. Thus conventionally arterial blood is red and venous blood is blue. In CYANOSIS tissues are bluish because their blood is deficient in oxygen.

Haemoglobin can also combine with CARBON DIOXIDE to form *carbaminohaemoglobin*, and this is one way in which this gas is carried round the body. The two gases have a complex chemical interaction with haemoglobin. When in metabolizing tissues carbon dioxide enters the blood, its combination with haemoglobin results in a weaker affinity for oxygen, which is split off and enters the cells. The reverse happens in the lungs. Temperature has a similar effect: if local temperature rises oxyhaemoglobin splits more easily. Both mechanisms help to match gas exchange to changing activity.

Red cells also contain *2,3-diphosphoglycerate* (DPG), a substance that increases the readiness with which haemoglobin gives up its oxygen. The DPG is increased in exercise and at high altitude, which facilitates the supply of oxygen to the tissues. Unfortunately this process takes several hours. Stored blood loses its DPG and is therefore less effective on transfusion than fresh blood, although there are ways to treat it that restore the DPG.

Although the haem is the essential part of the haemoglobin molecule to enable it to combine with oxygen, it is the four globin molecules which determine the amount of binding or affinity for haemoglobin and oxygen. The globins are identified by Greek letters, and a very large number have been discovered, many of them related to diseases of the blood. Healthy human adults have two α-globins and two β-globins. Fetuses have two α-and two γ-globins. As a result fetal haemoglobin has a stronger affinity for oxygen than does the adult form. When maternal blood flows through the placental circulation, oxygen diffuses across the placental barrier into the fetus and, because of the difference between the two haemoglobins, the fetus extracts a proportionally higher amount of oxygen. This success in parasitism is clearly to the advantage of the fetus. After birth the fetal haemoglobin is slowly replaced by the adult version.

In healthy humans, haemoglobin is only found in *erythrocytes*, the blood red cells. The advantage in confining the haemoglobin in cells is threefold. First, if the haemoglobin were free in solution it would give the blood a treacle-like consistency, and the heart would be unable to force it fast enough through the capillaries. Second, the chemical environment in the red cell, including for example the presence of DPG, allows the haemoglobin to take up and release oxygen with greatest efficiency. And third, if the haemoglobin were free in solution it would be excreted and lost in the kidneys. Patients with red cell breakdown, for example in malaria, pass haemoglobin into the urine, where it is broken down to the brown pigment *methaemoglobin*; hence one form of malaria is called 'black-water fever'.

A few animals — some of the worms mentioned earlier — do have free oxygen-carrying pigments in the blood, but their molecular sizes are 40 times that of haemoglobin, so they are not excreted. One species of antarctic fish is said to lack both red cells and haemoglobin, but it lives in a cold environment and its metabolism and oxygen requirement must be very low.

Human red cells live on average about 120 days in the bloodstream, and then they become fragile and are broken up, especially by scavenger cells in the spleen and liver. The haemoglobin is not released into the blood, but is immediately broken down into haem and globins. The haem is in turn split into iron, which forms chemical compounds as part of the

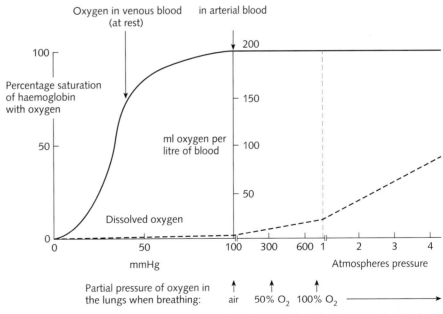

The way in which blood takes up oxygen, in relation to its partial pressure. The S-shaped curve on the left refers to the normal situation, when at rest: blood leaves the lungs with its haemoglobin saturated with oxygen; in the tissues 25% of the oxygen leaves the arterial blood; venous blood is 75% saturated. The graph is extended on the right to show the effect of breathing progressively higher percentages of oxygen, up to 100%: there is an increase only in dissolved oxygen (broken line).

blood iron pool available for future haemoglobin synthesis, and an amber pigment, *bilirubin*, which contributes to the pale colour of plasma. Bilirubin combines with albumin in the blood, and the large size of this combined molecule prevents it from being excreted in the kidneys. Instead it passes to the liver, where it is excreted in the BILE, contributing to its colour. When it reaches the intestines it is acted on by bacterial flora, and forms the brown pigment *stercobilinogen*. Most of the stercobilinogen appears in the faeces, giving it its characteristic colour (but not its odour), and the rest is reabsorbed into the bloodstream. Here a proportion recirculates in the bile but most, now called urobilinogen, is excreted in the urine. Thus not only does haemoglobin provide the colour of the blood, but its breakdown products are largely responsible for the colours of plasma, bile, faeces, and urine. JAUNDICE is due to an excess of bilirubin in the blood and tissues.

There are many diseases caused by abnormal haemoglobins. In all of them it is the globin part of the molecule which is abnormal. Not only may haemoglobin be unable to combine normally with oxygen, but since the haemoglobin is an integral part of the structure of the red cell, these cells may be deformed. An example is *sickle cell disease*, where the red cells become rigid and deformed and break down more readily, leading to anaemia. Another common disease is *thalassaemia*, where there is a defect in the synthesis of the β-globin chains. Less common conditions are the persistence of fetal haemoglobin long after birth, and abnormalities in the enzymes associated with haemoglobin (e.g. DPG) that affect its affinity for oxygen. JOHN WIDDICOMBE

See also ANAEMIA; BLOOD; BLOOD TRANSFUSION; CARBON DIOXIDE; CYANOSIS; JAUNDICE; OXYGEN; RESPIRATION.

Haemolysis
The breakdown of red blood cells. A normal occurrence, chiefly in the blood sinuses of the SPLEEN, when the cells are ageing after 3–4 months in circulation, but it can happen abnormally in the circulating blood, causing *haemolytic anaemia*. In either case, the cells become more fragile than normal, disintegrate, and shed their contents. Normally the haemoglobin is broken down and recycled, so its iron is not lost. When free haemoglobin is released in the plasma, some products are retained, but excessive amounts are excreted from the kidneys (*haemoglobinuria*). Fragility of cells in a blood sample can be assessed by placing them in a series of salt solutions of progressively lower osmolality than the blood itself, which causes them to swell, and finding the osmolality at which they burst. S.J.

See BLOOD; HAEMOGLOBIN.

Haemorrhage
is merely another word for bleeding or blood loss. The amount of a haemorrhage may range from the trivial, for example following minor injuries or a small nosebleed, to life-threatening emergencies. Sometimes the

haemorrhage and its extent are obvious, but often it may not be detected without careful examination or special tests. A fracture of the femur, for example, can result in very severe hidden bleeding into the thigh. Bleeding may occur slowly and persistently into the gastrointestinal tract from ulcers or tumours and only be detected by biochemical tests on the FAECES.

The effects of haemorrhage depend both on the amount and on the rate of the blood loss. Slow haemorrhages may not actually cause a substantial decrease in the volume of blood, as this may be replaced as rapidly as it is lost. However, the lost red blood cells and their pigment, HAEMOGLOBIN, may not be replaced and often the first signs and symptoms of severe chronic blood loss are those of ANAEMIA: tiredness, pallor, and breathlessness on exertion. People can tolerate quite rapid and relatively large losses of blood with little apparent effect. Healthy people often donate nearly a pint of blood and are unaware of any after-effects. When the volume of blood depleted from the body exceeds about 20%, or 1 litre in an average adult, BLOOD PRESSURE may fall when standing, due to the added effect of blood 'pooling' in dependent veins, and the person may faint.

A moderate blood loss results in a decrease in cardiac output (volume of blood pumped per minute by the heart) but no change or even an increase in arterial blood pressure. Because the amount of blood pumped at each heart beat is smaller, the pulse of the arterial blood pressure is diminished, and this provides a smaller stimulus to the BARORECEPTORS. The resulting response

is an increase in the degree of constriction both of resistance vessels and of some veins, and also stimulation of the heart. More severe haemorrhage (over about 30% of blood volume or 1.5 litres in an average person) usually leads to a decrease in blood pressure. Baroreceptor stimulation is much reduced and the sympathetic nerves are strongly stimulated. This results in powerful constriction of blood vessels, seen in the skin as pallor. Other effects of the sympathetic nerves are sweating and piloerection (hairs standing on end). The patient is in shock and is pale, sweating, and has a rapid, 'thready' pulse.

As well as evoking these rapid reflex responses, haemorrhage also results in increases in the blood concentrations of several HORMONES, in particular ADRENALINE and NORADRENALINE, which augment the effects of sympathetic stimulation; *vasopressin* (antidiuretic hormone), which causes the KIDNEYS to retain more water (urine volume decreases); and *angiotensin*, which in addition to constricting blood vessels causes secretion of another hormone, *aldosterone*, which acts on the kidneys to retain both salt and water (see figure).

Severe haemorrhage, if untreated, is a very dangerous condition. The normal compensating responses eventually fail, the sympathetic nerves cease to fire, and activity in the vagus nerve to the heart may increase. This results in FAINTING. If very low blood pressure and low flow persist they are likely to cause irreversible changes so that even replacement of all the lost blood does not restore blood pressure. The most common cause of death is kidney failure, because the inadequate blood flow can damage the tubules of the kidney.

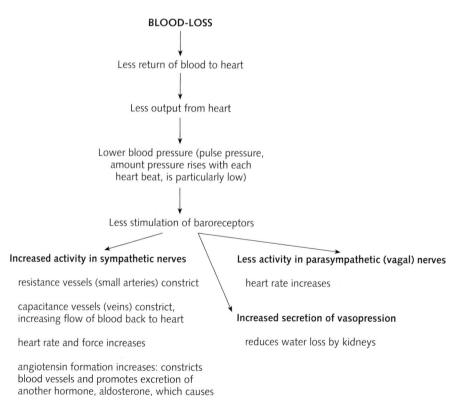

BLOOD-LOSS

↓

Less return of blood to heart

↓

Less output from heart

↓

Lower blood pressure (pulse pressure, amount pressure rises with each heart beat, is particularly low)

↓

Less stimulation of baroreceptors

Increased activity in sympathetic nerves

resistance vessels (small arteries) constrict

capacitance vessels (veins) constrict, increasing flow of blood back to heart

heart rate and force increases

angiotensin formation increases: constricts blood vessels and promotes excretion of another hormone, aldosterone, which causes kidneys to retain salt and water

Less activity in parasympathetic (vagal) nerves

heart rate increases

Increased secretion of vasopression

reduces water loss by kidneys

Other problems include *septicaemia* (infection in the blood) and HEART FAILURE. Severe haemorrhage must be treated by measures to stop the bleeding and by transfusion, ideally of blood, but if this is impossible suitable substitute solutions may be used.

Moderate or slow haemorrhages are compensated by the body. The sympathetic stimulation which constricts the arteries and arterioles (resistance vessels) cuts down the flow of blood into the capillaries. This decreases the pressure of blood which would tend to move fluid out through their walls, so that instead the osmotic pressure of the proteins in the blood is unopposed and draws fluid in from the tissues into the circulation. This can replace much of the lost circulating volume within a few hours. The protein constituents are replaced by the liver in days and, if sufficient iron is available, the bone marrow replaces the lost red cells in weeks.   R. HAINSWORTH

See also AUTONOMIC NERVOUS SYSTEM; BARORECEPTORS; BLOOD PRESSURE; INJURY; SHOCK.

Haemorrhoids (piles)

Haemorrhoids (piles) are swellings arising from the anus that may bleed or cause the area to be itchy or painful. They are a common condition and many of us will experience them to a certain degree at some time during our lives. They are especially common in women during pregnancy. The majority of haemorrhoids resolve spontaneously, but persistent symptoms, especially of bleeding in people over 50 years old, may need investigation as, rarely, they can mimic other more serious bowel disease such as cancer. Haemorrhoids are the most common cause of bleeding from the anus; the bleeding usually occurs after passing a bowel motion and will appear on the toilet paper.

Haemorrhoids have been recognized and treated for at least 4000 years. The term itself, as described by Hippocrates, comes from the Greek, *haema* — blood — and *rhoos* — flowing. Despite their common occurrence and extended history the exact cause of haemorrhoids is still unclear. In medieval times it was thought that haemorrhoids were enlarged veins that expelled superfluous melancholy humours. The concept of haemorrhoids as enlarged veins persisted until recently, when detailed anatomical studies demonstrated their soft tissue nature and the close association they have with the normal anus. Many long-held beliefs regarding the exact cause of haemorrhoids have been difficult to prove scientifically. Generally accepted associations are that haemorrhoids occur more frequently in those who are constipated, strain excessively when passing a bowel motion, or spend a long time sitting (especially on the toilet seat). In some cases a genetic component for the formation of haemorrhoids may well be responsible.

Haemorrhoids arise from the three cushions of tissue just inside the anus that normally function to give a watertight seal. These cushions may be damaged, bleed, or be pushed down by the passing bowel motion, thus forming a haemorrhoid.

If trapped outside the anus the haemorrhoid's blood supply may be disrupted, causing the severe pain of a 'thrombosed pile'.

The cornerstone of treatment and prevention of haemorrhoids is a high-fibre diet, producing a soft bowel motion that is easy to pass without straining. Combined with this it is important to avoid sitting for prolonged periods or excessive wiping of the anus after passing a bowel motion. Use of a moist cloth, wet wipe, or lying in a bath filled with lukewarm water are also helpful when the haemorrhoids cause symptoms. Historically, anaesthetic creams have been used to reduce the pain felt locally; however these may be irritating to the skin and should be considered secondary to other measures. If basic treatment fails, outpatient 'banding', injection, or freezing treatments can shrink the haemorrhoid, thus speeding resolution. Surgical treatment, where the haemorrhoids are removed at operation (*haemorrhoidectomy*) is used less frequently now, as outpatient treatment is very effective.   G. A. SMITH
P. J. O'DWYER

Hair

Hair is present in differing degrees on all mammals, and its most important function in those other than human is to conserve body heat by insulating against cold. Humans are the most hairless of all mammals, and yet hair occupies a central place in human development and sense of self. Whether it is the gradual decrease of hair leading to male BALDNESS, the loss of pigment leading to white or grey hairs and signalling the onset of middle age, or the adolescent desire for the pubic hair that signals approaching adulthood, hair often tells others something about our place in culture.

Hair types and styles have, at various times, in various countries and on various continents, come to be associated with definitions of race, the possibility of being or becoming the right kind of woman, with radicalism or revolution, and with the right to occupy a particular social space in a class hierarchy. While often discussed as a personal statement of style or FASHION, humanity's relationship to hair is far more complicated.

During the monarchy in France, the prince's hair, for example, was never cut — it was curled and pampered. Rastafarian followers of the early twentieth-century Ethiopian religious leader Haile Selassie not only refused to cut theirs, but were forbidden to comb it either. Early records indicate that the ancient Egyptians, men and women alike, shaved their hair off and wore wigs. Prostitutes in Nazi Germany were forced to shave off their hair so they could be easily identified and shamed. In the post-war period, women who had collaborated with the Nazis were similarly forced to shave their heads. Delila cut off Samson's long hair so that she could strip him of his fabled strength and power. As a sign of respect for the law and British custom, judges and lawyers during America's colonial period wore powdered wigs over their natural hair. Rapunzel let her hair cascade out of a window and down a tower so that Prince Charming might climb up and rescue her from imprisonment. Among the Yoruba people, hair signifies aesthetic value; and for East African pastoral peoples, such as the Pokot and Samburu, its styling indicates age status. A 1970s American Broadway musical, *Hair*, received numerous awards and set records for attendance.

Individual human hairs vary in colour, diameter, and contour. The different colours result from variations in the amount, distribution, and type of MELANIN pigment in them, as well as from variations in surface structure that cause light to be reflected in different ways. Hairs may be coarse, or so thin and colourless as to be nearly invisible. Straight hairs are round in cross section, while wavy hairs are alternately oval and round; very curly and kinky hairs are shaped like twisted ribbons. During the nineteenth century, renowned social scientists posited relationships between some of these variations in hair type and intelligence, or the potential for civilized behaviour, and indeed, in some instances, saw them as a marker of humanness.

In his 1848 *Natural History of the Human Species*, Charles Hamilton Smith, for example, suggested that hair type is crucial for defining the three typical 'stocks', or races, of mankind: the bearded Caucasian, the beardless Mongolian, and the woolly-haired Negro. His work included a chart which positions the 'woolly-haired' at the base of a triangular hierarchy and the Caucasians at the apex. Smith's 'woolly-haired race' became a metaphor for African physical traits which served prima facie as evidence of racial difference, such as mental 'lack', and as a justification for slavery and racial discrimination. The lingering effects of such pseudo-scientific theories may help to explain why people of African descent continue to spend billions of dollars each year trying chemically to alter the texture of their hair in order to make it straight, as opposed to 'woolly'.

Each hair grows from a *hair follicle* in the deep layer of the SKIN. There are different types of hair at different stages in life, and in different parts of the body. The first to develop is the lanugo, a layer of downy, slender hairs that begin growing in the third or fourth month of fetal life and are entirely shed either before or shortly after birth. During the first few months of infancy appears fine, short, unpigmented hairs called down hair, or vellus. Vellus covers every part of the body except the palms of the hands, the soles of the feet, undersurfaces of the fingers and toes, and a few other places. At and following PUBERTY, this hair is supplemented by longer, coarser, more heavily pigmented hair, called terminal hair, that develops in the armpits, genital regions, and, in males, on the face and sometimes on parts of the trunk and limbs. The growth and the distribution of hair are under the influence of the SEX HORMONES. The hair of the scalp, eyebrows, and eyelashes are of separate type and develop fairly early in life. On the scalp, where hair is usually densest and longest, the average total number of hairs is between 100 000 and 150 000. Human hair grows at a rate of 10–13 mm/month. While hair texture and type was of importance for nineteenth-century social scientists in the shaping of racial hierarchies, for middle-class women in Christian countries, hair length has been important in the shaping of hierarchies of femininity. In part due to a passage in the King James version of the Bible ('if a woman have long hair, it is Glory to Her' 1 Cor: 11–15), such women the world over have often been urged by society at large, and by patriarchs in their individual households, to wear their hair in long, precisely styled hair-dos that they refrained from cutting. During the Victorian period the long, elaborately-styled hairdos favoured by the middle classes signalled wealth, leisure time, and modesty (it was almost impossible for a woman to fix her hair in one of the fashionable styles without the paid help of a hairdresser, and the styling could often take three hours or more). During the 1920s, women who 'bobbed' or cut their hair to ear length caused a furore in Europe and the US. The new hair style, which went hand in hand with shockingly at, or above, the knee skirt lengths was seen as immodest and outside of prevailing standards of decency. This was true in part because bobbed hair was immediately favoured by women in the 'world's oldest profession' due to its ease of care.

By the late 1960s, long hair came to be back in vogue amongst male and female youth in America. However, far from being a return to the earlier ideals of propriety often associated with long hair, lengthy hair now denoted a counter culture or radical stance in both white and black communities. One of the surest ways for white teenagers and young adults to identify themselves as in rebellion against prevailing middle-class ideals and culture, and governmental political strategies, was to wear their hair in the long, straight styles favoured by hippies, flower children, and political activists. During this same period afros came to be a popular style in African–American communities. The afro was understood to denote black pride, which became synonymous with black nationalism, activism, and a radical political consciousness. This sentiment moved sharply against the prevailing integrationist ideology and evidenced a belief that the gains of the Civil Rights Movement were not broad-based enough, and was a style favoured by radical groups like the Black Panthers.

In addition to the presence or absence of hair, hair texture and styling have played a long and important role in human history. It is not clear just why hair has come to mean so very much to so many people, but there is no mistaking the important role that hair has played in the process of identifying a relationship to a particular culture or subculture. Hair can lead to acceptance or rejection by certain groups and social classes, and its styling can enhance or detract from career advancement. What many envision as a personal statement is also implicated in an intricate web of religious and social politics.

NOLIWE ROOKS

See also BALDNESS; SEX HORMONES; SKIN.

Hairdressing Whether ornate or simple, hairdressing has been employed by nearly every society from ancient time to the present. In 400 BC some Greek women dyed their hair; in the Roman period, dyeing and bleaching were common. Japanese women used lacquer (a precursor of modern-day hair spray) to secure their elaborate coiffures. Whatever the style, there have been groups of people who made their living and built their reputations by cutting, shaving, curling, and styling the hair.

Hairdressing is a profession that has appealed to both male and female practitioners. While in earlier periods, male hairdressers (often called barbers) mainly worked with male hair and women worked with women, during modern times, such distinctions have become less rigid. It is, however, still rare to find hairdressers who are willing to transgress racial boundaries in the styling of hair. Barbershops and beauty parlours remain amongst the most segregated of public spaces. Nonetheless, whatever the race or sex of the participant, a first trip to the hairdresser is often viewed as a rite of passage. A boy's first haircut is an event, a non-biological marker of movement from babyhood into childhood. A girl's first trip to the hairdresser marks her entrance from childhood into young womanhood. For both, the place where they encounter the hairdresser introduces them into what may become a significant social sphere in their lives. Barbershops and beauty salons have historically served as a primary site for gender-specific interaction, support, and nurturing.

Prior to the first few decades of the twentieth century, career choices were limited for all women, but particularly so for poor and migrant women, and those of ethnic minorities. Hairdressing has been a particularly attractive career option for such women because of the ease with which one may set up a business. A reputation as a sought-after hairdresser could lead to a career that was performed in the home, if one so chose, or in the more public setting of a shop, if resources allowed. In either case, hairdressing could support a family at monetary levels significantly higher than derived from domestic, factory, or agricultural work. Hairdressing did not require college training and one could have some control over working hours — making it an ideal occupation for women with small children to raise.

Beginning with the crude curling iron used by women of ancient Rome in creating their elaborate hair styles, hairdressing came to be associated with a variety of technological accoutrements, ranging from simple combs and hairpins to hold the hair in place to complex electrical appliances for drying and grooming the hair. In addition, chemical processes were used to tint, wave, curl, straighten, and condition the hair. By the twentieth century, hairdressing itself and the manufacture of materials and equipment had become an occupation and practical art of large proportions.

NOLIWE ROOKS

See also BODY DECORATION.

Halitosis, bad breath, or *foetor oris* (stench of the mouth) is an age-old and universal problem. Nowadays it is called *oral malodour*. But halitosis by any other name still smells as foul! Bad breath is mainly a social problem — a fact exploited by the cosmetics industry. Nearly 25 centuries ago, Hippocrates wrote that 'a pleasant odour is essential in any girl, and can be obtained and maintained by using a mouthwash containing anise, dill seeds, myrrh and white wine'. The Roman dramatist, Maccius Plautus claimed that his wife's breath was so foul that he would 'rather kiss a toad'.

Oral malodour is caused by nasty-smelling chemicals, such as hydrogen sulphide (H_2S) and methyl mercaptan (CH_3SH). These substances are by-products of protein breakdown by bacteria. In the case of oral malodour, these proteins are mostly derived from cells shed from the lining of the mouth. However, some cases may arise from dental plaque and from food debris trapped between the teeth.

In about 85% of cases, the malodour originates in the mouth. The commonest sources are the spaces between the teeth, around the gum margins, and at the back of the tongue. Dentures can sometimes be a cause, especially if these are not regularly cleaned. Malodours may also originate from the nose and throat. Unpleasant breath smells can occasionally occur after eating foods such as garlic, or in heavy smokers. Breath smells may arise from other organs, such as the gastrointestinal tract and lungs, or in metabolic disorders such as diabetes mellitus. But these are relatively rare causes of oral malodour.

People are not usually aware of the malodour. (A few people are obsessed about bad breath, even though their breath smells normal.) Just as beauty is in the eye of the beholder, so bad breath is in the nose of the receiver! In other words, we rely on others to tell us of any problem. This can be a source of embarrassment. Hieron of Syracuse allegedly reprimanded his wife for not informing him of his bad breath. She neatly avoided an awkward situation by replying innocently that she thought all men's breath must smell so foul!

People are unaware of their own breath, partly because senses adapt to a constant stimulus, but mainly because the air flow from the mouth does not enter the nose. We can detect malodours if we smell dental floss or woodsticks that have been used to clean between our teeth. Another way is to smell a spoon that has been scraped over the tongue surface. Devices are now available for detecting and measuring the chemicals responsible for malodour.

In most cases, the remedy is simple. Effective oral hygiene will remove the causative agents. This involves cleaning between the teeth and also brushing or scraping the surface of the tongue. Interestingly, the practice of tongue scraping was introduced in India many centuries ago. Mouthwashes can also be used, but are generally ineffective without the oral hygiene measures.

ROBIN ORCHARDSON

Further reading

Ratcliff, P. A. and Johnson, P. W. (1999). The relationship between oral malodor, gingivitis and periodontitis. A review. *Journal of Periodontology*, **70**, 485–89.

Rosenberg, M. (1996). Clinical assessment of bad breath: current concepts. *Journal of the American Dental Association*, **127**, 475–82.

Hallucination may be simply defined as the perception of an external object in the absence of a corresponding stimulus, yet such a simple definition obscures a whole series of conceptual difficulties which surround the medical and psychiatric use of the term. The range of conditions subsumed under this category is massive, and includes such varied phenomena as religious visions, PHANTOM LIMBS, TINNITUS, psychedelic 'trips', schizophrenic inner voices, the personal experience of DOPPELGANGERS, and a sceptical apprehension of the unreality of the outer world.

Such variety has naturally frustrated any attempt at providing a clear classification of the phenomenon. Attempts to distinguish the various forms of hallucination according to their origins, their content, their intensity, and the condition of their hosts have been largely unsuccessful. Most psychiatrists in Europe and North America have now adopted a fairly broad definition of the phenomenon, simply relying upon the distinction between ILLUSION, which resulted from the misinterpretation of an existing external object, and hallucination, in which the false perception is generated without any reference to the outside world. Even this definition, which was introduced by the French psychiatrist J. E. D. Esquirol in the early nineteenth century, fails to account for such borderline phenomena as synaesthesia in which the sensations provoked by an object become confused, so that the subject may taste colours or see sounds.

Alongside this ongoing contest over the definition and classification of hallucination there exists a more fundamental struggle over the meaning and significance of the phenomenon. Artists and mystics have long criticized the modern medicalization of hallucinations, portraying the process as a secularizing attempt to pathologize religious or spiritual experience. Certainly popular attitudes to hallucination have been transformed across the last thousand years. In the Platonic tradition of classical philosophy, the subjective vision was celebrated as a form of privileged insight beyond the phenomenal experience of the external world. Likewise in the Christian and Jewish religions the objective quality of the inner hallucination had long been regarded as a proof of its spiritual reality, although its origin could have been either demonic or divine.

These Platonic and Christian traditions were united in the work of the Primitive Church fathers. Their writing held up the visionary experience as a charism, a gift from God which allowed individuals to perceive some object which was normally invisible to men. This conception was further refined by St Augustine, who divided visions into three classes: the corporeal, in which an apparition of an object was presented before the individual's eyes through either natural or spiritual means; the imaginative, in which an image was supernaturally created in the host's mind; and the intellectual, in which sense of personal assurance was created directly by God, without recourse to implanted words or images.

This framework for interpreting the hallucinatory experience persisted into the nineteenth century. Many romantic writers, such as Coleridge and Wordsworth, complained that normal vision enslaved the mind to the mundane world of material object. In contrast, they proposed a 'Spiritual Optics' (to borrow Thomas Carlyle's phrase) in which the inner eye would be awakened to the creative inspiration of the spirit. Such a programme sat unhappily with contemporary medical investigations in this field. In the late eighteenth and early nineteenth centuries, many writers commented upon the correlation between hallucination, injury, and disease. This correlation suggested that the hallucination had a somatic basis, originating in either the disordered operations of the peripheral nerves or an aberrant psychological process in the brain.

This interpretation of hallucination as a symptom of organic nervous disorder persisted throughout the nineteenth century. In 1881 the Italian psychiatrist, August Tamburini, presented a coherent neurological model for the experience, arguing that hallucination was produced through a pathological excitement or EPILEPSY in the higher sensory centres of the brain. This materialist account did little to diminish the mystical celebration of hallucination. Writers influenced by spiritualism and the Swedish mystic Emanuel Swedenborg accepted the scientific identification of hallucination with organic disturbance, arguing that this identity provided strong evidence for the objective reality of visions.

The mystical assessment of the significance of hallucinations was undermined by a series of psychological surveys at the end of the nineteenth century. During the 1880s the statistician, Francis Galton, circulated questionnaires on mental imagery to schools and acquaintances. From the responses he was able to demonstrate a gradation between hallucination and the familiar acts of visualization which occurred in everyday life. Galton suggested that hallucination was not a distinct experience, but rather that it represented an extreme point on two axes representing the strength of the mental image and its resistance to conscious control. This statistical erosion of the boundary between normal visualization and pathological hallucination was reinforced in a more wide-scale survey published by the Society for Psychical Research (SPR) in 1892. The SPR's 'Census of Hallucinations' discovered 1684 cases of waking hallucination amongst 17 000 respondents. Further analysis suggested that hallucination was most prevalent amongst women, children, and the insane, although the experience could occur in almost any individual.

In the twentieth century the hallucinatory experience seems to have lost its spiritual significance. The popular use of hallucinogenic drugs, such as LSD and psilocybin, and increased understanding of the chemical mechanisms of their actions, has encouraged a more instrumental attitude towards the visionary experience. Hallucination is no longer seen as a gratuitous event except in pathological cases such as fever or schizophrenia. Rather it is a state which can be induced directly through chemical, electrical, or mechanical means. As the neurosurgeon Wilder Penfield demonstrated, intense mental images may be created through the electrical stimulation of a subject's brain. Likewise hallucinations of movement (see PROPRIOCEPTION) can be induced at a particular joint through the mechanical vibration of the muscles attached to it. Through such technical advances the meaning and cultural significance of hallucination has been transformed. The vision, which once revealed the mind of God to men, is now seen as a symptom revealing the disordered mind of man to others.   RHODRI HAYWARD

Further reading

Berrios, G. E. (1995). *The history of mental symptoms*. Cambridge University Press, Cambridge.

Critchley, M. (1987). *Hallucinations and their impact upon art*. Carnegie Press, Preston.

See also ILLUSIONS.

Halo The halo, usually represented as a luminous figure around the head of a god or holy person, appears in the iconography of a number of religious traditions. The indigenous civilizations of Central America depict agrarian gods with golden crowns or halos, suggesting an association of the halo with the sun. This is clearest in the Inca god, Viracocha, who wears a tiara that is also a sun. In other traditions, the connection to light symbolism is much more general, pointing to intellect, knowledge, or enlightenment. Within some Mahayana Buddhist texts, for example, *bodhisattvas* are described as having halos studded with 500 Buddhas, each attended by numberless gods. In this way, the halo points to the transcendent nature of the *bodhisattva*.

The halo is used in Hellenistic representations of gods and goddesses and those associated with them. Similarly, in Christianity, halos around the head of a figure mark it as divine or saintly. In the third and fourth centuries, the halo or nimbus (Latin: 'cloud' or 'mist') was used only for Christ and the lamb. In the fifth century and after, it was extended to the Virgin Mary, angels, and saints. By the eighth century, square halos were used to designate donors, bishops, and popes.

When used for human figures, the halo represents holiness or sanctity, and its iconography is developed to mark important distinctions between the figures represented. Square zones of light behind the head are used to show that the person was living at the time the painting was made. The square is inferior to the circle and is associated with the earth. Trinitarian figures often have three rays of light emanating from the head. The Virgin Mary always appears with a circular halo. A cross within the circle of light is used to signify Christ. Halos also appear around the heads of animals who symbolize a saintly or divine figure. A lamb with a circular halo within which the cross appears, for example, is a common figure for Christ.

AMY HOLLYWOOD

Further reading
Collinet-Guérin, M. (1961). *Histoire du nimbus des origines au temps modernes.* Nouvelles Editions Latines, Paris.

Hamstrings are the muscles of the back of the thigh: 'ham' being appropriate to describe the bulk of the muscles, and 'strings' to describe their TENDONS behind the KNEE. These muscles span both the HIP joint and the knee joint, because they are attached above to the pelvic bone, and below to the tibia. By virtue of these attachments they are the muscles that bend the knee, and they can also assist extension at the hip (backward movement of the leg). Stretching routines to encourage flexibility of the hamstring muscles therefore involve bending at the hip whilst straightening the knee. The *semitendinosus* (its lower half mostly tendon, hence the name) and the *semimembranosus* (its upper part a flattened tendon) form the hamstring tendons on the inner side; the *biceps femoris* forms the hamstring tendon on the outer side. These can be felt easily when the knee is bent.   S.J.

See PLATE 5.

Hands The major purpose of the forelimbs in most vertebrates is locomotion; humans are an exception. Bipedality freed the forelimbs and allowed development of the hands as highly specialized appendages with great dexterity. The hands and the brain are believed to have co-evolved, and both are associated with the appearance of language, tools, and other signs of advanced intelligence. Refinement and exploitation of tools required a hand that had both power and precision: a 'power grip' for grasping a branch or broom handle and a 'precision grip' for picking up small objects, or in writing or painting. The crucial evolutionary step in this regard was the arrangement of muscles, bones, and joints to allow the movement known as *opposition* — the ability to bring the thumb across to meet any of the fingers. Also in primates, the presence of nails rather than claws on the tip of the digits assists manipulation.

Structure and movement
Movements of each hand are initiated from a localised region of the opposite side of the BRAIN (in the grey matter of CEREBRAL CORTEX); thence nerve fibres pass down, cross to the other

side, relay, and emerge from the SPINAL CORD in the neck, and are distributed in the nerves of the arms to the muscles of the forearms and the hands. This is the means of activation, but the control of the movements depends essentially, like all movements, on sensory messages from the skin, the muscles, and the joints returning to the spinal cord and brain, as well as on the influence of other parts of the brain.

Muscles which have their main bulk in the forearm end in tendons (*sinews*) that reach across the wrist — back, front, thumb-side — to be attached to the bones of the WRIST, hand fingers, and thumb (*carpals*, *metacarpals*, and *phalanges*). Contraction of these different muscles can thus variously extend or flex the wrist, and straighten or curl up the thumb or the fingers. Personal observation will confirm that each finger cannot be moved entirely independently in this way, because of fibrous links between tendons where they traverse the hand. For the pull of the tendons to be effective, they must be held firmly close to the joints which they cross, or else they would spring out beneath the flexible skin; they also each require a frictionless tube in which to move — provided by a lubricated sheath of tissue which passes through the tough fibrous retaining tunnels at the wrist and all the way to the furthest bone of each finger. The strength of the grip depends essentially on the strength of the forearm muscles. The hand also has its own *intrinsic* muscles. The ones which flex the thumb and 'oppose' it to the fingers (for picking up and holding) lie at its base; their opposite number on the little-finger side flexes that finger and also takes part in cupping the palm and closing the grip. Deep in the palm there are other small muscles between the metacarpal bones. Blood vessels and nerves branch from the main ones at the wrist to supply the hand muscles as well as the joints and the skin.

The hands are exquisitely sensitive. It is common knowledge that they are the best tools for feeling texture, assessing temperature, or recognising objects by their feel when they cannot be seen; bad for the pain of a pinprick or insect bite but good for locating it exactly. This finesse and discrimination is due to the greater density of SENSORY RECEPTORS in the skin compared with other parts of the body surface, serving sensations of heat, cold, pressure, and pain, and to the disproportionately large area of the sensory cerebral cortex devoted to the hand. The skin is also well provided with sweat glands, especially on the palms.

The hand in history and culture
The hand was also a common unit of measure used by ancient Hebrews, Egyptians, Greeks, and Romans. The Egyptian hand was a subunit of the royal cubit (524 mm), the most widely used standard of measure in the ancient world. The basic subunit was the digit, presumably the width of a finger; four digits equaled a palm, five a hand. Based on a statue of King Henry VIII, the British

hand was established as four inches. The hand is still occasionally used today, most notably to measure the height of a horse from the ground to the high point of its back at the base of the neck.

The fingers bear unique and identifying marks, and FINGERPRINTING has been one of the most reliable forms of identification, used in China since 700 CE, and since the 1880s in Britain, mainly for criminal and police records. The patterns of whorls, arches, and loops on the ends of the fingers are unique to each person, and virtually indelible since superficial burns, cuts, or abrasions do not alter them. The hand- and footprints of infants may also be recorded for purposes of identification because they do not change with growth or age. A site of aesthetic expression, Ancient Egyptian women decorated their hands and also their feet with elaborate and intricate designs in henna. This practice is still part of Middle Eastern cultures today, particularly for special occasions such as weddings, when along with the bride, her mother, aunts, and friends will henna themselves as well. Recently, having one's hands decorated with designs in henna has become more popular in the United States.

Hand GESTURES, from sign language to the thumbs-up to seemingly universal obscene gestures, carry an infinite number of meanings. 'To lend a hand' means to help; 'to give a hand to' however, has an ambiguous sense of both to help, but also to applaud. An open hand is a symbol of generosity, and shaking right hands is a common greeting, especially among European and American men. The handshake, however, originated in seventeenth-century Holland, not as a greeting, but as a symbol of reconciliation. After a dispute had been settled by an official local arbiter, he would ask the parties involved to shake hands, as a sign that each regarded the other as an honest man and asked for forgiveness. As a gesture made between equals, the handshake was adopted by radical Protestant sects such as the Quakers who rejected traditional forms of greeting, like bowing, which stressed deference to social superiors. The handshake remains an egalitarian gesture of goodwill, though it was only during the nineteenth century that the handshake as a sign of greeting, friendship, or respect appeared in England and slowly spread throughout Europe. Traditionally, however, men did not shake, but kissed, the right hand of women in greeting.

The position of the hand, and especially of the fingers, is significant in religious practices, such as in Christian blessings, when one makes the sign of the cross, or raises the first two fingers when giving a blessing. Hands are often raised in prayer, the worshipper symbolically reaching toward heaven. The prayer position of both hands pressed together, pointing upward, is a symbol of the flame, and is used by Roman Catholics, Hindus, and Buddhists alike. The position of the hands also has significance in Hindu and Buddhist meditation (*mudrās*); for instance Buddhists sometimes assume the position of

Buddha when he called on the earth to witness his own enlightenment: left hand open in his lap, palm up, and right hand with the palm down, fingertips resting on the ground. In Buddhist iconography, the right and left hands joined together represents the union of wisdom and compassion.

The left hand has been associated with that which is base or evil. For instance, the left hand is considered dirty in Muslim and Hindu cultures, among others, as it is often the hand used to wash oneself after defecating. The left hand is associated with being 'sinister', which means both 'threatening evil' and simply 'on the left'. Thus, a left-handed compliment is one which conceals an insult. Until very recently, left-handedness in children was often discouraged, and even punished, by parents and educators.

Fingers are also the site of cultural expression, such as rings, which are worn both for decoration, but also as signs of status. In early modern Europe, a man's insignia, his seal, might be worn on a ring. Betrothal rings are believed to have originated in ancient Rome. The Roman Catholic Church still awards episcopal rings to bishops, and papal rings to popes and cardinals. These, and the rings of kings, are traditionally kissed in deference. Most common today are school rings, friendship rings, and wedding rings.

On a more sober note, in several cultures, particularly some Native Americans, Australian Aborigines, and African Bushmen, among others, the first joint, or sometimes the entire finger, is amputated, as a sign of mourning. It is often young girls and women whose hands are thus mutilated. European Palaeolithic cave paintings of hands without digits indicate that this practice may be very ancient. Some ancient law also required the amputation of the hand as punishment for theft;

this is still practised in some Islamic countries today. SARAH GOODFELLOW
SHEILA JENNETT

Further reading
Bremmer, J. and Rooderburg, H. (ed.) (1991). *A cultural history of gesture: from antiquity to the present day*. Polity Press, Cambridge.

See PLATE 5.

See also GESTURES; MOVEMENT, CONTROL OF; MUSICIANSHIP AND OTHER FINGER SKILLS.

Handedness

About 90% of us are better at doing things with the right than with the left hand. We write with the right hand, throw with it, and use it to hold implements such as scissors, a spoon, a knife, chopsticks, a sword, or a racquet. There are some activities that require both hands, but it is usually the right hand that plays the dominant role, as in threading a needle or unscrewing the lid of a jar. It is, of course, the greater skill of the right hand, in most people, that gives rise to the term DEXTERITY.

This dominance of the right hand is a characteristic of the human species. Other animals may show a systematic preference for one hand or paw when reaching for things, or using implements, but over the population of the species as a whole there is typically no overall preference for one or other hand or paw. Even individual mice typically show a systematic preference for one paw when reaching for food in a glass tube, and the preferred paw usually has the stronger grip; but there are as many left-pawed as right-pawed mice. Chimpanzees in the wild have been observed to use sticks to extract termites from their nests, and individual animals vary with respect to which hand they prefer to use to hold the stick, but again there appears to be no overall

preference. There is evidence for a slight majority of right-handers among captive chimpanzees for some activities, such as feeding, but the overall bias is only about 67%, significantly lower than the proportion of right-handed humans. The only species known to show a bias comparable to that in humans is the parrot, since roughly 90% of them prefer the *left* foot when picking up small objects or bits of food!

Right-handedness appears to be universal among humans. There is slight variation across cultures, but this is largely restricted to activities in which there are strong sanctions against using the left hand. For instance, in some traditional cultures it is forbidden to eat with the left hand, which in Hindu society, for instance, is regarded as 'the hand of the privy'. Until quite recently, there were strong pressures to force left-handed children to write with the right hand, although it is now generally recognized that this is likely to do more harm than good. Forced right-handers may be more than usually prone to stuttering, and may fail to realize their full potential for manual and verbal skills.

It was once thought that the ancient Israelites must have been predominantly left-handed because Hebrew is written from right to left. This Eurocentric view ignored the many other right-to-left scripts: until about AD 1500 there were about as many right-to-left scripts as left-to-right ones. The present-day prevalence of left-to-right scripts almost certainly owes more to European expansionism than to handedness. Again, it has been argued that the ancient Egyptians were left-handed, because Egyptian art typically portrays humans in right profile, whereas the natural tendency of right handers is to draw faces and bodies in left profile. But the preference for right-sided profiles in ancient

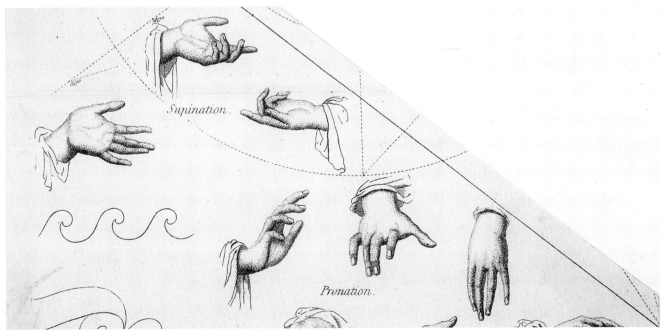

An assortment of hands. Mary Evans Picture Library.

Egypt was probably due to a belief that the left side of the body is inferior and should be hidden. Indeed, the very universality of such beliefs is testimony to the universality of right-handedness itself. Evidence from works of art suggests that the proportion of right-handers has been roughly constant for at least 5000 years. Close examination of the design and wear of ancient stone tools suggests that right-handers may have been in the majority throughout the Stone Age, going back two million years or more.

Given the overwhelming majority of right-handers, it is all too easy to overlook the left-handed, or to infer that left-handedness is in some way pathological. Yet there is virtually no indication that left-handers are in any way inferior in intellect or skill, and indeed they often seem to excel. The Italian Renaissance artist and inventor LEONARDO DA VINCI, one of the greatest geniuses of all time, was left-handed, and confused the right-handed world by writing, in mirror-image fashion, from right to left. Several US presidents, including Harry Truman, Gerald Ford, Ronald Reagan, and Bill Clinton, join such historical figures as Alexander the Great, Julius Caesar, Cicero, Charlemagne, and King David in being left-handed. Left-handers in the entertainment world include Charlie Chaplin, Harpo Marx, Rock Hudson, Paul McCartney, and Ringo Starr. A disproportionate fraction of prominent sportspersons have been left-handed, especially in sports involving racquets and bats: Rod Laver, Jimmy Connors, John McEnroe, and Martina Navratilova in tennis; Babe Ruth in baseball; David Gower in cricket.

It is not always clear whether the prominence of left-handers in some walks of life has some biological cause, or whether being left-handed simply makes people want to prove themselves in a right-handed world. The advantage they often seem to show in competitive sport may also be due to the unexpectedness, to right-handers, of their movements and actions.

It is sometimes suggested that the prevalence of right-handedness is simply due to environmental pressure. We live in a right-handed world. The location of door handles, the way pages are arranged in books, the construction of objects such as scissors, corkscrews, nuts and bolts, golf clubs, and even access to the zipper on men's trousers (to the wearer of the trousers, that is), are all designed for the convenience of right-handers and are a source of frustration to left-handers. But the very universality of right-handedness, extending to cultures that have been isolated for tens of thousands of years, suggests that causation is the other way round: it is the biological disposition toward right-handedness that is responsible for the cultural pressure. Moreover, the stubborn persistence of left-handers as a roughly constant proportion of the population in all human societies suggests that handedness may be under genetic control.

No one has yet located a gene for handedness, if indeed there is one (or perhaps there are several); but there have been reasonably plausible attempts to capture some of the facts about human handedness in terms of a hypothetical gene. Children are more likely to be left-handed if one or both of their parents are left-handed, but handedness does not 'breed true', since the proportion of left-handers born to two left-handed parents is somewhat less than half. It has therefore been suggested that the handedness gene does not simply determine whether one will be right-handed or left-handed. Rather, one form (or allele) of the gene, which we may call D for *dextral*, may code for right-handedness, while the other allele, which we may call C for *chance*, leaves the direction of handedness to chance. Different versions of this idea have been proposed by Marian Annett of the University of Leicester, and by Christopher McManus of the University of London. The chance element may also explain why some people are ambidextrous rather than clearly right- or left-handed. The children of left-handed parents would then have a chance of receiving two C alleles, one from each parent, which perhaps explains why only about 50% (or less) are left-handed. The C allele also helps explain why identical twins, like

Tweedledum and Tweedledee in Lewis Carroll's *Through the Looking Glass*, are often of opposite handedness, although other factors are likely to contribute as well.

Besides being right-handed, most of us are right-footed when kicking, right-eyed when aiming, and right-eared when listening on the telephone, and for most people it is the *left* side of the BRAIN that controls SPEECH and LANGUAGE. Since it is also the left brain that controls the right hand, this has led to the idea that the left side of the brain exerts a general dominance, especially over skilled actions like tool use or speech. This view has been tempered, however, by discoveries that the right brain is the more involved in other functions, such as spatial attention and orientation, and in non-verbal activities, such as art and music.

Nearly all right-handers are left-brained for language, suggesting that the D allele controls both handedness and brain dominance for language. Left-handers show a much more mixed pattern. Some are left-brained, some right-brained, and some appear to have speech represented on both sides. This is further evidence that the C allele, which is assumed to be present in the great majority of left handers, does not have a directional influence.

Throughout recorded history, and in virtually all human cultures, handedness has invited myth, superstition, and of course prejudice. One reason for this may be that handedness is not evident in the hands themselves. It is difficult to tell whether a person is left- or right-handed by physically inspecting the hands — although there may be some give-away signs like rings, or a watch, or differential signs of wear. Handedness is really only evident from the way people *do* things — a reflection of brain activity rather than of how the hands themselves are formed. The hidden sources of handedness may explain why it is often linked to supernatural or extrabodily sources. The right hand is often the hand of God or virtue, while the left hand is the hand of the Devil or wickedness. In the Bible there are over 100 favourable references to the right hand, and about 25 unfavourable references to the left.

The true nature of handedness is still not fully understood, and there is no reason to suppose that our modern theories are entirely free of age-old superstitions.

MICHAEL C. CORBALLIS

Further reading

Corballis, M. C. (1991). *The lopsided ape*. Oxford University Press, New York.

See also LANGUAGE AND THE BRAIN; SYMMETRY AND ASYMMETRY.

Hangover Suffering from a hangover — the after-effects of too much *alcohol* — is such a common experience that there has been little research on it. But most people know what it feels like! Kingsley Amis provides an evocative description of this undesirable state in his well-known novel *Lucky Jim*:

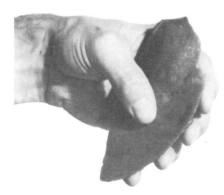
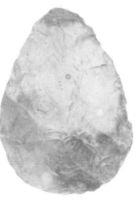
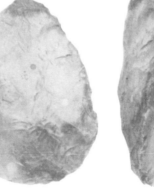

Evidence of handedness can be seen in stone age tools. The scraping implement held in a left hand was formed by careful chipping by a hammer stone held in a more dextrous right hand. The stone axe shows a twist suited to right-handed use. Less frequently left-handed tools are found.

He lay sprawled, too wicked to move, spewed up like a broken spider-crab on the tarry shingle of the morning. The light did him harm, but not as much as looking at things did; he resolved, having done it once, never to move his eyeballs again. A dusty thudding in his head made the scene before him beat like a pulse. His mouth had been used as a latrine by some small creature of the night, and then as its mausoleum. During the night too, he'd somehow been on a cross-country run and then been expertly beaten up by secret police. He felt bad.

The long list of *symptoms*, documented in numerous medical and literary sources and abundant in personal accounts, can be grouped into eight categories: constitutional (FATIGUE, weakness, and thirst); pain (HEADACHE and muscle aches); gastrointestinal (NAUSEA, VOMITING, and stomach pain); SLEEP and BIOLOGICAL RHYTHMS (less sleep, and more disturbed sleep); sensory (VERTIGO, and sensitivity to light and sound); cognitive (decreased attention and concentration); mood (depression, ANXIETY, and irritability); sympathetic hyperactivity (TREMOR, SWEATING, and increased PULSE rate and systolic BLOOD PRESSURE).

Some hangover symptoms are due to the direct effects of alcohol on the body — as a DIURETIC for example, increasing urination, dehydrating the body, and increasing thirst. Other symptoms result from the body's efforts to cope with the removal of alcohol and counteract its depressant effects on the central nervous system. Unpleasant sensations such as tremors, sweating, and rapid heartbeat plague the sufferer. Behaviours associated with the previous evening's drinking, such as eating too little, having less sleep than usual, or overdoing it on the dance floor, may also account for some of the aches and pains.

The experience of a hangover is not the same for everyone. If your hangovers seem worse than other people's, it may be because your personality or how you feel about your life is contributing to the symptoms. Researchers have suggested that personality traits, such as anger, defensiveness, and neuroticism, feelings of guilt about drinking, and experiencing negative life events (such as divorce, death, loss of employment, or other stressful events) can increase the experienced severity of hangovers. Other factors are involved too. We probably all know people who say they can drink certain kinds of alcohol without ill effect whereas other kinds result in misery the morning after. Red wine, for instance, is more likely to result in a severe hangover than white wine; bourbon and port are more likely to than gin or vodka. The 'culprits' responsible for these differences are known as 'congeners' — the toxins present in the organic chemicals used to colour and flavour alcoholic beverages (examples are methyl alcohol, aldehydes, and tannins). Research studies indicate that people vary in their *tolerance* of alcohol and of the congeners in different drinks, so that bodily reactions to 'detoxifying' — getting rid of poisonous substances — will reflect individual differences in the ways in which alcohol is metabolized and the body clears itself of toxins. Seasoned heavy drinkers may cope more easily with this process, possibly because their metabolism adjusts more quickly or because they have become less sensitive to the effects than the occasional or less heavy drinker.

So what can you do to enjoy the pleasures of alcohol and avoid the pain? There are steps you can take to alleviate the discomfort. Drinking plenty of water before going to bed helps counteract dehydration and dilutes the congeners; replacing lost fluids by drinking water, fruit juices, or tea the morning after might also reduce the intensity of a hangover. Although a strong cup of coffee will certainly not get rid of the alcohol in your body, CAFFEINE is a stimulant and might perk you up. If you can face it, bland foods such as toast or crackers may relieve feelings of nausea. Medication can provide symptomatic relief, but needs to be used with caution, since some kinds of medication are likely to exacerbate symptoms or add to the toxicity in the body, and other kinds appear to be ineffective in reducing headaches and other hangover symptoms.

Down the ages, there have been numerous 'folk' cures and remedies for hangovers, one of the best known being 'the hair of the dog that bit you' — another drink on waking. It is the likely base of the 'tissue restorer' favoured by P. G. Woodhouse's Bertie Wooster and prepared by his manservant Jeeves:

> He returned with the tissue restorer. I loosed it down the hatch, and after undergoing the passing discomfort, unavoidable when you drink Jeeve's patent morning revivers, of having the top of the skull fly up to the ceiling and the eyes shoot out of their sockets and rebound from the opposite wall like raquet balls, felt better.

The remedy works — temporarily! But the body still has to clear itself of the after-effects of the drinking bout, and morning drinks, if taken too often, can signal problem drinking. Time, sleep, and rest are the best 'cure' for a hangover.

B. THOM

Further reading

Rae, S. (ed.) (1991). *The Faber book of drink, drinkers and drinking*. Faber and Faber, London.

Swift, R. and Davidson, D. (1998). Alcohol hangover mechanisms and mediators. *Alcohol World Health and Research*, **22**(1), 54–60.

See also ALCOHOLISM.

Harelip
The description 'like the lip of a hare' was first applied (in Greek) by GALEN to a cleft or ridge in the upper lip which results from defective development during fetal life. The cleft in the lip may or may not be accompanied by a cleft in the palate. Such defects can now be satisfactorily repaired.

S.J.

See CLEFT LIP AND PALATE.

Harem
The arabic word *harem* derives its original spelling and meaning from the Egyptian word *harim*, meaning 'women'. Originally, it was in the women's part of a Mohammedan dwelling-house that its inhabitants and the place were seen as sacred.

The harem can also be referred to as a *seraglio* (meaning, 'the walled palace'), wherein the sultan's wives, children, divorced wives, concubines, slaves, and eunuchs might live. As Alain Grosrichard states in *Structure du serail* (1979):

> The order of the seraglio is set with the despot in view and according to his needs, and most of all for sexual pleasure which begins with the privilege of sight.

Though an isolated domain, harems in the nineteenth century became known to tradesmen and merchants who would wait outside the main gates for an invitation to show their wares to the women indoors.

The harem and the *odalisque* (a reclining female nude or semi-nude) have increasingly become North Africa's cultural icons, dominating visual perceptions in the European mind. Particularly influential in visually capturing such images in the nineteenth century were a group of French and British painters known as The Orientalists. Artists included Eugene Delacroix, Jean–Dominique Ingres, J–L. Gerome, and Frederick Leighton.

ANNE ABICHOU

Further reading

Alloula, M. (1987). *The colonial harem*, (trans. M. Godzich and W. Godzich). Manchester University Press, Manchester.

Badran, M. (1987). *Harem years: the memoirs of an Egyptian feminist*, (trans. Badran). Feminist Press, New York.

Harvey, William
William Harvey (1578–1657) was both a physician and a remarkable natural historian. His great achievement was the demonstration of the circulation of the blood, a discovery which replaced centuries of theory and speculation with knowledge firmly based on accurate observation and experiment. His work was of vital importance in illustrating the sequence of hypothesis, experiment, and conclusion which has governed all medical discovery since his time. He was the founder of modern PHYSIOLOGY.

Harvey was born in Folkestone in Kent on 1 April 1578, the son of a yeoman, James Harvey, and his wife Joane Halke. Aged ten, in the year of the Spanish Armada, he was sent to King's School, Canterbury, and from there to Cambridge University, being admitted to Gonville and Caius College on 31 May 1593. He graduated BA in 1597 and deciding to study medicine, travelled though France and Germany to Padua, where Galileo was then teaching. There is no evidence that Harvey ever met Galileo, nor of whether he believed in the heliocentric view of the universe. His own mentor was the great anatomist, Fabricius of Aquapendente, who maintained the traditions of VESALIUS at Padua. Harvey graduated MD in Padua on 25 April 1602 and returned to London, taking his Cambridge MD in that same year. Two years later he married Elizabeth Browne, daughter of Dr Lancelot

Browne, onetime physician to Queen Elizabeth. In 1607, he became a Fellow of the College of Physicians and in 1609 began his long association with St Bartholomew's Hospital, on appointment as assistant physician.

In 1615, Harvey was elected Lumleian Lecturer at the College of Physicians, and he delivered his first lectures in April 1616. The notes he used for these lectures not only illustrate his wide reading and knowledge of the classics, but also reveal some of the ideas that led him to the discovery of the circulation of the blood. For many years he gave the Lumleian lectures annually at the College.

His position as a physician was increasingly recognized in wider circles through these years. In 1618 he became physician to James I, initiating a link with the Royal family that persisted throughout his long life. In 1630, at the behest of King Charles I, he accompanied the Duke of Lennox on a European tour and two years later travelled with the King to Scotland. In the years before the Civil War he was in London, but he went to Oxford in attendance on the King in 1642. There, on 7 December, he was made MD of the University. He pursued his anatomical studies and dissections at Merton College. He was at the battle of Edgehill and is said to have had charge of the Prince of Wales and the Duke of York during the action. After the surrender of Oxford in 1646, he returned to London and there continued his scientific studies. He was active in the affairs of the College of Physicians, being elected President in 1654, an honour he declined because of his increasing years, being 76 years old. In that same year he donated his library to the College. He died on 3 June 1657 and was interred at Hempstead.

Harvey's monumental work *De Motu Cordis* was published in 1628. In his dedication to King Charles I, he likened the position of the monarch in his kingdom with that of the heart within the body. Until that time, medical opinion was governed by the views of the second century writer, GALEN, whose works had gained a position among learned physicians that was almost akin to holy writ. The Galenical view was that the blood was formed in the liver from nutrients derived from the intestine. It passed from there to the heart, where it was imbued with 'vital spirits', and then traversed the septum (which divides the right and left sides of the heart) through invisible 'pores'. The different functions of the veins and arteries were unknown and the blood was considered to ebb and flow in the veins to reach the tissues of the body.

Harvey's observations clearly showed the Galenical view to be erroneous. Using experiments in animals such as the snake, he demonstrated that the blood passed from the veins to the right side of the heart (the right ventricle), that the supposed pores in the septum of the heart did not exist, and that the right ventricle propelled the blood into the lungs. It then returned to the left side of the heart. The left ventricle was thicker and more powerful than its counterpart on the right side, because it pumped blood not just through the lungs but throughout the entire body. Harvey clearly demonstrated that blood in the arteries was always carried away from the heart, and how the valves in the veins, originally described by his teacher, Fabricius, ensured that the venous blood always flowed towards the heart. He calculated how much blood might be propelled from the heart with each heart beat and showed there was no likelihood that the liver could synthesize sufficient blood to enter the heart as proposed by the Galenists. From ingenious but classically simple experiments and observations, Harvey concluded that the only explanation for the heart's action must be that a defined amount of blood constantly circulated throughout the body.

Harvey's discovery, comparable to the anatomical studies of Vesalius, was of great importance in destroying the influence of Galen, whose dogmatic assertions had by then become pernicious. It was perhaps natural that so novel and original a discovery would generate controversy. On the continent, Leyden was the first university to accept Harvey's conclusions; in many other schools, particularly in Paris, it was a further half century before Harvey's work was fully appreciated. So important was his work, however, that by the beginning of the eighteenth century the great Dutch teacher of medicine in Leyden, Hermann Boerhaave, stated that nothing that had been written before Harvey was any longer worthy of consideration.

Harvey was interested in many other aspects of comparative anatomy and physiology, for example the problem of reproduction, then poorly understood. But his discovery of the circulation of the blood remains his lasting memorial. His death in 1657 preceded by three years the foundation, by Charles II, of the Royal Society of London. It was, however, in large part due to the influence of William Harvey that the Society chose as its motto 'Nullius in verba'.

C. C. BOOTH

Further reading

Keynes, G. (1978). *The life of William Harvey*. Clarendon Press, Oxford.

Whitteridge, G. (1976). *William Harvey: an anatomical disputation concerning the movement of the heart and blood in living creatures*. Blackwell Scientific Publications, Oxford, London.

See also BLOOD CIRCULATION.

Headache is arguably the commonest of the human ills, and perhaps, in proportion to its impact, one of the least well understood.

There are many different types of headache, whether considered as to how they behave or as to how they are caused. Headache may broadly be classified as primary or secondary: there are situations in which headache itself is the problem (*primary headache*), and others in which headache is a symptom of some other condition (*secondary headache*). Headache has been classified in detail by the International Headache Society, and whole textbooks have been written about it.

The main types of primary and secondary headache are listed in the table, which is based on a population survey. The main primary headaches are migraine (which is considered separately under that heading) and 'tension-type headache — which is the commonest of all. It is often dull, both-sided, mild but otherwise featureless. It is surprisingly poorly understood. One of the most severe forms of headache, and one of the most difficult to treat, is 'chronic daily headache', which involves having headache most days of the week for most of the day. This may be either a form of chronic migraine or of tension-type headache; it is probably experienced in some form by up to 4% of the population, and is often associated with *analgesic* (painkiller) overuse. The daily headache syndrome is often due in part to the constant cycle of taking painkillers and then having their effects wear off: so-called *rebound headache*. Regular use of painkillers, particularly those containing more than one ingredient, such as mixtures with codeine, CAFFEINE, or barbiturates, is a potent cause of difficulty in the treatment of headache. Also any regular intake of anti-migraine drugs, including ergotamine and triptans (sumatriptan and related compounds), may potentially cause or aggravate this problem.

Headache does not have any single cause. Just as there are many types of headache, there are many causes of the problem. With respect to the cause of the pain the mechanisms are much less well understood for the primary than for the secondary headaches. Whereas the pain due to injury to the skin, for example, is well understood as being due to stimulation of specific nerve endings in conjunction with local inflammatory events, it is not clear in primary head pain whether the nerves are firing normally or abnormally in response to various stimuli. Much work is to be to done, especially in regard to understanding tension-type headache.

Headache due to serious disease is rare, but a sufferer should be concerned about a headache when it has certain features. These include: sudden onset or sudden worsening, such as a severe headache never previously experienced; headache associated with fever, together with neck stiffness or altered consciousness, such as drowsiness; headache that is gradually worsening over a short period — say one to two months; or headache associated with pain in the temples, and pain on chewing, particularly if there is any visual disturbance. These latter symptoms are very important and a sufferer should seek immediate medical attention.

Most countries have established flourishing patient groups, which can be contacted by reference to telephone directories, such as the Migraine Trust in the UK and the American Council for Headache Education in the US.

PETER J. GOADSBY

See also MIGRAINE.

Type	Primary headache			Secondary headache
	Prevalence (% of all primary headaches)	Cause		Prevalence (% of all secondary headaches)
tension-type	69	systemic infection		63
migraine	16	head injury		4
idiopathic stabbing	2	vascular disorders		1
exertional	1	sub-arachnoid haemorrhage		<1
cluster	0.6	brain tumour		0.1

Types of headache. After Rassmussen, B. K. (1995) Epidemology of headache. *Cephalalgia*;**15**:45–68.

Further reading

Goadsby, P. J. and Silberstein, S. D. (ed.) (1997). *Headache.* Butterworth–Heinemann, New York. (Asbury, A. and Marsden. C. D. (ed.) *Blue books in practical neurology*, Vol. 17.)

Lance, J. W. and Goadsby, P. J. (1998). *Mechanism and management of headache*, (6th edn). Butterworth–Heinemann, London.

Headhunting

Few if any customs have the ability to conjure up the image of the exotic more evocatively than headhunting and its compelling souvenir, the shrunken head. This well-documented activity, as opposed to other former behavioural symbols of the 'primitive' such as CANNIBALISM or incest, has been discontinued due to Western contact, including colonial rule, and subsequently due to the activities of the independent state. As a result, and oddly enough, these relics of headhunting may now litter museums in our countries with greater abundance than in their native homelands. This Western interest in shrunken heads not only suggests cultural curiosity on our part, but also hints at cultural correspondences in the form of preserved body parts displayed as sacred relics, scientific remnants, and symbols of conquest. (In this context, some former colonies in Africa have had to request the return of the heads of historical figures involved in the resistance to colonialism from European museums where they have been on display.)

Despite the pervasive cultural impression of a generic exotic other, headhunting *per se*, as opposed to the world-wide distribution of trophy collecting as the result of combat, had a relatively limited cultural distribution. Taking heads, and their treatment for subsequent and often elaborate ritual attention, was limited in South-East Asia to scattered ethnic groups inhabiting parts of Indonesia (particularly Borneo), Malaysia, and the Philippines among the Ilongot. In Amazonian South America, the practice has been documented only for the Jivaro (also known as the Shuar) of south-eastern Ecuador, the Mundurucu of Central Brazil, and the nearby Tupi-Kagwahiv (also known as the Parintintin).

Anthropological attempts at interpreting the cultural significance of headhunting have been surprisingly limited. Explanatory efforts for the activity are characterized by projecting causation and meaning to the actors in question or alternately accounting for the function of the custom in a simplistic fashion. As a result, we learn from the literature that heads are taken for the sake of revenge or to garner supernatural power, and that it reduces the male population sufficiently enough to allow for polygyny. Such explanations may well be spurious. In attempting to gasp the significance of the custom it is best to adhere to what can be said with assurance.

In this context it should be noted — since it usually goes unmentioned — that the act of taking heads was restricted to adult males. However, it is clear from written accounts and museum collections that females, as well as children and the aged, could be the victims since they were presumed to offer the least threat to the headhunter. The reasons offered for engaging in the activity were varied, and usually explained by those involved in terms of a custom mandated by the ancestors. In addition, it has also been intimated that the taking of a head brought positive results to the community in the form of prosperity, fertility, and general well-being. On an individual level, the activity was rationalized in terms of the expiation of grief over the death of a loved one, revenge for a similar activity perpetrated by others, a mark of having achieved adulthood, or an attempt to impress a desirable female. The suggestion that headhunting in general was also a form of aggressive sacrifice has also been proposed, but this argument fails to correspond to the ethnographic facts for all implicated groups. Even the purported *sine qua non* of the headhunting complex, the subsequent ritual elaboration of the object, fails to garner universal inclusion, since among the Ilongot the perpetrator immediately disposed of the head where and when it was taken, in a moment of grief and rage.

The inability to isolate a set of consistent characteristics for headhunting, and the various interpretations offered by participants and external commentators alike, suggests parallels in other cultural settings. Thus, it may be best to consider headhunting as a particular cultural expression of a more widespread attempt at ritual communication through the use of human body parts. The fact that Western cultures also engage in the activity as broadly defined may well explain the relative lack of analytical detail on the subject. W. ARENS

Further reading

Hoskins, J. (ed.) (1996). *Headhunting and the social imagination in Southeast Asia*. Stanford University Press, Stanford CA.

Healing

The expectation of a cure for all ills among people in the developed world increases enormously with the growth of medical technology and with scientific exploration of the human body. In America, they say, death is optional, and indeed plastic surgery, organ transplants, heroic chemical therapies, and any number of diets and exercises almost make a joke seem reality, for the very rich at least. In countries with high living standards and universal health insurance, life expectancy is increasing among all social classes, and infant mortality is dropping to record lows. Hope for physical well-being has never been higher among the fortunate, and among the unfortunate, the conquest of DISEASE seems only a matter of time and money. And yet, everyone has died of something sooner or later, so far, and it would seem that just as one disease is conquered, another pops up, more dangerous and mysterious than the last. Equally as worrying for the wary consumer of health news are the conflicting reports of what one should do to stay well. Some fats are good but others will kill you; alcohol is bad except red wine; VITAMINS can prevent CANCER, or maybe not. The choices are staggering and the stakes are high. What we all need, whether to avoid illness or to be restored to health is a reliable source of learned advice. But where can such a source be found?

Philosophers (and politicians) advise self-reliance, but whether the vagaries of science or the caprices of the gods, the ways of healing are just too complex for most people to manage without help. The ill and the worried turn to books, television, physicians, quacks, relatives, priests, and neighbours, all in search for deliverance. Ultimately they fail, of course, but the quest is revealing of the many ways in which humans have regarded ILLNESS, and of the ways in which they have sought relief.

Spiritual or religious healing is found in most cultures. Even now some television ministers claim to cure sufferers if they touch the screen. We tend to sneer at such antics as the province of the ignorant lower classes, but in fact not until recently has any method of healing united every level of society. The Greek. god of healing was Apollo, who counted among his patients the Olympian gods themselves. His son, Asculepius, a demigod, became so proficient at the art of medicine that the poets report he angered Hades, the god of the underworld, who accused him of depopulating Hell. Zeus killed the doctor with a thunderbolt and he became a god himself, with a cult of priest–physicians at his service in temples scattered throughout ancient Greece. Temples to Asculepius, called Asclepia, were located in cities like Cos and Cnidus, later to become famous for the presence of Hippocratic philosophical physicians. The most famous of the Asclepia was at Epidaurus, a fashionable mineral spa, which was celebrated by some of the most famous gentleman writers of antiquity.

At the temple, the sufferers would be greeted by authoritative physician–priests, who assured them of the greatness of their god and of his many cures. Ritual purification followed, which consisted of soothing baths in the mineral springs, which were often themselves associated with divinities. Massages and animal sacrifice accompanied these rites, followed by the famous 'temple sleep', during which the afflicted had a dream or vision of the nature of the problem which suggested treatments. If they were very lucky, a sacred dog or even a snake would appear to them and lick the affected part. After relief was achieved, the gods were thanked, sometimes with the story of the cure inscribed on a tablet for the temple collection. Many such temples throughout the ancient world also are littered with images of body parts offered by the thankful, sometimes of arresting anatomical correctness, and often moulded in terra cotta.

The Old Testament of the Christian Bible recounted how the Children of Israel were cautioned to observe complex purification rituals after intercourse, childbirth, or menstruation, and were cautioned to eat only certain foods and avoid others, as a sign of their covenant with God. In the Gospel, Jesus commanded his followers to heal the sick. In one of the most impressive miracles recorded in the ancient world, Jesus caused devils tormenting two madmen living among the tombs to inhabit a herd of swine, who subsequently rushed into a lake and drowned (Matthew 8: 28–32). Elsewhere he healed lepers, caused the blind to see, and even raised the dead, usually by a simple word or touch. Anxious to demonstrate that these miracles were meant to teach and were not magic, Jesus often repeated that it was not he himself, but the faith of the sufferers or those surrounding them that accomplished the healing.

During the Christian Middle Ages the tradition of healing miracles was taken over into the cult of SAINTS. Monarchs, merchants, and peasants all sought out miraculous healing at the shrines of holy women and men. Certain saints specialized in healing certain ills. Mothers, lepers, even people with bones caught in their throats, all had patron saints. The body parts of saints were preserved in ornate boxes called reliquaries, often made of gold and studded with jewels. So widespread was the rage for collecting saints' relics that church legislation had to be enacted to prevent the faithful from boiling down the bodies of the saintly dead for their bones until a decent interval had elapsed. Raging disputes erupted over whether a holy person really were dead, which often lasted for days before putrefaction settled what theology could not.

The boundary between life and death in the medieval period was much more hazy than it is now. An interval of a year or more was not an unusual time to elapse before friends and relatives were satisfied the soul had left the body. Even learned university physicians visited the bodies of friends thought to have healing powers, confident that the personality of the dead person remained and might exert a helpful or comforting influence. Conversely, the recovery of

people from what we would call comas or deep sleep could be interpreted as an example of miraculous RESURRECTION, perhaps accounting in part for the enduring popularity of saintly healing.

The popularity of religious healing endures even today, especially when scientific medicine is not available, or when the sought-after cure lies outside the boundaries of scientific medical practice. Once the person in need of healing has accepted the authority of the god or gods to perform the healing, further advice is often not necessary. Usually communication between sufferers or their advocates and the divine is direct, or with few intermediaries. This is not often the case with the use of more familiar methods of healing like pharmacy and surgery, which are nearly the sole instruments of scientific medicine today.

Diet and pharmacy were almost indistinguishable in early medicine — foods could act as drugs and drugs could be nourishing. Dietetic medicine, which was developed by the ancient Greeks, emphasized the preservation of health and avoidance of disease much more than its cure. In order to accomplish this, the person was compelled to seek the advice of a philosopher–physician, who understood the client's place in the larger world, and could tailor that particular regimen of health to the particular individual. Every aspect of the client's 'lifestyle' — occupation, time of birth, habits, ancestry, gender, and class — all were important in dietetic medicine to preserve health and prolong life. Astrology was a useful tool to the dietetic physician, as was a knowledge of the broader world of nature and of how each person fit into it. When something went wrong, this was attributed to a falling out of harmony with nature. This imbalance could be corrected gently, over time, with mild remedies intended to purge offending substances from the body and restore its well-being. Such a system implied an excess of leisure, and certainly a great amount of faith in the practitioner, for a regimen of health is much more difficult and expensive to maintain than is taking a pill or two when something goes wrong.

An important break with the dietetic tradition in medicine came with the medical and religious reformer Paracelsus (1493?–1541). Paracelsus was one of the first exponents of chemical therapy. He believed that illness was not caused by disturbances in the entire complexion or constitution of the body that were peculiar to individuals. Instead, he argued that diseases 'attacked' the body from outside and were poisons, excited into action by chemical disturbances taking place among the stars. Healing was accomplished not by gradual readjusting of the humoral balance, but by using chemicals against the poisonous attacker which would act on the disease at its particular site. What is more, these chemical remedies worked the same for everybody, worked quickly, and did not need the complicated (and expensive) advice of the learned physician. It is little wonder that Paracelsus has

been called by some the Martin Luther (1483–1546) of medicine. Like Luther, Paracelsus wanted to 'eliminate the middleman' and make healing simple, quick, and mystical rather than logical.

Paracelsus and his followers ushered in what historians have called an age of radical medical interventionism. Chemical therapies like mercury for syphilis, surgical procedures like cutting for the bladder stone (without anaesthesia), and letting buckets and buckets of blood for fever, or nearly anything else, became the mainstays of medical therapy. Patients demanded these tortures, and submitted to them, because they thought they worked and because there seemed no alternative. By the nineteenth century, the discovery of anaesthesia allowed surgeons to take their time, and, more important for patients, allowed them to sever the experience of bodily suffering in hopes of a cure.

The development of bacteriology by Louis Pasteur (1822–95) and Robert Koch (1843–1910) revolutionized medical understanding of disease, and the invention of various antibiotics, beginning early in the twentieth century, revolutionized their cures.

Medical technology has enabled scientific medicine to vanquish its rivals in the medical marketplace in the quest for patient patronage and health insurance funds. A health care machine, centred in the hospital and university, is where we are born and where most of us will die. But as healing grows more complex, the knowledge required to make healing choices becomes more and more difficult to accumulate. Issues of trust and authority continue to challenge the suffering and the fearful.

FAYE GETZ

Further reading

Cook, H. J (1993). Physical methods. In *Companion encyclopedia of the history of medicine*, (ed. W. F. Bynum and R. Porter, Routledge, London and New York.

Finucane, R. C. (1977). *Miracles and pilgrims: popular beliefs in medieval England*. Rowman and Littlefield, Totowa, NJ.

Pouchelle, M. C. (1990). *The body and surgery in the Middle Ages*, (trans. R. Morris) Rutgers University Press, New Brunswick.

Temkin, O. (1991). *Hippocrates in a world of Pagans and Christians*. Johns Hopkins University Press, Baltimore.

See also DRUG; HEALTH; MEDICINE; RELICS; SAINTS; SURGERY; WITCH DOCTOR.

Health is commonly thought of as the absence of disease, and indeed it is difficult to discuss one without the other. Equally problematic is the consideration of the health of the body apart from the state of the mind or the spirit, because historically the topics were closely connected, especially before the seventeenth century. Even with these difficulties in mind, it is still possible to focus on certain notions about the health of the human body as a natural state and about how this natural state could be restored or maintained.

One idea about health that unites many cultures, from the classical Indian, Mesopotamian, Egyptian, ancient Greek, sub-Saharan African, Semitic, and native American, is the notion that there was a time when the human body existed in a perfect state of health and when no diseases beset it. People lived in harmony with nature, in a childlike state of material plenty and spiritual obedience. Bodily ills came into the world, so many stories go, when a 'sin', often one of disobedience, angered divine authority. One thinks of the myth of Pandora's box or the expulsion of Adam and Eve from the Garden of Eden, as told in Genesis, as examples, but other cultures provide many more such tales. Stories about original sin and the fall from grace are, in short, as common as creation myths in their explanations for why humanity no longer experiences natural health and, in some cases, long physical life.

Such myths carry in them crucial meanings for understanding the history of the body and its health that are with us still. The idea that there was a time when perfect health existed naturally is a powerful one. The author of Genesis wrote of painless childbirth before the Fall, and of, even after it, the remarkable age and sexual prowess of the Patriarchs. These stories also link health, or lack of it, to moral or religious conduct, and often join good health to a vigorous old age.

If perfect bodily health existed once, some argued, it could exist again. The restoration of balance and harmony with nature and with the divine was commonly offered as a way to achieve this restoration. Taoist thought sees good health as a balance between the opposing forces of Yin and Yang, which exist in the individual as well as in the world at large. The ancient Greeks viewed good bodily health as the duty of the aristocracy, along with military service and good governance. Medical texts are among the earliest surviving philosophical writings of the Greeks, indicating an eager audience for this type of advice.

Ancient Greek notions are perhaps the most important for defining how health would be regarded, at least in European and Islamic cultures. Most important is the nearly universal idea of microcosm and macrocosm. Very simply put, the body (microcosm) was thought of as a part of the larger world of nature (macrocosm). The four elements of nature: earth, air, fire, and water, and the four qualities: hot, cold, moist, and dry, found their counterparts within the body in the four humours: blood, which was hot and moist; choler, which was hot and dry; phlegm, which was cold and moist; and melancholy, which was cold and dry. Health lay in balancing these humours within the body through a regimen consisting of diet, exercise, and regulation of the emotions. Moderation and balance in all these natural factors was the road to good health and long life. Indeed, the Greeks counted gymnastics among the liberal arts, along with rhetoric and logic, as activities proper to a gentleman and ones leading to moral virtue.

Roman Stoic philosophers and Christian thinkers who followed after them held physical health in rather less esteem. Stoics sought to free themselves from bodily concerns by philosophical contemplation, while some Christians found value in mortifying the flesh, thereby turning their thoughts to the immortality of the soul. Medieval Islamic culture elaborated the Greek ideal of the healthy, happy aristocrat, and cultivated royal doctors famous for entertaining stories and jokes. It also promoted musicians, all to preserve the health of noble patrons. Medieval scholastic philosophers, rather surprisingly, took up another Islamic pursuit, alchemy. From the thirteenth century the Pope, who ideally ruled for life, patronized Christian alchemists. They argued that the recovery of knowledge about the philosophers' stone (which was known to the ancients) would not only make one rich, but return the body to its pristine state before original sin brought disease and the ravages of old age into the world.

The rage for medical alchemy, which only grew during the Renaissance, brought into focus the importance of philosophical thinking, drawing upon the ideas of many cultures, to the development of notions about bodily health. Rationality, a peculiar obsession of the Greeks, contributed to the separation of bodily concerns from those of the spirit. Although ancient Greek physicians called themselves philosophers, they excluded from philosophical/medical consideration supernatural causes of disease as being the province of magicians, because they were anxious to define their young profession as different, and better, than that of the faith healer. Medieval Christian and Islamic physicians admitted that lack of health could be associated with sin or magic, but dismissed these factors as outside the realm of Aristotelian medical practice. The seventeenth-century thinker Descartes (1596–1650), as part of a larger mechanical philosophy, made a separation between mind and body that was total. For Descartes, and other mechanists who followed after him, the healthy body was nothing more than a well-functioning machine, soulless and subject to chemical and mechanical remedies.

Cartesian medical philosophy not only excluded religious concerns from the proper duty of the learned physician, but also made easy the postulation of 'mental' illnesses and 'mental' health as being separate from the state of the body. Vitalist views of the body and health did not fade from consideration all at once. Individualized, pastoral-style medical care of the whole person experiences periodic revivals, especially when Westerners study subcontinental and far-Eastern methods of healing. But the notion of the body as a machine emphasized the sameness of all bodies rather than their uniqueness. The remarkable growth in medical technology from the end of the eighteenth century allowed medical scientists to 'look inside' the normal, living body and define its typical characteristics as never before. For example, the discovery of

auscultation and later the stethoscope made individual patient reports of symptoms less important than the physician's own collection of diagnostic signs. Doctors could listen to the internal sounds made by hundreds of healthy bodies and easily isolate the 'abnormal', leading to a kind of medical objectivity never imagined before. The modern diagnostic laboratory of today allows the isolation of ungendered, raceless, classless tissue samples from subjective judgement and, for better or worse, minimizes the patient's own assessment of his or her state of health.

Nostalgia for a lost golden age never disappears from the medical scene, of course. Nineteenth-century Romantic thinkers offered the 'noble savage' or the 'primitive' hunter-gatherer as an ideal of bodily (and sometimes of moral) health. Even today, experimental studies with animals suggest that living in a state of near-starvation the way our ancestors were forced to do would lead to longer life and greater health — as if such a life would be worth prolonging. 'Quality of life' considerations will always be foremost in the mind of the patient, and this is an aspect of health that technologically-based scientific medicine, almost by definition, may appear to neglect. But in the contexts of clinical trials and medical audit the profession increasingly acknowledges the importance of quality of life as a component of outcome assessment.

FAYE GETZ

Further reading

Ackerknecht, E. H. (1982). *A short history of medicine.* Johns Hopkins University Press, Baltimore and London.

Bynum, C. W. (1995). *The resurrection of the body in Western Christianity, 200–1336.* Columbia University Press, New York.

Temkin, O. (1991). *Hippocrates in a world of Pagans and Christians.* Johns Hopkins University Press, Baltimore and London.

See also CREATION MYTHS; ILLNESS; MEDICINE.

Health foods The importance of FOOD to good health is one of the oldest and most significant notions in human material culture. Obviously people must eat or they will die, but the concept of 'health food' carries with it moral, religious, and even political meanings that go far beyond mere nutrition. For most people just getting enough to eat can be a struggle. But for those living beyond the margin, the selection of what one ought to eat or to avoid to recover or to preserve health is profoundly revealing of cultural attitudes and of the relationship of the body to what enters it.

The biblical book of Leviticus offered a daunting array of dietary restrictions to the Jews, embedded among other laws they had to observe in order to keep their covenant with God. Much later commentary on the lists of forbidden foods notes, for example, that prohibition of pork was done for 'good reason', because pork would have carried an unusual amount of disease. Such logic does not, however, apply to the prohibition of rabbit, for instance, and we must look elsewhere for a better explanation of these enigmatic documents. Leviticus itself suggests an answer. After promising his people a land of milk and honey, God continued:

'I have made a clear separation between you and the nations, and you shall make a clear separation between clean beasts and unclean beasts and between unclean and clean birds …You shall be holy to me, because I the Lord am holy'

(Leviticus 20: 24–6).

If God's people obeyed his laws, which included eating certain foods and avoiding others, they would enjoy a life of plenty and would be holy before the Lord. If they polluted themselves, they would lose God's favour.

Many cultures throughout history have observed similar restrictions. Adam and Eve were told to avoid apples, which they did not. The Pythagoreans shunned beans. Hindus do not eat beef and Moslems avoid pork. History offers numerous examples of pious Roman Catholic women who claim to exist on the wine and bread of the Holy Sacrament alone. 'Health food', in this sense, implies certain dietary restrictions that affirm a person's place in the social order and assure them that they are doing something that will keep them from bodily or spiritual harm. The more positive approach — that certain foods actually are better for one than others — also has a long history.

The ancient Greek science of dietetics embraced not only what one ate but also one's physical activity and emotions. Each person's diet was individualized according to gender, class, age, and occupation. Healthy food was food that was peculiarly suited to one's unique constitution or complexion. Food was essential to keep the bodily fluids in balance and to maintain harmony with the world of nature. In the Greek system, which dominated medical philosophy in the West until the seventeenth century, the distinction between food and medicine was never clear. A disordered constitution, one affected by FEVER for instance, could be returned to balance with temperate foods that would have a moderating influence. The body would require a long time to return to normal, however, and this sort of medicine never dealt very well with acute conditions. By the seventeenth century, more radical treatments, often chemical, came into fashion and the gentle, gradual, and individualized diet fell out of favour.

A returning focus on food came when scientists began to study diseases that were caused by deficiency of nutriments, required in tiny amounts, that came to be called *vitamins*. Scurvy, which was revealed as a problem by long ocean voyages, was identified and treated by eighteenth-century naval physicians. By the 1880s, beriberi and other vitamin deficiencies were being identified, and by the 1920s most major VITAMINS had been identified and supplements like cod liver oil were being recommended, especially for children.

'Health food', in the modern sense of what one might buy in a health food shop, has its immediate roots in the nineteenth century. In the US, new Protestant sects like the Church of Jesus Christ of Latter-Day Saints (1830) and the Seventh-Day Adventists (1861) avoid tea, coffee, alcohol, and tobacco, believing that the body, as the temple of the soul, must be protected.

VEGETARIANISM in various forms is increasing in popularity even outside of religious groups. Many vegetarians avoid meat out of compassion for animals and because they believe animal products are unnecessary or unnatural. But some associate meat-eating with capitalism and the exploitation of the environment, and are making a political as much as a nutritional statement. The macrobiotic movement, which claims to have originated in mid-nineteenth-century Japan, returns to more ancient concepts of healthy eating. One popular regimen, lasting seven years, emphasizes cereal grains and the consumption of local and seasonal fruits and vegetables only, because only locally-grown produce can restore balance and harmony.

Popular interest in health foods is becoming more widespread, especially as scientists explore the importance of micronutrients in disease prevention. 'Whole foods' that have been minimally processed are recommended in the mass media as being more nutritious, as are 'natural' vitamins that are thought to be more complex and not chemically-produced. Health food restaurants and juice bars are no longer the sole property of fashionable parts of New York and California, and shops are crammed with 'lite' and 'no-fat' alternatives to butter, sugar, beer, and eggs. Health foods, ironically, are becoming less 'natural' and more 'processed' as science excites popular anxiety about proper nutrition and as eaters attempt to observe the rituals they think necessary for long life and good health.

FAYE GETZ

Further reading

Bynum, C. W. (1987). *Holy Feast and Holy Fast: the religious significance of food to medieval women.* University of California Press, Berkeley.

Cook, H. J. (1993). Physical methods. In *Companion encyclopedia of the history of medicine,* (ed. W. F. Bynum and R. Porter). Routledge, London and New York.

Douglas, M. (1966). *Purity and danger: an analysis of concepts of pollution and taboo.* Routledge, London.

See also CHOLESTEROL; DIETS; FASTING; FOOD; TABOOS; VEGAN; VEGETARIANISM; VITAMINS.

Hearing Sounds are rapid variations in pressure, which are propagated through the air away from a vibrating object, such as a loudspeaker cone or the human vocal cords. Our sense of hearing allows us to detect and identify the myriad sounds present in our environment, and to determine their whereabouts. In humans and other animals with a poorly-developed sense of smell, hearing plays a particularly important role

in alerting the listener to novel events in the environment. Through speech and music, human hearing also makes an extremely important contribution to social communication.

When the prongs of a tuning fork vibrate back and forth in a regular manner, a periodic sound is produced. For such a pure tone, the simplest type of sound, the pressure increases and then decreases following a smooth wave pattern (a *sinusoidal function*). The number of complete cycles per second is known as the frequency of the tone and is measured in *Hertz* (Hz). More commonly, natural sounds contain a number of different frequency components, the variation in intensity across the frequency range being referred to as the *spectrum* of the sound. The *fundamental frequency* of a complex tone corresponds to its perceived pitch, whereas the full spectrum determines the *timbre*, or sound quality. Thus, the same note played on two different musical instruments may sound different, as a result of differences in the additional frequencies in their spectra.

Young, healthy humans can hear sound frequencies from about 40 Hz to 20 kHz, although the upper frequency limit declines with age. Other mammals can hear frequencies that are inaudible to humans, both lower and higher. Some bats, for example, which navigate by echolocation, both emit and hear sounds with frequencies of more than 100 kHz. In general, there is a good match between the sound frequencies to which an animal is most sensitive and those frequencies it uses for communication. This is true in humans, who are most sensitive over a broad range of tones that cover the spectrum of human speech.

Compared with total atmospheric pressure, airborne sound waves represent extremely small pressure changes. The amplitude of the pressure variation in a sound directly determines its perceived loudness. Because the range of sound pressures that can be heard is so large, a logarithmic scale of *decibels* (dB) is used to measure sound intensity. On this scale, 0 dB is around the lowest sound level that can be heard by a human listener, whereas sound levels of 100 dB or more are uncomfortably loud and may damage the ears. At pop concerts and in discos the sound level can be much higher than this!

The design of the ear changed substantially between aquatic and terrestrial vertebrates, but has remained very similar among mammals (except for specializations for different parts of the frequency spectrum). The human ear is illustrated in the figure. It is subdivided into the external, middle, and inner ear. The visible part of the ear comprises the skin-covered cartilaginous EXTERNAL EAR. This includes the *pinna* on the side of the head and the *external auditory meatus*, or ear canal, which terminates at the eardrum. As they travel into the ear canal, sounds are filtered so that the amplitude of different frequency components is altered in different ways depending on the location of the sound source. These spectral modifications, which are not perceived as a change in sound quality, help us to localize the source of the sound. They are particularly important for distinguishing between sounds located in front of and behind or above and below the listener, and for localizing sounds if you are deaf in one ear, or when listening to very quiet sounds, inaudible to one ear. Because of its resonance characteristics, the external ear also amplifies the sound pressure at the eardrum by up to 20 dB in humans over a frequency range of 2–7 kHz.

Lying behind the eardrum is an air-filled cavity known as the *middle ear*, which is connected to the back of the throat via the EUSTACHIAN TUBE. Opening of this tube during SWALLOWING and yawning serves to maintain the middle ear cavity at atmospheric pressure. Airborne sounds pass through the middle ear to reach the fluid-filled *cochlea* of the inner ear, where the process of *transduction* — the conversion of sound into the electrical signals of nerve cells — takes place. Because of its greater density, the fluid in the cochlea has a much higher resistance to sound vibration than the air in the middle ear cavity. To avoid most of the incoming sound energy from being reflected back, vibrations of the eardrum are mechanically coupled to a flexible membrane (the *oval window*) in the wall of the cochlea by the three smallest bones in the body (the malleus, incus, and stapes — together known as the *ossicles*). These delicately suspended bones improve the efficiency with which sound energy is transferred from the air to the fluid in the cochlea and therefore prevent the loss in sound pressure that would otherwise occur due to the higher impedance of the cochlear fluids. This is achieved primarily because the vibrations of the eardrum are concentrated on the much smaller footplate of the stapes, which fits into the oval window of the cochlea. The smallest SKELETAL MUSCLES in the body are attached to the ossicles,

and contract reflexly in response to loud sounds or when the owner of them speaks. These contractions dampen the vibrations of the ossicles, thereby reducing the transmission of sound through the middle ear. As with the external ear, the efficiency of middle ear transmission varies with sound frequency. Together, these structures determine the frequencies to which we are most sensitive.

The inner ear includes the cochlea, the hearing organ, and the *semicircular canals* and *otolith organs*, the sense organs of balance. Both systems employ specialized receptor cells, known as *hair cells*, for detecting mechanical changes within the fluid-filled inner ear. Projecting from the apical surface of each hair cell is a bundle of around 100 hairs called *stereocilia*. Deflection of the bundle of hairs by sound (in the cochlea) or head motion or gravity (in the balance organs) leads to the opening of pores in the membrane of the hairs that allow small, positively-charged ions to rush into the hair cell and change its internal voltage. This causes a NEUROTRANSMITTER to be released from the base of the hair cell, which, in turn, activates the ends of nerve fibres that convey information from the ear towards the brain. Although there are some differences between the hair cells of the hearing and balance organs, they work in essentially the same way.

The mammalian cochlea is a tube which is coiled so that it fits compactly within the temporal bone. The length of the cochlea — just over 3 cm in humans — is related to the range of audible frequencies rather than the size of the animal. Consequently, this structure does not vary much in size between mice and elephants. It is subdivided lengthwise into two principal regions by a collagen-fibre meshwork known as the *basilar membrane*. Around 15 000 hair cells, together with the nerves that supply them and supporting

cells, are distributed in rows along its length. Vibrations transmitted by the middle ear ossicles to the oval window produce pressure gradients between the cochlear fluids on either side of the basilar membrane, setting the membrane into motion. The hair cells are ideally positioned to detect very small movements of the basilar membrane. There are two types of hair cells in the cochlea. The inner hair cells form a single row, whereas the more numerous outer hair cells are typically arranged into three rows.

In the nineteenth century, the great German physiologist and physicist Hermann von Helmholtz proposed that our perception of pitch arises because each region of the cochlea resonates at a different frequency (rather like the different strings of a piano). The first direct measurements of the response of the cochlea to sound were made by Georg von Békésy a century later, on the ears of human cadavers. He showed that very loud sounds induced a travelling wave of displacement along the basilar membrane, which resembles the motion produced when a rope is whipped. Von Békésy observed that the wave built up in amplitude as it travelled along the membrane and then decreased abruptly. For high-frequency sounds, the peak amplitude of the wave occurs near the base of the cochlea (adjacent to the middle ear), whereas the position of the peak shifts towards the other end of the tube (the apex) for progressively lower frequencies. This indeed occurs because the basilar membrane increases in width and decreases in stiffness from base to apex. These observations, which led to von Békésy winning the NOBEL PRIZE, established that the cochlea performs a crude form of Fourier analysis, splitting complex sounds into their different frequency components along the length of the basilar membrane.

More recently, much more sensitive techniques, which can measure vibrations of less than a billionth of a metre, have revealed that motion of the basilar membrane is dramatically different in living and dead preparations. In animals in which the cochlea is physiologically intact, the movements of the basilar membrane are amplified, giving rise to much greater sensitivity and sharper frequency 'tuning' than can be explained by the variation in width and stiffness along its length. This amplifying step most likely involves the living outer hair cells, which, when stimulated by sound, actively change their length, shortening and lengthening up to thousands of times per second. These tiny movements appear to feed energy back into the cochlea to alter the mechanical response of the basilar membrane. Damage to the outer hair cells, following exposure to loud sounds or 'ototoxic' drugs, leads to poorer frequency selectivity and raised thresholds of hearing. The active responses of the outer hair cells are probably responsible for the extraordinary fact that the ear itself produces sound, which can be recorded with a microphone placed close to the ear and used to provide an objective measure of the performance of the ear.

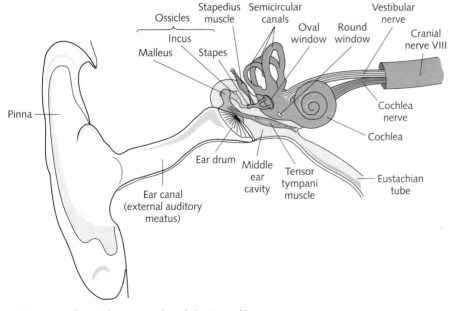

The human ear illustrated in a section through the temporal bone.

Vibrations of the basilar membrane, detected by the inner hair cells, are transmitted to the brain in the form of trains of nerve impulses passing along the 30 000 axons of the auditory nerve (which mostly make contact with the inner hair cells). Each nerve fibre responds to motion of a limited portion of the basilar membrane and is therefore tuned to a particular sound frequency. Consequently, the frequency content of a sound is represented within the nerve and the auditory regions of the brain by which fibres are active. For frequencies below about 5 kHz, the auditory nerve fibres act like microphones, in that the impulses tend to be synchronized to a particular phase of the cycle of the stimulus. This property, known as *phase-locking*, allows changes in sound frequency to be represented to the brain by differences in the timing of ACTION POTENTIALS and is thought to be particularly important for pitch perception at low frequencies and for speech perception. The intensity of sound is represented within the auditory system by the rate of firing of individual neurons — the number of nerve impulses generated per second — and by the number of neurons that are active.

Auditory signals are relayed through various nuclei (collections of nerve cell bodies) in the brain stem and THALAMUS, up to the temporal lobe of the CEREBRAL CORTEX. At each nucleus, the incoming fibres that relay information to the next group of nerve cells are distributed in a topographic order, preserving the spatial relationships of the regions of basilar membrane from which they receive information. This spatial ordering of nerve fibres establishes a neural 'map' of sound frequency in each nucleus. The extraction of biologically important information — 'What is the sound? Where did it come from?' — takes place in the brain. As a result of the complex pattern of connections that exist within the auditory pathways, many neurons, particularly in the cortex, respond better to complex sounds than to pure tones. Indeed, in certain animals, including songbirds and echolocating bats, physiologists have discovered neurons that are tuned to behaviourally important acoustical features (components of bird song or bat calls). But auditory processing reaches its zenith in humans, where different regions of the cerebral cortex appear (according to studies involving IMAGING TECHNIQUES) to have specialized roles in the perception of language and music.

The ability to localize sounds in space assumes great importance for animals seeking prey or trying to avoid potential predators, and also when directing attention towards interesting events. Although sounds can be localized using one ear alone, an improvement in performance is usually seen if both ears hear the sound. Such binaural localization depends on the detection of tiny differences in the intensity or timing of sounds reaching the two ears. At the beginning of the twentieth century, Lord Rayleigh demonstrated that human listeners can localize sounds below about 1500 Hz using the minute differences between the time of arrival (or phase) of the

sound at the two ears, which arise because the sound arrives slightly later at the ear further from the sound source. He also showed that interaural intensity differences, which result from the acoustical 'shadow' cast by the head, are effective cues at higher frequencies. Using these cues, listeners can distinguish two sources separated by as little as 1° in angle in the horizontal plane.

Studies in animals have shown that neurons in auditory nuclei of the brain stem receive converging signals from the two ears. By comparing the timing of the phase-locked nerve impulses coming from each side, some of these neurons show sensitivity to differences in the sound arrival time at the two ears of the order of tens of microseconds, whereas other neurons are exquisitely sensitive to interaural differences in sound level. As well as facilitating the localization of sound sources, binaural hearing improves our ability to pick out particular sound sources, which helps us to detect and analyze them, particularly against a noisy background (aptly termed the 'cocktail party effect').

ANDREW J. KING

Further reading
Moore, B. C. J. (1997). *An introduction to the psychology of hearing*, (4th edn). Academic Press, London.

Pickles, J. O. (1988). *An introduction to the physiology of hearing*, (2nd edn). Academic Press, London.

See also DEAFNESS; EAR, EXTERNAL; EUSTACHIAN TUBE; HEARING AID; SENSE ORGANS; SENSORY INTEGRATION; TINNITUS.

Hearing aid Artificial instruments to aid hearing have been in use for at least four centuries and may date back even longer. For example, the simple measure of cupping the hand behind the ear is referred to in ancient Roman medical documents. A variety of purely mechanical devices were used from the seventeenth to the nineteenth centuries to increase the size and capacity of the ear to conduct sound. In the twentieth century, these were surpassed by electric hearing aids, which also amplify and, in more recent devices, process sounds in an attempt to improve the perception and recognition of speech and other environmental signals.

Most non-electric aids to HEARING were portable so as to avoid restricting movement and were either worn or held by the listener. These included horn-like ear trumpets, which were made from wood, various metals, or even adapted conch shells, whose effectiveness in transmitting sound depended on their length and shape. Speaking tubes with funnel-shaped endings for the talker's mouth worked by attenuating sounds less than would be the case in the free field. A variety of artificial ears, including larger versions of the shape of the normal pinna, were also used in an attempt to improve upon the natural acoustical properties of the EXTERNAL EAR. In addition to devices that amplified airborne sounds, some instruments took advantage of the

fact that sounds can reach the inner ear, albeit much less effectively, by bone conduction. This was useful when middle ear disease was present, and involved connecting the hearing aid to the listener's teeth. Acoustical chairs and tables from which amplified sounds were conducted to the ears were also used in the eighteenth and nineteenth centuries. The most effective mechanical hearing aids tended to be large, conspicuous instruments. However, as with modern electric hearing aids, there was pressure to make these devices as inconspicuous as possible by reducing their size or by hiding them in beards, hairstyles, walking sticks, and fans. This inevitably led to a reduction in the benefit they provided.

The first electric hearing aids were developed in the US around the beginning of the twentieth century. Initially using radio valves, and then transistors, they essentially comprise three components. Sound waves are converted by a microphone into electrical signals that vary with the pitch and intensity of the sound. An amplifier is used to increase the gain of the signal, which is then reconverted into sound energy by a receiver and transmitted into the ear canal by a fine tube held in place by an individually moulded ear piece. As with the earlier mechanical aids, most receivers conduct amplified airborne sound, although a few devices, which may be used if there is a completely closed ear canal or if the ear is discharging chronically, work on the basis of bone conduction. Electric hearing aids are typically worn behind the ear, in the ear canal itself, or on spectacle frames. Body-worn aids are also sometimes used in the case of severely impaired individuals.

Hearing aids provide a personal amplifying system for the hard of hearing. In the case of a conductive hearing loss, the problem is lack of amplification. However, this form of DEAFNESS is often treated satisfactorily by drugs or surgery, and most people for whom hearing aids are prescribed actually suffer from a form of sensorineural hearing loss, where the intention is to make maximum use of residual hearing by boosting the input for the range of frequencies that are still audible.

Early electric hearing aids often distorted and restricted the acoustic information available, and sometimes actually made it harder for the listener to hear. However, the design and performance of hearing aids has greatly improved in recent years as a result of advances in signal processing. Individuals with poor hearing thresholds may exhibit normal sensitivity to more intense sounds. If this condition, which is known as *loudness recruitment*, is present, the gain of the hearing aid is adjusted automatically so that quieter sounds are amplified more than the most intense sounds. Modern hearing aids also provide an improved frequency response, which can be adjusted to suit the needs of individual hearing-impaired listeners, and, by including directional microphones, are beginning to enhance the listener's ability to understand speech in noisy surroundings.

Individuals with profound sensorineural deafness cannot be helped by conventional hearing aids because there are no or very few sensory cells left in the cochlea. However, the discovery during the past century that electrical stimulation of the surgically exposed auditory nerve results in the sensation of hearing has led to the development of electronic devices known as *cochlear implants*. Sounds are converted to electrical impulses by a microphone and processed by a control unit that is typically worn in the clothing. These signals are then transmitted to a radio frequency receiver implanted under the skin behind the ear and then to one or more electrodes inserted into the cochlea. The electrodes bypass the damaged or missing sensory hair cells and activate the remaining auditory nerve fibres directly. Initially, the implants comprised a single electrode. By varying the frequency of electrical stimulation, some individuals with single-channel implants can detect changes in pitch and, as long as deafness occurs after language acquisition, can even recognize simple melodies. Cochlear implants now include more than 20 electrodes, which, by stimulating selective groups of auditory nerve fibres, can elicit different sensations and therefore carry more information to the brain. Current work, including the use of animal models, is directed toward improving the way in which signals delivered to the electrodes are processed so that the patterns of nerve impulses generated in auditory nerve fibres are as close as possible to those that would normally be generated by acoustic stimulation.

Although the effectiveness of cochlear implants varies, they do restore some useful hearing that can enhance lip-reading and sometimes provide a good level of speech understanding, sufficient for conversing by telephone. Implants can also facilitate the acquisition of spoken language in profoundly deaf children.

ANDREW J. KING

Further reading

Killion, M. C. (1997). Hearing aids: past, present, future: moving toward normal conversations in noise. *British Journal of Audiology*, **31**, 141–8.

Moore, B. C. J. (1997). *An introduction to the psychology of hearing*, (4th edn). Academic Press, London.

Stephens, S. D. G. and Goodwin, J. C. (1984). Non-electric aids to hearing: a short history. *Audiology*, **23**, 215–40.

See also DEAFNESS; EAR, EXTERNAL; HEARING.

Heart

Heart Throughout human history the rhythmic beat of the heart has quintessentially represented life. Until the advent of the HEART–LUNG MACHINE, the lack of a heart beat, unless reversed within a few minutes, invariably signalled death. The beat of our own heart can be apparent to us in the pulse felt, or seen, at various parts of the body, occasionally heard or — because of an unusual rhythm or 'skipped' beat — noticeable in the chest.

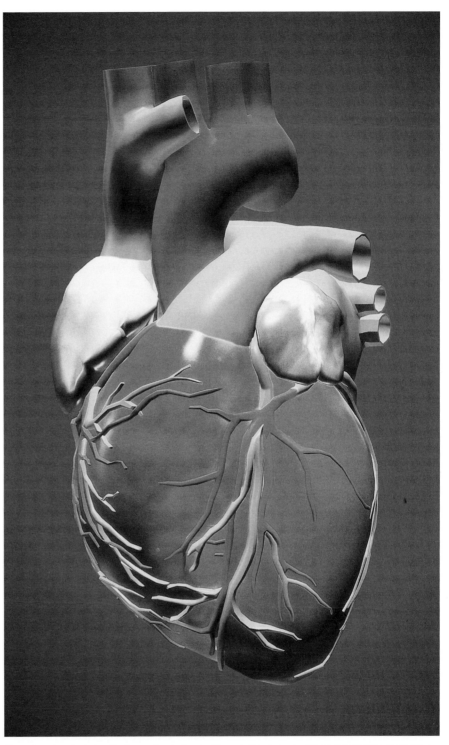

Computer artwork of a healthy human heart, showing the main blood vessels. Mike Agliolo/Science Photo Library.

The heart is a hollow muscular organ. It acts as the 'prime mover' for the circulation of the blood and the maintenance of the BLOOD PRESSURE. A certain *volume* of blood is delivered with each beat, and a further key aspect is the *pressure* at which this flow is delivered. Vital functions such as those of LUNGS and KIDNEYS, or the exchange of components of the blood and tissue fluid at the capillaries, are critically dependent on the pressure achieved within the circulatory system.

Anatomy

The heart comprises a series of blood-filled chambers; the walls are composed virtually entirely of muscle cells of a type unique to the heart (*cardiac myocytes*). The heart is actually

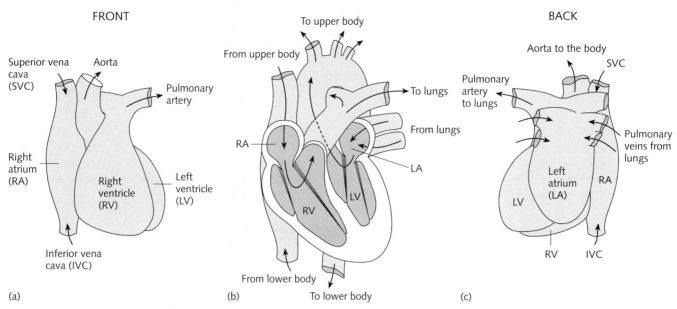

FRONT

BACK

To upper body

From upper body

Aorta to the body

Superior vena cava (SVC)

Aorta

To lungs

Pulmonary artery

Pulmonary artery to lungs

SVC

Pulmonary veins from lungs

From lungs

Right atrium (RA)

Right ventricle (RV)

Left ventricle (LV)

RA

LA

Left atrium (LA)

RA

LV

LV

RV

Inferior vena cava (IVC)

From lower body

To lower body

RV

IVC

(a)

(b)

(c)

Diagrammatic views of the heart to show the chambers and the direction of blood flow: a) from the front; b) cut away from the front; c) from the back.

two double pumps acting in series; there are four chambers in all. The right side receives blood returning from the entire body (in the great veins) and pumps it into the *pulmonary artery*, which supplies only the alveoli (gas exchange sites) in the lungs. The left side receives blood from the lungs and pumps it into the *aorta*, the largest artery. (The heart is generally illustrated as seen from the front, so 'left' and 'right' appear mirrored.) The aorta branches to form the arterial tree that supplies blood to the whole body. The heart, appropriately, is itself the first organ supplied with blood from the aorta. The *coronary arteries* open from the beginning of the aorta and take blood to all parts of the heart tissue. Each side of the heart has an upper chamber, the *atrium* (plural: 'atria'), into which the veins drain. They serve as antechambers to the respective *ventricles*, the thicker-walled chambers that lie below them.

Atria and valves The arrangement of one-way valves and the prevailing pressures mainly determine blood flow from vein–to–atrium–to–ventricle during the cyclic activity of the heart beat, but some pumping of blood by the atria into the ventricles also occurs. The valves preventing back-flow from ventricle to atrium are tough, parachute-like structures partly anchored in the connective tissue plate which forms the physical union of the ventricular and atrial portions of the heart. Their free edges are restrained by several *papillary muscles*. These are slim extensions from the inner wall of the ventricles, each with a tendinous end fused with the valve; acting like parachute cords, they prevent the valve being pushed through into the atrium as its flaps become filled when the ventricle contracts and puts pressure on its contents. The *mitral* (or *bicuspid*) *valve* on the left side has two flaps, and the *tricuspid valve* on the right has three. The 'parachutes' press together forming a complete closure preventing regress of blood into the respective atrium whence it came. Instead, when the pressure has risen sufficiently, blood is directed into the pulmonary artery and the aorta through one-way valves which separate them from, and prevent back-flow into, their respective ventricles (see Figure).

The heart beat

The heart beats between 60 and 220 times per minute in a typical young adult; 40 to 50 million beats per year. The rate alters, often rather obviously, according to one's state of physical and mental activity. This results in pumping over 3 million litres of blood (per year) through the body and an equal volume through the lungs. The pump work done by the heart is equivalent to lifting a 1 kg weight to about twice the height of Mount Everest each day. This level of persistent, rhythmic, and decidedly dynamic activity may provoke a sense of awe, although it is hardly more remarkable than the prosaic activity of every other organ — except in its absolute necessity to keep at it! We will first consider the electrical processes of the heart since, like many muscles, it is triggered into activity (contraction, the heart beat) by an electrical wave. This section is followed by consideration of contraction itself.

Electrical aspects The left and right atria beat virtually simultaneously and then, after a fraction of a second's delay, both ventricles contract. Electrical activity, as in most other muscles, triggers the contraction. This activity arises not from excitatory nerve fibres, but spontaneously within the heart itself from a small clump of PACEMAKER cells near the point where the vena cava joins the right atrium: the *sino-atrial (SA) node*. The electrical wave, or ACTION POTENTIAL, spreads across the heart from cell to cell. This spread is made possible because each heart cell is connected to its immediate neighbours at several contact regions which offer a relatively low resistance to the flow of electrical current. All the muscle cells of the heart are thus electrically linked together. This means that the activity spreads as a wave, its direction determined by the cell-to-cell couplings available. It also means that, as far as we know, every cardiac myocyte is active at some stage during every heart beat. The muscle cells of the atria and ventricles only make electrical contact in one small region, the *atrio-ventricular (AV) node* at the centre of the heart. Thus, activity follows a predictable, regular path — across the right and left atria, through the AV node, along specialized faster-conducting heart cells (*Purkinje fibres*) on the internal face of the muscular wall between the two ventricles (*interventricular septum*), and thence through the substance of both ventricles. Heart cells, like other electrically excitable cells, become inexcitable (*refractory*) for a brief period after each action potential. Consequently, once the wave has passed right through the ventricles it ceases, since there are no non-refractory cells available to excite. A new wave is spontaneously initiated at the pacemaker region.

Contractile (mechanical) aspects All the heart muscle cells are thus electrically excited and it is this that triggers them to contract. The wave of contraction, therefore, follows the same sequence: atria first, then ventricles. The electrical activity triggers an abrupt rise in the concentration of 'free' calcium ions inside the cells — a common feature in signalling contraction in muscle of every type. The calcium ions required are derived in part by influx from the extracellular fluid, in part by release from intracellular stores in the *sarcoplasmic reticulum*. The influx is through calcium-selective channels in the surface membrane which are opened by the depolarization. The influx itself transiently promotes further influx, and also triggers the release of more calcium from the intracellular store.

In each ventricle, as the muscular walls contract (develop tension and shorten) they press upon the blood they enclose. The pressure rises and the AV valve fills out and closes. At this stage of the cycle, the exit valve into the relevant artery (pulmonary artery or aorta) is also closed because the pressure in the arteries is higher than that in the ventricles. Temporarily, each ventricle is thus a closed chamber, it can neither lose nor gain blood, so pressure rises quickly until it exceeds that in the exit artery; the exit valve is then pushed open and blood is ejected, squirted from the ventricles as their muscular walls continue to shorten. The pressure at which the valve opens is much higher on the left side than on the right side, in accordance with the higher blood pressure in the aorta and its branches than in the pulmonary artery and its branches. The resistance offered by the lungs to blood flow is much less than that by the body generally; thus the pressures required of the right ventricle can be lower, yet achieve the same flow rate. Both ventricles eject the same volume of blood (the *stroke volume*): in the adult heart, about 70 ml (half a teacup) which is half or less of the volume it contained. As action potential finishes, the intracellular calcium concentration has already started to reduce again: some calcium is being 'pumped' back into the store, and some is leaving the cell by an ion exchange process. With the raised calcium concentration signal thereby removed, the force of contraction quickly wanes in the muscle, so ventricular pressure falls. The elasticity of the arteries, which were dilated when blood was ejected into them, now ensures that a higher pressure is sustained in them than in the rapidly relaxing ventricles (the 'garden hose' effect, familiar to those who have turned off a hose-pipe supply tap only to see water continue squirting as the elastic pipe collapses). The respective exit valves are thus pushed closed again, preventing reflux into the ventricles. Blood pressure, therefore, falls more slowly in the arteries than in the ventricles. At this stage about 90 ml of blood remains in each ventricle. Pressure continues to fall quickly until it is below that in the atria. Thus, the AV valves are pushed open, allowing blood to flow from the atria into the ventricles 'topping them up' with more blood. (Despite the appearance in some published schematic diagrams and 'cartoon' sequences, at all stages of the heart beat the chambers are 'full' of blood. It is the enclosed *volume* which changes, depending on the tension and elasticity of the muscular walls and the status of the inlet and outlet valves.)

The return of the ventricle to its 'resting' shape between beats is due to its own elasticity. Like a squeezed sponge or hollow rubber ball, this significantly 'sucks' blood from the atria, thereby contributing to its own filling. The reduction of this factor in old age or its enhancement by athletic training have a major effect on overall cardiac function. These effects are analogous to problems associated with 'stiff' inelastic valves which perhaps more obviously compromise effective flow in and out of the chambers of the heart.

The state when the heart is contracting is termed *systole* (sis'-toe-lee); the relaxed state is termed *diastole* (di-a'-stoe-lee).

Control of pump function

The *cardiac output* is the volume of blood pumped per minute by each ventricle — some 5 litres/minute at 'rest' — and is simply the product of heart rate and stroke volume. Cardiac output will thus alter if either varies. The stroke volume is in turn influenced by *cardiac filling* and by the *contractility* of the cardiac muscle itself — its intrinsic ability to contract (shorten and/or produce tension).

Heart rate The earliest human hunters will have noticed, like later horror film makers, that even when removed from the body, the heart continues to beat for a time. Other organs also continue to live, but their activity is hardly as impressive as that of the heart.

Because all the cells of the heart are electrically connected to their neighbours, the whole behaves as a unit. Most regions are inactive, unless artificially stimulated. The activity of the regions with the property of 'firing' spontaneously is conducted to all their inactive neighbours, so they act as *pacemakers*. The inherent pacemaker firing rate, typically about 100 per minute, is influenced by nerve actions of the AUTONOMIC NERVOUS SYSTEM: sympathetic nerves release NORADRENALINE which increases rate, and parasympathetic (*vagus*) nerve fibres release ACETYLCHOLINE which slows the rate. Heart rate typically varies between 60 per minute (in deep sleep) to approaching 200 per minute (during brief bursts of maximal exercise). The normal 'resting' rate while sitting, relaxed, is about 70 per minute, but shows wide variation amongst entirely healthy individuals. (In one university class of 350 twenty-year-old students, the range was 48 to 90 per minute.) One common feature is a marked variation within the breathing cycle: breathing in usually increases the rate. Physical fitness, particularly that associated with endurance rather than muscle strength, is often associated with a low resting rate. Extremes such as the tennis player Bjorn Borg, or the professional cyclist Miguel Indurain, with resting values in the low 30s per minute, are well known. Young children have higher resting rates; whilst still in the womb, a baby will have a rate of 120 to 160 beats per minute; it is often reported that rates above 140 indicates a female baby, but there are more reliable tests!

Cardiac filling 'Filling' reflects the flow of blood back into the heart (*venous return* from the lungs and the body). William Harvey observed that the presence of valves requires that blood in the larger veins can only flow towards the heart, the key to recognizing that blood circulates. Amongst other factors, the extent of muscular activity, breathing movements, and body positions (standing, lying, arms or legs raised) all affect the rate of return of blood to the heart. Cardiac muscle shows the unusual property that, within limits, it contracts more powerfully when starting from stretched lengths, so that the ventricle 'empties' more forcibly when it is 'filled' more than usual. This is achieved at trivial extra metabolic cost; the efficiency of pumping thus increases as output increases; surely a paradigm for 'productivity gains'. This property allows the heart to compensate automatically when the volume of blood within it at the start of the beat (the *end diastolic volume*) is greater than previously, by pumping more forcibly, thus ejecting a larger volume. This feature is termed Starling's 'Law of the Heart', after one of its discoverers.

Contractility It is obvious that an intrinsically stronger heart will be able to eject blood more forcefully and more completely. Unlike our voluntary (skeletal) muscles, the 'strength' of heart muscle can vary quickly, even from one beat to the next. This is because it is sensitive to chemical influences (especially of adrenaline/noradrenaline) and electrical influences that can rapidly modify the intracellular processes that underlie contraction. Additionally, as with voluntary muscle, the extent of growth and development of the heart muscle will affect the overall strength of the organ; athletes generally have thicker heart walls which match the larger muscles in their thicker limbs. A normal, sudden increase in contractility is associated with the onset of physical activity or even with its anticipation; this is signalled to the heart, along with the increase in heart rate, by activity in the sympathetic nerve fibres which release noradrenaline. The combination of higher rate and stronger, more rapid contraction tends to match cardiac output to the increased 'demands' for blood flow to the exercising muscles.

The heart of the matter and the matter of the heart

The control systems which influence the heart rate and strength of beating are the same as those implicated in such apparently diverse processes as blushing, breathing rate, sexual arousal, mental stress, or alertness. These links seem to have been recognized by our forebears in advance of the definitive precision of the discoveries of cardiovascular physiology. Poets report that hearts leap, hearts are strong, hearts are united, hearts are hot, heart strings are plucked, hearts are 'in the mouth', hearts become feeble, hearts are chilled, hearts tremble, and hearts are broken. In human history, the nature of the circulation of the blood and the (quite literally) central role of the heart in this system are still recent discoveries, even though they rank with the very earliest of the truly 'modern' scientific method. Nevertheless, the heart (with perhaps the eye) is the organ most quoted in literature and song to define the essential qualities of life and even its very presence. The ready perception of the action of the heart, its racing rate when we are excited or surprised, aroused or shocked, the shallow, rapid beat encountered in feverish poor health, the occasional irregularity of beat that can concern us all (often, thankfully, quite unnecessarily), together form the shared 'heart' experiences of mankind that writers and poets have ever drawn upon. We are generally blissfully unaware of the other hives of metabolic industry that contribute to our physiology. The liver, the thyroid, the hypothalamus, the pituitary, the spleen, the pancreas, not one of these is dignified with a property recognisable to their owners. It is surely the literal vitality of the heart's rhythmic beating, the recognition of its link to the movements of blood, the necessary identity between this continual activity and life itself (outside an operating theatre) that validates the continuing truth of poetic notions of 'heart'. DAVID J. MILLER

See PLATE 2.

See also AUTONOMIC NERVOUS SYSTEM; BLOOD PRESSURE; BLOOD CIRCULATION; BLOOD VESSELS; CARDIAC MUSCLE; HEART ATTACK; HEART BLOCK; HEART FAILURE; HEART SOUND.

Heartache

in its more physical sense, originates in heartburn, that is, the metastatic attribution of indigestion pains to the heart. In its more figurative sense it was coined at the beginning of the seventeenth century, in order to characterize the psychosomatic pain caused by loss or other distress due to love in its various forms. As such it becomes a core element in the anatomic vocabulary of melancholia in its cultural heyday. Not for nothing does 'heartache' figure amongst the afflictions to which the flesh of the arch-melancholic Hamlet is heir.

The heart is rhetorically made to ache like the head or the tooth, and this primarily in the metaphorical sense of the heart as the seat of love. The metaphor in question is, however, more properly a kind of metonym; a figure produced through a contiguous association. The ache is found with the heart. For the heart can, of course, ache almost physically in as far as it is indeed the seat and motor of the cardiac system, which registers the excitement of erotic and other passions, and is traumatized by aches and breaks when the passion is mortified or sickens and so dies.

As one part physical and several parts figurative, heartache has passed extensively into the currency of lyric poetry and from there to the stock of received ideas which are the stuff of more popular cultural lyrics, of Broadway musicals and Country and Western ballads. Common parlance in German recognizes the liability of heartache to become cliché by coupling heart ('*Herz*') with ache ('*Schmerz*') as a somewhat painful love-match of rhyme-words. The two parts of heartache thus seem to belong together, yet always as a combination which is not quite true to life. A. WEBBER

Heart, artificial

Since the 1960s there have been many attempts to develop implantable pumps to replace the function of the heart. These were initially evaluated in animals. Only in the past few years have the newer designs, refined in the light of experimental findings in animal trials, been used with reasonable success in humans. Improved materials as well as advances in electronics and mechanical engineering have also played a major part in making the artificial heart sufficiently safe and effective to allow limited clinical application.

In principle, the device consists of a rigid chamber, made of an inert material such as titanium, usually of hemispherical shape and about 7–8 cm in diameter, within which there is a moving polyurethane diaphragm which evacuates the contained blood. An inlet and an outlet valve ensure flow in one direction. Early models used an external pump to pneumatically displace the moving diaphragm. Recent designs have miniaturized electrical motors activating a pusher plate within the device, but connected to externally carried batteries by wire, or by a transcutaneous electrical energy transfer system. As the devices are not linked to any of the normal influences in the body which naturally control the output of the heart, there have to be control systems which modify the artificial pump's output and regulate the pressure of the blood flowing into the device.

Most causes of HEART FAILURE, for which use of an artificial device might be contemplated, affect the left ventricular pumping chamber. It is therefore possible to use a mechanical pump which takes its input of blood from the diseased left ventricle and returns the blood at appropriate pressure to the aorta — thus acting as a *left ventricular assist device*. It is this form of device which is presently showing most clinical success and has widest application.

For patients with both left and right ventricular failure, devices are available which have two parallel pumping chambers. This device is a true 'artificial heart', and is a mechanical alternative to a heart transplant.

The problems associated with artificial devices used to replace the heart are considerable. Clotting of blood within the device is a risk. Clots can immobilize the artificial valves and interfere with the pump itself, or can detach from the device to travel in the bloodstream. This results in clinical effects which depend on where the clot goes. If a clot enters the circulation of the brain the result is often a stroke. *Anticoagulant drugs* are required to minimize this risk, and anticoagulation itself carries risks of bleeding. Also, there is the risk of infection developing in the device; mechanical devices are liable to damage the blood, causing rupture of red cells and a risk of kidney damage due to the released haemoglobin from the red cells; and there is a need for regular changes of battery power source.

At present left heart assist devices will allow relatively normal life for many months, reversing many of the adverse effects on the body of long-standing heart failure. Most clinical use has been as a 'bridge to transplant', enabling ill patients to survive until a suitable heart becomes available for TRANSPLANTATION. Occasionally, use of a left heart assist device has been temporary, where the heart has been affected by a condition which is recoverable.

At present, the technology of artificial hearts is advancing rapidly, but the devices currently in use are not as satisfactory as the transplanted human heart. D. J. WHEATLEY

See also HEART FAILURE; PROSTHESES.

Heart attack

This term is most often used to describe the signs and symptoms associated with *acute myocardial infarction*, the sudden interruption or inadequacy of blood flow (*ischaemia*) to sections of the heart itself. If the inadequate blood flow persists for several minutes it can cause the affected section of heart muscle to die. The dead cells become replaced with scar tissue, and the dead area is known as an *infarct*. The immediate problem, however, is that the effectiveness of the heart's pumping action is abruptly reduced. Loss of function in any part of the heart will obviously reduce the strength of the pump. But a potentially greater threat is that damage, even to a small area, can induce within it erratic, spontaneous electrical activity. (Similar, but not dangerous, phenomena are sometimes seen in limb muscles when they twitch involuntarily if they or their associated nerve fibres, are underperfused with blood.) Since each heart cell is in electrical contact with its neighbours, the erratic activity is conducted to other, non-infarcted regions. If the electrical disturbance is serious enough, it can cause CARDIAC ARREST.

Heart attack is a distressingly common clinical problem in many (but not all) Western developed societies. The incidence in the UK is about 150 000 per annum, of which nearly half prove fatal. (This can be judged against a total UK mortality of about half a million per annum.) The major cause of myocardial infarction in Western society is progressive coronary artery disease. The coronary arteries are the first blood vessels to branch from the aorta (the large artery leaving the heart). Although only two coronary arteries arise directly from the aorta, these branch extensively, forming an intricate network of vessels supplying all areas of the heart muscle with oxygenated blood. The arrangement of this 'plumbing' system makes the heart peculiarly vulnerable to interruptions of supply. In most other tissues, there are significant alternative routes by which arterial blood can reach any one region; so-called collateral supplies. Thus the cells of the heart are like leaves on a tree; they are at the end of the furthest twigs of the supply system. By contrast, in other tissues, the supply is more like a road network; very few houses are at the end of cul-de-sacs, most can be reached from several directions. If the flow of blood is stopped in one of the branches in our 'tree' analogy, the heart cells downstream, beyond the block, will inevitably suffer. (It is sobering to note that many other mammalian species do not have their hearts 'plumbed' so extensively this way. But the pig and several breeds of dog do suffer the risks of this 'design flaw' much like us.)

Typical signs of coronary artery disease include a painful feeling of 'tightness' in the chest or 'heaviness' brought on by physical effort, heavy meals, cold weather, or emotional stress. The sensation starts behind the breast bone and radiates across the chest. The pain is frequently confused with that of severe indigestion. Frequently, it is associated with a leaden feeling in the arms. Occasionally the sensation may be perceived in more unusual sites (e.g. in the jaws or teeth). An abnormal sensation of breathlessness on effort or at rest can occur, known as *dyspnoea*. Patients often feel cool, yet clammy or sticky to touch, and sometimes have dilated hand veins. If the symptoms are relieved by rest then this tends to indicate a serious narrowing of the coronary artery circulation (*stable angina pectoris*) rather than actual blockage. If the symptoms occur whilst at rest, or are not relieved by rest, they could indicate a heart attack. The severity of the symptoms is often indicative; patients may report a sense of impending doom, the chest pains are severe, vice-like, and persistent; the attack itself may provoke collapse, often without warning.

Coronary artery disease, with its ultimate sequel of myocardial infarction, is almost always due to *atherosclerosis*. The initiating event in the development of atherosclerosis is thought to be damage to the layer of cells lining the inner surface of the artery. Such injury triggers bloodborne factors to stimulate proliferation of cells within the wall of the artery and deposition of protein and cholesterol, known as an *atheromatous plaque*, that narrows the artery. In the majority of cases, the cracking of the atheromatous plaque causing a sudden blockage of the artery is the event which results in progression from atherosclerosis to infarction. Only very rarely is a myocardial infarction produced by other factors (e.g. a spasm within artery). It should be clear that if ejection of blood from the heart is suddenly reduced for any reason, the heart itself will receive an inadequate supply which can precipitate heart attack. In this category comes a variety of causes such as drug overdose, major HAEMORRHAGE, electric shock, and so on.

Treatment of coronary artery disease, thereby reducing the risk of heart attack, has many elements. It involves alterations to lifestyle, exclusion or treatment of precipitating factors, drug treatment, and surgery if medical treatment fails. Alteration in lifestyle involves a reduction in physical activity in work and the home. It may require a change of job. SMOKING must stop and weight reduction may be required. Many socially related activities can be continued with medical treatment. The most important precipitating factors for coronary artery disease are high blood pressure, diabetes, and high cholesterol levels in the blood. These factors can largely be treated or controlled by diet and drugs; such treatment could prevent the progression of coronary artery disease to myocardial infarction. In the main, drug therapy involves drugs that act to dilate the

blood vessels or reduce the contractility (and thereby oxygen requirements) of the heart muscle receiving a reduced blood supply. Surgical approaches to coronary artery disease include CORONARY ARTERY BYPASS (where a vein is connected to the aorta and to the coronary artery beyond the narrowed region to improve blood flow) and coronary angioplasty (where a catheter containing a fine, elongated balloon is guided from the main leg artery into the coronary artery, positioned within the region of narrowing, and then briefly inflated, forcing open the narrowing).

DAVID J. MILLER
NIALL G. MACFARLANE

See also CORONARY ARTERY BYPASS; HEART.

Heart block

Heart block is an abnormal delay or, in extreme cases, complete block in the conduction of the electrical impulse from the atria to the ventricles (*A-V block*) or in the specialized conducting network supplying the ventricles (*bundle block*).

Gerbezius, an early eighteenth-century German physician, described the pulse of a man he attended as being 'so very slow, that before the subsequent pulsations followed that which went before, three pulsations would certainly have pass'd in another healthy person'. But it was two Dublin clinicians more than a century later who gave heart block and its effects the eponym Stokes–Adams syndrome. Adams and Stokes both reported patients with persistent pulse rates around 30. The exceptionally slow heart rates in these patients (and in others recognized subsequently) became from time to time even slower, causing them to pass out in a manner which could be confused with EPILEPSY or 'APOPLEXY'. Such a black-out became known as a 'Stokes–Adams attack', occurring because the brain was deprived of blood flow when a 'subsequent pulsation' did not follow for far too long.

The mechanism whereby, normally, the 'subsequent pulsation' follows after a proper interval of one second or less, depends on transmission

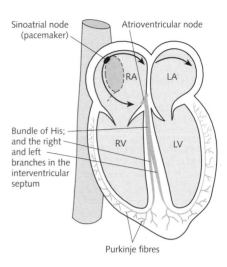

Fig. 1 Diagram of heart chambers showing spread of excitation and sites of heart block. (RA, LA: right and left atrium. RV, LV: right and left ventricle.)

of electrical signals from the heart's PACEMAKER, the *sino-atrial* (SA) node, through the atria to the only, and restricted, pathway through which it can reach the ventricles — via the *atrio-ventricular* (AV) node and thence along the rapidly conducting modified muscle cells known as the *Bundle of His* and its branching fibres, to spread through the whole ventricular muscle mass. Should the signal fail to get through, it cannot stimulate the ventricles to beat. But there are cells beyond the AV node which can take over as pacemakers, generating regular signals at a slower pace than that which is normally imposed. The SA node keeps firing off at its own faster rate, but to no avail as far as ventricular contraction is concerned. The ELECTROCARDIOGRAM (ECG) shows P waves and QRS complexes which are completely dissociated from one another. The QRS waves, and therefore the heart beats, are 40 or fewer per minute. This is the condition of complete, or third degree, heart block.

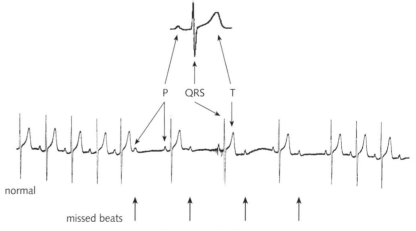

Fig. 2 ECG from a subject with partial heart block. The first five beats are normal. At the 'missed beats' the arrows point to P waves that are not followed by a QRS complex, indicating failure of transmission of activity from atria to ventricles. Each missed beat is followed by a normal one.

The importance of the normal sequence of activation lies in the fact that a wave of contraction is initiated first in the atria then, after a brief delay, in the ventricles. The relative timing of this sequence, as well as the sequence itself, are important determinants of the effectiveness with which the heart pumps the blood. Since heart block is a major disturbance to the smooth progress of the triggering wave, its consequences can be serious.

There are lesser degrees of block, where some activations get through and others do not (shown by the presence of any isolated P waves) and in its mildest form there is simply a slowing down of transmission from atria to ventricles (shown by a prolonged P–R interval). It is also possible for just one of the main branches of the Bundle of His to be blocked.

The cause of heart block is damage to the conducting fibres, by deprivation of blood supply picking out that part of the heart when there is coronary artery disease, or as a result of infection; it may also be congenital.

Nowadays, heart block can be treated by implanting an artificial pacemaker to drive the ventricles.

DAVID J. MILLER
NIALL G. MACFARLANE

See also ELECTROCARDIOGRAM; HEART; PACEMAKER.

Heart, broken

Heart, broken In Lewes on 18 January 1796, a servant girl dropped down whilst reading a letter, and instantly expired. It appeared to have been written by a young man, who had formerly been her fellow-servant and professed admirer, and it stated that he had lately been married to another woman. This story, reported in *The Gentleman's Magazine*, appears to be a classic, not to say extreme, account of a broken heart. The AUTONOMIC NERVOUS SYSTEM was probably responsible: the parasympathetic fibres of the VAGUS nerve, which normally respond to intense distress by slowing the heartbeat, presumably brought this girl's heart to a standstill and killed her outright. Traditional assumptions of a link between EMOTION and the heart find sad confirmation here.

The heart, considered as a physical organ, is seldom so obviously implicated in a reaction to grief. So why should the words 'broken heart' enshrine its status as an emotional centre? In fact, other ages and cultures have witnessed various distributions of thought and feeling within the body. According to Alexander Cruden's *Complete Concordance to the Old and New Testament* (1737), 'The Hebrews look upon the heart as the source of wit, understanding, love, courage, grief, and pleasure.' It 'dilates with joy, contracts with sadness, breaks with sorrow, grows fat, and hardens in prosperity.' But many tender emotions also resided in their bowels. Elaborately metaphorical use of language relating emotions to the body appears in *Deuteronomy* 10: 16: 'Circumcise therefore the foreskin of your heart, and be no more stiffnecked.' Ancient Greek and Roman

hearts were seats of feelings and thought, but livers were also sources of passion, especially love — a belief which survived into the Renaissance. Orsino, a romantic Shakespearean lover (in *Twelfth Night*) aspires to win his beloved's 'liver, brain, and heart'.

Heartbreak is not monopolized by the bereaved and conventionally lovelorn. When Shakespeare's Falstaff, a scheming old rogue, lies on his deathbed, emotionally shattered by the King's unexpected coldness, Pistol declares, 'His heart is fracted and corroborate' (*Henry V*). Nor is it invariably considered fatal: Ellie Dunn, heroine of Bernard Shaw's *Heartbreak House* (1919), finds it intellectually liberating. After humiliating military defeat at Prestonpans (1745), Sir John Cope announced, 'My heart is broke', then survived for years.

How should the heartbroken behave? Ostentatious lamentations may appear hypocritical, but restraint is dangerous. In *Macbeth*, Ross warns the bereaved Macduff that

'the grief that doth not speak
Whispers the oer-fraught heart and bids it break.'

In John Ford's tragedy, *The Broken Heart* (1633), the Spartan princess Calantha hears terrible news in the course of a ceremonial dance: her friend, fiancé, and father have died. She stoically continues the dance, then puts her affairs in order and dies, a pattern of dignified sincerity. Had she any chance of survival? The diagnosis, nature, and treatment of the interactions between mind and body associated with severe grief have been subjects of constant scrutiny, from Roberrt Burton's *Anatomy of Melancholy* (1621–51) to present-day medical research on bereavement and depression.

CAROLYN D. WILLIAMS

Heart failure

Heart failure The characteristic symptoms of heart failure are recognizable in writings at least as far back as the twelfth century, when the health problems of Alexius I (Comnenus), the Byzantine emperor, were documented by his physician. The 'failure' is manifest in the heart not providing sufficient output of blood to meet the 'demands' of the body. A useful term here is 'exercise intolerance'. A typical heart failure patient will have become accustomed to an inexorable decline in physical vigour. Activities such as climbing stairs, carrying a heavy load (perhaps a suitcase), even walking, far less running, and other such 'exercises' usually considered to be within the normal range become increasingly difficult or impossible. One key associated symptom is breathlessness, another is OEDEMA (the accumulation of fluid in the tissues) for example in the ankles. Both symptoms reflect raised pressure in the veins ultimately caused by the insufficient pumping action of the heart. The seriousness of heart failure is such that, at the time of writing, about half of the patients affected die within five years of the initial diagnosis. Of these fatalities, about half will suffer a major heart attack, the remainder will suffer a steady decline of heart function until

pump failure itself proves fatal. Against this gloomy scenario, new discoveries about the underlying causes, the development of new drugs to slow down, halt, and ultimately reverse the harmful aspects, and an increasing awareness of the value of lifestyle and dietary change promise to improve the prospects for the heart failure patient in the twenty-first century — even if too late for the Emperor Alexius.

The most common single cause in modern Western society, accounting for about half of the cases, is a HEART ATTACK. By killing one region, the attack leaves heart function compromised. Until the later decades of the twentieth century a very major cause was undiagnosed and untreated high BLOOD PRESSURE — the heart in this instance must work harder and harder to force blood into the arteries where the pressure is too high, and eventually 'tires'. Although long-term high blood pressure is still a contributor to heart failure, modern drugs have helped to reduce its significance. A range of other causes include the various heart valve malfunctions, certain infections, congenital structural abnormalities, genetically-determined disorders, and drug abuse. There is clear evidence that the factors that increase the likelihood of heart attack also contribute to the severity of the ensuing heart failure. These factors include high blood cholesterol, atheromatous vascular disease, sedentary lifestyle, and smoking. In third-World countries, infections such as the insect-transmitted trypanosomal Chagas' disease are among the main causes of heart failure. Even amongst economically advanced nations there are wide differences in the incidence of heart failure between, say, Japan (very low) and Western Europe and the US (high); nation-specific combinations of dietary and genetic factors are thus the target of much research into underlying causes. There is widespread agreement that taking regular exercise not only strengthens the heart and improves its own circulation (particularly by improving collateral blood supplies) but also that exercise is a very useful part of any rehabilitation regime designed to prevent the development of heart failure after a heart attack.

Heart failure refers to a characteristic pattern of features caused by an abnormality of the heart. It is a complex clinical syndrome resulting from the entanglement of cause and effect, of symptoms and compensatory changes. Several body systems and organs are involved, especially the lungs, kidneys, and blood vessels, their associated hormonal systems, as well as the heart itself. It is increasingly clear that many and varied patterns of disturbance to each of these systems can result in convergence into the full repertoire of malfunctions which together are termed heart failure.

In normal circumstances, the 'challenge' to the heart posed by 'demand' for increased blood supply is most obvious during exercise, however mild. The physiological challenge is similar when the heart is unable, by virtue of disease, to meet even normal requirements. In either case,

homeostatic mechanisms operate which promote the maintenance of two parameters of heart function: blood pressure and blood flow. An example of these compensatory processes is one promoting retention of water and salts by hormonal influences on the kidneys. This will increase blood volume and tend to keep up both blood pressure and cardiac output (the volume pumped). Unfortunately, in heart failure, the compensatory mechanisms prove clearly ineffective; they actually contribute to the symptoms observed (e.g. breathlessness and ankle swelling) and become important factors in the gradual worsening of the condition. The use of DIURETIC drugs (which stimulate kidney function and reverse fluid retention) is widespread in the treatment of heart failure. The heart itself generally responds to an abnormal workload by increased growth (hypertrophy), but the nature of the growth is abnormal in subtle ways, unlike the hypertrophy associated with general physical fitness which is positively beneficial. It is now known, for example, that a hypertrophied failing heart both contracts and relaxes more slowly, and is more prone to life-threatening electrical abnormalities.   DAVID J. MILLER
NIALL G. MACFARLANE

See also HEART; HEART ATTACK.

Heart–lung machine

Operating on the human heart poses problems which inhibited surgery on the heart until the early 1950s. Manipulation of the heart, and opening of its cavities' interferes with its function and its ability to sustain the circulation. The *heart–lung machine* is a system which takes over the function of the heart and the lungs with sufficient safety to maintain life while the heart is stopped or opened to allow surgery on the coronary arteries or the heart valves, or to allow repair of congenital abnormalities.

While in theory it is only necessary to bypass the function of the heart, it soon became apparent that in practice it is simpler to bypass the function of both the heart and the lungs. The main components of a heart–lung machine are a *pump* (to provide the driving force to the blood in the arterial system), an *oxygenator* (for exchange of oxygen and carbon dioxide), and a *heat exchanger* (to allow control of temperature of the body). The connecting tubing and filter are other components of the heart–lung bypass circuit.

Venous blood is siphoned from the body via a tube in the right atrium of the heart, or via two tubes in the major veins which converge on the heart. It is pumped through the oxygenator and heat exchanger, and returned via a plastic tube into the arterial system of the body — usually at the upper portion of the ascending aorta (see BLOOD CIRCULATION).

The design of *pump* which is in most common use today is the roller pump — a simple rotating arm carrying rollers which compress a loop of polymeric tubing against a solid surface. Speed of rotation of the roller-bearing arm is controlled to allow a pumping rate similar to that of the normal

heart at rest (about 2.4 litres/min/m² body surface — or typically about 5 litres/min in an adult).

There are two main types of *oxygenator* in use at present. '*Bubble oxygenators*' expose the passing blood to a stream of gaseous bubbles composed of 95% oxygen and 5% carbon dioxide. Gas exchange with the blood occurs on the surface of the bubbles and results in reasonably normal levels of oxygenation of the blood and maintains carbon dioxide in the normal physiological range. The bubble oxygenator has a sponge-like filter and reservoir to enable gaseous bubbles to be removed from the oxygenated blood before it is pumped back to the body.

Membrane oxygenators consist of a series of fine tubes which allow diffusion of oxygen and carbon dioxide between the blood flowing through them and the ventilating gas surrounding them (or vice versa).

The oxygenator also combines with a *heat exchanger* — a system of tubes through which the blood passes, surrounded by circulating water at controlled temperature. This allows the blood temperature to be maintained (counteracting the heat loss during the passage of blood through the heart–lung machine). It also allows deliberate cooling and subsequent rewarming of the blood, giving the surgeon the option of reducing, or even stopping, the circulation of the blood around the body for a period of time with safety, because the oxygen requirement of the body is reduced by hypothermia.

The connecting tubes, the oxygenator, and the pump tubing are all filled with a physiologically compatible fluid (priming fluid) prior to final connection with the circulation of the body. Avoidance of air bubbles in the heart–lung circuit is of vital importance. Exposure of blood to the foreign surfaces of the heart–lung machine initiates the natural clotting mechanisms of the body, and this must be inhibited by giving the drug *heparin* to the patient before allowing the circulation to be taken over by the heart–lung machine. Normal blood clotting is restored after the operation by the administration of protamine, which neutralizes the heparin.

The heart–lung machine has made virtually all the advances in cardiac surgery possible. With the function of the heart and lungs taken over temporarily by artificial means it is possible to stop ventilation of the lungs, and to stop the heart, and open the coronary arteries or the cavities of the heart for repair or replacement of the heart valves, or to undertake the correction of congenital abnormalities of the heart.

For periods of up to two or three hours (usually adequate for most surgery) the heart–lung machine is safe; beyond this time there is a risk of increasing damage to the red cells of the blood. Exposure of blood to the foreign surfaces of the artificial circuit initiates an inflammatory response throughout the body, and there is an impairment of function of many organs for a short period after surgery. Nevertheless, the heart–lung machine has become a safe and crucial

component of virtually all surgery on the heart and on the major blood vessels around the heart.
D. J. WHEATLEY

Further reading
Millner, R. and Treasure, T. (1995). *Explaining cardiac surgery: patient assessment and care.* BMJ Publishing Group, London.

Heart sounds

With an ear applied to the chest — or more usually, with a stethoscope — it is normally possible to detect two sounds in every heart beat, which are produced when the valves of the HEART close. The sounds arise from the brief turbulence of blood flow occurring just as a valve closes. The left side of the heart develops a higher pressure than the right side, which means that the sounds produced there, by the mitral (bicuspid) valve between atrium and ventricle, and the aortic valve at the exit from the ventricle, are generally louder and precede the sounds produced from the equivalent valves on the right side (tricuspid and pulmonary valves). The first heart sound is produced by closure of the two atrio–ventricular valves, when the ventricles start to contract. It is often described as '*lub*'; the '*l*' reflecting the louder mitral valve closure preceding the quieter tricuspid valve closure '*b*'. Deep inspiration widens the split between mitral and tricuspid closure: '*lu-ub*'. The second heart sound is produced by closure of the aortic and pulmonary valves (between the ventricles and their respective arteries), and is often described as '*dup*'; the '*d*' reflecting the louder aortic valve closure preceding the quieter tricuspid valve closure '*p*'. With experience, the two sounds can be distinguished by pitch and intensity; also at a resting heart rate there is a longer interval between beats than between the two sounds.

Heart murmurs are soft sounds, like those made during a forcible expiration with the mouth open. They are most often caused by any departure from the crisp sounds described here which reflect equally crisp function of the valves. Valves may become leaky, allowing backflow (incompetence), or they may become stiff and narrow (stenosis). Stenosis, for example, of the aortic valve leads to an abnormal turbulence during ejection of blood through it from the left ventricle, so it is a systolic murmur because it occurs during the phase of contraction (systole), preceding the second heart sound at the closure of the valve. Incompetence of this same valve allows some blood to flow back into the ventricle causing a diastolic murmur at the time of the second sound when it closes incompletely during ventricular relaxation (diastole). An incompetent mitral valve allows blood to regurgitate into the left atrium throughout ventricular contraction, causing a systolic murmur, whereas mitral stenosis causes a murmur as the blood flows from atrium to ventricle during diastole.

Other characteristic murmurs are caused by congenital defects, such as a hole in the ventricular septum, or a failure of closure of the connection between aorta and pulmonary artery which is present before birth (patent ductus arteriosus).

A murmur is classified with respect to its intensity (just audible, soft, moderate, or loud), the point on the chest wall where the murmur is heard best (which assists its localisation to a particular valve or part of the heart), and the timing of the murmur in the heart beat (in relation to the first and second heart sounds).

Not all murmurs signify abnormality of the heart. Systolic murmurs, due to normal turbulence during ventricular contraction and ejection of blood, may be present particularly in young people, and not uncommonly in exercise and in pregnancy.   DAVID J. MILLER
NIALL G. MACFARLANE

See also HEART; SOUNDS OF THE BODY.

Heartstrings

'Heartstrings' was first used in nonanatomical literature in the late fifteenth century to describe the nerves and tendons thought to keep the heart in place. The use of the term 'nerves' may be misleading and may have been occasioned by translating the Greek 'neuron', a term used by Aristotle in *Parts of Animals III* to describe sinews or fibres located in the heart, perhaps the chordae tendineae. The term 'heartstrings' has also been used synonymously with 'precordia', a term used incorrectly to refer to the PERICARDIUM.

In a symbolic sense, 'heartstrings' are the deepest or most intense EMOTIONS and affections. Edmund Spencer (1522–99) used the term figuratively in *Faerie Queene* (iv, vi) in 1597. In the *Timaeus*, Plato (427–347 BCE) located the spirited part of the soul, which governed behaviours we now term emotions, in the heart, and associated the throbbing of the heart in emotional situations with an intensification of the heart's heat. Galen (AD 129–216), whose physiology was influential until the Renaissance, accepted Plato's location of the spirited part of the soul. Passions were described in terms of heat or a lack of it, as illustrated in phrases such as 'surrounded by the warmth of love', 'the heat of anger', and 'cool disdain'. The standard medieval and Renaissance view that the heart is hot originated with Aristotle (384–422 BCE) and was accepted by Galen, William Harvey (1578–1657), and René Descartes (1596–1650). Furthermore, Aristotle believed that all animals possessed an innate spirit originating in the heart, the centre of the body. He asserted in *Parts of Animals III* that 'all motions of sensation, including those produced by what is pleasant and painful' begin and end in the heart. In *Movement of Animals* Aristotle likened the body's actions to those of a marionette, in that the bones correspond to the pegs and the sinews to the strings which cause movements. Therefore, as the locus of thought and sensation in Aristotle's philosophy, the actions of the heart could occasion considerable changes throughout the body, such as blushing, pallor, shuddering, or trembling — in short, manifestations of emotional reactions. It is now understood that the AUTONOMIC NERVOUS SYSTEM accelerates the heart rate and causes general bodily effects in emotional situations, thus explaining why such situations seem to 'tug at the heart strings'.   KRISTEN L. ZACHARIAS

See also EMOTION; HEART.

Heat exposure

Although the origins of human life were in the tropical regions, modern man is better able to cope with cold environments than with extreme heat. The SKIN and subcutaneous tissues of the body can function normally over a wide temperature range, and the temperature of the skin will generally follow the temperature of the surrounding environment. The deeper tissues, and especially the brain, however, must be maintained within a few degrees of the normal body temperature of 37°C if optimum function is to be maintained and irreversible damage prevented. Exposure to a high ambient temperature is a major challenge to the body's ability to keep its temperature within optimum working range.

Heat is exchanged between the body and its surrounding environment by physical transfer involving conduction, convection, and radiation. When skin temperature is higher than the environmental temperature, heat is lost by these mechanisms, but at high environmental temperatures, heat is gained. Heat exchange can be regulated to some degree by regulating the skin blood flow, which alters the effective insulation layer between the deep tissues and the surface, but behavioural mechanisms, including alterations in the amount of clothing worn and control of the environmental temperature, are more effective. Heat is constantly produced by the metabolic reactions occurring within the body. These are relatively inefficient, and about 75% of the energy appears as heat: this is about the same level of efficiency as the internal combustion engine. At rest, the rate of heat production is low (about 60 W — roughly equivalent to the heat output of a small domestic light bulb), but this rises dramatically during exercise, and the average marathon runner produces more than 1 kW of heat (similar to the output of a small electric fire). When the ambient temperature is low, this can be lost to the environment by physical transfer without any large change in deep body temperature.

When the ambient temperature is high, heat is gained from the environment by physical transfer, and metabolic heat production continues to add to the heat load. Heat loss is promoted by increasing the rate of blood flow to the skin: this allows skin temperature to rise and reduces the thermal gradient, reducing the rate of heat gain. In order to prevent a catastrophic rise in body temperature, an additional heat loss mechanism is invoked as body temperature begins to rise. This involves evaporation of water from the body surface, and active secretion of sweat onto the skin surface will be initiated. The latent heat of vaporization of water is high, and evaporation of this water is an effective way of removing large amounts of heat from the body surface. Water is also lost by evaporation from the respiratory tract, but this is much less important in humans than it is in those animals which have thick coats of hair or wool, as such coats prevent evaporation from the skin by restricting air movement and allowing the air to become saturated with water vapour. A similar problem arises when the humidity of the air close to the skin is high: this is why a hot, humid climate feels more uncomfortable than a hot, dry environment.

At rest, low sweat rates are sufficient to maintain body temperature, but the sweat rate rises dramatically during EXERCISE to balance the increased rate of heat production by the exercising muscles. Industrial workers in hot environments, or athletes competing in hot climates, can sweat at rates approaching 3 litres/hour. Prolonged exposure to these conditions results in dehydration, and there is a need for fluid replacement if the work is to be sustained. Some of the water lost in sweat is derived from the blood plasma, with the remainder coming from the spaces between and within the body cells. Large sweat losses cause the blood volume to fall by 10% or even more. The reduced blood volume challenges the body's ability to continue to supply sufficient blood flow to the working muscles to provide oxygen and nutrients and to remove waste products, including heat, as well as to supply a high rate of blood flow to the skin to carry heat to the body surface where it can be lost. Heart rate will increase in an attempt to maintain the cardiac output, but eventually skin blood flow will fall, and body temperature will rise.

If body temperature is allowed to rise above about 40°C, a variety of symptoms of heat illness will appear. These include nausea, headache, and dizziness, which should be seen as warning signs. A core temperature of about 42°C or more will result in loss of consciousness, circulatory collapse, and eventually COMA and death. The brain, liver, and kidneys, and the blood clotting mechanisms, appear to be particularly sensitive to rises in temperature. The danger of heat illness is obviously increased when both temperature and humidity are high, and is greatest when exercise has to be performed in these conditions. There have been many famous examples of athletes in endurance events collapsing in the later stages of an event, and these collapses normally occur only when the weather is unusually hot. The case of Dorando Pietri, who fell to the track close to the end of the 1908 Olympic Games Marathon held in London, is well known: Pietri was assisted to his feet, and staggered to the finishing line, only to be disqualified on the grounds that he had received assistance during the race.

Sweat contains a variety of salts (especially sodium chloride) as well as a large number of different organic molecules, and replacement of these salts as well as of water is necessary when large sweat losses are incurred. Humans have a limited appetite for salt compared with many animals, but it is normal to feel the need to add extra salt to food when sweat losses are high. Drinks taken to maintain hydration should contain small amounts of sugar and salt to stimulate water absorption in the intestine: this is the basis of the formulation of oral rehydration solutions developed for the treatment of the excessive rates of water loss caused by infectious diarrhoea. Sports drinks used by athletes are formulated along the same principles to achieve effective fluid replacement. The thirst mechanism is not normally sufficient to ensure an adequate rate of fluid to balance the sweat loss, and a conscious effort to drink beyond the level dictated by thirst must be made when sweating rates are high.

On repeated exposure to heat, the body adapts to increase its thermal tolerance. This is achieved by lowering the temperature threshold for the onset of sweating and increasing the sensitivity of the sweating mechanism so that a greater sweat rate is achieved for any given level of body temperature. There is also a more even distribution of sweating over the body surface, ensuring an effective rate of evaporation while minimizing the amount of sweat that drips from the body surface without evaporating. The salt content of the sweat is reduced to compensate for the increased sweating rate, allowing conservation of electrolytes to occur. These adaptations begin within one or two days of exposure to the heat, and the degree of adaptation is related to the amount of heat strain experienced. Adaptations occur more rapidly and more completely if exercise is performed during periods of heat exposure: passive exposure to heat is less effective. Adaptation is essentially complete after about 10–15 consecutive days of exposure to exercise in the heat. After adaptation, heart rate will be lower at any given level of thermal stress, and exercise tolerance is greatly increased. Even after a comprehensive programme of heat acclimatization, however, exercise performance remains impaired relative to that which can be achieved in cool conditions. On returning to a cool environment, the beneficial changes accompanying adaptation are gradually reversed.

R. J. MAUGHAN

Further reading

Maughan, R. J. and Shirreffs, S. M. (1998). Fluid and electrolyte loss and replacement in exercise. In *Oxford textbook of sports medicine* (ed. Harries, Williams, Stanish, and Micheli), 2nd edn pp. 97–113. Oxford University Press, New York.

Sutton, J. R. (1994). Physiological and clinical consequences of exercise in heat and humidity. In *Oxford textbook of sports medicine*, (ed. Harries, Williams, Stanish, and Micheli) pp. 231–8. Oxford University Press, New York.

Wenger, C. B. (1988). Human heat acclimatization. In *Human performance physiology and environmental medicine at terrestrial extremes*, (ed. K. B. Pandolf, M. N. Sawka, and R. R. Gonzalez) pp. 153–98. Cooper Publishing Group, Carmel.

See also BODY FLUIDS; METABOLISM; SWEATING; TEMPERATURE REGULATION.

Heatstroke A dangerously high body temperature (*hyperthermia*) — above 41°C or 106 °F — which may be accompanied by coma or convulsions, and requires emergency life-saving measures. The body has passed the limit of its heat-

losing mechanisms. It may follow from the less serious condition of *heat exhaustion* due to excessive sweating and dehydration during heat exposure, usually with heavy work or exercise in a hot environment. S.J.

See HEAT EXPOSURE; SWEATING.

Hedonism is derived from the Greek *hedone*, meaning 'sweetness', 'joy', or 'delight', and refers to theories about the nature and function of pleasure. Originally, *hedone* was the sort of sweetness that could be appreciated by taste or smell; then hearing was involved; finally, it was applied metaphorically to any pleasant sensation or emotion. The word's history reminds us that much pleasure is rooted in physical needs and desires.

'*Psychological hedonism*' attempts to explain human conduct, claiming that people are motivated solely by the desire for the maximum degree of pleasure, and invariably act on the stronger of conflicting desires. This need not mean that everyone automatically seizes the most immediately attractive opportunity: the principle of deferred gratification often comes into play, when people sacrifice a present pleasure in hope of greater pleasure to come. Nevertheless, this theory requires a very broad view of pleasure. Imagine, for example, a group of commuters shivering at a bus stop on a cold winter morning. Presumably they have all left their warm beds at the compulsion of some overmastering motive: duty, ambition, or fear of poverty. Yet if you told them they lived for pleasure alone, they might well invite you to redefine your terms. '*Ethical hedonism*' covers the doctrines that pleasure is the only ultimate good, and that everyone should live with that end in view, though they need not seek pleasure for themselves: thus 'ethical egoism' reconciles pleasure-seeking with altruism. Most discussions of pleasure cover both psychology and ethics. A closely-related subject is the examination of what pleasure actually is. This often involves philosophical attempts to decide whether pleasure can be distinguished from happiness, and, if so, to assess their relative merits.

The ancient Greek legacy

Hedonism's history is bedevilled by two false and damaging assumptions: that it advocates only bodily pleasures, and that they are invariably sinful and degrading. In fact, most philosophers seem to share this distrust of the body and advocate rational hedonism, regarding spiritual and intellectual joys as more lasting, and less likely to produce painful or inconvenient consequences. A rare exception is Aristippus (435–356 BC), a body-centred, radical hedonist who identified good and evil with pleasure and pain. He was frequently depicted as the embodiment of shameless, irresponsible sensuality. Epicurus (341–270 BC) also defined life's goal as happiness, but found it in tranquillity, arising from wisdom and virtue, rather than in active sensual enjoyment. He and his followers were often accused of bestial

devotion to bodily gratification and indifference to all other concerns; this probably arose from a wish to discredit his materialism, rejection of superstition, and denial that individual identity survived after death. Today, an 'epicure' is a gourmet, rather than a monster of indiscriminate depravity: this sense of the word was already developing in the description of the Franklin in the Prologue to *The Canterbury Tales* by Geoffrey Chaucer (*c.* 1340–1400). He was 'Epicurus' owne sone', believing that perfect happiness lay in pure delight, whose house was always full of food and drink, abundant in quantity and superb in quality — woe betide his cook if the sauces were insufficiently piquant! However, a more sinister image of Epicurean theory and practice was also in circulation: for example, in Shakespeare's *King Lear*, Goneril complains that her father's unruly knights have reduced her court to something like a riotous inn:

> 'epicurism and lust
> Make it more like a tavern or a brothel
> Than a grac'd palace.'

She certainly has no wish to imply that catering standards have risen under their influence. Epicurus' dubious reputation reflected the Christian tendency to regard earthly pleasures as the evil lures of the world, the flesh, and the devil.

As rational hedonists, Plato (*c.* 428–*c.* 348 BC) and Aristotle (384–22 BC) were less subject to misrepresentation. Plato's *Phaedo* depicts Socrates arguing that the true philosopher should study to separate his soul from his body by cultivating wisdom and weaning himself from physical pleasures. At death, it will join the gods in a happy state of immortal wisdom. The souls of those who have addicted themselves to sensual delights hover disconsolately about the tombs of their host bodies until they become reincarnated in animals: hardly encouragement to physical fulfilment! Although in later dialogues, like the *Philebus*, Plato allows pleasure a role in the good life, he stresses the importance of intellectual joys, and makes pleasure itself subordinate to other qualities, such as reason. The most obviously corporeal delights are dismissed as false pleasures, adulterated by the pains of privation and appetite. Similarly, Aristotle's *Nicomachean Ethics* recommends the pursuit of '*eudaimonia*', 'happiness', but advocates temperance in physical pleasures (especially those involving taste and touch) and places the greatest value on abstract contemplation.

Utopian synthesis

Rational hedonism acquired a new lease of life when classical learning, combining with Christian theology, engendered Renaissance humanism. Thomas More's *Utopia* (1516), first translated into English by Raphe Robinson, describes an ideal commonwealth whose philosophers believe that 'all our actions, and in them the vertues themselfes be referred at the last to pleasure, as their ende and felicitie.' Nevertheless, they rank pleasures in an order which gives low priority to the body:

'They imbrace chieflie the pleasures of the mind. For the delite of eating and drinking, and whatsoever hath any like pleasauntnes, they determyne to be pleasures muche to be desired, but no other wayes than for healthes sake.'

Any man who pursues bodily satisfaction for its own sake

'must nedes graunt, that then he shal be in most felicitie, if he live that life, which is led in continuall hunger, thurste, itchinge, eatinge, drynkynge, scratchynge, and rubbing. The which life how not only foule, and unhonest, but also how miserable, and wretched it is, who perceiveth not? These doubtles be the basest pleasures of al, as unpure and unperfect. For they never come, but accompanied with their contrarie griefes.'

In the sixteenth century, 'honest' meant 'respectable' and 'honourable' as well as 'virtuous', so Robinson's prose condemns bodily pleasures as vulgar and socially degrading. The moral connotations of 'base' and 'unpure' suggest that physical pleasures are not only unsatisfactory, but wicked and shameful. The best way to reconcile hedonism with virtue is to demonstrate that only virtuous thoughts and actions provide pleasant sensations. Unfortunately, this does not appear to be the case with most people, even in Utopia. More's philosophers tackle this difficulty by rejecting subjective experience in favour of intellectual and ethical standards as a means to establish the intensity, value, and reality of pleasures. They condemn as false such alleged enjoyments as pride in dress or ancestry, covetousness, gambling, and hunting. At first they make sensation the criterion of enjoyment: 'why sholdest thou not take even as much pleasure in beholdynge a counterfeite stone, whiche thine eye cannot discerne from a righte stone?' Subsequently, however, they concede that sensory gratification may arise from some false pleasures, but that does not prove their authenticity, for 'perverse and lewde custome is the cause hereof'.

Utopians maximise the benefits of deferred gratification. Life led according to nature, right reason, and virtue will inevitably foster the physical health which is necessary for all other pleasures. Generosity to others is trebly advantageous:

'For it is recompensed with the retourne of benefytes, and the conscience of the good dede with remembraunce of the thankefull love and benevolence of them to whom thou hast done it, doth bring more pleasure to thy mynde, then that whiche thou hast withholden from thy selfe could have brought to thy bodye. Finallye (which to a godly disposed and a religious mind is easy to be persuaded) God recompenseth the gifte of a short and smal pleasure with great and everlasting joye.'

This influential text airs many aspects of pleasure theory which were debated for ensuing centuries.

Pleasure and the enlightenment
Hedonistic theories proliferated spectacularly in the seventeenth and eighteenth centuries. Some were frankly materialistic, like the analysis of psychology, politics, and morality in Thomas

Hobbes' *Leviathan* (1651). He believes the fundamental law of nature is 'to seek peace, and follow it'; the 'Passions that encline men to Peace, are Feare of Death; Desire of such things as are necessary to commodious living', and 'a Hope by their Industry to maintain them'. His views, often condemned as atheistic, inspired *philosophes* like Claude–Adrien Helvétius (1715–71), Paul–Henri d'Holbach (1723–89), and Julien de la Mettrie (1709–51). As material prosperity increased, it became easier — and more necessary — to devise theories which demonstrated that human happiness was consistent with the order of the universe. The political economist Adam Smith (1723–70), champion of the unregulated *laissez-faire* economy, believed that the more its people were left to their own devices, the more prosperous and efficient a nation would become. British natural theologists, including John Ray (1628–1704) and Robert Boyle (1626–91), united science with religion in an attempt to show that happiness was part of God's plan. Drawing their evidence from observations on the world about them, they argued that God, having designed such a well-run, comfortable universe, must intend men to be happy, in this world and the next. This optimism was extended to psychology and morality by those who claimed that virtue and benevolence were not only profitable, but sources of pleasant sensations. The Revd Joseph Butler, in *Fifteen Sermons* (1726), Sermon Nine, expounds the paradox of hedonism: people intent on their own pleasures gain less gratification than those who care for others' interests. Anthony Ashley Cooper, third Earl of Shaftesbury (1671–1713), and Francis Hutcheson (1694–1746) argued for the existence of a 'moral sense'; David Hume (1711–76) declared it the sole criterion of ethical value. The full hedonistic implications lurking in Utopian accounts of virtue's benefits could be spelled out in embarrassing detail. Some philosophers cynically suspected that all actions were essentially self-gratifying. Did altruism really exist? Bernard Mandeville's *Essay on Charity* (1723) says, 'thousands give money to beggars from the same motives as they pay their corn-cutter, to walk easy.' Shaftesbury advocated the cultivation of virtue for its own sake, believing the introduction of any ulterior motive, like hope of heaven or fear of hell, rendered it 'illiberal and unworthy of any honour or commendation'. Christian apologists retorted that only the prospect of eternal pains and pleasures could ensure good behaviour among the population at large. A properly regulated hedonism must find moral approval from a viewpoint which regarded pleasure not only as a direct and indirect reward of virtue, but as proof of God's benevolence, if not his existence.

Even animals could benefit from divine goodness. The Revd William Paley, Archdeacon of Carlisle (1743–1805), in *Principles of Moral and Political Philosophy* (1785), claims that God enables every sentient being to experience an appropriate degree of bliss:

'When we are in perfect health and spirits, we feel in ourselves a happiness independent of any particular outward gratification whatever, and of which we can give no account. This is an enjoyment which the deity has annexed to life; and probably constitutes, in a great measure, the happiness of infants and brutes, as oysters, periwinkles, and the like; for which I have sometimes been at a loss to find out amusement.'

With God omitted from the calculations, the prospect of animal pleasure could still enhance a system of universal harmony: in *The Origin of Species* (1859), Chapter 3, Charles Darwin attempts to soften the harshness of natural selection by arguing that, for the successful, a sense of well-being is the order of the day:

'When we reflect on this struggle, we may console ourselves with the full belief, that the war of nature is not incessant, that no fear is felt, that death is generally prompt, and that the vigorous, the healthy, and the happy survive and multiply.'

Utilitarianism
Jeremy Bentham's *Introduction to the Principles of Morals and Legislation* (1789) shifted the emphasis from individual happiness to the good of society, announcing that all legislation should be designed to achieve 'the greatest happiness of the greatest number.' His hedonistic utilitarianism combines psychological and ethical approaches:

'nature has placed mankind under the governance of two sovereign masters, *pain* and *pleasure*. It is for them alone to determine what we ought to do as well as what we shall do.'

He was concerned with quantity rather than quality, defining 'utility' as

'that property in any object whereby it tends to produce pleasure, good or happiness, or to prevent the happening of mischief, pain, evil or unhappiness to the party whose interest is considered.'

In *Utilitarianism* (1861), Chapter 2, Bentham's disciple, John Stuart Mill, introduces a hierarchy of pleasures to defend the system against the traditional anti-Epicurean complaint that a life with no higher end than pleasure was 'worthy only of swine'. Mill points out that

'the Epicureans have always avowed, that it is not they, but their accusers, who represent human nature in a degrading light; since the accusation suposes human beings to be capable of no pleasures except those of which swine are capable.'

He claims that the 'higher', or intellectual, pleasures, are better in quality than 'lower', physical, enjoyments. He declares, with a touch of arrogance,

'It is better to be a human being dissatisfied than a pig satisfied; better to be a Socrates dissatisfied than a fool satisfied. And if the fool, or the pig, are of a different opinion, it is because they only know their own side of the question.'

Utilitarianism is perpetually controversial. What happens when the individual's interests conflict with those of the rest of society? 'Ideal utilitarians' question the validity of identifying the good with pleasure. Problems also arise from the difficulty of calculating consequences.

Should we be 'act utilitarians', always trying to do whatever will produce the greatest good on any occasion? Or should we become 'rule utilitarians', conforming to whatever behaviour would normally turn out best? Whatever the uncertainties about individual duties and gratifications, there can be no doubt that hedonist utilitarianism has extensive applications for society in general. With the rise of democracy and consumerism, pleasure must be acknowledged as a formidable economic and political force. Pleasure is not merely the preoccupation of frivolous moral weaklings; the founders of the world's most powerful nation held it self-evident that man had an inalienable right to the pursuit of happiness.

The science of pleasure

Important twentieth-century developments included psychological investigation of hedonic reactions (feelings of liking or disliking) to various stimuli, and neurological research linking responses associated with pleasure to specific areas and chemical reactions in the brain. Recent advances in pharmacology and technology have given new urgency to old problems. With the appropriate use of drugs and electrodes, attempts to assess the value of a life spent in constant pleasure, regardless of other considerations, might cease to be a matter of philosophical speculation.   CAROLYN D. WILLIAMS

Further reading

Annas, J. (1993). *The morality of happiness*. Oxford University Press, New York and Oxford.

Campbell, C. (1990). *The Romantic ethic and the spirit of modern consumerism*. Blackwell, Oxford.

Glover, J. (ed) (1990). *Utilitarianism and its critics*. Macmillan, New York: Collins Macmillan, London.

Porter, R. and Roberts, M. M. (ed.) (1996). *Pleasure in the eighteenth century*. Macmillan, Basingstoke.

See also PLEASURE; PLEASURE, BIOLOGICAL BASIS.

Heparin This, the body's natural anticoagulant, is a muco-polysaccharide of variable molecular weight (12 000–25 000) containing sulphate groups. Heparin is produced in the liver and stored there and in other cells, such as mast cells. The levels in circulating blood are very low in normal conditions. It is able to prevent blood coagulation by acting at three separate points on the 'cascade' of chemical events in the plasma that causes blood clotting. First it prevents the interaction of thrombin with fibrinogen, so that the conversion of the latter to fibrin, the basic structural element of a clot, is prevented. Second, it prevents the conversion of prothrombin to thrombin and causes the destruction of Factor Xa, an early factor in the cascade. Given intravenously or subcutaneously heparin can be used to treat deep vein thrombosis and acute arterial thrombosis.   ALAN W. CUTHBERT

See also BLOOD; BLOOD CLOTTING.

Herbal medicine Plants have been used for medicinal purposes for as long as history has been recorded. China, India, Egypt, and Assyria appear to have been the places which cradled the use of herbs, but herbalism was common in Europe by medieval times. Despite the progress in orthodox medicine, interest in alternative medicine, including herbalism, is on the increase in the West — and for 80% of the world herbal medicine is still the only kind to which ordinary persons have ready access.

A great variety of plants are used for medicinal treatments. Either the dried plant, or a specific part of it (root, leaves, fruit, flowers, seeds), is formulated into suitable preparations — compressed as tablets or made into pills, used to make infusions (teas), extracts, tinctures, etc., or mixed with excipients to make lotions, ointments, creams, etc. Few herbal drugs are subject to legislative control. Obviously control is needed for poppy capsules (which contain opium), belladonna, digitalis, nux vonica beans (which contain strychnine), and rauwolfia (which contains reserpine). Most herbal remedies are freely available, although rarely have any been investigated with the thoroughness of orthodox medicines. The claims made for many herbal remedies are for trivial or minor ailments, due partly to the strictures put on legal claims for efficacy, and partly because herbalists claim to treat the whole person to restore normal physiological balance, rather than to treat or cure a particular medical illness. Activities of herbal medicines are often described in very general terms — such as carminative, laxative, demulcent, antitussive, expectorant, sedative, antiseptic, or astringent. Unlike orthodox medicines, which usually consist of a single, isolated principle often synthetic), plants or extracts of plants contain multiple constituents, not all of them active. Herbalists often claim that the admixture of multiple constituents leads to synergism between the active moieties. Similarly, many consider that since plants are natural materials they are safer and will produce fewer side-effects than synthetic drugs. There is little substance or reason in either of these claims. For example, comfrey (*Symphytum officinale*) is considered a safe herb and is used as a demulcent. However, it contains pyrrolizidine alkaloids, which are toxic to the liver and can cause liver cancer. Media attention can often cause a major increase in the demand and use of herbal drugs — for example, evening primrose oil, feverfew, Ginko biloba, and ginseng. One of the problems with herbal drugs, especially those with active principles which have well-defined medicinal effects (e.g. digitalis), is that the amount of active principle(s) varies according to the location where the plant is grown, the prevailing weather conditions, etc., so it is vital in these instances that the crude material is assayed appropriately so that the dosage can be accurately controlled, especially where the therapeutic ratio is low. (Therapeutic ratio is the ratio of the dose causing toxic effects to that required for treatment.)

From time to time new drugs are discovered from herbal sources — for example, *taxol*, derived from the yew, is an important drug for some forms of cancer. The active principle is extracted and purified from plant material for as long as that process remains economically viable compared with chemical synthesis.

ALAN W. CUTHBERT

Hercules (Greek: 'Heracles') was the greatest hero of the Greek world, known for his feats of strength. His mother Alcmene was mortal, his father was the god Zeus. Even as a child, Heracles strangled serpents in his cradle. As an adult, after murdering his own children in a fit of madness caused by the goddess Hera, he was punished by having to carry out twelve labours, which included cleaning the stables of Augeas, capturing the man-eating mares of Diomedes, taking the belt of the queen of the Amazons, stealing the golden apples of the Hesperides, and chaining up Cerberus, the many-headed hound of Hades, who wags his tail when the newly deceased arrive but attacks and eats those who try to leave. These labours took him to the limits of the known world and, in the case of Cerberus, to the world of the dead. In art, he is represented with a lion-skin cape and hood (courtesy of the object of another labour, the Nemean lion), and carries a club and a bow and arrows.

He was finally defeated only by trickery. In the version given in Sophocles' play, *The Women of Trachis*, his wife Deianira gave him what she thought was a love potion, but was in fact poison given to her by the centaur who had previously tried to rape her. The poison was used to impregnate Hercules' robe, but it ate away his flesh, causing him unbearable pain.

A number of Greek rulers claimed descent from Heracles as a symbol of their power; these included the Macedonian royal family, whose most notable member was Alexander the Great. The cult of Heracles may have been the first foreign cult to be introduced to Rome; he was particularly popular with merchants, because of the amount of travel involved in his labours. Dogs were excluded from his sanctuary at Rome; maybe he had seen enough of them with Cerberus. In the later Roman Empire a number of emperors identified with Hercules and had themselves represented in statuary with his attributes — most notably Commodus, who issued a commemorative medal showing himself wearing Hercules' lion-skin, with the inscription 'To the Roman Hercules'.

Hercules' reputation as a strong-man derives in particular from his wrestling bout with the supposedly invincible Libyan giant, Antaeus. Knowing that Antaeus renewed his strength by physical contact with his mother, the earth goddess, Hercules held up his opponent so that his feet could not reach the ground, then crushed him to death. Another feat demonstrating his strength was the establishment of the 'Pillars of Hercules' at the limits of the known world — the Strait of Gibraltar.   HELEN KING

See also GREEKS.

Heredity In popular parlance, the word 'heredity' is used to explain the observation that every living organism gives rise, through reproduction, to a look-alike organism. In biology and medicine, it is a term refering to the biological information that is transmitted from parents to offspring in every generation. Nowadays, the field of genetics is responsible for the scientific study of heredity and its mechanisms, and the main focus of genetic research is the examination of the GENE as carrier of information on the structure, function, and biological attributes of the organism, and its transmission to subsequent generations.

The term 'heredity' was introduced into the English language in the 1860s from the French *hérédité*, as a noun referring to the properties and characters considered as hereditary. The term 'heredity' was preferred over the existing term 'inheritance' by biologists of the time, because it was not loaded with the Lamarckian overtones of the latter. Borrowed from landed gentry and used to refer to old family property as well as to

---

Cross between varieties displaying yellow (YY) or green colour (yy) seeds

---

P1 = parental generation;

F1, F2 = hybrid generations

Y = dominant yellow; y = recessive green

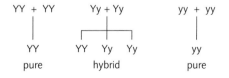

(in F1, all plants contained yellow seeds)

Crossing F1 with F1:

YY Yy Yy yy (F2)

(in F2 a 3:1 ratio was observed: of every four plants obtained, three contained yellow seeds (YY, Yy, Yy) and one contained green seeds (yy))

Self-fertilization within F2:

YY + YY   Yy + Yy   yy + yy
| | |
YY   YY Yy Yy   yy
pure   hybrid   pure

From this, Mendel confirmed the existence of three types of F2 plants: pure yellow-seeded, hybrid and pure green-seeded.

---

that acquired during a particular lifetime, the term 'inheritance' was associated with notions of acquired characteristics. Francis Galton, an active spokesman for the importance of heredity in the human make-up, and founder of the science of EUGENICS, claims in his autobiography to have been the first to use the term 'heredity' in the 1860s. However, other biologists, such as Charles Darwin, had started using the term some years earlier.

In 1900, Gregor Mendel's 1866 paper on the study of hybrids of the edible pea was independently 'rediscovered' in Europe. Although Mendel's experiments were part of his interests on the origin of new species by hybridization (rather than by variation), and were thus not directly concerned with the elucidation of the laws of heredity, they were interpreted in 1900 as the first systematic study unravelling the mechanisms of heredity.

Gregor Mendel (1822–1884), an Augustinian monk at Brno, Moravia (now part of the Czech Republic), performed his classic experiments using varieties of the edible pea (*Pisum sativum*) grown in the monastery garden. By artificial fertilization, he crossed two pure varieties of peas and followed the inheritance of seven pairs of character differences (yellow or green seeds; round or angular seeds; white or grey-brown seed coats; green or yellow pods; smooth or ridge pods; tallness or shortness; axillary or terminal flowers). He reported that, in the first hybrid generation (F1), only one character in each pair of character differences would be manifested. He used the word 'factor' to refer to the determing agent responsible for each character, and described their effects as either dominant or recessive. Through self-fertilization, he crossed the F1 to produce the second hybrid generation (F2) and reported the reappearance of the recessive characters in a 1:3 ratio. Mendel explained his results by describing the characters studied as distinct, stable factors, which were passed on independently and unchanged from parent to offspring. Although the recessive characters would be masked in the F1, their independent transmission from parent to offspring could be confirmed by observing their reappearance in the F2. The reappearance of hidden recessive characters in the F2 disagreed with prevailing notions on 'blending' inheritance, postulating the blending and dilution of parental traits in the offspring. Mendel also carried out the self-fertilization of the F2, from which he confirmed the existence in the F2 of three types of plants: two pure parental types and one hybrid type.

Mendel's hybridization experiments are theoretically formulated in the figure. As example, this shows the cross between two varieties of peas displaying seed colour as character difference.

In 1900, with the international recognition of Gregor Mendel's work as the basis for a new science of heredity, a new wave of experimentation with hybrid formation began that appealed to the breeding interests of botanists and zoologists. In 1906, the Cambridge zoologist William

Bateson introduced the word 'genetics' to refer to the expanding new field of research. Bateson became a vocal defender of the validity of Mendel's conclusions as the scientific foundation for the new discipline. He encouraged the use of Mendelian principles not only for the study of the plant and animal world, but also for the examination of heredity in humans. On February 1, 1906, he addressed the Neurological Society of London on the topic of Mendelian heredity and its application to man. In this lecture, Bateson presented to an audience of physicians a new picture of human heredity in which human physical traits were treated as Mendelian segregating characters, and he reformulated human hereditary disease as being caused by single genetic factors obeying Mendelian principles. He explained brachydactyly, congenital cataract, albinism, alcaptonuria, haemophilia, and colour blindness as being caused by Mendelian factors (dominant or recessive) of heredity.

Bateson spoke extensively about the behaviour of Mendelian factors, but was unable to provide a material mechanism guiding their operation. He refused to accept ideas associating the gene with a particular stretch of chromosomal material. However, between 1910 and 1915, Thomas Hunt Morgan and his students, working at Columbia University, New York, gathered enough data to support successfully the chromosomal theory of the gene, which firmly established the Mendelian genetic factors as material unities, or 'genes', embedded in the chromosome. The use of the chromosomal theory of the gene gave rise to a very productive area of experimentation, now known as 'classical genetics' which produced the first genetic maps, showing the relative positions of genes on the chromosome, and a gave clear notion of the nature of mutations.

Outside the laboratory, the concept of heredity occupied a crucial role in debates on the importance of nature over nurture and on the possibilities of using biological norms to guide social reform during the end of the nineteenth century and the first decades of the twentieth. Hereditarian theories, considering heredity as the central factor determining human character, were used by biologists, physicians, and social activists to explain human temperament, family pathology, and the structure of society. Francis Galton, a strong believer in the hereditarian position, founded the discipline of EUGENICS, which sought to improve the quality of human heredity by manipulating human reproduction. The field of eugenics developed into a breeding programme proposing a series of measures to prevent the reproduction of those labelled as 'unfit' or 'feebleminded'. As a counterpart, such programmes sought to promote the reproduction of those harbouring in their heredity 'superior' human qualities. Eugenic thought became highly influential during the first decades of the twentieth century in the US and in Britain, Germany, and other parts of Europe. It started losing its pre-eminence in the 1930s and 1940s, when it was highly criticized by scientists and the public for its scientific inaccuracy, for its class and race bias, and for the excesses to which it could lead, as exemplified by the horrors taking place during the implementation of state controlled reproductive policies in Nazi Germany.

SILVIA FRENK

See also EUGENICS; GENE; GENETICS, HUMAN.

Hermaphrodite

The idea of the hermaphrodite who has fully functioning male and female organs and is (theoretically) capable of self-fertilization is a myth, though a very persistent one, which has long exercised a fascination over the human mind. It provided a way of thinking about and transgressing the binary division between the sexes, and may have externalized and isolated less coherent ideas about the existence of contrary sexual characteristics in both sexes and about innate bisexuality.

Surprisingly, given the development of the male and female sexual organs from the same primitive gonad in the embryo and the possibility of errors occurring, various forms of hermaphroditism, though they do exist, are extremely rare. Like many rare conditions, however, it has had an interest for scientists inversely proportional to its frequency, because of the light such anomalies shed on the course of normal sexual development and the differentiation of the two sexes. There are many stages of development at which intersexuality can occur, from the chromosomal to the behavioural, but a hermaphrodite is usually taken to be an individual who has physically present both male and female gonadal organs and sexual characteristics, rather than someone, who, though to all intents and purposes of one sex, is chromosomally of the other, as in some rare genetic conditions.

In most cases a child born with ambiguous GENITALIA will be assigned to the most likely gender, with, possibly, some surgical tidying up. This may be a satisfactory solution if only the external genitals are effected, but in many cases of such ambiguity, external organs which are closer to those of one sex are found in conjunction with internal organs of the other. This may not become apparent until puberty, when the hormonal changes may lead to the 'boy' starting to menstruate, or having abdominal pains caused by obstructed menstruation, or the 'girl's' voice breaking and facial hair appearing. At this stage decisions may need to be taken as to whether the individual is 'really' of the gender of original assignment, and just needs some alien tissue removing, or whether they are 'really' of the opposite sex. The powerful influence of the need to categorize human beings as definitely either male or female is very apparent, even though it may necessitate surgery and hormonal treatment of the unfortunate individual who fits neither.

The idea of hermaphroditism has been invoked to explain homosexuality. Abandoning a simple physical explanation, nineteenth-century sexologists projected a disjunction between external appearance and internal sense of self. Thus (echoing Elizabeth I's claim to have the 'heart and stomach of a man' within the body of a 'weak and feeble' woman) the homosexual or 'invert' was believed to have the spirit of one sex inside the body of the other. The model constructed desire for the male as 'feminine' and for the female as 'masculine', thus preserving the notion of sexual difference.

If hermaphrodites did not exist, it would probably be necessary to invent them as a useful conceptual category. LESLEY A. HALL

Hernia

A hernia is where a part of the abdominal content protrudes or bulges through an abnormal opening in the inner layers of the wall of the abdomen. The hernial 'sac' usually contains either fatty tissue or a loop of intestine. Some common types are groin, umbilical, and incisional hernias.

Groin hernias

There are two types of groin hernia, *inguinal* or *femoral*, the former being far more common and making up 98% of all groin hernias. Inguinal hernias are common in newborn boys, where they arise as a result of a 'canal' normally present in the embryo between the inside of the abdomen and the scrotum, which fails to close. They are also common in adult life and increase in frequency as one grows older. Inguinal hernias are approximately twenty times more common in men than women, while, interestingly, femoral hernias are more common in women.

Usually a groin hernia presents with a lump in the groin, felt all the time or only when straining. It often causes a dull ache that is worse with activity. The lump may get bigger with coughing or straining and shrink or disappear with lying down. Not all hernias are easily felt, however. When the contents can be pushed back into the abdomen the hernia is said to be 'reducible' — and 'irreducible' if not.

Surgeons have been treating and repairing hernias for over 3000 years, with varying degrees of success. The Mummy of Pharaoh Merneptah (nineteenth dynasty, 1224–14 BC) showed a large wound in the groin, with the scrotum separated from the body indicating that crude surgery had been performed on an inguinal hernia that had passed down into the scrotum. Nowadays many hernia repairs are performed worldwide each year, some 80 000 in the UK alone. The repair is usually performed by reinforcing the defect with stitches or a plastic mesh, often as a day case procedure, using either a local or a general anaesthetic.

While most hernias are usually just troublesome, on rare occasions they enlarge quickly with a sudden intense pain and part of the bowel gets trapped and becomes blocked. This *intestinal obstruction* is an emergency situation and requires surgery to free the trapped piece of bowel or to excise it if irretrievably damaged by 'strangulation' of its blood supply.

Umbilical hernias

Up to a fifth of babies are born with a bulge through a defect at the site of the umbilical cord. The majority will close by themselves and they only occasionally need surgical repair if the hernia becomes excessively large or inflamed, or if it is still present by the age of about four. Adults also develop hernias in the region of the umbilicus (paraumbilical). These are often associated with obesity, can be uncomfortable, and may become irreducible. Again they are usually repaired as a day case or overnight stay procedure.

Incisional hernias

These occur months or years after abdominal surgery and are common after such procedures as large bowel surgery in either sex, or hysterectomy in women. They are more common in obese patients or following a postoperative wound infection. They may become very large and unsightly. Rarely they may cause the bowel to obstruct and require emergency surgery. Nowadays they are usually repaired with a large piece of mesh, as there is a high recurrence rate after a sutured repair. S. G. TAYLOR
P. J. O'DWYER

See also ALIMENTARY SYSTEM; SCROTUM.

Heroin

is a modified form of morphine obtained by acetylating morphine with acetic acid, so that both hydroxyl groups are modified. Chemically, therefore, it is *diacetyl morphine*. It is about three times more potent than morphine, and because of its increased lipid solubility it rapidly enters the brain. Addicts claim it gives a better 'rush' when injected intravenously. Heroin is now only rarely used to treat intractable pain, as appropriate dosing regimens can maintain analgesia using morphine or other drugs.

A. W. C.

See ADDICTION; ANALGESIA; DRUG.

Hiccough or hiccup

We are all familiar with the common occurrence of hiccup or hiccough. It consists of a series of forceful but abruptly blocked intakes of breath. Each abrupt blocking of inspiration gives rise to a characteristic sound. The condition is often triggered by gastric distension or alcohol intake, normally lasts for no longer than a few hours, and is either self-terminating or responds to simple folk remedies. However, on rare occasions hiccups can be present continuously for more than 24 hours or prolonged bouts may recur daily. Such cases of chronic hiccups may reflect a great variety of underlying disease processes. Chronic hiccups have been reported in association with disorders and lesions of systems as diverse as the gastrointestinal, hepatic, renal/urinary, and both the central and peripheral nervous systems. In addition, chronic hiccups can occur following the administration of certain drugs and as an accompaniment to psychiatric illness. The direct danger of severe hiccups, continuously present over a long period of time, is simply one of physical exhaustion, quite apart from any hazards relating to underlying disease or drugs.

A hiccup is produced by a sudden, forceful contraction of the DIAPHRAGM. This causes a rapid inspiration but the inflow of air through the LARYNX into the LUNGS is blocked by an almost immediate closure of the glottis, meaning that the vocal cords come together. This process has no known physiological function; in fact there is remarkably little information on the biology of hiccups. They can occur in a wide variety of circumstances, from those associated in the fetus with normal activity to those accompanying terminal disease. Some workers have suggested that there is a hiccup centre in the brain and experimental work in anaesthetized animals has located a region in the medulla which, when stimulated electrically, produces a powerful inspiration with sudden glottic closure. This can also be produced by mechanical stimulation of the back wall of the upper PHARYNX.

The general assumption is consequently that hiccups are due to activation of a REFLEX because of an adequate but abnormal or pathological sensory input, or because the threshold for the reflex is substantially lowered by excitation within the brain, or because an existing inhibition of the reflex is removed. It is difficult to envisage the circumstances in which such a reflex would have any utility. An alternative suggestion is that the condition is not a reflex but a *myoclonus*, which is defined in this context as a sudden, brief, involuntary movement, arising from abnormal spontaneous activity within the central nervous system, comparable to that occurring in EPILEPSY. Chronic hiccups have been associated with brain lesions in diverse areas including the temporal lobe, the thalamus, and understandably, the medulla.

Simple hiccups may respond to a variety of folk remedies, e.g. a sudden fright, breath-holding, or drinking a large glass of water without taking a breath. Most of such remedies have the common feature in that they interrupt breathing and so could increase the level of CARBON DIOXIDE circulating in the blood. An increased arterial carbon dioxide level in turn increases the drive to the respiratory system and the assumption is that this enables the medullary respiratory centre to suppress interruptions (hiccups) to its ongoing rhythmic activity. However, in the rare cases of chronic hiccups, attention has to be directed to diagnosis and treatment of the underlying disease state, to remove the triggering factors. If no underlying disease can be found, or if a drug is inducing the hiccups but that drug is essential to some other treatment, the condition may have to be treated symptomatically using an agent that will simply suppress it.

Despite many well-conducted investigations, the current state of knowledge of hiccups is still unsatisfactory. ALLAN THEXTON

Hinduism and the body

The name 'Hinduism' is a relatively recent term for a pluralistic religion and way of life whose origins lie in South Asia's ancient past. Its most sacred books are the four collections of hymns called Vedas, the oldest sections of which may date from as early as 1500 BC. These hymns, addressed mostly to powerful male deities of nature, are considered by Hindus to have been divinely revealed to seers of the nomadic, fair-skinned Aryan tribes who, entering first the north-west region (now Pakistan) from Central Asia, subjugated the dark-skinned indigenous peoples and eventually spread their culture over the whole of the subcontinent and beyond.

The hymns indicate, not surprisingly, that strength of body was highly regarded in a man. A girl with physical defects found it difficult to get a husband. Upper and lower garments were worn and the body was ornamented with bracelets, anklets, necklaces, and earrings. Dance was enjoyed. *Kāma*, the love between a man and a woman, who brought about all kinds of physical sensations, was deified, and men and women used charms to make their lovers' bodies burn for them. In one such charm (Atharvaveda 3. 25), Kāma is besought to release an arrow to pierce the object of a young man's desire. At its release her spleen would dry up, it would burn her body and dry her mouth so that she would run to him.

Diseases were believed to have been brought about by the curses of the gods, sin against them, violation of moral law, or *possession* by evil spirits. Priestly physicians attempted cures using charms, sympathetic magic, amulets, and medicines; the physician tried to bring his patient back to health irrespective of whether he was ill, dying, or had already died. Religious rites were performed before and during pregnancy to try to ensure the birth of a male child. Cremation was the usual means of disposing of the corpse. The god of fire was invoked to carry the body to the other world, keeping it intact and healing any injury caused to it by animal or insect. When the spirit had travelled by the path of the Fathers it was believed to unite with the glorious body and enter a life in highest heaven untroubled by bodily imperfections and frailties.

Philosophic speculation concerning the nature and origin of creation, and the search for a godhead, occurs in the late hymns: 'Who brought together the two heels of a person; by whom was his flesh assembled, his ankle joints, his clever fingers?' (Atharvaveda X. 2). A hymn of the Rgveda (X. 90) describes the world as coming into being through the sacrifice of a primaeval man whose parts, when cut up, became parts of the creation; the sun came from his eye, the moon from his mind, Indra (the war god) and fire came from his mouth, wind from his breath, air from his navel, the sky from his head, earth from his feet. In the early philosophic texts, the older Upanishads (c. sixth century BC), there arises the idea that the bodily parts of the cosmic person are identical to the bodily functions of the individual, and that 'Fire became speech and entered the mouth (of the individual), wind became breath and entered the nostrils, the sun became sight and entered the eyes' (Aitareya 2). The single divinity is identified as the self (*ātman*) of all beings. The individual self is further identified as being the same as the self of the entire creation,

Brahman, the Supreme Spirit. The body is known to be mortal, there is speculation that after death the indestructible self enters a new womb, desirable or undesirable according to the person's deeds, and that a perfected soul can escape the cycle of birth and death.

The centuries immediately preceding and following the beginning of the Christian era are notable for the production of an immense body of literature. All learning was collected into books called *śāstras*. The material in these texts is not dated, instead each branch of knowledge is given a mythical divine origin and, if possible, linked to one of the four Vedas, for in Hinduism there is no clear division between the religious and the secular. By this time the correlation of the *macrocosm* and *microcosm* was complete and the doctrine of *metempsychosis* fully formulated. Worship of a personal deity was believed to bring about the fulfilment of all desires, even *emancipation* from the cycle of birth and death. These fundamental beliefs have not since changed to any great extent.

The *Kāmasūtra*, the oldest surviving text of *Kāmaśāstra* (the science of sexuality), is instruction in how to attain the complete sexual satisfaction considered important for both sexes. Dance is not merely an art form but a means of achieving union of the individual soul with the divine. Its treatise, the *Nātyaśāstra*, describes gesture and movement so refined as to amount to a complete body language able to express story, thought, and feeling through the movement of the major limbs, the head, hands, chest, buttocks, abdomen, waist, and thighs, and the minor limbs, the eyes, eyebrows, nose, lips, cheeks, and chin. Detailed descriptions of the human body are found in the literature belonging to the classical system of Indian medicine called *Āyurveda* — 'knowledge for long life' (the word 'veda' in this context means 'knowledge'). The earliest of the texts which have come down to us are the compendia of *Caraka* and *Suśruta*, which probably date from the second century AD, but which contain some much older material.

Suśruta's compendium, which differs from that of Caraka largely in that it contains surgery, describes *dissection*, by means of a bamboo blade, of a body left to decompose for a few days in running water. It appears that this practice did not continue after Suśruta's time, probably because of opposition from the priestly caste. As might be expected, the particular weakness of the system is the lack of precision in the descriptions of the vessels and soft tissues of the body, whereas the description of bones is more accurate, although teeth, nails, cartileges, and protuberances were also included — Suśruta counts 300 bones, Caraka 360.

According to Hindu thought, the entire physical world is made of combinations of five great *elements*; ether, air, fire, water, and earth. The body is the sum of the modifications and combinations of the elements which have produced it. The elements are intimately connected with the five senses of the individual; ether with hearing, air with touch, fire with sight, water with taste, and earth with smell. At death the body returns to the elements, what is of ether to ether, air to air, and so on. The medical texts explain that modifications of the elements produce the seven essential constituents of the body, called *dhātus*, which are chyle, blood, flesh, fat, bone, marrow, and semen. (No particular mention is made of the woman's body, but some texts seem to propose breast milk as an equivalent for semen.) Each of these constituents arises from the previous one, the whole being dependent on the intake of food, or in the case of the fetus, the mother's chyle. The quintessence of all is *ojas*, a word which can be roughly translated as 'vitality', although *ojas* is said to be a substance, which is distributed around the body by the heart, the most important of the body's organs. Maintenance of the equilibrium of the *dhātus* is of vital importance for health, for when one or more is depleted or in excess, the body will exhibit symptoms of disease.

When healthy food and drink are taken into the stomach, they are digested by being 'cooked' by internal fire. Those parts which cannot be assimilated into the chain of production of the *dhātus* produce faeces, urine, ear wax, the secretions of the eye, nose, and mouth, sweat, hair, nails, etc., as well as the three HUMOURS of the body, wind, bile, and phlegm. The theory is that, in their right proportions, these are also maintainers of the body, and as such are also considered to be *dhātus*, but when they exceed or become less than their proper measure they become impurities, which pollute the body and may destroy it. By far the most important of them are the three humours.

Wind holds the dominant position as leader of the humours. It is dry, cold, light, subtle, mobile, and rough, and scatters everything in different directions. It carries the sensations of sound, touch, etc.; is the producer of speech; stimulates the body fire to promote appetite; and is the cause of the evacuation of urine, faeces, and other waste products, and of parturition. Bile is greasy, hot, sharp, fluid, and acrid. Its functions are to bring about coloration, digestion, heat, sight, hunger, and thirst, and the softness and radiance of the body. Phlegm is motionless, viscid, sticky, heavy, inert, cold, soft, and white. Its functions are viscidity, nourishment, the binding of joints, the solidarity of the body, and the maintenance of sexual vigour. Caraka says that from the time of the formation of the fetus these three are working, either in equal quantities or with different degrees of predominance. People with a predominance of phlegm are generally healthy, whereas those with predominance of bile or wind are always of indifferent health. The balance of the three in a person is his bodily nature. When the balance of one, two, or all three of the humours is disturbed they cause havoc in the body by invading each other's domain: this is the root of disease.

The semen of the father, the blood of the mother, and the past deeds of the individual determine the bodily features of the child. The behaviour, diet, and inclinations of the mother during pregnancy also have their effect. Equilibrium of the proper measure of the *dhātus* keeps the body in good health, therefore a person should take care that his behaviour, regimen, and personal hygiene are such that this balance may be maintained. Failure to do so, Caraka says, is an offence against wisdom.

Although speculation and debate concerning the details of anatomy and the working of the body continued, as is evident from the vast literature of *Āyurveda* produced during succeeding centuries, the fundamental scheme laid out in the early texts has not changed. Even today writers and commentators on *Āyurvedic* texts tend to absorb modern concepts into the system rather than discard the traditional scheme.

In general, the ideal male body is that of the hero; muscular, with broad shoulders, long arms, a neck shaped like a conch shell, a noble head with large eyes and a prominent chin, well-proportioned limbs, and a deep chest. The ideal female form emphasizes fertility: heavy breasts, narrow waist, large hips, tapering thighs — as well as a face as lovely as a lotus, fair skin, and dark hair — are features much admired.

Hinduism holds that for the ordinary person there are three aims of life: virtue, wealth, and fulfilment of desire. The ultimate aim, though, is *mokṣa*, liberation from the wheel of birth and death. The person who has this aim, which, it is believed, may take many embodiments to achieve, must undertake ascetic discipline to free himself from the notion that the world he has been born into is reality. The body is regarded by him as a temple or a city in which the Supreme Spirit dwells. Meticulous cleanliness is important. Special postures, regulation of breath, sexual continence, and restraint of the senses are practised in order to subdue the body, so that it will not disturb the mind in meditation. When all the bonds of phenomenal existence have been loosed, and there is union of the individual self with the Supreme Spirit, then for that soul, it is said, there is no further embodiment.

A. GLAZIER

Further reading

Dasgupta, S. (1932). *A history of Indian philosophy*, Vol. 2, Chapter XIII. Cambridge University Press.

Hume, R. E. (2nd edn, revised 1931). *The thirteen principal Upanishads*. Oxford University Press.

Sharma, R. K. and Dash, B. (1977). *The Caraka Saṃhitā* Vol. 2, *Sārīrāsthāna*. Chowkhamba Sanskrit Series, Varanasi.

Hip The hip joint is an example of a 'ball and socket' (*multiaxial*) type of joint, with the top (head) of the long bone of the leg (femur) being the 'ball' and the socket being a depression in the bone of the PELVIS known as the *acetabulum*. This arrangement permits movements in three planes — forwards and backwards (*extension/flexion*); inwards and outwards (*adduction/abduction*); and inward twist and outward twist (*internal and external rotation*). Combination of these movements also gives rise to 'circumduction', a circular movement of the whole leg which describes a 'cone' with the foot at the base and the hip at the apex. The joint is spanned by powerful muscles, which are required not only for postural control and movement but also to confer stability at the hip. The large muscles constituting the BUTTOCKS (gluteal muscles) are particularly important for maintenance of hip stability and for promoting a normal GAIT. The hip is one of

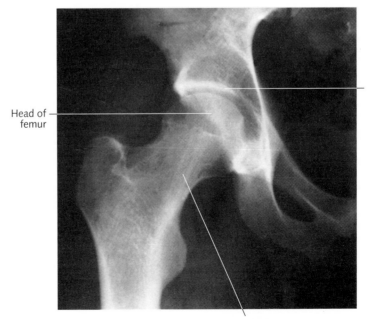

Head of femur

Acetabulum: socket in the pelvic bone

Neck of femur

X-ray of adult hip joint. Reproduced, with permission, from *Cunningham's textbook of anatomy*, (12th edn), OUP.

the most strong, secure, and stable joints in the body. This stability is due to the depth of the *acetabulum*; the powerful muscles surrounding the joint; and a strong, fibrous capsule reinforced by ligaments. Such securing of the joint is understandable when one considers the considerable strains placed on the hip during everyday activities such as walking, running, and particularly jumping. The hip is a large, weight-bearing joint which, because of the continued stresses placed on it throughout life, can develop *osteoarthritis* in later years. The cause of osteoarthritis is still poorly understood, but it may be the consequence of thinning of the cartilage covering the bones (acetabulum and head of femur), followed by bone overgrowth. This condition can be debilitating and can lead to severe pain and stiffness of the hip. One of the success stories of modern medicine is the surgical treatment of this condition by a hip joint replacement (*arthroplasty*). The technique, perfected by the British orthopaedic surgeon Sir John Charnley, involves an operation to remove the diseased joint and insert an artificial one made of metal and tough polyethylene. In this operation both the head of the femur and the acetabulum are replaced (total hip arthroplasty). Hip joint replacement can also be performed for other types of hip joint disease or malformations, and has been used after severe injury. These are sometimes sporting injuries, and there are recorded cases of individuals being able to return to sporting activities after successful operation.

The neck of the femur is a common site of fracture in the elderly, often resulting from a fall; the fracture is often called a 'broken hip'. This is more common in females, due to the greater thinning of bones with advancing years (*osteoporosis*) in women than in men. There is evidence to suggest that HORMONE REPLACEMENT THERAPY (HRT) after the menopause can slow the rate of bone loss. Treatment of a fractured neck of femur is usually by total hip joint replacement, as bone healing becomes poorer with advancing age and osteoporotic bone poorly supports metallic implants. The pelvis is wider in females than males because of the need to permit childbirth, and this results in the femoral heads being further apart. Consequently the thighs tend to be more sharply inclined inwards at the knees (*valgus*).

WILLIAM R. FERRELL

See also JOINTS; OSTEOPOROSIS; SKELETON.

Hip replacement

By the end of the twentieth century hip replacement had become the commonest major orthopaedic operation in the over-60 age group — and the most successful, by virtue of relief of pain, and restoration of mobility and independence for periods of up to 20 years.

Total prosthetic replacement of the hip joint involves substitution both of the socket in the pelvic bone and of the head of the femur, which rotates within it. This was first carried out in 1938, by Philip Wiles at the Middlesex Hospital, using all-metal replacement parts, secured by screws, as an advance on earlier procedures, which replaced only the head of the femur. This 'metal-on-metal' prosthesis was not successful because of the loosening of the metal parts, caused by high friction in the joint which the fixation screws were unable to withstand when the patient took full weight on the leg.

Following World War II, McKee of Norwich and Charnley of Wrightington developed further types of hip joint replacement. The major advance was the first use of methyl-methacrylate bone cement to fix the components into the bone of the pelvis and of the femur, based on pioneering work by Wiltse in the US. This prevented loosening of the components and gave immediate pain relief to the patient. The McKee–Farrar type was a chrome–cobalt metal replacement for both surfaces of the joint, whereas the Charnley type employed a high-density polyethylene cup for the socket and stainless steel for the femoral head. Charnley had demonstrated by wear-testing methods that friction was lower with a polyethylene cup articulating on metal. He predicted that it would not loosen and would last for 10–20 years.

If the technique for inserting the bone cement was not performed precisely, the cement was prone to fracture or to loosen in the bone, causing a recurrence of pain, and it was extremely difficult to remove. Hence, in the 1970s and 1980s, many experiments were directed towards hip replacements which did not require cement; instead they had a roughened surface which would encourage fixation by incorporation in the surrounding bone. A variety of porous coatings, employing metal beads or micromeshes, and more recently hydroxyapatite, were developed. Although these are being pursued in some centres still, the long-term results have not become comparable with those achieved by the original cemented hips.

As time passed it became apparent that the all-metal joint had some problems, in terms of friction and loosening, which were not present with the high-density polyethylene articulating on stainless steel. However, time has also shown that all prostheses are prone to wear. Moreover, the particles produced by wear from the polyethylene type of prosthesis eventually stimulate the formation of bone-destroying cells, which cause it to be loosened from the bone over a period of 10–20 years. Although it is possible to replace these hips a second time, the result of the operation is never so successful as the first.

Recently, new interest has been generated in improving the quality of the high-density polyethylene to reduce its wear by sterilizing it in an oxygen-free atmosphere to reduce cross-linking. At the same time, more precise engineering of the bearing surfaces of metal-on-metal hip joints has occurred, so as to maintain low friction with fluid-filled bearings; this may create a prosthesis which wears very little and will thus last longer than 20 years.

The results for relieving pain and improving quality of life in severe osteoarthritis of the hip have been dramatic, and the lives of many thousands of patients throughout the world have been transformed. Most patients walk with crutches on the day after operation and walk unaided 6–8 weeks later. In the late 1990s approximately 400 000 hip replacements were performed annually world wide: about 200 000 in the US, 50 000 in the UK, and 150 000 elsewhere). Between 5% and 10% require replacement of the opposite hip within 5 years — and that gives equally good results.

Prospective clinical trials on hip replacements have been few, although the establishment of the Swedish Hip Registry of all prostheses implanted has yielded extremely valuable information, from long-term follow-up studies, regarding the performance of the different types and the factors that contribute to success and failure. For example, out of 415 patients treated by cemented Stanmore and Charnley hip replacement at the Royal National Orthopaedic Hospital between 1982 and 1987, 96% of the replaced hips survived with good function for 10 years. Studies from other centres have indicated an advantage of cemented prostheses over uncemented designs.

The quest continues, however, for the everlasting hip. This may be achieved by the use of better articulating surfaces which do not wear, such as ceramic femoral heads articulating on high-density polyethylene or ceramic articulating on ceramic. The alternative may be the improvement of metal-on-metal articulations. However, it appears that all prostheses will wear in due course, and though improvement will be achieved, the everlasting joint seems unlikely.

GEORGE BENTLEY

Holism

'My body is not a machine!' 'Treat the whole person!' 'The whole is different from the sum of the parts.' 'Reductionism is wrong, because organisms possess properties at a certain level of organization that cannot be explained in terms of properties at lower levels.' 'How people work, love, or vote is not determined by our genes!' These are holist views.

The term 'holism' was coined in 1926, from the Greek *holos* (whole), by the South African statesman General Jan Smuts. But whilst the period between the World Wars was a heyday of holist creativity in biology and medicine, approaches that we can identify as holist are much older. Holism was the unquestioned orthodoxy of the Western tradition of practising medicine and investigating nature for the two millennia before the nineteenth century. The body was a complex system, in dynamic equilibrium with its environment, and disease a state of imbalance. Mechanistic approaches were canvassed in the seventeenth and eighteenth centuries, but they left this ancient model largely intact. By the end of the nineteenth century, however, it could be taken for granted no longer. From palatial new laboratories, mechanistic science reigned increasingly triumphant. Living organisms, once models for the entire cosmos, were now themselves modelled on industrial machines. The nervous system functioned like the telegraph, the eye like a photometer.

As the 'century of science' drew to a close, and especially after World War I, various scientists and intellectuals, professionals, and cultural critics pronounced a crisis of scientific confidence. They began to question the achievements of a science that was not just mechanistic but increasingly specialized and fragmented, industrialized and bureaucratic, and to express scepticism, unease, and even horror at its methods. Whilst the scientific factories efficiently probed and shocked, dissected and sliced, crushed and ground bodies into new facts, the most important problems of life, and of living, appeared to cry out for solution in vain. In reaction against 'machine science' holists produced new ways of knowing and healing, approaches that sought to respect rather than take apart and analyze the whole. This holism was a collection of self-consciously defensive or oppositional interventions by a wide variety of people, united — if at all — only by what they were against.

Many of the leading holists were themselves scientists. In answer to the general fragmentation of knowledge about the body, they preached synthesis and interdependence. Opposing the claims of mechanistic reductionism, they asked what kind of science could do justice to the complexity of living organisms and their purposiveness. Relativity and quantum theory were beating the old mechanistic physics on its own ground, they observed; surely it was *passé* still to be modelling animals on locomotives? Some embryologists, for example, followed Hans Driesch in arguing that no machine could compensate for loss of parts in the ways that embryos did. He embraced vitalism, teaching that the development of a harmonious whole embryo was guided by a nonspatial and immaterial 'entelechy' — but other biologists came up with organicist approaches that gave the whole embryo priority over its parts whilst remaining safely within materialist bounds. In academic psychology the Gestalt theorists, Max Wertheimer, Kurt Koffka, and Wolfgang Köhler, claimed that not atomistic sensations but structured wholes are the primary units of mental life. And, like many holists, they were not content to reform scientific theories but also took up the challenge of finding appropriate paths to knowledge in science. Gestalt experimentation in Weimar Germany investigated the variation among perceptions not between but within individual subjects, and so opposed the administrative, classifying style of science embodied in intelligence testing that was becoming dominant in the US. The Gestalt psychologists prided themselves on doing rigorous science, but some holists explored alternative ways of knowing, such as intuition, that to most scientists smacked of the irrational, of the frankly unscientific.

Especially in medicine, holists concentrated on setting acceptable terms for the relations between the new laboratory sciences and their professional practice. Early-twentieth-century medical élites,

for example, cultivated the clinical art as a mark of a gentleman. It would temper the cold precision of scientific medicine — and prevent the physician becoming a mere technician. Against the spectre of specialized and bureaucratic state medicine they defended traditional doctor–patient relationships and a medicine of the whole person. In many ways from the other side but also holistic, the mid-twentieth-century 'social medicine' of Oxford professor John Ryle criticized the dominant anti-bacterial and surgical strategies as narrow and blinkered. The social medicine movement showed the dependence of sickness on the social variables of lifestyle and environment, and called for medicine to move beyond the hospital and the laboratory. More widely, as people confronted the extension of mechanistic science and technology into their lives, many were moved to ask how they could avoid becoming mere cogs in its machines, and to wonder what new insights might re-enchant a world that science appeared to be emptying of meaning.

The political geography of twentieth-century holism was extremely complex. Conservatives and liberals, fascists and communists, feminists and male chauvinists, racists and internationalists were all known to help themselves to holist rhetoric. Variously opposing alienation, atheism, bureaucracy, democracy, free-market capitalism, industrialism, mass culture, and metropolitan life, some holists have sought to defend human individuality as an absolute, whilst others have subsumed individuals into groups, be they classes, nations or — as most notoriously in Nazi Germany — races. Holists have traditionally opposed the treatment of human beings as machines, but historian Jeffrey Herf has shown that in Weimar and Nazi Germany some reactionaries succeeded in reconciling their 'hunger for wholeness' with a cult of technology.

Holism was marginalized after World War II, but since the late 1960s holist approaches have attracted renewed interest. Many holists are outside and opposed to official science and medicine, especially in the alternative health, environmentalist, feminist, animal rights, and New Age movements. But, though generally elusive, much more holism can be found in mainstream science and medicine than their dominant reductionism would suggest. Scientists continue to model bodies on machines, but in the age of digital computers machines can do things of which turn-of-the-century holists never even dreamed. The language of DNA is among the most reductionist ever invented, but the intricacies of gene regulation can warm the cockles of a holist heart. Just as hard-headed reductionists have pragmatically factored in some complexity, so holists have typically had to accept some reductionist means. The very terms are treacherous — but the opposition endures.   NICK HOPWOOD

Further reading

Lawrence, C. and Weisz, G. (ed.) (1998). *Greater than the parts: holism in biomedicine, 1920–1950*. Oxford University Press, New York.

Homeopathy is a system of treatment evolved by a German physician, Samuel Hahnemann (1755–1843). Hahnemann carried out tests on himself with extracts of cinchona bark, which contains quinine, and found it caused fever. From experiments of this kind he formulated the major principle of homeopathy, 'similia similibus curantur' (like cures like) — that is, agents which cause symptoms in a healthy person will cure the same symptoms in a sick person. It is worth considering how such an unlikely hypothesis came to be made, especially when something as essential as a simple clinical thermometer was not available to measure body temperature. Hahnemann's idea is actually very old, with 'the hair of the dog that bit you' hypothesis for treatment going back to the time of Hippocrates. Also, Jenner, who was contemporary with Hahnemann, had shown that cowpox could provide immunity against smallpox, and Hahnemann may have misinterpreted this finding, by failing to realise that vaccination recruits the IMMUNE SYSTEM to achieve its effects.

Hahnemann found that some of the remedies when given in large doses may aggravate the symptoms they were designed to eliminate, and formulated a further principle, that of reducing the doses to minute proportions. It has been suggested that the reason for this was to reduce the likelihood of adverse effects, following litigation by dispensing chemists who feared for their livelihoods. Whatever the reasons, the use of dilute preparations has become part of the methodology of homeopathy. To prepare homeopathic remedies, the medicament is diluted with an *excipient* — usually *lactose* (milk sugar) for solids, or water for liquids — and triturated in a mortar (solids), or *decussed* (shaken) (liquids). Usually 1 part of drug is used to 100 parts of diluent. The resulting mixture is then diluted again as before, the whole process being repeated up to 30 times. It is claimed that the more dilute the preparation the more potent it is.

These unsual claims need further comment. Simple calculations, making use of Avogadro's number, confirm that in the more dilute preparations there is likely to be only one molecule of the medicament in a sphere the size of Saturn. The standard reply of homeopaths to this criticism is either that, in the process of preparation, special energies are released, and retained in the diluent, or that the molecules of the active principle leave their imprints on the diluents. These imprints, which are complementary in shape to the medicament molecules, may be the active moiety, as they counteract the effects caused by the medicament itself. These improbable mechanisms are not supported by any evidence, but if true would mean that most of what is known about the chemistry of molecules would have to be rejected. Homeopathic remedies often have fancy names going back to Hahnemann's time, when much of medicine was obscured by use of dog Latin. For example, some enormous dilution of *Nat. mur.* is a common remedy for a variety of simple complaints even today. *Nat. mur.* is short for natrium muriate, the sodium salt of muriatic acid, commonly known as ordinary salt. Body fluids contain around 150 mM salt, and most foodstuffs contain some salt, so the administration of an odd salt molecule as a form of treatment is surely nonsense.

Homeopaths claim to treat the whole person, so the prescribed treatment will depend on the totality of the person as well as the disease condition. For this reason there have been very few properly constructed clinical trials of homeopathic remedies. There is no scientific basis whatsoever to support homeopathy as a useful form of treatment. Most people get better from most things most of the time, and merely the belief that one is being treated can, through the placebo effect, at least cause the sense of feeling better. But if recovery is coincident with taking a homeopathic remedy then a causative relationship may be claimed, and knowledge of the magical properties passed on to others. Homeopathic remedies continue to be popular, as a result of concerns about side-effects of conventional, allopathic drugs, and patronage from prominent persons. While allopathic remedies require licensing by regulatory bodies, showing both safety and effectiveness, there is no such legislation for homeopathic preparations. The safety of these latter, because of their dilution, is not an issue, but their effectiveness is questionable.

ALAN W. CUTHBERT

Homeostasis

Homeostasis (Greek: staying the same) is a fundamental idea in our understanding of the workings of the body. The concept had its origin in the 1870s, when the French physiologist Claude BERNARD showed that, although the concentration of sugar in the blood could be raised or lowered by a number of processes, the net effect of these processes was to keep the concentration of sugar within certain limits. Bernard extended the idea to other constituents of blood — for which he had less evidence — and in a timeless phrase referred to the constancy of the internal environment ('*le milieu intérieur*'): '*La fixité du milieu intérieur est la condition de la vie libre, independante.*'

Bernard contrasted this constancy with that of the changeable world that surrounded the animal ('*le milieu extérieur*'). He likened the protective function of the internal milieu to that of a greenhouse, though to us this may seem rather an odd analogy. The constitution of the internal milieu (extracellular fluids, including blood and lymph) has been suggested to represent some primal sea in which vertebrates have evolved. It is a likeable hypothesis, but one which is rather difficult to test.

Bernard's proposal attracted little contemporary attention, which was hardly surprising, for it was about 50 years ahead of its time. But during the period 1915–35 two American physiologists, W. B. Cannon (1871–1945) and L. J. Henderson (1878–1942), revived it. Cannon was particularly concerned with demonstrating the importance of the AUTONOMIC NERVOUS SYSTEM in maintaining the constancy of the *milieu intérieur*: he realized that the constancy of BLOOD PRESSURE was an essential part of the maintenance. It was Cannon who actually coined the word 'homeostasis', and in his *Wisdom of the body* (1932) he described how several of the body's systems were involved in homeostatic mechanisms.

Cannon's fellow professor at Harvard, L. J. Henderson, analysed the way in which the body maintained the hydrogen ion concentration of body fluids (usually expressed as pH) within narrow limits. There is a short-term pH homeostasis which is a property of blood itself: a bicarbonate-buffering system. If this is not adequate, the KIDNEYS cope with any larger deviation. Henderson published his findings in a classic work, *Blood: a study in general physiology* (1928). The kidneys are, incidentally, the homeostatic organs *par excellence*: every renal activity is involved in maintaining the internal milieu, whether it is the concentration of ions in blood, blood volume, blood pressure itself, or the excretion of alien substances.

How do the body's systems actually maintain the constancy? The most conspicuous mechanism is generally known as 'negative feedback', illustrated below.

As an example, blood glucose concentration could be the 'regulated variable' in the diagram. The control system for the variable is the hormone INSULIN, whose main action is to accelerate the entry of glucose into many of the cells of the body, thereby lowering its plasma concentration. Insulin is released from cells in the Islets of Langerhans of the pancreas (the controller), the most important stimulus for its release being a rise in blood glucose concentration, as occurs after a meal ('disturbance' in the diagram). The reason for this being a 'negative' feedback system is that the action of insulin, by lowering the blood sugar, tends to remove the stimulus for its own release. Negative feedback is a ubiquitious principle in engineering and electronics.

It is clear from this example that the mechanism does not keep glucose concentration (the regulated variable) at a fixed level. The level oscillates, because there are delays in both arms of the system — it takes a finite time for insulin to lower blood glucose concentrations, and also for elevated glucose concentrations to increase the production of insulin from the pancreas.

Another regulated variable is carbon dioxide. The control of a constant partial pressure of CARBON DIOXIDE (PCO_2) in blood is a very precise feedback loop, and its control system is the act of BREATHING. The body produces the gas constantly, adding it to blood. The CO_2 sensor in this system consists of neurons in the medullary respiratory centre of the brain; the control system consists of motor nerves passing from the brain to the diaphragm and intercostal muscles. These nerves stimulate the act of breathing, which transfers carbon dioxide from blood into the lungs, lowers the blood PCO_2, and temporarily removes the stimulus to the medullary respiratory centre. Because the body is still producing carbon dioxide, the blood PCO_2 begins to rise again, the medullary receptors are stimulated, and the cycle repeats itself. A CO_2-sensitive electrode inserted into an artery shows small, regular oscillations whose frequency corresponds precisely to the act of breathing.

The speed of response of the carbon dioxide loop is far greater than that of the glucose loop, a difference that derives from nervous compared with hormonal mechanisms: the $PCO2$ varies by only about 10% around its average level, whereas glucose varies by about 40%. The concentration ranges of some other constituents of blood provide us with clues about the nature of the relevant homeostatic mechanisms. Sodium ions (135–145 mmol/litre) and chloride ions (95–105 mmol/litre) have narrow ranges; this is the result of a mixture of nervous and hormonal mechanisms; the range is wider for potassium (3.5–5.0 mmol/litre) which is adjusted by hormonal action in the kidneys. By contrast, the hormones that provide the control systems regulating these variables show far wider concentration ranges in blood, according to the changes in secretion rates stimulated by disturbances in the variable they control. Thus ACTH (adrenocorticotrophic hormone) has a range of 3.3–15.4 pmol/litre, aldosterone 100–500 pmol/litre, and insulin 0–15 mUnits/ml (unfed) and 15–100 Units/ml (after food).

Homeostasis can itself be reset or entrained by higher nervous centres. The diurnal variations shown by ACTH and cortisol demonstrate high concentrations between midnight and midday (cortisol concentration 280–700 mmol/litre) and midday and midnight (cortisol 140–280 mmol/litre). Similarly, on a longer time-scale, the

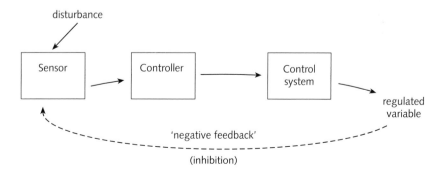

changes seen in the female reproductive cycle represent a 28-day cycle of entrainment. On a longer time-scale still, the growth and development of the child must represent the ultimate homeostatic entrainment by the brain. We might envisage old age as representing a genetically programmed deterioration of homeostasis.

Claude Bernard's intuition about 'le milieu intérieur' has come a very long way in a century. The mechanisms of homeostasis are so ubiquitous, their patterns so subtly intertwined, that we are tempted to produce a teleological question, and ask why. What *is* so useful to the organism about this precision? We do not have to look far, because the workings of every cell in the body depend on the maintenance of a negative potential inside the cell. In turn, this negative potential depends upon the relative concentrations of ions inside and outside the cell: a high sodium concentration in the extracellular fluid, and a high potassium concentration inside the cell, the gradients across the cell wall being maintained by ionic pumps within the CELL MEMBRANE. But these pumps could not begin to control this gradient if the ionic concentrations in blood (extracellular fluid) were not kept within narrow limits in the first place. The subject comes into sharp focus when we consider the situation in the heart, which is very dependent on a constant plasma potassium level, within the range of 3.5–5.0 mmol/litre. The elevation of this value by 1–2 mmol/litre constitutes a medical emergency: the excitable components of the heart begin to conduct nervous impulses spontaneously and, without treatment, death soon follows from uncoordinated contraction of different parts of the ventricles (*ventricular fibrillation*).

It soon becomes clear that the body's function involves countless homeostatic mechanisms, both within and outside cells. Not only are the mechanisms ubiquitous, but careful analysis often shows two or more feedback loops apparently serving the same function; a good example is the elaborate relationship that exists between the control of blood pressure and plasma volume. Perhaps the apparent redundancy provides the organism with back-up systems that improve evolutionary survival value. Improvement or not, such duplication makes the understanding of disease processes very much more difficult to disentangle. J. R. HENDERSON

See also ACID–BASE HOMEOSTASIS; BODY FLUIDS; HORMONES.

Homo sapiens
The species to which all living humans belong. The Latin meaning, 'wise man' reflects the greater endowment of the brain power compared to his predecessors. The species is defined in terms of anatomy, and the first member of the species is recognized from about 150 000 years ago. Compared to other members of the family Hominidae (all members of the human lineage since the divergence from the common ancestors with chimpanzees about 5 million years ago) and the genus Homo (larger brained hominids that appeared about 2 million

years ago), the species is characterized by a higher and more vertical forehead, a round and gracile cranium, small face and teeth, a prominent chin, and a more slender and elongated post-cranial skeleton. Early forms of Homo sapiens co-existed in some parts of the world with other hominid species such as Homo neanderthalensis until about 26 000 years ago. Although members of Homo sapiens may vary around the world, the species cannot be clearly divided into sub-species or races, and all living humans can inter-breed with each other and produce fertile offspring — hence their designation as a single species. ROBERT FOLEY

See also EVOLUTION, HUMAN; NEANDERTHALS; SKELETON; SKULL.

Hormone replacement therapy
Ovarian function starts to decline from as early as the twentieth week of embryological life, with oestrogen production falling to a critical level during a period known as the 'climacteric'.

De Gardanne (1816) coined the term 'La Menespausie' from the Greek *men* (month) and *pausis* (cessation). The MENOPAUSE is normally diagnosed when a woman has not had a period for 12 months. Aristotle (384–22 BC) recognized that MENSTRUATION normally stopped around the age of 40 years but that some women could continue with their periods until their fiftieth year. In the seventeenth century less than a third of women lived to experience the menopause. However, the increase in life expectancy in the twentieth century has meant that most women will spend a third of their adult lives in the post-menopausal years.

The menopause, now occurring on average at 51 years in developed countries, is associated not only with a cessation of menstrual periods but also a wide range of symptomatic and physiological effects. These include hot flushes, night sweats, loss of energy, urogenital atrophy, OSTEOPOROSIS, and ischaemic heart disease. A number of non-hormonal remedies have been used to treat menopausal problems, with varying degrees of success. GALEN (AD 129–216) advised phlebotomy so that any 'retained poisons' could be released; the use of purgatives and the application of leeches was popular in the sixteenth century. In 1777 John Leake recommended

'where the patient is delicate and subject to female weakness, night sweats or an habitual purging, with flushing in the face and a hectic fever: for such; ass's milk, jellies and raw eggs, with cooling fruits. At meals she may be indulged with half a pint of old, clear London porter, or a glass of Rhenish wine.'

Brown–Sequard (1889) is credited with pioneering the concept of hormone replacement therapy (HRT). He reported the rejuvenating effects of injections of testicular extracts, and postulated that ovarian extract would have the same effect. Two years later Murray developed the first effective form of HRT when he administered oral thyroid gland to treat myxoedema. The first three clinical trials of dried or fresh ovarian tissue to treat climateric symptoms were

published in 1896, and in 1912 Adler produced the changes of oestrus by injecting watery extracts of ovary into virgin animals. However, it was not until 1923 that Allen and Doisy isolated the ovarian hormone OESTROGEN. The first commercial preparations of HRT were based on the work of Zondek and Laquer and became available in 1926. Premarin, derived from pregnant mares' urine, was introduced in 1943 and is probably still the most widely used preparation. The publication of *Feminine Forever* in 1966 brought HRT to the attention of the public, with many demanding that it should be a NHS benefit. General practitioners were initially divided, with some prescribing it enthusiastically and others being completely dismissive.

The three natural oestrogens in women are oestrone (E1), 17-beta-oestradiol (E2), and estriol (E3). Free oestrogens are lipophilic and freely transverse CELL MEMBRANES, exerting their metabolic effect by binding to nuclear receptors. This stimulates the production of mRNA and hence protein production. E2, the most active oestrogen, because it binds to the receptor complex for the longest time, is found mainly before the menopause, as its serum concentration falls when ovarian follicular development ceases. E1 is the main postmenopausal oestrogen and is produced by conversion of adrenal androgens in peripheral fat. Oestrogens are conjugated in the liver and excreted in the urine or bile.

HRT can be administered orally, transvaginally, as an implant, or through the skin as a percutaneous cream, gel, or patch. There is clear evidence that it is effective in reducing the vasomotor symptoms of the menopause and enhances the quality of life. Skin, hair, and mood are also improved. Atrophy of the lower urogenital tract can be treated effectively with HRT, with many women finding a vaginal cream or oestrogen-releasing ring helpful. HRT is used for prophylaxis against a number of conditions as well as for treatment. The years immediately following the menopause are associated with an increase in bone loss, and by the age of 70 a woman may have lost 10–30% of her bone mass. HRT delays this period of accelerated loss: five years of treatment can halve the risk of osteoporotic fractures. This may be particularly important in thin women who smoke, take little EXERCISE, and have a family history of osteoporosis, as they are particularly at risk of this problem. The increased risk of cardiovascular disease after the menopause is also reduced, presumably because of the favourable effect of oestrogens on lipids and blood flow in the coronary arteries.

The main side-effect of HRT is vaginal bleeding in those women who still have a uterus. Unopposed oestrogen therapy leads to an increased risk of endometrial carcinoma (cancer of the lining of the uterus), so progestogen therapy needs to be given for at least 12 days each month, inducing a regular withdrawal bleed. However, recently the use of Tibolone, a synthetic compound which combines oestrogenic and progestogenic activity with weak androgenic properties, and other continuous preparations have helped to overcome this problem. There is also a slightly increased incidence of breast carcinoma for those women who take HRT for more than 10 years, but the beneficial effects in terms of a reduction in deaths from osteoporotic fractures and heart disease far outweigh the potential risks. HRT can therefore be given indefinitely.

LINDA CARDOZO

Further reading
Wilson R. A. (1966). *Feminine forever*. Mayflower-Dell, London.

See also BONE; MENOPAUSE; OSTEOPOROSIS; SEX HORMONES.

Hormones
Despite the advent of e-mail the majority of people still communicate by letter or telephone. Similarly there are two ways in which messages are sent round the body. The first is via the NERVOUS SYSTEM, which like the phone system is 'hard wired' and usually operates on a point to point basis. The second way is by means of hormones — chemical messengers — circulating in the blood, which effectively acts as a postal system. Just as, when someone sends out a circular in the mail, those who are interested act on the information and those who are not discard the letter, so when an *endocrine gland* secretes a hormone the appropriate cells respond while the rest are unaffected. Classically, hormones are defined as chemical substances secreted directly into the bloodstream that act on a distant target organ or type of cell.

Historical background
Diseases resulting from lack of a hormone (such as *diabetes mellitus*), or excess production (such as *thyrotoxicosis*), have been known for centuries, although the cause was not recognized. A nineteenth-century anatomist called Henle, after whom a section of the renal tubules was named, was the first person to describe glands without ducts that secreted their products directly into the bloodstream. Then in 1855 the Frenchman, Claude BERNARD, who laid the foundations of physiology, distinguished the products of these so-called ductless glands from those glandular secretions, such as saliva and sweat, which are effectively outside the body, by calling them 'internal secretions': hence the name 'endocrine' (*endon*: Greek for within) as opposed to 'exocrine' secretion (*ex*: Greek for outside).

The first person who tried to use extracts of endocrine glands for therapeutic purposes was Brown–Sequard, a French physician, neurologist, and endocrinologist, who in 1889 employed testicular extracts from animals to treat male ageing. A few years later, in 1902, Bayliss and Starling, working in University College London, prepared an extract from the duodenum which stimulated secretion of pancreatic digestive juices when it was injected into the bloodstream. They called the product 'secretin', and coined the term 'hormone', meaning 'to excite' or 'to set in

motion'. Since then a wide variety of hormones have been identified. The steps in identifying whether a given gland or tissue has an endocrine function are first to demonstrate changes on its removal and then to demonstrate reversal of those changes, either when the gland is reimplanted at any site where it can link up with a blood supply, or when an extract of the gland is injected into the blood. The active principle can then be isolated, purified, and the chemical structure characterized. Ways of measuring the identified hormone (*assays*) can be established, and finally one can confirm that venous blood leaving the gland has a higher concentration of the hormone than the arterial blood entering it.

The role of hormones
The major endocrine glands are the PITUITARY, the THYROID, the four PARATHYROIDS, the PANCREAS, the two ADRENALS, and the paired TESTES or OVARIES (See Plate 7). Hormones are also produced by organs or tissues whose function is not primarily an endocrine one: the digestive tract, the heart, and the kidneys all produce hormones. Even nerve cells produce them. For example, the hormones controlling secretion from the anterior lobe of the pituitary gland are synthesized in the HYPOTHALAMUS, but they are released into the local blood supply to the anterior pituitary, rather than entering the general circulation. These cells are said to have a neuro-endocrine function. Furthermore, it is now recognized that hormones need not even be released into blood vessels. The hormonal products of some nerve cells stimulate adjacent neurones and thus act as neuromodulators, while in the digestive tract hormones act on surrounding cells and are said to have a paracrine function (*para*: Greek for beside). Finally, some hormones, such as growth factors, can act on the originating cell itself; in this case they are described as exhibiting autocrine control. The classical definition has therefore been extended to include chemical messengers which are secreted by certain cells, and which reach and act upon cells which are receptive to them, whether local or distant.

Chemical nature of hormones
Chemically, most hormones belong to one of three major groups: PROTEINS and PEPTIDES, STEROIDS (fat-soluble molecules whose basic structure is a skeleton of four carbon rings), or derivatives of the AMINO ACID tyrosine, characterized by a 6-carbon, or benzene, ring. There are some hormones, such as melatonin from the PINEAL gland and the locally acting PROSTAGLANDINS, which cannot be included in any of these groups, but may share a number of their characteristics. The glands which produce protein and peptide hormones are the pituitary, certain cells of the thyroid, the parathyroids, and the pancreas. Steroids are produced by the cortex or outer layer of the adrenal gland and by the ovaries and testes. The tyrosine derivatives are the thyroid hormones, and the CATECHOLAMINES (adrenaline and noradrenaline) which are produced in the medulla of the adrenal glands.

Knowledge of the chemical nature of a hormone is important as it enables one to predict how the hormone is produced, how rapidly it can be released in response to a stimulus, in what form it circulates in the blood, how it acts, the time course of its effect, and the route of administration therapeutically.

Hormone synthesis and secretion
The mechanisms underlying the synthesis of *protein and peptide hormones*, such as GROWTH HORMONE and INSULIN, are just the same as the synthesis of any other protein, involving transcription of the gene and translation of a messenger RNA (mRNA). Generally the mRNA contains the code for a longer peptide than the normal form of the hormone. These extended forms are called pro-hormones and there may even be pre-pro-hormones, as for example pre-pro-insulin. The active hormone is cleaved from these molecules. The pro-hormone is stored in secretory granules, then released by a process of *exocytosis*, — the membrane of the storage granule fuses with the plasma membrane, which in turn parts, allowing the contents of the granule to be discharged.

Steroid hormones, such as cortisol and the sex hormones, are all synthesized from CHOLESTEROL, with a variety of enzymes mediating the transformations into the different products. Since they are fat soluble, and therefore readily cross membranes, they cannot be stored, but are synthesized as needed. Their release is therefore slower than that of peptide hormones.

The thyroid hormones are formed as part of a large protein, thyroglobulin, which can be stored, while the catecholamines are synthesized by a multi-enzyme process and are also stored in granules.

Neither the steroid hormones nor the thyroid hormones are readily soluble in water, and they circulate in the plasma in association with proteins. The importance of this is that the compound molecules are too large to be filtered out of the blood in the kidney and so are not lost in the urine, which is one of the reasons why they remain in the plasma for days. Peptide hormones, by contrast, disappear within an hour or so, because they are both broken down in plasma and tissues and also lost in the urine. Protein and peptide hormones have therefore to be administered more frequently if used therapeutically, although longer acting preparations are available. Another problem with the administration of these hormones is the fact that they cannot be given by mouth as they would be broken down in the digestive tract. This presents particular problems for diabetics, who have regularly to inject themselves, whereas people with thyroid hormone deficiency only have to take pills.

Hormone action
The chemical nature of the hormone also affects the mechanism of action. All hormones act on cells by way of their 'receptors'. Each hormone has its own receptor to which it binds, matching rather like a lock and key. This is why hormones

circulating throughout the body in the blood may leave capillaries to enter the extracellular fluid of many tissues, but act only on those cells which possess the appropriate receptor. Proteins and peptides cannot enter the cell and so act via cell MEMBRANE RECEPTORS, producing their effects by 'second messengers', which are activated in the cell as soon as the hormone binds to the receptor. Thus peptide hormones can produce quite rapid responses. Steroid and thyroid hormones, by contrast, can enter the cell and bind to intracellular receptors, producing their effects by stimulating the production of new proteins. There is therefore a relatively long lag period before the response to these hormones is seen.

Hormones produce a variety of responses throughout the body and may be grouped according to their actions, although there is overlap between the groups.

First there are the metabolic hormones which control the digestion of food, its storage and use. Such hormones include those produced by the digestive tract, which control secretion of digestive juices and activity of the muscle in the wall of the tract; also the hormones which regulate blood glucose, namely insulin, (which lowers it), and glucagon, growth hormone, the thyroid hormones, and cortisol, which all raise it.

Second are the hormones which regulate the composition of the blood, and hence of all the BODY FLUIDS. Excluding those that regulate the glucose content, these are: *aldosterone* and *atrial natriuretic hormone* (produced in the heart), which control the amount of sodium in the blood; vasopressin or antidiuretic hormone, which controls the amount of water; parathyroid hormone and vitamin D, which raise blood calcium; and calcitonin, which lowers blood calcium. It is perhaps surprising to learn that a vitamin can also be a hormone, but it is similar in many ways to the steroid hormones, and the active form is produced in one part of the body for action an another. The vitamin D taken in the diet or formed in the skin under the action of UV light is not the active form: this is produced after modification takes place first in the liver and then the kidney.

Next are the STRESS hormones, primarily adrenaline and noradrenaline, which are under the control of the AUTONOMIC NERVOUS SYSTEM: cortisol and a number of the pituitary hormones are also involved in the response to stress.

A further group are those responsible for growth, development, and reproduction. These include growth hormone itself, and the hormones controlling ovarian and testicular function (luteinising hormone, LH, and follicular stimulating hormone, FSH) — all of which come from the pituitary — and the hypothalamic hormones, which in turn control these pituitary secretions. Included also are the steroid hormones, produced by the ovaries (oestrogens and progesterone) and testes (testosterone), and those hormones involved in birth and lactation, chiefly OXYTOCIN and prolactin.

The final major group includes those hormones that control other endocrine systems, and therefore interact with the other groups. The

Principal hormones

Site of release	Name of hormone	Main 'targets'	Involved in regulation of:	Main mechanisms regulating secretion	Chemical nature
Anterior pituitary	Growth hormone	Most tissues	Growth and metabolism	Hypothalamic releasing or inhibiting hormones; negative feedback from levels of the relevant hormones in the blood.	
	Prolactin	Mammary glands	Milk production		
	Trophins: TSH	Thyroid gland	Thyroid hormone secretion		
	ACTH	Adrenal cortex	Cortisol secretion		
	FSH	Gonads	Germ cell maturation		
	LH		Gonad hormone secretion		
Posterior pituitary	Antidiuretic hormone (ADH)	Kidneys	Osmolality and volume of the blood	Hypothalamic osmoreceptors	
	= Vasopressin	Blood vessels			
	Oxytocin	Uterus, breasts	Labour and lactation	Reflex via hypothalamus	
Atrial wall	Atrial natriuretic hormone (ANH)	Kidneys	Osmolality and volume of the blood	State of stretch of the atria of the heart.	Proteins
Pancreas	Insulin	Most tissues	Blood level, storage, and cellular uptake of glucose.	Blood glucose level Sympathetic nervous system.	and
	Glucagon	Liver	Release of glucose		peptides
Gut	Gastrin	Gut, liver, gall bladder, pancreas: smooth muscle and secretory tissue.	Gastro-intestinal function: motility, digestion, absorption	Chemical and mechanical factors in the alimentary canal.	
	Secretin				
	Cholecystokinin				
	Vasoactive intestinal peptide and others				
Parathyroids	Parathormone	Bone, kidneys, gut	Blood Ca^{2+} via calcium and phosphate absorption, secretion, and turnover in bone	Negative feedback from concentration of Ca^{2+} in the blood.	
Thyroid	Calcitonin				
	Thyroxine (T_4) Triiodothyronine (T_3)	Most tissues	Cellular oxidative metabolism	TSH from anterior pituitary; negative feedback from blood hormone level.	Amino acids (iodinated)
Gonads testis	Testoterone	Genitalia and many other tissues	Reproductive function and sex characteristics	FSH and LH from anterior pituitary; negative feedback from blood hormone level.	
ovary	Oestrogens Progesterone	Uterus, breasts and many other tissues	Menstrual cycle; early pregnancy; lactation. (Placenta takes over secretion during pregnancy.)		Steroids
Adrenal cortex	Cortisol	Most tissues	Metabolism: response to stress	ACTH from anterior pituitary.	
	Aldosterone	Kidneys	Volume of body fluids, via salt concentration	Renin-angiotensin; blood levels of Na^+ and K^+	
Adrenal medulla	Adrenaline Noradrenaline	Heart, smooth muscle, glands	Cardiovascular and metabolic adjustments to activity and stress	Sympathetic nervous system	Catecholamines

pituitary hormones *adrenocorticotrophic hormone* (ACTH), *thyroid stimulating hormone* (TSH), and the gonadotrophic hormones LH and FSH control the release of some of the metabolic and stress hormones and of the reproductive hormones, whilst hypothalamic hormones in turn control pituitary function.

Regulation of hormone release

The commonest form of control in biological systems is *negative feedback*, and this forms the basis for the control of hormone release. In this type of feedback loop any perturbation of the controlled variable results in a response to return it to the pre-determined level. An example of this is the control of blood sugar concentrations. A rise in blood glucose (after a sugary drink or food) acts on the pancreas to stimulate insulin secretion, which in turn lowers blood glucose by storing it away inside cells.

A more complex system is seen in the control of pituitary hormone secretion. For hormones which control secretion from a target gland, there is simple negative feedback, with the target organ secretion inhibiting pituitary hormone release (for example, the secretion of thyroid-stimulating hormone is inhibited by a rise in circulating thyroid hormone). However there is also control from the hypothalamus via stimulating and inhibiting hormones. The hypothalamus receives a huge array of inputs originating both in the body and in the external environment, so that by this route a large variety of factors influence the output of the pituitary gland, and hence the other endocrine glands, which it in turn controls.

Endocrine disorders

In a such a complex regulatory system, one would predict that disordered function would have significant consequences. The most common endocrine disorder is diabetes mellitus, with disorders of thyroid function coming second. Endocrine disorders may stem from over- or undersecretion of a given hormone. Oversecretion may be due to a tumour either in the tissue normally producing the hormone or in one growing in an abnormal location — for example in the lung. It may alternatively be due to inappropriate secretion from the whole gland. There is, for example, an autoimmune disease of the thyroid: thyrotoxicosis or 'Grave's disease', in which antibodies stimulate the gland to oversecretion. Apparent underactivity of an endocrine gland may in fact be due to a failure of the target tissues to respond to a particular hormone. For example, those who develop diabetes later in life may have an elevated rather than a low concentration of insulin in the blood. This is because their tissues are relatively unresponsive to the hormone. There may even be failure to convert a hormone to its more active form. In the male some tissues are responsive to dihydrotestosterone rather than testosterone itself, and so a deficiency of the enzyme catalyzing this conversion produces the appearance of testosterone deficiency.

Most endocrine disorders can now be successfully treated. Diagnosis and treatment, however, require accurate measurement of blood hormone concentrations. Early assays were bioassays performed on animal tissue, and these are still used in checking the activity of hormone preparations made for medicinal purposes. However, routine determination in blood now involves the technique of *radioimmunoassay*; when care is taken in setting this up, even very low concentrations of hormone can be determined quite rapidly on a large number of samples.

So the days are past when diabetes mellitus led inexorably to coma and death; when a mother might decline with a mysterious illness after giving birth because of post-partum pituitary degeneration; or when a young woman could 'burn out' with thyrotoxicosis — to name but a few of the endocrine disorders which could be seriously debilitating or fatal before the twentieth century.   MARY L. FORSLING

Further reading

Rubenstein, E. (1980). Diseases caused by impaired communication among cells, *Scientific American*, March, 78–87.

Snyder, S. H. (1985). The molecular basis of communication between cells, *Scientific American*, October, 114–23.

See PLATE 7.

See also ADRENAL GLAND; GLANDS; HYPOTHALAMUS; INSULIN; PEPTIDES; PITUITARY GLAND; SEX HORMONES; STEROIDS; THYROID GLAND; WATER BALANCE.

Host

The host is the consecrated bread of the Eucharist; its Latin root, '*hostia*', meaning a sacrificial victim, suggests a theological understanding of the Eucharist as the sacrifice of the Body of Christ.

In the later Middle Ages, especially the twelfth century, the notion that the host is the body of Christ, developed in the doctrine of transubstantiation and expressed particularly in the establishment of Corpus Christ as a feast day, led to many rules and rituals to ensure the host was made and treated with proper respect. Human handling of the host meant that the threat of disrespect was always present. The bread was to be made of wheat because Christ compared himself to a grain of wheat; it should be whole and form a full circle, white, thin, and be inscribed with a cross, the letters IHS, or even (from the twelfth century) a crucifixion scene or lamb of God. This eucharistic bread was baked in appropriately reverent circumstances in religious houses.

Because the host was understood to be the body of Christ, it was important that no part of it be wasted, and so, in England especially, special 'houselling cloths' were used to catch crumbs dropping out of the mouths of lay communicants. Similarly, the consecrated host was to be kept in a fitting manner, in a *pyx*, a small box made of silver or ivory which could be locked. If the sacrament was to be reserved it was put in the pyx, which was usually draped with a cloth, and

hung over the altar or kept in a small cupboard in the north wall of the chancel. Taking communion to the sick, which meant taking the host out of the safety of the church, led in some places to elaborate processions every time the host was taken outdoors, and members of the laity were exhorted to join that procession by the ringing of bells, and to engage in reverential behaviour similar to their pious practices at the elevation of the host. The reception of the host by the sick person was also a cause of anxiety for the priest, for the sick person might have difficulty receiving the host. If the person had difficulty swallowing, the host was to be dissolved in the wine for them, and if the host was vomited back up by the sick person, it was to be crumbled in the wine and consumed by the priest.

It became the custom in the later Middle Ages that the laity should receive only the bread, not the wine (which was received only by the priest) and that they should receive communion infrequently: the fifth Lateran Council of 1215 established the principle that the laity should receive at least once a year, usually at Easter. The priest's role — as mediator of grace in the sacraments — was central, and his celebration and reception of the Eucharist every day was understood to be done on behalf of all Christians; his frequent communion was used as an argument for infrequent reception by the laity. His bodily gestures at the altar in presiding at the Eucharist, especially in consecrating the bread and wine, were important. The gesture of elevating the host signified the moment of consecration and thus for showing Christ's body to those watching. This central ritualistic moment appealed to all the senses: bells were rung, incense burnt, and candles lit, so that the layperson would see the elevation of the body of Christ, would bow in reverence, and be appropriately prayerful. In some places, the laity would rush towards the altar, at the moment of the elevation of the host, and in some towns, enthusiastic lay persons would go from church to church in order to witness the elevation of the host in as many places as possible in one day.

The host played an important part in the spirituality of some women religious, such as Hadewijch, Catherine of Genoa, and Catherine of Sienna, in the late Middle Ages: they fasted, surviving only on the consecrated host, thereby feeding only on the body of Christ. This use of the host indicates the strong connection between the (female) body and food, and an attempt by women to orient their spiritual practices and thereby gain access to spiritual power through that which was readily available to them as women — namely, food.

At the Reformation, the Protestant reformers gave both the bread and wine to the laity, and, in their rejection of the doctrine of *transubstantiation*, made the Eucharist a simple meal — the Lord's supper — rather than an elaborate ritual. Thus they abandoned the late medieval devotion to the host, and all the practices which had surrounded it.

The Roman Catholic Church has retained some of these practices, and the high Anglican ritualists of nineteenth-century England revived many of them in the Church of England (and they have consequently spread to other parts of the Anglican communion where Anglo-Catholicism has been influential). The Eastern Orthodox churches have always held the view that eating the Eucharist is a physical act which transforms and sanctifies the body. In the twentieth century, some Christians in non-Western parts of the world asked whether the host had always to be bread, especially if bread was a food not indigenous to their culture, and therefore whether they might use a local food such as rice instead. This raises interesting questions about the relationship between Christianity and culture; on the whole, Western Christians have not responded positively to such questions, and at the end of the twentieth century, Rome drew up guidelines making it clear that the host should be a certain kind of bread. JANE SHAW

Further reading

Rubin, M. (1991). *Corpus Christi. The Eucharist in late medieval culture.* Cambridge University Press.

See also CHRISTIANITY AND THE BODY; EUCHARIST.

Hottentot apron In 1815, French anatomist Georges Cuvier declared, 'there is nothing more celebrated in natural history than the Hottentot apron, and at the same time there is nothing which has been the object of such great argumentation.' The subject of speculation throughout Europe since the seventeenth century, the Hottentot apron has gone by many names: *tablier* and *joyeau* in French, *sinus pudoris* and *macronympha* in Latin, and in English, 'drape of decency' or 'curtain of shame'. These terms refer to the extended inner lips of the vagina, or *labia minora*, which can hang down several inches below the vagina, giving the impression of a flap of skin covering the genitalia. No longer recognized as an ethnic group, the Hottentots inhabited the southern tip of Africa, around the Cape of Good Hope, and were probably related to the Khoikhoi or Khoi-San of today. Though usually ascribed to Hottentots and Bushwomen, the apron can be found in several places in Africa.

The occasion of Cuvier's statement quoted above was the dissection of a woman widely known as the Hottentot Venus. We do not know her original name, but she was called Saartjie Baartman in Dutch and christened Sarah Bartmann in English. In 1810 her Dutch master brought her to Europe for his, and allegedly her, profit. An anatomical curiosity, she was to display to scientific and popular audiences her 'racial characteristics'. These were believed to be intimately and inseparably linked to her sexual characteristics and included not only the shape of her face, colour of her skin (which was described as yellowish, not black), and texture of her hair, but also her protruding buttocks and her genitalia. For centuries it had been reported that women from the southern tip of Africa had a special piece of skin which hung between their legs and covered their genitalia. The fact that Hottentot women reportedly also wore a 'flap of skin', i.e. a piece of animal hide, over their genitalia often made eyewitness accounts ambiguous, further confusing the question of whether the Hottentot apron existed at all. Thus, with the publication of his autopsy results in 1817, Cuvier was able to confirm that it did indeed exist and was not a unique anatomical structure, but rather an (over) development of the labia minora. It was, he claimed, 'an extraordinary appendage which nature had made a special attribute of her race'.

During the late eighteenth and nineteenth century, the Hottentot apron played a role in theories about race, SEXUALITY, and culture which were grounded in studies of comparative anatomy conducted by Cuvier, Henri de Blainville, and Geoffroy Saint–Hilaire, among others. Racial theorists linked moral and cultural status with biology, believing that signs of intelligence and sensibility were evidenced in physiology. At a time when crania were measured as an indication of intelligence, the Hottentot apron was analogously regarded as evidence of both bestiality and lasciviousness. Facilitating the dehumanization of native populations, theories of race in part justified nineteenth-century European imperial policies: the greater the physical differences between white Europeans and the 'lower' races, the less human they were. Enlarged genitalia could only be the product of a depraved culture with 'filthy habits', or, conversely, a retarded biology — each was indicative of the other: on the supposed Great Chain of Being, Hottentots were ranked below other Africans, occupying a liminal position between humankind and apes.

It is not coincidental that the Hottentot apron as a defining (and damning) racial trait was part of African female sexual anatomy. Recent scholarship has examined how, during the nineteenth century, the black female, and in particular the Hottentot, came to symbolize that which was primitive, animal, and sexual, the antithesis of 'civilized' Europe. The supposedly over-sexed African, and especially the female, was pathologized, functioning as the 'abnormal' against which to define (white European) 'normal' sexuality. The eminent French naturalist Georges Buffon, for instance, compared black female sexuality with that of the ape. The Hottentot apron became considered an 'abnormality' characteristic of bestial sexuality.

The origin of the Hottentot apron occupied European scholars into the twentieth century. According to Dutch ethnographer Sture Lagercrantz, as late as 1937 there was still no consensus as to whether the Hottentot apron should be regarded as a racial characteristic or cultural attribute. Labia stretching as part of a girl's passage into womanhood and sexual maturity is now known to be practiced in various cultures throughout Africa. SARAH GOODFELLOW

Further reading

Fausto–Sterling, A. (1995). Gender, race, and nation: the comparative anatomy of 'Hottentot' women in Europe, 1815–1817. *Deviant bodies.* Indiana University Press, Bloomington.

Gilman, S. (1985). Black bodies, white bodies: toward an iconography of female sexuality in late nineteenth-century art, medicine and literature. *Critical Inquiry,* **12**, 204–42.

Schiebinger, L. (1993). *Nature's body.* Beacon Press, Boston.

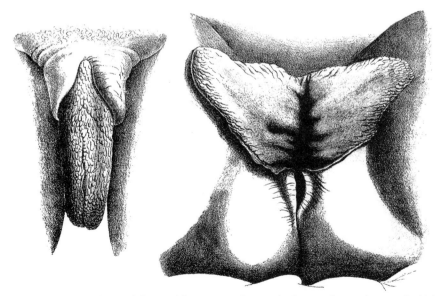

Hottentot apron, natural size. Left figure: adult woman standing upright, the apron hanging between the thighs. Right figure: adult woman lying on her back, the apron spread out to the sides. (Billroth, *Frauenkrankheiten,* Vol. 3.)

Humanism was an intellectual and cultural movement based on the recovery, interpretation, and imitation of Greek and Roman antiquity. It began in the fourteenth century and continued to flourish until the seventeenth, making an impact not only on scholarship but also on literature, art, and science. A variety of different attitudes towards the body can be found in the writings of humanists. What all these views have in common, however, is that they derive from the study of the classical past.

Many humanists were teachers, and in their pedagogical theory and practice they devoted attention to physical development as well as to intellectual formation. *The Education of Boys* (1450), for example, by Enea Silvio Piccolomini (1405–64), later to become Pope Pius II, is divided into two parts: the first concerned with the body, the second with the mind. Piccolomini stressed the necessity of developing a sturdy physique by avoiding feather beds, silk clothing, and other luxurious items which encouraged softness and effeminacy. Youths were advised to obey Plato's dictum, as recounted by St Basil, that the body should be indulged with food and drink only to the extent that it was of service to philosophy. Relying on the Roman rhetorician Quintilian and the Greek moralist Plutarch (to whom an influential pedagogical treatise was falsely attributed), Piccolomini counselled against *corporal punishment*, 'since boys must be led to virtue by rational arguments, and admonitions, not by wounds and blows'. He was nevertheless a keen advocate of energetic physical training and martial exercises, as practised by the ancient Spartans and described by the Roman military theorist Vegetius, since these helped to develop a strong and vigorous body, which his noble and princely students would need for future exploits in battle.

In addition to the pedagogical value of *physical exercise*, humanists took an interest in its health-giving benefits. The physician Hieronymus Mercurialis (1530–1606) drew on an enormous range of Greek and Latin texts in his *Six Books on the Gymnastic Art, Famous among the Ancients but Unknown in Our Times* (1559). Although Mercurialis wanted to revive this lost art, he recommended exercising only in the morning and taking a nap in the afternoon, because man's physical constitution had weakened considerably since antiquity on account of changed eating habits and daily routines.

For the French medical humanist Jacobus Sylvius (1478–1555), the difference between ancient and modern bodies was more than a matter of physical condition. A passionate defender of Galen, Sylvius argued that where the Greek physician's anatomical descriptions differed from those of his critic Andreas Vesalius (1514–64), which were based on dissection, it was due to the fact that the massive Roman frame had degenerated over the centuries into the puny body of contemporary man. Despite such cases of misguided devotion to antiquity, the philological study of Greek medical works,

many newly available in print in the Aldine editions of Galen (1525) and Hippocrates (1526), contributed in no small measure to the increasing knowledge of human *anatomy* in the first half of the sixteenth century.

Humanists also gained knowledge of the body through their study of Greek and Latin tracts on *physiognomy*, which taught them to infer mental and moral characteristics from corporeal signs. In *On Good Manners for Boys* (1530), Erasmus (*c.* 1469–1536) maintained that a smooth brow indicated a good conscience and that a well-ordered mind would reveal itself through calm, steady eyes. In addition, he showed how to decode *body language*: crossing one's legs when sitting was a sign of uneasiness, while standing with one's legs wide apart was the hallmark of a braggart. Among the bodily habits for which Erasmus laid down behavioural guidelines were spitting, nose-wiping, and answering the call of nature (to be done in private, but even so with modesty and decency, 'for the angels are always near').

Another ancient source from which humanists took ideas about the body was Greek *philosophy*. Marsilio Ficino (1433–99) translated all of Plato's dialogues into Latin, thus making generally available the Platonic belief that the body occupied the lowest level of reality, that it was the prison of the soul, and that the truly wise man would attempt to escape its material confines through contemplation of immaterial ideas, such as Truth and Beauty. From Epicurus, on the other hand, humanists such as Thomas More (1478–1535) learned to appreciate the value of *corporeal pleasures*. In his *Utopia* (1516) More imagined an ideal society, whose entirely rational inhabitants had a high regard for the stable and calm pleasures which derive from health, beauty, and strength, and even took unashamed delight in those which come by way of the senses.

A popular humanist genre was the praise of mankind, which usually included sections on both the body and the soul. The first book, for instance, of *On Man's Dignity and Excellence* (1452), by Giannozzo Manetti (1396–1459), is a hymn to the beauty, utility, and divine craftsmanship of the human body. Quoting long passages of Cicero's *On the Nature of the Gods* and Lactantius's *On the Handiwork of God*, Manetti lovingly describes each organ and limb, noting how man's erect posture, unique among all living beings, allows him to observe and contemplate the heavens; and how the placement of his eyes, ears and nose 'in the citadel of the head' is marvellously adapted to *sense perception*, while nevertheless keeping these delicate organs far away from the bodily equivalent of drains, which, as in the best-designed houses, are relegated to the rear.

Humanists uncovered a more inspiring parallel between buildings and the human body in the architectural treatise of the Roman author Vitruvius. He compared the symmetry of a temple to that of a well-proportioned man, who, with extended hands and feet, fits exactly into both a circle and a square, the two most perfect

geometrical figures. The famous drawing of 'Vitruvian man' (Venice, Accademia) by Leonardo da Vinci (1452–1519) is a good example of the way in which the humanists' study of ancient texts influenced the Renaissance perception of the human body.   JILL KRAYE

Further reading

Kraye, J. (ed.) (1996). *The Cambridge companion to Renaissance humanism.* Cambridge University Press.

Nutton, V. (1988). *From Democedes to Harvey: studies in the history of medicine.* Variorum Reprints, London.

Humans in research Experiments in man, and the concerns that relate to them, are largely phenomena which began in the twentieth century. To be sure, it could be argued that over the centuries any deviation from the standard treatment — an alteration in drug dosage, say, or a change in operative procedure — has always been an experiment. Also, several classic human studies were carried out before 1900: Sanctorius' (1561–1636) work on insensible losses from the body in himself started a whole line of self-experimentation, which continued into the twentieth century with J. S. Haldane's work on decompression and Werner Forssmann's on cardiac catherization; James Lind's (1916–94) on preventing scurvy in seamen on long voyages; and William Beaumont's (1785–1853) on digestion in the stomach as observed through a fistula in a patient with a gunshot wound, being well-known examples.

However, experiment here is used in the sense of research with an element of the unknown, undertaken to investigate a hypothesis completely anew or to confirm preliminary findings, and several events illustrate the heavy emphasis on man as the subject of large-scale research since 1900. In the US (where the bulk of this research has been done) the Rockefeller Institute for Medical Research and the Carnegie Institution of Washington were both founded in 1902; the National Institute of Health was established through the transformation of the Hygienic Laboratory in 1930; and the Committee on Medical Research arose as a subdivision of the National Defense Research Committee set up by President Franklin D. Roosevelt in 1940. Though the initial emphasis of all of these may not have been on clinical research, within a few years it was clearly a priority (as shown for example by the opening of the hospital attached to the Rockefeller Institute within six years of its opening).

Evolution outside the US

A similar evolution occurred in other Western countries. In Britain (probably the second country in terms of recent output), the Medical Research Committee, set up in 1913 largely to study TUBERCULOSIS, evolved in 1923 into the Medical Research Council, with a much broader remit. In 1935 the Postgraduate Medical School (with its heavy emphasis on research) was established at Hammersmith Hospital in London; and throughout the 1920s and 30s Sir Thomas Lewis, professor of medicine at University College Hospital, was popularizing his phrase 'clinical research'. The recent extent of this research is staggering, as can be illustrated for just the US and the National Institutes of Health (as it became in 1948). For 1946–94 the statistics show 109 474 principal investigators, 275 195 competing for awards worth $26.3 billion, and 786 444 awards of all types, worth $121.7 billion. Much of this was devoted to research in which human studies were involved.

From the beginning of the twentieth century, then, the explosive and sustained growth of such research has been underlined by the development of other new institutions and the expansion of existing departments to establish new programmes. Moreover, scientists recognised that the enterprise would be incomplete if they could not disseminate their results and discuss them with their peers. Hence not only did the existing societies expand their programmes, but new ones were formed as well — the path-breaking and broadly based American Society of Clinical Investigation in 1907, and the British Medical Research Society in 1930.

Importance of publication

Publication in journals played an equally important part. Throughout this period there were opportunities for this in the general science journals, such as *Science* and *Nature*. Over time the general medical journals, such as the *Journal of the American Medical Association* and the *Lancet*, also started to publish many more research-oriented articles, and new specialist journals were founded to accommodate the more recondite ones. The last were often associated with specialist societies — for example, the *Journal of Clinical Investigation* (founded in 1924), and *Clinical Science* (previously called *Heart*), were linked with the American Society for Clinical Investigation and the Medical Research Society, respectively. In addition, the specialty journals — such as those devoted to paediatrics, chest disease, or neurology — began to shift the emphasis of their contents from clinical case descriptions to reports of research based on human experiment.

Why did such an emphasis on experimentation in man occur at the turn of the century? The true medico-scientific revolution began largely in the nineteenth century, and was based mainly on studies either *in vitro* or in animals in the laboratory. Nevertheless, some studies, such as on SENSATION, clearly could not be done in any other way than on human subjects, while in Britain especially there was a growing opposition to vivisection, culminating in the Cruelty to Animals Act of 1876. The development of safer investigative techniques, such as ANAESTHESIA and antisepsis in surgery, must have been an additional stimulus to human research, aided finally by the tendency by the 1890s for most of the

principal academic medical centres in France and Germany to have their own research institutes. Touring Europe to study medical education at the beginning of the twentieth century, Simon and Abraham Flexner were to emphasize the importance of these institutes in their report, which was seminal in reforming medical education, principally in the US but also in Britain (particularly after William Osler had become Regius Professor of Medicine at Oxford in 1905). Thus, certainly by the end of World War II, several medical schools in the US had professorial clinical departments in which research was a key element, and, albeit haltingly, in the 1920s Britain followed suit.

Finally, three further stimuli to the expansion of clinical research should be mentioned, in the early, middle, and latter parts of the century. In 1901, under the will of the Swedish armaments manufacturer, Alfred Nobel. the NOBEL PRIZES FOR PHYSIOLOGY OR MEDICINE were inaugurated emphasizing the societal value of research. To take just the first three of these, given in 1901–3, is to show just how 'respectable' research targeted to the needs of patients had become: respectively, the prizes were awarded to Emil von Behring (diphtheria antiserum), Ronald Ross (mosquitoes and malaria), and Niels Finsen (ultraviolet light in lupus vulgaris). The second impetus came from the specific needs raised in both World Wars — to prevent tetanus in the troops fighting in the manure-contaminated trenches of Flanders, for example, or to find an effective substitute for controlling malaria when the Japanese captured the sources of quinine in 1941. After both World Wars techniques in medical research were to benefit from spin-offs in technological advances elsewhere (particularly instrumentation — a feature that continues to the present day, as, for example, the miniaturization of devices suitable for inserting into body cavities based on developments initially introduced in the space programme). Thirdly, starting in the late 1920s and early 1930s, statistics were introduced into research. Just after World War II this was to culminate in the randomized controlled trial, turning the screw of scientific rigour through a whole revolution.

Ethical aspects

Much space elsewhere in this Companion is devoted to descriptions of some of the important research studies in man and the researchers who conducted them. Hence for the remainder of this article I will concentrate on an issue that had always been in the background, but grew gradually from the beginning of the twentieth century until World War II, when it assumed the prominence it has never since lost — namely, the ethical aspects of human experimentation. Concerns over risks to the subjects of research which offered no direct benefit to them came into prominence at the turn of the century, with newspaper comment over Walter Reed's work on yellow fever, in which volunteers were paid $100 in gold for volunteering to be bitten by the

postulated vector, the mosquito, and another $100 if they developed the disease (given to the widow in case of death). In particular, the debate centred on issues of how truly *informed consent* could be obtained.

Thereafter, until the 1950s, the concern followed a sine wave course, tending to be neutralized by other events, and sometimes by action — which in the event was to prove ineffectual. Thus for yellow fever the research came to a quick close with the establishment of the postulated mechanism and the tragic death of one of the principal investigators. After this we can see five major episodes that provoked public scrutiny. In the first decade of the twentieth century there was a debate on the rights of inpatients in public hospitals (particularly paupers and children), with reports of procedures, such as lumbar puncture and radiological examinations, undertaken purely for research without any consent. Hospital physicians argued that admission to public hospitals automatically gave them the right to carry out what procedures they wished without consultation.

Informed consent

Public concern provoked sufficient anxiety among research workers that the American Medical Association established a special committee on the protection of medical research, with Walter Cannon as its chairman. A few years later, in 1914, this issued a statement to the editors of medical journals, urging them to check that informed consent was specifically mentioned in any paper accepted for publication in which human experimentation was mentioned.

Despite this, the second crisis occurred in 1916, with a published report on the transmission of syphilis from patients with general paresis into animals. Under local anaesthesia, burr holes had been made in the skulls of six living patients, and material was aspirated from their brains and then injected into rabbits. The animals developed a syphilitic infection, thus showing that the human infection was still active even at a very late stage of the illness. The professional and public rumpus over the lack of any informed consent in this work died down probably only because it took place at the time when the US declared war on the Central Powers.

The third episode happened in Germany in the late 1920s with the Lübeck disaster. A preparation of *Bacille Calmette Guérin* vaccine, used to immunize against tuberculosis, was contaminated with virulent bacilli, and 100 children died. The government responded by issuing official guidelines in 1931 on human research, which included emphasizing the importance of informed consent. Despite such guidelines, however, the fourth event provoking public concern also occurred in Germany: during World War II the Nazis conducted egregiously unethical research on Jewish and other prisoners in concentration camps — with (often lethal) experiments on hypothermia, explosive decompression, and iatrogenic infections.

Soon after the war the United Nations established the Nüremberg Code, reiterating the minimum conditions needed to make human clinical research acceptable. Nevertheless, ten years later an American anaesthetist, Henry K. Beecher, and an English physician, Maurice Pappworth, produced books and journal articles showing how widely, and dangerously, its provisions were being ignored in practice. This time, Western society was not prepared to leave matters alone, and in 1965 the World Medical Association, guided by Hugh Clegg (editor of the *British Medical Journal*) and Tapani Kosonen (Secretary General of the Finnish Medical Association), produced the Declaration of Helsinki. Its provisions are now universally observed in research laboratories and clinics all over the world, with the establishment of protocols, approval by research ethics committees, and provision for compensation for any subject still unfortunate enough to be injured despite stringent safeguards.

Thus, although long ago enlightened physician–scientists had recognized the need for informed consent (William Beaumont, for example, putting such a clause in his contract with Alexis St Martin, his patient with the stomach fistula), it took over another 100 years before subjects achieved parity with laboratory workers in what should have been an equal partnership from the beginning. STEPHEN LOCK

Humours For over 2000 years Western medicine and culture perceived the body and the mind in humoral terms. Some of the Hippocratic writers (*c.* 450–350 BC) developed physiological and pathological theories centred on the belief that the fluids in the body were its most significant constituents. In the Hippocratic treatise *On the Nature of Man*, blood, phlegm, yellow bile, and black bile were listed as the four humours or fluids, and these became the canonical four humours (early on water was considered a humour, but black bile replaced it). Blood and phlegm were clearly apparent, yellow bile was found in the gall bladder of animals and showed itself in jaundice, and black bile, which was supposed to be the heavier part of the bile, manifested itself in conditions where the skin became black.

Greek physicians came to believe that health occurred when the humours were in balance and illness when they were out of balance. The latter happened when there was an excess of a humour, or if a humour took on an abnormal quality — if, for instance, it became putrefied or too hot.

The relationship of humoral medicine with Greek natural philosophy was formalized by GALEN (129–216 AD). He wrote that the four humours were made up of the four *qualities*: hot, cold, dry, and wet. These qualities had been used by Aristotle (384–22 BC) as the building blocks of the four *elements*: earth, water, air, and fire, with which he explained the material nature of everything on earth and below the moon. The humours of the body and the elements of the

physical world thus shared a common qualitative nature, and the *microcosm* (the little world of the human body) and the *macrocosm* (the greater world) were related to each other.

The qualitative theory of humours and elements is shown diagrammatically in the figure.

The diagram shows, for instance, that the combination of hot and cold produces the element of air and the humour of blood. Blood predominated in spring, and a person with a natural excess of blood would have a sanguine physical and psychological humoral constitution, or temperament. In Greek medicine, physical and psychological aspects were believed to be causally interrelated, so the four constitutions expressed both physical and behavioural characteristics.

HEALTH and ILLNESS were conceived in terms of the overall balance of the humours and qualities, the idea of balance reflecting the Greek praise of moderation in all things. Therapeutics was concerned with restoring the equilibrium or healthy mixture of the humours. An excess of a humour could be eliminated by bleeding, purging, vomiting, or sweating, as could also a vitiated or unhealthy humour. Attention to diet, exercise, and other aspects of a patient's lifestyle would preserve a balanced constitution or restore it. Specific remedies — mainly based on herbs, though some minerals were also used by Greek, Roman, European medieval, and Renaissance practitioners — were employed on allopathic principles. It was believed that 'opposites cure opposites', so a cold remedy could cure a hot illness. Herbs and other drugs were given degrees of heat, moisture, etc. based on a sensory subjective assessment from one to four; this was especially popular in the Middle Ages and the Renaissance.

The humoral system was holistic. Illness was perceived as an internal disorder of the whole body, rather than being the result of specific external agents of disease such as bacteria.

However, the external, visible world was deemed to affect the body. Geography and climate shaped a nation's as well as an individual's humoral constitution. The Hippocratic treatise *Airs, Waters, Places* asserted that the races to the North of Greece were hardy and tough, whilst the Egyptians were soft, living as they did in a climate with little change and posing no hardships. The outside world and a patient's response to it, seen in their lifestyle (diet, exercise, the emotions), were viewed by Galenic physicians as key determinants of health. Humoral medicine related to the individual patient rather than to the disease. Each constitution was different — though lying within the four categories of sanguine, phlegmatic, etc. — for the circumstances that shaped a constitution varied with each patient. Advice on regimen and on treatment had to take into account the particular patient's constitution, lifestyle, and environment. In this way, humoral medicine was tailored to the individual. Not surprisingly, it was an expensive form of medicine, as, in theory at least, the practitioner had to spend a good deal of time listening to the patient's story and assessing his or her circumstances. A cheaper form of medicine was provided by practitioners who treated the disease rather than the patient, and who gave the same treatment to everyone suffering from the same disease. This was the practice of the empirical group of doctors whom Galen attacked for ignoring the patient, and for using the results of trial and error as the basis of their therapeutics. In the Middle Ages and the Renaissance, the 'learned physicians' who were taught Galenic humoral medicine in the universities labelled such doctors quacks, empirics, and mountebanks.

The humoral vision of the body lasted until the late seventeenth century in Europe. Then the 'new science' of Galileo, Descartes, Newton, and Boyle

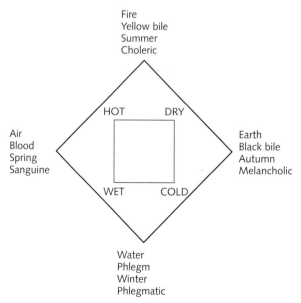

The humours and their qualities.

replaced Aristotelian qualitative natural philosophy with a mechanical, chemical, and mathematical vision of the world and of the body. Humoral medicine retained some influence in the eighteenth century. Therapeutic measures such as bleeding and purging, designed originally to get rid or excess or malign humours, continued to be used. The language of the humours was still employed to characterize people, and melancholy, especially, was a major category of mental illness into which the well-to-do, the sedentary, and the studious were even more liable to be placed in the eighteenth century than they had been in preceding centuries.

Today, the humours live on in traditional Arabic medicine, which is based on Galen via the writings of Avicenna. In India, as well as Arabic medicine, there still exists the ancient humoral and qualitative system of Ayurveda. In the West, the bacteriological and technological revolutions in medicine of the late nineteenth and twentieth centuries have all but obliterated the humours from orthodox scientific medicine. Now the emphasis is on the disease and on parts of the body rather than on the whole person and their lifestyle. Holistic medicine, which for centuries had been associated with the humours, still exists — though largely bereft of humoral theory — as alternative medicine. The irony is that the medicine that focused on the disease rather than the patient, which had been derided by the past orthodoxy of learned humoral medicine as quackery, has become, after various historical processes, the established medicine of the West.

A. WEAR

See also GALEN; HEALTH; ILLNESS; MEDICINE.

Hunchback

Hunchback According to the *Oxford English Dictionary*, Miss Mitford once said, 'The only bearable hunch-back of my acquaintance is Richard the Third.' When Anthony Sher was preparing to play this role, he did not wish to replay Charles Laughton's acclaimed film performance of Victor Hugo's hunchback Quasimodo. For him, this would have led to a portrayal of the King as having a head literally trapped inside his deformity. Seeking alternative models, Sher visited a number of patients suffering from spinal deformities, where he learnt about *kyphosis* and *scoliosis*. Kyphosis is characterized by a central hump, whereas in scoliosis the spine is twisted into an 'S' or 'C' shape, forming a side hump with one shoulder up and forward. It was the latter condition that Sher felt was most convincing for Shakespeare's representation of Richard III.

Before 1779, all sorts of curvatures of the spine were confused together. It was not until the pioneering work of Percival Potts (1713–88), the greatest surgeon of his day, that a clear distinction was made between curvatures caused by 'caries' and other kinds. *Spinal caries*, known as Pott's Disease, is TUBERCULOSIS of the spinal column. Once prevalent among children, it attacks the vertebral bones and inter-vertebral fibro-cartilages. The disease can advance to the extent that the affected parts disintegrate. The characteristic bunching up causes the spine to curve into a bow. A distinctive hump can also develop. This is now rare in the developed world.

Degenerative changes in the SPINAL COLUMN associated with OSTEOPOROSIS in older people can cause curvature and shortened stature. The spine can be affected indirectly by problems with other parts of the body, such as the HIP JOINTS, causing an abnormal stance and GAIT. Maintenance of a bad posture for sitting and walking can be responsible for causing minor irregularities of normal spinal curvature; physiotherapy, involving manipulation of the spine and exercise, can correct these problems. Such curves can present in adolescents or older children with no apparent underlying cause. A more severe form of scoliosis can occur — due to abnormalities such as spina bifida — which may be treated with a brace. Sometimes surgery is required, whereby metal rods are inserted into the back to straighten the spine.

Victor Hugo's *Notre Dame de Paris* (1831) is the most well-known novel about a hunchback, although this word did not appear in the original French title. It came to be included in later English translations. Film treatments from 1923 onwards have used the title 'The Hunchback of Notre Dame'. Laughton's sympathetic portrayal of the hunchback in 1939 contrasts with Shakespeare's representation of Richard III as a hunchback, who is demonized as 'a lump of foul deformity' by Lady Anne. The notion that this physical abnormality corresponded to Richard's moral deformity draws on the superstitious belief that it was a punishment for sin. In *The Man who Laughs* (1869), Victor Hugo advocates an acceptance and recognition of such abnormalities as a gateway to the sublime: 'Now you are ugly, but hideous. Ugliness is insignificant, deformity is grand. Ugliness is a devil's grin behind beauty; deformity is akin to sublimity.'

MARIE MULVEY-ROBERTS

Hunger

Hunger can have a variety of meanings. For example, to a nutritionist it may be used to describe starvation resulting from a lack of food. However, to most of us hunger refers to the sensations we feel when we need food, such as an aching, growling stomach, weakness, or a grumpy mood. Indeed, the *Oxford English Dictionary* defines hunger as 'The uneasy or painful sensation caused by want of food.' This sensation generally motivates an individual to find and to consume food.

Let us start our consideration of hunger with how it feels. Descriptions of hunger come from written reports consisting of checklists of particular sensations, or line scales on which the degree of a sensation is marked. Open-ended verbal reports in which the experience of hunger is described freely are of interest but difficult to quantify. Sometimes the emphasis has been on where in the body an individual experiences hunger. All of these different types of assessments agree that gastric sensations, such as an aching or growling stomach, are most commonly associated with hunger. Other sensations found to occur less frequently are weakness, headaches, pain, dizziness, anxiety, loss of concentration, food craving, thoughts of food, watering of the mouth, discomfort, dry mouth, nausea, and thirst. Large individual differences are seen in both the degree to which hunger is experienced and the way it is perceived. However, in general, when hunger is reported over the entire day it is seen to follow a cyclical pattern in which it rises gradually before meals and falls rapidly as eating proceeds.

An important issue is whether reported hunger can be used to infer how much a person would eat in a given situation. Investigators have found that in some situations hunger does correlate well with food intake, but often it does not. For example, regardless of how hungry someone feels, the amount consumed in a meal can be affected by the palatability, variety, and amount of food offered. The eating environment may also influence intake, in that people often eat more when they are with a group of friends than when eating alone.

Much research has been directed at discovering the role of hunger in the regulation of food intake and food selection. Since hunger is a subjective sensation, strictly speaking it can only be studied in humans. However, experimental animals, particularly laboratory rats, are often used in studies of hunger and the regulation of food intake. Thus, hunger has been defined in ways that do not rely on reports of subjective sensations. Hunger in animals is inferred and measured by the amount eaten. So, for example, if the time since the last meal affects the amount consumed, we assume that this is because food deprivation increases hunger. The assumption in both experimental animals and humans is that, when there is a need for food, the body senses this through a variety of physiological mechanisms, including changes in blood glucose and insulin, and metabolic signals from the liver, all of which are integrated by the brain. When the brain detects that the body needs fuel, a state of hunger develops and the animal eats an amount appropriate to reduce the hunger and reverse the deficit.

While hunger may relate to the physiological signals indicating the body's need for food, learning and environmental influences can influence it as well. A newborn baby apparently experiences hunger in response to cues signalling a need for food, and cries to be fed regularly every few hours. Gradually, through learning, this behaviour changes so that it conforms to imposed meal times. That these times vary widely between cultures — for example, dinner is eaten early in the evening in Norway and late at night in Spain — illustrates the impact of learning on the cyclical pattern of hunger over the day. Studies also indicate that people learn the types and amounts of food required to satisfy their hunger.

Sometimes hunger and food intake are unrelated to the body's need for food. For example, when we are bored or nervous, we may not feel hungry but will nevertheless eat to pass the time or to calm ourselves. Such inappropriate eating can become problematic and contribute to the development of obesity. Some behaviour therapies for obesity emphasize learning to recognize hunger sensations and to eat in response to them. However, some obese individuals complain that they never experience hunger. A critical question which has not yet been clearly answered is whether some overweight individuals have impairments in physiological systems that normally signal hunger.

It is also important to determine whether low food intake, or anorexia, can be due to impaired or reduced hunger in response to physiological needs. For example, hunger may be reduced in chronically ill patients and is reported to be low in individuals with anorexia nervosa. The challenge to their carers is how to induce them to eat. They may need to stimulate 'appetite' rather than hunger. While hunger refers to the need to eat, appetite relates to the pleasure of eating. It is appetite that steers us to particular foods. While hunger and appetite are often experienced together, when we are hungry and want a particular food, appetites for foods can occur in the absence of hunger. Thus, we may have an appetite for chocolate or ice cream at the end of a large meal when we are no longer hungry.

Like many other bodily systems, those underlying hunger and the regulation of food intake change with age. Many elderly people do not eat enough to maintain their body weight. While the low food intake may be due in part to poor appetite associated with decreased ability to smell and taste food, there are also changes in hunger. Older individuals not only may report decreased hunger, but studies show that many do not adjust intake appropriately to changes in bodily needs.

Studies of hunger are important clinically in that they may suggest an abnormality of physiological systems related to the detection of signals from normal metabolism of ingested food. Understanding both the biological and behavioural foundations of hunger may help to suggest therapies for inappropriate food intake. For example, some pharmacological agents can reduce both hunger and food intake, which is helpful in the treatment of obesity. When food intake is inappropriately low, treatment may involve stimulating appetite, for example, by increasing the variety and palatability of the available foods, which could increase food intake even when hunger sensations are depressed.

The sensation of hunger links our bodily needs to behavioural food seeking and ingestion. In the wild, animals would be unlikely to survive if the sensation of hunger were abnormal. However, in humans, food is often abundant and culture dictates when and how much should be consumed, so the sensation of hunger has become less crucial for survival. Nevertheless, the high incidence of disorders of body weight indicates that relying on these environmental cues rather than hunger to guide food intake is not an optimal strategy.

BARBARA J. ROLLS

Further reading

Bell, E. A. and Rolls, B. J. (2001). Regulation of energy intake: Factors contributing to obesity. In: *Present Knowledge in Nutrition*, 8th Edition. Eds B. Bowman and R. Russell. ILSI Press, Washington, D.C., pp. 31–40.

Rolls, B. and Barnett, R. A. (2000). *The Volumetrics Weight-Control Plan: Feel Full on Fewer Calories*. HarperCollins Publishers, New York.

See also EATING; EATING DISORDERS; OBESITY.

Hydrocephalus

Derived from the Greek for 'water' and 'head', hydrocephalus was recognized by Greek and Roman philosophers, including Hippocrates and Galen. Arabic medical scholars, like Albucasis, preserved and built upon the knowledge of the ancients, combining it with Arabic surgical expertise. One of the earliest illustrations of the condition, and a method of treating it, which involved opening the head and evacuating fluid, appeared in the fifteenth-century surgical manuscript by Sharaf ad Din. Nearly 200 years later, the Italian surgeon Marco Aurelio Severino depicted and described a case of infantile hydrocephalus in *De Recondita Abscessuum Natura Libri VII* (Seven Books on the Obscure Nature of Abscesses).

Hydrocephalus is sometimes called 'water on the brain', but the excess of fluid is in fact 'in' rather than 'on'. There is normally CEREBROSPINAL FLUID filling the CEREBRAL VENTRICLES — the cavities deep inside the brain — and hydrocephalus describes an increase in its volume, and therefore of the size of the ventricles. Cerebrospinal fluid (CSF) is continually produced by transfer of a watery solution from the blood into the ventricles, flowing slowly through these cavities, and into the *subarachnoid space*, to bathe the outside of the brain and spinal cord; thence it is continually reabsorbed into the bloodstream. Hydrocephalus occurs if the rate of absorption does not keep pace with production.

Most often the problem is a mechanical obstruction. This may occur before birth, due to a malformation in the brain, resulting in an enlarged head which can pose problems during delivery. In other cases, although caused by a congenital defect — often associated with *spina bifida* — hydrocephalus may develop only later during infancy. Up to the age of two, when the bones of the skull begin to fuse, hydrocephalus results in overall enlargement in the size of the baby's head.

Later in life, at any age, a tumour may block a narrow part of the ventricular system, so that the system above this block expands; or there can be blockage in the surface spaces due to adhesions following meningitis or haemorrhage.

Obstructive forms of hydrocephalus occurring after fusion of the skull bones result in increasing intracranial pressure, with headache, vomiting, and danger to sight, with eventual death if unrelieved. The block can be located by IMAGING TECHNIQUES (CT scan or MRI), which clearly show the shape and size of the ventricles. If it is not possible to remove the obstruction, the block may be bypassed by inserting a tube, with a one-way valve, leading from the ventricles either to the venous side of the heart or into the peritoneal cavity.

Hydrocephalus may result also from wasting away of the brain substance due to progressive disease such as Alzheimer's, or to sudden and massive insults such as those which lead to the vegetative state. There is no rise in pressure because the excess of 'water' simply takes up the space in and around the wasted brain.

KAROL K. WEAVER
BRYAN JENNETT

Further reading

Lyons, A. E. (1995). Hydrocephalus first illustrated. *Neurosurgery*, 37, 511–3.

Montagnani, C. A. (1986). Pediatric surgery in Islamic medicine from the Middle Ages to the Renaissance. *Progress in Pediatric Surgery*, 20, 39–51.

Hygiene

The word *hygiene* derives from the name of the ancient Greek goddess of healthful living, *Hygeia*. Initially worshipped in her own right, by the fifth century BCE in Athens Hygeia was instead depicted as a demi-god, the daughter or wife of the god of healing, *Asclepius*. While worship of Asclepius aimed at curing disease through divine intercession, worship of Hygeia emphasized obtaining health by living wisely in accordance with her laws. In contemporary Western society the concept of hygiene has become associated with standards of personal grooming which often have little effect on individual health.

Historical background

Hygiene in the earliest sense was not connected to *cleanliness* or personal grooming. Indeed popular attitudes in Western Europe and the US held that frequent bathing was dangerous to individual health. It upset the physical system, robbed the body of precious natural oils, and led to debilitating illness. Though individuals such as Benjamin Franklin urged cleanliness as a necessary component of healthful living, the plumbing technology required to make this easy was underdeveloped and expensive. Travellers in Europe and the US during the early nineteenth century frequently commented on the filthy conditions both of persons and households. One historian has suggested that, in a largely agricultural community, the dirt of honest labour was associated with both economic and physical well-being, an outlook that applied to both peasant cultures in Europe and yeoman farm life in the US.

Beginning in the early nineteenth century, the repeated onslaught of diseases such as cholera began to alter people's understanding of personal hygiene. Since orthodox medicine seemed powerless in response to these PANDEMICS, a variety of alternative medicines gained popularity. Many of these alternatives emphasized disease prevention through healthful living, which included diet and clothing reform, daily cold water bathing, exercise, regulation of bowel movements, and abstinence from coffee, tea, alcohol, and sex. In their attack on heroic medicine, reformers emphasized personal and domestic responses to health crises.

For these reformers, living hygienically was essential both because it led to physical well-being, and because it revealed proper moral character. Catherine Beecher, the most prominent domestic advice author of the mid-nineteenth-century US, propounded this view of hygiene. In *Letters to the People on Health and Happiness* she called her hygiene precepts, '… *laws of health and happiness*, because our Creator has connected the reward of enjoyment with obedience to these rules, and the penalty of suffering with disobedience to them'.

Florence Nightingale, in her efforts to reform English hospital care, provided the most cogent arguments linking personal and public hygiene with good health and morals. Like many of her contemporaries, Nightingale believed that unhealthy living made individuals susceptible to contagion. She rejected germs as a specific causal agent, however, asserting that dirt, sewer gases, and other environmental contagion produced illness. Nightingale's system for training nurses reflects this belief, and Nightingale nurses cleaned the patient and created order in the hospital. Nightingale is, therefore, a transitional figure linking the idea that the individual has a moral responsibility to live healthfully with a desire to control external threats to individual health.

As Western society became more urban and industrial, the disorderliness of city life seemed to threaten the health of even the most dedicated follower of Beecher's 'laws of health and happiness'. Gradual acceptance of the germ theory compounded the fear that right living alone could not prevent illness. The eleventh edition of the *Encyclopedia Britannica* reflects this attitude by asserting that hygiene embraces 'all the agencies which affect the physical and mental well-being of man.' Hygiene as a system included not only personal hygiene related to food, clothing, exercise, cleanliness, and sexual control, but also sciences such as engineering, meteorology, bacteriology, and public sanitation and waterworks.

Since social health required both environmental cleanliness and hygienic behaviour on the part of the masses, reformers sought to extend private middle-class standards of hygiene into the public arena by reforming garbage collection, water delivery, and sewage disposal. They also sought to change the behaviours of the lower classes. In the US the effort to transmit hygienic practices to the masses was inextricably linked to Americanization. The goal was to lift so-called 'dirty foreigners' to middle-class American standards. The lessons of hygienic living were first taught to women through 'settlement houses' and visiting nurses, but the most effective pedagogy of

hygiene targeted children in schools. Hygiene instruction prodded children to swat flies, refrain from spitting, brush their teeth and hair, clean their clothing, wash all of their body and not just the parts that showed, eat balanced meals, and abstain from alcohol, tobacco, and sex. Humiliation of children who did not meet the teacher's standards was frequently used to reinforce these lessons, and students were expected to carry the lessons home. African–Americans and immigrants readily embraced hygienic living as a means of uplift. Booker T. Washington, prominent leader of the African–American community and founder of the Tuskegee Institute, emphasized the 'gospel of the toothbrush'. Ironically, African–Americans, many of whom worked as janitors, maids, and laundresses, were viewed as indelibly dirty and diseased regardless of their adherence to the hygienic standards of the white middle classes.

Racial hygiene

The racism inherent in this evaluation of blacks and immigrants was at the root of the international EUGENICS movement, also known as the *racial hygiene* movement. Proponents of eugenics in the US, Great Britain, Australia, France, Germany, and Scandinavia maintained that social health and progress would arise from increased childbearing among presumably superior people and limitation of reproduction for genetically inferior people. The US led the way in passing legislation which allowed forced STERILIZATION of 'undesirables' in custodial care, such as the mentally ill, criminals, and racial minorities. By the 1930s, 2000–4000 operations per year were performed in 23 states, with nearly half of all sterilizations occurring in California.

In 1933 Germany followed the American lead with the passage of two sterilization laws patterned primarily on California's model. The chief difference was that the law in Germany standardized procedures for determining eligibility for sterilization and applied these rules to the entire nation, an 'advantage' much admired by many American genetic scientists and eugenicists. The Nazi use of showers as a façade for the gassing of millions of Jews, homosexuals, gypsies, and communists ironically underscores this perversion of hygienic practices.

Advertising cleanliness

The 1920s saw the introduction of a new corporate understanding of hygiene that wedded the educational approach of the social reformers to the methods of mass communication. Good hygiene became associated with good business. Metropolitan Insurance of New York and the Henry Street Visiting Nurses Association reached an agreement whereby the nurses taught Metropolitan clients to live hygienically. The Cleanliness Institute, founded by the Association of American Soap and Glycerine Producers, created lessons for teachers on personal hygiene. They also hired a popular children's author to create a series of five books with churlish characters called *goops*, including the unhygienic characters

of Hatesope and Rodirtygus who refused to bathe. The lesson of each of the tales was that no good child would behave like a goop. Since corporate promoters of hygiene had two aims, to draw new users into the market for their products and to encourage greater consumption of their products by current users, they added new diseases, such as HALITOSIS (bad breath) and *body odour*, to the list that good hygiene supposedly prevented. The introduction of these 'disease states' indicated a shift in the understanding of hygiene, which now emphasized a well-groomed personal image and social acceptability as important outcomes of what was once extolled as the harbinger of health. In the US this meant that hygiene now included removal of 'unsightly hair' from women's underarms (beginning in the nineteen-teens) and legs (after the 1940s).

Sexual hygiene

Attitudes on hygienic sexual practice paralleled the evolution of general understanding of hygiene. When healthful living and moral character were equated, good sexual hygiene meant abstaining from all sexual activities. William Andross Alcott, a prominent health reformer in the nineteenth century, warned that sexual activity, including frequent heterosexual intercourse and 'self abuse' or masturbation, led to poor mental and physical health, because it exhausted the body's vital energies. When proper hygiene was seen as a bulwark of social order and civilization, the American Society for Sanitary and Moral Prophylaxis and the American Social Hygiene Association promoted control of erotic impulses through publication of 'scientific' information on sex, and sex education in schools, which emphasized negative consequences of intercourse and was intended to prevent sexual experimentation among teenagers. In addition to supporting forced sterilization of 'undesirable elements', the early-twentieth-century sexual hygiene movement also aimed at eliminating prostitution and inculcating a single sexual standard for both males and females. The corporate approach to hygiene created an interesting paradox concerning sex. Consumers, particularly girls, were urged to engage in hygienic practices that would make them sexually desirable, while health educators warned that nice boys and girls did not engage in sexual activities outside of marriage. None the less, heterosexual relations within the bonds of marriage were seen as natural and healthy. In the youth rebellion of the 1960s hygienic teachings about grooming and abstinence became associated with the corrupt ways of bourgeois society. Ironically, the counterculture embraced both dirt and unrestrained sexual relations as a means of breaking from this corruption and creating a 'purer', more 'natural', and 'healthier' way of life.

Contemporary understanding of hygiene reflects the tensions inherent in its history. Hygiene has partially become a byword for the quaint sexual mores promoted in high school classrooms of the 1950s. Yet in a era of teenage pregnancy and epidemics of sexually transmitted diseases, schools and public health agencies are returning to the message that abstinence and sexual self-control are essential to continued good health. We also face the paradox that advertising and mass communication, which successfully used sex and social acceptability to sell hygienic practices to our grandparents and great grandparents, are now promoting images of health and beauty linked to epidemic levels of EATING DISORDERS.   JACQUELINE S. WILKIE

Further reading

Hoy, S. (1995). *Chasing dirt: the American pursuit of cleanliness*. Oxford University Press, New York.

Kühl, S. (1994) *The Nazi connection: eugenics, American racism and German National Socialism*. Oxford University Press, New York.

See also EUGENICS.

Hymen

The hymen, which medical descriptions depict as nothing more than a lunule or crescent-shaped membrane bordering the LABIA minora, is among the most meaningful of body parts. For much of history and in many parts of the world, the hymen has been valued as the sign and seal of a woman's VIRGINITY, even though medical authorities define it as merely a *partial* covering that many women are born without and that many others lose in the course of everyday activities. Nevertheless, the medical description and symbolic status of the hymen continue side by side. The OED, for example, defines the hymen as a mere fold or partial cover, but at the same time terms it 'the virginal membrane'. In her 1976 study of mariology (*Alone of All her sex*), Marina Warner described how convent schoolgirls are taught that, because the hymen closes the vagina, using tampons will irreparably damage their virginity. Moreover, hymen construction through plastic surgery is popular in Japan and India, among other places, where a high value is placed on female virginity in spite of changes in sexual mores.

Although the word 'hymen' is derived from the Greek term for membrane, ancient anatomy did not recognize a membrane covering the vagina as part of the normal female body. Nor did the Greeks associate the anatomical term '*hymen*' with the *hymenaios* or wedding song, or with the god of marriage. As Sissa notes in her essential study *Greek virginity*, '*hymen*' described a particular type of tissue, a membrane or light film that wrapped all vital organs and bones and was in no way specific to the virgin. Hippocratic nosography viewed a membrane over the vagina as an abnormality, classing it with membranes that harmfully covered other orifices — the anus or the penis, for example.

Although classic Greek medicine did not recognize a virginal membrane, evidence suggests a concept of the hymen as vaginal seal had developed at least by the second century AD. Sissa points out that such a belief was mentioned and contradicted by the Greek doctor Soranus, who taught medicine in Rome. In his *Gynaikeia* Soranus cited as an 'error' the opinion that a thin membrane grew in the middle of the vagina. We do not know the source of this 'error' or when belief in it began. However, we can be certain that by the fourth century a vision of the female body with a natural seal or hymen was central to Christian beliefs about the birth of Jesus and the status of Mary.

For Christians, the miracle of a VIRGIN BIRTH fulfilled the Old Testament prophecy: 'Behold a virgin shall be with child, and shall bring forth a son, and they shall call his name Emmanuel' (Isaiah 7:14). Ambrose, writing in the fourth century, found the hymen necessary for a correct interpretation of Scriptures; it is the physical detail that makes miraculous the virgin birth and places it outside of all natural occurrence. Physical virginity was central to the Marian cult from its official beginnings in Byzantium, and the Church proclaimed Mary's 'seal' as intact before, during, and after the birth of Christ. The second Council of Constantinople in 381 and the Council of Chalcedon in 451 affirmed Mary's perpetual virginity. Moreover, the importance of physical virginity as a model for all women was reiterated throughout the Middle Ages in writings like Peter Damian's 'Letter on Divine Omnipotence' (*c.* 1067). In arguing against Jerome's alleged remark that although God can do anything, He cannot restore a woman's virginity, Damian responded that God was capable of such a feat, but abstained from doing it because repairing the virgin seal, as he terms it, was not justifiable. For undervaluing a precious treasure God imposed a penalty, a lasting sign (the broken hymen) that would forever recall the transgression. Mary's virginity remained a model for Christian women, and during the sixteenth century the Council of Trent reaffirmed the doctrines surrounding the Blessed Mother's status as virgo intacta.

Literal interpretations of purity as physical virginity gave onto images of Mary as the enclosed garden, a sealed fountain, a '*porta clausa*'. Her unbroken hymen was likened to a pane of glass that the sun passed through without piercing. Paintings representing scenes from Mary's life, and in particular the Annunciation, often drew on these metaphors. They were especially popular with Northern painters of the fifteenth century, as, for example in Jan van Eyck's *Annunciation in a Church* (*c.* 1428; National Gallery of Art, Washington, DC) or in Roger Campin's *Mérode Altarpiece* (*c.* 1426; Cloisters Collection, New York). In each of these works the artist shows the Virgin placed near light rays, depicted as golden shafts, passing through a glass window pane. Also represented was a story from the *Apocryphal Gospels* in which the midwife Salome, who does not believe in Mary's virginity, examines her manually to ascertain if the hymen is intact. For her incredulity Salome is punished with a withered hand, and we see her so represented in Roger Campin's *Nativity* (*c.* 1420; Musée des Beaux–Arts, Dijon).

The unbelieving midwife who must physically touch Mary's hymen reminds us that midwives from the early Christian period through the Enlightenment laid claim to this procedure for testing virginity. These midwives were targets for doctors who disputed their ability, and (perhaps surprisingly) for the Church fathers who, despite their insistence on Mary's intact body, themselves doubted that the hymen provided incontrovertible proof. Ambrose, for example, sent an indignant letter to the bishop of Verona who allowed a midwife to examine a Christian virgin manually. Not only might such contact provoke the very catastrophe it pretended to determine, but, Ambrose noted, most learned physicians said physical inspections were not entirely reliable. Thus Ambrose, like Augustine and Cyprian after him, presses his belief in the hymen as the signaculum of woman's (and Mary's) virginity, and at the same time admits that medical science has shown the hymen an unreliable sign at best.

In the matter of the hymen, midwives were a particular target for the sixteenth-century physician Ambroise Paré who was disgusted that judges often relied on their untrustworthy testimony. He noted that although midwives will swear they can distinguish a virgin from a deflowered woman, their testimony is suspect since they cannot decide where the hymen is located: one says at the entry to the vagina; another in the neck of the womb; and a third in the womb itself. Against this ambiguous testimony Paré places the results of his practice; after examining girls between the ages of three and twelve under his care at the Hospital of Paris, he found no evidence of the alleged virginal seal. Paré, however, admits that some colleagues also believe in the hymen, as do entire peoples, such as the Africans of Mauritania who display the soiled bed linen after a nuptial defloration. Paré attributed the blood associated with first intercourse not to breaking the hymen, but to tearing little veins spread over the woman's reproductive organs.

By the eighteenth century many physicians such as Buffon rejected both the word 'hymen' and the image of a membrane stretched across the vagina. Buffon, instead, recognized a whole series of possibilities including the idea that a half-moon of skin grew around the vagina. Like Paré, he offered alternative explanations for phenomena (such as the shedding of blood on first intercourse) associated with the hymen. But perhaps more importantly, Buffon suggests a sociocultural origin for the hymen. Men, he argued, have always made much of whatever they believed their exclusive possession and this madness has made a real entity of the maiden's virginity. Buffon goes on to say that virginity, which is a virtue, has been transformed into a physical object and made a concern for all men.

As an object of concern for men, the hymen found itself in many places: religious treatises, court rooms, medical texts, and erotic novels like those of the Marquis de Sade in which the deflowering of a virgin — whose status is guaranteed by an intact hymen — produces an extra frisson of excitement. Paintings symbolized Mary's hymen as an unbroken pane of glass, and poems like Pope's *The Rape of the Lock* (1712–14) figured the maiden's maidenhead as fine, breakable porcelain. Although midwives could not precisely say in what part of the female body the hymen was located, it could be found in the *Encyclopédie*'s (published 1751–65) entry on virginity: 'Anatomy leaves the existence of the membrane known as the hymen totally in doubt.'

If a fantasy of the hymen had its uses for Christian theology, it has also been helpful to psychoanalysis. Sigmund Freud, whose theories of femininity remain influential today, argued in *The Taboo of Virginity* (1917) that the first penetration of a woman's genitalia destroyed an organ. Belief in the hymen-organ allowed Freud to depict woman's first act of sexual intercourse as leaving a physical wound, which then translated in her mental life as a blow to narcissism. The double wound produces the hostility that every woman, according to Freud, feels toward her first lover. That hostility he associates with penis envy, which in Freud's theory of femininity stands as a defining feature of woman's mental life. As in the case of the Church fathers, the hymen here operates as verification of some deeply held belief necessary to the workings of a system. Indeed, the history of the hymen points not to the physical actuality of an organ, but to the social and theoretical utility of a sign imagined as truly present in the female body.

MARY D. SHERIFF

Further reading
Sissa, G. (1990). *Greek virginity* (trans. A. Goldhammer). Harvard University Press, Cambridge, MA.

Warner, M. (1983). *Alone of all her sex. The myth and cult of the Virgin Mary*. Vintage Books, New York.

See also VIRGINITY; VIRGINITY TESTS.

Hyperbaric chamber

Hyperbaric chambers in industry

Although Henshaw, an English clergyman, constructed a pressurized chamber — or 'domicilium', as he termed it — in 1662, the technology which allowed the construction of large vessels capable of holding greater pressure developed in the early to mid nineteenth century, and was associated with the construction of bridges and tunnels. Water ingress was a major problem in such workings, and in 1830 Admiral Lord Thomas Cochrane patented the technique of using compressed air in tunnels and caissons to exclude water. In 1839 Triger used the technique during the sinking of a shaft through quicksand to a seam of coal at Châlons in France. The technique was successful, was applied elsewhere, and its use was soon followed by reports of decompression illness in the workers. In 1854 Pol and Watelle recorded the relief obtained by workers so afflicted who went back into compressed air, and the workers, finding this cure out themselves, voluntarily went back to the pressurized caisson to obtain relief when they got the 'bends'. These observations were strongly supported by Paul Bert's demonstration of the success of

recompression as a treatment in animals, but it was only after large projects, such as the New York tunnels under the Hudson and East rivers in 1889 and 1893, which caused more than 5000 instances of the disease, that the benefit of systematic recompression therapy for decompression illness was fully established. In order to avoid the inconvenience and danger of carrying patients back into the workings, special hyperbaric chambers were used at tunnelling sites. These were called medical locks, and the early ones were nothing more than boilers mounted horizontally with an airtight door at one end. The chamber formed could be divided by a bulkhead incorporating a door, and this formed a lock whereby the inner chamber could be entered without lowering its pressure. The chamber was equipped with electric light, bunks, and the necessary compressed air connections and controls. Following their development for compressed air workers, hyperbaric chambers were also widely used to treat divers and, later on, aviators with decompression illness.

Present-day hyperbaric chambers are categorized in terms of the number of locks that they contain, whether they can accommodate more than one person, and to what pressure they can be compressed. A chamber for one person is called a monoplace chamber, and these have only one lock or compartment. These chambers may be metal or even fabric, but are commonly constructed of acrylic tubes with metal end plates. They are now almost exclusively used for medical applications. Multiplace chambers accommodate more than one person and come in any number of sizes and pressure ratings depending on their purpose. They are equipped with pressure-proof windows and have a small interlock let into the hull which is used to allow the passage of small items, such as food and drink, without decompressing the main lock. They are used still in industry for the treatment of decompression illness, but the last 30 years has seen them used also as pressurized living habitats for divers working at great depths.

The hyperbaric chamber environment and saturation diving

As atmospheric pressure is increased in the chamber there is adiabatic heating and the atmosphere warms. This heat does disperse once a stable pressure is obtained, but during decompression the atmosphere cools, often to the extent that water condenses out and a fog appears. Gas density increases with atmospheric pressure; the partial pressure of the various gases in the atmosphere rises proportionately and their various toxic effects become manifest. At pressures over three atmospheres (more than three times the typical barometric pressure at sea-level) the NITROGEN in air exerts its anaesthetic properties, with gradual loss of mental ability and co-ordination, until at 10 atmospheres and above loss of consciousness occurs. The increased gas density can also cause underventilation of the lungs, and carbon dioxide

build-up in the blood. For these reasons the use of air in hyperbaric chambers is limited to six atmospheres, and usually three atmospheres are not exceeded. At higher pressures, chambers are usually compressed using helium, which is very much less narcotic and also less dense, although it does distort speech to the extent that special electronic equipment is required to make the speech to the divers comprehensible. As pressure is increased further with helium, the thermal capacity and thermal conductivity of the gaseous environment increase; conductive and convective heat loss increase, and the body loses the ability to control its temperature. At about 30 atmospheres the body is effectively poikilothermic (the body temperature changes with that of the environment). Chamber temperature under these conditions needs to kept at around 30°C to avoid HYPOTHERMIA in the chamber occupants, and much higher temperatures can cause hyperthermia.

The partial pressure of OXYGEN also gives cause for concern. At partial pressures much over 0.3 atmospheres, oxygen affects the lung, and at over 0.6 atmospheres it is frankly toxic, causing oedema and inflammation, although this takes some time to happen and the early effects are entirely reversible. At higher partial pressures, oxygen is also toxic for the brain, causing CONVULSIONS, and disturbs most other body systems. In hyperbaric oxygen therapy, not more than three atmospheres of oxygen are ever used, and then only within very strictly controlled schedules.

The increased pressure of oxygen and nitrogen increase the fire hazard in pressure chambers. Ignition temperature falls as the partial pressure of oxygen rises, and the rate of spread of fire increases as the partial pressure of nitrogen rises, since the atmosphere conducts heat more efficiently. In order to speed decompression schedules, and in medical applications, 100% oxygen is frequently breathed in pressure chambers. This is accomplished in small monoplace medical chambers by simply flushing the chamber with a high flow of oxygen. In large, multiplace chambers, the presence of high levels of oxygen in the atmosphere is considered to pose too great a fire risk, and the oxygen is dispensed from special breathing equipment, which allows the exhaled gas to be vented from the chamber. The problem of escape from the chamber and the rapid rise of pressure caused by the increasing temperature makes fire safety a primary concern in hyperbaric chamber operation.

The hyperbaric chamber is an enclosed space and so, as the occupants consume oxygen the level of this gas falls and the products of metabolism such as heat, carbon dioxide, water vapour, and other gaseous wastes build up. Compressed air chambers at low pressures can be ventilated, but as pressure increases this becomes more difficult because of the amount of gas required. Chambers compressed with helium, which is expensive, are not ventilated.

Oxygen can be added to the atmosphere and carbon dioxide removed using a chemical absorbent. If the chamber is to be occupied for some time then an entire atmosphere conditioning unit or life support system is required, which also controls temperature, humidity, and other contaminants. Oxygen levels are kept at or below 0.4 atmospheres. Needless to say these chambers are equipped with showers and toilets appropriately modified for the environment. Such systems are used for 'saturation' diving techniques, so-called because the partial pressure of inert gas in the divers' tissues equilibrates with that in the pressurized atmosphere. The divers live in a chamber, on a vessel or offshore structure, which is held at the same pressure as their underwater work site for periods of up to four weeks. They commute to and from their work in a pressurised diving bell. The time wasted by compression and decompression, and the associated dangers, are thus minimized, since the diver may only have to be compressed and decompressed once during the spell at pressure. Decompression, however, takes days rather than the minutes taken using conventional diving techniques.

Hyperbaric chambers in medicine

In parallel with the industrial use of hyperbaric chambers went attempts to develop more general medical applications. Between the years 1834, when Junod used compressed air to treat various pulmonary ailments in France, and 1928, when Cunningham constructed the largest pressure chamber of all in Cleveland, Ohio, compressed air therapy achieved some degree of popularity with the public, but never with any demonstrable medical benefit. Cunningham's chamber was six storeys high and 64 feet in diameter. It had all the facilities of an hotel, including carpeting, dining rooms, and a smoking room. Cunningham was unable to validate compressed air therapy for the general medical conditions that he treated, such as syphilis, diabetes, and cancer, and it was condemned by the American Medical Association and the chamber forced to close in 1930. Compressed air is no longer used as a medical treatment.

Nevertheless, hyperbaric chambers are still quite justifiably used in medicine to allow the administration of very high partial pressures of oxygen — so-called hyperbaric oxygen therapy. This technique has largely replaced recompression in air as the treatment of decompression illness, since it allows treatment in the absence of inert gas, which is accordingly excreted very much more quickly and effectively. Oxygen breathing at high atmospheric pressure increases the body's oxygen stores, and because of this it is possible to stop the heart, or cut off the blood circulating to an organ, for very much longer than otherwise possible. At three atmospheres pressure, enough oxygen can be dissolved in the plasma to support the oxygen demands of the body at rest in the absence of haemoglobin. Because of these effects, hyperbaric operating

theatres were developed in the 1950s and 60s to enable various cardiac and circulatory operations. However, since the development of the cardiac bypass apparatus this application has dwindled. Hyperbaric oxygen therapy can also stimulate new blood vessel growth and improve healing in hypoxic wounds. At present the generally accepted medical indications for hyperbaric oxygen therapy are acute CARBON MONOXIDE poisoning, gas EMBOLISM, gas gangrene and similar infections, and in the treatment of tissue damaged in the course of RADIOTHERAPY for cancer. There are a number of other less well-accepted indications and there is a thriving interest in the use of hyperbaric oxygen in alternative or complementary medicine for a number of conditions. These include multiple sclerosis, and unfortunately patients are treated without any real or objective demonstration of clinical efficacy.

Hyperbaric chambers are simple devices, but their operation can be far from straightforward either from the technical or physiological point of view. It is essential that they are well maintained and operated within the statutory guidelines and regulations by trained personnel.

JOHN A. S. ROSS

See also DECOMPRESSION SICKNESS; DIVING; OXYGEN.

Hyperglycaemia
An abnormally high concentration of glucose in the blood, most commonly due to DIABETES mellitus, when the normal regulatory action of INSULIN is missing — either because it is not being adequately secreted from the PANCREAS, or because its function — of promoting removal of glucose from the blood into body tissues for utilisation or storage — is compromised. When blood glucose concentration is normal, the kidneys retain it all, but in hyperglycaemia the glucose 'overflows' into the urine.

S.J.

See BLOOD SUGAR; INSULIN.

Hypertension
High BLOOD PRESSURE. There is no exact level of blood pressure which labels a person hypertensive, but values as high as 160 mm Hg/90 mm Hg (= systolic/diastolic; highest and lowest in the period of one heart beat) would generally be regarded as marginal in someone at rest. A systolic blood pressure higher than this is reached by healthy people in heavy exercise, and if the exercise is 'static' (isometric), both systolic and diastolic are higher; but 'hypertension' is a term usually reserved for abnormally high pressure at rest.

S.J.

See BLOOD PRESSURE.

Hyperthyroidism
The classic picture of excessive THYROID activity is that of a patient with *Graves' disease* — a form of *thyrotoxicosis*. Robert Graves was a renowned Dublin physician, whose bicentenary was celebrated in 1996. In addition to promoting a radical innovation in medical education — ward rounds with bedside teaching — he wrote in 1835 the first clear

description of this disease. In a short paper titled 'Palpitation of the heart with enlargement of the thyroid gland', he recognized the defining significance of a 'triad' of symptoms: goitre, protruding eyes, and palpitations.

In the UK about 2% of women will suffer from thyroid overactivity (hyperthyroidism). It is ten times less likely among men. The hyperthyroidism of at least 50% of the patients is due to Graves' disease — now known to be an autoimmune condition.

Normally, thyroid activity is subject to positive regulation by thyroid stimulating hormone (TSH), which is secreted from the pituitary and stimulates thyroid growth and function. Very rarely, thyrotoxicosis is caused by excessive production of TSH. Hyperthyroidism of non-autoimmune origin is usually due to either a *toxic nodular goitre* ('Plummer's disease', after a physician at the Mayo Clinic in the 1920s) or a *toxic adenoma* — a benign tumour in which the cells retain the follicular arrangement characteristic of the thyroid gland. In complete contrast, the overactivity encountered in Graves' disease is due to the aberrant production of autoantibodies, known as thyroid stimulating antibodies. These mimic TSH and persistently stimulate the thyroid follicular cells. These antibodies are unique in having a stimulating as opposed to a blocking action. They were first described in a classic series of studies conducted in the 1950–60s by Adams and Purves in the University of Otago.

Thyroid overactivity results in the secretion of excessive amounts of thyroid hormones into the bloodstream. As a consequence, the clinical symptoms are the exaggerated effects of thyroid hormones on peripheral tissues. The basal metabolic rate increases and the effects of some other hormones — notably adrenaline — are potentiated. The symptoms include persistent weight loss despite a healthy appetite, sweating, hand tremor, and often a GOITRE. The patient is agitated, fatigues easily, and is intolerant of heat. Adrenaline potentiation is most seriously manifested by atrial fibrillation (a fast, irregular heartbeat). Some symptoms are additionally indicative of an autoimmune origin of the hyperthyroidism — Graves' disease. These include eye signs, which range from protruding eyes (*exophthalmos*) to — in very rare cases — optic nerve compression with loss of vision. There can also be a characteristic thickening of the skin over the lower legs and on the tops of the feet or big toes. If there is a goitre, it is a diffuse enlargement and an isotope scan shows that the entire gland is uniformly overactive.

A hyperthyroid patient may be rendered *euthyroid* (hormone levels within normal limits) with antithyroid drugs, for example carbimazole, which inhibit the biosynthesis of thyroid hormones. After treatment for 12–18 months, spontaneous remissions occur in about half the patients with Graves' disease, so that if the antithyroid drugs are withdrawn the symptoms do not recur. This is typical of the 'waxing and waning' of some autoimmune conditions, and remissions were described without specific treatment in the early nineteenth-century reports. By contrast, spontaneous remission will not occur in patients suffering from hyperthyroidism of non-autoimmune origin. If remission is not achieved, long-term treatment usually requires partial or total elimination of the thyroid. This is achieved either by the use of radioiodine or by surgical removal (thyroidectomy).　　N. J. MARSHALL

See also GOITRE; HORMONES; HYPOTHYROIDISM; THYROID.

Hyperventilation The ventilation of the LUNGS is the volume of air breathed in (and out) per minute. Hyperventilation means that this volume is excessive, such that CARBON DIOXIDE is lost from the lungs at a greater rate than it is being produced by metabolism in the body.

The term 'hyperventilation' does not apply to the increases in BREATHING that meet appropriately the varying demands of movement, work, and exercise. In the alveoli, in the depths of the lungs, when breathing changes involuntarily to meet these needs, there is very little change in the average concentrations of OXYGEN and of carbon dioxide. These concentrations are such that the blood, after exposure to them, leaves the lungs with its oxygen topped up to full saturation (however much has been removed during circulation around the body) and its carbon dioxide reduced to the concentration which is normal for arterial blood (however much has been added).

Now, deliberately, take a few extra deep breaths: in the lung alveoli the concentration of oxygen is immediately increased, and that of carbon dioxide decreased. This cannot load more oxygen into the blood, because the oxygen concentration in the lungs was already sufficient to saturate the oxygen-carrying capacity of its HAEMOGLOBIN. However, what this over-breathing can and does do, very readily, is to remove more carbon dioxide. Then there is less of it in the blood leaving the lungs, and hence less in the arterial blood; and after a few more deep breaths, less everywhere in the body, because carbon dioxide diffuses readily in and out of body fluids and cells. But if attention is now diverted from breathing, any small decrease which has been imposed on the carbon dioxide level in the blood will have been detected by the chemoreceptors, leading to a reflex decrease in breathing which rapidly restores the blood carbon dioxide to its normal level.

What, then, happens if hyperventilation — deliberate over-breathing — is continued? The 'wash-out' of carbon dioxide progresses, from the lungs, and hence from the blood, and from the body tissues including, importantly, the brain. Carbon dioxide is a crucial variable in ACID–BASE HOMEOSTASIS; its reduction shifts the body fluids towards greater alkalinity (increased pH) and this has further knock-on effects. For one thing, it tends to cause constriction of some blood vessels, particularly those in the brain, reducing its blood supply and

therefore its oxygen supply. So, in what might seem the midst of plenty when an excess of air is being shifted in and out of the lungs, the brain can actually be short of oxygen. It is for this reason that persistent, vigorous over-breathing soon makes us feel faint and dizzy. Another result of the alkalinization of the blood may be TETANY: an uncontrollable twitching (caused by neuromuscular over-excitability consequent upon an increase in the binding of calcium ions to proteins in the plasma).

All of this implies that the measureable criterion of hyperventilation is lower-than-normal carbon dioxide in the blood. (This is usually expressed as the 'PCO$_2$', representing the partial pressure of carbon dioxide gas with which a sample of blood would be in equilibrium.) In most circumstances, in healthy people, the involuntary breathing control mechanisms keep the PCO$_2$ in arterial blood at the normal level, or bring it quickly back to that level following any disturbance.

There are, however, circumstances when other vital physiological adjustments take precedence over maintaining the normality of the arterial blood carbon dioxide. In these instances the body's reflex control of breathing itself results in hyperventilation. One of these circumstances is *high-altitude* HYPOXIA. When the pressure of oxygen in the inhaled air is too low to saturate the haemoglobin in the blood, an increase in breathing gains a little higher concentration of oxygen in the lungs, at the expense of decreasing the carbon dioxide. Some resulting disturbance of acid–base balance can be tolerated, and compensated for if exposure is prolonged. A second circumstance is an increase in blood acidity, such as occurs due to production of lactic acid in strenuous exercise, or of other acids in starvation. This disturbance is countered by reflex hyperventilation, causing a shift back in the alkaline direction by washing out carbon dioxide.

Short-term, minor degrees of hyperventilation can occur without conscious intention as an aspect of ANXIETY: adrenaline and other components of the stress response can also stimulate breathing. Airplane pilots, for example, have been reported to hyperventilate during landing procedure, and it is a common experience to be aware of overbreathing in some demanding situations. More seriously, full-blown 'panic attacks' are likely to be accompanied, and aggravated, and some would say caused, by hyperventilation.

There has been considerable medical interest, research, and some controversy in recent decades concerning the so-called *hyperventilation syndrome(s)*. Certainly some people hyperventilate habitually, for reasons that are usually unclear, but that have been linked to PSYCHOLOGICAL DISORDERS. A wide variety of mental and physical symptoms have been attributed to such hyperventilation and its consequences, simulating other medical conditions, and even surgical emergencies. Improvement of health and well-being can follow a training regime to bring the breathing pattern back to normal.

Deliberate hyperventilation before breath-holding can extend the time before the breaking point at which the urge to breathe can be resisted no longer. It seems obvious that this is to be expected, simply because the more oxygen has been taken into the lungs the longer it will last. But it is not as simple as that, and the complexities are relevant to the potentially dangerous situation of over-breathing before diving or swimming underwater. The predominant factor that ends a breath-hold, by causing an overpowering drive to breathe, is a certain trigger level reached by the rising carbon dioxide; after overbreathing it takes longer to reach this trigger, because the starting level was lowered. But the overbreathing has *not* stored extra oxygen in the blood, so that it now has a longer time in which to go on being depleted. The result can be faintness or even unconsciousness, before the swimmer feels the need to surface. Although the progressive oxygen depletion itself also contributes to the drive to breathe in this situation, those individuals whose reflex response to oxygen lack is relatively insensitive may be at risk.

SHEILA JENNETT

See also BREATHING; CARBON DIOXIDE; CHEMORECEPTORS; DIVING; LUNGS; OXYGEN.

Hypnosis as commonly conceived, is a sleep-like state, induced by monotonous stimulation and repetitive suggestions, in which the subject becomes abnormally responsive to suggestions (including therapeutic ones), and may display novel or enhanced abilities. The concept evolved from the 'animal magnetic' or 'mesmeric' movement of the period 1780–1850. Franz Anton Mesmer (1734–1815), a Viennese physician, studied the supposed healing properties of magnets, but eventually concluded that the healing effects could be equally well induced by application of the operator's hands. He developed a theory that maintenance of healthy function requires the circulation round the body, particularly the nerves, of a quasi-magnetic fluid, 'animal magnetism'. Any disturbance to this circulation is harmful, and causes disease, but can be corrected if a healthy operator 'magnetizes' the patient by making 'passes' with the hands over his body. Having fallen out with the Vienna medical faculty, Mesmer came to Paris in 1778 and established a highly successful clinic, where he treated all kinds of ailments (not just 'mental' ones).

The 'mesmeric passes' sometimes had side-effects, for instance CONVULSIONS or SLEEP. One of Mesmer's pupils, the Marquis de Puységur (1751–1825) discovered that certain subjects would pass through a sleep-like state into a state of 'somnambulism' (later called 'trance' or 'sleep-waking'). 'Somnambulic' subjects might converse with the operator; diagnose and prescribe for their own ailments or those of others; have visions of distant persons, places, and scenes; show enhanced powers of memory; and carry out prescribed actions, including postdated ones. Afterwards they would remember nothing of this until again put into the somnambulic state.

There were thus two therapeutic methods at the animal magnetists' disposal: the 'mesmeric passes', and the diagnoses and recommendations offered by magnetic somnambules. In the early nineteenth century these practices, and the associated theory of 'ANIMAL MAGNETISM', spread widely across Europe, and by the 1840s they had established themselves in Britain and the US. The movement reached its peak in the late 1840s when public attention was caught by numerous reports of major surgical operations carried out painlessly on patients put into a sleep-like state by mesmeric procedures.

Magnetic practitioners were mostly well-intentioned individuals, and sometimes medically qualified (though the medical profession was generally hostile). But there also appeared numerous public demonstrators who would put on mesmeric shows for the entertainment of large audiences. These popular demonstrators played a significant part in transforming the 'mesmeric' movement of the first half of the nineteenth century into the more respectable 'hypnotic' movement of the second. For a scientist or medical man might sometimes attend a public demonstration, and realize that, however implausible the fluidic theory, the phenomena required investigation and explanation. Among persons whose interest was thus aroused were James Braid (1795–1860), a Manchester physician, who introduced the word 'hypnotism', and Charles Richet (1850–1935), the French physiologist and Nobel Prize winner. Both influenced the hypnotic school which developed in the late 1870s at the *Salpêtrière* in Paris, under the leadership of J. M. Charcot (1825–93), the neurologist. Charcot held that fully-fledged hypnosis is a pathological state with physiologically definable stages initiated by specific physical stimuli. This view was undermined in the middle 1880s by the 'Nancy School' of hypnotists under A. A. Liébeault (1823–1904) and H. Bernheim (1840–1919), whose work brought about a widespread, though incomplete, convergence of opinion among interested scientists and medical men. The key term was 'suggestion'. Hypnosis is a state of partial sleep induced by repetitive sleep suggestions. Mesmeric passes in their setting constituted such suggestions, but sleep and other suggestions can more conveniently be given verbally. Part of the otherwise sleeping brain remains alert to the voice and commands of the hypnotist. Through this channel, ideas instilled by the hypnotist can take root and may develop with great rapidity and force owing to the quiescence of potentially competing brain systems. Hence 'good' subjects may be made to hallucinate, to obey commands automatically, to playact or regress to childhood, to remember some things and forget others, to block out pain, and to display transiently enhanced mental or even physiological powers. Neurotic disorders, which arise from self-suggestions, can be treated by countervailing suggestions, and sometimes physical disorders can be indirectly helped.

Views of these kinds, with their roots mainly in clinical observation and practice, held sway with many variations and some dissentients well into the twentieth century. But thereafter non-clinical influences became increasingly prominent. Experimental psychologists emphasized methodological problems. Many have questioned whether there is any 'special state' of hypnosis. No generally agreed objective markers of such a state (such as a certain EEG pattern) have been uncovered, and 'hypnotic' phenomena, it is claimed, can often be obtained with unhypnotized subjects when their motivational level and degree of 'imaginative involvement' are appropriately manipulated. Dispute continues. Methodological questions have also been raised over the supposed benefits of hypnotherapy. Few studies of the outcome of such therapy have utilized matched control groups or have correlated therapeutic success with patients' ratings on scales of hypnotic susceptibility. Thus, even when hypnotherapy is apparently successful, it often remains unclear what part has been played by the hypnotic procedures as such, though it does seem that they may particularly benefit certain psychosomatic disorders.

The methodological arguments have been linked to a multiplication of theoretical positions. The 'neodissociationist' view of Ernest Hilgard (b. 1904), which explains hypnotic phenomena in terms of the partly autonomous functioning of 'cognitive control systems' in the brain, has some dedicated followers, as does the 'socio-cognitive' school of Nicholas Spanos (1942–94), which holds that 'hypnotized' subjects use 'cognitive strategies' to enact the social role of 'good hypnotic subject'. However, many theorists present not so much a unitary theory of hypnosis as a multipronged approach to the phenomena traditionally labelled 'hypnotic'.

Meanwhile many hypnotherapists adhere to older paradigms (which patients can easily grasp), and continue to practice with little regard to recent methodological and theoretical arguments; but in this respect hypnotherapy is perhaps little different from other forms of psychotherapy.   A. GAULD

Further reading

Forrest, D. (1999). *The Evolution of Hypnotism.* Black Ace Books, Forfar.

Gauld, A. (1992). *A History of Hypnotism.* Cambridge University Press, Cambridge.

Hypochondria is a condition in which a person believes that he or she is ill when no objective signs of illness can be observed. It has an obsessive as well as a delusional component. Sufferers from hypochondria, or, to use the clinical term, *hypochondriasis*, remain convinced that they are ill despite reassurances, and often present themselves to their doctors over a long period of time as suffering from a series of different symptoms and diseases. The onset of hypochondria is frequently in the 30s in men and 40s in women. Those in sedentary occupations are notoriously liable to it, and, whilst medical students usually suffer only a transient bout of hypochondria, some doctors remain hypochondriacal throughout their career. Depression and alcoholism exacerbate the condition.

Originally hypochondria meant an illness of the organs lying immediately under the ribs and on each side of the stomach: the liver, gall bladder, and spleen. By the sixteenth century hypochondria had become an aspect of *melancholy* and was associated especially with the humour of black bile and with the spleen, the organ that was supposed to clear black bile from the body. A variety of somatic and psychological states were subsumed under hypochondria, and its modern sense was prominent. As Robert Burton pointed out in the *Anatomy of Melancholy* (1621), the belief in imaginary illness was an important aspect of melancholy; he wrote that the imagination could produce real illness, to the extent that fear of plague might lead to actual plague and death. In the next century George Cheyne in his *The English Malady* (1733), or the 'spleen', wrote that the vapours and hysterical and hypochondriacal disorders (the last two had overlapping meanings) were characteristic of the English upper and middle classes, and were brought on by the nation's prosperity and peculiar climate. However, even though hypochondria was a fashionable disorder in the eighteenth century, it had a strong stigma attached to it, and this has continued up to the present day.

Hypochondria today lies in the domain of psychology and psychiatry. It is a label that is largely unproblematic to everyone except the sufferer. But in some instances it has been used to hide medical ignorance. In the nineteenth century many sufferers from *multiple sclerosis* were diagnosed as hypochondriacal, and it was not until the discovery of signs such as Babinski's sign, in which an abnormal reflex of the great toe is elicited, that objective evidence supported what in the early stages of the disease are often subjective sensations such as paraesthesia (sometimes described as 'pins and needles'). It is possible that another instance of blaming the patient for medicine's lack of knowledge is *chronic fatigue syndrome*, which at present has few physical signs associated with it. The dispute between those clinicians who seek to give it organic causes and the psychologists who view it as a mix of depression and hypochondria is evidence that the diagnosis of hypochondria is not always unproblematic.   A. WEAR

Hypoglycaemia An abnormally low concentration of glucose in the blood. With regular meals, and despite an overnight fast, the level does not normally drop at any time below its range of 3.5–5.5 mmol/litre. Healthy people become hypoglycaemic only after a more prolonged fast, or heavy exercise without adequate intake. Severe hypoglycaemia can occur in people with DIABETES whose insulin dosage has been excessive relative to food intake. Because the brain depends exclusively on glucose for its metabolism, they may lose consciousness in *hypoglycaemic coma*, but wake up rapidly if glucose is infused into a vein.   S.J.

See BLOOD SUGAR; INSULIN.

Hypotension

A low arterial BLOOD PRESSURE. The range of blood pressure in health is quite wide, and the term hypotension is not applied simply to an individual whose blood pressure is habitually at the low end of the normal range (say, 110/60 mm Hg). Rather, it refers to some abnormal situation when the blood pressure falls, such as in FAINTING, after serious HAEMORRHAGE, in HEART FAILURE, or in SHOCK. *Postural hypotension* refers to a fall in blood pressure on standing up. Significant hypotension is that which deprives the brain of an adequate blood supply. The brain 'defends itself' against this by widening its blood vessels, but a profound fall in blood pressure (below about 70/40 mm Hg) is beyond the limit of this compensation, and consciousness is lost.   S.J.

See BLOOD CIRCULATION; BLOOD PRESSURE.

Hypothalamus

Although small, this is one of the most important parts of the GREY MATTER of the BRAIN, for it participates in a number of vital activities. It regulates a variety of hormonal functions by action on the PITUITARY GLAND, and it exerts magisterial control over the blood vessels and glands of the body via the AUTONOMIC NERVOUS SYSTEM. It is an integral part of the LIMBIC SYSTEM, which influences important aspects of our behaviour and even our very survival, regulating such functions as emotion, sexual and nutritional appetites, rhythms, and SLEEP cycles. Some cells of the hypothalamus detect changes in body temperature and chemistry, and participate directly in the control of our temperature and chemical balance.

The hypothalamus, as its name implies, is situated below the THALAMUS — a huge collection of nuclei in the centre of the cerebral hemispheres. It forms part of the walls and floor of the central chamber of the CEREBRAL VENTRICLES, called the *third ventricle*. Hanging on a stalk underneath the hypothalamus is the pituitary gland.

The hypothalamus receives many important sensory inputs, which include information from all the major senses, but especially from the TASTE AND SMELL receptors and from the viscera. It consists of a number of distinct nerve cell clusters or *nuclei*. The tiny *suprachiasmatic nucleus* receives axons directly from the *optic nerve*, carrying information from the eye, which is used to regulate sleep and other bodily rhythms. This nucleus controls a sympathetic pathway to the pineal gland, which plays its part in the 'biological clock' by secreting *melatonin* in amounts that vary with the time of day. This in turn affects a variety of body processes.

Our internal BODY CLOCK plays a large part in determining our cycles of sleeping and waking. The connection from the EYES to the suprachiasmatic nucleus is thought to reset the clock each day and hence to keep it locked to the periodicity of the world. If the clock could not be altered (albeit with some difficulty and delay) it would be impossible to adapt to night work or to overcome 'jet lag', which afflicts us when we fly to other time zones. Visual input to the hypothalamus also seems to play a part in determining mood. The continuous absence of natural light during the winter months at extreme latitudes can precipitate depression. This condition, which is called *Seasonal Affective Disorder*, can sometimes be reversed simply by exposing the sufferer to a high-intensity, full-spectrum light for a period of time each day.

Parts of the thalamus, and the frontal lobes of the CEREBRAL CORTEX that are important in controlling mood, also connect to the hypothalamus. Disturbances in these pathways are thought to result in abnormal affective (emotional) behaviour; some of the symptoms of schizophrenia may be related to this system. Axons of neurons in the hippocampus (a specialized part of the cerebral cortex involved in conscious memory) run in a tract called the *fornix*, which ends on neurons in the *mammillary bodies* of the hypothalamus. They then send axons to the thalamus. This circuit, crucially important for linking emotions to events in the outside world, is part of the limbic system.

Many nerve cells in the hypothalamus have a so-called '*neuroendocrine*' function — instead of producing transmitter substances that simply communicate directly with other neurons, they secrete chemicals that act as HORMONES, circulating in the blood and affecting other parts of the body. In the front part of the hypothalamus lie the *supraoptic* and *paraventricular nuclei*, which send axons down through the stalk of the pituitary gland and into its posterior lobe, called the '*neurohypophysis*'. These nerve fibres end in large swellings that release into the bloodstream the hormones OXYTOCIN (which causes contraction of smooth muscle in the uterus and breast) and *vasopression* or *antidiuretic hormone* (which makes blood vessels constrict and controls the salt balance of the body by reducing the loss of water in the urine). The disease *diabetes insipidus*, in which there is excessive production of urine, is due to damage to the vasopressin system.

Other neuroendocrine parts of the hypothalamus secrete specialized hormones, called '*releasing factors*', into the blood of small capillary vessels (called the *hypophysial portal system*), which run down into the anterior lobe of the pituitary gland, where they stimulate specialized cells to secrete other hormones that pass into the general circulation and affect remote organs. These include GROWTH HORMONE (which regulates growth), *prolactin* (which controls milk production in the breast), and *follicle stimulating hormone* (which acts on the ovaries). Two of the hormones of the anterior pituitary act on yet other endocrine glands: adrenocorticotrophic hormone stimulates the ADRENAL GLAND and *thyrotrophin* the THYROID. In these cases, the 'cascade' of chemicals (releasing factor, to anterior pituitary hormone, to target endocrine gland) amplifies the effect of the initial signal in the hypothalamus.

The great Oxford neurophysiologist Sir Charles Sherrington called the hypothalamus the 'head ganglion of the autonomic nervous system'. Anterior parts of the hypothalamus excite *parasympathetic* functions such as constriction of the pupils of the eye, stimulation of the gastrointestinal tract, salivation, and respiratory and cardiac depression. The posterior hypothalamus brings on sympathetic activity, such as dilatation of the pupils, inhibition of gastrointestinal function and salivation, and increased respiration, heart rate, and blood pressure. These effects are produced by fibres projecting from the hypothalamus to parasympathetic nuclei in the BRAIN STEM, and to sympathetic centres in the SPINAL CORD.   LAURENCE GAREY

See also AUTONOMIC NERVOUS SYSTEM; BODY CLOCK; BRAIN; THALAMUS.

PLATE 6.

Hypothermia

has been reported during marathons, on the mountains, in caving and canoeing, at work on land and at sea, and in and under water. It may occur, even during the summer, among the elderly and the very young, in the operating theatre, and in association with some medical disorders. Geographically hypothermia has in fact been recorded from most parts of the world even at low altitudes in the Sahara and from tropical Kampala.

Thermally the body can be divided into zones. The temperature of the 'core', including the vital organs, heart, and brain, is kept stable over a surprising range of environmental conditions. The 'shell' is superficial, and its size and temperature varies considerably. Hypothermia is defined as a core temperature below 35°C. However, hypothermia is not a diagnosis, but a sign that changes must have occurred in the body, which vary with the circumstances which have led to cooling. During COLD EXPOSURE the body 'burns' carbohydrate to generate heat and the amount of fuel left depends on the rate of cooling. Also fluid is lost through increased urine output, and there are complex movements of fluids in the body, related in magnitude to the duration of exposure to cold, which reverse during rewarming. There are therefore different types of hypothermia.

(i) In '*immersion*' *hypothermia* the cold stress is so great that the body's heat-generating capacity is overwhelmed and the core temperature is forced down. Because energy reserves are available, the person will have very little difficulty in rewarming once removed from the severe environment. Falling into cold water is the commonest accidental cause, and hypothermia deliberately induced for medical reasons is of this type.

(ii) In *'exhaustion' hypothermia* the body maintains the temperature until energy sources are exhausted. Then, since the heat-generating ability is reduced, even relatively mild cold exposure may cause continued cooling. Thermal protection must therefore take account of every avenue of heat loss, because even small variations of available heat may make the difference between life and death. This is the type most commonly found in mountaineers or hill walkers.

(iii) With *'urban' hypothermia*, the cold has been mild but prolonged. The core temperature remains normal (35°C or above) possibly for days or weeks, with massive fluid shifts. The temperature eventually drifts down, or faster cooling is precipitated by some other factor such as a fall. This is the most usual type found in the elderly or in association with malnutrition.

(iv) *'Submersion' hypothermia* occurs in people who have been totally submerged in very cold water. Recovery has been known even after 15–60 min (typical submersion survival is about 3 min). Survival, more likely in children, depends on resuscitation being started immediately on rescue.

The case history distinguishes the different types, though they may overlap. A climber in a snowstorm disabled by a broken leg will cool as rapidly as if immersed, because the shock of the injury increases the rate of heat loss, and the fracture prevents heat generation from voluntary activity or shivering. A deep diver may suffer 'immersion' hypothermia, even in a dry pressure chamber, because of the tremendous heat transfer capacity of the compressed oxyhelium gas mixture which he is breathing. A swimmer lost overboard in relatively warm water is a candidate for 'exhaustion' hypothermia. A middle-aged man or a child with severe malnutrition is likely to develop 'urban' hypothermia, whereas a fit 70-year-old out walking in the hills would be liable to 'exhaustion' hypothermia.

When a person is in a situation where hypothermia is imminent there is a great temptation to continue to move in order both to keep generating heat from the activity and to escape the situation. This may not be the best option for survival, since the activity increases the rate of heat loss and aggravates exhaustion. The best prospect of SURVIVAL AT SEA is not to try to swim but to stay with a capsized boat. Similarly in the hills in bad weather the macho response of trying to battle a way out has resulted in many deaths, whereas those who 'go to ground' — taking shelter until the weather improves — usually survive.

A variety of signs and symptoms of hypothermia have been described (see table). However there is great individual variation. For example, loss of consciousness may occur at a core temperature as high as 33°C, but in one case consciousness was still present at a rectal temperature of 24.3°C, and other causes of unconsciousness may confuse the issue. Shivering is

Signs and symptoms in hypothermia

Core temperature °C	
37.6	'Normal' rectal temperature.
37	'Normal' oral temperature.
36	Increased metabolic rate to balance heat loss. Breathing and pulse faster.
35	Shivering at a maximum. Reflexes exaggerated; speech disordered; thinking slowed.
34	Usually responsive; normal blood pressure. Lower limit compatible with continued exercise.
33–31	Retrograde amnesia; consciousness clouded; blood pressure low; pupils dilated; shivering usually ceased.
30–28	Progressive loss of consciousness; increased muscular rigidity; slow pulse and respiration; irregular heart beat. Susceptible to ventricular fibrillation if heart mechanically irritated.
27	Voluntary movement lost.
26	Pupillary light reflex and deep tendon and skin reflexes lost. Victims seldom conscious.
24–21	100% mortality in shipwreck victims in World War II
20	Heart standstill.
17	No electrical activity in brain.
14.4	Lowest known accidental hypothermic patient with recovery.
9	Lowest artificially cooled hypothermic patient with recovery.
4	Monkeys revived successfully.
1–7	Rats and hamsters revived successfully.

considered to cease usually at 30°C — but shivering has been recorded at a core temperature of 24°C. At the other extreme some experimental subjects can cool without shivering and many mountain rescue cases never shiver.

Diagnosis requires measurement of core temperature, usually rectal, but since this route may not be practical in the field, the person should be treated as a 'cold casualty' if the armpit feels 'as cold as marble' to the rescuer's hand. In hypothermia the diagnosis of other accompanying conditions is difficult. Slurred speech, staggering, incoordination or a change in personality may be due to hypothermia and not necessarily brain damage. In hypothermia the REFLEXES are affected and there is stiffness of the muscles; there are changes in the electrical and mechanical functions of the heart; and the lungs may show clinical and X-ray features similar to pneumonia, though these clear on rewarming. It is therefore important that the patient should be restored to normal body temperature before any diagnosis is made or any irrevocable treatment started.

If the heart stops, the lack of circulation, and therefore of oxygen supply to the brain would ordinarily cause permanent brain damage in about three minutes. Although hypothermia can give some protection for the brain by prolonging the time before oxygen lack causes permanent damage, it is cardiac function that is most important for survival. As the heart cools it becomes more susceptible to ventricular fibrillation (VF) (an uncoordinated electrical activity of the heart which produces no actual pumping of blood). This may be triggered by mechanical irritation (which may be as mild as rolling a patient for bedmaking), by hypoxia of the heart muscle, or by rapid changes in pH or electrolytes in the blood, or in temperature gradients within the heart muscle. Inappropriate rewarming techniques add to the hazard.

Rescue and care

Profound accidental hypothermia can be very difficult to distinguish from death. The only certain diagnosis of death in hypothermia is failure to recover on rewarming. However hypothermia is seldom present in isolation. Victims may also be injured or have some illness, possibly cold-related. In water, DROWNING may precede or follow cooling. If neither heart nor breathing activity can be detected and there is evidence that the person was alive within the previous two hours, the rescuers should start RESUSCITATION, though only if this can be continued until the casualty has been rewarmed or has reached hospital: otherwise members of the rescue team will become exhausted and may then become hypothermic casualties themselves. Also, the heart may occasionally still be beating and providing some circulation, even when this cannot be detected; the mechanical effects of active resuscitation attempts may trigger ventricular fibrillation, and the patient would then be in a worse state and needing continuing resuscitation.

EVAN L. LLOYD

Further reading

Lloyd, E. L. (1986). *Hypothermia and cold stress.* Croom Helm, London.

See also COLD EXPOSURE; NEAR-DROWNING; SURVIVAL AT SEA; TEMPERATURE REGULATION.

Hypothyroidism

Hypothyroidism is due to underactivity of the thyroid gland, and results from its failure to secrete sufficient thyroid hormones into the bloodstream.

For normal function, the thyroid gland relies upon stimulation by a hormone from the pituitary gland known appropriately as thyroid stimulating hormone (TSH). Primary hypothyroidism is due to failure of the thyroid itself, whilst secondary hypothyroidism occurs when the pituitary secretes inadequate TSH. Primary hypothyroidism is the usual reason for thyroid underactivity.

There are several potential causes of primary hypothyroidism. It may for example be due to insufficient intake of iodine in the diet, since iodine is an essential constituent of thyroid hormones. This is a major health problem in many regions of the underdeveloped world and ranks first as a global cause of thyroid deficiency. In contrast, congenital hypothyroidism is due to a rare failure of the thyroid gland to develop during fetal life. Another infrequent cause of hypothyroidism is a failure in the complex biosynthetic pathway which leads to the secretion of its hormones by the thyroid gland (thyroid dyshormonogenesis). But if there is sufficient dietary iodine, the most common cause of hypothyroidism is autoimmune destruction of the cells which make up the basic functional unit of the thyroid gland — namely, the thyroid follicle. The thyroid gland is particularly prone to autoimmune disorders. Thus in *Hashimoto's thyroiditis*, which in the UK afflicts about 1 in 10 women, but only 1 in 100 men, there is progressive hypothyroidism with declining secretion of thyroid hormones. The thyroid is gradually infiltrated by lymphocytes and the follicular architecture of the gland breaks down. At the same time, the overall mass of the gland can increase, and if untreated a large multinodular goitre sometimes develops. Hashimoto's thyroiditis is named after the Japanese surgeon who gave the first clear description of the condition in 1912. In 1956 it was demonstrated by Doniach, Roitt, and Campbell in London that Hashimoto's thyroiditis is further characterized by the presence in the circulating blood of thyroid autoantibodies (anti-thyroglobulin and anti-thyroid peroxidase).

Most of the symptoms of hypothyroidism in adults are the result of lowered cellular metabolism, due to the inadequate output of thyroid hormones. Typically, the patient feels cold, lethargic, and depressed. There is often weight gain, a puffy appearance (*myxoedema*), dry hair, and maybe a goitre. The pulse tends to be slow, cardiac output is reduced, and in women (the majority of sufferers) there may be menstrual irregularities. In children, since thyroid hormones are required for growth, there is stunted growth along with lethargy and obesity. One of the particular problems of this condition is that because hypothyroidism develops slowly these symptoms are insidious; they can go unnoticed or be wrongly attributed, for example, to the menopause or to natural ageing.

Inadequacy of thyroid hormones is particularly serious for the fetus, because they are required for the development of the nervous system *in utero*. In iodine-deficient regions of the world, this leads to the birth of neurological cretins, who have suffered major and irreversible damage to their central nervous system. It is estimated that, even in these days, 100 000 such cretins are born each year. In contrast, the incidence of neonatal hypothyroidism in iodine-replete Western society — a condition often referred to as 'sporadic cretinism' — is about 1 in 4000 live births; this is due to failure of the fetal thyroid to develop. This congenital hypothyroidism, unlike the neurological cretin, is amenable to treatment with thyroid hormones.

Hypothyroidism can readily be treated by oral thyroxine, which is one of the two hormones synthesized by the thyroid gland. This was first demonstrated by George Murray, a physician in Hartlepool. In 1891 he reported to the Newcastle Medical Research Society the beneficial effects of administering extracts of sheep thyroids to his profoundly hypothyroid patients. This was the first example of hormone replacement therapy.

N. J. MARSHALL

See also GOITRE; HORMONES; THYROID.

Hypoxia

Hypoxia means a shortage of OXYGEN — as compared to *anoxia*, which means a total lack of it. In common with other mammals, humans have evolved with a system of BREATHING and BLOOD CIRCULATION, which allows intake of oxygen from the air and its transport throughout the body. The tissues need to extract oxygen from the blood constantly at a basic rate for their METABOLISM, along with the extra needed for work and exercise, and also are accustomed to a certain level of oxygen in their immediate environment. The body can compensate to some extent for a decreased *level*, but life depends on maintainence of the *supply* of oxygen. Different organs and tissues can survive lack of oxygen for different lengths of time: the brain is the most rapidly and irrevocably damaged. Because the brain regulates breathing and the circulation — the means by which oxygen is supplied to the whole body, including itself — deprivation of the brain prevents restoration of the supply; a potentially lethal vicious circle.

Hypoxia occurs (i) when there is less than the normal amount of oxygen in the air inhaled; (ii) when BREATHING is obstructed, is inadequate, or stops; (iii) when oxygen is not transferred normally from the lungs to the blood; (iv) when the blood cannot carry its normal quota of oxygen; (v) when the flow of blood is inadequate, or stops.

The air inhaled may provide insufficient oxygen either because the atmospheric pressure is low (at high ALTITUDE) or when the supply of fresh air is restricted. At high altitude the air is 'thinner' in that every molecule of the gas occupies a larger volume. The blood leaves the lungs carrying less oxygen than normal, therefore the tissues are exposed to a lower oxygen level. If this is not too profound, they can still obtain oxygen at the required rate, at least for resting metabolism, because the rate of flow of blood can increase. The tissues are living at a lower *level* but are still getting a sufficient oxygen *supply*.

When the supply of fresh air is restricted — with a bag over the head, in a closed cupboard, or in a larger enclosed space crowded with people — oxygen is progressively depleted and exhaled CARBON DIOXIDE accumulates. In some circumstances there may be displacement of air by other gases, and the effect of irritant or toxic gases, such as smoke, chlorine, or sulphur dioxide, can complicate the effects of displacement of oxygen.

Disturbance of breathing Obstruction to breathing can occur either externally (smothering, strangulation, compression of the chest in a crowd disaster) or internally (choking, allergic swelling of the upper airways, asthmatic attacks). In other less drastic ways breathing can become inadequate to keep the oxygen level up to normal, and carbon dioxide down to normal, in the lungs and blood: when breathing becomes mechanically difficult in some types of lung disease; when there is damage to the BRAIN STEM or to the upper SPINAL CORD where the nerves arise which activate the muscles of breathing; or when the muscles themselves are weak. Breathing may be depressed by drugs acting on the control centres in the brain, and it may stop entirely in collapse from various causes (CONCUSSION, NEAR-DROWNING, HEART ATTACK, electric shock).

If obstruction or cessation of breathing is total, the condition is known as *asphyxia*: it rapidly causes death by depriving the brain of oxygen. A lesser degree of inadequate breathing is called hypoventilation, characterized by a lowered level of oxygen and a raised level of carbon dioxide in the lungs, blood, and tissues; a person suffering from chronic lung disease, for example, can live for many years in a state of moderate hypoxia. The term SUFFOCATION is less precisely defined, but is commonly applied either to obstructed breathing or to lack of fresh air supply.

Oxygen transfer from the lungs to the blood can be impaired in some types of lung disease because the barrier it has to diffuse across is thickened. So despite breathing as much or more than normal, the blood and tissue oxygen level is below normal, although, again, an adequate supply may be maintained by increased blood flow. There are also conditions (including some congenital heart defects) in which the blood is not routed properly through the lungs, so that some blood bypasses the oxygen supply, with the result that arterial blood is hypoxic.

In all the types of hypoxia described so far, the HAEMOGLOBIN in the arterial blood is less than fully saturated with oxygen. The redness of blood depends on this saturation. In hypoxia it becomes more blue, and CYANOSIS is the outward and visible sign of this when blueness tinges the skin.

The oxygen-carrying capacity of the blood is lowered when red blood cells, and haemoglobin, are in short supply (ANAEMIA): the blood carries less oxygen than normal, although there is sufficient oxygen in the air and in the lungs, and all available haemoglobin is fully saturated. There are also conditions in which the haemoglobin is not all in its normal form. CARBON MONOXIDE poisoning acts by combining with haemoglobin, making it unable to carry oxygen.

Deprivation of blood flow makes organs and tissues hypoxic: the state of 'ischaemia'. This can occur either as part of whole-body deprivation in HEART FAILURE, or locally where blood vessels are obstructed by arterial disease or by clots, or constricted as in the skin in COLD EXPOSURE.

Defences against hypoxia

The body has ways to defend itself against hypoxia at each stage of the process of oxygen acquisition: by breathing harder, to get more into the lungs; by crowding more red cells into the blood so that it can carry more in every circulating millilitre; by pumping the blood around at a greater rate; and by widening the blood vessels which supply the vital organs. Most of these adjustments can be made very rapidly.

When oxygen is low — but tolerably so — in inhaled air, and hence in the blood, the arterial CHEMORECEPTORS — minute structures in the neck — sense this and, via the brain, cause a reflex increase in breathing. This brings the oxygen concentration in the lungs closer to that of the outside air — it remains low, but not as low as it would be if the breathing did not increase. Stimulation of breathing occurs more dramatically when carbon dioxide is accumulating in the blood whilst oxygen is decreasing, such as in the example of breathing in a confined space.

If hypoxia of a tolerable degree is sustained for weeks, the bone marrow produces extra red blood cells, resulting in *polycythaemia*. The greater density of red cells brings the oxygen concentration in the blood back towards normal despite their haemoglobin carrying less than it ideally could. The down side is that the thicker blood gives extra work to the pumping heart. This defence mechanism cannot of course operate against anaemia, when the fault itself lies in a deficient production of red blood cells.

The heart compensates for hypoxia by pumping out more blood per minute so that the actual delivery rate of oxygen to the tissues can be kept up despite its lower concentration in the blood.

These automatic attempts at self-preservation operate unless the oxygen lack becomes too profound to sustain brain functions, including that of maintaining breathing itself. At worst, the heart weakens, the blood pressure falls, breathing stops, and cessation of the heartbeat soon follows.   SHEILA JENNETT

See also ALTITUDE; BREATHING; CYANOSIS; LUNGS; OXYGEN; SUFFOCATION.

Hysterectomy is the term used to describe an operation involving the removal of the UTERUS. This normally involves excision of the body of the uterus and the cervix (*total hysterectomy*). Occasionally just the body of the uterus is removed, leaving the cervix (*subtotal hysterectomy*). The OVARIES and FALLOPIAN TUBES may also removed during a hysterectomy (total hysterectomy with *bilateral salpingoopherectomy).*

Hysterectomy was first described in the fifth century BC when Soranus of Ephesus is said to have amputated a gangenous uterus through the vagina. Vaginal hysterectomy was reported in the medical literature sporadically over the next 2000 years. Perhaps the most famous of these was Faith Howard, who in around 1670 amputated her own uterus which repeatedly prolapsed out of her vagina. Not only did she survive this, but she went on to live for several years afterwards, despite having rendered herself incontinent from a hole in her bladder.

This operation was first established as acceptable practice in Britain by Isaac Baker Brown and Spencer Wells, surgeons working in London in the late nineteenth century. At this time vaginal surgery was considered the safest way for the operation to be performed, since abdominal surgery had a very high mortality rate and was to be avoided wherever possible. Abdominal hysterectomy was first described by Charles Clay in Manchester in 1843, when a massive fibroid uterus was mistaken for an ovarian tumour and an abdominal incision had already been made. Unfortunately this patient died, and it was another 10 years before a woman successfully survived this operation.

The advent of antiseptics and anaesthetics meant that abdominal surgery began to become safer, and the abdominal hysterectomy was established in the latter part of the nineteenth century, principally through Lawson Tait, Scottish gynaecologist working in Birmingham. In 1884 Tait published his series of 1000 abdominal operations including 54 hysterectomies, the first such report in the medical literature. Subsequently this has become the most frequently used route for this procedure, as it allows easier access, especially if the uterus is enlarged. Today the most common form of abdominal hysterectomy is performed through a transverse cut in the lower abdominal wall (bikini line incision). This approach allows easy removal of the ovaries, which is not always possible vaginally.

Vaginal hysterectomy is still used in around 1 in 5 hysterectomies in the UK, and allows a quicker recovery. This operation is usually preferred for prolapse or heavy periods where removal of the ovaries is not essential and the uterus is of normal size (although some surgeons will remove some enlarged wombs vaginally).

Hysterectomies are performed for a variety of benign (non-cancerous) conditions, most commonly including heavy, painful periods and prolapse of the uterus. The painful, heavy periods can be caused by a variety of conditions including endometriosis, fibroids, chronic pelvic infections,

and adhesions. A hysterectomy may also be advised when a woman has an ovarian cyst or where she has precancerous changes to the cervix that have not resolved with simple treatments.

A more radical type of abdominal hysterectomy, called a Wertheim's hysterectomy, is used to treat women with cancer of the cervix. (It was named after the Austrian gynaecologist who pioneered it in 1900.) This operation allows the wider removal of the tissue either side of the uterus and the removal of lymph nodes to check whether the cancer has spread. Hysterectomy is also used in the treatment of cancer of the uterus or ovary.

Over the last 20 years interest has grown in minimal access or 'keyhole' surgery. This led Dr Reich, a gynaecologist in Pennsylvania, to perform the first laparoscopic hysterectomy in 1989. This operation allows the easier removal of the ovaries vaginally at the time of the hysterectomy and the removal of a larger uterus vaginally. Total and subtotal laparoscopic hysterectomies have also been described, although none of these are commonly performed at the present time.

PHILIP TOOZS–HOBSON

LINDA CARDOZO

Hysteria Since the rise of the so-called '*psychodynamic psychiatries*' early in the twentieth century, hysteria has been regarded as a psychological malady *par excellence*. Through most of its long medical history, however, the concept was interpreted as a disorder purely of the body, with specific causes, symptoms, and treatments that were organic.

The modern English word 'hysteria' derives from the Greek '*hystera*' — uterus — which in turn derives from the Sanskrit word for stomach or belly. Inherent in these simple etymological facts is the meaning of the earliest views on the nature and origin of the disease. According to some historians, an Egyptian medical papyrus dating from around 1990 BC — one of the oldest surviving documents known to medical history — records a series of curious behavioural disturbances in adult women. As the ancient Egyptians interpreted it, the cause of these abnormalities was the movement of the uterus, which they believed to be an autonomous, free-floating organism that could move upward from its normal pelvic position. Such a dislocation, they reasoned, applied pressure on the diaphragm and gave rise to bizarre physical and mental symptoms. Egyptian doctors developed an array of medications to entice the errant womb back down into its correct position. Foremost among these measures were the vulvar placement of aromatic substances to draw the womb downward, and swallowing foul-tasting substances to repel the uterus away from the upper parts.

Hysteria in ancient history

This ancient Middle Eastern source furnished the basis for classical Greek medical and philosophical theories of hysteria. The ancient Greeks adopted the notion of the migratory uterus and embroidered upon the connections between hysteria and sexual dissatisfaction. In an often-cited passage in the *Timaeus*, Plato wrote colourfully about the vagaries of female reproductive physiology:

> 'the animal within them [women] is desirous of procreating children, and when remaining unfruitful long beyond its proper time, gets discontented and angry, and wandering in every direction through the body, closes up the passages of the breath, and by obstructing respiration, drives them to extremity, causing all varieties of disease . . .'

Various texts of the school of Hippocrates, from the fifth century BC onward, explain similarly that a mature women's deprivation of sexual relations causes a restless womb to move upward in search of gratification. As the female reproductive parts move or function irregularly — ascending or descending, convulsing or prolapsing — they cause dizziness, motor paralyses, sensory losses, and respiratory distress (including *globus hystericus*, the sensation of a ball lodged in the throat) as well as extravagant emotional behaviours. Ancient Greek therapies included uterine fumigations, the application of tight abdominal bandages, and a regular regimen of marital *fornicatio*.

Traditional historical accounts of the disease observe that ancient Roman physicians, too, wrote about hysteria. With the growth of anatomical knowledge, the literal hypothesis of the morbidly wandering womb became increasingly untenable. However, Roman medical authors continued to associate hysteria exclusively with the female generative system. The principal causes of hysterical disorders, they conjectured, were 'diseases of the womb' and disruptions of female reproductive biology, including amenorrhea, miscarriage, premature births, and menopause. GALEN of Pergamon formulated a particularly popular theory tracing the origins of the malady to the retention of excessive menstrual blood. Engraved in the *Corpus Hippocraticum* and the Galenic writings, these hypotheses formed a medical ideology that remained influential for millennia of medical history. Descriptive and theoretical details evolved, but the basic doctrine of *gynaecological determinism* — the crux of the classical heritage in the history of hysteria — endured until remarkably late into the modern medical period.

Christian attitudes

The coming of Christian civilization in the Latin West initiated a major paradigm shift in the history of hysteria. From the fifth to the thirteenth centuries, naturalistic pagan construals of the disease were increasingly displaced by supernatural formulations. In the writings of St Augustine, human suffering, including organic and mental illness, was perceived as a manifestation of innate evil consequent upon original sin. Hysteria in particular, with its shifting and highly dramatic symptomatology, was viewed as a sign of POSSESSION by the devil. The hysterical female was now interpreted alternately as a victim of bewitchment, to be pitied, or the devil's

soulmate, to be despised. No less powerfully mythopoetic than the classical image of the disease, the demonological model envisioned the hysterical anesthesias, mutisms, and convulsions as *stigmati diaboli* or marks of the devil.

This sea change in thinking about the disorder brought with it changes in treatment. The elaborate pharmacopeia of ancient times was now replaced by supernatural invocations — prayers, incantations, amulets, and exorcisms. Furthermore, with the demonization of the diagnosis came the widespread persecution of the afflicted. During the late medieval and Renaissance periods, the scene of interrogation of the female hysteric shifted from the hospital and sick bed to the church and the court room, which now became the loci of spectacular interrogations. Official manuals for the detection of witches, often virulently misogynistic, supplied instructions for the detection, torture, and at times execution of the witch/hysteric.

Early medical theories

The late Renaissance, which witnessed the height of the WITCHCRAFT craze in continental Europe, also produced in reaction several substantial efforts to renaturalize the idea of hysteria. Advances in understanding the structure and function of the human nervous system provided a new model for many previously baffling nervous disorders, including hysteria. Gynecological and demonological theories waned; in their place, new neurocentric theories combined with fashionable mechanical and iatrochemical ideas from the physical and chemical sciences.

In Britain, which dominated medical thinking about the subject during the early modern period, the neuroanatomist *Thomas Willis* propounded a theory according to which an excess of 'animal spirits' was released from the brain and carried by the nerves to the spleen and abdomen, where it entered the bloodstream to circulate through the body. Robert Whytt thought the disorder was caused by a weakness of the nerve fibres, and *William Cullen* attributed it to a slowing of the nervous fluids through the brain. In the 1680s, the famous physician *Thomas Sydenham* hypothesized that the condition was caused by an imbalance in the distribution of the animal spirits between body and mind, brought on by sudden and violent emotions, such as anger, fear, grief, and love. English and Scottish medical literature about hysteria during the seventeenth and eighteenth centuries offers memorable clinical descriptions of classic hysterical phenomena, including the hysterical attack in the arched back position and the *clavus hystericus*, or feeling of a nail being driven into the forehead. In the 1700s in particular, in France and Britain, these ideas provided the basis for an entire 'nervous culture' in which men and women of high society fashioned themselves as refined, sensible, and civilized.

The 1800s brought a multiplication of theories about hysteria, including new uterine, neurological, and characterological models. During the final quarter of the century — hysteria's

famous heroic age — the centre of attention shifted to France. In the 1880s, the Parisian clinical neurologist Jean–Martin Charcot, formulated a comprehensive, neurogenic model of 'the great neurosis'. For Charcot, hysteria was strictly a dysfunction of the central nervous system, akin to epilepsy, syphilis, and other neurological diseases. Like these ailments, hysterical neuropathy, he held, was the result of a lesion of an undetermined structural or functional nature that could be studied through the methods of pathological anatomy and that resulted from defective heredity. Charcot lavished his attention on the descriptive neurosymptomatology of his cases. He developed a schematized, four-stage model of the hysterical fit, and he mapped a series of 'hysterogenic zones' onto the body of the hysteric.

Emergence of psychology

Socially, the late nineteenth century witnessed the appearance of 'the Victorian nervous invalid.' Significant numbers of men and women modelled their sickness behaviour on the contemporary teachings of hysteria doctors like Charcot until these nervous disorders seemed to reach epidemic proportions. Culturally, the character of the nervous invalid figured prominently in fictional prose writing of the time. By the time of Charcot's death in 1893, medical thinking about hysteria had reached an impasse. The search for the missing lesion of hysteria, and therefore for its somatic basis, remained fruitless. As a consequence, physicians turned to alternative conceptualizations of these mysterious, multiform disorders, including to psychological theories.

The psychologization of the hysteria concept a century ago is associated foremostly with *Sigmund Freud*, who worked in Vienna in the late Victorian mould of the private nerve specialist. Psychoanalysis began as a theory and therapy of hysteria. In a series of essays and monographs written between 1885 and 1900, Freud radically reconceptualized hysteria. He reversed the previously projected direction of mind–body causality, claiming that hysteria was a psychological disease with quasi-physical symptoms. Furthermore, Freud placed the emphasis on the psychological mechanism of hysterical symptom formation. According to his formulation, hysterogenesis rests in the repression of traumatic memories. These memories are usually remote in the emotional past of the individual and invariably libidinal, or sexual, in content. Because these remembrances are painful or unpleasant, they are unable to find conscious psychological expression. Freud postulated further that the negative emotional energy, or 'strangulated affect', associated with these memories is then unconsciously converted into the somatic manifestations of hysteria. Moreover, in this process of hysterical *conversion*, symptoms are not arbitrary and meaningless phenomena but complex symbolizations of repressed psychological experiences. In psychoanalytic psychology, the body is the physical field on which the wishes, anxieties, and traumas of the hysteric are dramatized.

Recent trends

The most consequential development in the history of hysteria in the last century was the rapid decline in the medically recorded incidence of the disorder. In part, this diminution is due to the liberalization of gender norms, permitting freer social, emotional, and sexual expression among women. It also traces to a process whereby many symptoms and behaviours formerly constitutive of hysteria have been reassigned to other diagnostic categories, including organic disorders, psychoses, and psychoneuroses. Since the 1970s, hysteria as an independent diagnostic entity has been deleted from the official manuals of medical diagnosis. In Anglo–American psychiatry, much of what was characterized as conversion hysteria in psychodynamic psychiatry is now classified under the more scientific-sounding rubric of *somatization disorder*. An exception to this rule can be found in French medicine, which continues widely to employ the concept of hysteria in psychological theory and clinical practice.

Conclusions

Several conclusions may be drawn from hysteria's long and colourful past. First, it is most likely impossible in this instance to project a single, unchanging pathological entity through history. The clinical descriptions lumped under the heading through the ages have been highly diverse, and the theoretical structures for understanding these behaviours have varied enormously. Many different morbid phenomena have no doubt been gathered under the umbrella of 'hysteria'. Second, what has been called hysteria in the past may clearly be read as a kind of cross-gender portraiture in the field of medicine. To a very great extent, 'the history of hysteria' consists of a body of writing by men about women. Feminist-informed scholars of the later twentieth century emphasize that this literature often depicts, in the descriptive language of the clinic, features of the opposite sex that male élites in past patriarchal societies found irritating, incomprehensible, or unmanageable. Hysteria theory literally embodies these ideas, attitudes, and biases.

A third conclusion concerns the distinctive blend of science, SEXUALITY, and sensationalism in the story of hysteria. Given the extravagant physical symptoms, emotional outbursts, and erotic undercurrents involved in many cases carrying this label, it is hardly surprising that hysterics have often been forced into lurid roles and vaudevillian performances. In short, hysteria has been the vehicle for astute clinical observation, pioneering neuropathological research, and brilliant psychological theorizing; it has equally been the site of much misogyny, sensationalism, and mistreatment. Fourth and finally, hysteria's history may be read as an ongoing attempt to theorize the *mind–body relation* within the medical sciences. Is hysteria fundamentally a psychological disorder with physical manifestations; an organic disease with mental and emotional epiphenomena; or some inseparable intermixture of the two? Studying the subject through the ages has involved a continual, relational reconfiguring of the role of psyche and soma in human mental life. Within the clinical human sciences, hysteria represents the shifting and diversely theorized interface between the history of the body and the history of the mind.

Some scholars have argued that hysteria is the oldest and most important category of neurosis in recorded medical history. Similarly, perhaps no non-fatal disorder boasts a richer metaphorical and mythological past. Over the centuries and in many different cultures, thinking and writing about the subject has mirrored dominant attitudes about health and sickness, the natural and the supernatural, the sexual and the spiritual, mind and body, and masculinity and femininity. Now, it appears, hysteria — construed variously as a term, theory, and behaviour — is vanishing. Given the remarkable cultural indispensability of the concept in the past, readers can only speculate on what will take its place in the future.

M. S. MICALE

Further reading

Gilman, S. L., King, H., Porter R., Rousseau, G., and Showalter, E. (1993). *Hysteria beyond Freud.* University of California Press, Berkeley.

Micale, M. (1995). *Approaching hysteria: disease and its interpretations.* Princeton University Press, Princeton.

Veith, I. (1965). *Hysteria: the history of a disease.* University of Chicago Press, Chicago.

See also NERVOUSNESS; PSYCHOLOGICAL DISORDERS.

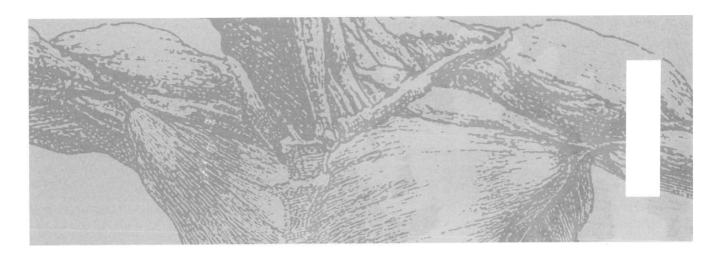

Iconography and the body

'Iconography', according to the *Oxford English Dictionary*, is a pictorial representation or description of something, a book or work in which such a representation appears, and/or the branch of knowledge which deals with such representations.

From Christian icons, through alchemical philosophy, up to the images on the British pound and the Nike 'swoosh', icons are supposed to evoke the presence and power of what they represent. Often, the distinction between the representation and the thing represented is ambiguous, particularly when the entity represented does not exist in corporeal form. Ancient Greek statues of gods, for example, were thought not only to represent, but actually to contain the deity. The representation of bodies in particular has been the subject of much recent scholarship. Influenced in part by studies in semiotics, art history, and cultural and women's studies, images of the body have come to be seen as one of the ways a society 'thinks' about those bodies and the individuals whom they represent.

Iconography as the study of representation, also called *iconology*, entered mainstream academia at the beginning of the twentieth century. This was when art historians began to analyse works of art in relation to the social and historical context in which they were produced, rather than discussing them purely in terms of transcendent aesthetic value. Before this time, iconographic studies, exemplified by Cesare Ripa's *Iconologie* (1644), consisted mainly of works listing the symbolic meaning of images from Christian and classical traditions. For instance, in early Christian art, Christ was often represented as a fish, and the Holy Spirit as a dove; in the fifteenth and sixteenth centuries, a SKULL represented the idea of mortality.

Iconography has been central to some of the oldest and most bitter conflicts in world history. Islam, for instance, forbids the graphic representation of any person, especially the Prophet Mohammed, and conservative Muslims find images of any living creature unacceptable.

Hinduism and Buddhism, in contrast, have extremely rich iconographies. The Hindu caste system, for example, is explained in reference to the body, and Hindu gods often appear in significantly altered human form; Shiva, for example, is blue and has four arms. Iconography has proved a source of controversy within Christianity, though the body of Christ, represented on the crucifix and invoked during the Catholic mass, is perhaps the most significant icon in the history of Western culture. During the Protestant Reformation the worship of icons, including saints and relics, was believed to be idolatrous.

From images on ancient Greek coins to Uncle Sam, iconography has a significant political dimension. Icons are not always meant to glorify their subject, as when the king is maligned in underground media as a representation of monarchy. That Roman emperors were depicted as gods, and Marie-Antoinette was portrayed as a harpy in the underground press during the French Revolution, are examples of how icons both reflect and form people's attitudes about the personae they represent.

Much recent scholarship on iconography and the body has focused in particular on the representation of women's bodies in Europe and the US during the eighteenth and nineteenth centuries. Supporters of democratic movements in this era frequently chose to represent their guiding principles — Justice, Liberty, Equality, etc. — in the form of female icons; entire nations came to be embodied in figures such as Marianne, Germania, Britannia, and Columbia. The irony that it was during this time, when equality itself was given female form, that women were explicitly excluded from the democratic public sphere, indicates that female icons do not, and are not intended to, represent real women. The ambiguity and potentially ironic multivalence of iconographic figures has been addressed by recent feminist scholarship, particularly with regard to these eighteenth- and nineteenth-century images. Marina Warner, for example, maintains that in Western cultures, the FEMALE FORM,

standing for both desire and chaste virtue, is perceived as generic and universal; the male form, on the other hand, is seen as an individual, even when used to express a generalized idea. Historian George Mosse proposes that these female icons stood for the eternal and immutable qualities of a nation, the static setting against which men would take political action.

In a similar vein, female icons have dominated scientific texts, personifying Truth, Reason, and Nature since at least the scientific revolution of the sixteenth century. Londa Schiebinger has discussed the way in which a certain style of scholarship came to be both associated with the feminine and excluded from scientific practice, while images of Scientia continued to be female. She proposes that these female icons are part of a Neoplatonic world-view where perfection is achieved through the union of the male and female. Thus, since the philosopher is male, his counterpart, Nature or Scientia etc., must be personified as female. During the nineteenth century, however, abstract scientific icons disappeared along with the gentle (wo)man philosopher, replaced by the professional, white-coated man of science and his image.

Iconography has been useful in the analysis of the cultural meanings ascribed not only to specific icons like Lady Liberty and Hercules, but also to bodies in general. Susan Bordo and others have analyzed how the generic young, toned, hard yet flexible body idealized in popular culture, including the popular media and advertising, can be seen as an icon representing the values of contemporary US culture.

Iconology, like the icons it studies, also has political and historical dimensions. For instance, some of the oldest known icons are of female figures, one of the most famous being the *Venus of Willendorf* (c. 25 000 BC), a small, round limestone figure of a nude, which has traditionally been regarded as a highly sexualized, even erotic, symbol of female sexuality and fertility. Recent interpretations have proposed that the *Venus* is not an eroticized fertility goddess, but perhaps a form of self-portraiture, and/or the product of a

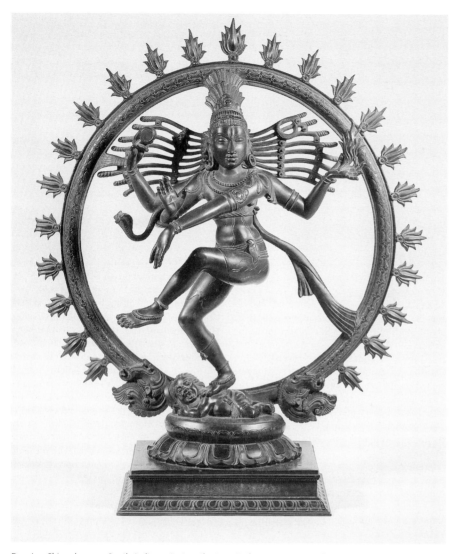

Dancing Shiva, bronze, South Indian, nineteenth– twentieth century. Oriental Museum, Durham University, UK/Bridgeman Art Library.

culture whose understanding of GENDER did not correspond to our categories of male and female.

SARAH GOODFELLOW

Further reading

Bordo, S (1993). *Unbearable weight: feminism, Western culture and the body*. University of California Press, Berkeley.

Mosse, G. L. (1985). *Nationalism and sexuality: respectability and abnormal sexuality in Europe*. H. Fertig, New York.

Schiebinger, L. (1989). *The mind has no sex? Women in the origins of modern science*. Harvard University Press, Cambridge, MA.

Idols 'Idol', from the Greek word *eidolon* (image), first takes on a religious meaning in the Greek translation of the Hebrew Bible known as the Septuagint (third to second centuries BCE), where it refers to physical representations of deities. It is used to translate a number of Hebrew words, among them *elilim* — weak, insignificant, nothing; *pesel* — free-standing

carved statue; and *tselim* — image. Throughout the Hebrew Bible, idol is given a pejorative meaning as it is used to describe non-Israelite or non-Jewish divinities considered to be false or alien gods. These are the gods of other nations from whom the Israelites are commanded to separate themselves. This meaning passes into New Testament usage in the Acts of the Apostles (7: 41; 15: 20), Pauline letters (Romans 2: 22; 1 Corinthians 8: 4, 7; 10: 9; 12: 2; 2 Corinthians 6: 16; 1 Thessalonians 1: 9), 1 John (5: 21), and Revelation (9: 20). Paul in particular makes it clear that idols are entities made and then worshipped by humans (Romans 2: 22).

Insofar as an account of idols can be derived from the Hebrew Bible, two related issues emerge: concern with the worship of alien gods and concern with the worship of images meant to represent Yahweh. Most prominent is the insistence that the Israelites avoid the worship of other, alien gods. Prophetic texts, in particular, warn the Israelites against turning to the gods of their neighbours or those of foreign queens (1

Kings 11: 7, 33; 13: 1–8). These deities, the prophets claim, are empty (Isaiah 44: 14–17), dead, or even demonic (Deuteronomy 32: 17).

Archeological and textual evidence suggests that use of images to represent the divine was the norm among Israel's neighbours in west Asia and along the Mediterranean basin. The statues, often life-sized, stood in temples or other sacred places. They were the recipient of sacrifices, libations, prayers, and votive offerings, were sometimes bathed and clothed, and in general had a 'living' quality that suggests the deity was understood to be present within them in some way. These practices mirror those found in a variety of African and American traditions, within Hinduism, and within some medieval and modern Catholic Christian communities.

There is evidence in the Hebrew Bible, moreover, that, despite prohibitions, representations of Yahweh were made. In Judges 17: 1–5, Micah makes a *pesel* and a *massekhah*, a carved image and idol of cast metal. After the schism of 935 there appears to have been a cult in the northern kingdom of Israel that worshipped Yahweh in the form of a bull (1 Kings 12: 25–33; 2 Kings 15: 24). In the post-exilic period (*c.* 539 BCE), the prophets, in line with the legal code's prohibition against making representations of the divinity (Exodus 20: 4–6; Deuteronomy 4: 15–19; 5: 6–9; Leviticus 26: 1), fight against the use of images and any tangible representations of the divine, insisting that these practices are empty, futile, and absurd.

By the New Testament period, idolatry seems to have ceased to be a problem, as it is not mentioned by the gospel writers. However, with the movement of the early Christian community into the gentile world, the prophetic denunciations return as early Christians confront Greek and Roman religious practices. In Galatians 4: 8, Paul argues that pagan gods have no substance, following the prophets who claim that idols are nothing but stone and wood (Jeremiah 16: 20) and utterly vacuous (Isaiah 44: 14–17). Paul argues in 1 Corinthians 10: 19 that in venerating idols one calls on demons.

Early Christian thinkers developed the claim that in worshipping idols one worships the demonic. According to Augustine, for example, by venerating part of the created realm as god, idolaters subvert the natural order and pay service to demonic forces. Rather than being mere stone and wood, these human fabrications are invested with demonic force by the perversion of human nature entailed in their worship. In this way both the Pauline texts and their elaboration by early Christian thinkers extend the notion of idolatry to include any created thing or being put in the place of the divine.

Similar prohibitions against idols are found in the Qur'an, where again the primary offence is the confusion of created things with God. All three of the major Western religious traditions, then, understand idols as created entities that are claimed, by their worshippers, to be divine. The shared assumption is that God is uncreated, immaterial, and disembodied.

The pejorative connotations of the term 'idol' were instrumental in Western, particularly Christian, encounters with other religious traditions. The images of divine beings found among the peoples of Africa and the Americas, for example, were understood to be not simply representations of deities, but themselves, as material objects, worshipped. Hence for European Christians encountering the religious practices of parts of Africa and the Americas, an idol was not merely an image of a deity, but itself reputed to be, and treated as, divine. In this way, Western monotheistic beliefs about the immateriality of the divine and the exclusiveness of their own deity were conflated, and the association of idolatry with materiality emphasized. The complex theophanic nature of images within Hinduism and many other traditions — despite occasional parallels with Christian practices, particularly in the medieval Catholic and Eastern Orthodox churches — is only beginning to be acknowledged and studied by Western scholars of religion.   AMY HOLLYWOOD

Further reading

Ackerman, S. (1998). Idol, idolatry. *The Eerdmans Dictionary of the Bible*, (ed. D. N. Freedman). Eerdmans, Grand Rapids, MI.

Eck, D. (1985). *Darsan: seeing the divine image in India*. Anima Books, Chambersburg, PA.

Ries, J. (1987). Idolatry. In *The Encyclopedia of religion*, (ed. M. Eliade) Macmillan, London and New York.

Ileum The section of the small intestine beyond the duodenum and the jejunum, and ending where it joins the caecum. Digestion is mostly completed before this point, but absorption into the blood of the resulting simpler substances continues here. The surface area of the lining is increased (though less than in the jejunum) by its folds and protrusions (villi). The last part of the ileum has a unique and essential function in the absorption of vitamin B_{12}, necessary for normal blood formation.   S.J.

See ALIMENTARY SYSTEM; PLATE 1.

Illness Concepts of illness cannot be understood just in terms of the absence of good health. Advances in the science of genetics are so persuasive to many apparently healthy people that they have agreed to allow double mastectomy or removal of the colon merely because the physician has advised them of the likelihood of cancer at some future date. Conversely, sufferers from conditions like chronic fatigue syndrome or Gulf War illness claim extreme disability in the absence of a proven organic cause and in the face of scientific denial that there is anything 'really' the matter save malingering or 'yuppie flu'. The desire by lawyers, especially in the US, to exculpate their clients has led to recognition of any number of novel illnesses, including battered spouse syndrome and junk food 'madness', which rely only on the ability of a lawyer to

persuade a jury of the 'reality' of an illness for the defence to be effective. The way in which medical care is funded has 'medicalized' a number of conditions once considered moral failings, including compulsive gambling, ALCOHOLISM, drug ADDICTION, and OBESITY. Finally, some illnesses seem almost to be the result of fashion trends, or to have their roots in the social stigma attached to a particular GENDER, race, or class. Some examples are chlorosis, hysteria, neurasthenia, 'reefer madness', shell shock, recovered memory, epidemic violence among black men, attention deficit disorder, and even alien abduction syndrome.

Attitudes to illness

In the developed world it is indeed science that holds principal authority over the patient's contested body, with respect to deciding about whether or not a person is 'really' ill, what sort of treatment is required, and who will pay for it. But other authorities are at work as well, including government bureaucrats, insurance companies, politicians, the media, history, the law, and even the patient, whose subjective judgements about his or her state of health hold greater or lesser sway according to any number of circumstances.

Other societies have respected, or even worshipped, other authorities, which have in turn shaped concepts of illness. Shamanistic cultures even today conceive of illness in ways that seem to us supernatural or magical. If a person has been cursed or has committed some transgression, the true nature of the problem is discovered and an appropriate remedy sought. Supernatural diseases require supernatural cures, which often involve consultation with a dead relative, who intervenes with the gods or with powers of Nature to restore health. All this is conducted quite publicly, often under the guidance of an experienced healer, who may supply a suitable story as to why an illness has occurred. The satisfactory nature of this system is attested to by its enduring popularity, even when scientific medicine is offered as an alternative. Illness in shamanistic societies can affect individuals, but also afflicts families or even entire villages. The cure in such cases often involves isolation of an offending individual from the group, at least until the situation returns to normal.

Ancient Greek physicians were among the first to distinguish themselves from what are usually called temple healers, that is, healers relying on resort to the gods. They did so not by offering better cures for illnesses, at least not by modern scientific lights, but by appealing to the fashion for rational philosophy among the upper classes of society. Hippocratic physicians debated with their rivals in the marketplace in the same way that philosophers did, and their writings are among the earliest testimonies to the Greek understanding of nature.

The Hippocratic corpus of texts, most of which date from between 430 and 330 BCE, were the work of many different authors. In a particularly significant text, *On the Sacred Disease*, the

writer dismissed the notion that EPILEPSY was caused by the gods or by supernatural influence. Every disease was in some sense divine, the writer argued, because nature itself was divine. But the proximate cause of the sacred disease and indeed of every disease was entirely natural and therefore by implication subject to natural remedies. Epilepsy was caused by a congestion of PHLEGM that stopped up the brain and made the sufferer fall down and lose consciousness. One could easily see this by examining the brains of goats, which were particularly subject to the condition and had very phlegmy brains. This is scientific nonsense, of course, but it is also totally rational, within its own terms of reference, and was based partly on observation.

Illness, for the Greek physician, was a lack of balance and harmony with nature. The physician was therefore a student not only of the individual body, or microcosm, but of its place in the larger natural world, or macrocosm. This sort of thinking is particularly apparent in another Hippocratic work, *Airs, Waters, Places*. In that treatise, the writer outlined how environmental factors dictated the sorts of illnesses people suffered from and how the physician, often an itinerant, had to study the environment of the ill person before treatment could be effective. The treatise is also intensely political. The traditional enemies of the Greek city states were characterized as flabby, lazy, and decadent, as a consequence of the hot eastern environment they inhabited, and were subject to diseases of sloth as a result.

Acceptance of science

It can be argued that, after the rebirth of science in the seventeenth century, the concept (and conquest) of illness marched forward quickly. Thomas Sydenham (1624–89), the English Hippocrates, revived rational observation and dismissed excessive theorizing about disease. John Snow (1813–58) demonstrated the waterborne nature of cholera with his study of the Broad Street pump. Louis Pasteur (1822–95) and Robert Koch (1843–1910) pioneered bacteriology, and science's triumph over disease seemed nearly complete. But in fact objections to rational or scientific concepts of illness have been strenuous throughout history. These attacks are characteristically levelled against medical 'experts' and are largely based on cultural conflict and the vast area of human experience that science-based medical practice appears to neglect.

The Roman gentleman Pliny the Elder, who died in the eruption of Mt. Vesuvius in AD 79, wrote one of the earliest and most influential attacks on rational Greek medicine in his encyclopaedia of natural history. For him, Greek physicians were not only foreigners, but murderers, preening sodomites and, worst of all perhaps, experts, who separated medicine from the general knowledge that a paterfamilias like Pliny believed was necessary to care for his estate, including its health. Greek physicians more than anyone were responsible, Pliny concluded, for ruining the morals of Rome. For aristocrats like Pliny, medicine need not be complicated. A proper regimen of health was really all that was necessary. Traditional folk remedies and rituals, like cabbage stew or inhaling the breath of farm animals, usually did the trick. These things could be learned from friends and relatives, or from reading the right kinds of books oneself.

Pliny's fulminations against medical experts enjoyed a wide audience especially among medieval and Renaissance humanists, who lauded not only the great encyclopedist's learning but also his advocacy of rural retirement and domestic economy as the road to good health and the way to avoid illness. The humanist poet Petrarch (1304–74) wrote a famous invective against learned physicians, directed at Pope Clement VI, advising him to dismiss his doctors, who did nothing but belch lies with their medicine-smeared tongues and waste people's time. Geoffrey Chaucer (?1340–1400), an open admirer of Italian humanism, echoed similar sentiments in his *Nun's Priest's Tale*, one of the *Canterbury Tales*. In this epic, the old widow who ruled the farm survived happily on very little money and needed only a temperate diet, exercise, and a glad heart to keep her healthy. Like a true Stoic, she expected to experience illness, old age, and death, but by careful living and above all by self-sufficiency she managed to be happy nonetheless without resort to physicians and medicines. Her chickens, vain to the last, believed otherwise and suffered for it.

Another sort of dissent came from religious and medical reformers like Paracelsus (1493–1541) and Van Helmont (1579–1644), who, like medical humanists, elevated folk practice, nationalism, and use of the vernacular in their medical ideas. Paracelsians and Helmontians objected to humoural explanations of illnesses. These explanations were based on the Greek idea that disease affected the entire body and was thus 'systemic' and individualized. Humoural illnesses required gradual treatment under expert guidance that could take weeks or even longer. The dissident Paracelsus and his followers argued otherwise. Often employing militaristic metaphors, Paracelsus argued for what would later be called the 'ontological' theory of disease — that is, the theory that diseases were caused by agents that attacked the body from outside and affected it only locally. Disease entities thus had a real existence outside the sufferer and affected similar people in similar ways. The purpose of therapeutics, then, was to apply counteragents, usually chemical ones, which would act quickly against the attacker.

Van Helmont elaborated on Paracelsus's hypotheses, as did others, and it is tempting to assume that the two men somehow prefigured the germ theory and modern medical chemistry. But Paracelsian and Helmontian world views undermined traditional medical authority much more radically than is immediately apparent. Like Pliny and like some Christian humanists, these medical philosophers argued that bodily ills were caused by occult and mystical influences. For them, the Greek idea of the natural cause of disease could explain very little. Paracelsus went further, to argue that ontological disease agents were poisons of sorts that were unleashed astrologically by chemical disturbances in the heavens. Exactly how this was accomplished remains unclear. But arguments like these crop up from time to time against totally materialistic explanations of the origin of bodily ills. A medical system that excludes from consideration notions of the mystical, occult, spiritual, or religious will never be entirely satisfying to many. To the understandable sufferer's question 'Why me? Why now?' the scientific physician might offer a statistical observation or simply deny that such concerns have anything to do with medicine. A medical astrologer could answer the sufferer very easily, as long as the patient believed in the validity of the explanation.   FAYE GETZ

Further reading

Bynum, W. F. (1993). Nosology. In *Companion encyclopedia of the history of medicine*, (ed. W. F. Bynum and R. Porter Routledge). London and New York.

Levi-Strauss, C. (1963). The sorcerer and his magic. In *Structural anthropology*. Basic Books, New York.

Lloyd, G. E. R. (ed.) (1978). *Hippocratic Writings*. Penguin Books, New York.

See also HEALTH; SHAMANS.

Illusions

We see far more than meets the eyes, though not always correctly, for we experience various phenomena of illusion — departures from physical reality. Although they are errors, illusions are useful evidence of how eyes and brains normally work.

But 'illusion' is hard to define adequately. If illusions are departures from reality, what is reality? This is difficult to answer, for we have many descriptions of reality, in science, in art, and so on. No doubt all are incomplete and perhaps largely wrong. Certainly physics frequently changes its mind. If we take the account offered by modern physics of matter as invisible atoms in violent motion, with weird effects of quantum mechanics, this is so different from how things appear that we might be tempted to say *all* perception is illusion! But this is not more helpful than to say that all perceptions are dreams.

We are pushed into thinking that illusions must be departures from quite simple-minded physics, as measured with rulers, protractors, and clocks. Illusions include distortions of length, angles, and time. There are also perceptual experiences that one might call 'ghostly fictions' (Table 1(d)). Some figures or objects appear impossible (Table 1(c)). Others seem to flip from one perception to another, though there is no change of the image at the eyes (Table 1(a)). These are weird and wonderful phenomena, which are central to art, but are hazards to the

Table 1 The skeletal Necker cube is perceptually ambiguous: it switches in depth; the upper line of the Ponzo illusion looks too long; the Tri-bar or 'Devil's Trident' looks impossible; the ghostly square (a Kanizsa figure) does not exist.

Kinds of language errors and illusions of vision

Classes	Language errors	Visual illusions
Ambiguities	'People like us'	(a) Necker Cube
Distortions	'He's miles taller'	(b) Ponzo illusion
Paradoxes	'Dark-haired blonde'	(c) Tri-bar
Fictions	'They live in a mirror'	(d) Kanizsa figure

physical sciences, and can be dangerous in every-day living. They are well worth explaining.

Explaining illusions

It seems useful to try to classify phenomena of illusions, as classifications are important for all science. Chemistry and biology were transformed by the Periodic Table of the Elements, and by names for species and varieties. How shall we start for illusions? It is suggestive that *illusions of seeing* correspond with *errors of language*. Appearances of illusions fall into classes which may be named quite naturally from kinds of errors of language — *ambiguities*, *distortions*, *paradoxes*, and *fictions*.

It is intriguing that these apply both to VISION and to LANGUAGE, for it is more than possible that language grew from pre-human classifications of objects and actions over millions of years. If the evolution of language were parasitic on these perceptual mechanisms, it might explain how language developed so rapidly for humans. It is a tricky question how much extra brain was needed for language, and how much language makes a brain more effective. This is rather like using any tool, such as an electric drill or a computer. One needs the skill to use it; but then the tool adds a lot of extra skill. Tools increase intelligence. Indeed our language, and tools of technology, are large parts of our intelligence, though we are never infallible.

Let us compare errors of language with kinds of illusions:

There seem to be four principal *causes* of illusions. The first is optical disturbance between objects and the eyes. The second is the physiological disturbance of signals in the 'peripheral' machinery of vision (in the retina and early areas of the visual cortex). The third and the fourth are extremely different — for they are *cognitive*. This is like mistakes of interpreting plainly visible words. This can happen by confusions of *meanings* (semantics), or by misapplied *rules* of grammar (syntactics). There are similar kinds of cognitive errors in vision and other perception, because perception is based on knowledge of the world and it works by applying general rules. Either kind of cognitive mistake can mislead, by not being appropriate to the situation. The same kinds of cognitive illusions can occur in computer vision.

Here is one example of each kind:
These are examples of false perceptions of different origin. In a looking glass, one sees onself *through* it, yet *knows* one is in front of it — doubled, yet one person! Pure, monochromatic yellow light cannot be distinguished from a mixture of red and green light because they cause the same activation of the three types of colour-sensitive cones in the retina. The café wall illusion looks like a chess board, but with alternate rows displaced sideways by half a square: the horizontal rows of squares appear like long wedges, converging towards one side or the other. If you stare at a rotating spiral it appears either to shrink or expand, depending on which way it is rotating. If you then look away, whatever you are now looking at appears to do the opposite — to expand or to shrink — an example of an *after-effect* that is probably due to 'fatigue' of neurons in the visual cortex. *After-images* are ghost-like blobs that move with each eye movement, resulting from over-stimulation of one region of the retina. The most familiar after-images are the dark blobs that persist after looking at a light bulb or a camera flashlight. But after-images (of complementary colour and brightness) can be caused by staring intently at any pattern of high contrast. What is 'figure' (or object) and what is 'ground' (the background between objects) is the most basic perceptual decision. In ambiguous situations (such as the famous Rubin picture, with two silhouette profiles of faces, staring at each other, creating a vase shape between them) perception can flip from one interpretation to the other (from faces to vase). Perspective illusions are distortions produced by converging lines, which signal depth (even when depth is not perceived), e.g. the Ponzo illusion in Table 1. 'Ghostly shapes' are perceptual interpretations that go beyond the immediate information in the retinal image, as in the Kanizsa figure in Table 1. Impossible objects are representations that are not compatible with sensible 'perceptual hypotheses', such as the Penrose impossible triangle, or the Tri-bar in Table 1. The inside of a mask (a hollow face) appears as a normal face, with the nose sticking out, presumably because the improbable interpretation of a true hollow face is rejected. Small objects feel heavier than large objects of the same weight — because large objects are expected to be heavier. The Magritte

painting shows a back view of a man looking into a mirror — but paradoxically we see the *back* of his head in the mirror. Faces-in-the-fire are fictional perceptual interpretations seen fleetingly in the flames of a fire.   RICHARD GREGORY

Further reading

Gombrich, E. (1960). *Art and illusion*. Phaidon, London.

Gregory, R. L. (1997). *Eye and brain*, (5th edn). Oxford University Press.

Robinson, J. O. (1972). *The psychology of visual illusions*. Hutchinson, London.

See also PERCEPTION; VISION.

Imaging techniques

In recent decades, technological advances in imaging of the body have been phenomenal. X-RAY photographic images (*radiographs*), with or without the use of contrast medium, became of major importance in medical diagnosis, from their invention at the end of the nineteenth century onwards. But traditional X-ray images have their limitations: there is no clue to 'depth' from a single image; the shape, site, and size of, say, a growth or infection showing a 'shadow' in a lung can only be assessed approximately by taking radiographs from different angles or by 'screening' the subjects as they move around.

Whilst plain radiographs remain the cornerstone of modern radiology, new imaging techniques have developed along with advances in physics — nuclear and otherwise — and in computer technology. Some utilise X-rays and others gamma rays from radioisotopes, with exposures to radiation too small and too brief to cause damage. ULTRASOUND uses high frequency sound waves and MAGNETIC RESONANCE IMAGING uses radio waves. All these are utilised for 'scans' in which a moving source provides information to be picked up by multiple detectors, computed to yield detailed 2-dimensional images, or 3-dimensional reconstructions.

CT scans

A new form of X-ray imaging, *computed tomography* (*CT scan*), was developed in 1972 by Sir Godfrey Hounsfield in the UK and Allan Cormack in the US. A narrow X-ray beam traverses the body in an axial plane (the anatomical term for a vertical plane dividing the body from front to back) and multiple detectors, surrounding the body, record the strength of the exiting X-ray. This data is analysed, integrated, and reconstructed by computer to produce images of cross-sections or 'slices' of an organ or region of the body. Using sophisticated software, 3-dimensional reconstruction images can be created to demonstrate specific organs.

The introduction of CT was one of the greatest advances particularly in neurological diagnosis, giving 2-dimensional thin section images or 'slices' of the brain or spinal cord, and allowing precise localisation of 'space occupying lesions' such as blood clots or tumours. CT was also a major advance in imaging tumours and other

Table 2 Classes of illusions and kinds of causes

Classes	Physical causes		Cognitive causes	
	Optics	Physiology	Rules	Knowledge
Ambiguities	Looking through mist	Pure yellow versus red + green	Figure–ground reversals	Hollow face
Distortions	Mirages	Café wall illusion	Perspective illusions	Size–weight illusion
Paradoxes	Looking glass	Rotating spiral after-effect	Impossible objects	Magritte's painting of the mirror
Fictions	Rainbow	After-images	Ghostly shapes	Faces-in-the-fire

abnormalities in almost any part of the body, often allowing their detection without resorting to exploratory surgery. The advanced technique of Electron Beam Computed Tomography (EBCT) has more recently become useful for cardiac imaging and identification of coronary artery calcification. Spiral CT is another new technique which gives very rapid multi-slice scans with fast image reconstruction, providing greatly improved anatomical definition of organs and blood vessels.

Digital subtraction angiography (DSA) is a
sophisticated method which improves on traditional X-rays for imaging BLOOD VESSELS following injection of a soluble radio-opaque substance. Using digitized images, computer analysis subtracts overlying and unwanted shadows of bones and soft tissues, giving greatly improved definition of blood vessels whilst minimising the radiation dose and the amount of contrast medium required.

Isotope scanning

Together with the application of radioactive isotopes in treatment (RADIOTHERAPY), diagnostic isotope scanning now constitutes the specialty of *nuclear medicine*. Following an intravenous injection, an isotope is taken up by different organs in varying amounts. The radiation emitted is detected by a scintillation counter (a *gamma camera*, invented in 1961) and the image recorded. Having a very short half-life, the radioactive isotope decays completely before it can cause damage. Different isotopes tend to concentrate in particular organs. Technetium-99m is most widely used, especially to investigate lungs and bone, whereas iodine-131 shows thyroid function.

Positron emission tomography (PET scanning) involves the emission of particles of antimatter (positrons) from an isotope incorporated in a tracer substance given by injection or inhalation; the positrons are neutralised by electrons within the body tissues, releasing energy in the form of radiation, which is detected and analysed to produce an image. This is used in neurological studies since it can map out blood flow and metabolic activity (oxygen or glucose usage) in the different areas of the brain in health or disease. For example *oxygen-15* (^{15}O) is a positron emitter, and can be used to label oxygen in the inspired air. The labelled oxygen, is transferred to the circulating blood and then passes into water when it is used in metabolism, multiple detectors around the head can provide computed tomographic images showing the relative degrees of oxygen uptake in all regions of the brain — and hence their level of function compared to the normal. Such methods can show localised increases in blood flow and metabolism accompanying specific tasks, such as speech, or finger movements, and can trace the pathways of cerebral activation. PET scans are available only where there is a cyclotron close by, because the emitters have a very short life: oxygen-15, for example, has a half-life of only two minutes.

Single photon emission tomography (SPECT)
is an alternative, less expensive but less quantitative method for obtaining two- and three-dimensional reconstructions of the distribution of brain blood flow, involving injection of a radionuclide and detection by a gamma camera rotating around the head.

Ultrasound scans (ultrasonography)

Originally developed from underwater sonar (used to detect fish and submarines in World War II), ultrasound moved from sonar and non-destructive industrial research into medical imaging in the 1950s and 1960s. Ultrasound waves are of a frequency at least a hundred-fold greater than that of the sound waves at the top of the range of human hearing. The waves are reflected from any barrier they meet in proportion to the 'acoustic impedance' of the substance. Pulses of high-frequency ultrasound, usually greater than 1 MHz, are emitted from transducers and traverse the body. Different tissue layers cause reflections. Analysis and digitization of the signals provides a greatly improved and clearly defined image. Many pioneers worldwide contributed to this new technology, the growth of its medical applications, and its involvement with manufacturers, leading to its present sophistication. Douglas Howry, a trainee radiologist, and Joseph Holmes, a kidney specialist, of Denver Colorado, along with Ian Donald, Professor of

Obstetrics in Glasgow, were among the earliest pioneers in clinical application.

Being quick, relatively inexpensive, and non-ionising, with no known biological hazard when used within the diagnostic range of frequency, ultrasound scans are a prime diagnostic method in obstetrics — monitoring pregnancy and imaging fetal development and the newborn brain. Ultrasound is also widely used to image stones in the GALL BLADDER, suspected abdominal tumours, or the thyroid gland, and for evaluating the heart by ECHOCARDIOGRAPHY. It is also used for BIOPSY guidance almost anywhere in the body.

Doppler ultrasound scan

Christian Doppler was an Austrian physicist who first described the *Doppler Effect*: that the apparent frequency of light or sound waves is affected by the relative motion of the source and the detector. This effect is applied in the detection and measurement of the velocity of flow in blood vessels. An ultrasonic beam with a frequency of 4–5 MHz is deflected by the flowing blood, causing a Doppler shift proportional to the flow rate; the resulting small modification of frequency can be detected and analysed. The combination of ultrasound images and Doppler blood flow studies is known as *duplex scanning* and is of considerable clinical value in diagnosing problems of blood flow, especially arterial disease and venous thrombosis.

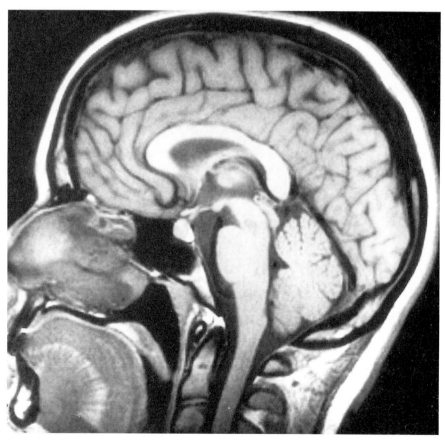

MRI scan of a normal living human brain.

Magnetic resonance imaging (MRI scan)

The patient is placed within a magnetic coil and radio-frequency energy is applied to the body. The harmless radio waves excite protons that form the nuclei of hydrogen atoms in the body. The protons give off measureable electric energy which with the aid of computation create an image. MRI provides a hazard-free, non-invasive way of generating images without using X-rays or gamma rays. In the late 1980s MRI proved to be superior to other imaging methods — and more expensive — giving outstanding definition especially in the brain and the skeletal system, as well as most other organs and tissues. *MRI angiography* is a unique non-invasive method of imaging blood vessels without using contrast medium. As in CT, three-dimensional reconstruction images can be created to demonstrate specific organs. J. K. DAVIDSON

See also RADIOACTIVITY; RADIOLOGY; X-RAYS.

Immaculate conception

The doctrine of the immaculate conception holds that Mary is the one fully human being preserved from original sin because she is the Mother of God. Grace intervened at the very instant in which her life began, preventing sin from touching her in any way, and so making her holy and immaculate from the moment of her conception. This made her worthy, and suggests that she was divinely chosen, to be the Mother of God. Christ preserved Mary from sin because she was his Mother; as Ambrose taught, 'Christ chose this vessel into which he was about to descend, not of earth, but of heaven; and he consecrated it a temple of purity.'

There is little scriptural basis for this doctrine because scripture does not speak explicitly about Mary's conception, and theological opposition to the doctrine might be found in the claim, in Romans 5, that all humans have shared in original sin. Nevertheless, the doctrine was important in the East, as theologians such as John of Damascus made it central to the idea of Mary as Theotokos, or God-bearer. Devotion to Mary spread to the West and the immaculate conception was increasingly debated in the later Middle Ages; some theologians, notably Aquinas, opposed it on the grounds that through natural (human) conception, original sin is transmitted, and therefore Mary cannot be exempt from the law of original sin, but the Council of Basle (1439) declared it in accordance with the Catholic faith, reason, and scripture.

The doctrine was increasingly depicted in woodcuts, paintings, and sculpture from the fifteenth century onwards, and was very popular with seventeenth-century Spanish painters such as El Greco. One popular image was that of the tiny Mary, visible in her mother Anne's womb, with rays of divine grace descending from God onto her. Another, frequently depicted, was of Christ and Mary trampling the serpent: this became especially popular with seventeenth- and eighteenth-century artists, and a variation on that theme, with Christ plunging a pointed cross into the mouth of the serpent, was much propagated by Franciscans and Jesuits.

The Roman Catholic Church continued to cultivate the doctrine, not least through its various religious orders. In 1476 Sixtus IV approved the feast with its own Mass and Office, and in 1708 Clement XI extended it to the Universal Church and made it a feast day of obligation (December 8). In 1854, Pius IX declared that the doctrine 'has been revealed by God and is therefore to be believed by all the faithful'. He thus exhibited the authority of the church's Magisterium, and that of himself as Pope, in interpreting divine revelation, in the case of a doctrine for which there was little evidence in the Scriptures, or even patristic evidence.

JANE SHAW

Immune system

Have you ever wondered why you are resistant to the colds that plague your friends, even though you have been exposed to the same environment? This is because you have an efficient immune system which is working overtime to identify and mount a reaction to 'invaders', including MICROORGANISMS capable of causing disease and foreign macromolecules like polysaccharides and proteins — a phenomenon known as *immunity*.

Historically, immunity referred to protection from infectious diseases, and the term was derived from the Latin word *immunitas*, meaning the exemption from civic duties and prosecution extended to Roman senators. However the concept of immunity existed long before, especially in the Chinese custom of making children inhale powders of crust of skin lesions of patients recovering from small pox. The first scientifically documented evidence of inducing immunity was the landmark work of Dr Edward Jenner, an English physician. He noticed that milkmaids who had recovered from cowpox were resistant to contracting small pox. When he injected the material from a cowpox pustule into a young boy, the boy did not develop small pox even when intentionally inoculated. Jenner published his findings in 1798 and laid the foundation for the future development of 'vaccination' (the Latin word *vacinus* means of or from cows) and other forms of IMMUNIZATION.

Two basic levels of immunity exist in healthy individuals to confer protection against microbes and other foreign bodies; the less perfect *natural immunity* and the more specific *acquired immunity*.

Natural immunity

Those defence mechanisms that exist prior to exposure to foreign substances, that are not enhanced by subsequent exposures, and that cannot discriminate between most foreign molecules, are categorized as natural or innate immunity. This includes the first line of defence — the protective barriers like the SKIN and the MUCOUS MEMBRANES lining the body tracts, which secrete acids and ENZYMES capable of digesting bacterial cell walls. Often a failure at this level may lead to fatal complications (such as in cystic fibrosis, where the mucus formed is not protective).

If this protective barrier is breached, the next lines of defence involve two components of natural immunity — the *humoral* (mediated by substances free in the body fluids) and the *cellular* (mediated by cells). A number of humoral agents are rapidly produced or activated to exert non-specific effects: that is, they are equally effective against multiple microbes. They include *acute phase proteins*, *serum complements*, and *interferons*. Interferons are vital mainly in controlling viral infections. At this time the cellular component also comes into play. Two types of phagocytic cells 'eat up' and destroy the foreign molecules. The first of these are the *polymorphonuclear neutrophil leucocytes* (white blood cells), which circulate in BLOOD and migrate to sites of microbial invasion; the second are called *monocytes* in the blood and *macrophages* in the tissues (they migrate between the two) — collectively, the macrophage–monocyte system. Humoral and cellular mechanisms interact: serum complements bind to the surface of the foreign molecule and increase the efficiency of phagocytosis by the cells.

Acquired immunity

By the time the components of natural immunity perform their act, more specific defence mechanisms are also mounted. These mechanisms are induced by exposure to the foreign molecules which are known as *antigens*. Besides amplifying the protective mechanisms of innate immunity, the specific immune system also 'memorizes' each encounter with a particular antigen such that subsequent exposure to that antigen leads to the development of 'active immunity'. Specific immunity can also be induced in an individual by transferring cells or serum (depending on the type of immune response, see later) from a specifically immunized individual, so that the recipient becomes immune to the particular antigen without getting an actual exposure to it. This form of immunity is called 'passive immunity', and often is a useful method for rapid conferring of immunity. This technique has helped in saving lives following potentially lethal snake bites, by the administration of antibodies from immunized individuals. Much more commonly, anti-tetanus serum has been widely used to confer passive immunity after potentially contaminated minor injuries.

Lymphocytes are the primary players in specific immunity. These are cells that are present throughout the body, circulating in the blood and lymph and organized in lymphoid tissues. They are produced in *primary lymphoid organs* — the liver in the fetus, the THYMUS, and the BONE marrow. Some lymphocytes pass through the thymus after release from the bone marrow, re-enter the circulation and then settle in *secondary lymphoid organs* like the spleen and the lymph nodes. During passage through the thymus these lymphocytes acquire *antigen specificity*, properties which equip them to act against a particular invader, and are thereafter known as *T-cells*. Other lymphocytes do not pass through the thymus, but settle directly in the secondary lymphoid organs where they mature and develop antigen specificity. These cells are called B-lymphocytes or *B-cells*; they carry on their surface a 'recognition molecule' or *antibody*, which acts as a receptor for an antigen.

Antibodies belong to a group of proteins called *immunoglobulins*. They are similar in their overall Y-shaped structure. The 2 arms form the part known as 'Fab', which binds with the antigen. Here the amino acid sequence varies widely; these regions determine the specificity of the antibody and also account for the diversity of immunity. In fact there are between 10 and 1000 *million* structurally different antibodies in an individual, each with unique amino acid sequences in the Fab region. The stem of the antibody determines its biological function, and its properties are used in classifying the immunoglobulins (IgG, IgM, IgA, IgD, and IgE.)

Humoral immunity is mediated by antibodies that are released into the circulation from B-lymphocytes, and can therefore be transferred to non-immunized individuals by cell-free components of blood. It is the principal defence mechanism against extra-cellular foreign molecules or their toxins because the antibodies bind to these and lead to their destruction. Intracellular antigens are handled by cell-mediated immunity, of which the main component is T-lymphocytes. This form of immunity can be transferred only through the cells of the blood. Humoral and cellular immunity are thus the two types of acquired or specific immunity.

Following exposure to an antigen, the specific immune response is brought about in a sequential manner, which can be divided into three phases: 'cognitive', 'activation' and 'effector'. During the *cognitive phase*, the antigen binds to specific receptors on mature lymphocytes of both types. The antibody on B-lymphocytes recognizes and binds foreign proteins, polysaccharides, or lipids in soluble form. Receptors on T-lymphocytes, on the other hand, can recognize only short peptide sequences in protein antigens present on the surface of other cells. In the technical jargon of immunology, the portion of an antigen that is specifically recognized by the antibody is called an 'epitope'.

Next, in the *activation phase*, the antigen-specific lymphocytes of both types proliferate by cloning, thus amplifying the immune response. Lymphocytes develop into cells whose primary function is to eliminate the antigen. All clonal B-cells secrete the same antibody, which combines with the antigen and initiates a sequence of events leading to destruction of that antigen. Subsets of the antigen-specific T-cell clones develop different functions; some activate PHAGOCYTES; others, called *T-cytotoxic cells*, directly break down cells that produce viral antigens; some regulate the production of antibody

by B-cells. Those T-cells, which promote the immune response, are called *T-helper cells*, while others that inhibit it as part of the self-limiting capability of the immune response, are called *T-suppressor cells*. Another subset, the *Tdth cells* (delayed type hypersensitivity) produce factors that modulate the functions of lymphocytes and macrophages.

A set of membrane proteins that are products of genes determining (in)compatibility of tissues between individuals are known as HLA (called *human lymphocyte antigens*, because they were first recognized on these cells, but they occur on other cells also). They regulate the T-cell activity in such a way that T-cells recognize other antigens only when they are associated with the HLA molecules. This system is highly variable in the human population and it is rare for two individuals to have the same HLA products. This is often the reason for transplant rejection due to an immune response, when the donor's proteins serve as antigens in the recipient. HLA typing and matching is thus an essential step before any transplant surgery to minimize the chances of an immune response.

Once the lymphocytes have been activated and the antigen has been presented to them, the immune response enters the *effector phase*. Few antigens bind directly to antigen-reactive T- or B-cells but are presented to the lymphocytes bound to other '*antigen presenting cells*' such as macrophages. The effector phase requires the participation also of other non-lymphoid '*effector cells*' such as *mast cells*, *eosinophils*, or *natural killer* (NK) cells, which act also as components of natural immunity. Antibodies bind to the antigen, and this promotes phagocytosis by neutrophils or other phagocytes. Antibodies can also activate the '*complement system*', generating proteins that cause INFLAMMATION, cell breakdown, and phagocytosis of the antigen. Some antibodies, like IgA released from mucous membranes, coat the antigen and prevent its docking on the epithelial lining of body tracts. T-cells also secrete chemicals called *cytokines*, which stimulate an inflammatory response and enhance the function of natural immunity. The antigen thus faces a barrage of defence mechanisms' which leads to its destruction.

Once the antigenic stimulation is removed, lymphocytes become quiescent and only some remain viable as *memory cells*. On a subsequent exposure to the same antigen these become rapidly activated and can mount a faster response than the first time, called the *secondary immune response*. A series of feedback controls also come into play, which makes the immune response self limiting.

One of the distinguishing and essential features of the immune system is its ability to discriminate between foreign and '*self-antigens*'. Immunity is unresponsive to molecules present in the individual that would be antigenic in another. This arises due to an acquired process called *self-tolerance*. Thus during the early stages of development, functionally immature 'self-recognizing' lymphocytes come in contact with

self-antigens and are prevented from developing to a stage where they can respond to self-antigens. However, in certain unfortunate conditions, abnormalities in induction or maintenance of self-tolerance may occur, which leads to the immune system acting against a normal component of the same body. This leads to the development of AUTOIMMUNE DISEASES.

SHILADITYA SENGUPTA
TAI-PING FAN

See also ALLERGY; AUTOIMMUNE DISEASES.

Immunization Immunization is the process of conferring increased resistance (or decreased susceptibility) to infection. The term '*vaccination*' is also used to describe this kind of protective measure, although, strictly speaking, this term refers only to the protection conferred against smallpox by material taken from a cow infected with *vaccinia* virus (which causes cowpox). *Inoculation* also is used synonymously for immunization, but less commonly nowadays.

The history of immunization goes back to early attempts to prevent smallpox by the Chinese; much later, in the eighteenth century, came the classical experiments of Edward Jenner in Gloucestershire, who induced protection in a child by the inoculation of material from a cow infected with cowpox.

Achievements in the history of immunization are summarised in Table 1. Although the early work to control infection was made before microbiological methods were firmly established, rapid progress was made, based on sound scientific principles, once modern bacteriology, and later virology, came on to the scene. For example, the isolation of poliovirus allowed for the development by Jonas Salk, and later by Albert Sabin in the 1950s, of highly effective poliovaccines, which led to a dramatic diminution in poliomyelitis. Before then, there were alarming outbreaks of this paralytic disease: over 8000 cases occurred in the UK in 1950. By the late 1980s, poliovirus capable of producing paralysis was still circulating widely in all continents of the world except Australia. But by 1998 the Americas were polio-free and elsewhere there is substantial progress being made towards the goal of worldwide eradication of this much dreaded disease.

Similarly, with measles the isolation of measles virus in 1954 made it possible to culture a strain which is now the basis of the measles vaccine in use today. Prior to the use of the vaccine, in the UK as many as 800 000 cases were notified annually, but its introduction has resulted in a dramatic decline.

Immunization is one of the most cost-effective public health measures available. But although it is possible to manufacture vaccines against a wide variety of viruses and bacteria, it is, of course, important to ensure that the introduction of a particular vaccine will always confer a major benefit to the population receiving it. Therefore certain broad principles are followed before a vaccine is recognised as being suitable

Table 1 Some important dates in the history of immunization

(?) BC	Early attempts in China to immunize against smallpox
1721	Introduction into Britain from Turkey by Lady Wortley Montagu of inoculation of material from smallpox patients into healthy persons (*variolation*)
1796	First vaccination against smallpox performed by Jenner
1880	Pasteur developed fowl cholera vaccine
1881	Pasteur, Roux, and Chamberland introduced anthrax vaccine
1885	Pasteur developed rabies vaccine
1895	Yersin produced plague vaccine
1898	Almroth Wright developed typhoid vaccine
1921	Calmette and Guérin introduced BCG vaccine
1923	Ramon developed diphtheria toxoid
1927	Ramon and Zoeller developed tetanus toxoid
1940	National immunization campaign launched in Britain by Ministry of Health; did not become widespread until 1942
1954	*Salk* (killed) polio vaccine introduced
1957	*Sabin* (live) polio vaccine introduced
1960	Measles vaccine developed by Enders
1962	Rubella vaccine developed by Weller
1967	Jeryl Lynn strain of live attenuated mumps vaccine licensed in the US
1968	Meningococcal (type C) vaccine developed
1968	Measles vaccine introduced on a national scale in Britain
1970	Rubella vaccine became available in Britain
1981	Hepatitis B vaccine licensed in US
1988	Measles, Mumps, Rubella (MMR) vaccine introduced into Britain
1992	Haemophilus influenzae b (HiB) vaccine introduced into Britain

for general use: (i) there should be a major risk of contracting the infection against which the vaccine is intended to protect; (ii) the vaccine should prevent an illness which (including complications and sequelae) is regarded as serious and especially if it can be fatal; (iii) the efficacy of the vaccine should be sufficiently high; (iv) any risk associated with the vaccine should be sufficiently low; (v) the procedures and the number of doses required for successful immunisation should be acceptable to the public.

An ideal vaccine should confer long-lasting, preferably lifelong, protection against the disease; it should be inexpensive enough for large scale use, stable enough to remain potent during transportation and storage, and have no adverse effect on the recipient. If the introduction of a vaccine is agreed upon at national level then a further decision has to be made as to whether it should be for general use (e.g. polio vaccine) or for specific use when exposure is possible (e.g. typhoid vaccine, given when travelling to regions where typhoid is endemic).

Vaccines may induce immunity against infection either actively or passively.

Active immunization

Active immunization is brought about by stimulating the individual's own immunity by introducing either *inactivated* (killed) or *attenuated* (live, but enfeebled) agents (Table 2). The protective response by the body is mainly expressed through: (i) specific antibodies, measurable by serological tests, which confer protection against many agents, particularly viruses and toxins. (ii) the cellular immune response, which involves both phagocytes and 'memory cells'.

Inactivated vaccines are prepared in three ways (examples in Table 2): (i) from killed whole organisms; (ii) from sub-units of the killed organisms; (iii) from the toxins which the organisms release, inactivated by formaldehyde (*toxoids*).

When the organisms have been killed there can be no multiplication within the body, and thus these vaccines cannot produce infection similar to the natural disease. On the other hand, local and whole body reactions may result from response to the organism or to foreign protein used in the vaccine. If the person has not previously been immunized, more than one dose is usually required, although some response can be produced by even a single dose. Protection often lasts for many years, although periodic 'boosts' by subsequent injections may be required to maintain immunity.

Attenuated vaccines are prepared from modified strains of the causal organisms or from related organisms. Because of this, some live vaccines may sometimes cause illness resembling the natural disease, but the symptoms are usually milder. In general, however, these vaccines have fewer side-effects than inactivated ones and the immunity usually lasts for many years.

Passive immunization

Passive immunization is obtained by giving preformed, antibodies. These are usually injected in the form of human immunoglobulin or, rarely, antisera prepared in animals. Protection is usually rapid, but the immunity derived is often short-lived, being limited to the time taken for the antibodies to be broken down in the body — from a week or so, with animal antisera, to about six months for protection against hepatitis A by human normal immunoglobulin.

Special risk groups include those persons particularly liable to suffer from complications of infection, for whom protection by appropriate immunization is therefore of particular importance: for example, those with chronic lung disease, asthma, congenital heart disease, Down's syndrome, or Human Immunodeficiency Virus (HIV) infection, and babies who are born prematurely or are 'small-for-dates'. Immunization of travellers to some countries overseas is often a particular problem, as the risk of certain infections may be especially high and it often has to be given when time is short.

Surveillance of immunization procedures is necessary. Immunization it is not without its occasional hazard and it is important that those involved should balance the risk of the disease against the possible risk of the vaccine. Surveillance measures should be aimed at assessing not only the application, utilisation, and effectiveness of vaccines in the control of infection, but also any side effects, so that rational decisions about whether to vaccinate can be made.

In conclusion, the achievements of successful immunization policies have been spectacular

Table 2 Examples of viral and bacterial vaccines

	Inactivated (killed)	Toxoids	Attenuated (live)
Viral vaccines	Influenza Poliomyelitis (Salk) Hepatitis A Hepatitis B		Yellow fever Poliomyelitis (Sabin) Measles Rubella Mumps Rabies
Bacterial vaccines	Typhoid Cholera Whooping cough	Diphheria Tetanus	BCG (tuberculosis)

when the ravages caused by vaccine-preventable infections in former years are compared with those of today. Smallpox has now been eradicated, and other greatly feared infections (such as poliomyelitis) are well under control. Because immunization can often be given quite cheaply and quickly to large numbers of people, it is a remarkably cost-effective measure, which has undoubtedly made a major (if not *the* major) contribution to the overall protection of the world's population against infection.

DANIEL REID

Further reading

Department of Health, Welsh Office, Scottish Home and Health Department (1996). *Immunisation against infectious disease.* HMSO London.

Nicholl, A. and Rudd, P. (ed.) (1989). *British Paediatric Association Manual on infection and immunizations in children.* Oxford University Press, Oxford.

Wiedermann, G. and Jong, E. C. (1997). Vaccine-preventable diseases: principles and practice. In *Textbook of travel medicine.* B. C. Decker Inc., Hamilton, Ontario.

See also IMMUNE RESPONSE; INFECTIOUS DISEASE.

Implant

Anything deliberately embedded in the body, other than an organ or tissue from another body (transplant). An implant may be a drug in 'depot' form, to provide gradual absorption over an extended period; or a man-made replacement for damaged tissue such as heart valves or major arteries; or a permanent electrical device such as a pacemaker for the heart or a stimulator for emptying the bladder. The computer chip age promises far-reaching developments in this last area. Artificial joints and screws and plates for fixing fractures are also implants, though not usually given that name.   S.J.

Implantation of an EMBRYO into the lining of the UTERUS occurs a week or so after an ovum has been fertilized in one of the FALLOPIAN TUBES. The uterine lining has been routinely prepared to receive it in the second half of the MENSTRUAL CYCLE, but the mother's body does not 'know' that there is an embryo on the way until it has become embedded and can send hormonal signals via the maternal blood to the OVARY whence its ovum came. This *chorionic gonadotrophin* makes the ovary continue to secrete PROGESTERONE, which in turn, via the blood, makes the uterus maintain its welcoming lining, avoiding the catastrophe (for an embryo) of MENSTRUATION. The embryo implants itself by passing though the outer cellular layer of the uterine lining, assisted by chemicals which it secretes. At this stage it is more or less spherical and covered with villi (frond-like protrusions); these provide a large surface area for exchange of gases, nutrients, water and waste with the maternal blood.   S.J.

See PREGNANCY.

Impotence In sexual problem clinics, men tend to present with problems about actually 'doing it' rather than failing to enjoy it. Impotence in the male is not simply the inability to achieve and retain ERECTION of the penis (erectile dysfunction): under this heading are commonly subsumed premature EJACULATION (precipitate emission of semen before the sexual act is fully completed), and retarded ejaculation, in which the man is either unable to achieve ORGASM and ejaculation, or else finds that this takes an exceedingly long time. The same individual may well experience different forms of sexual dysfunction at different times and on different occasions.

Erections of the penis occur for sexual purposes and also during the night during REM (rapid eye movement) sleep. Impotence is usually understood to mean a lack of sufficient firmness and stiffness of the penis at the time of sexual intercourse. For a normal sexual erection the following events must occur:

(i)   There needs to be sufficient sexual stimulus. This can be sexy mind pictures, seeing one's partner naked, the smell of one's partner or the touch of one's partner, and these stimuli are particularly intense with a new partner. Impotence often occurs at a time of life when these various stimuli are less attractive than before.

(ii) As the penis starts to become erect there is a relaxation of muscle fibres in the walls of the penile arteries, and as a result there is increased blood flow into the penis. In older men with high blood pressure and hardening of the arteries this increased blood flow occurs less readily.

(iii) At the same time as more blood enters the penis there is relaxation of muscle fibres inside the twin erectile bodies (corpora cavernosa) in response to nitric oxide released from nerve endings within them. As a result of the increased blood flow and relaxation of corpora cavernosal muscle there is an increased pressure within the erectile bodies, and this shuts off exit veins from the penis, thus the erect penis is firm and warm. We now know that the health of the erectile muscle is maintained by periodic perfusion with warm arterial blood. When the penis is soft and cold and containing only a little venous blood the oxygen tension within the corpora cavernosa is very low. If periodic erections do not occur there is progressive damage to the erectile muscle which is gradually replaced by fibrous tissue and becomes less responsive to nitric oxide. Thus, there is truth in the saying 'Use it or lose it'.

There are a number of physical causes for erectile failure. Damage to the local peripheral nerves or blood vessels, injury or disease of the spinal cord, ageing, conditions causing narrowing or obstruction of the blood vessels, neurological disorders, hormonal deficiencies, diabetes, and some drugs can all have this effect. Local conditions leading to impotence include *priapism* — a

persistent and painful erection, which may result for reasons not fully understood in permanent erectile failure — and Peyronie's disease, which causes the penis to bend to one side during erection. However, although it is now recognised that physical factors may contribute to a far greater number of cases of impotence than previously supposed, in many cases the aetiology is psychological. Like other apparently reflex physical actions, erection can be affected by the state of mind of the individual. Given that sexual interaction is an emotionally-laden area of life, impotence may occur especially in situations which are felt to be particularly stressful and in which there is considerable pressure on the male to 'perform', for example on the first occasion with a new partner. A considerable percentage of men experience intermittent and situational impotence.

Failure of sexual power is still regarded as a slur on the manhood of an individual and is very seldom admitted to, in spite of being perhaps one of the most common of sexual difficulties. So sensitive a subject is it that men tend not to take the problem to their general practitioners but seek out various forms of private assistance. The aid to failing manhood once offered by dubious quacks in newspaper small advertisements is now offered by 'Well Man' clinics and similar institutions via explicit advertisements in the quality papers covering several column inches, and indeed on World Wide Web pages.

There are a number of procedures which the physician can deploy to assess erectile function and to determine whether the failure is psychological in origin or whether there is some organic cause. Simple measures are ascertaining whether erections take place during sleep (using a mercury-in-rubber strain gauge) or in response to erotic materials, though the first is not always practicable and the second may not be personally or culturally acceptable. If erection occurs, this does not totally exclude physical causes, but strongly suggests psychological causation. Other means of investigation are seldom as non-invasive. Moreover, investigations into penile blood flow during erection and other vascular phenomena, and on the nerve system of the penis, show rather contradictory results, which limit their usefulness as tests.

Injections into the corpora cavernosa may be used as a diagnostic procedure to assess erectile response, and have been enthusiastically taken up by some practitioners as a treatment. This appears to be effective in cases where there is a neurological reason for erectile failure, and some cases of psychological origin also respond to this treatment, but there are problems in cases with severe damage to the blood supply.

For psychogenic impotence, or when there are contributing psychological factors, the central problem is usually to overcome the negative pattern established by performance anxiety. Use of 'sensate focus' techniques may be advised, encouraging the man to engage in various forms of pleasurable touching and stimulation without obligation to attain an erection and attempt penetrative intercourse. For premature ejaculation, the use of 'stop-start' (reaching a state of high arousal, ceasing stimulation, and then resuming) and 'squeeze' techniques (firmly squeezing the tip of the penis to prevent ejaculation), though requiring much repetition in order to break the old habit and establish the new, has been shown to be of some benefit. Sometimes the impotence is due to deeper and more long-standing problems for which psychotherapy may be advised.

Recently, various medicines have been found to exaggerate the nitric oxide stimulus that relaxes the corpora cavernosal muscle. The medicine in most general use in the UK in the 1990s was self-injection of PROSTAGLANDIN or alternatively a urethral prostaglandin pellet. However, oral tablets containing a phospho-diesterase inhibitor, sildenifil, (trade name *Viagra*) are nearly as effective and have become the first line treatment throughout the world. An interesting side-effect, experienced by 5–10% of men is an alteration in the perception of light and this is explained by sildenifil inhibiting also phosphdiesterase-6, which is found in cells in the retina of the eye. When men experience this side effect, light may appear brighter or objects may appear with a blueish tinge. In general, however, sildenifil has been shown to be very safe and although there has been a scare about heart attacks the numbers reported are no different from the numbers that would have been expected in a population of similar age who have not taken the drug. Another new tablet that is now available contains apomorphine, and in contrast to sildenifil works by influencing chemical pathways in the hypothalamus in the brain, again, like sildenifil, only in the context of sexual stimulation. There are several sildenifil-like and other tablets being developed and these and other so-called Quality-of-life drugs are causing major funding problems for health care systems.

If all else fails, there is the possibility of implanting a penile prosthesis — a simple plastic splint, or an inflatable implant, — but there is rarely a good case for this, certainly in no more than 1% of patients, and most of them would be paraplegic.

The problem of impotence is best — and most often — addressed in a multidisciplinary clinic, including psycho–sexual counsellors, psychologists, endocrinologists, and urogenital surgeons.

Impotence is often considered to be one of the prices paid for leading a modern, urbanised, and 'unnatural' life, and to bear some causal relation to the changing social role of women. Anxiety about the ability to manifest manhood by sustaining an erection, however, appears to have been prevalent throughout history, during which few women enjoyed anything like the social and economic power now delineated as so threatening. Accusations of manhood stolen by witchcraft and charms for its restoration suggest that in apparently 'simpler' societies erection was not necessarily a reliable biological reflex, and that impotence should, perhaps, be seen as one of the

prices humanity has paid for becoming self-conscious — indeed, human.   LESLEY A. HALL
TIM HARGREAVE

See PLATE 8.

See also COITUS; EJACULATION; PENIS.

In vitro fertilization (IVF) Fertilization of ova by sperm outside the body, in a 'test-tube' environment. The last resort in the treatment of INFERTILITY. OVA are removed from the woman's OVARY after preparation with hormone treatment, which stimulates the maturation of several ova at the same time, rather than the usual one per month. The ova are then exposed to seminal fluid. FERTILIZATION may be successful in some of the ova, and some of the fertilized ova may proceed through the normal first stages of cell division. The resulting embryos are observed during these earliest cell divisions before 'good' embryos (usually up to three) are transferred into the UTERUS. One or more of these embryos may successfully implant. The likelihood of achieving PREGNANCY is very variable — perhaps one in ten such attempts. Spare embryos may be frozen for repeated attempts. A more sophisticated technique attained in the 1990s is 'ICSI' — intracytoplasmic sperm injection — in which a single chosen SPERM is directly inserted into an ovum, leaving still less to chance. There are reports that this can be successful even with non-motile sperm, which could never make the *in vivo* journey on their own.   S.J.

See ASSISTED REPRODUCTION; INFERTILITY.

Incontinence — inability to contain oneself — may apply to many contexts of human function and behaviour. When applied literally to the body it means the uncontrolled leakage of excreta — or sometimes to unbridled sexual activity.

Urinary and faecal ('double') incontinence is of course universal in infants, common in debilitated or demented old people, and occasional between these extremes of age in some nervous system disorders. In all these instances the conscious brain has no dominion over the reflex emptying of bladder and bowel. Yet even with a normal nervous system and the best will in the world, other persons can suffer this ignominy for a variety of reasons. Faecal incontinence can happen to anyone if the 'call to stool' is precipitate in severe diarrhoea. Urinary incontinence in men may accompany abnormality of the penis or problems with the prostate. But incontinence, especially of urine, is most commonly a female affliction.

Incontinence of urine in women

Incontinence of urine in women is certainly common, although due to embarrassment, and the fact that some women regard it as the inevitable consequence of childbearing and ageing, the exact prevalence is uncertain: estimates suggest that at least 14% of women over 30, up to 50% of the elderly and infirm, and hence at least 2–3 million women in the UK are affected.

Incontinence impairs quality of life in a number of ways. Embarrassment may lead to withdrawal

from normal social activities, may cause difficulties with childcare or employment, and may interfere with relationships; nocturnal incontinence leads to disturbed sleep; caring for an elderly relative with incontinence can become intolerable, leading to institutional care. Embarrassment and isolation may lead to feelings of worthlessness and depression. In some cultures women suffering from incontinence are completely ostracised and forced to leave their community.

Continence of urine

Continence of urine is normally maintained by the BLADDER and urethra acting as a single unit with a dual role: holding urine until it is convenient to void, and then, at a suitable time, completely emptying the bladder under voluntary control. As a storage organ the bladder must relax to accommodate large volumes of fluid without any rise in pressure. This requires that the muscle of the bladder wall (the *detrusor*) remains relaxed and compliant and able to stretch. To prevent urine leaking during this storage phase there is a sphincter mechanism acting to close the neck of the bladder and prevent urine entering the urethra. This sphincter has a number of components, all of which contribute to continence and which may be disrupted in a variety of ways. The bladder and urethra are maintained in position by the muscles of the pelvic floor and by fibrous supporting ligaments; when held in its correct position within the pelvis any rise in the pressure within the abdomen, during physical activity or coughing, is also transmitted to the urethra, preventing urine leakage.

In a baby voiding of urine is via a spinal reflex, but brain control of this reflex is gained during 'potty-training' and the ability is developed to suppress bladder contraction until a convenient time. During normal voiding the detrusor muscle contracts and the muscles of the urethral sphincter and pelvic floor relax in a co-ordinated fashion to allow the bladder to empty.

Causes of incontinence

Incontinence of urine results from a number of underlying causes:

(i) genuine stress incontinence (urethral sphincter incompetence);
(ii) detrusor instability/detrusor hyperreflexia;
(iii) overflow incontinence, retention, voiding difficulties;
(iv) fistulae (abnormal openings into the vagina from the urethra, bladder, or ureter);
(v) congenital (abnormal development of the urinary tract);
(vi) temporary causes (urine infection, constipation, drugs);
(vii) functional (immobility, dementia).

Stress incontinence is a term coined in 1928 by Sir Eardley Holland and refers to the loss of urine on coughing or straining. *Genuine stress incontinence* (GSI) is incontinence believed to be due to weakness of the urethral sphincter after other causes have been excluded. Childbirth has a major influence: during PREGNANCY hormonal changes and the increase in pressure on the pelvic floor cause softening and stretching of the supporting structures of the bladder and damage may occur during delivery. Ageing results in a loss of muscle strength; also, after the MENOPAUSE the reduction in oestrogen levels causes loss of elasticity of the tissues of the urethra, bladder, and pelvic floor. There are racial and hereditary differences related to variations in posture, pelvic muscle strength, and collagen. OBESITY, CONSTIPATION, and chronic COUGH also increase pressure on the bladder.

These factors lead to weakness of the tissues supporting the bladder in its correct anatomical position and allow it to descend during straining. This, together with damage to the sphincter mechanism, prevents the normal transmission of intra abdominal pressure to the urethra and allows the leakage of urine during physical effort.

Treatment of GSI Pelvic floor exercises were first described and used by Kegel in 1948 and remain the first line of therapy: their aim is to improve the muscle strength and tone of the pelvic floor. Continence surgery is warranted when conservative measures fail or when incontinence is severe, but the fact that over 150 operations have been described suggests that no one single procedure is best. Most operations aim to restore the bladder to its normal anatomical position. *Colposuspension* has been shown to be one of the most effective of these with success rates in excess of 90%. Other procedures utilising synthetic or natural slings or laparoscopically placed sutures also have a place in certain circumstances. Surgically implanted artificial sphincters have also been tried, with varying success.

Detrusor instability is the second commonest cause of female incontinence; uninhibited contractions of the detrusor muscle lead to the need to void frequently and urgently and in severe cases to 'urge incontinence'. The cause is unclear, but may be due to the bladder 'learning' to empty frequently. It may be aggravated by tea, coffee, alcohol, and stress. Loss of the normal bladder control may also occur in neurological conditions such as multiple sclerosis and after spinal injury, leading to uncontrolled detrusor contractions, known as detrusor hyper-reflexia.

Detrusor instability tends to be a chronic condition and its management aims to alleviate, rather than cure, the symptoms. Bladder retraining is useful — increasing the times between bladder emptying by the clock — and there are drugs which can be employed to assist this process. As a last resort, for those with severe and intractable incontinence, surgery may be necessary, to make a new bladder or to divert the urine to an artificial reservoir.

Overflow incontinence implies incomplete bladder emptying, overflow, and constant dribbling. This can occur if the bladder has been overstretched, if there is obstruction to normal emptying in pregnancy or by an enlarged fibroid uterus, or in neurological conditions which interfere with the emptying reflex.

Fistulae The tissues of the lower urinary tract may be so damaged that a direct channel forms from the bladder to the vagina and urine can leak continuously. Historically this form of incontinence was the most important as fistulae formed after prolonged obstructed childbirth: such fistulae have been identified in Egyptian mummies. This is still the commonest cause of incontinence where modern obstetric facilities are not available; specialist 'fistula hospitals' have been set up in parts of Africa. Fistulae are unusual in developed countries but may occur following surgery or radiation therapy or in advanced cancer.

Many other conditions may lead to incontinence. Infection of the urine causes symptoms of urgency and sometimes leakage of urine. Fibrous scarring of the bladder wall after radiation therapy can lead to a shrunken bladder unable to hold sufficient urine. Lastly, anything which limits an older person's independence can precipitate incontinence, which will be transient if the circumstances are reversed.

To investigate the cause of incontinence, infection of the urine is first excluded by microbiological examination of a sample. For further study, more complex tests of bladder function are necessary. The bladder has been described as 'an unreliable witness' as symptoms alone do not always reveal the underlying cause. 'Urodynamic' studies can be employed, to measure urine flow and the pressures within the bladder during filling and emptying. IMAGING TECHNIQUES (X-ray, ultrasound, and magnetic resonance imaging) can reveal the anatomy of the pelvic floor and lower urinary tract, and the inside of the bladder can be visualised directly with a cystoscope.

In some women incontinence is intractable and the aim is to improve quality of life. Absorbent pads, indwelling catheters, hand-held urinals, commodes, and toilet adaptations can be supplied; continence may be improved by promoting mobility and making toilets more accessible. Changes in lifestyle and coping strategies may also help. Devices worn internally may help some women to remain dry without the use of surgery. Support is essential to help women cope with their problems, and Continence Advisors, usually specially trained nurses, are being increasingly employed. The outlook for sufferers has improved dramatically. Modern investigation and treatment seems likely to restore continence and relieve the misery of increasing numbers of women.
JOHN BIDMEAD
KELVIN BOOS
LINDA CARDOZO

See also BLADDER; DIARRHOEA; FAECES; PENIS; PROSTATE; URINE.

Indigestion a commonly used term which encompasses a wide variety of gastrointestinal symptoms, including abdominal pain, heartburn, acid regurgitation, belching, bloating, bad breath, and even excessive passage of flatus. Each of these symptoms may have one of many causes when present as an isolated symptom and indicator of a specific disease; or many of them may occur together and be indicative of one or more disorders. Doctors may discern from the detailed history of the symptoms of 'indigestion' whether they are likely to represent a disorder of either the upper or the lower gastrointestinal tract.

The term indigestion however, is most often used to describe the symptom consortium often referred to as 'dyspepsia' — commonly defined as upper abdominal or epigastric pain which may or may not be related to eating. Associated symptoms may include heartburn, upper abdominal bloating, or belching. This is an extremely common condition occurring at one time or another in 25% of the adult population. Dyspepsia may be categorised as 'organic dyspepsia', when there is a clearly definable cause and disease entity, or as 'functional dyspepsia' when the pathophysiology has not been defined.

Organic dyspepsia

Common causes include chronic peptic ulcer, gastro–oesophageal reflux with or without oesophagitis, symptomatic gallstones, chronic pancreatitis; and intra-abdominal malignancy. Rarer causes include metabolic disorders, such as the uraemia of renal failure and hypercalcaemia, and conditions such as diabetes mellitus which disturb the function of the autonomic nervous system and hence impair gastric emptying.

Functional dyspepsia

Many now regard this as part of a wider spectrum of functional abdominal disorders which includes irritable bowel syndrome. In many instances the symptom pattern resembles that of an organic dyspepsia, although 'alarm' symptoms and signs such as weight loss, gastrointestinal bleeding, enlarged lymph glands, or an abdominal mass are absent. The cause of functional dyspepsia has not been clearly defined but is thought to relate to disturbances of motor function of the upper gastrointestinal tract, possibly associated with abnormalities of visceral sensation. Psychosocial factors such as stress, life events, and disturbance of affect are thought by some to be permissive for symptom production, even though they may not be the primary cause of the problem.

People under middle age who have no 'alarm' symptoms are not routinely investigated and are likely to be offered symptomatic treatment, with a variety of approaches including dietary modification, antacids, cognitive therapy, and possibly anti-depressant medication when appropriate. For those with symptoms that suggest the presence of organic disease, and for older people in whom such disease is in any case more likely, further investigation is required, such as upper gastrointestinal endoscopy, abdominal ultrasound scan; and possibly abdominal CT scan. Specific therapy can then be directed towards the identified cause.
MICHAEL FARTHING
ANNE BALLINGER

See also ALIMENTARY TRACT.

Infant feeding

Mammals have existed on earth for around 200 million years. The first hominid mammals appeared about 5 million years ago, while the genus *Homo* is known to have existed for at least 2 million years. Our own species *Homo sapiens sapiens* appeared only in the last 150 000 or so, and some populations probably began the transition from hunter gatherer, hunter fisher to farmer during the last 12 000 years.

With animal husbandry came increased opportunities for feeding human infants on the milk of other mammals. Although it is likely that other lactating females in the tribe would provide for the needs of most orphaned infants, high maternal mortality would encourage the finding of alternative sources of milk. With the industrial revolution came increasing social pressures for women to work outside of the home and to use at first home made and subsequently commercially prepared substitute formulas for feeding their infants.

Earliest records of infant feeding practices date from about 3000 BC. The civilisations of Mesopotamia and Egypt were largely matriarchal and from the Old Testament Hebrew text we learn that the ability to suckle children was regarded as a gift from God. In the pre-Semetic Sumerian peoples of Mesopotamia the goddess Inanna was believed to protect the child throughout early life, and in ancient Egypt the goddess Isis is usually depicted nursing the infant king Horus. Much of our information about these early civilisations comes from the papyri of Ebers and Lesser Berlin (sixteenth century BC). Remedies recommended in these documents include rubbing the breasts with poppy plant whilst eating fragrant bread of soured Dourra to improve milk supply. To relieve breast pain it was recommended that a mixture of calamine, oxgall, fly dirt, and yellow ochre should be rubbed into the breast daily for four days.

Wet nursing

A Sumerian lullaby of the third millenium BC refers to the wife's nursemaid suckling the son of Shulgi, ruler of Ur. The Code of Laws of Hammurabi, Amorite king of Babylon, indicates that there were laws safeguarding arrangements between parents and employed wet nurses — probably one of the earliest examples of employment legislation.

From the Old Testament we learn that there was a search amongst Egyptian and Hebrew women for a wet nurse to feed the infant Moses rescued from his basket trapped in the bullrushes. We also learn that Deborah was the wet nurse to Rebecca and that Ruth gave her son to her mother-in-law Naomi to nurse.

Around the time of the birth of Christ it was clear from the contracts of wet nurses that they were usually, but not always, slave women. Some contracts specified for how long the child should be breast-fed by the nurse and from this information it was clear that up to 3 years was not uncommon but 16 months would be about the average length of contract. Hannah breast-fed her own son, Samuel, for three years and Isaac, son of Abraham, was weaned from the breast at 2 years. In Greek mythology Zeus was reported to have been suckled by the goat Amalthea, and Romulus and Remus, the founders of Rome in the eighth century BC, were thought to have been suckled by a she-wolf. Direct suckling from animals is well documented throughout recorded history and persisted in Europe into the twentieth century.

There is very little recorded about the views of Hippocrates, the father of modern medicine, on matters related to early infant feeding and it seems likely that records of his views on this topic have been lost or not recorded. Aristotle (384–22 BC), who was the son of a court physician but was not himself a physician, made several references to children and clearly indicated that breast-feeding should ideally commence on the first day, contrary to many earlier European and Asian reports which delayed suckling at the breast for 3–4 days. He also made the link between the duration of breastfeeding and menstruation; the longer the duration of suckling the greater the delay in the recommencement of menstruation (and therefore child-bearing). He also repeated the myth that breast milk (which was believed to be formed from menstrual blood diverted to the breast) produced after menstruation had recommenced was unfit for infant feeding. Soranus of Ephesus (AD 98–117) recommended that the newborn infant should be given boiled honey or honey and goat's milk during the first few days to help expel meconium from the infant bowel before giving the child to a wet nurse for feeding. He held the view that maternal milk was unwholesome for the first 21 days after birth. Galen (AD 130–200) recommended boiled honey for three days before allowing the mother to feed her infant, but only after she had expressed or allowed an older child to suckle her 'first milk'. Thus the meddlesome interference by men in the natural feeding processes of mother and infant has a long and sorry history.

Emperor Tiberius was a drunkard and Caligula a cruel thug. History relates their behaviour to the fact that Tiberius had an alcoholic wet nurse and that Caligula's was spiteful, blood-thirsty, and smeared her nipples with blood. These views on the transference of character through the breast milk persisted throughout medieval times. During the sixteenth to eighteenth centuries in Europe understanding about the transmission of what we now know as venereal diseases and tuberculosis gradually improved, although it was not until the nineteenth century that Koch and Pasteur began to clarify the nature and basis of infections.

Artificial feeding

Feeding vessels such as terracotta feeding horns and horns of sheep and goats have been identified in infant graves from about 4000 BC and shown to contain residues of milk. Since then most societies have used horns of animals with the tips cut off and covered with parchment, leather, sponges, and cloths for infants to suckle. A variety of shaped containers and feeding spoons and cups were manufactured for feeding artificial milks and weaning foods. Many of these vessels undoubtedly transmitted infections to the infants resulting in disease and death. Even with modern plastic bottles and synthetic teats failure of hygienic cleaning and contaminated water supplies can prove lethal.

The unsatisfactory nature of animal milks for the human infant led to many experimentations in attempts to 'improve' or modify animal milks. In an MD dissertation submitted in 1761 Thomas Young, later to become a Professor of Medicine in Edinburgh, reported on the admixture of alkali, gastric juices, and other chemicals to milk and the differences between fore-milk and after-milk. Pierre Budin in Paris in about 1860 used calf pancreatic extracts to 'digest' cow milk for feeding to the infants in his maternity hospital, as he was unable to obtain adequate supplies from wet nurses and the mortality from feeding untreated cow milk was horrendous. Infant morbidity and mortality in Europe during the late nineteenth century due to artificial infant feeding was similar to that found in developing countries today. Current commercially-produced infant formulas are subject to strict controls in terms of microbiological safety and chemical composition, but remain nutritionally inferior to the natural mother's milk in many respects. There are a number of identifiable health benefits to infants fed solely breast milk during the first months of life.

Weaning

A report on health and social subjects entitled 'Weaning and the Weaning Diet' published by a Working Group of the Committee on Medical Aspects of Food Policy of the Department of Health in England and Wales, defined weaning as the process of expanding the diet to include foods and drinks other than breast milk or infant formula. Weaning allows the infant to meet changing nutritional needs and to become less nutritionally dependent upon milk. In Egypt during Roman times weaning was usually commenced once the child was erupting teeth (6–8 months). Other foods, particularly animal milk and eggs, were introduced and the milk of camels, goats, sheep, and cows, together with fruit and vegetables, were the usual weaning foods. Corn and pulses are also mentioned in the Old Testament. Even in today's societies there are many different weaning practices dependent upon history, religious taboos, and the availability of nourishing foods suitable for infants. Continuation of breastfeeding during the weaning process contributes a degree of protection to the infant gastrointestinal tract whilst new foods and potentially infectious materials are introduced during the weaning processes. The modern view is that human milk is entirely nutritionally adequate for the first four to six months of life but thereafter other nutrients need to be introduced to the diet. The duration of breast-feeding is largely determined by the mother's and family's attitudes to child rearing and the financial, social, and educational status of the mother and society. The Department of Health report on Weaning and the Weaning Diet gives a view of the current weaning practices in the United Kingdom.

FORRESTER COCKBURN

Further reading

Fildes, V. A. (1986). *Breasts, bottles and babies.* Edinburgh University Press.

Still, G. F. (1996). *The history of paediatrics.* College of Paediatrics and Child Health, London

HMSO (1994). *Weaning and the Weaning Diet.* Report on Health and Social Subjects, Vol. 45. London.

See also BREAST; INFANCY; WET NURSE.

Infection
The normal human body is covered with billions of harmless MICROORGANISMS: indeed, we each carry more bacteria than the total human population of the world! These, together with the skin and the IMMUNE SYSTEM, serve to protect the body from invasion by harmful, or 'pathogenic' microorganisms.

If there is a breach in one of these lines of defence, these pathogens can gain access to the body. Entry may be, for example, via a skin wound, inhalation, ingestion, or sexual intercourse, and may be facilitated by immune deficiency or loss of the normal organisms living on the body, for instance after a course of ANTIBIOTICS.

As soon as the immune system detects the presence of a pathogen it mounts a response to kill it, which is highly successful in most cases in healthy people. On the rare occasions where it fails, or in people with poorly functioning immune systems, the organism may succeed in establishing itself and cause disease: an infection occurs. The term 'infection' therefore encompasses not only the classical 'INFECTIOUS DISEASES', but also such diseases as boils, thrush, urinary tract infection, and surgical wound infections.

The immune response produces a syndrome of INFLAMMATION at the site of the infection. This is characterised by redness, warmth, pain, and swelling, caused by extra blood supply to the area bringing white blood cells to fight the infection. Pus may be formed (a mixture of white cells, dead tissue, and organisms). Usually this stops the infection from spreading. However, if the organisms gain entry to the bloodstream, sepsis or 'blood poisoning' may ensue. In sepsis the body's white cells respond by producing vast amounts of chemicals which, as well as helping to kill the marauders, result in FEVER, flushing, shivering, low blood pressure, rapid heart rate, and, in severe cases, delirium. Sometimes this immune response is more harmful than the infection itself. Conversely, sepsis may be difficult to recognise in patients with suppressed immune systems who cannot mount such a florid response. Finally, some microorganisms are not easily recognised by the immune system at all, so that infection may have few if any symptoms until later in the course of the disease when damage to the body by the organism is well advanced. Examples are the human immunodeficiency virus which causes AIDS, and the PRION causing Creutzfeld-Jacob disease.

Hospital infection and antisepsis
For many hundreds of years, fevers and infections were believed to be caused by 'miasmas', or noxious air exuding from rotten materials. In the nineteenth century the most notorious, and perhaps the most tragic, manifestation of sepsis was puerperal sepsis, or childbed fever, in which the dangerous bacterium *Streptococcus pyogenes* (now known as the Group A streptococcus) gained entry to the bloodstream via the birth canal. It had a very high fatality rate and was responsible for the deaths of countless young mothers every year. Although well-recognised as a complication of childbirth, the cause was not understood. The Hungarian obstetrician Ignaz Semmelweis, working in Vienna in the 1850s, was particularly concerned by the high rate of childbed fever on one of his wards which was attended by medical students. On this ward nearly a fifth of his patients died of sepsis. On his other ward, attended only by midwives, the rate was only about 3%. He realised that the medical students came directly from the autopsy room to the obstetric ward and proceeded to examine the patients without even washing their hands in between. He insisted that each student should wash his hands with soap and water and then an antiseptic before entering the ward, and saw the mortality rate drop immediately to less than 2%. Thus he proved not only transmission by hand of an infectious agent, but also that it could be prevented by use of antisepsis.

This was a dramatic result, but despite this Semmelweis was ignored and even ridiculed. It was Joseph Lister, working in Glasgow in the late 1860s, who brought about the general acceptance of surgical antisepsis. He used carbolic acid to transform SURGERY from a highly dangerous last resort to the treatment of choice in many conditions. Florence Nightingale did the same for hospitals after the Crimean War, during which she had shown that cleanliness and hygiene were paramount in preventing injured soldiers from dying of infections — although, ironically, she never believed in the germ theory of disease, rather she believed that filth and dirt bred disease directly.

Since then the refinement of antisepsis before and during operations has been one of the most important developments in allowing the practice of surgery as we now know it. Even now, maintaining a low infection rate is one of the priorities of every surgeon. Low levels are attained by the use of 'asepsis' — that is, sterilising the instruments so that no microorganisms are present on them — and 'antisepsis' — the use of chemical solutions to decrease the number of the patient's and the surgeon's own microorganisms as far as possible. Nowadays, one of the greatest challenges facing hospital infection control is the prevention of spread of bacteria that are resistant to many antibiotics, such as methicillin-resistant *Straphylococcus aureus* (MRSA)

ANGHARAD PUW DAVIES

See also INFECTIOUS DISEASES; MICROORGANISMS.

Infectious diseases
are the result of damaging MICROORGANISMS obtaining access to the body, and not being repelled or destroyed by the immune system. Their relationship to man is that of parasite and host, and is continually adjusting. Numerous different types of BACTERIA, VIRUSES, and other organisms may cause disease, and infection may take place through close contact with an infected person, or through the respiratory, digestive, or genito-urinary systems, depending on the organism and the disease involved. Infection may also occur by transmission from an animal, or via an insect vector. Organisms can damage the body by their multiplication in or around its cells, or by the widespread poisonous effects of substances (toxins) which they release. Many infectious diseases are of a self-limiting character, ending in either full recovery or death. While certain of them may occasionally have long-term sequelae, the body, if its defences win, for the most part returns to normal, often retaining a lifelong subsequent immunity against that specific infection. Other infections, such as syphilis, are, however, chronic, and eventually fatal if untreated.

Diseases included in the category 'infectious' include colds and influenza; the familiar infectious illnesses of childhood, and the more serious conditions such as poliomyelitis, diphtheria and meningitis, typhoid, typhus, cholera, dysentery, and smallpox. TUBERCULOSIS is also an infectious disease, although its clinical progress is chronic rather than acute.

Most of these diseases have a very ancient history. While many only emerge as identifiable entities in the medical writings of the seventeenth and eighteenth centuries, others can be demonstrated to have been present in antiquity. Smallpox, for example, which was declared eradicated by the World Health Organisation in 1977, can clearly be identified by characteristic lesions on the mummified corpses of ancient Egyptians, while a stele of the same civilisation, dating from 1580–1350 BC, shows a young man displaying a withered and shortened left leg, held in the 'equinus position' characteristic of paralysis possibly caused by poliomyelitis. Infectious diseases also occur in the animal kingdom, and some, such as anthrax and yellow fever, are transmissible to man.

Understanding
While the closely allied concepts of infection and contagion (transmission of disease from one person to another by direct or indirect contact) are probably almost as old as mankind, it was only in the mid nineteenth century, with the development of accurate microscopes and of laboratory research, that these processes began to be scientifically elucidated. Several observers indicated the likelihood of microorganisms as causal agents of disease, and even detected their paths of transmission, such as the faecal–oral route for typhoid and cholera, but it was Louis Pasteur who, in the early 1860s, first gave a coherent account of the process of infection in what is popularly known as the *germ theory* of disease. In 1876, Robert

Koch identified the causal organism of anthrax, and within a few years had also identified the agents of tuberculosis and cholera. By 1900, the specific agents of numerous diseases had been identified, and the diverse routes of transmission — of infection and contagion — were beginning to be mapped out.

Infectious diseases are often 'crowd diseases', which depend for the most part on reservoirs of susceptible people to maintain themselves. Person to person infections, for example, are thought to have become more apparent between 3000 and 500 BC, when urban centres grew large enough to support them. These diseases soon established an *endemic* character in such centres, meaning that the diseases or infectious agents were constantly present in that area. City populations, exposed early in life, acquired high levels of immunity to them, compared with rural populations. Rapid and unregulated urban growth brought a great escalation in the incidence of and mortality from many of these diseases in Western Europe and North America during the nineteenth century, and several, including tuberculosis, typhoid, measles, and whooping cough, were responsible for much human misery and many thousands of deaths. Recurrent gastro-intestinal infections, in particular, helped to undermine the health, and natural resistance to infection, of babies and young children, and indeed of adults also. By 1830, annual death rates of over 30 per 1000 living persons were commonplace in Western cities, while infant mortality rates rivalled those of under-developed nations today.

Prevention

Beginning in the 1830s, public health movements began to develop in many Western states in response to this crisis of mortality. For example, in Britain — one of the first nations to begin to adopt public health measures — early reformers such as Edwin Chadwick stressed the enormous economic costs of such a wastage of life. At this period, notions of contagion marched in parallel with a belief that gases generated by rotting organic matter were productive of EPIDEMICS, and early attempts at preventing premature deaths focused on environmental improvement. Slowly and painfully, through the following decades, filtered and piped water systems, mains drainage, systematic scavenging, and slum clearance brought about cleaner, healthier urban environments, and disrupted the transmission routes of a number of important infections, notably of water-borne typhoid and cholera and of louse-borne typhus.

The development of specific methods of prevention came late in the history of the infectious diseases. Smallpox, one of the most ancient and most hideous diseases, was the first to be tackled in this way. At some point, the Chinese had discovered that by introducing matter taken from smallpox vesicles into a scratch on the normal healthy body, controlled, immunizing infections could be established. This method, the *inoculation* of material containing the living organism, itself was not foolproof, since it was not possible

to ensure a mild rather than a virulent infection, which might prove fatal. Nonetheless, knowledge of the technique spread along trade routes to Turkey, and thence to Europe in the early eighteenth century. In 1796, a Gloucestershire medical practitioner, Edward Jenner, picked up on local lore which suggested that infections with cow-pox would protect against smallpox, and demonstrated that this was indeed the case. This practice, vaccination (from *vaccinus*: pertaining to a cow) was later refined, and, encouraged by many European governments, the introduction of the modified or related organism displaced inoculation as the principal preventive against smallpox. At this stage, however, the processes and principles which made vaccination effective were still not understood.

Smallpox vaccination represented an ideal for disease eradication which provided an important model for future medical research. Louis Pasteur, for example, set out in his later career to investigate the principles of immunology with a view to understanding how vaccination worked. Pasteur's breakthrough with the principle of attenuating viruses — reducing their virulence — came in 1876. This meant that the body's immunity to subsequent infection by a virulent organism could be actively provoked in response to a non-threatening form of the same strain; Pasteur proceeded to develop immunizations against various animal diseases, including anthrax and rabies. It was his reluctant application of rabies vaccine to the boy Joseph Meister in 1883 that first alerted the general public to the eventual possibilities of immunology.

As the discipline developed through the work of Pasteur, his colleagues, and his successors, new therapeutic and preventive indications emerged. Early successes came for diphtheria in 1894 with anti-toxin therapy (the use of material produced by the inoculation of animals with toxins produced by bacteria), and for both diphtheria and tetanus with the development of active immunization (the production of protective antibodies by stimulating the body's immune system). In 1896, Almroth Wright succeeded in producing an anti-typhoid vaccine using killed bacteria, thus extending the theoretical options for vaccine development. In the interwar period, successful vaccines were developed against diphtheria and tuberculosis, and, in the years following World War II, they were developed against most of the principal childhood infections — whooping cough, poliomyelitis, German measles, and measles, and eventually against mumps and chicken-pox as well.

Since 1870, there has been an enormous decline in death rates from infectious diseases in developed countries. This decline has been hastened by the availability of immunizations, but in most cases had begun well before such protection was available. Rising living standards — including smaller families, better housing, improved domestic hygiene, a reduced incidence of gastro-intestinal infections, and better nutrition — together with public health measures contributed largely to

this reduction. Many childhood diseases remain serious in poor and under-developed countries. Immunization, although a valuable resource with some diseases, is by no means a viable prospect for all infections; despite decades of research, no vaccine has yet been approved for malaria, one of the world's most serious infections.

New infections

New infectious diseases are still emerging, and there is no room for complacency in this regard. The emergence of poliomyelitis as a serious killer and maimer between about 1911 and 1962 was partly attributable to improved hygienic standards in the West, which meant that children were no longer harmlessly exposed to the virus as babies. Lassa fever, exemplar of a whole new generation of sinister tropical fevers, emerged in Nigeria in 1969, while Legionnaires' disease was identified in the US in the 1970s. The rapid global spread of HIV infection since 1980 echoes that of syphilis in Europe in the fifteenth century. Epidemics of the terrifying Ébola virus in Zaire, and of bubonic plague in India in the early 1990s, indicate that both new and old infections retain the potential for major human tragedy. One consequence of global warming could possibly be the reappearance of malaria as an indigenous infection in parts of the world which have been free of it for many decades. Relentless human exploitation of tropical resources, uncontrolled human reproduction, increased travel, and unregulated technological development all create the potential for unleashing fresh manifestations of new and old infections by disturbing global environmental equilibrium.

ANNE HARDY

Further reading

Garrett, L. (1996). *The coming plague: newly emerging diseases in a world out of balance.* Penguin Books, London.

McNeill, W. H. (1979). *Plagues and peoples.* Penguin Books, Harmondsworth.

See also ANTIBIOTICS; EPIDEMIC; FEVER; IMMUNE SYSTEM; IMMUNIZATION; MICROORGANISMS; SEXUALLY TRANSMITTED DISEASES.

Infertility may be primary or secondary. Primary infertility is when no pregnancy has ever occurred. Secondary infertility is when there have been one or more pregnancies but a further pregnancy has proved impossible. It has been estimated that the chances of conception for a given couple having regular sexual intercourse without any contraception are 80% and 90% after 12 months and 18 months respectively. It is therefore usual to begin investigations after one year. At this time some problems may be discovered and it should be possible, the basic tests having been done, to offer a realistic prognosis and a possible treatment outline. It is important to discover if there are any obvious abnormalities because with the new methods of treatment that have become available over the last twenty years it is frequently possible to offer real hope of success.

Female physiology

The Fallopian tubes lead from the ovaries, where the eggs are made, to the uterus. Each month, around 12–14 days from the last menstrual period, an egg (OVUM) is released from the OVARY. The ovum passes down the tube and its passage is facilitated by the moving cilia of the lining cells, which waft the ovum along. If intercourse occurs around this time the SPERM swims up through the uterus to the tube and one of them joins the egg in the tube. The fertilized egg then continues down the tube to the uterus which has been prepared by hormones to receive the egg.

Causes of infertility

Unexplained	27%
Male factor	24%
Anovulation	21%
Tubal factors	14%
Endometriosis	6%
Sexual dysfunction	6%
Mucus hostility	3%

Unexplained infertility is not easy to define. The more investigations that a clinic is able to perform the lower is the incidence of unexplained infertility. Hopefully some time in the future all will be explained.

Male infertility It is not always recognised how commonly the male partner is the infertile one. The average amount of seminal fluid ejaculated each time is 2–5 ml. Persistent low volume may indicate an abnormality. If the number of sperm is less than 10 million/ml this makes fertilisation less likely. The mobility of the sperm is also a factor, as is the ability of the sperm to penetrate the egg. These factors can all be tested in the laboratory. An important cause of reduced sperm numbers is a history of mumps, as the testicles are damaged in some cases.

Anovulation means that for some reason no ovum is produced in each MENSTRUAL CYCLE.

Tubal factors The main tubal factor is blockage, which may result from infection from sexually transmitted disease or a previous miscarriage. The blockage prevents the union of sperm and ovum so that no pregnancy occurs. Sometimes, although the tube may not be blocked, the cilia, which assist the passage of the ovum down the tube, are damaged so that the ovum gets stuck in the tube and union with the sperm does not occur. Sometimes the sperm does manage to fertilize the stuck egg and this results in a pregnancy occurring in the tube — an ectopic pregnancy. As this pregnancy grows the tube may rupture, with serious consequences due to bleeding into the abdominal cavity.

Endometriosis is a condition where, for unknown reasons, portions of the lining of the uterus grow in other parts of the pelvis such as the ovaries. The reason why this causes infertility is not clear.

Sexual dysfunction occurs sometimes due to psychological factors that prevent proper intercourse.

Mucus hostility means that the secretion from the neck of the womb (cervix) is abnormal, and kills the sperm so that they cannot travel through the uterus to the tubes.

Investigations

At an infertility clinic both partners are given a full physical examination and a detailed medical history is taken.

In the *male* a good proportion of infertility is due to deficiencies in SEMEN, so a proper seminal examination is essential. This involves measurement of the volume of the ejaculate — the sperm count — which should be 20 million/ml or more; the swimming ability of the sperm; and the numbers of abnormal forms present. A history of mumps or sexually transmitted disease or genital trauma are important, as are previous hernia operations. A social history of drug and alcohol intake may be relevant, as may occupations involving working at extremes of temperature or at altitude. Physical examinations may reveal some testicular or penile abnormality.

There is still controversy as to what constitutes normal semen. With modern methods of assisted reproduction many men with very low sperm counts can produce enough sperm which can be used to fertilize eggs '*in vitro*' (IVF). Our ideas as to what constitutes an infertile male have radically altered in the last twenty years.

In the case of the *female* partner the occurrence of ovulation can be tested by Basal Body Temperature measurement (the temperature rises 1 degree following ovulation in the second half of the menstrual cycle) and by measurement of the female hormones, OESTROGEN and PROGESTERONE. The use of ULTRASOUND can visualise the ovum in the ovary, and taking a sample of the lining of the uterus can show whether or not the uterus is being prepared properly in each cycle for reception of a fertilised ovum. Assessment of the state of the tubes can be achieved by injecting dye through the cervix. This fills the uterine cavity, and, with the use of a small telescope (laparoscope) inserted into the abdomen, dye will be seen flowing from the tubal opening at the ovary if the tube is patent. If no dye is seen the tube is blocked. A newer method, falloscopy, involves the introduction of a tiny telescope (falloscope) into the tube through the tubal opening in the uterus and allows evaluation of the state of the tubal lining — so important for the transport of the egg. The mucus at the cervix can be sampled and tested to see if it kills sperm; if it does, there are methods of avoiding this.

A small telescope (hysteroscope) can also be used to examine the inside of the uterus to see if there any abnormalities of shape and to exclude the presence of tumours. All these tests are available at properly equipped infertility centres.

A history of pelvic infection may be relevant — perhaps after a miscarriage or previous abdominal operation, or due to sexually transmitted disease. An abnormal menstrual history may suggest a hormonal disturbance. Previous use of hormonal contraception (the Pill) can result in anovulation, and use of the intrauterine device can cause infection and blocked tubes.

The success of infertility treatment varies enormously depending on the cause. In the most favourable cases treatment may be 90% successful. In cases it may be quite unsuccessful. Nowadays, with proper investigation and treatment the results are incomparably better than a quarter of a century ago.

MALCOLM MACNAUGHTON

See also ASSISTED REPRODUCTION; FERTILITY; IMPOTENCE; MENSTRUAL CYCLE; OVUM; PREGNANCY; TESTIS.

Inflammation The word incorporates the Greek for flame, and indeed an inflamed body part may feel 'on fire'. In its traditional clinical description, inflammation has four characteristics: *calor* (heat), *rubor* (redness), *tumor* (swelling and *dolor* (PAIN). They are the manifestations of the body's defence against INJURY or against invasion by foreign material or MICROORGANISMS, including the means of removal or destruction of the offending agent, restriction of the spread of infection, and preparations for the healing process. But the IMMUNE SYSTEM that implements vital self-preservation may also sometimes cause inflammation by misdirected attack on some part of the body itself.

Inflammation can occur anywhere, acutely in the skin around a wound or a sting, or in less visible sites such as the lining of the middle ear, or of the bladder, or of the gall bladder. Chronically it can be related to persistent infection, ulceration, mechanical or chemical irritation, or AUTO-IMMUNE disease. Wherever inflammation occurs there are certain local mechanisms in common, despite differences in the precipitating factors and also in the relative prominence of the four cardinal features. Even with relatively minor and apparently localized problems, there are whole-body responses. Wherever inflammation is located, the condition is given a name ending in *-itis*, prefixed by the traditional name of the body part, such as arthritis for the joints, gastritis for the stomach, pericarditis for the membranes around the heart, ileitis for the small intestine, osteitis for bone, encephalitis for the brain.

Tissue damage results in the release by cells of various chemical agents, including PROSTAGLANDINS. Vasodilator substances relax the blood vessels in their vicinity and the resulting increase in blood flow accounts for the redness and heat; swelling follows from increased permeability of blood vessels. This all enhances the supply of factors normally present in the blood that are important for the inflammatory response, including white blood cells and certain proteins in the plasma. Locally released substances (*cytokines*), as well as bacterial toxins if there is infection, attract cells of the immune system — macrophages and lymphocytes.

The nerves that carry the signals, set up by chemical and mechanical stimulation of SENSORY

RECEPTORS, that we perceive as pain, themselves in turn promote an increase in local blood flow through the *axon reflex* mechanism. The nerve fibres (*axons*) give off branches back to their site of origin, and these release '*substance P*', a peptide that relaxes the vessel walls. This, together with prostaglandins and other substances released from damaged tissues and also from the macrophages that congregate at the site, increases the sensitivity of sensory nerve endings, enhancing pain.

The events are not confined to the focus of trouble. Cytokines circulating in the blood provoke diverse whole-body responses. A major site of action is the HYPOTHALAMUS, where they can affect its regulation of pituitary secretions, of sympathetic nervous system activity, and of body temperature. Whilst the resulting responses mainly promote the many aspects of defence, some also modify reactions that might otherwise be excessive: ENDORPHIN release modifies pain, and the increase in secretion of corticosteroids has anti-inflammatory effects, including toning down the activity of macrophages and interfering with prostaglandin synthesis.

The manifestations of inflammation vary greatly with the nature and severity of the insult and whether the process is rapidly or slowly developing. It can be simply *serous*, with fluid exudation, such as in a blister or a swollen joint, or in the *rhinitis* (of the nose) at the start of a common cold. With some types of infection it can be *suppurative*, where tissue and immune cell debris form a collection of pus; and chronic inflammation can be *granulomatous*, with nodules composed of packed inflammatory cells.

The phenomena of inflammation reflect an appropriate response to infection, or to mechanical damage either by acute injury or prolonged pressure or friction. When they occur inappropriately as a reaction against the body's own tissues the manifestations are similar. Thus conditions that might be called 'inflammatory' may refer to chronic infections, or to degenerative processes (as in osteoarthritis), or they may result from congenital abnormalities (as in cystic fibrosis) or autoimmune disease (such as rheumatoid arthritis or regional ileitis (Crohn's disease)).

It would be inappropriate to attempt by treatment to diminish the body's responses, in terms of both local and widespread effects, if and when they were entirely appropriate and necessary to contain or cure the condition. Alleviation of the pain of inflammation by analgesic drugs is clearly beneficial to the sufferer; otherwise the first concern of treatment is if possible to remove the cause (such as treating infection by ANTIBIOTICS, or removing foreign material). Other treatments in recent decades have been directed against inflammation itself, in conditions related to injury, 'wear-and-tear', and auto-immunity. Imitation and enhancement of the body's own anti-inflammatory corticosteroids became possible with synthetic STEROID preparations, but there are undesirable side-effects. Along with the

understanding of the role of prostaglandins in the mediation of inflammation and fever, a whole family of 'non-steroidal antiflammatory drugs' (NSAIDS) were developed, and they are widely used for a variety of muscle and joint problems, from accidental sprains to widespread arthritis. These drugs inhibit enzymes necessary for formation of prostaglandins, thus diminishing their local and general effects. (ASPIRIN was well known to be useful in this context long before it was known to act by this mechanism.) No evidence has emerged for any positive or negative effect on the progress of the underlying conditions themselves (as opposed to relief of the symptoms), supporting the notion that the body's inflammatory responses are not always useful. Symptoms may indeed be relieved, but there are side-effects of NSAIDS, particularly gastrointestinal complications, related to the inhibition of prostaglandin synthesis where and when it is normally needed.   SHEILA JENNETT

See also AUTOIMMUNE DISEASES; FEVER; IMMUNE SYSTEM; INFECTION; INFECTIOUS DISEASES; INJURY; PAIN; PROSTAGLANDINS.

Initiation rites are regarded by anthropologists as a special class of RITES OF PASSAGE, displaying a tripartite sequential form, dominated by the themes of death from one social position and rebirth to a new one. Well-known initiation rituals in Western society include initiations into craft guilds, Masonic lodges, and fraternities and sororities in American colleges, as well as into religious orders and cult groups. These vary from relatively spontaneous events to highly complex ceremonials where the testing of an initiate's worthiness is combined with the inculcation of esoteric knowledge and injunctions to secrecy. A similar range of rituals is found in traditional societies, with many of the more elaborate associated with entry into adulthood, which is also sometimes associated with membership of cults and secret societies. Such rituals commonly stretch over many months, or even over many years in cases where the initiation involves a progressive set of grades, such as those for initiation into manhood by Australian Aboriginal and New Guinea groups.

At the heart of all these is the right to membership of a tightly-defined community, to a distinctive identity and status. The individual is both 'tested' for his fitness and, in many rituals, transformed and made-over in line with cultural prescription. To some extent, the themes of hazing, humiliation of the novice, and the often dangerous ordeals — or ordeals which are made to appear dangerous to the initiand — play their part in this context. The submission of the individual to the authority of the group and its representatives is also an overt element. For example, among the Mende of Sierra Leone, boys must be initiated into the Poro Society before they are recognised as adult. To this end, they are 'eaten' by the Poro spirits, an act which is represented by the painful scarifications made upon their naked and prone bodies. This is followed by a prolonged period where the initiands must

fend for themselves, secluded for a year from the rest of the community. Submission to the spirits, impersonated by masked elders, is followed by a period of self-reliance, both qualities deemed necessary for successful adult life.

The particular form such ordeals take raises further problems of interpretation. Initiations into adulthood, as this example shows, often involve permanent forms of bodily mutilation, from the extraction or filing down of teeth, to scarification and TATTOOING, genital operations of many kinds, elongation of the earlobes or neck, and the insertion of facial or other bodily forms of ornamentation. All such practices leave visible and permanent marks of membership; literal inscriptions of the social onto the body. The question is, whether this is all? Is the form they take purely arbitrary, a matter for the free play of the cultural imagination, or do some of these mutilations betray ulterior motives? The issue has arisen in its most controversial forms with respect to genital mutilations such as CIRCUMCISION, for which, one might think, every possible 'explanation' has been advanced. It has been interpreted (amongst other things) as a substitute for human sacrifice and CASTRATION; as a hygienic measure; as a way of increasing sexual desire and/or FERTILITY or, alternatively, of decreasing it; as a way of enhancing the differences between male and female genitalia or, through its mimicry of female bleeding, a way of making them more similar — and so on. All of these may form part of local exegesis; the question of whether they have any wider or universal validity is today generally regarded as both unfashionable and unprofitable. Anthropologists, pointing to the extent of cultural variation, tend to insist on the importance of contextual understanding. The majority hold to the line originally advanced early in the twentieth century by Van Gennep, who wrote that culturally the body has been treated simply like a block of wood, which each has cut and trimmed to suit himself.

For many years the anthropological postulate of arbitrariness opened up a broad chasm between psychoanalytic and anthropological approaches to the subject, with the latter contesting the psychoanalytic view that genital mutilation is central to the development and purpose of such rites. Social function was stressed at the expense of sexual meaning and no essential difference was seen between genital and other bodily mutilations. Anthropologists tended rather to problematize the role of pain and trauma in such rites in terms of their capacity to forcefully impose social values, to leave indelible marks on the body and memory. Socialisation is also at issue in considering the stoic bravery expected of the novice in many rituals, often, though not exclusively, in those that extol martial values for their menfolk. Many such rituals invite comparison with modern forms of military training. For example, among the Gisu of Uganda, boys stand the ordeal of circumcision when they are between 18 and 24, in a public demonstration of courage where even involuntary movements of the body, such as blinking the eyes, are taken as a sign of cowardice. This is believed to give them a quality of manhood which differs in kind from that of men of non-circumcising tribes and which radically distinguishes them from women in the force of their anger and potential for VIOLENCE.

Nevertheless, with GENDER identity and PERSONHOOD so clearly at issue, the old divide between the disciplines is no longer so evident, as anthropologists have begun to explore the subjective experience of initiation as it is encoded in different cultural idioms. Initiations do not simply bestow a status in the sense of formally bequeathing it, but many aim at an active transformation of human potential. In her study of the *chisungu* rites among the matrilineal Bemba of Zambia, Audrey Richards directly addressed the question of what is taught during this girls' initiation ceremony. This ritual prepares a girl directly for MARRIAGE, yet, as Richards noted, although the girl is subject to repeated injunctions on her coming role as wife and mother, very little of this formal instruction goes beyond what she already knows from growing up in the society. But, through the elaborate ritual with its focus on fertility and its dangers, Richards argues that 'teaching' is still a relevant dimension to our understanding of the purpose of such rites. We should understand this as not about teaching *knowledge* but rather of teaching *attitudes* as Bemba women 'regrow' their girls. By undergoing the initiation, Bemba girls learn to experience themselves differently, and are made ready to cope with the coming dangers of fertility, in which they are responsible for protecting their home and hearth from the potentially polluting powers of SEXUALITY.

Regrowing in the context of the acquisition of adult gender identity is also at issue in male initiations in New Guinea, with their plethora of explicit sexual symbolism. For example, among the Sambia of New Guinea the initiation of boys into manhood begins at the age of around 8 and lasts many years. These years are dedicated to ridding the boys of polluting maternal influences and turning them into pure and fierce men. To this end, they are subjected to repeated painful episodes of bleeding, induced by inserting sharp grasses into their nostrils. This is held to release accumulated maternal blood. This is followed by repeated episodes of fellation by adult male initiators to 'feed' the boy masculinity, a masculinity which is associated with physical strength and military prowess. In these cases, anthropologists have usefully brought psychoanalytic forms of understanding to bear in understanding the dynamics of gender creation, though always in the context of local understandings of the person.

Studying the transformative powers embodied in such rituals is an eclectic venture, in which many forms of understanding are applicable to a comprehension of the potency of such ritual processes. Victor Turner, for example, was particularly concerned to explore the existential dimensions involved in the experience of liminality, occurring most usually in the mid-phase of such rites when the person is ritually dead to the world. He sees the key process here as one of ritual levelling, with the person stripped of social insignia and signs of secular status, and subject to humiliation by ordeal, test, and trauma. It is this humbling process which interests him, and he speculates that it contains a revitalising element for both the individual and the community. For the initiand, it reaffirms the bonds of essential humanity upon which the social order ultimately rests, uniting him closely with the others with whom he has shared the experience. Culturally, it seems to allow also of other possibilities. The ritual dissolution of normal social forms, as initiands are ritually refashioned, allows for a juggling of the normal factors of existence, a freeing of creative potential. The often monstrous nature of the sacra, of MASKS and EFFIGIES, and of contact with the normally forbidden, throw elements of the culture into relief by exaggeration, challenge, inversion, and paradox.

SUZETTE HEALD

Further reading

Herdt, G. (ed.) (1982). *Rituals of manhood: male initiation in Papua New Guinea.* University of California Press, London.

Richards, A. (1956). *Chisungu.* Routledge, London.

Turner, V. W. (1969). *The ritual process.* Penguin Books, Harmondsworth.

Van Gennep, A. (1960). *The rites of passage.* Routledge, London.

See also BODY MUTILATION AND MARKINGS; RITES OF PASSAGE; TABOOS.

Injury to the body can result from accidents, acts of violence, or surgery. This third category, inflicted by the medical profession itself, is often forgotten, but it does of course cause damage to body tissue — although hopefully the overall result of surgery will be of benefit to the patient.

Injuries can range from damage so minor as to be hardly noticed, to that which is so severe that it causes death or prolonged disability. The size of the problem becomes apparent when it is realized that almost a quarter of all deaths in Europe and the US are caused by injury, particularly to children and young people (six times as many children die from injury than from cancer). In Britain, road traffic accidents are the main cause of death from injury, but in the US gunshot and knife wounds kill more people every two years than the total number of fatalities in the whole of the Vietnam war, and in young black males gunshots at home are the single greatest cause of death.

Understanding the responses to injury (even when the injury is not severe) and developing treatments, is clearly very important. Research indicates that such responses are complicated and variable. They depend on the type and site of injury, the age and health status of the victim, and the time after the injury.

Our bodies can adapt extremely quickly to injury by activating a whole array of responses to limit damage. These occur not only at the specific site of the injury, but also involve most of the general systems in the body, including the heart and circulation, the endocrine, nervous and immune systems, and complex changes often called the 'defence response' or 'acute phase response'. All of these changes are directed towards helping the body to cope with damage, to keep functioning normally, and to start the processes of repair and recovery. However, sometimes, when injuries are severe, it is the body's own defence responses which can actually cause problems and even death, because they are inappropriate or excessive.

Within seconds of injury, responses start to be activated. The first of these — and the one of which we are most aware — is the sensation of PAIN. Nerve signals from the damaged tissue signal to the brain in fractions of a second a 'red alert' to move away from the source of pain and protect the injury. These nerve signals also have other functions. They activate a whole-body response, which has been called the 'fight or flight' response, because it involves many of the same changes which occur when we are fearful of danger or need to flee away from threats.

The 'fight or flight' response (which is seen even in very primitive organisms) means that the brain automatically activates our *sympathetic nervous system* to increase heart rate and blood pressure, to direct blood to important regions (the brain, the heart, and in this case the site of injury), and to stimulate release of specific HORMONES. These hormones tend to stimulate body functions which may be needed to fight off infection, support repair of injuries, and help the heart and other organs cope with the threat to survival. For example, the ADRENAL GLAND releases increased amounts of the steroid hormone *cortisol* (often used in medicines to reduce inflammation); the PANCREAS releases the hormone *glucagon*, which mobilizes glucose (needed as a rapid energy supply); and the sympathetic nervous system releases ADRENALINE and NORADRENALINE, which not only stimulate the heart and blood vessels, but also start to mobilize body fuels.

Another very important part of the body involved in injury is the IMMUNE SYSTEM, which acts locally at the site of damage and throughout the body. A group of proteins, called *cytokines*, are produced quickly by immune cells and injured tissues. They, together with other factors released by tissue damage, cause swelling around the injury, and stimulate immune cells in the blood to race into the wound and surrounding tissue. Cytokines also induce the LIVER to produce a second wave of proteins known as *acute phase proteins*; the endocrine glands to alter HORMONE release; the brain to cause changes such as FEVER and the general symptoms of illness; and many other organs and systems to make various changes. As with most responses to injury, cytokines can help to limit and localize damage and stimulate repair and recovery. However, it is now clear that overproduction of certain cytokines can cause problems, and severe cases may prove fatal, so there is intense research into ways of limiting the production of cytokines.

These general responses are common to many types of injury, but other changes in the body depend on the type or severity of the injury. For example, severe loss of blood (HAEMORRAGE) can actually cause a reduction in blood pressure and may result in 'SHOCK'. Severe pain or injury can also result in shock and loss of consciousness, and toxins released from bacteria in the gut after severe injury can result in a condition similar to severe infection. If this progressive deterioration goes unchecked, it can lead to a fatal condition known as *multiple organ failure*, where major organs such as the liver, kidney, heart, and lungs are unable to function.

Damage to the brain can be rather different to injury in other parts of the body, for several reasons. Nerve cells (neurons) in the brain, unlike other cells of the body, cannot regrow. Therefore, when they are lost, recovery is limited by the ability of existing brain to compensate, that is, the extent to which functions can be 'recovered' in other healthy areas of the brain. Secondly, quite minor damage to the brain can have very major effects on responses in the rest of the body and therefore on survival. For example, damage to very small parts of the lower, most primitive parts of the brain (the BRAIN STEM), which control the essential functions of breathing and the heart, can prove fatal, whereas quite severe loss of some other parts of the brain can be survived with only modest disability.

The responses to injury are often divided into *acute* (early and quite rapid) and *chronic* (prolonged and sustained). It is usually the early phase which is critical, but of course delayed and prolonged events in the body are also important. The mobilization of fuels necessary for the acute response means that body tissues (fat and protein resources) must be broken down. This, together with loss of appetite or inability to eat after injury, usually means quite significant weight loss. In otherwise healthy adults, this may not be a problem — though even patients who are overweight can have difficulties because protein (mainly muscle) is broken down as well as fat. The implications are much more severe in young, growing children and in elderly patients. Because old people are often underweight and not very mobile, loss of muscle, for example after breaking a leg, can be a real problem.

Finally, the injury itself must recover. This requires repair to the damaged tissue, and possible formation of a scar. SCARS are not just a cosmetic problem; they can reduce the normal function of some tissues (particularly the brain) and result in a focus for future problems. Again, research is starting to identify factors — particularly proteins known as *growth factors* — which can aid repair of injured tissues, and those which lead to scars. Considerable advances in understanding the processes which occur after injury and development of new treatments mean that we can now, with the right medical care, survive some injuries that would once have been fatal.

Physical repair may not of course be the end of the story for the injured person. The prolonged, varied, and complex psychophysiological after-effects of major injury, particularly from assault and violence, known as '*posttraumatic stress disorder*', have been — and continue to be — a focus of research, especially with respect to the aftermath of war and rape. As more becomes known about the mental and physical processes involved, there is hope for more effective assistance towards recovery.

NANCY J. ROTHWELL

Further reading
Rothwell. N. J. and Berkenbosch, E. (ed.) (1994). *Brain control of responses to trauma*. Cambridge University Press.

See also AUTONOMIC NERVOUS SYSTEM; HAEMORRHAGE; IMMUNE SYSTEM; PAIN; SHOCK; STRESS; WOUND HEALING.

Instinct The concept of instinct is an attempt to explain why some kinds of behaviour develop consistently in a given species across a wide range of environments. Each species of animal exhibits some characteristic forms of behaviour that have this developmentally robust quality. Bees, for example, dance to indicate the location of pollinating flowers, and they do this with no formal instruction. When a type of behaviour develops in this way, without the need for learning or any other environmental input beyond the bare minimum for physical survival, it is usually attributed to a strong internal force that pushes development in certain directions rather than in others. It is to this idea of a strong internal force that the notion of instinct refers.

Though popular in the nineteenth century, the concept of instinct fell into disrepute during the early decades of the twentieth century. The rise of ethology in the 1940s led to a resurgence of interest in the concept. Led by Konrad Lorenz and Niko Tinbergen, the ethologists argued that even learning — a paradigmatically non-instinctive kind of development — often required certain predispositions. The search-space of possible hypotheses was just too large to be explored successfully without the aid of some innate guide. The distinction between instinct and learning was not, therefore, an exclusive one: rather, many forms of learning required an instinctual support.

Though relatively uncontroversial for explaining animal behaviour, applying the notion of instinct to human behaviour has had a much more chequered history (see SOCIOBIOLOGY). Nineteenth-century thinkers such as Darwin and Freud were quite happy to explain some human behaviour in terms of instincts, but in the twentieth-century psychologists were much more reluctant to do so. This is because PSYCHOLOGY was dominated for much of the century by the view that the mind is a 'blank slate' upon which experience writes what it needs. It was not until cognitive scientists, such as Noam Chomsk, began, in the 1950s, to call attention to the problems with this view, that

psychologists again began to take seriously the idea of innate constraints on learning.

Chomsky did for LANGUAGE what the ethologists had done for learning in animals: he pointed out that learning a language would be impossible without some predispositions to learn certain things. The distinction between learning and instinct was once again shown to be more subtle than the way in which it was often presented. Language is a good example, because, although it has to be learned, the learning is guided by innate rules, unlike, say, learning to play chess. In Darwin's apt phrase, the ability of humans to learn language is 'an instinctive tendency to acquire an art'. The psychologist Steven Pinker has made this point vividly in his book *The Language Instinct* (1994).

The concept of instinct does not, therefore, entail an inflexible notion of development. On the contrary, it is quite compatible with the idea that developmental outcomes are contingent on environmental conditions, and with the idea that learning plays an important part in development. In contemporary cognitive science, developmental outcomes are seen as the result of a complex interplay of innate programs and environmental inputs. The innate programs do not take the form 'Thou shalt', but rather specify disjunctive rules such as 'if … then …'. The environmental inputs determine whether the rules are applied or not. In this model of development, the disjunctive rules correspond to instincts.

DYLAN EVANS

Further reading
Lehrman, D. S. (1953). Critique of Konrad Lorenz's theory of instinctive behaviour. *Quarterly Review of Biology*, **28**(4), 337–63.

Tinbergen, N. (1951). *The Study of Instinct*. Clarendon Press, Oxford.

Insulin Glucose, dissolved in the blood (BLOOD SUGAR), is one of the main sources of energy for the body. Different organs and tissues use other fuels to varying extents, but the brain uses glucose exclusively. To protect vital functions mammals have evolved a mechanism for keeping the concentration of glucose in the blood fairly constant — an example of HOMEOSTASIS. This includes diverse hormonal responses that *increase* the blood glucose concentration. Yet, in what seems a remarkable oversight of nature, the body relies almost entirely upon just one hormone, the protein INSULIN, to bring about a *decrease* in blood glucose. Insulin facilitates the entry of glucose from the blood into the tissues of the body.

It has been known since 1899 that removal of the PANCREAS from dogs led to DIABETES, with its characteristic persistent increase in blood glucose (*hyperglycaemia*) and presence of sugar in the urine (*glycosuria*). The fascinating saga of the eventual discovery of insulin by Banting and Best in 1921 is well known. They were able to show that injection of an extract from the pancreas of a healthy dog led consistently to a decrease in the amount of sugar in the blood and urine of diabetic dogs. They published their account, entitled 'The Internal Secretion of the Pancreas', in 1922. Their experiments, which were to prove life-saving, assured the insulin molecule a key place in medical history, and won a Nobel Prize for Banting and Macleod (in whose Canadian laboratory the work was done) as well as earning the grateful thanks of diabetic people in their millions around the world. It was some 30 years later that Frederick Sanger embarked on his painstaking but highly successful molecular dissection of insulin, which unravelled its precise AMINO ACID sequence. This was a landmark achievement, representing as it did the first successful sequencing of any protein molecule, and it earned Sanger his first Nobel Prize. With subsequent establishment of its three-dimensional structure, insulin was revealed as a vital protein of classic polypeptide design. Despite 300 million years of divergent evolution, the molecular form and function of insulin has been remarkably well conserved across the entire zoological spectrum.

The dynamic glucose–insulin system on which the body's METABOLISM so critically depends is controlled and modulated by various factors impinging on the 'β-cells', which are found in the pancreas in cellular nodules, the *Islets of Langerhans* — named after the German pathologist who described them in 1869, long before their function was known. These 'β-cells' detect glucose in the blood and secrete insulin in appropriate amounts in response to the meal-induced tidal changes in blood glucose level.

Insulin is normally quite rapidly removed from the blood and survives in the circulation for only 5–15 min, thus placing a continuing demand on the β-cells for the release of more insulin in order to establish an effective feedback control of blood glucose concentration. This moment-by-moment process requires, in the β-cells, mechanisms for the manufacture, storage, and rapid release of insulin. To replenish its insulin supply, the genes of a pancreatic β-cell switch on their protein manufacturing machinery, producing a much larger single chain precursor molecule, called pro-insulin, which contains the amino acid sequence of insulin. Successive and controlled proteolysis (breakdown of this protein molecule) finally leaves the 51 amino acid sequence of insulin itself, and ensures its correct folding to create the three-dimensional shape of the molecule. Once formed in the β-cell, insulin is stored in granules as a symmetrical hexagonal array of 6 insulin molecules combined in a stable crystalline structure with 2 atoms of zinc. When released into the circulation at effective concentrations, insulin is transported as, and normally acts as, a single molecule.

To exert its effects on target cells — muscle, liver, or fat cells — the insulin molecule must first be recognised by specific insulin-receptor protein molecules in the CELL MEMBRANES. Part of the insulin receptor spans the membrane, so that, when an insulin molecule binds to the external part of the receptor, a signal is transmitted across the membrane to other molecules, leading to a cascade of enzyme activity in the target cells.

Insulin resistance may occur when the blood glucose level is not well controlled, as in a type of diabetes which begins in adult life, where the pancreatic β-cells do not produce enough insulin. Not only does this lead to the appearance of the symptoms of diabetes, but the high level of glucose in the blood decreases the sensitivity of the target cell receptors for insulin and so makes the situation worse. It is possible to treat this type of diabetes by mouth with agents that boost the output of insulin from any viable β-cells that are present, or reduce the blood sugar by other means. If, on the other hand, pancreatic β-cells have all been destroyed, as in juvenile diabetes, then insulin must be injected daily as replacement therapy.

Unfortunately insulin cannot be given orally because it is a peptide and is therefore rapidly broken down by enzymes in the gut. Different preparations of insulin are available for injection, depending on the duration of action required. Insulin was originally extracted on a massive scale from the pancreas of animals (cows or pigs). It can now be obtained by genetic engineering of bacterial cells, causing them to express human insulin. It is noteworthy that insulin was the first protein to be commercially produced by such recombinant technology. Although this allows large scale production and isolation, pig pancreas remains the main source of insulin for human treatment: pig insulin differs from human insulin by only one amino acid.

Various insulin formulations may combine rapid-, medium-, or long-acting forms of crystalline insulin so that individual requirements for insulin can be matched to blood glucose levels following meals. Insulin has thus become firmly established in modern medicine as a remarkably effective therapeutic agent, but a whole life-time of constant injection is an unwelcome hazard for anyone suffering from juvenile diabetes. The design and production of a non-peptide, orally-active insulin analogue therefore remains a major goal of pharmaceutical research.

E. K. MATTHEWS

See PLATE 7.

See also BLOOD SUGAR; HORMONES; METABOLISM; PANCREAS.

Intelligence

What is intelligence? Ability to learn? Success in adapting to new situations? The number and originality of mental associations? Skill in reasoning or producing abstract ideas or problem-solving? All of these definitions have been proposed but none has yet become definitive, either for professional psychologists or for the lay public. In general, intelligence most often refers to practical problem-solving ability, verbal ability, social competence, and effective adaptation to one's environment and to new situations and changes within it. There is often a quantitative dimension as well: some individual or group or species has more or less of it than some other. Cross-cultural studies have revealed significant differences in the ways in which various groups define the sets of characteristics associated with something like overall mental ability.

And historically, even in the West, intelligence has meant a number of things. It was used most often until the twentieth century to refer simply to all the intellective functions of the mind, as distinguished from the will and the emotions, universal human properties little associated with measurable individual ability.

Francis Galton in England and Alfred Binet in France were among the most significant within psychology in developing the modern conception of intelligence. Beginning in the 1860s, Galton pursued a programme of investigating individual differences in mental ability by measuring reactions to various physical stimuli and then showing that those measurements were distributed, like height or weight, according to the normal or bell-shaped curve. Although Galton's anthropometric approach was soon abandoned, his insistence that intelligence was a biological entity that was inheritable, and normally distributed in populations, persisted, and became linked to a very different method of assessing intelligence devised by Binet. In response to a governmental education commission, Binet and his colleague Théodore Simon created a set of tests, individually administered, which were designed to track normal intellectual progress. Oriented toward the higher mental processes, the Binet–Simon Intelligence Scale (1905, 1908, 1911) was able to produce a number, the mental age (MA), that characterized the intellectual level of each child administered the examination. Not only did it allow test-takers to be ranked according to the level of their intelligence, but it suggested that intelligence itself was a discrete and measurable entity.

The Binet–Simon Intelligence Scale set the standard for all further developments in the field. Lews M. Terman's 1916 revision of the Binet–Simon scale, the Stanford–Binet, quickly became the benchmark instrument for the assessment of intelligence, and helped to introduce the concept of the intelligence quotient (IQ), a ratio of mental age to chronological age which was adopted from German psychologist Wilhelm Stern and designed to produce a measure of intelligence which was constant over time. Revised in 1937 and again in 1960, the Stanford–Binet has remained one of the pre-eminent individual measures of intelligence. Its main rivals have been the tests of child (WISC) and adult (WAIS) intelligence developed by David Wechsler, starting in the 1940s, which provide, in addition to an overall measure of IQ, individual assessments of verbal and non-verbal ability.

Wechsler's provision of two additional scores highlights one of the persistent theoretical issues pursued in studies of intelligence: whether it is one thing or many. Using factor analysis, British psychologist Charles Spearman (1904) argued that performance on intelligence tests could be explained on the basis of two factors, general intelligence (*g*) and task-specific abilities (*s*). Spearman's theory was challenged during the 1920s and 1930s, by L. L. Thurstone in the US and Godfrey Thomson in the UK, both of whom also employed factor analysis, but who used it to argue against *g* and in favour of the existence of a small number of relatively independent abilities. During the post-war period, Philip E. Vernon, among others, attempted to arbitrate between these competing theories using a hierarchical conception of intelligence, which depicted intelligence as extending from a single overall ability down to a large number of specific skills. This approach was rejected by Joy P. Guilford, however, who proposed instead a three-dimensional model that initially posited 120 independent mental factors and subsequently posited 150. Commencing in the 1970s, various cognitively-based models have been put forward, including most prominently those by Howard Gardner, with his seven discrete types of intelligence, and Robert J. Sternberg, with his triarchic theory of intelligence. These cognitive approaches owe a great deal to the influence of the psychometric tradition and also to developmental studies of intelligence, particularly those associated with Jean Piaget (stages of intellectual development) and Lev Vygotsky (social influences on intellectual development).

The second major theoretical issue in intelligence studies has been over the relative weights of nature and nurture. Galton's work on individual intelligence began with the assumption that intelligence was both biological and inheritable, a belief that ran strong during the heyday of EUGENICS (1900s–20s), and was used to support such programs as immigration restriction and STERILIZATION of the mentally deficient. Research during the 1930s and 1940s, however, especially at the Iowa Child Welfare Research Station, emphasized the importance of nurture: IQ, for example, was found to change when children were placed in different environments. After the war, studies continued to show the powerful effects of both nature and nurture on IQ. Research on identical twins has led some psychologists to conclude that at least 60% of IQ results from heredity. At the same time, a great deal of data has been collected indicating the influence of nutrition, kind of education received, and degree of sensory stimulation on IQ score.

The enormous professional interest in intelligence has been sustained by its many practical applications. As part of mobilization for World War I, American psychologists created new instruments that could be group administered, and tested approximately 1.75 million army recruits. This programme served to introduce the nation to standardized intelligence testing, and during the 1920s intelligence testing boomed, adopted by schools and industry as a means of efficient placement and assessment of students and personnel. Although some of the infatuation with testing receded by the end of the decade, intelligence and its measurement had by then become permanent features of the social and intellectual landscape. Debates over the provision of educational opportunities, the capabilities of various ethnic or racial groups, and the value of affirmative action have all been conducted at least in part through the language of native intelligence. However ill-defined, intelligence has become a concept of much consequence within the contemporary world.

JOHN CARSON

Further Reading

Ceci, S. J. (1996). *On intelligence: a bioecological treatise on intellectual development.* Harvard University Press, Cambridge, MA.

Sokal, M. M. (ed.) (1987). *Psychological testing and American society, 1890–1930.* Rutgers University Press, New Brunswick.

Intestines The whole of the gut or alimentary tract beyond the stomach. The *small intestine* comprises duodenum, jejunum, and ileum, and the *large intestine* the caecum, colon, and rectum. The functions of the intestine are summarised as completion of digestion (which started in the stomach); absorption of nutrients, minerals, and water; motility (the various types of movement which mix and move the contents); and defence against invasion by harmful organisms. To these ends, the lining secretes mucus, ENZYMES, and water, and has folds and protrusions that increase its surface area. The tubular wall has layers of SMOOTH MUSCLE and an intricate nerve network; ample lymphatic tissue provides defence responses; and non-pathogenic MICRO-ORGANISMS usefully inhabit the colon. S.J.

See ALIMENTARY SYSTEM; PLATE 1.

Intrauterine device (IUD)

Intrauterine devices have a long and controversial history, with their widespread acceptance being delayed until the later part of the twentieth century. Hippocrates has been credited with using a hollow lead tube to insert pessaries or other objects into the uterus over 2500 years ago, and Arabs and Turks are known to have placed stones in the uteri of their camels to prevent pregnancy while on long journeys. It was not until 1909 that Richter, a German physician, developed a looped aluminum–bronze wire spiral that could be placed in the human uterus. However, his results did not include details of pregnancy rates because of strict laws against birth control measures in place at the time. Twenty years later Grafenburg reported the use of an intrauterine silk suture, and then modified his technique by using a ring wrapped in wire that contained 26% copper. Early IUDs were associated with high rates of pelvic infection, septic ABORTION, and haemorrhage, particularly as they were also used by some to terminate pregnancies. A number of maternal deaths were attributed to their use and this led them into disrepute amongst both the medical profession and the general population. It was not until the first international conference on IUDs in New York in 1962 that they gained widespread acceptance. They are now the second most commonly used form of reversible CONTRACEPTION worldwide, mainly because they are so popular in China.

Intrauterine devices work primarily as a foreign body stimulating the IMMUNE SYSTEM into producing an excess of leukocytes and PROSTAGLANDINS. This creates a hostile environment in the uterus and fallopian tubes, making it difficult for FERTILIZATION to occur. In addition, the IUD creates a barrier to implantation of an embryo into the endometrium. Because the contraceptive effect may occur after fertilization some women find this form of family planning unacceptable. Most IUDs are now made of a plastic frame, with copper wrapped around them to increase their contraceptive action and therefore reduce the failure rate. Threads are usually attached to the lower end to facilitate removal. They are extremely reliable, with pregnancy rates of less than 1 per 100 women using them for a year. However, they are not very effective at preventing ectopic pregnancies which develop outside the uterine cavity. IUDs can also be used as 'emergency' contraception up to 5 days following the calculated date of ovulation.

Coils, as they are commonly known, are not usually recommended for women who have never been pregnant, as they are more difficult to insert and the slightly increased risk of *pelvic inflammatory disease* (PID) may impair future fertility. They are also unsuitable for women with a recent history of SEXUALLY TRANSMITTED DISEASE or multiple sexual partners. Women with an abnormally shaped uterus, possibly caused by fibroids, should use a different contraceptive technique as the risks of failure are much higher in this situation.

The recent development of progestogen-releasing IUDs has been an exciting new contraceptive advance. Difficulties associated with older generation coils, such as heavy and sometimes painful periods, promise to be overcome. They have also provided a new treatment option for women with heavy periods who no longer need contraception, perhaps because they have already been sterilised. This type of IUD can be used to oppose the unwanted effects of oestrogen on the endometrium in women receiving HORMONE REPLACEMENT THERAPY (HRT).

ANDREW HEXTALL

LINDA CARDOZO

See also CONTRACEPTION.

Ion channels

CELLS are enveloped in a lipid membrane that forms a barrier to the diffusion of ionized substances. Ion channels are specialized PROTEINS that sit in the membrane and form aqueous pores, through which ions can flow. Ion fluxes across the CELL MEMBRANE produce electrical currents, which cause changes in the membrane potential. Cells can generate a rich variety of electrical signals by the opening and closing of different combinations of ion channels. These signals are used for a multitude of different purposes. All of the sensory information we receive from the outside world, whether it be visual, auditory, olfactory, or mechanical, is processed and analysed using electrical signals. Nerve cells use electrical signals of approximately 100 mV in amplitude and 1–2 milliseconds in duration to convey information rapidly over distances of up to 1 m. These signals are called ACTION POTENTIALS, and they can travel at rates of up to 120 m/sec without diminishing in size. The HEART uses similar electrical signals to regulate the rate and force of the heartbeat. IONS that play a key role in the electrical excitability of nerve and muscle include potassium (K^+), sodium (Na^+), calcium (Ca^{2+}), and chloride (Cl^-).

Other ion channels found in electrically non-excitable cells have predominantly a transport role. For example, those in the KIDNEYS are important in regulating the levels of salts and water within the body, whereas those in the LUNGS regulate fluid secretion and absorption — when these channels are absent, as occurs in patients with *cystic fibrosis*, then the mucous lining of the airways becomes dehydrated.

The opening and closing of ion channels is highly regulated. Different types of channels respond to different stimuli, which can be chemical, electrical, or even mechanical. Those activated by a change in membrane potential are called voltage-activated, whereas those activated by an external chemical ligand (a molecule that binds to them) are called ligand-activated. Ion channels are selectively permeable to different classes of small ions; this is necessary for a channel to generate the electromotive forces needed for electrical signalling. Some ion channels discriminate only between cations and anions, whereas others are highly selective and can discriminate very effectively between ions that are similar. For example, many of the potassium-selective ion channels prefer potassium to sodium by a hundred-fold or more, and despite their discerning nature can conduct 10 000 000 potassium ions across the membrane each second through a single channel molecule. Ions move through the pore passively, and the direction of current flow depends only upon the difference in the internal and external ionic concentration and the potential across the membrane, so when the electrical force and chemical force acting upon an ion are of equal magnitude, but opposite in direction, then there is no current flow across the membrane.

In nerve, muscle, and endocrine cells, electrical signals are translated into a cellular response by the opening of voltage-activated, calcium-selective ion channels. The resting levels of calcium within cells is very low (less than 10^{-7} M), and the influx of calcium into the cell causes a rise in the internal concentration. Many cellular processes, including contraction of all types of muscle and the secretion of neurotransmitters and hormones, are regulated by internal calcium. Thus the influx of calcium triggers a response. Internal calcium also controls the 'gating' of some ion channels.

The idea that channels form aqueous pores in the membrane began in the 1950s, when Hodgkin and Huxley developed a method for clamping the voltage across the membrane of a giant *axon* (nerve fibre) taken from a squid,

whilst simultaneously measuring the current flow. The large size of the currents suggested that ions must flow through aqueous pores rather than be transported by a carrier mechanism. Hodgkin and Huxley measured inward currents carried by sodium ions and outward currents carried by potassium ions, and showed that these voltage-activated channels underlie the generation of action potentials in axons.

In the late 1970s and early 1980s, Neher and Sakmann developed 'patch clamp' recording methods, which enabled very small patches of membrane to be electrically isolated from the rest of the cell membrane. The tip of a glass micropipette (diameter 1 μm) is pressed against the cell and a seal is formed, between the glass and the membrane, which has a resistance of greater than 10^9 ohms. Currents flowing through *single* ion channels within the patch of membrane can be recorded, and the opening and closing of the channel is observed as step-wise changes in the current level.

Some of the most important advances in our understanding of ion channels in the last two decades have arisen from the development of *recombinant DNA techniques*, which have enabled the CLONING of genes that encode ion channel proteins. The first ion channels to be purified and cloned were an ACETYLCHOLINE receptor channel and the voltage-activated sodium channel from the electric organs of the marine ray and electric eel, by Numa and colleagues in the early 1980s. Similar channels were subsequently cloned from mammalian muscle. They are macromolecular complexes composed of several different protein subunits. Well over 100 ion channel genes have now been cloned, and from the predicted amino acid sequences it is clear that there are families of related ion channels that must have arisen from the same ancestral gene by the process of gene duplication and subsequent divergence of the sequence. Similar ion channel structures are found in cells from a wide variety of life forms, including animals, plants, paramecia, and bacteria, indicating that these channels appeared very early on during evolution.

In more recent years, molecular genetics has revealed an increasing number of hereditary diseases that we now know to be caused by mutations in genes that encode ion channels. One of the most well known is cystic fibrosis; others include muscle diseases such as (para)myotonia congenita and hypo- and hyper-kalaemic periodic paralysis. There are also hereditary kidney and heart diseases which are known to be caused by conductance defects. One of the challenges for the future is to develop gene transfer therapies to treat patients with these diseases.

RUTH MURRELL-LAGNADO

See also CELL; CELL MEMBRANE; GENETICS, HUMAN.

Ions carry an electric charge or charges. Those with one or more positive charges are called cations, whereas those with negative charges are called anions. The names arise from considering

what happens if a current is passed through an ionic solution; cations migrate to the cathode and anions to the anode, allowing current to flow through the solution. Common inorganic cations found in the body are sodium (Na^+), potassium (K^+), and calcium (Ca^{2+}), while common anions are chloride (Cl^-) and bicarbonate (HCO_3^-). Neither anions or cations can exist in isolation, as the total electrical charge must be in balance. A solution of sodium chloride will have an equal number of Na^+ and Cl^- ions, and a solution of calcium chloride will have twice the number of Cl^- ions as Ca^{2+} ions. Organic molecules can also be ionic. The neurotransmitter acetylcholine chloride will give, in solution, a positively charged acetylcholine moiety together with a chloride ion. Some organic molecules may carry a positive and a negative charge on different parts of the molecule and are known as *zwitterions*.   A.W.C.

See also BODY FLUIDS; COMPOSITION OF THE BODY.

Iron lung While 'iron curtain' has a provenance that is clear, the origins of the term 'iron lung' are uncertain. First records of its use surfaced in newspaper articles during the poliomyelitis epidemic of the 1920s, when reference was made to a rigid case fitted over the patient's body, used for administering prolonged artificial respiration by means of a mechanical pump. Yet already in 1670 John Mayow had advanced the concept that negative pressure draws air into the chest, and subsequently John Dalziel, a Scottish physician, described a negative pressure device which augmented respiration in his paper 'On sleep, and an Apparatus for Promoting Artificial Respiration'. The first practical demonstration of the technique was provided by Dr Woillez of Paris, who was awarded the silver medal of the 1876 Le Havre Exhibition of Life Saving Equipment for his hand-operated bellows, the *Spirophore*. He was to be followed some 40 years later by Dr Stewart in South Africa, who built a wooden box sealed at the shoulders and waist with clay. However, it was not until the polio epidemic of the 1950s that the use of such a device became commonplace.

In the 1920s experiments were being made on anaesthetised cats to record the positive pressure changes caused by inspiration in an enclosed chamber around the animal's thorax. The investigator's colleague, Dr Philip Drinker of the Harvard School of Public Health, acutely aware of the clinical problem at the nearby Children's Hospital, of respiratory failure in infantile paralysis, repeated the experiment with cats paralysed with curare. He found that animal could be ventilated and kept alive by the suction action of a syringe attached to the box enclosing the animal's body. Drinker sought and obtained funding from the Consolidated Gas Company of New York (who had previously sponsored a committee chaired by Drinker, which reported on improved methods of resuscitation in cases of gaseous poisoning), and with Louis Shaw he

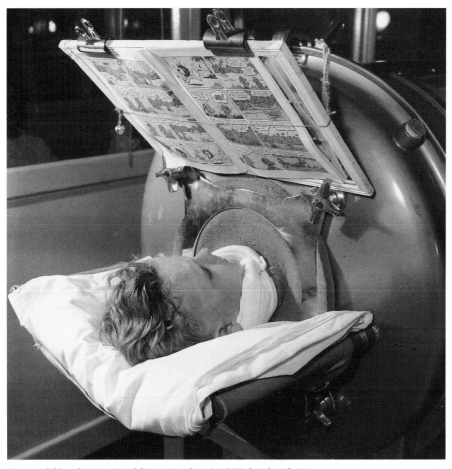

A young child reading a comic while in an iron lung (c. 1955).© Hulton Getty.

built a wooden cabinet, which opened and shut like a drawer, to contain the human torso.

In 1926 his first iron lung (perhaps named for the iron of the pump) was left at the bedside of an eight-year-old girl affected with respiratory paralysis due to polio. As she deteriorated she was placed in the cabinet, but the staff, unfamiliar with the device, feared to turn on the pump, which was left to Drinker himself. Within minutes the moribund young girl was revived, only to die soon after of pneumonia.

Thus it had been established that artificial respiration could maintain life, but little was known of the natural history of such respiratory paralysis. Would this mean the prospect of an entire lifetime in an iron lung? Although this was the case for some, the second patient to be treated, at the adjoining Peter Bent Brigham Hospital, recovered respiratory muscle function, and the era of LIFE-SUPPORT was begun.

In the 1930s, 'Drinkers' as they also became known, were found throughout the US; in the UK a cheaper alternative, designed by Both, an Australian, was also available, being paid for by the motor car manufacturer and philanthropist Lord Nuffield. By 1937, 965 of these were to be found throughout the UK and elsewhere. Improved access for patients was achieved with a hinged opening of the tank, like the jaws of an alligator (or Alligator tank) this time by Captain Smith-Clarke of the Alvis Motor Car Company. Cape Engineering company produced aluminum versions, of which 150 were sold between 1954 and 1967. An additional modification was introduced in 1961 by Dr W. Howlett Kelleher of the Artificial Respiration Unit at the, Western Hospital, Fulham. This was a rotating version of the Iron Lung, which permitted chest physiotherapy in all positions.

The non-invasive application of positive pressure through nose masks has largely superceded the iron lung in the treatment of respiratory failure, but the final chapter in the story of the iron lung is still to be written. In the UK a few patients remain ventilated for part or all of the day using the iron lung, and it is still used by some in the short term for people with acute exacerbations of chronic airways obstruction.

ADRIAN J. WILLIAMS

See also ARTIFICIAL VENTILATION; BREATHING; RESUSCITATION.

Islam and the body As was the case in other pre-modern societies, the peoples of the Middle East conceived of the body in various ways, reflected in both popular perceptions and the formulations of formal intellectual disciplines. In early Islamic times, in the seventh to ninth centuries, Muslims displayed far more systematic interest in the body in religious and legal terms than in strictly medical affairs, and by the time a formal medical tradition began to emerge in Iraq, in the mid ninth century, there was already a copious literature on the subject in the religious sciences of Islam. This material continued to be extremely influential throughout Islamic history and remains so today.

Religious views of the body

The scholars who formulated the religious thought of Islam had definite views on the body. In some respects these views were also shared by Christians and Jews, but for Muslims the agenda was to uphold a strict and pristine monotheism that they considered the older faiths of Judaism and Christianity to have abandoned.

Where the body was concerned, the central argument was teleological. All things come from God, including the human body, which must therefore reflect God's merciful and beneficent plan for mankind. If this is so, then the body must reflect a principle of harmony and order in keeping with the unity and omnipotence of its author. The human body, it was maintained, works in harmony for the sake of the whole: fingers, for example, do not exist for their own sake, but for the sake of the whole body, which benefits from the grasping and manipulative functions that fingers perform. Some parts of the body, it is true, are not essential to life — blindness is a disability, for example, but one suffering from it can still lead a fulfilling life. But nothing in Creation can be superfluous, not even barren deserts or seas full of salt water, otherwise God would be either a trifler or a faulty planner and orderer of His creation, both of which conclusions were of course impossible in a monotheistic context. Thus nothing in the body is useless; all parts have a function that can be related to the functions of other parts. This notion — the so-called '*argument from design*' — was of course already prominent in the traditions of peoples of the past. The Old Testament contains many examples of this, and in Greek medical thinking the idea is prominent in the works of the Hellenistic physician Galen 129–216 AD. But Islam promoted it in a major way, and his deployment of the argument from design, with a major role for the demiurge, was undoubtedly one factor that made Galen very attractive in the heyday of the translation movement (ninth to tenth century), when Greek texts were being rendered into Arabic as much for their disputational and didactic utility as for their medical content.

Islamic views of the body were also shaped by the fact that Islam, in contrast to Christianity, had no doctrine of original sin. The Qur'an states explicitly that all souls are Muslims from the moment of Creation — it is errant upbringing in human society that turns them to other religions. The God–man relationship is therefore an essentially positive one; man is fickle, weak, and unmindful and forgetful of his duty to God, but he is not encumbered by the burden of the sin of Adam.

The implications of such formulations for notions of the body were significant. Islamic social sensibilities and law have always placed heavy emphasis on the ritual purity (*tahara*) of the body and its preservation from pollution. A Muslim's preparations for prayer always include ritual washing, and the pristine state thus produced remains only so long as one avoids contact with ritually unclean things, such as blood, urine, faeces, semen, and unclean animals. On the other hand, illness in Islam does not imply sinfulness on the part of the sufferer, nor disapproval of him by God; on the contrary, the Qur'an repeatedly states that in the sick, the blind, the lame, and the weak 'there is no fault', and recommends visitation to those who are ill. In extreme cases, such as death from plague or in childbirth, sayings attributed to the Prophet Muhammad state that the victim's suffering earns him or her God's mercy and direct entry into Paradise. Law and society in the Islamic world have traditionally adopted an essentially lenient and compassionate attitude toward the ill. The madman, for example, was not held accountable for his actions since he was not in control of them, and the ill were excused from religious requirements, such as fasting during the month of Ramadan and attendance at Friday prayers. In most cases (leprosy being a notorious exception) physical illness did not result in ostracism from society, and the scenes that still appear in Mecca and Medina every year, when the pilgrims rally around the infirm and the elderly to assist them in their performance of the various rites of the pilgrimage, illustrate the extent to which medical disadvantage could make one a focus of communal solicitude.

A similar solicitude was also extended to children. Childhood was recognized as a period of growth and maturation distinct from adulthood, the transition to the latter for the most part being identified in and recognized through physical changes in the body. The Qur'an specified when a child should be weaned, and children seized as captives in war were not to be taken away unless they were a certain height ('five spans of the hand' was the measure most commonly cited). Children were expected gradually to assume more of the responsibilities of adulthood, such as attendance at prayers, but until sexual maturity they were not held legally or morally accountable for them. Once able to father or give birth to children, however, one became a full member of adult society and was responsible for his or her actions. Daughters were married off at a young age, based on the precedent of Aisha, who as tradition had it had been married to the Prophet Muhammad at the age of 9 (though it was apparently rare for girls to enter a consummated marriage at this age). Young men were regarded as adults at the age of 15 (made the 'standard' age for maturity already in early Islamic times), and it was not uncommon for youths to rise to great power: the author of the early Islamic conquests in India, for example, was Muhammad ibn al-Qasim (*d. c.* 717), who personally led and directed the campaigns at the age of 17.

If Islamic law and social norms allowed the adult man instant and almost unlimited leeway for advancement, it also held him entirely responsible for the actions of his body. This was often enforced in a most particularist fashion. The canonical punishment for theft was amputation of a hand, for example, and the utterer of blasphemy could have his tongue cut out. The bodies of executed criminals were often subjected to further humiliation through public display of their remains, or dispatch of heads to the offended ruler, often with public processions along the way. Fire was believed to consume the soul as well as the body, and was in any case a punishment normally reserved for God to inflict through condemnation to Hell; but in extreme cases rebels and heretics were burned alive for their transgressions, the ultimate crimes being punishable by the ultimate act of destruction that could be visited upon the body.

There have at times been major trends toward the renunciation of the body. Extreme asceticism has never found particular favour in Islam, but various mystical and ascetic movements have viewed the body as a vehicle for the function of the senses and appreciation of the pleasures of the physical world, and hence as distractive of man's attention from God. A wide variety of trends collectively referred to as Sufism thus arose to address the problem of how this distraction might be suppressed or removed. Answers ranged from collective meditations and devotions in groups, sometimes involving swaying or whirling of the body, to extremely austere seclusion away from human society. A special sanctity often attached to religious hermits and saintly ascetics, who were revered for their piety and sought out for the healing abilities of the blessed power (*baraka*) attributed to them.

Social background

The religious manifestations of concern for the physically disadvantaged (children, the old, the ill, the insane, and so forth) are related in important ways to social considerations. Among the most important of these is the central role of the extended family, which is extremely solicitous of the welfare and reputation of its members. In time of illness, it closes around the sufferer for support and encouragement: an ill person is a family responsibility and concern, and to fail to offer assistance in any way possible would be to fail in a central obligation of kinship and call into question the honour and reputation of the family as a whole. It comes as no surprise to find that, in the medieval Islamic world, deathbed scenes and accounts of the demise of known individuals never took place in a hospital, which seems primarily to have been the recourse of those without family to attend to them — travellers, visiting merchants, and the poor. In modern times the same attitude can be seen in the generally negative attitude toward placement of the elderly in retirement and old-folk's homes. Threats to the body of the individual, in other words, comprise challenges to the body of the family.

The interplay between social and religious factors can be seen in the special status accorded in Islam to the dead. Death of the physical body called for specific rites of ritual purification involving washing and shrouding, and essentially inspired by references in the Qur'an to the 'torment of the grave', it was discussed whether or not a person can continue to feel pain after death. It was believed that on the Judgment Day the dead will be raised in their physical bodies, and in the condition in which they had passed from the physical world. A famous example is the tradition of the Prophet stating that those who die in the holy war (*jihad*) will appear before God still bearing their wounds, which will, however, smell as sweet as musk. A special problem was posed by the cases of those who had died in such a way that no physical body would remain to be called forth (e.g. a victim of a fire, or one drowned at sea and so presumably eaten by the fish). Like victims of plague or childbirth, these too were deemed to have won immediate entry to Paradise, thus precluding any need for a physical body for Judgment.

Such sensitivities over the dead, and considerations of what would occur after death, discouraged actions that involved the dismemberment of the body. Some were uneasy about amputations of limbs, even if necessary to save life, since one would still appear before God eventually, but bearing the proof of an earlier effort to escape His will. The mutilation of criminals certainly had this point in mind, and it is likely that it also discouraged an interest in autopsy or dissection of cadavers for medical purposes, which seems not to have been regarded by doctors as a source of useful information in any case.

There was also an important magical dimension to the body in Middle Eastern society. Continuing an age-old tradition of such beliefs, Muslims, Christians, and Jews all considered it a manifest fact that spirits of various kinds could and did interfere with human affairs and affect the body. Apart from the evil eye — a disembodied but willing malevolent power that could bring misfortune, once attracted to a victim by ostentatious good fortune or boasting, or by the jealousy or malice of others — there was a wide range of demons and spirits with which to contend. The most important of these were the *jinn* (sing *jinni*, hence the English 'genie'), who, like man, were mortal beings and part of the physical world: human beings could benefit from their help or suffer from their mischief; see, talk with, and even intermarry with them, and outmanoeuvre and defeat them. Protection against such potential sources of harm was sought through sympathetic MAGIC. Amulets or charms were calculated to defeat spirits in various ways, and were worn or kept on the body as protection. Illnesses in particular were regarded either as communicated to man by spirits, or as animate entities that could be tricked or compelled to leave the body.

Perceptions of the human body have also been profoundly influenced by a more general social attitude toward women which manifested itself at many other levels as well. As in other traditional societies, women have been regarded as weaker than and inferior to men, and are subject to male guardianship — either father, male relatives, or husband — at all times. A woman grew up under the authority of her father and moved to that of her husband upon marriage; if her father died she was subject to the supervision of her other male relatives, and if divorced she moved back to the home of her family or a male relative. A woman lived on her own only in the most extraordinary circumstances, and to choose to do so would have invited suspicion and gossip as to her moral character and would have brought her family into disrepute. Men enjoyed wide latitude in exercise of their authority over women, including beating (sanctioned in the Qur'an), but excesses and brutality were deemed reprehensible and in extreme cases comprised grounds for divorce.

The female body was primarily associated with childbearing; MENARCHE marked the passage to full adult status, and society expected that as soon as she was able to do so a woman would marry and bear her husband's children. The role of motherhood was absolutely crucial. A barren wife was subject to summary divorce, and a woman who died a virgin was often considered a martyr since she had not fulfilled herself by bearing children.

As these examples indicate, the position of women was closely linked to that of SEXUALITY in Islamic society. Intense sensitivities about nakedness and the honour of the individual and the family did not prevent the rise of a lively and often quite open attitude toward sexuality, at least among men. Sexual jokes and anecdotes, hilarious and often quite graphic, appeared in even very respectable literary texts, and sexual poetry was highly developed. Guides and advice manuals on sexual intercourse, many of them illustrated, were popular, and medical compendia routinely contained chapters advising on how to prolong or maintain erection, heighten sexual pleasure, and intensify orgasm. In general, the quest for sexual fulfillment lay within the purview of men, from whom vigorous sexual activity was anticipated as soon as maturity had been attained. Prostitutes, slaves, and concubines were all readily available; homoerotic experience was well known, and while they were frowned upon in some quarters as demeaning to one's manhood, no shame necessarily attached to homoerotic acts so long as one was the active partner. For women, however, sexual activity outside of marriage was entirely taboo, and much anxiety and effort was devoted by men to ensuring that the conduct of their womenfolk gave not the slightest grounds for suspicion. While there is no reason to believe that women were any less aware of their sexuality than men, overt interest in such matters by a woman was widely regarded as suggestive of promiscuous inclinations, and female circumcision — as opposed to male, which was performed for reasons of ritual purity — was often employed in efforts to curb sexual desires.

Developments in modern times

The Islamic views of the human body in social, religious, and legal terms prevailed in various forms until the nineteenth century. The steadily weakening situation of Islamic regimes throughout the Middle East, however, was highlighted by Napoleon's invasion of Egypt in 1798, and Muslim rulers adopted varying degrees of Westernization in order to confront the threat of economic and political domination by Europe.

Views of the body have been no less subject to radical change than other aspects of traditional life. Western dress, beginning with military uniforms but spreading quickly to other areas, including the attire of women, has challenged centuries-old norms and sensitivities concerning the body. The sanctions of Islamic law and religious norms concerning the body have been undermined by modern law codes, and have been called into question more generally by endless exposure to Western values via media such as radio, film, television, and the press.

These challenges have never passed unanswered, and in the past twenty years particularly vigorous efforts have been made to revive traditional ways. Islamic dress, for example, has been promoted as an assertion of identity and a symbol of personal commitment to the faith, and in some countries Islamic law pertaining to the body — amputation of a hand as punishment for theft, for example — has been revived. Social and legal expectations of women have in some ways become more restrictive.

Informing all of these activities is a general awareness that the physical entity of the body is hedged about by, and ultimately is only meaningful in terms of, an enormous range of constructs defined, upheld, and promoted by the society in which one lives and to which one belongs. The current dialogue between Western and Islamic views of the body in the Middle East and the rest of the Islamic world, or wherever Muslims live as a community, essentially arises from a desire to benefit from Western advances in knowledge while still preserving the Islamic body both as an achievable reality and as a symbol of how the genuinely religious life should be lived.   LAWRENCE I. CONRAD

Further reading

Gil'adi, A. (1992). *Children of Islam: concepts of childhood in medieval muslim society.* Macmillan/St Antony's College, Oxford, Basingstoke.

Malti-Douglas, F. (1991). *Woman's body, woman's word: gender and discourse in Arabo-Islamic Writing.* Princeton University Press, Princeton.

Winter, M. (1995). Islamic attitudes toward the human body. In *Religious reflections on the human body.* (ed. J. M. Law). Indiana University Press, Bloomington.

See also BUDDHISM AND THE BODY; CHRISTIANITY AND THE BODY; ISLAMIC MEDICINE; HINDUISM AND THE BODY; JUDAISM AND THE BODY; RELIGION AND THE BODY.

Islamic medicine
Medicine played a prominent role in science and culture in the pre-modern Middle East. It arose as a formal discipline in the wake of an ambitious movement, in the ninth century, to translate Greek texts into Arabic, and prevailed for nearly a millennium thereafter.

Medical theory and the human body

Islamic theoretical formulations about the human body were founded on those of classical Greek philosophy and Graeco-Roman medicine, elaborated and developed by individual authors in the Arab Islamic tradition, not always in agreement with one another. In anatomical terms, the various parts and organs of the body were conceived of as comprising interrelated physical systems: skeletal, nervous, circulatory, and reproductive. The functions and activities attributed to these systems, however, and the connections drawn between them, often betrayed the limited extent to which empirical data could be collected and verified in the pre-modern age.

A good example is thinking on the circulatory system. Veins were identified as single-walled vessels that carried nourishment from the intestines to the liver, and then carried blood from the liver to feed the rest of the body. Arteries, on the other hand, were double-walled vessels carrying a finer kind of blood and *pneuma*, a sort of actualizing vapour, to the rest of the body. In this schema, circulation was entirely centrifugal: blood moved only outward from the heart and liver to the various parts of the body, where it was consumed for nourishment. Nothing travelled back to the heart and liver, which had constantly to replenish and renew the supply of blood outward to the rest of the body.

Arab–Islamic medicine, like Greek medicine before it, attributed key roles to certain major organs, each of which performed a specific vital function. The heart was the source of the 'innate heat' that sustains life. Body temperature was seen as a product of innate heat, the loss of which must invariably result in death. Anger was also a product of innate heat, which excitement and emotion agitated and caused to rise to the surface from the heart. The liver was the seat of the natural faculties of conception, growth, and procreation, which were carried throughout the body by the veins. A child was conceived, for example, when the procreative faculty carried to the uterus by the veins produced a fetus from the male sperm and the female menstrual blood. Bones grew because the faculty of growth was carried to them by the veins.

The brain was the seat of the psychical faculties — reason, imagination, thought, memory, and sense perception all had their origin here. The brain was also recognized as the source of voluntary movement: psychical *pneuma* passed through the nerves from the brain to the limb that was to move.

All of the above are part of what Islamic medicine called the 'naturals': the humours; the basic qualities of hot, cold, wet, and dry; personal temperament, and the faculties and *pneumata* — in sum, all that human beings really are. In addition, there were two other sets of factors that were deemed to affect the body, but that were not regarded as part of it. These were the 'extra-naturals' by which was meant illness and its symptoms, and the 'non-naturals' — six things external to the body, but vital to the preservation or restoration of health.

The doctrine of the non-naturals had been vital to GALEN's system of medicine, and in Islamic medicine these were constantly stressed and elaborated. The first of the non-naturals was the consideration of air: good air encouraged and maintained good health, while corrupt air could throw the humours out of balance and cause illness. Epidemics, for example, were routinely attributed to bad or corrupt air.

The second was movement. Islamic medicine placed great stress on the role of exercise in maintaining health, and prescribed it in moderation as part of a recuperative routine. The third was eating and drinking: these were divided into categories of regular foodstuffs, foodstuffs with a remedial function, drugs, and poisons. Diet was a paramount consideration in both maintenance of health and recovery from illness. This category also covered matters of attire. One should dress warmly enough to maintain the innate heat, but not so excessively as to cause overheating.

Another of the non-naturals was sleep, along with wakefulness. Sleep was deemed to help digest food and mature humours, since it allowed innate heat to spread through the body. Wakefulness was also important, since too much sleep dulled the mind and could also cool the body.

The fifth non-natural was excretion and retention: this not only had to do with digestive function, including constipation and diarrhoea, but also covered intercourse and bathing. There was a voluminous literature on intercourse, which for many medical writers was linked to the quest for pleasure, since, as one author noted, most human beings and all animals engaged in intercourse for enjoyment and not for offspring. Again, the theme was moderation. Too much sex could weaken one's other faculties, it was warned, since blood was drawn away from other organs in order to produce new semen. Too little, however, could result in melancholy as vapours from retained semen reached the brain and disturbed it — the orientation toward male sexuality here is of course to be noted.

The last of the non-naturals was psychical states, illustrating how mental function was integrated into the physical and how it was recognized that this could have a decisive impact on one's physical well-being. Medical works cautioned that tendencies to be overly suspicious, fearful, angry, shy, or morose had to be regulated, as they could throw the body out of balance and produce illness. Conversely, psychical states could be controlled by reason.

The doctrine of the non-naturals highlights the themes of moderation and balance that dominated medieval Islamic thinking on the healthy body. Health itself was defined as a natural state of balance that was specific to oneself; there was no universal paradigm — variety was what made people individuals. In order to treat patients successfully, the physician had to be able to recognize the temperaments and natural states of each individual.

A special problem was posed by the female body. Islamic medicine usually regarded the female body in terms of gynaecology and obstetrics, and chapters on women's health and illness more often than not discussed nothing else. Diagnosis and therapy made major assumptions about the female body that reflected the more general views of a society dominated by men. Following the Greeks, Islamic medicine held that women were too cold in temperament to produce sperm, and too weak to grow proper male genitalia. They possessed weaker constitutions than men, became ill more quickly, and could not bear medications in the same way that men could. They were also inclined to emotional extremes and hysteria.

Diagnosis and therapy: practical aspects of the medical body

It is important to bear in mind that in medieval Islamic times the *medical body* (as conceived of in medical theory and practice) was in important ways something apart from the human body. Medicine as an intellectual discipline dealt with subjects such as HEALTH, ILLNESS, and HEALING as theoretical abstracts; aspiring physicians learned these, for the most part from books and often with little or no experience with actual cases, but then eventually had to apply them to human beings, where the ideas they had absorbed (e.g. the actions of humours) were not immediately visible or evident.

Assessment of an ailing patient's condition involved questioning the victim and relatives and associates who might have important information, and examining the patient's body. In both of these areas certain sensitivities had to be overcome. Nakedness, for example, was religiously disapproved, and there was a pronounced emphasis on individual privacy and modesty.

In examining a patient the physician devoted considerable attention to personal constitution and temperament — that is, to determining where along the continuum the patient's natural state of health might be. Physical signs were also examined; the physician sought to determine whether the patient was hot, or sweaty, or pale or flushed in the face, and so forth. Manual manipulation and palpation were likewise employed to check for broken bones, determine if internal organs were overly hard or soft, or identify the location and status of tumours and swellings.

Over and above all these other diagnostic techniques, however, physicians relied on examination of PULSE and URINE. There was a voluminous literature on the pulse, largely inspired by Galen (130–210 AD), whose works on the subject, as on so many others, had been translated into Arabic in early Islamic times and promoted to a position of practically unassailable authority. The pulse was assessed not only in terms of whether it was weak or strong, slow or fast, regular or irregular, but also, for example, whether it was large or small and hard or soft. From such examination, physicians considered that they could identify problems ranging from jaundice to dropsy, diphtheria, pregnancy, and anxiety.

Again, there was an extensive literature on the urine, inspired and defined by the works of Galen. Urine was subjected to minute discussion and classification. Great importance was attached to its colour: varying shades of yellow, colourless, or tinged with green, red, or black. Thinness or viscosity, odour, 'touch', clarity, foaminess, and probably taste, were all considered. Sediment in urine was broken down into numerous categories: sandy, greasy, flaky, hair-like, ash-like, and so forth. These properties revealed much about a patient's state of health. Mental dysfunction, for example, produced blond urine with a wine-like foam; red urine was regarded with alarm and taken as a sign that death was probably near; black urine was associated with liver problems and at the beginning of an illness it meant certain death; viscous cloudy urine meant that a headache was imminent.

Despite the impression in the medical literature of close contact between doctor and patient, there is clear evidence that the physical presence of the patient was not deemed absolutely necessary for an accurate diagnosis. A family member with no medical background could describe a relative's illness, or bring a written account or a urine sample to the doctor, who would identify the problem and prescribe a therapy without direct recourse to the patient. One may conclude that the medieval physicians were supremely confident in their theoretical constructs and diagnostic techniques.

The theoretical dimension of Galenic medicine was decisively systematised by Avicenna (d. 1037), and its practical side was advanced in various areas (such as pharmacology, ophthalmology, and surgery). However, as an explanation for physical dysfunction it comprised a closed system already able to account for every problem. Divergence from the views of Galen was exceptional.

For all their confidence in their system, physicians were acutely aware of its limitations; this expressed itself not only in a widespread feeling that physicians would never be able to command all that the great Galen had known, but also in an emphasis on public health and preventive medicine as opposed to therapeutics.

This sense of limitation was nowhere more evident than in the field of SURGERY. This was highly developed in Islamic times, in terms of both instrumentation and technique, and procedures of great delicacy — such as repair of inguinal hernia and cataract surgery — were successfully performed. But the range of surgical expertise dealt largely with the surface of the body: for example cautery, BLOODLETTING, and draining boils and abscesses. More problematic were matters requiring invasion of the body cavity. After injuries exposing internal organs, the physician might do whatever he could to repair the damage, clean the exposed parts, and close the wound. But this was done with little hope of success, and the risk of fatal infection — of which the true causes were then of course unknown — was simply too great to allow exploratory or remedial surgery on the physician's own initiative.

The limited use to which knowledge of internal anatomy could be put, combined with the overarching authority of the results already achieved by Galen, and social sensitivities over treatment of the dead, dictated that there was little interest in AUTOPSY or DISSECTION. The diagrams of the 'Five-Figure Set', a collection of anatomical drawings which appeared in Islam for the first time in manuscripts of a Persian surgical text written in 1396, seem not to reflect any special attention to internal anatomy. They are paralleled by similar drawings in medieval Western texts and probably originate with late antique models taken up from Greek texts translated in early Islamic times but since lost. There are occasional references to dissection of apes and efforts to confirm or test Galenic anatomy, but as the prospects for applying such knowledge remained so bleak, these explorations were doomed to remain sporadic and of little practical importance.

Developments in modern times

The efforts of Islamic regimes to cope with the challenge of the West included major programmes of modernisation in medicine. Egypt, invaded by Napoleon in 1798, was the scene of pioneering developments under the energetic leadership of Muhammad Ali, and it was there, in the early decades of the nineteenth century, that the first real, modern medical schools and hospitals in the Islamic world were established. Since then, Western bio-medicine has everywhere come to prevail as the authoritative interpretation of the medical body.

The adoption of modern Western medical science and technology on a massive scale has had a dramatic impact. Infant and child mortality have dropped sharply, and life expectancy has risen considerably. Prestigious medical centres in national capitals successfully perform complex and costly operations (e.g. heart transplants); but such institutions are largely irrelevant to the vast majority of the population of the country, who often live far from the capital, and suffer most from basic problems of poor public health. The goals and priorities of medicine have thus been areas of particularly vigorous discussion.

There have also been activities on other fronts. Books promoting the practical and herbal remedies of the so-called 'medicine of the Prophet' have proliferated, and enjoy a brisk market, and there has also been a marked revival in the role of healers who use religious spells and incantations to exorcise demons and spirits from the body. There are also healers who attract patients for consultations with spirits, whom only the healer can see or hear and who recommend therapies and predict the outcome of serious cases. Dabbling in communications with the spirit world, however, is disapproved — often vehemently — as blasphemy, by some religious authorities. Still, the magical interpretation of problems concerning the body is clearly on the rise, and not just among the poor or in rural areas.

There has also been a marked trend toward the promotion or revival of Galenism as a formal medical system. In India and Pakistan, where it never declined so precipitously as it did in the Arab world, it survives under the name *Unani Tibb* ('Greek medicine') and is officially sanctioned and supported by government.

In the Arab lands, the dialogue between Western and traditional views of medicine and the body takes the form of debate over properly Islamic medical ethics. A vast array of subjects is covered. Medical issues concerning sex and reproduction, such as SEX CHANGE operations, AIDS, MENSTRUATION, ABORTION, MASTURBATION, artificial insemination, sperm banks, and COSMETIC SURGERY, have provoked great interest and heated debate, as also have euthanasia and post-mortem examination.

Implicit in all these debates, as in discussions involving the body in other fields of endeavour, is an effort to maintain the social and religious norms of Islam in the face of challenges posed by foreign structures of science and technology based on other assumptions.   LAWRENCE I. CONRAD

Further reading

Conrad, L. I. (1995). The Arab–Islamic medical tradition. In L. I. Conrad *et al. The Western medical tradition: 800 BC to AD 1800*. Cambridge University Press.

Rispler-Chain, V. (1993). *Islamic medical ethics in the twentieth century*. Brill, Leiden.

Rosenthal, F. (1990). *Science and medicine in Islam*. Variorum, Aldershot.

Ullmann, M. (1978). *Islamic medicine*. Edinburgh University Press.

See also GALEN; HEART; HUMOURS; ISLAM AND THE BODY; MEDICINE; PULSE.

Isokinetics A form of STRENGTH TRAINING in which the person works against a machine which automatically varies its resistance to allow the same angular velocity to be maintained throughout the range of movement.   N.C.S.

Isometrics A form of STRENGTH TRAINING in which muscles are contracted strongly without producing significant movement, by opposing themselves against a fixed object or, more commonly, the same action of the opposite limb or the antagonist muscles of the same limb. The term is derived from the muscle physiologist's adjective, 'isometric', describing a contraction in which the muscle does not change length. Contrast 'isotonics' and 'isokinetics': both of these develop strength over the whole range of joint angles, which isometrics cannot do.   N.C.S.

Isotonics A form of STRENGTH TRAINING in which a given weight or resistance is moved through a wide range of limb angles. The term is derived from the muscle physiologist's adjective, 'isotonic', describing a contraction in which the muscle exerts a constant force while it changes length.   N.C.S.

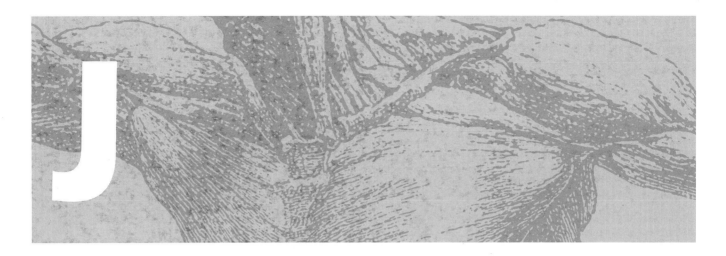

Jaundice The occurrence of jaundice — the yellow discolouration of skin, the sclerae of the eyes and other heavily perfused tissues — is well recorded in ancient writings, including those from Assyria, where epidemic jaundice was first described. In these ancient times, however, jaundice was considered a disease in itself, rather than a sign of an underlying disorder. It was Baillie, a Scottish physician in the early 1800s, who first linked the occurrence of jaundice to cirrhosis of the LIVER. Shortly afterwards, Bright (the Guy's Hospital physician most famous for his description of kidney disease) distinguished four hepatic causes of jaundice: 'hepatic congestion', 'biliary obstruction', 'chronic changes in the liver' and 'acute, diffuse inflammation of the substance of the liver', which would either resolve or progress to chronic disease.

Accumulation of the pigment *bilirubin* in the bloodstream, leading to jaundice, may result from either overproduction of bilirubin or impaired hepatic metabolism of this substrate. About 80% of the bilirubin normally circulating is derived from the continual turnover of red blood cells, which become senescent when they reach their normal lifespan of approximately 120 days. Destruction of these cells releases haem from their HAEMOGLOBIN, which is quickly metabolised in the liver to biliverdin and, in turn, to bilirubin. The remaining 20% of circulating bilirubin is derived either from the destruction of maturing blood cells in the bone marrow or from the metabolism of various haem-containing enzymes. The liver plays an essential role in the metabolism of bilirubin and the excretion of its metabolites into the BILE. Jaundice usually becomes clinically evident only when the level of bilirubin in the serum increases to at least twice the normal upper limit.

In practical terms, therefore, jaundice is the consequence either of abnormal HAEMOLYSIS, when excessive destruction of red blood cells releases increased quantities of bilirubin, overwhelming the liver's metabolic reserve; or of liver cell or bile duct disorders, in which the hepatic uptake, metabolism, or biliary excretion of bilirubin is impaired. Common examples of these latter disorders include disturbance of liver cell function by acute hepatitis and obstruction of the bile ducts by impacted GALLSTONES. Mild elevation of the bilirubin level in the blood, especially evident during fasting or any general illness, and usually to less than twice the upper limit of normal, is most often due to 'Gilbert's syndrome' — described by this French physician in 1900 and later explained as a benign genetic variant in which the activity of a liver enzyme called 'glucuronyl transferase', is reduced. Normally this enzyme converts bilirubin to a water soluble conjugate prior to excretion in the bile. Gilbert's syndrome is present in at least 1% of the normal population and is not associated with either liver disease or haemolysis.

STEPHEN M. RIORDAN
ROGER WILLIAMS

See also BILE; HAEMOGLOBIN; LIVER.

Jaw The 'jaw', in everyday language and in descriptions of facial characteristics, commonly refers to the lower jaw that gives the CHIN its shape. The word is derived from the Anglo-Saxon for 'chew' and is properly applied to both participants in this function: the upper as well as the lower jaw. Jaw movements are fundamental to the processes of both eating and speaking.

In mammals, the upper jaw or *maxilla* is one of the bones forming the facial part of the SKULL; the lower jaw or *mandible* forms a joint with the skull (temporo-mandibular joint) and is suspended by a set of jaw-closing muscles, attached to the temple and to the cheek bone as well as to the maxilla. Forceful jaw closure is a function of these muscles; the *masseter* that runs from the cheek bone to the angle of the jaw can easily be felt bulging and hardening when the TEETH are clenched.

Below the mandible on each side there is a Y-shaped set of muscles. The two upper arms of the 'Y' are attached respectively to the mandible in front and to the base of the skull above and behind. The stalk of the Y is attached to the sternum (breastbone) below. The small U-shaped hyoid bone, which lies below the mandible at the base of the TONGUE, is at the junction of the three arms of the 'Y' on each side. In effect both mandible and hyoid are suspended within a chain of muscles. Lowering of the jaw is produced by contraction of the muscles forming the front upper limb of the 'Y' only if the other muscles of the 'Y' are contracting and thus fixing the hyoid; if the other muscles of the 'Y' are relaxed, the hyoid will be moved forwards.

The posture of the jaw at rest depends on the length of the jaw elevator muscles, and the factors determining this are similar to those controlling posture in the body generally. Muscle length depends upon the operation of muscle-length detecting receptors (*muscle spindles*) that reflexly cause a proportionate muscle contraction if the muscle is stretched. Jaw-closing MUSCLE TONE is thus maintained so that, while awake, gravity does not pull the mouth open. The muscles passing from the mandible to the hyoid and to the tongue are of importance in maintaining tongue posture and airway patency, so jaw position is a factor in keeping the airway open. The converse is that restriction of the nasal airway results in a mouth-open posture.

Conscious or voluntary jaw movement is produced by activity in the primary motor cortex that projects directly to the MOTOR NEURONS of the jaw muscles in the BRAIN STEM. The automatic, rhythmic jaw movements of feeding are, however, produced by a *central pattern generator* (CPG) in the brain stem that can be activated by pathways descending from the motor cortex and/or by sensory input to the brain stem from the mouth. The activity of the CPG then produces a sequential activation of the motor neurons of the jaw opening and closing muscles as well as activation of other muscles involved in feeding.

In normal function, the movements of the jaw vary directly in magnitude with the hardness of the ingested food while the extent of tongue movement varies inversely. Consequently, as hard food is converted into a soft bolus in the mouth, the amplitude of jaw movements reduces while the amplitude of tongue/hyoid movement increases. There is, consequently, evidence for sensory feedback from the mouth influencing the expression of the activity of the CPG.

The teeth are supported in their sockets by the periodontal ligament that transmits the jaw-closing force to the teeth. Sensory nerve endings in this ligament detect the loading and produce neural signals proportionate to the load. These signals cause reflex inhibition of jaw-closing motoneurons and have been considered to represent a device for preventing excessive forces being applied to any individual tooth.

ALLAN THEXTON

See also MOVEMENT, CONTROL OF; PHARYNX; SKULL; TEETH; TONGUE.

PLATE 1.

Jejunum The part of the small intestine next beyond the duodenum, and leading to the ileum. Its lining has an enormous surface area, by virtue of folds, projections (villi), and microvilli on the villi. Enzyme secretion and digestion, started in the stomach, continue here, and absorption of the products begins — of glucose and amino acids into blood capillaries and of fats into lymph capillaries (lacteals). S.J.

See ALIMENTARY SYSTEM.

Joints '… the thigh bone's connected to the knee bone, the knee bone's connected to the leg bone … O hear the word of the Lord.' … or marvel at the evolution of the superb engineering and biological 'servicing' throughout a human lifetime whereby these connections are combined with mobility, and the moving parts kept intact and well 'oiled' — if we are lucky.

Joints evolved in animal bodies along with skeletons, whether external (insects) or internal (vertebrates). Clearly a bony core would not be compatible with movement without joints, not only for running, climbing, and flying but also for the limbless propulsion of snakes and fish.

A study of the bare bones of the human SKELETON reveals the shape of the surfaces of the bones where they move on each other at joints, and gives some indication of the direction and range of movement which those shapes will permit. Also, in the living joint, the structures that connect the one to the other vary in being appropriately loose or tight to allow or restrict movement. The movement itself also depends on the arrangement of the MUSCLES and of their TENDONS which span the joint.

Joints first appear during the sixth week of fetal life, and develop from embryonic mesoderm, the precursor of connective tissue. By the ninth week discernable joints are present, which by the twelfth week are well developed and can be moved by muscle contractions. By the sixteenth week such fetal movements are just perceptible to the mother.

This account will describe the features common to all joints in the body, the different types in mechanical terms, the tissues that form them, and the means whereby their living structure is maintained and repaired. As well as the examples which illustrate these features, details about the main individual joints and the muscles which control movement at them can be found under their own names.

General features of joints

Freely movable joints are referred to as synovial joints. The whole joint region is enclosed by a 'capsule' of CONNECTIVE TISSUE, which is firmly attached to the bones beyond the surfaces involved in the joint itself. The opposing surfaces of bone have a covering of CARTILAGE, a tough material but with more resilience than bone itself, which acts as a 'shock absorber'. (This cartilage is different from the various specially shaped 'cartilages' which are present, for example, in the knee). In most joints the lubrication necessary for these covered surfaces to move smoothly against each other is provided by synovial fluid, so called because it resembles egg white (derived from 'syn' meaning 'with' and 'ovium' meaning 'egg'). This is secreted from a thin lining layer on the internal surface of the capsule. This forms the completely enclosed 'cavity' of the joint — though cavity is not quite the right word, since it is really a potential space lined by a thin film of synovial fluid. This fluid, which is derived from the blood flowing to the joint, has another important function of providing nutrition to cartilage, which is devoid of blood vessels. When the joint is injured or inflamed excess synovial fluid may be formed (an effusion), leading to swelling of the joint.

The joint capsule contains SENSORY RECEPTORS which, when appropriately stimulated, give rise to nervous impulses which the brain interprets as a sensation. PAIN is an important sensation which is associated with most forms of joint injury or disease (arthritis). Although normally pain plays an important protective role to warn of tissue injury or damage, it is debilitating in chronic arthritis. A less obvious but ever-present sensation derived from joints is the 'sixth' sense called PROPRIOCEPTION — the conscious awareness of joint position and movement. This sensory feedback is vitally important in the development of the control of the musculature which is reflected in the smoothness and co-ordination of movements.

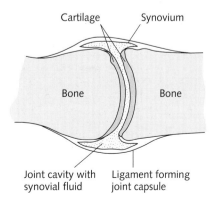

Diagram of a synovial joint.

Types of joint

A few personal observations reveal the different mechanical nature of the main joints of the limbs: ELBOWS and KNEES have no side-to-side movement and a range approaching a half-circle; these and the finger and toe joints work like hinges. The restrictions are imposed mainly by the shape of the bones at the elbow, and by ligamentous connections between them at the knee. At the SHOULDER, by contrast, the arm can be wielded in all directions, implying something like a 'ball-and-socket' — though the socket has to be shallower than that in a car-to-trailer joint which allows movement only in the horizontal plane. This arrangement makes the shoulder more liable than any other joint to dislocation — the ball at the top of the humerus slipping out of its socket on the scapula (shoulder blade). The HIPS also have a ball and socket structure, with a somewhat deeper socket in the ilium (pelvic or hip bone) for the head of the femur (thigh bone). The wrists have an intermediate freedom of movement; the 'hinging' is wider in range than side-to-side movement. The ankles are essentially hinge joints; the side-to-side movement of the foot relative to the leg is achieved at joints beyond the ankle joint itself.

In both the HANDS and the FEET there are joints among the small bones of the carpus (beyond the wrist joint) and tarsus (beyond the ankle joint), and between these and the five metacarpals and five metatarsals, each of which is jointed to the bones of the digits (fingers and toes) themselves. Within each digit, there are a further two joints between the three bones (phalanges) — crucial of course in the hand for fine manual skills, but of only vestigial importance in the toes.

Some individuals have a larger than normal range of movement at their joints and are sometimes referred to as being 'double-jointed'. Of course, this is not literally the case, it is simply that these individuals have 'looser' joints. This is more properly called joint hypermobility, and some individuals with this condition find employment as contortionists.

Movements at many other joints are less easy to observe, though at least as important for posture and movement. Each of the separate bones of the spine (the vertebrae) has joints with its neighbours above and below, allowing bending and rotation; at the top end, the highest of the cervical (neck) vertebrae (the 'atlas' — compare he who supported the world) has joints with the SKULL which support it and allow nodding movement; also the head can turn from side to side because this 'atlas' forms a rotating joint with an upward protuberance on the next below — the 'axis' vertebra. Near the lower end, the sacro–iliac joints link the SPINAL COLUMN to the PELVIS — in this instance, forming a relatively rigid connection rather than allowing a range of movement. Since the two iliac bones are bound strongly together at the centre front, the bony pelvis (sacrum and iliac bones) can only be tilted as a whole by movement at the hip joints and by bending the spine. There are thus strong links

413

between the lower limbs, via the hip joints, to the spinal column — very necessary for upright posture and movement. The upper limbs by contrast are not linked by joints to the spine. The shoulder 'girdle' from which the arm is suspended, incompletely encircles the upper torso and consists of clavicles (collar bones) jointed to the sternum (breast bone) at the front, and scapulae (shoulder blades) which are relatively freely mobile.

There are joints in the chest which are crucial for breathing movements. The 'rib cage' is lifted and enlarged by muscle action when we breathe in, assisting the filling of the lungs. It can change shape in this way because of the small joints which link the back end of every rib to the vertebral column, and the front end of all but the lowest ribs to the sternum.

Problems with joints

Minor injuries are often called 'sprains': this may involve tearing of some fibres of the joint capsule or ligaments; there may 'be swelling' due to soft tissue damage outside the joint itself or to an increase in the production of synovial fluid inside the cavity (effusion).

Dislocation occurs when the bones become displaced from their proper position in the joint, due to a strong jolt which forces an unnatural direction of movement. Weakness of the relevant muscles can make it more liable to happen. Shoulders, fingers, and toes are the most liable to this type of injury, and the displacement can usually be reversed without serious damage. Dislocations in other joints, and ones which are more serious, can along with fractures of the limb bones.

Displacement of other components of joints include the common sports injury to the knee, when the flat horseshoe-shaped cartilages which lie on the upper end of the tibia slip out of place or are torn. More seriously in the knee, the cruciate ligaments can be damaged; these join the tibia to the femur, at angles which prevent over-extension (forward bending), so the knee becomes unstable if they are ineffective. Then there is the notorious 'SLIPPED DISC' in the spine: the joint between the main bony bodies of adjacent vertebrae consists of an 'intervertebral disc' which has a soft but not liquid centre. 'Slipping' means that this soft substance bursts through the fibrous membrane around it, protruding to where it can irritate a nearby nerve root where it leaves the spinal canal, leading to pain being felt in the territory innervated by that root. The pain of 'sciatica' can be felt in the leg or even the foot, although the actual site of nerve irritation is close to the spine.

Arthritis is a general term for different types of disorders affecting joints. The commonest, osteoarthritis, often referred to as being a 'degenerative' condition is associated with wearing down of the cartilage, particularly of the weight-bearing joints, which becomes progressively more common with increasing age. Other types include rheumatoid arthritis which is an AUTOIMMUNE

DISEASE process affecting any joint, and which occurs in younger individuals but has a long time course. It is often associated with severe deformity of the hands. Infections with bacteria or viruses can give rise to an acute inflammation of a joint (septic arthritis).

When joints are badly damaged and painful, usually as a result of chronic disease, a very successful treatment performed by orthopaedic surgeons involves complete replacement of the joint with an artificial one (arthroplasty). However, these never last as long as the joints we are born with, and further, more difficult, operations (revisions) may be necessary.

WILLIAM R. FERRELL

SHEILA JENNETT

See also ANKLE; ELBOW; HIP; KNEE; SPINAL COLUMN; WRIST.

Judaism and the body

The association of the 'Jews' with the healthy and the ill body is a long-standing one in the West. Within traditional (Orthodox) Judaism as a religious practice there are complex rituals concerning the body, ranging from infant male CIRCUMCISION to the ritual washing of the CORPSE (Halacha). These rituals are commented on in the Talmud, the commentaries and explanations of Biblical rituals. Such traditional views have their mystical parallel in the Zohar's image of the body of God and the role of the body in ritual dance and movement in Jewish mystic groups, such as the Chasids. In the Western image of the Jew, on the one hand, we have the image of the medieval Jewish physician who was claimed to have a special knowledge of the most efficacious medicine (obtained from Greek sources, read in Arabic). On the other hand, there are medieval and early modern images of the Jews as the source of all EPIDEMICS from the Black Plague to syphilis. The Jews were even accused of spreading illnesses by which they themselves remained untouched. Both of these fantasies about Jews and illness had real results in the real world. On the one hand Jewish doctors were particularly sought by non-Jewish patients; on the other, entire communities of Jews were murdered. The association of Jews with illness and the HEALING art remains powerful even today. The dehumanizing image of the 'dirty Jew' — carrier of illness, ugly, destructive — is also countered by the philo-Semitic (and equally fantastic) image of the 'beautiful Jew', 'der shejne Yid' (a proverb in Yiddish) — intelligent, strong, and moral.

The image of the 'Jewish body' does not merely rest on the fantasy of Jewish difference as represented in the non-Jewish world. 'Real' Jewish physicians, from Maimonides in the Golden Age of Spanish Jewry, to the German physician Tobias Cohen, whose 1707 book on medicine began the Haskalah, the Jewish Enlightenment, in Germany, to the Viennese neurologist Sigmund Freud, and beyond, had to deal with the particular association of 'Jews' with illness and the healing arts. The Jewish healer is

assumed to have a special relationship to his/her patient. The appeal of Sigmund Freud and the rise of the talking cure, in contrast to the cold and harsh manner commonly used to treat psychiatric patients of his day, is rooted in the simple fact that Freud and the psychoanalysts actually listened to their patients. Thus the perceived 'Jewishness' of psychoanalysis was both a pejorative label (as in C. G. Jung's words) and also an acknowledgment of the belief that Jewish doctors were more empathic.

The images of the healthy and the ill Jewish body shaped, and were shaped by, the existence of 'real' Jewish doctors and 'real' Jewish patients. These real Jewish doctors and their patients, such as the 'Jewish Patient', Franz Kafka (the title of Sander Gilman's book on Kafka) were also impacted by fantasies about the Jewish body.

The association of the Jews with moral cleanliness led to the creation of the first programs for social work in Germany to rescue young Eastern European Jewish women from the brothels; at the same time the association of the Jewish with SEXUALLY TRANSMITTED DISEASE became a hallmark of anti-Semitic rhetoric. The Third Reich's pseudo-documentary The Eternal Jew (1941) portrayed Jews as being like rats spreading disease across Europe. Zionist ideology from the same period stressed the need to transform weak (and ugly) Jewish bodies into the strong (and beautiful) bodies of the Kibbutzniks. The ideology of sick and healthy bodies can be seen to have a specific focus in the representation of the 'Jew'.

Central to this discussion is the antithesis perceived between the 'social' and the 'biological' body of the Jew. Religious ritual becomes translated into racial biology: Jews, who ritually circumcise their male children, are claimed in the medical literature, beginning in the eighteenth century, to have a higher rate of male children who are actually born circumcised! Biological differences, such as the real or perceived higher (or lower) rates of illness such as HYSTERIA or CANCER, are read as having either racial, biological, or social causes. Jewish scientists, such as the founder of the Sociology of the Jews, Artur Ruppin, or the Zionist–physician Max Nordau, seek a biological understanding of the ill and corrupt Jewish body and find it in the experience of the Jew 'who has lived 2000 years in the ghetto'. Socio-biological change, the creation of a 'new muscle Jew', will enable the Jews to become new people in a new land. In the 'old land', Jewish institutions ranging from hospitals to sanatoria to gymnastic societies had as their goal the amelioration of human suffering and the reconstitution of the healthy body, but in complex and different ways.

The gendering of the Jewish body into female and male is a complicated element in the construction of the image of the healthy and the ill Jewish body. The gendering of the Jewish body and the meaning of SEXUALITY are of course linked. The idea of Jewish males and females as different from non-Jews begins with the medieval

Christian discussion that male Jews menstruate! — and therefore that they need the blood of Christian children to cure their female woes. This initial image of the diseased Jewish male body raised the meaning of the Jewish male as a potential 'third sex'. The reinterpretation of circumcision as CASTRATION in the eighteenth and nineteenth centuries feminizes (or at least de-masculinizes) the male Jew. Thus there is a discussion of the number of Jewish homosexuals in the medical literature of the nineteenth century. Here images of ritual murder and circumcision can be linked. The works of Magnus Hirschfeld (who was Jewish and gay), at the turn of the century, link Jews and gays in interchangeable categories. The universal modern definition of the human body (defined as the masculine body) as strong and healthy, places the female body as its antithesis, weak and ill (because her reproductive functions are seen as illness). It is little wonder that the juxtaposition of Aryan (masculine) and Jewish (feminine) is a standard trope of the visual arts of the nineteenth and twentieth centuries.

From the writings of the early Church to the anti-Semitic writings of the Aryan Nation, the Jewish body has been labeled as ill and deformed because it is truly the body of the Devil incarnate. The image of the Devil's goat-foot becomes the flat foot of the prototypical Jewish draft dodger in the anti-Semitic art of the twentieth century. But even more so, 'Satan's Synagogue' becomes an image of the Jew and his ritual practices. It is not merely that the Jew, like the Devil, is deformed; the stereotypical Jew will deform the rest of humanity out of inherent hatred and malice.

Historically the juxtaposition of the tortured and treated Jewish body provides a set of contradictory images from the Middle Ages to the twentieth century. The concentration and death camps of the Third Reich saw the Jewish body as the object of torture because of the differences attributed to the 'essence'. Children at Hohenlychen were experimentally infected with tuberculosis and later murdered so that the experiment would not be discovered by the approaching Allied forces. With such acts, the mythological discussion in the nineteenth century of Jewish immunity to tuberculosis has its horrible end. But the counter to this image can be found in the work of Ludwick Fleck, the famed physician and philosopher of science, who worked as a physician on a typhus vaccine in the death camps, and refused to give it to the Nazis.

The realities and the fantasies of the 'Jewish body' as a different body are linked in modern understanding of the Jew as a different being.

SANDER L. GILMAN

Further reading

Biale, D. (1992). *Eros and the Jews: from biblical Israel to contemporary America.* BasicBooks, New York.

Boyarin, D. (1997). *Unheroic conduct: the rise of heterosexuality and the invention of the Jewish man.* University of California Press, Berkeley.

Eilberg-Schwartz, H. (1990). *The Savage in Judaism: an anthropology of Israelite religion and ancient Judaism.* Indiana University Press, Bloomington.

Gilman, S. L. (1991). *The Jew's body.* Routledge, New York.

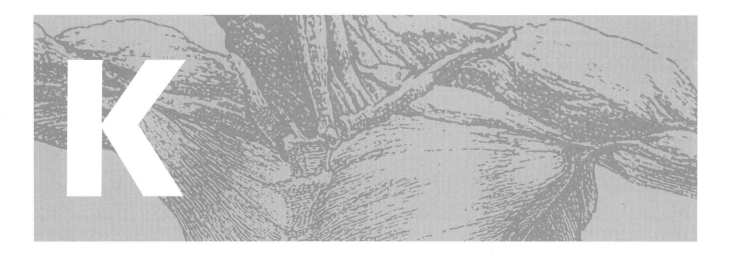

K

Ketosis is recognisable by the smell of acetone (as in nail varnish) on the breath. It occurs when the body's processing of nutrient materials for the release of energy depends predominantly on the use of FATS. In the absence of a dietary carbohydrate supply for maintaining blood sugar, or if sugars cannot be utilised normally, fuel must come from stored fat and muscle protein. This can occur in previously healthy people during prolonged FASTING or STARVATION, after persistent VOMITING, or on a very high fat and low carbohydrate diet; or it can occur because of disordered hormonal control of metabolism in DIABETES mellitus. The high rate of breakdown of fatty acids by the LIVER produces the 'ketone bodies', acetoacetate and β-hydroxybutyrate, which are released into the blood. Some of the acetoacetate is converted to acetone — another 'ketone body' — mainly in the lungs, and this becomes noticeable on the breath.

The physiologically useful consequence is that ketone bodies, which are made only in the liver and exported from it, can be used by other tissues for energy production. During starvation even the brain, which normally uses only glucose, can adapt to utilising ketone bodies.

In diabetes, the fault lies in the absence of the effects of INSULIN. Normally, this hormone acts to restrain mobilisation of AMINO ACIDS from muscle protein and their conversion to glucose in the liver, and to restrain the mobilisation of FATTY ACIDS from lipid store in adipose tissue. Without this restraint, the liver not only overloads the blood with glucose, which most other tissues cannot take up and use without the action of insulin, but also overloads the blood with ketone bodies as a by-product of its excessive use of fatty acids. If the condition is uncontrolled — as it used to be before the days of insulin treatment — increasing ketosis leads to progressively more harmful acidosis, diabetic coma, and death.

SHEILA JENNETT

See also ACID-BASE HOMEOSTASIS; FATS; INSULIN; LIVER.

Kidneys The kidneys are situated on each side of the vertebral column, at the level of the last (twelfth) rib. Each kidney is about 12 cm long and weighs about 150 g — about the size of a fist. Despite their small size, the two kidneys receive an enormous blood flow — about 1.2 litres/min in an adult — which is a quarter of the total output of the heart (5 litres/min).

One of the main functions of the kidneys is the removal from the body (EXCRETION) of waste products such as urea, uric acid, and creatinine. However, the kidneys' role is not merely excretion. They are also regulatory organs, controlling the volume and the composition of the BODY FLUIDS and maintaining the correct osmolality, ion concentrations, and acid–base status of the body.

Each kidney is bean-shaped, with a slit opening — termed the *hilus* — through which pass the renal artery and vein, the renal nerves and lymphatics, and the ureter, which connects the kidney to the bladder (Fig. 1). A tough connective tissue capsule covers the outer layer of the kidney, the cortex. The deeper part of the kidney, the medulla, consists of a number (6–18) of conical pyramids, the tips of which (*papillae*) project into the funnel-shaped urine collectors — the renal calyxes (calices) — which merge to form the funnel-shaped upper end of the ureter — the renal pelvis. (Renal, pertaining to the kidney, from its Latin name, *ren*.)

The *nephron* is the functional unit of the kidney. (*Nephros* is the Greek for kidney.) Each kidney has about one million nephrons, and the total length of the nephrons in the body is about 100 miles!

The nephron begins as a Bowman's capsule — the blind end of the nephron — invaginated by a knot of capillaries, the *glomerulus* (glomerular capillaries). A Bowman's capsule and its glomerular capillaries are together termed a *renal corpuscle*. Sir William Bowman, British surgeon and histologist, described this in 1842.

The rest of the nephron consists of the proximal convoluted tubule, proximal straight tubule, loop of Henle, and distal convoluted tubule. The distal tubules join to form collecting tubules which in turn join to form collecting ducts, which open at the tip of the renal papilla (Fig. 2).

The Bowman's capsules, proximal tubules, and distal tubules are situated in the renal cortex, whereas the loops of Henle and the collecting ducts extend down through the medulla.

The function of the kidneys is to produce urine, a fluid of variable volume and composition (within limits), depending on the need of the body to excrete or conserve water or solutes. The first step in the production of urine is the filtration of plasma passing through the kidney. This filtration (sometimes called *ultra*filtration as it occurs at the molecular level rather than gross particle level) occurs from the glomerular capillaries into the Bowman's capsule to form tubular fluid. The glomerular filter prevents plasma PROTEINS from passing into the nephrons, but is permeable to all other plasma constituents (such as ions, glucose, amino acids, urea, etc). Thus filtration in the kidney is essentially *non-selective* — substances which the body needs to retain are filtered, as well as those substances which need to be excreted.

Filtration is the *bulk flow* of water through a *semipermeable membrane* (filter), carrying with it those solutes which can pass through the filter. As mentioned above, the glomerular filter only excludes plasma proteins. Water moves by bulk flow through the filter as a consequence of pressure gradients. Immediately upstream and downstream from the glomerular capillaries, there are blood vessels which have smooth muscle in their walls, so that they can constrict or dilate, and so alter the resistance to the flow of blood. These vessels are, respectively, the afferent and efferent arterioles. They permit precise regulation of the hydrostatic pressure of the blood in the glomerular capillaries, which is maintained at a higher level than in capillaries in other parts of the body. This force drives plasma from the glomerular capillaries into the nephrons. However, two forces work in opposition to this movement. One is the osmotic pressure exerted by the plasma proteins, which increases as filtration proceeds and the

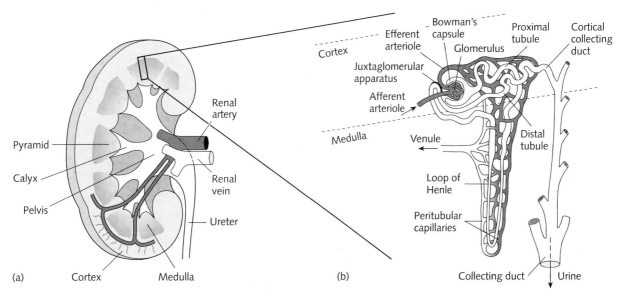

Fig. 1 Diagrammatic cross section of the kidney.

Fig. 2 Enlarged nephron showing blood supply.

proteins, because they are not filtered, get more concentrated. The other force opposing filtration is the hydrostatic pressure within the Bowman's capsule. The resultant is a net filtration pressure which diminishes as blood flows through the glomerlus. The amount of filtration that actually occurs is known as the glomerular filtration rate, or GFR. It is about 120 ml/min (180 l/day). This seems an enormous volume — and it *is* an enormous volume — but it is important to realise that it is only a small fraction of the total plasma delivered to the kidneys in the blood. In this respect, the kidneys are rather different from our everyday experiences of filters. For example, when we make filter coffee, we pour water over coffee in the filter, and essentially all the water goes through the filter, leaving a 'sludge' of coffee grounds in the filter. If all of the plasma delivered to the kidneys passed through the glomerular filters into the nephrons, the filters would be clogged with a 'sludge' of red cells, white cells, and plasma proteins. This is prevented because only 20% of the plasma arriving at the filter actually passes through. The remaining 80% continues into the efferent arterioles.

The volume of plasma in the whole of the circulating blood is only about 3 litres, yet we filter 180 litres per day of it. This apparently paradoxical situation is possible because, after filtration, almost all (99%) of the plasma is reabsorbed along the nephron, so can be filtered again and again (60 times a day!). The selectivity of the kidney — how it is able to conserve some substances and excrete others — is due to the transport processes (reabsorption and secretion) which occur along the nephron, modifying the composition of the glomerular filtrate.

In the nephrons, the terms '*reabsorption*' and '*secretion*' indicate the direction of movement. Reabsorption is movement of a substance from the tubular fluid, through the tubular cells or between them and thence into the blood. Secretion is movement in the opposite direction.

If a TRANSPORT process is directly linked to the consumption of metabolic energy, it is termed '*active*'. In the kidney, the quantitatively most important active transport process is the reabsorption of sodium ions (Na^+). Up to 80% of the kidneys' oxygen consumption drives this process, and because the energy comes from the breakdown of ADENOSINE TRIPHOSPHATE (ATP), Na^+ active transporters are termed ATPases. There are many other transporter molecules in the nephron cells, many driven by gradients (e.g. for Na^+) set up by active transport. Such transport is termed '*secondary active*' for example, glucose reabsorption is via a transporter which also carries Na^+ into the cell, with the driving force being the Na^+ concentration gradient set up by the active transport of Na^+ out of the cell. In addition to ATPases and transporter molecules, nephron cell membranes also contain proteins which constitute 'channels' for the passage of ions, neutral molecules or water.

The proximal tubule reabsorbs about 70% of the filtered Na^+, 70% of the filtered water, and, normally, 100% of the filtered glucose and amino acids. *Diabetes mellitus*, the condition in which glucose is excreted in the urine, is caused by the failure to maintain the normal plasma level of glucose. In diabetes mellitus the plasma glucose concentration is increased, so the filtered load of glucose is increased; if the increase is big enough the nephrons are unable to reabsorb it all, and some appears in the urine.

The sodium which is reabsorbed in the ascending loop of Henle is not accompanied by water, since this part of the nephron is impermeable to water. Consequently, Na^+ transport at this site lowers the solute concentration of the tubular fluid, and raises that of the fluid in the interstitial space of the medulla, which surrounds the tubules. This high medullary concentration is the osmotic driving force for water reabsorption in the collecting tubules under the influence of ADH (see below).

Just how efficient the kidneys are at controlling our body fluid volume is demonstrated by the constancy of the body weight from day to day. Even if you spend the evening in the pub and drink a couple of kilograms of beer, your body weight will be back to normal the next day!

The volume of URINE excreted by the kidneys can vary between 400 ml/day, and about 25 L/day. The main determinants of urine volume are the osmotic concentration of the body fluids, and the effective circulating volume (the volume of blood circulating around the body in the vascular system). These regulate the urine volume primarily by affecting the release or production of HORMONES which control renal function.

If our fluid intake is less than the fluid loss, the body fluid osmotic concentration (*osmolality*) increases — the solutes of the body are in a smaller volume than normal, so their concentration is higher. This increased osmotic concentration is detected by 'osmoreceptors' in the brain, and these lead to the release, from the posterior PITUITARY GLAND, of the peptide antidiuretic hormone (ADH), also called vasopressin. This hormone circulates in the blood and binds to 'V2' receptors on the cells of the kidneys' collecting tubules. It causes them in effect to become more permeable to water, by incorporating water channels in their cell membranes. Because there is always an osmotic gradient tending to move water out of these tubules into the fluid around them and thence into the blood, more water is reabsorbed, the volume of urine is decreased and it becomes more concentrated. The raised osmolality of the body fluids is thus corrected. Because of this continual homeostatic mechanism, the urine volume, which can range from 400 ml/day to 25 litres/day is primarily determined by the level of circulating ADH. A typical volume is 1.5 litres/day.

Decreases in the effective circulating volume also increase ADH release, but in addition such decreases increase the release of *renin* from the

417

juxtaglomerular apparatus of the kidney (a region of each nephron where the afferent arteriole and distal tubule are in contact). Renin is an enzyme, which acts on a plasma protein (α_2 globulin) to release a 10-amino acid peptide, angiotensin I. This in turn is converted, by an enzyme present in blood vessel walls, (ACE — angiotensin converting enzyme), to an 8 amino acid peptide, angiotensin II.

Angiotensin II increases nephron Na^+ reabsorption. Since water follows Na^+, water reabsorption also increases, and urine volume falls. Angiotensin II acts directly on the nephrons, and also causes ADH release and the release of another Na^+-retaining hormone, *aldosterone*.

Another important regulatory function of the kidney is the control of ACID–BASE HOMEOSTASIS. In general, the metabolism of the body produces excess H^+, and this is secreted into the urine by the nephron cells. The pH of the blood and extracellular fluid is kept constant at 7.4, but to achieve this, the kidneys can vary the urine pH from 4.5–8.0.

Kidney function may become impaired, leading to renal failure. There are many potential causes of renal failure, including reduction of the renal blood supply (e.g. as a result of major HAEMORRHAGE), toxins and disease organisms, and blockages of the urinary tract. If the kidneys fail, one of the first signs is the accumulation of urea and other nitrogenous waste in the blood — *uraemia*. This may require treatment by DIALYSIS or by organ TRANSPLANTATION. However, other problems associated with failing kidneys relate to the fact that the kidneys are themselves important endocrine glands. They produce the hormone *erythropoietin*, which stimulates bone marrow to produce red blood cells, and also convert the precursor form of vitamin D to the active form. Both of these functions can be disrupted in renal failure, leading to ANAEMIA and to disturbance of CALCIUM supply to the bones.

If just one kidney fails, or is surgically removed, then changes take place in the remaining one to enable it to maintain homeostasis. Although the number of nephrons in the surviving kidney does not increase, the glomerular filtration rate of each individual nephron increases, so that the overall glomerular filtration rate increases to approach that which was previously achieved with two kidneys.   CHRIS LOTE

Further reading

Lote, C. J. (2000). *Principles of renal physiology*, (4th edn). Kluwer, Amsterdam.

See also ACID-BASE HOMEOSTASIS; DIALYSIS; URINE; WATER BALANCE.
See PLATE 8.

Killing
Throughout the history of humankind, acts of killing have been used not only to regulate the LIFESPAN, but also to place social value on particular kinds of bodies. While almost all civilizations have outlawed MURDER, certain forms of killing, like the murder of slaves and enemies, have been tolerated and indeed sanctioned by various societies at different historical moments.

Even before birth, the body may be killed through induced ABORTION and other types of feticide, such as stabbing the fetus in the womb. Although the abortion of nonviable fetuses is legal in most industrialized nations and is considered part of women's reproductive freedom, religious groups espousing fetal rights and the sacredness of human life contend that abortion is still murder. Shortly after birth, human life is also subject to termination through infanticide. Socially and legally reprehensible in many cultures today, infanticide was widely practised for eugenic purposes in ancient Greece and Rome, and, more recently, in Nazi Germany. In antiquity unhealthy, deformed, and sometimes normal, but female infants were abandoned or drowned, while in Nazi Germany defective infants were poisoned, gassed, or starved.

Over the course of the lifespan, an individual can become the victim of manifold other types of homicide (the killing of one human being by another). Acts of killing performed without malice, such as deaths resulting from drunk driving, or other accidents, are classified as manslaughter, whereas deaths stemming from intentional injuries are considered murder. To deter and punish deliberate homicides, many governments have instituted capital punishment, executing CRIMINALS who have transgressed the socially decreed boundaries of acceptable killing. Nonetheless, members of various groups have often enacted private or vigilante justice, in which they have created their own criteria and circumstances for killing. The history of homicide in the US, for example, contains numerous instances of vigilantism and group terrorism, ranging from outlaw justice on the antebellum frontier, to nineteenth-and early twentieth-century lynchings in the South, to present day inner-city gang warfare. More widespread and socially devastating than any form of vigilantism or individual homicide, however, is systematized, state-sanctioned warfare. With the shift away from politically and territorially based victories in the nineteenth century, modern warfare has made its chief objective the destruction of enemy bodies and resources. During the period of World War II, in the wake of the Nazi holocaust, the term GENOCIDE was introduced to describe the intentional, systematic slaughter of a racial or cultural group.

At the end of the lifespan, one way that the body may be killed or that natural death may be hastened is through EUTHANASIA. Generally performed to avoid unnecessary or prolonged suffering, euthanasia can take the form of physician-assisted suicide, passive euthanasia, or active euthanasia (sometimes known as 'mercy killing'). Like infanticide, euthanasia was practiced in Greek and Roman antiquity as well as in Nazi Germany to end the lives of the chronically sick and those deemed 'lives not worth living'.
      CHRISTINA JARVIS

See also EUGENICS; EUTHANASIA; GENOCIDE; MURDER; WAR AND THE BODY.

Kinaesiology
the study of movement and the structures involved — mainly used in the US (*kinesiology*).   N.C.S.

See MOVEMENT, CONTROL OF.

Kiss
To kiss — to make contact with the lips — is often a sign of friendship or affection. In this respect it is seen as a Western gesture of intimacy and is not, therefore, observed in all cultures.

The target of the kiss is not of course restricted to the mouth and can be directed to any part of the body, with varying pressure. There are different types of kissing behaviour, such as mouth-to-mouth, French kissing, and cunnilingus. The '*French kiss*' is a type of sexual arousal in which two people kiss with their mouths open so that the tongues can touch. This is sometimes also called 'soul kiss' or 'tongue kiss'. *Cunnilingus* is another type of sexual kissing whereby a person stimulates the external female genital organs (vulva, clitoris) with the mouth or tongue. The word '*cunnilingus*' is derived from the Latin *cunnus* meaning 'vulva, vagina', and *lingua* meaning 'tongue' (or *lingere* 'to lick up').

The use of the kiss can also be seen as a religio-erotic symbol in the West. One of the most famous of all kisses was the kiss of betrayal: Judas' kiss. In the Christian tradition, Judas betrayed Christ with a kiss and in doing so brought death and treachery to an act that was associated with peace and unity. St Augustine later warns against the misuse of the physical kiss, especially if the heart is full of deceit and dishonesty. That Judas betrayed his master with a kiss was accounted by Christians as a betrayal of the kiss itself as well as of the Lord. In the early Christian centuries the kiss was a mystic symbol imbued with powerful feelings such as peace, union, and love. As Nicolas Perella states in *The Kiss Sacred and Profane* (1969): 'The repeated use of this formula and the contexts in which it occurs suggests that the kiss was quickly institutionalized in the young Christian community as a mystic symbol both in liturgical and non-liturgical ceremony'.

In the early centuries it was the practice of Christian ICONOGRAPHY to borrow motifs from well-established pagan myths; especially in the case of sarcophagi designs. Among the motifs applicable in this way were those connected with the myth of Psyche and Eros; one of the most favoured by the Christians of Rome was the image that showed a pair embracing and kissing. Psyche — the human soul of the departed, and Eros — always a powerful god of love. Nicolas Perella suggests that this was acceptable to the Christians because it could well depict a wedding union in heaven. It is Eros who bestows the kiss, with all the suggestion that he is infusing the spirit of new life into Psyche. Thus the adoption of the 'kissing couple' is understandable.

The *kiss of life* and the *kiss of death*, are the extreme life forces which have become powerful symbols for writers and artists. The breath or spirit of God has always been seen as a life-giving act, and the Holy Spirit can be given in the form of a kiss. For example, the Virgin Mary was *kissed* by the Holy Spirit so that she might become impregnated. The iconography of a kiss often portrays both ecstacy and death simultaneously. The *kiss of death* is at its most obvious when we see Judas kiss Jesus; this is both a physical and metaphorical manifestation, which results in a corporeal death.

By the sixteenth century, authors were using the kiss and death as sexual metaphors. The kiss, both given and stolen, is romanticised in poetry and prose. The traditional medieval motif, for example, of the poet seeking solace from his lovesickness is disguised in the wantoness of his lover's kisses. The poet was often chaste where his love and kisses were concerned; the Metaphysical poets, in particular, wrote of the constant turmoil where sexual and platonic love were concerned.

Another method of inviting a kiss, though not necessarily of giving one, can be found in the 'language of the fan' in the eighteenth century. Though used as a form of concealment, the fan, when pressed to the lips, indicated the anticipation of a kiss. The pressure of the fan on the mouth would often indicate the level of sincerity and passion involved.

A number of modern-day artists and writers have used kissing as a powerful and symbolic form of friendship, intimacy, and sexual activity. The well-known Parisian artist Auguste Rodin (1840–1917), for example, immortalised a man and a woman coming together in this way when he produced a life-size sculpture in marble, entitled *The Kiss*, in 1886. By contrast, in 1897 the French anthropologist Paul d'Enjoy remarked on the horror of the Chinese at seeing mouth-to-mouth kissing by Westerners.

Another way of using the kiss as a dramatic and controlling device can be seen as a power play between the two sexes, especially in the guise of fairytales. Twentieth-century notions of the male as hero, waking up and resuscitating the 'sleeping' female with his kiss' have been challenged by feminist writers such as Simone de Beauvoir. Myths of 'The Sleeping Beauty', 'Snow White', and 'Cinderella' that are handed down from generation to generation, usually to girls, depicting the all-embracing *kiss*, are being reassessed in the wake of feminist theory.

ANNE ABICHOU

Further reading

Beauvoir, S. de (reprint 1970). *The second sex.* Bantam Books Inc., New York.

Kolbenschlas, M. (1979). *Goodbye Sleeping Beauty. Breaking the spell of feminine myths and models.* The Women's Press, Dublin.

Liggett, J. (1974). *The human face.* Constable, London.

Perella, N. J. (1969). *The kiss sacred and profane. An interpretative history of kiss symbolism and related religio-erotic themes.* University of California Press, Berkeley and Los Angeles.

See also BODY LANGUAGE; GESTURES.

Knee The knees and kneeling have many cultural and social associations. The joints themselves reveal mechanical and physiological features superbly appropriate to their crucial role in the standing or moving body — but susceptible eventually to wear and tear.

The knee joint is functionally a hinge joint, which principally allows movements of the lower leg forwards (*extension*) and backwards (*flexion*), although a limited degree of rotation is also possible towards the end of extension. Extension is achieved by a group of four large

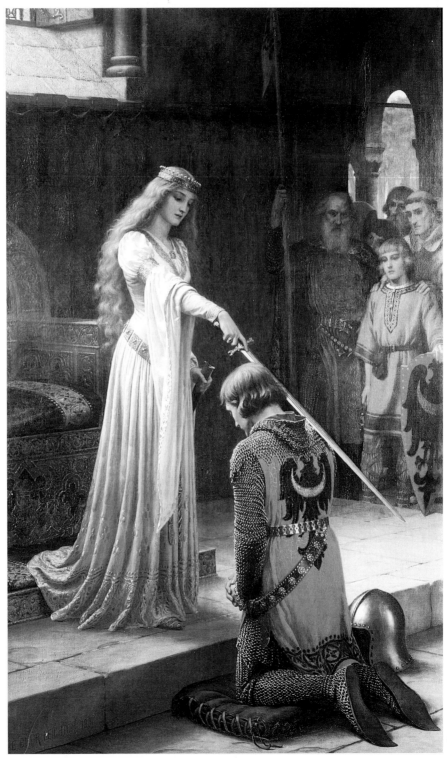

Kneeling. The Accolade by Edmund Blair (1853–1922). The Bridgeman Art Gallery.

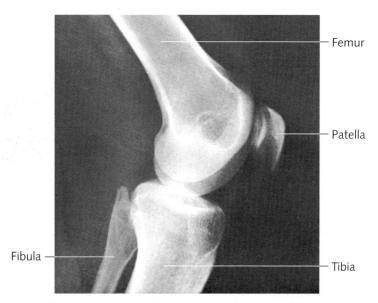

Femur

Patella

Fibula

Tibia

Lateral X-ray of adult knee joint. Reproduced, with permission, from *Cunningham's textbook of anatomy*, (12th edn), OUP.

muscles at the front of the thigh (QUADRICEPS), whilst muscles at the back of the thigh (HAMSTRINGS) produce flexion. The lower end of the femur articulates, through two *condyles*, with the top of the tibia, which is shaped rather like a plateau. In addition to the CARTILAGE covering the surfaces of these bone-ends, there is another piece of cartilage (*meniscus*) separating them on each side. These can be torn by rotational injuries, particularly in football and rugby players, a condition commonly referred to as *torn cartilage*.

This hinge joint is a less stable arrangement than a 'ball and socket' joint like the hip, and the stability of the knee is achieved by a combination of tough ligaments, the extensor and flexor muscles spanning the joint, and the fibrous capsule of the joint. The *cruciate ligaments* (so called because they cross over within the joint) are of particular importance as they prevent fore and aft instability. These ligaments are a common site

of damage — again, in contact sports such as football and rugby — and damage can sometimes end a lucrative career despite reconstructive surgery. Lateral stability is achieved by the ligaments on each side of the knee. When it is injured or inflamed, excess fluid can collect in the joint (*effusion*) making it swell and stiffen. As the knee is relatively accessible, this fluid can be removed (*aspirated*) and drugs (often STEROIDS) injected directly.

The stresses on the knee, as a large weight-bearing joint, make it a major site for development of *osteoarthritis* in later life. This can be treated by complete joint replacement (*total knee arthroplasty*).

Because it is the largest joint in the human body, which sustains some of the greatest stresses and which is seriously injured with relative ease, the knee is traditionally and symbolically a site of vulnerability. 'Kneecapping', for instance, is a practice associated with terrorists and organized

crime groups; it involves destroying the kneecaps, either by shooting someone in the knees or by shattering them, typically with a baseball bat. The result is not life-threatening, but extremely painful and permanently disabling. To be 'brought to one's knees' is to be in a position of submission and desperation; to be 'cut off at the knees' is to be humiliated and disabled.

To kneel voluntarily is to submit symbolically to a higher authority. Kneeling during prayer, bowing to social superiors, and getting on one's knee to propose marriage or to be knighted, are all expressions of reverence or humility. In Japanese tea ceremonies, guests greet one another with a kneeling bow. Before it became an expression of humility, however, kneeling in prayer was a way of indicating one's proximity to the underworld. Today, Christians kneel when receiving a blessing or the Eucharist, and Muslims kneel in prayer facing Mecca; Jews did not reject kneeling in worship until after Christians adopted it as part of their practice.

As a symbol of vulnerability, the knee has also been a point of erotic encounter, especially as the place where the first touch between two people occurs. Playing 'kneesies', for instance, meant rubbing or touching knees in a flirtatious and surreptitious manner, especially while seated where such activity would be concealed, as under a dining table. Eric Rohmer's film *Claire's Knee* tells the story of an older man infatuated by a younger woman; her knee is the first focus of his desire when he encounters her on a ladder in an orchard. Fashions which exposed women's knees were considered daring and *risqué* in the 1920s — a sign of new freedoms; however, by the 1940s short pants were acceptable for both men and women.

In ancient Greece, for something to be 'on the knees of the gods (*theón en gounasi*)', meant that it was totally beyond human control or knowledge.

WILLIAM R. FERRELL
KRISTEN L. ZACHARIAS

See PLATE 5.

See also CARTILAGE; JOINTS; SKELETON; RELIGION AND THE BODY.

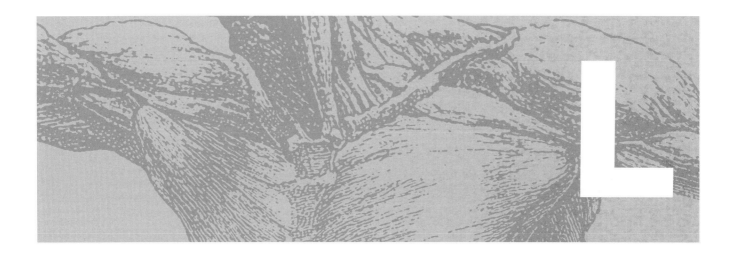

Labia Although the term 'labia' can refer to the fleshy, liplike edges of any organ or tissue, it more specifically describes the outer (*labia majora*) and inner (*labia minora*) folds of the VULVA. Woman's genital lips are now the focus of a new symbolics articulated by French feminist philosopher Luce Irigaray, who seeks to re-metaphorize the female body and free women from negative conceptions of their SEXUALITY. It is through the labia that Irigaray theorizes woman's autoeroticism and sexual pleasure in a way significantly different from Freud and his French interpreter Lacan. In their psycho-analytic accounts, woman's sexuality is marked by her lack of a penis and by her position as passive object of desire. In contrast to psycho-analytic theories that imagine and valorize the male genitals as closed, singular, and whole, Irigaray revalues the openness that allows the woman's two lips to be separate, but also in constant contact. She argues for a vision of female pleasure that is multiple and mutual, tactile more than visual. Speaking of woman's autoeroticism, Irigaray writes that woman touches herself in and of herself, without any need for mediation. In her pleasure woman is both active and passive, both the one touching and the one being touched. Mastery of one by the other is not necessary to this feminist vision of female sexuality.

The two lips become for Irigaray the basis for theorizing a *parler femme*, a speaking as a woman. Contact again becomes a key idea, as *parler femme* relies on the contiguity of language, the closeness of words in their signification and sound. Such contiguity produces a speech in which one element slips into another, and Irigaray conceptualizes a feminine syntax that does not reduce the meaning of words and language to a single truth. As in her conception of female sexuality, doubling and multiplying are associated with the feminine. To speak as a woman is not to invent a new language, but to exploit the possibilities within existing systems and to disrupt the hierarchical logic of either/or propositions.

In associating woman's two sets of lips, Irigaray reworks an idea present in the Western tradition since the Greeks. Comparing the lips to the labia was common in Hippocratic medicine, which perceived the upper and lower portions of the female body as symmetrical and used the same term, *stoma* or mouth, to describe them. The mouth from which speech flowed corresponded to that of the uterus. Both were lined with lips that opened and closed. But this synonymy between the female lips was used to woman's disadvantage in antiquity. From Plato to Plutarch, the female mouth, like the female genitals, required strict legislation. A woman who conversed with men other than her husband was suspected of loose morals and potential infidelity. Hence the garrulousness of the mouth pointed to an improper activity of the nether lips.

The association between the two lips continued through the Middle Ages, exploited especially in the French *fabliaux*, verses of comic and/or moralizing content performed in the thirteenth and fourteenth centuries. As E. Jane Burns has pointed out in analyzing the *fabliaux*, their invocation of a 'vaginalized mouth' derives from the similarity between the lips of the mouth and the genital labia. In *Le Fabliau du moigne*, a monk searching for the ideal 'cunt' rejects one whose lips are too thin and whose form is not sufficiently mouthlike. And in *Du Chevalier qui fist les cons parler* a young knight about to be seduced asks that the maiden reveal her motive by speaking through her labia, rather than through her potentially deceitful lips. The idea of the talking vagina was not lost to the French tradition, and Diderot calls it up in *Les Bijoux indiscrèt* (1748). The plot centres on a magic ring that makes women reveal their sexual exploits not with their lying lips, but through their most honest and experienced parts — their genitals.

Irigaray's invocation of the labia, therefore, erodes from within a tradition that stresses woman's susceptibility to loose talk and sex. As well as challenging psychoanalysis, Irigaray's stress on woman's difference counters anatomical texts that present the female body as an inferior version of the male. Thomas Laqueur provides a history of such reasoning in his *Making sex*, and cites Gaspard Bauhin (1560–1624), professor of anatomy in Basel, who argued that the tendency to see all genital organs with reference to man was deeply embedded in language. Bauhin cited among the words for labia the Greek *mutocheila*, meaning snout, or more explicitly, penile lips. It was common, moreover, for anatomical texts to liken the labia to the foreskin; examples include writings by Mondino de Luzzi (1275–1326), Jacapo Berengario da Carpi (1522), and Josef Hyrtl (1880).

Most recently, *The Complete Dictionary of Sexology* (1995) records that 'The labia majora are homologous to the male scrotum.'

If one tradition views the labia as homologous to male parts, another uses them to distinguish women of different racial types. Eighteenth-century travellers to southern Africa, such as François Le Vaillant and John Barrow, described what became known as the 'HOTTENTOT APRON', a hypertrophy of the labia minora caused by manipulating the genitalia. European scientists believed the Hottentot apron to be an innate characteristic of the black female body, and as such it fascinated medical professionals and lay-men. Carl Linnaeus mistakenly supposed it was characteristic of all African women, and like other naturalists believed it a vestige of the Hottentot's animal origin. More sympathetic observers like Peter Kolb suggested that as a natural fig leaf it modestly concealed the female genitals. Still others compared it to female artifice and believed it formed through manual manipulation. Writers commonly linked it to the over-development of the clitoris, and to the notion, common since the eighteenth century, that such overdevelopment led to lesbian love, or 'trib-adism' to use the earlier term. Perversion thus became attached to the African genitals in a scientific account that reinforced stereotypes of the over-sexed, promiscuous black woman.

MARY D. SHERIFF

Further reading

Irigaray, L. (1991). *This sex which is not one*, trans. Catherine Porter. Cornell University Press, Ithaca, N.

Schiebinger, L. (1992). *Nature's body. Gender in the making of modern science*. Beacon Press, Boston.

See also GENITALIA; HOTTENTOT APRON; SCROTUM; VULVA.

Labour Birth is a remarkable and explosive event that occurs usually between 35 and 39 weeks after conception (37–41 after the mother's last menstrual period). It is typified by painful contractions of the UTERUS (womb), progressive dilation of the cervix (the lowermost part of the uterus), and descent of the presenting part of the baby through the mother's birth canal (uterus and VAGINA). There are three stages of labour. The first lasts until full dilation of the cervix, the second until birth of the baby, and the third ends with delivery of the PLACENTA.

The processes that initiate normal physiological labour in humans are poorly understood. The sheep has provided the most useful experimental animal model for the study of the fetus and has provided many important insights into human pregnancy. In the sheep, labour is initiated by the fetus, which starts the process by producing a surge of corticosteroid hormones from its ADRENAL GLANDS. This results in a change in the balance of steroid SEX HORMONES (oestrogen and progesterone) in the ewe which, in turn, encourages the production of prostaglandins in the membranes attached to the placenta. PROSTAGLANDINS (so called because they were first discovered in prostate glands in men) stimulate contractions of the uterus, thus initiating labour. It is an attractive concept that the baby should orchestrate the timing of labour and birth when it has reached sufficient maturity to be ready for life outside the uterus. The process is not, however, so clear-cut in humans, although prostaglandins do seem to be important. In many women, changes take place over days or weeks before labour proper starts, including some opening of the cervix and increasing *Braxton Hicks contractions* (non-painful, non-regular 'hardening' of the uterus), which are named after the nineteenth-century London obstetrician who first described them.

The first sign of labour is usually that uterine contractions become increasingly painful or frequent, although labour may sometimes start with rupture of the placental membranes and release of the amniotic fluid that surrounds the baby throughout pregnancy. In later labour, the contractions occur every two or three minutes. With each contraction, the blood supply to the placenta is cut off, stopping the supply of oxygen to the baby. Well-grown babies have more than sufficient reserves to deal with this potential stress, but poorly-grown babies with low metabolic reserves may become rapidly and seriously distressed. It is, therefore, important to monitor the heart rate of the baby during labour to check for distress. This may be done by listening through the fetal stethoscope (named after the French obstetrician, Adolphe Pinard), or by electronic methods — although the simplest and oldest method was to place the ear directly on the abdomen.

As the contractions pull against the cervix, already softened by the effect of prostaglandins, it dilates. Once it is completely open, the presenting part of the baby is propelled downwards by the contractions, deeper into the mother's pelvis. In 96% of babies at term (after 37 weeks), the presenting part is the head; in 3% it is the rump (breech). As the head reaches the funnel-shaped muscles of her pelvic floor, the mother feels an urge to push, and her efforts add to the impact of the contractions. The head rotates and emerges through the lower end of the vagina, to be followed by the rest of the baby.

Sometimes it proves necessary to deliver the baby by CAESAREAN SECTION during labour, notably because of signs of distress in the baby or a failure to make progress — either because the baby's head is too large for the mother's PELVIS, or because the uterine contractions prove inadequate. When such problems occur during the second stage of labour, birth can be hastened by application of obstetric forceps or the vacuum extractor. Forceps were first constructed and used by the Chamberlens, a Huguenot family who fled to England during the sixteenth century. By discreet use of the instruments under sheets they kept their secret hidden for decades. The first practical vacuum extractor was made by the nineteenth-century Scottish obstetrician, James Young Simpson; further refinements occurred during the twentieth century.

Simpson's other contribution to the care of women in labour was of still greater significance. At a famous dinner party in Edinburgh in 1847 he proved to himself (and to his accommodating guests) the pain-relieving power of chloroform. His advocacy of chloroform as an ANALGESIC during labour met vigorous opposition, backed by citation of the Bible, for God had reportedly said to Eve, after she ate the forbidden fruit:

> I will greatly multiply your pain in childbirth. In pain you shall bring forth children (Genesis 2: 16).

Public opinion in Britain was changed by Queen Victoria's use of chloroform during one of her many labours; the acceptance of pain-relieving measures as legitimate was thereby ensured. Labour is a painful experience for most women and options that are available nowadays include opiate drugs, inhalation of NITROUS OXIDE gas, transcutaneous nerve stimulation (TENS), and EPIDURAL anaesthesia. A hot bath helps with many types of pain and has become popular during labour; indeed some women now like to give birth in water. However, access to any such facilities is denied to very many women world-wide, many of whom do not have the availability of even very basic clinical care. The consequences are dramatically and tragically illustrated in the developing world where, in rural areas far from clinical facilities, women may labour for days. In these communities, adolescent girls are especially at risk of obstructed labour because the pelvis is both incompletely grown and also often stunted because of chronic undernutrition. Prolonged obstructed labour typically results in death of the baby, and often in death of the mother from INFECTION or, if she survives, in vesico–vaginal fistula — a channel between bladder and vagina that causes chronic INCONTINENCE of urine, social ostracism, and great misery. The ability to transform the lives of these young women by successful surgery has been demonstrated by the famous fistula hospital in Addis Ababa, Ethiopia. However, prevention is, as always, better than cure, and the 'partogram', a graphical representation of the progress of labour developed by Professor Hugh Philpott in Zimbabwe, gives early warning of obstructed labour and is now widely used throughout the world. Women who have had babies previously suffer a different consequence of neglected obstructed labour: rupture of the uterus, with severe internal HAEMORRHAGE and high risk of death.

The challenge for obstetricians and midwives providing care for women in labour in more affluent settings is to ensure safety for mother and baby whilst avoiding meddlesome and unnecessary clinical interventions and allowing the women free choice of possible options which would include, for example, her favoured position at birth, or delivery at home. High rates of Caesarean section, induction of labour, and continuous electronic fetal heart monitoring suggest, to some, that the balance is not yet right.

JIM NEILSON

See also BIRTH; DEVELOPMENT AND GROWTH: INFANCY; PREGNANCY.

Lactate threshold Intensity of exercise above which lactate accumulates increasingly in the blood; traditionally ascribed to shortfall in oxygen supply to muscles, requiring some energy to be supplied by anaerobic metabolism — hence also known as '*anaerobic threshold*'. Recent research challenges this; lactate can be produced by fully-oxygenated muscles, as a result of processes driving the *oxidative* processes faster. Only above the maximal rate of oxygen uptake does lactate accumulation unequivocally indicate that significant energy is being supplied anaerobically.

NEIL SPURWAY

See also BREATHING DURING EXERCISE; EXERCISE; FATIGUE; METABOLISM.

Language may be the most appropriate trait by which to classify humans within the order of nature, even more so than rationality (*Homo sapiens*) or technology (*Homo faber*) — and not only because language is less honorific than rationality and more intrinsic than technology. In a sense *Homo loquens* trumps all other terms, since the very act of definition is itself a move within language. Speculation that all three species-specific capacities — reasoning, tool use, and language — were bound together in an evolutionary nexus is supported by recent pale-oanthropological evidence that the beginnings of language were linked to the sociability of hominids and the growth of co-operative tool production. Localized brain mechanisms correlate with the lateralization of the neo-cortex and are common to both SPEECH and manual skills.

Evolution of language

There is now more scholarly interest in the origin of language than at any time since the eighteenth century, although among linguists, anatomists, and anthropologists no consensus has emerged as to its timing and nature. When over the course of the nineteenth century no evidence of any 'primitive' languages was found, discussion of origins was for a long time officially proscribed. One current view has it that an explosion of cave art and symbolic behaviour some 40 000 years ago coincided with the abrupt extinction of Neanderthals, and was causally related to the emergence of language. But this is probably based on an illusion of synchronicity. The adaptation of the vocal tract for speech production — in particular the lowering of the larynx — seems to have been complete at least 125 000, and perhaps 200 000 years ago. This would seem to support a much earlier origin for language; some form of proto-language may well have been present in the earliest hominids.

The question — which exercised Charles Darwin — as to whether there is evolutionary continuity between animal signalling systems and human language, has prompted, over the last thirty years, a number of widely publicized experiments involving attempts to teach human language to apes. Some of the early efforts foundered on the fact that other primates do not have the anatomy necessary for human speech production; later attempts using sign language seemed to fare better. The enduring ambiguity of the results lies not only in the slippage around definitions of language, but also in the tendency of primatologists, as linguistic creatures, to impute sense to their subjects, and to project the human world onto the realm of nature. The assumption of cross-species continuities and homologies with respect to language, implicit in the methods of ethologists and behaviourists working on very old associationist principles, was flatly rejected in a notorious 1959 polemic by the linguist Noam Chomsky, who argued that human language was based on entirely different principles from animal communication. Some detected, in this unqualified assertion of the absolute uniqueness of the human language faculty, an echo of the Victorian geologist Charles Lyell's remark, when he told Darwin that, despite being a supporter, he was unable 'to go the whole orang'.

The power of the language faculty, however it came to be part of the species endowment, is acknowledged across all human cultures. The first words of a child are universally recognized as a momentous threshold; for an adult to have speaking privileges, or to decide who may talk or not, is a sure sign of social power. Those without language, infants (from the Latin *infans*: 'non-speaking') and domestic animals, as well as those denied language — the shunned, the gagged, the silenced — are in real ways disabled members of a community. Speech impairment typically results in discrimination; despite the partial success of the disability rights movement and the recognition that signing is no less a linguistic system than spoken language, 'dumb' is still widely unchallenged as a term of abuse.

It has often been claimed that in GESTURE lies the origin of language, but, if so, speech very early achieved primacy, perhaps because a vocal-auditory system had crucial advantages: no mutual visibility was necessary between speaker and audience, the mouth was otherwise unoccupied except when EATING, and the hands were freed for other employment. The language faculty co-opted brain and body structures (mouth, ear) that had been developed for other functions (BREATHING, eating, BALANCE). Spoken language makes use of sound carried on out-breathed air from the lungs, which is modulated by articulators (TONGUE, lips, etc.) to produce the vocal repertoire of a natural language. No single language uses anything like the full range of sounds of which humans are capable, and certain classes of sound — for example, clicks and implosives, where the airstream is reversed and moves inwards — are rare in the world's languages.

Grammar and the body

The discovery and analysis of the fundamental unit of spoken language, the *phoneme* (which had been intuited in antiquity by the Levantine inventors of the alphabet, and which corresponds roughly with the letter) was facilitated by formalist experiments in the disintegration of sound and meaning in certain centers of European modernism following World War I, in particular Moscow, Prague, Paris, and Geneva. Notwithstanding the interest of avant-garde poets in the sounding body, the legacy of Cartesian rationalism and the privileging of mind cast a long shadow far into the twentieth century. Indeed, the dominant traditions of inquiry into language continue to discount the body by way of an implied hierarchy in which speech is only the (more or less) imperfect performance of an abstract system, whose formal and logical structure it is the task of linguistic science to reveal. Such abstraction, idealizing away to a genderless speaker-hearer and relegating gesture, posture, and expression to the limbo of 'paralanguage', has led to far-reaching insights into grammatical theory. But the body lay hidden in the closet. That is to say, after all the abstraction, there remains a residue — or rather a core — of human language that cannot be reduced to context-free formulation. The phenomenon that linguists call 'deixis' ('pointing' in classical Greek) sets limits to the decontextualization of language; even so austere a logician as Bertrand Russell acknowledged that the body could not be eliminated in the analysis of language, and that 'deictic' categories such as personal pronouns (I, you), demonstrative (this, that), and adverbs (here, now) depend for their interpretation upon the relative, and reflexive, positioning of bodies in space and time.

The body and meaning

Anthropocentrism is deeply embedded in the fabric of language, which reflects the shape and properties of the body, which in turn grounds the linguistic encoding of social relations — from empathy and solidarity to politeness and deference. The physical experience of gravity and the asymmetries of the human anatomy establish the meaning, for example, of 'up' and 'down', 'front' and 'back', 'right' and 'left'. (More than one science fiction plot has turned on the problem of conveying the concepts of 'right' and 'left' to an alien being whose body does not share with humans the necessary asymmetry.) Nor is it arbitrary that 'up' and 'front' tend to be positively valued relative to 'down' and 'back', since upright, confronting encounters are taken as the norm for humans in speech situations. Modernity's array of communications media — radio, film, television, video, the internet — are greatly extending what the invention of writing first set in train, namely, the uncoupling of language in complex ways from its primordial face-to-face matrix. It is hardly clear what will be the outcome of the new relations of virtuality, but human meanings will necessarily continue to rest on embodied understandings, however much they are mediated. Indeed, such is the power of gesture that a wink or a sarcastic intonation inevitably reframes and inverts the 'literal' meaning. The classic studies by the sociologist Erving Goffman of the management of daily encounters show how centrally the body is involved in the making of meaning; they reveal the significance and complexity of sight and touch in the business of opening, organizing, and closing conversations — synchronizing turns at speaking by gesture and GAZE, assessing one's reception through visual back-channel cues, and helping to 'perform' talk.

More recently, the linguist George Lakoff, collaborating at the intersection of cognitive linguistics, computer science, and neurology, likewise contends, from a quite different perspective, that meaning is grounded in the body. He makes a radical break with the rationalist tradition of his teacher, Noam Chomsky, by asserting the centrality of metaphor and by claiming that it is only through the body that concepts can be formed, since the human conceptual system grows out of the sensorimotor system.

Discourse and the body

Conversely, understandings of the body and its conduct are largely mediated through language and metaphor. Metaphors, moreover, are never innocent; they have cognitive, affective, and political import. The human body is truly the trope of tropes; body parts ('head', 'foot', 'face') are everywhere mapped onto nature's body — head of the river, foot of the mountain, face of the deep. Bodily functions are a universal reservoir for terms of profanity and scatological abuse. When the body is in distress, the power of language to organize its experience is attested in those HEALING traditions where speech is focal; 'a disease named is a disease half cured'. In all cultures linguistic taboos circumscribe the body; where the naming of certain body parts in front of doctors may involve a loss of 'face', figurines have been used, allowing the patient to point to the affected part without showing or naming it.

The deportment of bodies in social space, and the gearing of language into the infinite variety of improvised and ritual encounters, show that humans converse as 'communities of co-movers'. But no community is homogeneous, and speaking takes place in a discursive forcefield constituted through a pragmatic negotiation that registers asymmetries of power in the bodily movements and speech of those co-present. 'Voice quality', for example, is an unavoidable accompaniment to the act of speaking, and conveys culturally coded, and often finely textured, meanings about the speaker's identity in multiple intersecting dimensions — age, class, sex, gender, region, subculture, ethnicity, nationality, and so forth. The existence of etiquette and elocution manuals, and the importance of diplomatic protocols, suggest that such 'signs' are partly, but only partly, under the control of the speaker. Reading (and writing upon) the body has taken on fresh meaning in the late twentieth century, with the penetration of advertisements onto personal clothing, and the related vogue for inscriptions on the body surface itself.

The language animal

The practice of inscribing the body is at least 40 000 years old — no surprise, perhaps, for the primate that speaks. Language seems to have been the evolutionary Rubicon for *Homo sapiens*, though the Berkeley paleolinguist Johanna Nichols rejects the notion of linguistic monogenesis implicit in the image of a single crossing over into language. She believes it happened many times, and that hundreds of distinct languages were already being spoken in the Rift Valley of East Africa — as many as are spoken today in Papua New Guinea — before humans had fanned out on the way to planetary hegemony, armed with the mythomanic power of speech. The scandal of representation once prompted the critic Kenneth Burke to summarize the species in his own wry definition: 'the symbol-using animal, inventor of the negative, separated by instruments of his own making, goaded by the spirit of hierarchy, and rotten with perfection'. IAIN BOAL

Further reading

Foley, W. (1997). *Anthropological linguistics.* Blackwell, Oxford.

Lakoff, G. and Johnson, M. (1999). *Philosophy in the flesh.* Basic Books, New York.

Lieberman, P. (1984). *The biology and evolution of language.* Harvard, Cambridge, MA.

See also EVOLUTION; HUMAN; GESTURE; SPEECH; VOICE.

Language and the brain

Injury to the brain caused by STROKE or trauma can disrupt a person's ability to speak, to understand language, or both. Language disorders known as *aphasias*, resulting from neurological damage, led researchers to examine the relationship between language and the brain. Clinicians and scientists throughout history have observed that language impairments generally result from damage to particular areas of the left cerebral hemisphere, and have suggested that specific parts of the hemisphere are involved in producing and comprehending language.

Early studies of aphasia

One of the most celebrated proponents of this view was the French surgeon Paul Broca. In 1865, Broca published a case report of a patient known as 'Tan', who had suffered a stroke that damaged the inferior frontal gyrus of the left hemisphere (now referred to as *Broca's area*). This region is adjacent to areas of the brain that control the movement of the facial muscles and muscles of SPEECH. Tan had a severe impairment in the production of speech; he was able to utter only a single word, 'tan', which he pronounced with great effort. Broca concluded that this brain region was responsible for the production of speech sounds. The aphasia characterized by hesitant, effortful speech, but relatively normal comprehension of language, is now referred to as *Broca's aphasia*.

Shortly after Broca published his study of Tan, German psychiatrist Carl Wernicke reported cases of two patients with damage to the left posterior temporal lobe adjacent to the primary auditory area of the left hemisphere (now referred to as *Wernicke's area*). These patients were able to speak fluently, but the language they produced was nonsensical, and they had great difficulty understanding what was said to them. Thus, unlike Tan, these patients could produce the movements of speech, but were unable to comprehend or formulate spoken language. Wernicke proposed that they had lost the sound patterns associated with spoken language. Wernicke called this disorder '*sensory aphasia*', and claimed that the damaged region of the temporal lobe was responsible for storing the sound representations of speech. The aphasia characterised by fluent, disordered speech and severely impaired comprehension is currently referred to as *Wernicke's aphasia*.

The apparent anatomical separation between the production and comprehension of speech led Wernicke and others to suggest that language might be represented in the brain in terms of a set of discrete 'centres', each with its own specific function. In 1885, Ludwig Lichtheim proposed that spoken language was subserved by three interconnected centres: a motor centre (M) responsible for the movement patterns of words; an auditory centre (A) for the sound patterns of words; and a conceptual centre (C) for the meanings of words and the formulation of ideas. According to Lichtheim's *Connectionist Model of language* (which was elaborated by Norman

Geschwind in the twentieth century), each of these centres was associated with a specific brain area. Damage to an area, or to a connection between two areas, would produce an aphasia. Lichtheim's model not only accounted for the aphasias reported by Broca and Wernicke, but it predicted the existence of aphasic disorders that had not yet been reported. For example, the model predicted that damage to a connection between the auditory and motor areas of the brain would result in an inability to repeat spoken words, without difficulty in producing or understanding them. This disorder, called *conduction aphasia*, was later observed in a number of patients and is associated with damage to the *arcuate fasciculus*, a tract of fibres that connects Broca's and Wernicke's areas.

Although the Connectionist Model provided a compelling and powerful account of aphasic disorders, the approach was criticized by a number of clinicians and researchers in the late nineteenth and early twentieth centuries. French neurologist Pierre Marie studied numerous cases of speech impairment resulting from neurological damage, and observed that many patients with apparent Broca's aphasia had suffered damage to regions other than Broca's area, and that damage to Broca's area did not always result in classical Broca's aphasia. British neurologist John Hughlings Jackson criticized the methods and assumptions of the Connectionist approach, and argued that 'to locate the lesion which destroys speech and to locate speech are two different things.' Hughlings Jackson also questioned the model for its separation of language from other cognitive functions, and proposed that language and intellectual ability are inextricably linked. A similar view was adopted by British neurologist Henry Head, who favoured the investigation of both linguistic and non-verbal abilities as a means of examining the nature of language impairments in aphasic patients. Despite these criticisms, the conception of the brain as a set of discrete centres continues to influence models of language to the present day, and concerns about the localization of function and the relationship between language and more general cognitive processes remain active debates in current research.

Clinical and psychological approaches

Clinical studies of aphasic patients over the past century have attempted to establish a more detailed description of the language impairments observed in particular aphasic groups by systematically examining various aspects of language processing in individual patients. Comprehensive batteries of tests have been developed to provide quantitative measures of fluency and comprehension and to assess a range of linguistic abilities. The classical disorders of Broca's and Wernicke's aphasia are now well-defined clinical syndromes. Broca's aphasia is characterized by a disturbance in the articulation of speech with comprehension relatively spared, coupled with a phenomenon known as *agrammatism*: individuals with Broca's aphasia tend to omit or substitute grammatical function words and markers in their spontaneous speech, and they have difficulty producing and comprehending complex sentences. In contrast, Wernicke's aphasia is characterized by fluent articulation coupled with severely impaired comprehension. The speech of Wernicke's aphasics tends to be nonsensical, and typically includes *jargon* (utterances that are not actual words in the individual's native language, e.g. 'habe') and *semantic paraphasias* (substitutions of a word of similar meaning for an intended word, e.g. 'cat' for 'dog'). The clinical definitions of the syndromes of Broca's and Wernicke's aphasia have formed the basis for subsequent research into the nature of language processing in these patient groups.

Psychological investigations of aphasic disorders have examined the basic components of language, and have attempted to incorporate advances in linguistic theory into the study of the neural bases of language. A number of researchers have assumed a *hierarchical model* of language, in which linguistic information is processed in a series of discrete stages. The first stage in the hierarchy is the processing of *speech*, which involves the discrimination and identification of speech sounds (*speech perception*) and the planning and implementation of articulatory movements (*speech production*). Sheila Blumstein has examined the perception of speech sounds in aphasic patients and found that many individuals with aphasia have difficulty discriminating and labelling speech sounds. However, Blumstein and her colleagues have not observed a consistent relationship between deficits of speech perception and higher-level language comprehension impairments, including the comprehension deficit observed in Wernicke's aphasia. This finding calls into question the classical account of Wernicke's aphasia as an impairment in the ability to perceive the sounds of speech. Blumstein has also examined speech production in aphasia, and has observed that Broca's aphasics are impaired in the timing and co-ordination of speech-motor movements, whereas Wernicke's aphasics are impaired in the planning of sequences of speech sounds.

The next stage in the hierarchical model of language processing is the 'mental dictionary' or *lexicon*. The lexicon is thought to contain information about words, including *word form* (the sequence of sounds that uniquely characterizes a word) and *lexical-semantics* (the meaning of the word and its relationship to other words in the lexicon). Many aphasic patients have difficulty comprehending word meanings and producing word forms. For example, Wernicke's aphasics and other fluent aphasics tend to produce semantic paraphasias in their spontaneous speech, and have difficulty judging semantic relationships between words and sorting words into meaningful categories.

These observations have led researchers to suggest that Wernicke's aphasics may be impaired in the processing of lexical-semantic information. In addition, certain types of aphasics have particular difficulty producing the names of objects,

and these naming deficits can be specific to particular classes of objects, such as animals or tools. Hannah Damasio has found that patients who are impaired in naming animals tend to have suffered damage to brain regions associated with the processing of finely detailed visual information. In contrast, patients who are impaired in naming tools tend to have suffered damage to the intersection of brain regions associated with visual processing and the implementation of motor movements. The results suggest that the perceptual properties of particular objects may have influenced the neural organization of the mental lexicon: animals may be identified primarily on the basis of their visual features, whereas tools may be identified in terms of both their functional properties and their visual characteristics.

The next stage in the hierarchical model is the *grammar*, which is responsible for the production and comprehension of sentences. Grammatical relationships between words in a sentence can be expressed in two ways: *syntax* (the order that words occur in a sentence) and *morphology* (grammatical markings on the words themselves). A number of researchers, including Harold Goodglass, Alfonso Caramazza, Edgar Zurif, and David Caplan, have systematically examined the production and comprehension of grammatical information in Broca's aphasia. These investigations have revealed that Broca's aphasics are impaired in the generation and interpretation of morphological endings (e.g. forming the past tense 'jumped' from 'jump') and complex syntactic structures such as passives ('The boy was kissed by the girl') and embedded clauses ('The boy that the girl kissed is tall'). However, Broca's aphasics have no difficulty using word meaning to determine who did what to whom in sentences such as 'The apple was bitten by the boy', indicating that Broca's aphasics are able to use word meaning, but not syntax, to interpret complex sentences. David Caplan has proposed that there is a component of working memory that is responsible for deriving meaning from syntactic structure, and that this component is damaged in Broca's aphasia.

Theoretical perspectives

The results of these studies suggest that damage to particular brain regions may result in the disruption of specific aspects of language processing. Linguist Noam Chomsky proposed that the brain contains a 'language organ' that is specialized for the representation of linguistic information. This claim has been extended by theorists such as Steven Pinker, who have proposed that language is organized in terms of a set of domain-specific *modules*, each of which may be associated with distinct neural mechanisms. This approach is supported by the apparent separation between the lexicon and the grammar suggested by the disorders of Wernicke's and Broca's aphasia. However, recent studies have revealed that the language impairments associated with particular aphasic groups may not be as clear-cut as was originally believed.

For example, when a variety of different measures are used, lexical and grammatical impairments are typically observed in both Broca's and Wernicke's aphasias.

A number of theorists have suggested that the apparent domain-specific language deficits in aphasia may in fact reflect impairments in more general language processes. For example, Sheila Blumstein and William Milberg have proposed that the language impairments observed in both Broca's and Wernicke's aphasia result from disturbances in the activation of words in the lexicon, which may also interfere with the construction of sentence-level meanings. Further, Elizabeth Bates has observed that the syntactic structures that are most commonly impaired in aphasia are also disrupted in neurologically intact individuals under general cognitive stress, suggesting that grammatical impairments do not necessarily result from damage to a grammar module. It is hoped that future research into the nature of the language impairments observed in aphasic patients, coupled with advances in brain imaging techniques, will shed new light on the relationship between language and the brain.

JENNIFER AYDELOTT UTMAN

Further reading

Caplan, D. (1992). *Language: structure, processing, disorders*. MIT Press, Cambridge MA.

Sarno, M. T. (1991). *Acquired aphasia*. Academic Press, Inc., San Diego CA.

See also SPEECH; STROKE.

Large intestine The part of the gut between the small intestine and the anus: caecum, colon and rectum. 'Large' because it is a wider tube, although much shorter, than the 'small' intestine. From the caecum, low on the right side (from which the appendix arises), the ascending, then the transverse, then the descending parts of the colon lead to the rectum, low on the left side. Water is progressively absorbed as the contents are moved onwards for storage in the rectum.   S.J.

See ALIMENTARY SYSTEM; PLATE 1.

Larynx The larynx is the 'voicebox', the organ in the neck that plays a crucial role in SPEECH and BREATHING. The channels for air and for food, which share the PHARYNX at the back of the NOSE and MOUTH, diverge at this point, leading respectively to the trachea and to the OESOPHAGUS. The opening for air through the larynx is known as the *glottis*, and the EPIGLOTTIS, below and behind the TONGUE, plays a necessary part in closing off the glottis during SWALLOWING.

The larynx has three important functions: control of the airflow during breathing, protection of the airway below it, and production of sound for SPEECH. The main part of the framework of the larynx is the *thyroid cartilage*, and it is the front part of this that can easily be seen and felt as the 'Adam's apple'. The larynx rests on the ring-shaped *cricoid cartilage*, and below this is the trachea. Above, and attached by ligaments to the larynx at the front, is the U-shaped *hyoid bone* that provides support and moves upwards with the larynx during swallowing. Halfway down the larynx the paired vocal folds (commonly known as the *vocal cords*), formed by ligaments covered with mucous membrane, project inwards from its wall. The vocal folds form a 'V' shape, open towards the back. At the rear end of each vocal fold are the small *arytenoid cartilages*. Many small muscles are attached to these, and their action can vary the size of the aperture, by pulling the arytenoids apart or drawing them nearer together, widening or narrowing the 'V'. This movement occurs rhythmically during inhalation and exhalation in regular quiet breathing. Closure of the glottis occurs only momentarily during swallowing; abnormally, near-closure (*laryngospasm*) seriously obstructs breathing and causes *stridor* — high-pitched and noisy breathing.

During speech, SINGING, or playing a wind instrument, the size of the aperture is narrowed and varied, to produce sounds of different pitch. This increased resistance to airflow out of the lungs converts the flow to a rapid pulsation as it passes between the vocal folds; this produces sound that is then modified by the upper vocal tract.   MARJORIE P. LORCH

See PLATE 3.

See also BREATHING; SINGING; SPEECH; VOICE.

Laughter and humour

Charles Darwin noted in the 1870s that certain bodily movements and FACIAL EXPRESSIONS occurring during emotional states are similar in people around the world, independent of cultural or other differences. Laughter, a behaviourally stereotyped, staccato vocalization, is a case in point. Laughter emerges by around 4 months of age, long after the ability to smile or cry, and eventually co-occurs with speech. As an overt behavioural marker of humour, laughter signals an affective state of mirth or joy, although it does not exclusively signal this state: it may also signal anxiety or embarrassment (as in nervous laughter), derision, or even agreeableness (as in polite laughter at Oxford high tables). Uncontrolled, involuntary bouts of laughter in situations in which laughter would be inappropriate have occasionally been reported in patients with certain kinds of brain injury — especially injury to the parts of the frontal lobes.

Mirthful laughter is triggered by a variety of verbal and non-verbal situations. What may strike one person as extremely funny may be perceived by another as only mildly so, if amusing at all. In part because of the extreme variability of stimuli and response, the phenomenon of humour has not, until recently, been studied experimentally, despite being a long-standing interest among philosophers, writers, psychoanalysts, and sociologists. Indeed the very complexity of the phenomenon has led to a recognition that an adequate understanding of what makes something humorous will require a joint consideration of at least three levels of analysis:

the cognitive, the social, and the affective. On the cognitive end, the notion of incongruity, or what Arthur Koestler has termed 'bisociative thinking' has been seen as central to humour perception. That is, humour is thought to involve an abrupt realization that a particular belief or expectation about a situation is not the only way of perceiving the situation. While incongruity recognition is thus seen to be necessary for humour to be perceived, it is not sufficient: for something to be perceived as humorous, rather than as threatening, the new interpretation should be seen to have trivial rather than terrifying implications, and should bring in absurd, playful, and/or indiscreet elements into an otherwise 'serious' scenario. Thus, the affective aspect of humour stems both from the pleasure of 'getting' the joke and the relief from the recognition that it is, after all, only a joke — that the danger is not real. Finally, the social aspect of humour resides in the fact that what is considered laughable will depend on shared beliefs and implicit norms, concerning the extent to which these beliefs can be temporarily called into question and subjected to a reinterpretation through humour. Indeed there may be no better way to 'calibrate' the social mores of a new group you are introduced to than by telling them jokes.

There can be both physiological and psychological benefits from laughter. It requires the coordinated action of 15 facial muscles and the thoracic cavity. It produces spasmodic SKELETAL MUSCLE contractions, tachycardia, changes in BREATHING pattern, and an increase in CATECHOLAMINE production. Hearty laughter increases heart rate, BLOOD PRESSURE and respiratory rate, and muscular activity. Many of the physiological changes associated with laughter are beneficial ones. For example, the increased ventilation and clearing of mucus may aid patients with chronic respiratory conditions such as emphysema. The increased heart rate and blood pressure that accompanies laughter can exercise the myocardium and increase arterial and venous circulation. It has been suggested that this in turn allows an increased movement of OXYGEN and nutrients to tissues and facilitates the movement of immune elements and PHAGOCYTES, thereby aiding the body in fighting infections. The enhanced venous return helps to reduce vascular stasis and may lower the risk of thrombus formation. Muscle relaxation following bouts of hearty laughter may break the spasm–pain cycle in patients with neuralgias or rheumatism. A reduction in laryngeal muscle tension associated with laughter may help patients with vocal fold pathology to produce a more relaxed voice. Laughter also appears to aid the recovery of phonation in patients with psychogenic dysphonia, a puzzling disorder characterized by an inability to phonate during speech despite intact articulation and no identifiable pathology of the larynx. Finally, the increased catecholamine levels associated with laughter may be responsible for beneficial effects of humour on mental functions, such as alertness and creativity. (But despite the far-reaching claims, these appear

to be nonspecific 'benefits' and it is not clear why laughter should be any more beneficial in this regard than playing cricket.)

A number of psychological benefits have also been claimed for laughter and humour. Humour is said to loosen boundaries between strangers and strengthen bonds between friends and intimates. It provides a way of allowing people to mask deficiencies or disclose vulnerabilities. It is also thought to increase flexibility in thinking, foster solidarity and intimacy, and provide an alternative to despair.

Theories about the functional significance of humour have ranged from psychoanalytic, through social/anthropological, to cognitive, and even metaphysical accounts.

Psychological theories
According to Freud, humour makes possible 'the satisfaction of an INSTINCT (whether lustful or hostile) in the face of an obstacle that stands in its way'. Thus, the PLEASURE in a joke arises from the savings in psychic energy made possible by the relief from conscious monitoring. The association of humour with aggressive or sexual impulses has also characterized many subsequent accounts of humour — fuelling debate over whether hostility is an inherent element. Proponents of the so-called *superiority theory* (Aristotle, Plato, Hobbes, and Bergson) view humour as reflecting a moral stance on the part of the humorist. As described in Hobbes's *Leviathan*, 'The passion of laughter is nothing else but sudden glory arising from a sudden conception of some eminency in ourselves by comparison with the infirmity of others, or with our own formerly.' Superiority may be revealed not just by laughing at others' deficiencies but also by showing that one can laugh at (and rise above) one's own imperfections. For Henri Bergson, humour 'consists in perceiving something mechanical encrusted on something living'; laughter asserts the human values of spontaneity and freedom and thus erupts whenever a person behaves rigidly, like an automaton.

Social/Anthropological theories
The social significance of laughter and humour has been emphasized (for example by Konrad Lorenz). Laughter has been regarded as a marker of group membership and solidarity for those who share a joke, and of exclusion for those who are the 'butt' of the joke, thus providing a means of maintaining social control and group cohesiveness.

Cognitive theorists
Cognitive theorists of humour include Kant and Schopenhauer (two singularly humourless German philosophers) and the Gestalt psychologist Norman Maier. They have focused on describing the mechanisms that underlie humour processing. From a cognitive perspective, humour is thought to arise from a sudden 'paradigm shift' — a restructuring of an internal mental model upon recognizing some ambiguity, inconsistency, or contradiction in a situation. That is, we experience humour when we become

aware of a discrepancy between what is expected and what is experienced — but only if that discrepancy turns out to be non-threatening.

Evolutionary hypotheses

Evolutionary hypotheses have speculated on the possible adaptive significance of human laughter and humour. They fall into five groups:

Humour as a temporary disabling mechanism laughter disrupts the status quo. While laughing we, quite literally, are rendered incapable of thinking of, let alone doing, anything else. This may have been evolutionarily useful in that it gets us out of a routine or fixed way of thinking, thus enabling a creative approach to problem solving.

Humour as social learning the origins of humour have been traced to the laughter of young primates and children in response to tickling and play. Thus Weisfeld notes that 'the pleasure of humour motivates us to seek out fitness-enhancing input' and that laughter is 'a pleasant social signal that prompts the humorist to persist in providing this edifying stimulation'. However the proposition that participating in play and humorous interactions in fitness-relevant situations (such as sexual, aggressive, or other social interactions) aids in social learning, does not explain why humour (rather than, say, gossiping, or fantasizing) is necessary for such instruction.

Humour as status-manipulation the notion that mirthful laughter creates and strengthens group boundaries is at the centre of a theory of humour proposed by Alexander; humour developed as a form of ostracism, providing a means of manipulating status within a group. Ostracism in turn has repercussions for reproductive success. According to this view, humour functions primarily as a means of creating solidarity among some members of a group by excluding or demeaning others. These notions echo those described above under social learning, since they suggest that humour is a form of social scenario-building, providing an edge in learning how to negotiate in 'fitness-relevant' domains. However, the question remains as to why humour *per se* is necessary or useful in accomplishing the goal. Why are humorous put-downs needed when direct criticism or insults could suffice?

Humour as vocal grooming the theory of language as a vehicle for social bonding through its origins in grooming and gossip has interesting implications for an understanding of humour. Inasmuch as LANGUAGE facilitates social bonding, humour in language may offer a shortcut to forming deep, affectional ties with those with whom one discovers and tacitly cultivates a common ground. 'Finding the same thing funny is not only a prerequisite to a real friendship, but very often the first step to its formation' (Konrad Lorenz). The fact that much of conversation is punctuated by laughter and that laughter releases endogenous opiates suggests that humorous discourse may have arisen as a means for eliciting more laughter, in the service of social bonding.

Laughter at a false alarm the present author has proposed that laughter allows the individual to alert others in a social group (usually kin) that a detected anamoly is trivial, that there is no real danger and therefore nothing to worry about. The laughter (and its spread within the group) announces that there has been a false alarm, that the rest of the community need not waste precious energy and resources responding to a spurious threat. In this view, an individual's nervous laughter may be seen as an internalized reaction to stressful situations: a way of distracting oneself from one's anxiety by setting off one's own false-alarm mechanisms. Similarly, the smile may be seen as a weaker form of laughter — an aborted orienting response, signalling 'I know you pose no threat'. The same line of reasoning may explain why people laugh when tickled: a potential threat turns out not to be one.

Clues to the neural mediation of laughter and of humour have come mainly from clinical reports of their disorders. Patients with damage in the right cerebral hemisphere show preserved sensitivity to the surprise element of humour but a diminished ability to establish narrative coherence. Disorders of humour such as foolish or silly EUPHORIA and a tendency toward making inappropriate jokes have also been reported in patients with damage to the frontal lobes. Deficits in humour appreciation are more common in patients with right frontal damage, supporting a view that the right frontal lobe serves an important role in responding to 'anomalies'. Disorders of laughter can occur independently of disorders of humour. They are most commonly associated with the type of STROKE known as *pseudobulbar palsy*, when laughter can be intermixed with crying. A sudden display of laughter has been reported to precede acute strokes. And 'gelastic' (laughing) seizures originating from the left hemisphere (typically resulting from a rare tumour in the hypothalamus) are another manifestation of pathological laughter. Although infrequent, disorders of laughter are almost always associated with abnormal activity in, or damage to, parts of the brain that are components of the LIMBIC SYSTEM; given the well-known role of the limbic system in producing an orienting response to a potential threat or alarm, it is not altogether surprising that it is also involved in the aborted orienting reaction in response to a false alarm — namely, laughter. There is also evidence that particular regions of the cortex of the temporal lobe are associated respectively with the affective side of laughter (the feeling of merriment that accompanies it), whereas others are involved in the motor act of laughter itself.

Research on the brain bases of humour and laughter has depended largely on the study of clinical cases. Whilst this is provocative, there is clearly also a need for experimental research to examine more fully the neurophysiology and neuropsychology of laughter and humour.

J. VAID
V. S. RAMACHANDRAN

Further reading

Morreall, J. (1983). *Taking laughter seriously*. State University of New York Press, Albany.

Ramachandran, V. S. (1998). The neurology and evolution of humour, laughter, and smiling: the false alarm theory. *Medical Hypotheses*, 51(4), 351–4.

Vaid, J. (1999). The evolution of humour: do those who laugh last? In *Evolution of the psyche* (ed.) D. Rosen and M. Luebbert), pp. 123–38. Praeger, Westport CT.

Weisfeld, G. (1993). The adaptive value of humour and laughter. *Ethology and Sociobiology*, 14, 141–69.

See also EMOTION; FACIAL EXPRESSION; PLEASURE; SMILING.

Learning disabilities

Learning disabilities What connections exist between the body and 'learning disability' or 'mental retardation'? We assume that there is a realm of mental nature separable from physical nature, at least for investigative purposes; we also often see mental disorders as being analogous to physical ones, or physical conditions as causing mental ones. We assume that mental ability or disability is a part of an individual's make-up, and therefore that what is congenital is also largely incurable. All these assumptions are modern, in the historian's sense of the term: they belong to the last three centuries.

According to GALEN, the supreme medical authority before modern times, human reason was activated by 'animal spirits' which moved around the brain and, if sluggish, caused *amentia* (mindlessness); however, any normal individual could experience this condition temporarily. Sometimes a landowner's heir might suffer from congenital incompetence, but this was a problem for lawyers, not doctors; it was not distinguished from the assumed incompetence of the entire labouring population, and where people did not own property there was no problem. Nor was congenital incompetence necessarily permanent: God might cure it providentially. People whom we might now call 'learning disabled' were depicted by artists; but neither their behavioural gestures and bodily features, nor their social role, were clearly distinct from those of jesters and professional fools whose minds were perfectly sound. Medical writers did not research the causes of mental (or physical) monstrosity, since these were God's responsibility; rather, monstrosity demonstrated His marvellous creative powers. Only mavericks among them, such as astrologers or followers of the derided Paracelsus, had a specifically medical interest in connections between the body and permanent lack of reason. Even for them, reason tended to mean divine illumination rather than the personal mental equipment described by modern psychology.

In the seventeenth-century roots of that psychology we begin to find a learning disabled type recognisable to ourselves, defined by the purely mental characteristics of an individual. The influential philosopher John Locke summarized these as a lack of ability to think 'abstractly', and psychology has refined this picture very little since then. However, the approach to physiological phenomena associated with 'idiocy' (as it was then technically known) has changed frequently. These changes have social and political connections. Locke was also a leading Whig theoretician, and saw idiots as people who lacked the mental equipment needed to exercise their individual autonomy, the basis of the new Whig political philosophy of government by consent. As a medical practitioner himself, he thought this lack might be caused by their having different bodily mechanisms. He did not investigate further, possibly because the discipline of anatomy was controlled by his political opponents. His Tory contemporary, Thomas Willis, believed there was an anatomical distinction between the brains of 'stupid' and 'mad' people, although he also continued to believe Galen's hypothesis of slow-moving 'animal spirits'. Descartes's discussion of the mind (one of the sources for modern accounts of a distinctly human psychology) located the reasoning soul in the PINEAL GLAND, which previously had been merely a valve controlling the flow of animal spirits. Anatomists under Descartes's influence, dissecting the corpses of mad people and idiots, claimed that the former possessed excessively flexible pineal glands, the latter excessively rigid ones.

Eighteenth-century medical theorists opened up an empire of the mind, developing psychological classifications in terms similar to those of bodily disease. At the same time their interest in the physiology of idiots largely reverted to external characteristics, particularly facial features (*physiognomics*) and skull shape (PHRENOLOGY). In the mid nineteenth century, with the rise of colonialism and ANTHROPOLOGY, theories of idiocy and race were united. The mental characteristics of idiots were identified with the alleged psychological inabilities and corresponding external physical characteristics of non-whites. Fetal development was thought to retrace the primitive stages of human history which the non-white races still exhibited; sometimes development was arrested, a notion embodied in the 'mongol', whose facial features apparently betrayed a low level of psychological competence comparable with that of the mongoloid races. Segregated institutions and then sterilization programmes arose from this culture, with the aim of improving the health of the race. Administered largely by practitioners of physical medicine, they appeared first in the Anglo-Saxon countries; in Germany the same culture led to mass exterminations of learning disabled people at the end of the 1930s.

Since then a rapid refinement in the diagnostic technology of chromosomes and genes has renewed our interest in internal bodily causes. There has been a correspondingly rapid increase in the number of psychological labels attached to syndromes (e.g. 'fragile X'); the human genome project now promises to locate DNA markers for the lower band of a socially determined 'normal IQ'. This profusion of learning disabled conditions has interacted with rapid changes in their

social status and acceptance. Pathology advances in some directions while retreating in others. At the time of writing, for example, genetically-related autism has fanned out into an autistic 'spectrum', annexing and reinventing 'Asperger's syndrome' as a mild variant which may affect the apparently normal population. Its socially segregating effects are inseparable from the diagnosis itself, by which autistic people are said to belong mentally in a separate world from others; this notion reinforces a separate professional specialization, creating more research and labelling. In a simultaneous but contrary tendency, numbers of prospective parents reject termination after a positive test for Down's syndrome, partly because children and young adults with this condition have become increasingly integrated in the community.

People began by wanting a physical diagnosis of learning disability, for various religious and political reasons, in the seventeenth century when biochemistry was inconceivable. But whatever the precision of today's diagnostic techniques in this respect, it has not been matched, either in psychology or in cognitive and behavioural genetics, by a corresponding precision in the diagnosis and description of the 'mental' aspects; these remain as fluid and subject to social context as ever. CHRISTOPHER GOODEY

Further reading

Wright, D. and Digby, A. (1996). *From idiocy to mental deficiency: historical perspectives on people with learning disabilities*. London.

Trent, J. (1994). *Inventing the feeble mind: a history of mental retardation in the United States*. Berkeley.

See also INTELLIGENCE.

Legs

Physically, human legs, along with the feet, are the primary means of both support and locomotion. Symbolically they suggest mobility or stability. As such, the balancing of weight on the legs and the qualities of a stride are both legible as forms of nonverbal communication, or body language.

The English language contains many phrases that suggest the importance of legs as a means of support. To 'stand on one's own two legs' is to take or retain control or independence; to 'find one's legs', especially 'sea legs' or 'land legs', is to gain control and ability. Similarly, to be 'on one's last legs' or to 'not have a leg to stand on' suggests failure or the losing of support or independence. To 'pull one's leg' is to fool someone, to bring them off-balance. Some phrases have been transmuted through the replacement of 'legs' with 'feet': 'to stand on one's own feet' or 'again' 'to have one's feet on the ground'.

There are fewer common phrases that use legs as symbolic of mobility, but the value Western culture places on mobility renders legs symbolic of freedom or independence. If something 'has legs', it has worth and is 'going somewhere'; asking someone to 'shake a leg' is asking them to hurry. The importance of legs as both symbols and

mechanisms of mobility has created an interesting split within the making of prosthetics, where one can have either a *visual prosthetic* (a leg that looks real) or a *mobile prosthetic* (a leg that works well).

The physicality of legs is often gendered. Muscled legs are often seen as masculine, while slender legs are attributed to femininity. The US takes it further yet; gender roles there demand adult women shave the hair from their legs, making them appear pre-adolescent or doll-like, and exaggerating the relative smallness and smoothness of women's legs. Many cultures frown on the display of bare legs, especially in formal settings; women who wear skirts in business contexts are often still required to wear stockings or tights. Other cultures require long skirts or trousers to cover the legs, on the assumption that they are erotic and titillating.

In anatomical terms, the legs are built around three bones. The *femur*, in the thigh, articulates at the HIP joint with the pelvic girdle, linking the legs to the vertebral column via the sacro-iliac joints. The lower end of the femur articulates at the KNEE joint with the *tibia* (shin bone); the *fibula* lies beside the tibia on the outer side of the lower leg. These two bones together link the leg to the foot at the ANKLE joint, although it is the tibia which carries all the weight. Here, at the sides, their lower ends form the protuberances known as the *malleoli*, which 'clasp' the sides of the *talus* bone of the ankle, on which the leg hinges. The strong muscles of the BUTTOCKS (*glutei*) span the hip joints, and are crucial to support and stability. The fleshy mass of the QUADRICEPS ('four-headed') muscle in the front, and the HAMSTRINGS in the back of the thigh span both the hip and the knee; when the hip is stabilised, they respectively extend and flex the knee, or, with a straight knee, they take part in movement at the hip. The lower, tendinous portions of these muscles help to encapsulate the knee joint, and the central component of the quadriceps forms the strong *patellar tendon*, connected to the knee cap. In the lower leg, the calf muscles (*gastrocnemius* and underlying *soleus*) attach to the heel via the strong *Achilles tendon*, and lift it from the ground during walking and running. Other muscles in the back and in the front of the lower leg act at the ankle and also, by means of long tendons spanning the ankle, are the main means of moving the toes, and of modifying the shape of the foot — e.g. by tensing the instep — during WALKING. In these functions they are assisted by the several layers of small muscles in the sole of the foot itself. The *tibialis anterior*, that can be felt on the front beside the shin when the foot is lifted, is particularly important for this action during walking: 'footdrop' is the consequence of damage to its nerve supply.

The nerves to the legs come from the spinal nerve roots that form the *lumbar plexus* and the *sacral plexus*, and which lie deep against the back of the abdomen and the pelvis. Here the motor and sensory nerve fibres that connect with the lumbar and sacral segments of the spinal cord are variously rearranged to emerge and to proceed to the legs, as the main nerves — the *sciatic* to the back, and the *femoral* to the front. Some smaller nerves, and the branches of these two main ones, supply the whole of the legs and the feet.

The main arterial blood supply to each leg is the *femoral artery*, which can be felt pulsating in the groin — and which can readily be used as a 'pressure point' in first aid, for HAEMORRHAGE anywhere in the leg except the upper part of the back of the thigh, which is served by other vessels. At the back of the knee, in the hollow called the *popliteal fossa* (where it is also accessible for pressure), it changes its name to *popliteal artery*, and ends by branching below that into a main stream on each side. Veins run both deep in the legs and superficially under the skin. It is a penalty of the upright posture that pressure in the leg veins is high. The return of blood to the heart against gravity is assisted by the presence in them of valves, preventing backflow, and by the contraction of the leg muscles, which tends to 'milk' the blood upwards; if the valves are damaged, the irregular bulges of VARICOSE VEINS become all too obvious.   JULIE VEDDER
SHEILA JENNETT

See PLATE 5.

See also ANKLE; HIP; KNEE.

Leisure

Leisure The release of the body from the tension and strain of work may be understood as a natural physical response to FATIGUE. Yet RELAXATION as a regulated right of human labour in the Western world emerged only in the nineteenth century, and ever since has been repeatedly checked by anxieties about mass leisure and by the dynamics of economic growth.

Many cultures share a 7-day cycle of 6-days' work with one day's rest and societies break up routinized labour with festivals. In medieval Europe, 100 holidays per year was common. Over time, holidays were extended with the addition, for example, of half-day 'preparations' preceding feast days. Workdays varied in length with daylight, weather, and the task to be done. The average was probably about 10 hours. As late as the eighteenth century, economists assumed that workers would work less if given increased wages, preferring more leisure to higher incomes.

Yet this image of a pre-industrial 'leisure ethic' must be qualified. Most festivals corresponded to lulls in seasonal work cycles, usually tied to agriculture. This explains, for example, the long season of holidays between October and February. Even holidays like midsummer (late June) and the English Wakes' Week (August) coincided with breaks in the farming work cycle. These holidays did not conform to the need of the body for rest. And many work-free saints' days and even Sunday were more of a privilege than a right, bestowed on the skilled and politically powerful urban male trades.

The growth of markets and mechanized production gradually undermined the traditional leisure culture but also established conditions for regular relaxation as a right. Religious reformers attacked both the length and unruly practices of festivals like Mardi Gras, especially from the second half of the sixteenth century. During the 1650s, English Puritans attempted to replace the irregular festival calendar with the weekly and subdued Sabbath rest. The attempt of the first French Republic in 1793 to create a 10-day week to replace the 'Christian' 7-day week and festival calender was merely an extreme example of a common effort of market-oriented reformers to increase the regularity of work. In the eighteenth and nineteenth centuries, long festival seasons (like the week between Christmas and New Year) were reduced to single holidays. Employers also suppressed the informal practice among mostly privileged male trades of 'Saint Monday' — extending the Sunday rest into Monday. By the 1820s, by taking advantage of gas lighting, employers lengthened workdays in textile factories to 12 and 14 hours. They increased working hours in order to meet competition and to make efficient use of expensive machinery.

The demands of a market/mechanized economy for a more disciplined workforce led élites to attack the anarchic character of much of festival leisure. They opposed the release of physical and psychological tensions in bursts of boisterous play (drinking, gambling, and violent sport) that was common in the festival play of the popular classes. Wealthy English gradually withdrew their patronage of local festivals and even blocked access to popular sports fields and walking paths. Authorities outlawed violent, chaotic inter-village sporting matches and tried to license ale houses and other drinking places in hopes of reducing gambling, blood sports like cock fighting, and too-ready access to drink.

By the 1830s, more positive notions of relaxation were beginning to appear when reformers (doctors, clergy, politicians, and even some factory owners) began to recognize the social, biological, and cultural costs of overwork. The revival of the Anglo-American Sabbatarian movement was an attempt to prevent work and the market from invading the sanctity of Sunday rest and religious observance. And by the 1850s, factory owners in Britain were beginning to grant women workers a Saturday half-holiday in hopes that this would give them time to shop and clean in anticipation of a restful family Sunday.

In the 1830s and 1840s, reformers found the increased intensity, regularity, and length of worktime in mechanized textile jobs to threaten the education and growth of children. Long, exhausting hours for women seemed to undermine the female's 'duty' to produce children and to care for the family. These concerns culminated in the English 10-hour day law of 1847 for women and children in textile factories. American and European employers and governments only grudgingly granted the right to leisure, applying it in stages, first to children, then to women, and then to men in dangerous or especially fatiguing trades (like mining).

Victorian reformers also promoted new forms of leisure in 'rational recreation'. The ideal was a leisure designed to restore the body, improve the mind, and compensate for the loss of domestic life due to the separation of work from home caused by industrialization. Among its many forms were the public parks intended to encourage family promenades on Sundays, the homelike atmospheres of YMCA reading rooms, and even 'rationalized' SPORTS like soccer controlled by strict rules and referees that minimized injury and violence.

These ideas about recreation emerged from the middle classes. Although they trickled down to labourers, working-class leisure retained many aspects of the traditional festival culture. Rational recreation was best expressed in the suburban ideal of the bourgeois family home that had clearly emerged by 1850. There, parlour board games, oral reading of new family magazines, and outdoor sports like croquet could bind the family, sheltered from the disorder of the urban crowds.

Despite the success of the Ten-Hour Law, intellectual and business élites continued to fear that a legal limit to the workday would force businesses into costly investments in machinery and inventory, make industry less competitive in expanding markets, and undermine employers' social control over workers. Late Victorian and early twentieth-century intellectuals like Le Bon, Durkheim, and Freud were obsessed that freedom from work would unleash the passions of urban crowds.

Still others argued that regular relaxation should be a fruit of increased productivity and a necessity of more intense work. Scientific management, pioneered by the American Frederick Taylor in the 1890s, found that new pay and work methods and reorganized factories could increase individual output and make it possible to reduce daily working hours. Especially after 1912, trade unionists and reformers proposed a trade off of more intense and strictly managed work for an 8-hour workday. Beginning with Herman von Helmholtz in the 1860s, scientists began to understand the working body as a 'motor' with a measurable capacity for work and the need for regularly spaced rest. This concept challenged the view that the natural 'laziness' of workers could be overcome only by applying external discipline. Work scientists like Angelo Mosso believed that output could be optimized if exhaustion was avoided. Overwork reduced longevity, decreased fertility, stunted the growth of youth, produced insomnia and NERVOUSNESS, and encouraged ALCOHOLISM and torpor. Efficiency in the human motor required daily and weekly rest breaks and even regularly spaced rests within the workday. The sophistication of work science grew during World War I, providing a powerful support for the 8-hour, 6-day week which became common in 1919.

In the 1930s, Western European workers won an annual paid holiday and Americans won a 2-day weekend. After World War II, these reductions made possible working-class tourism (especially in Europe) and suburbanization (especially in the US). In the postwar generation, a 'perfect' balance of work and leisure seem to have been achieved in the US, ideally based on wage-earning husbands working 40 hours a week supported by a home-making wife in the suburbs.

Since the 1970s, complex economic and social trends have reversed the historical trend toward increased leisure time. Increased speed of communications and transport along with the rise of global competition have created the 24-hour economy and, with it, work at all hours. Economic maximizing and consumerism have induced workers not only to opt for overtime but to choose timesaving devices to aid in their leisure. This has meant a saturation of free time with leisure goods and their maintenance, thus creating what Staffan Linder calls a 'harried leisure class' of consumers. Decline in the rates of growth in the West from the 1970s and the rise of the Pacific Rim economies, where leisure time still does not match Western standards, has weakened the influence of Western labour and efforts to reduce worktime. The more than doubling of the rate of married women in the work-force since the war (from 25% to 61% between 1950 and 1981 in Britain) has undermined the domestic culture upon which family leisure was formerly based and has created serious pressures on women to stretch time between wage and caring work. Many two-income couples, especially those unable to purchase personal services, have experienced a 'domestic speedup' when the traditional realms of personal life — family care and leisure — are crammed into shorter periods of the week. Relaxation is an elusive goal, despite the increases in productivity that should make it attainable for all.   GARY CROSS

See also RELAXATION; SPORT.

Leonardo da Vinci (1452–1519)

Leonardo was renowned in his lifetime as a painter, sculptor, architect, musician, engineer, and cartographer, but the degree of awareness of his anatomical work among his contemporaries is a mystery. Almost everything that we know today about his researches is contained in 200 sheets of drawings and notes housed in the Royal Library at Windsor Castle.

As a young artist in Florence, Leonardo absorbed the prevailing theoretical interest in a quasi-scientific basis for painting. This included the study of superficial anatomy, through life drawing and attendance at the public dissections that were occasionally held by the medical schools. There is no evidence that he was interested in deep anatomy until the late 1480s, by which time he had moved to Milan. There he outlined a plan for a treatise on the human body, covering not only anatomy but also conception, growth, proportion, the emotions, and the senses. A number of sheets from around this date comprise syntheses of animal dissection, surface observation, and traditional beliefs, though Leonardo does not seem to have pursued his

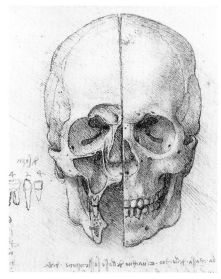

studies systematically. He reportedly compiled a manuscript treatise on the anatomy of the horse, now lost; his human material was primarily skeletal, most notably a series of highly accurate drawings of the skull, sectioned in an attempt to locate the sites of the mental faculties.

Due to other obligations, Leonardo's anatomical work ceased from about 1493 till around 1504, when in connection with the abortive *Battle of Anghiari* mural in Florence he systematically surveyed the superficial aspects of man. An interest in hydrodynamics soon led him back to a study of the deeper systems of the body, for he now had some access to corpses in the hospital of Santa Maria Nuova. In the winter of 1507–8, Leonardo was present at the peaceful demise of an elderly man, prompting him to perform an autopsy 'to see the cause of so sweet a death'. The resulting drawings and notes include the first records of the appendix, cirrhosis of the liver,

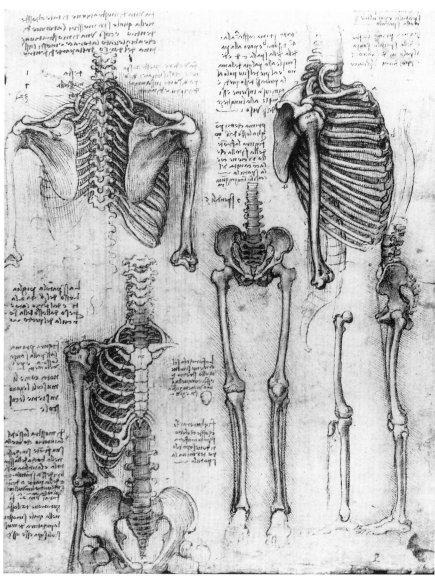

Drawings by Leonardo da Vinci. Above: *The skull bisected and sectioned* (1489). Below: *Orthogonal views of the skeleton* (c 1510–11). (Collection of Her Majesty the Queen).

arteriosclerosis, calcification of vessels, and coronary vascular occlusion. He also returned briefly to an investigation of the structure of the brain, making a wax cast of an ox's ventricles.

Shortly afterwards Leonardo's interests changed fundamentally. A beautiful and highly accurate series of drawings, datable to the winter of 1510–11, concentrate on the mechanics of the osteological and myological systems. His methods of illustration were particularly inventive: the bones of the thorax drawn orthographically; the cervical vertebrae in an exploded view; the hand through six stages of dissection; the shoulder muscles reduced to lines of force to depict the whole system in a single drawing; the arm in seven views through 180 degrees; and so on.

This change in approach seems to have been due to a collaboration with Marcantonio della Torre, the young Galenist and professor of anatomy at the university of Pavia. Leonardo now had much greater access to human material: the number of dissections he claimed to have performed grows from 'more than ten' around 1509, to 'more than thirty' towards the end of his life. This was the only phase of his researches when he achieved a working compromise between coverage and detail, for it was still his intention to publish a treatise, and, after Marcantonio's death in 1511, Leonardo concentrated primarily on cardiology and embryology.

Leonardo dissected a fetus of about six months, studying the relative sizes of the viscera, though his understanding of the structure of the human placenta was coloured by observations made in an earlier dissection of a gravid cow. More rewarding was his work on the bovine heart. He identified the auricles and described the movements of diastole and systole; he constructed a glass model of the aortic valve and, observing the vortices in the sinuses, he correctly deduced the exact mechanism of closure of the valves. Leonardo was on the verge of discovering the circulation of the blood, but he could not abandon the ancient belief in the independence of the arterial and venous systems, and he modified his results to accommodate this.

In late 1513, Leonardo moved to Rome, where he conducted research in the Ospedale di Santo Spirito, though few resulting drawings can be identified. In 1515 he was accused before Pope Leo X of unspecified sacrilegious practices and was barred from the Ospedale. The following year he went to France, dying there without resuming his anatomical work, and without having completed the treatise that he had planned for thirty years. Leonardo's papers passed to a pupil, Francesco Melzi, at whose villa near Milan they were occasionally seen by visitors, but they were not widely known until the publication of a series of facsimiles around 1900.　MARTIN CLAYTON

Further reading

Keele, K. and Pedretti, C. (1979). *Corpus of the Anatomical Studies in the Collection of Her Majesty The Queen at Windsor Castle*. Johnson Reprint Co., London and New York.

O'Malley, C. D. and Saunders, J. (1952). *Leonardo da Vinci on the human body*. H. Schuman, New York.

See also ANATOMY; DISSECTION.

Leprosy Leprosy may briefly be defined as a chronic, potentially disabling disease, mainly affecting the nerves, skin, and eyes, caused by a bacillus, *Mycobacterium leprae*, which microscopically resembles the organism of TUBERCULOSIS. However, a better understanding of this complex disease calls for attention to (i) the long incubation period (usually 2–5 years); (ii) the remarkable diversity of clinical findings, apparently related to the level of immunity of different individuals; (iii) the frequency of adverse (damaging) immunological reactions, based on either cell-mediated or humoral (antigen–anitbody) mechanisms (iv) its propensity to produce disability and deformity, which in some cases may be severe and widespread, affecting eyes, face, or limbs; and (v) the social and psychological consequences of leprosy for the patient, the family, and the community, sometimes leading to outright stigmatisation and rejection.

Leprosy is generally believed to have originated in Asia. From India, it probably spread to China in about 500 BC and then to Japan. It may have been carried from India in the fourth century BC by returning soldiers and camp followers of the Greek wars of conquest in Asia. In Europe, leprosy was active between the tenth and fifteenth centuries and then, for reasons largely unknown, steadily declined. Fear, stigma, and awareness of the disease also declined, but reappeared a few centuries later when the imperialist and colonialist activities of the countries in Western Europe revealed large numbers of cases in Africa, Asia, and Polynesia. *Chaulmoogra* (hydnocarpus) oil was introduced as treatment in the nineteenth century, but its beneficial effects were short-lived and it was not until the 1940s that effective CHEMOTHERAPY became available. Dr G. H. Faget of the National Leprosarium at Carville, Louisiana, US, showed that a sulphone, '*Promin*' (glucosulphone sodium) was effective intravenously in the treatment of leprosy, and this led to the use of *dapsone* (diamino di-phenyl sulphone), given as tablets by mouth, on a wide scale.

The number of registered cases in the world has decreased from 5.4 million in 1985 to 700 000 recently. They are mainly in South and Cental America, Africa and the Far East. These remarkable changes have come about largely as a result of the widespread implementation of regimens of multiple drug therapy for all cases of leprosy as recommended by (WHO) in 1982. The enormous success of these regimens led to the establishment by WHO in 1994 of an *Action Programme for the Elimination of Leprosy*, aimed at reducing the prevalence of leprosy worldwide to less then one case per 10 000 of the population, and thus eliminating the disease as a public health problem.

A glance at the world map of prevalence suggests that the current distribution is somewhat tropical, but in the past leprosy has been quite widespread in Europe, Scandinavia, China, Korea, and Japan. The likelihood is that its development and spread are favoured by poverty and a range of poor socio-economic conditions, including over-crowding, malnutrition, illiteracy, lack of clean water, and inadequate (or non-existent) basic health services, including IMMUNIZATION.

For reasons which are not understood and which are in stark contrast to the situation with tuberculosis, the current HIV/AIDS pandemic has not, as yet, had an adverse effect on diagnosis, clinical management, treatment, or the control of leprosy. Coincident cases (HIV infection and leprosy in the same patient) have been reported from various countries, but there is no general evidence that HIV infection alters the clinical course of the disease or response to treatment.

Despite much research through the years, it is still impossible to grow the causative organism, *Mycobacterium leprae*, in laboratory culture in an artificial medium. A breakthrough was however achieved by Charles Shepard of the US Public Health Service in 1960, when he demonstrated that the bacillus could be grown in the foot-pads of laboratory mice, thus providing for the first time a model to establish the biological identity of the bacillus, assess the value of new drugs, and study drug resistance. In 1971, Eleanor Storrs and Waldemar Kirchheimer in the US reported that the 9-banded armadillo, *Dasypus novemcinctus Linn.*, was susceptible to inoculation with bacilli of human origin, and the model was rapidly developed in the US and elsewhere to provide enormous numbers of bacilli for vaccine research and other projects. Although these endeavours have not entirely escaped the attention of animal rights activists, the general public has remained sympathetic to the importance of research and the use of animal models in order to pursue studies aimed at the prevention and treatment of leprosy in human beings.

Somewhat disappointingly, no specific vaccine against leprosy has yet been developed. It has, however, been shown that armadillo-derived, killed leprosy bacilli, in combination with BCG (Bacille Calmette-Guérin, the standard antituberculosis vaccine) offers a high degree of protection, as shown in field trials in India, though not confirmed in trials in Venezuela and Malawi. Despite impressive progress, much remains to be done in the 'final' push towards elimination. The WHO has recently summarized the situation as follows:

'Leprosy elimination stands at a critical and extremely difficult juncture. This is partly because the commitment to eliminate leprosy in many endemic countries is beginning to slacken (among decision-makers and in the field). Moreover, those areas that are easy to reach and to work in, have been effectively covered. The residual problem is far more difficult — from all perspectives — and is further complicated by structural inadequacies in local health services. Even today, people in many areas do not have ready access to diagnosis and MDT (including those with long-standing disease). Therefore, achievements will no longer be sustainable if significant numbers of hidden cases remain undetected and accessibility to treatment services remains difficult'

A. COLIN MCDOUGALL

Further reading

Action Programme for the Elimination of Leprosy. *Status Report, 1996.* WHO/LEP/96.5 World Health Organisation, Geneva, Switzerland.

Hastings, R. C. (ed.) (1985). *Leprosy,* 'Medicine in the Tropics Series'. Churchill Livingstone, Edinburgh, London, Melbourne, and New York.

Jopling, W. H. and McDougall, A. C. (1996). *Handbook of Leprosy,* (5th edn) CBS Publishers and Distributors, 4596/1-A, 11-Daryaganj, New Delhi, 110002, India.

Lesion A structural abnormality of any type in some part of the body. A lesion may be congenital (present from birth) or subsequently acquired. Within the acquired category a lesion may be traumatic (wound, burn, fracture), inflammatory (infective or toxic) degenerative (e.g. osteoarthritis, arteriosclerosis), or neoplastic (benign or malignant growth). S.J.

Leukaemia Leukaemia is a general neoplastic condition of the tissues that form white blood cells (*leucocytes*), such that abnormal white cells accumulate in vast numbers. They accumulate first in the organs of origin (for example, *granulocytes* in bone marrow and *lymphocytes* in lymph nodes); circulate in excessive number in the BLOOD and collect in the rest of the body, resulting in organ dysfunction. The various types of leukaemia may take an acute or chronic form. The causes of leukaemia are unknown and clusters of cases sometimes occur in children. Claims have been made that these clusters are caused by exposure to RADIATION, but infection by an unknown VIRUS is a more likely cause. Many leukaemias can now be successfully treated by chemotherapeutic agents. A.W.C.

Libido Libido, like so many words associated with the sexual sphere, has a variety of meanings both popular and technical. On the most simple colloquial level it may be used as a synonym for the sexual drive, and various remedies are advertised as the surest way to revive a flagging libido, even perhaps incorporating 'libido' in the name (e.g. Dr X's Libido Energiser). The word is of much later derivation than the term 'libidinous' — from the Latin for lust, meaning characterised by excessive sexual desire. Libido was first brought into usage by Freud as a term which would express for the sexual instinct what 'hunger' did for the instinct of nutrition, and which did not have the duality of meaning (both desire and its satisfaction) that pertains to 'lust' in German.

Freud made the startling statement about this quality that, though generally assumed to be absent in childhood, to become manifest at PUBERTY, and to develop fully in maturity under the influence of irresistible sexual attraction between the opposite sexes, it was in fact present from birth and far less simple in its progression towards the end decreed by social convention. The infant's libido, he argued, was first directed to itself and the pleasures it could obtain from its own body. Thus the libido was initially directed towards the mouth and the oral pleasures of sucking, then to the anal region, and only subsequently to the genital organs. However, eventually the libido would become invested in (cathected towards) external objects. The first external object to which the libido became attached was the mother; it would attach to the father much later.

The popular assumption was that, following puberty, the libido would 'naturally' be turned as it awoke towards an eligible member of the opposite sex. However, if the libido had been in existence since birth, and had already become attached to various organs or objects, it might, Freud claimed, for various reasons, have become fixated at one particular level, which would create problems in turning in the direction of a more appropriate object. This could have disastrous effects for later sexual life. The individual would have no conscious awareness of the nature of the fixation, but the libido would constantly turn away from the possibility of satisfaction in reality, towards a fantasy gratification.

Freud has been criticised for his identification of the infantile (pre-pubertal) libido as male, so that the female child's sexuality, focussed on the clitoris, was defined by him as an immature masculine stage. As she developed, the female was supposed to make the transfer from clitoral to mature womanly vaginal satisfaction. However, given the importance which Freud attached to the pre-genital elements in the development of the libido, and his suggestion that only at puberty did a male–female polarity occur, it is possible to read the libido as a much less gendered force which, even in the male child, may not have an assertive and phallic quality.

Freud (*Libidinal Types*, 1931) suggested that the direction of the adult libidinal urge fell into three broad categories, according to whether the instinctual id, the super-ego, or the ego predominated in the individual's make-up. The '*erotic*' type, swayed by the 'elementary instinctual demands of the id', was mainly interested in love, and being loved was more important than loving. The '*obsessional*' type, ruled by the super-ego, was ruled by fear of the naggings of conscience. And the '*narcissistic*' type did not have the tension between the requirements of the ego and the demands of the super-ego manifested by the obsessional type, was mainly interested in self-preservation, and in erotic life was more concerned with loving than being loved. However, these types were seldom found unmixed, and usually two were found in combination. Freud suggested that, while theoretically possible, it was

almost a jest to posit the threefold mixture, erotic–obsessional–narcissistic, but a serious one since this was an absolute norm, an ideal harmony. However, although there were these three ways of deploying the libido, one or two were almost certain to predominate in any particular individual at the expense of the alternative possibilities.

In his later writings, and in particular following his identification of a 'death instinct', Freud positioned the libido as the characteristic energy of the life instincts. However, he never went as far as Carl Jung, for whom the libido was the manifestation of general psychic energy, which might be expressed through sexual channels but was not in itself sexual. Jung saw the libido as flowing between the opposite poles of the conscious and the unconscious, the outer and inner life, in a continuous cycle of progression and regression.

Other psychoanalysts and psychoanalytic schools also advanced differing views on the nature of the libido. The 'Neo-Freudians' (Adler, Rank, Horney, Sullivan, and Fromm, to name the best-known theoreticians of this school) rejected the theory of instinctual drive embodied in classical Freudian libido theory, and emphasized the significance of interpersonal relationships in structuring the psyche, replacing the primitive drives of the libido with the idea of a healthy striving towards 'self-realisation'. Ronald Fairbairn (1889–1965), who had a significant influence on the British 'object relations' school, saw the object as the aim of the libido: it was a movement from the ego towards an object rather than an inherent quality, but did, however, most easily pass via the erotogenic zones. For Fairbairn, the libido, being concerned with the formation of a satisfactory emotional contact with an external object, was generated by the ego, whereas for Freud it was an impersonal force gushing out of the well of primitive passions, the id. At the other extreme, Wilhelm Reich reified the libido as an actual physical force grounded in the body, 'orgone energy', rather than a powerful metaphor for shifting and mutable sexual interest.

Freud's conception of the libido as a mutable, slippery, constantly transforming force is, it is apparent, reflected in the changing meanings which have been assigned to this concept.

LESLEY A. HALL

See also EROTICISM; SEXUALITY.

Life-support Given that the HEART is beating, and that metabolic processes in the body organs and tissues are intact, continuation of life depends on there also being effective exchanges with the external world: BREATHING, food and water intake, and output of waste. Damage may necessitate artificial take-over of one or more of these functions. Such take-over has become possible by virtue of medical technology.

'Life-support' describes any continuing medical treatment necessary for survival, as distinct from the short-term interventions involved in

RESUSCITATION, which are life-*saving* rather than life-*sustaining*. Very often, however, such life-sustaining measures become necessary after the initial success of a life-saving intervention.

The commonest forms of life-support are mechanical ARTIFICIAL VENTILATION and ARTIFICIAL FEEDING through a stomach tube. Such support may be required only for a period of weeks or months until recovery of the lost function occurs, but continued survival for some patients depends on permanent life-support. In that event the patient usually remains in hospital, but sometimes arrangements can be made to manage permanent life-support systems at home. Long-term DIALYSIS for kidney failure is another form of life-support.

Sometimes a decision is made to discontinue life-support and let the patient die. This is most often in the first few days after resuscitation, when it becomes clear that there is no prospect of survival and that treatment is futile because it is merely prolonging the process of dying. Occasionally life-support is withdrawn after months or years, as when a patient on dialysis who develops new complications requests its withdrawal, or when a brain-damaged patient is diagnosed as in a permanent vegetative state and it is decided to stop tube feeding.

BRYAN JENNETT

See also ARTIFICIAL FEEDING; ARTIFICIAL VENTILATION; DIALYSIS; RESUSCITATION; VEGETATIVE STATE.

Lifespan

Of all the land mammals, humans have the longest lifespan. The documented record holder for being the longest-lived person was Madame Jeanne Calment, a French woman who died in 1997 at the age of 122. Of the other mammals, the Bowheaded whale and the Asiatic elephant come close, but the really long-lived species tend to be cold-blooded or plants, for example the Pacific clam and Galapagos tortoise live to more than 200 years, while the Bristlecone pine is reputed to grow for up to 5,000 years and is the world's oldest organism.

All living creatures eventually die (with the possible exception of some single-celled organisms) and several factors are related to the lifespan of each animal species; longer-lived animals tend to be larger, have a bigger brain in relation to body size, and have a slower metabolic rate (this gives cold-blooded animals the advantage). Though humans are not large compared with elephants and whales our larger brain seems to offer the advantage, possibly by allowing us to adapt to change, and use reason to avoid danger and find food, so helping prehistoric humans to live longer. A large brain also means it takes longer for infants to develop, adulthood is delayed, and parents must be present to teach their offspring — so longer-lived parents were necessary for the next generation to survive. These changes have occurred over the last 1.5 million years, during which time both maximum lifespan and the numbers of neurons in the brain have almost doubled.

From earliest recorded history the ancient Egyptians suggested maximum lifespan was 110 years, and Roman funeral records describe people of over 100 years old. Although these early records may have been exaggerated it is likely that many people did at least reach their 70s and 80s in Biblical times, as noted in the Psalms:

> 'The days of our years are threescores years and ten; and if by reason of strength they be fourscore years, yet is their strength labour and sorrow; for it is soon cut off, and we fly away'

(Psalm 90:10, King James Version).

But for most people in history old age was not a possibility. On average the ancient Greek population (around 1100BC) lived 35 years, and on the whole this remained the average lifespan in Europe up to the nineteenth century. Even as recently as 1901 the average life expectancy in England was only 47 years. The fast rise in life expectancy, to the present 76 years, is due almost entirely to reduction of infant and childhood deaths in the early to mid twentieth century. As Fred Astaire remarked, 'Old age is like everything else. To make a success of it you've got to start young', and this is as true of health, as any other part of life. Improvement has come about through better nutrition, HYGIENE, and housing, and medical advances in immunization and ANTIBIOTICS removing the past childhood killers, tuberculosis, pneumonia, diarrhoea, and a host of INFECTIOUS DISEASES (e.g. typhoid, scarlet fever, diphtheria, measles).

Present medical research is concentrating on improving health in later life by treating what are now the major fatal diseases—STROKE, heart disease, and CANCER—and the increasing risk of DEMENTIA. Because of this, the average lifespan is predicted to rise to 83 years by 2030. Some small groups of people already have a longer than average lifespan, for example the 7th Day Adventists in the US, and Japanese priests, who have a low disease rate through healthy living (no smoking, alcohol, or meat) and active lifestyle.

In spite of the obvious increases in average life expectancy, there is very little evidence to suggest that humans can increase their maximum lifespan much beyond 120 years. To do that would mean halting or slowing the complex AGEING process, which involves continuous random damage to all cells and their DNA from the by-products of metabolising oxygen and glucose — paradoxically essential for life. Lifespan is also influenced by genetics — for example, long-lived parents produce long-lived children, and women live approximately 6 years longer than men, mostly due to cardiovascular protection by female SEX HORMONES. These factors must be accounted for before the limits on lifespan can be understood and breached.

Fashions in wonder drugs, DIETS, and EXERCISE to promote immortality come and go, although so far only 'dietary restriction' has proved effective in mammals. This involves reducing calorie intake by half while maintaining all the other nutrients at normal levels. Using this strategy rats and mice can live up to 40% longer and have fewer diseases associated with old age. It remains to be seen if this could also apply to humans, but for now a more realistic aim is to improve health at all ages, and not to strive for immortality. As George Bernard Shaw, who lived to age 94, wrote. 'Do not try to live forever. You will not succeed.'

JANE E. PRESTON

Further reading

Smith, D. W. E. (1993). *Human longevity*. Oxford University Press.

See also AGEING.

Ligament

From the Latin for a bond or tie. A sheet or band of tough, inelastic, fibrous CONNECTIVE TISSUE. Around JOINTS, ligaments form a cuff or 'capsule', along with additional strengthening bands outside it (e.g. spanning the sides of the KNEE), or they link the ends of the bones inside a joint (e.g. the *cruciate ligaments*, joining the tibia and femur in the knee joint). The edges or ends of such ligaments are fused with the relevant bones. (Not to be confused with TENDONS, which extend SKELETAL MUSCLES to their attachments.) Supports in other sites include the *broad ligament* for the UTERUS and FALLOPIAN TUBES, which attaches them to the pelvic wall, and the *suspensory ligaments* for a variety of organs (e.g. eyeball, breast, penis).

S.J.

See also CONNECTIVE TISSUE; JOINTS.

Limbic system

The term 'limbic system' (from Latin *limbus*: edge) was first used by MacLean in 1952 to describe a set of structurally and functionally related structures of the brain bordering the midline, inner surface of each cerebral hemisphere. These structures were considered to be evolutionarily ancient. MacLean called them the '*visceral brain*' and suggested they mediate behaviourally 'primitive' functions inherited from lower mammals, particularly emotion and motivational behaviour. Although such *phylogenetic* arguments (based on comparison between species) are now commonly rejected, the concept of the limbic system survives and has since grown to be highly influential yet controversial.

First, there is no consensus over exactly which structures comprise the limbic system. Most schemes, however, consider it to consist of various parts of the cerebral cortex forming a set of 'rings' on the inner surface of each hemisphere, linked to a central core of structures lying below the CEREBRAL CORTEX. The cortical areas include the cingulate cortex, hippocampus, parahippocampal cortex, and rhinal cortex. The various subcortical areas included in the limbic system extend down through the core of the brain to the upper part of the BRAIN STEM.

Second, there is considerable debate over what the function of the limbic system is. In addition to early ideas relating the limbic system to emotion and motivation, it has also now been implicated in the processing of sensory (especially olfactory) and cognitive information, learning and MEMORY, sexual function (as part of a reward system serving emotional reactions), and motor functions. Most intriguing is the suggestion that the limbic system is concerned with mental integration of all functions related to personal 'experience'.

As the number of brain areas said to belong to the limbic system has grown, its proposed functions have, not surprisingly, proliferated. It has been argued that such a heterogeneous collection of structures and functions can no longer be defined by a single general criterion and that the concept of the limbic system has become incoherent, even meaningless. An alternative view is that a quantitative approach (a 'fuzzy limbic system'), in which different brain regions are described as having a certain degree of 'limbicness', would avoid the problem of having to define precise boundaries.

Despite controversy, the popularity and universal recognition of the term cannot be denied. This may be due partly to the very vagueness of the concept, which has often been used by authors as a convenience to refer to particularly poorly understood areas of the brain.

MARK J. BUCKLEY

Further reading

Kotter, R. and Meyer, N. (1992). The limbic system: a review of its empirical foundation. *Behavioural Brain Research*, 52, 105–27.

See also BRAIN; CEREBRAL CORTEX; EMOTION; MEMORY.

Lip-reading
The common understanding is that lip-reading is trying to understand SPEECH by watching the lip and mouth movements of someone speaking when the normal accompanying speech sounds cannot be heard. This has led to the general assumption that lip-reading is, by and large, a preoccupation of the deaf and hard-of-hearing. But psychological and psychophysical studies, together with modern brain IMAGING TECHNIQUES, have shown that there is more to lip-reading than meets the proverbial eye.

In 1880, the World Congress of Educators in Milan resolved that deaf children everywhere should be taught to lip-read. The decision was predicated on the belief that a speaking face provides sufficient linguistic information to permit speech comprehension, and that practice is all that is necessary to effect skilled performance. In recent years, however, it has become apparent that, for a child who becomes deaf before learning to speak, speech recognition through lip-reading alone is an ability slowly mastered, accompanied often by delays in acquiring an understanding of LANGUAGE and impaired communication skills later in life. And yet infants who can hear normally learn to speak more quickly than blind children, and this is probably because they can also see movements of the faces and lips of other speakers. So how can such apparently contradictory observations be resolved, and how should we properly conceive

of the information conveyed visually? A clue is provided by the detailed analysis of how lip-reading is possible at all.

The ability to extract verbal information from the speaker's face relies on the fact that the configuration of the visible articulators, primarily the lips, teeth, and tongue, shapes the simple resonances of the vocal track to modulate the emitted sound. Visual speech cues permit the discrimination of the place of articulation of certain consonants (e.g. 'p' can be distinguished from 'v'), as well as the identity of different vowels. However, some parts of the acoustic speech signal are generated by movements within the oral cavity that cannot be seen and are consequently indistinguishable visually (e.g. visual perception of 'ga' and of 'ka' are virtually identical). Thus, visible speech cues provide some, but not all, of the linguistic information that acoustic signals offer, necessitating a certain amount of 'guesswork' to fill in the gaps when sound is absent. In fact it turns out that these visual cues provide information about precisely those parts of speech that are most difficult to discriminate by ear alone. Lip-reading, therefore, directly complements auditory speech perception: speech comprehension is very much an audio-visual activity. To conceive of lip-reading as a cognitive ability in isolation from auditory speech perception is to misunderstand the nature of its contribution to human communication. Lip-reading, it seems, is useful to all sighted people, including those with normal hearing.

From early infancy, human beings are predisposed to put together what they see and what they hear. Even at the age of 4 months, infants presented with two video displays of a person articulating different vowels, while listening to a tape recording of one of the vowels, attend selectively to the video of the vowel that can be heard. The early development of this capacity to link sound and sight may relate to the fact that, especially for infants, heard speech is usually accompanied by the sight of the speaker. By the time we reach maturity, the visual information emanating from a speaker's mouth and face during normal conversation plays a significant role in influencing the perception and understanding of spoken language. This is particularly apparent in noisy surroundings, such as a crowded party, where *seeing* a speaker can improve intelligibility to a degree equivalent to increasing the intensity of their voice by about 15 decibels. Nevertheless, we are usually unaware of the influence of visual

cues on heard speech. They become apparent only when they contradict the auditory information. This happens, for example, when watching a poorly dubbed movie: the late or early onset of the speaker's lip movements hampers our ability to hear what is otherwise a clean auditory signal. The potency of the influence of vision on what is heard was graphically demonstrated by psychologists Harry McGurk and John MacDonald in the 1970s. They artificially induced a mismatch between the auditory and visual channels by dubbing the sound of a spoken syllable onto a videotape of someone mouthing a different syllable, and demonstrated that the *seen* syllable reliably influenced what viewers heard (even if they knew exactly what was going on). For example, pairing an auditory 'ba' with a visual 'ga' generally induced the perception of something intermediate, typically 'da'. Instructing subjects to attend solely to the auditory signal made no difference to their report, as long as their eyes were open. This suggests that the visual processing of speech is a significant, and perhaps mandatory, part of the speech process when the speaker is in sight. But how do these visual speech cues help us to hear what is being said?

In 1997 a team of scientists used the novel brain imaging technique, called 'functional magnetic resonance imaging', to try to discover where in the BRAIN the sight of someone speaking might influence the perception of that they are saying. When normal, hearing people looked at a video of someone speaking, with the sound turned off, areas in the occipital lobe of the CEREBRAL CORTEX, long known to be involved in processing visual information, became active. But, surprisingly, so did cortical areas that are normally activated by listening to speech (including the primary auditory region, thought to be involved in rather simple processing of sound). This visual activation of auditory areas even occurred when the video showed someone silently mouthing incomprehensible nonsense, but did *not* happen if the face was simply moving without the lips being opened — suggesting that visual signals are sent to the auditory cortex whenever they look like vocalizations, but that this process happens relatively automatically, without actual recognition of speech. These findings point to a physiological explanation for the subjective experience that you can *almost* hear what's being said when you watch someone speaking in a silent movie. If the effect of visual speech cues broadly equates to turning up the

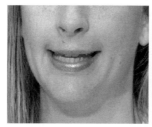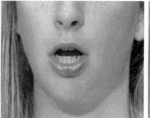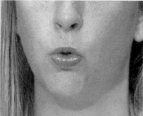

Can you hear the sounds?

volume knob, small wonder that George Bush famously told US voters: 'Read my lips'!

GEMMA CALVERT

Further reading

Dodd, B. and Campbell, R. (1987). *Hearing by eye*. Lawrence Erlbaum Associates, London.

See also CEREBRAL CORTEX; DEAFNESS; HEARING; IMAGING TECHNIQUES; LANGUAGE; SENSORY INTEGRATION.

Liver The concept that certain organs, such as the liver, brain, and heart, enjoyed a higher status than others was first proposed and accepted in the earliest days of medical thought. Indeed, the Babylonians considered the liver to be the seat and mirror of the soul and, as a consequence, this organ became the focus of divination ceremonies, in which the livers of sacrificial animals were carefully inspected by priests for signs of damage prior to being offered as gifts to the gods (see figure). The observed condition of the excised organ was taken to portend the future and, especially, to predict whether or not conditions were favourable for battle. Prayers at these solemn ceremonies were even inscribed on tablets shaped like livers, many of which were subsequently recovered from countries bordering the Mediterranean, far beyond the limits of Babylon.

It was the Greeks who first abandoned superstition in favour of an approach to the understanding of the body based on anatomy and physiology, and it is in the writings of Aristotle where the first attempts to describe animals' livers based on dissection are to be found. However, because of his great influence, Aristotle also helped to perpetuate the notion that human emotions were controlled by four cardinal 'HUMOURS', two of which — yellow bile and black bile — emanated from the liver. These liver-derived humours were held to be responsible for choleric and melancholic moods, respectively. The coming of the Renaissance age and the scientific revolution put paid to the notion that body organs exist under a hierarchical structure, and the fallacy of the four humour theory was exposed. Rather than denigrate the importance of the liver, however, advances in anatomy and physiology over the years have instead highlighted how important the liver is for normal bodily function.

Anatomy

The liver — the largest internal organ of the body — weighs approximately 1200–1500 g or, on average, one fiftieth of the total adult body weight. It is relatively larger in the infant, comprising approximately one twentieth of the birth weight. Situated in the upper abdomen, beneath the right rib cage and separated from the chest cavity by the DIAPHRAGM, the upper border of the liver lies approximately at the level of the nipples. Largely composed of cells known as hepatocytes, which are involved in a multiplicity of synthetic, metabolic, and biotransformatory processes, the liver is unusual in that it is perfused with a dual blood supply. The portal vein carries blood from the SPLEEN and INTESTINES and accounts for approximately 75% of the liver's blood supply, whilst the hepatic artery, which arises indirectly from the aorta, delivers the remaining 25%. Owing to the higher oxygen content of arterial blood, oxygen delivery to the liver is about equally derived from the portal vein and hepatic artery. There is continuous exchange between hepatocytes and the perfusing blood, as various chemicals delivered to the liver from elsewhere in the body by the bloodstream are taken up for degradation and further metabolism, whilst others produced by the liver are, conversely, exported from it. An alternative pathway for dispersal of substances produced in the liver is through secretion into an extensive system of minute canals which eventually form the bile ducts draining into the intestine.

Functions

A multitude of functions of the liver have already been well described, and there are many more of which relatively little is currently known. One of the most important — and easily recognisable when deranged — is the metabolism of the pigment, *bilirubin*, a chemical predominantly derived from products released during the normal destruction of senescent red blood cells. Yellow discolouration of the eyes and the skin (JAUNDICE) ensues when overproduction of bilirubin exceeds the liver's metabolic capability or when hepatic metabolism of bilirubin is impaired.

Another important function of the liver is the synthesis of *bile acids*, which are then transported via the bile ducts into the intestine to aid in the digestion of fatty foods and the absorption of certain fat-soluble VITAMINS, particularly vitamins A, D, E, and K. These vitamins are important for night vision, building strong bones and maintaining normal skin integrity and nerve function, as well as for ensuring normal clotting of the blood. CHOLESTEROL and phospholipids — each of which are important constituents of all cell membranes — and triglycerides — which contain a variety of FATTY ACIDS and act as an important storage form of energy — are also synthesized in the liver.

The liver is the main site for the metabolism of a vast range of chemical substances produced as a result of the digestion of food in the intestine. For example, ammonia, produced by digestive processes and by the action of intestinal bacteria on dietary protein, is absorbed into the bloodstream. Ammonia in high quantities interferes with normal brain function — an eventuality prevented by its conversion in the liver to the non-toxic compound, urea. Many other AMINO

Inscribed model of the sheep's liver, probably used for instructing pupils in divination. Each box explains the implications of any surface markings apparent at the corresponding position on the liver of the sacrificial animal. Probably from Sippar, around 1700 BC. Reproduced with permission from: Reade, J. (1996) *Mesopotamia*. British Museum Press, London.

ACIDS — the building blocks for protein synthesis — which are derived from the diet and from tissue degradation, are also carried by the bloodstream to the liver. Once there they are metabolised to various PROTEINS with a wide range of important functions, including the prevention of fluid accumulation within the tissues and the binding of potentially toxic compounds, such as copper and iron. The liver has a remarkable capacity for such tasks. Under experimental conditions, at least 85% of the liver must be removed or damaged before protein synthesis is substantially impaired.

The liver also plays a key role in CARBOHYDRATE metabolism, resulting in the synthesis of glucose for energy and the generation of body heat. Excess quantities are stored as GLYCOGEN, which can subsequently be mobilised as required. There is also a complex system of ENZYMES which function to convert a myriad of DRUGS and other toxins, including alcohol, to non-toxic metabolites. The activity of these enzyme systems may be modified by various factors. For example, the capacity of the liver to metabolise alcohol is increased by a steady high level of drinking but markedly impaired by alcohol binges.

Another important function of the liver is performed by so-called 'phagocytic' Kupffer cells, which line the vascular networks. These cells play an important role in the prevention of systemic infection and inflammation, by extracting and destroying particulate matter, such as pro-inflammatory bacterial cell walls, as it passes through the liver via the bloodstream.

Advancing age has various effects on the liver. Liver weight and blood supply are each reduced in the healthy elderly subject, but most functions of the liver are well maintained. However, the metabolism of certain drugs may be impaired and this may be at least partly responsible for the increased sensitivity to drugs and possibly also for the high prevalence of adverse drug reactions in this group, especially when multiple drugs are ingested.

Disorders

Any or all of the various liver functions outlined above may be disturbed to varying extents in acute liver disorders, such as acute viral hepatitis. Most such episodes resolve spontaneously without sequelae, owing to the great capacity of liver cells to regenerate. Chronic liver disorders, such as cirrhosis, in which fibrosis and nodule formation occur as the common end result of many disorders causing destruction of hepatocytes, may have more serious consequences. Over the past thirty-five years, liver TRANSPLANTATION has grown from a largely experimental procedure to become a well-established treatment option, not only for that subgroup of patients who have advanced cirrhosis and an otherwise poor prognosis, but also for those patients with the less commonly encountered acute liver failure or liver-based metabolic disorders. Over 650 liver transplantations are performed annually in the UK alone, with over 70% of recipients making a full recovery.

It is clear that, even though ancient cultures were mistaken as to the functions of the liver, they were certainly correct in attaching so much importance to it. Indeed, the maxim that 'life depends on the liver' is as pertinent today as ever before.
STEPHEN M. RIORDAN
ROGER WILLIAMS

See PLATE 1.

See also BILE; GALL BLADDER; JAUNDICE.

Lobotomy, frontal

'Lobotomy' means cutting a lobe of the BRAIN. It is synonymous with *leucotomy* (from the Greek '*leukos*', 'white' and '*tome*','cut') — that is, cutting tracts of nerve fibres (*white matter*) that connect different regions of the BRAIN. Lobotomy of the frontal lobe is an operative procedure used to alleviate symptoms of mental illness. Currently, it is used more commonly in North America than elsewhere.

On 12 November 1935, a Portuguese neurosurgeon, Almeida Lima, performed the first human lobotomy, using alcohol injections to destroy the brain tissue. This procedure had been proposed by his Nobel Prize-winning colleague, Egas Moniz, as a result of hearing a lecture by the American neurologist John Fulton earlier that year. Fulton had described a chimpanzee that became much calmer after surgery destroying the connections between the frontal lobe and areas below the cerebral hemispheres, which are concerned with the EMOTIONS. Lima operated on a total of 20 patients, all of whom survived. Seven were considered to have made a complete recovery and an equal number were described as having markedly improved.

Encouraged by these findings, Walter Freeman and James Watts modified Moniz's technique and introduced 'frontal lobotomy' into the US. This operation, also called *prefrontal leucotomy* or *standard lobotomy*, was performed widely, and soon its beneficial as well as its detrimental effects became apparent.

Like other brain operations, frontal lobotomy was associated with risks of INFECTION, bleeding, and an increased likelihood of developing seizures. In addition, it also became evident that it altered the behaviour and personality of patients, and this gradually limited its use, which further declined in the 1960s because of the development of pharmacological means of treating mental illness. Nevertheless, the use of neurosurgery for treating mental disorders has continued to the present day and is still available in several centres worldwide.

Earlier operations underwent many modifications, as neurosurgeons sought to reduce their damaging and irreversible side-effects. 'Open' procedures gave way to 'closed' ones, in which the neurosurgeons operated through small holes in the skull, and free-hand operations were replaced by stereotactic procedures, which allowed the neurosurgeon to site lesions with great precision. These changes and developments resulted in the neurosurgical procedures that are currently in use today. The four procedures available worldwide aim to interrupt key connections

between specific parts of the frontal lobe and other areas of the brain. Lesion sites vary, and the surgeon's blade is no longer used; instead lesions are created using controlled radiation, or burning or freezing of tissue.

As more operations were performed it gradually became apparent that the patients that benefited most had primarily mood and ANXIETY disorders as opposed to schizophrenia. Hence, the aim of current procedures is to destroy those areas of the brain thought to be important in the regulation of emotion and anxiety.

Psychosurgery, the treatment of mental illness by neurosurgical procedures, has been criticised because it has developed empirically more than on rational grounds, and because of a lack of 'scientific' evidence supporting its purported therapeutic efficacy. However, the operations are offered only to those patients with severe intractable illnesses who have unsuccessfully tried all reasonable alternatives. In order to evaluate the effectiveness of these procedures accurately, a closely-matched, comparative group of patients would need to be studied, and this would be extremely difficult. Furthermore, it is not ethical to deny patients an operation altogether or to withold information concerning treatment options for the purposes of research, and this also limits the feasibility of conducting a 'clinical trial'.

One novel neurosurgical technique, developed in New York, is of particular interest, since it allows surgeons to conduct a double-blind therapeutic trial of psychosurgery, comparing a mock procedure and the genuine operation. This technique is performed without a general anaesthetic and relies on the combined effect of more than 200 precisely-focused beams of cobalt-60 gamma radiation. As there are no significant adverse effects, it is possible for all patients to undergo both a mock procedure and the real operation but be unaware of the order in which these are administered. Hence currently a 5-year, randomly assigned, double-blind study is being carried out to evaluate this particular procedure in the treatment of intractable obsessive—compulsive disorder.

Open, uncontrolled studies, of which there are many, have repeatedly shown that these procedures are effective in alleviating the symptoms of obsessive–compulsive disorder, anxiety states, and major depressive disorder. In most series nearly half the patients have recovered and the majority have experienced some benefit, although there is often a need for continuing medication, and in some cases the operation has to be repeated in order to extend the size of the lesion. The results are impressive, especially when one considers that these patients are treatment-resistant and have not responded to all other available therapeutic measures.

For many people the term 'lobotomy' conjures up images of disturbed beings whose brains have been damaged or mutilated extensively, leaving them at best in a VEGETATIVE STATE without a personality or feelings. This was never true, even in the case of prefrontal leucotomy, and is certainly not the case for the modern stereotatic procedures. Indeed, even in the classical case of Phineas Gage, who in 1847 through an industrial accident suffered severe damage to his prefrontal brain, there was no evidence of impairment of intellect or memory.

The term *psychosurgery* has had years of bad press and is now wrongly associated with only the adverse effects and negative outcomes. It has been suggested that such terms should no longer be used to describe the sophisticated procedures in use today and that, in the new millennium, a simple descriptive term, '*neurosurgery for mental disorders*' (NMD), be adopted, in the hope that the prejudices associated with this treatment can be forgotten. It is only then that NMD will be thoroughly evaluated and its place in the management of mental illness ascribed.

GIN MALHI

Further reading

Malhi, G. S., Bridges, P. K., and Malizia, A. L. (1997). Neurosurgery for mental disorders (NMD). A clinical worldwide perspective: past, present and furture. *International Journal of Psychiatry in Clinical Practice*, **1**, 119–29.

See also PSYCHOLOGICAL DISORDERS; PSYCHOSIS.

Lungs The name 'lungs' is derived from their lightness in weight, since they contain air, and the butcher refers to them as 'lights' for this reason. Adult lungs will float in water, but lungs from a fetus who has not breathed will sink. 'Pulmonary', from the Latin, refers to the lungs and is used in medical terminology, as in *pulmonary function tests* or *pulmonary disease.*

When the lungs are taken out of the chest they partially collapse. This is because they contain elastic fibres in the walls of the airways and *alveoli* (air sacs); open a festive balloon and it will empty itself. In addition, a thin layer of liquid lining the alveoli exerts surface tension, tending to collapse the lungs, although this surface tension is greatly decreased by the presence of SURFACTANT. A soap bubble will collapse when pricked, although it has no elastic material; the surface tension of the film provides force enough.

The function of the lungs is to provide an enormous surface for gas exchange, with OXYGEN entering the body and CARBON DIOXIDE leaving it. The surface has to be protected against physical and environmental assault, in this respect resembling the internal gills of fishes and differing from the external gills of, for example, tadpoles. Thus the lungs are encased in structures — the chest wall and DIAPHRAGM — which will also provide the means of its VENTILATION. Amphibia inflate their lungs by pumping air in from the mouth; mammals, far more active and usually much larger, suck air into the lungs by muscular effort which creates a negative pressure around them.

Our knowledge of the structure and function of the lungs has depended on two major

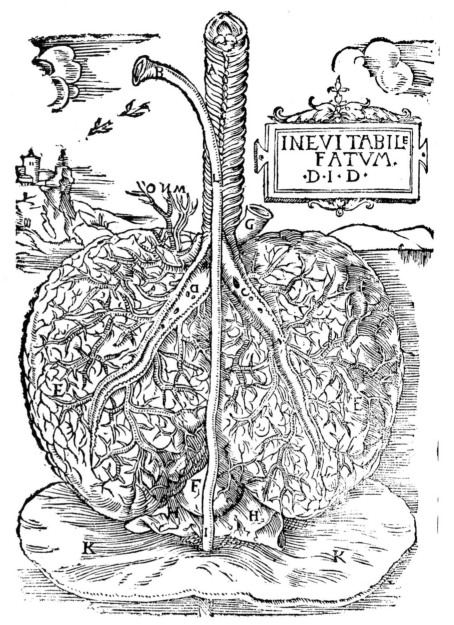

Lungs: woodcut from Mundinus *Anatomica*, Marburg, 1541. Wellcome Institute Library, London.

technological advances over the past three centuries: the light microscope and, later, the electron microscope. For almost two thousand years it was thought that the lungs were generally similar in structure to the liver, spleen, and pancreas, the only important difference being that air could enter the lungs through the trachea to mix physically with blood, cooling it by passing into the blood vessels. The superb anatomical dissections of LEONARDO DA VINCI (1452–539) and VERSALIUS (1514–64) were regarded as consistent with this view. It was the use of the microscope by Malpighi (1628–94) that demonstrated for the first time the air-filled alveoli, the blind ends of the air passages into the lungs. He described them as 'an almost infinite number of orbicular bladders'. Malpighi also showed that

the blood capillaries in the lungs were vessels with walls that separated blood from gas, and allowed the passage of blood through the lungs, as deduced but not demonstrated by William Harvey. However, Malpighi knew nothing of gas exchange and thought the function of *alveolar ventilation* (the flow of air in and out of the alveoli) was to stir and mix the blood in the capillaries. From the 1950s onwards, the electron microscope displayed in detail the structures of the walls of the alveoli and of the tracheobronchial tree, extending to 'ultrastructure' within cells, knowledge of which had advanced meanwhile as light MICROSCOPY improved.

The airways below the LARYNX consist of (i) the *trachea*, a tube that extends almost to the middle of the chest; (ii) the *bronchi* (bronchial tree), formed by the trachea splitting into two and then each branch dividing again; (iii) the *bronchioles* — thin and short distensible airways that again divide many times to form (iv) the *alveolar ducts* from which (v) the *alveoli* arise. This multiple division results in about 23–5 generations of airway, with geometrically increasing numbers and total cross-sectional areas, and decreasing diameters. For example, from one trachea with a diameter of about 180 mm in an adult, by the tenth generation we have 1000 bronchi, each with a diameter of about 1.3 mm; by the twentieth generation we have 1 million bronchioles, each with a diameter of about 0.5 mm; and right at the end there are about 300 million alveoli. The diameter of the alveoli, like that of the bronchi and bronchioles, varies with the degree of lung inflation, in the range 0.1–0.3 mm. The alveolar surface area may be 30–100 m^2 — often described as the size of a tennis court.

In the human embryo the lungs first begin to develop at about 3 weeks after fertilization. The alimentary tract develops earlier, and a 'bud' from its ventral surface progressively extends into the chest to form the airways and lungs. This common embryological source of the lungs and gut is reflected in adult structure and function; thus there are similarities in that both have smooth muscle in their walls, glandular secretion of mucus from their linings, and a nerve supply from the AUTONOMIC NERVOUS SYSTEM, although of course other differences in structure and function are considerable. At about 16 weeks alveoli begin to appear, looking rather like glands with thick walls. Only at about 20–25 weeks does the lung begin to resemble the adult tissue. Even at full-term birth the lungs, although functionally adequate, are not fully developed anatomically, having fewer bronchial branches and a far smaller alveolar surface area than they eventually acquire.

The airways: trachea, bronchi, and bronchioles

These are the conducting airways, and do not take part in gas exchange. Their function is to condition the air we breathe in and to conduct it to the alveoli. If inspired air reached the alveoli directly, if it were cold it would cool the tissue, if hot it would heat it, and if dry it would parch and destroy the alveolar walls. Only if we breathed air at 37°C and 100% humidity — a rare occurrence — would we avoid tissue damage. When we breathe through the mouth, as in exercise or with nasal blockage, we have eliminated the air conditioning role of the NOSE, and the MOUTH is much less efficient for this purpose. If the inspired air is cold and dry it will be raised to body temperature and full humidity by the first few generations of bronchi. This makes the airway lining itself (the *mucosa*) cold and dry, but protects the alveoli. On breathing out the mucosa will take up heat and water vapour from the expired air, restoring it to

normal. Not only are the alveoli protected, but loss of heat and water from the body as a whole is minimized.

The walls of the trachea and bronchi have several layers. On the inner lining surface, the 'luminal' side, there is a layer of EPITHELIUM as a kind of skin. Most of the epithelial cells are ciliated, with microscopic 'hairs' (cilia) that continuously sweep any surface material towards the larynx, where it is coughed up or swallowed. This is the '*ciliary escalator*'. Other cells secrete mucus, the slimy liquid that constitutes PHLEGM and lies on the cilia. Just under the epithelium is a dense blood capillary network that provides nutrition for the epithelium and glands, and may be the site of uptake of inhaled pollutants and drugs. Deeper in the wall are the *submucosal glands*, the main source of the mucus that lines the airways. The glands are stimulated to secrete by many factors, the most important being pollutants, including cigarette smoke, and viral or bacterial infections of the airways. Smoker's COUGH brings up the mucus thus secreted, and in chronic bronchitis there is the overproduction of mucus that characterizes the disease and is due to local pathological changes. The secreted mucus normally has several important defensive effects. It will create a barrier and take up soluble pollutants and smoke particles, slowing down their entry into the body and protecting the epithelium from their harmful effects, and eliminating them via the ciliary escalator. It will stimulate cough as an even more rapid means of their removal. In health the mucus sheet is very thin and difficult to measure; it is probably about 0.02–0.05 mm thick. Even in disease when the output of mucus is greatly increased, it remains too thin to block the airways, unless there is associated inflammation.

Deeper in the airway wall there is CARTILAGE and SMOOTH MUSCLE. The cartilage stabilizes the airways and prevents their collapse during vigorous acts of breathing, such as coughing. The smooth muscle has not been shown to have a physiological role, unlike that in the intestines, which is responsible for the squeezing movement of peristalsis, but possibly it adjusts the diameter of the airways to make them optimally efficient for conducting gas to the alveoli.

The trachea and bronchi contain many sensory nerves, in general of two types. In the smooth muscle are receptors that signal the degree of stretch and therefore of inflation of the airways and lungs, and control the pattern of breathing — its rate and depth, probably to make it as efficient as possible. If the vagus nerves that carry sensory information from the bronchi are cut, in most animals the breathing becomes slow, deep, and mechanically inefficient. Secondly, in the epithelium there is a network of fine nerve fibres, with finger-like projections reaching almost to the airway lumen, that respond to inhaled pollutants and inflammatory mediators and set up a range of reflex responses. The most striking is the cough, but there is also reflex mucus secretion

and smooth muscle contraction. The nerves look like, and act as, tripwires and sensing rods just under the surface, ready to respond to any adverse intruder.

The smallest air-conducting vessels, the bronchioles, are distinguished by having no cartilage in their walls, no mucus cells in their epithelium, and few or no submucosal glands. When the lungs inflate they probably distend equally with the alveoli, but there is little gas exchange in them. If they are inflamed, as in bronchiolitis, the alveoli they supply collapse, with a stiffening of the lungs and a failure of gas exchange.

Because the airways take no part in gas exchange, they are sometimes referred to as the 'anatomical deadspace'. At rest their volume is about 150 ml in a healthy adult. If an average tidal volume of 500 ml is inhaled, at the end of inspiration only 350 ml will have entered the alveoli, and 150 ml will remain in the airways. The ventilation used for gas exchange will be only 350/500ths — or 70% — of the total ventilation. The rest could be called wasted ventilation but, as described earlier, it has an essential function in conditioning the inspired air. When we breathe out, the first 150 ml is unchanged 'fresh' air, followed by 350 ml of air from the alveoli, rich in carbon dioxide and partly depleted of oxygen.

Asthma

In asthma the contraction of bronchial smooth muscle can have a profound effect by narrowing the airways; a greater muscular effort is then required to inflate the lungs. The smooth muscle contracts in response to two main stimuli, chemical and nervous, and either can cause the wheezing associated with asthma. Most types of asthma involve INFLAMMATION, with release of chemical mediators like histamine, bradykinin, and substance P, which diffuse to the smooth muscle and make it contract. In addition, nervous signals can come down from the brain via the vagus nerves, when asthma and wheezing are induced by emotional factors in susceptible subjects.

It used to be thought that asthma was solely due to smooth muscle contraction narrowing the airways. This view was supported by the effectiveness of treatment by smooth muscle relaxants such as salbutamol. But asthma is now considered to be an inflammation of the airways, with multiple effects that all narrow the airways: smooth muscle contraction, thickening of the mucosa by OEDEMA because of leaking blood vessels, and secretion of mucus into the airway lumen. The use of anti-inflammatory drugs has become general.

The alveolar ducts and alveoli

Here gas exchange takes place. There are about 15 million alveolar ducts, and each gives rise to about 20 alveolar air sacs. Each of these alveoli is surrounded by a network of blood capillaries — a bit like a balloon in a close-fitting string bag except that the alveoli are not spherical, and they

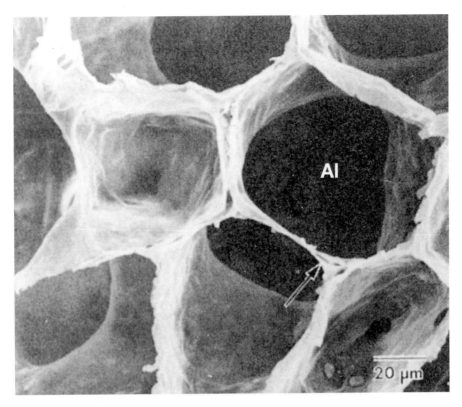

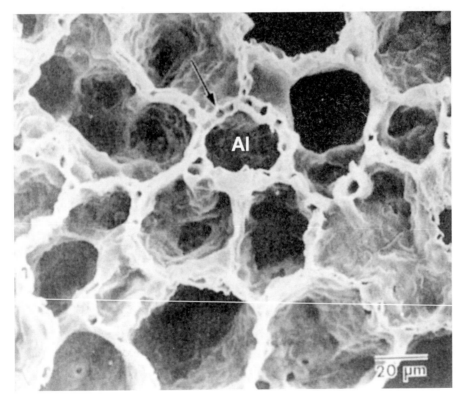

Scanning electron microscope view of lung alveoli, magnified × 750, showing the way in which their shape is retained as their size alters with changes in lung volume. (a) At full capacity (b) At the volume representing the end of a normal expiration. Note that the alveoli are not circular in section but have flat walls, common to adjacent alveoli, with curvatures at the junctions. Compare the capillaries in the stretched alveolar walls in (a) with the rounded capillaries in (b). Adapted from Albertine, K.H., Williams, M.C., and Hyde, D.M. (2000). Fig. 1.22, p. 17. In *Textbook of respiratory medicine*, 3rd edn. (ed. J.F. Murray and J.A. Nadel). W.B. Saunders, Philadelphia.

share the 'string' with the adjacent alveoli all around (see figure for shape in cross-section). The entire output of the right heart goes through the alveolar blood vessels and then into the left heart. The enormous alveolar surface, up to 300 m², promotes gas exchange between blood and air, since the rate of diffusion of a gas depends on the surface area, the thinness of the diffusion barrier, and the solubility of the gas (*Fick's Law*). The alveolar wall is extremely thin, from 0.2–0.5 μm, depending on the degree of inflation of the lungs. The barrier to diffusion has three components. On the surface of the alveoli is a thin layer of secretion, containing surfactant, the detergent phospholipid that lowers the surface tension of the lungs and allows them to be stretched by relatively low pressures. The surfactant layer is about 0.15 μm thick. Then there is the epithelial cell layer of the alveoli. This consists of two types of cells, those which mainly provide a mechanical sheet (*type I*) and those that secrete surfactant (*type II*). Together they constitute the lining 'skin' of the alveoli. The capillary endothelium is the third component of the barrier. Cells of a different type, the alveolar macrophages, are found within the cavities of the alveoli; their function is to ingest and remove solid particles, such as those of smoke.

Carbon dioxide is over twenty times more soluble than oxygen in body liquids, and diffuses twenty times more quickly out of the body than oxygen enters. In any diseases where alveolar gas exchange is decreased, for example when the alveolar wall is thickened by alveolitis, the first changes in blood gas transfer will be with oxygen, and the patient may develop quite severe hypoxia before the blood carbon dioxide begins to increase.

For many years at the beginning of the twentieth century there was intense scientific dispute as to whether the alveoli of the human lungs could secrete oxygen into the bloodstream. The argument was that at high altitudes the oxygen pressure was so low that it could not maintain blood oxygen pressure without active transport through the epithelium. Perhaps the indirect methods to test the problem were not sensitive enough for a clear solution — and it was known that some fishes could actively secrete oxygen into their swim bladders, taking advantage of the properties of their haemoglobin that did not seem to apply to human haemoglobin. The problem was finally solved when more sensitive analysis showed that human lungs, and presumably those of other mammals, could *not* secrete oxygen and that all gas exchanges could be explained by passive DIFFUSION. Even in the absence of oxygen secretion, some climbers can just get to the top of Mount Everest without added oxygen.   JOHN WIDDICOMBE

See PLATE 3.

See also BREATHING; CARBON DIOXIDE; DEVELOPMENT AND GROWTH: BIRTH AND INFANCY; OXYGEN.

Lymphatic system This comprises a body-wide network of branching *lymphatic vessels* (carrying the fluid *lymph*); the *lymph nodes* and other *lymphoid tissue*; the *lymphocytes* (in the circulating BLOOD); the SPLEEN, the BONE marrow, and, in early life, the THYMUS.

That blood circulates is common knowledge. The less dramatic circulation of lymph is less well known, but although its interruption has less immediately hazardous consequences, it is physiologically essential. Also, the lymphoid tissue is a vital component of the body's IMMUNE SYSTEM.

All blood capillaries are to some extent leaky, though the leakiness varies between different organs and tissues. The hydrostatic pressure inside the capillaries is greater than that in the tissues, pushing fluid out. The fluid that leaks out into the interstices among the cells is a little of the watery part of the blood plasma, with all the substances it contains except for the larger proteins. Conversely, some water moves into the capillaries because of the osmotic pull of those proteins. Normally, there is a small net loss from the blood. This fluid movement has the effect of refreshing the tissue fluid in the immediate environment of the cells. Fluid does not accumulate in the tissues, but moves away by entering the blind ends of microscopic lymphatic channels, which are present in all organs and tissues except the CENTRAL NERVOUS SYSTEM. These vessels drain into progressively larger ones, and they have valves which maintain flow towards the chest. *En route*, lymph vessels encounter *lymph nodes* or other *lymphoid tissue* such as the patches which lie behind the lining of the large intestine, and the *tonsils* and *adenoids* at the back of the throat and nose. The lymph passing through these is exposed to PHAGOCYTES which pick up any foreign material, notably bacteria, and take part in the processes of the IMMUNE SYSTEM mediated by the lymphocytes which populate the lymphoid tissue. Thus any invader which gets further than the point of entry, and travels in the lymph, will be 'challenged' at the first lymph node it reaches; for this reason an infection for example in a finger may give rise to an inflamed lymph node at the elbow, or if it gets past there, in the armpit; or a sore throat or mouth ulcer can cause tender swollen lymph nodes in the neck. The lymphoid tissue in the wall of the large intestine performs a similar function for any bacterial or other invasion from the faeces.

The lymph nodes are outposts of the immune system, well placed to challenge bacterial invaders. CANCER cells gain access to lymphatic vessels in tumour tissue, and spread by this route; further spread may be initially forestalled at the lymph nodes. For this reason, surgical removal of a malignant tumour may also involve a clearance of the lymph nodes to which its vessels drain. If lymph vessels draining a part of the body (such as an arm) are blocked or removed, there will inevitably be a collection of excess fluid in the catchment area of those vessels: this is one cause of OEDEMA.

The lymph from the whole body (except the central nervous system) finally drains into vessels at the base of the neck (the major one is the *thoracic duct*) and flow through these into the venous blood stream, on its way to the heart. Thus the fluid lost from the blood capillaries is recycled. Overall, the rate of flow is about 4 litres in 24 hours.

The lymph drained from the small intestine has an additional function: it carries the fats absorbed from the food. Because of this, the lymph in the thoracic duct (known as CHYLE) has a high fat content; it also has a high protein content because although a very small fraction of the plasma proteins escape from blood capillaries in the tissues, the amount collected from the whole body is significant.   SHEILA JENNETT

PLATE 4.

See also BLOOD; IMMUNE SYSTEM; OEDEMA; THYMUS.

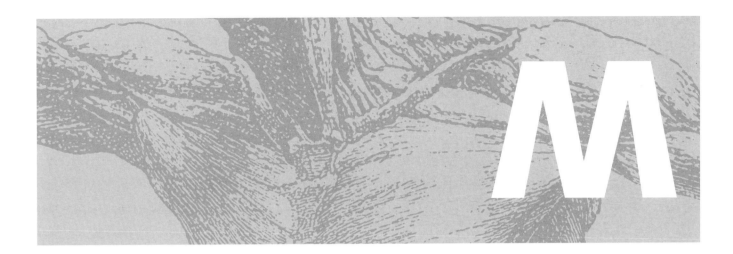

Magic During its long history as a European and Western concept, magic has had two principal meanings. (Its use as a label to describe non-European and non-Western beliefs and practices has been seriously misleading and is now usually avoided.) Firstly, it has signified the pursuit by adepts of a highly elevated and esoteric form of wisdom based on the perceived presence in the world of mystical patterns and intelligences, possessing real efficacy in nature and in human affairs. Secondly, it has been applied as a term of disapproval by theologians and other intellectuals and professionals wishing to condemn various popular practices and techniques because of their perceived *in*efficacy in nature and human affairs. In the first context, important from antiquity down to the high Renaissance, magic was *magia*, the highest form of (natural) philosophy; in the second, important from medieval times through to the nineteenth century, it was tantamount to superstition.

In *magia* the human body, as material substance, was something to be transcended. Even when the Renaissance Neoplatonist Marsilio Ficino talked about the health of the scholar he meant to refer to the state of his *spiritus*. Nevertheless, in this tradition man was thought of as a microcosm and the proportions and harmony of his body were therefore assumed to resemble those of the universe. Hence the well-known depictions of the human frame with the arms and legs outstretched to meet the circumference of a perfect circle. Another Renaissance *magus*, Heinrich Cornelius Agrippa, wrote that every part of the human body corresponded to 'some sign, some star, some intelligence, some divine name.' This tied medicine closely to the practice of astrology, with body parts linked to the various zodiacal signs. By correspondence too the hand or face might indicate the whole person, providing the basis for palmistry and physiognomy. A further derivation from *magia* was natural magic, the study of nature's most hidden and secret processes. Among the 'occult qualities' that, in medieval and early modern medicine, were thought to govern the workings

of the body, were those to do with the spread of contagions, the effects of poisons and their antidotes, the properties of narcotics, the behaviour of allergies, and the relief of ailments by purgatives. Many diseases were thought to have 'occult' causes, and many other aspects of the body's behaviour could be explained in terms of the appetitive aspects of natural action known as 'sympathies' and 'antipathies'. The doctrine of 'signatures' also provided the physician with magical remedies — substances derived from plants and minerals that had their properties and uses stamped on them by heavenly influence. In all these various contexts, however, the magical aspects of the human body and of medical practice were thought of in what were then regarded as naturalistic terms — as part of the workings of nature. Thus, for a practitioner like Paracelsus, magic represented the highest level of medical efficacy.

This was not the case with the 'magic' condemned by disapproving intellectuals and professionals faced with the vast array of traditional 'folk' practices to do with healing, protecting, and preserving the body (many of which Paracelsus himself admired). The practitioners concerned presumably did think that they worked in a straightforward causal way: that they were not magical at all, but were simply techniques. But from the time of St Augustine onwards it was usual for them to be dismissed as having no natural efficacy. As long as such judgements were tied to religion, this type of magic remained irreligious, even demonic; when they were secularized, it became bad science or just foolishness. A great many types of popular diagnosis and treatment fell into this category, as well as traditional notions of how the body worked, how it might be harmed and how that harm might be avoided. Typical instances are diagnosis by measuring a person's belt or girdle; healing by charms or other forms of words or by symbols (especially the misuse of religious words or symbols); healing by wearing amulets; the belief in the 'evil eye' and in illness by bewitchment or by being touched; the attribution of various powers

to body parts or substances (notably blood and semen); many practices to do with determining the sex of a child during conception; the opening of chests or doors to relieve labour pains; and the curing of a wound by treating the weapon that inflicted it. Such practices were popular among all social groups in pre-modern times; it was religious doctrine, then scientific orthodoxy, together with the professional and institutional interests these served, that deemed that they should be disallowed as spurious. In this sense too, the magic of the human body has been culturally constructed, there being nothing in our attitudes to it or ways of dealing with it that is inherently magical.   STUART CLARK

Further reading
Thomas, K. V. (1971). *Religion and the decline of magic*, chapter 7. Weidenfeld and Nicolson, London.

Wilson, S. (2000). *The Magical Universe: Everyday Ritual and Magic in Pre-Modern Europe*, parts II–III. Hambledon and London, London.

Magnetic brain stimulation
refers to a technique for electrical stimulation of part of the brain, through the intact skull, by the principle of electromagnetic induction.

The fact that the brain can be excited by electric current was first demonstrated by David Ferrier in England, and by Fritsch and Hitzig in Germany in the early 1880s. They removed part of the skull of anaesthetised dogs and monkeys, in order to expose the surface of the CEREBRAL CORTEX, and then applied small electrical shocks to what is now termed the motor cortex, which is a strip of cortex running down the side of the cerebral hemisphere. Stimulation produced twitches in muscles on the opposite side of the body — in the legs if the electric shock was given near the midline of the brain, in the forelimbs if the stimulus was more lateral.

Mapping the brain in humans
Neurosurgeons, operating on human patients to remove tumours or areas of abnormal brain tissue giving rise to epileptic seizures, are obviously

anxious to avoid unnecessary injury to particularly important regions of the brain, such as the motor cortex, damage of which causes permanent paralysis. In the 1930s, the Canadian surgeon, Wilder Penfield, exploited the technique of electrical stimulation of the exposed cortex to map the location of the motor cortex. The operation could then be conducted in such a way as to avoid this area if at all possible. Since the brain itself has no direct pain sensation, this kind of mapping was usually carried out under local anaesthesia, so the patient could also report any sensations that were produced. This enabled Penfield to explore many of the sensory areas of the cortex. For instance, he found that stimulation of the strip of cortex directly behind the motor cortex (the *post-central gyrus*) produced curious sensations (*paraesthesiae*) in skin and deep tissues of parts of the body, forming a 'map' of the body lined up with the neighbouring motor map. This was the first proof that the post-central gyrus is the location of the primary somatic sensory cortex in humans. In the same way, Penfield discovered that electrical stimulation of the visual or auditory areas of the cortex gave rise to corresponding sensory HALLUCINATIONS, and stimulation in the lower part of the temporal lobe could elicit whole episodes of experience, involving many different sorts of sensory experience.

The barrier of the skull

Being able to define the motor cortex and other regions before surgery is extremely valuable. But, despite the extensive use of electrical brain stimulation in experiments on anaesthetized animals and during human neurosurgery, it was assumed that the overlying skull had to be removed in order to apply current to the brain. Then electroconvulsive therapy (ECT), developed in the 1930s for treatment of depression, showed that the brain could be stimulated by applying electric current through the skull. However, this technique is hardly amenable for application to people except for therapeutic reasons: the stimulus is not focal, it provokes seizures, and is nowadays always performed under general anaesthesia.

Apart from a very small number of largely unsuccessful attempts to refine the parameters of electrical stimulation and to make it more focal, the concept of transcranial stimulation was virtually forgotten for the next fifty years. The problem is that the high resistance of the scalp and skull prevents all but a fraction of the current applied to electrodes on the scalp from reaching the brain. Most of the current flows along the skin, causing local pain and contraction of scalp muscle. The solution came in two stages. First of all, in 1980, Merton and Morton found that it was possible to use a single high-voltage electrical pulse, applied through small scalp electrodes, to stimulate the motor cortex in conscious subjects. Because the stimulus was very brief, the pain was reduced. This technique rapidly became a standard way of testing the integrity of the nerve pathway from the motor area of the cerebral cortex to the motoneurons in the SPINAL CORD. Damage to the pathway was indicated if the size of the resulting muscle twitch was smaller than usual, or if the delay between stimulation and contraction was unusually long. Nevertheless, because the stimulus also caused a large twitch in the scalp muscle and considerable discomfort, the range of applications was limited.

In 1985, a new development occurred that solved this problem. Barker and colleagues in Sheffield had developed a magnetic stimulator that they had tested successfully by using it to stimulate peripheral nerves through the skin. It relied on the principle of electromagnetic induction, and consisted of an insulated coil of copper wire connected to a large electrical capacitance. The capacitance was charged up to a high voltage and then short-circuited through the coil. A current of several thousand amps flowed for about 1 millisecond and generated a magnetic field at right angles to the coil. Like the current in the coil, this field changed rapidly, being zero before the pulse was given and reaching a strength of 1–2 Teslas (several million times the earth's magnetic field) after 0.5 milliseconds or less. According to Faraday's laws of electromagnetic induction, a changing magnetic field can induce electric current to flow in any conductive structure nearby. The saline environment of the body is no exception to this, so the magnetic field induced an electrical current inside the body, and it was this that stimulated the peripheral nerves. In effect, the magnetic field acted as a 'carrier' of an electrical stimulus from the external coil into the body tissues.

Because magnetic fields can penetrate BONE as readily as any other body tissue, Barker and colleagues thought that their stimulator might be an ideal way of overcoming the problem of scalp pain with transcranial electric stimulation. They therefore brought the first version of their magnetic stimulator to London in 1985 so that Merton could test it out on his own head. On the very first occasion, the magnetic stimulator activated the motor cortex through his scalp and caused a twitch of the hand on the opposite side of his body. Better still, the scalp sensation was minimal, because there was no impedance to the passage of magnetic field into the brain. The electric current induced on the surface of the skin was similar to that induced in the brain, rather than being 10–100 times larger, as with the electrical method.

Applications

The magnetic technique is now the method of choice for all investigations (both clinical and experimental) using transcranial brain stimulation. However, there are two limitations: first, the stimulus spreads out some distance from the coil, so that several square centimetres of tissue may be stimulated at the same time; second, the effectiveness of the stimulus falls off rapidly with distance, so stimulation of deep brain structures is not possible at the present time.

The principal clinical application is to measure conduction in the corticospinal pathway from motor cortex to spinal cord. However, there is now speculation that the technique can be used therapeutically. New stimulators that can deliver repeated stimuli up to 50 times a second are available, and this has given rise to speculation that they could produce persistent changes in the strength of SYNAPSES between nerve fibres and nerve cells in the cortex. Such repetitive stimulation has been shown, in extensive studies on animals, to change the amount of NEUROTRANSMITTER released by the fibre or the number of receptors in the receiving cell's membrane, altering the effectiveness of the synapses — long-term potentiation or depression. The hope is that, by applying repeated stimuli to a cortical region, it may become possible to encourage changes in protein synthesis that affect receptor sensitivity or transmitter release at cortical synapses. Trials are presently being conducted to test the effectiveness of the method in treating patients with depression.

Finally, the ability to stimulate the brain in conscious human subjects is proving to be a remarkable experimental tool that can complement other methods of human brain imaging. For example, PET and fMRI are IMAGING TECHNIQUES that provide information about which areas of brain are active in a particular task, but give no information on whether a particular area is essential for performance of the task, or just associated with it. Similarly PET and fMRI provide poor information about the timing of events in the brain. Regions of activity are mapped out, but the precise sequence of events cannot be demonstrated. Both points can be addressed with magnetic stimulation. A single stimulus to any area of brain disrupts function in that area for a tenth of a second or so. Thus if an area is essential to a particular task, a magnetic stimulus will disrupt performance if applied at the appropriate time.

J.C. ROTHWELL

See also BRAIN; CEREBRAL CORTEX; IMAGING TECHNIQUES; MEMORY.

Make-up, or cosmetics, along with clothing fashions, jewellery, body piercing, TATTOOING, and hair adornment, is one of the many forms of BODY DECORATION regularly practised around the world. Like hairstyles and clothing fashions, make-up is usually a temporary form of adornment, one that can be washed off and changed at will. Make-up usually involves painting or dyeing the skin of the face, hands, feet, or other body part in normative patterns and colours, which vary across cultures and time periods. Western make-up since about the time of the Roman Empire has had two main purposes: to remedy some deficiency of nature, supposed or actual, and to keep up with contemporary fashion.

Current Western body ideals emphasize high cheekbones, bright eyes, smooth skin, and full lips. Women use foundation or concealer to diminish fine lines and hide blemishes, FRECKLES, or other skin markings in order to make facial skin appear young, fresh, and pure. Blusher is often applied in successively darker shades beneath the cheekbone to create the appearance of high cheekbones, while eyeshadow, eyeliner, and mascara outline and deepen the eyes, making them appear brighter and more distinct. Lips are lined and painted to make them appear fuller and darker. All of these techniques help to accentuate what we see as women's sexual cues and increase a woman's sexual desirability — assuming, of course, a moderate application.

Although we often think of make-up as something which serves to extend natural possibilities of the body, FASHION often dictates make-up trends which differ markedly from subtle enhancement. Green, white, or black lipstick, blue mascara, body glitter, and stark applications of strong shades highlight both the artificiality of make-up application and its trendiness. Make-up can thus serve to indicate membership in social subcultures, such as Goth or rave culture, or to advertise a person's identity as fashionable or hip.

Make-up has a long history, both as a fashionable marker and as a highly marketed commodity. Ancient Egyptians had a highly developed art of make-up, especially for the ruling class; different shades of eyeshadow were appropriate to different times of year, and different times of day called for different tones to complement the strong desert light. Make-up was so important, in fact, that mummies were often buried with make-up for the afterlife. While early saints condemned women for cosmetics, European noblewomen frequently painted their faces; Elizabethan court women used pastes of white lead and vinegar to create a very pale face (as well as significant health problems), and vermilion, a mercuric sulfide, to create very red cheeks and lips. Later Englishwomen followed different make-up fashions that often included very pale skin of varying shades, and bright cheeks and lips; this palette of red and white was established in the medieval period over other popular colours such as green.

While the east Asian cultures of Japan and China produced make-up traditions that were similar to those of Europe, other non-Western cultures frequently used make-up in ways that did not mimic natural bodily forms. Middle Eastern women have historically used henna to paint designs on their hands and feet, while also rimming their eyes with kohl to reduce the glare of the equatorial sun. South Pacific islanders painted their faces and bodies with ochre, while ancient Britons of both sexes stained their skin with woad (a blue dye). Hair dyeing in colours of blue, green, orange, or purple was also common in different cultures. One explanation for the dramatic face-painting of many diverse cultures was that the 'devil masks' scared away evil spirits who might otherwise do harm. Another was that certain patterns and colours resonated with cosmological figures who might then bestow beneficence.

Today we associate make-up primarily with women, but historically men also used cosmetics. Besides the face-painting of warriors in a wide range of cultures, Western noblemen, especially kings, practiced an art of make-up that included face-painting and the blackening of eyebrows and moustaches with burnt cork. Even when fashionable, men's make-up has often been judged frivolous and demeaning; privileged young men or dandies of the seventeenth and eighteenth centuries were called 'Macaronis' (hence the lyrics to 'Yankee Doodle Dandy').

Make-up's dramatic transformative properties are best on display in the work of stage and screen make-up artists, who use a variety of make-up supplies and techniques to change a given actor or actress into a particular character, altering age, ethnicity, and sexual identity at one stroke. While this allows convincing portrayals of a wide range of characters, and even monsters of

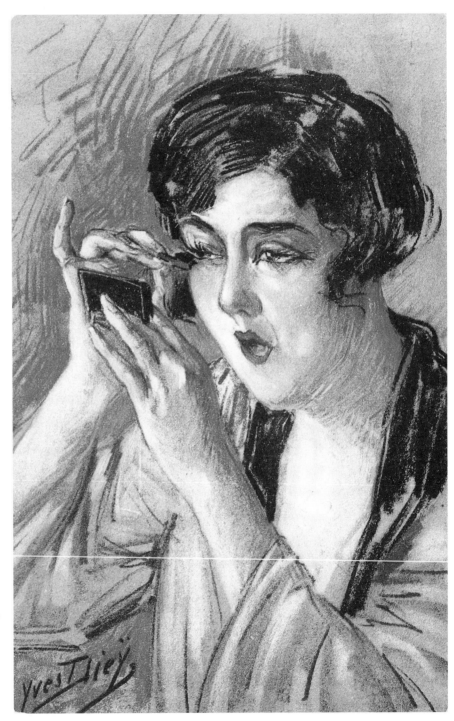

'Le rimels' ('mascara'). Postcard by Yves Diey. Mary Evans Picture Library.

various sorts, it also highlights the ways in which make-up is used as a way to present an identity to the world at large. Stage make-up is necessarily heavy, in order to be seen, and seen as natural, by the audience. Outside of a dramatic context, however, heavy make-up is usually associated with prostitution, and even light make-up was long associated with the courtesan. Jezebel, in the Old Testament of the Bible, was perhaps the first 'painted lady' but royal mistresses in England and France often led make-up trends, and even an Aztec father admonished his daughter, 'Never make up your face nor paint it; never put red on your mouth to look beautiful. Make-up and paint are things that light women use — shameless creatures.' Both make-up and prostitution are associated with a heightened sexuality; while we expect adults and even teens to wear some make-up, make-up on young girls, unless clearly in the context of make-believe and dress-up, is often seen as shocking and irresponsible. It seems natural and obvious today that make-up is used to bolster the natural attributes of a female face to make her more desirable. Make-up's long history, however, suggests that it can be, and often is, used for very different purposes.

JULIE VEDDER

Further reading

Angeloglou, M. (1970). *A history of makeup*. Macmillan, New York.

Wykes-Joyce, M. (1961). *Cosmetics and adornment: ancient and contemporary usage*. Philosophical Library, New York.

See also BODY DECORATION; BODY MUTILATION AND MARKINGS; FACE; FASHION.

Mandrake,

Mandrake, or mandragora, or Satan's apple, is the plant *Atropa mandragora*, a native of Southern Europe. Its mystical and magic properties date back into the mists of time, where APHRODISIAC and FERTILITY qualities were accorded to it. Indeed, a reference to the cure of sterility can be found in Genesis 3: 14. In the time of Pliny (23–79 AD), pieces of root were given to patients to chew before surgery. The root, which is rather toxic, has anodyne and soporific properties. In larger amounts it causes delirium and madness. The name 'Satan's apple' derives from the yellow fruit, which resembles a small apple, and causes poisoning in cattle when eaten — indeed, the Arab name *mandragora* means 'hurtful to cattle'.

It is probable that so-called 'mystical' properties were attributed to mandrake mainly because of the form of the parsnip-like root system, which usually divides to give 'arm and leg' appendages to a human body form, which can take either female or male characteristics. Many have claimed that the plant shrieks when it is pulled from the ground. Pulling it by hand is considered an ill-advised thing to do. Rather, the plant should be tethered to a dog to pull it out of the ground, for anyone hearing the shriek would certainly perish. The root of the plant was commonly used for its medicinal properties, as an emetic and purgative, and for expelling demons. Mandrake was an important component for lunar rituals and was needed to produce moon water. To do this small pieces of root were placed in a chalice of water and exposed to moonlight each night until the moon became full. Chemical investigation has shown that the plant contains alkaloids — all of which can cause the pupils to dilate, of which the predominant one turns out to be madragorine, shown to be identical to ATROPINE, which is found in belladonna plants. As both plants are from the same family the coincidence is not surprising. In 1526, Peter Treveris, in the *Grete Herbal* poured scorn on all the mandrake legends, stating 'all which dreames and old wives tales you shall henceforth caste out your bookes of memories.' In spite of this early, and undoubtedly correct, denouncement, the tales and myths linger still.   ALAN W. CUTHBERT

Manikins and mannequins

Manikins and mannequins A variant of 'mannequin' is 'manikin' and the latter's definition might well describe the present day role of the international fashion model: 'one of the small gaily-coloured birds of the passerine family inhabiting tropical America'. Mannequin, manikin, and model are all terms which suggest a creature designed to be seen rather than heard and the origins of the contemporary 'mannequin' (a word now rarely used) are to be found in the dual worlds of fine art and FASHION.

Artists' models of the human variety have a long history, but the small, jointed figures found among the stocks of artists suppliers also date back several centuries. A number of examples survive from the eighteenth century, including the articulated lay figure used by the sculptor Louis-François Roubiliac, which is in the Museum of London collections. This small, androgynous creature with its box containing both male and female clothing can be transformed into a fashionable miniature artist's model by the addition of wig, hat, and garments. The 1771 inventory of the artist Louis-Michel van Loo's possessions lists '*des mannequins et leurs habits*'. Other artists used life-sized lay figures on which garments of distinguished sitters could be arranged to ensure that no mistake was made when painting the details of state robes, orders etc. In many respects such full-scale models must have resembled the life-size effigies carried on the coffins of the great; examples of these can be seen in the museum attached to Westminster Abbey.

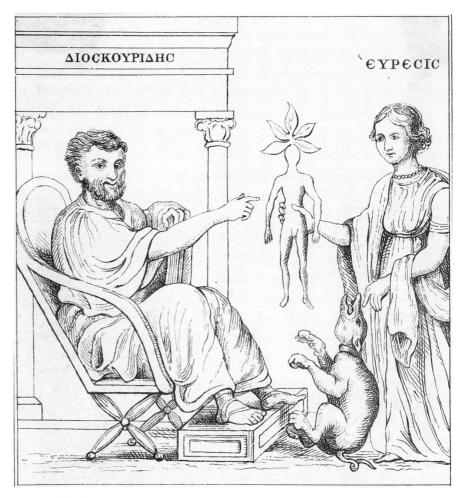

ΔΙΟϹΚΟΥΡΙΔΗϹ   ΄ΕΥΡΕϹΙϹ

Euresis, goddess of Discovery, giving a mandrake root to Dioscorides. The dog who pulled it out of the ground dies in consequence. From a fifth century edition of Dioscorides' *Materia medica*. Mary Evans Picture Library.

Fashion dolls also have a long history, and their origins can be traced back to the fourteenth century. These carefully dressed miniatures wore the latest fashions and, although fragile, were transported throughout Europe and to the New World to display the latest fabrics, styles of dress, accessories, and HAIRDRESSING. They were despatched to milliners and dressmakers prepared to pay, and be paid in return by their customers, for the privilege of displaying the latest fashions from London or Paris. By the end of the eighteenth century, fashion journals had replaced these travelling mannequins (the term used in French, alongside *poupée* (doll) to describe both artists' miniature figures and fashion dolls).

It is not known exactly when and where a dressmaker decided to demonstrate new fashions to customers by displaying them on a young woman whose height and physique would show the design to advantage. As with many other innovations, the credit for the idea is given to the first great couturier, the Englishman Charles Worth. He used his wife to model his latest creations both within his salon and in the fashionable meeting places of second empire Paris. In fact, as Diana de Marly's *History of Haute Couture* (Batsford 1980) makes clear, when Worth worked at Gagelin, the Parisian mercer's, from the late 1840s until 1858, the silk shawls and mantles which they sold alongside rolls of fabric were modelled for potential customers over plain dresses worn by *demoiselles de magasin*, one of whom, Marie Vernet, became Worth's wife. This practice had probably evolved naturally as an element in persuasive salesmanship, particularly in regard to the latest styles. The advantage of house mannequins was that young women of the physique which reflected the current ideal of fashion provided human forms on which new ideas could be tried without argument or discussion.

Paul Poiret, a couturier of considerable influence in the ten years before 1914 was inspired to create clothes which suited his wife Denise, a slender woman quite unlike the statuesque beauties usually associated with that period. His designs were much admired and copied and it is, in part, from him that we can trace the origins of narrower lines worn by graceful, slender mannequins. He was also a powerful self-publicist, taking his clothes, mannequins and even an early film 'on tour' to major European capitals in 1912 and to New York in 1913. His mannequins were also photographed in his latest designs, but they competed with society figures and actresses who more readily personified the current ideals of beauty and physique.

Lucile, an English couturier, claimed the credit for introducing fashion shows in her salon in London; she employed tall, buxom mannequins of nearly six foot to impress her customers. Two of them became so celebrated that they were known by name: Dolores and Hebe. Fashion shows became so popular in Europe and America that by 1913 *The Daily Express* reported that they were 'rivalling in popularity the ordinary theatre play'.

Many of the elements: theatrical display, exquisitely crafted garments, memorable young mannequins (the term '*model*' did not start to replace the word mannequin until the 1920s), publicity through photography and in magazines, have changed little since that period. However, for a long time modelling was a badly paid, often boring occupation. Until the 1950s there were no model agencies to advise and develop the careers of young entrants to this field. Couturiers, department stores, and magazines could provide work, and finishing schools and charm schools taught the rudiments of grooming and movement, but the assessment of a model's abilities and whether she should work in a salon, on the catwalk, in a photographic studio, or could combine all these elements was immeasurably assisted by the introduction of agencies.

A spurious glamour surrounded the work even when it was poorly paid; models wore beautiful clothes, travelled to faraway locations, and married rich men, or so it was thought. Some inspired great designers, such as Lulu de la Falaise at Yves Saint Laurent; others, like Twiggy, signalled the importance of the youth market, with clothing designed to be fun, cheap, and disposable, not exquisite and expensive. By the 1980s and 1990s the most successful models were known by name, highly paid, travelled to the most glamorous cities and resorts in the world and had become, in some instances, even more famous than the designers whose clothes they modelled. The shadow side of this evolution from anonymous mannequin to celebrity model can be found within the powerful fashion industry. For what had begun as a means to show clothes to advantage within a couturier's salon developed into an internationally promoted but often unrealisable ideal of female perfection which has spawned diets and EATING DISORDERS with occasional tragic consequences for impressionable women.　　VALERIE CUMMING

Further reading

Garland, M. (1957). *The changing face of beauty*. Weidenfeld and Nicolson, London.

McDowell, C. (1984). *McDowell's directory of twentieth century fashion*. Frederick Muller, London.

Ribeiro, A. (1984). *Dress in eighteenth century europe, 1715–1789*. Batsford, London.

Ribeiro, A. (1995). *The art of dress, fashion in England and France 1750–1820*. Yale University Press, New Haven.

See also FASHION; MODELLING, FASHION.

Marriage
Since the nineteenth century, complex issues in the study of marriage have involved the productive and reproductive powers of the body. In the late nineteenth and early twentieth centuries, many scholars, such as Lewis Henry Morgan, Sigmund Freud, and James Frazer, viewed evolution in sexuality and family life as a crucial dynamic in the history of human civilization, asserting an evolutionary development from primitive promiscuity and group marriage to modern constraint, monogamy, and patriarchy. In the 1920s and 1930s, the increased practice of fieldwork — the extended practical observation of everyday life in societies — induced specialists in this ethnographic discipline, such as the anthropologist Bronislaw Malinowski and his students, to abandon the 'conjectural histories' of the evolutionists. Rather, they developed a view of sexual constraint and individual marriage — as opposed to promiscuity and group marriage — as common elements in many different types of societies. This new method, described in its earliest form as functionalism but modified considerably over time, has become a mainstay of the modern social sciences; it stresses the crucial significance of marriage for many aspects of group structure in all societies, including patterns of descent, residence, alliance, and classification of kin.

Definitions

These perspectives share a concern to define marriage, whether as a means to trace the evolutionary development of its different types or as a prelude to the identification of its distinctive functions in society. Many attempts have been made to identify the essential nature of marriage and to list its purposes, a project often as revealing of the observer's assumptions as of the observed practices. Across cultures, the ceremonial and social phenomena conventionally defined as marriage assume myriad forms and serve varied purposes, yet marriage is usually defined as the formal ideological recognition of a sexual relationship between one man and one woman (*monogamy*); among one man and two or more women (*polygamy: polygyny*); or among one woman and two or more men (*polygamy: polyandry*). Because sexual intercourse is approved in this relationship, the children of a marriage usually possess a status superior to children born beyond its boundaries.

In an argument against such essentialism, the anthropologist Edmund Leach rejected universal definitions and instead approached marriage as a 'bundle of rights'. Among the classes of rights allocated by institutions 'commonly classed as marriage', Leach noted that in different societies 'marriage' may serve:

(i) to establish the legal father of a woman's children;

(ii) to establish the legal mother of a man's children;

(iii) to give the husband a monopoly in the wife's sexuality;

(iv) to give the wife a monopoly in the husband's sexuality;

(v) to give the husband partial or monopolistic rights to the wife's domestic or other labour services;

(vi) to give the wife partial or monopolistic rights to the husband's labour services;

(vii) to give the husband rights over the property of his wife;

(viii) to give the wife rights over the property of her husband;

(ix) to establish a joint fund of property, a partnership, for the benefit of the children of the marriage; and

(x) to establish a socially significant 'relationship of affinity' between the husband and his wife's brothers.

Leach's essay, and the debate it provoked in the late 1950s, had a seminal influence on approaches to marriage as an ethnographic problem, as a culturally specific set of beliefs, practices, and institutions. Because marriage did not establish *all* of these types of rights in any known society, Leach concluded that the 'institutions commonly described as marriage do not all have the same legal and social concomitants' and that the meaning of marriage in any society could emerge only from detailed investigation of its ethnographic context. At the same time, Leach's essay typified an approach that has focused on how marriage may structure relationships between individuals and among groups, and has stressed the interrelationship of principles of descent, rules of residence, and issues of power over property.

Yet such jural approaches have serious ethnographic limitations, as even the basic conditions of sex between spouses and reproduction of legitimate offspring are not invariably present in relations understood as marriage. A form of woman-to-woman marriage among the Nuer in eastern Africa, observed in the 1930s, created conjugal relationships that furnished heirs for barren women but excluded the sexual partner of the child-bearers from the marital relationship. Nuer also practised a form of 'ghost marriage' between dead men and living women — marriages undertaken by the male relatives, usually younger brothers, of men who died heirless — in order to preserve the names of the deceased in their lineages. In this context, the jural marriage existed between the living and the dead, not between the sexual partners. Furthermore, in several European states and in the US, weddings are performed for lesbian and homosexual partners and also for heterosexual partners who are incapable of sexual intercourse. The meanings and experience of marriage elude persistent efforts to define the custom in terms of legitimate sexuality, the approved reproduction of children, or other sets of formal 'rights and duties'.

Recent trends

Two important recent developments in work on marriage have been the feminist critique of jural approaches and the revival of the broad historical and comparative perspective of the late nineteenth century, without its 'conjectural histories' and flawed evolutionist designs. A feminist perspective on marriage has suggested that the stress on 'rights and duties' too narrowly subsumes women's experiences under juridical issues and obscures the reciprocity between husband and wife and the informal power women wield within marriage. These insights have been useful in the analysis, for instance, of the competition for power among male heads of households and co-wives in polygynous marriage systems.

A second recent development in the study of marriage has revived the project of comparative social science as a complement to the ethnographic discipline of fieldwork. Avoiding what Jack Goody has styled 'the ghastly warning of what can go wrong' in the work of the earlier evolutionists, this approach uses ethnographic data, Goody's 'clusters of interacting variables', to address 'problems of comparison and long-term change' in social institutions. A major focus of comparison has been the correlation of marriage practices, patterns of inheritance, and other aspects of social systems, such as divisions of labour and forms of economic production, in the societies of Africa, Asia, and Europe. This comparative method has resulted in appropriately qualified correlations among (i) monogamy, dowry, status endogamy (like marrying like in class terms), and forms of plough agriculture in many Eurasian societies, producing more stratified social systems; and (ii) polygyny, bridewealth, exogamy, and horticulture in African societies, resulting in more open and interrelated social systems. Furthermore, a distinctive European pattern of marriage and inheritance has been identified, developing after the fourth century CE and marked by 'extensive prohibitions' of close or cousin marriage; abolition of the *levirate and sororate* (customary unions with the wife of a dead brother or the sister of a dead wife) and an increase in widows who did not remarry; the limitation of adoption; and the proscription of concubinage. More controversially, it has been suggested that this pattern resulted from the Christian Church's use of its power over laws of marriage and family to secure property for its temporal purposes.

DAN BEAVER

Further reading

Evans-Pritchard, E. E. (1951). *Kinship and marriage among the Nuer.* Clarendon Press, Oxford.

Goody, J. (1983). *The development of the family and marriage in Europe.* Cambridge University Press, Cambridge.

Rosaldo, M. and Lamphere, L. (ed.) (1974). *Woman, culture, and society.* Stanford University Press, Stanford.

Martial arts The martial, or fighting arts are among humankind's oldest avocations. The urge to fight and compete, whether between individuals or groups, arises with every new generation, and becomes channelled or sublimated in various ways in different cultures. In earliest times tribes fought with each other, invading and defending territories; individuals within tribes fought for leadership, prestige, goods, and mates. As societies became larger and more complex, the importance of warriors and military effectiveness increased. Children mimicked martial heroes (just as in modern times children's games have included cowboys, cops and robbers, spies, space warriors, computer combat, and so forth), and successful warriors often went on to become kings or nobles.

Martial arts also lie at the root of competitive SPORTS, whether sanitized by erecting a barrier between players to eliminate physical contact while hitting a ball as a substitute for pummelling blows (tennis, volleyball, baseball), or intellectualized in a game like chess in which the armies of two kingdoms seek to kill each other until 'checkmate', — an Anglicization of the Arabic *sheikh mat* ('the sheik is dead'). As in war, success in sports requires strategy and tactics. The very same skills that can mean the difference between life and death in combat — speed, agility, strength, determination, reflexes, stamina, timing, vigorous training, and surprise — spell success in sports.

Outside today's military, martial arts are still cultivated for physical and even spiritual improvement. Martial competitions have become sporting events, where one puts one's body and sometimes even one's life on the line, though there have been many attempts to transform sports such as BOXING, wrestling, judo, and karate into safer events where points, rather than lasting bodily damage, determine the winner. The Japanese, for example, differentiate between *jutsu* and *do*, the former designating a fighting art, such as *ju-jutsu*, and the latter its modification into a sport form, such as *ju-do*. In modern Chinese the term for martial arts, '*wushu*', implies demonstrations of movements, often closer to DANCE or GYMNASTICS than fighting.

Many ancient cultures extolled martial arts, whether in epics (the Iliad or Mahâbharâta) or in artifacts (Egyptian tomb paintings or the vast life-sized terracotta army buried with China's first Emperor, Shi Huangdi, in the third century BCE. From India's warrior caste arose such spiritual progenitors as the Buddha and Mahâvira (putative founder of Jainism) and the mythical Arjuna, hero of the *Bhagavad Gitâ*. The warrior's existential proximity to death could engender deep philosophical and religious reflections on the meaning of life. Hence the most prominent patrons of Zen Buddhism, when it was imported to Japan, were the samurai, primarily due to the fearlessness toward life or death displayed by many Zen masters.

The origins of East Asian martial arts are murky. The ancient Chinese produced an extensive literary tradition of martial classics on strategy and tactics, the most famous work being *Sunzi* (Sun Tzu), attributed to a military genius of the sixth to fifth centuries BCE. It applied principles similar to those found in early Daoist works, such as the *Laozi* (Lao Tzu), to military matters like the deployment of troops, adapting to terrain, using spies, how a smaller force can overcome a larger force, and so on. Daoist notions, such as the soft or gentle overcoming the hard, became foundational martial principles.

They underly the judo axiom, 'use the opponent's force to overcome him', or the Taijiquan axiom, 'four ounces overcomes a thousand pounds.'

Chinese martial arts apparently disseminated elsewhere into Asia during the Tang dynasty (649–712) since an early Korean martial art is called Tang Su do (Way of Tang Boxing). Another Korean style, Tae Kwon Do, with some of the most powerful kicks of any martial art, developed later. Tang Su was introduced to Okinawa, where the Chinese characters were pronounced Kara-te (kara = *Tang*; te = *su*: 'hand, fist, boxing'), which meant 'Chinese boxing'. In 1922, in an effort to nationalize the art and strip it of its Chinese origins, the Japanese substituted another character, also pronounced kara, meaning 'empty', so that *Karate* came to mean 'empty fist' rather than 'Tang hand' (or boxing). Many Japanese karate *katas*, or sets of practice movements, still resemble those used in Tang Su do. In Japan the newly nationalized Karate was one of several new sport forms: judo and aikido (grappling and locks) developed from ju-jutsu (holds and throws) in 1882 and 1925 respectively. Kendo, a sport version of ken-jutsu (swordsmanship), began roughly a century earlier, swords often being called the soul of the samurai and the soul of Japan. Sumo wrestling and a host of weapon jutsus (halberd, staff, etc.) have an older history, many going back to the tenth century. In Asian cultures, where martial arts have long been considered national, even religious treasures, demonstrations of martial art prowess by individuals, groups, and children are often integral parts of religious and national festivals. Chinese customs such as lion dances, in which one or more people perform acrobatically while shrouded in a lion costume, were originally martial displays.

In the first half of the twentieth century, Westerners became aware of Asian fighting arts, mostly in their Japanese forms, as popularized by the ju-jutsu in Mr Moto movies (starring Peter Lorre) and the fierce karate techniques of Japanese soldiers during World War II. Breaking boards and bricks with bare hands seemed impressive, almost magical. Sailors brought kick-boxing techniques back to Mediterranean ports, labelling the 'new' sport Savate. It was not until the 1970s, with the international stardom of Bruce Lee, that Westerners gained an appreciation for the Chinese martial arts. Today many Asian styles of martial arts are practiced in the West, including Thai boxing, Chinese Taijiquan, Burmese Bando, and even several rare arts from India, such as Binot. By the end of the twentieth century American Yokozunas (Sumo Grand Masters) — such as the Hawaiians, Akebono and Musashimaru — began to emerge: a shock to Japanese sensibilities since Sumo is intimately associated with the imperial prestige of the Emperor.   DAN LUSTHAUS

See also BOXING; KILLING; SPORT; WAR; WRESTLING.

Martyrdom

From the Greek word meaning 'witness', the term was originally used within Christianity for the Apostles — that is, those who had witnessed Christ's life and RESURRECTION. As Christians came to be persecuted in the pre-Constantinian period, it was used first for those who underwent hardship for the faith, and then only for those who died for the faith.

The suffering body plays an important role in the martyrdom accounts of the early Church. In that act of suffering TORTURE and enduring death, the martyr defeated the enemy (identified with the devil) and imitated the suffering and endurance of Christ on the Cross. The idea of patience ('*patientia*') was important, for, in the practice of patience, a person became the master of their body and could battle their persecutors. Cyprian, Bishop of Carthage, martyred in 258, preached on this in his sermon 'On the Good of Endurance', three years before his own martyrdom. Thus developed the notion of active resistance through the 'patience' of the body, and martyrdom narratives stressed both the physicality of the Christian's suffering, and the dignity of the Christian's bodily gestures. In the account of Polycarp's death, his age and stamina, his composure despite a scraped shin, his upright stance in the flames (with no need of being tied to the stake) are all emphasized by the narrator.

Martyrs were portrayed as overcoming worldly concerns in their endurance, as seen, for example, in female martyrs who were represented as being as strong as men in their endurance, to the extent that they could overcome worldly notions of gender. Blandina, one of the third-century martyrs of Lyons, was both a woman and a slave and yet bore her tortures like a 'noble athlete'. Perpetua, who wrote part of her martyrdom account herself before she died at Carthage in 203, wrote of a vision she had just before her death in which she had to fight an Egyptian: when she stripped for combat she discovered she had become a man; she defeated the Egyptian easily and trampled on the head of a serpent. Both she and Felicitas, who died with her, were mothers: Perpetua weaned her baby while in prison, and Felicitas gave birth almost on the eve of her death. Their martyrdom account speaks frankly of the physical aspects of their being mothers and martyrs, Perpetua commenting on the absence of pain in her breasts when she stopped nursing her child, and a comparison being made between the blood of Felicitas giving birth and the blood of martyrdom.

The bodies of martyrs quickly became sacred, and their relics were sought. As early as the mid second century, Christians were trying to reclaim the martyr's body after death — as in the case of Polycarp (who died in 155 or 156 AD), but in that case they were frustrated by the Nicetes and the Jews and had to be content with the ashes of the cremated Polycarp. A martyr's RELICS were collected and kept at the tomb, and, from the end of the second century, the anniversary of a martyr's death was kept as a feast, often with a liturgical celebration at the tomb. Later, in the post-Constantinian era, churches and cathedrals were often built on the sites of these tombs and the martyr's relics — which were thought to have great holy power — were kept under the altar. This practice continued in the Roman Catholic church up until 1969, for until then relics of martyrs had to be contained in every consecrated altar. Martyrs' days are still kept in the Roman Catholic and Anglican liturgical calendars, when the priests' stoles and chasubles are red to signify the martyrs' blood shed for the faith.

In the Reformation period, *The Bloody Theatre*, or *The Martyrs' Mirror* (a set of documents about Anabaptist martyrs collected in the seventeenth century by the Dutchman, Thieleman Van Braght), and the Protestant John Fox's *Book of Martyrs*, stressed, like early Christian martyrdom accounts, the endurance and heroism of those who were persecuted and died for their faith. Amongst twentieth-century Christian martyrs might be included Dietrich Bonhoeffer, Oscar Romero, and Martin Luther King.

In JUDAISM martyrdom is seen as obligatory — the path to be taken rather than breaking the laws of idolatry, unchastity, or murder. The history of Jewish martyrs goes back to the Hellenistic period (as evidenced in the Books of Maccabees). It has included those such as the scholar Akiva, who died in revolts against the Romans in the second century CE; those who died in periods of persecution and in pogroms in Europe in the medieval and modern periods — such as the Jewish scholar and physician, Ibn Daud, who died in Toledo in the late twelfth century; and continued into the twentieth century with the millions who died in the Holocaust, from 1933 to 1945.

The Arabic term for witness is '*Shahid*', and has come to mean 'martyr'. In Islamic tradition, one who dies in battle against the infidels is promised great rewards in paradise. Being already pure, these martyrs' bodies are not washed before burial and may be buried in their blood-stained battle clothes. Shi 'a Islam places a particular emphasis on martyrdom. The death of the prophet al-Husain in the Karbala tragedy in the seventh century, an event which became a founding event for Shi 'a Islam, made al-Husain the chief of martyrs. Followers who engage ritually in an imitation of his sufferings perform severe self-flagellation and, sometimes, the re-enactment of his life and death.

Sikhs who have been martyred for their faith — '*sahid*' in Hindi — have included, recently, those who died at the hands of the British in the twentieth century, and earlier, those who chose torture rather than accept Islam — some of whom suffered particularly gruesome deaths, including being sawn in half, being boiled to death, being roasted alive in an oil-soaked cloth, death on a wheel, and scalping.

JANE SHAW

Further reading

Shaw, B. D. (1996). Body/power/identity: passions of the martyrs. *Journal of Early Christian Studies*, 4(3), 269–312.

Masks The word 'mask' is related to a *masque* or *masquerade*, which was a courtly performance popular during the Renaissance and the seventeenth century. Characterized by masks worn by the players, the entertainment was derived from their dancing and acting in a dumb show. The wearing of masks was part of a religious and liturgical tradition, linked to the thespians of ancient Greek THEATRE. Later, these masks were adopted and adapted for the Roman amphitheatre. Mapped onto the mask is a human EMOTION, belonging to a cast of theatrical conventions, which is more stylised than realistic. By 1705, Joseph Addison drew attention to the limitations of the mask, by asking: 'Could we suppose that a Mask represented never so naturally the great Humour of a Character, it can never suit with the Variety of Passions that are incident to every single Person in the whole Course of a Play.'

Another important theatrical tradition is that of Japanese mask-making in relation to Noh dramaturgy, the ceremonial art of the Samurai warriors of the early sixteenth century. Noh theatre can be traced back to the Gigaku and Bugaku forms of mask DANCE drama, which originated in Korea in the seventh and eighth centuries and then went to China. These masks are a synthesis of Iranian, Indian, Indonesian, Manchurian, and Indo-Chinese traditions.

The first Japanese mask-makers were influenced by esoteric Buddhist sculpture and drew on imagery of the guardian spirits of Buddhism. Entering into an almost trance-like state, the artistry of the mask-maker lies in getting under the skin of the mask. The Japanese Noh masks express not only eternal beauty and human emotion, but also the inner mind. Through the Noh theatre, it was believed that the gods made themselves manifest through the mask. For this reason, it is forbidden to touch its face. In order to make the eyes, before the mask-maker bores through the finest Japanese cypress wood, out of which the mask is made, he must utter a prayer. According to tradition, it is at the point of being pierced that the mask becomes imbued with life and spirit.

The mask, as a sacred object endowed with magic powers, was a feature of the mask rituals of Mexico. The vestiges of such beliefs have been revived by the mask-maker, El Zarco Guerrero, the creator of the contemporary *Nagual* mask, which is central to the masked dance that takes place during the *Dia de Los Muertos* Festival in Arizona.

By contrast, in eighteenth-century England the mask was associated with degeneracy. Attributed with aphrodisiac properties, it was associated with prostitutes, as illustrated in Hogarth's moral cycle, *The Harlot's Progress*, of 1732. Masquerade was a licence for debauchery in Restoration and Georgian England. According to the anonymous author of *Short Remarks upon the Original and Pernicious Consequences of Masquerades* of 1721, the masquerade was nothing less than a '*Congress to an unclean end*'. Its carnivalesque and liberating anonymity is captured by eighteenth-century novelists such as Defoe, Fielding, and Smollet. Women, in particular, were released from moral constraints by the mask, which also served to protect their blushes.

From the way in which P. B. Shelley uses the trope of the mask in his social protest poem, *The Mask of Anarchy* (1819), to Jim Carrey's social comedy in the feature film, *The Mask* (1994), it is apparent that this is an artefact which continues to fascinate. The reason may not simply be that masks are representations of the universal aspects of ourselves, but also the recognition that what they hide beneath is a revelation of our inner self.   MARIE MULVEY-ROBERTS

See also THEATRE.

Massage broadly construed as therapy by touching, is one of the oldest and most widespread of medical practices. Although massage has been used to treat a number of bodily and mental illnesses, it has always been popular with the healthy to promote feelings of 'well-being'. Massage is a common accompaniment to sexual activity, and attempts at 'professionalization' have suffered from massage's association with male and female PROSTITUTION. Other health care-related professions incorporate massage, including nursing, physical therapy, CHIROPRACTIC, and OSTEOPATHY.

Some forms of therapeutic touching rely on what might be called a transfer of force or power from the operator to the patient. The Gospel reports that Jesus took a dead girl by the hand and revived her. At the same time a woman was healed of a twelve-year haemorrhage by touching Jesus' robe. He then caused two blind men to see by touching their eyes (Matthew 9: 18–31). During the Middle Ages and until the eighteenth century, the skin condition scrofula, or king's evil, was thought to be healed merely by the royal touch. *Mesmerism* in eighteenth-century France and *magnetic therapy* in nineteenth-century America both relied on the special power of the operator to stimulate the subject, often in a sensational public spectacle. From the early seventeenth century medicinal flogging was a popular form of therapy, especially for sexual difficulties and later for various types of mental illnesses.

Massage that would be recognized as such by readers of today had its origins in the Swedish court of Charles XIII, who opened the Central Institute of Gymnastics in Stockholm in 1813. Under the director, Pehr Henrik Ling (1776–1839), a system of 'active massage' or medical GYMNASTICS known now as *Swedish massage* was developed. What distinguishes Swedish massage from other forms is the resistance the patient was expected to exert against the manipulation of the operator. Massage and exercise in Swedish therapy are therefore combined. Romantic interest in classical statuary seems to have stimulated this growing interest in physical culture and in an association of a sound body with morality. Nineteenth-century scientists also began to compile any number of measurements and statistics which allowed them to postulate an 'ideal' body type, making people exceedingly conscious of any deviation from it.

Passive massage, which is perhaps more popular, has an important place in the medical professions, especially in physical therapy and in nursing. By World War I, distinctions were being made between various forms of passive massage, including kneading, stroking, rubbing, and tapping, each with its own purposes and rules. In general, passive medical massage was thought to improve the circulation of blood and lymph, to release waste material from the muscles, and to improve nutrition within the muscle itself. This was especially important for the polio victim, who could not exercise wasted muscles. Medical massage textbooks advised that the male or female operator be very physically fit and above all have a glowing good character, due to the intimate nature of the activity.

Nowadays most people do not think of massage as a medical activity supervised by doctors and nurses in a hospital, although in this context it is one of the techniques important in physiotherapy. Most massage takes place in the private commercial sphere of the marketplace and is seldom covered by health insurance unless part of physical therapy for an injury. Some commercial massage, Swedish or sexual for instance, are offered to patrons because it feels good, whether one is ill or not. More interesting are the sorts of passive massage that purport to treat various complaints outside the realm of traditional medical practice. chiropractic and osteopathy are two medical disciplines involving bodily manipulation that have fought long and hard for respectability within the health care system. Osteopathy had its origins in the efforts of Andrew T. Still (1828–1917), who formulated a medical system in Kansas and Missouri, US, in the 1870s, based on his belief that disease was caused by 'lesions' that impaired the flow of blood and lymph. Osteopathic therapy consists of the removal of this lesion by manipulation, and not by surgery or drugs. It also insists on corrective hygiene, diet, and good mental and physical regimen. Osteopathy is widely recognized in the American Midwest and is also practised in Canada and in Europe.

Chiropractic was developed at the end of the nineteenth century in Davenport, Iowa, US, by a non-traditional healer, Daniel David Palmer, who began his career by using his 'personal magnetism' to cure by touch. Palmer theorized that many diseases could be treated by 'freeing the nerve flow' from blockage by spinal manipulation. Like osteopathy, chiropractic believes that the body possesses the innate power to heal itself, and that the operator helps restore balance and harmony by physical manipulations. Chiropractic has spread worldwide, especially to Japan. Like osteopathy it is a licensed and examined medical speciality.

Other forms of massage derive from an Oriental and Indian system of healing that comes ultimately from China. *Shiatsu*, or finger pressure, is a Japanese system of massage. Its theoretical basis is like that of ACUPUNCTURE or acupressure: disease comes from an obstruction in the flow of 'ki' (chi) along the meridians of the body. The operator is instructed to gather information about the patient by touching, listening, looking, and asking questions. The patient must trust the operator because, unless that happens, important information and illnesses will be hidden and treatment will not be successful. The operator applies finger pressure to the patient for the purpose of freeing the flow of ki to restore health and prevent disease. REFLEXOLOGY is similar to chiropractic in that it relies on the manipulation of one part of the body to restore balance and harmony in remote parts. The purpose of reflexology is to relieve 'congestion' and 'tension' all over the body by selective massage of the foot. Reflexologists claim their art has its origins in ancient India, China, and Egypt.

Commercial massage obviously meets the needs of large numbers of people who enjoy the experience, or who suffer from complaints not recognized by traditional scientific medical practice. The refusal by many massage practitioners to separate mental from physical well-being no doubt appeals to many clients. Such massage therapies seem to be following the development of other medical professions. In many countries they are licensed and board-certified.

FAYE GETZ

Further reading

Bloch, M. (1973). *The Royal Touch*. Routledge, London.

Cook, H. J. (1993). Physical Methods. In *Companion encyclopaedia of the history of medicine*, (ed. W. F. Bynum and R. Porter). Routledge, London and New York.

See also CHIROPRACTIC; OSTEOPATHY; PHYSIOTHERAPY.

Masturbation

There are many expressions for this practice, including auto-eroticism, self-abuse, the solitary pleasure, and onanism (incorrectly; the sin of Onan in Genesis was practising coitus interruptus, not masturbation). According to George Ryley Scott's *Encyclopaedia of Sex* (1939), it is 'as old as the world itself . . . the vice of all races, classes, and ages', and has been observed in animals as well as humans. The Greek Cynic philosopher Diogenes remarked that it was a pity that the pangs of hunger could not be assuaged as easily as the pangs of lust, simply by rubbing the affected part. The early-twentieth-century Viennese satirist, Karl Kraus, remarked that one met a better class of partner in masturbatory fantasy. Nonetheless, it has been abhorred as a vice for centuries and is still somewhat stigmatised. Even in the 1990s, when the AIDs epidemic placed safe sex high on the agenda, advocating this safest of practices led to the dismissal of a US Surgeon-General. No questions on it were included in the British survey sponsored by the Wellcome Trust, published in 1994 as *Sexual Behaviour in Britain. The National Survey of Sexual Attitudes and Lifestyles*. If no longer regarded with horror and loathing, it may be considered the resort of the sad loser unable to find a suitable partner.

This stigmatisation seems particularly odd for what is probably the most universal of all sexual practices, at least among men. The evidence accumulated by surveys since Kinsey suggests that over 90% of men masturbate at some time during their lives, although the figures for women are significantly lower, at around 50–70% according to different surveys, and the frequency of masturbation in women is around half that in men. There is some evidence that the practice has become more common among women but still not as near-universal as it is among men.

Masturbation has not been the subject of legal regulation, though at least one British case is recorded of a man arrested for 'procuring an indecent act with himself': an element of exhibitionism would appear to have been present. The stringent objections advanced about the practice have been both moral and medical. On moral and religious grounds masturbation has been regarded as a sin of lust. As a non-procreative act, in medieval Christian theology it counted as an act against nature, more serious than adultery or rape.

On health grounds, it has been regarded as leading to depletion of the energies contained in the seminal fluid; in ancient Chinese medicine various practices were resorted to in order to conserve vital yang energy by avoiding EJACULATION. In the West, the major medical case against masturbation emerged in the eighteenth century. Following Tissot, authorities declared it to be a habit leading to a gothic plenitude of ailments, physical, mental, and moral, with repercussions not only upon the individual himself but his offspring. This belief in the debilitating effects of masturbation (rather than its being something morally deleterious which it might benefit the soul or character to struggle against) led to the introduction of various stringent means of preventing it (and even of preventing involuntary nocturnal emissions).

Although it is often supposed that infantile masturbation was the focus of these anxieties, it is clear from the literature that it was young men at puberty and in the years immediately following who were the group at which much of the agitation against self-abuse was directed. The perception of the dangers of masturbation and the outcries against its practice have been directed overwhelmingly towards men. Although there have been occasional diatribes against masturbation in women, this never generated the virtual industry of pamphlets and preventive and curative prescriptions dealing with the apparent epidemic of sexual debility caused by 'the secret vice' in males. During the heyday of belief in a clear distinction between immature clitoral and mature vaginal orgasm, masturbation was supposed to interfere with women's capacity to achieve the correct kind during intercourse. However, being neurotic and immature, though deplorable, was hardly as serious a threat as the major mental and physical debilitation men allegedly risked. These proliferating fears around the sexuality of young men from the mid-eighteenth century may bear some relation to the increasingly late age of marriage. Many authorities even believed masturbation to be a far greater danger than intercourse with prostitutes (even though these might well be diseased). There is indeed some evidence of fornication being recommended as a 'cure' for masturbation during the nineteenth century. When, from the early twentieth century, sex educators began to disseminate reassuring messages that masturbation would not cause consumption, tabes dorsalis, or insanity, the practice was still said to be best avoided and not indulged to excess. From being physiologically damaging it became an indicator of some psychological defect, neurosis, immaturity, or an inability to form proper interpersonal relationships. At a half-folkloric, half-joking level, the belief that it causes hair to grow on the palms of the hands is still bandied about.

The false etymology deriving the term 'masturbation' from '*manustupration*' — from the Latin meaning to defile with the hand — alludes to the commonest, but by no means the only, method of self-stimulation. Much of the fear around self-abuse was exacerbated by this awareness that the means was always to hand. However, some men masturbate by rubbing or thrusting against something, or by using vibrators, inanimate objects with holes in, or water jets. PORNOGRAPHY in its various forms may also be regarded as an appurtenance to masturbation. In women, in spite of the long historical tradition of dildos, the preferred method is direct stimulation of the CLITORIS, occasionally with additional vaginal stimulation. Some women are capable of achieving orgasm simply by squeezing their thighs together. Of recent decades masturbation has been recommended to women as a means of familiarising themselves with their own sexual responses in order to overcome difficulties in achieving orgasm. And of course, more recently, it has had advocates as a safe form of sexual activity which does not transfer bodily fluids.

LESLEY A. HALL

Medicine

according to *The Shorter Oxford English Dictionary*, is 'the science and art concerned with the cure, alleviation, and prevention of disease, and with the restoration and preservation of health'. From its ancient origins as a barely-tolerated trade on the margins of early human society, medicine has grown in stature and status to become a vast, professional enterprise that commands increasing proportions of the resources of modern, developed countries. The main driving force behind this process has been the claim by the medical profession to possess unique, privileged knowledge of the human body, of its functioning in HEALTH and DISEASE, and of the ways in which natural healing processes can be imitated, accelerated, or augmented.

In modern Western medicine, the conventional way of acquiring medical knowledge about the body involves the telling and retelling of patients' stories (the history), and the gathering of physical evidence, both immediate (the examination) and hidden (the further investigations). From this information, patients' conditions are given names (the diagnosis) or, if their doctors cannot be specific, several possible names (the differential diagnosis). Armed with a DIAGNOSIS, doctors can inform their patients about what will happen to them (the prognosis), and begin treatment.

History

Even in the age of high technology medicine, nothing improves the efficiency and efficacy of medical intervention more than an accurate and complete history, detailing a patient's medical problems, past and present, their family's medical history, and their social circumstances. Histories, however extended and refined, have been an integral part of Western medicine for 2500 years. The works ascribed to the Greek physician Hippocrates (sc. 460–370 BC) notably include the *Epidemics*, in which the author notes details of patients' circumstances before and during their illness, as well as the presence and nature of any change in their condition, mental or physical. These works may have been little more than an aide-memoire for the author in his practice, or possibly in his teaching, but, as the author of the first book of *Epidemics* describes, 'learning from the common nature of all and the particular nature of the individual, from the disease, the patient, the regimen prescribed and the prescriber' allowed him to make more accurate judgements about the likely outcome of the case. Case histories are written repositories of the collective experience of the medical profession.

The ultimate purpose of the history is to understand the patient, their environment, and their place in society. At various times in history it has been considered important to know where patients live (Hippocratic doctors believed that each locality was prone to particular diseases because of its climate); when they were born (Arabic and medieval Western medicine placed much emphasis on the astrological portents accompanying illness); or what their job is (many occupational diseases have been identified since the English surgeon Percival Pott (1714–88) first described cancer of the scrotum in chimney sweeps).

Besides being good listeners, doctors are also natural storytellers. Recent scholarship by physicians, literary critics, and anthropolgists has drawn attention to the narrative structure of medical knowledge, in particular how patients' endlessly varied and complex 'stories of sickness' are translated into more strictly regimented 'doctors' stories'. Medical students are taught to ask specific questions in order to elicit information for all the categories of the ideal case history: the presenting complaint, the history of that complaint, the patient's past medical history, their past medications and allergies, their family history, and their social circumstances (including their smoking and drinking habits). They are taught to interpret patients' symptoms and organize them into systems — cardiovascular, respiratory, gastrointestinal, nervous, and so on. As critics of medicine have pointed out, the resulting narrative bears little resemblance to that presented by the patient, and there is a danger that the story may lose something — the patient as an individual — in translation if the doctor is not alive to that possibility. The taking of accurate and full histories is vital for the science of medicine; the art of medicine is to construct, within the bounds of accepted form, a vibrant history which retains the concerns and character of the patient while stressing those aspects of the illness which are amenable to medical intervention.

Examination

Clinical examination of patients' bodies creates, not least by the symbolism of laying on of hands, a special relationship between doctors and their patients. Clinical examination, like history-taking, has a long history. The author of the *Epidemics*, for example, paid as much attention to the physical state of his patients' bodies as to the symptoms of which they complained. He regularly noted the presence of fever, jaundice, or enlargement of the spleen, and the character of any sputum, urine, and faeces. Many other Hippocratic texts record physical findings, such as the sweet taste of diabetic urine. Indeed, Hippocratic medicine was based around semiotics — the recognition and interpretation of signs — and it is startling to realise that these skills were for the most part held in abeyance by the medical profession for over 2000 years, until the creation of clinical medicine in the late eighteenth century. Social mores conspired to keep doctors away from the body, though such TABOOS did not apply to substances excreted from it. While the doctor would often be limited in his examination to feeling the patient's PULSE, he usually had free access to the urine, faeces, and other excreted matter. The interpretation of pulses and urines became highly refined skills: Chinese doctors, for example, used a silk thread held between the thumb and forefinger to feel the oscillations of six pulses in the wrist, each one of which was thought to correspond to a specific internal organ; medieval Western doctors carried specially designed urine bottles, and charts showing the colours and character of morbid urines.

At the end of the eighteenth century a new form of medicine was created in European hospitals. Clinical medicine required immediate access to patients' bodies, both in life and after death, in order to elicit signs of disease and to correlate those signs with morbid changes seen *post mortem*. The egalitarian hospitals of Paris, crowded with soldiers returned from the Napoleonic wars, proved an ideal environment in which this new approach to the body could flourish. Old, rarely used skills, such as percussion (first described in the 1730s by the Austrian physician Leopold Auenbrugger (1722–1809), were rediscovered and refined. New skills were introduced, most notably AUSCULTATION of patients' hearts and lungs by means of the stethoscope, an instrument which has become emblematic of modern medicine. The stethoscope signifies both doctors' intimacy with, and their detachment from, their patients' bodies: immediate auscultation — putting one's ear directly to the patient's chest — was often physically unpleasant or socially unacceptable. Mediate auscultation (listening to the chest through a tube), invented by the French physician René-Théophile-Hyacinthe Laënnec (1781–1826) in 1816, spared the sensibilities of both doctors and their patients, as well as improving the acoustics of the technique.

Modern doctors are heir to the spirit as well as the skills of the first clinicians. Medical students learn, and repeatedly practice, the four central skills: inspection, palpation, percussion, and auscultation. The spirit of clinical examination was captured by the English surgeon George Humphry (1821–96) in the aphorism 'eyes first and most, hands next and little, tongue not at all'. Of these perhaps the most important is the first. Few diseases produce pathognomonic signs — the 'spot diagnosis' beloved of senior students and junior doctors — but experienced clinicians can sometimes determine much of what they need to know about their patients' health simply by observing them carefully. Arthur Conan Doyle (1859–1930) modelled his fictional detective Sherlock Holmes, the epitome of skilled observation, on the Edinburgh physician Joseph Bell (1837–1911), a doctor of tremendous clinical acumen who insisted that successful diagnosis was due to the 'precise and intelligent recognition and appreciation of minor differences'.

Investigations

Clinical medicine, created at the end of the eighteenth century, enjoyed a golden age in the flourishing hospitals of the nineteenth century. Yet doctors still had to cope with the unyielding complexity and variability of the human body, and the fundamental uncertainty of medical practice. In their quest for certainty, doctors in Europe and the US turned to science for answers. Science itself was a new, fragile discipline at this time: experimental physiology, pathology, and pharmacology first flourished in Berlin and Paris in the 1820s. As scientists delved ever deeper into the ANATOMY and PHYSIOLOGY of the human body, they devised new methods of investigation, which soon entered medical practice. Chemical tests for the presence of sugar or protein in urine, supplanting previous methods such as close inspection or tasting, entered practice in the 1840s and 1850s, at a time when the chemical study of biological processes was being pioneered by the German chemist Justus Liebig (1803–73). The investigation of blood and other tissues under the microscope became necessary in the context of the cell theory, first propounded in 1838 by the German physiologist Theodor Schwann (1810–82) but vastly extended and modified by the German pathologist Rudolf Virchow (1821–1902). With the advent of the germ theories of disease — created and implemented by the French chemist Louis Pasteur (1822–95) and the German bacteriologist Robert Koch (1843–1910) — finding, fixing, and staining bacteria became part of standard medical practice. By 1914, public institutions and private companies were providing extensive diagnostic laboratory services for doctors throughout Europe and the US.

The discovery of X-RAYS, in 1895, by the German physicist Wilhelm Röntgen (1845–1923), was immediately exploited by the medical profession to examine areas of the human body which were previously inaccessible in life. X-rays proved especially useful in diagnosing fractures and chest diseases. Since World War II several new IMAGING TECHNIQUES have been developed: ultrasound began to be used to diagnose diseases of the brain, heart, and abdomen in the 1950s; computerized axial tomography (the CAT scan, now known simply as computed tomography, or CT), invented by the British electrical engineer Godfrey Hounsfield (1919–), was introduced commercially into practice in 1972; more recently still, magnetic resonance imaging (MRI) and positron emission topography (PET) technology are providing detailed information about the anatomy and physiology of the body.

Imaging technology primarily provides information about the structure of the body. Information about its function comes from other investigations, the earliest and most widely used of which is the ELECTROCARDIOGRAPH (ECG), which records the electrical activity of the heart. The ECG was first described in 1903 by the Dutch physiologist Willem Einthoven (1860–1927). Similar technology was applied to the recording of brain waves when in the 1930s the American physicist Alfred Loomis (1887–1975) and his colleagues showed that ELECTROENCEPHALOGRAPH (EEG) recordings varied during a night's sleep.

Patients entering hospital today, for whatever reason, can expect to have blood taken for simple tests, their ECG recorded, and a chest X-ray taken. Those with suggestive findings in their histories or examinations may then have more complex investigations undertaken. In many cases these investigations will allow a firm diagnosis to be made; in others they may simply confirm a diagnosis already arrived at by clinical reasoning, while giving some indication of the prognosis of the individual patient's illness; in yet others they may provide little or no information to confirm or rule out a diagnosis. Despite the enormous incursion of science into medicine over the last two hundred years, medicine remains an enterprise best characterized by the Hippocratic aphorism, 'Life is short, the art long, opportunity fleeting, experience treacherous, judgement difficult'.

Diagnosis, prognosis, and therapy

And what do doctors do when they have taken their patient's history, examined them, and made all the necessary investigations? In modern medicine the goal of all these activities is the making of a diagnosis and, ideally, the implementation of therapy. Diagnosis is so central to modern medicine that it is difficult to believe that in earlier eras it could be a matter of little or no interest. The goal of Hippocratic medicine, for example, was to establish the patient's prognosis, that is, the likely future course and outcome of their illness given their past course and present state. Prognosis was important for the Hippocratic doctor, partly because he would only take on cases that he thought would recover (his reputation and even his life being in danger if his patient died), and partly because he had little to offer his patients in the way of specific treatment for disease, believing that diseases arose from an imbalance within the body, or between the body and its environment. Very occasionally some surgical manipulation was indicated, usually to replace a dislocated or broken bone, but otherwise Hippocratic therapy required a change of regimen (in modern terms, lifestyle, including food, drink, and exercise, both physical and mental) to restore the lost equilibrium.

In those cases which Hippocratic doctors did take on, the goal of therapy was to cure the patient completely. This remained the sole goal of therapeutics until the late eighteenth and early nineteenth centuries. Specifics — single drugs which cured specific diseases, hence their name — were highly valued and very rare. As doctors, and in many cases their patients, became increasingly sceptical about the value of long-used remedies, new schools of thought both within and outside the medical establishment began to preach that nature alone cured disease, and that doctors could at best hope to treat the patient by promoting and aiding nature's best efforts. Within orthodox medicine this sceptical attitude fostered experimental research into the actions of drugs: in the 1820s, for example, the French physiologist François Magendie (1783–1855) and pharmacist Pierre-Joseph Pelletier (1788–1842) isolated strychnine from *nux vomica*, morphine from opium, and quinine from Peruvian bark; around 1900 the German pharmacologist Paul Ehrlich (1854–1915) investigated hundreds of chemicals in his search for antimicrobial agents, before the 606th (christened 'Salvarsan') proved to be effective against the spirochaete that caused syphilis; and in 1941, the Australian pathologist Howard Florey (1898–1968) and the British biochemist Ernst Chain (1906–79) purified penicillin from the *Penicillium* mould first described in 1928 by the British physician Alexander Fleming (1881–1955). Today, new drugs are evaluated in thousands of patients at dozens of hospitals, the results of trials being subjected to sophisticated statistical analysis on powerful computers. Armed with these results, however, an individual physician must still decide whether they apply to each individual patient; often a policy of watching and waiting, without giving drugs may be the most appropriate. Outside orthodox medicine a natural scepticism reached its acme in the doctrine of homœopathy, invented by the German physician Samuel Hahnemann (1755–1843), according to which diseases are treated with drugs at infinitesimal dilutions.

SURGERY — which prior to the nineteenth century had hardly been regarded as part of medicine at all (in mediaeval times surgeons shared their guild, and their work, with barbers) — flourished as pills and potions fell out of favour. The development of ANAESTHESIA by the American dentists William Morton (1819–68) and Horace Wells (1815–48), and its rapid uptake by surgeons across the world, revolutionized surgical practice, allowing longer and more complex operations to be carried out. This however was of little importance if the majority of those operated upon died of infection soon afterwards; the introduction of antiseptic technique by the Scottish surgeon Joseph Lister (1827–1912), and the subsequent development of aseptic operating theatres, was of equal importance in raising the prestige and effectiveness of surgical treatment of disease. By providing a scientific basis for personal hygiene, these developments also transformed preventive medicine by adding new weapons to its previous armoury of quarantine and sewers.

The contributions of scientific research to medicine in the twentieth century were legion, but scientific progress has often brought with it new ethical, social, and financial dilemmas for medicine. In cardiology, for example, the development of basic and advanced life support techniques, and of new drugs designed to prevent and treat heart disease, have significantly reduced the chances of dying from a HEART ATTACK. But the cost of the equipment needed for advanced life support, and of drugs (such as those that lower CHOLESTEROL in the blood) that improve survival, mean that these therapies are largely confined to well-funded hospitals in wealthy countries. Again, one of the most significant discoveries of all occurred in 1921 when the Canadian physiologists Frederick Banting (1891–1941) and Charles Best (1899–1978) isolated the hormone INSULIN. At last it seemed that there would be a cure for *diabetes mellitus*, a disease recognised since Hippocratic times. But seventy-five years of experience with insulin has taught us that it does not cure the disease. The pancreatic β-cells whose destruction is the defining stage in the disease are not restored by giving insulin. Instead, insulin allows diabetes to be managed, a difficult, time-consuming, often frustrating process that requires doctors and their patients to co-operate over long periods. Nothing could demonstrate the difference between the science and the art of medicine more clearly: scientists push on, trying to understand the pathological processes that take place in the body of a patient with diabetes, elucidating the genetics of both common and rare forms of the disease, and

producing new therapies such as recombinant human insulin; doctors, meanwhile, continue to wrestle, as their ancestors did for thousands of years, with the complexity, variability, and uncertainty of their patients' bodies, and their patients' minds.　　MARK WEATHERALL
D. J. WEATHERALL

See also DIAGNOSIS; DISEASE.

Meditation

Meditation as covered by this entry refers primarily to Buddhist meditation, that is the set of techniques within Buddhism known by the Sanskrit term *bhāvanā* and its cognates. These techniques are varied, and mostly involve both 'mind' and 'body' in Western terms. Thus 'mental' imagery may be used to affect the 'body', and 'bodily' techniques such as breath control may be employed to calm or direct the 'mind'. All these techniques have come to be known in modern English as 'meditation', while equivalent techniques in Hinduism are more frequently referred to as *yoga*. In fact, present-day Hindu and Buddhist practices have many similarities, both going back to a common body of Indian ascetic procedures. The term '*yoga*' is used within some Buddhist traditions, and some modern Hindu teachers use the term 'meditation' (e.g. the Maharishi Mahesh Yogi's 'transcendental meditation'). Related techniques are also found in East Asia (*qigong*, etc.), in Islam (among the Sūfis), and in Judaism and Christianity.

As with other aspects of Buddhism, one can make a general distinction between the Southern (Theravāda) schools (found today in Śrī Lanka and South-East Asia), the Northern schools (Tibet and Mongolia), and the Eastern Schools (China and East Asia). Theravādin Buddhist societies tend to use relatively simple methods, and place emphasis on breathing practices and body mindfulness. Codified by the fourth-to fifth-century author Buddhaghosa in the *Visuddhimagga*, they were mostly not taught to lay people until modern times. Tibetan methods employ the full range of 'Tantric' yogic practices, involving complex imaginal transformations of the self and environment and the use of ritual formulae (*mantra*) and gestures (*mudrā*). Tibetan Tantra also includes procedures involving visualized and actual use of sexual intercourse, but these have never been common in Tibet or Mongolia, since most practitioners are monks and such practices are believed to require a very high degree of mind–body training for successful performance.

Tantric techniques are known in East Asia (e.g. Shingon in Japan), but the most common form of meditation in East Asia, known in Chinese as *Ch'an* (Japanese *Zen*), involves simple sitting for prolonged periods and, in some traditions, contemplation on paradoxical statements (Japanese *kōan*); both are intended to force a breakthrough to non-conceptual insight. While Theravādin meditation traditions were practised primarily in monastic and ascetic contexts until the growth of lay meditation centres in the twentieth century,

Tibetan meditation has a longer tradition of lay involvement, going back to the early days of Buddhism in Tibet. East Asian traditions, which represent a synthesis of Buddhist and indigenous (Daoist, etc.) meditation tradition, have been incorporated to some degree into martial arts and other aspects of secular life, although the 'Zen' nature of Japanese flower-arranging, tea ceremonies, etc., has been exaggerated by Western popularizers.

Two terms widely used in both Theravādin and Tibetan contexts are *śamatha* (Pali *samatha*) and *vipaśyanā* (Pali *vipassanā*). They may be translated roughly as 'calm meditation' and 'insight meditation'. *Śamatha* meditation is directed at the attainment of a series of mind–body states (*dhyāna*, Pali *jhāna*; also *samādhi*) characterized by calmness, reduction of involvement with sensory input, one-pointedness of mind, etc. *Vipaśyanā* is aimed at insight into the true nature of reality, ultimately leading to the duplication of the enlightenment or awakening (*bodhi*) of the historical Buddha. *Śamatha* is regarded as a necessary precursor to *vipaśyanā*, but it may also be practised for its own sake, since it is held to lead to the attainment of *siddhi* (psychic or magical powers).

Dominant forms of Theravāda meditation in the West today emphasize *vipaśyanā* and downplay *śamatha*, but monastic and recluse traditions in South-East Asia employ complex *śamatha* practices which are associated with the ascription of magical powers to highly-attained monk meditators. In the Tibetan context, *śamatha* and *vipaśyanā* are usually regarded as preliminary practices to Tantra. The contrast between the attainment of specific mind–body states and the attainment of insight into reality nevertheless forms part of Tantra too. There is a great elaboration of specific states associated with particular Tantric deities and practices, often intended to bring about specific this-worldly results (health, protection, prosperity).

Skilled meditators can undoubtedly develop a high level of conscious control over bodily processes (e.g. body temperature, breathing process). Indigenous theoretical models treat body–mind processes as aspects of a single whole, and may provide useful pointers to the direction a Western scientific understanding of these processes might take.

GEOFFREY SAMUEL

Further reading

Beyer, S. (1973). *The Cult of Tārā: magic and ritual in Tibet.* University of California Press, Berkeley.
Nyanaponika, T. (1969). *The heart of Buddhist meditation.* Rider, London.

See also BUDDHISM AND THE BODY; RELAXATION; RELIGION AND THE BODY; YOGA; ZEN.

Melanin

Melanin a brown pigment in the SKIN and elsewhere. It is made in *melanocytes*, which are cells in the deepest layer of the epidermis, and these distribute granules of pigment to the other

skin cells. Synthesis is stimulated by sunlight, and also by a hormone from the anterior PITUITARY GLAND. This is the pigment in simple moles and freckles, and in the areolar of the nipples; melanocytes are the cells which become cancerous in a *malignant melanoma*. Other sites are in HAIR, behind the retina of the EYE, and in part of the ADRENAL GLAND.　　S.J.

See PIGMENTATION; SKIN.

Membrane receptors

Membrane receptors are specialized protein molecules in the membranes of cells, to which external molecules (hormones, neurotransmitters, drugs) attach, triggering changes in the function of the CELL. This process is called *transduction*: the external signal is transduced into action. Hundreds of receptors are known and there are undoubtedly many more yet to be discovered. Many drugs exert their therapeutic effects by activating or blocking membrane receptors.

Membrane receptors were postulated to exist long before there was any direct evidence for them. The first evidence came from work by the English physiologist Langley on nerve SYNAPSES, as long ago as 1889. He painted a solution of the drug NICOTINE on to ganglia (nodules on sympathetic nerves, containing synaptic connections between axons from the CENTRAL NERVOUS SYSTEM and nerve cells whose postganglionic fibres run out to innervate organs such as the heart, eye, and gut). Langley noted that the nicotine caused excitation, then inhibition, of the organs innervated by the postganglionic nerves, implying that it had activated and then blocked the nerve–nerve junctions in the ganglion. Similarly, when nicotine was put on to the junction between motor nerve endings and SKELETAL MUSCLE fibres, the muscle fibres twitched, suggesting that it mimicked chemical signals released by motor nerves.

When the VAGUS nerve is stimulated, the heart slows, and Dixon suggested in 1907 that something was set free from the nerve endings to combine with a 'body' in the CARDIAC MUSCLE. The demonstration of chemical transmission had to await the Nobel prize-winning discovery of the German pharmacologist Otto Loewi, reported in 1921. Following an idea for an experiment that he had in a dream, Otto Loewi set up 2 perfused frog hearts such that the perfusate from the first flowed over the second. When the vagus nerve attached to the first heart was stimulated that rate of beating slowed; after a few seconds so did that of the second heart. Some substance (which Loewi called '*Vagusstoff*'), liberated from the first heart, flowed to the second and caused the equivalent of nerve stimulation. Thus the idea was born that there exist receptive sites to receive chemical signals (although this experiment did not prove that the effector substance came from the vagus nerve itself).

Identification of binding sites

Not until the 1950s were attempts made to look for specific binding molecules in cell membranes.

Waser used radioactively-labelled CURARE — which is known to block the receptors for ACETYLCHOLINE, the neurotransmitter released by motor nerves in skeletal muscle — and showed, by *autoradiography* (photographic detection of radioactivity), that the material was bound to the muscle at the NEUROMUSCULAR JUNCTION, exactly where the nerve fibres contacted the muscle.

In another seminal study, the British pharmacologists William Paton and Humphrey Rang used radioactive ATROPINE to bind to smooth muscle membranes, where atropine was known to prevent the action of acetylcholine at parasympathetic nerve endings. They detected specific binding molecules of finite size and were thus able to quantify, for the first time, the number of acetylcholine receptors (known here as the muscarinic type) present in SMOOTH MUSCLE.

The naturally-occurring 'messenger' substances that bind to receptors on cell membranes are not all neurotransmitters released from nerve endings. Some are HORMONES, secreted by endocrine glands, and circulating in the blood, which leave through capillary walls to gain access to tissue fluids around their target cells. Others are released by cells to act on other neighbouring cells, as 'local hormones' or *autacoids*.

In general, each receptor is the product of one gene. By now, many receptor genes have been cloned and much is known about the molecular structure and mechanism of the receptors.

Agonists and antagonists

Any substance that binds to a receptor is known as a *ligand*: those ligands that activate receptors are called *agonists*, while *antagonists* occupy receptors without activating them and thereby prevent the action of agonists. In normal circumstances, the ligands acting on our receptors are 'endogenous', i.e. they are substances produced within the body itself. However, many drugs cause their therapeutic actions on the body by specifically binding to particular receptors. These drugs are generally not themselves identical to the endogenous ligands, rather they are different substances, extracted from plants or other animals, or synthesized, which act as 'exogenous' ligands. There are two reasons for not using endogenous substances as therapeutic drugs. Firstly, many agonist drugs are actually much more effective at activating their receptor than the naturally-occurring endogenous ligand. Secondly, in the case of drugs that work by preventing overactivity of bodily systems, what is needed is an antagonist that binds to the receptor, blocking the action of the endogenous ligand.

You may wonder if all drugs that work by stimulating receptors have equivalent endogenous ligands — in other words, whether the drugs are all reinventions of our own internal chemistry. Consider the pain-relieving drug morphine; it is of plant origin and has a formula unlike anything found in the body. Hans Kosterlitz, working in Aberdeen in the 1970s,

maintained that for each non-endogenous agonist there is indeed a corresponding endogenous ligand. He went on with his co-worker John Hughes to discover the *enkephalins*, the body's natural analgesics, which are the endogenous ligands for the opiate receptors on which morphine acts. The same argument now appears to be true for the *cannabinoids*, found in marijuana, and the *benzodiazepines* (such as Valium), which relieve anxiety. There are still many drugs that are thought to act on naturally-occurring receptors for which there are no known endogenous ligands: such receptors are known as 'orphan' receptors.

The transduction process

There are important generalizations to be made about receptors and how they transduce their effects. The first consideration is *specificity*. The body needs to be able to turn on and off specific processes as they are needed. If you are frightened and fleeing from an attacker you do not need to salivate or digest your last meal, but you do need to mobilize all the mental and physical energy you can. Yet there are only a few ways in which a cell can switch on or off a process. Receptor activation by a 'first messenger' (hormone or neurotransmitter) can in turn activate key ENZYMES in the cell or change the concentration of intracellular ions (particularly CALCIUM ions), which act as 'second messengers' within the cell, triggering specific processes.

The body achieves specificity by having many 'first messengers' and many sorts of receptors and by arranging their disposition. For example there are two types of histamine receptor, H1 and H2. H2 receptors are confined to a few sites, including the stomach, where they are involved in acid production, explaining why the antihistamines that block only the H1 receptor (used to treat allergies) do not prevent gastric acid formation. Different types of cells are programmed by their genes to make only some receptor types and to locate them appropriately. In this way the body is able to respond in a very specific way to different situations.

How do receptors transduce? Clearly, if a receptor is to receive an external chemical signal, part of the protein molecule must be outside the cell. This is the recognition site, which binds specifically with the messenger molecule. When antagonists are bound, the recognition site is blocked and nothing further need happen. Normally antagonists have a high affinity, so that they bind tightly to the receptor for a long period of time. When endogenous or exogenous agonists bind to the receptor then something further must happen in order to transduce the effect. There is, in this situation, a 'conformational change', which means the three-dimensional structure of the receptor protein is altered to activate the next stage. While agonists have a high specificity for the binding sites, their affinity is low, so they are soon released to allow further activation by another agonist molecule. For example, when you walk, many groups of muscle

fibres in the legs, arms, and torso undergo rapid contractions and relaxations: if the chemical messenger at the receptors were to act for long periods this would be impossible. However, when an anaesthetist wants to relax your abdominal muscles for surgery, a long-acting blocker (an antagonist) is used.

The *recognition site* in each receptor is joined to the rest of the protein molecule by the *transmembrane domain* — a chain of AMINO ACIDS that crosses back and forth across the membrane, ending up with an *intracellular terminus*. The number of membrane crossings is variable, between as few as two and as many as twelve.

Types of receptor

There are three main receptor families:

G-protein coupled receptors account for 80% of receptors. Here, the intracellular domain of the receptor is bound to one of many sorts of G-protein (G-proteins are so-called because of their high affinity for guanine nucleotides). The conformational change brought about by the agonist causes release the G-protein, which in turn initiates complex interactions, notably the formation of 'second messengers'.

In *ligand-gated ion channels*, binding of the agonist causes a structural change in the transmembrane domain, creating a 'channel' through which particular ions can flow, into or out of the cell. For instance, *nicotinic receptors* in muscle form channels that allow sodium ions to enter the muscle when activated by the neurotransmitter *acetylcholine*, released by motor nerves (or by nicotine). Similarly, so-called *GABA receptors* on neurons in the brain act as chloride ion channels when stimulated by the inhibitory neurotransmitter *GABA*.

Tyrosine kinase-linked receptors 'dimerise' (forming pairs) when activated by a ligand. In this state they can stimulate *tyrosine kinase enzymes* in the cell, leading to further effects. The hormone insulin acts on cells in this way.

ALAN W. CUTHBERT

See also CELL SIGNALLING; HORMONES; NEUROTRANSMITTERS.

Meme The term 'meme' was coined by Richard Dawkins in his 1976 book *The Selfish Gene*. Memes are habits, skills, songs, stories, or any kind of behaviour that is passed from person to person by imitation. Like genes, memes are replicators. That is, they are information that varies and is selectively copied. While genes compete to get copied when plants and animals reproduce, memes compete to get stored in our memories and passed on to someone else.

On this view our minds and culture are designed by the competition between memes, just as the biological world has been designed by natural selection acting on genes. Familiar memes include words, phrases, and stories; TV and radio programmes; chess, bridge, and computer games; famous symphonies and mindless jingles; the habits of driving on the left (or the right), eating with a knife and fork, wearing clothes, and shaking hands. These are all different kinds of information that have successfully been copied from person to person. Without them we would not be fully human.

The idea of memes is highly controversial. Critics argue that memes have not been proved to exist, cannot be identified with any chemical or physical structure as genes can, cannot be divided into meaningful units, provide no better understanding of culture than existing theories, and undermine the important notions of free will and personal responsibility. Proponents respond that memes obviously exist, since humans imitate widely and memes are simply defined as whatever they imitate. Also, the demand for a physical basis is premature. The structure of DNA was not discovered until a century after Darwin, so we may be in the equivalent of the pre-DNA phase in the new science of memetics. The question of units is tricky for genes too, and we can study memes by using whatever unit is replicated in any given situation — which may be anything from a few notes to an entire symphony, or a few words to a whole story.

More important is whether memetics really can provide new insights into human behaviour or culture. One example is Dawkins's idea of religions as viruses of the mind. A biological virus is a small package of information that uses someone else's copying machinery for its own replication. An equivalent in memes might be a chain letter or e-mail virus. For example, you might receive an e-mail message that says 'A deadly virus called "Happy Birthday" is circulating by e-mail. IBM and Microsoft warn that it is powerful and untreatable. It will destroy all the information in your computer. Pass this warning on to all your friends immediately'. This little piece of information is a complete lie but by using threats (to your computer), promises (you can help your friends), and an instruction to pass it on, it thrives. Religions, argues Dawkins, have a similar structure. They use threats (hell, damnation, and horrible punishments), promises (heaven, salvation, and God's love), and instructions to pass them on (teach your children, read the texts, pray, and sing in public). Moreover, they use other tricks to protect themselves from scepticism. A child who asks why she can't see God is told to have faith, not doubt.

This approach also explains something that is inexplicable in biological terms — the celibate priest. A true celibate cannot pass on his genes, but having no children means he can devote his time and resources to spreading more memes. So the meme for celibacy succeeds. Apart from religions, other viral memes include alternative therapies that don't work, new age fads and cults, and astrology, which is immensely popular even though most of its claims have been tested and found to be false.

Of course, not all memes are viruses. Indeed the vast majority are the foundation of our lives and cultures, including all of the arts and sports, transport and communications systems, political and monetary systems, and science. And note that science has a very different structure from religion. Both are 'memeplexes' (groups of memes that work together), and science certainly contains viral memes such as false theories and fraudulent claims, but the very basis of science is the method of testing all claims. This means that science eventually throws out ideas that prove useless or false.

LANGUAGE is another important example. Although humans appear to have an innate tendency to learn language, the words we use are learned by imitation (i.e. they are memes). Blackmore has argued that once early humans became capable of imitating sounds, memetic evolution drove the gradual improvement of language, and with it the restructuring of our brains to be especially good at learning language. In a similar way she argues that our big brains were driven by, and for, the memes. Any of our early ancestors who had slightly bigger brains and were therefore slightly better at imitation would have been at an advantage because they could pick up and use the latest memes — whether these were ways of hunting, cooking food, wearing clothes, or dancing and singing. These people would therefore have attracted more mates and had more offspring. Therefore, as the memes spread, so did genes for having big brains capable of spreading them, and (perhaps more importantly) of selecting which memes to copy and which to reject. If this is so, the whole of human evolution has been shaped by the successful memes of the past, and we are products of two sets of replicators, memes and genes, not just one.

There are several mysteries about human nature that might potentially yield to a memetic explanation. Humans are far more co-operative and altruistic than any other species. Indeed, in those cultures with the best communications and hence the most memes, many altruistic ideas thrive — such as pacifism, vegetarianism, charity work, recycling, the Green movement, and the caring professions. Many people put enormous efforts into helping others who are not their relatives (i.e. do not share their genes) and who are unlikely or unable to reciprocate in the future. In other words, these behaviours are hard to explain in biological terms. The memetic approach is to ask why these particular memes spread. Perhaps we spend more time with the most altruistic people and so their memes get more chances to spread, including their altruistic memes. These are testable ideas which might, in the future, allow memetics to be found useful or to be rejected.

Human CONSCIOUSNESS is perhaps the greatest mystery of all. According to the American philosopher, Daniel Dennett, humans are a particular sort of ape infested with memes, and human consciousness is itself a huge complex of memes. He argues that the brain builds multiple drafts of what is happening at any time, and one of these drafts is the story we tell ourselves about a self who is in charge. In other words the self is a kind of 'benign user illusion' of the human brain.

Blackmore suggests it is not benign at all. In her view the self is the root of human suffering, yet it is a collection of memes that have come together for their own mutual protection and propagation. Ideas that become 'my' beliefs, or 'my' hopes or intentions, are at an advantage and survive. They then carry with them the idea of a self that not only has beliefs and opinions, but free will and consciousness. All this, argues Blackmore, is illusion. Our actions are the result of memes and genes competing to be copied in a complex environment, not of a self with free will. In this view human consciousness is distorted by the false idea of a self, and can be changed by practices like meditation, which undermine the idea.

This is where the moral objections of critics come to the fore. They argue that without a sense of self with free will and personal responsibility, we could not have effective legal systems and could not expect people to behave morally and co-operatively. Memetics clearly strikes at the heart of human nature. Yet if the theory of memes is right we cannot reject it on those grounds, and we may have to rethink many of our most precious ideas.

According to memetics that rethinking is urgent. Communications systems are rapidly expanding to spread more memes. Satellite systems, mobile telephones, and e-mail mean that everyone spreads more memes than ever before, even if this does not necessarily improve their lives and may burden them with information overload. The Internet is a vast playground for memes, many of which will propagate a round the world without any human having control over them or even noticing them. If we are to understand this rapid change, we may need a much better theory of memetics.

SUSAN BLACKMORE

Further reading

Blackmore, S. J. (1999). *The meme machine*. Oxford University Press, Oxford.

Dawkins, R. (1976). *The selfish gene*. Oxford University Press, Oxford. (New edition with additional material, 1989.)

Dennett, D. (1995). *Darwin's dangerous idea*. Penguin, London.

Memory Life is unpredictable. But memory provides organisms with the ability to learn — to modify their behaviour in the light of experience — and hence to reduce their uncertainty about the world. This is clearly an important behavioural adaptation, from the point of view of EVOLUTION. Indeed, most animals exhibit some forms of learning and memory, ranging all the way from gradual weakening (habituation) or strengthening (sensitisation) of simple reflex actions, to conscious recollection of personal experiences.

We can remember a telephone message for the few seconds it takes to write it down. But we can also remember things over very long periods of time. For example, adults may still remember some of the things they were taught at school —

both general abilities, such as how to add numbers together, and specific things, such as the translation of 'la plume de ma tante'. Additionally, we can also remember (though unconsciously) many of the skills attained through life, such as how to ride a bicycle or play the piano. There are many different ways in which humans and other animals remember things. It follows that memory cannot be conceptualized simply and that there are likely to be a variety of different, interacting memory systems.

Much of our sense of who we are as individuals depends on a particular kind of memory, involving recollection of our own past experiences, feelings, and relationships. One only has to imagine not being able to recall what has happened in one's past, or whether or not one even has family and friends, to realise how disruptive and distressing severe AMNESIA (such as occurs in Alzheimer's disease) can be, both to the patients themselves and to those close to them.

Psychologists have long drawn distinctions between different types of memory systems and memory processes. As early as 1890 William James distinguished between 'primary memory' (information one is presently aware of) and 'secondary memory' (information in the psychological past). Current ideas still maintain a distinction between short-term memory and long-term memory, evidenced by impairments of one or the other in brain-damaged patients. However, early 'multistore models', which proposed separate short-term and long-term memory stores, have now been discredited as being too simplistic.

The idea of a unitary short-term store has now largely been replaced by the concept of 'working memory'. The working memory system is concerned with both active processing and short-term storage of information and allows one to plan for the future and to bring together thoughts and ideas. Damage to the frontal lobes seems to impair working memory: patients with such damage function rather normally apart from being impaired in the use of stored knowledge to guide appropriate behaviour. Experiments on monkeys have shown that individual nerve cells in certain parts of the frontal cortex not only fire impulses when certain objects are seen by the monkey but continue to respond when the object disappears from view, as if holding a memory of the object. Furthermore, studies on the effects of damage of the frontal lobes in monkeys suggest that different forms of working memory can be localized to specific regions of the prefrontal cortex — the front part of the frontal lobes.

The concept of a single long-term store has also been replaced, by the view that there are several interacting long-term memory systems. There have been many attempts to subdivide long-term memory, but none has proved entirely successful. Another early distinction was between 'episodic memory' and 'semantic memory'. Episodic memory is autobiographical recollection of personally experienced events (such as what you had for breakfast), whereas semantic memory is general knowledge about the world, factual information and its meaning (such as the fact that breakfast is a kind of meal). Despite a clear conceptual difference, there is less evidence that these two types of memory rely on different memory systems in the brain. Indeed, semantic and episodic memory would appear to be strongly interdependent. For instance, retrieving semantic information may depend upon recalling the particular episodic event or events during which the semantic knowledge was gained. Likewise, it has been argued that recalling an episodic event (for example, remembering seeing an elephant at the zoo) depends on intact semantic memory (the definition of an elephant). Both types of memory may therefore rely on common underlying neural structures.

An alternative distinction was made between 'declarative memory' and 'procedural memory'. Declarative memory refers to knowing 'what', and includes both semantic and episodic information, whereas procedural memory refers to knowing 'how', and relates to skilled behaviour without the need for conscious recollection, such as the ability to remember how to drive a car. Support comes from observation of certain patients with amnesia who seem to have relatively intact procedural learning abilities (they can still learn how to do things) in the face of impaired declarative learning (e.g. not remembering where they are). However, the distinction between declarative and procedural knowledge is imprecise and many kinds of behaviour involve aspects of both. Furthermore, some patients with severe amnesia are capable of certain feats of memory (such as learning new factual information) that cannot be explained by procedural learning alone.

A further theoretical distinction was made between 'explicit memory' and 'implicit memory'. Explicit memory is said to be involved in tasks that require conscious recollection of previous experiences, whereas tasks that are facilitated in the absence of conscious recollection are said to depend on implicit memory. Many traditional methods used to test memory involve the person being asked to remember specific experiences, and are therefore measures of explicit memory. For instance, the memory of a previously-seen list of words could be tested by free recall ('Tell me the words that were on that list you saw earlier'), by recognition ('Was this word among the list you saw?'), or by cued recall ('Complete these letters to form a word that occurred on the list').

To demonstrate implicit memory it is necessary to show that a person has a long-term memory of a past experience although they can't consciously recall it. For example, the perceptual identification of words presented extremely briefly is easier if the words have previously been seen. Amnesic patients perform relatively normally on such 'repetition priming' tasks, as well as being able to acquire new motor skills, yet they are impaired on most tests of explicit memory. However, the distinction between explicit and implicit memory is again rather general and does not account for all of the patterns of long-term memory performance in amnesic subjects. Furthermore, the theory does nothing to address the fact that amnesic subjects can still form conscious short-term memories, which clearly involve explicit learning.

Observations that amnesic patients can retain some information briefly but not for long periods of time led to the development of the 'consolidation theory'. This suggests that immediate experiences are somehow crystallized into long-term memory, and that this process is disrupted in amnesia. The theory also maintains that the process of memory consolidation occurs over a period of time, during which memory traces are particularly vulnerable to permanent disruption by such things as a blow to the head, certain drugs, electric shock to the brain, etc. However, consolidation theory cannot account for the fact that apparently lost memories can sometimes be retrieved subsequently.

'Context-dependent theories' on the other hand propose that each memory trace (for instance of a particular person) is encoded together with information about the associated context (where you met the person), and that subsequent retrieval of the memory may be facilitated by reinstating the context. (Everyone is familiar with the fact that it is difficult to remember the names of even close friends when you meet them in unexpected places.) This theory is supported by the remarkable observation that divers recall more words learnt underwater when subsequently tested underwater than when tested on land, and vice versa. Learning while under the influence of certain drugs is also context-dependent, being better recalled when the same drug is administered.

Related 'state-dependent theories' maintain that agents or procedures that induce amnesia do not permanently disrupt memories but rather 're-encode' the memory traces in association with the brain state induced by the amnesic agent or procedure. Patients who have electroconvulsive shock (for instance, to treat depression) often complain of loss of memories; and this procedure indubitably disrupts long-term memory when given experimentally to rats. But rats can retrieve their lost memories after a subsequent shock, because this puts the brain back into the condition in which the information was 're-encoded', thereby providing an additional cue to aid remembering.

Although it is hard to verify whether a deficiency of memory reflects re-encoding or permanent memory loss, the importance of forgetting should not be underestimated. Although the brain has a huge capacity for memories, it must be finite. Since the brain appears to be able to form associations between disparate stimuli very easily, so it is important for it to be able to forget meaningless or arbitrary associations and remember only those associations that prove consistent or relevant. It has been theorized that inappropriate associations in the brain may specifically be weakened during the phase of SLEEP in which rapid eye movements and vivid dreams occur (REM sleep).

It is intuitively obvious that memories of all sorts involve functional changes in the brain, sometimes occurring remarkably quickly. Much of what we know about learning and memory has been gained from clever experiments involving the training of animals, both intact and with brain damage, as well as from studies of normal and amnesic human beings. But over the past few decades neurophysiologists and molecular biologists have made great strides in their understanding of the cellular mechanisms of learning and memory. One fruitful approach has involved examining basic forms of learning in animals with relatively simple nervous systems, such as the marine snail *Aplysia*. This animal withdraws its gill apparatus reflexly when the 'mantle' around it is touched, and the circuit of sensory and motor nerve cells responsible for this has been defined. This reflex is subject to habituation (if the touch to the gill is repeated time after time), and to sensitisation (if the touch is coupled with other stimulation). It turns out that these simple forms of short-term implicit learning involve changes in the effectiveness of synaptic transmission (mainly changes in the amount of transmitter substance per nerve impulse released at a particular SYNAPSE in the circuit). Longer-term memory requires new protein synthesis and the growth of new or larger synapses.

More complicated forms of learning may involve elaboration of a common set of molecular mechanisms. For instance, most animals can learn to associate one stimulus with another (such as the association formed between the sound of a bell and the sight of food in PAVLOVS' famous experiments on classical CONDITIONING). The underlying neural change, just as for sensitisation in *Aplysia*, is thought to involve increased release of transmitter substance at synapses in the circuit associating the two forms of stimulation.

In recent years, attention has focused on a primitive part of the CEREBRAL CORTEX called the *hippocampus*, which is tucked inside, under the lower edge of the temporal lobe of the cerebral hemispheres. Extensive damage to this general region in humans can cause devastating retrograde amnesia, which virtually eliminates the capacity to form new long-term conscious memories, while leaving old semantic and personal memories relatively intact. Traditionally, the hippocampus itself has been considered the seat of human episodic memory. However, recent research with monkeys has revealed several, functionally dissociable memory systems in this region of the temporal lobe. These include the *perirhinal cortex*, for object memory, and the *amygdala*, for memory for the emotional significance of stimuli and events. These individual areas, each with its different specialization, may then contribute to a broader-based temporal lobe memory system providing the basis of both episodic and semantic memory. The monkey's hippocampus may have a relatively restricted role in memory for spatial location.

In rodents, the hippocampus certainly seems particularly involved in spatial memory: when it is damaged, rats and mice cannot remember their way around mazes. It turns out that the connections between certain nerve cells in the hippocampus are remarkably 'plastic'. Synapses can be strengthened simply by a brief burst of nerve impulses, so that single impulses will subsequently (and for very long periods of time) evoke much bigger electrical responses in the receiving cell. Much is now known about the molecular basis of this phenomenon, called *long-term potentiation*. This mechanism may provide the basis of, or at least contribute to, many forms of learning, in several different regions of the brain, ranging from perceptual learning in young animals to human explicit memory.

Memory is central to the human condition and has been investigated at many levels. Neuroscientists have studied the molecular and cellular mechanisms of memory in animals and humans, and psychologists have contributed to our understanding about the different kinds of processes involved in memory through research with amnesic patients and normal subjects. Temporal lobe dysfunction is commonly associated with declarative or explicit memory impairments. However, since most amnesic patients either exhibit diffuse brain damage (*Korsakoff's syndrome*) or have focal damage to a range of different structures, our present understanding of which particular neural systems are important for different memory processes has come predominantly from animal 'models' of human amnesia.   MARK J. BUCKLEY

Further reading

Bolhuis, J. (2000). *Brain, perception, memory: advances in cognitive neuroscience*. Oxford University Press.

Eysenck, M. W. (1995). *Cognitive psychology: a student's handbook*, (3rd edn). Erlbaum, Hove.

See also AMNESIA; BRAIN; CEREBRAL CORTEX; LIMBIC SYSTEM.

Menarche The first MENSTRUATION which occurs at puberty. The majority of girls (95%) reach menarche between 11 and 15 years of age, the average being about 13 years. Ovulation can occur at the time of menarche but usually this does not happen for several months or even up to 2 years later. Thus the first few menstrual cycles are often anovulatory and hence infertile.   S.A.W.

See MENSTRUAL CYCLE.

Meninges is the plural of *meninx* — Greek for membrane. The term encompasses a group of three membranes that provide mechanical protection and support to the delicate tissue of the CENTRAL NERVOUS SYSTEM — the BRAIN and the SPINAL CORD. Moving inwards from the skull towards the brain, or from the vertebral canal towards the spinal cord, the three meninges are: *dura mater* or *pachymeninx* (Greek *pachy*, meaning thick), *arachnoid mater*, and *pia mater*. Arachnoid and pia are also called *leptomeninges* (thin membranes).

The dura consists of an outer layer, rich in blood vessels and nerves, and an inner layer, firmly attached to the arachnoid. At some sites within the SKULL, these two layers are separated, forming channels for blood draining from the brain into the veins — the *venous sinuses*. The sagittal sinus, for example, curves from front to back over the midline of the brain — 'in the line of an arrow' (Latin *sagitta*, an arrow). The dura also extends into membranes that subdivide the cranial cavity into compartments: the central, vertical *falx cerebri* (Latin *falx* — a sickle — which describes its shape), which separates the cerebral hemispheres, and the *tentorium cerebelli*, a 'tent' stretched over the cerebellum, forming the roof of the *posterior fossa* of the skull, which contains the CEREBELLUM and BRAIN STEM. The free front margin of the tentorium fits closely round the back of the brain stem; the brain stem can be damaged, for example if a tumour growing above or below the 'tent' encroaches on this narrow space. The dura also forms a diaphragm above the PITUITARY GLAND, through which passes the pituitary stalk, joining the gland to the HYPOTHALAMUS.

The blood supply to the dura is provided by an artery (*middle meningeal*) that is vulnerable to laceration by fracture of the skull; this can cause an EPIDURAL haemorrhage between the skull and the dura.

The dura of the brain is in continuation with the dura of the spinal cord, which is separated from the *periosteum* (the covering of the vertebral bones) by a narrow epidural space. Epidural anaesthesia to eliminate sensation from lower regions of the body, especially in childbirth, involves injection of drugs into this space. The dura tapers at the lower end of the spinal cord, forming a sheath around its thin remnant (the *filum terminale*). At the gaps between the vertebral bones, on each side, the dura forms a sleeve around the nerve roots that carry sensory and motor information to and from the spinal cord down its whole length.

The arachnoid surrounds the brain (bridging the *sulci* — the furrows on the surface of the cerebral cortex), and also the spinal cord and the cranial and spinal nerves. The space between arachnoid and pia is called the *subarachnoid space*, and contains the CEREBROSPINAL FLUID (CSF), which drains out of the CEREBRAL VENTRICLES. The space is narrow over the convexity of the brain and wider below and around the brain stem, where large spaces are formed, called *cisternae* by obvious reference to water cisterns.

The subarachnoid space surrounds the spinal cord and extends beyond its lower end, forming a 'cistern' that extends from the upper lumbar to the sacral part of the bony canal. This provides a site from which CSF can be sampled through a hollow needle for diagnostic purposes — the so-called *lumbar puncture*.

The subarachnoid space contains arteries and veins, which can be the site of abnormalities such as *cerebral aneurysms* — 'blow-outs' of artery walls, or malformations of the blood vessels.

Rupture of these is the cause of *subarachnoid haemorrhage*.

The subarachnoid space is continuous with the cavities of the cerebral ventricles. The rate of formation of new CSF within the cerebral ventricles is matched by a continuous flow through the subarachnoid space, back into the bloodstream. The route for this is provided by protrusions of the leptomeninges into the sagittal venous sinus. These protrusions are the *arachnoid villi*. They act as passive, pressure-dependent valves that discharge the CSF from the subarachnoid space into the sinus.

The innermost meningeal layer, the pia mater, is closely applied to the surface of the brain tissue and carries many small arteries and veins. The pia and arachnoid follow the branches of the surface blood vessels where they penetrate the brain tissue, so that a microscopic CSF-containing space surrounds them as far as the capillaries.

Meningitis — inflammation of the meninges — can be a dramatically severe and dangerous illness if due to infection by meningococcus bacteria — but is often relatively innocuous when (now most commonly) caused by one of many possible virus infections.

FRANCESCO SCARAVILLI

See also BLOOD–BRAIN BARRIER; CEREBROSPINAL FLUID; CEREBRAL VENTRICLES.

Menopause This is defined as the cessation of menstruation that occurs at the end of a woman's reproductive life. However, since menstrual periods can become very irregular towards the menopause, it is difficult to know which menstruation will actually be the last. Women around the age of 50 are usually considered to be past their menopause if menstruation has not occurred for a year. A variety of terms are associated with that of the menopause: premenopausal, peri-menopausal, post-menopausal. The 'climacteric' or more popularly 'the change of life' refer to the physical and psychological symptoms which occur in the peri-menopausal years. The menopause normally occurs between the ages of 45 and 55, although occasionally women may undergo a premature menopause much earlier in their reproductive lives. An 'artificial menopause' may be brought about by HYSTERECTOMY. When only the UTERUS is removed in a pre-menopausal woman, the cyclical changes continue in the OVARIES and the subsequent decline of ovarian hormone secretion takes its natural course. However, if the ovaries are removed at the same time, which is often advised in the late forties, the full menopausal condition is precipitated, and HORMONE REPLACEMENT THERAPY is likely to be required.

The natural menopause occurs because all the egg-containing follicles left in the ovary ultimately degenerate and so there are no follicles which, under the influence of gonadotrophins, will develop and begin secreting OESTROGEN. Ovulation will not occur and there will be no formation of a corpus luteum to secrete PROGESTERONE and oestrogen. Thus the body becomes deprived of the female SEX HORMONES normally produced by the ovaries. Since these have previously had a negative feedback effect on gonadotrophin secretion by the pituitary, this secretion increases dramatically. There remains only a limited source of female sex hormones after the menopause, by conversion of androgens secreted by the adrenal cortex. This does not compensate for the 'oestrogen deficient' state of the post-menopausal woman whose ovaries have ceased to function. If a woman lives to 90 she will spend nearly half of her life in an oestrogen-deficient state.

The loss of oestrogen secretions has several profound effects, not only physically but also psychologically. Some of these symptoms are limited to the peri-menopausal period when a woman is adjusting to the loss of her hormones. Others may become manifest at the menopause but can have serious consequences in the long term. Common symptoms associated with the peri-menopausal period are hot flushes and night sweats, vaginal dryness, and depressive episodes. There is evidence that oestrogens can affect dilatation of arterioles, and thus symptoms, like flushes, linked with altered control of blood flow during oestrogen withdrawal are not surprising. Loss of oestrogen also leads to the thinning of the vaginal walls and loss of vaginal secretions. This causes vaginal dryness, and sexual intercourse can become painful.

Psychological symptoms are often linked with the menopausal years, particularly in those women who have a history of depression. However, it is difficult to determine to what extent these are due to social changes (such as children leaving home, marriage becoming dull) and negative cultural influences (AGEING and loss of reproductive status and SEXUALITY). Nevertheless some women do suffer from tiredness, lack of concentration, ANXIETY, tearfulness, and loss of interest in sex.

After the menopause there is an increased loss of bone mass (OSTEOPOROSIS). In both men and women peak bone mass is usually achieved between the ages of 30 and 40 years and thereafter there is a gradual age-related loss in both sexes. In women, after the withdrawal of oestrogens at the menopause this bone loss is accelerated for several years, thereafter continuing at a similar rate to men. The result is that the age at which bones become so brittle that they are likely to fracture without any major trauma is, on average, much earlier in women than men. Thus women are far more likely than men to suffer from fractures related to osteoporosis. Common fractures are those of the wrist, hip, and spine (vertebrae). Indeed, fractures of the vertebrae can occur without trauma, and the resulting compression can cause the loss of several inches in height. Hormone replacement therapy (HRT) can stop the acceleration of bone loss, but when the therapy is withdrawn the usual rate of bone loss will recur. There is, however, considerable individual variation in bone loss, which may well be affected by lifestyle: exercise, especially if it involves 'impact', has been shown to decrease the rate of bone loss.

The other major long-term adverse effect of the menopause is on the cardiovascular system. The loss of sex steroids changes metabolism so that there is an increase in the amount of fats in the blood. This can increase the risk of arteriosclerosis (narrowing of the arteries by fatty deposits), which can lead to coronary artery disease and stroke. Thus pre-menopausal women are to some extent protected against cardiovascular disease by their sex hormones, as are women taking HRT. After the menopause, or after withdrawal of HRT, their risk of developing cardiovascular disease becomes the same as that of men.

There is no doubt that the loss of female sex hormones, notably oestrogens, can have profound effects on physiological functions in women. There is also little doubt that cultural influences can affect the way in which women experience and cope with menopausal symptoms. Western women live in a society in which social influences on the menopause are largely negative and there is a tendency for women to feel that they are left with the choice of being 'saved' by HRT or becoming old, sexless, and useless members of society. In contrast, in cultures where menopausal women achieve status and social advantages the reported incidence of menopausal symptoms is often negligible or even absent. For example amongst the Rajput of Northern India, women who are past their menopause are no longer in purdah and are able to move freely within their community. This has a positive effect on their outlook. Similarly the New Zealand Mayans view their post-menopausal years as a relief from child-bearing, and thus the menopause is an attribute. Japanese women report a lower frequency of menopausal symptoms compared with American and Canadian women, and the same is true for the Navajo Indians.

But all is not gloom and doom, even in Western society. The increasing presence of women in responsible posts in political, business, and professional life, and the acceptance in general of their employment outside the home enhances the prospect of rewarding and indeed more energetic activity without the inconveniences of the menstrual cycle and of potential pregnancy; employment of mothers also enhances the scope of the traditional role of the grandmother in the extended family. Thus, while the menopause can be considered as the beginning of an oestrogen-deficient state which may become an increasing health problem as longevity increases, there are clearly large cultural influences which can affect the way women experience this change of life.

SAFFRON WHITEHEAD

Further reading

Greer, G. (1991). *The change: women, ageing and the menopause*. Fawcett Books, Greenwich, CT.

Mackenzie R. (1984). Menopause. Sheldon Press, SPCK, London.

See also HORMONE REPLACEMENT THERAPY; HYSTERECTOMY; OVARIES; SEX HORMONES.

Menstrual cycle

Menstrual cycle Throughout a woman's reproductive life — from PUBERTY to the MENOPAUSE — the ovaries are programmed to produce a mature egg (OVUM) approximately every 28 days and to prepare the UTERUS (womb) for implantation of an embryo if the egg becomes fertilized. To achieve this reproductive competence the OVARIES must receive the correct hormonal signals from the brain and the pituitary gland. These signals stimulate the production of female SEX HORMONES and the cyclical changes which occur in the ovary during each normal menstrual cycle. In turn the sex steroids released by the ovary induce changes in the lining of the womb and other parts of the female reproductive tract. The system is subtly regulated and fine-tuned by feedback effects of the ovarian steroid hormones on hormone secretions from the HYPOTHALAMUS and PITUITARY GLAND, so there is a complex interplay of hormones and feedback signals which ultimately controls female fertility. Collectively these events constitute the menstrual cycle.

The first day of the menstrual cycle is defined as the first day of menstrual blood loss. This is when the uterus begins to shed its lining and bleeding occurs. At this time the secretion of hormones (oestrogen and progesterone) from the ovaries is at a minimum. This diminishes the braking effect that circulating ovarian hormones have on the secretion of the *gonadotrophic* hormones from the pituitary gland, namely *luteinizing hormone* (LH) amd *follicle stimulating hormone* (FSH). As a consequence these pituitary secretions increase and stimulate a new wave of activity in the ovaries.

Early in the cycle, FSH stimulates growth of a few follicles (egg-containing 'sacs') in each ovary. By about day 10 the ovaries contain several follicles with a diameter of 14–21 mm. As mid cycle approaches, all but one of these degenerate, and only the 'dominant' follicle becomes fully mature, with a diameter of 20–25 mm. What determines which follicle becomes the dominant one, and in which ovary, remains speculative. Local hormones or other factors acting within the ovaries may play an important role. This first half of the ovarian cycle is known as the *follicular phase* and is characterized by increasing secretions of oestrogen from the developing follicles; this is released into the bloodstream, reaches the uterus, and causes its lining to thicken: the glands enlarge and it becomes richly supplied with blood vessels: the *proliferative phase* of the uterine cycle.

In most normal human menstrual cycles only one follicle reaches full maturity, to be released at ovulation, on about day 14. The occasional release of two accounts for non-identical TWINS, and fertility drugs can increase the number of follicles reaching maturity at mid cycle. These drugs are either pituitary gonadotrophins, or synthetic chemicals which interfere with the negative feedback loop in such a way as to promote an increase in the release of these hormones from the pituitary gland itself. In

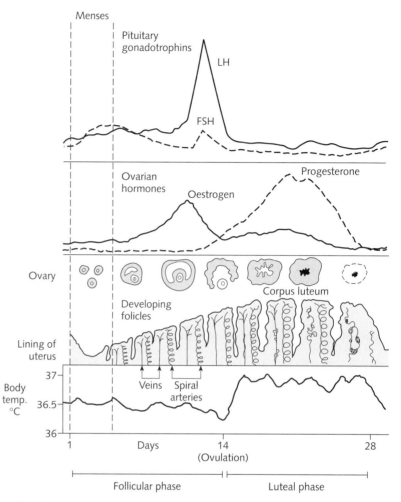

Changes of hormone concentrations in the blood during a 28-day menstrual cycle, and the associated changes in follicular development and ovulation (*follicular phase*), formation and degeneration of the corpus luteum (*luteal phase*), cyclical growth and degeneration of the endometrium of the womb, and changes in basal body temperature.

both cases the ovaries receive an increased 'drive' for follicular development, and thus several follicles will mature. Such drugs are used for treating certain types of infertility, and are given to women undergoing *in vitro* fertilization (IVF) treatment. If the result is multiple ovulation, the chances of fertilization are increased or, in the case of IVF, more than one mature egg can be recovered for external fertilization and subsequent implantation.

At mid cycle there is a dramatic change of events. There is a high blood concentration of oestrogen, but this ceases to have a braking (*negative feedback*) effect on the pituitary hormones. About 24–48 hours after the peak of oestrogen production a surge of the gonadotrophins occurs — especially of luteinising hormone. This is one of the rare biological examples of a *positive feedback* action. The surge causes the mature 'dominant' follicle to rupture and release its egg within 9–12 hours. Indeed, one way of predicting ovulation is by the detection of the increase in luteinising hormone in the blood, which is reflected in the urine. This is the scientific basis for the kits

which are commercially available to identify the most likely time for conception.

At the time of ovulation there is a small rise in body temperature. This is thought to be due to the action of rising progesterone in the blood, resetting in some way the 'thermostat' in the brain which controls our body temperature. This small rise can be used to indicate when ovulation occurs, but obtaining reliable temperature measurements is difficult, making the method often unsatisfactory. Some women feel mild pain in the abdomen around the time of ovulation, lasting from a few minutes to a couple of hours. Known as *Mittelschmerz* (German for 'midpain'), it is probably caused by irritation of the abdominal wall due to blood and fluid escaping from the ruptured follicle. Changes in the cervical mucus also occur about the time of ovulation.

After ovulation the empty follicle left behind in the ovary is remodelled, and it plays an important role in the second half of the menstrual cycle, known as the *luteal phase* of the ovarian cycle. The cells remaining in the ruptured follicle proliferate rapidly and form the *corpus luteum*.

This 'yellow body' produces increasing amounts of progesterone and some oestrogen, and these hormones act on the lining of the womb — it becomes thick and spongy and its glands secrete nutrients that can be used by the embryo if fertilization has occurred: this is the *secretory phase* of the uterine cycle. The high progesterone level in the blood, together with oestrogen, also exerts negative feedback effects, which decrease the secretion of the gonadotrophin-promoting secretion by which the hypothalamus influences the pituitary. Small amounts of gonadotrophins nevertheless continue to maintain the function of the corpus luteum — but if fertilization does not occur, towards the end of the cycle this support fails and the corpus luteum breaks down. The precise mechanisms which induce this degeneration are unknown, but the consequences are that progesterone and oestrogen secretions decline, the hormonal support of the uterine lining is lost, the spiral arteries contract, and the lining cells, starved of their blood supply, break away. Menstrual bleeding ensues. A new cycle begins.

While the average time for each menstrual cycle is typically depicted as 28 days, cycles do vary considerably in length, ranging from 25 days to 35 days. It is usually the length of the first (follicular) phase of the cycle that accounts for most of the variation. The luteal phase is more likely to last the typical 14 days, with ovulation occurring two weeks *before* rather than after the onset of menstruation, so it is unpredictable. Furthermore, the luteal phase in some women can also vary. This variability clearly makes 'safe period' birth control unreliable.

SAFFRON WHITEHEAD

Further reading

Jones, R. E. (1997). *Human reproductive biology*, (2nd edn). Academic Press, New York.

See also MENSTRUATION; PREMENSTRUAL TENSION; OVA; OVARY; SEX HORMONES; UTERUS.

Menstruation is the periodic shedding of the endometrium (lining of the uterus) accompanied by blood loss, that identifies the reproductive years of a woman's life. The first menstruation (menarche) usually occurs at puberty (typically between the ages of 11 and 16) and menstrual periods continue until the menopause around the age of 45–50. However, menstruation does not occur during PREGNANCY and can be suppressed or disrupted in women who are breast-feeding. This was noted by the scientist and philosopher, Aristotle (384–22 BC), who believed that pregnant women did not menstruate because the seed of the male caused blood to coagulate into an egg from which the fetus developed. Milk was also thought to be formed from menstrual blood because of the absence of menstruation in lactating women.

The old ideas as to why women menstruate stemmed from the teachings of Hippocrates (*c.* 400 BC) who believed that health was governed by the balance of the four body fluids or HUMOURS — blood, phlegm, black bile, and yellow bile. Thus menstruation was seen as a means of getting rid of excess blood to prevent the body filling with this humour, upsetting the balance and causing illness. This theory was finally disproved by John Davidge in 1814, who pointed out that a woman might only lose a few teaspoons of blood in a typical menstrual flow, while the loss of a much greater amount of blood through blood-letting (cutting the veins) did not prevent menstruation. He concluded that menstruation, rather than being a means of getting rid of excess blood, could be attributed to some odd condition of the ovaries which excited the blood vessels of the womb. In essence his premise was correct.

Menstruation is the culmination of a complex series of hormonal events associated with the cyclical production of a mature egg within the ovary and the release of this egg for fertilization. In the first half of the menstrual cycle, ovarian follicles, containing an egg, develop, and produce increasing amounts of OESTROGEN. This sex hormone stimulates a build-up of the lining of the womb and the growth of spiral arteries into this thickened lining. After ovulation, which occurs around day 14 of the cycle, the empty follicle in the ovary becomes a corpus luteum. This produces high concentrations of PROGESTERONE and some oestrogen. The progesterone further increases the thickness of the uterine lining and causes it to secrete a fluid which will nourish a fertilized egg and encourage implantation of the embryo. If fertilization does not occur the corpus luteum breaks down towards the end of the cycle and so the endometrium loses its hormonal support from the ovary. As a consequence the endometrium literally dies, and the cells of this lining are shed along with some loss of blood from the spiral arteries which have grown into the lining of the womb. Menstrual bleeding usually lasts 3–7 days, although endometrial regeneration can begin as early as the third day after the beginning of menstruation. Interestingly, only in man, apes, and Old World monkeys is the endometrium shed. In most other mammals the endometrium is resorbed at the end of each cycle and there is no bleeding — this is probably related to the absence of spiral arteries.

While the shedding of the uterine lining actually signifies the end of each reproductive cycle, the first day of menstruation is defined for convenience and accuracy as the beginning of a new menstrual cycle. Typically each cycle lasts between 25 and 34 days in 95% of women, with 28 days being the average. Hence the term 'menstruation', since it tends to recur at monthly intervals. Total blood loss during each menstruation varies from cycle to cycle, and in different women at different stages of their reproductive life. However, the average blood loss is about 50–60 ml (a teaspoon holds about 5 ml), although it can vary from about 10–80 ml. Excessive loss of blood (menorrhagia) can lead to iron-deficiency ANAEMIA.

Many myths, legends, and TABOOS have grown up around menstruation throughout the centuries, but all with the underlying sentiment that menstruating women are unclean and capable of producing bad effects on the world about them. It became a focus of religious observance. For example, Hindu women are not supposed to prepare their husbands' food when they are menstruating. Those Moslem women who are normally allowed to pray in a Mosque may not do so during menstruation. Some Buddhists think it is wrong to enter a temple during menstruation and Jews are supposed to refrain from sexual intercourse during this time. In medieval times menstruating women were excluded from going to church and the Church of England has a service for 'The Churching of Women', a ceremony to be performed when a woman has had her first menstruation after the birth of a child. And so from the early teaching of Hippocrates, right through the centuries menstruation has been seen as a way of getting rid of something undesirable, unclean and potentially harmful. No wonder such derogatory terms as 'the CURSE' came into existence.

SAFFRON WHITEHEAD

Mermaid The mermaid is one of the most popular figures in world folklore. Her characteristic appearance is as a nubile young girl, with long hair and a fish tail, carrying a comb and a mirror. Unlike the other part-human, part-animal creatures of myth and folklore, mermaids have been the object of many sightings up to the present day; it is as if there is a desire to prove the reality of mermaids, which makes them closer to creatures such as the Loch Ness monster and the Yeti than to centaurs and sirens. Another expression of this desire to believe can be found in the many fake mermaids, usually made of the upper torso of a monkey and the tail of a salmon, which have been exhibited in fairs and circuses. In the age of trade and exploration, seeing a mermaid was an almost essential part of travelling to new worlds; Christopher Columbus saw three off Haiti, Sir Richard Whitburne sighted one when discovering Newfoundland in 1610, and Henry Hudson's crew saw a mermaid off Nova Zembla in 1625. In each case, the surviving accounts consciously compare what has been seen with the dominant images in art — Columbus finding his mermaids less pretty and more masculine than he expected. The most famous mermaid to have been captured, the 'mermaid of Amboina', was found off the coast of Borneo in the eighteenth century and is said to have lived in captivity for four days. She refused to eat, and made plaintive sounds like those of a mouse. The account given of these events in 1754 suggested that dead mermaids were never found because their flesh rots particularly rapidly.

Where do the myths of mermaids come from? Somewhere in the later Middle Ages, the fish-woman mermaid supplanted the bird-woman siren as the creature believed to lure sailors astray, although in many languages words based on 'siren' continued to be used for the fish-woman. The shift to fish-women as the danger facing mariners may be related to an increasing ability to travel to the open sea, where mermaids live, out of sight of the coastal rocks where sirens had been thought to perch. Both sirens and mermaids have musical talents; bird-sirens sing and play the pipes and the lyre, whereas mermaids rely on their voices to entice sailors to their death. Mermaids can raise and calm storms at will and, like the Sphinx, they can trap men with questions and riddles. In nineteenth-century Greek folklore, sailors in the Black Sea may meet the fish-woman Gorgona, who asks, 'Does Alexander live?' If they do not give the correct answer, 'He lives and rules the world', Gorgona will raise a storm and kill all aboard.

Mermaids combine the beauty of a young girl with a repulsive, fishy lower body. Physically, the problem this poses is how the men whom they target are supposed to have sexual intercourse with them. Some medieval representations get around this problem by showing the mermaid with a forked tail, but perhaps the whole point about the mermaid is that she is sexually unattainable except through death. As popular songs of the nineteenth century remind us, a man who marries a mermaid can never leave her, as there is no divorce court 'at the bottom of the deep blue sea'. An unusual solution to the problem of the sexual availability of mermaids is found in Magritte's *Collective Invention* (1935), which shows a beached mermaid with the upper half of a fish and the lower half of a woman. A related problem is how mermaids themselves reproduce; male mer-people, or tritons, are shown in art, particularly in the Renaissance, but again they may miss the point. Matthew Arnold's poem *The Forsaken Merman* (1849) is a rare example of the treatment of mermen in literature; it reverses the common pattern of a mortal man loving a mermaid but being deserted by her, to imagine a mortal woman being called back from the mer-world by the distant sound of church bells.

Modern literary representations of the mermaid are dominated by the influential *Little Mermaid* of Hans Christian Anderson. Here the mer-world is a systematic inversion of our own, in which not birds, but fish, fly in through open windows. Rather than causing shipwrecks, the little mermaid saves the life of a shipwrecked prince, then makes a bargain with the sea-witch, exchanging her tongue for a pair of human legs. Every step she takes causes her terrible pain, and her feet bleed. Unable to win the love of the prince without her voice, she rejects the chance to kill him and thus return to her life as a mermaid, but instead dies when he marries someone else. Feminist interpretations of this story suggest that the little mermaid's surrender of the power to speak in order to enter the prince's world is an image of women giving up their own voices if they are to be accepted within patriarchy. Anderson's own message was that, by her love for the prince, the mermaid gained the chance of winning the immortal soul she most craved.   HELEN KING

See also CHIMERA.

Metabolism According to the Shorter Oxford English Dictionary, the term metabolism is defined as 'the chemical processes by which nutritive material is built up into living matter, or by which complex molecules are broken down into simpler substances during the performance of special functions'. The various reactions which involve the synthesis of complex molecules can be grouped under the heading of *anabolism*, whereas the breakdown of complex molecules is known as *catabolism*. As might be expected, both anabolic and catabolic processes include a vast number of different chemical reactions, but there are a number of common features. Most of the metabolic processes occur inside the cells of the body, mainly in the cytoplasm, but also inside intracellular organelles such as the mitochondria. Anabolic and catabolic reactions involve the action of ENZYMES and the utilisation of energy. In some cases the metabolic processes are regulated locally, i.e. by the cell itself, but often the metabolism of the whole body is controlled in an integrated fashion by the action of hormones and/or the nervous system.

Anabolic processes

These mainly involve the use of the carbohydrates, fats, proteins, and minerals consumed in the diet to synthesize complex molecules — such as the structural material of the SKELETON, CONNECTIVE TISSUE, and CELL MEMBRANES; nutrient stores for later use; and HORMONES and PROTEINS which are secreted from cells into the blood or into the digestive tract. In order for these anabolic processes to proceed efficiently, it is essential that the cells are provided with the correct raw materials (and are able to extract them from the blood) and that the appropriate enzymes are present within the cells. Obviously, these enzymes will have been synthesized within the cells, as a result of activation of the appropriate genes in the cell nucleus.

Catabolic processes

These can be classified into a variety of categories, including the breakdown of energy-containing components of the diet (or their storage forms) to make energy available for the cells; the removal and breakdown of potentially toxic substances in the bloodstream; and the breakdown of damaged cells and tissues with the re-use of many of the components. These catabolic processes require the presence of the appropriate enzymes; many also require OXYGEN to be available, and the waste products to be removed from the tissues by the blood.

In many cases the processes of anabolism and catabolism occur coincidentally. A good example relates to the protein in the body, which is in a constant state of flux. Every day some of the body protein undergoes catabolism and is replaced by new material. Thus, there is a constant turnover of protein in the body, which requires a continuous supply of protein in the diet, and which also uses a substantial amount of energy.

Control of metabolism

For the body to function efficiently, there has to be an effective means of controlling and integrating the metabolic processes occurring in all the cells, tissues, and organs. This integration and control is mainly achieved by circulating hormones, with their release being regulated in turn partly by the nervous system and partly by direct effects of substances in the blood on the endocrine glands. An example of this integrated control of metabolism is the way in which blood glucose concentration is regulated to ensure an adequate supply of glucose to the brain. After meals, the hormone INSULIN acts to promote storage of glucose in the form of GLYCOGEN in the liver. The brain continuously extracts glucose from the blood to use as a fuel for its metabolic processes. In the periods between meals, this continued use of blood glucose causes the concentration to fall, which could impair brain function. However, a fall in blood glucose is detected in the PANCREAS and leads to the release of the hormone GLUCAGON, which acts on the liver to cause breakdown of glycogen and release of glucose into the blood. In addition, if blood glucose falls sufficiently to affect brain metabolism, the sympathetic nervous system is activated, causing the adrenal gland to release ADRENALINE, which also stimulates the release of glucose from the liver; also the individual feels hungry and is prompted to eat.

Energy metabolism

A fundamental feature of both anabolic and catabolic processes is the utilisation of energy. Almost all of the chemical reactions in the body require the expenditure of energy, which is made available mainly by the catabolism of the 'macronutrients': fats and carbohydrates (particularly glucose), and (to a small extent) proteins. This utilization of energy can be compared with the use of fuel for cooking or for generating electricity. In these two cases, the combustion of a fuel (coal, gas, or oil) produces carbon dioxide and water and releases heat which is used to warm the food (often causing chemical changes in it) or to generate steam to drive turbines. In the body's metabolism, the energy released from the oxidation of the macronutrients is used for a series of chemical reactions, instead of being released only as heat.

The main way in which the energy contained in the macronutrients is used in metabolism is via the substance ADENOSINE TRIPHOSPHATE (ATP). Cells require energy for their metabolic processes, so they contain the enzymes and organelles needed to produce ATP from the catabolism of fats, carbohydrates, and/or proteins. In most cases, the production of ATP occurs in association with the oxidation, so that the final products are ATP, carbon dioxide, and water, as illustrated below for the oxidation of glucose ($C_6H_{12}O_6$):

$$C_6H_{12}O_6 + 6O_2 = 6CO_2 + 6H_2O + ATP$$

This is an example of *aerobic metabolism*, requiring the supply of oxygen and the removal of carbon dioxide from the cells by the circulating blood. Thus, in order for this predominant type of metabolism to proceed effectively in the whole body, there needs to be integration of the respiration, circulation, and supply of nutrients.

In some situations, *anaerobic metabolism* can occur — ATP is produced without the use of oxygen — but the energy-releasing capacity of these systems is very small compared with that of aerobic metabolism, and the anaerobic reactions lead to the production of waste products such as lactic acid which impair cell function if they are present in high concentrations.

ATP is the single most important molecule for the metabolism of almost all the cells of the body. It is used to release the energy needed for muscles to contract, for chemical bonds to be made during the synthesis of complex molecules, and for other bonds to be broken during catabolic processes. Cells do not store large quantities of ATP, but rather produce it when it is needed. Thus, most cells of the body need to regulate the concentration of ATP within them. This occurs via the effects of ATP, and its immediate breakdown product ADP (adenosine diphosphate), on the enzymes responsible for synthesizing ATP: when more ATP is used, its concentration falls, and that of ADP rises, leading to the activation of the enzyme which synthesizes more ATP. This in turn requires more oxygen to be used, and nutrients to be broken down.

An example of the complex integration of metabolism is provided by considering the processes involved in muscle contraction during EXERCISE. This involves the brain and other parts of the nervous system in the initiation of voluntary muscle contraction and movement. Contraction can occur only if ATP is available within the muscle cells. As the ATP already present is used, so the concentration of ADP will rise, which stimulates more ATP production. At the same time the contraction of the muscles stimulates the breakdown of the intramuscular glycogen, and may also stimulate the uptake of glucose and fatty acids from the blood. The increased availability of these fuels is accompanied by stimulation of their oxidation, so the ATP concentration is maintained, and muscle contraction continues, supported by an increase in aerobic energy metabolism. For this to be possible, it is also necessary for the supply of blood to the muscles to increase, in order to deliver more oxygen and carry away more carbon dioxide and heat; the action of chemical products of local metabolism, which dilate local blood vessels, effectively links flow to requirement.

The above examples illustrate the complexity of metabolism in the human body, and show that for normal function it is essential that local processes are co-ordinated and integrated throughout the body.   I.A. MACDONALD

See also BLOOD SUGAR; EXERCISE; HUNGER.

Metals in the body There are no metals normally present as such in the body, except those put there during surgery. Tantalum is used for sutures, and steel in artificial hip joints. Some children with congenital heart abnormalities have fine tungsten spirals inserted into the heart to plug small holes between the cavities of the two ventricles. The spirals are inserted, using fibre optic and catheterisation techniques, via the femoral artery; the probes are fed through the circulation until the heart is reached. Fibrous growth around the spirals then seals the hole. People with artificial PACEMAKERS have an electrode — which delivers the pulses — inserted into the heart, connected to a control unit placed under a skin flap in the abdominal region. The casing of the control unit is made of the finest steel and sealed to prevent attack by body fluids. In all instances the metals used in these artificial devices needs to be non-toxic, non-corrodable, and long lasting. The devices become part of the person and they forget about their presence, only to be reminded when they pass, for example, through metal detector screens at airports, where an artificial hip joint or a pacemaker control box will set off the alarm.

Three-quarters of all the hundred-odd elements that exist in the environment are metals. It is not surprising, therefore, that many of these metallic elements are found within the body, though mostly only in small amounts. Some of these are described as *trace elements*, vital for some body function. They do not exist in the body as elemental metal but as metal salts, or complexed with some organic component. An example is iron; complexed with haem it forms an essential component of HAEMOGLOBIN, the oxygen carrier that gives red blood cells their colour. Many of the metallic elements exist in the body, without any function but at levels low enough to be tolerated. For example, 54 different elements exist in sea water, and people who live near the coast have detectable traces of all of these. Sometimes man does things that raises the levels of metal elements in the body to those which are unacceptable, and correction is needed. The yellow lines painted at the edges of roads to indicate no parking for vehicles originally contained bright yellow compounds of chromium, which has no known bodily function. The dust created by moving vehicles crossing the lines led to rising levels of chromium in the air and the practice was abandoned, non-chromium substitutes being found. After the Chernobyl disaster in Russia, sheep grazing in parts of Scotland were found to have raised levels of uranium in their bloodstreams. Uranium salts had been carried in the air and fell in rain on the Scottish highlands, becoming incorporated into the grass upon which the sheep grazed. For a while sheep from this region could not be used for food products. In a similar way many people in Europe stopped using dairy products in the Sixties at the time when atomic tests were carried out in remote parts of the world, because detectable amounts of radioactive strontium-90 could be detected in milk.

Which of the metal elements are essential for our existence? The list includes sodium, potassium, CALCIUM, magnesium, manganese, iron, cobalt, copper, zinc, and molybdenum. In addition, small amounts of other metals are found which are unavoidably present, but have no known function. These include lead, aluminium, arsenic, mercury, cadmium, gold, bismuth, antimony, and beryllium. It is important to realise the extreme range of concentrations that exist among the metal elements found in the body — if the amount of arsenic equalled that of magnesium then you would have expired long ago. Perhaps the easiest way to consider the range is to give the value of 100 to sodium and potassium, then calcium and magnesium will have the value 1–2 (ignoring bone) and manganese, iron, cobalt, copper, zinc, and molybdenum will be in the range 0.1–0.001 (ignoring red cells). For all the others listed above the content will be even less. Beryllium, for example, is lethal at one part in a million of body weight. It is possible to have toxic effects even from those metallic elements which are essential for body function. For example, excessive intake of iron, often in those who self-medicate in the belief they can build up their strength, can lead to an abnormally high level in the blood, followed by deposition in the liver, pancreas and skin. Cooking in iron pots, as by the Bantu people, sometimes leads to iron intoxication.

How does the body use the metallic elements? The salts of sodium and potassium are the main providers of the osmotic strength of body fluids. It is not surprising that the compositions of body fluids are not unlike the milieu from which life evolved, namely the oceans. Yet the strength of sea water is far greater than that of blood. However, the sea has become increasingly salty over aeons of time as the rains have washed the soluble salts down from the mountains. Many sea creatures have evolved intricate mechanisms to keep the composition of body fluids constant in the presence of the increasing tonicity of their environment.

Calcium and magnesium are among the most abundant elements on earth, so they are imbibed as drinking water and as milk. Calcium is essential for the structure of bones and teeth, where it is kept in a highly insoluble form, and in milk production. It is an essential 'second messenger' in cell signalling and a requirement for muscle contraction and for BLOOD clotting. If blood levels of calcium fall then calcium is withdrawn from bone, resulting in osteomalacia and osteoporosis. All phosphate-transferring enzymes, like those used in carbohydrate metabolism, require magnesium. Magnesium salts (e.g. magnesium sulphate, known as Epsom salts) were formerly used as osmotic purgatives. Our intake of manganese is through plants, spinach being a particularly rich source. This may explain why the well-known cartoon character Popeye and his companion Olive Oil always downed a tin of spinach before embarking on some heroic act. Manganese is an

461

essential co-factor for many enzymes, and without it the growth of many green plants would fail and spinach would not exist. The body contains about 5g of iron, three-quarters of it in red cells complexed in haemoglobin, with half the remainder stored in the liver, kidneys, bone marrow, and spleen.

Cobalt is an essential part of the vitamin B_{12} complex, which in turn is essential for red blood cell formation. B_{12} cannot be made in the body and we depend on the diet for its supply, liver being the richest source. Cobalt is also a necessary activator of some important enzymes. Eating liver or shellfish gives us our intake of copper, essential for the synthesis of haemoglobin. Excess copper is excreted, but when copper handling is disrupted, copper is deposited in the eyes. In treating the rare condition of Wilson's disease, where there is an excess of copper, penicillamine is used to form a soluble complex with copper, which can then be excreted. Both zinc and molybdenum are necessary for the functions of many different enzymes.

What can be done if the concentration of metallic elements rises above the toxic threshold, particularly those that have no known function in the body? Some of these have been deliberately used as POISONS, much beloved of Victorian melodramas, such as *Arsenic and Old Lace*, in which two seemingly sweet spinsters ran a boarding house, poisoning the lodgers with arsenic to relieve them of life's struggles. Yet some rather toxic metals, albeit in insoluble form, have been used as medicaments: Bismuth, for example, as an antacid. Yet others were intended to be absorbed; lithium salts for schizophrenia, antimony salts for protozoal diseases, mercury for syphilis. Other metallic elements have been inbibed *en passant* over a lifetime: lead, for example, picked up from old water pipes, and aluminium, from saucepans, the latter connected by some with Alzheimer's disease. Little can be done to reverse degenerative changes that have occurred consequent upon low level intake over many years. However, heavy metals can be removed from the body, whether they have accumulated chronically or by acute exposure. For this purpose *chelating agents* have been developed, some rather specific for certain metals. 'Chelate' means 'to claw', and it does exactly that: one or more chelate molecules combine with the metal atom to form a complex, with the metal held in the pincers of the claw. Chelates are generally very water soluble, so that the chelating agent containing the offending metal is excreted in the urine.

There are traces of many other metals in the body, and some of them will likely turn out to have essential functions in yet undiscovered bodily processes, but the amounts required will be infinitesimally small.   ALAN W. CUTHBERT

Metamorphosis is a feature of myth, whereby social, cultural, and species boundaries that are usually fixed are able to become flexible. In particular, it refers to the process of changing bodily shape, sometimes permanently, but more commonly as a temporary shift by a god, another divine being, or someone using magical powers. For instance, in Hindu myth, Ganesha acquired his elephant head after being decapitated by his father Shiva and therefore needing a replacement. In many cultures, divine figures share human and animal attributes; for example, the Celtic horse goddess Epona and the horned god Cernunnos.

Stories of such transformations were very popular in the Hellensitic period; several authors are known to have complied collections of them, although all such collections are now lost, with the exception of some excerpts which have survived under the name of a writer of the early Roman empire, Antoninus Liberalis. However, the Roman poet Ovid collected about 250 transformation stories, which survive as the *Metamorphoses*. In Apuleius' book of the same title, more commonly known as the *Golden Ass*, the hero Lucius tries to uncover the secrets of witchcraft but is transformed into an ass. After a series of adventures, he is restored to human form by the goddess Isis. In all these stories the theme of metamorphosis is used to question the established boundaries between human and beast, god and mortal, animate and inanimate, thus becoming a way of exploring the limits of what humanity can do.

The following accounts of metamorphosis are best known from Ovid, and are also common in Renaissance as well as classical art. Daphne was a river nymph who was chased by the god Apollo; she asked her mother, the earth goddess, to change her form, and became a laurel tree, thus escaping the god's advances. Callisto was a princess or a nymph, who was seduced by Zeus. In some versions of her myth, she was transformed into a bear so that this could take place, but in others her metamorphosis is a punishment for her pregnancy, and she gives birth to a human son while she is a still a bear. Her son later kills her by mistake when hunting. In a particularly violent myth of transformation, Tereus leaves his wife Procne and rapes her sister, Philomela, telling Philomela that her sister is dead. To ensure Philomela's silence, he cuts out her tongue. Philomela discovers the truth and sends her sister a message woven into a tapestry; Procne then kills her son by Tereus and serves his flesh to his father. When Tereus pursues the sisters threatening to murder them, they ask the gods for help; all three are transformed into birds, Tereus becoming a hoopoe, Philomela a nightingale, and Pronce a swallow. The order of the last two is reversed by some ancient writers, because an alternative version has Procne as the victim of Tereus' silencing, and the bird forms are significant; the hoopoe, being a crested bird, is 'royal', while whichever sister loses her tongue must be the one who becomes the bird with the power of song who, in the words of T. S. Eliot, 'Filled all the desert with inviolable voice' (*The Waste Land*).

In all these stories, violent attempts to transgress the boundaries of the female body by rape act as the catalyst for the dissolution of the boundaries between humans and the rest of the natural world. It is, however, not only women who are the subjects of metamorphosis in a sexual context. A myth concerned with the preservation of the boundary between gods and mortals tells how, when the hunter Actaeon accidentally came upon the goddess Artemis bathing, she turned him into a stag and he was then torn apart by his own hunting dogs. In some artistic representations of his metamorphosis, seen as a particularly cruel one because he did not intend to disturb the virgin goddess, the still-human Actaeon is shown in the process of sprouting horns. Some versions of the myth take his violation of Artemis' chosen isolation further by suggesting that he wanted to marry her. In a further story of metamorphosis in the context of sexual transgression, the mortals Atalanta and Melanion make love in the sanctuary of a god, and are then punished by being turned into lions.

As well as the human/animal boundary, that between male and female is also vulnerable; in classical myth, Caenis was a girl who was loved by the god Poseidon, who changed her into the boy Caenus at her request as a gift. Myths that describe transgression do not, however, serve to sanction it in real life. The Oedipus myth, with its central character unwittingly killing his father, then marrying his mother, only to blind himself when the truth comes out, acts as a warning of what can happen if social boundaries are crossed. The fact that Oedipus puts out his own *eyes* when he 'sees' the truth is only one example of the connection in ancient myth between physical blindness and moral vision; other expressions of this are the tradition that the poet Homer was blind, and the myths of the blind seer Teiresias.

In Greek mythology, several gods had the power to change shape. For example, Dionysos was able to do this, while when the deities Poseidon and Demeter slept together they took the respective forms of a stallion and a mare. But most frequently it was the supreme god, Zeus, who used metamorphosis in the course of finding ways of disguising himself when seducing mortal women; he took Leda in the form of a swan, Europa in the form of a bull, and Danae in the form of a shower of gold. As well as confusing the objects of his sexual interest, Zeus' power of metamorphosis was supposed to protect them. One of Zeus' mortal lovers, Semele, was tricked by Zeus' jealous wife Hera into testing him by demanding that he should appear to her in his true shape; this immediately killed her, since Zeus appeared as a thunderbolt.

Some mortals have also been thought to possess the power to change shape by witchcraft or by other methods, sometimes deliberately, sometimes against their will.

HELEN KING

See also GREEKS; MYTHOLOGY AND THE BODY; WEREWOLVES; WITCHCRAFT.

Metaphor

Ordinary language is saturated with corporeal metaphors. We frequently speak of 'the lip of a cup', and 'the legs of a table', and use expressions like 'the walls have ears', 'the interviewer kept me on my toes', and 'let's get to the heart of the matter'. Not only are many of our metaphorical expressions rooted in the body and our experiences of it, but metaphors, in turn, significantly shape our cultural perceptions of the body.

Definitions and interpretations

From the Greek word '*metaphora*' meaning 'transference', a metaphor has generally been understood as a figurative expression which interprets a thing or action through an implied comparison with something else. Aristotle, who is usually considered the originator of 'comparison' theories of metaphor, described metaphors in the *Rhetoric* as elliptical similes — comparisons of 'things that are related but not obviously so' without using 'like' or 'as'. According to Aristotle, the best or 'most well liked' type of metaphor transfers its meaning from one subject or 'register' to another through the principle of analogy. As Aristotle observes in the *Poetics*, these metaphors often depend on logical relationships between multiple terms. The metaphor 'old age is the evening of life', for instance, relies on the relation between a set of terms describing day and another set describing age.

Aristotelian approaches to metaphor remained largely unchallenged until 1936, when I. A. Richards offered what philosopher Max Black has termed an 'interaction' view of metaphor. Critiquing both Aristotle's notion of metaphor as special or ornamental use of language, and his assumption that metaphor involves the mere substitution of one term for another, Richards claimed that metaphor relies on a complex interaction of thoughts, rather than a process of linguistic substitutions. To explain how a metaphor functions as a 'double unit', Richards introduced the terms 'tenor' and 'vehicle', which refer to the 'principal subject' and the name of the figurative term itself, respectively. (In the metaphor 'Juliet is the sun', for example, 'Juliet' would be the tenor and 'sun' the vehicle.) Richards' theory of metaphor as the product of an interaction between vehicle and tenor was later refined by Max Black in his 1962 book, *Models and Metaphors*. In this volume, Black suggested that a metaphor acts as a 'filter' in which two or more subjects interact according to a 'system of associated commonplaces' (a shared set of cultural responses) to produce new meanings for the entire phrase or sentence. In the metaphor 'Tom is a fox', then, not only is 'Tom' viewed in terms of cultural associations of foxes as sly creatures, but 'fox' is also reinterpreted through its juxtaposition with a human male.

In the late 1970s, John Searle rejected both interaction and comparison theories of metaphor, and offered an understanding of metaphor based on the 'speaker's utterance meaning'. In *Expression and Meaning*, his 1979 study of speech act theory, Searle criticized earlier approaches to metaphor on the grounds that they tried to locate the meaning of metaphors in the sentences or metaphorical expressions themselves. Instead, Searle suggested, we must examine the slippage between the speaker's meaning and the sentence or word meaning. In other words, metaphorical utterances work not because a certain juxtaposition of words produces a change in the meaning of the lexical elements but because the speaker's meaning differs from their literal usage. Thus phrases like 'It's getting hot in here' or 'Sally is a block of ice' function as metaphors only in certain contexts with specific truth conditions: there is no single principle according to which metaphors operate.

Despite divergent theories of the ways in which metaphors operate, twentieth-century approaches have almost uniformly attempted to broaden traditional conceptions of metaphor as special use of language, offering an understanding of metaphor as a fundamental cognitive process or structure. In short, metaphor came to be seen as 'the omnipresent principle of language' (Richards), as a basic pattern of organizing and concertizing experience. No longer simply the domain of rhetoric or literary studies, metaphor has, over the past three decades, become a central topic of debate for fields like psychology, linguistics, philosophy, and the cultural studies of science.

Bodily metaphors

Throughout the latter half of the twentieth century, scholars have shown that many of our metaphorical expressions (along with much of thought itself) develop from our perceptions and experiences of the body. In her 1956 volume on reading poetry, *Modern English and American Poetry*, Margaret Schlauch suggested that one of the most basic types of metaphorical transfer is the naming of a new object through its resemblance to part of the body. Citing such examples as '*head*land', '*foot*hill', 'the *face* of a watch', and '*blind* alleys', Schlauch offered a comparison view of corporeal metaphor in which meaning is transferred from bodily parts and sensuous experiences to other objects on the basis of similarity.

Paul Ricoeur's 1978 essay, 'The Metaphorical Process as Cognition, Imagination, and Feeling', likewise claimed that the body should play a key role in our understanding of metaphor. In accordance with his view that there is a 'picturing function' of metaphorical meaning, Ricouer suggested that the term 'figure of speech' is rooted in our very understanding of the body as a figure. Just as the body twists and changes position, so, too, do metaphors, which 'turn' or 'twist' standard meanings through particular usages of words or phrases. According to Ricouer, figures of speech such as metaphor provide language with a 'quasi-bodily externalization'; in making abstract or foreign concepts more tangible, metaphors 'embody' ideas, offering a 'figurability to the message'.

The body's role in shaping metaphors and cognition was expanded and refined in Mark Johnson's 1987 book, *The Body in the Mind*. Breaking with objectivist views on metaphor and meaning, Johnson asserted that human embodiment is central not only to metaphorical projection, but also to our most basic processes of developing and articulating meaning. Johnson argued that metaphor, one of our primary cognitive structures for ordering experience, stem from fundamental embodied schema relating to the body's movements, orientation in space, and its interaction with objects. The body's general upright position in space, for instance, creates a 'verticality' schema, which influences numerous metaphors. When we speak of 'upscale living', and use expressions like 'she's on top of it' or 'he was down on himself', we are using metaphors based on a hierarchy derived from the body's orientation in space. The body's interaction with objects likewise contributes to the general metaphorical correlation of 'up' (as opposed to 'down') with 'more'; as we observe through our bodily interactions, when we add liquid to a container or magazines to a pile, the level increases. Thus even phrases like 'falling stock prices' and 'rising costs' derive their abstract representation of quantity through basic bodily experience. Other embodied schemata that are projected through metaphorical networks include: balance, in/out, front/back, contained/uncontained, and force or weight. Although revolutionary in its examination of the ways in which human embodiment is encoded into metaphor, Johnson's work has been critiqued by feminist scholars like Katherine Hayles for its failure to account for individual and cultural bodily specificities like gender, ethnicity, and physical ability.

In addition to influencing the names we give to objects and basic patterns of metaphorical thought, the human body has also had an impact on many of the metaphors we employ to describe society. Perhaps the most prevalent of these bodily metaphors, the *body politic* has contributed to our understanding of institutions like the state and church since the age of Pericles in ancient Greece. Whether in Plato's *Republic*, where the problems of the *polis* are metaphorized as diseases, or St, Paul's writings, in which the Church is compared to a human body with unified 'members', the metaphor of the body politic has shaped the way scholars have envisioned the hierarchies and interrelationships between various elements of society. Indeed, we still speak of 'heads of state', 'governing bodies', and crime as 'a social disease'.

Metaphors for the body

Just as the body has played a crucial role in influencing our metaphorical networks, so too have metaphors shaped our understanding of the body. Metaphors for the body are as diverse as the cultures and civilizations that have created them; however, several key metaphors can be identified as central to Western thought. Dating back to Plato's *Cratylus*, the metaphor of the body as a prison or house for the soul has influenced philosophical, religious, and other cultural attitudes toward the body — especially the mind/body dualism. At the heart of Plato's metaphor is the notion that the true essence of human beings lies in their soul or spirit; the body is alien, brute matter, a vessel for the soul/mind. The metaphor of the body as dungeon or house took on particular gendered implications with Aristotle's writings on the *chora* and reproduction, which contend that the mother merely 'houses' the child, providing the shapeless matter, while the father provides the form or shape. In the New Testament and other early Christian writings, the body was again conceived of as a house or temple, offering the distinction between the immortal, god-given soul and the mortal, corruptible body in which it dwells.

Another primary metaphor in Western perceptions of the body and the mind/body split is the Cartesian metaphor of the human body as a machine. Intervening in the mechanism versus vitalism debate, René Descartes suggested that the body (*res extensa*) could be understood as a self-moving machine composed of separate mechanisms that function according to the laws of nature. Descartes' metaphor of body as machine and its association of bodies (but not minds) with nature was fundamental in positioning the body as a universally knowable subject fit for scientific investigation. In the twentieth century, fields like art history and medicine used the body as machine metaphor in interesting new ways. Within the art world, the metaphor intersected with modernist theories of aesthetics, as artists like Fernand Léger and Marcel Duchamp depicted the body in an increasingly mechanized fashion. Drawing on earlier notions of a mechanistic body, and an understanding of the Fordist mass production system, the medical community utilized new cultural perceptions of the body through its metaphorical elaborations of the 'Fordist body'. As described by Emily Martin in '*The End of the Body?*', the Fordist body functioned according to principles of 'centralized control and factory-based production'. This metaphorical conception of the body not only created a hierarchy among bodily organs, with the brain (centralized control) at the top and the other organs below, but also caused the body to be considered in terms of productivity and efficiency.

Central to much recent work on embodiment is the metaphor of the body as a text or surface upon which our cultural and personal identity is written. Though widely used by many body theorists, the metaphor is most often associated with Michel Foucault. Drawing from Nietzschean notions of the body as a site of social incision, Foucault described the body as 'the inscribed surface of events' ('Nietzsche, Genealogy, History') and as an 'object and target of power' (*Discipline and punish*). For Foucault, the body became a text or a medium on which power operates, producing culturally and historically marked subjects.

Thus, as various feminist scholars have noted, cultural gender norms are 'written' on female and male bodies through diet, make-up, exercise, dress, footwear, and other practices. We should be careful, however, not to see the body solely as a blank slate awaiting cultural markings; as feminist philosophers Susan Bordo and Elizabeth Grosz point out, the materiality of the 'page' (the body itself) must be taken into consideration when we examine the ways in which bodies are culturally or otherwise inscribed.

The relationship between metaphor and the body is quite complex. Not only do metaphors affect our cultural perceptions of the body, but many of our metaphors and patterns of metaphorical cognition are shaped by our understandings of the body and embodiment. Thus, as science studies scholar Gillian Beer observes in '*Problems of description and the language of discovery*', metaphors are both descriptive and productive. As they move from level to level, cutting across disciplines with free movement and flexibility, metaphors become an important 'resource for discovery'; they become sites for reconceiving and recreating the body in new and exciting ways.

CHRISTINA JARVIS

Further reading

Grosz, E. (1994). *Volatile bodies: toward a corporeal feminism*. Bloomington and Indianapolis.

Johnson, M. (1987). *The body in the mind: the bodily basis of meaning, imagination, and reason*. Chicago and London.

Lakoff, G. and Johnson, M. (1980). *Metaphors we live by*. Chicago and London. Sacks, S. (ed) (1979). *On metaphor*. Chicago and London.

Metastasis Transfer of disease from one part of the body to another. The term is most commonly used in relation to tumours, when cancerous cells from the primary tumour break away, are carried in the blood or lymph, and lodge elsewhere, where a secondary tumour then forms.

A.W.C.

See CANCER.

Meteopathy or 'weather sense', is a word only recently introduced into English (from the French *météopathique*, Italian *meteopatico*, the nearest equivalent of which, in common parlance, is the expression 'under the weather').

Most people who live in urban societies claim to be unaffected by the weather. But for a minority, the approach of bad weather may be accompanied by unpleasant symptoms (headaches, limb pains, nausea, etc., depending on the individual), and of vaguer feelings better described as changes of mood (lethargy, uneasiness, irritability, depression). Conversely, when meteorological conditions improve, these individuals experience a sense of well-being and the adverse symptoms disappear. Although still not entirely scientifically respectable, there is interest in the biological basis of such phenomena. Indeed, a serious academic organ, the *International Journal of Biometeorology*, publishes research in this field.

Of particular interest, given the medical and economic consequences, is the Föhn effect (or Föhn illness) affecting people living in Geneva and southern Germany, where the Föhn winds, in their passage over the Alps, become electrically charged. At least one regional newspaper (the *Münchner Merkur*) carries a 'Bioweather' (*Biowetter*) forecast alongside the daily weather map. Similar geography produces an excess of positive over negative ions in Canada's chinook winds. The symptoms of so-called 'Pos-Ion' sufferers range from mild headaches to suicidal tendencies. The Meteorological Office, UK, does not measure atmospheric charge.

Rather little is known of the physiology or the functions of our 'weather sense'. The best physical predictor of meteorological change is atmospheric pressure, but sensory receptors responding to this stimulus have not been identified in the body of any animal. On the other hand, 'weather', as distinct from climate and season, is not so much a physical as a perceptual concept — made up of local phenomena that alter from day to day and hour to hour. The changes in temperature, humidity, air movement, and light produced by a rise or fall of the barometer can all be picked up, consciously or unconsciously, by traditional sense organs. The EYE, acting as a light meter, by way of the small number of optic nerve fibres that run directly to the HYPOTHALAMUS, can monitor the drop in light intensity as cloud cover builds up. The SKIN, with its hair follicles and many free nerve endings, might be responsible for 'Pos-Ion' sensitivity and for sensing the excess of negative charge associated with good weather.

Neural centres for integrating such diffuse information, and perhaps for altering sensitivity to pain and other stimuli, are likely to be in the parts of the brain responsible for sleep, wakefulness, and motivation. Like the weather states they mirror, the moods of meteopathics vary over a wide range.

The experiences of meteopathics are usually explained away in pathological terms (as disturbance of normal functioning). But that overlooks a possible biological function: a 'predictive' role essential for the survival of our hunter-gatherer ancestors. Great adaptive value would attach to any and all senses that altered mood and motivations in advance of a storm or to prepare for a spell of fine weather. The same would hold for other animals. Pathological consequences of our 'weather sense' may arise from man-made environments that inadvertently mimic certain weather conditions. This might account for so-called 'Sick Building' syndrome.

Conversely, the view that meteopathy is evolutionarily adaptive may be extended to some of the manifestations of the condition called Seasonal Affective Disorder (SAD). A craving for carbohydrates, weight increase, hypersomnia, mild depression, and inertia, which trouble some people, especially women, during the autumn months, have all been regarded as the body preparing itself for the 'natural' hardships of winter. The fact that bright light is effective in treating SAD, especially if delivered in the morning (10 000 lux for half an hour, or lower intensities for much longer, irrespective of wave length), supports the hypothesis that SAD is triggered by a decline in the amount of daylight in northern latitudes during the latter part of the year. Phototherapy, with light influencing the PINEAL GLAND, probably via the optic nerve fibres that run to the hypothalamus, alters the production of the chemical transmitters, melatonin and serotonin, which, in turn, influence bodily rhythm and mood. Perhaps the pineal gland, that ancient third eye, considered by René Descartes to be the seat of the soul, had the more prosaic but still somewhat intangible function of keeping the body in harmony with the seasons, much as neighbouring parts of the brain kept it in tune with the weather. ANDREW PACKARD

See also BODY CLOCK; BRAIN STEM; HYPOTHALAMUS; PAIN; PINEAL GLAND; SLEEP.

Microorganisms

These are microscopic forms of life which are ubiquitous in the environment and on the human body. They were first detected in 1675 by a Dutch draper, Anthony van Leeuwenhoek, who noticed tiny 'animalcules' in droplets of rainwater under his microscope. He went on to discover that they were present in dental plaque, faeces, and many other substances.

Most microorganisms are harmless or even beneficial to man. Only a minority cause disease in healthy humans (although many more may do so in patients with damaged immune systems). Thus it may not be so surprising that it was another 112 years after van Leeuwenhoek's discovery before it was shown that these minute creatures were also under certain circumstances the agents of disease: this was first demonstrated by Agostino Bassi in 1835 for a bacterial infection of silkworms. The German Robert Koch was the first to prove that a bacterium could cause a human disease, namely anthrax, in 1876. Naturally this discovery aroused huge scientific and public interest, although of course there were those in both the lay and the scientific communities who were opposed to the new theory of infection. This is the subject of Ibsen's play *An Enemy of the People*, in which the town doctor learns that the presence of bacteria in the water supply might transmit diseases such as typhoid and cholera. He campaigns to have the water cleaned, but the whole idea of tiny invisible 'animals' is met with ridicule by the community and his career is ruined.

The study of microorganisms is known as microbiology and not surprisingly much of the study is directed at those organisms which do cause human disease. It is now realized that not only are microorganisms responsible for what are conventionally considered 'INFECTIOUS DISEASES' but they may also contribute to such diverse illnesses as peptic ulcers, angina, and cervical cancer. There is no doubt that in the future microorganisms will be found to be involved in many more 'non-infectious' diseases. However, they are also essential to human life. Every square inch of our body surface is colonized by many thousands of organisms which help to protect the body from invasion by other potentially harmful organisms. If this normal 'flora' is damaged, for instance by a course of antibiotics, it leaves the way open for the harmful organisms to get a foothold and establish themselves instead. Microorganisms are also employed in a wide variety of home and industrial processes. For example, yeasts are essential for making bread rise and for the process of alcohol fermentation; genetically engineered bacteria are used to make insulin and in the production of genetically modified foods.

Microorganisms are classified into BACTERIA, VIRUSES, fungi, and PARASITES. PRIONS, which are thought to be infective protein particles rather than live organisms, are included also in the field of microbiology. These groups are totally unrelated to one another, the only common factor being that they are all microscopic.

Bacteria

These are single-celled organisms, usually either rod-shaped or roughly spherical. They are classified according to their reaction to Gram's stain: those that go blue with this stain are termed Gram positive, those staining red are Gram negative. This reflects a fundamental difference in the structure of their cell walls. They are responsible for diseases ranging from typhoid, plague, cholera, meningococcal meningitis, tuberculosis, tetanus, gonorrhoea, and syphilis, to the more mundane urinary tract infections, boils, and acne. They are killed by antiseptics and by boiling, although they may produce toxins which are not destroyed. Many were originally sensitive to antibiotics such as penicillins, but overuse of these drugs has resulted in many multi-resistant bacteria. The most notorious is multi-drug resistant tuberculosis. In terms of numbers, however, the greatest problem in the UK has been methicillin resistant *Staphylococcus aureus*, or MRSA. Although often it merely colonizes the skin and causes no harm, it can cause a wide range of infections and is difficult to treat. Great attempts have been made to limit its spread in hospitals, for instance by placing patients carrying the organism in isolation rooms.

Viruses

These are even tinier than bacteria and cannot be seen through a light microscope: electron microscopy is required. Their name comes from the Latin for 'toxin'. Their existence was first suspected when it was found that some infectious agents could pass through a fine filter, unlike bacteria, which were too large. They are very simple life forms, often consisting simply of a DNA or RNA core and a protein coat. They cannot reproduce except inside another living cell, which they must hijack in order to do so. They are susceptible to heat and to some antiseptics.

The most high-profile virus of recent years has been the human immunodeficiency virus — HIV — which causes AIDS. Other viral illnesses include influenza, the common cold, Lassa fever, and ebola. There have been few anti-viral drugs available, and the main line of defence has been vaccination, which has eradicated smallpox and may do the same for polio in the near future. Unfortunately, many viruses, including those causing HIV and the common cold, have a very high rate of genetic change so that they can evade the immune system, which makes the development of vaccines extremely difficult. Recently there have been great advances in the treatment of HIV with the development of 'triple therapy', or 'highly active anti-retroviral therapy' (HAART). This consists of the use of three or sometimes more drugs together to combat the infection, and has been highly successful in slowing the progression of the disease to full-blown AIDS. The use of the combination of drugs prevents the virus from becoming drug-resistant so rapidly.

Fungi

Like bacteria, microscopic fungi are everywhere. They may be yeasts or moulds. Yeasts have been used for centuries by peoples worldwide to ferment sugar to alcohol; the drug penicillin was found in a mould. They have a very resilient cell wall, which makes them difficult to treat. The commonest fungal infections are vaginal thrush, which often occurs after a course of antibiotics has destroyed the normal vaginal bacteria, and nail and skin infections such as 'ringworm'.

In the UK more serious fungal infections are generally only found in seriously immune-deficient patients, such as leukaemia or AIDS patients. However, in other parts of the world there are fungi which can cause severe disease in healthy individuals.

Parasites

These are organisms which live in or on the body of another known as the 'host'. The host may provide a source of nutrients or a safe haven in which to reproduce. They range in size from single cells, like the malaria parasite, to tapeworms which may reach thirty feet in length and hence are not microscopic at all! Parasites are mainly a problem of developing countries, although some, such as thread worm, are also common in the UK.

Prions

These are the simplest infectious particles known, now widely accepted as the cause of a group of degenerative diseases of the brain that includes Creutzfeld–Jacob disease (CJD) in humans, bovine spongiform encephalopathy (BSE) in cattle and scrapie in sheep. Since the BSE epidemic in Britain in the 1980s there has been concern that a new variant of CJD may be transmitted to humans who eat the meat (specifically nervous tissue) of infected cattle. Prions are thought to consist merely of a protein with no DNA or RNA so in this sense are not 'live'. They are nonetheless infectious because when the abnormal prion protein comes into contact with a similar but normal protein it causes a change in the way the normal protein molecule is folded up. This turns the normal protein into another abnormal protein, which alters other nearby proteins in turn, and so on until disease is evident. No treatment is available for prion diseases; also prions can withstand heat, desiccaion and conventional antiseptics, making safe disposal of infected material very difficult.

In the 1960s and 70s the rapid expansion in the number of antibiotics being developed led man to believe that he had won the battle against infection with microorganisms, but it is now evident that this is far from being the case. The emergence of new viruses and prion diseases, together with ever more antibiotic-resistant organisms, makes the study of microorganisms as urgent as ever.   ANGHARAD DAVIES

See also EPIDEMICS; IMMUNIZATION; INFECTIOUS DISEASES; PRIONS.

Microscopy
A microscope is an instrument that enables one to observe objects too small to be seen clearly by the naked eye. The microscope that is most familiar and most widely used for biomedical examination is the optical or light microscope, typically using visible light to study a transparent specimen mounted on a glass slide, which produces an optical image directly on the retina of the observer.

History
The use of light microscopes for biological studies was pioneered by the English scientist Robert Hooke (1635–1703), who first used the term 'cells' to describe the cavities he saw within sections of cork, and by Antoni van Leeuwenhoek (1632–1723), a Dutchman who created single lens microscopes of extraordinary resolving power unequalled by the later compound microscopes until the mid nineteenth century. Using these, he was the first to describe red blood cells, sperm, protozoa, and even bacteria.

Between the early eighteenth century and the mid nineteenth century, increasingly elegant and sophisticated compound light microscopes were developed; these involved separate lenses at the eye (eyepieces) and above the specimen (objective lenses). But since lens design was an empirical art, with little understanding of the optical principles governing image resolution, these microscopes were of little use for serious scientific research, and largely remained the playthings of gentleman naturalists.

Modern light microscopy can be dated from 1866, when Carl Zeiss (1816–88), a microscope manufacturer in Jena, Germany, invited a young physicist named Ernst Abbe (1840–1905) to join him as research director. Over the next decade, Abbe determined the principles of image formation in compound light microscopes, and the Zeiss workshop started producing rather plain-looking optical microscopes of exceptional optical performance and resolving power, equipped with objective lenses of near theoretical perfection. Subsequent advances in optical microscopy

have principally been concerned with the development of novel contrast generation techniques.

The twentieth century also witnessed the invention of many other ingenious forms of microscope, employing electrons, sound, X-rays, surface probes, or electromagnetic radiation outside the visible spectrum to generate their images. Since the human eye can only image visible light, the images generated by these other types of microscope must all be converted into some form of optical image in order to be perceived.

Microscope design and image formation
All microscopes fall into one of two classes. The first, the 'full field' microscopes, include conventional light microscopes, ultraviolet and infra-red microscopes, and transmission electron microscopes. In these, the entire field of view of the specimen is simultaneously illuminated by the incident radiation, and this radiation, after being modified in some way by the specimen, is focused to form a real image which is then observed. The other class is that of the 'point scanning' microscopes, in which the specimen is interrogated point by point, by moving a focused incident beam of illumination or a physical scanning probe line by line along a regular roster through or across the surface of the specimen. In this way, the resulting image is built up point by point, usually electronically on a video monitor or similar display device. Microscopes in this class include the scanning electron microscope, the acoustic microscope, the confocal light microscope, and a wide variety of scanning probe microscopes, including the scanning tunnelling microscope and the atomic force microscope, in which a physical probe is moved over the surface of the specimen.

The characteristics of microscope imaging systems
Whatever the microscope type, the imaging system has three characteristics that the user must understand in order to appreciate the significance of the image formed, which differs from the specimen itself in significant ways. The first and most obvious of these is the *magnification*, which can range from as little as ten times in a binocular dissection microscope used to observe structures in the millimetre range, to more than a million times in electron microscopes used to observe individual metal atoms about 0.15 nanometres ($1 \, nm = 10^{-9}$ metres) in diameter.

The second characteristic is the *minimum resolvable distance* (also referred to as the *resolution* or *resolving power*) of the microscope, defined as the distance separating two point objects within the specimen that can just be distinguished from one another in the image. In a high quality light microscope employing an oil immersion objective lens of the highest numerical aperture (NA 1.4), with which the image quality approaches theoretical perfection, the minimum resolvable distance is a little less than half the wavelength of the illuminating light employed, thus being about 240 nm for green

light of wavelength 546 nm. In contrast, the magnetic lenses of even the best electron microscopes are far from perfect, with low numerical aperture and severe lens aberrations, limiting the minimum resolvable distance to about 0.1 nm, many times the wavelength of the electrons employed. For the scanning electron microscope and the confocal light microscope, the minimum resolvable distance is determined in part by the diameter of the focused electron or light beam striking the specimen, while with scanning probe microscopes the resolution is a function of the sharpness of the scanning tip employed. Magnification and image resolution are related in the sense that the image must be sufficiently enlarged for the eye to be able to appreciate the fine details that are resolved within it. However, magnification beyond this range is termed 'empty magnification', since it reveals no further detail in the specimen.

The final characteristic of the imaging system is the most variable, both between different types of microscope and also within a single type. This is the *contrast generation mechanism*. In the light microscope, for example, images can be formed by absorption contrast using stained or naturally pigmented specimens, by polarization contrast using birefringent specimens, or by fluorescent emission from autofluorescent or fluorescently labelled specimens. They can also be formed by dark ground illumination, by reflection techniques such as reflection interference contrast microscopy, or by a variety of interference techniques. In these, cunning optical tricks are performed with the light that is transmitted by the specimen, enabling refractive index changes in transparent and otherwise almost invisible specimens (including living cells) to be converted into intensity variations within the image. Other forms of microscopy measure different properties of the specimen. The acoustic microscope, for example, can be used to image changes in the mechanical properties of the specimen, including the elastic modulus, viscosity, thickness or density, enabling one, for example, to distinguish bone from cartilage. Contrast within transmission electron microscope images directly reflects the distribution of atoms within the specimen, particularly atoms of high atomic number that are often used to stain regions of the specimen selectively. These scatter electrons beyond the limiting angle of the objective aperture, leaving fewer to contribute to the image of that region, which thus appears dark. While transmission electron microscopy requires an extremely thin specimen, typically only 100 nm thick — one ten thousandth of a millimetre! — scanning electron microscopy and the various scanning probe microscopies measure various characteristics of the surface of the specimen, which may therefore be thick and opaque.

Three-dimensional imaging in microscopy
While most microscopic images are two-dimensional, one of the most rewarding characteristics of many types of microscope is their ability to

provide three-dimensional information about specimens. The scanning probe microscopes can measure surface topology to high precision by recording the vertical excursions of the probe as it is scanned at a constant distance above the specimen surface. A transmission electron microscope image is an in-focus projection through the specimen. By recording multiple projection images while tilting the specimen in the electron beam, or alternatively by mathematically combining the images obtained from numerous identical objects observed in different orientations, the 3-D structures of such specimens can be determined. While the light microscope can be used to look within transparent specimens, the images conventionally obtained are combinations of in-focus information arising from the focal plane with out-of-focus information contributed by the regions of the specimen lying above and below this plane. This out-of-focus blur is one of the limiting factors of conventional light microscopy of thick specimens, particularly in fluorescence mode. However, the confocal fluorescence microscope avoids this problem by scanning the image point by point, while excluding light from out-of-focus regions by a simple optical device, the *confocal imaging aperture*, thus generating a blur-free optical section. By systematically changing the focal plane between successive acquisitions of such digital images, a set of optical sections can be non-invasively obtained which constitute a three-dimensional image of the transparent specimen. If this procedure is repeated at regular time intervals on a *living* specimen, a sequence of 3-D images may be obtained, forming a four-dimensional image with the dimensions of *x, y, z,* and *time,* enabling, for instance, dynamic cellular processes to be observed.

Such techniques, together with *cryo electron microscopy* — a method whereby thin aqueous specimens are vitrified by ultra-rapid cooling, and then observed in the hydrated vitreous state while maintained at below −100°C on the cold stage of a cryo electron microscope — have revolutionized biomedical microscopy in the last two decades, enabling us to determine the 3-D structures of virus particles, crystalline membrane proteins, and macromolecular complexes such as ribosomes, to study changes in the 3-D distribution of known proteins within living cells, and to image cellular physiological responses such as fluctuations of ionic concentrations and membrane potential. For these reasons, microscopy remains the most powerful and versatile of all biomedical research techniques. DAVID M. SHOTTON

Further reading

Royal Microscopical Society's *Microscopy Handbooks Series.* Oxford University Press and Bios Scientific Publishers, Oxford.

Celis J. E. (ed.) (1997) *Cell biology: a laboratory handbook,* 2nd edn, Vol. 3. Academic Press, San Diego.

For examples of images see BLOOD VESSELS; DEAFNESS; GLYCOGEN; LUNGS; MYELIN; NEUROMUSCULAR JUNCTION.

Migraine Migraine comes from the Greek 'hemicrania', or half-sided HEADACHE, and is in essence a form of 'primary headache', which is to say that the headache is itself the disorder and is not secondary to some other process, such as infection or injury. Migraine has been recognized throughout recorded history and there are reasonably clear descriptions that date back to Sumarian times. Migraine is as real as high blood pressure or a broken bone. It is an important, biologically-based disorder that should never be thought of as psychosomatic. Migraine is characterized by episodes of often severe, usually one-sided, frequently throbbing or pounding pain, associated with other features, such as nausea or vomiting, sensitivity to body movement, sensitivity to light (*photophobia*), or sensitivity to sound (*phonophobia*).

Migraine is probably best viewed as an inherited tendency to have headache, or perhaps *headacheyness,* rather than just the limited view of episodes of severe headache. Certainly many migraine patients suffer very severe, disabling headache that does not shorten life but can make it virtually a living hell. However, a broader view is necessary to explain everything that the physician encounters, and other aspects of the problem may dominate in the individual.

The frequency of migraine varies greatly between individuals — occurring almost every day, once or twice a year over many years, or just a few times in a whole lifetime. The biology of migraine does not always obey the rather strict rules that have been evolved to describe it: although these are very useful for research, one should not be a slave to rules for a problem with such a complex biology.

The cause and incidence of migraine

Migraine is probably for the most part inherited. It is thought to be *autosomal dominant* (see GENETICS, HUMAN), which means that about half the children of an affected parent will carry the genes irrespective of sex. Its expression in any one patient varies and so while most migraine sufferers will have an affected relative this is not always the case. Migraine can start at almost any time in life but the peak incidence is in the 20s and 30s. About 4–6% of children are affected, slightly more boys than girls, and about 10% of most adult Caucasian populations that have been studied. Probably fewer people are affected in African populations, and fewer still in oriental Asian populations. At puberty, with the onset of menstrual periods, the prevalence (number of people with the problem) of migraine increases in females and remains greater than in males right up to the 80s. The peak prevalence is about the age of 40; in this age-group about 1 in 5, or 20%, of adult Caucasian women have migraine. This is an enormous public health issue that has barely been addressed, yet has been with humans for several millennia.

Migraine aura — the flashing lights and zigzags

Migraine aura is a very special part of the problem that affects only about 20% of sufferers. It consists of zigzag flashing lights, loss of vision, bright sparkles, pins and needles over the face or arms, or even weakness, speech problems, or balance problems. Aura usually comes at the beginning of an attack and lasts about 30 min; less commonly it can occur during or even after the headache; it very rarely lasts more than an hour. It has two very important features: firstly, it moves slowly across the field of vision, or up or down the limb, almost never moving suddenly; and secondly, it is completely reversible — it always gets better. Changes to such symptoms should result in prompt medical review. Recently, the nature of a very special, rare form of aura, called *hemiplegic aura,* involving complete loss of use of the limbs on one side, has been elucidated. It is often due to a mutation, a change in the gene for a particular protein that allows electrically charged chemicals into body cells and controls the release of messenger molecules in the brain. These mutations on chromosomes 1 and 19 are pointing to ways in which we might understand how ordinary migraine starts: this is an active area of research.

The pain of migraine

This does not have a single explanation, which is perhaps why it has been difficult to characterize precisely. The PAIN in migraine involves abnormal signals in nerve fibres from the large blood vessels in the head — both from those within the skull (brain blood vessels) and also some from outside the skull, as well as from the protective covering of the brain, the MENINGES, particularly the tough fibrous part, the *dura mater.* The brain does not feel pain itself but because of an episodic defect in the nerve systems that control pain and other signals coming into the brain, normal or somewhat abnormal signals are amplified. So a normal or slightly dilated blood vessel gives a pounding or throbbing pain, often in time with the pulse. The pain is felt on the forehead, behind the eyes, over the top, around the sides, or over the back of the head, because the nerves that take pain signals from all over the inside of the skull go to the same place in the brain stem, to the *trigeminal nucleus.* Just as it can be impossible to locate the source of pain arising from organs in the body cavities — the abdomen or the chest — so migraine pain can be all over the head, or just on one side, or just in one place, wherever the source of the signals. Pain location in migraine, particularly over the back of the head, does not therefore necessarily implicate that area as diseased. This applies, for example, to the neck, which is often blamed for migraine but is seldom the true cause. The poor location of pain from within body cavities, referencing it elsewhere, is called *referral of pain,* and is a well-established, important concept that also applies to migraine. Referral of pain takes place because pain fibres from a deep structure, (such as, in this case, a brain blood vessel), and a superficial structure (such as the skin), both project to the same nerve cell in the trigeminal nucleus. The body cannot thus distinguish where the signal comes from, and wrongly attributes, or 'refers', the pain to the skin or other superficial structure.

The other symptoms of migraine can be thought of broadly as sensitivities to various things: movement, noise, light, smells, even something in the stomach to cause nausea (although we currently think that nausea has an important component from connections of the pain nerves with nausea cells in the brain). The areas in the human brain that have been shown to be active in migraine have two very interesting roles in normal physiology. One area in the brain stem controls, 'gates', or modulates incoming sensory information. It allows us to concentrate on something and to ignore irrelevant noise or even tactile (feeling) information. It is likely that this area, called the *nucleus locus coeruleus*, dysfunctions in migraine so that normal light or sound are perceived by the brain as too bright or loud, or normal smells as unpleasant. Many migraine sufferers report that their brain seems clouded, they cannot concentrate, and their thought processes are just not right. It seems likely that it is abnormalities in the locus coeruleus and associated areas that form the basis of the biology of these very real symptoms. One of the areas shown by imaging techniques to be active in migraine is also active during sleep induction, so it is no surprise that migraine sufferers for thousands of years have appreciated the benefit of sleep.

Much has changed in our understanding of migraine in the last decade, such that sufferers can now be given a reasonable explanation of most of their symptoms and thus be optimistic that soon their disease will be even better understood.

Meanwhile, the main thing that sufferers can do is to understand their limits. Many triggers for migraine can be identified, such as STRESS. (However, stress can trigger just about any type of headache, and there can therefore be no distinct thing called *stress headache*.) Environmental situations, some chemicals and foods, and a host of other situations are patient-specific triggers. These triggers have one general theme. The migraine sufferer is less tolerant of altering circumstances — such as skipping meals or eating late (and this is particularly true of children). They may not tolerate stress but, in an apparent paradox, may also get headache when they relax, or when they over-sleep or under-sleep, or when they exercise too much or not enough. In short, the migraine sufferer must be a little more careful with their life and think out what situations they can avoid; this may apply particularly to women during the menstrual cycle.

The remedy then is to exercise, eat, and sleep regularly and perhaps, oddly enough, always have a little stress! If one has headaches on Saturday mornings, is it just because of 'sleeping in', or because of the sudden relaxation at the end of a hard week, or even a change in caffeine consumption? Often a simple solution is to get up at a similar time to the weekdays and organize something to do. A trap for people to watch out for if they suffer headache regularly — and perhaps particularly migraine — is that of analgesic over-use. Over time, many patients increase their use of over-the-counter or even prescribed medications to a point where they get a 'rebound headache': as the dose of the headache medication wears off the headache comes back and more medication is taken. A vicious cycle commences that may require medical intervention.

A doctor who is consulted about migraine will want to take a medical history to be sure of the diagnosis, compared with other forms of headache, and to make a full clinical examination. The approximate rule for headache action is that new or changing headache, especially of sudden onset, requires urgent attention, while persistent long-standing headache requires time, patience, and thought when planning management. Among the many other questions that might be asked, one of the most important pieces of information can be what medication has been used in the past, in what amounts, and for how long.

With detailed information from the patient about the nature and pattern of the pain, and with knowledge gleaned from experimental work from the last ten to fifteen years, migraine is now relatively well understood and can be better managed than at any time in the last 4000 years. Treatments include preventative medicines and those for use in acute attacks. The preventative medicines are drawn from a number of other areas of medical practice; migraine is not *caused* by high blood pressure, depression, or epilepsy, but the drugs used in treating these conditions work also in migraine and should be viewed as anti-migraine drugs. (Thus they include β blockers, serotonin blockers, antidepressants, or anticonvulsants.) For acute attacks, there are the common pain-killers such as aspirin or paracetamol, together with an anti-sickness tablet, such as domperidone, or so-called Non-Steroidal Anti-Inflammatory Drugs (NSAIDs), again with an anti-sickness medicine. There are also drugs specific for migraine, and for a rare form of headache called cluster headache, but not generally useful for other headaches, there are the *ergot* derivatives, and the family of *triptans*. The triptans were developed specifically for migraine and are certainly the most effective and best studied medicines for the condition.

There is currently considerable research into the condition. It is better understood than it has ever been, and this level of knowledge deepens with time. As understanding improves so does treatment.   PETER J. GOADSBY

Further reading

The Migraine Trust and Migraine Action Association (UK) and The American Council for Headache Education (USA) publish various information for sufferers and doctors.

Goadsby, P. J. and Silberstein, S. D. (ed.) (1997). *Headache*. Butterworth-Heinemann, New York.

Lance, J. W. and Goadsby, P. J. (1998). *Mechanism and management of headache*, (6th edn). Butterworth-Heinemann, London.

See also HEADACHE.

Mind–body interaction The assumption that there is an identity of, or a close link between, mind (*psyche*) and body (*soma*) is as old as Western medical thought. This link underlies much of the understanding of madness and its somatic basis in the modern age. But this tradition has its roots at the very beginnings of modern thought about the body and the psyche. Greek humoural theory, as presented in the Hippocratic corpus, postulated a relationship between the vital fluids and the manifestations of mind and character. Thus the dominance of blood presented a sanguinary humour; of phlegm, a phlegmatic one; of bile, a bilious one; of black bile, a melancholy one. It was not that the vital fluids generated the character, but that the character and the humour were vitally linked. Thus childhood and its mindset was the age in which blood dominated; youth, that of bile; adulthood, that of black bile; and old age, that of phlegm. Imbalance of the humours resulted in various temperaments, thus the dominance of black bile causes melancholy; blood, sanguine temperament; phlegm, a phlegmatic temperament; or yellow bile, a choleric temperament. Such a conception of the relationship between the mind and the body informs many different discourses — medical, philosophical, and cultural.

The medical views of the Greeks came to be recycled in complex ways in eighteenth-century Europe. They helped shape the views, for example, of the *physiognomists*, such as the eighteenth-century Swiss divine, Johann Caspar Lavater, who believed that character and the body were one. Philosophical approaches in the seventeenth century, such as those of René Descartes and Gottfried Wilhelm Leibniz, provided models for the relationship between the mind and the body. *Monistic* theories, such as those of Descartes, saw the mind and body as one unit, with all aspects of one present automatically in the other. Leibniz's views were not quite as schematic, yet he believed that each aspect of the human being was necessarily linked in a 'predisposed harmony' with other aspects. Such views attempted to bridge long-held dualistic views that mind and body were separate entities that bore little or no relationship one to the other. Such theories saw 'madness' as a sign of imbalance.

The modern medical view was set at the turn of the eighteenth century with the rise of the concept of PSYCHOSOMATIC ILLNESS — illness that arises in the mind but has bodily as well as psychological symptoms. Building on German Romantic thought, psychiatrists, such as Johann Heinroth and Karl Wilhelm Ideler, evolved complex ideas of the relationship between illnesses of the mind and the state of the body. Your body is what your mind deems it to be. Mental illness, illness of the psyche, could also be illness of the body. These followers of the 'psychic' theory assumed the primacy of the mind over the body. Such views ran parallel to the views of materialist physicians of the time, the so-called 'somaticists', such as Wilhelm Griesinger, who, seeing the mind (and mental illness) as a product of the brain, argued that 'mind illness is brain illness'. All assumed that 'mental illness' (always differently defined) was the core phenomenon that would prove their views. The former gave rise to the theories of *psychosomatic* illness; the latter to theories of *somatopsychic* illness.

If one could show that the ill mind could create pathological effects in the body in the form of specific and definable symptoms, or the other way around, one could move to treat one aspect of the monistic body/mind by treating the other. Mental illness was the means by which the physician could show the relationship between the ill body and the ill mind: *Mens non sana in corpore insano.*

It was not by chance that this view began to dominate the understanding of the body with the German Romantics at the beginning of the nineteenth century. The fascination with the 'nightside' of life, with the ill and the corrupt as well as with the psychologically unstable, became one of the hallmarks of Romantic fantasy. The philosophical question came to be about where the interaction between mind and body took place. Carl Gustav Carus, in his book *Psyche* (1846), stated that the 'unconscious was the key to the knowledge of the conscious life.' This view dominated anti-materialist European medicine during the closing decades of the nineteenth century. Even materialists came to be influenced by this notion. Jean Martin Charcot, the leading neurologist of nineteenth-century Paris, thus moved from an interest in the somatic results of brain lesions to an understanding of the physical nature of hysterical symptoms as the result of some hidden physical trauma.

When Sigmund Freud came to study with Charcot during 1885–6, it was to learn more about juvenile neurological problems. In Paris he was confronted with Charcot's hysterical patients and their physical symptoms, and he returned to Vienna convinced that the hidden truth was somewhere between Carus and Charcot. During the 1880s and 90s Freud developed a complex theory of psychosomatic illness, locating in the unconscious the illness process that produced physical symptoms, such as the *globus hystericus* (inability to speak). His interest before 1895 focused on the conversion of psychological trauma into specifically related physical symptoms.

Freud's interest in psychosomatic illness lessened after 1895, and he abandoned his trauma theory, but he inspired a long line of psychoanalysts (from Georg Groddeck to Alexander Mitscherlich) to examine the questions of the origins of physical illness in the psyche. Of all the psychoanalysts to write on psychosomatic illness, none was more influential than the Berlin/Chicago psychoanalyst Franz Alexander.

In Alexander's work one can see the refining of Freud's views in Alexander's own distinction between conversion neurosis, functional illness, and psychosomatic illness. His most important work in this regard is *The Medical Value of Psychoanalysis* of 1936.

Other approaches, such as the return of the Hippocratic 'characters' in the form of the 'constitutional types' of Ernst Kretschmer, in the 1920s, led to work on a clinical theory of constitutions. Here the work of Friedrich Curtius on the psychosomatic basis of colitis and asthma is typical of the application of a twentieth-century theory of 'types' as a means of understanding how physical predisposition relates to mental and physiological states.

Of the early twentieth-century philosophers whose work served as an underpinning for much of the work on psychosomatics, none was more important than Victor von Weizsäcker, specifically in his 1898 study of *Pathophysiology*. For von Weizsäcker, illnesses differ from individual to individual, since each patient provides a different structure for his/her illness. Each illness is influenced by the psychic structure of the patient. These variations on the model of psychosomatic illness provide a wide range of positions for its possible interpretation.

The wide acceptance of the psychosomatic model was such that a whole range of popular as well as medical adaptations of it appeared during the mid-twentieth century. Thus in 1979 Norman Cousins, the former editor of the American *Saturday Review*, published what became a best-selling account of his overcoming of a collagen disease through his positive attitude under the title *Anatomy of an Illness as Perceived by the Patient: Reflections on Healing and Regeneration.* Such texts of self-help to overcome somatic illness through the improvement of attitude have become a staple of the English-language reading public. They rely on the audience's acceptance of a psychosomatic model that would imply conscious control over somatic illness and its psychological results. Be happy and you will not be sick, is their motto.

Conversely, the 'somatopsychic' model is closely related with theories of physical therapy (such as that of Moshe Feldenkrais) for the relief of psychic discomfort. Here the view is that a healthy body makes for a healthy psyche.

The rejection of mind–body dualism in the twentieth century was virtually total. Yet the problems of understanding how the 'mind' and the 'body' function remain. Indeed, the very continuation of a bipolar (if interconnected) model for 'mind' and 'body' suggests a continuing understanding of these as two different sites for illness and healing.   SANDER L. GILMAN

Further reading
Gilman, S. L. (1996). *Seeing the insane: a cultural history of psychiatric illustration.* University of Nebraska Press, Lincoln.
Shorter, E. (1993). *From paralysis to fatigue: a history of psychosomatic illness in the modern era.* Free Press, New York.
Shorter, E. (1994). *From the mind into the body: the cultural origins of psychosomatic symptoms.* Free Press, New York.

See also PHILOSOPHY AND THE BODY; PSYCHOLOGICAL DISORDER; PSYCHOSOMATIC ILLNESS.

Mind–body problem
The relation between mind and body lies at the heart of much philosophy.

Action, which (it seems) originates in the mind and results in bodily movements, raises many questions, most notably that of free will. It may be that every physical event is the inevitable result of past circumstances together with the laws of nature (*determinism*). If so, how could it ever be up to us, who have no control over the past or the laws of nature, what we do? As it happens, the behaviour of subatomic particles appears to obey only statistical laws, analogous to those governing games of chance; and so most physicists nowadays reject determinism. But it is no more evident how we could affect the paths of elementary particles via our intentions than it is how we could affect the distant past or laws of nature. A perennial philosophical research project is to try to explain what it is to have a choice about what one does that is compatible with determinism and other physical theories.

Another traditional problem about mind and body is what it takes for us to persist from one time to another: what makes some past or future being *you*, rather than someone else? (What would it take, say, for you to continue to exist after your biological death?) One answer is that you are that past or future being that has your mind — roughly speaking, the one whose life you can remember, or who can remember your life. A rival view is that our identity through time consists in some physical relation not involving the mind: you are that past or future being that has your body, or that is the same biological organism as you are. If your mind were destroyed in a way that left the rest of you relatively intact — if you were to lapse into a persistent vegetative state, for example — then according to the bodily approach the resulting being would be you, whereas on the psychological approach you would cease to exist.

But the paradigmatic 'mind–body problem' has to do with the nature of the mind itself. In particular, are mental phenomena in any sense physical? Do human beings think and feel solely by virtue of the workings of their brains and other organs? If so, *how* do thought and consciousness arise out of that biochemical machinery?

Mental phenomena are thought to have features that resist explanation in physical terms. For example, we know about our own sensations in a way that no one else possibly could, whereas physical phenomena are always publicly accessible, at least in principle. Some mental states seem to have an essentially subjective character that no physical state could have. Thought is intrinsically purposeful in a way that physical phenomena, which are fundamentally mechanical, could not be. And so on.

One response to these convictions is to deny that any physical body could be the subject of thought: mentality is an entirely non-physical phenomenon. You and I, since we do think, are therefore immaterial things (or at least have an immaterial part). On this view, associated with the French philosopher René Descartes (1596–1650), a perfect physical duplicate of you, with a brain identical to yours, might fail to be conscious, or even to have any psychological features at all, for such features reside in an immaterial thing that even the most sophisticated physical object might lack.

Cartesians have found it difficult to explain how the mind relates to the physical world. One problem is how something with no physical properties could affect, or be affected by, physical objects, as appears to occur in action and perception. Another is that having psychological features seems to admit of degrees, whereas something either definitely has or definitely lacks an immaterial part. Thus, there seems to be no principled way of saying when, in the development of a human being from an embryo, the organism comes to be associated with a Cartesian soul, or what animals besides human beings have one. And Cartesianism makes it surprising that damage to the brain should cause unconsciousness, rather than merely preventing one from moving or perceiving anything. Quite aside from these difficulties, Cartesians are as much in the dark about *how* non-physical things manage to think and feel as their opponents are about how physical things can do so.

Some anti-Cartesians deny that the mind exists at all. Logical behaviourists claim that when we use the language of psychology we are merely talking about how people are disposed to act, and not about any internal states. Eliminative materialists argue that the 'folk theory' of belief, sensation, consciousness, and other familiar mentalistic concepts is fundamentally mistaken and will one day be replaced by a science of behaviour that bears no more resemblance to traditional psychology than modern chemistry bears to alchemy.

Most of those working on the mind–body problem today believe that the mind is in some sense physical; but there is much disagreement about what this comes to. One view (the so-called *mind–brain identity theory*) is that psychological states are simply special physical states: for example, pain was once thought to be the firing of C-fibres. A more popular strategy is to identify mental features with functional properties: what makes something a pain is its characteristic causes (injury) and effects (groaning, worry, actions one believes will alleviate it) — much as what makes something a carburettor is the role it plays in the functioning of an internal combustion engine. Thus, pain might be a different state, as it were, in different creatures.

Others argue that, although mental phenomena are produced by the brain (and not by anything immaterial), they cannot be explained in physical terms, or at least not in the terms of current physical science. One intriguing suggestion is that the human mind is simply incapable of understanding itself, though there is nothing *intrinsically* mysterious about it.

ERIC T. OLSEN

Minerals Minerals are specifically inorganic compounds occuring naturally in the Earth's crust or lithosphere. They consist of a metal element in the form of a salt or oxide and are often crystalline in nature and usually highly insoluble, the more soluble salts having been washed from the land into the rivers and seas. Consider, for example, three calcium minerals; the fluoride, the phosphate, and the carbonate. The first, calcium fluoride or fluorspar, exists as beautiful crystals, often seen in caves, and is highly insoluble. However, in regions where it is found sufficient fluoride enters the drinking water to prevent dental caries, making fluoridation unnecessary. The second, calcium phosphate is modestly soluble, and may originate from the decayed teeth, bones, and sea shells of living creatures accumulated over aeons of time. It, together with calcium carbonate, or the chalk of limestone deposits, is what makes water 'hard' and furs up the kettle. Thus through the drinking water, even in those who do not consume dairy products (the major dietary source), the intake of calcium can be assured. Only in special circumstances is supplementation of calcium intake required, as in pregnancy. However, there is recent evidence that for the avoidance of osteoporosis in later life it is important for school-age girls to increase their calcium intake above the usual norm.

All the essential elements that are needed by the body in inorganic form have minerals as their source of origin, although many will be derived through the intermediacy of plant or animal material in the diet. For example, our small but essential need for manganese is satisfied through leafy vegetables, such as spinach. Where the mineral intake is inadequate we seem to know, adding that extra sprinkle of salt on our meals. Trace elements such as copper, molybdenum, and iodine, and even the somewhat larger requirement for iron, may be satisfied through the drinking water, but this has a geographic dependency, requiring that the water passes over appropriate minerals before entering the domestic supply. The THYROID GLAND needs iodine to make the hormone thyroxine. If the iodide content of the blood is too low the gland in the neck swells to produce a GOITRE. In the county of Derbyshire in England the local rocks are such that the iodide content of the drinking water is very low indeed, so that goitre was common in the region, where it was known as Derbyshire Neck. Goitre has now disappeared, as most table salt is iodised, either because sodium iodide is added to the sodium chloride in the preparation of table salt, or more generally because salt deposits containing traces of sodium iodide are used without attempting to remove the iodide. A more likely source of minerals other than

drinking water is provided by the food we eat, in which plants and animals have already accumulated what is necessary. Thus a healthy diet is one which contains all our needs, and we have presumably evolved so that all our mineral requirements are met in this way. Strict vegetarians and vegans are probably more aware of these requirements as, for example, it is difficult on a purely vegetable diet to maintain an adequate intake of vitamin B_{12}, with its essential cobolt mineral component. In this instance supplementation of the diet with cobalt salts does not help, as man cannot make the vitamin: it has to be supplied in the diet.

Our intake of iron is essential for maintaining red blood cell formation. Women have a higher requirement than men because of the monthly blood loss through menstruation. Many animal foods, such as liver, are a rich souce of iron, although iron supplementation in the aged and those who are slightly anaemic can be achieved with the mineral itself, in the form of iron sulphate tablets. Until the 1950s, and into the 1960s, iron tonics were popular over-the-counter products bought in chemists shops. One called 'Dr Parrish's Chemical Food' was particularly popular. The way it was made is of interest. Pure iron wire was weighed out and the calculated amount of phosphoric acid added, just sufficient to dissolve the wire. The resulting fluid was then mixed with syrup, and red colouring added to produce the tonic. In the eyes of the public it clearly contained real iron and would certainly give them strength. It was as if some believed that the wire was reconstituted in the body, adding some sort of steely structure to the human frame.

Today, in the developed world, it is difficult to be mineral deficient while eating a normal, balanced diet. However, in Victorian times it was common among the wealthier classes to visit health-giving spas in order to 'take the waters', which meant drinking quanties of water directly welling up out of the earth. The spas were often associated with hot water springs where the visitors would immerse themselves in pools. Some spas are of great antiquity, such as those started by the Romans all over Europe. The waters were often sulphurous and smelt rather badly of rotten eggs. The benefits of visiting spas probably owed more to a placebo effect than for any other reason. Even today many no longer drink tap water; bottled mineral water is the fashion. The labels on the bottles give long lists of the mineral contents. One well known brand of mineral water used to include on its label the amount of 'radioactivite'. Often hot spring waters come from great depths and are in contact with radioactive minerals, which impart traces to the water. In recent times the amount of 'radioactivite', which was in any event miniscule, has disappeared from the label. The reason that mineral water is popular today is less because of its mineral content but rather to avoid contaminants in tap water. The contaminants are usually the result of the use of agrochemicals, fertilizers, and sprays used to increase crop yields, which then get washed into rivers and reservoirs and hence into drinking water. The most common culprit is inorganic nitrate. Those who feel they are mineral deficient can avail themselves of numerous products in health shops, where tablets containing all the needed minerals in the correct ratios can be found.

ALAN W. CUTHBERT

See also COMPOSITION OF THE BODY; METALS IN THE BODY; SALT.

Mirrors Mirrors answer the desire to behold one's own image — to see oneself as others do. Optically speaking, a mirror is a reflecting surface that forms an image when light rays deflected by an object fall upon it. Nature provided the model: the reflective surface of still water, into which Narcissus so famously gazed. Both the absorption of Narcissus in himself — his vanity — and his fascination with himself as other are central to the mythology of mirrors. When mirrors allow us to see ourselves as others do, they are capable, at best, of initiating a sense of self and identity in the world (as per the psychoanalyst Jacques Lacan, who developed the theory of the 'mirror stage' of human development) — and, at worst, of engendering that self-reflexive form of love called vanity.

The earliest known man-made mirrors, circular discs of highly polished obsidian, were discovered in a Neolithic settlement in Anatolia, Turkey, and date to about 6000 BCE. Subsequently, discs made of copper and bronze — some with handles, some with stands — made their appearance throughout the Near East. Many of the mirrors of antiquity that have been unearthed appear to have served a religious purpose. The handles of several bronze and silver mirrors dating to *c.* 2000 BCE were papyrus-shaped, and resemble the handles of divine standards. Other handles are carved in the form of deities or, as in the case of several Late Period (*c.* 750–332 BCE) gilded-silver mirror handles, of four goddesses encircling a papyrus-shaped column.

The ancient Greeks developed the stand mirror — the bottom of whose handle was large enough to serve as a base — and the box mirror, the prototype of the twentieth-century powder compact. The lids of the latter type were frequently decorated with mythological and/or erotic scenes. The glass wall mirror seems to have gained popularity among the Romans around the first century BCE. Through trade with the Roman Empire, mirrors found their way to the Indian subcontinent.

In China, mirrors came into use around 2000 BCE. Like those of Egypt and Greece, early Chinese mirrors are typically round, made of bronze, and decorated on the back. Throughout much of Asia, mirrors were and still are thought to have the power to avert evil. As a result, mirrors were often buried with the dead, and mirrors are still to be seen on the exterior of South Asian temples: hideous demons, catching sight of themselves, will flee in fright.

In the Christianized West, on the contrary, soulless beings—vampires, werewolves, demons, and the like—were thought to show no reflection in a mirror. The reverse of this superstition was the belief that, after a death in the house, mirrors could hold the souls of the living and detain the soul of the deceased in its flight from the body. Enlightened physicians refused to be daunted, and it became a tradition for a mirror to be placed close to the mouth or nose of a moribund person to determine, by the misting of the mirror, whether the person was still breathing. A mirror–soul link persists in the taboo on breaking a mirror, which is popularly believed to bring seven years of bad luck. In some cultures, placing the shards in running water is thought to mitigate the harm.

In Europe throughout the Middle Ages, the possession of mirrors was limited to those of great wealth or high station. Various reflecting surfaces were used: polished metallic rocks such as obsidian, pyrite, and iron; rock crystal; and an alloy of rose copper and tin, plus an alchemical brew consisting of white arsenic, red tartar, and nitre. Meanwhile, artisans explored the effects of altering the surface, from flat to concave or convex. The Dutch painter Jan van Eyck (*c.* 1390–1441) incorporated a wall-mounted convex mirror to stunning effect in his double portrait, *The Arnolfini Wedding* (London, National Gallery), painted in 1434. The reflection serves not only to capture elements of the interior not otherwise in view (for example, the backsides of the couple, who face the viewer) but also to document the presence of two additional figures just visible in the reflection (one of whom is presumed to be the painter himself) as witnesses to the event taking place in the painting, which is thought to be the betrothal of the Arnolfini couple. Mirrors were subsequently included in numerous Flemish paintings, as homage to the naturalism of van Eyck, and to its capacity to replicate the surfaces of the visible world.

During the latter half of the fifteenth century, the glassmakers of Venice developed a clear, colourless glass called *cristallo*, which, backed with a coating of tin or mercury, provided a clearer reflection than previous mirrors. By the seventeenth century, Venice and the island of Murano were exporting mirror glass throughout Europe and as far east as the Indian subcontinent. The rage for mirrors reached an apogee in the construction of the great Hall of Mirrors at Louis XIV's palace at Versailles, completed in 1678; here the Sun King's magnificence could be endlessly reflected.

Throughout the later Middle Ages and the Renaissance, numerous books carried the word mirror in their titles (much as newspapers still do today—*The Daily Mirror*, or the *Tagesspiegel*), and the mirror also acquired a certain iconographical power in the visual arts. Mirrors were employed as symbols of truth, of deception, and of vanity. In all three cases, the mirror is thought to bear a particular relation to appearances, which may or may not be deceptive. In recent times, too, much has been made of over-investment (particularly by women) in the image of oneself encountered in the mirror. Deception by mirrors has a basis in optical principles, in so far as reflections in mirrors do not correspond wholly to the objects that caused them. This can easily be demonstrated by tracing the contour of the reflection of one's head in a mirror; the reflection may correspond in proportion, but will generally be half in actual size. Moreover, mirror images are two-dimensional; bodies are not.

The craft of mirror-making has made prodigious strides since the days when the Murano glassmakers painstakingly ground and polished glass until the surface was completely smooth, or for a convex mirror (such as the one whose properties van Eyck explored) carefully cut from a blown bubble as it was hardening. While fine mirrors are still made by these methods, most mirrors are made of 'float glass', a ribbon of glass that is run out of the furnace along the surface of a bath of molten tin. By controlling the temperature of both elements, both surfaces can be made perfectly flat. Generally speaking, there are three types of mirrors: the plane — which has a flat surface, the convex, and the concave — the latter two known collectively as spherical mirrors, because their surfaces are usually part of a sphere. Amusement park mirrors exploit the properties of spherical mirrors, bloating or shrinking and otherwise distorting the figures reflected in them.

The invention of the reflex camera in which a mirrored surface allows one to see exactly the image that will be captured on film, was a monumental advance, as it allows for the production of photographic images that actually correspond to what is viewed through the lens of the camera. Another technological application of mirrors, in telescopes, has allowed for enormous expansion of our visual horizon. Human interest in mirrors ultimately depends on cultural and technological faith in images, and the ability to correlate our understanding of things as they are with things as they appear.

CLAUDIA SWAN

Miscarriage The common term for what is technically known as *spontaneous abortion*. A pregnancy may be lost for many different reasons and most often the cause is elusive, without a definable abnormality of either the fetus or the womb. The popular fictional instances of a shock or an accident precipitating miscarriage are rare in real life. The commonest time is at around three months of pregnancy, when the fetal tissue of the placenta is completing the takeover, from the ovary, of the production of hormones necessary to maintain the quiescence of the muscle of the womb.

S.J.

See ABORTION; PREGNANCY.

Model, artist's Although models have been used since classical times, it was only with the establishment of life-drawing academies in the sixteenth century that working from the living

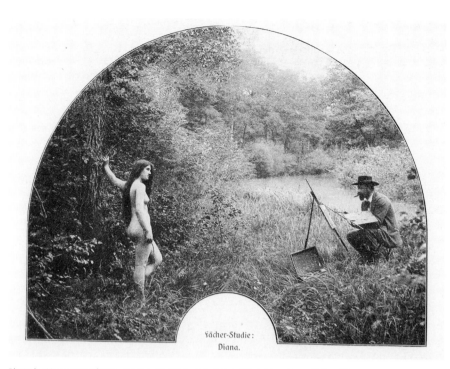

Photo by Hermann Ludwig von Jan in Weibliche Schrönhat, 1904. Mary Evans Picture Library

human figure became a staple activity of artistic training in the West. Male academic models comprised most of the profession until the nineteenth century, when female models, hitherto privately hired, were first permitted to pose in state-sponsored academies in Europe and the US. The figure of the nude model achieved an apotheosis during this period. With the ascendancy of the female model the nude took on a number of cultural meanings: having embodied the lofty purities of unmediated nature or classical formalism, and the frail contingencies of innocence or desire, the model also came to represent the gritty freedom of bohemia, and the stylish glamour of fashionable society.

In the art of the abstract, commercial twentieth century, models have resumed their two basic functions: presenting visual information about the body, and conveying visual effects with the body that will stimulate work in an artist. The method, however, varies greatly. In a drawing class, where the primary aim is to study the figure, models usually make their own poses, in accordance with an instructor's agenda. A sculptor working alone might position a model's body very precisely to study a particular visual phenomenon: light falling on a muscle insertion, a proportional relationship. Models can also be called upon to embody moods or ideas. An abstract painter might observe a model moving autonomously through a sequence of gestures from which to derive non-figurative images. The work ranges from that of a movie stand-in, who replicates a pre-existing image and sustains it for the purposes of observation, to a dancer, who enacts drama and composes space by means of bodily expression. Artists' models thus inhabit a rather curious intersection of seemingly

contradictory modes of embodiment: stasis and movement, activity and passivity, authority and submission. Physically, they have to exert themselves in order to remain motionless. As a performer, the model also projects a self-image that is thoroughly convincing and yet fulfills other people's imaginative demands. The job of posing is unquestionably gruelling and mundane: the most creative and spontaneous session is always ultimately a matter of endurance, flexibility, and timing. Yet the intimacy of the studio and the aspiration lurking in even the humblest forms of artistic labour are likewise undeniable, as are the potent and intricate politics of looking and showing. The artist demands a pose, the model complies; but once the model assumes the pose, the artist must pay attention. Nude or clothed, the model's motionless body becomes the prime mover of the artist's eye and hand. However engulfed in the quotidian they may be, artist and model relations are susceptible to inflections of eroticism, idealism, or romance.

ELIZABETH HOLLANDER

Further reading

Borel, F. (1990). *The seduction of Venus: artists and models*. Albert Skira, Geneva.

Borzello, F. (1982). *The artist's model*. Junction Books, London.

Modelling, fashion

Fashion modelling refers to the practice of displaying trends in costume, beauty, and grooming using human subjects or the human form. These displays may be performed as live fashion shows; they may be photographed and placed on billboards or in magazines; or they may be recorded as commercials or as television programmes.

Fashion modelling has existed for more than four centuries. Books of engravings — illustrating ancient, foreign, and contemporary fashion — became available with the invention of printing in the mid fifteenth century. In the seventeenth century, wooden DOLLS dressed in the most popular styles were sent to wealthy women in major European cities to entice them to purchase popular styles. The dressmaker of Marie Antoinette continued to exhibit her handiwork in this manner up until the end of the eighteenth century. At that time, the first fashion magazines, highlighting creations for royal courtiers, appeared and the fashion plate, or picture dedicated to showing the very latest mode, came into existence. Eventually, the term 'fashion plate', would describe both a fashion illustration and a woman who ostentatiously purchased fashionable costumes. Fashion PHOTOGRAPHY made its début in 1840 and ultimately replaced line drawing as the dominant way to depict current fashions.

In the 1850s, Charles Worth popularized the use of live models to sell clothes when he encouraged his wife to wear his creations and show them off to his clientele. The use of live models continued, and the runway (or 'catwalk') appeared in 1914 at a Chicago fashion exhibit. The runway allowed customers to inspect clothes while being entertained by extravagant fashion spectacles created by the hottest names in couture.

Modelling agencies (businesses that arrange contacts between models, designer, and sellers) owe their existence to the ingenuity of John Robert Powers, an out-of-work American actor of the early twentieth century. Powers realized a profit could be made by matching up attractive men and women with photographers and advertising companies. Modelling agencies, like Elite, Ford, and John Casablancas, still dominate the world of fashion. The twentieth century also witnessed the creation of the 'supermodel' — the highly paid paragon who displays not only coveted fashions but an enviable lifestyle as well.

The influence of modelling reaches far beyond the world of fashion. Many argue that female models do not serve as good examples for women to follow. The rail-thin appearance of many models has been cited as a factor contributing to EATING DISORDERS, such as anorexia nervosa and bulimia. Critics directed bitter attacks against the 'elegantly wasted' look (often achieved through extensive use of drugs) in vogue in the early nineties and embodied in the body of Kate Moss.

Male modelling has not been studied as extensively as female modelling. The research that has been done suggests that in the last three decades, with the increasing fashionability of sportswear for men, physical fitness and good health have become important ideals for the male body. Thus male models are not held up to the same standards of beauty and thinness that have dominated female modelling.

KAROL K. WEAVER

See also FASHION; FEMALE FORM.

Modesty Etymologically linked to the Latin *modestus*, 'keeping within measure', this term originally signified moderation, as in Cicero's 'golden mean of living'. Gradually, modesty took on the gendered connotation of a sexual virtue particularly important for women. Sixteenth-century writers commonly portrayed women as more lustful and unruly than men, but Christine de Pisan and other early feminists countered such misogyny with evidence of feminine modesty drawn from the historical record and from the female physique: women were by nature more modest than men because their private parts were covered with hair and did not require handling for urination.

Enlightenment theorists maintained such physical rationale and added a political resonance to the modest woman. According to Jean-Jacques Rousseau, modesty was a necessary virtue in women because of their physical and sexual weaknesses: only shame could save women from their 'insatiable desires'. If trained properly as demure wives and mothers, however, women could attain self control and contribute to national unity by channelling their husbands' drives into socially useful pursuits.

In the 1870s, Charles Darwin conceived a theory of female modesty to resolve an enigma left unsolved by his work on natural selection. Long puzzled by the brilliant plumage of male birds and the dowdiness of females, Darwin deduced that such splendour must be necessary to prompt the female to reproduce. Drawing an analogy between human morality and animal behaviour, Darwin concluded that since females are less lustful and more discriminating, males have to be more beautiful. The interval before the modest female surrenders to her preening suitor contributes to the evolution of the species, necessitating an exercise in cultural improvement that favours aesthetic display.

For nineteenth-century sexologists, modesty was a crucial key to female psychology. Many held that women's apparent lack of interest in sex was due to their innate passionlessness or 'sexual anaesthesia'. Havelock Ellis, on the contrary, claimed that, under her modest façade, every woman held the capacity for sexual feeling — modesty was merely a delaying device to arouse male desire. With an adept partner, any woman might be drawn out of her habitual reticence into the active enjoyment of SEXUALITY.

Standards of public honour, like fashions of dress, have changed dramatically over time. According to early Christian thinkers, the importance of bodily modesty originated in the Book of Genesis. After eating of the fruit of the Tree of Knowledge, Adam and Eve knew that they were naked, and thus made themselves aprons of leaves. The injunction to cover the body initially applied only to men, because only in men is sexual arousal obvious. But the Church Fathers soon extended the rule to women as well, for their ability to arouse was feared to lead men away from the spiritual. These religious teachings had a direct impact on bodily conduct: from the beginning of the Christian Era until the fourteenth century, European clothing was largely monochromatic and devoid of ornamentation. Both men and women dressed in full-length tunics or robes designed to conceal the body from sight.

But in the middle of the fourteenth century, the rising commercial classes embraced a new style that hugged the body and celebrated its physical attributes. The Renaissance styles — emblematized by the masculine vogue for the short fitted jacket, tight hose, and prominent codpiece, and the snug busts and daring décolletages of women's clothing — symbolized a shift from the medieval preoccupation with the spiritual to an interest in worldly matters. Such sartorial expressivity — associated with aristocratic splendour — would remain popular until late in the eighteenth century, when the political values of the aristocracy were widely denounced. Breeches, the style of trousers favoured by the wealthy because they revealed the shape of the leg, were then rejected in favour of long trousers that symbolized activity and utility. Male attire became desexualized and austere; colour and ornamentation were relegated to women's clothing.

In the nineteenth century, men who wore artistic, expressive clothing were denigrated as dandies and social parasites. Napoléon III decreed that the only attire appropriate for men was the English gentleman's business suit, the riding habit, or the military uniform. The task of expressing the opulent spirit of the age was thus carried out through female fashions. This era heralds the ideal hourglass figure, which required tightly bound corsetry that caused constant discomfort and wreaked irreparable damage on women's bodies.

Standards of female modesty have undergone countless redefinitions over the years, in response to cultural, political, and economic factors. In recent years the concept has been reinterpreted to reflect women's increasingly prominent role in the public sphere and the problematic morality associated with working mothers. Ruth Rubinstein has shown that in eras when women attain public power, female fashions are dominated by elaborate artifice that masks the sites of feminine sexuality and projects a larger-than-life body image. The 'power suit' adopted by working women in the 1970s can thus be seen as a modern-day version of the stiff, high-necked masculine bodices and voluminous skirts favoured by sixteenth-century noblewomen in imitation of Catherine de Médicis and Elizabeth I.

Concepts of modesty are determined by cultural as well as historical factors. The reports of missionaries and anthropologists who have lived among 'primitive' or nonliterate groups offer many cases of peoples who walk around naked and seem to feel no shame or guilt. Australian Aborigines, for instance, appear indifferent to nakedness but are deeply embarrassed if seen eating. If caught in the fields without her veil, a peasant woman in some Arab countries will throw her skirt over her head, thereby exposing what to the Western mind is a much more embarrassing part of her anatomy.

JULIA DOUTHWAITE

Further reading
Laver, J. (1969). *Modesty in dress.* Houghton Mifflin, Boston.

Rubinstein, R. P. (1995). *Dress codes: meanings and messages in American culture.* Westview Press, Boulder, CO.

Yeazell, R. B. (1991). *Fictions of modesty: women and courtship in the English novel.* University of Chicago Press, Chicago, IL.

See also CLOTHES; MORALITY; SEXUALITY.

Molecular biology is a branch of biological science that investigates how genes govern the activity of CELLS, tissues, and organisms. It evolved by the coming together of the sciences of GENETICS, BIOCHEMISTRY, and CELL BIOLOGY. Its cardinal rule is that *DNA makes RNA makes protein.*   A.W.C

See CELL; GENETICS, HUMAN.

Monsters The meaning of the word 'monster' has undergone drastic variations throughout history. The word involves a twofold Latin root — '*monstrum*', from *monere* (to warn) or *monstrare* (to exhibit) — and was in principle the equivalent of the Greek *teras*, meaning sign or warning. The 'monsters' of the classical world were thus those signs, not necessarily of human or animal origin, that were clearly identifiable as such, and *teratology*, the science that studied those signs, was simply a different form of divination. It must be emphasized that it was precisely because of their unusualness that monsters were defined as being clear and distinguishable warnings.

It is important to take into consideration that during the Middle Ages a distinction was drawn between monstrous individuals and monstrous races or species, and that the members of these particular groups, who were first given a systematic classification by Pliny the Elder (23–79 AD), qualified as 'monsters' mainly as a consequence of their unusualness. They were monsters not so much because they were deformed, but because they were rare and extraordinary. From this point of view, a monster was a curiosity, a portent, an unusual sight.

The Renaissance saw the first serious attempt to bring the ambiguous nature of the word 'monster' to an end, and to bring the study of teratology within the scope of anatomical investigations. In sixteenth- and seventeenth-century treatises on monsters the senses of 'monster' both as a divine or unnatural sign or omen, and as an unusual or curious phenomenon, were seriously challenged. According to Martin Weinrich, a German naturalist who wrote a treatise on monsters at the end of the sixteenth century, not every phenomenon that threatened the natural order could legitimately be called 'a monster'. Teratology, on the other hand, could no longer be defined as a discourse related primarily to unusual events. It was suggested, by the French surgeon Jean Riolan and the Italian naturalist Ulysses Aldrovandi, that the new teratological science claimed to understand monstrosity exclusively in terms of physical deformity. By defining monsters as natural beings, it became possible to establish a classification of potential deformities based, for the first time, on anatomical criteria. But this new attitude towards the realm of monsters was not without its difficulties. First, seventeenth- and eighteenth-century anatomists, naturalists, and surgeons proposed so many different definitions of the word 'monster', on many occasions upon examination of a single and isolated case, that far too often there was no possibility of reaching a consensus about a 'monstrous' nature. Second, in order to separate the study of monsters from the popular imagery — still anchored during the Enlightenment in medieval and Renaissance sources — the enlightened teratologist understood that abnormalities had to be established as fact before any further investigation could legitimately take place. This lack of agreement in the definition of the term 'monster' helps to explain why the study of physical abnormalities was almost strictly confined to a collection of examples or instances during the eighteenth century. For example, in the *Philosophical Transactions* of the Royal Society between 1665 and 1780, there were over 100 communications regarding forms of 'monstrosity', and the French Academy of Sciences published another 130 papers on the subject between 1699 and 1770.

A transition from the understanding of monsters as beings 'from outside' to seeing them as 'deviations from within' led in the mid nineteenth century to teratology becoming a modern science, whose main concern was no longer the enquiry into the nature and origins of monsters but the study of major physical abnormalities or malformations in humans or animals. In fact, when the French naturalist Geoffroy Saint-Hilaire published his *Traité de Teratologie* — the first important milestone in the contemporary history of teratology — in 1832, he explicitly mentioned that this new teratological science should refrain from using the word 'monster' to describe its new object of study. From the mid nineteenth century, those who suffered from major or minor physical abnormalities, no matter how serious or unusual their condition, were no longer termed 'monsters' in scientific literature. However, many of these, like SIAMESE TWINS for example, were still referred to as 'monsters' in the 'freak shows' and circuses popular during the nineteenth and the early twentieth centuries.

JAVIER MOSCOSO

See also CONGENITAL ABNORMALITIES; FREAKS.

Moon

The moon is the most 'human' of the heavenly bodies, since its phases and the shadows on its surface give it a face, encouraging the popular lore about the 'Man in the Moon'. Belief that the moon has a special influence on human affairs has been universal. Because of its phases, it has been linked to the rhythms of life and to nature's cycles: water, rain, and FERTILITY. 'The moon has great influence in vulgar philosophy', observed Samuel Johnson, touring the Scottish Highlands, 'In my memory it was a precept annually given in one of the *English Almanacks, to kill hogs when the moon was increasing, and the bacon would prove the better in boiling'.*

Many religious beliefs have been woven around the moon, which has commonly been personified as a goddess. She is *Ishtar* to the Babylonians, *Asthoreth* to the Phoenicians, and, to the Greeks, *Artemis* (Roman *Diana*), the chaste huntress who cruelly punished those who failed to worship her.

Three main connotations have been ascribed to the moon. It has stood for the feminine principle. Being smaller than the sun and reflecting its light, the moon has been taken to represent female dependence and passivity. In Taoist terms, the moon is thus *yin*, being receptive, relative to the sun's *yang*. Amongst the Inca, the moon was the sun's wife, and hence the goddess of women. Its waxing and waning has also served as an analogue for supposed female fickleness.

The moon has also been regarded as controlling MENSTRUATION. According to the eighteenth-century physician, Richard Mead, 'everyone knows how great a share the Moon has in forwarding those evacuations of the weaker sex.' The very word menstruation means 'moon change', while in France it is called 'le moment de la lune'. In Saibai and Yam, two islands off Australia, it was believed that menstruation was caused by the moon, who came as a man to seduce the pubescent girl.

Menstrual seclusion rituals are thus commonly governed by the lunar phases. The Juluo of East Africa believe that menstruation comes with the new moon and that only then can women become pregnant. There have been evolutionary speculations that since the lunar and the menstrual cycles each are of approximately 28 days' duration, menstruation is causally related to the action of the moon on the tides, somehow dating back to the time when we were all sea creatures.

Finally, the moon has been judged to be the cause of madness, the term 'lunacy' deriving from the Latin *luna*, meaning moon. Hippocrates, Pliny the Elder, Plutarch, and the Bible all affirmed its harmful influence. Aretaeus of Cappadocia and Rhazes held that epileptic seizures were governed by the moon, while Hildegard of Bingen deemed that 'a male born on the seventeenth day of the Moon will be an idiot.' Shakespeare affords many references to the Moon as the 'sovereign mistress of true melancholy':

> It is the very error of the moon,
> She comes more near the earth than she was wont
> And makes men mad. (*Othello*)

As late as 1791, the French psychiatrist Joseph Daquin wrote in his *Philosophie de la Folie* that 'it is a well established fact that insanity is a disease of the mind upon which the moon exercises an unquestionable influence.' His younger contemporary, Jean Esquirol, concluded that the moon affected the insane through its light, which excited some and terrified others. Although such beliefs have waned, many modern studies have investigated the significance of the phases of the moon in relation to SUICIDE, MURDER, mental hospital admissions, VIOLENCE, MIGRAINE, ANXIETY, childbirth, and marital breakdown.

ROY PORTER

Morality

Morality refers to ethical issues — principles of right and wrong conduct — as well as instances of real behaviour — the manner in which individuals comply more or less fully with such standards. Based on the Latin *mor* — 'a manner, custom' — this term covers all kinds of human actions, although it is often associated specifically with virtue in sexual conduct. To encourage moral conduct, early theological representations of sin and evil highlighted the body's capacity for suffering. *Luxuria* or lust was commonly represented as a nude woman whose past misconduct prepared her present torture — in some church statuary snakes devoured her breasts and vulva, or toads issued from her mouth. In the medieval and early modern ages, morality referred to a religious framework; through diet and bodily maintenance, the individual was expected to defend himself against the temptation of the flesh.

Codes of morality have evolved in keeping with larger cultural, historical, and economic currents. PROSTITUTION had long been considered wicked and detrimental to the commonweal, but it was not until the nineteenth century, when national interests were linked directly to commercial economies, that this practice became known as 'the social evil'. More than other traditional targets of moral reform, such as the drunkard or blasphemer, the prostitute was vilified because of her unproductivity; she partook of sexuality without repaying the nation with the commodities it needed most — citizens and domestic stability.

In modern industrial societies, the body has largely lost its connotation as a vessel of sin and has become increasingly involved in the secular mechanisms of consumption and display. The 1920s were crucial for the formation of the modern-day body ideal; by the end of the decade, women, under the combined impact of the cosmetic, fashion, and advertising industries, had for the first time in large numbers put on makeup and rayon stockings, and abandoned CORSETS for rubber girdles. The rage for sunbathing in the interwar years further legitimated the public display of the body. Whereas Christian religious traditions aimed to subordinate the body to 'higher' spiritual ends, modern consumer culture works to release the naked body from shame and guilt. The individual's primary responsibility shifts from his soul to his health, body shape, and appearance. Since the 1960s the ideal of the youthful body has dominated Western culture; fitness and slimness have largely replaced spiritual goals as indicators of human worth. But the opprobrium inflicted on the immoral remains powerful: those who do not maintain standards of bodily maintenance are considered lazy, self-indulgent, even a burden to national well-being.

While age-old controversies regarding homosexuality, PORNOGRAPHY, drinking, gambling, and other 'immoral' practices remain current today, they are perhaps less compelling than the dilemmas created by recent innovations in medical technology. The availability of techniques to alter the beginning of life (through fertility drugs, surrogacy, or prenatal testing) and the end of life (through doctor-assisted suicide or machine-enhanced existence) has prompted the growth of a new morality — the ethics of medical intervention on the human body.

JULIA DOUTHWAITE

Morning sickness

Almost three-quarters of women are troubled by NAUSEA and/or VOMITING in early PREGNANCY. This usually stops at around 14 weeks of pregnancy and the cause is attributed to human chorionic gonadotropin, a hormone produced in large amounts by the PLACENTA early in pregnancy. Nausea is more troublesome in multiple pregnancies and where there is overgrowth of the placenta (*hydatifidiform mole*). Occasionally, nausea and vomiting may be so severe (*hyperemesis gravidarum*) that care in hospital proves necessary. The Greek physician, Soranus, described accurately the time-span of morning sickness in the second century AD and he advised giving 'little and easily digestible food, like a soft boiled egg or a porridge, and not some very fat fowl'. This advice holds well today.

JIM NIELSON

Motion sickness

At some point in their lives, most individuals experience motion sickness, in one form or another, while being transported in moving vehicles. There is a wide variability in susceptibility, with a greater prevalence in females than males, and in children between 3 and 12 years of age. It is characterized by initial feelings of DIZZINESS, general discomfort, pallor, and cold sweating, followed by NAUSEA, VOMITING, and apathy. It has been given many specific names relating to the mode of transport involved (such as sea-, air-, space-, or even camel-sickness), but all forms are thought to arise from the same basic cause.

The first known report of sea-sickness was by Hippocrates, and the word 'nausea' actually derives from the Greek for ship (*naus*). The precise cause has been difficult to establish, although it has long been realized that it is associated with stimulation of the VESTIBULAR SYSTEM of the inner ear. Thus, motion sickness is never experienced by individuals who have no vestibular function. Older texts often suggest that the cause is over-stimulation of the vestibular system, but current opinion favours an explanation in terms of what has been called the *sensory conflict theory* of motion sickness. This is

based on the notion that the stimuli which cause motion sickness are those that generate sensations that do not conform with a repertoire of expected sensations that has been built up and stored in the brain on the basis of past experience of the sensory stimulation associated with motion.

Two major sources of sensory conflict are recognized: intra-vestibular and visual–vestibular. Intra-vestibular conflict arises from the fact that there are two types of sensory organ in the vestibular system, the semicircular canals, which respond to rotation, and the otolith organs, which respond to linear motion and to changes in orientation with respect to gravity. If a rotational movement of the head is made, such as pitching the head forward to look down at the ground, the otoliths and canals independently give signals about the magnitude of the movement during and after the motion. Because such head movements are made very frequently, an internal representation of the association between these two signals is built up, so that they are then accepted as compatible. However, if the same head movement is made in a different context, the signals may become incompatible. For example, if such a head movement is made during prolonged rotation on a fairground carousel the sensation of head rotation will be influenced by the rotation of the carousel, resulting in a conflict with signals arising from the otolith organs. Equally, head movements made in space, where gravitational acceleration is almost eliminated, will elicit sensations of turning from the canals, which are not matched by the normal otolithic signals.

Visual–vestibular conflict may arise from the fact that the vestibular stimulation experienced with head motion stimuli is normally associated with a compatible visual impression of movement. If the motion of the visual scene is modified, as it is for example when viewing the world through binoculars from a moving vehicle, the incompatibility between the vestibular sensation and the visual motion sensation may be sufficient to induce motion sickness. Viewing the horizon from the deck of a ship on a rough sea helps to reduce motion sickness because the vestibular sensation is compatible with a stable visual world, whereas viewing the wave motion of the sea itself is likely to generate conflict. Apparent motion of the visual world, as generated by large, projected moving images (e.g. cinerama), in the absence of the head movement that would normally occur when seeing such images, may also provide sufficient conflict to induce motion sickness.

Associated with the concept of the sensory conflict hypothesis is the notion that continued exposure to new combinations of visual and vestibular motion stimuli should lead to adaptation of the internal model and thereby to reduced susceptibility. This is supported by the observation that individuals may initially experience motion sickness on a sea voyage, but quickly adapt and gain their 'sea-legs' within a period of 3–6 days. For those susceptible individuals

who are continually exposed to provocative motion stimuli it is possible to carry out a process of adaptation based on this principle. For more limited periods of exposure there are some anti-motion sickness drugs (scopolamine, dimenhydrinate) that are effective in preventing the onset of sickness, at least for the period of the journey.

GRAHAM BARNES

See also VESTIBULAR SYSTEM.

Motor neurons

Two way communication between individuals, or, stated differently, between their NERVOUS SYSTEMS, is entirely dependent on muscular contraction. This is so because although information concerning the external world is received and processed through our senses, the resulting percepts and mental (cognitive) activities remain entirely private within one's own consciousness. They remain so unless communicated to others by movement, whether through an infant's cry, a Gallic shrug, or an aggressive or submissive posture; whether through writing a poem, a philosophical work, or just graffiti; but above all through vocalization, whether simply as an approving grunt, or linguistically refined by articulation into speech or song; and for the deaf by hand signing. Even when disease has resulted in a major loss of muscle, as in motoneuron disease, communication remains possible providing that a single tiny muscle remains under conscious control, so that either its contractile force or associated electrical activity can be used in a prosthesis to control a typewriter, or to generate artificial speech. This is no better instanced than by the remarkable feat of communication by the mathematician Professor Stephen Hawking in explaining his reasoning about the origin and nature of the universe to the rest of us who dwell within it.

Skeletal (voluntary) muscles normally contract only in response to commands from the CENTRAL NERVOUS SYSTEM (CNS). With its cell body within the SPINAL CORD or BRAIN STEM, and its emergent process, the *axon*, innervating a group of muscle fibres known as the *motor unit*, the motor neuron forms the interface between the sentient, perceiving, and thinking human nervous system and the external world; it is, therefore, of paramount importance as the key structure mediating communication between individuals. Its importance was clearly recognized by Sir Charles Sherrington who, at the beginning of the twentieth century, designated the motor neuron as 'the final common path' from the CNS to the muscles. (These are now also called *alpha motor neurons*, because since Sherrington's time another type has been described, the *gamma* or *fusimotor* neurons; the specialized muscle fibres which these innervate do not directly contribute to force production and external work. Instead they control the discharge properties of the *muscle spindles*, receptors in the muscle that signal information about length and about the velocity of changes in length.

The spinal and cranial alpha motor neurons are among the largest neurons in the CNS, many having cell bodies in excess of 50 μm in diameter. From the cell body extend 5–7 long processes, the *dendrites*, and the axon, an extra-long process, which arises from a conical bulge known as the *axon hillock*. The axon innervates muscle that can be more than a metre away in the case of muscles moving the toes. The surface membrane of both the cell body and the dendrites is covered with microscopic structures of button-like shape, the '*synaptic boutons*'. These are formed by the axon terminals of other neurons, and indicate the sites at which information is transferred to this one neuron from many others. Such transfer is not achieved by cellular continuity — a matter of fierce debate in the late nineteenth century; instead, it is mediated by a process which Sherrington, by deduction from the properties he disclosed through studies of spinal REFLEXES, conceived as a functional though flowing discontinuity between neurons. That time discontinuity at the junction was attributed to a 'SYNAPSE', which he named from the Greek word for 'clasp'. The delay is now understood to be due to the process of chemical transmission, following the release of a transmitter substance 'presynaptically' when a nerve impulse invades an axon terminal at a synapse with another neuron. The transmitter diffuses across the narrow gap, some 0.1 μm wide, between the terminal and the motor neuron dendrite or cell body, where it acts 'postsynaptically' by briefly altering the membrane potential of the motor neuron. It may either decrease it (depolarization) or increase it (hyperpolarization), thereby enhancing or depressing the motor neuron excitability. These brief unitary events, the *excitatory and inhibitory synaptic potentials*, respectively, have a triangular shape, taking about 1–2 milliseconds (0.001 sec) to rise or fall to their peak value and declining over 10–15 milliseconds. They have the property of summation when they overlap in time; thus the motor neuron (and most other neurons) can be described as integrating the information it receives moment by moment via its presynaptic inputs. Here a sense of scale has to be introduced. There is an estimated total of 30 000–50 000 boutons of different types across the entire surface. On average perhaps five of them are formed by the branching of each presynaptic axon, (analogous to the branching of the motor neuron axon that forms the motor unit within a muscle). In order for a motor neuron to discharge repetitively, say at rates typically between 5–20 impulses/sec, the motor neuron surface has to be exposed to a barrage of synaptic inputs (excitatory) with a net rate of approximately 12 000–20 000 inputs/sec. Then the summed activity lowers the membrane potential sufficiently to trigger a sustained discharge of the motor neuron in the region of the axon hillock. If each presynaptic input itself fired at 100/sec then it would require the co-operative but random activity of 150–200 individual neurons to provide the necessary excitation; and such steady state firing underlies the maintenance of POSTURE. For rhythmic or strongly phasic movements, the presynaptic inputs themselves become progressively more synchronized, to generate the time course of the intended movement. The fastest, such as those that move the eyes rapidly from one target to another, are called *ballistic movements*. But willed movements rarely achieve the speed of pathological ones, for example the jerks typical of 'myoclonic' EPILEPSY or, for that matter, the speed of normal ones as in the knee-jerk reflex.

When the patellar tendon at the knee is tapped, the motor neurons that innervate the quadriceps muscles (many thousands of neurons in the grey matter of the spinal cord) are subjected suddenly to a highly synchronized synaptic input from the several hundred nerve fibres from muscle receptors which were briefly stretched by the tap. The synaptic potentials all occur at much the same time, because the receptors project directly to the motor neurons to form a 'monosynaptic' pathway. Temporal and spatial summation therefore is great indeed. This causes the depolarization to reach the firing threshold for a substantial fraction of the quadriceps motor neurons, and their combined axonal discharge leads to the rapid muscle twitch that extends the leg at the knee joint. At the other extreme of quadriceps activation is the steady discharge of motor neurons that underlies the holding of a posture. Between these extremes is a whole range of movements at different velocities and with varying time course in relation to their force, as required for example for the diverse finger movements in playing a musical instrument, a 'stop volley' in tennis, or for increasing one's walking pace. Each participating motor neuron receives a time-varying pattern of excitation and inhibition such that its output pattern of discharge acts in concert with others to produce the desired movement. It is not surprising therefore that when the capacity to perform movements is impaired by one of the motor neuron diseases, such as amyotrophic lateral sclerosis, which specifically destroy motor neurons, or others that affect them, such as poliomyelitis, without impairing intellect, the effects are so catastrophic for the patient.   TOM SEARS

See also CENTRAL NERVOUS SYSTEM; NEUROTRANSMITTERS; REFLEXES; SYNAPSE; SKELETAL MUSCLE.

Mouth The poetic (and biblical) view of the mouth and lips is almost entirely romantic and idealised — '. . . the lips of a strange woman drop as a honeycomb, and her mouth is smoother than oil . . .' (Proverbs), although an occasional writer illustrates the downside — 'I've a head like a concertina, I've a tongue like a button stick, I've a mouth like an old potato, and I'm more than a little sick . . .' (Kipling).

It is a rather unromantic fact, however, that the mouth is functionally the first part of the gastrointestinal tract — one end of the nutritional tube which starts there and ends at the anus. Because of its position it has acquired many other complementary functions — as a part of the respiratory system, for instance and as a most important part of the SPEECH mechanism — but these are secondary to its main function. In the human embryo the first sign of the potential mouth (or oral cavity) occurs in the fourth week of development and is a small depression in what will become the skin of the face. The depression deepens and quite rapidly meets up with the developing upper part of the gastrointestinal tube. The separating tissues disappear, and the embryo mouth is left in continuity with the rest of the gastrointestinal tract. The oral MUCOUS MEMBRANE includes many specialized features; the salivary glands, large and small, are derived from it, and it contains numerous sensory endings of various types. These include those in the taste-buds, the structures which are responsible (together with those in the nose mediating the sense of smell) for the recognition of flavour. Other types of nerve endings in the oral mucosa include those concerned with the sense of touch, recognition of temperature changes, and so on. In appropriate situations these provide signals to other parts of the body, stimulating the secretion of SALIVA, inducing gastric activity, initiating sexual awareness, and carrying out many other functions.

The bony structures within which the soft tissues of the mouth are contained are essentially the JAWS (the mandible and the maxilla, including the palate) which, together with the precursors of the TEETH, are formed as a later part of the developmental process described above. The system of embryonic structures involved in the formation of the mouth, lips, and jaws is complex, and the possibility of developmental errors occurring during this process is well known. In this highly visible and emotionally significant area of the body, failure of the normal processes, with resulting cleft formation, may be a highly traumatic matter for the individual involved. The integrity of the oral cavity and its relative proportions to the nearby structures, such as the nasal space and the sinuses, also largely determine the nature of speech, as the oral cavity is one of the series of resonators distributed about the base of the skull, which are greatly involved in modifying the primary speech (and song) sounds produced in the LARYNX.

In almost all of the functions of the mouth, the tongue and the teeth are closely involved. Perhaps less evident is the role of the saliva in this respect. As a lubricant with AUTONOMIC NERVOUS SYSTEM control of its flow (who has not had a dry mouth when subjected to almost any form of STRESS?), an adequate salivary flow is an absolutely vital factor for the success of most of the functions performed within the oral cavity.

The superficial margin of the mouth is marked by the lips — essentially the functional sphincter structure which seals off the mouth from the external environment, but with the ability to perform complex and sophisticated movements which quite transcend this simple function. The ring of individually controlled muscles in the substance of the lips, together with others in the facial structure, some of which are concerned predominantly with opening and closing the jaws, make up a highly complex system of control for the mouth, the lips, and the face in general. These include the group of the 'muscles of expression', which work with an integrated nerve supply to provide this vitally important mechanism of communication and of expression of EMOTION.

The mouth is, quite clearly, a primary ERO-GENOUS ZONE. In itself it is not a particularly attractive structure, but the lips are a different matter. The smile is on the *lips* of the Mona Lisa — at least in the popular view, although quite clearly the facial expression as a whole is involved in such aesthetic assessments. 'Thin lipped', 'thick lipped' and similar characterizations depend on the description of only one feature of a face, but evidently a crucial one.

When things go wrong in the mouth the emotive effect may be disproportionally high. The mouth and lips are of great importance aesthetically, sexually, and functionally. Perhaps because of this, the area is also the site of many well-recognised psychogenic disorders involving unexplained pain and unusual sensations. Because of the duplex origin of the oral mucous membrane, diseases both of the skin and of the gastrointestinal tract, as well as those of more localised origin, may manifest in the mouth. Many of these cause pain, and the impact on the individual may be very significant — speech, eating, and the other functions in which the mouth is involved may all be affected, and the overall effect may be disproportionately great. Even minor conditions affecting the lips may be particularly troublesome — the simple cold sore causes distress, not only because of the irritation, but also because of its very visible site.   WILLIAM TYLDESLEY

See also AUTONOMIC NERVOUS SYSTEM; CLEFT LIP AND PALATE; FACE; SALIVA; TASTE AND SMELL; TEETH; TONGUE.

Movement, control of
While walking to the station with a companion, we walk, navigate obstacles, maintain balance, carry objects, talk, and gesticulate. The performance of these multiple motor tasks is seemingly effortless, although they involve the co-ordinated activity of thousands of motor units in dozens of different muscles. By contrast, after damage to the brain's motor control system, the performance of even simple movements can be very exhausting and difficult; lesions of different parts of the system leave us with characteristic and often devastating deficits. We are unaware of much of the finer aspects of our own motor co-ordination and in fact have very little insight into how we perform a complex skilled act, such as riding a bicycle. We can conclude that for effortless performance of habitual tasks, our motor control system is much more sophisticated than one requiring constant supervision by the conscious brain. The distributed nature of the motor control system reflects the complexity of human movement, and this system comprises many different structures

within the brain and spinal cord. The control system must ultimately act through the '*final common path*': the discharge of MOTOR NEURONS in the BRAIN STEM and SPINAL CORD, and the mechanical response of the muscles they innervate. The interface between the neural 'command', ultimately expressed in terms of the pattern of motoneuronal discharge, and the mechanical response of the skeleto-muscular apparatus is a complex one. In engineering terms, understanding the motor system requires how the 'controller' delivers these neural commands to the 'plant'; namely, the muscles, tendons, ligaments, bones, and joints. The enormous variety and type of human movement, including our unique capacity to speak, must all be performed with the same 'plant'; although the number of muscles is large, the enormous motor repertoire must be a reflection of the flexibility of the motor control system. This repertoire can be greatly expanded and refined by training and practice — as demonstrated, for example, by musicians, athletes, artists, and surgeons.

The process of motor control
Consider the act of reaching and grasping a glass of water, raising it to the lips, and drinking. Models of motor control envisage the process as three different stages: the *idea* or plan of action to achieve a motor goal; the *programme* required to bring this plan about; and, finally, the *execution* of the movement. In the example given, the idea describes the objective or goal of the movement: acquiring the glass of water. This could be achieved in a variety of ways: with either arm, or by gripping the glass between the teeth. Thus the *idea* of the movement is quite general and does not need to be mapped out in terms of specific muscles or joints. It is known that some parts of the brain involved in motor control, such as the posterior parietal lobe of the CEREBRAL CORTEX, are more concerned with the idea or plan, than with the selection of which limb or set of muscles to use. The Russian cyberneticist Bernstein, one of the pioneers of the study of human movement, recognized that when an action is carried out, then some feature of the plan will be present irrespective of the particular effector used to perform it. This common plan is assumed to underlie the phenomenon of *equivalence of movement*, by which a movement pattern, such as your own signature, is preserved whether you write it with the pen held in the dominant or in the non-dominant hand, by the foot or even the mouth. The programme of the movement must control the entire motor act: once the plan has been adopted then the whole sequence of movements is expressed. The reaching movement might employ the right hand, passing along a straight line path towards the glass. To programme this movement, it is proposed that the brain has to solve the inverse kinematics problem, calculating the timing and scale of changes in angle of appropriate joints (shoulder, elbow, and wrist) that will be needed to make the hand follow the selected path of movement. Once the desired angular

changes are specified, the programme must define how the muscles are to produce them. This is not a trivial problem, since the torque that contraction of a muscle exerts at a joint will, in general, also have mechanical influences on remote joints (look at what happens to your wrist during rapid elbow flexion, for example). Thus the solution of this inverse dynamics problem is exceedingly complex. The forces and movements resulting from a neural command to contract a given muscle will vary greatly depending, for instance, on the length of the muscle, the speed at which it is shortening, and the contractile state of other muscles acting with it (its *synergists*) or against it (its *antagonists*). The execution of the movement requires the activation of selected sets of muscles in a manner that will achieve the objective of the programme. This may require co-ordination of groups of muscle synergists within one limb, or between several limbs, trunk, head, and eyes. The POSTURE at the onset of the movement (for example, your arm resting on the table before reaching for a drink) must be taken into account, as must the desired velocity, acceleration, and deceleration of the movement, such that your hand arrives accurately at the glass, rather than under- or over-reaching it, or knocking it over.

Importance of sensory input
An important aspect of motor control is the incorporation of sensory input into the different parts of the idea–programme–execute sequence. Sensory inputs from the eyes, from the ears, and from skin, muscle, and joint receptors can characterize the location, size, shape, weight, and texture of the object forming the goal of the movement (in our example, the glass of water). Our perception of the expected attributes of the task can exert a powerful influence over performance (as, for example, in the size–weight illusion). There is increasing evidence that while some movements may rely on *sensory feedback* for their control, most rely on a '*feedforward*' mechanism — a neural process based entirely on an 'internal model' within the brain of the required movement: that is, the entire motor action has an internal representation. Feedforward mechanisms are evidently essential for rapid movements (in which there is no time for feedback to play any part) and predominate in the execution of highly predictable and well-practised movements. They are also critical for movements of the eyes, such as *saccades* (very small 'scanning' movements), where no external loads or disturbances are likely to impede the production of the desired movement.

However, it is important to realise that sensory feedback must be used to create the brain's internal model of the movement in the first place. Feedback is important for updating and refining the model and for controlling unpredictable or novel movements (e.g. reaching out and lifting an object while underwater), and this process contributes to the acquisition of new motor skills. Through disease, some individuals completely lack any SOMATIC SENSATIONS — they have no incoming information from the body — but retain a normal motor innervation. They can perform complex movements under continuous visual control, but have great difficulty in doing so. In normal subjects, any movement generates a large amount of sensory feedback and an important function of the internal model may be to predict the type and time course of this movement-induced sensory input or 'reafference'. For example, the model could cancel the predicted cutaneous inputs experienced when the hand first contacts the glass of water. If the glass is unexpectedly slippery, warm, or heavy, an error signal will arise between the predicted and actual sensory input, and this will generate a corrective action. Some movements, such as those that occur during tactile exploration of an object, are carried out in order to generate such reafference and provide further information about the physical properties of the explored object.

The 'degree of freedom' problem

There are very many different muscles in the body and this means that the control system could adopt a very large number of possible solutions to achieve its goal. Bernstein recognized that the adoption of functional muscle synergies helps to solve this 'degrees of freedom' problem. These synergies are a well-recognized and important part of our motor control system, and are used for the co-ordination of activity within a limb (such as stabilization of the elbow joint while moving the wrist and fingers), between limbs (such as weight-bearing by one leg during walking), and for the co-ordination of eye, head, and body movements during orientation to a visual or auditory stimulus of interest (for example, when someone calls your name). Perhaps the most impressive example is the co-ordination of muscles in the face, mouth, tongue, larynx, chest, and abdomen during speech. Interestingly, many central motor structures, including the primary motor cortex and CEREBELLUM, appear to have a motor representation that involves control of muscle groups, rather than single muscles. All purposeful motor acts involve the contraction of multiple muscles.

The motor network of the CNS

The different parts of the central nervous system concerned with movement control are organized in a distributed fashion and are generally considered to act in a parallel rather than in a hierarchical fashion: damage to individual structures, such as the lateral cerebellum or motor cortex, does not abolish the capacity to move. Mechanisms within the spinal cord and brain stem are concerned with reflex activity and integration of spinal and supraspinal control. Complex patterns of movement, such as locomotion and swallowing, are encoded within specific groups of connected interneurons referred to as 'central pattern generators' (CPGs). The CPG contains the complete spatio-temporal pattern of

the complex act, and although it can act independently of peripheral sensory inputs and of descending motor pathways, these can influence and modulate the activity of the CPG. Descending motor pathways from the brain stem, midbrain, and cerebral cortex exert specific influences over groups of interneurons and motor neurons concerned with trunk, shoulder, pelvic girdle, and distal limb (hand or foot) movements. All of the higher order motor centres, including the cerebellum, BASAL GANGLIA, and cerebral cortex, must exert their respective influence through these pathways. The human corticospinal tract is derived from extensive regions of the frontal and parietal lobes of the brain (including the primary motor and premotor cortex, and the supplementary motor area); it also includes input from part of the limbic system, associated with innate and emotional behaviour, and from the sensory cortical areas. Measurement of regional cerebral blood flow (by the IMAGING TECHNIQUES of positron emission tomography (PET) or functional magnetic resonance imaging (fMRI)) show that some or all of these areas mentioned are active in human volunteers performing a variety of complex movements. The corticospinal tract is the largest single descending nerve pathway from the brain down to the spinal cord. Its nerve endings at synapses within the spinal grey matter enable the control of sensory input and the modulation of reflex activity as well as the generation of movement. The human corticospinal tract, like that in other primates, is characterised by direct, single nerve fibre-to-nerve cell (monosynaptic) connections with the spinal motoneurones, which go out to all the voluntary muscles, and this is thought to be of particular importance for the capacity to perform skilled hand and finger movements.

Interaction among cerebellum, basal ganglia and cerebral cortex

The motor areas of the cerebral cortex also influence sub-cortical structures from which other descending motor pathways arise (e.g. from the vestibular apparatus and from the brain stem to the spinal cord). The organization of the motor system is characterised by 're-entrant loops'. This means that the output of a particular structure is sent to a number of other regions which process this information and then feed it back, directly and indirectly, to the structure from which it originated. The two most important loops are those linking the areas of cerebral cortex concerned with movement with the cerebellum and basal ganglia; wide regions of the cerebral cortex send nerve fibres to these structures and the motor areas of the cerebral cortex receive a massive returning input from them via relays in the thalamus. There is detectable activity in the brain as much as a whole second before the onset of a voluntary movement; this is a long period with respect to nerve conduction velocity, so there is time to process information through these loops several times before the final command goes out. Transmission of information is altered by training and practice; pathways in the

cerebellum have been shown to exhibit considerable plasticity — forging new connections — and the cerebellum has an essential role in the learning and co-ordination of movement.

Damage to the different levels of the motor system hierarchy causes characteristic changes in movement performance: for instance, patients with damage to the basal ganglia may exhibit paucity or slowness of movements, also associated with rigidity and tremor (*Parkinson's disease*), while in other conditions there may be uncontrolled and involuntary movements, called *dyskinesias*. Patients with cerebellar damage show deficits of timing and co-ordination. Damage to the primary motor cortex and its descending motor pathways often results in the complete loss of skilled hand movements, whilst disturbances of head and body posture result from lesions of other descending pathways, such as the vestibulospinal tract. These results can best be interpreted in terms of the site of termination of the different motor pathways within the spinal cord.

Neurophysiological recordings in experimental animals show that neurons in different parts of the motor system are active before and during movement and that their rate of discharge can encode the different parameters, such as the force or direction of the intended movement. These same neurons often respond to afferent feedback from peripheral receptors. The encoding of movement parameters at the single cell level is not sufficiently precise to explain the accuracy of movements such as pointing to a target, and it is probable that whole assemblies of neurons co-operate for this purpose. There is also evidence that neurons show task-specific activity, and, in some of the 'higher' cortical areas, they can encode complex sequences of movement.

R. N. LEMON

Further reading

Porter, R. and Lemon, R. N. (1993). *Corticospinal function and voluntary movement*. Oxford University Press.

Rosenbaum, D. A. (1991). *Human motor control*. Academic Press, San Diego.

Rothwell, J. C. (1994). *Control of human voluntary movement*. Chapman and Hall, London.

See PLATE 6.

See also BASAL GANGLIA; BRAIN; BRAIN STEM; CEREBELLUM; CEREBRAL CORTEX; MUSICIANSHIP AND OTHER FINGER SKILLS; SKELETAL MUSCLE; PROPRIOCEPTION; SPINAL CORD.

Mucous membranes

are the moist linings of the orifices and internal parts of the body that are in continuity with the external surface. They cover, protect, and provide secretory and absorptive functions in the channels and extended pockets of the outside world that are incorporated in the body. This applies to: the whole of the *alimentary tract* from the mouth to the anus; the *respiratory tract* from the nose through the larynx, trachea, and bronchial tree leading to the microscopic millions of 'blind ends' at the lung alveoli; the *urogenital tract* — vulva, vagina, uterus, and Fallopian tubes in the female, urethra and bladder in both sexes reaching to the kidneys via the ureters, and the vas deferens and tubules reaching into each testis in the male. The linings of all of these are EPITHELIA and most are known as mucous membranes.

Although all these linings are moist, this is by no means everywhere related to the presence of mucus. Actual mucus-secreting cells are scattered among other cells of many mucous membranes, particularly in the intestines and the upper part of the respiratory tract. They are known as 'goblet cells' because of the shape of the globule of mucus which may be seen under the microscope inside the cells or discharging through a disrupted cell membrane.

The nature of the cells forming a particular mucous membrane (or *mucosa*) reflects the specialized function at that site. All these functions are related in some way to interaction between the internal and external environments of the body: nutrition, gas exchange, excretion, or the intrusions and extrusions required for reproduction.

The lining layers are of varying depth. In the areas which are closest to the transition from the skin — in the mouth, anus, and vagina — there are layers of thin cells, like those of the skin, but without the thickened protective outermost layer. In most other sites there is a single layer which may consist of tall 'columnar' cells, flat 'squamous' cells, or intermediate 'cuboidal' cells — again according to function. Many mucous membranes have GLANDS whose ducts dip from the surface to clusters of secretory cells in the deeper layer of tissue (*submucosa*).

In the alimentary tract, from the mouth through to the end of the small intestine, the glands of the mucosa produce enzymes and other chemical substances necessary for digestion. In the intestines, although the lining is a single-layered sheet of cells, it is thrown into folds, and also has frond-like protrusions (*villi*), which enormously extend the surface area available for absorption, particularly in the small intestine; here also, the surface of each cell has thousands of *microvilli*. There are goblet cells scattered throughout, but they become more dense in the large intestine, where lubrication by mucus becomes more necessary as the faeces become more solid.

In the respiratory tract, including the NOSE and PHARYNX, and the EUSTACHIAN TUBES that connect it to the middle ears, and down all the branching airways of the lungs as far as the small bronchioles, the cardinal feature of the cells of the mucous membrane is that they are *ciliated*. The beating movement of the cilia helps to shift upwards and outwards any foreign particles which adhere to a layer of mucus secreted from interspersed goblet cells. (In the finest tubes of the bronchial tree the cells become progressively flatter, until in the alveoli they form the thinnest lining of any epithelium anywhere in the body, facilitating diffusion of gases — no longer called a mucous membrane.)

In parts of the genital tracts also, the lining cells are ciliated, assisting movement of an ovum down the FALLOPIAN TUBE, or movement of SPERM along the tubules of the epididymis, from testis to vas deferens. There are glands in the mucous membranes of the Fallopian tubes, UTERUS, VAGINA, and VULVA, whose secretions all facilitate the reproductive process, from COITUS through FERTILIZATION to PREGNANCY; it is the mucosa of the uterus (the endometrium) which thickens and grows new glands monthly in anticipation of possible pregnancy, and which is shed if this doesn't happen, or develops further if it does. In the male, the glands of the mucosa of the genital tract secrete substances which provide an appropriate environment for sperm on their journey from the testes, and the components of the seminal fluid which accompanies them to their potential destination in the female tract.

In the urinary tract, the mucous membranes that line the urethra, BLADDER, and ureters are several cells thick, allowing, especially in the bladder, for expansion; the particular protection required here is against the acidity of the urine. (These linings are in continuity with that of the 'pelvis' of the kidney and in turn the ducts and tubules leading to the thin membranes at the glomeruli, which filter the blood.)

SHEILA JENNETT

See also ALIMENTARY SYSTEM; EPITHELIUM; LUNGS.

Mulatto The word 'mulatto' is derived from the Arabic *muwallad*, which originally referred to persons who were not 'genuine' Arabs, especially individuals born of black–white 'misalliances'. With the beginning of the transatlantic African slave trade in the fifteenth century, the word mulatto first found its way into Portuguese, and then into almost all European languages, as the term for offspring of mixed European (Caucasian) and African (Negroid) parentage. (Only Afrikaans used the word 'Bastard' for such persons.)

The social position of these 'half-breeds' varied from place to place and over time. On the sugar plantations of Latin America, in several Caribbean colonies, and in southern and western Africa, where white masters faced an overwhelming number of black workers in bondage to them, the mulatto and his or her descendants formed a buffer zone between blacks and whites that was indispensable for maintaining the authority and prosperity of the Europeans. Colonial masters assigned members of this group certain tasks that they would not themselves assume, but could not entrust to blacks, and in exchange granted to mulattos privileges which were denied to black workers on principle. As a result, such 'half-breeds' lost almost any incentive to ally themselves with blacks, while at the same time they sought to move closer to the white ruling class, which purposely permitted them such approaches — although always ranking them according to their ostensible percentage of 'white blood'. Much as would later be the case

with Jews in Nazi Germany, *sang-mêlés* were classified by degree of mixed parentage. A 'quarter-white' was thus a *sambo*, a *mulatto* was 'half white', a *quadroon* was 'three-quarters white', and a *mestizo* was 'seven-eighths white'. In the French colony of Saint-Domingue there were 128 such categories! People of 'mixed blood', who believed that, despite discrimination, such a system contained at least the promise of equality with Europeans for their descendants, and who therefore intentionally chose 'whiter' mates in hope of bearing 'fairer' children, of course found themselves disappointed. Entry into the caste of whites was prohibited to the offspring of mulattos even after many generations; a person whose blood contained a ratio of 127 white ancestors to one black was still a *sang-mêlé*, still a 'coloured'. As the intermediate class between blacks, with whom they did not *want* to be linked, and whites, with whom they *could* not be linked, people of 'mixed blood' thus achieved social permanence.

On the North American continent, in contrast to the aforementioned regions, there was no separate intermediate class of 'coloureds'. Here the whites enjoyed such a preponderance that they could dare to assign people of 'mixed blood' the same social and legal basis as their slaves. To be sure, there was a differentiation according to the amount of 'mixed blood', but its aim was to eliminate from the ruling caste of whites all 'half-breeds', even those with a truly minuscule portion of black ancestry, and thus incorporate them into a work force held in bondage. The word 'mulatto' has thus never been common usage in the US, and the word 'coloured', although a widespread term until the middle of this century, was synonymous with 'black', which even today includes all shades of the African-American population, from 'racially pure' blacks to almost 'racially pure' whites. Reports of 'white' slaves, male or female, have always been able to arouse the latent sadism in some people. (In contemporary Australia, Pauline Hanson and her 'One Nation Party' have taken the opposite tack and in order to further the interest of their white countrymen want to recognize only 'pure bloods' and 'half-casts' as true Aborigines, thereby depriving all others of any reparations by the Commonwealth of Australia.)

In Europe, with its ample reservoir of white labourers — in contrast to colonies dependent on enforced labour of imported workers or 'natives' — not only the ruling class but also the entire society tried to remain unsullied by 'black blood'. By the end of the nineteenth century, the constant threat of mass unemployment served as the background for the campaign against admitting members of 'alien races' as a 'ruinous contamination of the white race', and the number of mulattos was considered a measure of physical and psychological decay. Predicting the fall of Western civilization, right-wing ideologies in all parts of Europe proclaimed that the several hundred 'half-breeds' born of 'coloured' French auxiliary forces during the occupation of the Rhineland (1919–29) were the catastrophic result of a 'blood warfare' analogous to a 'gas warfare' and directed not only against Germany, but against the whole of the white race. Hitler, too, constantly referred to the ostensibly imminent 'peril' of a 'mulattoization' of Europe; after 1933, his party saw to it that corrective measures were taken: the 'Rhineland bastards' were forced to be sterilized.   PETER MARTIN

See also RACISM; SKIN COLOUR.

Murder

Murder The act of murder is unique to humanity. While animals kill outside of their own species for food, and may fight, wound, or very occasionally kill within species for territory, it is only within mankind that one person — out of malice or rage, for gain or revenge — takes another person's life by violent means. Though most religions and cultures have gone out of their way to define murder as unnatural (the very use of the words 'cold blooded' denotes our need to see it as less than human), its continued presence within our history might, if we were more honest, suggest the opposite.

As a central element in the drama of human life, murder has always figured powerfully within culture, but it is only in the last hundred years or so that it has itself become a recognizable art form: the murder mystery. The timing is interesting. It is surely not coincidental that at the same time as medical advances were lengthening human life, writers were finding themselves more and more obsessed by stories about shortening it. Or that as science was chipping away at the notion of God, the murder mystery was busy perfecting itself as a form which, by definition, always answered certain key questions about the mysteries of life: why is it this person who dies rather than another? And — the biggest question of all — who did it? Murder, the most violent of human activities, became in some ways the most reassuring of reads.

Increasingly, science has been playing an ever more powerful role in solving murder, both real and fictional. Where once the art of detection was as much about intuition as about the careful consideration of evidence (the archetypes here are Miss Marple versus Sherlock Holmes), scientific and forensic advances are now the name of the game. DNA testing is just one of a whole series of breakthroughs that have made the laboratory as important as the scene of the crime and the corpse as communicative as any witnesses. While the question 'why?' may still be the preserve of the traditional detective, the 'who?' and the 'how?' are now being answered by men and women in white coats, and their fictional equivalents, a whole rash of hero/heroine pathologists, are becoming the new superstars of the genre. Through them the dead speak. Which, in its own way, is a kind of resurrection of the body. Maybe that explains why, while as a society we fret continually about rising levels of violent crime, culturally speaking we can't seem to get enough of a good murder.

By definition, a murder is a *homicide* (the killing of one human being by another) that is committed intentionally, or with malice aforethought. All legal codes classify it as a crime; where the element of intent exists and there are no extenuating circumstances, the penalty may be death or life imprisonment. It is thus important that doctors and legal investigators — those routinely confronted by cases of sudden and unexplained death — have some way to determine whether they are dealing with murder, suicide (self-murder), or an accident.

The problem of determining the cause of sudden or accidental death is one of the most important functions of *forensic medicine*, the application of medical knowledge to the service of the law and the administration of justice. It is a subject which draws upon a wide understanding of the medical, surgical, and scientific consequences of violent assault, POISONING, and other criminal offences against the person. In cases where the victim has died and a charge of murder may be brought, the law relies upon a detailed forensic examination of the corpse (and the crime scene) by trained experts. A careful medicolegal *autopsy*, performed by a forensic pathologist, can accurately reveal the sequence of events leading up to death, while forensic scientists are able to link the suspect to the victim on the strength of evidence from bloodstains, fibres, hairs, weapons, wounds, etc. Every contact between victim and murderer leaves a physical trace.

Forensic examinations were performed in medieval China and Europe, where surgeons noted the distinctions between fatal and non-fatal wounds, and those made before and after death; the depth, direction, and location of cutting wounds helped to distinguish between suicide and murder. The differences between burning, hanging, and submersion inflicted before and after death were known, but the principal symptoms and internal signs of poisoning were easily mistaken for those of disease. Despite the growing corpus of medical knowledge, however, courts relied for centuries on crude methods of establishing the guilt of accused murderers, who were subjected to trial by ordeal, or tortured to extract confessions. Cruentation — the supposed bleeding of the wounds of a corpse in the presence of the murderer — was popularly accepted as a proof of guilt until the nineteenth century.

Today, murder is assumed if a corpse shows injuries that raise suspicion or give obvious evidence of criminal violence, as in deaths from gunshot or stab wounds, burning, and bludgeoning. When an individual is battered to death, there will be a lot of blood at the scene and defensive wounds on the victim's arms. The instrument used will often leave a discernible pattern on the body. Murder by burning — which is rare — causes contraction of the muscles; the presence of soot or carbon monoxide in the lungs indicates that the victim was alive when the fire began. Stab wounds show the type of blade used and its length; extensive superficial wounding usually indicates suicide. Bullet wounds can indicate the distance and position from which a gun was fired, thus determining whether a death was murder or SUICIDE. If a weapon is not found at the scene there is a strong presumption of murder, but sometimes the most severe wounds do not cause instantaneous death; suicides are occasionally able to walk some distance before collapsing.

When signs of mortal wounding are lacking, asphyxiation (resulting from inhalation of noxious fumes or smoke, DROWNING, hanging, smothering, or strangling) and poisoning are considered. Murder by strangulation is done with the hands or with a ligature (throttling). In both cases bodies exhibit blue lips and tiny haemorrhages on the face and eyes (petechiae). Victims strangled by hand have 'fingertip' bruises on the throat, and fractures of the hyoid bone of the voice box, while in throttling deaths the ligature is either present or will have left a distinctive groove on the neck. Self-throttling is possible, but self-strangulation by hand is not. Murder by hanging rarely occurs, but bodies are sometimes suspended after being murdered, to simulate suicidal hanging (which is common); when this is the case there will be other marks of violence on the corpse. Signs of vital reaction around the constriction mark on the neck indicate that the victim was alive when hanged. When neither is present, a medical opinion may be difficult to reach.

Drowning deaths are diagnosed by the presence of froth in the air passages, water in the stomach, and ballooning of the lungs; circumstantial evidence is required to distinguish between murder, suicide, and accident. The presence of microscopic algae (diatoms) in the circulatory system and internal organs can help to locate where the victim died, as they vary from place to place. No diatoms are found in the bodies of individuals murdered and then thrown into water. Smothering deaths leave few traces, but there may be evidence of pressure on the face and bloodstained froth from the nostrils; fibres found in the airways of the victim may prove that a specific soft object was used to prevent breathing. Deaths resulting from inhalation of irrespirable gases are usually suicides or accidents; circumstantial evidence may indicate murder. Lastly, only a small percentage of modern murderers use poison, which can be detected by chemical analysis (*forensic toxicology*).

If a murder victim remains unidentified, so does the murderer. But it is possible to gain a great deal of information from a dead body, or from parts thereof. When all that remains is a SKELETON, its age, sex, height, and race can be determined. Bones will show evidence of physical deformities, right- or left-handedness, and sometimes diseases or other medical conditions. Teeth are nearly impossible to destroy, and are thus an ideal means of identification. When murder is suspected only after burial, it is possible to prove even after a number of years have elapsed. Some details will be lost (for example, putrefaction and time destroy all evidence of death from drowning), but cause of death can

usually be determined following exhumation and forensic autopsy. In essence, dead men do tell tales.   SARAH DUNANT
                                      KATHERINE D. WATSON

See also AUTOPSY; DROWNING; POISONING; SKELETON; STRANGULATION; SUFFOCATION.

Muscle is the body's contractile tissue. 'Contraction', in the physiological sense, may involve shortening and change of shape, or it may generate force without any change in length. All contraction depends on physicochemical alterations in the molecules of protein filaments within the cells, resulting in the generation of force at linkages (*cross-bridges*) between two different kinds of filament. The main proteins involved, in the respective filaments of all types of muscle, are *actin* and *myosin*; and in all muscles the process is powered by breakdown of *adenosine triphosphate*, during which chemical energy is converted by the interactions between these proteins into the mechanical energy of contraction. To initiate the process, muscle cells require excitation, which leads to contraction by a sequence that crucially involves an increase in the concentration of free CALCIUM ions inside the cell — a sequence termed *excitation– contraction coupling*.

There are three main types of muscle in the body: skeletal, cardiac, and smooth. When SKELETAL MUSCLES contract they either move parts of the body via their attachments to bones, or produce tension to oppose stretch or even to allow controlled lengthening. CARDIAC MUSCLE and SMOOTH MUSCLE, by shortening, reduce the capacity of hollow organs and tubes: thus cardiac muscle ejects blood from the HEART; smooth muscle ejects urine from the BLADDER or the fetus from the UTERUS, moves the contents of the gut along, and influences the flow of blood to different regions by varying the diameter of BLOOD VESSELS.

Skeletal and cardiac are together known as *striated* muscles, because their fibres have a striped appearance under the microscope, due to the orderly arrangement of alternating ranks of interdigitating actin and myosin filaments within their cytoplasm. Smooth (*unstriated*) muscle does not show this: the two types of filament are mingled throughout the cytoplasm of the cells. Whilst cardiac and skeletal muscle have a structural resemblance, skeletal muscle can be under conscious control and is therefore also known as *voluntary muscle* whereas cardiac muscle and smooth muscle share the designation *involuntary* because their actions are never under direct conscious control. (In certain contemplative regimes, the subtle influence which may be achieved — such as on the heart rate — is an indirect consequence of a profoundly disciplined emotional state.)

The voluntary/involuntary distinction implies differences also in control of the three types of muscle. Skeletal muscle is controlled through pathways in the nervous system that can be consciously activated, cardiac and smooth by the involuntary or 'autonomic' pathways. Each

skeletal muscle fibre is called into action by release of transmitter from a terminal branch of a single axon from a motor neuron in the SPINAL CORD; the point at which this nerve terminal contacts the muscle fibre is a specialized SYNAPSE, the NEUROMUSCULAR JUNCTION. All muscle fibres controlled by this nerve are recruited together, and the grouping of a motor neuron plus its family of muscle fibres is said to comprise a 'motor unit'. When transmitter is not being released, the muscle fibres are relaxed. Individual cardiac muscle cells by contrast are activated by electrical transmission of excitation from their neighbours; this excitation originates rhythmically at a PACEMAKER, even in the absence of nerve action, although normally the rate of firing is modulated by the release, close to the pacemaker site, of transmitters from autonomic nerves. Smooth muscles differ again: in some, notably in the uterus at term, excitation is electrical, starting at pacemaker sites, much as in the heart. In others, such as those controlling the diameter of a large blood vessel, excitation is by NEUROTRANSMITTERS released from autonomic nerve endings close to the cells, but not with structured synapses. The contraction/relaxation state of smooth muscle can also be modified by chemical agents other than neurotransmitters, released from neighbouring cells or circulating in the blood. In the autonomic control of involuntary muscle, there is at many sites the possibility of either excitatory or inhibitory neural action, according to the particular transmitter released, resulting in a two-way control system analogous to accelerator and brake. The heart, for instance, is slowed by one transmitter, yet speeded up by another; the stomach wall is contracted by one and relaxed by another.   NEIL SPURWAY
                                      SHEILA JENNETT

See PLATE 5.

See also AUTONOMIC NERVOUS SYSTEM; CARDIAC MUSCLE; MOTOR NEURONS; SKELETAL MUSCLE; SMOOTH MUSCLE.

Muscle tone When muscles contract and develop force they do so because nerves leading to them become active; the messages result in electrical activity in the muscle which can easily be detected by electromyography (EMG). For much of our lives, however, our muscular capacity is grossly underused. In the course of a normal day, the average sedentary person uses perhaps only 10% of the force-generating potential of the muscles of his limbs. In the past it has been assumed that the passive force in resting muscle could be ignored, but it is now apparent that it may contribute importantly to the stabilization of posture that we take for granted; this is because resting muscle shows thixotropic properties. Thixotropy is a property displayed by many systems, particularly those with complex molecules with long chains, familiar objects being tomato ketchup and thixotropic paint. Tip up a bottle of ketchup and nothing comes out; shake it and it will flow freely. Leave it on a shelf

for some time and it stiffens again. Similarly, if there is no movement, muscle stiffens considerably, and much of this change takes place quite rapidly, say within two seconds. This property is one aspect of muscle tone and also contributes to the tone assessed as 'normal' for a muscle at rest during a neurological examination. The medical person moves the limb to and fro slowly to estimate resistance. Sometimes further information can be gained by moderate shaking: the limb should not flail excessively.

Muscle properties are influenced by temperature. When the fibres are warm they work faster. People who are cold often complain that their muscles are stiff, and athletes and pianists 'warm up' before starting their activities. This may well be due to the well-documented effects that temperature has on muscle thixotropy. When cold it is difficult or impossible to 'shake out' the stiffening due to enhanced thixotropy. Some treatments used by physiotherapists may be effective through such mechanisms; deep warmth, as by diathermy, and passive stretching will both have the effect of reducing this resistance.

When a limb is held stationary against gravity, inactive muscle fibres will exist alongside the active ones; the proportion of each depends on the total mass supported, with the active fibres in steady contraction. When sitting, the head is held up by the contraction of muscles at the back of the neck. If someone drops off to sleep in the sitting position, this activity is lost and the head slumps forward. Again, our mouths are normally kept lightly closed by contractions which counteract the action of gravity on the mass of the lower jaw.

Some muscles may be excessively active, resulting in unusual, if not ungainly, postures; in some people when nervous this may be expressed through the facial muscles as a grimace. Sometimes muscles which act against each other contract simultaneously; when severe this can result in spasm or CRAMP. But even when mild, such spasm can be undesirable, as in writer's cramp or the analogous problems for musicians. Awkward positions, such those inevitable in playing the violin, are particularly likely to generate difficulties.

Most people can relax fully without any special training: if a limb is supported, the muscle action switches off almost at once. 'Relax' is used in two senses: mechanical, referring to a reduction of muscular action, and metaphorical, a reference to mental tranquility. The physiological basis of procedures sometimes advocated to achieve such RELAXATION is often obscure.

Muscle tone, even in healthy people at rest, is thus dependent on quite complex mechanisms. However, it becomes even more difficult to describe under conditions of movement where parts of the body are accelerating and decelerating. For this reason it is usually preferable to speak only of 'resting muscle tone'.

The word 'tone' has the same root as the word 'tune', and the tension in the tendon of a muscle can be likened to that in the string of a guitar.

Based on these considerations, muscle tone in the resting state can be measured by applying rhythmic forces and observing at which rate of application the motion is the greatest. This is the 'resonant frequency'. Tone is related to the square of the resonant frequency.

At times the level of tone becomes set incorrectly. The body may be abnormally floppy — a state referred to as 'hypotonia' and children may be born with the 'floppy child syndrome'. But in some relatively common diseases the tone is increased and the limbs are unusually stiff. There are two main types of this hypertonia:

(i) *Spasticity* may follow injury to a main pathway for messages from the brain downwards. On manipulation of the limb the excessive tone may easily be felt, but the extent of this depends of the rate at which the limb is passively moved; there may be only a little extra resistance if the motion is slow. Stretching a muscle normally causes a reflex contraction; spasticity results when sensors in the muscle responsive to stretch become more than usually effective in causing this reflex contraction. These numerous receptors are important in the regulation of normal POSTURE; it is their unrestrained effects that cause difficulties such as may arise after a STROKE, or in children following birth injury (one cause of CEREBRAL PALSY).

(ii) *Rigidity* is distinct from spasticity. In this the resistance is independent of the rate at which the limb is manipulated by the examiner, and indeed, in extreme cases, it leads to a maintained postural abnormality described as *dystonia*. Such rigidity is one of the signs of Parkinsonism. Occasionally other disturbances are found. Thus someone may have the misfortune of suffering from an involuntary contraction of muscles of the neck so that the head is held in a quite abnormal posture. The medical term for such a 'wry neck' is *torticollis*.　　E. GEOFFREY WALSH

See also CEREBRAL PALSY; SKELETAL MUSCLE.

Further reading
Walsh, E. G. (1992). *Muscles, masses and motion.* MacKeith/Cambridge University Press.

Muscle wasting
A wasted muscle is one that has become thinner. It is a sign that all is not well with the motor nerve that innervates it, because a muscle depends on its motor nerve for survival and will die when it is permanently separated from it. A wasted muscle will be weak, and if separation from the motor nerve is complete, so will be the paralysis.

A muscle is composed of a large number of individual muscle fibres and its motor nerve contains a large (but smaller) number of individual nerve fibres. This smaller number is because an individual motor nerve fibre branches many times within the muscle, each muscle fibre receiving only one branch at its neuromuscular junction. Each individual nerve fibre is the axon of a motor nerve cell in the anterior horn of grey matter in the spinal cord, known as a *lower motor neuron* or *anterior horn cell*. The anterior horn cell, its *axon* (nerve fibre), and all the *muscle fibres* it innervates (there can be 100 or more) constitute a *motor unit*.

Causes of muscle wasting can be focal or localized, when only one motor nerve is affected, or generalized, when a disease process affects many motor nerves or lower MOTOR NEURONS. One of the commonest causes of focal muscle wasting is trauma to a motor nerve. For example, a laceration at the wrist can sever the *ulnar nerve*, which innervates many of the small muscles in the hand, leading to pronounced wasting (and also to sensory loss, because the ulnar nerve contains sensory nerves as well as motor nerves). If the nerve is not surgically reconnected, the muscle fibres will die, muscle wasting will be permanent, and the muscles it supplies will be totally paralysed. A similar pattern of wasting can occur when the ulnar nerve is damaged at the elbow, perhaps because of a fracture there. Other types of mechanical trauma have more insidious effects, by the slow compression of nerves, such as in the *carpal tunnel* on the front of the wrist, or with protrusion of an intervertebral disc, when wasting may accompany pain, due to simultaneous damage to both motor and sensory nerve fibres. Another example of focal wasting occurs with a 'Bell's palsy' (an inflammatory paralysis of the facial nerve on one side). This results in inability to wrinkle the forehead muscles of that side, to close the eye and mouth, or to smile normally. This syndrome also illustrates the capacity of motor nerves to recover and to *reinnervate* the denervated face muscles. The new nerve fibres slowly extend down the nerve, although not always reaching the same muscle that they originally innervated. Thus a motor neuron that is active during blinking may come to innervate the muscles around the mouth, so that the mouth contracts with each attempted blink. This process of re-innervation rescues the muscle fibres from death.

Muscle wasting will also occur when a disease process affects motor nerves generally, a condition known as a peripheral neuropathy. Long nerves usually show signs of dysfunction before shorter nerves; thus wasting and weakness is usually first evident in the lower leg and in the hands. Among the many causes of peripheral neuropathies are *toxic substances* (organophosphates, for example); *metabolic conditions* such as diabetes; *malnutrition* leading to vitamin deficiencies; *acute inflammatory neuropathies* such as the Guillain–Barré syndrome, in which the motor nerves are attacked by cells of the IMMUNE SYSTEM; and *genetic disorders* in which mutations lead to structural defects in the nerve. Some of these conditions are irreversible, but others, such as the Guillain–Barré syndrome, can partly or completely recover.

Finally, wasting can result from diseases that affect the anterior horn cells themselves. The commonest cause worldwide is the *poliomyelitis* virus, which is now partly controlled by IMMUNIZATION programmes. Those who survive the initial paralysis are left with varying degrees of muscle wasting, and in children this can interfere with growth, leading to limb shortening and spinal deformities. *Motor neuron disease* is a relatively rare cause of muscle wasting that is often accompanied by spontaneous muscle twitching (fasciculations). It usually affects individuals in middle or later life, but sometimes, especially in the very rare familial form of the disorder, may affect young people. *Spinal muscular atrophy* is a genetic disorder in which anterior horn cells fail to develop normally, leading to wasting and paralysis which in some forms are associated with death in infancy.

　　　　　　　　　　　　J. NEWSOM-DAVIS

See also CENTRAL NERVOUS SYSTEM; MOTOR NEURONS; MUSCLE.

Music and the body
Historical roots
From the very earliest relics we find examples of the link made by humans between music and the body. A corpse found in Poland, dating back to the eight century BC, was buried with nine musical bone pipes, thought to symbolize the man's shamanic wisdom and magical powers. Since ancient times, music has served many ceremonial functions, ranging from tribal circumcision to marriage and death. The ancient Egyptians depicted scenes on their sarcophagi of people playing instruments, to show their belief that music accompanied the body to its final meeting with the gods. So this recognized not only that music was created and performed by humans, but that it would assist them to transcend their bodily confines after death. Particularly in aboriginal culture, we see the strength of the link between music and the body. In this oldest living culture, surviving relatively unchanged for over 40 000 years, virtually all aspects of human behaviour have an intrinsic link with music: eating, hunting, love-making, birth, marriage, and death are all music-filled activities. The music of the Australian aborigines is heavily based in song, and so is linked to the most fundamental human instrument of all, the voice. Aboriginal songs include many kinds of vocalisations ranging from growling, grunting, and shrieking to bitonal syllabic chanting. This music demonstrates how human communication has evolved from survival function through to the engagement in singing for artistic pleasure. Of course, any communication involves the processes of both perception and response.

Music perception and response
In the case of Jeanne d'Albret, mother of King Henry IV of France, 'sweet' music was played to her every morning during her pregnancy in the belief that the fetus could hear the music, and that the music would help to mould the baby's temperament. Historians of the day reported that Henry IV was always in good spirits, as a direct consequence of this procedure. It was demonstrated only in the 1980s that the human cochlea (the organ of hearing) functions as early as the twentieth week of gestation, that the fetal world is a noise-filled one, and that new-borns

show familiarity with musical stimuli they have been exposed to six weeks before birth. So perception begins early, and audition is a significant fetal experience with aural learning occurring *in utero*. Indeed, arguably, much of what the fetus hears is essentially musical. Amniotic fluid attenuates sound; therefore the mother's voice, the sounds of her body such as heartbeat, and sounds from the outer world are only partially heard. Only the basic sound pattern of the mother's voice will be heard, stripped of its semantic content: the speech patterns are heard *in utero* as a series of undulating and related pitches. These patterns derive meaning for the fetus from the shape, speed, volume, and pitch height, and are associated with elements similar to those of a musical melody. Sounds are also experienced physically through the acoustical vibrations in the fluid, and so are directly related to bodily sensations. Thus, the sounds and feelings correspond closely to experiences of music in the external world.

Observation and reporting have widely indicated that from very early childhood music elicits bodily experiences linked to the experience of emotion: the enharmonic key changes in tonal music are often associated with 'shivers down the spine' or 'goose bumps', reflecting psychological states such as excitement, joy, or sadness. Linking back to the fetal experience of Henry IV, it would follow that the content of the music he was hearing may indeed have had some emotional effect, this in turn arguably having an impact on his personality state of general good spirits. Personality is, of course, a complex phenomenon, with many innate, stable components as well as emergent and changing aspects. Yet, research has suggested that amongst musicians very particular personality characteristics are evident, reflecting emotional qualities such as great sensitivity.

In the pre-natal experience, much is also mediated by the mother: in addition to the fetus's own direct responses to the music, it will have been receiving information about the mother's moods and emotions, conveyed through chemical and physiological changes, such as increased heart rate. Therefore, Henry IV was likely to have been heavily influenced by how his mother responded to the music as well as having his own perceptions. So, from the earliest exposure to musical stimuli, it appears that our responses are rooted in bodily sensation.

An example of music and its bodily origin is found in the way in which individuals perceive and respond to musical rhythm. It is known that we possess an innate ability to estimate intervallic relations. Indeed, when we listen to musical stimuli, we use the musical information already heard to provide a reference for ongoing perception. We are able to anticipate regular events (demonstrated by anticipatory body movements) — and react to a disturbance of these events. We find this intrinsically pleasurable, and our bodies are highly responsive. There is now ample evidence that fast musical pulses increase our heart rate and can make us drive faster, eat more quickly, make love more vigorously, and so

on. By contrast, slow musical rhythms provide relaxation, promoting rest: lullabies soothe, and assist sleep as the heart rate slows.

In the first year of life, it has been demonstrated that motor activity most typically occurs in rhythmical bursts. The rhythmical nature of these bursts is believed to have a key role in general motor development, giving the child a repertoire of motor routines that are practised to become increasingly fine-grained and specific. An example of this practice is how an infant's burst of rhythmical leg activity develops into walking in toddlerhood. From this base, it is possible to understand how motor skills for the performance of musical rhythms develop: initially, there will be bursts of activity that are not necessarily close to the musical rhythm, and, over time, increasingly controlled and accurate movements will develop that can be both predictive of a regular pulse, and able to adapt to disturbances in it.

There may be a direct link between physical movement and rhythmical expression in music. For example, the shape of a musical phrase moving from low to high or slow to fast is similar to the running-walking-stopping-walking-running patterns of speeding and slowing of bodily movement cycles.

Of course rhythm is not the only musical parameter which has an effect on the body: melody, harmony, and timbre (the tone colour of a particular note) all interact. In the case of timbre it is well reported that certain tone colours create bodily reactions: sharp, metallic sounds or smooth deep sounds, for instance, elicit specific physiological responses. Timbres often also allude to bodily tension. For instance, tightly squeezed string sounds can sound like some sort of bodily pressure. A study was undertaken where people were asked to select their favourite rendition of the Queen of the Night's aria from Mozart's opera *The Magic Flute*. Amongst the selection of voices there was a synthesized version, perfect in every way: accurate breathing, even frequency of vibrato on the tone, and effortless pitching of the high notes. Yet none of the listeners enjoyed the performance. They all commented that there was no physical effort involved, therefore it sounded 'disembodied', and as such was of no interest.

Musical performance

The influence of the performer's tension and effort is not always as positive as in the case of the Queen of the Night's aria. In performance, the adrenaline rush of the performance situation can lead to negative and increasing physiological and psychological effects on the performer: bow tremor or acute self-doubts, for instance. In extreme cases this performance stress can wreck a career if the musician becomes physically and psychologically blocked. Good teaching obviously looks carefully at the interaction of mind and body in the production of a performance, and every effort is made to assure confidence, skill, and control in both. Of course, the benefit from receiving the adrenaline rush of the performance

situation is to sharpen the senses and heighten the physical and mental potential of the performer. This enhancing interaction of physiological and psychological responses to performance is often a high source of motivation for individuals to engage with the long hours of mundane practice that are involved in acquiring musical skills.

The production of music obviously requires the development through practice of increasingly refined motor skills, which become in large part automated so that the body is able to execute the performance task without conscious attention having to be paid to every single component of the movement.

Vocal skill development is an interesting example, for there is no obvious visible or easily manipulable body part engaged in the activity. The vocal cords can neither be easily moved into place nor seen, unlike fingers in piano-playing. Trained opera singers learn to use their voices by experimenting with the physical sensations specific vocal sounds make. Once a sensation has been felt and understood, the means by which it is found is then generalised to other areas of vocal production. For instance, a sung 'ng' directs the vocal sound to the front of the face, and so into the nasal and sinus resonators. This produces a greater volume of sound. The singer learns to feel through the body where to 'place' the voice with this particular 'ng' sound, and then is able to transpose the 'ng' sensation to all other vocal sounds to achieve evenness in volume irrespective of what kind of vowel or consonant is being sung. Related to this, the pitching of particular notes can be achieved through physical sensation: a very particular feeling of vibrations, in the chest or elsewhere, can be linked directly to the production of a specific musical note.

Musical instruments and musical expression

Anecdotal reports claim that certain physical types are best suited to playing certain kinds of musical instrument. Specific physical features may predispose individuals towards particular instruments (strong front teeth for clarinet playing, large hands for the piano, long arms for the trombone), but there are many highly successful players who do not possess these apparent physical advantages; it is more likely that motivation, commitment, and creativity will determine engagement with an instrument rather than physical features. The deaf percussionist Evelyn Glennie is testimony to the possibility of achievement against heavy physical odds. It is certainly the case that individuals can adapt to playing a whole range of instruments. Some children who begin playing very successfully on one musical instrument can completely change the type of instrument (say from brass to strings) and continue to develop performance skills.

Of course, there are many inescapable physical demands on the player in the interface between body and instrument. Added to these are cultural rules about how, when, and why music should be played. Ethnomusicologists have been quick to study this complex relationship, and have shown how the development of the structures of a variety of musical styles can be traced quite directly to ergonomic factors associated with the instruments on which the music has developed. For instance, the English ethnomusicologist John Baily has shown how the music of the dutar, a stringed instrument from Herat, in Afghanistan, evolved from music associated with a neighbouring instrument, and in the process acquired characteristics that were specifically related to the ergonomics of the dutar itself.

In Western art music, the link between body, musical style, and expression has been discussed in many pedagogical texts. In 1834, for example, Balliot, a violinist and professor at the Paris Conservatoire, wrote a treatise on violin playing which suggested that performers could employ different types of body movements to perform music at different musical speeds. He remarked that the adagio speed requires 'more ample movements' than the allegro, where notes are 'tossed off', whereas in presto there is 'great physical abandon'. Recent empirical studies have convincingly demonstrated that, beyond technically executing the music on the instrument, information about both structural features of music (harmony, speed, melody climaxes and so on) and expressive intention (what the performer wishes to convey about the music) is also contained in a musician's body movement. The present author has proposed that, although body movements can be imposed onto a performance in the manner suggested by Balliot (and there are indeed a whole range of specific gestures that players use for particular dramatic effect, like saxophone players raising the bell of their instruments to demonstrate great intensity and effort), many of the expressive movements performers make are entirely unconscious. The movements originate in the mental intention to communicate the music rather than to make a specific gesture. In this way the resulting movements can neither be added to nor removed from the performance: rather, they are integral to the execution of its expressive component. Indeed, so intrinsically linked are these movements to the technique of playing that the two become inseparable. For instance, pianists do not move their hands mechanistically from one key position to another. Rather, they move smoothly, often lifting the hand between the two points of key contact, creating an arc gesture as the hand moves through the air. This movement relates directly to the time interval available between the two points of key contact, and to the mood of the sounds that are created.

The body in music

From all the discussion above, it is evident that the body has an integral role in specifying the key components of music itself. As we listen and respond to music, profound effects on our physical/emotional states occur. In performance, the character and style are shaped by the body as the music is produced. But finally, it is worth considering a range of instruments that have been developed in the West in recent years for the purpose of creating music with and through our bodies. These instruments do not require a skilled technique, rather they depend on the natural everyday movements of the body itself. The first is the Theremin, which uses a loudspeaker and radio-frequency oscillators. Changing frequency occurs as the 'player' moves his/her hand around a stick-like antenna. The moving hand can create variations in the pitch, volume, and speed of the music being produced. People report that Theremin playing is extremely pleasurable as there is such a direct sound-movement-space link. Other such instruments include Sound Beam, for which a three-dimensional space is filled with sensors that have musical sounds attached to them, so when someone interrupts the sensor path by walking through its beam, a musical sound is created. Again, pitch height, speed and volume, even timbre can be affected by the rate at which the body moves in the beams. The final example of a body instrument is the MIDI glove. Attached to a computer, the glove is filled with sensors which stimulate the production of many different sounds. A single hand gesture can create a huge symphonic swell of multiphonic chords.

Although body instruments like these may not be mass market items yet, perhaps there is a blossoming future for them as they appear to satisfy the human desire to make music of bodily proportions.

JANE W. DAVIDSON

Musicianship and other finger skills

Human beings have the potential to develop many skills, a versatility far greater than that of any other animal. For certain skills a phase of learning is enough to develop an aptitude which lasts a lifetime and needs perhaps only slight practice thereafter. Thus children learn to tie laces at first with difficulty but later the procedure can be repeated easily. Learning to tie a tie, a bow, a knot, and do up buttons is similar. The years needed to learn writing need little reinforcement by later activity. The complex procedures required to ride a cycle, or to swim, are only lost with ill health. Artistic skills are multiple; people may be painters, engravers, etchers, or sculptors. Their abilities, difficult to measure meaningfully, need practising for good results. Often skills are said to be 'context sensitive'; a professional pianist may have difficulty with typing shoelaces. Practice of one set of movements may not result in a general increase of finger dexterity.

Some people are clumsy and not at all adept at using their hands, they may say for example that they 'cannot draw a straight line' or 'cannot use a screwdriver'. Inability to execute an intended action is known as *apraxia*, slowness and difficulty in doing it is *dyspraxia*.

Professional musicians train extensively and their skills reach levels of control far beyond those of many others. Some musical instruments usually have a one-to-one relationship between the finger movement needed and the intended note or notes. This allows measurements of the intended accuracy to be made. Musical performance involves muscular action and, with woodwind and brass instruments, careful breath control. Without doubt, especially during training, aural and other forms of fine sensory feedback are needed.

The human being, by adopting an upright stance, liberated the hands and arms from their role in supporting the body whilst the retention of thumbs and fingers in evolution has allowed the use of hands for a great variety of skilled activities.

Prehistoric human beings developed the skills needed to shape stones. The finding of arrowheads has enabled studies of this activity, 'knapping', to be undertaken; one hand, usually the right, held the flint and the other struck it with another stone. The skills needed would not have been easy to acquire. Sometimes in prehistoric sites hollow bones are found into which holes have been drilled suggesting that they were used as flutes.

Sign language is another ancient skill. There are one-handed and two-handed deaf and dumb alphabets but these are slow as words need to be spelt out letter by letter. Quite different are complex sign languages. In some religious communities silence was enforced but monks in the time of the Venerable Bede in the seventh century learnt to communicate by means of finger signs. Sign languages of the North American Indian tribes and aboriginal Australians have been studied in detail; abstract ideas and poetry are not beyond the capabilities of some.

The thumb in medical and scientific studies is referred to as 'digit 1' and the index, middle, ring and little fingers as 2, 3, 4, and 5. Modern piano music also uses this convention, but for the violin and other instruments where the thumb has only a supportive role, the index finger is '1'. The thumb is proportionally larger in man than in apes and a specialization of great importance is that the thumb is 'opposable', meaning that it can be brought across the palm to, or towards, any finger. This enables the use of a great range of grips; rather than a mere clenching of the fingers to hold an object, which may be about all some monkeys can achieve. The hand is therefore adaptable to hold, push and pull in a great range of different ways. The word 'manipulate' takes its origin from Latin, *manus*, a hand. In many mammals, for example the horse, cow, and pig, the number of digits is reduced from the arrangements in the reptilian ancestors whereas in the human hand the arrangements remain basically the same. The capabilities of the horse, cow, and pig, are inevitably very limited in manipulative skills using the legs. In these animals food is investigated by the nose and mouth whilst the human being lives a 'hand to mouth' existence, food being taken to the mouth by the hand.

Some finger movements depend mainly on activity of muscles in the forearm, the 'long flexors' and 'long extensors', but there are also a number of small muscles in the hand lying

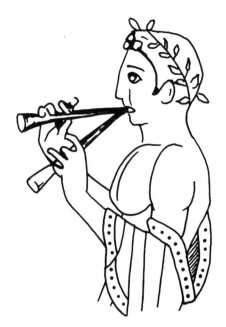

An Aulos Player. This reed instrument was widely used by the Ancient Greeks. It is related that the high notes sounded like squawking geese, and the lower ones like buzzing wasps. It was very loud and a player was said to charge one drachma to play but four drachmas to stop.

between the bones which play important roles in the control of individual fingers.

All muscles take significant times to contract and to relax so there is a limitation of the speed with which they can generate repeated movements. Few people can tap more rapidly than about seven per second. Such limitations, a result of muscle properties, apply to a violinist's vibrato and the beats of a drummer.

For about a hundred years the principal method of long distance communication was by telegraph. In the Morse code letters and numerals are sent by sequences of dots and dashes, the dashes being three times as long as the dots. The traditional Morse key, used for sending, has a metal lever which when depressed, makes an electrical contact. When the pressure is released the lever is raised by the action of a spring. The rate at which messages could be sent was of great economic importance but because of the limitations of muscle properties few operators could send more rapidly than about 25 words per minute. Morse operators were prone to suffer from 'Telegraphists Cramp'.

In states of excitement, often associated with the liberation of the hormone adrenaline, there is a change in muscle properties and the hands and fingers may shake. Such a TREMOR, if significant, constitutes part of stage fright and can seriously impair the performance of a musician. Its rate is usually about 10 per second.

In handwriting the small muscles of the hand are in constant activity in holding the pen or pencil between the thumb and index finger often with further support from the middle finger. Other activity is called for to make the strokes;

the time taken for these is quite variable but is often about a tenth of a second. The hand has also to be moved from left to right and the forearm must be rotated, 'three quarters prone', finally to start a new line the hand must be moved from right to left. There is probably no muscle between the shoulder and fingers which is not involved. When numerous people were employed as clerks there were often cases of 'Writers Cramp'.

In typing, two-finger typists use the 'hunt and peck' method but skilled typists read the material in advance of the keystrokes. The information is taken into a 'short term memory store'. The fingers are normally in motion towards more than a single keystroke simultaneously; as one finger approaches its target another is moving to operate the next key. Some typists can reach speeds of over 100 words per minute, whilst an office typist, typing at 60–80 words per minute, is averaging 5 to 7 key strokes per second.

Attempts to replace the 'QWERTY' keyboard, which arose historically with early typewriters, have made comparatively little headway and this arrangement is now widely used in computers. More than half the work is performed by the left hand. A typist needs to know, from the feeling in his fingers, that the key has been operated. There may be a hard stop, the key 'bottoms out' and stops moving at the point of actuation; this calls for the use of excess force. In other systems the force needed to push the key down decreases as soon as the contact is completed.

In musical performance much depends on accurate movements. Information is needed by the brain as to the position and movement of the hand and fingers; if this is lost there arise great difficulties in regulating movements. The trombone slide has seven positions, and finding them depends on the judgement and experience of the player. The cello is more demanding. An octave jump may cover a distance of, say, 30 cm, and the tolerance with good players is about ± 0.5 mm. The final position cannot be obtained by successive approximations or an intolerable 'miaowing' would result. The corresponding movement on the violin is 10 cm.

In some musical instruments most of the skill is needed by one hand or the other. For trumpeters the left hand acts merely as a clamp holding the instrument whilst the three valves are operated by fingers of the right hand. For the French horn the control of the valves is a function of the left hand. For the violin and its larger relatives the two hands have complementary complex tasks, the right hand controlling the bow, the left hand the stopping of the strings.

Some people are 'double jointed', their joints are significantly less limited in the range of possible positions than others. They may be able for instance to squat in the 'Lotus position' with the legs crossed and the soles of the feet pointing upwards. This 'hypermobility' shows ethnic differences, Caucasians being stiffer than Indians. Hypermobility can be found also in the hands and fingers. The virtuoso violinist, Niccolo

Paganini (1782–1840), showed an extreme degree of this condition, and it enabled him to play his instrument with unrivalled skill.

In woodwind instruments, such as the recorder or flute, the pitch of the note depends on the length of the closed tube. Pitch is lowered if, by closing holes or valves, the length is increased; it is raised if the length is reduced. The player is repeatedly called upon to make these adjustments, this is done by the fingers. The human hand is well provided with mechanisms for moving fingers in the same direction accurately at the same time. Simultaneous bending (flexion) or straightening (extension) of two fingers, either of the same or of opposite hands is accomplished easily by most people with errors of only a few thousandths of a second. Such small errors will not be expected to have detectable effects on the quality of the music that results. Fairly often however the requirements of the score are more demanding. It is often necessary to lift one or more fingers whilst lowering another or others. If this is not neatly done, with small errors, the quality of the resulting sound may be expected to vary. The errors of moving two fingers in opposite directions simultaneously are sometimes quite substantial. They are certainly large in children of primary school age who are commonly taught the recorder. There is usually no problem in getting fingers down onto holes of a recorder at the right time, but difficulties may arise because another finger is lifted too late. Professional woodwind players such as flautists, clarinettists, oboists are in general more skilled in this regard than violinists, pianists and accordion players. A very accurate group are the players of the Scottish Highland bagpipes. These musicians practise extensively, perform repeated grace notes, and the instrument is very responsive so that smallish errors will be apparent.

For acceptable musical performance the lengths of the resonant tube must be adjusted appropriately. The spacing between the fingers is often not well suited to this accomplishment. Some Indian bamboo transverse flutes have holes so far apart that they cannot be properly played by a Westerner. Because of these limitations the instrument maker, Theobald Boehm (1793–1881) invented a system of mechanical linkages allowing the 'holing' to be separated from the 'fingering'. This system is widely used in flutes and other woodwind instruments. In playing the flute only light pressure is needed to operate the valves but the musician cannot know that the hole is closed until the valve 'bottoms out'. An inexperienced player may use excessive force.

For pianists, the relative merits of having long or short fingers and a broad fleshy or slender bony hand have been debated; but at times hands which look unpromising can perform feats of extreme virtuosity. Beginners are taught standard fingerings. More advanced players may fall back on these when sight reading but may also become skilled at bending the rules and using the many opportunities for alternative fingering to advantage. In playing at a relatively advanced level the musician needs to take into account not only the immediate phrase but he should allow the fingers to be in an advantageous position for the execution of the next part of the score. Any of the ten digits may in principle be used to strike any key. Everything depends on the context in which the note is found. In arpeggios in Romantic music there is a successive playing of parts of a chord; they are usually played in order of ascending pitch and the highest note carries the melody, the tones are sustained by the use of the damper pedal.

There are anatomical linkages of tendons between some of the fingers and this can be a limitation to performance. Some players have had these connections severed surgically to increase the independence of finger movements that is possible. Such a procedure should only be undertaken, if at all, with the greatest caution. In the nineteenth century devices were invented to strengthen or increase the mobility of the fingers, but they are no longer used. In some of these the fingers were exercised against springs, in others wedges were used to force the joints into extreme positions and the consequences could be serious. Musicians are liable to suffer from cramps and a number of other 'upper limb disorders'. For a professional player, especially, the consequences can be serious and medical advice should be sought at an early stage.   E. GEOFFREY WALSH

Further reading

Boehm, T. (1964). The flute and flute playing. Dover.

Cole, J. (1995). Pride and the daily marathon. MIT Press, Cambridge, MA.

Shivas, A. A. (1988). The art of tympanist and drummer. Edinburgh University Press, Edinburgh.

Walsh, E. G. (1997). Synchronization of human finger movements: delays and sex differences with isotonic antiphase motion. *Experimental Physiology* **82**, 559–65.

Walsh, E. G. (2000). Mathematical analyses of telegraphic signalling. *Morsum Magnificat* **72** 8–15.

See also EVOLUTION, HUMAN; HANDEDNESS; HANDS; MUSCLE TONE; TREMOR.

Mutation is a change in the structure of the genome by alteration of the DNA. Alterations in the DNA sequence can arise when mistakes made during *replication* (copying of the DNA) cause the insertion or omission of a base (*point mutation*) or the removal or inversion of larger segments of DNA. Mutations can also be caused by radiation or by some chemicals (*mutagens*). The consequences of mutations are variable; if a mutation occurs within a gene then the composition of the *gene product* (a protein) will be altered and may affect its function. The evolutionary process depends on mutations in DNA.
A.W.C.

Myelin Myelin is the fatty insulating layer that surrounds many *axons* (nerve fibres) in both the *central* and *peripheral* NERVOUS SYSTEMS (CNS and PNS respectively). Nerve cells, with their

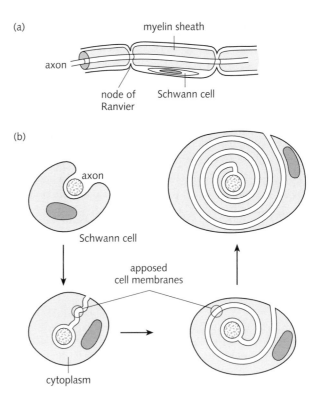

Fig. 1 (a) A myelinated axon in the peripheral nervous system and (b) its development. Each Schwann cell myelinates a single axon, to which it is directly apposed. During development (anticlockwise) Schwann cells loosely ensheath axons and the myelin sheath grows around the axon to form concentric layers, which become tightly apposed.

axons, and GLIA are the two major cell types of the nervous systems. Myelin is formed from membranous sheets that are elaborated by glial cells: *Schwann cells* in the PNS and *oligodendrocytes* in the CNS. A major difference between these two is that Schwann cells each myelinate part of a single axon, whereas oligodendrocytes can myelinate as many as thirty axons in the CNS. Also, whereas Schwann cells are directly associated with their myelin sheath (Fig. 1), oligodendrocyte cell bodies connect by thin, tenuous processes to their multiple myelin sheets, each of which may be some distance from the cell body (Fig 3a).

Along the axons, myelin sheaths are arranged in segments that are separated by narrow regions of naked *axolemma* (the cell membrane of the axon) called *nodes of Ranvier*; these are the sites of action potential generation in myelinated axons (Fig. 1a and 3a). Nodes occur at regular intervals ranging from 0.3–2.0 mm, according to axon size. The myelin acts as a layer of high electrical resistance and low capacitance, facilitating the rapid *saltatory* (jumping) conduction of electrical impulses from node to node for long distances along axons that may be up to 1 m in length. Perhaps the most striking evidence of the importance of myelin comes from human demyelinating diseases such as *multiple sclerosis*, which specifically attacks oligodendrocytes. The subsequent loss of myelin causes the conduction block that underlies the crippling clinical symptoms of the disease.

Myelin is a complex structure that shows in cross-section as spirals around the axon to form a sheath made up of concentric layers (*lamellae* Fig. 1b, 3b). The number of lamellae (N) determines the insulating properties of the sheath, whereas the intersegmental length (L) — the distance between nodes — determines the speed of conduction: since both N and L are directly and positively related to axon diameter, larger axons conduct faster than smaller ones. If unwrapped, a single myelin sheath would be seen to be a spade-like or trapezoid sheet of membrane, extraordinarily large relative to the axon it surrounded: in the order of 7 mm² (for a 15 μm diameter axon) or 0.4 mm² (for a 5 μm diameter axon); as though, say, a large handkerchief were wound around a length of thin string (Fig 3b). Thus, each myelinating cell maintains a myelin volume of 50 000–150 000 μm³ — according to axon diameter — an order of magnitude greater than its own volume. It is evident that the support of such a large volume of myelin places a considerable metabolic load on the myelinating cell, so, bearing in mind that each oligodendrocyte supports multiple sheaths, it is perhaps not surprising that oligodendrocytes have this exclusive function in the CNS. Moreover, myelin is continuously turned over and replaced by the myelinating cell.

It is difficult to imagine how the complex structure of myelin is formed. However, if the myelin sheet is envisaged as a flat layer of cytoplasm bounded by plasma membranes and then if the (a)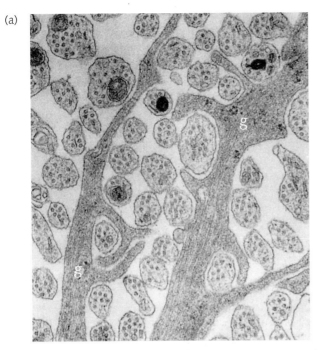

(b)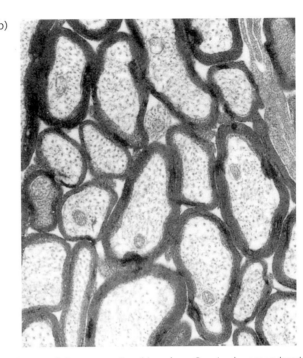

Fig. 2 Development of myelinated axons in the central nervous system, as seen by electron microscopy in transverse section. (a) newborn. Occasional axons are loosely ensheathed by primitive, undifferentiated glial cells, g, but myelin is not yet present. × 40,000. (b) Adult. The axons are fully myelinated. × 20,000.

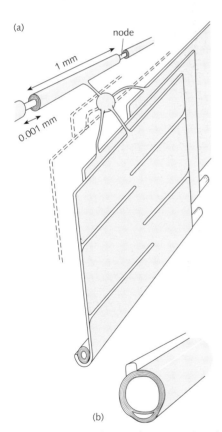

Fig. 3 Myelination in the central nervous system. A single oligodendrocyte myelinates numerous axons (a) and, in section, concentric layers of myelin are seen to spiral around the axon (b). Myelin sheaths are arranged along axons in segments 1 mm long separated by short nodes, and would appear as large sheets if they were unwrapped from around the axon.

cytoplasm is extruded so that the two plasma membranes are directly opposed to one another, then this is essentially a single lamella of compacted myelin (Fig. 1b). Since each plasma membrane consists of a double phospholipid layer, the myelin sheet comprises two double fatty layers wrapped concentrically round the axon and it is these that give myelin its excellent insulatory properties. Antibodies to one of the lipids in myelin have been used to study oligodendrocytes.

In addition to the lipids, there are a number of proteins that are enriched in myelin and are specific to it. Some proteins are believed to be important in communication between the axon and the inner lamella of the myelin sheath; others fuse and stabilize the layers. Their importance is made clear when mutations of the genes that determine their formation cause loss of one or more of these proteins, resulting in the unravelling of myelin; demyelination; hypomyelination; loss of axonal function; and ensuing clinical symptoms, such as tremor and paraplegia.

ARTHUR M. BUTT

Further reading

Ransom, B. R. and Kettenham, H. (ed.) (1995). *Neuroglia.* Oxford University Press.

See also ACTION POTENTIAL; GLIA; NERVES; WHITE MATTER.

Myopia or short sight is the inability to see distant objects clearly, because the eyeball is too long for the power of its own optical system (the cornea plus the lens). Hence, images of the outside world come to focus in front of the retina, even when ACCOMMODATION (the focusing mechanism of the eye) is completely relaxed. Consequently, the 'near point' of the eye (the closest distance at which objects appear sharp) is closer to the eye than normal. The higher the degree of myopia the closer is the near point. Myopia is partly genetically determined but can possibly occur as a result of concentrated close work when young, interfering with the normal growth of the eye. Myopia is corrected by wearing glasses with concave lenses, with negative power.

C.B.

See EYES; EYE MOVEMENTS; ORTHOPTICS; REFRACTIVE ERRORS.

Mysticism is frequently defined as an experience of direct communion with God, or union with the Absolute, but definitions of mysticism (a relatively modern term) are often imprecise and usually rely on the presuppositions of the modern study of mysticism — namely, that mystical experiences involve a set of intense and usually individual and private psychological states. While figures such as Teresa of Avila, Bernard of Clairvaux, and John of the Cross are seen to be paradigmatic mystics of the Christian tradition, no 'mystics' would have defined themselves as such before the twentieth century. Furthermore, mysticism is a phenomenon said to be found in all major religious traditions — though the common assumption that all mystical experiences, whatever their context, are the same cannot, of course, be demonstrated.

Mysticism involves the practice of contemplation both in the philosophical sense of the contemplation of truth and in the 'supernatural' sense of having knowledge of God via a life of prayer. Nevertheless, the 'mystic way' is primarily practical, not theoretical, and is something in which the whole self is engaged; the great

Christian mystics have spoken of how they acted rather than how they speculated. St Mechthild of Magdeburg wrote that the writing of her book had been seen and experienced in her every limb, seen with the eyes of her soul, and heard with the ears of her eternal spirit. Sharing the mental and physical suffering of Christ, in the meeting of the spirit with evil, is described by some mystics as central to their experience. Teresa of Avila warned her nuns that the trials given by God to contemplative could be intolerable, and that they might not be able to endure their sufferings for as long as a day. Images of action — battle, pilgrimage, search — are used to describe the mystic's inward work, which is, paradoxically, sustained by the outward stillness of contemplation.

Some have placed a particular emphasis on certain altered states, such as visions, trances, levitations, locutions, raptures, and ecstasies, many of which are altered bodily states. Margery Kempe's tears and Teresa of Avila's ecstasies are famous examples of such mystical phenomena. But many mystics have insisted that while these experiences may be a part of the mystical state, they are not the essence of mystical experience, and some, such as Origen, Meister Eckhart, and John of the Cross, have been hostile to such psycho-physical phenomena. Rather, the essence of the mystical experience is the encounter between God and the human being, the Creator and creature; this is a union which leads the human being to an 'absorption' or loss of individual personality. It is a movement of the heart, as the individual seeks to surrender itself to ultimate Reality; it is thus about *being* rather than *knowing*. For some mystics, such as Teresa of Avila, phenomena such as visions, locutions, raptures, and so forth are by-products of, or accessories to, the full mystical experience, which the soul may not yet be strong enough to receive. Hence these altered states are seen to occur in those at an early stage in their spiritual lives, although ultimately only those who are called to achieve full union with God will do so.

In Jewish mysticism, embodied in the collected teachings known as the Kabbalah, God is perceived as one who both reveals and conceals himself but who can be perceived through the practice of contemplation and resulting illumination. Because mystical knowledge can easily be misinterpreted, traditionally only people of a certain age and educational level, and usually men, were allowed to engage in mysticism. The role of the 'pure' and 'impure' body, and the place of gender relations, in Jewish mystical experience are illustrated by the story of Rabbi Nehunya ben Hakkanah, told in the sixth- or seventh-century *Hekhalot Rabbati*. The rabbi was in a mystical trance, at the sixth heaven but about to enter the seventh heaven, when the people with him wanted to ask him about his vision when he was speaking out loud to them while in his trance. They were faced with the question of how to get him out of his mystical trance, so they laid a piece of cloth on his knees which had been touched by a woman who had completed her menstrual cycle, had purified herself the first

time, but not the second, and was therefore not quite pure. When the cloth touched his knees the rabbi came out of his trance immediately so they were able to ask him the question, and then he went back into his trance.

In the late nineteenth century mysticism became the object of much research, partly because of the development of psychology and partly because of the new comparative study of religion by which phenomena were observed and compared across cultures. Key figures in this scholarship were Evelyn Underhill and Friedrich, Baron Von Hugel, though their analysis of mysticism was not theological. Von Hugel emphasized the Transcendent, the 'wholly other' as a fact of religions across cultures and thus he influenced thinking about the mystic's union with that Transcendent being. Underhill in particular saw mysticism as a process or way of life and as a cross-cultural phenomenon, and thus envisioned the 'mystic way' as a series of psychological states which could be found in mystics across different religions, times, and places. While Underhill insisted that a feature of mysticism was the abolition of individuality, the new emphasis, also found in the work of the philosopher William James, on the psychological states of the mystic led to an assumption that mystical experience is an essentially private and subjective matter. It did not involve, for example, questions of social justice — though mystics have long claimed that the mystical experience is proven 'true' in its effects or fruits, such as greater humility, acts of charity, and love of others. James associated the mystical with subjective states of feeling and the notion of mysticism as 'private' remains in most subsequent philosophical treatments of the subject. Both Underhill and Von Hugel made it clear that mysticism was an essential element in all religion, but never claimed it to be the whole content of any religion. However, some Protestant theologians, such as Emil Brunner and Reinhold Neibuhr, came to reject it as anti-Christian, considering it to be too Neoplatonic, while others, including Anglicans like W. R Inge, Dean of St Paul's, went to the other extreme and saw mysticism as the essence of Christianity.

Michel de Certeau's work, in the latter part of the twentieth century, has compared the procedures common to both mysticism and psychoanalysis, suggesting that the body, far from being ruled by discourse, is itself a symbolic language, and that in both psychoanalysis and mysticism the body is perceived as responsible for a truth of which it is unaware. Thus the body holds the 'key' to the 'truth' of the 'space' represented by the mystical or unconscious. This has caused the modern study of mysticism to focus, like psychoanalysis, on the bodily manifestations of the psyche's or soul's condition in order to understand the 'truth' of that condition. Perhaps the ultimate example of this is Jacques Lacan's attempt to locate the apparent impossibility or unknowability of female desire in the mystical experiences of Teresa of Avila, as depicted in Bernini's sculpture

in Rome; he states that on looking at that statue it is immediately clear to us, if not to Teresa, that she is experiencing an orgasm. Luce Irigaray, a feminist psychoanalyst, has appropriately responded (in *This Sex Which is Not One*) to this collapse and merging of female sexual desire and religious experience thus: 'In Rome? So far away? To look? At a statue? of a Saint? Sculpted by a man? What pleasure are we talking about? Whose pleasure? For where the pleasure of Teresa is concerned, her own writings are more telling.'

JANE SHAW

Further reading
Underhill, E. (1995). *Mysticism*, (15th edn, revised). Bracken Books, London.

Mythic thought
In mythic thought, the mythological 'message' can be repeated many times using different symbolic codes — most commonly sexual and dietary. For example, in myth, Thyestes sleeps with his brother's wife, thus becoming 'too close' sexually, and is punished by finding he has eaten the *flesh* of his own son, a further expression of becoming 'too close'. Here transgression is followed by appropriate retribution, moving from the sexual to the dietary register. Marcel Detienne has shown how the myths surrounding the young god Adonis, whose precocious sexuality was cut short by his death, only serve to emphasize the accepted social norms of the proper use of sex in legitimate marriage.

Mythic modes of thought can be used in other types of knowledge, for example geography and ethnography. In the classical world, as in many cultures, it was thought that the further one travelled from 'home', the more strange would be the customs encountered. The Greek historian Herodotus listed the bizarre habits of the non-Greek peoples, focusing on their practices with regard to food, sexuality, and the treatment of the dead. The last two categories were conflated in the practice of necrophilia with corpses selected for their beauty, for example, by the Egyptians responsible for mummifying the dead. In his work *Natural History*, the Roman writer Pliny codified some of these beliefs in his influential account of the monstrous races; including the Blemmyae, who have their faces on their chests, and the Straw-Drinkers, who have no nose or mouth. Here, at the limits of the known world, the body has confounded its own categories. Fear was expressed that even a civilized person might fall short of accepted behaviour when travelling to the limits of the world; Roman anxieties, for example, centred on the harmful effects of adopting foreign lifestyles and eating foreign foods.

HELEN KING

See also GREEKS; MYTHOLOGY AND THE BODY.

Mythology and the body
The human body is essential to human myth and storytelling, as it is the first reference point, the original source of sensation and apprehension that gives rise to all questions and all attempts to

answer them. Certain popular and deep-seated metaphors and symbols — images used for understanding and expressing human beliefs and situations, such as ACHILLES' HEEL and ADAM'S RIB — are taken from myths associated with the body. Other myths are concerned with the categories of the natural and the supernatural, and employ a bodily vocabulary of missing, or extra, body parts, and creatures whose identity hovers between human and beast, mortal and immortal, physical and spiritual. The winged angel, the centaur, the griffin, the sphinx, and the various demons and divinities with animal attributes, from ibis-headed Thoth to goat-headed Satan, are such hybrids, whose physical forms embody paradox and impossibility.

Mythic opponents are often represented with unusual numbers of body parts; the Irish Fomoire had only one leg and one arm, the Greek Cyclops one eye. Gods and other 'good' characters in myth may also have a less than perfect physical form; the Greek Hephaistos was born lame and is known as 'the limping god', while the Irish hero Nûadu lost his arm in battle but was given a silver prosthetic arm to replace it. In ancient Egyptian myth, the body of Osiris was torn into fourteen pieces by his wife's brother Seth, and scattered across Egypt; his wife Isis reassembled the parts, but was unable to find Osiris' penis, which had been eaten by fish. However, she made him a new one by magic, and restored him to life.

The normal human experiences of the life cycle were dramatized in, and experienced through, myth. For example, in ancient Greece the goddess Artemis had a special concern for the young, and presided over the transition to adulthood. Girls dedicated their childhood toys to her as they entered puberty, and women made offerings to her at marriage and after childbirth. However, the gods of many different cultures were themselves fixed at a particular age, missing out certain stages of the life cycle completely.

The story of Achilles' fatal weak spot, in his otherwise invincible body, describes how his mother, Thetis, the sea goddess, bestowed bodily immunity upon him by dipping him in the sea as an infant: the only part of his body not to touch the strengthening waters was his heel, by which she held him. The position of this flaw, in the lowliest and most disregarded portion of the body, synonymous with ignominy and debasement, reflects the earthbound nature of human weakness, as it is perceived in classical and Western thought. The heel, which touches the soil, and the head, which looks toward the sky, form a paradigm for the most basic of hierarchies, the one that values the vertical above the horizontal, and values that which is further away from the earth above that which is close to the earth. The logical extension of this pattern is found in the separation and elevation, in Western philosophy, of the mind over the body.

One of the most frequently found notions in mythology concerning the body is the association between earth and the female. The Mesopo-

tamian myth of a cosmos whose lower portions formed the female earth deity called Ki; the Greek earth goddess Gaia; and the Mayan female Earth Monster, are a few examples of this phenomenon. Mythology reveals a widespread, though not universal, identification of the earthly processes of growth and fruition, necessary for human nourishment and survival, with female bodily properties of fertility and barrenness, and the processes of gestation and childbirth. A Zuni myth from the present-day south-western US describes the beginnings of the world as a series of four wombs, in which the created beings developed before emerging, through a birth canal in the earth, into the light of day. The Japanese creation myth, on the other hand, held that the eight islands of Japan were themselves born from a female heavenly spirit, who not only produced the earth, sea, seasons, winds, trees, fields, and mountains, but from her vomit created metal; from her faeces, clay; and from her urine, hot springs.

While myths like these explain natural phenomena, or the existence of the world, by reference to human reproduction, there are also myths that account for the phenomenon of procreation itself. Sometimes the discovery of sexuality is presented as a fortuitous occurrence, an account that stresses the teleology of nature, and of genitalia. In the Japanese myth referred to, the original procreating pair observe of their own bodies that, while on one of their bodies the flesh in a certain part protrudes, in the corresponding part of the other the flesh is split in half. The pair then decide to put the excessive and defective parts of their bodies together — thus procreation is initiated, cued by the design features of male and female bodies.

Plato's *Symposium* posits a different source for human sexual drives as well as sexual differentiation. It states that such desire stems from the fact that, in the beginning, humans beings were each as large as two are now, as round as tree trunks, with two heads and two sets of everything else: some with two sets of male members, some with two sets of female parts, others with one of each. The gods Zeus and Apollo, fearful of these beings' strength, divided each in half, and since then, people have felt a longing to be united with their other half, to which end they strive and strive, some yearning after members of their own sex, others after those of the opposite sex.

The biblical story of the Fall makes a long-enduring and highly influential link between SEXUALITY, knowledge, and sin, in which the bodily act of EATING, and the bodily state of nakedness, are employed as emblems of human disobedience and shame. When Eve, tempted by the serpent, tastes of the fruit of the Tree of Knowledge, and tempts Adam to do likewise, the first knowledge they experience is of their own nakedness, and their loss of innocence — or of ignorance of good and evil — is demonstrated in their new feeling of shame at the sight of their own bodies. As the body was the vehicle for their transgression, so it becomes the vehicle

for their castigation. Fallen from the state of grace of blissful ignorance, and cast out of the timeless bounty of Eden, the first humans are condemned to knowledge of hunger, desire, pain, and loss; to process and change, growth and decay. They work out their sentence in producing food, and bringing forth children, by bodily toil and suffering.

The Christian solution to the problem of human fallibility demonstrates the peculiarly body-centred nature of this religion. Every nuance and aspect of the Christian moral universe is articulated through the body. As the fall of humankind, the exchange of innocence for experience, was brought about by Eve, and her wilful ingestion of divine knowledge, so the redemption of humanity was accomplished by the submission of the Virgin Mary to the will of God, and the impregnation of her body by the Holy Spirit. Adam's violation of the Tree of Knowledge is redeemed by the crucifixion of Mary's son, Jesus, upon a second 'tree'; the taste of the Edenic fruit on Adam's lips is transmuted into the bitter cup drained by Christ in another garden. The natural cycle of life, death, birth, and sexuality initiated by Eve is interrupted by Mary's miraculous virgin birth, and humankind is released from temporal death and decay, first visited upon Adam, by the miraculous resurrection of Christ.

The position of Christ on the ladder of existence as a being part human, part divine, or the divine embodied in the human, finds rough parallels in other mythologies. The Aztec god Quetzalcoatl, lord of life and death, is a composite figure, an intermediary between creatures. Like humans, he stands midway between the gods and the beings below, with the attendant dilemmas and possibilities of that position. He is the soul taking wings to heaven, and he is matter descending to earth as the crawling snake; he is the 'plumed serpent', emblematic of the human condition.

Thus mythology uses the body as the vehicle for demonstrating or expressing the underlying tensions, contradictions, problems, and dilemmas we face as conscious living beings inhabiting an alternately bountiful and hostile physical world.
HELEN KING
NATSU HATTORI

Further reading

Burland, C., Nicholson, I., and Oxborne, H. (1970). *Mythology of the Americans*. Hamyln, London.

Buxton, R. (1994). *Imaginary Greece*. Cambridge University Press.

Campbell, J. (1960–5). *The masks of God*, (Vols 1–3). Secker and Warburg, London.

Davidson, H. R. E. (1982). *Scandinavian mythology*. Hamlyn, London.

Jordan, M. (1993). *Myths of the world: a thematic encyclopaedia*. Kyle Cathie Ltd, London.

Willis, R. (ed.) (1993). *World mythology: the illustrated guide*. Simon and Schuster, London.

See also ANTHROPOMORPHISM; CREATION MYTHS; GREEKS; METAMORPHOSIS; MYTHIC THOUGHT; REPRODUCTION MYTHS.

489

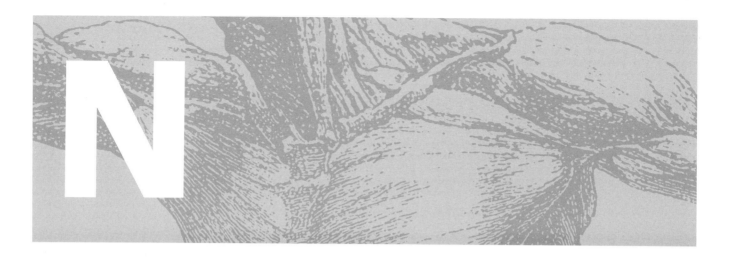

Naevus A purple/red area of skin, due to an overgrowth of blood vessels (haemangioma), usually congenital — a vascular BIRTHMARK. At best, a small red 'BEAUTY SPOT' and at worst the severe disfiguration known as a 'port wine' naevus. A 'strawberry' naevus is a different type which grows and reddens after birth, and usually regresses later. 　　　　　　　　　　　　S.J.

See BIRTHMARK.

Nails The replacement of sharp claws with flattened nails in primates is considered part of the evolutionary development of a HAND able to grasp objects. The nails start to develop in the fetus by the end of the third month, and are formed from the same epidermal tissue as the skin. They reach the ends of the fingers and toes about a month before birth.

The mature nail is a plate of the protein keratin which is also present in hair and skin. The pale 'half-moon' at the base — often exposed above the nail-fold only on the thumbs and big toes — marks the area of the bed of the nail where its substance is formed and from which it grows — the germinal matrix. The rest of the nail bed provides a surface for the growing nail to slide over as it advances at the rate of about 0.1 mm/day. The germinal cells continually divide to replace those which generate, and disappear into the non-cellular substance of the nail. This proliferation can be interrupted by injuries or acute illnesses, leaving grooves across the nails which gradually grow out.

The decoration of both toenails and fingernails for aesthetic purposes dates back at least as far as Ancient Egypt, where henna and other products were applied to colour the feet and hands as well as the nails. Growing long fingernails has also been practised in Chinese and Hindu cultures, in part as a sign of leisure and status, since many forms of manual labour are difficult or impossible with long fingernails. Well-groomed nails have been a sign of cultivation and cleanliness for both men and women in American and European cultures as well. As a 1952 etiquette guide pronounces, 'A fastidious man . . . keeps his nails clean and short with the cuticle pushed back. If he has his nails professionally manicured, they may be buffed but should never have any coloured or even colourless polish applied'. Coloured and clear nail enamel, or 'polish', became popular for women in the early twentieth century, and often replaced the literal polishing of nails with a buffer. False and elaborately painted nails are also now popular among some cultural groups.

In folk beliefs, the nails are often said to continue to grow after death. For instance, long fingernails, or sometimes no nails at all, are characteristic of VAMPIRES, revenants, and other beings of 'undead' status. In fact, in decomposition the tissues of the body dehydrate and contract, giving the appearance that the nails, hair, and teeth have 'grown'. Sometimes the nails are sloughed off with the outer layer of skin, leaving exposed what appears to be new skin or nails, another sign of preternatural 'life' in a CORPSE. This same phenomenon is also the explanation for stories of dead bodies supposedly having come to life in the coffin and having either chewed off their nails in anxiety, or having scraped them off trying to escape. To keep the nails in place, Ancient Egyptian embalmers sometimes either tied the nails to the fingers and toes, or covered them with metal thimbles. 　　　SARAH GOODFELLOW

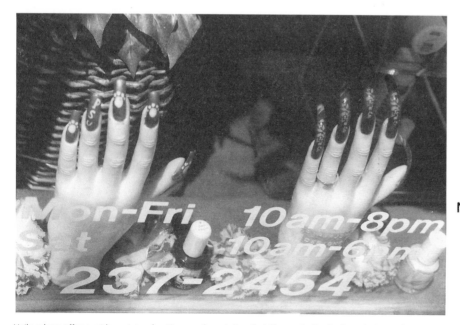

Nails salons offer a wide variety of options — from bejewelled flowers to the trademark. Pennsylvania State University. Nittany Lion paw print.

Narcissus Narcissus, from whose myth narcissism has been named, was the son of the river god Cephissus and the nymph Liriope. He fell in love with his own image reflected in water, pined away, and was transformed into the flower which bears his name. According to the Roman poet Ovid, the metamorphosis of Narcissus was a punishment for having rejected the nymph Echo, who fell in love with Narcissus but who was unable to speak except by repeating his words. The geographer Pausanias gives another version in which Narcissus fell in love with his twin sister; when she died, he thought he had found her again in his reflection.

Perhaps because of its contribution to debates about the nature of representation and the relationship between what is seen and what is real, the myth has been very popular as a subject in art, both during and since the classical period. About fifty murals depicting Narcissus survive from Pompeii alone. The best-known work from the modern period representing the myth is probably Salvador Dali's *Metamorphosis of Narcissus*. It is also a significant myth in psychological work. Narcissus' love for his own reflection is the origin of Freud's idea of narcissism as a stage in the development of the ego. Lacan saw primary narcissism as concerned with the creation of awareness of the body as body; he also drew attention to the fragmentation of the body in this myth, with Echo as voice alone, and Narcissus as the gaze. Derrida suggested that Freud was himself Narcissus, the man fascinated by his own image. HELEN KING

See also MYTHOLOGY AND THE BODY.

Narcosis From the Greek word meaning 'to benumb'. A soporific or insensible state; a state produced by a narcotic drug. Regrettably the word 'narcotic' has been misused, especially in the US, where various narcotic agencies seem to call all drugs of abuse 'narcotics', whether they be HEROIN or COCAINE, though the latter produces a state opposite to narcosis. A.W.C.

See ANALGESIA; DRUG; OPIATES AND OPIOID DRUGS.

Nausea The unpleasant sensation vaguely located in the upper abdomen and chest which heralds VOMITING or FAINTING, but which may also occur without dramatic issue. Nausea is well known to accompany strong negative EMOTION — disgust, fear, horror — or severe PAIN; also a side-effect of some drugs and of CHEMOTHERAPY and RADIOTHERAPY, and a feature of a variety of gastro–intestinal and other diseases. Its physical basis is the AUTONOMIC NERVOUS SYSTEM and the associated *visceral afferents* (nerves bringing in information from the gut); there may be nervous inputs from a diseased or insulted stomach or intestine, with appropriate reflex responses, or the system may be activated 'inappropriately' from higher regions of the brain. S.J.

See VISCERAL SENSATION; VOMITTING.

Neanderthals The Neanderthals (*Homo neanderthalensis*) were a separate species, or possibly a race, of 'archaic' humans who occupied Europe and the adjacent parts of western Asia from around 300 000 to 30 000 years ago. They probably descended directly from the earlier *Homo erectus* populations of the same areas. Discoveries of buried skeletal remains (mostly in caves) show that they were heavily built, muscular individuals, with heavy-browed faces, large noses and jaws, and receding chins. They seem to have been adapted partly to survive in the cold conditions of the last two European glacial periods, and partly to a strenuous lifestyle with a much more limited technological repertoire than that of *Homo sapiens*. Their brains were of similar size to ours (about 1400 ml on average), but could well have been differently organized. They were clearly proficient at the manufacture of quite complex stone tools (mostly from flint, quartzite, and similar rocks) and the production of certain wooden tools, such as spears. But, unlike their *Homo sapiens* successors, they produced virtually no recognizable tools in bone or antler. Most striking of all is the virtual absence of any evidence for artistic representation, or the use of 'ornamental' items, among the Neanderthals. All of this has been interpreted to mean that the Neanderthals had a very limited capacity for 'symbolic' or abstract thought, and either no formal LANGUAGE or a significantly simpler form of language than that of modern humans. The disappearance of the Neanderthals around 30 000 years ago was probably mainly due to competition with the rapidly expanding populations of anatomically and behaviourally 'modern' humans (*Homo sapiens*), which seem, from recent studies of DNA patterns, to have originated and dispersed from Africa shortly before this time. A sample of mitochondrial DNA recovered from bones of an original Neanderthal SKELETON (found near Dusseldorf in Germany) is so different from that of modern Europeans that it suggests that there was very little if any interbreeding between the 'native' Neanderthal populations of Europe and the new, intrusive *Homo sapiens*. However, a few skeletons have been found that have been claimed to show a mixture of Neanderthal and modern features — as in the case of a recently-discovered skeleton from Lagar Velho in Portugal. Periods of overlap between the Neanderthals and modern humans of up to 5000 years have been documented in some areas of Europe, during which the final Neanderthals apparently adopted or copied some features of more 'modern' behaviour. PAUL MELLARS

Further reading

Mellars, P. (1996). *The Neanderthal legacy: an archaeological perspective from Western Europe.* Princeton University Press, Princeton, New Jersey.

See also EVOLUTION, HUMAN.

Near-death experiences People who come close to death and survive often report remarkable experiences. Feelings of peace, happiness, and even joy are common, which seems paradoxical in the circumstances. Many survivors report having rushed down a dark tunnel towards a bright light — although the tunnel itself can look like anything from tiny stars or spirals of light, to the inside of a sewer pipe or an underground cave. In one study, about a third of near-death survivors reported out of body experiences, in which they seemed to leave their body and were able to watch what was happening from a distance, as though as an impartial observer. Less often they recalled leaving the scene of (near) death and travelling elsewhere. Finally, some people report wonderful heavenly scenes, peopled with angels, spiritual beings, or deceased friends and relatives. Less commonly they arrive at some kind of barrier and have to decide to return, or not. A small proportion report a 'life review' in which scenes from their life flash before their inner eyes, often all at once, or with no sense of passing time. This life review is sometimes remembered as an ordeal, with religious figures making judgements in a great book, but it can be purely personal, leading to calm acceptance and a re-evaluation of one's life and deeds.

After a near-death experience many people report that their whole attitude to life is changed. They are less concerned with material things and more interested in helping others. Research confirms these changes but it is not clear whether they are a consequence of the experience itself or just of having been so close to death.

Not all near-death experiences are blissful, and recent research has discovered an increasing number of hellish experiences — although just how many is hard to estimate, since people may be less likely to report them, and more anxious to forget. In many religions suicide is treated as a sin, so believers might expect those who attempt suicide to be especially likely to have hellish experiences. In fact they mostly report blissful or peaceful feelings, and the effect, far from encouraging another suicide attempt, seems to be a renewed enthusiasm for life.

The term 'near-death experience' became popular only after Raymond Moody's best-selling collection of accounts in 1975. However, similar reports had previously been collected from people who subsequently did die (i.e. deathbed experiences). In fact, reports of such experiences are widespread in many ages and cultures, and in literature, art, and film. Plato describes one in the *Republic*, Tibetan Buddhist literature includes the 'returned from the dead' writings, and there are myths from as far apart as ancient Greece, nineteenth-century native Americans, and Lithuanian folklore. In contemporary research, similar reports have been collected from Iceland, Britain, America, and India. In these accounts the basic features tend to be similar (including tunnels, lights, out-of-body excursions, and visions) but the details vary. For example, religious figures are often seen, but usually of the person's own religion. No Hindu is known to have seen Jesus, nor any Christian to have seen Hindu gods.

A few sceptics attribute the experiences either to wishful thinking or to taking drugs. This seems most unlikely, given the cross-cultural findings, and research showing that most drugs tend to reduce the clarity and complexity of near-death experiences. The important question is therefore why these experiences occur in a similar form all across the world.

The main contenders are either that near-death experiences are a glimpse of life after death, or that they are the effect of changes in an almost dying brain. The after-death hypothesis cannot be proven. If there is life after death, these experiences may tell us what it is like, but since none of the people concerned actually died we can never be sure. The closest we come to evidence is the claim that, during the experience, some people were able to see events at a distance that they could not possibly have known about or guessed. These claims are few, and none is substantiated by independent witnesses or physical evidence, although the best examples are probably those in which patients were able to describe complex medical procedures that occurred while they were comatose or even clinically dead.

There are several theories to explain how coming close to death can give rise to near-death experiences. Lack of OXYGEN is often implicated, although many near-death experiences occur when people are not deprived of oxygen, as in falls from mountains, during suicide attempts by jumping from heights, or after accidents. In such situations, however, the production and actions of various HORMONES and NEUROTRANSMITTERS may be affected. There are theories based on stimulation of receptors in nerve cell membranes called NMDA receptors, on the effects of the neurotransmitter SEROTONIN, and on the level of ENDORPHINS (the brain's own morphine-like chemicals). Endorphins are known to produce positive emotions and reduction of pain, and may be responsible for the blissful feelings in the midst of pain and fear. Disruption of the brain's neurotransmitters can produce random or excessive firing of neurons and this, depending on where it occurs, may produce the other experiences. For example, electrical stimulation of the temporal lobe of the cerebral hemispheres can produce life reviews and sensations of floating or flying, while random firing in the parts of the visual cortex (which also occurs with drugs such as LSD) causes the perception of lights, tunnels, and spirals.

These physiological explanations can account for much of near-death experiences, and may in time provide a complete account. Even so, they can never disprove the possibility of life after death. Some people may still prefer to believe that the experience is a glimpse of the next world rather than the product of the dying brain.   SUSAN BLACKMORE

Further reading

Bailey, L. W. and Yates, J. (ed.) (1996). *The near-death experience: a reader.* Routledge, New York and London.

Blackmore, S. J. (1993). *Dying to live: science and the near death experience.* Prometheus, Buffalo, NY.

Moody, R. A. (1975). *Life after life.* Mockingbird, Atlanta, GA.

Near-drowning Human beings have escaped drowning by surviving extraordinary periods under water. The longest documented was a young child, submerged for 40 minutes beneath the icy waters of a frozen lake. Breath cannot be held for much more than 2–3 minutes, so how could a child possibly have survived all that time without brain damage? Dolphins, seals, and whales, all air breathers like us, manage to remain submerged on a single breath hold for anything up to 40 minutes, and yet they are just as dependent on oxygen as we are. To understand how they are able to do this, it is necessary to consider some of the physiological principles at play.

Certain tissues of the body are much less sensitive to OXYGEN starvation than others. For example, BLOOD (which carries the oxygen) can be shut off from an arm or leg, and, provided the limb is being rested, the muscle can survive without its blood supply (and therefore without oxygen) for well over half an hour. It does so by drawing on its store of glucose, which it converts to lactic acid. This is known as anaerobic respiration, and muscle has a large anaerobic reserve. The BRAIN, though, has no such reserve, and any interruption to blood running up the carotid arteries results in unconsciousness almost at once, with permanent damage occurring after 2–3 minutes. The HEART is also vulnerable to oxygen starvation, because, unlike the muscles of the arms or legs, it can't be rested, and must go on beating, rapidly using up its anaerobic reserve.

So the strategy for a diving mammal is clear: its precious oxygen pool (carried by the red blood cells) must remain the sole preserve of the brain and heart, while the rest of the body can do without. This is achieved by reflex constriction, all blood vessels with the exception of the carotid and coronary arteries, stimulated by the effect of cold water touching the nose and face, and also by the very act of breath-holding. With only the brain and heart arteries to supply, the heart rate can slow right down, and drops to around 10 beats per minutes.

Evolution has robbed terrestrial mammals of the diving reflex, of which just a vestige remains, detectable only in the first few months of infancy. So, if, it is not the diving reflex influencing survival, then what? The answer lies with the temperature of the water. This is best explained by reflecting on the history of SURGERY. With the discovery of anaesthesia, surgeons found that they could operate on almost any part of the body, but they couldn't operate on the heart while it was beating. To stop the heart for anything more than a few minutes meant risking brain damage, so there was insufficient time for surgery.

However, animals appeared to recover fully from heart surgery with the circulation stopped, provided that their bodies had been cooled down a little first — the theory being that reduced body temperature meant a lower metabolic rate and so less oxygen consumption by the brain.

The cooler the animal, the longer the circulation could be stopped without obvious harm. The first heart surgery to be performed on a human subject took place in 1954. The patient was a child with a hole in the heart. Circulation was stopped for 15 minutes while surgeons repaired the defect. The operation was a complete success.

Of course, now that the work of circulation and breathing can be done by heart/lung machines, the cooling process can be controlled much more easily, and it is possible to take body temperature as low as 18°C. At that temperature, blood flow to the brain can be stopped for up to 60 minutes before tissue damage (such as a stroke) begins to show itself, though re-warming must be taken very slowly.

The analogy between cerebral protection with deep hypothermia, and cold water submersion, now becomes obvious. The chance of survival is increased in those whose brains have become coolest before the heart stops beating. It would be expected that very small children or infants submerged in ice cold water should have the best chance of all, because their rate of cooling is highest: this is indeed the case. So the clinical approach to resuscitation of these very cold individuals might logically be to reverse the cooling procedure used in heart surgery, and use the heart/lung machine to support circulation while re-warming. And remarkable results have indeed been achieved at centres where these facilities are available.

To summarize; experience in the use of deep HYPOTHERMIA in cardiac surgery has provided insight into the physiological principles governing survival after very long periods spent under water. Furthermore, these principles have been applied to the techniques used to resuscitate victims of near-drowning.   MARK HARRIES

See also COLD EXPOSURE; DROWNING; HYPOTHERMIA; RESUSCITATION; SURVIVAL AT SEA.

Necrophilia Since strictly speaking the word means 'love of the dead', it could be applied to anyone who persists in devotion to a dead spouse or lover over a prolonged period. Perhaps the most outstanding manifestation of such devotion is the Taj Mahal, erected by the Mogul emperor Shah Jehan as a tomb for his dead wife. However, necrophilia is usually taken to describe a rare, or at least, rarely reported, manifestation of the sexual instinct operating at a much lower and less idealistic or spiritual level.

In some cases the use of dead bodies for the purposes of sexual gratification is purely opportunistic, an activity encountered among those who have professional dealings with corpses in the course of their daily work, for example undertakers and morgue attendants. The practice was rumoured to be prevalent among the embalmers of ancient Egypt to such a degree that the bodies of highly-born women were not embalmed immediately after death but allowed to become slightly putrid as a deterrent. There is, however, no evidence that a desire for sexual relations with corpses leads individuals into these professions. Those who come into constant routine contact with corpses soon acquire a familiarity with them which might lead to using them as what could be considered an extremely bizarre masturbatory aid.

There are, however, those who are particularly excited by dead bodies and seek them out for sexual purposes. Accounts can be found — in the pages of the great collators of sexual deviance in its manifold forms, such as Richard von Krafft-Ebing — of individuals who even went so far as to disinter corpses in order to have intercourse with them or to perform sexually motivated mutilations. Krafft-Ebing suggested that the attraction was to a human form absolutely devoid of will, incapable of giving resistance. He also cited the case of an individual who required a prostitute to be made up to mimic a corpse and laid out on a bier, and there is anecdotal evidence to suggest that some brothels included this among their specialities.

This peculiarity segues into the related phenomenon of lust murder. The motivation of individual sexually motivated murderers would appear to vary. Some rape their victims and then kill them, others apparently find gratification in the actual act of murder, and others gain some form of sexual gratification with the body. Thus lust-murder and necrophilia are not identical but overlapping phenomena.

While most of the stigmatized sexual alternatives (SADOMASOCHISM, even PAEDOPHILIA) have their champions, defenders, and advocates, who claim them to be not only less deleterious than popularly imagined but positively benign and healthy, there does not seem to be any organization dedicated to promoting the Joy of Dead Sex, or Necrophile Liberation. However, a number of special interest webpages and discussions devoted to the subject have emerged in recent years.   LESLEY A. HALL

Neoplasm From the Greek 'new' and 'form': an abnormal growth of tissue, or *tumour*. A neoplasm can be benign or malignant. The name given to any particular tumour is an indication of the type of tissue from which it arises, plus the ending '-oma'. Benign growths range from small warts to huge ovarian cysts; they include fatty lumps (*lipomas*), bony excrescences (*osteomas*), and many others. Malignant growths (cancers) are broadly classified according to the type of cells they arise from as either *carcinoma*, from epithelial sites — body coverings or linings (e.g. skin, breast, colon) — or *sarcoma*, from deeper tissue (e.g. bone or muscle). Malignant neoplasms are characterized by being locally invasive and by forming *metastases* — seeding in other parts of the body via lymphatic or blood vessels. A malignant growth may therefore be primary — at the original site — or secondary, metastatic.   S.J.

See also CANCER.

Nerve gas The term 'nerve gas' implies substances manufactured with the intent of killing populations or decimating armies in time of war. They have never been used as such in a major world war. The idea that an enemy could stealthily pollute the air with a gas that when breathed would cause death, without affecting property, is horrific and the use of poisonous gases in this way is rightly banned by international treaty. Nevertheless the whole population of Britain, including children and babies, were issued with respirators ('gas masks') in World War II. Chlorine gas shells were used by the German Army in World War I, but it proved a hazardous business as wind changes often blew the gas back across the lines from where it came. Chlorine is not a nerve gas, and many soldiers survived the attacks, but were left with lifelong bronchitic type conditions because of the damage to the lungs.

The nerve gases are not really gases, and were designed to be sprayed as aerosols over enemy territory, the fine droplets being absorbed through the skin following contact, either directly from the air or by touching surfaces on which the droplets rested. Thus 'gas masks' were of no use, as the fine droplets of poison could easily be distributed without detection and persisted for some time after the air raid. The principle upon which the nerve gases worked was to inhibit a particular enzyme in the body, namely *acetylcholinesterase*, which rapidly breaks down the neurotransmitter, ACETYLCHOLINE. Acetylcholinesterase is associated with many nerve endings, both in the brain and in the periphery. Acetylcholine is the neuromuscular transmitter at motor nerve endings in SKELETAL MUSCLE, in ganglia (the relay stations of the AUTONOMIC NERVOUS SYSTEM), and at all parasympathetic nerve endings on the tissues they affect. The parasympathetic nervous system controls many vegetative functions of involuntary organs and is active under normal sedentary conditions, promoting secretions for example of saliva, and the digestive enzymes in the gut, and also, through the vagus nerve, serving to slow the heart rate and lower the blood pressure. If the enzyme which destroys the transmitter is itself inhibited then the transmitter will persist for much longer, so that overactivity at all situations where acetycholine is involved will be apparent. The consequences therefore are increased salivation, tears, and gastrointestinal and bronchial secretions; bronchoconstriction; slowing of the heart and a fall in blood pressure; constriction of the pupil; and a fall in pressure in the eyeball. Effects caused within the brain lead eventually to CONVULSIONS, loss of consciousness, and respiratory failure. It is of course possible to treat some of these symptoms and it is particularly important to give an atropine-like drug (which counteracts the effects of acetylcholine) to prevent the heart stopping altogether.

The nerve gases, and there are many of them, are pentavalent phosphorus compounds (known as organophosphorus compounds), such as *dyflos* (di-isopropyl fluorophosphonate) and *parathion*, which react irreversibly with acetylcholinesterase,

so the effects are long-lasting, requiring the body to synthesise new enzyme, which takes several weeks. The reason is that the organophosphorus compounds transfer a phoshate group to the enzyme, making it inactive. A little later there is a ageing process when the phosphorylated enzyme changes its structure. It is only before the ageing process occurs that it is possible to remove the phosphate group with nucleophilic drugs, such as pralidoxime. Clearly, treatment of any kind would be unlikely during a nerve gas attack with thousands of people affected.

Nerve gases have proved to have important peacetime uses. They are widely used as insecticides. The compounds can penetrate the insect cuticle as they can human skin. Occasionally farmers contaminate themselves when diluting the concentrate for spraying and need to be treated as described above. Dyflos is used in eyedrops to treat glaucoma (raised intraocular pressure); applied locally in the eyes it produces no effects elsewhere in the body.
                    ALAN W. CUTHBERT

See also CHEMICAL WARFARE; POISONS.

Nerve impulses are electrical signals, known technically as ACTION POTENTIALS, which transmit information along nerve fibres.
                    F.M.A.

See ACTION POTENTIALS.

Nerves The word 'nerve' is used in a variety of ways. In classical anatomy, nerves are tough, whitish threads and cables that are found throughout most of the tissues of our body. They form great, tree-like networks that can be traced back to the SPINAL CORD or BRAIN. Like the trunks, branches, and twigs of a tree, the further away a nerve is from the CENTRAL NERVOUS SYSTEM, the smaller it is, in general (from more than 1 cm, down to much less than 1 mm in diameter). The role of nerves in communicating information is obvious to anyone who has cut a nerve in an accident. Sensation may be lost in the skin and other tissues to which the severed nerve connects, or there may be spontaneous pain in the affected region; and if the damaged nerve is connected to muscles, they become weak or paralysed. Perhaps the best-known nerve is the *sciatic nerve*, which when inflamed or under pressure causes pain, tenderness, and weakness in the back of the leg (*sciatica*). All such nerves are part of the *peripheral nervous system*.

Such a peripheral nerve contains microscopic fibres called *axons*. Groups of a few axons are wrapped together in a delicate fibrous sheath, and bundles of such bundles are again enclosed in a fibrous sheath to form the whole nerve.

Axons are also known as nerve fibres. They are long *processes* (thin extensions from the main cell body) of neurons, the cells of the nervous system, which, to complicate things further, are also known as 'nerve cells'. Axons conduct brief electrical pulses called 'nerve impulses' (technically, ACTION POTENTIALS), which originate in the sensitive nerve endings in

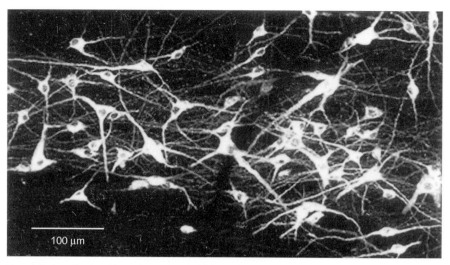

Nerve cells from the dorsal horn of grey matter in the spinal cord. They are involved in the transmission of nerve impulses that give rise to pain, and their axons ascend to the brain stem. Courtesy of Dr Andrew Todd, University of Glasgow.

the skin or other tissues, or at the cell body of a neuron. Impulses convey sensory messages in these *afferent* fibres into the central nervous system, and motor commands in *efferent* fibres from central neurons out to muscles and glands throughout the body.

Axons conduct impulses at speeds from about 0.5–100 m/sec. The velocity increases with the diameter of the axon (typically between 0.1 and 2 μm) and is even further speeded up if the axon is covered (as many of them are) by insulating fatty material, called a *myelin sheath*. In general, axons run uninterrupted along the entire length of a peripheral nerve as well as some distance inside the central nervous system. Thus they can be extraordinarily long. For instance, sensory axons extend from the skin of the big toe to the base of the brain; and motor axons run from the motor cortex of the cerebral hemispheres right down to motor neurons at the bottom of the spinal cord.

Nerve cells share many basic features with cells elsewhere in the body. They have a *cell body*, with a *nucleus* containing genetic information, in the DNA of the chromosomes; and *cytoplasm* containing *organelles*, which are involved in metabolism and the production of specific proteins necessary for the proper functioning of the neuron; all covered with a thin membrane. They differ from other cells in having two types of fibre-like processes. The cell body is surrounded by a bush of up to ten or so *dendrites* (Greek *dendron*: wood or tree), but typically has only one *axon*, which may have many branches. Axons are specialized not only for the conduction of impulses but also for the secretion, at their tips, of chemical messengers that affect the cells that they contact (muscle or gland cells, or the dendrites or cell bodies of other neurons).

The junction between the terminal of an axon and the membrane of another neuron is called a SYNAPSE, with a very narrow *synaptic cleft* between the two. The axon terminal contains many tiny droplets called *synaptic vesicles*, close to the zone of contact. A chemical NEUROTRANSMITTER (sometimes more than one kind) is stored in these vesicles and is released into the cleft when an action potential invades the terminal. This released transmitter then binds to *receptors*, specialized protein molecules in the membrane of the next cell, ultimately causing electrical excitation or inhibition of that cell. There are many different transmitters, but the most widespread excitatory ones are *acetylcholine, noradrenaline,* and *glutamate; glycine* and *gamma-aminobutyric acid* (*GABA*) are the major inhibitory transmitters.

Finally, the term 'nerves' has a colloquial usage, denoting ANXIETY or apprehension, or as an 'explanation' of unusual behaviour. While this adds further to the ambiguity of this over-used word, it is at least a popular recognition of the role of the nervous system in determining such 'mental' functions as the emotions and character.

LAURENCE GAREY

See PLATE 6.

See also GREY MATTER; NERVOUS SYSTEM; WHITE MATTER.

Nervousness is an early modern concept, although it has correlatives from the time of the Greeks in allied concepts of STRESS, debility, appetitive, and saturnine behaviour. Up to the late eighteenth century the word was imbued with mechanical meaning as the body's physical condition derived from its anatomical nerves. It gathered terrific significance in the mid seventeenth century under the weight of Descartes' physiological revolution and, even more emphatically, in Thomas Willis' system of neuroanatomy. Willis, an Oxford physiologist and practising physician who possessed profound clinical and empirical skills, wrote treatises on the nerves and brains of living creatures. He maintained that the body's degree of nervousness influenced human health more than had been appreciated and therefore merited as much clinical attention as the blood, lymph, or individual organs. Time has proved Willis right. Even in his own era his authority carried much weight, especially among disciples including Sydenham, Locke, and other early members of the Royal Society, and subsequent generations were impressed by his neurological theories, believing that more research was necessary. The result was the notion that living creatures could be measured according to the degree to which they partook of 'nervousness'. Therefore, whatever nervousness may have been historically, it came into its own approximately at the end of the seventeenth century.

Nervousness, as a social phenomenon rather than a physical state, underwent rapid proliferation in the mid eighteenth century: among individuals, in towns and cities under urban sprawl, and even among the branches of government; the earliest social scientists were thus enabled to configure the first models of nervous societies along lines of the old body politic and mind–body dualism.

After Willis, doctors continued to explain nervousness, especially when writing didactically rather than when presenting case studies, but they had little sense of the ways nervousness pervaded particular social groups or societies at large. For example, Dr James Makktrick Adair, one of the most fashionable 'nerve doctors' of Georgian England, whose patients sought him out to treat their nervousness, wrote that Dr Robert Whytt's 1764 treatise on the nerves (*Observations on the nature, causes, and cure of those disorders which have been commonly called nervous*) had such influence on the public that 'before the publication of this book, people of fashion had not the least idea that they had nerves.' Afterwards, everyone fashionable was pronounced nervous: a word resounding through the boroughs but not as yet gendered as it would become among women in the next century. The dissemination, according to Adair, was as if, almost with a magic wand, a single word possessed transformative power. Hence the rise of authoritative 'nerve doctors' both in Britain and Europe. Their ranks were equalled by marginal figures, if not blatant quacks, who also meddled in nerves through mesmerism, hypnotism, and erotic life therapies.

After this late-eighteenth-century development it was inevitable that nerves would become the most fashionable of upper-crust insignia: for the rich and famous, the glamorous and glittering, rather than the working-class poor. There emerged the profile of a languishing and delicate creature, male as well as female, too refined for ordinary work, too sensitive to cope with mundane matters. By the time Thomas Trotter published his *View of the Nervous Temperament* in 1807 or Jane Austen her novels a decade later — embodying nervous heroines like Marianne Dashwood and Fanny Price — this nervous type had become recognizable to the reading public. Its popularity grew with theories of physiognomy, craniology, and, later, phrenology. A century later, D. H. Lawrence firmly established his famous dichotomy between 'nervous' and 'sexual' loves, infinitely elevating the latter at the expense of the former. In these and many other paradigms of nervousness, the term became a catchall for all human states extending beyond the ordinarily perceptible. It designated some higher, sensual, almost physiological utopia in which the nerves, like violin strings, would be tuned to a pitch that maximized higher understanding. Down through the nineteenth century, doctors diagnosed one condition after another as diseases of damaged nerves, and critics claimed that creative geniuses suffered from them as well. Therapies and cures varied, but pre-eminent were addictive drugs and potions such as opium, laudanum, and numerous herbal preparations, as well as the panaceas of rest, recreation, solitude, travel, and a change of climate and scenery.

Nervous exhaustion

'Nervous exhaustion' (also called by other names) had been a topic of constant concern, since c 1740, especially for the health of women. It was the prospect of imminent collapse owing to the taut state of the nerves, and almost every doctor, and even philosophers as diverse as Carlyle and William James, harboured an explanation. The main line was a defect in the nervous constitution itself — its fibres and tissues: what we would designate as genetic make-up. In France, Lamarck's evolutionary theories also supported the belief that nervousness had evolved just as all other physical characteristics, and in 1859 this argument was reinforced by Darwin's *Origin of Species*. Concurrently a new myth flourished about the degeneracy of the nerves along hereditary lines, as in Bénédict Auguste Morel's *Traité des dégénérescences* (1857). A parallel myth about hysteria's nervousness had also developed, implicating the anatomical nerves. Its nineteenth-century legacy was a strengthening of the hereditary theory, as in Charcot's famous *Lectures on the Diseases of the Nervous System* (1879), which argued that hysteria and heredity were inextricably linked.

Meanwhile, theories of degeneracy and sexuality proliferated, almost always implicating nervousness as a sign, so that when Cesare Lombroso, the Italian jurist, adumbrated his theory of criminal degeneracy in *L'uomo delinquente* (1876), he could not omit the nerves as the veritable prime movers of pathology. Likewise, Richard von Krafft-Ebing, a leading German sexologist, claimed in his *Pyschopathia Sexualis* (1882) that synapses in both men and women were the most important clue in sexual deviation and linked heredity to virtually all the sexual disorders, especially inversion or homosexuality. Many of these works aimed to identify the physical basis of neurasthenia, despite the Victorian suppression of explicit discussions of the body, including its taut or flaccid nerves.

Female nervousness

As a result, neurasthenia was underdeveloped as a concept until late in the nineteenth century. A private discourse of nerves had arisen — partly behind bedroom doors in view of its delicate topics; all this while late Enlightenment classifications of neurosis (still meaning nervous, rather than deviant in Freud's sense) were being used for narrative purposes by all manner of novelists, despite the lack of research into nervousness. But as taboos about the body gradually lifted and the human sciences advanced, the knowledge of nervousness slowly changed. The American physician Dr Weir Mitchell's prescribed 'rest cure' ironically resulted in Charlotte Perkins Gilman's *The Yellow Wallpaper*, a literary account documenting her reversal of her doctor's orders not to do anything. At stake was the female's nervous deterioration, subsequent neurasthenia, and eventual dysfunction. Gilman landed upon a 'writing cure' as the only road to recovery.

Allegedly at fault was an inferior female nervous system, prone to such chronic neurasthenia. Doctors tried everything possible to strengthen it, including exercise and diet, but resorted especially to superior education, as Sir James Paget advocated in his 1867 *Clinical Lectures*. George M. Beard, a prominent New York physician, popularised neurasthenia as the hallmark of the woman, and was followed by dozens of doctors on both sides of the Atlantic by the time Freud published his *Studies on Hysteria* in 1895. Lists of excessively nervous patients included almost half the literate of England, and such American notables as Theodore Roosevelt, Henry Adams, Edith Wharton, and Emily Dickinson. Leaders were particularly vulnerable. Beard's group consisted mostly of 'brain workers': persons sedentary, creative, educated, professional, devoid of strenuous physical exercise, and tainted with creative feminine psychologies and responses. Prescribed paramedical panaceas of electrotherapy, massage, and isolation foreshadowed our contemporary treatments that range from aromatherapy to stress reductions.

Creative nervousness

Meanwhile, social conditions were altering and creating new mass stress. Writers and artists displayed an interest in these subjects and even took sides in the debates over the effects of excessive strain, and the rest cure, as did Henry James in *The Ambassadors* and Eugene Wister in *The Virginian*, both in 1903. Theodore Dreiser made the case for creativity as explicitly 'nervous' in *The Genius* (1915): the story of Eugene, who is artistic, feminine, creative, eugenically unfit to survive in the modern world; who suffers breakdown and finds cure in the opposites of rest and exertion. Virginia Woolf reflected on her own neurophysiology in the act of writing, claiming in her diary that 'it calls upon every nerve to hold itself taut.'

But twentieth-century nervousness has been construed even more ambiguously than these extremes suggest and has given rise to new paradigms — genetic, biochemical, neuroanatomic, synaptic. The debates in our generation encompass healthy and pathological stress and anxiety, and they now extend to the creative acts themselves: to the condition of the nerves at every stage of the creative process. It is debated, for example, whether a different set of synapses permits concert artists to perform. Of concern is the degree to which the capability lies in predetermined neuroanatomical and neurochemical structures, enabling certain physiological processes. These issues now extend to virtually every aspect of neuronal and brain function, including image formation and production of impressions and ideas, as well as short and long term memory. The subject is so complex and immense that it would be hard to identify any more influential concept in describing human motive and human behaviour than 'nervousness'.

GEORGE ROUSSEAU

Further reading

Lawrence, C. (1979). The nervous system and Society in the Scottish Enlightenment. In *Natural Order: historical studies of scientific Enlightenment*, (ed. B. Barnes and S. Shapin). Sage Publications, Beverly Hills.

Lutz, T. (1991). *American nervousness, 1903: an anecdotal history*. Cornell University Press, Ithaca.

Rousseau, G. S. (1989). Discourses of the Nerve. In *Literature and science as modes of expression*, (ed. F. Amrine). Kluwer Academic Publishers, Dordrecht.

See also ANXIETY; HYSTERIA; PSYCHOLOGICAL DISORDERS; STRESS.

Nervous system There are probably more than 100 000 million nerve cells in the body. The nervous system is the sum total of all these, together with their nerve fibres, which ramify throughout the body, and the various supporting components of nervous tissue.

The nervous system is subdivided into the CENTRAL NERVOUS SYSTEM (CNS) and the *peripheral nervous system* (PNS). Basically, the BRAIN and *spinal cord* form the CNS, while the rest is PNS. The CNS is well protected inside the skull and vertebral column. The PNS is essentially the NERVES, which run through most of the tissues of the body. The function of the nervous system is to collect information from the body and the outside world, through the sense organs, to process it in the CNS, and to distribute relevant commands to the muscles and glands throughout the body.

Like other body tissues, the nervous system is composed of *cells*, similar in general form to other cells in the body, but with some important modifications. One might imagine that *nervous tissue* consists of nerve cells and very little else. In fact a multitude of other components are essential to proper functioning of the nervous system, and form an integral part of it. Still, the most important cells of the nervous system are the nerve cells (neurons). Their most distinctive feature is their thin processes, called fibres or axons, which transmit impulses (ACTION POTENTIALS) and which contact muscles or glands, or, in most cases, other nerve cells. So the nervous system can be looked upon as an enormous series of 'chains' or circuits of neurons, each receiving excitatory and inhibitory messages from other neurons, and each sending impulses along its axon if the balance of incoming signals is in favour of excitation. A typical neuron in the brain may receive 10 000 terminals from incoming axons.

Many other cell types are necessary to support the neurons. BLOOD VESSELS supply blood to the nervous tissue and drain it away into the major veins. A large percentage of the human race will die from diseases associated with cerebral blood vessels, while many more people will be permanently handicapped, especially by STROKE (blockage or rupture of blood vessels).

The most important — certainly the most numerous — other supporting cells in the nervous system are the glial cells, or GLIA (from the Greek for glue). Amazingly, there are about 10 times as many glia as neurons in the nervous system. The most distinctive glial cells in the PNS are the *Schwann cells*, which wrap themselves around peripheral nerves to produce the fatty, insulating sheath called MYELIN. In the CNS various types of glial cells are involved in myelination, the transfer of nutrients from capillaries to neurons, and are also components of the defence system of the CNS, protecting against infection and helping remove degenerated neurons.

In the PNS, groups of, usually, a few hundred axons form bundles, several of which are united into a *nerve trunk*. Individual axons are well protected and peripheral nerves are fairly flexible. They even stretch somewhat, which is necessary if they run near a limb joint, or when a surgeon wishes to suture together two divided nerve stumps. Larger nerves have their own tiny blood vessels.

The nervous system also includes the *special sense organs* (eyes, ears, etc.) and sensory axons throughout the body. The essential feature of a SENSE ORGAN is the specialized neurons, called receptor cells, whose membranes include molecular mechanisms for detecting particular events outside the cell (such as the presence of particular chemicals, or light, or pressure on the membrane). Receptor cells 'transduce' the energy of these events into electrical changes inside the cell, which eventually produce a set of nerve impulses that race along axons towards the CNS. In the skin there are *free nerve endings*, specialized to signal touch, pain, and temperature. *Muscle spindles* and *Golgi tendon organs* are receptor organs found inside SKELETAL MUSCLE, which are stimulated by stretch of the muscle or tension on the tendon. They help inform the CNS about the state of activity of the muscles and therefore the position and balance of the body. Such information can either be conscious (involving signals reaching the CEREBRAL CORTEX of the brain) or unconscious (being used for example in spinal REFLEXES).

In the special sense organs, such as the eye and the ear, highly specialized receptors respond to light and sound. Sensory information also comes from the viscera and blood vessels. Although

viscera can produce conscious sensation, such as pain when they are distended, VISCERAL SENSATION is mainly used unconsciously by the AUTONOMIC NERVOUS SYSTEM.

The autonomic nervous system has both central and peripheral components. It is concerned with the automatic control of bodily function. It is subdivided into *sympathetic* and *parasympathetic* portions. To some extent, these two systems have opposing actions. For instance, sympathetic activity classically prepares for 'fight or flight', raising blood pressure and heart rate, facilitating breathing, dilating the pupils, and deviating blood from the skin and gastrointestinal tract to skeletal muscles. Parasympathetic activity, in contrast, adapts the body for rest and digestion. Cell bodies of sympathetic neurons are in the middle levels of the spinal cord. Their axons leave the cord and end on nerve cells in the *sympathetic trunk*, a long nerve tract beside the vertebral column. Thence the axons of these relaying nerve cells join, and are distributed with, other nerves of the peripheral system, to reach glands and blood vessels in all parts of the body (except the CNS itself). Others run to the eyes, to the heart and lungs, and to the abdominal and pelvic organs. Parasympathetic cell bodies are in the BRAIN STEM, with axons running in the tenth cranial (VAGUS) nerves, reaching glands around the mouth and throat, and extending down to the heart and lungs and to most of the abdominal organs. There is a second set of parasympathetic nerve cells in the lowest segments of the spinal cord, that send out fibres to the pelvic organs.

Thus the nervous system is responsible for rapid conduction of information throughout the body. Neurons are highly differentiated and, except in early fetal life, are generally incapable of division or *mitosis* to reproduce themselves. This means that if lost through disease or injury they cannot be replaced. On the other hand, axons regenerate readily in the PNS (as anyone who has cut a cutaneous nerve knows). One of the most important goals of neuroscience research in the years to come will be to understand why this is, and whether damaged neurons in the CNS can be persuaded to repair themselves.

LAURENCE GAREY

See PLATE 6.

See also AUTONOMIC NERVOUS SYSTEM; BRAIN; CENTRAL NERVOUS SYSTEM; NERVES; NEUROTRANSMITTER; SYNAPSE.

Neuromuscular junction
The body contains over 600 different SKELETAL MUSCLES and each consists of thousands of muscle fibres ranging in length from a few millimetres to several centimetres. The motor nerve fibres innervating them, which arise in the SPINAL CORD, can be more than 1 m in length. However, the area of apposition between the terminal tip of each nerve fibre and the 'endplate' of each muscle fibre is usually less than 50 μm (1/20 mm) in diameter. This particular type of SYNAPSE is called the

neuromuscular junction (see figure). In order to generate the complex and finely controlled movements that we all take for granted, there has to be a very efficient, fail-safe, and one-way transmission between the nerve and the muscle that ensures that muscle contractions faithfully follow commands from the CENTRAL NERVOUS SYSTEM. Such neuromuscular transmission depends on the release from the motor nerve terminal of the chemical ACETYLCHOLINE (ACh), and its binding to a protein receiver on the surface of the muscle, called the acetylcholine receptor (AChR).

When a nerve impulse reaches the motor nerve terminal, specialized proteins forming ION-CHANNELS in its CELL MEMBRANE open transiently, allowing a short-lived entry of calcium into the terminal. Stored inside the nerve terminal, and attached to special sites on the inside of the cell membrane, are small round vesicles filled with ACh. The sudden inrush of calcium causes some of the vesicle membranes to fuse with the nerve terminal membrane, and to release their contents into the *synaptic cleft* between the nerve and the surface of the muscle fibre (see figure (d)).

ACh diffuses rapidly across the ultramicroscopic 50 nm gap and binds to the AChRs that are very densely packed on the tops of the synaptic folds on the muscle fibre (see figure (c), (d)). When two ACh molecules bind to each AChR, its central pore (*channel*) opens, allowing small positively charged ions, mainly sodium, to enter the muscle, resulting in a local reduction in the potential across the membrane (*depolarisation*). The release of many ACh-containing vehicles by a nerve impulse leads to a large depolarisation called the *endplate potential*, which in turn opens the voltage-sensitive sodium channels situated at the base of each synaptic fold (see figure (d)). These are responsible for starting an 'all or nothing' action potential that is propagated along the muscle fibre in each direction and initiates muscle contraction.

After about a millisecond, the AChR pore closes and ACh unbinds and is broken down by an enzyme, ACh esterase (AChE), that sits in the synaptic cleft (see figure (d)). Choline is then taken back into the nerve terminal by special transporters, and used to make more ACh; this is stored in newly-formed synaptic vesicles, themselves made up of recycled nerve terminal membrane. The whole sequence of events, from the inrush of calcium to the initiation of the action potential, takes place in less than two milliseconds.

Many of the earliest studies on chemical synaptic transmission began with the AUTONOMIC NERVOUS SYSTEM, but they were soon extended to skeletal muscles when Dale and his colleagues (1936) showed that stimulation of motor nerves released ACh, and that ACh can induce muscle contraction. The action of ACh could be increased by using a drug, eserine, that inhibits the ACh esterase, and the action of ACh on the muscle could be blocked by the arrow

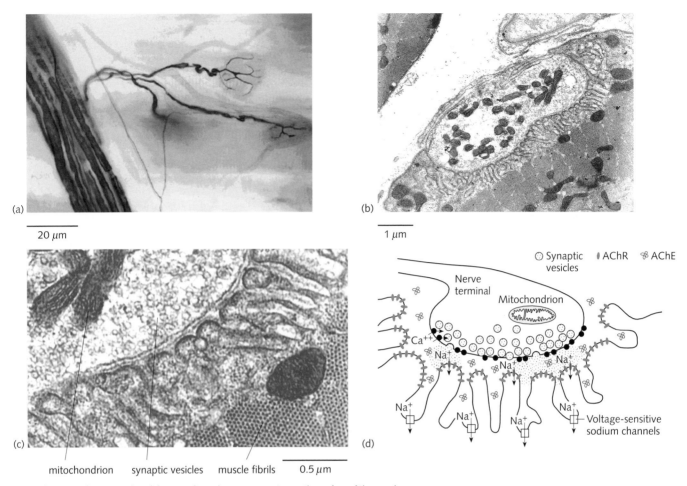

(a)

20 μm

(b)

1 μm

○ Synaptic   ▮ AChR   ⊗ AChE
vesicles

Nerve
terminal   Mitochondrion

Ca++

Na+   Na+

Na+   Na+   Na+   Na+ ─ Voltage-sensitive
sodium channels

(c)

(d)

mitochondrion   synaptic vesicles   muscle fibrils   0.5 μm

(a) A silver-stained nerve trunk and three myelinated nerves synapsing on the surface of the muscle.
    Each myelinated nerve ends as a series of fine, unmyelinated terminals that spread out over the neuromuscular junction.
(b) An electron micrograph of a single nerve terminal and the adjacent muscle fibre.
    There are many mitochondria in both the nerve and the muscle. The surface of the muscle fibre apposed to the nerve terminal is thrown into a series of folds.
(c) A higher magnification of part of (b). The nerve terminal contains many synaptic vesicles. At the top of the muscle folds the membrane is strongly stained because of the
    high density of AChRs. Just beneath the folds the muscle fibrils, which are responsible for muscle contraction, can be seen in cross-section.
(d) A diagram depicting the main components of neuromuscular transmission and their roles (see text).
    (a), (b), and (c) courtesy of Dr Clarke Slater, University of Newcastle.

poison, curare. Katz and his co-workers subsequently used intracellular micro-electrodes to measure the endplate potentials and showed that these followed the release of many vesicles of ACh, and that a similar depolarisation of the muscle occurred when ACh was applied directly onto the neuromuscular junction with a micropipette.

The neuromuscular junction, unlike most of the nervous system, is accessible to factors circulating in the blood. This can be both an advantage and a disadvantage. For many surgical operations, one of the important roles of the anesthetist is to relax the patient's muscles using an intravenous injection of the otherwise poisonous curare-like drugs — whilst taking over artificially the muscular function of breathing. Similarly, many species of venomous animals, such as snakes and scorpions, make toxins that paralyse their prey, and in some parts of the world this can also be a serious hazard for

humans. Such toxins are rapidly absorbed and carried to the neuromuscular junction where they bind with extraordinary efficiency to the AChRs and other ion channel proteins, leading to muscle PARALYSIS which can prevent breathing. Another important toxin is botulinum, which is produced by bacteria contaminating certain foods. Botulinum toxin blocks the release of ACh from the motor nerve terminals, and can cause fatal paralysis in babies; on the other hand it has recently found use as a treatment by local injection into muscles that are subject to uncontrollable severe spasm.

These neurotoxins have also provided marvellous tools for investigating function. For instance, a particular snake toxin, alpha-bungarotoxin, binds very strongly to AChRs and has been of immense use in the study of diseases that affect neuromuscular transmission. In myasthenia gravis (*mys*: muscle: *aesthenia*: weakness), the patient suffers from serious weakness and fatigue

that can be life-threatening if it involves swallowing and breathing muscles. Myasthenia was first described in 1672 by the very distinguished London physician and anatomist, Thomas Willis. Over three hundred years later, Jim Patrick and Jon Lindstrom at the Salk Institute in California induced a myasthenia gravis-like disease in rabbits by injecting them with AChR protein purified from the electric organs of certain fish. The rabbits responded to the 'foreign' protein by making antibodies to it, but these antibodies gained access to the rabbits' neuromuscular junctions, recognised the muscle AChRs, and reduced their function, producing muscle weakness. Following these experimental observations, radioactively-labelled alpha-bungarotoxin was used to show that patients with myasthenia have reduced numbers of AChRs at their neuromuscular junctions, and subsequently that this is caused by serum antibodies that bind to AChRs — just as in the rabbits. Drugs that inhibit the ACh esterase enzyme cause clinical improvement because they prolong the action of ACh, as first demonstrated in 1934 by Mary Walker, a young doctor in London, but nowadays the most important treatment is to reduce the circulating antibodies that bind AChR.   ANGELA VINCENT

Further reading

Hughes, J. T. (1991). *Thomas Willis 1621–1675. His life and work*. Royal Society of Medicine Services Ltd., London.

Katz, B. (1966). *Nerve muscle and synapse*. McGraw Hill, Inc., New York.

Vincent, A. and Wray, D. (1992). *Neuromuscular transmission: basic and applied aspects*. Pergammon Press, Oxford.

See also SKELETAL MUSCLE; SYNAPSE.

Neuroscience
is the study of all aspects of nerves and the nervous system, in health and in disease. It includes the anatomy, physiology, chemistry, pharmacology, and pathology of nerve cells; the behavioural and psychological features that depend on the function of the nervous system; and the clinical disciplines that deal with them, such as neurology, neurosurgery, and psychiatry.   L.J.G.

See NERVOUS SYSTEM.

Neurotransmitters
After Galvani had shown, in 1742, that electrical stimulation of the nerve to the muscle of a frog's leg caused the muscle to twitch, the idea gained ground that transmission from nerves to the 'end organ' was an electrical process. Today we know that only in very rare instances is transmission across a SYNAPSE — that is, between the end of a nerve and whatever it innervates — an electrical event. Virtually all neurotransmission is chemical. Nerves release one or more neurotransmitters, which act chemically on receptors in the membrane of the cells across the synaptic cleft. To detect neurotransmitters is a difficult task as the amounts released are minute and mechanisms exist that quickly remove the transmitter, leaving the system in a state of readiness for the arrival of the next nerve impulse. The first steps came from finding chemicals which could mimic the action of neurotransmitters. *Muscarine* was able to mimic the effects of stimulation of the HEART by the vagus nerves, and its actions were blocked by atropine. Similarly, *nicotine* mimicked the effect of stimulating motor nerves to SKELETAL MUSCLE, and this was blocked by curare.

Du Bois Reymond, in 1877, declared that chemical or electrical transmission were the only two real alternatives, although there was no data to decide unequivocally between the two. In 1904 Elliot suggested that adrenaline might be the transmitter in the sympathetic nervous system, and in the next year a nicotine-like substance was postulated by Langley as the transmitter in motor nerves to muscles. Dixon, in 1907, tried to extract from a heart the neurotransmitter released by the vagus, measuring the effect of the extract on another heart, but reached no conclusions. It was

1921 before Loewi performed the celebrated experiment in which two beating frog hearts were superfused in series, the perfusate of the first flowing over the second. Stimulation of the vagus nerve to the first heart caused its beat to slow and, after a brief interval, the second heart slowed too. While this experiment did not prove that the substance flowing over from the first heart was released from the vagus nerve, clearly something chemical rather than electrical slowed the second heart.

In the 1930s Dale and his school in England showed that ACETYLCHOLINE was the transmitter at motor nerve endings in skeletal muscle (NEUROMUSCULAR JUNCTIONS) and Cannon and his colleagues in the US demonstrated that an adrenaline-like substance was the transmitter in the sympathetic nervous system. These discoveries depended on the development of sensitive bioassays for transmitter substances. Dale was not convinced that the sympathetic neurotransmitter was ADRENALINE itself, because he demonstrated subtle differences between the responses to the transmitter and to adrenaline. Von Euler, in 1946, finally showed that the sympathetic neurotransmitter was NORADRENALINE (non-methylated adrenaline).

After this period there was a lull in which many thought that acetylcholine and noradrenaline were the only two neurotransmitters. After all, the transmitter at the neuromuscular junction in skeletal muscle, in the synapses in ganglia of the autonomic nervous system, and at the ends of parasympathetic nerve fibres was shown to be acetylcholine, and noradrenaline was the transmitter at sympathetic nerve endings. So all types of synapse appeared to be accounted for. There was also evidence that acetylcholine was a transmitter in the brain. Furthermore, by then, criteria for showing that an agent was a neurotransmitter had been laid down and these were quite difficult to fulfill, especially in complex situations like the neural pathways in the brain. These five criteria are demonstrations that show:

(i) the putative transmitter is released when the nerve trunk is stimulated;

(ii) application of the transmitter to the postsynaptic structure causes the same effect as nerve stimulation;

(iii) the nerve fibres have a mechanism for making, storing, and releasing the transmitter;

(iv) a mechanism is present for rapidly terminating the actions of the neurotransmitter; and

(v) an appropriate antagonist is equally effective at blocking both neurotransmission and exogenous application of the neurotransmitter.

Consider how these criteria are met for acetylcholine and for noradrenaline. We have already seen that these two substances were detected by sensitive bioassays in perfusates from neuronally-stimulated systems. To meet the second criterion it is necessary to show identity of action of the neurotransmitter and exogenously-applied

transmitter substance. While this was straightforward with acetylcholine, Dale's insistence that adrenaline was *not* the neurotransmitter was based on differences between the responses to adrenaline and to nerve stimulation. This was an essential step leading to the discovery of noradrenaline.

The third criterion is satisfied because nerves that release acetylcholine (*cholinergic nerves*) have an enzyme (*choline acetyltransferase*) in the nerve terminals that synthesizes acetylcholine from choline, while *noradrenergic nerves* have a series of enzymes that synthesize noradrenaline from the amino acid tyrosine. The enzymes are produced in the nerve cell bodies and pass down the axon to the nerve terminals in the so-called *axoplasmic flow* (they can travel a considerable distance — for example, from the spinal cord to the foot muscles).

With respect to the fourth criterion: after release of acetylcholine from the nerve terminals it is attacked by *acetylcholine esterase*, which breaks down the neurotransmitter to choline and an acetate group, thus quickly terminating its action at the muscle membrane receptors. The choline is taken up into the terminal and recycled.

The mechanism for terminating transmitter action is different in the noradrenergic system. Seventy per cent of the released noradrenaline is taken back up into the nerve terminals and stored for later reuse. The rest is metabolized either extracellularly or after uptake into the end organ.

We have seen earlier that there are specific antagonists for acetylcholine, which also antagonize the effects of cholinergic stimulation. Similarly there are antagonists, such as the β-blockers, which block both noradrenaline and noradrenergic stimulation, thus meeting the fifth criterion.

In 1934 Dale enunciated a principle which stated that a nerve liberates the same neurotransmitter at all its terminations. Thus if a nerve branches, each branch will release the same neurotransmitter. This principle has remained a truism and it would be difficult to imagine a nerve cell that could exclusively send a different set of synthetic enzymes, in the axoplasmic flow, down different branches. However, until relatively recently it was assumed that any one nerve produced only one type of neurotransmitter. As usual in science, advances arose when observations were made which failed to fit the established dogma. It was recognized that in some systems antagonists that were able to block exogenously applied transmitter were not able to block nerve stimulation completely. There was a residual activity with nerve stimulation that was resistant to the block. The term *NANC transmission* was coined, standing for 'nonadrenergic non-cholinergic transmission'. As the responses to nerve stimulation were partially blocked by antagonists with known specificities, the corollary was that the nerve must liberate more than one transmitter, but would do so from all its branches. Thus the concept of *co-transmission* was born, in which nerve stimulation could, in some instances, co-release more than one transmitter. In the peripheral autonomic nervous system — at the site where the nerves reach the tissue that they act upon — a great number of NANC transmitters have been claimed including, among others, ATP, VIP (vasoactive intestinal peptide), 5-HT, GABA, and DOPAMINE. Undoubtedly some of these substances are transmitters, but few have yet met all the five criteria required to confirm their bona fides.

What advantages might accrue from co-transmission? First, the small molecular weight transmitters (amine transmitters) and one of the peptide transmitters are likely to have very different kinetics (fast and slow effects). Secondly, the receptor targets for the two transmitters may have different locations, for example one on the end organ and the other on the nerve terminal itself, allowing feedback control and finally 'traffic neuromodulation'. This last results from the different ways in which the peptide transmitters and amine transmitters are handled. The 'machinery' needed to synthesize peptides like VIP is considerable. Consequently, these transmitters are synthesized in the nerve cell body and pass to the terminal in the axoplasmic flow, where they are stored ready for release. If there is heavy traffic in the nerve then the supply of the peptide neurotransmitter will soon be depleted. It is more difficult to deplete the supply of amine transmitters, which are made in the nerve terminal itself, so the ratio of the two transmitters released by nerve impulses will change.

While the criteria for proving that a chemical agent acts as a neurotransmitter in the periphery are not easy to achieve, the technical difficulties in the brain and spinal cord are much greater. Here there is a mass of neural tissue with intricate interconnections and ramifications within the brain, as well as the connections made with incoming and outgoing neural pathways. However, there is overwhelming evidence for many neurotransmitters in the central nervous system, even though not all the five criteria above have been satisfied. Histochemical methods have been used to demonstrate the localization of neurotransmitters in particular types of nerve cells, coupled with electrophysiological methods in which the physiology of a single identified cell is studied with microelectrodes. Finally, it is now possible to suck a few nanolitres of intracellular substance (cytosol) from a single, identified neuron in a brain slice and to determine which genes are activated, including those coding for proteins associated with neurotransmission (receptors, enzymes, etc.). Useful information can also be obtained by a study of disease states. For example, there can be no doubt that a lack of dopamine transmission gives rise to Parkinson's disease. Evidence from post-mortem brains and comparison of the dopamine concentrations in normal and diseased brains locates the dopaminergic pathways involved in the disease.

A potential forty neurotransmitters have been postulated to exist in the brain, of which ten are of the amine type with a small molecular weight.

The amine types include acetylcholine, noradrenaline, dopamine, 5-HT, and histamine, and there are also excitatory and inhibitory amino acids. Glutamate and aspartate are the principal fast-acting excitatory transmitters in the brain, while GABA and glycine are the main inhibitory transmitters. Initially there was great reluctance to accept that these simple amino acids could act as neurotransmitters. Identified neurons were excited or inhibited when these amino acids were squirted onto them from very fine micropipettes. However, the presence of a pharmacological response does not prove physiological relevance. The development of selective agonists and antagonists has, subsequently, established that the four amino acids are true neurotransmitters. The remaining thirty-odd neurotransmitters in the central nervous system are mainly peptides, but much more evidence is needed before their true roles are unravelled.   ALAN W. CUTHBERT

See also AUTONOMIC NERVOUS SYSTEM; NEUROMUSCULAR JUNCTION; PEPTIDES; SYNAPSE.

Nicotine is a simple alkaloid produced by the tobacco plant. The history of chewing and smoking tobacco, and of taking snuff, is of great antiquity. All the acute effects of the tobacco habit are dependent on nicotine, which has complex actions, both on the central nervous system and in the rest of the body. Nicotine acts on certain cell membrane receptors, which were therefore given the name nicotinic receptors. Nicotine was found to mimic the actions of the neurotransmitter ACETYLCHOLINE at these sites: at the NEUROMUSCULAR JUNCTIONS in skeletal (voluntary) muscle; at the SYNAPSES in the relay stations (the ganglia) of the AUTONOMIC NERVOUS SYSTEM; and in various parts of the BRAIN and SPINAL CORD. In many situations nicotine first activates the nicotinic receptors and then by its continued presence desensitizes them. Normally, at these nicotinic synapses, the transmitter (acetylcholine) is rapidly destroyed by the enzyme cholinesterase, so its action is evanescent; this is not the case with nicotine.

Nicotinic receptors are proteins which span the CELL MEMBRANE (e.g. of a muscle cell or neuron) and when activated by acetylcholine or by nicotine undergo a conformational change that creates ION CHANNELS in the membrane. These channels allow the passage of sodium ions inwards and potassium ions outwards through the membrane, leading to excitation of the cell.

Increased levels of nicotine can be measured in the blood up to one hour after a cigarette. Nicotine-taking, in whatever form, is for self gratification and reward, requiring reinforcement at intervals. If nicotine is withdrawn, irritability and failure to concentrate is the result. The actions of nicotine are caused by effects in the brain. Repeated intake of nicotine leads to increased numbers of nicotinic receptors in the brain, which might be expected to reduce the need for nicotine rather than increase it. But it seems likely that many of the receptors are in a

desensitized form and that the number of functional receptors is reduced, so that the addict requires increasing and repeated doses to maintain the effect. The claims that nicotine increases concentration, learning ability, and retention of learned information are well founded — numbers of performance tests have confirmed this. Nicotine produces a sense of alertness, but nevertheless of calm. This seems to be due to inhibition of reflex nerve loops in the spinal cord, with the effect of causing muscular relaxation.

The above actions all take place in the central nervous system. The effects of nicotine in the rest of the body are due to actions on the ganglia of the autonomic nervous system, predominantly on the sympathetic ganglia. Mimicking the effects of physiological sympathetic stimulation, they include increases in heart rate, cardiac output, and blood pressure, and reduction in gut motility and digestive functions. Because the adrenal medulla is a modified sympathetic ganglion — with secretion normally stimulated by acetylcholine — ADRENALINE and NOR-ADRENALINE are released by the action of nicotine; these are likely to be responsible for most of the cardiovascular effects. Nicotine also releases antidiuretic hormone from the posterior PITUITARY GLAND, hence reducing the formation of urine.

Nicotine is not used therapeutically, except for nicotine patches and chewing gum, which are used to help smokers give up the habit. They do not have the dangers associated with constituents of tobacco smoke.

For some time nicotine enjoyed popularity as an insecticide. However, in its concentrated form it is highly poisonous, and it can be absorbed through the skin, so is no longer used for spraying on plants. Lobeline, another plant alkaloid from Lobelia species, has very similar actions to nicotine.   ALAN W. CUTHBERT

See also ACETYLCHOLINE; AUTONOMIC NERVOUS SYSTEM; NEUROTRANSMITTERS; MEMBRANE RECEPTORS; SMOKING.

Nipples The nipples are the pigmented erectile tips of the mammary glands or BREASTS, and are present in both male and female mammals. Usually conical in shape, nipples can also be everted, flat, or, more rarely, inverted. They are encircled by a pigmented ring called the areola, and surrounded by nerve endings and blood vessels. When stimulated by touch or friction, or through sexual arousal, blood flowing through the vessels causes the nipples to become erect. Although stimulation of the nipples is usually pleasurable, both males and females vary greatly in the degree of sensation they experience. In women, nipples bear the openings of the lactiferous ducts through which milk is secreted when breast-feeding. During pregnancy and lactations, the woman's nipples become enlarged and her areolae darken in colour.

Like the female breasts, the nipples have historically been viewed in relation to woman's utility, PLEASURE, and BEAUTY. Differences between the beautiful and useful nipple are strikingly portrayed in Lehmann's late sixteenth-century portrait of Gabrielle d'Estrées, mistress of Henri IV, with her two sons and their WET-NURSE (Chateau d'Azay-Le Rideau). Gabrielle is shown seated in her bath, naked to the waist; behind her the elder child reaches toward a fruit bowl, while further back a wet-nurse holds d'Estrée's swaddled infant at her breast. The nurse's nipple contrasts with those of the King's favourite; where Gabrielle has small, pink nipples with little trace of pigmentation on her white breasts, the nurse's are large and brown, with the surrounding areola darkened in colour. The baby actively sucks at this working nipple, whose size and shape echoes the fruit in the bowl before her. In their configuration Gabrielle's nipples are nearer the pearls that ornament her hair, and in colour they resemble the pink flowers that surround her. The nurse here sets off the idealized body of the aristocratic mother whose nipples are ornamental, like the jewels and flowers to which they are compared. Of particular importance is the rosebud with its pink tip pointed towards Gabrielle. In France, the beautiful nipple was compared to a rose, since the word 'bouton' meant both nipple and rosebud. Dennel's later engraving of *The Comparison of the Nipple to the Rose* (1761) makes the connection explicit as a young girl holds a rosebud to her breast and assesses her beauty by comparing its size, shape, and colour to her nipple.

Although the portrait of Gabrielle d'Estrées shows wet nursing as an accepted practice, some doctors during this time encouraged mothers to nurse their infants by stressing the pleasures of breastfeeding. Ambroise Paré believed that nursing provided women a 'delicious stimulation' of the nipples, and that the nursing 'gently titillates them with tongue and mouth.' Paré argued that the nipples were sensitive not only because of their many nerve endings, but because of their affinity with the genitals. That this latter belief permeated popular thought is, evident when considering further the colloquial meaning of 'bouton', which besides referring to rosebud and nipple, also signified the clitoris.

By the eighteenth century those who encouraged maternal breastfeeding censured women who refused to nurse their infants for fear of disfiguring their breasts and nipples. Although Jean-Jacques Rousseau was the most influential advocate of breastfeeding, many others in the medical professions took up the cause. Doctors connected problems with breastfeeding to women's fashions. In 1706 Edward Baynard, a Lancashire physician, complained about women who wore corsets that squashed and flattened their nipples. Similarly, Dr Charles White of Manchester argued that the small, flat nipple buried in the breast was caused by the tight dress, 'which has for some centuries been so constantly worn in this island by the female sex of all ages and of almost all ranks.' By being continually pressed, the breast and nipple are deprived of their beauty and use.

For women living before the age of antibiotics, however, breastfeeding was actually a greater threat to their nipples than fashion. Nipples sore or cracked from nursing were easily infected; they could become ulcerated, obstructed, or deformed by scar tissue. Sometimes the nipples were so damaged that after nursing her first child the woman could not breastfeed the next; sometimes they were completely destroyed. To solve the problem of sore nipples and to aid in preventing or healing infections, women often used nipple shields. In basic design, the nipple shield has varied little from the sixteenth century to the present day. Worn over the nipples, these shields mimic their shape and size, and the tips are perforated to allow milk to flow through them. The primary difference between older and more recent versions is the material used in their manufacture. From the sixteenth to the nineteenth century, shields were made of tin, pewter, lead(!), horn, ivory, wood, silver, glass, or wax. Although the rubber nipple was patented in 1856, it did not come into widespread use until well into the twentieth century, because early versions were deemed foul smelling, bad tasting, and liable to contamination.

While the dangers of breast-feeding for the mother's health have been significantly reduced in the twentieth century, tensions between the erotic and the nourishing nipple limit women's opportunities for breast-feeding, especially in the US. In the 1990s, the many cases of security guards who harassed women for breastfeeding in public places led state lawmakers to enact legislation that excepted from public nudity laws a woman nursing a baby 'whether or not the nipple or areola is exposed during or incidental to the feeding.' That so many of these laws explicitly mention the nipple suggests that this part of the breast is especially charged as an erotic zone, and that exposing the nipple is tantamount to exposing the genitalia. Glorifying the breast as a sexual object led Americans to stigmatize its natural use by deeming public breast-feeding indecent. Only now are they belatedly undoing this latest damage to the breast.   MARY D. SHERIFF

Further reading

Baumslag, N. and Michels, D. (1995). *Milk, money, and madness. The culture and politics of breastfeeding*. Bergin and Garvey, Westport, CT and London.

Fildes, V. (1986). *Breasts, bottles, and babies. A history of infant feeding*. Edinburgh University Press.

See also BREAST; INFANT FEEDING; WET-NURSING.

Nitric oxide Two strands of research in the late 1970s led to a revolution in biology. Robert Furchgott was unravelling a paradox concerning the well-known neurotransmitter ACETYL-CHOLINE: when injected intravenously it lowers blood pressure, showing that the body's BLOOD VESSELS are relaxing, but when applied directly to blood vessels in isolation, outside the body,

acetylcholine normally makes them contract. Furchgott showed that the response of blood vessels depended critically on the innermost layer of cells lining the vessel — the *endothelium*. When the endothelium was present, acetylcholine relaxed blood vessels, but when it was removed they contracted. Acetylcholine was shown to cause the release of a diffusible factor from endothelium, and it was this *endothelium-derived relaxing factor* (EDRF) — its nature then unknown — which relaxed the blood vessels.

Meanwhile, Ferid Murad was investigating how blood vessels are relaxed by the nitrovasodilators (e.g. glyceryl trinitrate, amyl nitrite) used in the treatment of angina. He found that these compounds increase the levels of cyclic GMP (known to promote relaxation) inside the smooth muscle cells of the vessels, probably by generating the substance nitric oxide (more correctly called nitrogen monoxide; NO).

It was soon shown that EDRF also increases the levels of cyclic GMP in smooth muscle, and the two lines of research converged when it was found that various agents, including haemoglobin and the dye methylene blue, inhibit the action both of EDRF and of the nitrovasodilators. By 1987, Furchgott and Louis Ignarro were suggesting that EDRF and NO were one and the same. This was confirmed by Salvador Moncada, who showed that NO is synthesized from the dietary amino acid L-arginine.

It then became evident that the endothelium of blood vessels was not the only site where NO is made. The enzyme nitric oxide synthase (NOS), which uses L-arginine, oxygen, and cofactors to make NO, exists in three forms: *neuronal NOS* (nNOS), from nerve cells; *inducible NOS* (iNOS), in inflammatory and other cells when the body's defence mechanisms are activated; and *endothelial NOS* (eNOS). nNOS and eNOS are 'constitutive' enzymes — that is, they are always present in their cells — and they are activated by increases in the intracellular concentration of calcium ions. iNOS is produced in many cells in response to bacterial infection and other circumstances (such as rheumatoid arthritis) when the IMMUNE SYSTEM is activated; it is not regulated by calcium.

Nitric oxide is a tiny molecule. It is a gas, but dissolves in the fluids in and around cells. It is a free radical (sometimes denoted •NO to show that it has an unpaired electron, which makes it react very readily with other molecules). In particular, NO reacts with the radical anion, superoxide ($•O_2^-$), to form peroxynitrite ($ONOO^-$), which can damage cellular DNA and hence cause cell death. Thus, excess NO can cause damage to cells. In some situations this is valuable: for instance, cells of the immune system use NO to kill invading bacteria. However, it can also be dangerous. After a STROKE, for example, the nerve cells that have been deprived of oxygen fail to control their intracellular CALCIUM; this rises and triggers a massive synthesis of NO by nNOS activation, leading to peroxynitrite production and the death of surrounding neurons.

Peroxynitrite also oxidizes low density lipoproteins (LDL), which carry cholesterol in the blood, and oxidized LDL promotes atherosclerosis of blood vessels.

In septicaemia (blood poisoning), bacteria circulate in large numbers in the blood, and, in response, much NO is produced by many types of cells, including the muscle cells of the blood vessels this causes the blood vessels to relax. This leads to a severe fall in blood pressure, *septic shock*, which is difficult to reverse with agents such as adrenaline and dopamine, which normally increase blood pressure by constricting blood vessels. Septicaemia causes many deaths each year, and inhibition of NO synthesis appeared to be a promising treatment. But early attempts using inhibitors of NOS were largely unsuccessful. However, these were not selective for the relevant type (iNOS) and simultaneous inhibition of eNOS was deleterious to organ function. The increase in iNOS activity in inflammation can be inhibited by glucocorticoids (e.g. prednisolone, corticosterone), which explains part of their anti-inflammatory action, but they have no effect on the level of enzyme once it has been made. Thus the search is on for selective iNOS inhibitors which will leave nNOS and eNOS uninhibited.

NO has a good side and a bad side. While excess NO in septicaemia, inflammation, and stroke causes severe damage, localized production of small quantities of NO is essential for normal body function. Endothelial NOS maintains blood vessel function, and inhibition of this enzyme increases blood pressure. Indeed, hypertension is associated with decreased effectiveness of endothelial NO mechanisms. In blood vessels NO also regulates multiplication of muscle cells. Coronary artery bypass surgery sometimes fails because of narrowing of the newly replaced vessels; this is caused by thickening of their walls through muscle cell proliferation — thought to be due to decreased local production of NO as a result of endothelial damage during the surgery.

NO acts as a NEUROTRANSMITTER in nerves involved in controlling a number of 'vegetative' functions, including operation of the sphincters in the gut and ERECTION of the penis. *Viagra* (Sildenafil) works by prolonging the actions of NO released from penile nerves. In the brain, NO could even be involved in the formation of MEMORY. 'Long-term potentiation' — the increase in strength of synapses in the hippocampus, as a result of strong stimulation which is thought to underlie certain forms of memory — is blocked by drugs that inhibit NO synthesis.

This small inorganic molecule, which was probably best known to the general public as a pollutant in car exhausts, became the biological molecule of the 1990s. Its importance was recognized by the award of a Nobel Prize to Furchgott, Ignarro, and Murad in 1998 'for their discoveries concerning nitric oxide as a signalling molecule in the cardiovascular system'.

C. ROBIN HILEY

See also BLOOD VESSELS.

Nitrogen Four-fifths (79%) of the air we breathe consists of nitrogen, nearly all the rest being OXYGEN. It was known in the late seventeenth century that breathing air with its oxygen removed resulted in death, but only in 1772 did Rutherford isolate nitrogen; soon after, Lavoisier showed that pure nitrogen could not support life, although he misnamed it mephitic or 'smelly' air. It is odourless.

The nitrogen we breathe is chemically inert and takes no part in the chemical or metabolic reactions in the body. In this respect it resembles the 'inert gases' such as argon and neon which are a small part of the atmosphere. Nitrogen is poorly soluble in water and body liquids, and there is virtually no exchange between the nitrogen we breathe into the lungs and the body itself. However the chemical combinations of nitrogen are crucial for life. It is a definitive component of PROTEINS and their constituents, AMINO ACIDS. It is present in innumerable other essential chemical components of the body, from VITAMINS to HORMONES to ENZYMES and many other vital molecules; in recent years the ubiquitous importance of NITRIC OXIDE (NO) in physiological function has been recognized. It is no exaggeration to say that life only became possible by the creation of nitrogen-containing chemicals. But these chemicals reach their sites in the human body not from inhaled nitrogen, but from ingested plant and animal materials. Only plants (including some bacteria) can convert atmospheric nitrogen to the organic compounds needed for animal life, so plants are the ultimate source of all nitrogenous chemicals in the body.

In proteins nitrogen occurs mostly in amino- (-NH2) groups. During metabolic breakdown of these and other nitrogen-containing substances the nitrogen is not converted to its gaseous form for excretion in the lungs, but forms mainly urea, a small molecular-weight waste product that, as its name implies, is excreted in the URINE. Although the metabolism of proteins provides some energy for the body, this is normally far smaller than that due to burning carbohydrates (that contain no nitrogen), and fatty substances (most of which contain no nitrogen). Rather, the amino acids derived from the dietary proteins are taken up by body cells for use in the turnover of their own proteins, which they need to synthesize continually: for their growth and repair, cellular enzymes, secretions and so forth. In health, the necessary daily intake of nitrogen to balance inevitable losses is estimated at about 12 g, which would be contained in about 75 g of protein. In starvation or in the aftermath of serious injury or infection requiring rebuilding of tissues, protein is depleted, mainly from muscle, and is used for the production of glucose by the liver; only adequate nutritional supplements can avoid a state of 'negative nitrogen balance', with wasting and weakness.

Although nitrogen is poorly soluble in water, so that little is normally dissolved in body liquids, it is more soluble in fats, which accounts for its role in 'bends' or DECOMPRESSION SICKNESS, seen when deep-sea divers breathing air ascend too rapidly to the surface. After a significant time underwater the nitrogen will first have dissolved in the blood, since its pressure is high in the lungs, then passed into the tissues, particularly fat; on rapid ascent ('*decompression*') it comes out of solution to form bubbles in nerves and round joints, causing the characteristic pain of the bends. In practice air is nowadays never used in deep diving, the nitrogen being replaced by helium, which is far less soluble in fat.

Nitrogen under pressure will also cause psychological and neurological disturbances. This condition is called nitrogen narcosis, but long before actual narcosis (sedation and anaesthesia) occurs the nitrogen exerts toxic effects. These include euphoria, fixed and complacent ideas, uncontrollable laughter, and neuromuscular incoordination. Scuba divers may suffer from this, and it has been called the 'rapture of the depths'. It is not due to any chemical reaction of the nitrogen, since it can also be caused by 'inert' gases such as argon, but probably by the solution of the pressurized nitrogen in fatty substances such as the membranes of nerve cells in the brain. Possibly also the nitrogen attracts water to form hydrated forms which disrupt brain cell function. Although nitrogen narcosis may have the same physicochemical basis as decompression sickness, its clinical manifestations are quite different. In many respects it resembles the psychological and neurological effects of acute lack of oxygen, but the mechanisms are probably very dissimiliar.

JOHN WIDDICOMBE

See also AMINO ACIDS; DECOMPRESSION SICKNESS; DIVING; GASES IN THE BODY; PROTEINS.

Nitrous oxide (N$_2$O), commonly called 'laughing gas', was discovered in 1776 by Priestley. He inhaled the gas and noted that it caused confusion and analgesia. Later, in 1799, Humphry Davy suggested its use in surgical operations. However for the next forty-five years nitrous oxide was used only for entertainment, in which respectable persons were shown to lose their usual demeanour, breaking into laughter, often accompanied by singing and dancing or aggressive behaviour. Unwary persons were encouraged to volunteer for these exhibitions, particularly at fairgrounds. In 1844, Horace Wells, an American dentist, used the gas for tooth extraction, and two years later an American surgeon, William Morton, carried out major surgery under its influence. Nitrous oxide is not a very potent anaesthetic; it was sometimes used at 100% for rapid induction of anaesthesia, with subsequent addition of oxygen to avoid hypoxia.

Nitrous oxide continues to be widely used along with oxygen as a 'carrier gas' accompanying other inhalational anaesthetic agents. Its main advantage is that it has an *analgesic* (pain-relieving) effect, so that less of the main anaesthetic drug needs to be given. As '*entonox*' it is also used, mixed with air, as an analgesic during LABOUR. The common earlier use for dental extractions has diminished, with new regulations restricting the use of general anaesthesia for this purpose to special centres.

ALAN W. CUTHBERT

See also ANAESTHESIA, GENERAL; ANALGESIA; DENTISTRY; LABOUR.

Nobel Prize in physiology or medicine

The Nobel Prizes were established in 1901 by the Nobel Foundation, which was endowed by the Swedish industrial chemist and philanthropist, Alfred Bernhard Nobel (1833–96).

Alfred was born in Stockholm, the son of an industrialist and inventor Immanuel Nobel, who used explosives extensively in his construction business. After schooling and private tutors in Stockholm and St Petersburg, where his father moved after a business failure, Alfred travelled extensively in Western Europe, learning languages and attending chemistry lectures and demonstrations. Throughout his life he was to retain a special fondness for English literature and poetry. He returned to St Petersburg just before the Crimean War (1853–56), and worked in the family's munitions company, manufacturing naval mines that prevented the British Navy from entering St Petersburg. Immanuel went bankrupt in 1859, and the family returned to Sweden. During the next few years father and son both worked on the newly-discovered explosives, gun cotton and nitroglycerin. A tragedy hit the family in 1864 when their nitroglycerine factory blew up, killing several people, including Alfred's younger brother. From that time on, Alfred Nobel tried to devise a safer way to deal with nitroglycerine, and in 1867 patented 'dynamite', a more stable form of the chemical. Further developments and inventions, including synthetic rubber and artificial silk, contributed to Alfred Nobel's personal wealth, and by the time of his death he held over 350 patents.

After his death his Will of November 27, 1895 specified that the bulk of his estate should be deposited in a fund, the interest from which should be divided into five parts to be used for five annual Prizes, in Physics, Chemistry, Physiology or Medicine, Literature, and Peace. A close friend, Countess Bertha von Suttner, had become increasingly critical of the late nineteenth-century arms race, and correspondingly active in the peace movement, and she may well have influenced Nobel's decision to include in his Will an award to individuals or organisations who promoted peace. In 1905 Bertha was awarded the Nobel Peace Prize. Perhaps not surprisingly, several of Nobel's relatives contested the Will.

One of the five shares was to be awarded to the person 'who shall have made the most important discovery within the domain of Physiology or Medicine'. The Royal Caroline Medico-Surgical Institute in Stockholm, today the Karolinska Institute, was entrusted with the task of selecting the winners of the award. Why did Nobel select this field for attention? During much of his life, he had suffered from poor health, complaining of indigestion, headaches, and the occasional bout of depression. He was known to be interested in medical science and was absolutely fascinated when the medical use of nitroglycerine became well known for relieving pain in angina pectoris. In 1890 his own doctors suggested its use, which prompted Nobel to write to a friend 'isn't it the irony of ironies that I have been prescribed N/G 1 [nitroglycerine], to be taken internally.'

The awards became newsworthy almost immediately — their monetary value was substantially more than any other prize, and even at the end of the twentieth century, when other sources of spectacular awards are more common, a Nobel Prize carries unique cachet and prestige. Some of the greatest names in twentieth century medical science have received awards. Conversely, other great names have not. The restriction that the award can be shared by a maximum of three individuals in any one year, and cannot be awarded posthumously, has helped to fuel some bitter controversies over the apportioning of credit and priority for discoveries.

E. M. TANSEY

Further reading

Fox, D. M., Meldrum, M., Rezak, I. (ed) (1990). *Nobel Laureates in Medicine or Physiology: a biographical dictionary.* Garland Publishing, New York.

Sohlman, R. (1983). *The legacy of Alfred Nobel.* The Bodley Head Ltd, London.

Zuckerman, H. (1977). *Scientific elite: Nobel laureates in the United States.* The Free Press, New York.

See also the web site of the Nobel Foundation at: *http://www.nobel.se index.html*

Noradrenaline

(syn. *norepinephrine*) is the NEUROTRANSMITTER of the peripheral sympathetic nervous system, responsible for so-called *adrenergic neurotransmission*, at nerve endings in the heart, in smooth (involuntary) muscle, and in many glands. It is one of the CATECHOLAMINES. *Tyrosine*, an amino acid present in body fluids, is taken up into the adrenergic nerve terminal where it is acted upon by an enzyme, *tyrosine hydroxylase*, to form DOPA; this is converted to DOPAMINE and in turn to noradrenaline. The neurotransmitter is stored in small vesicles, awaiting release. Arrival of the impulse at the nerve terminal releases vesicles, freeing the noradrenaline to exert its effects. To terminate the action of the transmitter, some noradrenaline is oxidized to inactive material, but most is taken back up into the nerve terminal and stored for later use. There are two types of cell MEMBRANE RECEPTORS with which noradrenaline interacts, termed α and β, each group having several subtypes. Activation of β-receptors in smooth muscle causes relaxation, while activation of α-receptors causes contraction of SMOOTH MUSCLE, except for that in the intestine. Activation of β-receptors in the HEART causes an increase in both the force and rate of contraction. Noradrenaline is also an important transmitter in many parts of the CENTRAL NERVOUS SYSTEM, where it is involved in arousal, blood pressure regulation, and mood.

ALAN W. CUTHBERT

See also CATECHOLAMINES; HEART; SMOOTH MUSCLE; SYMPATHETIC NERVOUS SYSTEM.

Nose

The nose is at the centre of attention when we examine the FACE. One can read the culture of the nose and its central place in the study of physiognomy. One can stress that the face is the part of the modern body (along with the hands) which is uncovered, unveiled, and therefore available for analysis. A society in which all of its members wore MASKS could stress the imagined nose, much as Western society stresses the imagined breast or buttock. The West 'sees' the nose: it is 'real' and therefore immediate and concrete, and the more it becomes a place for fantasy the more real it seems.

Noses are loaded with multiple layers of meaning. As Charles Darwin noted in *The Descent of Man and Selection in Relation to Sex*: 'As the face with us is chiefly admired for its BEAUTY, so with savages it is the chief seat of mutilation'. This focus on the beautiful face is understood by Darwin as a quality of the modern world. Noses define civilization. Oswald Spengler, writing in his study of *The Decline of the West* in 1918, called this fascination a sign of the triumph of the 'science' of PHYSIOGNOMY and the movement toward a 'single uniform overarching physiognomy of all human beings'. The face and the sciences which contribute to its reading are given specific priority as signs of the modern.

The history of the nose is written as part of the history of the face. And we have a long tradition in the West of giving meaning to the face and its parts. One could say that the nose defines the human face. It is central to the face. The face, in terms of the psychology of PERCEPTION, is not a face without a nose. In the first modern history of plastic surgery (1838), Eduard Zeis commented that 'The eye is so used to seeing a nose on a human face, that even an ugly one is preferable to one that is partly or completely missing . . .' It is of little wonder that the classic image of the 'death's head' is one without a nose. Historically, anxiety about the loss of the nose is tied to stigmatizing diseases — LEPROSY and syphilis. The syphilis epidemic of the sixteenth century makes the 'lost' nose a sign of moral decay. In another context, the focus on Black slavery and the condition of the Black in the Enlightenment, associates the form of the Black's nose with defences of slavery; it becomes a sign of the 'primitive'. The Dutch eighteenth-century anatomist Petrus Camper presents criteria for the beautiful face in his study. Indeed, he defines the 'beautiful face' as one in which the facial line creates an angle of 100 degrees to the horizontal. According to the contemporary reading of Camper the African is the least beautiful — and therefore the least erotic.

The too-long nose comes to be read as a physical sign for the identification of the Jews as

Monk at the statue of Lord Bahubali, Jain festival, India. Joerg Boethling/Still Pictures.

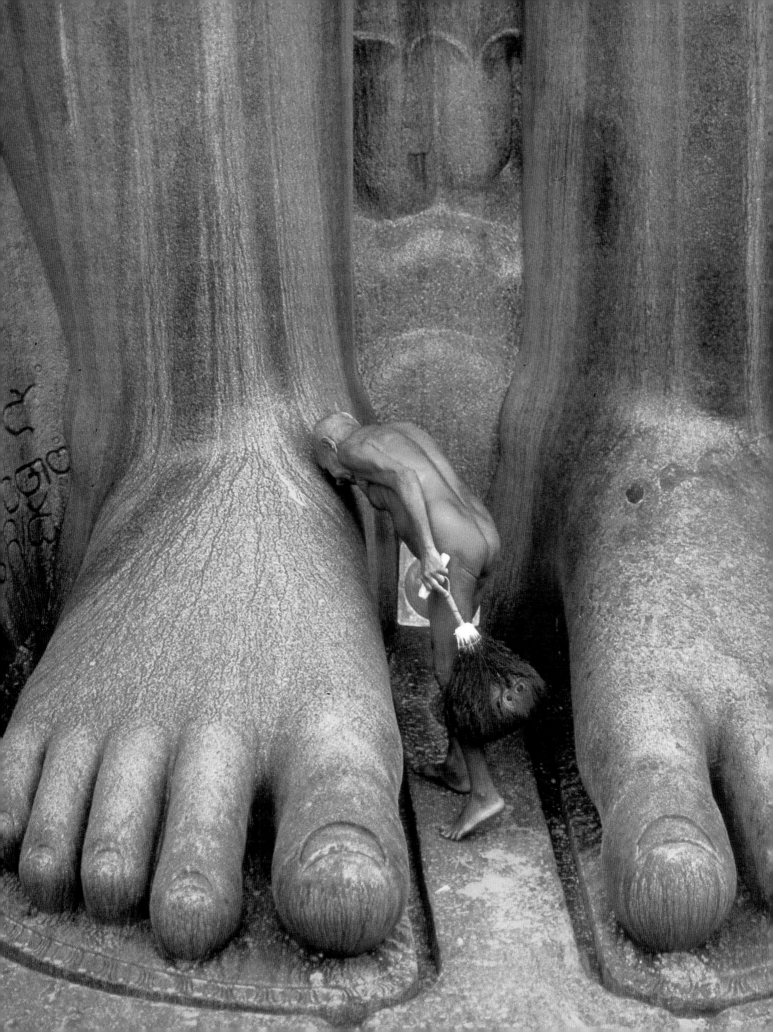

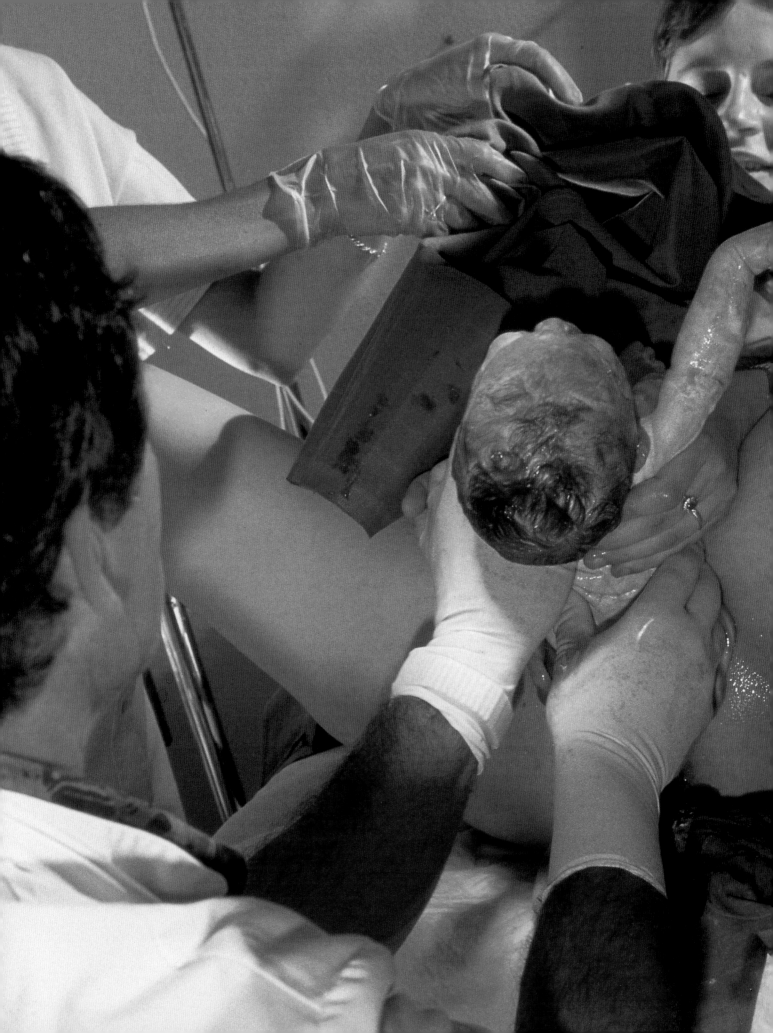

essentially different from all others in the modern state. George Jabet, writing as Eden Warwick, in his *Notes on Noses* (1848) characterized the 'Jewish, or Hawknose', as 'very convex, and preserves its convexity like a bow, throughout the whole length from the eyes to the tip. It is thin and sharp.' Shape also carried here a specific meaning: 'It indicates considerable Shrewdness in worldly matters; a deep insight into character, and facility of turning that insight to profitable account.' Noses become a sign of character, both good character and bad character. But they are always a sign of immutable character. All of these ideas of the nose exist simultaneously; it was only a question of emphasis and priorities — by a nose.

In functional terms, the nose is the route whereby aromas reach the nerve cells — in the upper part of its lining — whose fibres enter the brain through perforations at the base of the skull, and serve the sense of smell. The broader associations of this function are embedded in the language — to have a nose for something, to nose it out, or simply to be 'nosey', imply the ancient fundamental link in the animal kingdom between smell and appraisal of the outside world.

The nose is also the channel for quiet BREATHING. The nostrils have a greater resistance to airflow than any other part of the route into the lungs, contributing to the optimal mechanical balance which makes quiet breathing a negligible effort. (When we are pushed into breathing vigorously, the flow is diverted to the wider mouth.) The other highly effective function of the nose is as an air conditioner — a heat and moisture exchanger. Air enters dryer and cooler (usually) than the inside of the body. The moist and blood-warmed surface formed by the mucous membrane lining is much larger than the outside of the nose, because it is folded around three thin, curved sheets of bone (*conchae*) that project into the cavity on each side, as well as covering both sides of the central septum. In passing through this maze, the air is warmed and moistened — conditioned to do no damage to the lungs. Then, on its way back out, now saturated with water vapour and at body temperature, the air does not escape in that state; the membrane that it had cooled and dried automatically retrieves much of the heat and water. Thus in cold conditions, when heat and water conservation can be of major importance, the nose is a crucial protective tool. The normally beneficial divisions and restrictions of space within the nose are all too apparent when the lining is swollen by inflammation with the common cold, and obstructs the flow of air. Opening into the nose are conduits from the sinuses within the skull bones; also the ducts that drain the continuous eye-moistening secretions from the lachrymal glands, preventing overflow as tears, unless overloaded by the excesses of WEEPING. At the back in the *nasopharynx* the cavity of the nose communicates with the cavity of the middle ears through the EUSTACHIAN TUBES. This enables the equalization of pressure between the ears and the outside air via the nose, assisted by swallowing or by blowing against closed nostrils when external pressure alters, as in a descending aircraft.
                                SANDER L. GILMAN
                                SHEILA JENNETT

Further reading

Holden, H. M. (1950). *Noses*. World Publishing Co., Cleveland.

Romm, S. (1986). *Noses by design*. National Museum of American History, Washington, DC.

See PLATE 3.

See also PHYSIOGNOMY; TASTE AND SMELL.

Nosebleed Nosebleeds are common, particularly in children. They may be alarming but are very rarely ominous. The bleeding is usually from the septum of the nose — the central partition — and sometimes follows crusting and picking, or a minor injury. It usually stops quite quickly if the nostrils are compressed so that breathing is through the mouth; the clotting process can then proceed undisturbed. Various myths and old wives' tales are associated with nose-bleeding, such as the notion that a cold key placed on the back of the neck helps to stop it.

Rarely, nosebleeds may be a sign of a condition which causes a generalized tendency to bleed, such as a shortage of PLATELETS in the blood, or treatment with anticoagulant drugs. In the elderly, the bleeding may be from further back in the nose, and less easy to stop without medical attention. Contrary to popular belief, people with high blood pressure probably do not have nosebleeds more often than others of similar age, but when they do, the high pressure does make bleeding more profuse.
                                SHEILA JENNETT

See also BLOOD; HAEMORRHAGE.

Nucleus From the Latin for 'a little nut'. A rounded body found in all animal and plant cells. It contains the *chromosomes*, which in normal cell division duplicate themselves so that each daughter cell has a complete set contained within its nucleus. A chromosome consists of a gigantic linear DNA molecule wrapped around large globular proteins, rather like a string of beads. *Chromatin* is the name for the complexes of these proteins (called *histones*) with the DNA.

The term 'nucleus' (pl. *nuclei*) is also used to describe discrete islands of grey matter — clusters of nerve cells — in the brain, for example in the cerebellum, in the hypothalamus, or in the brain stem. These are relay stations for incoming or outgoing nerve fibres or the sites of origin of the cranial nerves.   A.W.C.

See CELL; DNA; GREY MATTER.

Nudism Being nude, not to be confused with naked, is to be without one's clothes. Nudism has a number of connotations: it can mean an individual's intolerance to CLOTHES; it can refer to a cult of nudists or naturists, who believe that society should discard its clothes; or it might be the visual representation of a nude in the form of a painting or a sculpture. More often than not 'the nude' is placed in a public setting.

There are various current theories that try to decode what nudism actually represents. The 'back-to-nature' philosophy is perhaps a rebellion against Victorian MODESTY. In psychiatry, a male's need for exhibitionism could be seen as a reaction against CASTRATION anxiety. And, in socio-sexual power play, a female's wish to display her body might be a means of demonstrating her ability to attract men. One could argue that the first nudes were Adam and Eve, who, knowing themselves to be naked, hid themselves with fig leaves.

Twentieth-century discourse surrounding ideas of the nude and the naked examined the complex relations between the spectator and the nude. Art historians and writers have tried to unravel the complex nature of nudism. Historically, the nudism represented visually by artists has nearly always been the female nude. Kenneth Clark's *The Nude* (1956) is a testament to a traditional and chronological approach to looking at male and female nudes, from the Greeks to the modern day. The nude, for Clark, is a symbol of truth and perfection. He writes: 'we remember that the nude is after all, the most serious of all subjects in art.' This is one approach. Clark unfailingly assumes a binary position, that of female nude and male spectator. And he asserts that the naked is, in fact, inferior to the nude: 'To be naked is to be deprived of our clothes and the word implies some of the embarrassment which most of us feel in that condition. The word nude, on the other hand, carries in educated usage, no uncomfortable overtone.'

Conversely, art historian T. J. Clark's reading of Manet's painting of a reclining female nude (a prostitute), entitled *Olympia* (1865), states that nakedness represents material culture and social class; whereas, nudity on the other hand, is a set of beliefs that the body is ours. Manet represented a turning point in modern art, for the traditional female ideal was broken and *Olympia* was the realism of the naked avant-garde. Kenneth Clark in contrast, maintains that to be naked is simply to be without clothes, whereas the nude is a form of art.

Helen Cixous talks at length of self-reappropriation and the traditional historic male culture:

> 'I found myself in a classic situation of women who at one time or another, feel that it is not they who have produced culture . . . Culture was there, but it was a barrier forbidding me to enter, whereas of course, from the depths of my body, I had a desire for the objects of culture. I therefore found myself obliged to steal them . . . but it is always there in a displaced, diverted, reversed way. (*Entretien avec Francoise van Rossum-Guyon*, 1977.)

In his book *Ways of Seeing* (1972), the writer and commentator John Berger, alongside others, explored the roles of the voyeur and the nude. Berger offers a way forward in culturally redefining the roles that men and women assume.

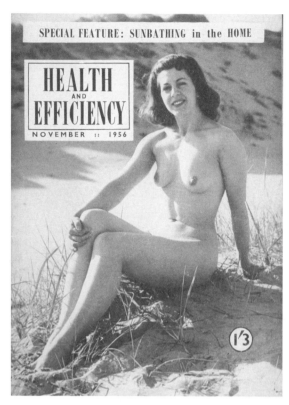

Health and Efficiency magazine cover from 1956. The Advertising Archive Ltd.

He acknowledges at the outset that the social presence of a woman is different from that of a man. The 'promised power' Berger talks of refers to the man's moral, physical, temperamental, economic, social, and sexual standing in the world. It is always external to him. In opposition to this, a woman's presence expresses her own attitude to herself, which unwittingly defines what can and cannot be done to her. She is constantly being surveyed both by men and by herself.

Susan Suleiman's *The Female Body* (1986) maintains that women have for centuries been the objects of male theorising, 'male desires, male fears and male representations'. Consequently, they had to discover and 'reappropriate themselves as subjects')

This ongoing debate concerning the nude and the naked has been taken up by a number of feminist writers (both male and female) for whom the traditional reading of a nude female by a male viewer has been re-evaluated. It is no longer merely a question of accepting the non-gendered understanding of a female without clothes on.

ANNE ABICHOU

Further reading

Berger, J. (1972). *Ways of Seeing*. BBC and Penguin, Harmondsworth and London.

Cixous, H. (1977). Entretien avec Francoise van Rossum-Guyon. *Revenue des Sciences Humaines, 44* (168), 479–93.

Clark, K. (1956). *The nude: a study of ideal art*. John Murray, London.

Clark, T. J. (1984). *Painting of modern life: Paris in the art of Manet and his followers*. Thames and Hudson, London.

Suleiman, S. R. (ed.) (1986) *The female body in Western culture — contemporary perspectives*. Harvard University Press, Cambridge MA and London.

See also ART AND THE BODY; FEMALE FORM.

Nutrition The origin of the term nutrition, and of 'nutrients', refers to all substances necessary for growth and for the maintenance of life and health of the body tissues. In this sense, not only FOOD but also water and oxygen can be called nutrients, and their provision can be called nutrition. But in common usage, nutrition means provision of substances in food and drinks. These include the 'fuels' for metabolic energy production and the raw materials necessary for growth, repair, and maintenance of the body's fabric — CARBOHYDRATES, PROTEINS and FATS — and also the VITAMINS and MINERALS essential for these processes.

S.J.

See DIETS; FOOD.

Nystagmus is a disorder of EYE MOVEMENTS, when they show involuntary, rhythmic oscillations. The name is from the Greek, depicting the slow nodding of drowsiness accompanied by irregular, quick raising of the chin. Clinically, most nystagmus is horizontal in direction, but vertical and torsional forms can occur. It usually presents a diagnostic challenge and special tests are used to induce nystagmus and elucidate the neurological cause. Two major groups are recognized: *jerk nystagmus*, with oscillations that are faster in one direction than in the other, creating a jerky rhythm; and *pendular nystagmus*, with oscillations that are roughly equal in speed to either side.

Jerk nystagmus is named according to the direction of the fast phase, although the slower, return movement that regains and holds ocular fixation is more important functionally. Such movements are easily seen in someone looking out of a moving train who is trying to count the railway sleepers in the adjacent track. The fast phase is in the direction of travel of the train. Such *opto-kinetic nystagmus* (OKN) can be demonstrated by rotating a cylindrical drum painted with black vertical stripes in front of the subject: the eyes will move in the direction of drum rotation, followed by a quick return to fixate on the next moving stripe. The urge to follow these movements is so powerful that OKN can even be used to prove vision in someone claiming to be blind.

Jerk nystagmus can also result from stimulation of the semicircular canals of the VESTIBULAR system. There are two groups of three canals that lie in three planes at right angles to each other in either side of the skull. Stimulation of these canals by head movement causes ocular movements that maintain the eyes' positions in space and so stabilize the field of view. If the head movement causes the eyes to reach the limit of comfortable sideward gaze the eyes make a fast, compensatory movement to the central position. Careful testing with OKN and vestibular-induced nystagmus can be used to pinpoint the site of neurological defects in some disease conditions.

Pendular nystagmus is found with loss of central, detail vision, such as occurs with bilateral macular lesions present from birth in albinism, aniridia (absence of the iris), or total colour blindness. There are rapid, pendular eye movements in *miners' nystagmus*' and the condition was attributed to defective illumination in mines. This occupational nystagmus has now been effectively eliminated by adequate lighting underground.

Congenital nystagmus can occur without other defects. The nystagmus appears pendular in straight-ahead gaze and becomes jerky on side gaze. Although visual acuity in the distance is always reduced, and usually to levels below the legal requirements for driving, reading can be surprisingly good, provided that the patient is allowed to hold the book in the preferred position. This may be closer than normal and with the head turned to one side. Parents of a child with congenital nystagmus may gain some comfort from the descriptive term 'dancing eyes' and from the knowledge that, with understanding teachers, education at a normal school followed by university is achievable.

PETER FELLS

See also EYES; EYE MOVEMENTS; VESTIBULAR SYSTEM.

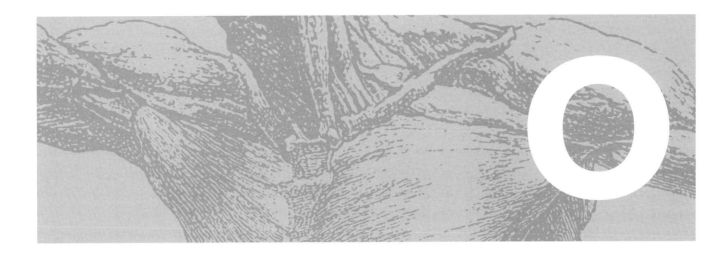

Obesity is most commonly defined as a condition of weighing at least 20% over ideal body weight, where ideal BODY WEIGHT is determined in the US by the 1959 or 1983 Metropolitan Life Insurance Company Tables. Like many aspects of obesity, use of life insurance tables as the sole indicator remains controversial. These insurance charts do not take into account the changes in ideal weight with age or provide information on body fat distribution; nor do they base measurements on all ethnic groups and those of the lower socioeconomic classes. To counter such biases, obesity can be determined by body mass index (which relates weight to height) and the percentage of body fat.

The causes of obesity continue to be debated and studied. Though it has long been considered the simple result of too little EXERCISE and too much EATING, new research suggests there may also be some hereditary influence, and particularly that the genetic tendency for obesity may be correlated to the mother's weight. Relatively unusual causes include adult-onset diabetes, deficient thyroid hormone secretion, and, very rarely, tumours of the adrenal gland, pancreas, or pituitary gland. Unexplained abnormal function of the brain's appetite control centre may also play a role. Researchers are particularly concerned about the increasing number of children and adolescents who are overweight in the US and Europe.

Obesity may cause a variety of health complications. Most clearly, overweight has an adverse effect on life expectancy. In general, the greater the degree of overweight, the higher the mortality or excess death rate. Obesity may be associated with elevated blood CHOLESTEROL, and has been linked to HYPERTENSION, diabetes, CANCER, coronary artery heart disease, degenerative arthritis, gall stones, SLEEP DISORDERS, and depression.

For many the 'psychological burden' of being obese in Western cultures, which prize slenderness, particularly in women, is an additional adverse effect. Prior to the nineteenth century, overweight and fatness stood as a sign of health and prosperity, and conveyed social esteem. By the mid and late nineteenth century, a new ethos emerged which championed slenderness as a sign of both beauty and physical health. By the early twentieth century, on the other hand, obesity became associated with laziness, gluttony, and the lower classes. As Keith Walden has written, 'females who stayed slim demonstrated that they had the money and sense to buy nutritious foods and eat balanced meals, and that they had the time to exercise. They did not have menial jobs which required substantial brawn to perform.' In twenty-first-century Western culture, especially for whites, and the middle and upper classes, the abhorrence of fat and obesity continues. As Anne Beller describes it, fat is suicidal: a sin at best and at worst a sort of felony. Yet for many African Americans and Hispanics, as well as other ethnic groups, a larger body still holds positive social value.

Suggested treatments for obesity range from a plethora of rarely successful fad diets to medical procedures such as stapling the stomach to reduce intake or shortening the intestines to curtail absorption. The most tried and true method remains adjustment of the energy balance — decreasing caloric intake while increasing energy usage. Vigorous exercise not only 'burns' nutrient stores but is also shown in some situations to increase metabolic rate for up to 15 hours after activity. Those with a hereditary tendency toward obesity find it more difficult to lose weight, due to a lower resting metabolic rate and possible complications in appetite regulation. In this regard, and in evolutionary terms, a tendency toward obesity can actually have survival value — a lower metabolic rate and a substantial fat store would allow one to live longer in times of famine. But in the contemporary West, where food is relatively plentiful and slenderness highly prized, it works to one's disadvantage.   MARGARET A. LOWE

Further reading

Beller, A. S. *Fat and thin: a natural history of obesity*. Farrar, Straus and Giroux, New York.

Walden, K. (1985). The road to Fat City: an interpretation of the development of weight consciousness in Western society. *Historical reflections*, **12**, 331–73.

See also BODY COMPOSITION; DIETING; ENERGY BALANCE; WEIGHT.

Oedema is an excess of fluid in the interstices of body tissues. It can happen anywhere, but swelling of the ankles is the commonest example, although not all 'thick' ankles are oedematous. To qualify as true oedema, the swelling must be capable of indentation by pressure from the fingers, known as 'pitting'. Also, oedema of the ankles, because it is enhanced by gravity, improves when the you 'put your feet up'.

This 'waterlogging' of the tissues comes about when the balance of forces tending to move water to and fro across capillary walls is disturbed. Blood capillaries in most sites are normally leaky. Because the hydrostatic pressure is greater inside them than outside, some water from the plasma, with its dissolved particles, moves out into the tissue (*interstitial*) fluid which everywhere bathes the cells and fills any gaps among them. But because plasma protein molecules (of which albumin is the most important in this context) are too large to escape readily from the blood, there is also an osmotic force tending to pull water back in. Usually there is a net loss into the tissues, and this is drained away by lymph vessels to re-enter the blood stream along with the rest of the lymph from the whole body.

It follows that tissue fluid may accumulate excessively if (i) capillaries become more leaky; (ii) pressure is abnormally high inside the capillaries, or low outside them; (iii) plasma proteins are deficient or diluted; (iv) lymphatic drainage is blocked.

Leaky capillaries are caused by chemicals released in response to tissue damage — hence, for example, the swelling around a wound or sting.

Pressure inside capillaries is raised by back pressure in the veins which drain them. In the legs this can be a complication of VARICOSE VEINS, when damaged valves fail to prevent distension of the veins below them. Even with normal veins, prolonged standing or sitting makes upward movement of the blood sluggish, and can result in ankle oedema. When the right side of the heart, which receives venous blood from the whole body, is not pumping effectively, pressure in all veins is raised but oedema is most evident in the dependent limbs because of the effect of gravity; likewise someone with right heart failure lying in bed will have oedema on the back and buttocks.

It is not only in the outward and visible parts of the body that oedema occurs. When venous pressure is high, fluid collects easily in the potential space of the peritoneal cavity, causing *ascites*: the equivalent of oedema fluid in tighter tissues.

In the lungs, a serious problem can arise if the left side of the heart stops pumping effectively, causing back pressure and excessive leakage from the lung capillaries, which can interfere with the transfer of oxygen to the blood. This *pulmonary oedema* can also occur at high ALTITUDE, because the HYPOXIA has the effect of raising the blood pressure in the lungs.

Pressure is lowered outside capillaries when the ambient pressure is lower than normal, enhancing a tendency to oedema for example during a prolonged flight (see FLYING, G AND G SUITS).

The concentration of proteins in the plasma falls when they are lost in the urine in kidney disease, or if they fail to be produced by the liver. They can be diluted by excessive saline infusions. Since their contribution to the osmolarity of the blood plasma is the component which normally keeps it higher than that of tissue fluid, a decrease in plasma proteins reduces the 'pull' of water into the blood from the tissues. This results in generalised oedema — or 'dropsical effusion' as it was called in the 1820s by Richard Bright, in his classic description of chronic nephritis (*Bright's disease*).

Lymphatics can be blocked by cancerous or parasitic invasion or interrupted by surgery: clearing the armpit of affected tissue when breast cancer has spread to the lymph glands can result in oedema of the arm.   SHEILA JENNETT

See also BODY FLUIDS; CIRCULATION OF THE BLOOD; LYMPHATIC SYSTEM; PLASMA.

Oesophagus

Oesophagus (esophagus), from the Greek for gullet, refers to the muscular tube, with a mucus-secreting lining, that leads from the mouth via the PHARYNX, down through the neck and the thorax, and through the DIAPHRAGM to the stomach. In the neck it lies behind the air passages — the lower end of the LARYNX and the upper part of the trachea. In the thorax, it continues behind the trachea and the heart, to pass into the abdominal cavity through a gap in the muscle of the diaphragm; less than an inch below this, it opens into the stomach. When SWALLOWING occurs, food is pushed into the top of the oesophagus, and is then propelled onwards by waves of circular muscle relaxation below it and of contraction above it: the *peristalsis* that occurs throughout the gut. This process can if necessary

defeat gravity; food, and even liquids, can be swallowed even standing on one's head, though clearly this is not generally attempted except as a remarkable demonstration. Muscle encircling the oesophagus at the top and bottom provides sphincters that, respectively, prevent air being sucked in during inhalation, and regurgitation of stomach contents.   S.J.

See ALIMENTARY SYSTEM; SWALLOWING; PLATE 1.

Oestrogens

Oestrogens Steroid SEX HORMONES, derived from cholesterol, which are produced mainly in the OVARIES and PLACENTA. This group of hormones, which includes oestradiol (the most active female hormone), oestriol, and oestrone, not only promote maturation of the female reproductive system but are important for controlling the MENSTRUAL CYCLE, production of OVA, and maintenance of PREGNANCY.   S.A.W.

See SEX HORMONES; STEROIDS.

Omnivore

Omnivore strictly means one who eats all things (Latin *omni*: all), but is used to describe those people or communities whose diet is not restricted to either animal or vegetable sources.   S.J.

Opiates and opioid drugs

Opiates and opioid drugs Opium is a crude extract of the seed capsules of the poppy, *Papaver somniferum*, which contains the opiate alkaloids *morphine* and *codeine*. Opioid drugs are synthetic derivatives that act in a similar manner to morphine. The earliest written records of the profound recreational and medicinal effects of opium date from approximately 4000 BC. There is also considerable reference to these effects in Greek and Roman mythology. In the late seventeenth century the physician Thomas Sydenham wrote:

> '*Amongst the remedies it has pleased Almighty God to give to man to relieve his sufferings, none is so universal and so efficacious as opium.*'

The recreational use of opium was popularised in the early nineteenth century by such writers as Thomas De Quincey (*Confessions of an English Opium Eater*) and Samuel Taylor Coleridge (*Kubla Khan*).

Morphine, named after Morpheus, the Greek god of dreams, is the prototypic opioid drug. HEROIN, a close structural analogue of morphine, is more lipid-soluble than morphine and rapidly penetrates the brain. This accounts for reports that the euphoric experience (often referred to as the 'rush' or 'buzz') following heroin administration is more intense. In attempts to exploit the desired therapeutic effects of morphine, but to avoid its unwanted effects (see below), a vast number of opioid drugs have been designed, synthesized, and tested. Some have been introduced into clinical practice. After centuries of research and drug development, and despite the undesired responses they evoke in man, morphine and heroin still remain major therapeutic agents in the treatment of severe PAIN states.

Both the naturally occurring plant-derived opiates and the opioid drugs exert their profound actions on the body by interacting with specific MEMBRANE RECEPTOR proteins on nerve cells (described as acting as *agonists* at these receptors). So also do the body's internally generated endorphins. There are three well-documented forms of these receptors, which are referred to by the Greek letters μ, σ, and κ. In addition, a new, closely related receptor, the *ORL1 receptor*, has recently been identified. Each of these receptors binds drugs in a specific manner and the binding of the drug to the receptor evokes a change in nerve cell activity. The different profile of responses mediated by the different receptors results from their differing distributions throughout the CENTRAL NERVOUS SYSTEM. Most of the therapeutically useful opioid drugs produce their effects by acting as agonists at the μ receptor, although some also have activity at the κ receptor. The therapeutic potential of the δ receptor awaits exploitation. *Antagonist* drugs such as naloxone can block the actions of opioid agonists. Such antagonists are useful in the treatment of opioid overdose.

Opioid agonist drugs produce a number of therapeutic responses. Pain relief (ANALGESIA) results from inhibitory actions in the spinal cord and in the brain. Whilst opiates are long-established as generally useful in suppressing severe pain, there are some pain states, such as trigeminal neuralgia, in which they or the opioid drugs are often ineffective. Opioids used to be referred to as narcotic drugs because they induce sleep. Opioids cause profound CONSTIPATION and can be used to treat severe states of DIARRHOEA. However, the constipating effect of opioids is undesired in the treatment of pain, especially if the drug is administered over a prolonged period. Codeine and some other agents are used as cough suppressants, but this action may not be mediated through the classical opioid receptors. In the treatment of pain states associated with terminal illness, opioid-induced EUPHORIA would appear to be of potential benefit, but there is some controversy over whether opioids induce even mild euphoria in patients suffering from severe, chronic pain.

Unfortunately opioid agonist drugs also have a number of unwanted actions. They depress RESPIRATION and this is usually the cause of death in overdose. Some individuals experience nausea and vomiting. Opioids can cause itching, by releasing histamine from mast cells. Also blood pressure may fall, heart rate may slow, and bronchoconstriction may be produced especially at high doses. Constriction of the pupils is a characteristic effect that can be used to diagnose opioid overdose, since other agents that induce COMA more commonly dilate them.

On repeated administration, the degree of effect induced by opioids declines, as the person becomes tolerant. This means that to obtain the same level of response the dose of the drug has to be increased. The intense euphoria that results from opioid administration, especially following intravenous injection, smoking, or sniffing, is the reason opioids are abused (taken for non-medicinal purposes). This results in the development of psychological dependence, which is manifest as craving for the drug. Such craving can last for many months after the last drug experience. Opioid-induced euphoria results mainly from an enhanced release of the neurotransmitter DOPAMINE from dopaminergic neurons that terminate in the region of the forebrain known as the *nucleus accumbens*. Other euphoric agents, such as NICOTINE and COCAINE, also enhance dopamine release at this site, but by different mechanisms. Opioids also induce physical dependence. On cessation of drug administration or on administration of an opioid antagonist, physical dependence is manifest by a withdrawal or abstinence syndrome characterized by fever, sweating, nausea, diarrhoea, insomnia, muscle cramps, and erection of hairs. This *piloerection* causes the goose pimples that explain the origin of the term 'cold turkey', and the muscle cramps have given rise to the term 'kicking the habit'. However, patients in severe pain do not appear to develop marked tolerance or physical dependence on opioids.

In summary, the site of action of opiates, which are the derivatives of plant-derived opium, and of the drugs that have been synthesized to imitate their effects, has been shown to be at specific cell membrane receptors, hence named *opioid receptors*, which also bind the body's own endorphins. All these agents may therefore be known generally as *opioids*.

GRAEME HENDERSON

See also ANALGESIA; DRUG ABUSE; ENDORPHINS; PAIN; RECEPTORS, MEMBRANE.

Optician A person who makes or deals in optical instruments, including SPECTACLES. A *dispensing* optician makes up and dispenses spectacles and other corrective lenses. An *ophthalmic* optician measures several aspects of VISION, in particular the refractive power of the eyes, and provides spectacles with lenses to correct REFRACTIVE ERRORS. The word 'optician' is becoming obsolete, being replaced by the American term, *optometrist*. P.F.

See OPTOMETRY; REFRACTIVE ERRORS; SPECTACLE.

Optometry (meaning *measurement of sight*) is the science of measuring visual acuity to determine REFRACTIVE ERRORS of the eyes, and prescribing and fitting appropriate corrective lenses (in SPECTACLES or as CONTACT lenses). The term 'optometrist', imported from the US, has virtually displaced the original word 'optician' in the UK.

Optometrists also have to deal with patients who have poor vision for whatever reason, prescribing special lenses or low-vision aids, which help them to lead independent lives. This is essential work in a world increasingly dominated by the visual image in television, films, advertising, and the Internet.

Certain occupations require legally-defined minimum acuity levels, particularly those concerned with flying, or driving trains, cars, heavy goods vehicles, buses — or any public service vehicle. In some cases, public service drivers with refractive errors are obliged to wear glasses, not contact lenses, so that an inspector can tell at once if corrective lenses are in use.

When the National Health Service (NHS) was inaugurated in Britain in 1948, the Supplementary Ophthalmic Service (SOS) was also started, with the intention that eventually all the sight testing would be done in hospitals. In 1958 the Opticians Act established the General Optical Council (GOC), which included a few doctors but was not part of the NHS. The GOC is the statutory body for opticians/ optometrists, with regulatory functions concerning approval of training courses, qualifications, registration, and discipline, similar to those of the General Medical Council for doctors. By 1968 it was apparent that the SOS would never be integrated with the NHS as previously hoped, and the General Ophthalmic Service (GOS) replaced the SOS. Family doctor committees now control the provision of relevant services by dentists, pharmacists, local general practitioners, and the GOS.

Optometry courses lasting three years are taught in eight university departments and schools in the UK. Subjects taught for the BSc degree include anatomy, physiology, visual optics and perception, binocular vision, occupational optics and lighting, clinical practice, pharmacology, microbiology, ocular disease, communication skills, and professional and legal matters. After a pre-registration year and pre-qualifying examination, the student must become a member of the College of Optometrists, the professional body, to start in practice.

The vast majority of sight tests are performed by optometrists. These include measurement of visual acuity and refraction, visual field screening, measuring intra-ocular pressure, and ophthalmoscopy (viewing the interior of the eye with an ophthalmoscope), as and when required. It is a matter of political decision as to which groups of patients may be entitled to a free sight test.

In some areas of the UK, special, shared care clinics to deal with the visual problems of diabetes and glaucoma have been set up to provide the optometric expertise required for hospitals and general practices. Simple consideration of the fact that there are approximately ten times as many optometrists as consultant ophthalmologists in this country, combined with increasing prevalence of these diseases, confirms the need.

Finally, a small but growing number of optometrists forsake the commercial world and work in university departments of visual science, gaining higher degrees and doing valuable research on vision, the optics of the eye, contact lens design, and related topics. PETER FELLS

See also EYES; REFRACTIVE ERRORS.

Organ The body's organs are discrete aggregations of different types of cells and connective tissue, formed into integrated structures with dedicated functions. Thus for example the heart has muscle, valves, electrically active pacemaker cells, and conducting fibres, all co-ordinated for pumping action; the eye has a 'window', a lens, and a retina, co-ordinated in the function of focusing images and relaying information about light and colour. The thoracic organs are the heart and lungs; the abdominal organs are the liver, spleen, kidneys, stomach, and intestines; the pelvic organs are the bladder and rectum, plus the uterus, tubes, and ovaries in the female, or prostate and seminal vesicles in the male. All body components are covered by the terms 'organs and tissues'. S.J.

Organ donation The donation of human organs and tissues is essential to sustain human TRANSPLANTATION, which is an increasingly important treatment for certain severe medical conditions, and for individuals with irreversible organ failure. Organs currently in demand for transplantation include the heart, kidneys, liver, lungs, intestines, and pancreas; tissues include corneas, heart valves, blood vessels, skin, and bone.

Legally, organ donation can take place from living, genetically-related individuals; from living, unrelated individuals in special circumstances where no unauthorized payment is made to the donor; or from cadavers. Live donation of a single kidney was the first of all (in 1954), but live donation of parts of other organs is a relatively recent innovation in the 1990s. As a source of organs this has a limited impact on availability.

To date the major source of organs and tissues in the West has been from cadaveric donors. Living tissue deteriorates rapidly when it loses its blood supply, and organs need to be cooled and transported for implantation into the recipient within a limited number of hours. Short transfer time, entailing removal of organs from 'beating heart' donors, was made possible by the acceptance of 'brain stem death' as death. Traditional death, with cessation of breathing and heartbeat, was all that was recognized until the late 1950s. The condition of brain stem death came as a consequence of technological advance, when it became possible to sustain the functions of the major organs with the help of ARTIFICIAL VENTILATION. There was a need to distinguish between those patients who could recover and those who had suffered brain damage so severe as to be incompatible with life. Mollaret and Goulon (1959) first described BRAIN DEATH in their classic work, '*Le coma dépassé*' — a state beyond COMA.

Brain death criteria were initially discussed by the Ad Hoc Committee of Harvard Medical School (1968). Subsequent recommendations equated brain stem death (or brain death) with traditional death, UK criteria being formally adopted in 1976. The principles of the Harvard criteria have been accepted in many countries and form the basis of the current diagnosis of brain stem death.

The ability to diagnose brain stem death, for an individual maintained on artificial ventilation, in turn maintaining the heart and circulation, allowed organs to remain perfused until a suitable recipient could be identified. Together with the development of drugs to prevent transplant rejection, this meant that transplantation of many organs became a viable medical treatment.

Worldwide, the demand for organs is growing, as the supply of organs and tissues for transplantation has not kept pace with demand. In the UK only approximately 900 individuals become organ donors each year, while over 6000 people are waiting for suitable organs. In the US much the same situation exists, with 70 000 presently on the waiting list and only approximately 5500 cadaveric donors per year. In part, the shortfall in donations reflects an increase in the number of individuals who could benefit from a transplant, but sub-optimal use of the available donor-organ pool; the problems that the acceptance of brain stem death, and the agreement to donate organs and tissues, pose for families also impinge. The often tragic and sudden nature of donors' deaths may be difficult for families to reconcile, especially as donors are previously healthy, relatively young, and robbed of a future. Families are necessarily approached about organ donation when their grief may be all-encompassing, with thinking and concentration a problem. However, if donation is to take place families need to make a number of decisions on behalf of their deceased relative. These decisions may be problematic, as they concern an operation on another's body; yet the time to debate the issues is constrained.

Relatives are asked to accept a non-stereotypical death, brain stem death, as death. The implications of brain stem death transcend the usual experience of the lay individual. The imagery of the brain stem dead is unfamiliar to society's expectations of the dead body, being conceived to be still, pale, and cold. The potential donor maintained on a ventilator may not look dead, and often has no external manifestations of injury, tending to be unscathed, resting, warm, and florid; their chest moves as if they are breathing, and they may even move occasionally if a spinal reflex is activated. Their time of death becomes an arbitrary decision made by the attending physicians, depending upon completion of the required tests. Not only are relatives asked to accept this situation as death, but also they are asked to agree to the removal of the very vital organs that normally would maintain life. They have to contend with accepting the operative mutilation of the body, saying goodbye to a loved one who does not appear to be dead. They have to come to terms with disposing of a body when their loved one's organs are responsible for improving the quality of a recipient's life.

Presently three major legal frameworks govern the donation of organs worldwide. The UK, along with a number of European countries, e.g. Germany and Italy, and Canada, Australia, and New Zealand have 'opting-in' systems. This means that the person in lawful possession of the body may authorize the removal of organs and tissues. In practice donation is usually requested from the next-of-kin of the deceased. Many other countries, including e.g. Austria, Belgium, and Singapore, have introduced 'opt-out' or 'presumed consent' systems that assume individuals have granted permission for their organs to be donated, unless they specify otherwise, in advance of their death. 'Required request' or routine enquiry of the next-of-kin of a potential donor, forms part of state law in the US. It provides for hospitals that fail to adopt 'required request' polices to be denied support from healthcare funding agencies.

None of the major world religions oppose the donation of organs. However, the Japanese culture which is underpinned by Shinto religion believes that if the 'itai', or bodily remains, are harmed then the soul of the dead is believed to be unstable and unhappy and to have the capacity to bring misfortune to the surviving relatives. Therefore, even with the recent acceptance of the brain stem death law Japan, unlike other countries, has chosen to support a system of predominantly living donations.

The shortage of human organs for transplantation has led scientists to explore techniques to facilitate the use of organs from animals (*xenotransplantation*), particularly the pig.

MAGI SQUE

Further reading

New, B., Solomon, M., Dingwall, R., and McHale, J. (1994). *A question of give and take: improving the supply of organs for transplantation.* King's Fund Institute, London.

Sque, M. and Payne, S. A. (1996). Dissonant Loss: the experiences of donor relatives. *Social Science and Medicine*, **43** (9), 1359–70.

See also BRAIN DEATH; LIFE SUPPORT; TRANSPLANTATION.

Orgasm
The term 'orgasm' — derived from 'organ', meaning to grow ripe, swell, or be lustful — is applied equally to the sexual climaxes of women and men. The medical lexicon distinguishes orgasm from EJACULATION; the latter term specifically describes a sudden spurt of fluid released in response to sexual excitement. The distinction arises partly because there is some question about whether female orgasms may result in an ejaculation, and partly because males can experience orgasms without ejaculation. (Pre-adolescent males and some adult males can apparently reach orgasm without the emission of semen.)

Poets have long sung of the pleasures of orgasm. Perhaps the most common literary trope for orgasm is that which likens the experience to dying; orgasm became, for seventeenth-century poets, *la petite morte*. (The historian and philosopher Michel Foucault famously punned on this relationship between *l'amour* and *la morte*.) Thus, in *Imperfect Enjoyment*, even while bemoaning the problem of premature ejaculation, Etherege looked with pleasure on that moment 'When, overjoyed with victory, I fall/Dead at the foot of the surrendered wall.'

Sexologists in this century have struggled to put the orgasmic experience into more precise, clinical terms. Probably the simplest description comes from Alfred Kinsey, the American human-sex researcher, who, in his classic 1948 study, *Sexual Behavior in the Human Male*, suggested that 'the most important consequence of sexual orgasm is the abrupt release of the extreme tension which preceded the event and the rather sudden return to a normal or subnormal physiologic state after the event.' Kinsey's description of orgasm in his 1953 *Sexual Behavior in the Human Female* was a bit more dramatic: 'This explosive discharge of neuromuscular tensions at the peak of sexual response is what we identify as orgasm.'

In short, sexologists of today have only confirmed what the poets of yesteryear knew — that sexual climax and dying share some key physiological similarities, not the least of which is the occasional loss of consciousness. Wrote Kinsey, 'Some, and perhaps most persons may become momentarily unconscious at the moment of orgasm, and some may remain unconscious or only vaguely aware of reality throughout the spasms or convulsions which follow orgasm.' Pleasurable? Kinsey wondered, on noting the intensity of experience, so similar to epileptic fits and physiologic responses to electric shock. 'In the most extreme types of sexual reaction, an individual who has experienced orgasm may double and throw his [or her] whole body into continuous and violent motion, arch his back, throw his hips, twist his head, thrust out his arms and legs, verbalize, moan, groan, or scream, in much the same way as a person who is suffering the extremes of torture.' Kinsey could only conclude, 'this makes it all the more amazing that most persons consider that sexual orgasm … provide[s] one of the most supreme of physical satisfactions.'

Satisfying indeed, but to what end? Two questions pervade two millennia of medical constructions of the orgasm: 'Can you suffer from too few or too many?' and: 'What purpose does the female orgasm have?'

Aristotle worried that the wombs of overstimulated women would become slippery and inhospitable to fetuses, but generally early anatomists were relatively unobsessed with questions of frequency. Humoral theories tended to require, for health, some periodic release of 'seed' (or at least a careful diet which would reduce production of the excitable stuff). Humoral theory held that semen was made up of phlegm — interestingly, the same stuff as the brain. (Upon opening, post-mortem, the head of a particularly lecherous fellow, an early-modern anatomist noted, without surprise, that there wasn't much brain left.) To relieve pressure, early-modern English medical texts recommended regular intercourse or even occasional episodes of masturbation. But too much activity was thought to risk the health or production of offspring, as well as one's own health.

The nineteenth century saw much bile spilled over the concern that people were excessively spending their energies on sexual gratification. Many Victorian physicians, enamoured of a conservation-of-energy approach to physiology, warned that frequent orgasms would only drain the life from the body and leave the other systems wanting. (A far less happy sex-and-death link.) This essentially constituted a new version of the old bodily-economy trope. Inventors designed devices to discourage erections (these tended to involve sharply-barbed clamps), and many physicians recommended clitorectomies for 'hysterical' women, particularly those who enjoyed too much sex or sex with other women. Even well into this century, versions of this dire belief — that one's bodily supply of energy could be squandered by sexual emissions — hung on. Most male athletes are familiar with the aphorism which prohibits 'spending' oneself before a match.

On the heels of the Victorians, Sigmund Freud invented new ways to worry about (or worry about worrying about) sexual gratification. Most infamous among feminists is Freud's belief that truly mature women achieve vaginal orgasms, not clitoral ones. Laqueur aptly notes that, 'prior to 1905 [the publication of Freud's theory], no one thought that there was any other kind of female orgasm than the clitoral sort.' In his *Three Essays on the Theory of Sexuality*, Freud argued that, while pre-pubescent girls might enjoy clitoral orgasms, clitoral stimulation in the adult woman was only meant to '[transmit] the excitation to the adjacent female sexual parts', namely the VAGINA, 'just as — to use a simile — pine shavings can be kindled in order to set a log of harder wood on fire.' If a woman could not move her seat of excitation to her vagina, she would only wind up frigid. Meanwhile, Freud argued that the very transfer of excitation from CLITORIS to vagina over the course of a woman's maturation left her prone to HYSTERIA.

Kinsey's studies did much to dispel the vaginal-orgasm dogma of Freud. Indeed, Kinsey, who saw vaginal orgasm as a 'biological impossibility', took Freud to task for leaving thousands of women in a well of frustration and shame. Masters and Johnson's 1966 tome, *Human Sexual Response*, and *The Hite Report* of 1976 confirmed Kinsey's findings: most women do not experience orgasms directly from intercourse, and female orgasms originate from stimulation of the clitoris. By the 1960s, so fascinated with orgasms had the populace become that the British writer Malcolm Muggeridge declared in 1966, 'The orgasm has replaced the Cross as the focus of longing and fulfillment.' Popular quasi-medical texts today offer clues about how to achieve more, better, and better-timed orgasms.

Freud's impetus towards vaginal stimulation did not die away after Kinsey, Masters and Johnson, and Hite. Sexologists continue to investigate the sensitivity of the vagina and the ability of certain women to achieve orgasm without direct clitoral stimulation. Reports of a 'G spot' — a zone of high sensitivity in the vagina — are yearly put forth and summarily condemned. (Beverly Whipple and John Perry named the 'G spot' after the gynecologist Ernst Graefenberg.) Some researchers posit that stimulation of a vaginal 'G spot' can lead to ejaculation.

Perhaps because science has been mostly a male sport, few scientific minds have pondered the question of the purpose of the male orgasm, but many a man (and a few women) have contemplated the point of the female orgasm. Early anatomists, who presumed essential similarities between men's and women's bodies, figured that, if men's orgasms were needed for reproduction, so were women's. Thomas Laqueur, in his historical study of sex, imagined the logic of Hippocrates: 'Like a flame that flares when wine is sprinkled on it, the woman's heat blazes most brilliantly when the male sperm is sprayed on it … She shivers. The womb seals itself. And the combined elements for a new life are safely contained within.' Aristotle figured that, if a woman did not climax, she would not become pregnant. These ideas led to some curious (and ineffective) attempts at birth control.

Well into the early-modern period, the assumption stood firm that woman's well-timed orgasm was necessary to CONCEPTION. Patricia Crawford has argued that, in early-modern England, this belief had both good and bad implications for women. On the one hand, men who wanted heirs would have worked harder for their partners' satisfaction. But 'if a rape were followed by pregnancy, the law deemed it no rape because the woman had, by definition, enjoyed the encounter.'

Once it became clear that women's orgasms were in fact unnecessary for PREGNANCY, the question of their purpose attracted the attentions of evolutionists. (That women can have multiple, closely-timed orgasms particularly bothers certain theorists.) Sarah Blaffer Hardy, Randy Thornhill, and other sociobiologists have offered reasons for why the female orgasm might be (or have been) functionally adaptive in evolution — that is, why female orgasm would be conducive to a lineage's life. (Thus sociobiology tries to translate the female's *petite morte* into the species' *grande vie*.) Other evolutionists, like Stephen Jay Gould, have argued alternatively that female orgasms have no adaptive purpose — that they are just a pleasant side-effect of the fact that human males and females share embryological roots: the clitoris and the penis are embryological homologues, so it makes sense that the clitoris would be super-sensitive and able to be stimulated to climax. Gould has sensibly noted that many non-scientists really don't care all that much *why* orgasms exist.   ALICE DREGER

Further reading

Gould, S. J. (1987). Freudian slip. *Natural History*, **96**, 14–21.

Laqueur, T. (1990). *Making sex: body and gender from the Greeks to Freud*. Harvard University Press, Cambridge, MA.

Porter, R. and Teich, M. (ed.) (1994). *Sexual knowledge, sexual science: the history of attitudes to sexuality*. Cambridge University Press, Cambridge.

See also COITUS; EJACULATION; FERTILITY; SEXUALITY.

Orthoptics

Orthoptics is the science concerned with ensuring that patients' EYES develop their full visual potential and keep working together throughout life.

During the latter part of the nineteenth century, Javal, in France, started using ocular exercises and training methods for SQUINTS, which were very time-consuming but sometimes effective. After many years, in 1896, Javal wrote, 'The first time that I revealed my methods to von Graefe (the foremost ophthalmologist of his day) he astounded me by saying that people are not worth the effort. Life's experience has shown me that von Graefe was correct.'

In London, at the start of the twentieth century, Worth, an eye surgeon, used a modified stereoscope (*amblyoscope*), which presented separate images to each eye via two tubes so that the angle between these two images could be varied in an attempt to stimulate their fusion — again time-consuming. Maddox, working in Bournemouth with various ophthalmic instruments he had devised himself, found a new solution to the ever-increasing time needed to examine patients. He solved this problem by teaching his daughter Mary, who was already working as receptionist/secretary in his consulting rooms, to use the amblyoscope and other special tests for orthoptic assessment and treatment. Miss Maddox opened her own private clinic in 1928 and was soon joined by Sheila Mayou to form the Maddox–Mayou Orthoptic Training School. A year later Miss Maddox was invited to open an orthoptic clinic at the Royal Westminster Ophthalmic Hospital (which became the High Holborn branch of Moorfields Eye Hospital in 1947). The increasing numbers of orthoptists in training led to the Orthoptic Board being formed in 1934 to provide a syllabus and code of conduct. In 1937 the British Orthoptic Society was founded, with Miss Maddox as president and Miss Mayou as chairman.

By the late 1930s, the belief that orthoptic training methods could overcome the problems of faulty visual development in squinting children was being revised. It was proposed that squint resulted from a series of obstacles to the normal development of fusion and binocular single vision. Orthoptics was no longer presented as the definitive cure for squints, but as offering diagnosis and treatment for specific types of squint and visual impairment. Patching the preferred eye to stimulate vision in the deviating or lazy eye had been introduced to England empirically by Erasmus Darwin (Charles' grandfather) by 1801. Such occlusion therapy was widely applied after 1930, but it was not until the 1960s that its neuro-physiological basis was established.

A course in orthoptics takes three years of study. As well as optics and refraction it includes anatomy, physiology, neurology, and child development, ensuring that orthoptists are particularly suited to examine vision in very young children. This is necessary to allow appropriate therapy to be started within the sensitive period of visual development for optimal results.

Orthoptists are often a young child's first contact with medical personnel or hospitals, and it should be a happy occasion and one which the child will be eager to repeat. Visual acuity can be assessed at only a few months of age by special tests where the infant turns to look at a target of broad black and white stripes in preference to a uniformly grey target of equal luminosity. The width of the black and white stripes is successively reduced until the infant ignores the target. Young children, before they can read, can point to a letter on a card that matches one held up by the orthoptist. The familiar 'Snellen' letters are used for acuity testing in older children.

REFRACTIVE ERROR can be measured by orthoptists, but the prescribing of corrective lenses has to be done by the ophthalmologist or optometrist. Ocular movements are noted and the angle of squint measured. Convergence is checked, and an assessment is made of the quality of fusion of the two images and of stereopsis (detailed depth perception). Areas of fusion and of diplopia can be charted, and an accurate and repeatable graphic record can be made of defective ocular rotations. These basic tests, together with more specialized ones, allow diagnoses to be made and therapy started. Orthoptists supervise occlusion therapy for amblyopia, and teach exercises to improve binocular control and poor convergence. In latent squint, where the eyes cannot maintain binocular fixation under the stress of illness or tiredness, the tendency for the eyes to deviate can be controlled with prisms should ocular exercises prove insufficient.

Once qualified, orthoptists have a number of additional courses available. These include visual field and intra-ocular pressure measurements in glaucoma; biometric assessment with ultrasound of eyes for cataract extraction, so that the correct power of replacement intra-ocular lens is used; photography of EYE MOVEMENTS; and fluorescent photography of ocular blood flow. Many of these supplemental skills are also exercised by optometrists; indeed some pre-and post-qualification courses are shared by orthoptists and optometrists. Nevertheless, when it comes to gaining the confidence and co-operation of infants and very young children during testing, the orthoptist reigns supreme.   PETER FELLS

Further reading

M. J. Revell (1971). *Strabismus — a history of orthoptic techniques*. Barrie and Jenkins Ltd., London.

See also EYE; EYE MOVEMENTS; OPTOMETRY; SQUINT.

Osmosis A term describing the movement of fluid (usually water) across a semipermeable membrane. The membrane is described as semipermeable because it allows water, but not dissolved substances, to cross it. Water moves across the membrane from where the concentration of dissolved substances is lowest to where it is highest. Thus, water moves down its concentration gradient from high concentration to low concentration. The process continues until the concentration of solutes is the same on both sides of the membrane. The nature of the dissolved substances is unimportant, other than their not being able to penetrate the membrane. The membranes of most living CELLS are semipermeable, and cells swell if they are placed in a solution containing less dissolved substance than blood (*hypotonic*), and shrink in more concentrated (*hypertonic*) solutions. Hydrostatic pressure can be applied to oppose fluid movement; the pressure required to oppose the movement exactly is the 'osmotic pressure'. Thus cells can act as osmometers, by changing shape when the tonicity of the bathing solution changes. In the HYPOTHALAMUS are cells which are very sensitive to osmotic changes in the blood. If, for example, blood becomes hypertonic, as in thirst, the cells respond by sending impulses to the posterior pituitary to release antidiuretic hormone, which prevents further fluid loss by the kidneys. Alternatively, if large amounts of fluid (beer, for example) are imbibed, antidiuretic hormone is cut off and diuresis ensues.

                    ALAN W. CUTHBERT

See also BODY FLUIDS; CELL.

Osteopathy first developed from the 1870s onwards in America, under the initial inspiration and guidance of Andrew Taylor Still (1828–1917), who claimed to have discovered a revolutionary new system of HEALING and an associated therapeutic philosophy. These were based upon two related principal elements; that the healthy body already contained all the relevant capacities for maintaining itself, and that it thus did not need the drug-based remedies of the day. These views at that time were not original, but they were combined with Still's description of 'osteopathic lesions'. These lesions, unless treated through his system of manual manipulation, were said to disturb the necessary internal balances of the body. Their occurrence became the controversial cornerstone of a distinctive osteopathic pathology. They were thought to be morbid alterations in tissue: muscular, osseous, visceral, ligamentous, or a combination of some or all of those in individual cases. In particular, osteopathic lesions were linked to inadequate articulation of the various parts of the musculoskeletal system, particularly regarding the condition of the spinal vertebrae. In Still's view, improper articulation produced a disposition to various types of disease, by affecting the neurological system and the circulation of blood and body fluids which were essential to good health.

The social context of the latter decades of nineteenth-century rural America provided a supportive background for Still's beliefs and his related therapeutic evangelism. He was an 'untrained' medical practitioner by modern standards, but, as was common in his day, learnt medicine through apprenticeship to his father. He was in practice for many years in Missouri before becoming increasingly interested in bone setting in the 1870s in Kirksville. This was an ancient craft, and the prevailing medical ridicule of it had recently been brought into question. The distinguished London surgeon, Sir James Paget, had published an article, 'On the Cases that Bone Setters Cure' in the British Medical Journal. This was followed by Wharton Hood's book *On Bone Setting* (1871), published in Britain and America. Hood, a general practitioner, was interested in the movements of flexion and extension, combined with external pressure, used by bone setters for back injuries. As Gevitz, a noted historian of osteopathy, points out, at that time Still may have picked up and refined elements of practice which existed in his environment. At this historical point many of the more drastic drug and surgical remedies of conventional doctors did not inspire public confidence, and Still with his 'new' methods worked within a tradition of bone setting which was at least familiar to his rural patients. His mechanical theory of health and disease, of aligned and misaligned parts, akin almost to malfunctions of farm machinery, dovetailed nicely with the cultural beliefs of Still's patients.

However, this period was only the starting point of osteopathy's subsequent growth as a rival and different system of practice to medicine in the twentieth century. Still founded a school in 1892 in Kirkville, Missouri, and from this a small group of graduates went on in 1911 to found the British Osteopathy Association. In both countries decades of medical professional opposition to osteopathy followed, but these disagreements had very different outcomes in the two countries, both for medicine and for osteopathy. In the American case, conflict has led eventually to a kind of integration: a movement by practitioners from their initial adherence to Still's beliefs to broadly accepting those of orthodox medicine. Indeed, by the turn of the century the first osteopathic colleges were already teaching some of the medical pharmacopoeia of the day, and gradually pharmacology was brought into osteopathic education and practice. By the 1960s all restrictions on osteopathy as a one-time marginal cult were disappearing, leading to eligibility for medical residencies, and appointment to hospital medical staffs and to positions in the military and public health services. In this gradual process of absorbing and sharing of notions of scientific practice with orthodox medical practitioners, American osteopathic practitioners made manipulation a part rather than the core of their practice.

In Britain and its Commonwealth, professional developments between the two groups have been somewhat different, reflecting in turn their varying social and legal contexts. In Britain osteopaths sought in the 1920s and 30s to secure from the Government the right to practise as independent but different medical practitioners. Eventually this pressure led in 1935 to a Parliamentary Select Committee enquiry into their case, conducted adversarially between two different systems of philosophy and treatment. Eight hundred leading allopathic medical and biological scientists asserted that osteopathy disputed the very basis of modern medical and surgical practice, and that in particular osteopathic lesions could not be affirmed by any objective scientific scrutiny. The osteopaths were not successful in their case for licensing or state registration. Thus they practised under marginalized conditions outside of the National Health Service for forty years after its inception in 1948. By the early 1990s, however, much had changed. Osteopaths had practised successfully for decades as private practitioners; back problems were a major cause of absence from work and were recalcitrant to conventional treatments, and furthermore medical and public attitudes had changed. British osteopaths now presented themselves as complementary practitioners specialising in biomechanics and the manipulation of the musculo-skeletal system. Although extensively trained in basic medical sciences, they did not claim the wider competence of conventionally trained doctors regarding treatment as in earlier decades. In 1993 osteopaths in Britain gained state registration and formal recognition, not so much as an adjusted part of medicine as in America, but as skilled colleagues, akin to physiotherapists, specialising in rather than diminishing the role of manipulation in the treatments they offered.   GERRY LARKIN

Further reading

Gevitz, N. (1982). *The D.O.'s: osteopathic medicine in America.* John Hopkins University Press, Baltimore.

Wardell, W. (1994). Alternative medicine in the United States. *Social Science and Medicine,* **38** (8), 1061–8.

Osteoporosis

Osteoporosis is a condition in which the BONES become porous and weak, and therefore fracture easily. The bone tissue is normal with a normal shape but it has lost mass and density and so lacks sufficient strength to withstand the forces which normally occur in daily life. There are no symptoms initially and the condition is often diagnosed only when a bone fracture occurs unexpectedly. These fractures occur in a third of all women and in one in twelve men. Post-menopausal and senile osteoporosis are recognized. The former is due to loss of oestrogen, the latter includes a time-dependent loss of bone common to men and women. Osteoporosis also occurs as a side-effect of some drug treatments, with oral corticosteroids for example, and occasionally, in a severe and little understood form at much younger ages.

Osteoporosis is often confused with osteoarthritis, another chronic problem of later life.

However, osteoarthritis is a disease of the joints which is rare in those who have osteoporosis (unless they have been treated with corticosteroids).

Osteoporosis is not a disease like those caused by viral or bacterial infection, but a long term consequence of a small imbalance in the natural process of bone remodelling. Bone is a living tissue which constantly remodels itself through a process of resorption and formation known as bone turnover. Most processes in the body slow down as we grow older but bone turnover speeds up and the balance tips in favour of resorption, resulting in net bone loss. A greater imbalance develops in some people than in others and they are the ones who will suffer from osteoporosis, especially if they began with relatively low bone mass in middle age. This variation is to a large extent genetically determined, but lifestyle factors also contribute, including smoking, lack of EXERCISE, low dietary CALCIUM intake and, in the elderly, lack of vitamin D. Individuals who are small and thin are at greater risk because of their low bone mass compared with heavier individuals. Women who had an early MENOPAUSE, or whose menstrual periods failed when they were young perhaps due to anorexia, are also at increased risk because the skeleton has had more prolonged exposure to a low OESTROGEN level. Although the process of resorption and formation is at the root of the osteoporotic condition, it is nevertheless a useful process which ensures that bone can repair minor damage and remodel itself in response to changing mechanical loads. It means that bone can respond positively to exercise and to drug treatments. Most of the effective drugs, such as bisphosphonates and HORMONE REPLACEMENT THERAPY (HRT), act by slowing down resorption and therefore slowing the rate of loss of bone or tipping the balance in favour of formation.

The sites most commonly affected by osteoporosis are the wrist, the vertebrae in the spine, and the top of the femur (the hip). Vertebral fractures lead to collapse of the vertebrae which results in substantial loss of height or marked curvature of the spine (the Dowager's hump) and sometimes severe pain. Hip fractures occurring in the elderly in Britain cost the NHS nearly £1 billion in 1997 and the fracture rate has been rising faster than the increase in the number of elderly people in the population. The mortality rate following hip fracture is high and survivors usually suffer loss of independence and mobility. Both of these manifestations of osteoporosis were considered to be part of the normal ageing process until the middle of the twentieth century, and it was not until 1986 that the National Osteoporosis Society was established to provide support for sufferers, and advice and reliable information about the disease, which are still not widely available.

The osteoporotic condition develops slowly until so much bone has been lost that a threshold of vulnerability is reached and irreversible damage is likely. Preventative strategies are needed

before this fragile state is reached. HRT is particularly useful for preventing post-menopausal loss in potentially vulnerable women. Adequate dietary calcium is essential. Dairy products such as cheese, yoghurt, and milk are rich in calcium. A pint of skimmed milk contains 700 mg which is the daily intake recommended in Britain. SMOKING should be avoided, including passive smoking: it is known to interfere with the effect of oestrogen on bone. Excessive amounts of alcohol or caffeine (in tea, coffee, and coke) are also associated with a higher risk of osteoporosis.

The natural stimulus for bone to maintain its functional strength is the loading which results from gravitational forces and the tensions exerted by muscular activity. Astronauts lose bone while floating in space and so do patients who are confined to bed for long periods. Conversely, physically active people have higher bone mineral density compared with those who are sedentary. Exercise therefore has a role in reducing the long-term risk of osteoporotic fracture. The most effective exercise provides a regular series of varied short sharp loads to the sites which are most vulnerable for fracture. Brief exposure such as running up and down stairs a few times each day may be enough. Intermittent jogging ('scouts' pace') is useful, and so is weight-training, provided that over 70% of personal maximum effort is used in lifting slowly with few repetitions. Research is still ongoing to find the best prescriptions. Improvements can probably occur at any age, but the increases appear to be largest before adolescence, and in later life vigorous exercise is obviously only safe for those who still have a robust skeleton. Bone changes slowly, improvements take months, and if the exercise is discontinued they are gradually lost again. In older people moderate exercise may prevent further loss of bone, and since fracture risk is only likely when bone density has fallen below a threshold value, maintenance is useful.   JOAN BASSEY

Further reading

The National Osteoporosis Society publishes booklets. Helpline 01761 471771.

See also BONE; HORMONE REPLACEMENT THERAPY; MENOPAUSE.

Out-of-body experiences

Out-of-body experiences (OBEs) occur when an individual's direct perception of the world seems to originate from a point outside their physical frame. Such perceptions usually engender the idea that the subject's consciousness or soul has become detached from the body, and thus released to fly freely throughout space. A typical example was reported by the author, Ernest Hemingway.

Hit by shrapnel during a battle in the 1917 Italian campaign, the writer reported an intense sensation of 'my soul or something, coming right out of my body, like you'd pull a silk handkerchief out of a pocket by one corner. It flowed around and then came back and went in again.' These brief ecstatic transports are an almost universal phenomenon. Similar experiences have been reported within most of the world's cultures and by people of all ages. They are not tied to any physical state nor any emotional situation. Surveys carried out by the University of Virginia in the 1970s suggest that OBEs occur in around 20% of the general population, with the incidence rising to almost 50% amongst marijuana users.

Despite the relative commonness of OBEs, they have traditionally been credited with a deep religious significance. In the Hindu *Upanishads*, the soul's flight in the sky appears as one of the six *siddhis* or supernormal powers attained by the enlightened. In Tibet, there is a separate designation (*delog*) for those who can detach themselves from their physical bodies. Similarly, the shamans of Siberia and North America achieve their special status through starvation and self-persecution rituals, which allow the adept to enter trances from which they can project their souls to distant places. Likewise the Yaqui sorcerer Don Juan, whose teachings were popularized (or possibly fictionalized) in the novels of Carlos Castaneda, claimed that out of body experiences could be controlled and promoted through the use of hallucinogenic drugs.

Although the Bible makes little explicit reference to OBEs its theology has provided the central framework for understanding these phenomena in the West. The episode in Acts 8: 39, when the Spirit of the Lord 'caught away Philip' from Gaza and placed him in Azotus, is sometimes understood as an OBE. Likewise, Paul's reference in Corinthians II 7: 2–4 to the convert 'caught up in Paradise', who heard unspeakable words, is seen as another example. These events map on to a division that has been central to Christian theology: the Pauline distinction between man's spiritual body and his fleshly self. Within the Christian mystical tradition, OBE has been interpreted as a moment of grace, which allows the individual to escape the restrictions of the sinful flesh. Moreover the experience of OBE did seem to provide immediate evidence for St Paul's division between the spiritual and carnal bodies.

With rise of Theosophy in the late nineteenth century, a more instrumental attitude to OBEs emerged. Drawing upon a mixture of Eastern mysticism and North American spiritualism, the theosophists developed a many layered model of man, gradating between the material and the astral selves. Authors such as Annie Besant and C. W. Leadbeater claimed that occult technique and meditation would allow the astral body to journey away from the physical flesh, joined only by a delicate silver cord. In the twentieth century, this model of 'travelling clairvoyance' or 'astral projection' was widely promoted in practical 'How To' books, such as Sylvan Muldoon and Hereward Carrington's *The projection of the astral body* (London, 1929).

Alongside the voluntary practice of astral projection, OBEs have also occurred spontaneously to individuals in situations of extreme stress or suffering. In 1918 Jack London published *The Star Rover*, a semi-fictional account of astral travelling based on the case of Edward Morell, a prisoner who repeatedly experienced OBEs whilst being tortured in Arizona State Penitentiary. On a larger scale, the Austrian psychoanalyst, Bruno Bettelheim, documented the incidence of OBEs amongst prisoners tortured and suffering in the concentration camps. More recently there have been minor epidemics of spontaneous OBEs unconnected to either stress or suffering. In America, the current wave of reports of alien abduction bears a strong resemblance to out of body experiences. In the UK house music scene, recreational users of the anaesthetic drug ketamine have reported a typical 'trip' in which the dissociated consciousness seems to travel from the prone body to a distant white room.

The pharmacological encouragement of OBEs provides strong anecdotal evidence for the idea that astral projection has a neurophysiological basis. This folk evidence has been reinforced by laboratory research carried out by Michael Persinger in Toronto and Susan Blackmore in Bristol. These psychologists have been able to simulate OBEs in subjects held in a state of sensory deprivation, through the electrical stimulation of the brain's temporal lobes. Persinger and Blackmore suggest that images witnessed during astral projection should be seen as makeshift mental models, made by the brain in order to orientate itself in the absence of sensory inputs. Within the framework of this research, the OBE does not reveal the soul's precarious connection to the body, rather it demonstrates the fragility of those models through which the brain normally makes sense of its place in the world.

RHODRI HAYWARD

Further reading
Blackmore, S. (1982). *Beyond the body: an investigation of out-of-the-body experiences.* Granada, London.

Crookall, R. (1961). *The study and practice of astral projection.* Aquarian Press, London.

Ova An ovum (plural ova) is a mature egg released at ovulation. In humans only one egg is normally shed, from one of the OVARIES, about 14 days after the start of each 28-day menstrual cycle. This contrasts with the massive output of sperm from the testes, which begins at puberty and continues throughout life. Thus females have a different approach to processing germ cells for fertilization — a process known as *oogenesis* (see figure).

In both male and female fetuses 'primordial germ cells' migrate from the yolk sac into the site where the gonads will develop; this process is complete about 30 days after conception. In a female fetus, in the absence of male SEX HORMONES, the 'indifferent' gonad develops into an ovary and the primordial germ cells begin to divide by a process of *mitosis* giving rise to oogonia (compare spermatogonia in the TESTES). This phase of mitotic proliferation, in which daughter cells have the normal 23 pairs of chromosomes (including the X-sex chromosomes), begins at 25–30 days of fetal life and continues almost up until the time of birth. Once the oogonia have been formed they begin their first meiosis. This type of cell division is also known as *reduction division*, because it gives rise to two 'haploid' daughter cells containing half the normal number of chromosomes — 23 single ones instead of 23 pairs. However, as the oogonia embark on this process, they become surrounded by a layer of ovarian cells, forming 'primordial follicles', and the meiosis is arrested: the oogonia do not actually divide, and are now called primary oocytes. At birth each ovary contains about 200 000 primary oocytes and by puberty this number is reduced to about 40 000. Throughout life there is a continual degeneration of ova and their follicles, and during a woman's reproductive years less than 400 mature eggs will ever be released from the ovary at ovulation. Just before ovulation the ovum completes its first meiotic division which may have begun two, three or four decades earlier. This ends with the most extraordinary inequality. Half of the chromosomes but almost all of the cellular substance (cytoplasm) goes to one cell, which becomes the secondary oocyte. The other half of the chromosomes are discarded in a very small bag of cytoplasm and form the polar body. However, unlike the male, where this type of division results in one cell containing an X-sex chromosome and the other the Y male-determining chromosome, both the oocyte and the polar body contain an X-sex chromosome.

The secondary oocyte and the polar body remain surrounded by the zona pellucida and the cumulus oophorus. Almost immediately after this event the secondary oocyte begins its second meiotic division but, just like the first meiotic division in the fetus, this process is arrested. The follicle ruptures and the secondary oocyte, surrounded by cumulus cells, bursts from the follicle. The ovulated egg plus cumulus is picked up from the peritoneal cavity by the nearby finger-like projections which extend from the open end of the Fallopian tubes. It is in the Fallopian tubes that fertilization takes place, and it is not until fertilization has occurred that the ovum completes its second meiotic division with the formation of a second polar body.

SAFFRON WHITEHEAD

See also MENSTRUAL CYCLE; OVARIES; SEX HORMONES.

Ovaries The ovaries lie one each side of the peritoneal cavity, just above the brim of the pelvis. Each is close to the open, fringed end of a FALLOPIAN TUBE, leading to the UTERUS which lies between and below them. The ovaries are whitish and ovoidal (3 cm × 2 cm × 1 cm) and weigh 5–8 gm. At birth each ovary contains about 200 000 eggs, each enclosed in a single layer of cells: these are the *primordial follicles*. Unlike the TESTES, where there is continuous production of sperm after puberty and throughout life, the

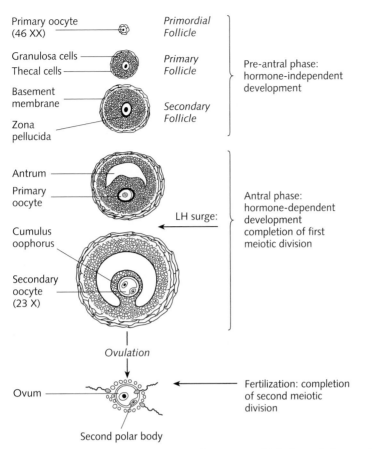

Primary oocyte
(46 XX)

Primordial Follicle

Granulosa cells
Thecal cells

Primary Follicle

Pre-antral phase: hormone-independent development

Basement membrane

Zona pellucida

Secondary Follicle

Antrum

Primary oocyte

LH surge:

Antral phase: hormone-dependent development completion of first meiotic division

Cumulus oophorus

Secondary oocyte
(23 X)

Ovulation

Ovum

Fertilization: completion of second meiotic division

Second polar body

The process of oogenesis, from a primary oocyte to a secondary oocyte, and folliculogenesis, from a primordial follicle into a mature Graafian follicle containing the secondary oocyte or ovim ready for fertilization.

ovaries do not produce any more eggs and women are born with all the eggs they will ever have.

Each ovary is enclosed in a tough, fibrous capsule and consists of an outer cortex and an inner medulla. The cortex is essentially the working part of the ovary containing all the follicles and remains of ruptured follicles embedded in vascular fibrous tissue. The medulla is where the blood vessels, lymphatics, and nerves enter the ovary. The appearance of the ovaries varies with the age of the woman. Before puberty they are smooth and rather solid in consistency. Between puberty and the MENOPAUSE their surface becomes more corrugated in appearance due to the activity during each monthly ovarian cycle. After the menopause the ovaries shrink and by then are covered with scar tissue where month after month a follicle has ruptured and released its mature egg.

Development of the follicles

Spontaneous growth of primordial follicles to primary and secondary follicles continues from birth to the menopause though many of these follicles never get past the first stage of development. The first stage is characterized by an increase in the size of the primary oocyte although meiosis is not reactivated. As the oocyte enlarges the cells surrounding it (granulosa cells) divide rapidly and

produce a protein material that forms a coating round the oocyte known as the zona pellucida. Contact between the oocyte and the granulosa cells is maintained by cytoplasmic processes of the granulosa cells that penetrate this barrier. At the same time ovarian cells condense on the outside of the follicle wall and form a loose network of spindle shaped cells known as the thecal cells. They are separatd from the granulosa cells by a basement membrane. This first phase of follicular development is independent of any hormanal stimulation. Nothing further can happen without the increased secretions of luteinizing hormone (LH) and follicle stimulating hormone (FSH) from the PITUITARY GLAND that occur at puberty and normally initiate cyclical ovarian activity and menstruation. At a critical stage of development the secondary follicle becomes sensitive to FSH and LH, enabling follicles to continue their (hormone-dependent) development. This is thought to occur over a period of three menstrual cycles during which time many of these follicles will degenerate. Of those that enter their final development stage at the beginning of the last of these cycles only one will normally be selected and recruited for releasing its egg. This is known as the dominant follicle. The rest simply degenerate, the eggs die and the follicle is invaded by white blood cells and becomes scar tissue. At the beginning of this second phase of development the 'thecal' cells

become richly supplied with blood vessels and the underlying layer of 'granulosa' cells, which surround the egg itself, rapidly divide. LH stimulates the thecal cells to produce progesterone and androgens; the androgens diffuse into the inner layer where the granulosa cells convert them to oestrogens under the influence of FSH. As the follicle grows it secretes increasing concentrations of oestrogen, and the inner part of the follicle becomes filled with fluid (*follicular fluid*); at this stage is called a *Graafian follicle* (after de Graaf, a Dutch anatomist and physician who described the maturing ovarian follicle in a major work on the female reproductive cycle published in 1672 — a year before he died of the plague aged 32).

The dominant follicle and ovulation

At the beginning of each menstrual cycle several follicles will have reached a certain size and maturity that would allow them to undergo their final stage of development so that a fully mature ovum could be released mid-cycle. For some unexplained reason normally only one follicle becomes more successful than the others and towards mid-cycle this dominant Graafian follicle rises to the surface of the ovay. At mid-cycle the granulosa cells become responsive to LH and a surge of LH secretion circulating in the blood from the pituitary gland reaches the ovary via the circulation. This LH surge stimulates the egg (the *primary oocyte*) to complete its first meiotic division into secondary oocytes. This means that the primary oocyte, containing 46 chromosomes, produces two daughter cells, each with 23 chromosomes, one of which is the X (female) sex chromosome. The second meiotic division is initiated but (unlike sperm) is not completed until and unless fertilization has taken place. Under the further influence of the LH surge, the mature follicle now ruptures and releases the egg, enclosed in its encircling cell layers (the *cumulus oophorus*), into the Fallopian tube.

The corpus luteum

The cells left behind in the lining of the ruptured follicle then proliferate rapidly, forming a *corpus luteum* (from Latin, 'yellow body'). Under the influence of LH and FSH the corpus luteum grows and produces progesterone. Unless fertilization occurs, it begins to degenerate after about 10 days, along with the decline in pituitary gonadotrophin secretion towards the end of the cycle; it becomes a fibrotic '*corpus albicans*', and finally all that is left of the follicle's life is scar tissue. If fertilization and PREGNANCY ensue, the corpus luteum is saved from decay by gonadotrophins secreted by cells of the implanted embryo itself, and its secretion of progesterone in turn maintains the requisite uterine conditions for early pregnancy. This ovarian secretion remains vital for the pregnancy in the first three months, until the fully developed PLACENTA takes over the secretion of progesterone and other hormones which support gestation.

At the menopause the ovaries become completely redundant. The remaining egg-containing follicles, which have been inactive since birth, simply degenerate, and all that is left of past activity in the ovaries are the scars from dominant follicles which have reached full maturity, ruptured, and released an egg for possible fertilization. SAFFRON WHITEHEAD

See PLATE 8.

See also MENSTRUAL CYCLE; OVA; SEX HORMONES.

Oxygen is the most common of all chemical elements on earth, being found in water, air, and most mineral and organic substances, including most compounds in the human body. It combines with almost all other elements, and is so reactive that it was given the Greek name 'oxygen', meaning acid-forming. However, most of the compounds it forms are not acids. Its chemical reactions usually form heat (as in the animal body) and sometimes light (as in candles).

It has always been known that animals cannot live without air, but in 1674 Mayow showed that only one part of the air, about one-fifth, is essential for life, and named it 'vital air'. A hundred years later Priestley isolated this part, oxygen; Lavoisier purified oxygen and its properties began to be studied.

Atmospheric air contains 21% oxygen, at a pressure of about 150 mm Hg varying with barometric pressure and to a small extent with humidity. It enters the LUNGS during BREATHING and is absorbed into the blood passively by diffusion, combining with HAEMOGLOBIN and being carried in the bloodstream to all parts of the body. There it is used to metabolize or 'burn' foodstuffs in the cells, especially FATS and CARBOHYDRATES, providing heat and creating new chemical compounds, water, and the waste product CARBON DIOXIDE. Tissues and organs vary in the length of time they can survive without oxygen, according to their provision for anaerobic metabolism. The BRAIN cannot survive without oxygen; the cessation of breathing will cause unconsciousness in a few minutes, and death soon afterwards. Other tissues such as SKELETAL MUSCLE can continue to work for a limited time, when glycogen stores are broken down without oxygen to provide energy; lactic acid is a by-product that leaks into the blood and makes it more acid, but can be recycled into carbohydrate stores in the liver.

In quiet breathing at rest we absorb about 0.2–0.3 litres/min of oxygen (depending on body size), but in vigorous EXERCISE this can go up to over 2 litres/min. This increase is accomplished by increased breathing (which supplies oxygen to the lungs at a greater rate), increased CARDIAC OUTPUT and flow of blood to the muscles, and greater extraction of oxygen from the blood by the muscles. If the oxygen supply to the muscles is inadequate then the anaerobic threshold is passed and anaerobic metabolism takes place,

with production of lactic acid. After the exercise additional oxygen is needed to convert the lactic acid back to GLYCOGEN, and breathing remains enhanced while the oxygen debt is repaid.

The supply of oxygen to the body depends not on the percentage in the air breathed but on its tension or pressure. At high ALTITUDE, say 5000 metres above sea level, the percentage of oxygen is still 21%, but because atmospheric pressure is halved, the oxygen pressure is half that at sea level — 75 mm Hg rather than 150 mm Hg. A person may as a result suffer from hypoxia — a lack of oxygen.

High oxygen pressures can be harmful and cause oxygen poisoning, including lung damage and brain dysfunction. In nature high oxygen pressures only exist in deep water diving, and mankind has not had to evolve ways of combating them. Once scientists had purified oxygen it became possible to administer it to patients; this has life-saving possibilities, but care has to be taken not to exceed the toxic level.

Some compounds rich in oxygen, such as the pollutant ozone (itself a molecular form of oxygen), and hydrogen peroxide, can react with cells to produce strongly reactive forms of oxygen. *Superoxide anions* and unstable oxygen FREE RADICALS (such as hydroxyl and hydroperoxy radicals) can be toxic to cells, by way of excess lipid peroxidation. These are implicated, for example, in damage following the restoration of blood flow (*reperfusion*) after the blockage which causes HEART ATTACKS or STROKES, and in a variety of other disease processes. However the body does have inherent enzymatic defences against free radical accumulation, and there are antioxidants, such as uric acid, ascorbate, and glutathione, which can inactivate them. Free radicals are likely to contribute also to the AGEING process: the very substance by which we live may itself limit our LIFESPAN. Thus oxygen, like most good things, can be dangerous in excess.

Mankind evolved to live close to sea level. Climbing mountains (causing hypoxia) and deep-sea diving (causing nitrogen narcosis or oxygen poisoning) can both be dangerous, in the absence of the right precautions.

JOHN WIDDICOMBE

See also BREATHING; DIVING; FREE RADICALS; GASES IN THE BODY; HYPOXIA; RESPIRATION.

Oxytocin is one of the two major hormones secreted from the posterior lobe of the PITUITARY GLAND, the other being vasopressin, the antidiuretic hormone. The posterior pituitary itself largely comprises endings of nerves whose cell bodies lie in the brain in the HYPOTHALAMUS. Its hormones are extruded from the nerve endings directly into blood capillaries and thence into the general circulation. Oxytocin is a relatively small peptide hormone, composed of only

9 amino acids. It is synthesised in nerve cells in the hypothalamus in the form of a larger, precursor molecule, which is transported down the nerve fibres through the pituitary stalk to the posterior lobe. The active hormone is cleaved from the precursor during this process.

Oxytocin was the first hormone to have its structure identified and to be synthesised in the laboratory. This was achieved in 1953 by two groups, one working in France and the other in the United States. The hormone plays an important role in birth and in feeding the infant. It has two major actions, the first being to promote contractions of the UTERUS, an action which is used in obstetric practice when the hormone is infused if LABOUR is protracted. The second action is to cause contraction of the muscular elements surrounding the alveoli and milk ducts in the BREASTS, thereby helping to expel the milk (milk let-down). Oxytocin is also found in men, but its role is not clear, although it has been suggested that it aids sperm transport during mating. The stimuli for release reflect the actions of the hormone and its actions are rapid because they are evoked by sensory nerve impulses which communicate with the hypothalamic nerve cells. Thus it is released during vaginal stimulation, so that during the process of birth, as the infant enters the birth canal, oxytocin is released and in turn causes increased uterine activity, allowing the process to proceed more rapidly. The oxytocin released at this time may also cause milk ejection, a response known as Ferguson's reflex. This reflex was first described in 1942, although herdsmen had been aware of it for centuries and had used it as an aid to milking; in the second century AD, Galen, the Greek physician and prolific writer, described how herdsmen would blow into the vagina of mares to improve milk yield. Oxytocin is also released in response to suckling and many other stimuli associated with breast feeding, such as the sight and sound of the infant. If the mother is not relaxed, this may act via the hypothalamus to inhibit oxytocin release so that problems with breast feeding may arise.

Interestingly, there have been no descriptions of clinical conditions associated with over- or underproduction of this hormone. Recent work with genetically modified mice which are unable to produce oxytocin indicates that the hormone is essential for lactation, but not for parturition.

Oxytocin exemplifies interplay between hormonal and neural systems: unlike most hormones, it is made in nerve rather than glandular cells. Sensory nerves stimulate the nerve cells to activate its extrusion into the blood so that — like other hormones — it reaches the 'target' site via the circulation. This is an example of a 'neuroendocrine' secretion. MARY L. FORSLING

See also BIRTH; BREAST; HORMONES; INFANT FEEDING; PITUITARY.

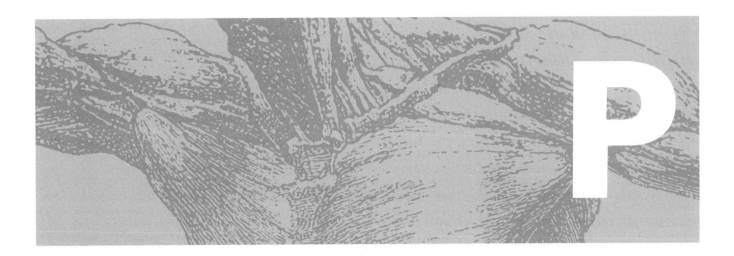

Pacemaker In the healthy HEART the cells of the *sino-atrial (SA) node* constitute the natural pacemaker, generating regular electrical signals which spread through the heart and cause it to beat. An artificial pacemaker is required if for any reason, usually HEART BLOCK, this natural system is compromised, resulting in an irregularly or consistently slow heart rate (*bradycardia*).

An artificial pacemaker contains a battery and circuitry which produces electrical pulses of short duration capable of stimulating the heart. The device was invented by Wilson Greatbatch of the USA and patented in 1960 after surgeons in New York had made the first clinically successful implant in a 77-year-old man. The pulses are delivered via an electrode which makes direct contact with the heart muscle. Pacemakers can be made to stimulate the heart at a fixed rate irrespective of the intrinsic heart rate, or a *demand pacemaker* may be used which is capable of sensing the native rhythm and pacing the heart only when the sensed rate falls below a certain value. Recent advances in design have produced pacemakers that are capable of re-synchronizing atrial and ventricular activity, thus functioning as a DEFIBRILLATOR.

A *temporary pacemaker* can be fitted by placing the pacing electrode within the right ventricle. The electrode is introduced through a needle inserted into a large vein in an arm or the neck. The electrode is advanced, under X-ray monitoring, within the vein following its course back to the heart. Once the electrode is in contact with the inner surface of the heart it is connected to the pacemaker, which remains outside the body. A temporary pacemaker may be required in the short term for certain individuals after a heart attack, during cardiac surgery or general anaesthesia. A *permanent pacemaker* is fitted in people requiring long-term pacing. The electrode in a permanent pacemaker is also introduced into a vein, but the vein in this case is surgically exposed. The permanent pacemaker is sufficiently small to be placed in a small pouch formed within the muscle under the skin; it is connected to the pacing electrode. Less commonly,

pacemakers may be implanted that can detect the onset of abnormal tachycardias (fast heart rate). The pacemaker can stimulate the heart in competition with the abnormal beat in an attempt to return it to a normal rhythm. More recently, power supplies capable of delivering high energies for defibrillation have been introduced. The pacemaker may last five to fifteen years, depending on the lifetime of the battery and the frequency of stimulation. More modern versions can retain a microchip memory of their activity for periods of up to a year; this information can then be routinely 'downloaded' for analysis so that the physician has access to a detailed electrical history of the patient's heart. Pacemaker batteries can usually be recharged via an induction coil outside the skin so no further surgery is required. Modern pacemakers thus have increasingly sophisticated microprocessor-controlled 'brains'. Like all such equipment, there is a risk of electrical interference by very powerful electrical devices; these risks are often signposted.

DAVID J. MILLER
NIALL G. MACFARLANE

See also DEFIBRILLATOR; HEART; HEART BLOCK.

Paedophilia The sexual interest of adults in children has been of recent years a subject vociferously discussed, and one which arouses very strong feelings. The image of the 'dirty old men' lingering around children's playgrounds and trying to lure little girls with sweeties, as the stigmatized image of the paedophile, is no longer the only or even the major picture conjured up. Sexual abuse of children within the family, once a subject concealed in a conspiracy of silence, has become widely publicized. Such sexual abuse is perhaps not quite the same as paedophilia, however, relating to issues of power and gender within families rather than being a question of SEXUAL ORIENTATION as such.

On an entirely different level, claims are made for the existence of well-organized rings of paedophiles operating internationally. There is some evidence for this in recent cases involving well-to-do persons of considerable social

influence who have extensive collections of child pornography. Concerns have been voiced over the role of the Internet in disseminating child PORNOGRAPHY and facilitating international contacts between paedophiles. Also, the global development of sex tourism relates to the low age of consent — or lack of age of consent legislation — in certain countries, facilitating sexual relations with children. While there is undoubted cause for concern there seems also to be an element of moral panic, in which the paedophile has become a demonised figure embodying complex anxieties of modern Western culture about changing sexual mores, the status of children, the altered role of women, and so forth. The furore caused by the supposed existence of Satanic covens of ritual abusers evokes long-standing images of dangerous and subversive cults, as described in Norman Cohn's *Europe's Inner Demons*. However, a problem does undoubtedly exist: in the UK cases have recently come to light where men with criminal records for child sexual abuse had managed to obtain positions with unsupervised access to children, and some child care institutions have been riddled with a culture of sexual abuse.

The concept of paedophilia, and its designation as one of the most antisocial of perversions, is a product of changing attitudes towards childhood and the status of children. Sexual relations with children may not ever have been precisely an accepted or approved practice. However, when children lacked many of the protections now assumed to be desirable, cultures in which there was general brutality towards children and in which they were often exploited as part of the labour force might well have included casual sexual abuse. Cases are recorded, late into the nineteenth century in Britain, of intercourse with children due to a folk belief that this would cure venereal disease. Even when an age of consent existed, in many countries this was set very low, and did not necessarily bear any relationship to nubility, given that menarche in girls often did not occur until relatively late in what would now be considered adolescence.

Early sexologists such as Krafft-Ebing (1840–1902) saw paedophilia as predominantly the last resort of the jaded debauchee in search of new sensations, and also a practice of young men frightened of the adult female and weakened by masturbation, or else a manifestation of mental deficiency. Krafft-Ebing differentiated 'violation' from rape as such, applying it to various forms of sexual assault without penetration. He considered that some cases manifested a particular psychopathology, sometimes due to drunkenness or epilepsy, but that in a few instances it was an actual perversion brought about by a morbid disposition.

René Guyon (1876–1963), a French legal scholar and philosopher of sexual relations, made a case in his works on sexual ethics that children not only were not injured by sexual activity but that it was actually beneficial, arguing that the repression of children's SEXUALITY had deleterious effects in later life. Like later apologists for paedophilia, he elided the desirability of children not being traumatically punished for their own sexual explorations, and the need for them to have some form of sex education, with the rather different issue of adult sexual access to children. The relationship between children and adults is not an equal one, given that adults are physically larger and stronger and have power and authority over them. It is questionable whether behaviour perceived by adults as sexual and seductive has such a meaning for the child.

The actual prevalence of sexual abuse of children is hard to estimate. More cases are known to the police than ever result in conviction, and probably the majority of cases are not reported. The incidence of reported cases of incest and unlawful sexual intercourse with girls under 13 in England and Wales remained relatively constant between 1946 and 1985 at a few hundred a year, although the incidence involving girls between 13 and 16 increased considerably. Approximately twice as many incidents involve girls rather than boys. Various surveys have investigated the frequency of the problem, but the figures are not consistent. Commonly cited statistics, such as one in three women having been subjected to sexual abuse in childhood, conflate single incidents, not necessarily involving contact (such as 'flashing'), with persistent and brutal abuse within the home.

The vast majority of known adult sexual abusers of children are men (over 90%), and in many cases are known to their victims rather than random strangers. While penetrational intercourse does occur, the majority of sexual activities involved are either touching and fondling, or exhibitionism. The characteristics of offenders are varied, and include the mentally handicapped, the mentally disturbed (for example elderly men in the early stages of dementia), the indiscriminately opportunistic seeker of sexual gratification, as well as those whose primary sexual orientation is towards children. It is argued that paedophilia may be caused by an inability to form sexual relationships with adults

(although this may be the result rather than the cause), or by a quasi-fetishistic fixation on an early type of sexual experience or partner. Its aetiology is obscure, and, as with other sexual classifications, may be an umbrella term covering several distinct phenomena.   LESLEY A. HALL

See also SEXUAL ORIENTATION.

Pain The International Association for The Study of Pain has provided the following definition of pain, which is used world-wide amongst scientists and clinicians interested in pain.

Pain is 'an unpleasant sensory and emotional experience associated with actual or potential damage, or described in terms of such damage. Pain is always subjective. Each individual learns the application of the word through experiences relating to injury in early life'.

Noxious stimulation of a part of the body gives rise to electrical activity in the nervous system, extending from the periphery to the brain. Receptors and pathways dedicated to the nerve impulses giving rise to pain are described as components of SOMATIC SENSATION and of VISCERAL SENSATION. That activity is modulated within the CENTRAL NERVOUS SYSTEM, both within the dorsal horns of the grey matter of the spinal cord and at higher levels. In this manner the input to the brain generated by noxious stimulation peripherally may be enhanced, diminished, or even, under certain circumstances, abolished — for example, in the heat of battle or a game of football. Thus, although noxious stimulation occurs, pain may not be felt at the time; such a mechanism clearly has value for survival of the individual in certain cases.

Our understanding of the physiology of pain control owes a great deal to the work of Melzack and Wall of some thirty-five years ago. Respectively a psychologist/physiologist and neurophysiologist, they proposed *the gate-control theory* of pain, which brought together previous work on the role of the nervous system in the generation of pain. They stated that within the dorsal horn of the SPINAL CORD there are transmission cells ('Trans cell' in the figure) and that, as a result of tissue damage and stimulation, nerve impulses pass to those cells, which project further nerve impulses to the brain, where pain is experienced. The level of activity of the transmission cells is controlled by small adjacent cells which either excite or inhibit them. In turn the level of activity of the smaller cells is determined by the extent to which they are stimulated by nerve impulses from the body or the brain. Large diameter nerve fibres (beta fibres), which are stimulated by touch, excite the small inhibitory cells (white circles in the figure) adjacent to the transmission cells. In contrast, tissue injury excites other (A delta and C) nerve fibres. The former are large diameter fibres which conduct rapidly and the latter are small diameter fibres which conduct slowly. Both stimulate the transmission cell and small excitatory cells (black circles in the figure). Therefore in an acute injury,

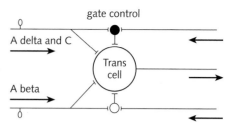

Gate-control theory of pain: the nerve pathways involved (see text)

for example when the thumb is struck by a hammer, the A delta and C fibre activity exceeds the activity in beta fibres and pain is felt. When the injured part is rubbed vigorously the pain lessens and it does so because rubbing the skin stimulates beta fibres to the point where their level of stimulation of the small inhibitory cells exceeds that of the stimulation by the A delta and C fibres of the small excitatory cells. As a result, the activity of the transmission cell is reduced or ceases. This mechanism is involved when clinicians use *transcutaneous electrical nerve stimulation* (TENS) to relieve pain. Neurons descending from the brain may also excite or inhibit activity of the transmission cells within the spinal cord by influencing the small adjacent excitatory and inhibitory cells. For example, in states of emotional calmness, inhibition of transmission cell activity occurs, and less pain is experienced than in states of anxiety, when the activity of the transmission cells is increased by stimulation of the small excitatory cells.

In some situations pain may be felt when part of the body is missing, for example after the amputation of a limb or breast. Such 'phantom pains' are located in the absent part at a site where pain may have been felt before the part was lost. How then can pain, which is at times chronic and excruciating, be experienced in a limb that does not exist as a physical reality? The answer lies in the way the brain functions. Activity in areas of the brain concerned with sensory activity in the missing limb continues despite the absence of the limb, and gives rise to a phantom. If in addition central pain processes are active, phantom pain is experienced in the PHANTOM LIMB. Such pain may be eliminated by stimulation of the sensory cerebral cortex but not by the division of nerves or the spinal cord. This supports the view that, although most people believe that pain actually exists at a site in the body that hurts, it is in fact a part of consciousness and the result of brain activity.

Until recently it was thought that the sensory and emotional elements of pain experience were linked solely to specific areas of the brain, namely the sensory and the emotional cortex, respectively. However, recent work using non-invasive brain imaging techniques — for example positron emission scanning — has revealed this model to be too simple. It is true that within the brain there is a degree of functional specialization for pain, but this is only part of the story. For example, damage to one half of the cerebral cortex does not necessarily abolish pain sensations from the opposite side of the body, and damage to areas of the brain associated with EMOTION does not necessarily remove the emotional component of pain. The reason for these apparent anomalies seems to lie in the fact that pain is generated within a widely distributed system or neuronal network. In this way, the brain detects tissue injury even when there is considerable damage to the nervous system. The brain functions as an active system, which filters, selects, and integrates sensory input against the background of lifelong experiences, both physical and emotional, which are preserved in the systems devoted to memory. One brain output from this process is pain.

Pain therefore occurs only in the conscious individual, and it is essential for survival. A small but unfortunate number of people are born without the capacity to feel pain. As a result they suffer horrific injuries in childhood and die young as a result of accidents or undiagnosed disorders, which in normal people give rise to pain.

In everyday life pain is recognised in two forms, namely acute pain and chronic pain. The former has a protective function. It alerts us to damage to the body, it increases our level of arousal, it directs our attention to the cause of the pain, and generates behaviour that leads to an escape from it. The chief emotion associated with acute pain is ANXIETY, and this subsides when pain is relieved and the cause is understood. In contrast, chronic pain does not appear to the sufferer to have any purpose and indeed has negative qualities. It gives rise to feelings of anxiety and at times of depression. The behaviours generated include withdrawal from social activities and a search for relief. The latter may well lead the sufferer to move from one doctor to another and to non-medical practitioners in the hope of pain relief. At times that process itself may generate more physical suffering through unnecessary investigation and the end result is pain, despair, and depression.

Both acute and chronic forms of pain are familiar, but in addition pain occurs in two other, quite different situations. It may occur as a symptom in a depressive illness. In other words it is not, as is commonly thought in such situations, that depression has developed because pain is being experienced but, in fact, the pain is part of a primary depressive illness. Up to half of those who develop depressive illnesses experience physical symptoms unrelated to any obvious underlying pathology, and of those symptoms pain is the most common. The failure of doctors to appreciate this fact does occasionally lead to a prolonged search for a physical cause for pain because its presence overshadows other features of a depressive illness.

Pain occurs in individual's experiencing anxiety, or emotional tension. For example, tension headaches are very common. The presence of anxiety in a pain sufferer tends both to increase

the severity of pain experienced and to reduce the individual's tolerance or ability to cope with it.

Pain may occur in the absence of an obvious physical cause and where the features of a mental illness are not detectable. Individuals with this type of pain may have had a trivial injury but the level of pain and disability with which they present is out of all proportion to the severity of that injury. In addition, the behaviour shown by the sufferer reveals considerable dependence upon others, loss of willingness to take responsibility for themselves, their home, and their work, and a preoccupation with a search for a 'cure' for the pain, which they regard firmly as physical in origin.

Consideration of pain problems in which an underlying physical cause is either minimal or absent highlights the fact that when trying to understand pain it is necessary not only to consider its sensory aspects, but also its emotional ones. Indeed it has been said that to ignore the emotional aspects of pain is to look at only one part of the problem, and probably not the most important part at that. The definition of pain given earlier reinforces this point.

As a consequence of the need to encompass the physical, psychological, and social aspects of pain experience, clinicians and pain researchers have developed what is known as the *biopsychosocial model* of pain. It is based upon what we know about the generation and control of pain within the nervous system, and also its psychological aspects and the social factors that influence the thinking of individuals about pain and their behaviour. This approach to pain has lead to the development of powerful psychological tools for pain management, which come under the broad heading of cognitive–behavioural theory and practice.

Consideration of socio-cultural and learning factors reveals that learning about pain takes place within a definite social context, and the way each of us behaves when in pain reflects that fact. At a national level it is customary in general for those who are from Northern European countries to regard complaints about pain, especially amongst men, as a weakness of character. In contrast, in Southern European countries to complain about pain is regarded as beneficial to the sufferer. These are very broad generalizations but do have some basis in fact. An important psychological mechanism by which we learn the behaviours we exhibit when in pain is defined as *operant learning*. It is a process by which overt behavioural responses to a stimulus are significantly influenced by their consequences, including the responses of others to them.

Operant learning is well illustrated by the effects of a simple injection upon a child. The sight of the needle and the pain experienced is an 'unconditioned stimulus' and as a response to it the child cries. On the next occasion the child cries at the sight of the syringe and needle, which have become 'the conditioned stimulus'. If crying leads to the abandonment of the injection the

child has developed a 'conditioned escape response'. Seeing another child crying before an injection which is then not given leads to another type of learning — 'an observational learning model'.

In some individuals such mechanisms lead to the development of pain behaviours that have a negative effect upon their lives — for example, the excessive use of rest to relieve pain, or the abuse of powerful narcotic-related drugs may actually lead to increasing chronicity of pain and disability. To counter such developments psychologists have developed techniques based upon *operant conditioning*, which are designed to reverse maladaptive pain behaviours and to replace them by adaptive behaviours. In other words, their techniques involve the use of learning of behaviour designed to lead to coping with pain and everyday life rather than withdrawing from them. Put in simple terms, 'good behaviour is rewarded and bad behaviour is punished'.

Operant conditioning has been criticized on the grounds that it does not take sufficient account of mental activity. In other words, individuals have thoughts about pain and attitudes towards it. They draw on memories of past experience when in pain, and this leads to thinking and behaviour, which is the result of those experiences. Such thoughts and attitudes, or cognitions, as they are called, cannot be ignored when a clinician is evaluating a person in pain and planning their treatment. For this reason, a purely behavioural approach has been replaced by a cognitive–behavioural approach to pain analysis and management. The main cognitive elements that have been identified include beliefs about pain and its causes, beliefs about the extent to which the individual feels he or she has control over pain, and the extent to which individuals believe that they are able to function despite pain. Therefore, self-efficiency is a significant factor in determining ability to cope.

People in pain often develop what are described by psychologists as 'cognitive errors'. For example, they may indulge in what is known as 'catastrophizing'. In other words they develop an unnecessarily negative view of their condition and its likely outcome. In such a state they tend to focus to a extent upon the negative features of their disorder. It has been demonstrated that negative qualities of thought, and catastrophizing in particular, are consistently linked to the development of depression in chronic pain disorders. The manipulation of coping mechanisms is of great significance when considering the management of pain and especially of chronic pain. We are all familiar with coping strategies, some of which are regarded as active — for example, indulging in active and distracting behaviour, whereas others are passive — for example, taking rest or medicines. If the strategy used maximizes function in the presence of pain and reduces anxiety, then it is said to be adaptive. On the other hand, if the strategies used involve too much rest, too great a dependence on medication or on others, or conversely too much activity which provokes excessive pain, they are maladaptive. Cognitive therapies involve changing thoughts and attitudes about pain with a view to changing self-management in the direction of adaptive behaviour: a change which often leads to a lessening of pain.

MICHAEL R. BOND

Further reading

Gatchell, R. J. and Turk, D. C. (ed.) (1996). *Psychological approaches to pain management.* The Guilford Press, New York and London.

Main, J. C. and Spanswick, C. C. (2000) *Pain management: an interdisciplinary approach.* Churchill Livingstone, Edinburgh & London.

Wall, P. (1999). *Pain; the science of suffering.* Weidenfeld and Nicolson, London.

See also ANALGESIA; CENTRAL NERVOUS SYSTEM; ENDORPHINS; OPIATES AND OPIOID DRUGS; SOMATIC SENSATION; VISCERAL SENSATION.

Pain, social perception

The word 'pain' is used frequently in Western society, yet it is difficult to define, because it covers so many feelings and situations. It may be physical or mental, acute or chronic, caused by body damage or created in the mind. It may be punishment (as in Hell) or perception (including the common slang usage that describes someone or some situation as 'a pain'). It may be a symptom, an isolated feeling, an indication for treatment (lobotomies have been done for intractable pain, both physical and mental). It can be a treatment in itself, as it was in Benjamin Rush's 'tranquillising chair', said to have been an adaptation of the Inquisition's 'witch chair', the revolving chair that drenched patients with more than two hundred pails of water at one sitting. More recently forms of aversion therapy and mental pain have been recognized in many psychiatric procedures.

Many aspects of pain are subjective, and therefore difficult to define and perhaps impossible to measure. There are also objective aspects. These include watching people in pain — and the idea that, since hell was eternal pain, heaven would be watching the damned burn. Watching executions was once a popular amusement (and still is, where they are held in public), indulged in even by so-called civilized people such as Pepys and Evelyn.

Pain can be inflicted for punishment, sport (stag- or fox-hunting), or amusement (bear- or badger-baiting, dog- or cock-fighting), or as an overt outlet for energy or sadistic gratification. Sadistic doctors (especially psychiatrists) are popular in fiction and films. They aren't supposed to exist in real life.

Pain of one sort or another is the commonest symptom for which people seek relief from doctors, either as a sign of body damage or as a 'cry for help' from a distressed mind. Doctors often try to solve the problem by turning it into an objective study. It can be an intellectual challenge, something to be reconstructed in a 'scientific' manner, reduced to something that can be measured. It can also be a challenge, a manifestation of power, part of some kind of progress, perhaps a gauge of medical progress or of civilization, or even a means of empire-building.

Michael Balint, who probably did more than anyone to teach general practitioners how the mind influences the body, wrote in his book *The Doctor, His Patient and the Illness*:

> Every doctor has a set of fairly firm beliefs as to which illnesses are acceptable and which not; how much pain, suffering, fear and deprivation a patient should tolerate and when he has the right to ask for help or relief … These beliefs are hardly ever stated explicitly but they are nevertheless very strong.

Pain can also be studied as a historical phenomenon. There have been enormous changes in public attitudes to pain during the last two hundred and fifty years. This was so striking that, at one time, the American physician Weir Mitchell thought that the physiology of pain had changed during the nineteenth century. There was a marked shift in attitude, from the belief that pain was a punishment for sin and should be borne with fortitude with the aid of the Church, to the belief that it was something to be conquered and cured and that this conquest was for doctors to achieve. Some came to believe that this was the sole purpose of doctors, their *raison d'etre*, a belief and attitude that is common today.

Although there have been attempts to overcome pain as long as there has been civilization, there seems to have been no concerted effort to do this until the mid nineteenth century. This can be seen in the lack of interest in or acceptance of ANALGESIA and ANAESTHESIA, despite the fact that they were known. God put Adam to sleep when he created Eve from his rib. Opium was known to virtually all civilizations. Paracelsus prepared ether or some such anaesthetic, which he called 'sweet vitriol' and said: '… it quiets all suffering without any harm, and relieves all pain, and quenches all fevers and prevents complications in all illnesses', but he dared not use it on humans for fear of offending the Church.

The Church was powerful in imposing attitudes towards pain. Christianity had no tradition of relieving pain. When chloroform was introduced it was bitterly criticised as immoral — because it relieved pain. Pain was not regarded as a physical malfunction but as part of the universe. It was what Dr Johnson called 'the pain of being a man', perhaps God's punishment. For some believers, such as Descartes, pain was a self-protective mechanism that taught the soul to avoid further damage to the body.

In 1800 Humphry Davy published the results of his experiments with NITROUS OXIDE and suggested that it might be used for anaesthesia, both in alleviating the pain of inflamed gums and 'during surgical operations'. Yet no one seems to have been interested in this for nearly half a century, despite the considerable increase in surgical knowledge and skill during that period. Even after anaesthesia had been accepted, it had little immediate effect on the practice of surgery or on the number of operations performed. The nineteenth century was an age of secularization and of increasingly humanitarian sentiments. Inevitably ideas about pain were part of these. In 1853 a medicine labelled as a 'painkiller' was marketed for the first time. Since then there has been decreasing emphasis on a world made bad by sin and increasing emphasis on a world made bad by suffering and pain. Progress in civilization has come to mean reduction of the sum of human suffering, even if the world does not comply. It may be because we can now envisage and even experience a pain-free existence (which would have been impossible before) that we are so horrified by the widespread infliction of pain in the modern world.

ANN DALLY

Palate

The colloquial link of 'palate' to taste, and thence more generally to fancy, liking, and pleasurable sensation, has a reasonable basis: the presence of SENSORY RECEPTORS for TASTE. There are however many more of these on the tongue than on the palate, and many of the subtleties of 'taste' are in fact dependent upon the sense of smell.

The palate is defined anatomically as the roof of the mouth. Its 'hard' component is part of the skull: a shelf of bone which separates the mouth from the nasal cavity, covered by MUCOUS MEMBRANE. The 'soft' component extends back and downwards, to a free edge with the uvula at its centre; it consists of muscle 'sandwiched' within mucous membrane. The muscle takes part automatically in the complexities of SWALLOWING.

An intact palate is necessary for speaking normally — as witness the interference with speech in the condition of 'cleft palate' — a congenital defect which goes along with harelip, representing a failure of embryonic tissues to join up appropriately.

SHEILA JENNETT

See also CLEFT LIP AND PALATE; EATING; SWALLOWING; TASTE AND SMELL.

Palmistry

is the best known of all the names relating to the reading of hands. The use of the word is comparatively modern for a practice that extends back through the centuries since time immemorial. *Cheiromancy* was formerly the predominant name for hand reading, used since classical times until palmistry usurped it in the seventeenth century.

Hand reading is found in many cultures; Greek, Roman, Arabic, Indian, Chinese, and Japanese among others. In the Orient palmistry is still highly respected and openly practised on the street. By contrast, within European culture the practice is much more subdued; formerly the practice was suppressed by the Church due to its links with astrology, while latterly science has largely spurned it as a subject unworthy of serious investigation.

The premise of hand reading rests upon the outer form and structure of a person's hand being visualized as the expression of the inner temperament and psyche. The skill of hand reading lies in being able to observe the minutiae of

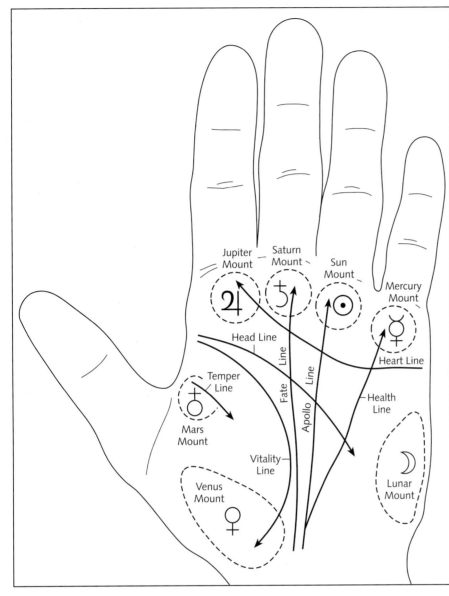

The main lines and other features used in palmar reading.

The *head line*, which runs across the palm between the vitality and heart lines, reflects a person's thinking skills and ability to communicate, along with their capacity to make plans and take decisions.

The *Apollo line*, which runs from the palmar base to the ring finger, reflects a person's creative expression; the brilliance of their talents and the fame achieved through them.

The *health line*, which runs from the little finger to the palmar base, reflects a person's health, intuition, inventiveness, and business sense.

Ideally a line should have a good length, and be clearly formed and free from markings. Whenever it is well formed it shows that the vital energy is flowing smoothly within the person and indicates that the corresponding area of a person's life is functioning soundly. For example, a clear head line indicates someone who can communicate their ideas well.

By contrast, markings such as islands, chains, bars, crosses, breaks, and forks all show interruption to the energy flow and indicate discord. For example, a head line with several islands indicates someone who is uncertain and has difficulty in communicating their ideas. Markings are often descriptive of particular experiences and can be timed coinciding with specific events in a person's life.

A skilled hand reader seeks to illuminate the sources of conflict as reflected in the markings of the lines, to assist the person to resolve them. Once conflict is overcome then the lines change and show signs of enhancement to the energy flow. Change to the palmar lines is normally gradual, taking months or even years to observe. However, the impact of sudden traumatic events can be reflected in the palmar lines within six weeks.

Despite acknowledging the importance of the development of the hand to our human evolution, science has generally viewed palmistry with great suspicion. This is largely because of the belief that the lines are crease marks in the skin related to the mechanical folding of the hand. The very idea that these 'crease' lines could be intricately linked to the consciousness of the person, and therefore relate to specific events and experiences in their life, has been regarded as nonsense. However this is refuted by palmists on the grounds that the lines develop on the fetal palm between the seventh and tenth weeks of embryological development, whereas it is only by the twelfth week that the muscles are sufficiently developed to begin the first primitive movements of the hand; thus the lines are clearly present on the palm two weeks before movement of the hand is possible.

Today, in a world where people are feeling alienated in an increasingly technological environment, more and more are rediscovering the cultural importance of hand reading for providing inner meaning to their lives. At a time when science is increasingly investigating the interrelationship of consciousness with matter, the study

each hand and to interpret what the specific formations mean in the life of its owner.

For many people palmistry is thought to be solely linked to interpretation and prognostication from the lines on the palm, but this is not strictly true. A complete reading of the hand considers its overall shape, the texture of the skin, the divisions of the palm into four quadrants, and the development of the thumb and each individual finger in turn, as well as an intricate inspection of all the palmar lines.

In all main traditions of hand reading the lines are seen as formations resulting from the flow of vital energy passing through the skin. This flow of vital energy is visualized as being synonymous with the flow of energy through the psyche, that fluctuates with every emotional experience. The sum total of all emotional experience is thus etched into the palm, resulting in lineal patterns that are unique to each person.

Accordingly every palmar main line is linked to a different area of experience; to use the palmist's nomenclature:

The *vitality line*, which curves around the thumb, reflects a person's vitality and physical constitution, the influence of the family, and their capacity to earn money and derive security.

The *temper line*, located in the angle of the thumb within the vitality line, reflects a person's physical strength, their resistance to illness, and their drives and sexual potency.

The *heart line*, which runs across the palm from underneath the little finger to the index finger, reflects a person's emotionality; their ability to express feelings and share them with others.

The *fate line*, which runs up the palm from the palmar base to the middle finger, reflects a person's application and concentration on their work or career and consequent achievement of success in life.

of hand reading could significantly enrich scientific investigation.

Due to the suppression of hand reading within European culture, its history is obscure. However, notable palmists include Napoleon Bonaparte, Alexander the Great, Homer, Hippocrates, Galen, Paracelsus, and Robert Fludd.   DYLAN WARREN-DAVIS

Further reading
Warren-Davis, D. (2001). *The hand reveals*. 2nd edn. Chrysalis Books Ltd., London.

See also HAND.

Pancreas
The pancreas (from the Greek meaning 'all flesh') is a pale, rubbery gland in the upper part of the abdomen, responsible for the production of digestive juices and HORMONES. The juices pass into the cavity of the duodenum (an example of *exocrine secretion*) while the hormones pass into the circulating blood (*endocrine secretion*). By means of these products the pancreas is essential to the proper processing of food, through digestion to absorption, storage, and utilization of nutrients.

Early authors found great difficulty in ascribing a function to the organ, as its rather evasive name implies. The rubbery texture suggested to some that the gland might be a shock absorber preventing the stomach from damaging itself on the vertebral column. It was not until the nineteenth century that any firm ideas of its function evolved. It was known that a small tube (the 'duct of Wirsung', described by him in 1642) connected the gland with the duodenum; in 1664, de Graaf inserted a wild duck's quill into the duct of a dog and collected a clear fluid, which he examined and decided was acidic. He had no idea of the fluid's function — and we now know that pancreatic juice is unambiguously alkaline, because the cells lining the duct system secrete bicarbonate ions.

Exocrine function
The function of the digestive juices became known long before hormones were recognized. The advances in chemistry in the nineteenth century led the way to understanding the process of digestion. It became clear that pancreatic juice contained agents — 'ferments' (subsequently renamed ENZYMES) that were capable of breaking down the three major components of food: carbohydrates, fats, and proteins. Many of the molecules in our diet are large, having been synthesized by the plant or animal being eaten. These large molecules are then reduced in size by the enzymes from the pancreas — continuing the digestive process already begun in the stomach; only small molecules can be absorbed from the intestines. CARBOHYDRATES are broken down to simple sugars (mono- and di-saccharides) by *pancreatic amylase*, fats to glycerol and fatty acids by *pancreatic lipase*, and PROTEINS to AMINO-ACIDS and small PEPTIDES by a variety of *proteolytic enzymes*. The French physiologist Claude BERNARD showed in the 1840s that both pancreatic juice and BILE (from the LIVER) were

necessary for the absorption of FAT. These two fluids enter the duodenum together where their main ducts converge. We know now that bile, by a detergent action, converts fats into tiny particles (*micelles*), and it is only when the surface area of the fat has been increased in this way that the lipase in pancreatic juice can break the fats down to fatty acids and glycerol. Probably to prevent the pancreas from digesting itself, proteolytic enzymes are secreted by the gland as 'pro-enzymes'. These molecules are inactive at digesting protein until they reach the cavity of the duodenum, where they are rendered active by another enzyme (*enterokinase*). Chronic disease of the exocrine component of the pancreas often results in a deficiency of pancreatic enzymes, giving rise to poor absorption of foodstuffs: the excretion of fat in faeces (*steatorrhoea*) provides the most conspicuous feature of this malabsorption. Microscopically, the gland is divided up into units known as *acini* (*acinus*: Latin for 'berry'). Each acinus is spherical, with the enzyme-secreting cells surrounding a central space (remarkably, every enzyme-secreting cell synthesizes *all* the pancreatic enzymes). The enzymes pass into the centre of the acini, whence they enter the narrowest ducts of the branching secretory system, and then pass by larger and larger ducts to the single pancreatic duct itself. The cells lining the duct system secrete water and bicarbonate ions and add them to the enzymes; the final juice is consequently alkaline.

The volume of juice secreted precisely neutralizes the acid contents of the stomach as they both enter the duodenum. This remarkable feat of homeostasis is brought about by acid in the duodenum causing release of the hormone secretin from cells in its wall; this secretin passes into the bloodstream and stimulates the production of water and bicarbonate ions from the duct system of the pancreas. Hence the greater the volume of acid gastric juice passing into the duodenum, the greater the volume of bicarbonate-rich juice produced by the pancreas. This tends to keep the contents of the duodenum neutral — the pH at which the pancreatic enzymes are most effective. *Secretin*, a protein hormone, was first demonstrated by Bayliss and Starling in London in 1902 — the earliest recognition that such 'chemical messengers' existed.

A similar mechanism exists for the enzyme component of pancreatic juice. Another hormone, CHOLECYSTOKININ (literally 'gall-bladder mover') is synthesized in the wall of the duodenum and jejunum, and is released in response to the presence of amino acids and fatty acids as partly-digested food starts to arrive from the stomach. Cholecystokinin passes round the circulation and causes enzyme secretion by the pancreatic acinar cells, thereby increasing the ability of the juice to break down more fats and proteins. Cholecystokinin also causes contraction of the gall bladder, providing bile that promotes the absorption of fatty acids and glycerol. About a litre of pancreatic juice is secreted each day in a person with typical eating habits.

Endocrine function
The main 'internal' secretions of the pancreas are the hormones INSULIN and *glucagon*. These are necessary for the regulation of storage, release, and utilization of fuels for METABOLISM. Insulin has a well-known association with sugar (glucose) in the body, because of its role in DIABETES.

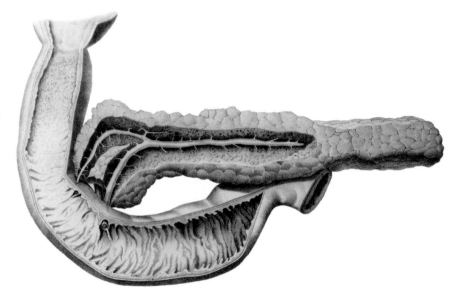

The pancreas and duodenum of a man (an executed criminal). Both organs have been dissected to expose their structure. The lobulated pancreas rests on the curved duodenum. The pancreatic duct runs through the centre of the gland, and divides before it enters the duodenum — an upper accessory duct runs parallel with the main duct before both ducts enter the duodenum. The main duct enters at the same point as the bile duct (glimpsed as a dark tube behind the pancreas) at a double opening known as the Ampulla of Vater. An accessory duct is common in mammals and occurs because the pancreas originates embryologically as two separate glands, which subsequently fuse. (From Claude Bernard's *Memoire sur le Pancréas*, 1856.)

Insulin lowers the BLOOD SUGAR, and glucagon raises it; but these hormones are also important in the body's handling of nutrients derived from fat and protein, as well as carbohydrate.

Among the acini and ducts which secrete enzymes and bicarbonate there are small clumps of cells which do not connect with a duct system. These account for a small fraction of the bulk of the pancreas, but their function is vital. They were first described by Langerhans, in his MD thesis in 1869. A clue to their function came twenty years later, when Mering and Minkowski, in Strasbourg, removed the pancreas from dogs under surgical anaesthesia, and found that they developed the features of human diabetes. At the turn of the century, Opie, at Johns Hopkins University, reported degeneration of the 'islands of Langerhans' in the pancreas of people who had died from diabetes. In 1916, the English physiologist Sharpey-Schafer linked these observations and proposed that diabetes was due to the lack of an internal secretion — a hormone — from the 'islets'. All this provided the background and the impetus for the accelerating and better known part of the story: the preparation in 1921 by Banting and Best, in Macleod's laboratory in Toronto, of an extract of pancreatic tissue, which reversed the rise in blood sugar in dogs whose pancreas had been removed. Next, the biochemist Collip prepared a refined extract, which was first used to treat human *diabetes mellitus* in 1922. Thus it was proved that the pancreas had an internal secretion — and it was named insulin from Latin *insula*; an island. The 'islets' were later shown to have two main types of endocrine cell, one producing insulin (beta cells) and the other producing glucagon (alpha cells). In the liver, the two hormones influence in opposite directions the balance between the storage of glucose (as glycogen) and its release into the blood; and they have contrary effects on new formation of glucose from amino acids. In fatty tissue they likewise have opposing effects on storage versus release of fuels. Insulin facilitates the uptake and usage of glucose by body tissues, notably muscle. In these ways the two hormones have opposite effects on the level of glucose in the blood.

The insulin: glucagon (I:G) ratio is therefore important and variable. By this balance, blood glucose level in particular is maintained for supplying the brain, nutrient supply in general is matched to the immediate needs of the body's tissues, and surplus is stored. When nutrients flood into the blood after digestion of a meal, insulin takes precedence, facilitating uptake and storage: the I:G ratio is high. When use of fuels for energy is at a peak during muscular work, glucagon promotes release of glucose and of fatty acids into the circulating blood, from liver and adipose stores: the I:G ratio is relatively low. In FASTING, and its extension to STARVATION, glucagon is of major importance, along with others of the body's hormones.

The regulation of these counterbalancing secretions is mainly by direct response of the secretory cells to the levels of glucose and amino acids in the blood supplying the pancreas: for example, a rise in blood glucose affects cell membrane receptors on beta cells, resulting in enhancement of synthesis and extrusion of insulin.

In recent years it has become clear that the islets secrete several more hormones (apart from insulin and glucagon). These include *gastrin* and *pancreatic polypeptide*. How these interact with insulin and glucagon is the subject of much current research.

Autonomic effects

As well as the hormonal and chemical mechanisms for regulating the exocrine and endocrine functions of the pancreas, the AUTONOMIC NERVOUS SYSTEM plays a faster, and even anticipatory role — preparing the pancreas to deal with food which is on its way. Parasympathetic fibres from the VAGUS NERVES stimulate enzyme secretion in response to EATING, before ever the meal reaches the duodenum, and branches from the network of autonomic nerves in the nearby gut send signals related to events in the stomach and duodenum. The hormone-secreting cells also are supplied by nerves from both the sympathetic and the parasympathetic systems, which respectively inhibit and promote insulin release, and have the reverse action on glucagon. These actions accord with nutrient mobilization from body stores during EXERCISE and STRESS, and on the other hand, the need for storage after digestion of a meal.

The pancreas is thus vital for the proper 'feeding' of the body tissues. Without its exocrine function, the digestion and absorption of foodstuffs is deranged. Without its endocrine function, untreated, we cannot long survive the inability to organize the use or storage of nutrients after their intake to the bloodstream.

JOHN HENDERSON
SHEILA JENNETT

See also ALIMENTARY SYSTEM; BLOOD SUGAR; INSULIN.

Pandemics INFECTIOUS DISEASES and their causal organisms survive alongside mankind in the relationship of parasite and host, and in stable, populous societies achieve an equilibrium in which acquired immunities in the settled population mitigate the worst ravages of the infections. Pandemics, by contrast, occur when an infection escapes from its endemic habitat to reach populations without a specific acquired immunity. By definition, pandemics are distinct from EPIDEMICS: they sweep out to affect a whole country, or one or more continents, or the whole world. Epidemics may involve a much smaller community — one family; a school; or a village, town, or county. Pandemics may thus be characterized as epidemic disasters, involving disease and usually death on a massive scale.

Early pandemics

While new infectious diseases emerge from time to time as a result of human contact with normally elusive animal reservoirs of disease (Lassa fever, for example, was discovered in 1973 to have originated among rodents in Nigeria), they require special circumstances of human activity to achieve pandemic status. Human mobility — notably migration and warfare, but also exploration, travel, and trade — has played a key role in past pandemics. It is likely that pandemics have occurred periodically since the establishment of the earliest civilized, urban societies between 3000 and 500 BC, but the surviving historical records do not permit conclusive distinctions between pandemics and epidemics until late in human history. It is clear, however, that epidemic disaster struck the Roman Empire in AD 165–80, and again in AD 251–66, with an unidentifiable infection breaking out in different cities year by year, and sometimes returning. It is possible that one or both of these pandemics were due to smallpox, or even measles.

Smallpox was (the WHO declared it eradicated in 1977) a very ancient scourge related to, and possibly deriving from, one of the various animal poxes. It may have originated in India, where ancient temples still survive to Sitala, the Hindu goddess of smallpox, and where smallpox in recent times retained very much the character of an endemic disease. One attack of smallpox conferred a lifelong immunity, which permitted it eventually to establish itself as an endemic disease in the urban societies of Europe and elsewhere. It was one of the disease which, imported into the Americas by Spaniards in the fifteenth century, caused terrible devastation among the native populations, and facilitated the European conquest.

The best attested pandemics belong to relatively recent history, and to three diseases in particular: bubonic plague, cholera, and influenza. Bubonic plague, which devastated medieval and early modern Europe with successive pandemics between 1346 and the early eighteenth century, caused alarm worldwide with another pandemic between 1894 and 1900. The Black Death of 1346–50 remains the classic pandemic of popular memory.

Cholera

Since bubonic plague, cholera in the nineteenth century, and influenza in 1918, have both achieved classic pandemic status, even though their full horror has not remained in popular memory. Cholera, like smallpox, has its natural home in India, in the delta of the Ganges river. The cholera bacillus is extremely sensitive to heat and humidity, but can survive almost indefinitely where the conditions are right. In the early nineteenth century, the activities of British traders and troops in India led to its breaking out of its historic heartland in the Ganges delta, and moving beyond its established epidemic hinterland in India and neighbouring areas. Between 1817 and 1823, travelling both by land and by sea, the disease reached out through south-east Asia, China, and Japan, and through Arabia to

Africa, the Persian Gulf, and southern Russia, before being cut short, perhaps by the very severe winter of 1823–4. The rapid development of trade and travel at this period ensured further pandemics of increasing geographical range.

Cholera infection is spread by food and water via the faecal–oral route, and is especially explosive when it enters a widely-distributed water supply. In the great, insanitary cities of newly industrializing Europe and America, opportunities for infection were legion. Six pandemics of cholera swept out of India between 1817 and 1923: 1817–23, 1826–37, 1846–62, 1864–75, 1883–94, and 1899–1923. The second pandemic was perhaps the most severe, with succeeding pandemics having a more variable global impact. Britain, for example, as a result of improved surveillance systems and public health reform, experienced no epidemic after 1866, while the 1866 epidemic was largely centred on London, and in particular in the water field of the East London Water Company, which had distributed contaminated supplies.

Cholera's ability to travel the nineteenth-century world was the result both of military activity and of the human and commercial interests which impelled ever-increasing numbers of people to travel or to migrate long distances. The disease regularly travelled the long-established trade-route across Russia, for example, and the 1893 epidemic at Hamburg was introduced by Russian Jews fleeing from persecution at home to a new life in the US, and who sought to travel on the regular migrant ships that sailed out of Hamburg port.

Both cholera and bubonic plague are example of diseases whose pandemic potential was eventually broken by patient observation and public health responses. Although it is likely that the cessation of plague pandemics was multicausal, the transmission routes of both diseases made them relatively susceptible to public health interventions. Infections which spread by direct contact, or the respiratory route, present a more serious challenge to human societies. The great influenza pandemic of 1918–9 illustrates the potential which such infections still have to devastate human populations.

Influenza

Influenza assumes many degrees of severity. It is caused by a notoriously unstable virus, which spreads with great speed and facility, and leaves only a brief immunity. Although it is another old disease, and although the evidence suggests some sixteen pandemics between c. 1100 and 1900, on the scale of global epidemic problems it was not highly rated by public health authorities before 1918. The pandemic of 1918–9 was a very different matter: with a death toll of more than 21 million persons worldwide, it was quite simply the worst disease pandemic ever experienced by human populations — a human catastrophe equalled only by the carnage of World War II. The disease strain was a particularly virulent one, and was especially lethal to young adults in the age group 20–40, although no age group was immune. Originating in America in the spring of 1918, the disease was rapidly disseminated through Europe by American troops arriving in support of the Allied armies for the final offensive against Germany, only assuming its extreme lethal character in the autumn of that year. In the climax of local outbreaks, public services broke down entirely, medical services were unable to cope with the numbers of sick and dying, and burial services were overwhelmed by the number of bodies needing interment. Those who survived often acknowledged it as one of the most profound experiences of their lives. The American writer Katharine Anne Porter spoke for many when she said of it that 'It just simply divided my life, cut across it like that.'

Sexually transmitted diseases

The airborne nature of influenza gave the 1918 pandemic its peculiarly immediate, universal, and devastating quality. The global pandemic of HIV infection which has spread out of the US since 1980 has less of this character and more in common with the pandemic of syphilis, which spread across Europe in the late fifteenth and sixteenth centuries, and whose initial characteristics were far more florid and alarming than those which it has subsequently manifested as an endemic disease. Both HIV and syphilis are essentially sexually-transmitted diseases, slower in manifestation and spread than airborne influenza. Nevertheless, the relatively rapid global spread of HIV as the result not only of late twentieth-century sexual mores but also of the ease and speed with which humans travel across the globe, taken together with the experience of 1918, affords some indication of the likely devastation should another lethal airborne — or easily transmitted — infectious disease acquire pandemic impetus.

ANNE HARDY

Further reading

Garrett, L. (1996). *The coming plague. Newly emerging diseases in a world out of balance.* Penguin Books, London.

McNeill, W. H. (1979). *Plagues and peoples.* Penguin Books, Harmondsworth.

See also EPIDEMICS; INFECTIOUS DISEASES.

Panting has more significance in furry animals than it has in people. It is their main mechanism for losing excess heat, whereas we can lose it through the skin in a regulated fashion by bringing heat to the surface with boosted blood flow, and by the evaporation of secreted sweat. The hart may pant 'for cooling streams', but it is the panting which will cool it more effectively than a cold dip.

When BREATHING increases for whatever reason, the greater the volume breathed in and out, the more heat is lost from the body. The inhaled air is automatically warmed and moistened on its way into the LUNGS (provided that the atmosphere is cooler than body temperature and is not already fully saturated with water vapour) because it passes over moist and warm surfaces, particularly in the NOSE. On its way out, some of the heat and water in the exhaled air is retrieved by the surfaces which were cooled and dried during inhalation, but a greater fraction is lost to the atmosphere.

Panting apart, the depth and rate of breathing normally vary according to the body's changing requirement for intake of OXYGEN and excretion of CARBON DIOXIDE. An increase in this gas exchange during EXERCISE, for example, is achieved by greater ventilation of the whole of the lungs: breathing more deeply as well as breathing faster. Such an increase causes a greater rate of heat loss than when the body is at rest, and assists disposal of the extra heat generated by the working muscles. But if a body needs to lose excess heat by this route when *not* exercising — when no additional oxygen–carbon dioxide transfer is needed — it would be not only unnecessary but also undesirable to over-ventilate the depths of the lungs, because of the deleterious effects of excessive wash-out of carbon dioxide. Panting is therefore different: it is rapid and shallow, whereas breathing in exercise may be rapid, but is also deep. Because it is shallow, not much of the extra to-and-fro of air actually reaches the depths of the lungs (the alveoli), instead it shuttles in and out of the upper air passages and the bronchial tree (known as the 'dead-space' because no gas exchange takes place here).

This route of heat loss is reflexively called into play in humans if body temperature keeps rising because the mechanisms for losing heat from the skin are already fully active, or ineffective. Curiously, and with no apparent physiological utility, immersion in cold water also stimulates rapid breathing of the panting variety.

Very heavy and sometimes distressed breathing during or after a bout of heavy work or exercise may sometimes be described colloquially as 'panting', though in the physiological sense it may be related more to the metabolic requirement of the muscular activity than to heat loss. Rapid shallow breathing may also occur in states of anxiety; although there may be a predominance of 'dead-space' breathing, HYPERVENTILATION is likely, with washout of carbon dioxide and its consequences.

In the literary sense, panting is also associated with all kinds of yearnings, as in the analogy of the dog with its tongue hanging out, panting and eager with desires and thirsts. Because water loss accompanies heat loss, causing concentration of the body fluids, panting does indeed lead to thirst; so the hart that was heated in the chase may well be needing the cooling streams for a drink.

SHEILA JENNETT

See also BREATHING; HYPERVENTILATION; SWEATING; TEMPERATURE REGULATION.

Paralysis implies motor weakness, and can be partial or complete. It can result from dysfunction at any point in the motor system, and the level at which this occurs determines the characteristics of the paralysis.

Movement is initiated by specialised motor nerve cells, the *upper motor neurons* (sometimes called pyramidal cells, because of their shape). These cells are situated in a special part of the cerebral hemispheres, the *motor cortex*, and are arranged in a 'somatotopic' manner — which means that motor neurons subserving a particular part of the body are clustered together, and are always found in that same place. Upper motor-neurones destined to serve movements of the leg, for example, are located nearer the midline than those destined for the arms. On each side of the BRAIN, the axons from these motor neurons converge as they leave the cerebral cortex, and pass down the BRAIN STEM as separate tracts. Just before they reach the SPINAL CORD, most of the fibres from one side cross to the opposite side. This means that upper motor neurons on one side of the cerebral cortex control movements principally on the other side of the body. In the spinal cord they descend as a tract in the outer side part of the cord, and fibres leave the tract progressively to reach and to act on *lower motor neurons* (anterior horn cells), either directly or via intermediary neurons. Those destined to activate arm muscles, for example, synapse with lower motor neurons in the cervical part of the cord. From there, axons of the lower motor neurons form the motor component of the peripheral nerves, finally reaching the muscle for which they are destined. In the muscle, each nerve fibre divides into a large number of branches. A single branch innervates an individual muscle fibre at a specialized structure, the NEUROMUSCULAR JUNCTION. The signal is finally passed from the nerve to the muscle by the release of a chemical substance, ACETYLCHOLINE, which diffuses across the narrow gap between nerve and muscle and reacts with specialised acetylcholine receptors on the muscle fibres. This reaction leads to a local electrical potential that triggers muscle contraction.

Upper motor neuron paralysis is characterized by stiffness of the affected muscles (*spasticity*); weakness of the muscles that extend the arm and of the muscles that flex the leg; drooping of the lower part of the face; increased *tendon reflexes* (the response that muscles make when their tendons are briefly tapped); and a positive *Babinski* (extensor plantar) reflex response, in which the toes move upwards when the side or sole of the foot is stroked.

A common cause of an upper motor neuron paralysis is a 'stroke', in which either *infarction* (loss of blood supply) or haemorrhage in one cerebral hemisphere disrupts the motor neurons destined for the opposite half of the body. *Hemiplegia* is the term for such one-sided paralysis. Other causes include head injury, cerebral tumours, cerebral abscess, and also cerebral palsy in which damage occurs around the time of birth. The extent of the weakness can range from a slight interference with walking, to a paralysis so profound that the patient is chair-bound.

Upper motor neuron fibres can be damaged in their course between the brain and their lower ends by spinal cord injury: a broken neck may cause paralysis of all four limbs as well as the muscles of the torso; or a broken back, paralysis of the legs. *Paraplegia* is the term for such paralysis on both sides.

Lower motor neuron paralysis has a different set of characteristics, comprising MUSCLE WASTING and weakness, loss of muscle tone, and depressed tendon REFLEXES. The cause can be damage to the anterior horn cells themselves (as in *poliomyelitis*); spinal injury in the lower back, where the motor nerve roots run down inside the vertebral column after leaving the spinal cord; or damage to the motor fibres in the nerves running from the spine to the muscles.

Weakness can be due also to a disorder at the neuromuscular junction. In this instance it has a characteristic 'fatiguable' quality, in which the more the muscle is used the weaker it becomes. The muscles are not wasted. The commonest disease causing a neuromuscular transmission disorder is *myasthenia gravis*, in which the IMMUNE SYSTEM makes antibodies to the acetylcholine receptors on the muscle fibres. The *toxins* of certain snakes (e.g. the banded krait) and of BACTERIA (e.g. *botulinum* toxin) also block neuromuscular transmission and paralyse their victim. CURARE and the contemporary drugs developed from it cause paralysis by acting at this site: originally an arrow poison, but now a feature used to good effect (and of course reversibly) in anaesthetic practice

Paralysis can also be due to muscle disease (*myopathy*). The weakness here usually principally affects the shoulder girdle muscles (making it difficult for the patient to elevate their arms) and the muscles of the pelvis (thereby interfering with walking). Rising from a chair or climbing stairs can be particularly difficult. Muscular dystrophies are genetic disorders, usually progressive, which can lead to profound paralysis. Other causes include inflammatory disorders (e.g. polymyositis), metabolic conditions, and toxic substances.   J. NEWSOM-DAVIS

See also MOTOR NEURON; MUSCLE WASTING; STROKE.

Parasites Like many words in the English language, 'parasite' has its origins in ancient Greek, where its full meaning was 'one who eats at the table of another'. With the growth of knowledge of infectious agents, worm infestations, and general microbiology in the eighteenth and nineteenth centuries, the term became eventually identified with organisms, whether of plant or animal origins, living in or upon others ('host' organisms), from which they derive nutriment. Bacteria and viruses qualify for inclusion in this definition; but once bacteriology and, later, virology, acquired their own academic disciplines and terminologies from the late nineteenth century onwards, 'parasite' in common usage came to refer, more often than not, to the larger and more or less visible organisms preying on human and animal bodies either externally (mites and ticks, fleas and lice) or internally (the large, multicellular *helminths* — i.e. worms or 'flukes' — and the unicellular protozoa).

External parasites as disease vectors

Mites, ticks, and lice have a long history as true parasites, as well as carriers of infections, notably of typhus (the body louse identified as carrier by Charles Nicolle in 1909), of African relapsing fever (carried by a spirochete, Dutton and others in 1904), and of Rocky Mountain spotted fever (carried by the wood tick, as shown by H. T. Ricketts in 1907). The demonstration by Theobald Smith of transmission of the protozoon, *Pyrosoma bigeminum*, of Texas fever of cattle by the cattle tick *Boöphilus bovis*, in 1893, was a milestone in the history of the study of disease transmission by ticks and insects. Insects rarely parasitize mammals, having originated in the Palaeozoic with a long period of adaptive evolution long before the arrival of mammals. Far more important is their role as vectors, transmitting some of the most serious tropical diseases such as yellow fever.

Although a nuisance rather than a serious threat to general health, scabies is the best known of the diseases in man which are caused directly by mites. The itch mite acarus (*Sarcoptes scabiei var. hominis, a.k.a. Acarus scabiei*) is ubiquitous, but outbreaks of scabies vary in frequency, both seasonally and geographically. Historically, it may or may not have been described in Biblical texts, but Hildegard of Bingen certainly referred to itch mites (*suren*) in her *Physika*, published in the twelfth century. Five centuries later, Cestoni of Leghorn and Giovanni Bonomo famously provided in 1687 the first complete evidence for the causal role played by the mite in scabies in man. Noted by Francesco Redi in the same year, the acarus mite and its biology and pathology were used from then on as model systems for smaller organisms — visible only with the help of microscopes — as responsible for development and spread of 'contagious' diseases. First introduced by C. F. Cogrossi in his *Pensieri* in 1713, this use of scabies and its pathogenesis as a favourite paradigm for the cause and spread of infections was to last well into the nineteenth century.

Anthony van Leeuwenhoek, using one of his own early microscopes, had found the ciliated protozoon *Giardia lamblia* in his own stools during an attack of DIARRHOEA in 1681. Today giardiasis is an increasing, if relatively innocuous threat to local populations and travellers in the tropics and the Western world.

Helminths

Worms are more easily recognized, even with the naked eye, in bodily fluids and waste products, and have been associated with disease in man and his domestic animals since the seventeenth century. 'Worms' and 'insects' were used as convenient synonyms for what were then unknown agents of 'contagion' of any kind, even when no such outward signs were observed. Scrutiny of the Ebers papyrus (1550 BC), and evidence from tissue samples of Egyptian mummies, have suggested that infections caused by the common roundworm (*Ascaris lumbricoides*), tapeworms, the guinea worm (*Dracunculus medinensis*), and the African schistosome (*S. haematobium*) were present in Egypt long before. More recent results also point to the presence of *Trichinella spiralis*, the nematode worm of global distribution whose pathology may have been responsible for the Jewish kosher taboo on the eating of pork products. In our own century, *trichinosis* has been prevalent in Germany and Eastern Europe — and in settlers from those countries on the North American continent — because of habits of using undercooked meat in sausages etc.

Another nematode worm, the humble hookworm, played a major role in the formation of the public health policies of disease control and prevention, which began in Europe and the US at the turn of the century, and were to grow into campaigns with worldwide concerns and consequences throughout the twentieth century. Hookworm disease in man (*Ancylostoma duodenale* and *Necator americanus*) had long been considered characteristic of tropical latitudes without any understanding of its epidemiology, until an outbreak among workers on the St Gotthardt Tunnel in 1880 forced the Italian medical authorities to review the situation. In spite of work by G. B. Grassi and E. Perroncito, little progress was made until Arthur Looss's discovery, at the turn of the century, of the ability of infective hookworm larvae to penetrate intact skin. This opened the way to introduction of control measures, at first tested in the early years of the twentieth century in mines in Belgium: the use of sanitary buckets, regular testing and treatment of infected miners, and instruction in personal prophylaxis. By then it had also been noted by Perroncito that salt was toxic to hookworm larvae, and that miners working in areas with a high salt content, in Poland, France, and Cornwall, showed resistance to infection. Scattering of salt around mines was recommended, but implementation was slow, and only became standard practice in South African gold mines more than twenty years later. Meanwhile, John D. Rockefeller had been persuaded to launch his philanthropic work by giving financial support to the Sanitary Commission's Hookworm Eradication Campaign, envisaged by C. W. Stiles, in the southern US, where the debilitating effects of hookworm disease had long been a threat to poor working populations. Although full eradication was never achieved, a satisfactory measure of control was reached after four years.

After that, the Rockefeller Foundation set its sights on wider targets: it was the beginning of the Foundation's concerns with the improvement of public health on a global scale. As a byproduct, it also paved the way for Rockefeller support for expansion of Patrick Manson's London School of Tropical Medicine into a full-scale school of public health concerned with temperate as well as tropical localities.

Among helminths classed as trematodes, the schistosomes occupy an important position as agents of the disease formerly called *bilharzia* (after Theodor Bilharz), now professionally referred to as *schistosomiasis*. The worms (*vesical blood flukes*) of the disease develop through stages in intermediate hosts via life-cycles as complex as those of many protozoa. Different species of schistosomes use different species of water snails as intermediate hosts. The *cercariae* emerge from their snail host into the water (river, rice field, etc.), and from there penetrate the skin of persons unlucky enough to swim or wade in contaminated water. If the disease remains undiagnosed and untreated, what initially appears in patients as merely vague feelings of being 'below par', leads at best to years of reasonably well tolerated infection with occasional acute episodes of decreased working capacity, at worst to liver failure or involvement of the central nervous system.

Parasitic zoonoses

Other parasitic zoonoses (parasites involving animals as primary or intermediate hosts of disease in man), rare but closer to home, include infestation with tapeworms of dogs and cats transmitted by the human flea *Pulex irritans*, and with *Toxocara canis*, sometimes transmitted via dog faeces to children, either playing in public parks or otherwise in contact with puppies. Unhappily this parasite can cause serious disease, including impairment — at worst, total loss — of sight. Such tragic consequences of local nematode infections are rare in the West; but in parts of Africa, *Onchocerca volvulus*, transmitted by the blackfly *Simulium damnosum*, continues to cause thousands of cases a year of 'river blindness' in Kenya's 'Valley of the Blind'.

Among parasites causing diseases regarded as largely tropical, three have been subjects of intense research from the beginning of the twentieth century: the plasmodia of malaria; the trypanosomes of African sleeping sickness (*Trypanosoma gambiense* and *rhodesiense*); and that of Chagas' disease in South America, *T. cruzi*. Yet they were not described, let alone linked to the serious diseases they cause, until the late nineteenth and early twentieth centuries.

Malaria (Italian: *mal aria*, 'bad air', named at a time when miasma theories of contagion prevailed) has a long and colourful history, which, in spite of real advances in understanding of its aetiology, and past and present hopes of the therapies, and lately of effective vaccines, still shows no firm promise of nearing an imminent conclusion. Malaria is caused by infection with one of four species of *Plasmodium* (*P. falciparum*, *P. vivax*, *P. malariae*, *P. ovale*) and transmitted by female anopheline mosquitoes, again of different species; the life cycle of malaria parasites is complex and the disease caused by *P. falciparum* is the most severe — in recent years increasingly so. It is now eradicated in Europe: it disappeared from northern latitudes early in this century, and a determined campaign saw it finally eradicated in

Italy after World War II. There were high hopes of eradication in Africa, India, and the Far East following the discovery of DDT and the synthesis of new anti-malarial compounds. These hopes were dashed when the mosquitoes developed resistance to DDT, and the *Plasmodium* parasites to new synthetic drugs, in step with their development. Additional problems include serious side-effects caused by synthetic quinine substitutes. Malaria ranks second only to the diarrhoeal and respiratory diseases in terms of global morbidity and mortality.

African sleeping sickness, like a number of other tropical diseases caused by protozoa, is almost invariably fatal unless promptly treated with drugs, which were introduced shortly after the trypanosomes were discovered in the first decade of the twentieth century. Transmitted by tsetse flies, in which the trypanosomes of African sleeping sickness develop, they enter their human host by the bite of the fly. The American form of trypanosomiasis, (*Chagas' disease*), is transmitted through the faeces of insects of the family *Reduviidae* ('assassin bugs') often infesting walls in dwellings in poor and remote areas of South America, making attempts at eradication difficult.

Humans and parasites have coexisted uneasily for centuries; only in the latter half of the twentieth century, following the end of hostilities after World War II, did hope burgeon for well-organized scientific control. Supported by the WHO and various private foundations, this might at last win the battle with parasites in tropical and temperate zones worldwide. The best hope lies in vaccine development. Advances in this area, especially against malaria and schistosomiasis, are not yet conclusive, but give cause for more optimism than before.

LISE WILKINSON

Further reading

Donaldson, R. J. (ed.), (1979). *Parasites and Western man*. MTP Press Ltd. Lancaster.

Warren, K. S. and Bowers, J. Z. (ed.), (1983). *Parasitology. A global perspective*. Springer-Verlag, New York etc.

Englund, P. T. and Sher, A. (ed.), (1998). *The biology of parasitism. A molecular and immunological approach*. Alan R. Liss, Inc., New York.

Parathyroid glands These small but vitally necessary groups of cells, usually four of them, lie on the back of the THYROID gland in the neck. They are endocrine glands — meaning that they deliver their secretion directly into the passing blood. The peptide parathyroid hormone (or *parathormone*) will therefore reach the whole of the rest of the body, but attaches only to those cells which have receptors for it. The activities which it then modifies in these 'target' cells all work towards an increase in the concentration of CALCIUM ions in the extracellular fluid compartment of the body — the blood plasma and the tissue (interstitial) fluid. It is necessary for a great variety of physiological functions — indeed for virtually all of them — that this concentration remains within quite narrow limits.

Where and how, then, would a hormone need to act in order to promote the addition of calcium into the body pool?

(i) Calcium from food is absorbed from the intestine: parathyroid hormone promotes conversion of Vitamin D to its active form; this in turn enhances intestinal absorption of calcium.

(ii) Calcium is stored in bone mineral: parathyroid hormone stimulates resorption from BONE into the blood by activating the *osteoclasts*, which break down bone and mobilize the minerals from it.

(iii) When the blood passes through the KIDNEYS some of its calcium ions escape into the urine: parathyroid hormone enhances reabsorption by acting on the renal tubule cells.

An appropriate concentration of calcium ions in body fluids is necessary for every transfer of a stimulus from nerve to muscle, and for the contraction of muscle of all types, including the beating of the HEART and the regulation of the diameter of BLOOD VESSELS. The translocation of calcium in and out of cells, and in and out of storage by chemical binding within cells, is also crucial for the secretory activity of glandular cells, producing both external and internal secretions — sweat, milk, saliva, insulin, cortisol, and all the rest, including parathyroid hormone itself.

The parathyroid glands 'know' how much hormone to secrete, because their activity is regulated by the concentration of ionized calcium in the blood that flows through them: a rise in calcium inhibits secretion of the hormone and vice versa (a *negative feedback* mechanism).

Parathyroid hormone thus keeps calcium concentration up — otherwise known as a *hypercalcaemic* effect. There is also another hormone keeping calcium down: *calcitonin*, secreted by the 'C-cells' within the thyroid gland.

Parathyroid deficiency is rare; it can occur acutely if the glands are inadvertently removed along with the thyroid or with cancerous neck glands. Rarely also, a parathyroid tumour can cause excess of the hormone, resulting in decalcification and cysts in the bones, and kidney problems due to the high concentration of calcium in the filtered blood.　SHEILA JENNETT

See also CALCIUM; HORMONES.

Parthenogenesis is a type of asexual reproduction in which the offspring develops from unfertilized eggs. It is particularly common amongst arthropods and rotifers, can also be found in some species of fish, amphibians, birds, and reptiles, but not in mammals. Parthenogenetic development also occurs in some plants species, such as roses and orange trees.

Most animal species that reproduce parthenogenetically also display a phase of sexual behaviour and sexual reproduction. In most cases, parthenogenetic reproduction occurs when environmental conditions are favourable and there is plenty of food that can sustain the generation of large numbers of individuals in a short period of time. When external conditions change and food supplies become less abundant, or when the environment becomes unpredictable, these species shift to a sexual mode of reproduction. Although sexual reproduction is considerably slower and generates fewer organisms, it gives rise to individuals containing variations in their genetic material. Some of these individuals might be at an advantage over their predecessors, because they might be more able to adapt to new conditions.

In some species of insects, such as the aphids, parthenogenetic reproduction occurs in the spring and summer, when conditions are favourable for rapid population growth. As time goes by and conditions become less favourable, the parthenogenetically born individuals mate and lay fertilized eggs. These eggs hatch the following spring, when conditions are again favourable for another cycle of parthenogenetic reproduction.

In some species of ants, bees, and wasps, the ability to reproduce both sexually and asexually is part of the mechanism establishing sexual differences. Usually, females develop from unfertilized eggs, containing only half of the genetic material of the mother, whereas males develop from fertilized eggs, containing the genetic contributions of both mother and father.

In other species of insects, such as the rotifers, females produce unfertilized eggs that develop into females during the spring and summer. This process goes on for several generations. During the autumn, smaller eggs are laid, which develop into individuals lacking a digestive system, but capable of secreting sperm. These individuals mate with females, who then produce highly resistant, fertilized eggs that remain viable during long periods of unfavourable conditions. These eggs hatch in the following spring, giving rise only to females, who then engage in a new period of parthenogenetic reproduction.

SILVIA FRENK

Pavlov, Ivan Ivan Petrovich Pavlov (1849–1936) was a Russian physiologist who won the Nobel Prize in Physiology or Medicine in 1904 for his work on the physiology of gastric secretion. However he is more famous for his subsequent studies on REFLEXES and for laying the foundations of the field of behavioural PSYCHOLOGY.

He was the eldest of eleven children of a Russian orthodox priest, and entered the theological seminary in his home town of Ryazan, in provincial Russia, with the intention of following his father's profession. In later years he recalled to colleagues that it was seeing an illustration of the gastrointestinal tract in a book by the English writer George Henry Lewes, *The Physiology of Common Life*, that persuaded him to leave the religious life to study the natural sciences. This drawing of the ALIMENTARY SYSTEM was based on the physiological research work of Claude BERNARD, and the complexity of it challenged Pavlov to explore its intricacies further.

Pavlov entered the university of St Petersburg in 1879 to study medicine, and, after graduating, obtained his doctorate in 1883 from the Medical Military Academy, also in St Petersburg. As a student he had been particularly influenced by, and collaborated with, the physiologist Elie Cyon, and on Cyon's advice he studied the nerves to the PANCREAS, and identified those which stimulated the secretion of its digestive juices; for this he was awarded the University's gold medal. It was thus a natural progression for him to travel abroad to study with two of the greatest living physiologists, Carl Ludwig in Leipzig and Rudolph Heidenhain in Breslau. Soon after returning to St Petersburg he was appointed Professor of Physiology at the Medical Military Academy, in 1890. He remained there until 1924, when the newly-created Soviet Academy of Sciences established a special Institute of Physiology for him.

Pavlov's work can be divided into two distinct phases: earlier work on digestion, and later work on the conditioned reflex. He was a noted experimenter and renowned surgeon, and, using anaesthetized experimental animals, usually dogs, he created several 'windows' in the body through which the secretions of the stomach, salivary glands, pancreas, and intestine could be collected. Of particular value was his ability to bring the stomach out through the body wall with its nerve and blood supply intact, so that he could observe its functions in a conscious dog, behaving normally. He also made an artificial hole in the oesophagus (gullet) so that food taken into the mouth escaped before it reached the stomach. Together, these allowed him to show that gastric juices were secreted in anticipation of receiving food from the mouth, and also to collect and study the secretions uncontaminated by food particles. His techniques led to the discovery and identification of several key ENZYMES and mechanisms that occur in normal digestion. This work had commercial spin-offs: from 1898 onwards Pavlov's lab contained a 'gastric acid factory', the acid produced by the dogs being collected and sold as a remedy for DYSPEPSIA, and by 1904 the project was contributing over 65% of the laboratory's budget.

Perhaps the most influential observation he made was in the early years of the twentieth century, when he noticed that even the mere sight and smell of food could stimulate the anticipatory production of salivary and gastric secretions in his experimental dogs. Further systematic experiments on this phenomenon revealed that if the appearance of food was repeatedly preceded by the ringing of a bell, then eventually the dog would produce secretions after hearing the bell, and before or without the appearance of food. This encouraged Pavlov and his co-workers to turn their attention to the activities of the higher nervous system and to the further study of such responses, which he originally called a 'conditional reflex', because 'their inclusion as reflexes had for him a conditional character'. To

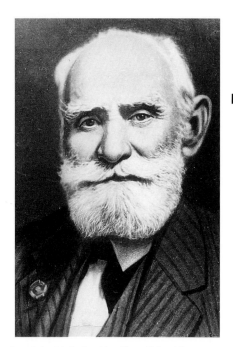

Ivan Petrovich Pavlov. Mary Evans Picture Library.

English speakers the expression has now become known as 'conditioned reflex', although the French still refer to 'le réflexe conditionnel'. His work from then onwards focused on links between nervous activity and behaviour, extending into observational and theoretical work on human behaviour. Many of his views were rapidly absorbed into psychological and psychiatric practice and teaching.

By the time of the Russian and Bolshevik revolutions in 1917, Pavlov was a world-renowned scientist. He was subsequently courted by the new regime, which wanted to build up Soviet science. In the years immediately after the revolutions Pavlov frequently denounced the Bolsheviks and their ideology, and at one period considered emigrating. He was, however, offered privileges for himself and his colleagues that permitted him to continue working, and by the 1930s had apparently reconciled himself to living in Soviet Russia, particularly through his friendship with Nikolai Bukharin. He continued nonetheless to be a critic of the government, and was subject to secret police surveillance for many years up to his death in 1936.

E. M. TANSEY

Further reading

Brown, E. M. (1990). Ivan Petrovich Pavlov. In *Nobel Laureates in Medicine or Physiology: a biographical dictionary*, (ed. D. M. Fox, M. Meldrum, and I. Rezak). Garland Publishing, New York.

Todes, D. P. (1995). Pavlov and the Bolsheviks. *History and Philosophy of the Life Sciences*, 17, 379–418.

Todes, D. P. (1997). Pavlov's physiology factory. *Isis*, 88, 205–46.

Todes, D. P. (1997). From the machine to the ghost within: Pavlov's transition from digestive physiology to conditional reflexes. *American Psychologist*, 52, 947–55.

See also CONDITIONING.

Pelvis The term 'pelvis' comes from the Latin meaning 'a basin'. It is formed from the two *innominate* (hip) bones that join to each side of the *sacrum* at the back, and with each other at the front of the body. The upper part, or *false pelvis*, houses the lower abdominal viscera, whilst the truly basin-shaped lower part houses and protects the urinary BLADDER, rectum, and internal genitalia. The innominate (derived from the Latin *in nomen*, meaning 'unnamed') is a large, irregular shaped bone which has been likened to an aeroplane propeller. In the adult, it is formed from the fusion of three separate bones — the *ilium* above, the *ischium* below and behind, and the *pubis* below and in front. These bones fuse in the region of the hip socket (the *acetabulum*) towards the end of puberty. Typically the female innominate has reached adult form by between 11 and 15 years of age whilst the male takes approximately two years longer to reach maturity. There is only a small temporal window of some 18 months for the female pelvis to transform completely from its juvenile to its final, adult, childbearing form. Such extensive alterations to a skeletal complex arise due to a massive influx of female SEX HORMONES concomitant with puberty. Therefore, those of us with teenage daughters should perhaps try to understand not only the psychological and physiological effects but also the anatomical implications brought about by that raging sea of hormones.

The articulation at the front between the innominate bones is known as the *pubic symphysis*, and this is a particularly useful area for identifying both the sex and the age at death of skeletal remains, whether they are archaeological or forensic in origin. The articulations between the innominates and the sacrum are at the *sacroiliac joints* and, with advancing age, they can *synostose* (fuse), although this only tends to occur in the elderly male. There appears to be a defensive mechanism in the female that protects the joints of the pelvis in particular and ensures that they

remain unfused and able to allow some degree of movement, which can outlast the advantage of this when giving BIRTH. Prior to childbirth, a female hormone called '*relaxin*' is produced, which serves to loosen both the sacro-iliac joints and the pubic symphysis to permit a few extra millimetres of mobility. This extra room helps the fetal head to squeeze through more easily — although it is still a very tight fit.

Certain clinical conditions, such as rickets, can permanently alter the shape of the pelvis and so have the potential to affect drastically the outcome of childbirth. In periods of history such as the industrial revolution, rickets was rife and as a result feto-maternal mortality was high. It must be remembered that, in the days before anaesthesia and asepsis allowed safe CAESAREAN SECTION, the only way to expel a fetus was by the natural pathway (*per vaginum*). If the fetal head could not pass through the pelvis (*cephalopelvic disproportion*) then labour could last for days and frequently neither the mother nor the baby survived. Some of the more educated women of the time knew that their chances of surviving childbirth were slim at best and so they resorted to many wildly inventive means of preventing pregnancy or, failing that, to ensure abortion of the fetus. It is interesting to note that today, in many of our densely urbanized areas, there is a resurgence of rickets.

The morphology of the pelvis is particularly important in the investigation of human evolution, as it clearly reflects the uniquely bipedal form of locomotion. The junctional position of the pelvis between the trunk above and the legs below ensures that it is intimately involved in the transfer of body weight from the upper body to the ground. This is essential for a bipedal animal, but the female has had to take into account the secondary function of the pelvis, which is, of course, to house a fetus. Not only does the fetus have to be provided with a safe environment for its development, it must have an unobstructed exit that is large enough for its entry into the world. The increased encephalization of the human fetus — the size of its brain and therefore its skull — compared with any other animal has meant that the female pelvis has had to expand even further to ensure safe passage. Therefore the

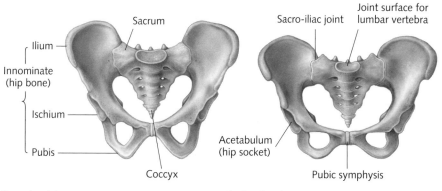

The male pelvis — Sacrum, Ilium, Innominate (hip bone), Ischium, Pubis, Coccyx

The female pelvis — Sacro-iliac joint, Joint surface for lumbar vertebra, Acetabulum (hip socket), Pubic symphysis

female pelvis is a functional compromise between providing on the one hand the necessary framework for attachment of the muscles that facilitate bipedal locomotion, and on the other a large enough birth canal. The male pelvis does not, of course, have to make any such functional compromise, and it is these fundamental differences between the sexes (*sexual dimorphism*) that permit the reliable identification of sex from the pelvis.

In the hands of an experienced observer, over 90% of skeletons will be assigned to the correct sex when the innominate bone alone is examined. In fact, not even the entire bone is required for such a degree of reliability. Whilst the front part is the most dimorphic, unfortunately it does not tend to survive burial as successfully as the back part of the bone and so the latter is much more commonly available for the identification of sex. However, a word of caution is needed before relying solely on the innominate for sex determination. Certain racial groups do not exhibit high levels of pelvic sexual dimorphism — for example the Dutch. In this group, the female pelvis is very masculine in appearance and so forensic anthropology achieves a very low level of correct identification. Dutch women are of large body size and so their ancestors have not invested heavily in the remodelling that occurs during puberty. It is interesting to note, however, that the babies born to them are no larger than the European average and hence these mothers enjoy the enviable position of having the lowest level of obstetrical complications in Europe.

SUE M. BLACK

Further reading

Aiello, L. and Dean, D. C. (1990). *An introduction to human evolutionary anatomy.* Academic Press, London.

Gebbie, D. A. M. (1981). *Reproductive anthropology — descent through Woman.* J Wiley and Sons Ltd., Chichester.

See also BIPEDALISM; EVOLUTION, HUMAN; HIP; LABOUR; SKELETON.

Penis In 1672, the anatomist Regnier de Graaf declared, 'the names of this organ ... are almost too many to count, and more are invented every day by after-dinner speakers and by men with time on their hands and a penchant for venery as well as by lascivious poets.' Things have not changed much since the seventeenth century; a recent survey of American college students pinpointed 144 alternative names for the penis among men and 50 among women. The word 'penis' is probably derived from the verb *pendere*, meaning 'to hang', but hundreds of euphemisms have arisen for reasons of propriety and comedy. The most traditional English-language synonyms include yard, phallus, and manhood.

The penis is undoubtedly the centre of much linguistic, artistic, scientific, and erotic attention because of its association with procreation, sexual pleasure, and prowess. An anatomically complicated and versatile organ, the penis, as De Graaf noted, 'consists of diverse parts which nevertheless all skilfully cooperate in making it able to stretch and relax.' This changeable nature is key: 'It would be unseemly and disgusting and it would totally impede one's conduct of worldly affairs to be like the Satyrs and have a penis always erect. On the other hand to have one always loose and floppy would incommode successful conduct of the affairs of Venus.' Much medical attention has been paid to the latter problem, namely impotence. Partly via research into impotency, we now know that erection derives from a complex system involving multiple psychological and physiological factors. The proximate cause of erection is an increase of blood supply to the spongy tissues of the penis.

Decorative codpieces and mythological tales have long encased the 'male organ'. Perhaps the best known penis-centred tale is that of Osiris, the unlucky Egyptian god who had his body chopped into parts and scattered about. Isis, Osiris's wife and sister, managed to locate all except the penis. Ever since, stories have abounded of penises which seem to enjoy virtually independent existences and wills.

Phallic worship has often centred around disembodied penises. Some native Peruvian peoples, for example, worship and seek strength from the 'phallus tree', the branches of which look like penises. Phallic worship generally speaks to issues of fertility (agricultural and human) and power. Thus, while testicles have been represented as the loci of maleness, the penis has also traditionally and cross-culturally signified virility and power. (What else but an attribution of power to the penis could explain the continuing fascination with the posthumously disembodied and preserved penis of Napolean Bonaparte? Having passed through at least nine sets of hands since Bonaparte's death, the emperor's penis now allegedly belongs to an American urologist.)

While the power of a penis — real or representative — has frequently been judged by the penis' size, Aristotle assumed that too large a member would actually render a man relatively infertile: 'Those who have a very big penis are less fertile than those with an average-sized one, because cold semen is sterile and what has to travel any great distance gets cold.' By contrast, today we find in Western popular culture a virtual obsession with penis size because of the equation of penile mass with prowess. In the US, a fast-rising number of men are seeking 'penile augmentation' surgeries designed to make their penises look longer or be wider. These procedures, which include tissue grafts and injections of fat, are not widely tested or approved and come with serious risks. Some men instead follow the 'low-tech' techniques of the sadhus, Indian ascetics who stretch their penises through the use of hanging weights.

Ornamentation of the penis is common in many cultures and involves lengthening, piercing, dressing, and TATTOOING. These cosmetic alterations often carry spiritual significance. At one time, the practice of circumcision (removal of the foreskin) was confined mostly to Jewish males, but early in this century, Western physicians became convinced that a circumcised penis is a healthier penis. (Infections may occur less often in circumcised penises, and penile cancer, although in any case very rare, is virtually unknown in circumcized penises.) The rate of circumcisions consequently soared. Lately, the number of male circumcisions done for 'medical' reasons has tapered off, as the foreskin's perceived value has again risen.

In spite of folk tales that a man's penis size can be guessed by the size of his nose or feet, penis size does not correlate with these other measurements, nor is post-puberty penis size easily predictable from pre-puberty size. Size may be considered critical, and boys born with a condition known as *micropenis* are sometimes raised as girls — but definitions of micropenis vary. With respect to general appearance, boys may be born with *hypospadias*, in which the urethral opening is on the underside of the penis rather than on the very tip of the 'head' or 'glans', but this is not often severe enough to require correction. So, while relatively strict criteria of penile normality may be held in Western popular culture, in fact penile anatomy varies considerably. Minor variations are common and do not require surgical attention.

The present-day criteria for penile 'normality' arose in part from the conviction among male psychoanalysts that the penis is critical in the development of male and female identities. Thus, while Sigmund Freud attributed a necessary 'penis envy' to women, his successor Jacques Lacan posited a multidimensional 'phallus'. Lacan's 'phallus' refers to representations of the penis; the phallus becomes a 'privileged signifier' taking precedence over all others. Pre-modern anatomists often likened the male penis to the female VAGINA, but it is in fact homologous to the CLITORIS.

ALICE DREGER

See PLATE 8.

See also CIRCUMCISION; COITUS; EJACULATION; PHALLIC SYMBOL.

Peptides are short chains of AMINO ACIDS linked together. If there are only two amino acids then the peptide is a *dipeptide*. Similarly there are *tripeptides, tetrapeptides,* and so on. If the number of amino acids in the chain reaches around ten or so, such substances are called *polypeptides*, while large polypeptides are called PROTEINS. There is no particular agreed size at which a large polypeptide becomes a small protein, but generally polypeptides have molecular weights of a few thousand, while proteins have molecular weights of tens of thousands. Depending on which amino acids are involved, between seven and ten amino acids will add about 1000 to the molecular weight.

Protein molecules in the diet are digested by ENZYMES (which are themselves specialized proteins), that break them down into smaller and smaller lengths, the breakage occurring at the peptide bonds. Peptides and amino acids are thus the final cleavage products of protein digestion. Amino acids are the main protein breakdown product absorbed from the gut, but some di- and tri-peptides are also absorbed, there being specific carrier systems in the cells lining the small intestine to transport these small peptides from the lumen to the blood.

The dipeptide *carnosine*, formed from the amino acids alanine and histidine, was identified in muscle a century ago, but only recently has research revealed its properties and the likely variety and significance of its functions. It is known to be present also in the BRAIN, where it may act as a NEUROTRANSMITTER. In muscle it is likely to be important in making the contractile filaments more sensitive to CALCIUM ions and in controlling the internal acidity of these fibres. It has been suggested that it may also be a scavenger of FREE RADICALS. Its strong binding with zinc may be important in co-absorption from the gut of this essential trace element; and physiologically significant interactions between carnosine, zinc, and HISTAMINE are being discovered.

The tripeptide *glutathione* (glutamic acid-cysteine-glycine) is an important co-factor for many enzymes, increasing their activity.

Polypeptide hormones

Polypeptides control or trigger a great many bodily functions, acting close to or at a distance from the site at which they are produced and released. The table below gives a few examples, giving the site of production, the number of amino acids, and an indication of the functions that the polypeptides promote.

Proteins usually fold to form particular three-dimensional shapes (which determine their actions), but polypeptides are not so structurally constrained, so in solution they can adopt many conformations. For example, OXYTOCIN and vasopressin have about a thousand different conformations in solution, all in dynamic equilibrium one with another. How is it therefore that they specifically attach to their receptors, with the requirements for specific shape and charge distribution? The answer is that some part of the polypeptide attaches to the receptor, while adjacent parts turn and rotate until the correct shape is reached. Thus the polypeptides use a 'zipper' mechanism to attach to MEMBRANE RECEPTORS.

Neuropeptides

There are many different peptides in neurons, released along with other neurotransmitters. Some peptides that were originally identified as HORMONES, thought to be produced at one particular site and to act at certain 'target' sites, have more recently been found to be made elsewhere also, and to have other functions. The body utilizes the same peptide for different purposes. This is true, for example, of CHOLECYSTOKININ (CCK), a 33-amino-acid polypeptide that was known for many decades as a hormone that originated in the duodenum and caused emptying of the GALL BLADDER. Since the 1980s it has been revealed to be a modulator of neural activity, produced by many nerve cells, widespread in the nervous system. Likewise, *corticotrophin releasing factor* (CRF), with 41 amino acids, was originally known to be made and released by a group of neurons in the HYPOTHALAMUS, passing to the PITUITARY GLAND and there stimulating the secretion of ACTH (adrenocorticotrophic hormone). But it too has been found to be a neuromodulator produced by neurons in many parts of the brain.

A family of peptides called *opioid peptides* or ENDORPHINS, found in the brain and elsewhere in the body, are responsible for the modulation of PAIN sensation. One group of these, the pentapeptide *enkephalins*, are released as neurotransmitters by nerve cells in certain parts of the brain and spinal cord. They bind to opiate receptors (the membrane receptors on which opiate drugs act) on other nerve cells in the pathways that mediate pain, hence acting as 'endogenous' (internally generated) ANALGESICS.

ALAN W. CUTHBERT
SHEILA JENNETT

See also AMINO ACIDS; HORMONES; OPIATES; OPIOIDS; PAIN; PROTEINS.

Perception Our senses probe the external world, and they also tell us about ourselves as they monitor the positions of our limbs and the balance of our bodies. Through PAIN they signal INJURY and ILLNESS.

How we experience and know about external objects is a question that was discussed by the Greek philosophers and has been ever since. Planned experiments on perception, in the spirit of the physical sciences, were hardly attempted before the mid nineteenth century. They have revealed a surprising complexity of physiological and cognitive (knowledge-based) processes, of which we are normally unaware, though many can be demonstrated simply and dramatically, especially through the phenomena of illusions.

There is a long-standing tradition in philosophy that perception, especially touch and VISION, gives undeniably true knowledge. For philosophers have generally sought certainty and often claimed it, whereas scientists (who are used to their theories being upset by new data) are more ready to settle for today's best bet. Many scientific instruments have been developed because of the unreliability or inadequacy of perception.

Perceptions are separate, and in several ways different, from *conceptual* understanding, for perception must work very fast (whereas we may take minutes or hours to 'make up our minds', and years to form new concepts). Also, it would be impossible for perception to draw upon all of our knowledge; and perceptions are of individual objects and events in present time, while concepts are abstract and generally timeless.

The evolution of mechanisms for the perception of objects and events at a distance (most completely through vision and hearing) freed organisms from the tyranny of reflex responses to immediate situations, and no doubt was a necessary precursor of all intelligence. It is a fairly new notion that perception itself is an intelligent activity, requiring still only partly understood problem-solving to *infer* the objective world from sensory signals. Earlier accounts, especially British Empiricism, portrayed sensory perception very differently, as a passive, undistorting window, through which the mind accepts sensations

	Amino acids	Origin	Action
Hormones			
Oxytocin	9	Posterior pituitary	Uterine contraction and milk ejection
Vasopressin	9	Posterior pituitary	Antidiuretic (water-retaining) action in kidneys
Glucagon	29	Endocrine pancreas	Increases blood sugar
ACTH	39	Anterior pituitary	Stimulates release of cortisol from adrenal glands
Gastrin	17	Stomach lining	Stimulates gastric acid secretion
Angiotensin	8	From precursor in the blood	Regulation of body fluid volume and circulation
Local agents			
Bradykinin	9	In tissues	Dilates blood vessels, stimulates secretions
Endothelin	21	Endothelium	Constricts blood vessels
Neuropeptides/hormones			
CRF	41	Hypothalamus and many other brain regions	Promotes release of pituitary and other hormones, and stimulates sympathetic nervous activity
Substance P	11	Nervous system, gut, inflamed tissue	Vasodilator; neurotransmitter involved in pain sensation
CCK	33	Duodenal lining; peripheral nerves and many brain regions	As hormone, stimulates gall bladder contraction and pancreatic secretion; neurotransmitter in brain

directly from objects. This is not consistent with physiological knowledge of the senses and the brain, nor with many phenomena, such as ILLUSIONS of vision and hearing and touch. The notion of 'direct perception' is, however, still maintained by some followers of the American psychologist J. J. Gibson, perhaps by taking this aspect of his important writings too literally. Perception is not traditionally thought of as an intelligent activity; though the power, especially of vision, to probe distance gains the time needed for intelligent behaviour and for the intelligence of perception itself.

Are perceptions simply *picked up* by the senses passively, or are they *created* actively by the brain, or mind? This issue between passive or active perception is a long-standing debate, with significant implications, such as: what is 'objective' and what 'subjective'? The philosopher John Locke (1690) suggested that there are *primary* characteristics, such as hardness and mass and extension of objects, in space and time — in the world before life, existing apart from mind — and *secondary* characteristics, created in minds or brains. Thus colours are not in the world, but are created within us, though related in complex ways to light and to the surfaces of objects. Sir Isaac Newton (*Opticks*, 1704) expressed clearly that red light is not itself red, but is: 'red-making':

> ... there is nothing else than a certain power and disposition to stir up the sensation of this or that colour. For as sound in a bell or musical string ... is nothing but a trembling motion.

Then (in Query 23 of *Opticks*) Newton speculates on something like a neural mechanism of vision:

> Is not vision perform'd chiefly by the Vibrations of this (Eatherial) Medium, excited in the bottom of the eye of Rays of Light, and propagated through the solid, pellucid and uniform Capillamenta of the optic Nerves in the place (the 'Sensorium') of Sensation?

The Empiricist school (of which, in their different ways, Locke and Newton were founders) also rejected the notion that minds can receive knowledge by direct intuition quite apart from sensory experience. Mind was now regarded as essentially isolated from the physical world — linked only by tenuous threads of nerve and by fallible inferences of what might be 'out there'. Some people find this too unsettling to be true. But it is now generally accepted that perception depends on active, physiologically based, intelligent processes. This is not intuitively obvious, since perception seems so simple and easy and we know nothing of the processes in our brains by introspection. Seeing happens so fast and so effortlessly that it is hard to conceive the complexity of the processes that we now know are needed to interpret the nature of the visual world from sensory signals — processes that remain largely beyond the capabilities of the most advanced computers.

Paradoxically, this takes us to concepts familiar to engineers and useful for physiology. We may describe the organs of the senses as 'transducers', which accept patterns of energy from the external world, signalling them as coded messages to be read by the brain, which uses these patterns to *infer* the state-of-play of the surrounding world, and something of the body's own states. Another useful engineering concept is that of 'channels'. The various senses feed specialized 'brain modules' through neural channels, discovered by physiological and 'psychophysical' (perceptual) experiments. Thus, as Thomas Young suggested in 1801, colour vision is created from information about the wavelength of light transmitted through three channels, red, green, and blue, responding to light of long, medium, and short wavelength, respectively. All the hundreds of colours we can see are interpretations by the brain of the relative activity of these three colour channels. The three colour channels correspond, initially, to three kinds of light-catching photopigment in the photoreceptors, called *cones*, in the retina.

There are similar neural channels representing the orientation of lines and edges, and for movement, as first shown by direct physiological recording from nerve cells in the visual cortex of cats by the physiologists D. H. Hubel and T. N. Wiesel in 1962. There are channels for many other visual characteristics: stereoscopic (3-D) depth, texture, spatial size, etc. The ear has many different frequency channels, and there are scores of channels for the sense of 'touch', including those for various kinds of pain, for tickle, and for monitoring the positions of the limbs and the stretch of muscles in order to control movement. We are unaware of activity in these sensory channels themselves. Somehow outputs from the many channels are combined to give consistent perceptions. Small discrepancies — such as the delay in sound between seeing a ball hit a bat and hearing the impact — are rejected or pulled into place to maintain a consistent world. Equally, whole objects are somehow assembled from the many signals in different sensory channels that define them. But how this ('*the binding problem*') is done is not understood.

The theory that perception is 'cognitive', depending on inferences from essentially inadequate sensory signals, was first clearly proposed by the German polymath physicist, physiologist, and psychologist, Hermann von Helmholtz (1821–94). He called perceptions 'unconscious inferences'. We might say that they (our most intimate experiences and knowledge) are simply *hypotheses*, essentially like the predictive hypotheses of science — though not always agreeing in particular accounts.

More recently, attempts to program computers to see (an important component of artificial intelligence) has shown how hard it is to infer objects from sensed data. The most influential attempt, by physiologist David Marr, suggested that object shapes are derived from the retinal images via three essential stages:

(i) the 'primal sketch(es)', describing intensity changes and locations or critical features and local geometric relations;

(ii) the '2½-D sketch', giving a preliminary analysis of depth, surface discontinuities, and so on, in a frame that is centred on the viewer;

(iii) the '3-D model representation', in an object-centred co-ordinate system, so that we see objects much as they really are in 3-D space, though they are presented from just one viewpoint. Marr supposed that this last stage is aided by restraints on the range of likely solutions to the problem of what is 'out there'. These information-processing constraints are set by assuming typical object shapes; for example, that the shapes of many objects, such as other human beings, are modified cylinders. Interestingly, the painter Paul Cézanne came close to this notion in 1904:

> Treat nature by the cylinder, the sphere, the cone, everything in proper perspective so that each side of an object or a plane is directed towards a central point ... nature for us men is more depth than surface.

David Marr stressed the importance of immediate, passive processing of sensory signals, over active, cognitive 'top down' application of knowledge gained from the past. This is a central controversy, currently moving towards greater cognitive 'top down' contributions, especially for vision. When computers (or the form of computing known as 'neural nets') can access vast amounts of knowledge appropriately, in real time, they might share our miracle of perception.

Artists and scientists can teach each other secrets of perception (as by Gombrich, 1960), though such cross-cultural communication is not easy for most of us.

RICHARD L. GREGORY

Further reading

Gibson, J. J. (1950). *Perception of the visual world.* Houghton Mifflin, Boston MA.

Gibson, J. J. (1966). *The senses considered as perceptual systems.* Houghton Mifflin, Boston MA.

Gombrich, E. (1960). *Art and illusion.* Phaidon, London.

Gregory, R. L. (1966, fifth edn 1998). *Eye and brain.* Oxford University Press.

Hubel, D. and Wiesel, T. N. (1962). Receptive fields, binocular interaction and functional architecture in the cat's visual cortex. *Journal of Physiology*, **160**, 106–54.

Marr, D. (1982). *Vision.* W. H. Freeman, San Francisco.

Zeki, S. (1993). *A vision of the brain.* Blackwell, Oxford.

See also ILLUSIONS; SENSATION; SENSES, EXTENSIONS OF; SENSORY INTEGRATION; VISION.

Perfume is used for a wide variety of purposes: aesthetic, religious, culinary, and medicinal, among others. Traditionally perfumes were made from plant and animal substances and prepared in the form of waters, oils, unguents, powders, and incense. This last method of fragrancing gives us our word 'perfume' which means 'to smoke through'. Most modern perfumes are alcohol-based and contain synthetic scents. While the term 'perfume' usually refers to fragrances in general, in the more technical language of the perfumer, a perfume must contain over 15% of fragrance oils in alcohol. Eau de parfum, eau de toilette, and cologne contain lesser amounts of fragrance oils in alcohol diluted with water.

The preferred fragrances for perfumes are by no means universal, but differ according to cultural dictates and fashions. In the sixteenth century, for example, pungent animal scents such as musk and civet were very popular. In the nineteenth century, by contrast, such animal scents were generally considered too crude, and light floral fragrances were favoured.

Perfumes were held in high esteem and widely employed in the ancient world. The wealthy would perfume not only their own bodies, but their furnishings and their favourite horses and dogs. On ancient altars perfumes were offered to the gods, while in the kitchens of antiquity the same scents — saffron, cinnamon, rose, myrrh — might be used to flavour food and wine.

With the rise of Christianity, perfumes became associated with a decadent lifestyle which catered to bodily desires rather than to spiritual necessities. Many of the early Church Fathers condemned the use of perfume as 'a bait which draws us into sensual lusts'. While disdaining the use of perfumes, however, the Church employed metaphors of fragrance to refer to the spiritual life. Prayer, for example, was presented as a symbolic form of incense, while the Christian soul was a 'perfumed garden' of grace. Such metaphors acquired a certain physical reality in the phenomenon of the 'odour of sanctity', whereby holy persons were believed to exhale a divine fragrance.

By the end of the Middle Ages, perfumes were once again enormously popular in social life. Those who could afford it perfumed their clothes, as well as their bodies, and wore gloves and shoes made out of perfumed leather. Even jewellery might be perfumed, or else fashioned of beads of hardened perfume. In the sixteenth and seventeenth centuries the Puritans and other Protestant reformers, following the ascetic doctrines of the early Christians, denounced this indulgence in scent as contributing to an immoral lifestyle and disguising an underlying stench of sin.

Along with offering pleasing scents, perfumes had many practical uses in premodernity. Perfumes were believed to play a role both in preserving health and curing disease. Thus the ancient poet Alexis decreed that 'the best recipe for health is to apply sweet scents unto the brain.' The ancients employed a variety of herbal scents to treat different ailments. The fragrance of mint, for example, was thought to ease a stomach ache. Perfumes might also be applied directly to a wound to relieve inflamation and counter the ill odour of decay.

In the Middle Ages and later perfumes played a particularly important role during periods of plague. According to contemporary theories, plagues were caused by corrupt air, and transmitted from person to person through smell. The best ways to prevent such olfactory contagion were to avoid coming into contact with infectious odours and to counter the odours of disease with other pungent smells, such as perfumes and incense. The pomander — a small perforated container filled with spices and herbs and worn on the body — was meant to provide a continuous fragrant shield against disease.

In the late eighteenth and nineteenth centuries, however, many of the hitherto practical uses of perfume fell out of favour. As bathing became more popular, perfumes were no longer needed to mask stale body odours. The medicinal value of perfume was also questioned. Perfumes, in fact, were sometimes decried by physicians as actually leading to disease by clogging pores, or by enfeebling the mind and body through their vapours. The development of germ theory in the late 1800s largely put to rest the age-old idea of corrupt odours as agents of infection. Perfumes, consequently, were no longer considered by the medical profession to either prevent or cure disease.

The aesthetic use of perfume also declined during the same period. This was due in part to a backlash prompted by the French Revolution against the perfumed, luxurious lifestyle of the aristocracy. Furthermore, the rise of industrial capitalism encouraged the accumulation and display of tangible goods. In this culture of the concrete, the evanescent nature of perfumes made them a 'bad buy'. Countering this materialist trend were various nineteenth-century artistic and literary movements, notably that of the Symbolists, which lauded perfumes as stimuli to the imagination.

During the nineteenth century, perfumes, which had previously been worn by both sexes, became increasingly restricted to women. The supposedly frivolous nature of perfume was deemed to make fragrance more suitable for 'frivolous' women than for 'serious' men. Sweet floral scents, in particular, were considered appropriate for women, while men, if they wore any scent at all, were offered woodsy or spicy fragrances.

In the late twentieth century a number of developments have influenced the cultural role of perfumes. The growth of 'consumer capitalism', with its emphasis on enjoyment, rather than mere accumulation, of goods, has led to a surge in perfume use. While perfumes are still considered primarily the domain of women, the market for men's perfumes is continually expanding. Research is also being undertaken on how the selective employment of fragrances may influence behaviour, stimulating office workers to work more effectively or shoppers to buy more products. Finally, the medicinal use of perfume has made a comeback in the contemporary practice of aromatherapy, which utilizes fragrant essential oils to treat a range of physical and psychological ailments. These trends towards increased perfume use, however, are currently being combatted by an anti-perfume movement, which argues that many people find perfumes irritating and allergenic, and agitates for an 'odour-free' environment.

CONSTANCE CLASSEN

Further reading
Classen, C., Howes, D., and Synnott, A. (1994). *Aroma: the cultural history of smell.* Routledge, London.

Pericardium A conical bag which holds the HEART. There is an outer fibrous covering, and within this a more delicate membrane: a closed sac, into which the heart is invaginated from behind, so that the two layers of membrane are in contact with each other. There is thus a potential space between the layers, which may be expanded with fluid in the condition of *pericarditis*, or with blood in penetrating injuries; since there is no exit, accumulated fluid interferes with the pump action, and needs to be aspirated.   S.J.

See HEART.

Perineum The anatomical name for the 'crotch' region, including the anus and VULVA in the female and extending from the anus to the SCROTUM in the male. At a deeper level, layers of muscle and connective tissue form the 'floor' of the pelvic cavity which is penetrated by the anal canal (from the RECTUM) and urethra (from the BLADDER), and by the VAGINA in the female. The bony limits of the perineum are the pubic symphysis, in front (where the two pelvic bones join), and the coccyx behind.   S.J.

See PELVIS; PLATE 8

Peritoneum A membrane which lines the inside of the abdomen and covers its contents. The peritoneal *'cavity'* is an enclosed sac between the lining and the contents, and normally contains only sufficient fluid to lubricate the movement of the loops of the intestines, allowing them to slide freely over each other and against the inside of the abdominal wall. Disease of the stomach, intestines, or appendix which causes leakage or rupture (*perforation*) can result in dissemination of infected material throughout the cavity, causing *peritonitis*. Accumulation of fluid in the peritoneal cavity (*ascites*) occurs along with generalized OEDEMA in conditions such as heart failure or kidney failure.   S.J.

Personality The story of personality is, in many ways, the story of the secularization of the human soul. From early in its history, the term has been closely linked to notions of what it means to be a person. Before the middle of the nineteenth century, however, the connotations were distinctly non-psychological: personality referred to the distinction between persons and things, and it was the theological and ethical dimensions of PERSONHOOD that were paramount. Individual differences in preferences were discussed largely in terms of temperaments; personality, on the other hand, referred rather to what was deemed to be fundamental and universal, the moral and rational nature of the human subject. As the importance of religion within Western culture waned, however, the meaning of 'personality' shifted. In the wake of Romanticism's celebration of idiosyncratic individuality and the growing psychological/psychiatric interest in naturalistic investigations of mental abnormality, the term became reoriented decisively toward the individual and psychological.

By the turn of the century, the new clinically inspired theories of Emil Kraeplin, Sigmund Freud, Théodule Ribot, and Pierre Janet had made personality a concept of great interest, both within certain specialist circles and for the public at large. Adopted by the general public in the 1900s and by mainstream academic psychology in the 1920s and 1930s, the meanings of the term sedimented around the notion of personality as those qualities of an individual that persist across time and contexts and that distinguish that person from all others. Americans have been particularly fascinated with the composite nature of personality, its malleability, and its dynamic relations to the social environment; Europeans, on the other hand, have been more concerned with deep structures, fundamental continuities, and the internal aspects of its development.

For all of the differences in orientation, most personality research has been guided by the same fundamental questions: Is personality one thing or many? Is it relatively constant or does it vary across situations? Does it result from internal drives or external pressures? How does personality develop and how can it be changed? What are the relative influences of conscious and unconscious processes? And how does personality become pathological? Although the responses to these issues have been, and continue to be, extremely varied, they have tended to cluster around two poles associated with two different types of investigative sites: personality as a collection of distinguishable traits analysed via techniques drawn from the experimental laboratory, and personality as a holistic assessment of an individual's overall make-up, determined through close observation in a clinical setting.

Holistic depictions of personality received their most influential modern articulation in the psychoanalytic depth psychology of Freud and his followers. For Freud, individual personality is developmental, indeed almost archaeological; the accumulated product of an ultimately unresolvable conflict, beginning in infancy, between deep-seated sexual and aggressive drives associated with the id, and various defences against them arising from the ego and superego. Developed out of Freud's psychopathological work and oriented towards the ideal of the integrated personality, psychoanalytic theory stresses

the role of the unconscious and of repression in the formation of personality. Because of the presumed intransigence of the unconscious to reliable self-knowledge, psychoanalytic theory has relied for most of its data on clinical observation, although projective techniques, such as the Rorschach inkblot test, have also been developed to supplement direct analysis. In the hands of other depth psychologists — Carl Jung and Alfred Adler, among others — psychoanalytic theory has been pushed in a number of directions, mostly by shifting emphases from the sexual to other drives, from the unconscious to the conscious, or from the inner to the outer. Nonetheless, all have remained committed to the notion that personality as an integrated entity exists and that it can be causally explained within a framework that unites biological and psychosocial forces.

Counterpoised to these holistic approaches to personality have been various composite theories, arguing that personality is a collection of discrete traits which vary in degree from person to person and/or from situation to situation. Interest in trait theories has been high since the 1930s–40s, when factor analytic statistical techniques, and the development of assessment instruments such as the Minnesota Multiphasic Personality Inventory (MPPI) and the Myers-Briggs Type Indicator, allowed researchers to isolate and intercorrelate particular personality variables. Studies by Raymond Cattell and Hans Eysenck have been particularly prominent in this regard, and have helped produce the current consensus around a five-factor model of major personality elements: neuroticism, extraversion, agreeableness, conscientiousness, and openness to experience. While most researchers have assumed that personality traits such as these are *nomothetic* (equally applicable to all individuals) and vary only in degree, some recent work has argued for an *idiographic* or *contextualist* approach, seeing traits as individual- and situation-specific, with behaviour the product of environmental influences interacting with underlying characteristics.

Three other approaches to personality within psychology also bear mention. Physiological or biological theories have accounted for personality primarily on the basis of physical factors, such as body type (Ernst Kretschmer, William Sheldon) or genetic make-up (Dean Hamer). Stimulus–response or learning theories, including those of B. F. Skinner and Albert Bandura, have taken an opposite tack, explaining personality on the basis of external stimuli and the individual's responses to them. Within these theories, patterns of behaviour are believed to develop as the result of reinforcement of personal experiences or imitations of others, and differences between individuals derive from the varied sets of stimuli experienced from early childhood. Finally, in recent years the cognitive revolution has engendered social–cognitive theories that explain behaviour on the basis of internal representations of context-specific situations.

Behavioural consistency (personality) exists because most individuals operate on the basis of a small repertoire of interpretive schemas or scripts, which they then use to guide action in a wide variety of particular circumstances.

These academic constructions of personality, however, do not exhaust its post-Enlightenment resonances. Coming into vogue as part of a reaction against the heavily freighted Victorian conception of character, personality came within popular culture to signify more external affect than internal essence. In this guise, while personality has been in one respect understood as synonymous with identity, at the same time it has also been indicative of a kind of surface feature, a way of being seen by the external world rather than a reflection of an internal self. This tension between the internal and the external, and between the persistent and the contextual, visible as well within psychological theory, continues to characterize notions of personality up to the present day.

JOHN CARSON

Further reading

Danziger, K. (1997). *Naming the mind: how psychology found its language*. London.

Harré, R. and Lamb, R. (1986). *The dictionary of personality and social psychology*. Cambridge, MA.

Personhood Though often taken to be innate and intuitively obvious, the European concept of personhood is neither. The Western idea of the 'self' as a whole and independent entity developed over time, and was influenced by particular philosophical, legal, and religious traditions. 'Personhood' is not found in many dictionaries or reference works. *Manhood* is a much older term, signifying adulthood, maturity, virility, and legal independence. *Personhood*, as a genderless form of the same concept, is a relatively new category.

What constitutes and defines a person varies greatly from culture to culture, entailing different rights, duties, kinship bonds, and titles. Most attempts to define personhood recognize that the human person must extend beyond a merely biological basis to include some form of consciousness or rationality. In Western political and social discourses, we distinguish persons from animals and inanimate objects (rocks and computers, for example). This raises metaphysical questions about the identity of consciousness over time, about the identity of states of consciousness with particular bodies, and about how we differentiate ourselves from what is not ourselves. It also raises ethical questions. The concept of personhood allows us to isolate appropriate objects of moral concern — persons, as opposed to anything else, deserve or require moral recognition. The notion of personhood also allows us to differentiate amongst those that are appropriate, in so far as personhood may admit of degrees. One human being might be more or less a person than another. Hence a comatose patient could be considered less a person than an alert one, while a fetus might be thought of as less a person than an infant. Some people reject this last view, arguing that by any definition of 'person', a fetus qualifies. According to this argument, one can be a potential person.

Many cultures — the Kwakiutl Indians, Heiltsuk, and Bellacoola, among others — mark each stage of life with a new identity, a new name, and new relationships to the clan. Taoism and Buddhism emphasize the individual as a composite and historical being. Hindu and Buddhist cultures are among the many that believe in reincarnation, where a person is reborn as another person or animal after death. Many Native American cultures also believe that a person is the incarnation of his or her ancestors and animal spirits. Personhood in these traditions is more a process than a state or category of being. The person as actually embodying part of his or her ancestral past is foreign to Christian tradition. Modern gene theory posits a literal continuation between generations in a family. The idea of a spiritual continuation, however, is not part of the Western European tradition, which believes each SOUL to be individual and unique, the inhabitant of only one body.

The idea of a person as having an inner life and inner CONSCIOUSNESS arose largely through a Christian tradition, which held that every person has a soul, regardless of legal or social status; a serf, who had very little autonomy, still possessed his or her soul and was solely responsible for its salvation or damnation. Christianity thus helped to establish the idea of the person as not only a legal, but a moral entity. Protestantism emphasized the autonomy of the individual in relation to God. Interestingly, there have been debates throughout European history as to whether various groups, including Native Americans and women, have souls.

The Western legal concept of a person as a citizen of the state with both legal rights and responsibilities originated in ancient Rome. In Latin *persona* originally meant 'mask'. The term came to imply an identity, but one which was assumed, external, not entirely identical with the individual who wore it. A *persona* was a legal entity, someone with specific rights and responsibilities to the state. Slaves, for instance, were not 'persons' in ancient Rome. Where and how they worked, ate, and lived (and died) was determined by their owners. Nor were slaves considered to have ancestors or any form of property. The status of an enslaved woman's children has frequently been an issue throughout history, but is almost always determined by her owner or the laws of the ruling elite. John Locke, at the end of the seventeenth century, proposed that all people, by birth, were entitled to certain 'natural' rights of life, liberty, and property. This was a radically egalitarian notion, and much of European history since then can be seen as working out who is entitled to such 'personhood'.

Personhood and civil rights in the West are and have been associated with physical characteristics such as sex and race. The perceived physical inferiority of women, Jews, blacks, and Native Americans, among others, has served as the basis for denying these individuals the right to participate in legal society as full persons. Modern legal definitions of personhood include states of semi- or potential personhood. During the eighteenth century, for instance, the Three-Fifths Compromise in the Constitution of the United States posited that a slave counted as three-fifths of a person for purposes of representative government; and European laws of coverture maintained that women, children, and the mentally handicapped and insane, were legally represented or 'covered' by their guardians, husbands, fathers, and so forth. During the last two centuries, more and more of these categories of 'person' have been awarded legal and civil rights. Homosexual activists presently lobby for full civil rights, including the right to legal marriage. Few would now argue that homosexuals are not people, but the status of the fetus as a person is more controversial and has been the focus of much debate in the latter half of the twentieth century. In the case of ABORTION, an abstract and theological conception of personhood, specifically Aquinas' theory of the 'mediate animation' of the fetus, has been used in order to restrict the rights of pregnant women, who should also be considered persons. The right to life, be it the mother's or the fetus', is often considered paramount to all other rights.

Personhood is no doubt an open-ended concept that defies philosophic analysis in unclear cases. Given the cultural diversity and philosophical confusion surrounding the concept, some contemporary philosophers have questioned whether the notion of personhood is useful, or whether its definition is merely the product of prejudice and parochialism.

SARAH GOODFELLOW
ASHLEY E. PRYOR
BENJAMIN S. PRYOR

Further reading

Carrithers, M., Collins, S., and Lukes, S. (1985). *The category of the person: anthropology, philosophy, history.* Cambridge University Press, New York.

Perspiration
Evaporation of water from the skin surface, without the active secretion of sweat. This *insensible perspiration* is continuous and inevitable unless the environment is very humid, and in typical temperate zones it accounts for a loss of 300–400 ml daily in the average adult. Colloquially, the word perspiration is used euphemistically to avoid the smellier implications of sweat.
S.J.

See BODY FLUIDS; SWEATING.

Perversion
Sexual perversion is usually implicitly assumed to mean some kind of unnatural, abnormal form of sexual behaviour. As such, its meaning is particularly fluid, depending on the position of the person using it, and their assumptions about the natural and the normal. While there would probably be a fairly broad consensus in favour of declaring necrophiliac CANNIBALISM to be a perversion, very few forms of sexual practice have *not* been defined by someone, somewhere, as perversion.

Act versus object
Perversity can be broken down into two categories: perverse acts and perverse objects. Acts which involve some other use of the genitals beyond the insertion of the PENIS into the VAGINA followed by EJACULATION have often been categorized as perversions. MASTURBATION, either mutual or solitary, comes into this category, as does oral sex. The use of CONTRACEPTION to thwart the reproductive purpose of intercourse has also been defined as perverted. It might be supposed that the one act which can always be defined as the normal, natural thing is sexual intercourse intended for the begetting of children (or at least, without the deliberate interposition of means to prevent this happening) between two persons of opposite sexes married to one another. At least in the abstract this is the case, but when it comes down to the practical, even the most reproductively intentioned married couple may be engaging in something which someone could define as perversion. The very position which one society regards as almost too natural even to think about may be regarded by another as an obscene variation calculated to inflame sensuality.

Acts which may in themselves be regarded as either perverse or bordering upon perversity may, however, be considered permissible if they conduce to better reproductive sex between married couples. Catholic confessional manuals, and twentieth century works on MARRIAGE advice, have licensed practices such as clitoral titillation or oral sex, or variations in sexual position, provided these were performed with the intention of rendering intercourse either more likely to be fertile, or (in the latter example) to induce better bonding between the couple thus improving the stability of the institution of marriage. The manifesto for such attitudes was proclaimed by the Dutch gynaecologist Theodor Van de Velde in his *Ideal Marriage* (1926): 'Ideal Marriage permits normal, physiological activities the fullest scope, in all desirable and delectable ways', while banishing 'All that is morbid, all that is perverse'. The 'full range of contact and connection between human beings, for sexual intercourse' was clearly marked as pertaining 'exclusively to normal intercourse between opposite sexes'. Thus Van de Velde was able to provide detailed instructions for preliminary 'love-play' and for variant positions suitable for different occasions, while firmly closing the door on the 'Hell-gate of the Realm of Sexual Perversions'.

While this does open up the possibility of acts being (perversely) indulged in for their own sake as a means of selfish gratification rather than the enhancement of a relationship, it also moves the question from the issue of the acts to that of the object. Perversity thus becomes not merely a matter of using the genitals in a 'wrong' way, but also of experiencing sexual feelings towards some object considered to be unnatural: for example, the body of an individual of the same gender, an animal, or some item of apparel, which are, under the rubric of 'the natural', not supposed to be endowed with erotic allure. However, even this became an area open to finesse: with the rise of the notion of 'congenital inversion' (an inborn homosexual tendency), sexologists made a distinction between 'inverted sexual practices' innately normal to those engaging in them, and 'perversions' indulged in for sensual variety by those who had no such excuse. Some cultures permit certain forms of homosexual interaction, and even ritualize these to some extent, while not having any category for homosexual relationships outside those bounds. This can be seen, for example, in societies where there is an accepted role of effeminate male homosexual, or which accept age-differentiated relationships between men and adolescent boys with an assumed pedagogic purpose. Behaviour which transgresses these structural norms, however, may be stigmatized.

The perverse and 'normality'

A perhaps more 'modern' way of considering perversion has been to place the defining barrier around the quality of the relationship. Something which leads to a reciprocal and mutually meaningful relationship between two individuals (whatever their gender and practices) may be regarded as natural and healthy. Impersonal acts and those unlikely to result in the formation of a pair-bond are thus still assigned to the realm of the perverse. The implicit model remains, of course, heterosexual matrimony.

Early sexologists both created and tried to defuse the question of the perverse by differentiating practices which were a distortion or a corruption of the sexual instinct from those which were (however deplorable), an exaggeration of 'natural' tendencies. This latter category could include manifestations of excessive sexual desire, exhibitionism and voyeurism, and the milder forms of fetishism and sadomasochism (particularly where the latter fitted received notions of male aggression and female passivity). However, as pioneer British sexologist Havelock Ellis pointed out, nearly all so-called perversions were capable of being interpreted as exaggerations of some tendency within 'normal' SEXUALITY.

Most of the practices defined as perverse have been and are still found either exclusively or much more commonly among men. This may represent women's lack of opportunities, since, in most societies throughout history, if not confined to marriage and motherhood, their only other role has been that of prostitute, indulging male quirks of desire rather than manifesting their own. Some female 'perversions', such as desire for clitoral stimulation, have been quite clearly defined by male assumptions about the appropriate form of female sexual satisfaction: indeed active sexual desire in the female has been interpreted as 'perverse'. Since discussions

of sexuality have often focused on women, it is therefore interesting to note that descriptions of 'perversion' are more likely to deal with men.

LESLEY A. HALL

See also FETISHISM; SADOMASOCHISM; SEXUAL ORIENTATION.

Petit mal is a specific form of EPILEPSY, characterized by a transient, subtle impairment of consciousness, occurring mainly in children. By contrast with *grand mal*, it does not involve complete loss of consciousness, falling, and whole body convulsions. The condition is perhaps best epitomized by its alternative name, *absence seizure*. This denotes the period of some 3–30 seconds duration in which ongoing motor activities such as talking, eating, or walking cease and the sufferer stares ahead, seemingly unseeing, unhearing, and uncommunicative, and there may be automatism consisting of repeated but aimless movements; the eyelids may flicker at about three cycles per second. The actual level of awareness within episodes and between patients may differ, from one of total unresponsiveness to questions, to a limited ability to repeat number strings or names or a familiar recitation but no recollection of this at the end of the episode. In excess of thirty such 'absences' can occur in a day but may go unrecognized even by parents until such inattention becomes noticed at school.

A remarkable, in fact diagnostic, feature of petit mal is the generalized electrical seizure of the CEREBRAL CORTEX that is detectable in the electroencephalogram (EEG) (or in its recent counterpart the ELECTROMAGNETOGRAM) recorded from electrodes on the overlying scalp. Unlike the normal, low amplitude rhythms of 20–50 microvolts, such as the alpha rhythm with a limited spatial distribution on the scalp, the electrical seizure is detected all over the scalp, is several fold greater in amplitude, and consists of bilaterally synchronous 'spike and wave' complexes repeating at about three times per second, with the spikes more prominent in the frontal regions. As well as accompanying an attack, brief episodes of such activity lasting 1–2 seconds can occur without overt behavioural signs, except brief hesitancies in counting that an investigator would seek to detect. The condition is of unknown cause and thus described as one form of *idiopathic epilepsy*; its onset is typically in childhood or early adolescence, the frequency of the episodes declining in adulthood, often to be replaced by more generalized CONVULSIONS.

TOM SEARS

See also CONVULSIONS; EPILEPSY.

pH The negative logarithm of the hydrogen ion concentration [H^+] in mols/litre. Lower pH therefore means greater acidity, and vice versa. Extracellular fluid (ECF), including the blood, is normally at a pH close to 7.4 which means [H^+] = $10^{-7.4}$ mols/litre, or 40 nanomoles/litre. At body temperature, neutral pH would be approximately 6.8; body fluids are therefore on the alkaline side of neutral. Control mechanisms

normally keep ECF pH within 0.04 of the norm either way. The pH inside cells is more acid, and more variable, related to metabolic activity.   S.J.

See ACID–BASE HOMEOSTASIS.

Phagocytes In the 1880s, Metchnikoff, a Russian zoologist, gave the name *phagocytosis* (Greek *phago*; to eat) to the way in which a single cell organism, such as an amoeba, takes into it a solid item from its environment by extending '*pseudopodia*' (false feet) that engulf it. He saw that some 'white' cells in the blood of animals ingested bacteria comparably, and that there was more of this going on in animals who had a recent infection. He proposed that these 'phagocytes' were the essential means of defence against invaders. In the first decade of the twentieth century, Metchnikoff was to share a Nobel prize with Ehrlich for work on immunity, whilst George Bernard Shaw took the theory on stage in *The Doctor's Dilemma* with the physician declaring 'we must stimulate the phagocytes'!

Metchnikoff was right to assign importance to the phagocytes, as part of the IMMUNE SYSTEM as it is now understood: they are confirmed to be unique among body cells in their function as 'killers'. But Shaw also anticipated later knowledge: part of the immune response does indeed involve 'stimulation' of phagocytes, in the sense that they kill under orders from the lymphocytes that identify the invader.

The cells whose main function is phagocytosis arise initially from the bone marrow. There are two main groups: the type of white blood cells known as *polymorphs* (polymorphonuclear leucocytes — those with multi-lobed nuclei); and *macrophages* that derive from the *monocytes* in the blood. Cells of the monocyte–macrophage system can move in and out of the circulation by squeezing between the endothelial cells that constitute capillary walls. Substances released at sites of INFECTION or INJURY attract such cells by chemotaxis: many different types of cells can produce a variety of related proteins known as *cytokines* and these in turn mediate a variety of inflammatory and defence mechanisms, including the attraction of both types of phagocytes. Phagocytes themselves also secrete cytokines, which influence the behaviour of other cells.

When a phagocyte ingests a potentially dangerous MICROORGANISM, it is dealt with in a set of compartments within the cell, equipped with enzymes and other substances that take hold of it, distort it, release lethal FREE RADICALS, and break down the remains.

Polymorphs mostly ingest bacteria, gathering at the site of localized infections such as pustules and abcesses; when pus forms, it is a collection of phagocytes which have died in the defence against more widespread invasion. Their numbers increase in the circulating blood during most types of more generalized bacterial infection.

Macrophages do not only ingest and destroy bacteria, viruses, inorganic foreign particles, and cellular debris. Some also act as 'antigen presenting cells', when peptide components of invaders are recognized on their surface and locked onto by antigen-specific lymphocytes; they provoke both the cellular and humoral components of the *immune response*. They also serve to pick up debris from the normal turnover of body cells, and dust particles inhaled into the lungs.

As well as the polymorphs and macrophages, there are cells that do not originate in the bone marrow, nor travel in the bloodstream, which can also act as phagocytes. Cells that line blood vessels and the blood sinuses of the liver and spleen (*endothelial cells*), and supportive (*reticular*) cells in lymphoid tissue, can all ingest foreign particles and cell debris. This dispersed group of cells gave rise to the term *reticuloendothelial system*.   SHEILA JENNETT

See also BLOOD; IMMUNE SYSTEM; INFECTIOUS DISEASES; LYMPHATIC SYSTEM.

Phallic symbol

'The derisive remark was once made against psychoanalysis that the unconscious sees a PENIS in every convex object and a VAGINA or anus in every concave one,' observed the Hungarian psychoanalyst Sandor Ferenczi, adding, 'I find this sentence well characterizes the facts.' For large sections of the lay public, and particularly for its opponents, psychoanalysis, from its earliest days, has indeed seemed to rely almost exclusively on sexual and genital symbolism. With the passing of psychoanalysis as a central mode of psychotherapy, jokes about shrinks seeing a phallus in every cigar have become rather less topical. For those seriously interested in the theories and techniques of psychoanalysis, however, the interpretation of symbols remains important and it is, of course, crucial for those interested in approaching literary or artistic works from a classical psychoanalytic angle. Even for historians and others who are interested in psychoanalysis only from a scholarly perspective, Freudian symbolism is a rich source of insights into the psychoanalytic *Weltanschauung*.

The subject of psychoanalytic symbolism is vast and, contrary to popular ideas, not all psychoanalytic symbols are necessarily sexual. According to Freud, dream-symbols refer to 'the human body as a whole, parents, children, brothers and sisters, birth, death, nakedness'. Sex, however, *is* of cardinal importance to psychoanalysts, and sexual symbolism (especially the symbolism of the male genitalia) has preoccupied a large number of practitioners.

As defined by Freud, a symbol is sensorial and concrete in itself, although the idea(s) it represents may be relatively abstract and complex. A symbol has multiple meanings and some resemblance to what it is supposed to represent, which in most cases is an unacknowledged idea or one the individual is not conscious of. Symbols appear in thought most readily when the individual is tired, experiencing neurotic problems, or dreaming. Dreams, Freud believed, represented the royal road to the unconscious, and 'symbolism', he asserted, 'is perhaps the most remarkable

chapter of the theory of dreams.' It is in the interpretation of dreams that psychoanalytic symbolism has been most prominent, most colourful, and, for the hostile or the flippant, most risible. 'The range of things which are given symbolic representation in dreams', Freud pointed out, 'is not wide ... but the symbols for them are extremely numerous.' The most apparently diverse dream-imagery, therefore, often turned out to indicate the same thing.

In recent years, psychoanalysis has been described as phallocentric and there is much evidence for this in Freud's discussion of dream-representations of the penis, which he described, seemingly without a trace of irony, as 'the more striking and for both sexes the more interesting component of the genitals.' The most basic phallic symbols in dreams were those resembling the organ in shape: sticks, umbrellas, posts, trees. Another kind of phallic symbol was provided by objects that could penetrate or injure: knives, daggers, or spears. Firearms belonged to both sets because of their shape and because they could injure. Other symbols of the phallus were provided by 'objects from which water flows' (taps, fountains, watering-cans) or by 'objects which are capable of being lengthened', which Freud exemplified with hanging lamps and extensible pencils.

Yet other symbols that the penis could be represented by were 'balloons, flying-machines and most recently by Zeppelin airships' because they all shared the 'remarkable characteristic of the male organ ... to rise up in defiance of the laws of gravity'. The same symbolic relation was expressed when the individual dreamt of flying: here, the phallus was treated 'as the essence of the dreamer's whole person' and the individual became one giant, flying, erection. Why, then, did women have dreams of flying? 'Remember', Freud urged, 'that our dreams aim at being the fulfilments of wishes and that the wish to be a man is found so frequently, consciously or unconsciously, in women. Nor will anyone with a knowledge of anatomy be bewildered by the fact that it is possible for women to realize this wish through the same sensations as men. Women possess as part of their genitals a small organ similar to the male one; and this small organ, the clitoris, actually plays the same part in childhood and during the years before sexual intercourse as the large organ in men.'

Symbols that were, according to Freud, unquestionably phallic but could not be easily classified into a group were hats, overcoats, neckties ('which hang down and are not worn by women'), cloaks, reptiles, fishes, 'and above all the famous symbol of the snake'. Woods and bushes, predictably enough, symbolized pubic hair in both sexes.

For comparative purposes, it might be appropriate here to briefly list the symbolic representations of the female genitalia. 'The complicated topography of the female genital parts', observed Freud, 'makes one understand how it is that they are often represented as landscapes, with rocks,

woods and water, while the imposing mechanism of the male sexual apparatus explains why all kinds of complicated machinery which is hard to describe serve as symbols for it'. The female genitals could also be represented by 'all such objects as share their characteristic of enclosing a hollow space which can take something into itself'. Pits, cavities, vessels, bottles, boxes, jewel-cases, trunks, pockets, ships, cupboards, rooms, and, by slight extension, churches and chapels all fell under this category. (Keys opening locked rooms, however, were definitely male.) Among animals, 'snails and mussels at least are undeniably female symbols' and among bodily parts the mouth represented the genital orifice. The BREASTS were commonly symbolized in dreams and 'these like the larger hemispheres of the female body, are represented by apples, peaches and fruit in general'. Flowers, however, always indicated the female genitals and often the idea of VIRGINITY; so did gardens. Sometimes in dreams, female symbols could represent the male genitals and vice versa; only the most clearly differentiated symbols (weapons, pockets, or trunks) were used constantly without any ambiguity. Sexual intercourse itself was not very prominent in the symbolic world, being represented by images of rhythmic activity (such as dancing or riding), violent experiences (being run over), being threatened with weapons, or climbing ladders or stairs.

What was the epistemic basis of these interpretations? The patient, after all, usually had no idea about the symbolic dimensions of his dreams and one could suspect that the analyst was dreaming up the interpretations.

Characteristically refusing to restrict himself to lofty medical or psychological discourse, Freud declared that the meanings of dream-symbols were far from imaginary: similar but far more easily understood symbols were found in fairy-tales, myths, jokes, idioms, sayings, songs, and folklore. 'If we go into these sources in detail, we shall find so many parallels to dream-symbolism that we cannot fail to be convinced of our interpretations.' There is certainly a grain of truth in this claim and, whatever one might think of the truth of psychoanalytic doctrine, one would probably acknowledge that the folklore of most cultures as well as their popular discourses were often crowded with genital symbolism. Such symbols are continually added to the cultural repertoire and used in ever more imaginative or ludicrous ways. Some of the more modern instances have been influenced, explicitly or unwittingly by psychoanalysis. Although Freud was none too pleased with the French Surrealists' interest in psychoanalysis in the 1920s, quite a large proportion of Surrealist imagery — one thinks, for instance, of the phallic neckties of Breton, the noses of Dali, and the bones of Tanguy — derived from Freudian symbolism. In a broader cultural sense, Freudian symbolism and, in particular, interpretations of phallic imagery, have become pervasive in fiction, the arts, and the media to the point of banality.

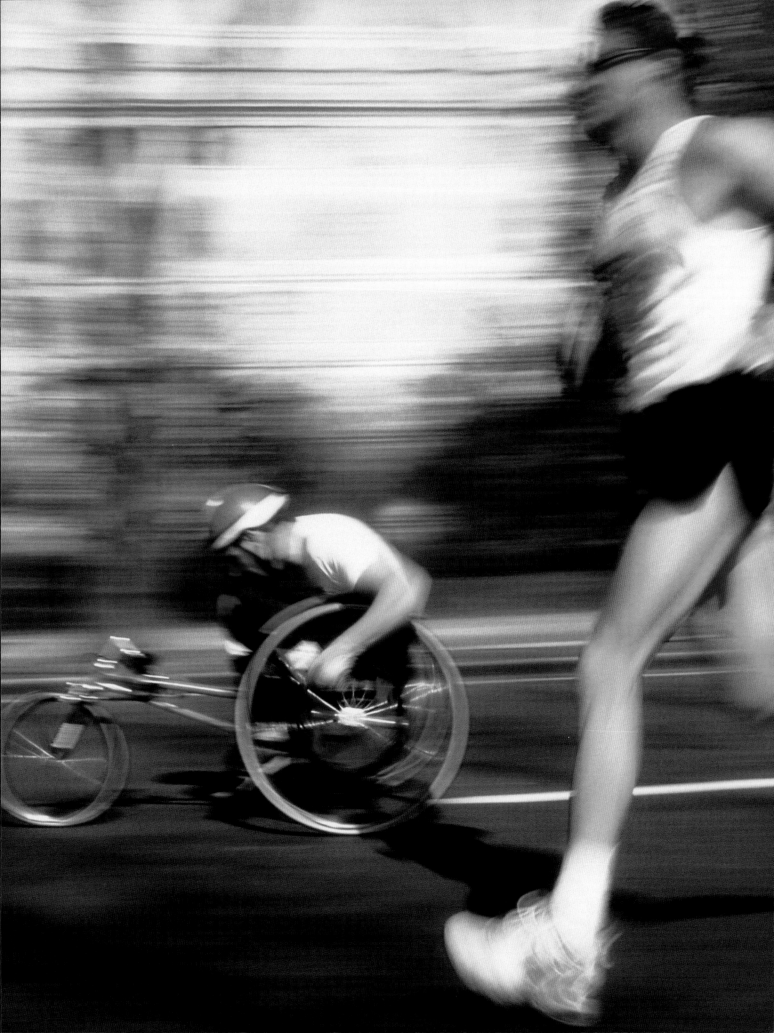

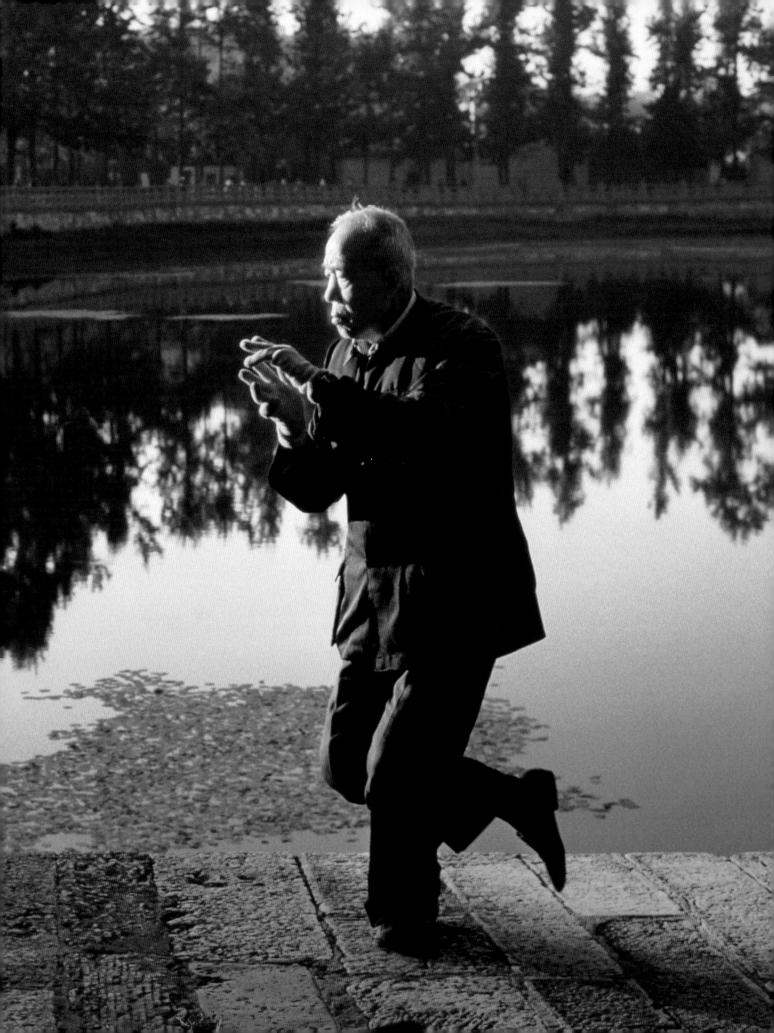

'Sometimes', Freud is supposed to have warned, 'a cigar is only a cigar!' The attribution of that story is dubious; its moral is not.

CHANDAK SENGOOPTA

Further reading
Freud, S. (1900/1953). The interpretation of dreams. In *The standard edition of the complete psychological works of Sigmund Freud*, Vols 4, 5 (ed. J. Strachey *et al.*). Hogarth Press, London.
Freud, S. (1915–16/1961) Introductory lectures on psycho-analysis. In *Standard Edition*, Vol. 15, (ed. J. Strachey *et al.*). Hogorth Press, London.

See also CLITORIS; DREAMING; PENIS.

Phantom limb

After loss of a limb more than 90% of patients experience a vivid illusory persistence of the limb in the form of a 'phantom'. The phantom appears immediately in the majority and after a delay of a few days or weeks in the rest. It can then persist for months, years, or even decades.

The phantom often has a 'habitual' position (for example a phantom arm may be partially flexed at the elbow with the forearm pronated) but spontaneous changes in its posture are common. The extent to which voluntary and involuntary movements occur in the phantom varies from patient to patient.

Phantoms can appear not only for a limb, but for almost any body part: breast, penis, face, jaw, or even for internal organs. Patients can experience phantom menstrual cramps after hysterectomy, the spasmodic pain of appendicitis after appendectomy, or ulcer pains after gastrectomy; even phantom erections have been reported after the penis is removed.

The term 'phantom limb' was coined in 1872 by Silas Weir-Mitchell, who published the first paper on this subject anonymously for fear of ridicule by his peers. Since then a fascinating clinical lore has built up and there have been hundreds of case studies. But a systematic scientific study began only towards the end of the twentieth century. Animal studies have combined with systematic psychophysical testing and brain imaging in human amputees, to move the study of phantom limbs from vague clinical phenomenology into an era of experimental research.

The phantom is enhanced by the presence of referred sensations: stimuli applied to other parts of the body that are experienced as arising from the phantom. For example, after arm amputation, touching the face will often evoke precisely localized sensations in the phantom fingers, hand, and arm. The points that evoke such sensations are topographically organized (consistently 'mapped') and the referral is modality-specific, meaning for instance that heat on the face will elicit heat in the phantom digits and that vibration is felt as vibration. This face-to-phantom-hand referral probably occurs because the face is right next to the hand in the complete map of the whole body's skin surface on the somatosensory region of the CEREBRAL CORTEX (described as a result of electrical brain stimulation studies by neurosurgeon Wilder Penfield in the 1930s).

The sensory input from the face skin ordinarily activates only the face area of the cortex, but if the adjacent hand cortex is denervated (cut off from any sensory input), then the input from the face starts activating the original hand area as well. This is a striking demonstration of plasticity in the adult human brain: that new neural links can be made. The observation also implies that even though the hand area is now being activated by sensory input from the face skin, higher brain centres still continue to interpret the signals as arising from the hand. Changes in somatosensory cortex topography — occurring over distances of 2–3 cm — have also been shown in the same patients using functional brain imaging techniques — especially magnetoencephalography (MEG); this allows researchers to correlate perceptual phenomena described by the patient (such as referred sensations) with the anatomical sites of activity.

These demonstrations of 'plasticity' in the adult brain can also be seen in monkeys in which one arm has been deafferented (all sensory nerve pathways interrupted). Indeed, the human studies were inspired by the animal experiments.

Sensations may also be referred the other way around between the hand and the face, after the trigeminal nerve that supplies the face is cut — an occasional last resort for severe neuralgia. The patient then has a map of the face on the hand. Again, after leg amputation, stimuli applied to the genitals are referred to the phantom foot. This is consistent with the representation of the foot next to the genitals in Penfield's original maps of the somatosensory cortex.

Vivid 'movements' in the phantom are reported by some patients. These sensations are very 'real' to the patient — so much so that volitional movements of the phantom hand can interfere with a dissimilar movement performed by the normal hand, in a manner identical to the interference between hands that occurs in normal people. The patient cannot for example rub his belly with his real hand while 'tapping his head' simultaneously with the phantom. These movement sensations in the phantom probably arise from 'feed forward' or corollary discharge: when the motor areas of the patient's cerebral cortex send a command to the missing arm, a copy of the command is sent to the cerebellum and parietal lobes so that intention can be compared with action. These commands may initially be experienced as movements, but the prolonged absence of visual confirmation, and of sensory input from muscles and joints of the missing arm, may lead eventually to a 'paralysed' phantom that the patient can no longer move.

Sometimes the phantom will develop a painful clenching spasm and the patient cannot voluntarily 'unclench' his imagined fist even with intense effort. If a mirror is propped up vertically on the table, in the plane that separates the right from the left half of the body, and if the patient views the reflection of his normal hand in the mirror, the reflection of the hand is seen superimposed on the felt position of the phantom — giving the visual illusion that the phantom has been resurrected. If he now moves the normal hand the phantom is suddenly 'animated' and is vividly felt to move. Sometimes this can lead to the unclenching of a previously clenched, painful phantom, suggesting a promising new therapeutic approach for phantom pain. The usefulness of the procedure requires detailed evaluation, but the illusion suggests that a great deal of interaction can occur between visual sensations and those from the limb.

Phantom limbs are also seen in a small percentage of patients with congenitally missing arms or legs, suggesting that at least the basic scaffolding for one's body image may be innately specified. Indeed, the phenomenon provides a valuable opportunity to investigate how nature and nurture interact in the construction of body image by the brain. A patient with leprosy whose hand gets whittled away gradually with progressive sensory loss does *not* have a phantom hand. But if the stump is then amputated, what emerges is not a phantom stump but a whole phantom hand. It is as though the original image of the hand had survived but was inhibited by the stump, only to be resurrected when the stump is amputated!

In summary, at least four factors seem to contribute to the vividness of the phantom: *stump neuromas* (nodules of scar tissue and curled up nerve endings); remapping of somatosensory areas in the brain leading to referred sensations; a genetically-specified 'body image' that partially survives limb loss; and monitoring of corollary discharge associated with motor commands sent to the phantom. The combination of systematic psycho-physical testing with brain imaging techniques in human amputees, together with animal studies on somatosensory remapping, has rapidly advanced the study of phantom limbs. Such research will allow investigation not only of how the brain remodels itself continuously in response to bodily injury, but also how the activity in the brain somatosensory 'map' leads to conscious experience of body image and somatic sensations.

J. VAID
V. S. RAMACHANDRAN

Further reading
Melzack, R. (1992). Phantom limbs. *Scientific American*, **266**, 120–6.
Ramachandran, V. S. (1998). The perception of phantom limbs: the D. O. Hebb lecture. *Brain*, 121, 1603–30.

See also AMPUTATION; BODY IMAGE; CEREBRAL CORTEX; MAGNETIC BRAIN STIMULATION; PAIN; PROPRIOCEPTION; SOMATIC SENSATION.

Phantom pregnancy

or *pseudocyesis*, is a well-known phenomenon to dog owners. It may be observed also in humans, though rarely. Women with phantom pregnancies stop having periods, have enlarged breasts and a distended abdomen, and may complain of nausea. It may be more common in cultures in which there are especially strong social pressures on women to produce babies.

J.N.

Elderly man practising Tai Chi by Green Lake, Kunming, China. Stone.

535

Pharmacology deals with all aspects of the actions of drugs on living tissues, particularly their effects on man. Drugs' actions, both at the molecular level (interaction of drug molecules with receptors) and also at the macroscopic or whole-body level (such as drug effects on the cardiovascular system), are considered. The subject can be divided into two main sections; *pharmacodynamics* and *pharmacokinetics*. The first is concerned with how the effects of a drug are generated, while the second is concerned with how drugs are distributed around the body, how they are metabolized, and how they are finally excreted or eliminated from the body. Discovery of new drugs proceeds by considering how chemical agents can be used to potentiate, inhibit, or modify some cellular or bodily process.   A.W.C.

See DRUGS.

Pharmacy derives its name from the Greek root *pharmakon*, a drug. Pharmacy is concerned with the manufacture, formulation, quality control, and dispensing of medicaments used to treat disease. The majority of modern medicaments consist of tablets, capsules, and injections, all produced under stringent conditions. Usually only a tiny part of the product is active drug, the rest being the 'excipient' which provides an appropriate vehicle for delivery to the patient. Many old-fashioned forms of medication — such as mixtures, tinctures, decoctions, elixirs, emulsions, and syrups — have now virtually disappeared, reducing the requirement for extemporaneous manufacture of products by dispensing pharmacists.   A.W.C.

See DRUGS.

Pharynx Derived from the Greek for throat, the pharynx is the continuous space behind the nose and the mouth that leads down both to the passage for food and to the passage for air. It has three parts; nasal, oral, and laryngeal. As well as being open to the nose, the *nasopharynx* is connected to the middle ears by the eustachian (pharyngotympanic) tubes. A passage behind the soft palate leads down to the oral part. When looking at the back of the throat, the arch that can be seen behind the uvula centrally, and behind the tonsils at the sides, is a muscular fold around the opening into the *oropharynx*. Further down behind the base of the tongue, where the epiglottis stands guard in front of the entry into the larynx (the glottis), the *laryngeal* part of the pharynx leads down behind that opening to reach the oesophagus. In the wall of the pharynx there are pairs of muscles that join at the centre back and encircle it to reach various attachments in front, including the hyoid bone at the base of the tongue and the cartilage of the 'Adam's apple'. These muscles can constrict the passages, change the shape of the spaces, or help to close off the different apertures in the various ways that are necessary, for example, during swallowing, speaking, singing, or blowing.   SHEILA JENNETT

See PLATE 3.

See also EPIGLOTTIS; LARYNX; NOSE; SWALLOWING; TONGUE.

Phenotype *Pheno* derives from the Greek for *display*: the phenotype is the manifestation of the genetic make-up of the individual.

'Old Blue Eyes' was the name given by many to Frank Sinatra. Having blue eyes is a trait that was part of his phenotype and is genetically determined, dependent on the genetic material derived from both parents. Of course a person's parents do not necessarily both have the same coloured eyes, and an individual may receive eye colour genes specifying different colours from their mother and father. In this situation one gene has *dominance* over the other gene, which is said to be *recessive*. Recessive genes can of course be passed on to progeny, and may be expressed in the next generation if dominance is not present.

Eye colour and hair colour are simple traits, but much more complex traits, such as general body form and appearance, result from the complex interplay of many genes derived from both parents. Many children grown up to look very like their mother or father, while most resemble neither very closely because of the considerable mix of the genetic material. *Nuture* is also able to modify the phenotype — for example, someone with the genetic make-up to express an obese phenotype would not do so if malnourished.

Some *diseases* that have a genetic basis give rise to unusual phenotypes. For example, children born with cystic fibrosis have inherited an abnormal gene from both parents that results in inappropriate secretions in many hollow organs, such as the lungs, intestine, gall bladder, or pancreas. This abnormal phenotype is usually not expressed by either of the parents, each of whom has one normal gene which is dominant and one abnormal gene which is recessive. The child receiving a set of two abnormal genes, one from each parent, will express these and show the abnormal phenotype.   ALAN W. CUTHBERT

See also GENETICS, HUMAN; HEREDITY.

Pheromones like HORMONES, are secretions that act as chemical signals. While hormones change the behaviour of target cells elsewhere in the body, pheromones are odours that 'carry stimulation' (from the Greek *phero* and *horma*) and change the behaviour of other creatures of the same species that pick up the scent. Pheromones are widespread in the animal world, from the single-celled amoeba to human beings. A classic example is the pheromone emitted by female gypsy moths, which can be detected by SENSORY RECEPTORS on the antennae of a male moth 1 Km or more away, enabling it to home in on the female. Unspayed female dogs can attract males from a similar distance. Ants have a 'lexicon' of different pheromones, which they use to elicit attacks on or flight from predators, to mark trails, and so on. Territorial mammals often mark their territory with pheromones in their urine, or rubbed on to 'scenting posts' from glands in their skin. There seems to be genetically determined variation of pheromones among individuals of some species, enabling them to recognise mates, offspring or intruders on their territory. Although humans appear to have lost much of the olfactory sensitivity of their mammalian ancestors, recent research suggests that body odours, not necessarily consciously perceived, play an important role in social interaction. Human sweat acquires a distinctive odour at puberty, but urine, as well as genital secretions, may also contain pheromones. The well-known synchronization of the menstrual cycles of nuns and girls at boarding school is probably mediated by odour, and there is evidence that smell enables mothers to distinguish their own children's clothing from that worn by others. Sexual preference is certainly influenced by smell: love may indeed be largely a matter of 'chemistry'.

COLIN BLAKEMORE

See also BODY ODOUR; TASTE AND SMELL.

Philosophy and the body The human body occupies an ambiguous, even a paradoxical role in cultural categorizations — from the cosmologies of the archaic societies to the concepts and practices of modern Western civilization. It is the most obvious and familiar visible 'thing' perceived, and yet tends to disappear in the very act of perception of, or relation to, the outside world. The ambiguous nature of the body may be formulated in a number of binary oppositions. The body is both the Same and the Other; both a subject and an object of practices and knowledge; it is both a tool and a raw material to be worked upon. The body appears to oscillate between presence and absence, most paradoxically in intense feelings — feelings as sensations and feelings as EMOTIONS. The body seems to be simultaneously the subject of highly articulated utterance and yet at perpetual risk of disappearing from our awareness.

As an element in cultural categorizations, the role of the human body goes far beyond its concrete physical boundaries. It acts as the basic model for cosmological schemes. This is obvious in the overt ANTHROPOMORPHISM of 'primitive' cosmologies. Less obviously, however, it may be detected in the basic scheme by which the order of the outside world is related to that of the inside in the macrocosm–microcosm model which has been so central in Western cultural tradition since Greek antiquity.

Body and …

From the start, the human body as a topic of both religious and philosophical thought has been structured in terms of distinction and difference — which derives from the very intellectual act of defining the body as an object of knowledge. Thinking about the body necessarily implies a vantage point which lies outside the body and is not identical with it. All the dualistic conceptions of the 'body and x' (where x = spirit, soul, mind, reason, psyche, or self) — prominent in the Western tradition — have their roots in this basic constellation, which allocates the vantage point to a perceiving and comprehending CONSCIOUSNESS viewing the body from a position which is logically, if not always spatially, detached.

This consciousness cannot grasp its own end (death), despite being fundamentally consciousness of death's inevitability. Consequently, even the prehistoric peoples believed in an aspect distinct from the body and residing in it: a spirit or soul which, according to an anthropomorphic scheme, was projected to all beings of the world. In animistic thinking, all these beings (humans, animals, trees, and stones) had a 'soul' or 'spirit' (*anima*), and thus they conceived of these beings as 'living'. However, the fixed point of anthropomorphism was located in the mystery of the life and death of the human body. Following E. B. Tylor it could be said that the distinction of body and 'soul' is determined in the relationship between the animate and the inanimate body. The soul is the outcome of the subtraction between them.

This is the basic distinction which is not yet linked to the distinction of material versus immaterial. Actually, in animistic thought the spirit was conceived of as a material (fluid) substance. Traces of this mode of thinking are found even in the EUCHARIST formula equating the two distinctions of body/soul and body/blood of Christ. Such 'materialism' is characteristic of the earlier stages of the Christian tradition — from the early Hebrews, who apparently had a concept of the 'soul' but did not separate it from the body, to the subsequent Old Testament formulations of the soul relating it to the concept of BREATH. Breath and blood are the two essential remainders of the live/dead subtraction, and it is worth noting that the term 'breath' in many languages refers also to 'spirit', which, not by accident, also indicates a fluid consistency.

The basic live/dead distinction does not necessarily imply the distinction of mortal versus immortal, even though the impossibility of comprehending the discontinuity of consciousness — while witnessing the decay of the body — involves a strong tendency to make such a connection. Both the difference between these two distinctions and their close relationship was manifested in the ancient Egyptian and Chinese ideas of a dual soul. The Egyptian *ka* (breath) survived death but remained near the body while the spiritual *ba* proceeded to the region of the dead. Similarly, the ancient Chinese distinguished between a lower, sensitive soul, which disappears with death, and a rational principle, the *hun*, which survives and joins the realm of ancestors.

Even the Old Testament — relating the soul to breath — lacks a distinction of the ethereal soul and the corporeal body: the strong formulation of a body/soul dichotomy actually originated with the ancient Greeks and was introduced into Christianity by St Gregory of Nyssa and St Augustine in the fourth and fifth centuries. In fact the major Greek influence on Christianity was Plato's and the Neo-Platonists' understanding of the soul as immaterial and incorporeal substance. This was the junction in which two of the aforementioned distinctions merged: the duality of material versus immaterial was linked to the duality of temporal (or discontinuity) versus eternal (or continuity). This is where the 'body vs. x' dualism — x being either soul, spirit (now immaterialized), or mind — is constituted in a stronger sense; it recurs thereafter in a variety of formulations within the Western philosophical and religious tradition.

However, this is not to say that the variety of attempts to solve the metaphysical 'body vs. x' dilemma did not include a number of reductionistic 'solutions' in which the other pole of the dualism is brought back to or subsumed under its opposite, which is thus defined as the primary being or substance. Such solutions were proposed within both idealist and materialist traditions, but more obviously in the latter (crudely: from Epicureans to behaviourists). On the other hand the philosophical tradition also contains attempts to overcome the dualism — while at the same time maintaining it — by means of a third entity which brings the two poles together, into a unity.

From body-mind dualism …

Thus it was, for example, when the paradigmatic figure of the body/mind dualism, René Descartes (1596–1650), formulated the absolute distinction between mental and material substance. The characteristic of the former was consciousness or 'thinking' (*res cogitans*) while the characteristic of the latter was that of occupying space (*res extensa*). He still needed a third entity to bring these two poles together: God. Then again, it should be noted that the Cartesian body/mind dualism defines the latter pole (mind) in a manner which distinguishes it both from the older idea of an immaterial soul and from the sense of the term 'mind', referring in broader terms to the whole human psyche, which was formulated and taken into use from the nineteenth century onwards. Descartes' concept of the 'mind' includes the acts of pure intellect and of will but excludes all the other aspects of the psyche — sensations, imagination, and emotions — which are located in the body and operate in the interactive and intermediate realm, bringing the body into a close relationship not only with the mind but also with the external world. So separate status is given only to the pure thought of the individual capable of controlling himself through acts of will — and being linked to the body only via the third entity (God). All the other dimensions of the mind — in the contemporary, broad sense — are conceived of both as bodily processes, in a manner corresponding to the materialism of humoral medicine, and as components involved in the interaction between the mind and body. In this respect Descartes' interactionist stance differs from some later Cartesian formulations, according to which there can be no direct interaction between mind and body and any instances of mind affecting body or vice versa must be explained as a result of God's intervention on the specific occasion.

Benedict Spinoza (1632–77) modified the Cartesian metaphysics of body/mind duality by replacing the idea of two distinct substances with the 'double-aspect theory'. This supposed a single substance (God or Nature) possessed of infinite attributes, of which the mental and the material are knowable to human beings. According to Spinoza, whatever manifested itself under one attribute had its counterpart in all the others; this implied — when reduced to the two knowable aspects — that to every mental event there was a precisely corresponding physical event, and vice versa.

In Spinoza's double-aspect theory (as also in later versions of neutral monism) the third element, which should dissolve the duality into a unity, is located at the level of substance, while the dual opposition is transferred to the realm of attributes. However, such a modification does not solve the problem concerning the relationships between the defined entities any more than the Cartesian abstract synthesis solved it by means of God. Yet Spinoza's reformulation was a step towards thematizing the body/mind relationship — and especially the influence of the body on the mind — more systematically than Descartes had done.

… to brain-mind reduction

Nevertheless, body/mind duality still remains in such neutral monism. Only if the common substance is interpreted in materialist terms — reducing mind into matter and, thus, reducing one of the poles in the duality to the other — is there a 'solution' concerning the relationship, albeit a reductionistic one. Here the third (uniting) element is rendered useless inasmuch as matter and its motion is given the quality of 'the eternal', of which mind is a specific temporal manifestation. It is temporal both as structured materiality, the brain (which we would now regard as a product of EVOLUTION), and as functioning mind (thinking, feeling, etc.). Actually, such a materialism tends to replace the older psycho-physiological parallelism (represented by Spinoza) — the body/mind relationship — with a narrower one — a brain/mind relationship in which states of mind, from emotions to thoughts, are reducible to motion in the brain. Materialism of this sort is not merely pure philosophical speculation. It figures in some fields of practical research, pursuing the detection of ever more subtle one-to-one relationships between the processes of brain and mind, which are strong in contemporary NEUROSCIENCE and in biologically-oriented psychiatry. On the other hand, even though modern neuroscientific research may very well find new correspondences between the actions of brain and mental phenomena, the problem of duality remains, simply because there is a systemic difference between action in the brain and the dynamics of the mind. To take a simple example, even though all the neurological mechanisms involved in the act of seeing could be defined, the fact that 'I see' still remains an unsolved mystery. Explicating the latter presupposes an essential shift in register. Specifically, we may speak of the psychodynamics of the process, which is not only located in the body but at the same time transgresses the bodily boundaries and is a central aspect of relatedness to other body/minds (= selves) and thus to the shared 'third world', which we may now (following Karl Popper, 1902–94) characterize as society, culture, and LANGUAGE.

However, even though the mind is re-defined in a broader sense which extends beyond the Cartesian mind as reflective reason, and even though it is granted a certain autonomy with a dynamics of its own, the MIND/BODY PROBLEM still prevails — in so far as the mind is still conceived of as self-consciousness and the latter is equated with the constitution of the subject. Such a conception of the self-conscious subject not only figures in Cartesian rationalism ('I think, therefore I am') but is a much more general characteristic of the Western philosophical tradition from Plato onwards. Even more generally, it is a characteristic of the whole Judaeo-Christian tradition and the ascetic ideal it cherishes, privileging soul over body, mind over senses, duty over desire.

Psychoanalysis and phenomenology

The latter interpretation was made by Friedrich Nietzsche (1844–1900), whose philosophy could be characterized as a critique of the philosophical and religious tradition which cast the body in an inferior and objectified position relative to the disembodied soul, mind, and consciousness. Nietzsche pursued the opposite direction by privileging the body over the soul, or better, by embodying the spirit (*Geist*) and arguing that the 'spiritual' should be understood as the 'sign-language of the body'. In other words, Nietzsche emphasized the bodily origins of the spirit — 'or the soul or the subject' — thus formulating an idea suggestive of the subsequent Freudian concept of 'sublimation'. In the same vein, Nietzsche shifted the focus from the conscious to the 'dark side' of the human mind, from the rational to the non- and irrational layers, thus anticipating the later psychoanalytic interpretation of the *unconscious*. Nietzsche's philosophical reflections on the human body, and his pursuit of going beyond the dualistic schemes in which the body had been imprisoned in the Western philosophical tradition, remained primarily at a programmatic rather than a systematic level. Nevertheless his thought has surely had an essential influence on later theorizing of the bodily themes, especially on the ideas of the French 'post-structuralist' Michel Foucault (1926–84), but the more systematic elaborations related to the problem of body/mind dualism and aiming beyond it are located primarily in two, partially interrelated, thought traditions: Freudian psychoanalysis and phenomenology, the latter especially represented by the work of Maurice Merleau-Ponty (1908–61).

The psychoanalytical approach from Sigmund Freud (1856–1939) onwards, in different variations, introduces a new formulation of the human mind which acknowledges its relative autonomy and its own specific dynamism and, furthermore, locates within it an 'other scene', the unconscious. Relating to the body/mind problem, the unconscious may be conceived as an intermediate realm constituting a continuity both between the body and the mind and between the mind/body unity and its social context or the cultural 'third world', especially as shared language.

The former link is emphasized in the formulations introduced already by Freud himself: 'The ego is first and foremost a bodily ego; it is not merely a surface entity, but is itself the projection of a surface.' In other words, the ego, and thus also the distinction between the ego and the id (involving the acknowledgment of the unconscious), are seen as deriving from the bodily being-in-the-world or, as Freud puts it, 'from bodily sensations, chiefly from those springing from the surface of the body'. Thus the formulation both establishes a 'body–mind' continuum and restructures the 'mind' by introducing its unconscious components. On the other hand, the bodily being-in-the-world implies always a relatedness to a socially constructed reality and thus the unconscious can act also as an opening and link to this shared realm. This latter link is emphasized especially in a more recent reformulation of the concept of the unconscious by the French psychoanalyst, Jacques Lacan (1901–81).

The other central attempt to go beyond body/mind duality, and the intellectualist and empiricist stances it involves, is made by Maurice Merleau-Ponty in his project on the phenomenology of the body. At the outset Merleau-Ponty rejected not only Cartesian dualism but also both psychoanalytic and structuralist approaches. In his view — especially in the earlier stages of his project — psychoanalytic conception of the human mind (unconscious included) reduced the human body to a mere mental representation (body-image), neglecting its actual bodiliness. So his starting point was in the sensory and experiencing body 'before' the reflective consciousness, as it were, from which he proceeded to the more complex form of relatedness of the body-subject to the world of objects and other people. According to Merleau-Ponty the emergence of the more complex forms of relatedness did not imply the marginalization of the human body into a mere abode of the mind but, on the contrary, the 'higher' functions, including thought itself, should still be regarded as bodily functions referring not only to the human brain but to the whole body in its relational being-in-the-world. Consequently, for Merleau-Ponty the speaking subject is still first and foremost a body-subject: 'authentic speech is the presence of thought in the world — not its garment, but its body.' In his latest writings, just before his death, Merleau-Ponty was revising his relationship to psychoanalytic thought, and his formulations approached the psychoanalytic conception of the unconscious.   PASI FALK

Further reading

Falk, P. (1994). *The consuming body*. Sage Publications/TCS, London.

Johnson, M. (1987). *The body in the mind.* University of Chicago Press.

Leder, D. (1990). *The absent body*. University of Chicago Press.

Merleau-Ponty, M. (1968). *The visible and the invisible, followed by working notes*. Claude Lefort (ed.). Northwestern University Press, Evanston.

See also MIND–BODY PROBLEM; PERCEPTION.

Phlegm is the mucus which we can cough up from the lungs. In the mouth it mixes with SALIVA (spit) to become sputum, which is then expectorated: phlegm plus saliva equals sputum, which is commonly studied by doctors to give signs of what is happening in the lungs.

In health the output of phlegm is too small to be measured accurately, but estimates give values of 15–50 ml/day, a minute amount. This is carried up to the LARYNX by the 'ciliary escalator', the wave-like movement of the hairs on the cells lining the trachea and bronchi. Once in the larynx, the phlegm is either coughed out, or more usually swallowed with, at the most, a throat-clearing 'huff'. In disease, excessive production of mucus in the airways is characteristic of illnesses such as chronic bronchitis, usually diagnosed by the large production of phlegm; the mucus stimulates nerve receptors in the lining of the airways, which excite COUGH, and this leads to the removal of the phlegm. The commonest causes of phlegm production are airways infections, such as influenza, and cigarette SMOKING. Smokers' cough is due to the irritation of smoke stimulating mucus output from the glands in the trachea and bronchi. At night this mucus stays in the lungs, and when the smoker gets up in the morning the accumulated mucus is coughed up. The greatest output of phlegm is seen in a rare condition, bronchorrhoea, in which as much as two litres/day of sputum may be produced.

Analysis of sputum can indicate what disease process may be present in the lungs. If it is white or yellow, there may be pus and bacterial infection in the lungs: viral infections usually leave the sputum translucent. Green sputum may point to an infection with a bacterium, *Pseudomonas pyocyanea*, common in cystic fibrosis. Red colouration indicates lung haemorrhage. Black sputum is a sign of inhalation of particles, usually from cigarettes, but classically from coal dust in miners. Occasionally, jelly-like casts of the bronchi are seen in severe chronic asthma, and even parasitic worms can be coughed up from the lungs. Detailed analysis of the chemistry and types of cells in sputum is increasingly being used to help precise diagnosis of lung diseases.

Hippocrates listed phlegm as one of the four HUMOURS, that which was cold and watery. Here is a paradox, because in its Greek origin phlegm means 'heat' or 'burning', which is consistent with its appearance in lung infections and inflammation; Galen claimed that there was an excess of phlegm in fevers. But phlegm has come to symbolize a cold clamminess and, in its relation to human personality, coldness and dullness of character. It is the humour of the winter, when we have coughs and colds and expectoration. Hippocrates believed that EPILEPSY was due to an excess of phlegm blocking the airways so that the body became convulsed in an effort to free itself from the obstruction; but we now know that, although too much phlegm may be a sign of infectious lung diseases, and can cause violent coughing, it certainly does not cause epilepsy.

Coughing up phlegm is always a sign to be taken seriously, although it could be due just to a common cold or to a smoky environment.

JOHN WIDDICOMBE

See also COUGH; LUNGS.

Photography

When photography was announced to the world in 1839, almost immediately three relationships to the body were established. The most pervasive of these was its use to produce PORTRAITS and snapshots that have served as surrogates, even fetishistic tokens, of the human body. As new technologies made photography progressively cheaper throughout the nineteenth century, photographic portraiture, produced in the studios of trained technicians, worked its way down to ever lower classes of society. Photographic portraits made present to broad classes of people images of the bodies of family members who had emigrated, gone off to war, died, or otherwise absented themselves, a privilege enjoyed previously only by the rich. For the last third of the nineteenth century photographic portraits were also collected and assembled into albums as a way for the public to see the leading political, artistic, and literary figures of the day.

As a different kind of surrogate, photography itself extended the reach of the body's comprehension of the world. Doing so more insistently than did other forms of mimetic representation, photography seemed to stand in for the direct, bodily experience of the individual, its lens becoming the roving eye of the beholder. Most obviously one sees this in travel and expeditionary photographs of the nineteenth century, for which skilled professionals travelled forth from Western Europe and the eastern USA to record and bring back views of sites as various as India, the American West and the Middle East (Fig 1).

Finally, photography played a role in the nineteenth-century comprehension of the body itself within the emerging sciences. Ethnographers saw in photography the potential to prove theories of racial difference, using photographs showing faces and full (frequently unclothed) bodies that had been produced both for the tourist trade and specifically for ethnographic study. Early investigators of psychiatry and EUGENICS considered the medium an objective tool of research, finding evidence in straightforward face shots as well as those that had been manipulated. Studies of PHYSIOGNOMY and the EMOTIONS were illustrated with photographs of faces stimulated by electrical charges, while eugenicists sought to arrive visually at average 'types' by exposing a single piece of photographic paper to multiple portrait negatives, one on top of the next, so that only the most commonly held traits appeared in the final picture. Within criminology, photographic 'mug' shots fixed the identities of convicted CRIMINALS, while detailed pictures of ears and other body parts enabled a crude method of tracking suspects, as today fingerprints and DNA are used. Physiology was advanced by studies of motion in the 1870s and 80s, which fixed the positions the body held through the course of a variety of activities. Using light waves beyond the visible spectrum, the invention of the X-RAY toward the end of the century let physicians study internal body parts.

At the end of the nineteenth century, photography's relationship to the body changed with the invention and mass marketing of George Eastman's Kodak, the first snapshot camera. The ease of use and mobility of this hand-held camera ('you push the button; we do the rest,' boasted the ads) made it an extension of one's own body. Already a 'point and shoot' camera, this early Kodak allowed individuals to take over many of the functions previously performed by professional photographers. Ever-growing masses of people could now make portraits and travel views of their own, with a camera handily carried anywhere. Within the snapshot photographs that emerged, the body itself was recorded in increasingly common and casual ways.

Also beginning at the end of the nineteenth century, mass reproduction of photographs

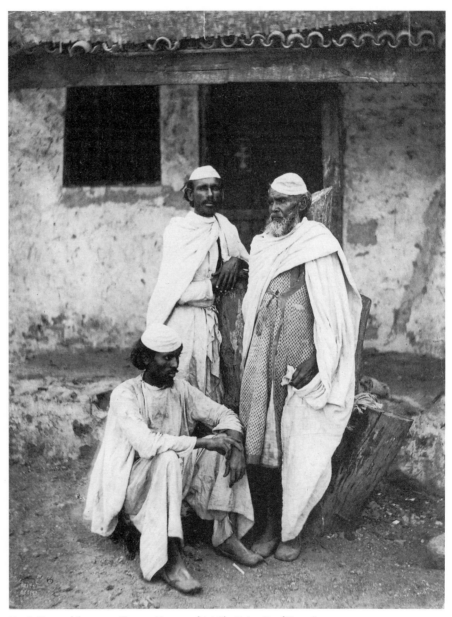

Fig. 1 Group of three men. (Spencer Museum of Art, The University of Kansas).

through new printing technologies expanded the audience for documentary and journalistic photography, which depended for its claim to veracity upon the imagined elision between the human EYE and the mechanical camera (an idea manifested in the title of a play based on Christopher Isherwood's life in Berlin in the 1920s, *I Am A Camera*). Major examples within this genre in which the body itself figured prominently are the documentary photographs produced for the Farm Security Administration, part of the USAs efforts to ameliorate the ravages of the Depression of the 1930s, and the surrealist-inspired work of photographers working in and around Paris in the 1930s, such as Hans Bellmer (Fig. 2).

Almost from the time of its invention, photography included the production of erotic imagery as a covert subset of its representations of the body. In the nineteenth century as well as the twentieth, such imagery often finessed the fine line between art and PORNOGRAPHY. Nineteenth-century photographers of the (usually female) nude included among their customers both artists seeking escape from the expense and possible tedium of working from live models and a more general public seeking this imagery for its potential EROTICISM. In the first third of the twentieth century, many photographers (mostly male) turned to the female nude body as a subject that would align their work in this new medium with the more traditional arts.

In the decades after World War II, photography of the body within the burgeoning mass media largely reinforced gender differences the war had momentarily eased. Fashion magazines returned in their imagery to a level of elegance and fancy dress not seen since the 1920s. Advertising photography, now in its heyday, constructed safely differing roles for men and women through images in which body posture, facial expression, grooming, and dress figured prominently. In the same postwar years, photographers working outside the commercial realm made pictures in which the body revealed strains on social relationships, as the dominance of straight, white males was questioned by new roles for women, greater freedom for people of colour, and an incipient visibility for gays and lesbians.

In the 1960s photography made evident the centrality of the body to radical changes in society. While battlefield corpses had figured prominently in photographs from the American Civil War, government censors successfully ruled out any large-scale photographic representation of battle carnage until the Vietnam War, when widespread disapproval of the war propelled photographers to defy censors. Not only did journalistic pictures record the carnage brought to the body by the war in Southeast Asia and the protest against it in Europe and America, but artistic pictures seemed to reflect symbolically the psychic stress of world events on otherwise normal bodies.

In the 1970s photography and the body intersected in new ways. No longer considered a transparent record or means of abstraction, as it had been for much of its history, photography was now seen as marking the extent to which the world is mediated, coming to us already as a representation. Using photography this way, artists explored the social and cultural bases of such attributes of the body as GENDER, race, class, and SEXUAL ORIENTATION. Artists used photography to document artistic performances that used the body in a very physical way to redefine

experience. Feminist artists employed photography as a means to record and comment upon transformations to which they submitted their bodies.

Postmodern artists in recent decades have followed the lead of these artists of the 1970s to make photographs of the body that are explicitly political, dealing with problematic notions of sexuality and self identity. In these works bodies are embedded in society, entering clearly defined social discourses at the time of their making. Photographers show the gay male body at

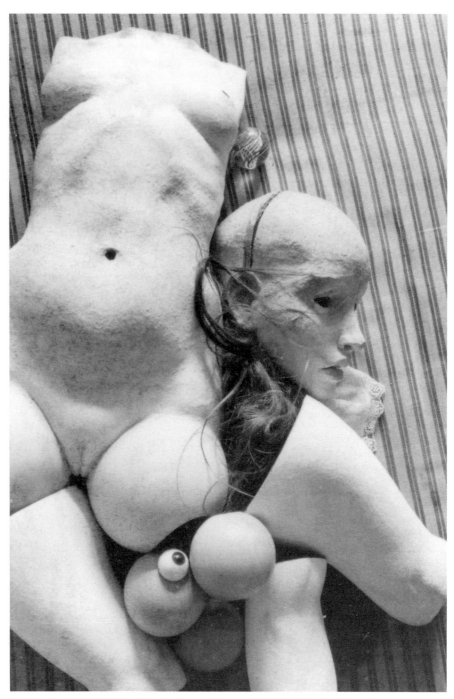

Fig. 2 *La Poupée* (c. 1935) Hans Belluvek. (Spencer Museum of Art, The University of Kansas).

precisely the time that the AIDS epidemic has made consensual invisibility no longer viable. Other photographers act out assumed or fictive roles, refusing to seek any 'true' or 'real' self. Still others have explored the social dimensions of race and racism by referring back to nineteenth-century photography that sought to define racial difference, thus recycling the history of photography's involvement with the body. JOHN PULTZ

Further reading
Pultz, J. (1995). *Photography and the body.* Everyman Art Library, London.

See also ART AND THE BODY; CINEMATOGRAPHY.

Phrenology

As the first biological science of mind, phrenology became an ubiquitous feature of nineteenth-century medical and natural philosopical thought, and of popular culture. Breaking down the distinction between mind and body, phrenology exemplified the shift from the speculative means of studying the human psyche as a metaphysical entity, which characterized Enlightenment thought, to the empirical methods introduced by the new scientific naturalism. Condemned in establishment social and scientific circles as an atheistic, materialist pseudo-science, phrenology was consistently accorded marginal status, a position reflected in historiographies aiming to document science as a story of progress. Recently, however, historians connecting science, medicine, and culture have begun to recognize phrenology's significance as a medium through which a number of naturalistic and functionalist concepts reached a wide and popular audience.

Phrenology's innovative principles were first enunciated in Vienna and Paris, around the turn of the nineteenth century, by the physician, Franz Joseph Gall (1758–1828). Significant variations were later introduced by Gall's assistant, J. G. Spurzheim (1776–1832), who applied the neologism, 'phrenology', to the doctrine, and by the prolific Edinburgh phrenologist, George Combe (1788–1858). Gall established that the BRAIN was the organ of mind — then a contestable view — and that it was composed of all the faculties that made up the human character. Using the analogy of the anatomical constitution of the body, he argued that the faculties were embodied in discrete cerebral 'organs', which were innate and inheritable, and that individual differences derived from variations in the physical organization of the brain. The principles underlying these hypotheses later became widely accepted. Two additional 'craniological' hypotheses, however, rendered the science empirically vulnerable, at the same time as they formed the basis of its popularity. Gall contended that the power of each faculty depended upon the size of the 'organ' which embodied it; and that the cranium reflected the form of the underlying cerebrum. Accordingly, character could be 'read' from the shape of the head. A primary task for *craniology* (Gall retained this term, along with

'cranioscopy' and 'organology') and phrenology was the 'discovery' and systematization of the faculties. Although Gall was a renowned cerebral anatomist, he insisted that the quasi-physiognomical method of correlating observed behaviour with variations in head shape was more revealing than DISSECTION. Indeed, phrenologists consistently repudiated animal experimentation involving surgical trauma, for ethical as well as scientific reasons.

As the prototype for a normalizing physical ANTHROPOLOGY, however, phrenology, with its value-laden stereotyping psycho-techniques, introduced new ethical problems. Gall's curiosity had initially been aroused by the differences he had noticed amongst individuals, but he subsequently began to compare CRIMINALS, lunatics, non-European 'races', and other 'deviant' groups with the gendered and Eurocentric norms that his craniological discourse was designed to construct. Indeed, the definition of normality was one of phrenology's major projects. As Spurzheim argued, this was a specifically medical project, for physicians had to understand the normal before they could recognize and cure the pathological. Spurzheim's phrenological modifications supplied people with new techniques both to construct normality and to achieve it in their own lives. Invoking the analogy of the GREAT CHAIN OF BEING, he grouped the faculties into separate lobes of the brain, placing the 'higher' intellectual organs in the forehead, the sentiments — including 'veneration' — at the summit, and the 'lower' animal faculties (for example, sexuality and mothering) at the base of the brain. Henceforth, human types could be constructed according to the predominance of various groups of cerebral organs. With their Baconian faith in generalization from an accumulation of facts, phrenologists collected large numbers of representative SKULLS and busts. They established societies and museums, and entered educational institutions, where these reified racial, sexual, and class stereotypes were exhibited for all to absorb, where people could learn the art of head-reading for themselves, and whence phrenological character analysis would begin to enter the domain of popular culture.

Phrenology was given an additional impetus when Spurzheim and George Combe, invoking the Laws of Nature, effected its transformation into a moral and meritocratic science of self improvement and social reform. Spurzheim introduced the element of cerebral functionalism with his theory of the complex interaction of the faculties. Opposing Gall's deterministic conception of each faculty as either good or bad, Spurzheim argued that all of them were intrinsically good, abnormal behaviour resulting from imbalance, when the superior intellectual and moral organs had failed sufficiently to direct the 'inferior' organs. Although natural endowment was determined by heredity, appropriate 'exercise' — that is, behaviour — could strengthen the good faculties and weaken the bad: hence phrenology's

application to criminal and lunacy reform. Moreover, the health and well-being of both the individual and the race could be improved by eugenic manipulation. For Spurzheim, the latter meant selective breeding, through the choice of marriage partners with propitious cerebral and physical constitutions. George Combe, however, later extended the eugenic theme with his addition of the Lamarckian theory of inheritance. In his best-selling tract, *The Constitution of Man* (1828), Combe popularized these hereditarian theories, providing a comprehensive explanation of the working of the 'organic laws', along with advice on how to obey them by applying phrenology to 'the practical arrangements of life'.

Although phrenology never lacked vociferous opposition, its impact remains indisputable. Its vocabulary infiltrated the language, and its naturalistic character analysis and positivistic conceptual framework, employed by novelists and poets (including Honoré de Balzac, Charlotte Brontë, George Eliot, and Walt Whitman) entered the popular imagination. If by the 1840s neurophysiological experimentation had fatally undermined the specific details of its cranial cartography, phrenology's underlying principles had been absorbed by many of the progenitors of the human sciences, and incorporated into the new disciplines of functional sociology, differential psychology, neurophysiology, physical anthropology, and evolutionary theory. As the comparative anatomist, J. F. P. Blumenbach, once declared in relation to phrenology, these disciplines thus contained 'much which is new and much which is true, but the new is not true and the true is not new'. JAN WILSON

Further reading
Cooter, R. (1984). *The cultural meaning of popular science. Phrenology and the organization of consent in nineteenth-century Britain.* Cambridge University Press.

Young, R. M. (1970). *Mind, brain and adaptation in the nineteenth century. Cerebral localization and its biological context from Gall to Ferrier.* Clarendon Press, Oxford.

See also CRANIOMETRY; SKULL.

Physiognomy

The study of expression, primarily of the emotions, and principally via the face, has a long and complex history. From Aristotle onwards, physiognomy has been the means of reading and judging character based on the expressions of the FACE. In sum, physiognomists recognized the face as an index of EMOTION and (moral) character; and physiognomy offered a way of conceptualizing these particular observations in terms of general categories or theories. The purpose of physiognomy was to identify and to describe the common forms that organized the diversity of appearances, and, as such, it functioned in a profoundly normative manner — as the determinant of what was common to all people and all things in the physical world. At best, physiognomy provided an explanation of human nature in terms of a uniform order of types or kinds, which worked by translating particular observations into general theories of character and emotion. At worst, it was disparaged as a mystical and highly deterministic practice, more akin to fortune-telling than to science, and cast as a poor resemblance of its family relation, PHRENOLOGY.

A number of thinkers have attempted to describe and explain how the desire to see the workings of the mind, and ultimately the soul, through the face answers these questions about man, mind, and nature. Aristotle, Charles Le Brun, Johann Caspar Lavater, and Charles Darwin are the most notable. The challenge they faced was how to establish the grounds upon which their teachings could be viewed as true or rejected as false. One of the earliest philosophical treatises on physiognomy, and the first attempt to present physiognomy as a hermeneutic, and possibly scientific, method, was a work thought to be written by Aristotle, *Physiognomica*, which identified three categories of physiognomic judgement — the zoological, the ethnological, and the pathognomical. Yet what emerges after Aristotle is a complex relationship between the classical mode of reading and judging character — physiognomy — and the rise and triumph of inner, scientific understandings of expression based on PHYSIOLOGY. Such a relationship originates with the work of Charles Le Brun, who believed an understanding of expression was the key to discerning the passions or the activities of the mind (SOUL). Based on Descartes' theory of the passions, Le Brun's *Conférence sur l'expression générale et particulière* (1668) sought to present a rational and coherent theory of expression. Le Brun wanted to demonstrate the necessary and natural correspondence between the movements of the passions and the movements of the facial muscles, and, from this, to deduce the laws of expression. A knowledge of the principles, psychological and physiological, which directed these activities and their external appearance would, he claimed, release the artist from simply copying nature and allow him to create his own images, which would be directed by, and maybe even improve on, the processes of nature.

This notion of 'improvement' was of crucial importance to Johann Caspar Lavater in his *Essays on Physiognomy* (1789–93). In his hands, each and every attempt to read and judge character was a means of ascribing an essence to human nature that imagined there was something hidden from external appearances, which, once discovered, made them more purposeful and more substantial. One could arrive at a definition of man by imputing a certain kind of 'spirit' from the 'surface' appearance of an individual. But the point was that Lavaterian physiognomy enabled the impressions of sense to be translated into common sense, which comprehended order and unity from the appearances of things. The appeal of essentialism for Lavater lay in its capacity to validate a 'science' of man based on a theory of natural kinds. But the problem of

essentialism for physiognomy was that it imagined its 'science' as the result of an intuitive understanding of the intrinsic properties and purposes of things. So, whilst essentialism underwrote Lavater's 'science' of man, it was also, and not incidentally, the cause of its many inconsistencies.

There is no doubt that Charles Darwin was sceptical about the claims of physiognomy with regard to expression and emotion. Nonetheless, it is interesting that his study of expression makes a number of contradictory claims about the possibility and plausibility of conducting a scientific analysis of expression. Darwin's oft-neglected work, *The Expression of the Emotions in Man and Animals* (1872), was self-consciously presented as the cornerstone of his evolutionary theory — the means of demonstrating once and for all that man was not a separate and divinely created species but continuous with other species. An evolutionary account of expression was not concerned with teleological explanations of physical attributes; rather, it was directed towards finding a means of understanding the process through which expressions are acquired. The result was a study of expression that tried to identify specific mental and emotional states as well as their corresponding expressions (by concentrating on their motor activity), and then map their common descent through groups of related organisms. If this could be done, then human feelings like love, anger, fear, and grief could be treated as habits and shown to have clearly recognizable parallels, perhaps even origins, in the animal world.

The rise and triumph of these inner, scientific rationales for the expression of the emotions placed the study of expression on new ground. Indeed, the evolutionary explanation of expression given by Darwin (and taken to its logical, albeit odious, conclusion by Francis Galton, father of eugenics) is both the long-term outcome of physiognomical teachings and the reason for their dissolution. As we reflect on the impact of physiognomy, there is much to suggest that its demise is no bad thing.

LUCY HARTLEY

Further reading

Darwin, C. (1998). *The expression of the emotions in man and animals,* (ed. P. Ekman). Harper Collins, London.

Evans, E. C. (1969). Physiognomics in the ancient world. *Transactions of the American Philosophical Society,* **59,** 5–97.

Lavater, J. C. (1789–93). *Essays on Physiognomy; for the Promotion of the Knowledge and Love of Mankind; Written in the German Language by J. C. Lavater, and Translated into English by Thomas Holcroft,* (trans. T. Holcroft London).

Montagu, J. (1994) *The expressions of the passions: the origin and influence of Charles Le Brun's 'Conférence sur l'expression générale et particulière'.* Yale University Press, New Haven.

See also FACIAL EXPRESSION; PHRENOLOGY; SMILING.

Physiology is defined by dictionaries as 'the science of the normal functions and phenomena of living things'. The physiology of animals emerged in Europe out of the Renaissance nterest in the experimental method, as exemplified by the work of William HARVEY (doctor to Charles I). Harvey's book of 1628 on the Motion of the Heart, '*Exercitationes Anatomicae de Motu Cordis*', brilliantly analyses structural and functional observations (quantitative as well as qualitative), which remorselessly led him, and similarly lead the present day reader, to the conclusion that the blood circulates, in man as well as in other animals. This volume remains central to our current understanding of the word 'physiology' because of its emphasis on experiment, data analysis, and hypothesis testing. Harvey's work also exemplifies the natural symbiois between physiology ('function') and ANATOMY ('structure'), a science from which physiology was to emerge as a separate discipline in the second half of the nineteenth century. Harvey's book also connects physiology to MEDICINE. Understanding of every disease follows from combining knowledge of the relevant normal physiology to the way in which it is perturbed in the particular disorder ('pathophysiology').

Historically, the subsequent meaning of 'physiology' is well illustrated by the way in which the word is used in the two following quotations. The first is from 1704 (J. Harris, *Lexicon Technica*): '*Physiology*, is by some also accounted a Part of Physick' (i.e. Medicine), 'that teaches the Constitution of the Body so far as it is sound, or in its Natural State; and endeavours to find Reasons for its Functions and Operations, by the Help of Anatomy and Natural Philosophy'. The second (a definition of Charles Darwin's colleague T. H. Huxley), 150 years later, is virtually identical to current usage: 'whereas that part of biological science which deals with form and structure is called Morphology; that which concerns itself with function is Physiology'.

It was the experimental work of Claude BERNARD in France in the mid nineteenth century that led to the profound insight that HOMEOSTASIS is central ot the success and survival of any organism. This implies that physiological systems must necessarily function in such a way as to regulate their internal environment, by means of what we now call 'feedback'. A homeostatic mechanism requires, at a minimum, a set of sensors to measure the relevant variable (e.g. body temperature), feeding back 'error signals' to an integrator (the brain), which controls an effector mechanism to adjust that variable (sweating, shivering, etc.). Such a negative feedback control system will act to return the variable towards the non-perturbed state. Such ideas of control and order are central to understanding and defining the discipline of physiology, whether it be in MICROORGANISMS, plants or animals.

The significance of physiology as the key science underpinning HEALTH and DISEASE (human and veterinary) accounts for the nomenclature adoped in 1900 by the Nobel Foundation. To recognise key developments in this field, the relevant NOBEL PRIZE is still awarded in 'Physiology or Medicine', although many Nobel prize-winners in this category (working in such fields as immunology, MOLECULAR BIOLOGY and bioengineering) would not readily have identified themselves as physiologists. But many would have done so. For example: in cardiovascular physiology, Krogh (for his studies of capillary function), Einthoven (who described the ELECTROCARDIO-GRAM) and Forssman (who developed cardiac catheterization); in neurophysiology, Sherrington (who conceived the idea of SYNAPSES), Adrian (responsible for our original understanding of coding of information by patterns of nerve impulses), and Hubel and Weisel (who worked out how the visual areas of the CEREBRAL CORTEX analyse specific features of the image); in endocrinology, Banting (INSULIN) and Guillemin and Schally (identification of the hypothalamic peptides that control the PITUITARY GLAND).

The interface between physiology and chemistry led directly to the emergence, in the first half of the twentieth century, of the major new discipline of BIOCHEMISTRY. Hence, such Nobel laureates in 'Physiology or Medicine' as Warburg (respiratory enzymes), Krebs (metabolic integration), Brown and Goldstein (CHOLESTEROL) and Sutherland (cyclic AMP) would probably not have thought of their scientific research as being part of 'physiology'.

Another science that grew out of physiology concerns nutrition; yet another is PHARMA-COLOGY, whose foundations arose from the experimental studies of physiologists such as Loewi (the discoverer of the transmitter substance ACETYLCHOLINE) and Dale (chemical transmission between nerve cells). Despite the natural and deepening methodological and cultural divergence, over time, of both biochemistry and pharmacology from physiology, they all share the goal of explaining the functions of the body. Moreover, now that the concepts of genetics and the power of molecular biology pervade the whole of biology, the communality of physiology, pharmacology and biochemistry has re-emerged. This is well illustrated by the recent discovery of Furchgott (another Nobel prize winner) and others, that NITRIC OXIDE, a tiny gaseous molecule, can convey information between cells simply by diffusing through their membranes.

Harder to define, yet critical to the discipline of physiology, is the term 'general physiology'. This subject emerged originally from the convergence of nineteenth-century physical chemistry with experimental biology. It was founded on quantitative studies of plant and animal cells. Because of its reductionist goal, general physiology was an obvious forerunner of what is now described as cell and molecular physiology. However, more than this, it attempted to use the theoretical insights gained from the 'hard sciences' (physics and chemistry) to provide a rational basis for analyzing living matter, and was thus eager to embrace and test theory quantitatively. An outstanding example of the success of this approach is the experimental analysis of the resting potential and the ACTION POTENTIAL (nerve impulse) by Hodgkin and colleagues in the late 1940s. Indeed, successful analysis of 'bioelectricity' is one of the factors that led to the foundation by physiologists of yet another off-shoot — biophysics. Although there are still (notably in North America) a number of distinguished university departments of Biophysics, growth of this subject as an independent discipline has been hampered somewhat by its failure to meld its 'physiological' roots with its links to biological physics (especially X-ray crystallography). However, the work of Nobel laureates Neher and Sakmann provides a spectacular example of how electrophysiological analysis can give biophysical insight not available through other means. These scientists, through clever technical developments, were able to design experiments that allowed structural, and hence functional, changes in single protein molecules (membrane ION CHAN-NELS) to be followed in real time by recording the flow of ionic current through them. By tightly sealing a fine, fluid-filled capillary tube to an extremely small part of a CELL MEMBRANE, and linking it to a sophisticated amplifier ('patch clamping'), they were able to measure the current through individual channels, flicking quickly from closed to open states. This physiological insight has very recently been matched by structural studies by MacKinnon and colleagues on membrane channels at atomic resolution.

Physiology has a complex, deep relationship with the approach of reductive science. This is in part because 'function', particularly 'interesting' or unexpected function, emerges from interactions that can be found only in relatively complex systems; hence physiologists are unlikely (unless they are working on essentially trivial problems) to find that molecular structures in isolation give more than partial insight into the problem under attack. 'Explanations' of physiological questions seem more likely to arise from combining such reductionist approaches with, on the one hand, thermodynamics and, on the other, control systems theory. Life depends on 'non-equilibrium' properties — i.e. on complex interactions that require the constant expenditure of energy to maintain them. And networks of information and control (the NERVOUS SYSTEM, HORMONES etc.) are central to the development, function, and probably the evolution of complex biological systems.

Seen in this way, the information encoded in the genes provides a very challenging experimental opportunity for physiologists. To have read the sequence of DNA is only a small step on the route to understanding how and to what extent our genes build and control our bodies, and cause disease. Genes do just one thing: they translate their information into proteins. To understand how the products of genes work individually and together to create the magnificent complexity of a whole organism is part of the exciting challenge that faces the revitalised science of physiology in the twenty-first century. Indeed, the prospects for physiology are wider still: it will ultimately need to link such understanding 'upwards' to such disciplines as experimental psychology, ecology and human biology.

RICHARD BOYD

Further reading

Hodgkin, A. L. (1977). *The pursuit of nature.* Cambridge University Press, Cambridge.

Boyd, C. A. R. and Noble, D. (1993). *The logic of life: the challenge of integrative physiology.* Oxford University Press, Oxford.

See also BERNARD, CLAUDE; BIOCHEMISTRY; BIOTECHNOLOGY; HARVEY, WILLIAM; MOLECULAR BIOLOGY; PHARMACOLOGY.

Physiotherapy The modern development of physiotherapy as a branch of professional health care began to take shape in the last few decades of the nineteenth century. Earlier physical treatments — in particular hydrotherapy, EXERCISE, and MASSAGE — in Europe have their roots in antiquity and the baths and gymnasia of ancient Greece and Rome. In this sense physiotherapy drew upon varying themes of physical health stretching back into the mists of time, but the late-nineteenth-century advent of modern scientific medicine and related new skills had a particular impact. Lay practitioners of ancient skills such as bone setting, herbalism, and a range of physical therapies lost place to a medical profession fortified by accumulating scientific techniques of diagnosis and safer interventions. New ancillary occupations, such as radiography and laboratory science, were developing, thus expanding the division of labour beyond that of doctors and nurses, through a process of specialization that continues to the present day.

In changing circumstances the more traditional therapists faced a choice, either to continue as part of a broader world of physical culture and practice, or to seek a niche within an increasingly professionalized health care system. Their position was somewhat different, however, to the other emergent occupations associated with particular modern techniques of diagnosis and treatment. Traditional therapists had to find a place within modern medical practice without being a central part of the scientific transformation which was gathering particular force in the latter part of the nineteenth century. Their skills were manual, drug free, and external to the body. Moreover, they were linked to a physical regime of treatment and exercise which was part of the spa culture of the past rather than any clearly new professional domain. They were not, however, anti-scientific, and played a role in the nineteenth-century revival of a general interest in exercise. The Stockholm Central Gymnastic institute and the Ling movement were influential in Britain, and increasingly linked to modernized understanding of physiology. Indeed, Swedish-inspired GYMNASTICS began to influence the curriculum of British schools from the 1870s onwards, but as part of general educational rather than specifically medical developments.

Within this general context the modern emergence of physiotherapy came not through any particular therapeutic revolution, but in effect through a professionalizing stratagem of 'moralizing' massage in the 1890s. 'Rubbing' had long been recognized as a valuable aspect of nursing practice, and doctors involved in mobilizing patients after injury and surgery were looking increasingly for assistance from nurses with these skills. However, 'massage' as more widely practised had acquired a lurid and sexual connotation, as highlighted in a British Medical Journal campaign from 1894 onwards against 'massage centres' — understood in reality to be brothels. In response to requirements for further training and a morally managed context for sound practice, a number of forward-thinking nurse-masseuses banded together in 1895 to found a Society of Trained Masseuses. They set out to accomplish two linked ends; to organise the training of legitimate masseuses, and to secure the approval of the medical profession for their standards of education and practice. 'Rubbing' as traditionally practised and the corruptions of improper 'massage' were to be transformed by respectable women trained in ANATOMY and PHYSIOLOGY, working with and through the medical profession.

Establishing respectability for physical treatments in the early years involved more than a proper ethical training for practitioners. Many doctors were critical of the therapeutic value of treatments offered by masseuses, and indeed of those medical practitioners working with them. Dr James Mennell, for example, a leading physical medicine specialist and far-sighted advocate of the mobilizing and gentle massage of patients soon after injury, recalled in later life the opposition of his colleagues. Massage and manipulation to assist healing remained for many doctors outside the pale of medical science, which for them centred on drug-based and surgical interventions. The other dimensions of early physiotherapy practice — heat, electrical, and water-based applications to aid muscle and joint movement — were equally thought to be reminiscent of charlatans and exhibitionist 'healers' who exploited both the desperately ill and the gullible well by useless practices and machinery. Mennell, closely associated for some three decades with physiotherapy in Britain, was approached as a young doctor by a delegation of his colleagues who asked him not to degrade his profession 'by studying such a very doubtful branch of medical practice'.

The 1914–18 war had a dramatic effect on the status of physiotherapy, in both Britain and North America. An earlier rule prohibiting female practitioners from treating male patients was swept away by the number of casualties. Men were not allowed to join the main professional association until after the war, and thus were trained and examined separately at this time. Leading masseuses founded the Almeric Paget Massage Corps to co-ordinate services through the War Office, hospital services, and other governmental agencies. In the context of war, the social status, value, and purpose of physical treatments changed considerably in public and professional perception. Consequently, in 1920 the earlier, small 'Society of Masseuses' became by royal recognition the 'Chartered Society of Massage and Medical Gymnastics'. A similar expansion of practitioners and changing medical requirements and attitudes in the US led in 1921 to the founding of the American Physical Therapy Association.

The efforts of early physiotherapists to secure medical professional approval brought benefits to physiotherapy's development, but also substantial tensions which have been mainly resolved only from the 1970s onwards. These tensions related to autonomy in treatment procedures and the degree of medical professional supervision required. Over time, the debates on these issues were complicated by the therapeutic eclecticism and swings of fashion at the centre of physical treatment, ranging across massage, hydrotherapy, electrotherapy, exercise machines, ULTRASOUND, and heat treatments in varying combinations and emphases. An early position was set out in 1917 by Dr J Mennell in his influential *Massage, its Principles and Practice*, and was based upon a clear model of professional subordination. Essentially, within this model the doctor was the thinker — diagnosing, prescribing, and monitoring — whilst the physiotherapist was the technician or assistant working to instruction. Physiotherapists were banned from seeing patients directly without medical referral and prescription. Internal debates over these requirements within physiotherapy, and between physiotherapy and medicine, routinely broke out throughout the first half of the twentieth century. Within the physiotherapy profession, private practitioners broadly chafed at medical restraints on their practice, whereas, at least up to World War II, hospital-based physiotherapists appeared less concerned about medical dominance.

During the first half of this century the profession was prevented from throwing off medical tutelage, however much resented by some practitioners, by an overall need to retain its practical advantages. Medical recognition gave access to hospitals, the focus of modern medicine, but also helped in establishing stable frontiers with other trained and untrained health care occupations. In Britain, for example, mergers have sometimes been discussed with occupational therapists, given that there are overlaps between the two groups. In the market-place, historically anybody could legally claim to be a physiotherapist and engage in practice. Equally, hospital employers could employ untrained workers in the absence of strongly organized, validated, and widely-supported certificates of competence. In practice, in many countries, along with other professions, physiotherapists have seen medical control as a step towards securing state licensing or recognition in their own right. After decades of pressure this has usually been attained, provided that local and national medical associations were not antagonistic towards such developments.

The earlier period of medical professional monitoring and supervision was characteristic of the first half of this century, and has now passed away under changing historical circumstances. Across time, physical medicine as a speciality area of practice for physicians had become increasingly a very minor part of medical specialization. In practice the everyday medical supervision of physiotherapy treatments had become nominal prior to its formal end in a number of countries. Physiotherapists now see patients with a wide range of conditions, both independently and by medical referral, when ILLNESS, INJURY, or DISABILITY inhibit normal movement. Their techniques include exercise and movement therapy, hydrotherapy, massage, and manipulation, and more recent complementary therapies. Physiotherapy has become one of the specialist professions of health care rather than an ancillary or supplementary occupation. This change has to be placed in a broader context of inter-professional relationships in health, moving from hierarchical to more co-operative models of practice. Furthermore the development of all professions in healthcare has been influenced by international social changes.

In particular, the wider relationships between gender, status, authority, and work have been changing. At one point, for example, physiotherapists were mostly female, whilst doctors were mostly male. This gender composition and balance has been changing for some decades, alongside wider social challenges to male-oriented dominance within many occupations. Another major change of recent decades, of very notable significance for many health professions, including physiotherapy, has been the educational shift from apprenticeship in the workplace to education in the modern university. This development is likely to foster the growth of a particular scientific knowledge base for physiotherapy practice. Finally, physiotherapy, after a century of modern practice, is in ever greater demand, due to epidemiological and demographic changes. The relatively successful treatment of infectious diseases, and growing life expectancy, have highlighted the prevalence of chronic conditions. At the same time, social expectations of full function and mobility in later life have grown. Thus, in changed but continuing ways, the fundamental rationale for physiotherapy — of finding and applying means of retaining, restoring, and where possible expanding physical function and mobility — remains as relevant at the end as it was at the beginning of this century   G. V. LARKIN

Further reading

Larkin, G. V. (1983). *Occupational monopoly and modern medicine*. Tavistock, London and New York.

Barclay, J. (1994). *In good hands, the history of the Chartered Society of Physiotherapy 1894–1994*. Butterworth-Heinemann, Oxford.

See also MASSAGE.

Pigmentation in the body is due to different forms of *melanin*, the name for a group of closely related substances, of different shades of black and brown, that are synthesized in body cells (*melanocytes*), mostly from the AMINO ACID *tyrosine*. The most widespread type of melanin is responsible for SKIN COLOUR; the melanocytes, deep in the epidermis, make it, and transfer it into the keratin cell layer of the skin. In 'white' skin, FRECKLES and moles are areas of concentrated pigmentation; exposure to sunlight results in stimulation of the melanocytes and hence to a 'tan'. Excessive stimulation can sometimes produce a *melanoma*, which can have serious consequences if not recognized and treated at an early stage.

Variations in EYE and HAIR colour are due to different types of melanin. As well as the visible sites, there is also melanin pigmentation in the choroid coat of the eye, the vascular layer that invests all but the front part of the eyeball, behind and around the retina; also in the cochlea and vestibule of the inner ear, variably in the ADRENAL GLANDS, and in the substantia nigra of the brain. It is normal for pigmentation to increase during pregnancy, particularly in the areola of the NIPPLES, and in the 'stretch marks' on the abdomen.

Abnormalities of pigmentation are of interest in understanding its normal significance. *Vitiligo* is a relatively common autoimmune condition, in which melanocytes are patchily destroyed, causing totally white areas in the skin. Provided that sun creams can be used for protection, the problem is only — though disturbingly — a cosmetic one, seriously so for dark-skinned people; small patches of depigmentation can also occur in the iris. In ALBINOS, pigmentation is defective everywhere: not only in the skin, hair, and iris but also behind the retina, with associated visual problems; melanocytes are present, but melanin synthesis is impossible due to congenital lack of the enzyme tyrosinase.

Excessive pigmentation can be caused by oversecretion of *adrenocorticotrophic hormones* (ACTH) and an associated *melanocyte-stimulating hormone* (MSH) from the PITUITARY GLAND. In 1855 Thomas Addison, physician at Guy's Hospital, London, reported '… a peculiar change of colour in the skin, occurring in connection with a diseased condition of the "supra-renal capsules"'. It was some considerable time before this link between pigmentation and disease of the adrenal glands was to be explained. We now know that if the adrenal cortex fails to maintain its normal output of hormones (notably cortisol), the low levels in the blood are detected in the HYPOTHALAMUS, through the normal feedback mechanism, and 'interpreted' as requiring a stimulus to action; thus the anterior pituitary is signalled to release more ACTH, which vainly flogs the dying horse. Whenever ACTH synthesis and secretion are increased, there is linked release of the closely associated MSH, and hence an increase in melanin production in the skin. This explanation is confirmed by observation of excessive pigmentation in other conditions in which ACTH secretion is excessive, and absence of such pigmentation when failure of the adrenal cortex is secondary to a failure of ACTH secretion itself. Primary disorder of the adrenal cortex — hypoadrenalism or 'Addison's disease' — was formerly most often due to TUBERCULOSIS; it is now rare, and usually the result of autoimmune destruction of the hormone-producing cells.

The link between these abnormal situations and the physiological significance of melanin secretion seems at first sight obscure. Whereas ACTH, and the adrenal secretions that it promotes, have now for long been recognized as counteracting the consequences to the body of actual or potential damage or STRESS, more recently it has been shown that there is a range of associated substances released from the pituitary gland along with ACTH, which may all contribute, one way and another, to protective responses. Melanin in the skin is best known for its protection against UV light; it does this by taking up 'FREE RADICALS'. Since these are released in a variety of other potentially harmful situations, not just in exposure to sunlight, melanin may have additional protective functions.

SHEILA JENNETT

See also ADRENAL GLAND; ALBINOS; EYE; FRECKLES; HAIR; PITUITARY GLAND; SKIN; SKIN COLOUR; SUN AND THE BODY.

Pineal gland This is a small structure, about the size of a pea, situated approximately in the centre of the head. Because it is one of the few obviously unpaired structures in the brain, the seventeenth-century French philosopher René Descartes (1596–1650) suggested that it was the seat of the soul, mediating subjective experience and intervening in the machinery of the brain in situations of free will and moral choice. In reality, the pineal gland is essentially part of the visual system. In mammals it responds indirectly to light because it receives messages along fibres from nerve cells of the *suprachiasmatic nucleus* of the HYPOTHALAMUS, which themselves receive signals from the EYE via fibres of the optic nerve. The suprachiasmatic nucleus is the body's major rhythm–generating centre — the heart of the BODY CLOCK. In lower vertebrates the pineal gland is itself a 'clock' and its cells respond directly to light. The main output of the pineal gland is the 'darkness' hormone *melatonin*, which is normally made at night. Melatonin, by the duration of its secretion, serves to indicate to the body both darkness and the length of the night. This signal is used to regulate the timing of biological rhythms.

JOSEPHINE ARENDT

Further reading

Arendt, J. (1995) *Melatonin and the mammalian pineal gland.* Chapman and Hall, London, New York.

See also BIOLOGICAL RHYTHMS; BODY CLOCK; HYPOTHALAMUS; MIND–BODY PROBLEM.

Pituitary gland This gland, also termed the *hypophysis cerebri*, lies in a bony cavity, the *sella turcica*, so called because it was thought to resemble a Turkish saddle. It lies under the part of the brain known as the HYPOTHALAMUS (whose location gives rise to its name, derived from the Greek, *hypo* meaning under and *phyen* to grow). It is connected to the hypothalamus by the pituitary stalk and in man is divided into two lobes, the anterior and the posterior, which develop in the embryo from completely different types of cell. The anterior lobe arises from below — from the same source as the mouth — and is made up of hormone-producing cells; the posterior lobe is developmentally a downward extension of the brain, and contains the endings of nerve fibres that arise from nerve cell bodies in one of two groups of cells ('nuclei') in the hypothalamus.

The existence of the pituitary gland was known before the time of Aristotle (384–22 BC), but it was only in the twentieth century that its true function was identified. Galen, the Greek physician and dogmatic teacher whose writing dominated Byzantine, Arabic, and medieval medicine for a millennium, thought the *pituita*, one of four HUMOURS, passed from the brain to the nasal cavity. Vesalius (1514–64), a Belgian anatomist, was of a similar opinion, believing that waste material produced in the formation of the vital spirit was drained from the brain via the pituitary gland. This view was challenged in the seventeenth century and debate about its function continued through the eighteenth and into the nineteenth century. It was only at the end of the nineteenth century, when clinical disorders were recognised as being associated with pituitary tumours, that its real function as an endocrine organ was established.

The anterior pituitary contains five different types of cell, each of which produce one particular hormone, with the exception of the 'gonadotrophs' which produce two: namely luteinising hormone (LH) and follicular stimulating hormone (FSH). All the hormones are peptide or protein in nature, varying in size from 39 amino acids (ACTH) to 204 amino acids (LH and FSH). The hormones fall into two groups: the first contains the four *trophic hormones* (from the Greek for nourishment), which control other endocrine glands; the second contains prolactin and GROWTH HORMONE, which have more widespread effects in the body.

The trophic hormones act to stimulate secretion of hormone from the target gland and to maintain its function and, if present in high concentrations, will cause the gland to enlarge. They are:

(i) thyroid stimulating hormone (TSH), which stimulates the secretion of the thyroid hormones;

(ii) adrenocorticotrophic hormone (ACTH), which acts on the ADRENAL CORTEX to promote the release of cortisol;

(iii) gonadotrophins LH and FSH, which act on the OVARIES and TESTES. They are however

545

named after their effects in women; FSH stimulates growth of the ovarian follicle containing the ovum or egg and LH stimulates production of oestrogen and progesterone from the ovary. The actions in the male are analogous; FSH stimulates sperm production and LH stimulates testosterone production by the testes.

Prolactin acts chiefly to cause milk production in the breasts.

Growth hormone has widespread effects, necessary not only for growth itself but also for metabolism throughout life.

Because the pituitary controls so many endocrine functions in the body it has been called 'the conductor of the endocrine orchestra', but more recent discoveries suggested that this term more properly belongs to the hypothalamus, with the pituitary being comparable to the leader of the orchestra. Since the nerves going to the anterior pituitary only supply the blood vessels there was some debate as to how the gland was controlled. It is now known that the hypothalamus produces stimulatory and inhibitory hormones, and that these reach the anterior pituitary via a network of small blood vessels or capillaries. The hormones are produced in nerve cells whose endings abut on the capillaries at the top of the pituitary stalk. This control of the pituitary by the central nervous system allows blood concentrations of the hormones to respond to a variety of external stimuli including STRESS. It also allows for complex patterning of release. Pituitary hormones in general are released in a pulsatile fashion, with many pulses during the day, and they can also show 24 hour (diurnal) rhythms. The gonadotrophins, linked into the human MENSTRUAL CYCLE, show a 28 day rhythm, while in animals which are seasonal breeders prolactin shows a seasonal rhythm. Blood concentrations of pituitary hormones are controlled not only by the hypothalamic hormones but by feedback, usually negative, exerted by target organ hormones such as cortisol or progesterone.

The posterior pituitary

Two hormones are released from the posterior lobe, *oxytocin* and *vasopressin (syn. antidiuretic hormone)*. These, like the releasing hormones that reach the anterior lobe, are produced within nerve cells in the hypothalamus. But in this case the axons travel right down the pituitary stalk, and the nerve endings release the hormones directly into the bloodstream (see Plate 7). The activity of the posterior pituitary hormones was established around 1900 in the UK by Schafer (a physiologist) and his colleagues working on what proved to be the actions of vasopressin, and Dale, a pharmacologist and Nobel Prize winner working on oxytocin. Vasopressin plays a role in water balance and the maintenance of blood pressure, normal circulating concentrations causing water to be retained by the kidney and higher concentrations causing blood vessels to constrict, thus raising blood pressure. As with the anterior pituitary,

control via the hypothalamus means that release of posterior pituitary hormones can be regulated by a variety of nervous inputs; the main stimuli for vasopressin release are an increase in the concentration of the blood plasma and a decrease in circulating blood volume, both of which reflect a fall in total body water. Oxytocin is important for the birth of an infant and for delivery of the milk supply.
MARY L. FORSLING

See PLATE 7.

See also GROWTH HORMONE; HORMONES; HYPOTHALAMUS; OXYTOCIN; PEPTIDES; WATER BALANCE.

Placenta The placenta forms from both embryonic and maternal tissues, and hosts an astonishing array of hormonal, nutritional, respiratory, excretory, and immunological functions. It is expelled after the baby as the 'afterbirth'.

When the developing, fertilized egg at the '*blastocyst*' stage becomes implanted in the lining of the UTERUS, it develops '*villi*' — fine, frondlike cellular projections from its outermost layer, the *trophoblast*. It is initially through these villi that nutrients are absorbed. Then, as the embryonic circulatory system develops, blood vessels grow into the villi on the implanted side of the embryo; this becomes the fetal component of the placenta. The nutritional functions of the placenta become concentrated in the *intervillous space*, which is bathed by the mother's blood from the *spiral arteries*, which are branches of the arteries to the uterus. The spiral arteries are converted in early to mid pregnancy, by trophoblast (placental) cell invasion, to become blood vessels that more resemble veins than arteries. (If this process does not occur, then the pregnancy may become complicated by *pre-eclampsia*, a condition characterized by high blood pressure and protein in the urine.) Normal, converted spiral arteries ensure steady supply of blood in a low-

resistance circulation. Glucose and amino acids in the mother's blood pass to capillary blood vessels in the fetal villi that dangle in the intervillous space, covered only by a thin membrane, and from them pass to the fetus, through the umbilical vein in the umbilical cord, to be used as building blocks for intrauterine growth.

At this same interface between mother and fetus, gas exchange occurs, with passage of OXYGEN to the fetus, and CARBON DIOXIDE to the mother. Thus, the placenta fulfils in intrauterine life the functions of the lungs after birth. A low concentration of oxygen in fetal blood encourages this direction of transfer, together with the particular nature of fetal HAEMOGLOBIN.

Similarly, the placenta has equivalent functions to the kidney after birth in permitting the excretion of the biochemical waste products of metabolism. There are fetuses that develop without kidneys (a condition known as *renal agenesis*). Because of the function of the placenta they often survive until birth, although they cannot survive long thereafter.

Although one might expect the placenta to be rejected by the mother's IMMUNE SYSTEM, because the fetal component is 'foreign', this does not happen, because of the presence of unique antigens on the cell surfaces.

In addition to these functions of exchange between the two individual blood streams, the placenta also produces an extensive array of HORMONES. These include *human chorionic gonadotropin* (HCG) produced by embryonic tissue right from the time of implantation: this promptly protects the embryo from rejection, by acting on the ovaries, causing them to sustain the hormone production that supports pregnancy. The presence of HCG also acts as the basis of PREGNANCY TESTING. After the third month, hormone production by the placenta takes over the pregnancy-supporting role from the ovary, by virtue of progressively increasing secretion of OESTROGENS and PROGESTERONE.

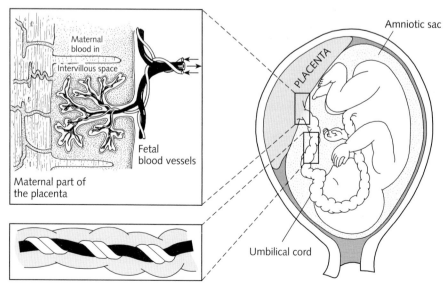

The placenta. The fetal (umbilical) arteries and their branches are shown white, and the vein and its branches black.

Growth of the fetus may be impaired if the placenta malfunctions. If the degree is severe, oxygenation may also become impaired, ultimately with death of the fetus and stillbirth. Other clinical problems associated with the placenta are *placenta praevia*, in which the placenta is located below the fetus, and *placental abruption*, in which the placenta separates prematurely from the wall of the uterus. Both of these conditions may be associated with brisk haemorrhage.

The placenta is ejected during the third stage of labour. JIM NEILSON

See also ANTENATAL DEVELOPMENT; LABOUR; OVARY; UTERUS; SEX HORMONES.

Plasma

Plasma is the liquid component that accounts for about 55% of the volume of BLOOD and in which are suspended the 45% taken up by cellular elements. When the two components are separated by centrifuge, using a test tube sample of blood treated to prevent clotting, the plasma separates as a yellowish layer. Plasma is different from *serum* — the fluid which is extruded when blood is allowed to clot — because some plasma constituents take part in clot formation. Plasma is about 95% water, with dissolved or suspended substances ranging from simple chemicals to complex protein molecules and fat particles. Its osmolarity (close to 300 milliosmoles/litre) and pH (close to 7.4) are closely controlled; likewise the main anions (chloride, bicarbonate) and cations (sodium, potassium, calcium, magnesium) and the major PROTEINS (albumin and globulins). Nutrients (glucose, FATTY ACIDS, AMINO ACIDS) and the nitrogenous waste product urea, vary more in their concentration, along with meals and metabolic activity. Other substances in much smaller concentration are equally important, such as the HORMONES, factors required for coagulation, and trace elements. Plasma is continually exchanging its constituents, apart from the large proteins, with all tissue fluids across capillary walls; it is also continually 'sampled' and its composition corrected by the KIDNEYS, which partially filter it off from the blood at a rate of 2–3 times the whole 2–3 litres of circulating plasma every hour, process it, and restore it to the circulation — except for about 1% which forms the urine. S.J.

See BLOOD; BODY FLUIDS; KIDNEYS.

Platelets

Platelets are small fragments of cellular material in the blood. They originate by splitting off from large cells in the bone marrow. Platelets have essential functions. They are necessary for the process of clotting when BLOOD VESSELS are damaged, both by providing crucial chemical substances and by physically plugging the hole — hence their other name: *thrombocytes*. That they have also a continuous rather than only an emergency function is shown by the effects of an abnormal shortage, known as *thrombocytopenia*; this leads to multiple tiny bleeds into the skin (*purpura*). S.J.

See BLOOD.

Pleasure

Pleasure Several philosophical movements have been explicitly directed towards pleasure, treating it as an end in itself rather than as the consequence of some higher ideal, such as virtue, knowledge, or faith. These include Epicureanism, Utilitarianism, and psychoanalysis. All three systems evaluate human behaviour in practical terms: what matters is not whether a given action is right or wrong, but whether it is conducive to happiness. Pleasure philosophies tend to be empirical and materialistic, taking SENSATIONS as a starting point and referring only to lived experience. Not surprisingly, they all evolved in opposition to the dominant world view.

Epicureanism arose in Greece in the fourth century BC. The school's founder, Epicurus, was trained in the Platonist tradition then popular in Athens, but came to reject Plato's philosophy because it undervalued day-to-day life. In place of the abstract reasoning which emphasized thought over feelings and subordinated worldly concerns to pure ideas, Epicurus taught that nothing exists beyond the realm of sensations. Nature is the best guide to behaviour; by appreciating our human instincts, and learning how best to satisfy them, we ensure that our lives will be happy.

Epicureanism has been misrepresented as favouring physical pleasure over other modes of experience. In fact, the greatest good to the Epicurean was not ecstasy, the gratification of the senses alone, but tranquility or peace of mind. Recognizing that physical pleasure is fleeting and may ultimately entail pain, Epicurus encouraged his followers to strive for the more durable happiness that would result from selecting intelligently among competing pleasures. Not only physical sensations but EMOTIONS, dreams, memories, fears, and fantasies affect our feelings in painful or pleasurable ways. The trick is to cultivate a state of mind that minimizes the painful while enabling us to experience pleasure as fully as possible.

The Epicurean way of life put happiness within everyone's reach. Also appealing, and absolutely unprecedented, was the egalitarianism of the community Epicurus established, where slaves and women, including prostitutes, were full-fledged participants. Following his death, the movement spread throughout the Greek world, as far as Egypt and Asia. It endured into the Roman era and coexisted with Stoicism and Christianity, was revived by humanists during the Renaissance and was espoused by the *philosophes* during the Enlightenment. What later admirers found so congenial was the Epicureans' realism. Their avoidance of the supernatural and the stress they placed on the material world were compatible with the more secular and scientific outlook that came to characterize the modern mind.

These currents fed into the movement known as *Utilitarianism*, which developed in nineteenth-century Britain. Utilitarians assumed that the amount of pleasure intrinsic to any course of action can be precisely calculated, making it possible to choose between rival activities according to the degree of happiness each is likely to produce. In the words of the school's founder, Jeremy Bentham, 'quantity of pleasure being equal, pushpin (a children's game) is as good as poetry.' Abstract considerations do not enter into the equation; the principle of utility implies neither moral nor aesthetic judgments. In the end, all that counts is whether the outcome is pleasurable or painful.

Consistent with the egalitarian spirit of Epicureanism, Bentham's goal was the greatest happiness of the greatest number. Here lies the originality of Utilitarianism: its definition of happiness is formulated in social, not personal terms. What is good for the individual should benefit the community as a whole. John Stuart Mill developed this doctrine into a total ethical philosophy, an alternative to the Christian reliance on duty. Mill saw no contradiction between the pursuit of self-interest and advancing the common good. Pleasing ourselves necessarily involves pleasing others, he believed, since the best way to achieve happiness as an individual is within a truly democratic society, one in which the needs of every member are met.

Utilitarianism had radical implications for political and legal reform. For Bentham, the best institutions and laws were those that increased pleasure and decreased pain, a proposition he set out to prove by drafting a model civil and criminal code. Underlying this system is the assumption that men and women are rational agents capable of recognizing their true interests and pursuing these at all times. To the objection that rational motivations alone do not determine behaviour, however, the Utilitarian had no reply.

Understanding the non-rational component of human experience (behaviour that seems to contradict our best interests) was the project of Sigmund Freud. *Psychoanalysis* began with pleasure. Indeed, Freud viewed the instinct for pleasure as the primary incentive for all activity. But he also saw that the way in which we achieve pleasure is neither a simple nor a straightforward process. Religious prohibitions, cultural institutions, and social structures — the parameters of the environment we inhabit — all serve to thwart the gratification of our desires, and this frustration causes pain. In response, we develop strategies for avoiding pain, not all of which are productive.

Psychoanalysis judges behaviour in purely functional terms. Those strategies which permit people to obtain fulfilment are good or healthy; bad or unhealthy behaviours prevent us from living comfortably in the world. By making us aware of the origins of our unhealthy behaviour, psychoanalysis helps us to adapt to external reality. But in the end, it is the individual who must decide which compromises to make.

In his later years, Freud devoted much effort to exposing the negative impact of civilization on human development. The experience of World War I also prompted him to modify his theory, leading him to postulate the existence of a destructive impulse in perpetual conflict with the instinct for pleasure. This critical tendency within Freud's thinking lent a pessimistic cast to his writing and probably accounts for the hostility with which his ideas were greeted. Nevertheless, psychoanalysis has exerted a significant influence on the twentieth century. Like other pleasure philosophies, it equips individuals with a sense of their own potential, instilling them with greater acceptance of themselves and tolerance for others.

LISA LIEBERMAN

Further reading
Gay, P. (ed.) (1989). *The Freud reader*. W. W. Norton and Company, New York and London.

Pleasure, biological basis

Pleasure might be defined as a subjective state associated with a reward. Termination of punishment or the omission of expected punishment may also produce pleasure. A reward is anything that we will work to obtain; a punishment anything that we will work to avoid or escape from. Reward has an important function in EVOLUTION, for it produces responses that usually help to adapt the organism to its particular environment. Natural selection has presumably favoured those genes that influence the organization of the brain so as to produce adaptive behaviour.

One example of pleasure is the TASTE AND SMELL of food, which we find particularly rewarding and pleasant when we are hungry. Water too produces more pleasure sensation when we are thirsty. These examples make the point that some types of pleasure are modulated by internal need states, so that behaviour is appropriately regulated and directed. They also show that pleasure can be selectively reduced. For example, the flavour of a food that we have eaten until satiated becomes less desirable, while other foods that we have not just eaten can remain pleasurable. The advantage of this sensory-specific decrease in the pleasantness of the taste of a much-eaten food is that it encourages us to consume a variety of different foods, and hence to obtain a wider range of nutrients. More generally, this tendency for initially pleasurable stimulation to become less pleasant if repeated is that it encourages exploration of different potential rewards. This modulation of reward represents a mechanism for enabling other behaviours to have their turn, and perhaps prompts us to explore a wide variety of different stimuli in the environment, which could enhance survival.

For many animals, pleasure is presumably solely associated with sensory stimulation. For human beings, and possibly other primates, mental reflection can excite pleasure. A good example is *Schadenfreude* — taking pleasure in someone else's misfortune. Why should we find this rewarding? It may be that we have developed mechanisms that can recognize when we are more likely to succeed than someone else. At a more abstract level, the pleasure associated with solving difficult mental, social, or intellectual problems may represent mechanisms by which our genes have built our brains so as to favour problem solving.

Touching and being touched can produce intense pleasure, presumably homologous with the evident pleasure that many animals experience as a result of being groomed by another individual. The pleasure associated with touch may relate, in part, to its adaptive value in reproductive behaviour, and in maintaining stable social communities (in that taking time to touch someone else implies an investment by one human in another).

It is more difficult to give a simple, scientific account of the aesthetic pleasure associated with many visual and auditory stimuli that are not obviously biologically adaptive, although sociobiologists have been ingenious in their efforts to provide such explanations. Flowers, for instance, give pleasure, because they are predictors of fruit later in the season. The waist-to-hip ratio that defines feminine BEAUTY might serve as a marker of youth and reproductive potential. Features that make men attractive to women might be produced by wealth and social status, as markers of the ability to provide resources. The pleasure produced by music may be related to the fact that *prosody* (the rhythmic aspect of speech), as in lullaby, can reduce activation and STRESS (or, in the converse, can produce martial behaviour). The arts and cultural activities, so extensively developed by human societies as a source of pleasure, may tap into evolutionarily ancient links between EMOTION and adaptive behaviour.

The brain has specialized systems for evaluating the reward value of sensory stimuli, and this evaluation normally occurs after the stimulus has been identifed and recognized. For example, in the parts of the CEREBRAL CORTEX devoted to taste and to VISION, the firing of neurons seems to represent the identity of the taste or the seen object, independent of whether the taste is pleasant or the object seen is associated with reward. But once an object has been identified by this preliminary stage of analysis, information is sent to the LIMBIC SYSTEM and related areas of the brain, including the amygdala and orbitofrontal cortex. Here, the reward value of the taste is determined, in conjunction with, from other brain areas, information about the state of HUNGER; and any reward associated with a visual object is decoded by reference to evidence that this stimulus has previously been associated with a rewarding situation.

This separation in the brain of the representation of what we taste and see from whether it is pleasant enables us to perceive and learn about objects (e.g. where they are) independently of their current reward value. In that emotions can be defined as states elicited by rewards and punishments, those brain regions (such as the orbitofrontal cortex and amygdala) which analyse whether stimuli are rewarding or punishing are centrally important in emotions, including pleasure.

EDMUND T. ROLLS
GEMMA CALVERT

Further reading
Rolls, E. T. (1999). *The brain and emotion*. Oxford University Press.

See also BRAIN; CEREBRAL CORTEX; EVOLUTION; LIMBIC SYSTEM; SOCIOBIOLOGY.

Pleura

A thin membrane which lines the inside of the chest cavity and also covers the LUNGS. The two '*pleural cavities*' are enclosed compartments, with normally only a film of fluid between the layer lining the chest (*parietal pleura*) and the layer covering the lungs (*visceral pleura*). The two layers continually tend to pull away from each other, because of the stretched elastic condition of the lungs — an important factor in the mechanics of BREATHING. If the chest wall is penetrated by a wound, air is readily sucked into the pleural cavity, separating the two pleural layers and collapsing the lung. S.J.

See BREATHING; LUNGS.

Poisoning

'Poison is in everything, and no thing is without poison. The dosage makes it either a poison or a remedy.' These words are attributed to Paracelsus (1493–1541), the Renaissance scholar and physician. The words are undoubtedly true, even for common substances, such as SALT or water, which under appropriate conditions can be poisonous. Modern medicines, useful and therapeutic in the prescribed doses, can be lethal when taken in excess; witness the number of suicides by overdose of sleeping pills. But these examples are not what is usually meant by poison. Poisons are agents that bring about the destruction of life when taken in small quantities. Further, if they are undetectable by their taste, smell, or colour their attractiveness as poisons is enhanced.

Poisonings can be accidental or deliberate. Accidental poisoning by plants, animals, or substances found around homes or places of work are not rare, especially among children, who may eat attractive berries from poisonous plants or mistake someone else's tablets or pills for sweets. In tropical countries, accidental poisoning from bites and stings of snakes, frogs, insects, or shellfish can be a major danger. Such areas usually have centres for the production of antidotes for the common animal poisons found there.

Deliberate poisoning on a grand scale, such as the use of poison gases in warfare is uncommon and contravenes international law. Deliberate poisoning of an individual by a poisoner has a long and fascinating history. It could be said that the most successful poisons (and poisoners) are by definition unknown, although it seems doubtful that such knowledge could remain undetected for long. All manner of means have been devised for delivering poison, the most common being to dissolve it in drink or mix it with food. Poisons that can be absorbed through the skin can be delivered through contaminated gloves or other clothing articles that make close contact with the skin. The mucous membrane lining the nose is highly vascular and a good site for absorption; poisons have been given by this route by incorporation into scents and nosegays. In fiction, at least, poison has been delivered to a victim when an envelope was licked. In an actual recent case in the UK the poison was applied to a door handle. Putting poison on one face of a carving knife blade delivers poison to the slice being cut or onto the next slice. By skilful use of such knives, which sometimes had small cavities to hold the poison on one side of the blade, a host could poison his guest victim while eating the same food. Alternatively, knives were designed where the slightest pressure on the blade caused the emergence of a poisoned barb from inside the handle. The minor prick might even go unnoticed by the victim, who would later become ill and die. Delivery of poison by manipulation of cutlery is of great antiquity and was apparently in use before Christ. In the Middle Ages the Borgias were said to have used this method.

Some poisons take a very long time to exert their lethal effect. In a remarkable case in modern times, an East European radio broadcaster working in London was, apparently accidentally, jabbed by a man carrying an umbrella while on the crowded underground railway system. The incident was soon forgotten, but in the days and weeks following the broadcaster became more and more ill, and eventually died. At post mortem a small, metallic hollow sphere that was filled with ricin was recovered. The gradual release of toxin was the cause of death. Poisons that take a long period to work offer advantages to the poisoner. He or she may be long gone and therefore unassociated with the demise of the victim; alternatively, time to create the impression of chronic illness can deceive the physician. At the other extreme, one of the most rapidly acting poisons is cyanide, acting within a few seconds; it was originally made from peach stones but now potassium cyanide is a common chemical used in many industrial processes and great care is needed to prevent accidental poisoning.

In early writings poisons were often catalogued along with drugs. The discovery of poisonous plants was attributed, by the Greeks, to the goddess Hecate, but it was the Arabs who turned poisoning into a specialist activity. Aconite was a commonly used poison, and under Roman Law it was illegal to grow the plant. It was, of course, a poisonous plant, hemlock, that gave Athens its state poison, used for the execution of Socrates.

Early European works on poisons were based on classic works of Galen, Dioscorides, and Nicander and those from Arabic sources. Petri de Abano in the fourteenth Century included mercury, copper, lapus lazuli, arsenic sublimate, litharge, nux vomica, laurel berries, and hellebore in his *De Remedis Venenorum*. In the *Book of Venoms*, 1424, Magister Sautes de Ardoynis listed arsenic, aconite, hellebore, laurel, opium, bryony, mandrake, leopard's gall, and menstrual blood. Books on poisons often gave recipes to be used, for example, for killing mad dogs or as

insecticides, but clearly many recipes had more sinister purposes, ending with a comment such as 'should kill within a day or so'.

In medieval times it was possible to hire a professional poisoner, as in Marlowe's *Edward the Second*. Poisoning of individuals in the Middle Ages was nearly always for political advancement or financial gain, and became such a hazard among the powerful and wealthy that they employed tasters. Other devices were to insist on drinking from Venetian glass, which was reported to explode if poison was added, or drinking from a vessel made from unicorn horn, which would neutralize the poison. Knowledge about poisons was common at this time, and detailed descriptions of poisoning appeared in literature. For example, a description of arsenic poisoning occurs in Shakespeare's *King John* (Act V, Scene 6) and *Henry IV* (Part 2, Act I, Scene 1). In an account of the history of Scotland, Macbeth's soldiers are reported to have massacred the invading Danes with belladonna (deadly nightshade).

The family most clearly connected with poisons is undoubtedly the Borgias. They arose in the fourteenth century in Spain and spread into Italy in the fifteenth and sixteenth centuries, with eleven cardinals, three popes, a queen of England, and a saint. Four members of the family are remembered for their scheming and intrigue, including murder by poison. They were two popes, Calixtus III and Alexander VI; a cardinal, Cesare Borgia; and his sister Lucrezia. Lucrezia Borgia has been cast in the role of the arch female poisoner, but the evidence for this view is thin.

ALAN W. CUTHBERT

See also CHEMICAL WARFARE; POISONS.

Poisons A poison is any substance that, by chemical action, is capable of killing or injuring living organisms when ingested or absorbed in small amounts. Poison is a quantitative concept, since virtually every known substance is harmful at some dose, but harmless in smaller quantities; the probable lethal dose can vary from a mere taste of those that are supertoxic (cyanide and strychnine, for example) to about a litre of those practically non-toxic (such as chemicals like lanolin and glycerin). All human beings vary in their response to drugs and chemicals, however, and some people can survive a dose generally regarded as fatal. Similarly, individuals may be more susceptible at some life stages than others — primarily infants or the elderly.

The route of administration influences the degree of poisoning that occurs. The major routes by which poisons gain access to the body are through the MOUTH or LUNGS, and less commonly by injection or by absorption through the SKIN. Inhalation is often the most serious type of exposure, as substances are absorbed into the body very effectively through the lungs. Once absorbed, they travel in the circulation and can cause adverse effects at sites remote from that of entry. Most affect one or two organs — the target organs of toxicity of a particular poison.

The CENTRAL NERVOUS SYSTEM is most frequently affected by poisoning, and muscle and bone the least. Some substances have a mainly local effect, the damage depending on the route of administration. Corrosives (mineral acids, alkalis, phenols) are in this category. They destroy any tissues with which they come into contact. They burn and erode skin and, if inhaled, damage the bronchi and lungs. When swallowed they produce inflammation and ulceration in the mouth, throat, stomach, and intestines.

Whenever poisoning occurs, death results when the extent and duration of bodily dysfunction has proceeded so far that treatment fails and recovery becomes impossible. A large group of drugs — general anaesthetics (ether, chloroform), barbiturates, opiates (morphine, codeine), and others — cause central nervous system depression, leading to COMA and respiratory and circulatory failure. The chlorinated hydrocarbons and certain heavy metals (including arsenic and antimony) cause liver injury and toxic hepatitis. Mercuric salts and ethylene glycol (antifreeze) damage the KIDNEYS. Inhalation of CARBON MONOXIDE produces ANOXIA (lack of oxygen for cell respiration) by binding to haemoglobin and preventing oxygen transport in the blood. Strychnine, atropine, COCAINE, certain snake venoms, and other poisons cause CONVULSIONS, resulting from altered nerve conduction in the brain and spinal cord. Organophosphorus compounds, the basis of 'nerve-gas', now used, with appropriate safeguards, as agricultural and horticultural pesticides, disturb function at nerve endings in the muscles and in the AUTONOMIC NERVOUS SYSTEM.

Poisoning may be acute or chronic. Acute poisonings usually follow a single large dose, and are characterized by a sudden onset of symptoms that run a short course not necessarily leading to death. By contrast, chronic poisonings develop after repeated exposures to small doses. Symptoms emerge gradually, often with remissions and recurrences, as the toxic agent accumulates in the body. Chronic lead and mercury poisoning, for example, follow this course (the term 'mad hatter' arose from the deranged behaviour of workers exposed to mercury compounds in the preparation of felt). Cumulative effects are not always associated with repeated exposure, however: carbon monoxide, for example is 'washed out' when oxygen or air is breathed, although smokers can have persistently raised levels in their blood. Chronic poisoning is often associated with occupational and environmental exposure, and identification of the specific agent can be difficult.

For many poisons, the effects of acute and chronic poisoning are very different. Acute benzene poisoning, for example, causes depression of the central nervous system, but chronic benzene poisoning can cause leukemia. In fact, chemical carcinogenicity appears to be a variant of chronic toxicity. Prolonged exposure to substances like asbestos and cigarette smoke can lead, often after many years, to the development of characteristic CANCERS.

Treatment of acutely poisoned patients requires the maintenance of respiratory and circulatory functions, and elimination of the poison from the body. Absorption of swallowed poisons can be interrupted or prevented by gastric lavage (washing out the stomach), induced vomiting, or administration of an adsorbing substance (for example activated charcoal or Fuller's earth). Specific antidotes are infrequently available. In cases of chronic poisoning, removal from the source of exposure and general nursing are most effective. The body may either recover fully, or sustain irreversible damage to some tissues.

During the nineteenth and early twentieth centuries there were many celebrated poison trials, whilst at the same time the science of toxicology (the study of poisons and poisoning) began to develop. For reasons partly connected with availability and partly the result of a continuously developing capacity to detect poisons in the human body, homicidal poisonings are now extremely rare. Figures for 1995 indicated that fewer than 0.5% of fatal poisonings in Britain and the US were proven homicides.

Today, the vast majority of people who suffer acute poisoning are victims of either accidental self-poisoning or SUICIDE attempts. Carbon monoxide (mainly from exhaust fumes or faulty heating systems) accounts for a sizeable proportion of poisoning deaths; children are particularly vulnerable to this and to accidental intake of medicines or household products. Fatal poisonings often follow overdoses of SEDATIVES, tranquillizers, antidepressants, painkillers, and 'social' drugs (alcohol, and illegal substances such as heroin and cocaine). It seems likely that acute and chronic accidental poisoning will continue to represent a significant health hazard for as long as vast numbers of toxic substances — including drugs, industrial chemicals, fuels, pesticides, paints, and household cleaning fluids — remain in daily use.   KATHERINE D. WATSON

See also CHEMICAL WARFARE; DRUG ABUSE; ENVIRONMENTAL TOXICOLOGY; TOXICOLOGY.

Pornography is notoriously hard to define.

The word comes from the ancient Greek *porne* (whore) and *graphien* (write), so pornography is 'writings by/or about whores'. Contemporary dictionaries give a very different definition: today pornography is considered 'obscene material whose intention is to provoke sexual arousal'. Problems remain: how are we to define 'obscene'? Are both James Joyce's *Ulysses* and Larry Flynt's *Hustler* 'obscene'? The US government has thought so. At what point does explicit SEX become 'pornography'? One is tempted to agree with US Supreme Court Justice Potter Stewart who concluded: 'I know it when I see it.'

The category 'pornography' is relatively recent and postdates modern European obscenity by at least two hundred years. The first obscene book, *The Raggionamenti*, was composed by Renaissance Humanist, Pietro Aretino (1492–1556) between 1534 and 1536. *The Raggionamenti* is both a bawdy dialogue between two whores and a biting satire of Renaissance church and state. For the next three hundred years, obscene texts usually included anti-clericalism, religious skepticism, and political satire. During the eighteenth century, pornography played a particularly important role in intellectual life: dirty books were among the century's best-sellers and obscene pamphlets spread the spirit of criticism from the intelligentsia to a small, literate public. Late in the century, Donatien-Alphonse-François, Marquis de Sade (1740–1814) perfected the themes of eighteenth-century pornography in a series of violent and explicit novels that advocated a thorough rejection of all norms, be they political, moral, or religious.

The content of pornography changed in the early nineteenth century: political obscenity vanished to be replaced by a fantasy world or what Steven Marcus calls, in *The Other Victorians* (1966), 'pornotopia'. The audience for obscenity, however, remained the rich: a paper-wrapped, unillustrated book cost a Victorian reader twenty guineas. The leather-bound, illustrated, limited editions printed for rich bibliophiles were even more expensive. Because it was limited to the elite, pornography had a kind of back-door respectability. Obscene texts could be found on the shelves of the British Museum and the Bibliothèque Nationale, but only in special, locked cases — the British Museum's Private Case and the Bibliothèque Nationale's Enfer — which were off-limits to working-class men, women, and children.

Rising literacy rates and the advent of national education made European elites anxious lest pornography made its way into the hands of the masses. To forestall such a possibility, governments in Europe and the US enacted the first anti-obscenity laws: the French laws of 1819, the US Customs Act of 1847, and the British Obscene Publications Act of 1857. All these acts were directed against materials cheap enough to reach 'persons of all classes, young and old'. In the US and Europe, private crusaders like New York's Anthony Comstock (1844–1915) and France's anti-obscenity leagues railed against the evils of 'smut'. Still, pornography proliferated: in France the number of obscene texts multiplied thirteen-fold in the latter quarter of the nineteenth century, and new pornographic media — newspapers, brochures, and naughty postcards — brought obscene images to the masses.

1910 constituted a turning point. In 1913, British and US courts admitted defeat and created a new obscenity standard. Price no longer mattered; only the 'harm' done by pornography. Because they sought to improve society or elevate the human spirit, 'science' and 'art' escaped the charge of obscenity. Only 'smut for smut's sake' (to paraphrase US Judge Curtis Bok) constituted pornography. Legal tolerance (especially of written materials) continued to grow in Britain and the US. In 1967, American courts finally lifted the ban on John Cleland's *Memoirs of a Woman of Pleasure or Fanny Hill* (1749). An American attorney observed that 'there is no longer any obscenity law as far as writing is concerned.'

However, writing was no longer the principal form of obscenity. The image replaced the word, and obscene magazines, video strips, and films were sold in bookstores, specialized cinemas, and arcades. Even the local convenience store stocked explicit magazines, making pornography available to more consumers than ever before. In response, British, Canadian, and American governments formed special commissions in the 1970s and 80s to deal with the 'pornography issue'. In 1968, US President Lyndon Johnson established the Commission on Pornography and Obscenity, which was followed shortly thereafter by the British Home Office Departmental Committee on Obscenity and Film Censorship (better known as the Williams Committee) and the Canadian Special Committee on Pornography and Prostitution. In 1985, distressed by the liberal recommendations of the Johnson Commission, President Richard Nixon established a second anti-pornography commission, the Attorney General's Commission on Pornography, commonly known as the Meese Commission.

The Commissions introduced two new voices into the pornography debate: feminism and social science. In the US, author Andrea Dworkin and lawyer Catherine MacKinnon argued that pornography hurt women by condoning the objectification of women, and RAPE. In 1975, Women Against Pornography, or WAP, was formed and a few feminists served on the 1985 Meese Commission. Meanwhile, social scientists brought laboratory studies to bear on the question of 'harm'. Psychologists concluded that extended exposure to violent pornography produces a 'desensitization effect', or an appetite for increasingly violent sexual media. The social scientists also concluded that only males already predisposed to antisocial behaviour were likely to commit rape after viewing pornographic films.

What is the future of pornography? Pornography continued to move from the margins to the mainstream of twentieth-century life. Home videos and the Internet have made seedy bookstore and sordid 'porn' theatres obsolete. Now consumers can experience 'hardcore' films in the safety and discretion of their own homes. Pornography can be acquired more easily and discreetly than ever before, which argues that pornography will stay with us in the twenty-first century.   KATHRYN NORBERG

Further reading

Hunt, L. (1993). *The invention of pornography: obscenity and the origins of modernity, 1500–1800.* Zone, New York.

Kendrick, W. M. (1987). *The secret museum: the history of pornography in literature.* Viking, New York.

See also SADOMASOCHISM.

Portraits The term 'portrait' generally designates the identifiable representation or likeness of an individual. Portraits may be painted, engraved, photographic, written, or otherwise manufactured records of the individuals or groups of individuals they portray; what characterizes the portrait as such is its capacity to convey the identity of its subject. Portraits represent their subjects by signification, rather than by metonymy or the presentation of actual remnants, for example. A lock of one's grandmother's hair does not a portrait make; nor are saint's remains portraits. Consequently, a verbal description of an individual might also constitute a portrait. In Western culture, however, portraits tend to be conceived and celebrated as durable likenesses, records that commemorate and immortalize. Whether painted or photographic, portraits serve to represent individuals (sometimes groups of individuals, hence 'group portrait') in their absence; they preserve the appearance or likeness of the living even after death.

The inversion of conventional expectations of portraiture in Oscar Wilde's *The Picture of Dorian Gray* (1891) is telling. In this novel, the character Dorian Gray miraculously retains his youthful appearance, while his painted portrait undergoes a gradual (human) ageing process. Generally speaking, portraits preserve the likeness of an individual at a specific moment in time. Whether they take visual or verbal form, portraits are structured to convey an individual's identity, and the media in which they usually do so — stone, as in carved portraits and portrait busts; metals, cast or carved, as in coins; paint; paper, from drawings to printed paper money; photographic film — are intrinsically incapable of representing subjects over time. It could be argued that, given the temporal flexibility of the medium, a written description of an individual could express change over time. But the extent to which portraiture is conventionally and historically associated with visual media (and not as yet with video or film) relates to Western tendencies to favour notions of fixed identity and, thus, to favour fixed representations thereof.

The origins of portraiture are bound up with the origins of naturalistic representation in the West. Classical accounts have it that a young woman of Corinth traced the outlines of her lover's shadow on a wall; this momentous pictorial event is said to have taken place on the eve of his departure for war. Not only did this line drawing capture the identifying features of the young man's PHYSIOGNOMY; it preserved them in his absence. One of the most resilient types of the portrait of Christ, the frontal image of his face called the *vera icon*, is derived from the impression of Christ's features on the handkerchief offered him by St Veronica on the way to Calvary. The question of whether a profile portrait in outline or a full frontal portrait most accurately captures an individual's appearance has undergone much discussion in the West. Coins tend to bear profile portraits; painted portraits tend, with important exceptions, to be frontal or three-quarter, and in varying lengths (bust-portrait, half-length, full-length, for example); the authority of these types and their respective capacity to convey social standing as well as character have shifted with time. Physiognomics, based on the premise that character is revealed by external features, has been popular since antiquity; by the nineteenth century, it had acquired the status of a science. Physiognomics is one of the means by which portraiture is 'guaranteed' to reflect the identity of its subjects. The rank and social standing of the subjects of portraiture are also expressed by conventions, which shift with time. The carved bust was the standard type for Roman imperial portraiture; equestrian portraits, whether cast in bronze or painted, have served for centuries to reflect a ruler's dominion; in the seventeenth-century Netherlands, pastoral portraits of burghers in shepherd and shepherdess costumes were all the rage. In a number of instances, the choice of the artist commissioned to produce a portrait is as significant as the portrait's format or composition.

St Luke became the patron saint of painters because he is reputed to have been inspired to become a painter when the Virgin Mary appeared to him in a vision, and he painted a portrait of her. The rise of portraiture as a central genre in the fifteenth century in Europe has a great deal to do with investment in the capacity of images to substitute, by mimetic means, for what they represent. In this regard, the humanist Leon Battista Alberti plays a key role. In his influential treatise *On Painting and Sculpture* (1435), Alberti argued that 'Painting contains a divine force which not only makes the absent present … but moreover makes the dead seem almost alive. Even after many centuries they are recognized with great pleasure and great admiration for the painter.' Indeed, the great portraits painted by Raphael, Rembrandt, Rubens, Gainsborough, and even Van Gogh are celebrated as much for preserving the likenesses of the sitters as for the hand of the artists responsible. The fact that van Gogh's portraits are capable of fetching record prices at auction surely has less to do with art collectors' interest in the figures van Gogh recorded than in the artistry of the works as such. Nonetheless, for several centuries portraiture was deemed lower in aesthetic value than other genres of painting, such as narrative religious or mythological compositions. Likeness was not, after all, considered morally edifying.

We speak of faithful, and unfaithful portraits. The latter type is held accountable for a betrayal that amounts to failing to represent the subject of the portrait (the 'sitter', in cases of painted portraits) accurately. The accuracy of a portrait is, in the limited sense, mimetic and, in the broader sense, judged according to the extent to which the portrait captures its subject's character. An image might conform to the external appearance of an individual in its aggregate details, but if it stops short of conveying the presence of a unique individual, we hesitate to deem it a portrait. Conversely, we might comfortably call an image a portrait, even if it does not bear witness to the shape of an individual's eyebrows or the exact curvature of her neck, where it does nonetheless embody a recognizable aspect of the sitter's personality or character. To the accusation that his painted portrait of Gertrude Stein (1906), the image by which Stein is still most widely known, did not resemble the sitter, Picasso famously responded, 'That's alright; she will come to resemble it.' And Stein herself is reputed to have added, 'I was and still am satisfied with my portrait, for me, it is I.' Above and beyond capturing likeness, portraiture can serve to construct individual or collective identities, whether in the case of family snapshots or royal, imperial, or presidential portraits.   CLAUDIA SWAN

Further reading

Brilliant, R. (1991). *Portraiture*. Harvard University Press.

Pope-Hennessy, J. (1979). *The Portrait in the Renaissance*. Princeton University Press.

Woodall, J. (ed) (1997). *Portraiture. Facing the Subject*. Manchester University Press.

See also ART AND THE BODY; PHOTOGRAPHY; SCULPTURE AND THE BODY.

Possession The altered state of consciousness known as 'possession' has been, and remains, extraordinarily widespread in societies and cultures across the globe. Typically it involves the occupation of human beings (although animals, too, can be possessed) by spirits who act and speak 'through' their hosts' minds and bodies. Instances abound of powers, deities, devils, or ancestors possessing the living in this way, and of ritual and ceremonial procedures for identifying them, communicating with them, interpreting their pronouncements and demands, and getting them to depart. In many cases, possession is associated with CULTS and occupies a highly significant place in the life of a culture or community — as it does, for example, in the Haitian folk religion of *vodou*. Hosts come to have a privileged social position as spirit mediums and often acquire therapeutic and other thaumaturgical powers. In these circumstances, spirit possession may be a highly desirable and voluntary experience and bring all sorts of communal benefits.

In the past, anthropologists have viewed such benefits in social–functionalist terms, interpreting possession as a form of conflict resolution, as a means for absorbing innovative forces or deviant persons into familiar frameworks, and as a way of enhancing the status of deprived or marginal groups and individuals. A much-discussed suggestion is that possession is a strategy for redressing the frustrated ambitions of female hosts, who otherwise experience only subservience and affliction. Alternatively, possession has been seen in terms of the psychodynamics of intrapsychic tensions and multiple personality disorders, as well as the physiology and epidemiology of trance states. More recently, the tendency has been to read possession for its symbolic meanings and its importance as a cultural resource and as learned behaviour. Here the stress is on the beliefs and values that support it, the codes and conventions in terms of which it is structured and modelled, and the opportunities it provides for communication between the spirit and human worlds and for negotiating questions of identity and selfhood.

In Christianity, possession has usually meant involuntary occupation of the body by the forces of evil. Possessing devils and other 'unclean spirits' were frequently the subject of Christ's own miracles, and the power to cast them out was devolved on his disciples and their followers (Matthew 10: 1; Mark 16: 17). This made exorcism simultaneously a much sought-after therapy and a powerful means of religious propaganda, since the true Church was defined and marked out by its successful use of the exorcistic powers proffered in the gospels as legitimating signs. It has been said that exorcism lay at the heart of the early Christian communities, and it featured prominently in medieval hagiography as the occasion for victories over devils by saints, either personally or at their shrines. Thereafter, formal rituals of exorcism were adopted by the Church throughout the medieval centuries.

When, on the other hand, the Protestant and Catholic Reformations brought deep religious division to Europe in the sixteenth and seventeenth centuries, exorcism naturally became contested. At the same time, demonic possession increased dramatically, probably because demonism in general and WITCHCRAFT in particular were preoccupations of the age. Northern Germany was particularly affected, with possessions becoming almost epidemic after about 1560, but cases are recorded from all over Europe, with female 'demoniacs' predominant. France in particular became notorious for the collective possession and exorcism of entire communities of nuns — notably at Loudun in 1634 and at Louviers in 1643–7. There was even a ministry of exorcists in Rome, and most Catholic clergymen were expected to free demoniacs of their devils by performing either the official Roman ritual or one of the many unofficial exorcisms that circulated in Catholic Europe. In this respect the Protestant clergy were at a disadvantage; they attacked Catholic possessions as fakes and the Catholic ritual of exorcism as a form of magic, but their own parishioners were just as likely to demand help for the same affliction. Eventually, possession again became a powerful propaganda weapon, with Catholic priests urging devils to make anti-Protestant statements and driving them out of their hosts by using Catholic sacraments — above all, the Mass. This often happened in front of substantial crowds and with a good deal of ecclesiastical drama, as in the cases of Nicole Obry at Laon in Picardy in 1565–6 and of Laurent Boissonet and others at Soissons in 1582. In effect, the early modern possessed became sites of confrontation, ostensibly between devils and exorcists but also between different churches.

In addition to these high-profile occasions, ordinary men and women would often become possessed and be diagnosed as demoniacs by their own families or by local village healers. Countryside exorcists were much in demand throughout Europe. The case-notes of the seventeenth-century English astrological physician Richard Napier mention patients of his who attributed 'troubles of mind', temptations, suicidal thoughts, religious anxieties, and hallucinations all to possession. The more spectacular symptoms of the condition, as established by sixteenth- and seventeenth-century physicians and theologians, included wild physical contortions, superhuman strength, speaking in unknown languages, and reacting adversely to holy words and objects. Possessed individuals often took advantage of their situation to blaspheme or behave in shockingly immoral fashion. Generally, they were not regarded as guilty of any sin or crime but as innocent victims of demonic attack; however, in several cases demoniacs did claim that they had been possessed as the result of witchcraft. This happened notably in 1692 at Salem, where the famous witchcraft trials and executions originated in the possession of a group of young and adolescent girls.

The principle that devils might inhabit humans was not abandoned by a substantial portion of the literate classes of Europe, including the medical profession, until the eighteenth century and beyond. In 1737 Isaac Newton's successor at Cambridge, William Whiston, was still saying that possession was as reliable a phenomenon in nature as gravity. But the seventeenth century was marked by considerable controversy surrounding the subject, with some physicians already arguing for a purely pathological, non-demonic explanation of the symptons and others suggesting that many cases were fraudulent — as indeed they were. Thus, Sir Thomas Browne, writing in 1646, allowed that 'the devil doth really possess some men; the spirit of melancholy others; the spirit of delusion other.' In modern times, disease and deception have naturally become the preferred categories for possession in the West, although exorcism is still available as part of the Catholic Church's rituals. During the nineteenth century a favoured approach — adopted particularly by the pioneers of French psychiatry, Louis Calmeil and Jean-Martin Charcot — was to assimilate possession naturalistically to HYSTERIA, and this too has become a common theme in the recent historiography of the subject. Meanwhile, speaking in tongues and other more positive aspects of possession have become features of Pentecostalism and other forms of charismatic religion, notably in America.   STUART CLARK

Further reading
Bourguignon, E. (1976). *Possession*. Chandler and Sharp Publishers, San Francisco.

Walker, D. P. (1981). *Unclean spirits: possession and exorcism in France and England in the late sixteenth and early seventeenth centuries*. Scolar Press, London.

See also WITCHCRAFT.

Posture The human body, like that of any other vertebrate animal, is a very flexible structure, the bones of the SKELETON being linked by almost frictionless JOINTS. In all conditions except that of free fall, a live body can be distinguished from an inert structure by the relative disposition of the body parts, its 'posture'. This is because, during waking life, most of the body is held clear of the ground. Because the body is flexible, appropriate forces have to be developed across each of its joints to support the weight of those parts that are not themselves directly in contact either with the ground or with some other structure supported on the ground. It is these forces that are responsible for the arrangement of the body parts that constitutes the *live* posture.

Muscle force
The source of the necessary forces is the muscular tissue forming the separable muscle masses that are given individual anatomical names. These recognizable '*muscles*' each contain a large number of individual muscle fibres, each in turn dependent for its activity on the arrival of impulses in the motor nerve fibre to which it is connected. When a muscle fibre is made active, it will do one or more of three things, depending on the conditions: it will shorten if it can; it will develop a tension against a resistance; it will show an increased resistance to extension. Since each motor nerve fibre serves a number of muscle fibres, all of these will be active together as a *motor unit* when the nerve fibre is active. The results depend on what else is going on at the time. The control of the forces needed for postural adjustment thus involves organizing the precise timing of the activities of each of the various motor units in the body — a quite formidable task, there being something like a hundred thousand of them in all.

Pulling and pushing
The only type of force that a muscle cell can exert is a tension — whereas, for many postural purposes, what is required is a thrust. The necessary transformation is provided by the leverage of muscles pulling on the jointed skeleton. Force can be transmitted from one place to another through a triangulated lattice structure where each triangle consists either of two ties and a strut or of two struts and a tie. (A *strut* pushes, and a *tie* pulls.) The muscles and tendons can act only as ties, while a bone can act either as a strut or as a tie. Since the combined action of a tension and a thrust applied at different places at one end of a bone can cause that bone to exert transverse thrust at its other end, a bone can also be made to act as a lever. These two mechanisms, the triangle and the lever, serve to supply the necessary forces to produce all the required movements of the parts as well as to maintain the jointed body in its various postures when apparently at rest. The relevant patterns of motor unit activation are idiosyncratic as well as habitual. In consequence, the resulting posture, even at rest, is often highly characteristic of the individual. A 'good' posture

is not only elegant and aesthetically pleasing to the onlooker; it is one in which the body is resilient, ready to undertake any movement that may be called for. This implies that none of the joints, especially those in the back and neck, is at the limit of its range of free movement. As a result, none of the ligaments that restrict joint movement are put under continuous strain.

Movement

In principle, the relative motion between any two objects has six *degrees of freedom*, three directions of linear motion, and three directions of rotation. In the body, however, the relative movement at any joint between two bones is limited in several respects by the ligaments. There are, nevertheless, few joints in the body that act as simple hinges, with only a single degree of freedom. In consequence, when an extremity such as a finger is to be moved from one place to another, there are several different ways in which the movement can be executed even without much change in the trajectory of the extremity itself. Any relative movement of a body part, even of a finger, calls for readjustments at all the joints in the body. All are affected because the change in the distribution of the weight alters the relationship between the position of the centre of gravity of the body as a whole and the disposition of the available supports, and to maintain balance a different pattern of force generation is now required.

Sway

Muscle force is required, not only to support the weight of the body and its parts, but also to set them into motion and to bring them to rest thereafter. Small adjustments in posture are required all the time, to avoid the body being overbalanced by the continual movements of the ribcage in breathing and by the pumping action of the heart. These adjustments affect the position and direction of the resultant supporting thrust (see BALANCE), and result in a continual postural swaying movement as successive incipient topplings in one direction or another are arrested and corrected. Larger changes in muscular activity are required for the voluntary movements of locomotion and for reaching, catching, throwing, and striking.

Where a linear movement is involved, the amount of force that has to be developed by the muscles depends on the linear inertia (or *mass*) of the part that is to be moved. For a rotation, a different measure, the *moment of inertia*, is involved. This measure takes account not only of the mass that is to be moved, but also of the distances of each part of that mass from the axis of rotation.

Preparation for action

Many voluntary actions are performed in two phases. There is a preliminary setting up, followed by the main part of the action. The success of the action is often greatly influenced by the nature of the preparation, e.g. the take-back or back-swing before the strike, or the enhanced

sway required to move the weight off one foot to allow the other to be lifted ready to perform a step. Because the moving parts gain momentum in this preparatory direction and this momentum has to be absorbed before the main movement can start, the activation of the muscles that are to produce the main movement occurs when they are being stretched. The force that a muscle can develop depends on what is happening to its length. It develops more force if it is being stretched than it can while it is shortening. There is thus a significant advantage in the preparatory movement in what appears, at first sight, to be in the wrong direction.

Aiming, throwing, and catching

Any form of voluntary action involves aiming — that is to say, some sort of goal to be achieved by the action — together with some mechanism for indicating a successful outcome. The various modes of locomotion involve throwing and catching the body as a whole by adjusting the forces between the limbs and the available supports, in magnitude, in direction, and in point of application. Too small a supporting thrust will allow the body to fall, while a thrust against the ground greater than that needed for support at rest will throw the body upwards. A horizontal component of thrust at take-off allows the body to move over the ground during the free-fall phase before landing. The body acquires momentum from gravity during the fall and this extra momentum has to be absorbed by extra force at the point of landing, with careful adjustment of the direction of thrust to avoid overbalancing. In some cases the unwanted momentum is absorbed by the stretching of ligaments and tendons. These are elastic structures that can store strain energy, like a spring. The stored energy can be recovered later, during the recoil phase, to generate new momentum in a different direction. This mechanism plays an especially important role in the bounding progression of the kangaroo.

Moving vehicles

When a person is travelling in a moving vehicle, which is changing its momentum under the action of stress forces — as in starting, changing speed, stopping, or being steered into a curved path — appropriate stress forces have also to be applied to the person's body if it is to keep its station within the vehicle.

This requirement does not apply if the vehicle is a spacecraft in orbit. The curvature of the orbital path is attributable to the unopposed action of gravity. The spacecraft together with all its contents, including the passengers, is effectively in free fall. Everything in the spacecraft is accelerating in the same way under the action of gravity, so all retain their relative positions without any support force against the floor or walls of the spacecraft being called for. The condition is referred to as WEIGHTLESSNESS. It is not correct to refer to it as a 'condition of zero gravity', since the orbital path itself is produced by the action of

gravity on the tangential speed of the spacecraft acquired during its launch.

Skills and gestures

In sporting activities the appropriate adjustment of the muscle forces required is clearly a matter of acquired skill, depending on assiduous practice. It is not usually realised that the more everyday activities of sitting up, standing, and moving about are equally dependent on acquired skill, as are also the small movements of the face, larynx, and chest-wall involved in the production of SPEECH. We start learning the necessary skills in early infancy and continue the process throughout life, adjusting our behaviour to suit the various new tasks that we encounter each day. Some of the resulting changes in habitual posture can be interpreted as the BODY LANGUAGE indicating changes in mood. Other changes are used as gestures in deliberate communication with other people, as in adding emphasis to the spoken word. All changes in posture depend ultimately on the same general pattern of neural organisation, namely the control of the detailed timing of the separate activations of each one of a large number of motor units in muscles distributed throughout the body.

Motor control

Attempts to account for the control signals in terms of engineering models usually depend upon the notion that the NERVOUS SYSTEM detects the sort of variables that an engineer designing a robot would use transducers to provide. However, none of the SENSE ORGANS in the body deliver signals corresponding to the simple continuous variables that are required for such models. All sensory messages consist only of irregular sequences of nerve impulses, and any coding that could be devised to correspond to the transformation at the receptor, from stimulus condition to successions of impulses, is unlikely to survive transmission across the SYNAPSES of the central nervous system. These engineering schemata must therefore be regarded as not directly relevant to the way the body actually works. A better understanding of the way the nervous system actually organizes its control of the body musculature should have profound implications, both for the management of clinical disabilities, and for the design of self-adapting machines to take over, in hazardous conditions, certain skilled tasks that at present can be carried out only by a human operator.   T. D. M. ROBERTS

Further reading
Roberts, T. D. M. (1995) *Understanding Balance.* Chapman and Hall, London.

See also BALANCE; MOVEMENT, CONTROL OF; WALKING.

Potty-training
Chinese toddlers often wear split pants, so that they can be held out to relieve themselves on to the ground without soiling their clothes. In the West, however, babies wear

nappies or diapers until they learn to use a pot. For many parents, the learning process becomes a battleground.

There are three probable reasons why young babies cannot learn to use pots. First, their sensory nerves (or the interpretation of their signals by the brain) are not well enough developed for them to know when they have excreted, let alone when they are ready to do so. Second, they do not know how to control their sphincters; so they can't perform on cue. Third, even though the thought of a wet or dirty nappy is horrible to the parents, most babies do not mind it at all.

Some parents try desperately to potty-train their children much too young, and may think not only that they have succeeded, but also that they, the parents, have made a great achievement. But then at the age of 3 or even 4 the children suddenly realize they have a wonderful weapon at their disposal, and start performing at the most inconvenient moments — in the supermarket, for example, or in the middle of lunch with Grandma …

A 1989 survey in Minneapolis reported that three-quarters of parents started potty-training when the child itself was apparently ready; 30.5% between 18 and 23 months, 42.6% aged between 24 and 29 months. The average age for completion was between 24 and 27 months.

Advice to mothers has gradually softened during the last two centuries. Pye Henry Chavasse suggested in 1839 that the baby should be held out over a pot at least a dozen times a day at 3 months old; if this were done, there need be no more nappies at 4 months!

Around the turn of the century, the now less-influential Sigmund Freud regarded sphincter control as part of the second, or 'anal' phase of development, and Freudians suggest that babies become aware that what they produce is theirs, comes out of their bodies and is part of them. Therefore it does not belong to the mother, and should not necessarily be given to her, let alone thrown away in the lavatory. Since then, psychoanalysts have suggested that much of our behaviour stems from the way we were toilet trained. To take just one example, a 1992 paper suggested that François Mittérand's toilet training accounted for his stiffness, obstinacy, shyness, anxiety, attitudes towards money and time, ambivalence, hesitations, contradictions, and desire for power.

In 1912 Edward Mansfield Brockbank said that 'After the second month, the baby can be held … in a sitting position, with some weight on the chamber. … It should be put on the chamber before, during, and after each meal …'

In 1939 Marie Stopes wrote, 'When a baby has responded to the touch of the chamber and passed either water or a motion, he should be rewarded by an expression of pleasure by nurse or mother. "That's right. Good baby" … On the other hand it is a cruel mistake to show signs of displeasure or annoyance about wet or soiled nappies.'

Many clever devices are available to help anxious mothers and encourage the babies, including a musical potty, marketed with the slogan 'Make toilet-training fast, easy, and fun!'. When gold-plated sensors register moisture they trigger one of sixteen cheerful tunes, including Yankee Doodle, Little Brown Jug, and Chim-Chim-Cheree.   ADAM HART-DAVIS

Pregnancy The biological event of pregnancy is established when a fertilized egg successfully implants itself in the lining of the UTERUS, about a week after conception.

The *corpus luteum*, which formed in the OVARY when it released the egg, secretes hormones that keep the uterine lining in a suitable state for implantation; if fertilization had not occurred, this hormone secretion would have ceased, and the uterine lining would be shed after two weeks. The hormonal 'message' from an implanted embryo via the mother's bloodstream to the ovary prevents its own rejection.

Early pregnancy continues to be maintained by the hormones produced by the corpus luteum in the ovary that produced the egg; but later, when the PLACENTA has fully developed (by about 3 months), this takes over the maintenance function through its own hormone production.

Pregnancy produces profound changes in the mother, which may be detected from early stages. There is a marked rise in the output of the heart by 3 months, and it rises further as pregnancy advances, reaching 30–40% above the non-pregnant level by the end. This rise is mainly due to an increase in output with each contraction of the heart muscle (stroke volume), although the heart rate also increases. The volume of BLOOD in the circulation also increases, with a greater increase in plasma volume than in red blood cells, producing the so-called 'physiological anaemia of pregnancy'. Although these changes in the circulation can produce serious consequences for pregnant women with certain types of heart disease, they are necessary to deal with the demands of the growing fetus, placenta, and uterus, and have no deleterious effects in healthy mothers.

There are changes in the BREASTS from an early stage of pregnancy; they enlarge, and surface blood vessels become prominent, reflecting preparation for eventual lactation. Hormonal changes cause development of the glandular tissue: the potential milk-secreting cells and the ducts to the nipples. Although the hormones which cause milk production (*prolactins*) are produced during pregnancy, the actual secretion of milk is suppressed by other hormones until after delivery.

Other changes include a laxity of the JOINTS, which ultimately may assist LABOUR and birth, and increased brown pigmentation of the skin ('*chloasma*' if in the face). *Stretch marks* are other hallmarks of pregnancy in the skin. The mother has increased blood flow to the KIDNEYS, and therefore increased urine production, and this results in more frequent visits to the toilet — a common symptom of early pregnancy. The placenta produces large amounts of the hormone PROGESTERONE, which appropriately prevents the uterine smooth muscle from contracting, but also relaxes smooth muscle throughout the body. This results in many of the so-called minor symptoms of pregnancy, including CONSTIPATION and heartburn, and it may exacerbate VARICOSE VEINS.

The mother's appetite usually increases — but the extra energy requirement for the *whole* pregnancy is not more than about 60 000 Kcal — or 20–24 extra days' worth of food intake. Where there is abundance of food, excessive eating and undue WEIGHT gain are not uncommon, although there is in fact a normal physiological tendency to lay down more fat stores in the earlier months. Appetite for particular foods and drinks, or rejection of others, can be capricious. Occasionally the nausea of morning sickness, which is common in early pregnancy, may extend to other times of day, may be more severe than usual, and may be accompanied by vomiting or may be prolonged into later pregnancy.

The uterus enlarges considerably to accommodate the growing fetus. It emerges from the pelvis at around 12 weeks, reaches the navel at around 22 weeks, and the ribs at around 36 weeks.

Pregnancy normally reaches its dramatic conclusion with the onset of labour, between 35 and 39 weeks after conception.

The establishment of antenatal care to detect problems during pregnancy, and to attempt to ensure that women were in good health at the time of delivery, is generally credited to J. W. Ballantyne, an Edinburgh obstetrician, who took the first step towards this at the beginning of the twentieth century. Clinics became established in major centres in the UK, the US, and Australia by the time of the first World War.   JIM NEILSON

Pregnancy: the cultural context

Pregnancy occupies potent symbolic space in cultures around the world. As both the development of a life and a significant transitional event within the woman's lifespan, pregnancy becomes the focus of cultural desires and anxieties around gender, power, selfhood, and even nationhood. Medical technology has increasingly refigured the physiological possibilities of pregnancy, especially through ASSISTED REPRODUCTION for the infertile, its extensions to surrogacy and older-age pregnancy, and through genetic testing.

One of the most common cultural mythologies about pregnancy is that it is evidence of full womanhood. Because mothering is so closely tied into cultural GENDER roles, to be pregnant is to fulfill one's gendered destiny. Although this emphasis on pregnancy emerges from culturally-specific definitions of femininity and womanhood, many people see the urge as instinctive and the process itself as natural, even as industrialized countries increasingly rely on medical technologies to avoid, create, sustain, and complete pregnancies.

Differential worldwide rates of FERTILITY, infant mortality, and maternal mortality have led the World Health Organization to focus attention on women's differential access to services and opportunities with respect to men as well as between different countries and regions. At least partly because of this focus, all three of these rates dropped by about one-third over the twenty years up to 1998, when overall fertility rate was 2.7 births per woman; Europe was lowest at 1.6, while Africa remained highest at 5.4. Infant mortality rate world-wide was 57 deaths per 1000 live births, whereas highly industrialized countries such as the US and the UK had rates as low as 7 deaths per 1000. Maternal mortality rate (expressed as deaths per 100 000 births) in the UK showed a dramatic drop from the 1930s onwards, whereas until then it had been essentially unchanged at around 500 for 100 years; in the 1980s it was below 10. By the end of the twentieth century, according to the World Health Organization, developed nations averaged a rate of 27 deaths per 100 000 live births. This contrasts with 480 on average in developing nations (comparable to Victorian Britain), with some regions as high as 1000. The global average was 430. While these numbers are specific to pregnancy, and associated with disparities in medical services and supplies, they may also reflect the status of girls and women in different cultures, and their relative power in their societies.

Pregnancy, in the natural order of things, becomes possible and physiologically appropriate as soon as ovulation is established after the MENARCHE, usually during the teens, or even earlier. But in modern developed societies, the issue of teenage pregnancy is increasingly a concern to both moral leaders and health educators. In the UK the rate has been rising: in 1997, under-16s accounted for over 8% of all known conceptions in the under-20 age group; meanwhile rates declined in other European countries and in the US there has been some reduction since the late 1980s. The spectre of the pregnant young girl is often cited as a wake-up call for issues as diverse as promiscuity, health education, and the viability of the welfare state.

Young women who maintain pregnancies are less likely to finish or continue their education, face greater marital instability, have fewer life-long assets, and have lower incomes later in life than women who did not become pregnant young. Yet pregnant teenagers have become symbolic more of the decline of social morality than of the lack of resources granted to young women worldwide.

Teenage and unmarried pregnancies have always existed, but the advent of new methods of CONTRACEPTION in the twentieth century has changed the significance and experience of pregnancy for hundreds of millions of women worldwide. Before these methods were widely and legally available, pregnancy often signified the end of a woman's career choices, if not her need to work; closely successive pregnancies, when timing could not be controlled, often led to early death, as it still does in many places worldwide today.

Female-directed methods, such as the modern INTRAUTERINE DEVICE (IUD) and hormonal control by the Pill or by long-lasting implants, have allowed women to choose not only the occurrence but also the timing of pregnancy. Earlier barrier methods of contraception had allowed women to control their pregnancies somewhat, although they also required them to negotiate with their husbands. Hormonal contraceptives have changed many women's relationship to pregnancy by putting the choice in their own hands. Indeed, world health leaders are calling for this globally as a step towards women's liberation from socially imposed controls.

As women have been afforded more control over pregnancy, they have also been granted more responsibility for the outcomes. European societies of the seventeenth and eighteenth centuries often assumed that strong maternal emotions would mark the fetus; disfigured babies were blamed on maternal viewing of disfigured persons or other disturbing events. Modern versions of maternal responsibility relate to the links between birth outcomes and maternal behaviors, such as drinking alcohol, SMOKING cigarettes, or taking DRUGS (licit or illicit). Whilst high risks for fetal abnormality are established for some maternal excesses (e.g. alcohol, COCAINE), for specific nutritional deficiencies (some VITAMINS and trace elements), and for certain prescription drugs, prohibitions and exhortations may often be overstated. While women around the world and through time have made sacrifices and

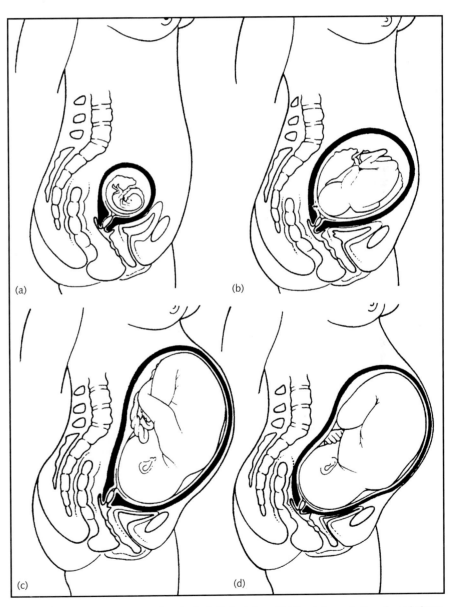

Relative size of the uterus at the end of (a) the third; (b) the sixth; and (c) the ninth month. Near the end of pregnancy the head usually sinks down into the pelvis (d); this is called 'lightening'. Reproduced, with permission, from Youngson (1995), *Encyclopedia of family health*, Bloomsbury Publishing.

personal changes for the good of the fetus, this modern focus on risk and risk management has defined what constitutes 'the good of the fetus'. The rights of women to bodily integrity and self-determination seem sometimes to be undermined by a society's concern to protect the fetus from any possibility of harm.

In the latter half of the twentieth century also, medical technologies began to address INFERTILITY, and to develop methods of assisted reproduction. These have not only benefited childless couples, but have also resulted in extensions of pregnancy in two other contexts. Surrogacy, the creation and carrying of a pregnancy for another woman or couple, has gained both prominence and notoriety in recent years. The practice has spawned high-profile custody cases, the most famous of which is the Mary Beth Whitehead case, as well as more prosaic cases of women carrying babies for their sisters, daughters, and friends — as demonstrated in *Sisters*, US television drama. While this has created legal disputes about the relative importance of genetic parenthood over physical parenthood, it has also enabled infertile couples, including lesbian couples, to create genetically-connected families.

The medical procedures involved in surrogacy — hormone treatments, ova extraction, in-vitro fertilization (IVF), and gamete intrafallopian tube transfer (GIFT), for example — have also allowed post-menopausal women to bear children. A number of cases have recently occurred in the US, where several women in their 50s and 60s have given birth. These events touched off a national debate about appropriate motherhood and the dual pressures towards a career and a family that modern women often face.

Even routine pregnancies in industrialized countries are increasingly technological, as couples are offered genetic counselling, and ultrasound scans and amniocentesis have become commonplace. While these procedures can sometimes highlight problems that medical technology can successfully address, they may create anxiety through false positives, nebulous results, and the construction of pregnancy as problematic, instead of generally successful. While technology has long been able to transform, and has often usefully assisted the procedure of birth, these diagnostic procedures have only recently allowed the medical profession immediate and even cellular control over the management of pregnancy.

Pregnancy is essentially a personal event, but international attention is currently focusing on pregnancy around the world. While the World Health Organization is focused on lowering rates of fertility, infant mortality, and maternal mortality in order to improve the lives of women and children, national concern for differential pregnancy rates frequently betrays racist undertones; industrialized countries, and well-off populations within them, worry about how 'they' will outnumber and overtake 'us'. Although often categorized as a 'woman's issue', pregnancy and the social attitudes towards it thus highlight important cultural issues, such as the relationship between life and technology, the definitions of gender roles in a given society, and the relationship between nations and their citizens.

JULIE VEDDER

See also ANTENATAL DEVELOPMENT; ASSISTED REPRODUCTION; BIRTH; CONTRACEPTION; FERTILITY; INFERTILITY; LABOUR; OVARIES; PLACENTA; SEX HORMONES; UTERUS.

Pregnancy tests

The cardinal feature of pregnancy is of course the cessation of menstruation. But some women have irregular MENSTRUAL CYCLES, and there are many other possible causes of amenorrhoea. The early signs of breast changes, urinary symptoms, and 'morning sickness' can confirm a suspicion within a few weeks of conception, but there may be a more urgent desire or pressure to be certain. For a variety of social, cultural, and sometimes legal reasons, there has no doubt been a very long history of tests for pregnancy. One such is recorded in the Ebers papyrus (about 1350 BCE): 'a water melon is pounded, mixed with the milk of a woman who has borne a son, and is given to the patient to drink. If she vomits she is pregnant, if she has only flatulence she will never bear again.'

Modern pregnancy tests are based on the detection of *human chorionic gonadotropin* (HCG), a hormone unique to pregnancy that starts to be produced by the embedding 'chorionic villi' of the embryo as soon as it becomes implanted in the uterus. The hormone can therefore reach the mother's bloodstream within days of conception, and is excreted in the urine. Tests for its presence by *immunoassay* on samples of urine or of blood are nowadays very sensitive and rapid.

Earlier methods of *bio-assay* for identifying HCG in the mother's urine depended on the use of mice or frogs. In the pregnant woman, the hormone acts on the ovaries so as to maintain the secretion of the ovarian hormones that in turn make possible the continuation of pregnancy; without them, there would be menstruation. If injected into animals, gonadotrophin stimulates the ovaries and ovulation occurs.

Ascheim and Zondek were the first to show, in Berlin in 1927, that pregnancy could be confirmed even before the first missed period, by injection of an extract of the mother's urine into immature female mice. The ovaries were stimulated, causing enlargement with development of eggs that could be seen in the abdomen when the animal was killed after a suitable interval. In 1933, a successful pregnancy test was achieved by Shapiro and Zwarenstein in Cape Town, using a particular variety of frog (*Xenopus*), which had been shown to respond to injection of gonadotrophins by ejecting visible eggs from the body. This *Xenopus test* was refined over succeeding years and in the 1940s the Cape Town laboratory reported >98% correct results. Reporting the history of the test in 1985, Zwarenstein put on record a letter from a family doctor who wrote: 'Thank you for your report on the pregnancy test on Mrs X. You may be interested to know that of one GP of many years' standing, one specialist gynaecologist and one frog, only the frog was correct.' The bio-assay methods continued until the late 1960s, when immunoassay took over.

SHEILA JENNETT
E. M. TANSEY

See also ANTENATAL DEVELOPMENT; PLACENTA; PREGNANCY; SEX HORMONES.

Premenstrual tension

The first 'modern' account of premenstrual tension (PMT) was published in a medical journal in 1931. Feelings of tension, self-deprecation, and even severe depression experienced by women in the 7–10 days preceding MENSTRUATION were accurately described. By the 1950s the list of symptoms reported by women in the premenstrual period had increased, and there was a growing realization that so-called 'tension' was just one aspect of the problems. In a paper published in 1953 the term 'premenstrual syndrome' was introduced to encompass the extending list of symptoms. The name eventually stuck, and the problem is now often referred to as PMS.

The symptoms of PMS include not only anxiety, irritability, and depression but also constipation, food cravings, sleep problems, tiredness, and a feeling of bloatedness, particularly in the abdominal area (due to water retention). These are just a few of the common complaints, and in fact it has been mooted that when all reported symptoms of PMS are added up the total can reach the unbelievable number of 160.

The incidence of PMS ranges from 5% to 95% according to different surveys which have been undertaken. For example, in a survey by Woman's Own magazine in 1993, nine out of ten women claimed to suffer from at least some of the symptoms. A study in the early 1980s by the World Health Organization reported that the incidence of premenstrual mood changes varied between 23% amongst Sudanese women to 73% amongst Muslim women in the then Yugoslavia. Thus one is left with the conclusion that women can and do suffer from PMS irrespective of culture and society. However, such a wide variation in the estimated incidence can either fuel the sceptics or suggest that *not* suffering from PMS is abnormal. In whatever way it is viewed, it is quite clear that many women do experience symptoms associated with their changing hormone levels during their MENSTRUAL CYCLE, and there is now growing awareness that symptoms described by patients as PMS are not always limited to the premenstrual period; they can extend into the menstrual period itself.

The causes of PMS remain unknown. It is generally believed that symptoms result from the waning hormone secretions from the ovaries as the corpus luteum begins to degenerate towards the end of the menstrual cycle. At this stage concentrations of PROGESTERONE and OESTROGEN in the circulating blood decline, and this is thought to precipitate the various symptoms. How the loss of these hormone secretions results in the physical, behavioural, and psychological symptoms ranging, for example, from abdominal bloating to food cravings and lethargy remains unknown, as does the question as to why some women should suffer from PMS while others do not. Theories have been proposed regarding the ratio of oestrogen to progesterone secretions or the absolute concentrations of these hormones, but these have not been consistently validated. More likely, the cause is an individual's response to her changing hormone secretions, which may be exacerbated by social and/or cultural influences.

There is no doubt that SEX HORMONES can influence brain function. It has long been recognised that they can affect the NEUROTRANSMITTERS which transmit neural signals within the brain, and also the receptors on nerve cells which recognize these neurochemicals. Recent work has suggested that the specific receptors for SEROTONIN (otherwise known as 5-hydroxy-tryptamine) are increased by oestrogens but decline when secretions of this hormone are reduced. A deficiency of this same neurotransmitter, or a loss of its receptors, has also been linked with food cravings. Thus it is possible that many of the symptoms of PMS may be caused by the loss of hormone secretions and a consequent reduction in some aspects of brain chemistry. It follows that treatment of symptoms with drugs that can increase serotonin activity, including vitamin B_6, can alleviate the symptoms of PMS.

However, the question still remains: can PMS be defined as a pathological condition or is it a 'normal' consequence of changing hormone secretions? In this respect it is interesting to note that women who are prone to suffer depression are more likely to suffer from PMS than those who do not. Perhaps one should consider that whether or not one suffers from PMS will very much depend on the 'background' of brain chemistry against which the hormones (or lack of them) are working. SAFFRON WHITEHEAD

Further reading

Dalton, K. and Holton, D. (1994). *PMS*. Harper Collins, London.

See also MENSTRUAL CYCLE.

Prions (rhyming with aeons) is an acronym for 'proteinaceous infectious particles'. The term was coined in 1982 by Stanley B. Prusiner, a neurologist at the University of California at San Francisco, who proposed that a new type of pathogen consisting solely of PROTEIN is responsible for a school of deadly neurodegenerative diseases called Transmissible Spongiform Encephalopathies (TSEs). These include scrapie in sheep, bovine spongiform encephalopathy (BSE or 'mad cow disease') in cattle and Creutzfeldt-Jakob Disease (CJD) in people.

Inheritance and infection

TSEs come in an array of strains and types, each causing a distinct pattern of brain damage and clinical signs. The 'drowsy' and 'hyper' lines of sheep scrapie first alerted researchers to such variations in the 1950s. In the late 1970s a type was discovered in North American captive elk that causes a wasting disease. In some human strains, such as CJD, symptoms progress from disturbances of balance and co-ordination to blindness and deep DEMENTIA. Others produce sleep disorders.

Some TSEs look like genetic conditions. For example, the very rare human TSE Gerstmann–Straussler–Scheinker Syndrome (GSS) appears to be strictly familial, striking distant cousins on opposite sides of the globe with eerie similarity. By contrast, other TSEs can clearly be the result of infection. Pioneering work by French veterinarians in the 1930s and 1940s illustrated that scrapie could be spread between sheep and goats by injection.

Among humans, the disease kuru, found in the south Pacific, was also shown to be transmissible. In the 1950s, it was the leading cause of death in the Fore-speaking tribe of the Eastern Highlands of Papua New Guinea, until an international team of researchers discovered that it was spread by funeral rites in which the dead were revered by eating or handling their organs. The West suffered cases of what experts came to dub 'high tech cannibalism': since the 1970s, corneal transplants, dural grafts and contaminated human GROWTH HORMONE extracted from cadaveric pituitary glands have all been shown to be potential vectors for the spread of CJD.

Mechanism of infection

TSE infection has some very odd features. Victims mount no obvious immune response, and the agent responsible is extraordinarily resilient. The solvents used for the storage of pituitary glands for production of growth hormone should have killed all known pathogens. The infectivity of brain matter from scrapie-positive sheep survives exposure to formaldehyde and even ultraviolet radiation. The latter observation prompted a suggestion by British researchers that the scrapie agent, unlike VIRUSES and BACTERIA, might not contain nucleic acid (DNA or RNA), since this would have been destroyed by ultraviolet radiation. Prusiner cited this evidence when he proposed the prion model in 1982.

Since then, Prusiner and supporters of his ideas around the world have tackled TSEs with a series of dramatic experiments using the latest molecular techniques. They have treated diseased brain tissue with detergents and centrifuges and harvested the encrusted, suspect prion. After several groups determined the genetic sequence of that protein, Prusiner realised that it was a fragment of a normal protein (prion protein or PrP), the function of which is still uncertain, which is found in healthy nerve cells. They have gone on to argue, but not to prove, that once mutated, this protein becomes an aberrant prion, e.g. PrP (Scrapie), which might then convert similar healthy protein to the diseased form through a domino-style process that Prusiner calls 'conformation'. This conversion can be sparked, Prusiner speculates, in three different ways: a person can inherit 'weak' proteins genetically inclined to mutate; a person's natural prion protein can spontaneously mutate; or the mutated form can be transmitted through food, surgery, or drugs, seeding the transformation of the host animal's natural protein.

Continuing controversy

In 1997, Prusiner was awarded the Nobel Prize for Physiology or Medicine for elucidating an 'entirely new genre of disease-causing agents'. However, for UK government scientists at the coalface of the British BSE crisis, and other TSE specialists in the United States, the award was premature.

Prions, they observed, had never been shown to cause disease. Only four days before Prusiner's Nobel Prize was announced, the prion scarcely merited a mention in an article in the journal *Nature* by the leading researcher Moira Bruce of the Neuropathogenesis Unit (NPU) in Edinburgh. Bruce described evidence that the same agent that had infected more than a million British cattle was responsible for the variant form of CJD (vCJD), which had started to strike young Britons. Two groups of test mice experimentally infected with either diseased cattle brain or human tissue from victims of vCJD, had very similar patterns of brain damage after very similar incubation times. In presenting her evidence, Bruce only once mentioned the word prion, and couched it in a distancing pair of quotation marks.

Bruce insists that the TSE agent 'behaves exactly like a virus', though her group thinks that it may be an unconventional sort, which they call a 'virino'. The argument between the virus/virino and prion camps is built on styles of investigation that could scarcely be more different. Bruce's group is inheritor of a line of research founded on traditional biological observation. Much of what we know about the pathogenesis of these diseases comes from this group, and the Institute for Animal Health in Compton, Berkshire.

They inoculated mice with extracts of brain tissue from sheep with scrapie, then observed the emergence of infection over two years or more. They established that the strains of scrapie can be recognized by the incubation time and pattern of brain damage in such host mice. They detected the presence in the test mice of a gene that clearly affects incubation times, which they named Sinc, for 'Scrapie Incubation'. It turns out that Sinc is the PrP gene.

They also discovered that the host animal must have a *healthy* IMMUNE SYSTEM for infection to take hold. Infection somehow rides the organs of the immune system and eventually floods out into the CENTRAL NERVOUS SYSTEM, proceeding up the spinal cord to the brain, causing holes and protein deposits (plaques).

In 1993, presenting her findings to the Royal Society in London, Bruce demonstrated that when another species (monkey, sheep, antelope, cat) has been infected with material from a cow with BSE, the infectious material from that new species still exhibits the characteristics of BSE in her strain-typing tests. The prion conformation model has yet to cope adequately with this finding.

All the other species have very different natural prion proteins. The conformation and thus progression of the disease should logically vary according to the particular chemical composition of the victim's own prion protein, which is supposed to be transformed into an aberrant prion by the initial infection. To Bruce, the obvious explanation for the persistent properties of BSE in so many different species was that the BSE agent is a virus-like agent, possessing its own DNA or RNA, which, as in a viral infection, causes the production of more infectious agent just like itself.

To Prusiner, the failure of the opposition to isolate a virus or a nucleic acid is critical. He and his collaborators have shown that mice genetically engineered to stop them producing their own PrP cannot be infected with TSEs from other animals. To them, this is evidence that the protein is the agent. The virus camp sees PrP as a receptor for a foreign agent.

Prusiner and his supporters come back to the toughness of the aberrant protein and its resilience in the face of enzymes, radiation, formaldehyde, and heat. However, prion-sceptics point to work from 1991 indicating that TSE agents are probably not indestructible, just devilishly tricky to get at. And other viruses can survive formaldehyde. During rendering, autoclaving and hormone extraction, protein fragments toughen and aggregate. Whether it is this toughening, or native impenetrability, that protects the TSE agents, their inactivation remains a key challenge in agriculture and medicine.

The most important inroads paved so far by prionism have come in the field of molecular genetics. Prionists have found mutations in the PrP gene that point to genetic susceptibility to TSEs. Neurologist John Collinge, of Imperial College London, with Prusiner in the early 1990s, discovered the PrP mutation involved in the seemingly familial prion disease GSS.

It turns out that the natural prion protein usually carries two delicate tree-like carbohydrate structures, called glycoforms. Prusiner and collaborators in Oxford and Ohio have observed that glycoforms change during disease. Prionists construe the change as a destabilizing part of the protein conformation process. The viral camp sees it as a classic side-effect of a foreign agent getting inside a cell and disrupting protein glycosylation.

Whatever causes the change, pathologists around the world now use glycoform analysis to help them determine the strain of TSE they are seeing in patients. Not enough is known about the protein-sugar variation to determine whether or not it can serve as a stand-alone test to, say, distinguish scrapie from BSE.

The prionists even claim to have demonstrated the conformation process in a test tube, by mixing normal PrP with the aberrant scrapie version, although only limited amounts were converted before the process fizzled out.

Despite impressive progress for the prion model the scientific case is not proven. Bruce's group still believes that the tough protein revealed by Prusiner's research simply cloaks and protects an independent nucleic acid, making up a virino. The prionists, they argue, have not adequately accounted for strain variation in scrapie, or the persistence of a particular TSE's characteristics, whatever its host.

What began as an obscure argument over a rare class of neurological diseases, and continues as an intense scientific controversy, is now at the heart of a world-wide public health crisis. Estimates of the number of Britons likely to succumb to vCJD now swing from hundreds to hundreds of thousands. And the rest of Europe is now battling to stem BSE in its own herds. A current challenge is development of reliable tests that can quickly detect the difference between normal and diseased prions, for screening of food and blood. EMILY GREEN
COLIN BLAKEMORE

Further reading

Collinge, J. (2000) *Concise Oxford Textbook of Medicine* Chapter 13.17 Oxford University Press, Oxford, 855.

Farquhar, C. F., Somerville, R. A. & Bruce, M. E. (1998) Straining the prion hypothesis, *Nature* 391, 345–346.

Prusiner, S. B. (1982) Novel Proteinaceous Infectious Particles Cause Scrapie, *Science*, 216: 136–144.

See also DEMENTIA; INFECTION; MICROORGANISMS; VIRUS.

Progesterone One of the progestogens, steroid SEX HORMONES, which are synthesized in the initial steps in the biosynthetic pathway in the gonads that converts cholesterol to androgens and to oestrogens; or any natural or synthetic steroid having a progesterone-like action. Progesterone is the main progestogen produced by the ovaries, particularly in the second half of the MENSTRUAL CYCLE after ovulation has occurred and the empty follicle has formed a *corpus luteum*. They are also important hormones in PREGNANCY and secreted in increasing concentrations during gestation. S.A.W.

See SEX HORMONES.

Proprioception How do you know where your fingers are, or how much force your muscles are exerting? The terms *proprioception* and *kinaesthesia* cover these sensations. The terms were coined in the late nineteenth century, and evolved to be synonyms, despite their different historical backgrounds. They refer to neural signals which have access to CONSCIOUSNESS and which can contribute to controlling the MOVEMENT and POSTURE of the body. These signals arise from peripheral sensors and from internally generated 'commands' to move. The former arise from inputs to the CENTRAL NERVOUS SYSTEM from specialized receptors, which respond to forces and length changes in MUSCLES, JOINTS, and LIGAMENTS, and in the SKIN. Not surprisingly, all these classes of specialized receptors can change their discharge during voluntary movement and muscle contractions. This finding has been confirmed in conscious human volunteers by recording the discharge of single nerve fibres from these receptors with a microelectrode inserted into a peripheral nerve. This technique is termed *microneurography*. Perceived signals of 'motor commands' arise within the brain and are related to the timing and effort involved in deliberate muscular contractions.

Proprioception is not a single sensation but a group of sensations. It includes the sensations of position and movement of joints (loosely termed 'joint position sense' by neurologists), sensations of muscular force and effort, sensations related to the perceived timing of contractions, and sensations related to the body image. As well as this diversity in the various sensations making up proprioception, even for an individual component more than one mechanism can operate. From an evolutionary point of view this redundancy is not surprising: it ensures that crucial elements in the control of movement are not dependent on a single channel of information.

Clinicians frequently assess a patient's sensation of *passive movement* of a joint. If it is unimpaired, they then know that some peripheral receptors, their links to the spinal cord via peripheral nerves, and their ascending pathways to the thalamus and then to specialized regions of the cerebral cortex, are all intact. Controversy has dogged understanding of this aspect of proprioception, because researchers have often emphasized the role of one category of input and appeared to deny the role of other inputs. However, it is now clear that input from muscle, joint, and skin receptors can provide perceived signals that joints have moved, and in which direction.

Signals from the sensory endings within the main receptors in muscles, the *muscle spindles*, probably play an important role in signalling the direction of passive movements and their velocity. Muscle spindle endings respond to very small changes in muscle length, and the gain of their input can be affected by the specialized motor output from the SPINAL CORD to the spindles, termed the *fusimotor system*. Specific signals from muscle spindle endings are interpreted centrally in the light of the fusimotor output to them, along with signals from antagonist muscles, joints, and nearby skin. Most *joint receptors* discharge towards the extreme end of a range of movement, while some local and more remote *cutaneous receptors* discharge as the skin is distorted by movement of nearby joints.

The force of a muscle contraction, and the apparent heaviness of weights actively lifted by the limb, are encoded by sensitive tension receptors (*Golgi tendon organs*). They are connected between the muscle fibres and intramuscular extensions of the tendon, and they respond to global forces generated actively by the muscle. However, a potent additional mechanism dominates judgements about force and heaviness: signals of motor command or effort are critical. An abnormal increase in motor command or effort can explain why weights lifted by fatigued or pathologically weakened muscles feel heavy despite the fact that their physical weight is unchanged. In an experimental situation subjects can distinguish between the signals of central command and those of peripheral force. However, this distinction is less obvious when lifting a heavy suitcase at an airport — it still seems to get heavier.

For the various sensations comprising proprioception, acuity is not necessarily identical at all joints of the body. As examples, detection of passive movements applied to the terminal joint of the big toe over a range of velocities is comparatively poor, while, for judgements of force, accuracy is comparatively high across a wide range of forces for the terminal joint of the thumb.

Rather like the judgements of force, the proprioceptive mechanisms that determine the perceived timing of muscle contractions have both a 'peripheral' and a 'central' component. Subjects can attend to either a central signal associated with the motor command to move, or one arising from muscle, joint, and skin receptors *after* the muscle contraction has begun. Clearly the former signal is generated without a peripheral input, because it arises *before* movement occurs. Furthermore, subjects can accurately attend to signals about the size and destination of motor commands, particularly those directed to the intrinsic muscles which move the fingers and thumb.

The importance of input from proprioceptors is highlighted when peripheral nerve damage (such as a severe sensory neuropathy), or damage within the brain (such as a STROKE), eliminates sensations based on signals from specialised muscle, joint, and cutaneous receptors. When this occurs there is marked impairment of tasks requiring manipulative skill and the co-ordination of multiple muscle groups, such as walking. It also becomes difficult to sustain a steady muscle contraction. More restricted losses of proprioceptive inputs, such as those following surgical replacement of joints, produce only minor impairment to proprioception.

SIMON GANDEVIA

Further reading

Gandevia, S. C. (1996). Kinesthesia: roles for afferent signals and motor commands. In *Handbook on integration of motor, circulatory, respiratory and metabolic control during exercise*, (ed. L. B. Rowell and J. T. Shepherd), pp. 128–72. American Physiological Society.

McCloskey, D. I. (1978). Kinesthetic sensibility. *Physiological Review*, **58**, 763–820.

See also BALANCE; JOINTS; MOVEMENT; SENSORY RECEPTORS; SKELETAL MUSCLE.

Prostaglandins

are a group of biologically active compounds with a plethora of different actions and produced in virtually all tissues of the body. Unlike most *autacoids* (substances formed by cells themselves, which act as 'messengers' to other cells) they are not synthesized and stored ready for use. Rather, they are produced on demand in response to a great variety of stimuli. They have a major role in the mediation and modulation of inflammatory states — from the response set up around a splinter lodged in a finger to involvement in a major asthmatic attack or in anaphylactic shock. Many drugs which can be bought over the counter in pharmacies are anti-inflammatory agents, from lowly ASPIRIN to many more modern remedies. All these so-called NSAIDs (*non-steroidal anti-inflammatory drugs*) have their effects by reducing or preventing the actions of prostaglandins.

The name 'prostaglandin' was coined after it was found that SEMEN contracted the smooth muscle of the uterus. It was considered that the substance in the semen responsible for this effect came from the PROSTATE GLAND. There are many different prostaglandins and related substances, and the nomenclature is complex. All are derived from a membrane lipid called *arachidonic acid*, which has 20 carbon atoms and 4 double bonds. The substances derived from this acid are more properly called *eicosanoids* (eicosa-20; enoic-double bonds). There are three main groups of eicosanoids — prostaglandins, *thromboxanes*, and *leukotrienes*. The first two, prostaglandins and thromboxanes, are sometimes called prostanoids.

Arachidonic acid is part of some membrane phospholipids. Phospholipase enzymes liberate the arachidonic acid from its linkage to the phospholipid. (Anti-inflammatory STEROIDS, such as cortisol, prevent this liberation and hence relieve inflammation.) The free arachidonic acid then undergoes a complex series of biochemical transformations, to produce the prostanoids (PGE_2, PGD_2, $PGF_{2\alpha}$, PGI_2 (prostacyclin)) and the thromboxanes (TXA_2 and others). The cyclo-oxygenase enzymes are involved at this stage, and it is these that are inhibited by NSAIDs, including aspirin.

Bergstrom and Samuelsson, in Sweden, worked out the complex chemistry of arachidonic acid and its products, and Vane and colleagues, in England, showed that aspirin inhibited the cyclo-oxygenase system. Together they shared a Nobel Prize in 1982 for their work on the prostanoids. There is an alternative pathway for metabolism of arachidonic acid using lipoxygenase enzymes, rather than cyclo-oxygenase; the end products are a family of leukotrienes (B_4, C_4, D_4, E_4, and F_4).

The whole eicosanoid cascade is set off by a great variety of different types of stimuli. Three examples are these: following the action of thrombin on platelets during the clotting process; by the actions of *kinins* released on INJURY; and following the reaction of antibodies with antigens on the surface of cells, as in an allergic response.

Not all eicosanoids are produced in all tissues. For example, prostacyclin is produced predominantly from the cells lining BLOOD VESSELS: this causes vasodilatation and inhibits platelet aggregation. On the other hand, the thromboxane TXA_2 is formed in platelets and causes vasoconstriction and platelet aggregation. Because the enzymes used in the production of prostacyclin and TXA_2 are different, a small daily dose of aspirin is able to prevent TXA_2 formation without affecting prostacyclin formation. This is therefore an effective way of preventing intravascular thrombosis, and thus reducing the risk of STROKES and HEART ATTACKS. Many people now follow this simple routine. The prostanoid PGE_2 is effective in inhibiting gastric secretion and stimulates mucus secretion in the stomach; it is also a mediator of FEVER. Many prostaglandins have bronchoconstrictor actions. Leukotrienes generally cause bronchoconstriction and vasodilatation (except for the coronary arteries, which are constricted); they are important mediators in all types of inflammation, and responsible for the slow, second, histamine-resistant phase of anaphylaxis.

ALAN W. CUTHBERT

See also ALLERGY; ASPIRIN; FEVER; INFLAMMATION.

Prostate

The prostate gland surrounds the urinary passage at the exit of the male BLADDER. The gland is very small in babies and grows at the time of puberty in response to TESTOSTERONE secreted by the testicles. The function of the prostate is to secrete fluid which together with secretions from the seminal vesicles makes up most of the volume of the seminal fluid. The functions of seminal fluid are incompletely understood and more than a hundred compounds have been isolated from it. The gland has given its name to the group of substances known as PROSTAGLANDINS, first identified at this site, but now known to be present throughout the body; prostaglandins in the seminal fluid may cause contractions of the female genital tract, facilitating transport of sperm through the UTERUS to the FALLOPIAN TUBES. The fluid also helps with the nutrition of SPERM and defence against infection. The ejaculate forms a clot which sticks to the mucus of the cervix, enabling the passage of sperm into the mucus, through which they can travel to enter the uterus. An enzyme called prostatic specific antigen (PSA) then liquefies the sperm clot and the seminal fluid subsequently seeps out of the vagina. PSA is produced by the lining cells of prostate ducts and a small amount can be detected circulating in the blood. Any condition that increases prostate cells, such as benign enlargement of the prostate, or CANCER, or any condition which causes leakiness of the cells such as prostatitis, results in increased levels of PSA in the blood. Very high levels of PSA usually indicate cancer, but moderately raised levels may indicate a whole variety of prostate disorders. There is worldwide research on the merits of PSA estimation as a screening test for prostate cancer but because increased levels may occur in a number of prostate disorders it can never be a perfect test.

Most men remain unaware of their prostate until late middle age when enlargement interferes with urination by constricting the urethra and reducing urine flow. This is often associated with the need to rise at night and pass urine more frequently. For more minor symptoms, there is effective drug treatment. When the symptoms become sufficiently disabling the usual treatment is an operation. The current life-time chance of requiring a prostate operation is about one in ten. Prostate cancer is very common in elderly men and is a significant cause of pre-mature death, but the paradox is that many more men have prostate cancer than die of it. Benign enlargement of the prostate and in some cases, cancer, can be treated by operations to remove part, or in cancer cases, the whole of the prostate. Many men fear these operations will result in IMPOTENCE. In most cases of benign enlarge-ment of the prostate there is no danger of impo-tence. Removal of part or all of the prostate does however result in a lack of external EJACULATION because the junctions between the genital and urinary tracts lie within the prostate. In opera-tions to remove the gland completely, it is possi-ble for the nerves to the penis to be damaged, since they run close to the prostate. For many men with prostate cancer, total removal by oper-ation is not feasible and the mainstay of treat-ment is to give hormones. Both the normal and the cancerous prostate grow in response to testosterone and the strategy of hormone treat-ments is to deprive the cancer of male hormone. This can be done in a number of different ways, both by blocking production of testosterone and by blocking its action. Hormone treatments are not curative but they may remain effective for many years.   TIM HARGREAVE

Further reading

Rous, S. (1995). *Prostate book*. Norton, New York.

See PLATE 8.

See also EJACULATION; SEMEN; SEX HORMONES.

Prostheses A prosthesis is an artificial replace-ment for a missing or non-functioning body part. It can be either functional or cosmetic, and can be attached to the body externally or implanted surgi-cally. Probably the best known images of prosthe-ses are fictional: from the fearsome hook and peg-leg of the seafarers of old (*Captain Hook* and *Long John Silver*) to the modern prosthetic supermen of television and film (the *Bionic Man* and *Robocop*). In the broadest sense, the area of prosthetics includes not only artificial limbs, JOINT replace-ments, HEART valves, and dentures, but also HEARING AIDS of various kinds, PACEMAKERS, and breast and penile implants. The medical reasons for prosthesis use include congenital absence of body parts, other birth defects, trauma, AMPUTATION, radical surgery (often for cancer), disease, burns, and arthritis.

External prostheses have a long history. The *Rig Veda*, an ancient collection of hymns and one of the foundations of the Hindu religion, tells of Vispala, to whom the gods gave an iron prosthe-sis when she lost her leg in battle. According to Herodotus, the soldier Hegistratus of Elios used an artificial foot. Pliny, in his *Natural History*, writes of Marcus Sergius, who, during the Second Punic War, went into battle with an iron hand, fashioned to hold a shield, tied to his arm. Most prostheses of the early modern era were

custom-built by armourers for their warrior masters. The German imperial knight Götz von Berlichingen, who in 1509 lost his hand in the Battle of Landshut and in 1773 was immortal-ized in a play by Goethe, commissioned an iron hand, which had four fingers and a thumb. This mechanical masterpiece was copied many times over the following two hundred years.

Advances in surgery, such as the use of ANAES-THESIA and the tourniquet, eventually meant that a large number of patients could live through an amputation procedure, although surviving the almost inevitable INFECTION afterwards was another matter. A significant market for limb prostheses was created by the first example of truly modern warfare, the American Civil War (1861–5), and by the US Government's commit-ment to supply prostheses to war veterans. From this time, companies began to supply limbs made from wood, metal, and leather. With simple con-struction and operation, these devices could be quite reliable. Feet were generally single units, usually with a simple hinge joint at the ankle. Knees locked when weight was placed upon them, and otherwise swung through when the wearer moved his hip forward. Many prosthetic hands were simple clamps or hooks driven by cables attached to harnesses slung across the shoulders and back of the wearer. Other hands had anatom-ic shapes but were of cosmetic value only.

The first externally powered prosthetic limbs were built in Germany around 1915, although it was not until the 1950s that electrically and pneumatically powered devices appeared for general use. The need to care for large numbers of amputee casualties from World Wars I and II led to significant advances in the field of pros-thetics, especially in Europe, as later did the sudden temporary increase in babies born with limb abnormalities (resulting from maternal treatment with the drug thalidomide). Current motivations for further improvements in pros-thetics include the need to help those suffering from traumatic loss of limbs caused by land mines and other explosive devices, and a desire to meet the ever-increasing demands of prosthesis

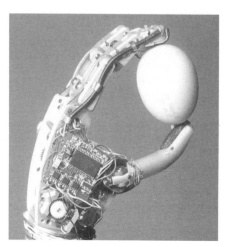

Prosthetic hand. (Photo Peter J. Kybert.)

users, many of whom wish to hold physically demanding jobs or to take part in sports.

The first use of a microprocessor in an external prosthesis occurred in the 1990s in a device that controlled the speed that an artificial knee could swing forward during walking, automatically matching the wearer's pace. More complex devices are now possible, due to a broad range of improvements in materials and electronics. Direct attachment of external prostheses to the skeleton has recently been achieved; this allows forces and vibrations to be transmitted directly to the bones, enhancing what the user can feel through the prosthesis, so-called *osseo-perception*.

Along with limb replacements, dentures, although kept within the mouth, are another form of external prosthesis with a long history. It is thought that the first set was made more than two thousand years ago by the Etruscans. In the modern era, a famous denture-wearer was the first President of the US, George Washington, whose dentures, although rumoured to be made of wood, were manufactured from hippo-potamus ivory and cow's teeth, along with some metal and springs. By the late eighteenth century, porcelain had replaced ivory as the material of choice for teeth in dentures. It is now possible to be fitted with replacement teeth that sit on titani-um posts implanted directly into the jaw bone. An important aspect of this and many other implant procedures is *osseo-integration*, or the achievement of firm fixation of the implant within bone.

The development of implantable prostheses is linked to advances in surgery. Until Lister intro-duced aseptic surgical techniques in the 1860s, infection after surgery was a great hazard, espe-cially if any foreign material was inserted into the wound. By using carbolic acid to cleanse open wounds, Lister was able to achieve healing in cases where previously amputation was the only treatment. His techniques also made it possible to limit infection after an open operation. This paved the way for surgically implanted prosthe-ses, although it was not until alloys, plastics, and ceramics with adequate inertness and mechani-cal properties were produced that real advances were made. This requirement of 'biocompatibili-ty' of implant materials, in which the material exists in close harmony with the body without the bodily environment adversely affecting the material or the material adversely affecting the body, reduces the potentially usable implant materials to only a few dozen.

Even before Lister, orthopaedic surgeons were experimenting with metal wires and pins for repairing broken bones. In the first half of the nineteenth century, some of the first animal experiments to determine the suitability of materials for use in the body were carried out in dogs. After Lister's advances, widespread clinical investigations and further animal experiments were conducted to study the reactions of the soft tissues and bones to the presence of a foreign material in the body. It gradually became clear that steel possessed the best properties for highly stressed applications, although it was not until well into the twentieth century, with the introduction of stainless steel (containing molybdenum), Vitallium (an alloy of cobalt, chromium, and molybdenum), and tantalum, that implant surgery was truly able to advance.

Joint replacement by prosthetic means is one of the most successful operative procedures in modern medicine in terms of number of patients treated and quality-of-life improvement. The hip has historically received the greatest attention. In 1946, the Judet brothers introduced a hip prosthesis (replacing the upper part of the femur alone), which was the first femoral prosthesis designed on biomechanical principles and used on a widespread basis. It was also the first mass-produced surgical prosthesis in which a thermoplastic was used. Over time it suffered from serious problems of material degradation and inadequate fixation to bone, but it nevertheless stimulated considerable effort towards the improvement of joint replacement. In the 1960s, hip replacement was put on a firm basis by Charnley, who used polymethylmethacrylate cement to fix both the metal femoral component and the plastic pelvic component of the prosthesis into bone. It is now possible to replace almost all the joints of the body, including hips, knees, elbows, shoulders, ankles, and fingers.

Work on cardiovascular prostheses began after World War II, when techniques were developed to maintain circulation of oxygenated blood through the body during open-heart surgery. The main technical problems to be overcome are the tendency of blood to clot on a foreign surface and the need to maintain natural blood flow rates through the prosthetic devices. The first clinical use of a mechanical heart valve prosthesis was reported in 1954, but it was not until the 1960s that the caged-ball type valve (metal cage and rubber ball) met with major clinical success. Pivoting disc valves with pyrolitic carbon discs and bileaflet designs are now also on the market. The first report of a synthetic vascular graft appeared in 1952, when Voorhees described his initial work in dogs. Arterial prostheses made of Dacron became commercially available in 1957, while expanded polytetrafluoroethylene (ePTFE) grafts were introduced in the 1970s. In 1969, Cooley performed the first total artificial heart implantation in a human. However, despite early optimism, the rate of progress in this field has been disappointing. The primary use of the total artificial heart today is as a temporary support to allow some recovery of function or until a donor heart can be found.

Much of the progress in the field of prosthetics over the last fifty years has been due to cooperation between prosthetists, surgeons, engineers, and materials scientists. Replacement of almost every part of the human body has been attempted. The next generation of 'spare parts' will depend on the development of new materials which can adapt to the demands placed on them and on collaborations with cell biologists so that hybrid artificial organs made of both living elements and synthetic materials can be developed.

The real challenges lie in replacing complex organs, such as the heart, lungs, kidneys, liver, and pancreas, and in being able to design prostheses that will last for decades.

AMY B. ZAVATSKY
PETER J. KYBERD

Further reading

Atkins, D. J. and Meier, R. H. (ed.) (1988). *The comprehensive management of the upper-limb amputee.* Springer-Verlag.

Black, J. (1999). *Biological performance of materials: fundamentals of biocompatibility.* Marcel Dekker, New York.

Childress, D. (1985). Historical aspects of powered limbs prostheses. *Clinical prosthetics and orthotics*, 9(1), 2–13.

Schurr, D. G. and Cook, T. M. (1990). *Prosthetics and orthotics.* Appleton and Lange.

Silver, F. H. (1994). *Biomedical materials, medical devices and tissue engineering: an integrated approach.* Chapman and Hall.

Williams, D. F. and Roaf, R. (1973). *Implants in surgery.* W. B. Saunders Company Ltd., London.

See also BODY DECORATION; COSMETIC SURGERY; DENTISTRY; HIP REPLACEMENT.

Prostitution is widely described as the world's oldest profession; the practice of selling sex for cash or other immediate compensation has existed across cultures and times from the ancient Greeks, through religious servitude, to today's madam scandals that have rocked the British Parliament, America's Hollywood, and America's east coast Blue Bloods. Prostitution also crosses class lines, from the poor 'streetwalkers' with their stereotyped drug habits and abusive pimps to the high-class brothel and escort service workers with their designer clothes and stylish apartments.

While the prostitute technically sells a service, namely sexual intimacy, the ways in which prostitution is discussed suggest that, at least to modern sensibilities, she or he is selling far more than that. Common euphemisms for prostitution in English include 'selling her body' and 'selling herself': conflating the body and the self with sexual intimacy suggests that sexual intimacy both defines and controls the body and the self. What one does, then, defines who one is. A whore is always a whore.

A common misconception of prostitution is that a significant majority of prostitutes are women. While women's prostitution is far more easily talked about, male homosexual prostitution has existed alongside female heterosexual prostitution at least since the time of the ancient Greeks, but it is rarely discussed or studied. Nearly all of prostitution, however, serves the sexual needs of men; very little prostitution services women of any class.

Most analyses of prostitution suggest that both men and women enter prostitution, either professionally or temporarily, as relative amateurs, for economic and monetary reasons.

Certainly, through most of history there were few professions open for women, especially if they had little family support or they lacked the education or class status to aspire to the few professions that respectable women could participate in. Conversely, many people who are advocating a departure from the shame culture surrounding sex in a variety of arenas, including sex work, argue that some prostitutes work in order to challenge repressive GENDER roles which restrict women's SEXUALITY to a romantic ideology and oppressive patriarchal MARRIAGES. As these activists are also working to change women's opportunities and thus eliminate prostitution as a forced, last-ditch option for staying alive, they are not simply romanticizing prostitution but complicating it by forcing the world to consider the positive choices of sex workers.

The economic argument, however, has been boosted in the past two decades by the development of the East Asian sex trades, which form significant portions of the economies of countries such as Thailand. American military installations during the Vietnam War helped begin the sex trades as military officials organized R&R for their soldiers. As the global economy forced previously agrarian cultures to move towards a capitalist, cash-based system, the sex trades boomed as young girls were sold or forced into urban prostitution in order to support families in more rural areas. Currently, it is common for men from First World countries to join tours in East Asian countries that consist entirely of patronizing the sex industry.

Although the East Asian sex industries have brought the issue to prominence recently, the issue of child prostitution has always been a rallying cry for those interested in eradicating sex work. The mythologies surrounding VIRGINITY — including the regenerative powers of having sex with a virgin, the idea that virgins could cure SEXUALLY TRANSMITTED DISEASES, and the thrill of the power differential between an experienced man and a young, inexperienced girl — have always ensured that young girls, sometimes as young as six, will be included in the sex industry. As prostitution frequently involves an economically exploitative relationship with a pimp or a madam, young girls are at even higher risk of abuse and exploitation than their older counterparts.

Forced prostitution, beyond families selling their girl children into sexual servitude, has also become a political issue recently as the Korean women forced to serve as 'comfort women' for Japanese troops in World War II have demanded restitution and apology from the Japanese Government. Repeated RAPE as a form of terrorism and war crime often blurs the line between rape and prostitution as women are forced to provide sex to ensure their very lives.

Social tolerance for prostitution has varied widely; some cultures and times have accepted it as a natural part of life, regulating it to prevent the spread of disease or illness, and to prevent the abuse of women. Other cultures and times have turned a blind eye, criminalizing it but not enforcing the law. Still others, notably Victorian England and contemporary America, have actively worked to eliminate the practice altogether through raids, undercover police work, moral exhortation, and prosecution. While prostitution necessarily involves two people, elimination efforts have focused on the prostitutes themselves, and not their customers.

International feminist coalitions are working to eliminate prostitution on the grounds that sex work is an extreme manifestation of patriarchally-enforced gender roles, whereby women's social position is necessarily one of subservience to men, and women's work is often connected to the sexual or domestic servicing of men in order to achieve financial and social support. Further, prostitution helps to maintain the old dichotomy of the good girl/bad girl; women are either asexual, moral creatures, above reproach, or they are the sexual and dirty things that men go to for the relief of unbearable urges. These feminists argue that the elimination of prostitution would allow women to renegotiate gender roles and sexual experience because they would have a valuable bargaining chip.

Whores' rights activists cite the same problem 'the virgin/whore dichotomy' but argue that legitimizing sex work undermines the distinction by highlighting the ways in which women's gender roles are based upon sex as a valuable commodity. They also argue that sex work provides a valuable service that should be granted more respect. Groups like COYOTE (Call Off Your Old Tired Ethics) are interested in changing the moral value of sex, and thus the moral value of prostitution as well, while at the same time undermining the idea that consenting adults are any more exploited than they would be in another industry.

While activists and politicians today disagree about whether sex work between consenting adults is legitimate, there is little question on the official level that child prostitution and forced prostitution should be eradicated.

JULIE VEDDER

Further reading

Barry, K. (1995). The prostitution of sexuality. New York University Press.

Evans, H. (1979). *Harlots, whores and hookers: a history of prostitution.* Taplinger Publishing Company, New York.

See also PAEDOPHILIA; SEXUAL ORIENTATION.

Protective clothing might be anything from
a fig leaf to protect against embarrassment to a medieval knight's ARMOUR to ward off swords, arrows, and lances, or something in between.

The term 'protective clothing' covers a wide range of products, including high visibility garments for workers amongst traffic; flame-proof coveralls for racing drivers; flame and heat resistant turn-out suits for firemen; gas, liquid, and dust proof suits for the chemical industry's workers; chain-mail gloves for butchers; chainsaw stopping trousers for forestry workers; hard hats and hard-toe boots for building workers; welders' UV protective gloves and goggles; hearing protectors, immersion suits, and buoyant garments for workers on water; rescue harnesses and fall arrest systems; bullet proof vests; and a wide range of sports equipment from fencing masks to ice hockey goal keepers' whole body coverage with impact absorbing padding.

Viewed simply, protective clothing is something an individual places between themselves and a hazard in order to stay in the vicinity of the hazard with a reduced risk of injury.

It is better to reduce the hazard than to wear protective clothing

The recognition of the need to use protective clothing is an admission of failure to find another way of carrying out the task that eliminates the hazard or removes the worker or sportsman from the vicinity of the hazard. During the industrial revolution many industries produced uncontrolled hazards such as the dust from cotton spinning and weaving. When the resulting fire risks and illnesses were recognized, regulations and ventilation were introduced to control the dust. Modern protective clothing could allow workers to work in the cotton dust, but the appropriate solution is still to control the dust. Similarly, highly carcinogenic dyestuffs can be handled safely, but it is better to replace them by less dangerous ones.

There remain, however, many situations in which the people cannot be or even do not wish to be separated from the hazard, so apart from using protective clothing increased safety can only be achieved by ending the activity. Cricket would not be the same game if the ball was so soft it could not cause injury. The batsman's pads, gloves, and helmet are the protective-clothing response to the hazard of the high speed hard ball. Health care workers cannot be separated from the infectious patients they treat. They therefore need clothing that is a barrier to BACTERIA and VIRUSES. Motorcyclists will remain at high risk of severe and fatal injuries from road and vehicle impacts, until they all drive cars. Helmets and leathers are worn to reduce the severity of the injuries in the inevitable accidents that occur.

Is discomfort the penalty of protection?

Naturists regard all clothing as an unnecessary impediment to the enjoyment of life and freedom of expression. All clothing has mass and bulk, so it inevitably impedes movements and the free exchange of energy with the environment. In a hot humid climate any clothing is a burden and we would be better off wearing none. However, when the sun shines clothing is a beneficial barrier against radiant heating and ultraviolet burning.

An individual's choice of what regular clothing to wear depends on its availability and cost, changing FASHIONS, cultural conditioning, desire to project a particular image, and perception of comfort. Comfort is a person's subjective evaluation of satisfaction with prevailing conditions, including external physical factors, internal physiological responses, and psychological and emotional state. It is well known that a lot of physical discomfort is acceptable if the right image can be projected. On the other hand, desire for comfort may well have led people to develop clothing that provided a high level of protection long before such a concept was coined. The Inuits' traditional caribou skin garments protect against severe cold, and a cowboy's chaps protect against thorny vegetation.

Protective clothing is primarily developed to prevent a particular hazard causing harm to the person in the clothing. Developers seek materials and construction methods expected to resist the hazard. They consider which parts of the body are most at risk and seek to cover these. If the hazard is a dust or gas they may have to design for total enclosure. Consideration of the wearer's comfort, mobility, dexterity, and level of physiological stress tends to come after the desired protection level has been achieved. Not surprisingly, users complain that this is the wrong way round.

Discomfort is the major unsolved problem with protective clothing. As greater mass and bulk are added to provide specific protection, discomfort escalates. Soldiers may be quite comfortable in a range of conditions wearing underclothing providing soft skin contact and a battle dress designed to keep them dry, warm, clean, and inconspicuous. However, they soon become very uncomfortable wearing a flak jacket and ballistic helmet as well. Add an NCB coverall (nuclear, chemical, and biological protection) and a respirator, and major physiological strain occurs on exercise. Add climatic conditions such as those in Saudi Arabia and it is obvious that the essential protective clothing is going to become a very big problem to its wearer.

Re-thinking the job may reduce the need for protection and therefore discomfort

Sometimes a radical re-evaluation of a job results in alternative solutions to the use of protective clothing. Work on the sea bed used to be done by divers in rigid, steel pressure-resisting suits with atmospheric pressure inside. Their capacity for work was very limited. Now divers are compressed in HYPERBARIC CHAMBERS to the pressure at the depth at which they will work, and breathe special helium/oxygen mixtures to prevent subsequent DECOMPRESSION SICKNESS. When at depth they are at the same pressure as the sea water, so they can wear light, non-pressure-resisting suits and do much more work. The disadvantage is that they have to remain compressed for many days and nights, and have to go through a long decompression process before they can safely leave the chambers.

Developing better protection and barrier systems for use in protective clothing may directly and indirectly cause problems. Firemen used to stand back from fires and direct their hoses at the burning buildings. This was not very effective. Modern practice is to get inside the building, and as close to the seat of the fire as possible, and to extinguish it directly. Much higher resistance to flames and to the transmission of heat is therefore needed in the firemen's clothing, and this has progressed from colourful uniforms, through heavy woollen fabrics, to the current multilayer non-flammable thermal barrier systems. The closer the fireman gets to the fire the greater is the need for a thermal barrier, and it is this that causes most problems, because it prevents the fireman's own metabolic heat being lost whether he is near a fire or not. Heat stress is an almost inevitable result. In addition, more mechanical protection is needed close to the fire due to the hazards of collapsing buildings and explosions; this adds to the weight, bulk, and stiffness of the clothing and hence to harder work with a higher heat output by the fireman.

Standards for the performance of protective clothing

Protective clothing can be regarded as an aspect of occupational health. It is worn to prevent injury or ill health due to contact with a hazard. The performance of the clothing when it is needed may be critical, but its ability to deliver the performance may not be obvious to potential users. Therefore there has been extensive activity to produce standards for protective clothing so that purchasers can be told what the clothing should do. This work received great impetus with the publication of Council Directive 89/686 of 21 December 1989, by the European Union Commission. The Directive covers all personal protective equipment (PPE), including clothing, and it lists certain basic health and safety requirements that protective clothing must meet. The response of industry, Standards authorities, Test Houses, and users' organisations has been to work on harmonizing the protective clothing standards existing in European countries, and to develop new standards. The work is now usually being done with ISO (the International Organisation for Standardisation) resulting in worldwide participation and application. By 2001 over 250 PPE standards had been published and 100 were under development. It is only through the application of standards and the mandatory provision of understandable information to users that people will be able to make rational decisions about the protective clothing they need, and to identify it.

Standards for the ergonomics of protective clothing

As with the development of protective clothing itself, early standards concentrated on test methods and specifications for the protection offered. The physiological needs of the users were largely ignored. The ergonomics of the PPE were not taken seriously. Partly this was because it is much more difficult to specify and measure the lack of hindrance to movement, or to define methods for measuring discomfort, than it is to measure, say, the rate at which toxic chemical penetrates the coating on the fabric.

Partly it is also because traditionally only the protection was specified.

The main ergonomic problems identified so far are that protective clothing is too heavy, too bulky, too hot, too ill-fitting, too tiring to wear, and too ugly. The subjectivity of these characteristics makes standards hard to define. What is too heavy? For whom is it too heavy, and when? Furthermore, the results of the use of test panels of subjects to evaluate comfort are generally too imprecise and unrepeatable for certification to standards.

Though most people can recognize symptoms of discomfort and over heating, they will not realize their own deterioration in mental performance, so in relatively familiar surroundings heat strain can develop with fatal consequences. It is said that up to one in a hundred workers in some industries suffer heat strain each year. Certainly some sportsmen and soldiers are known to die of heat strain. It is obvious that

their protective clothing could be a contributory factor and that they need better information about the hazard of over heating.

Thermal effects of clothing on users are related to the weight, the bulk, the sweat impermeability, and the basic thermal properties of the fabrics. Both thermal effects on users and the thermal properties of clothing can be measured, so standards are being developed in this important area.

Ventilated, refrigerated, or liquid-cooled suits are means by which extreme environments can be survived, but they are hugely expensive and often impractical. In reality options are limited in many sports and in industry. Therefore heat stress will occur. The main contributory factors are high air temperatures, high radiant heat absorption by the clothing, high humidity, low air velocity, high clothing insulation and coverage, high metabolic heat production, and long duration of exposure. The last

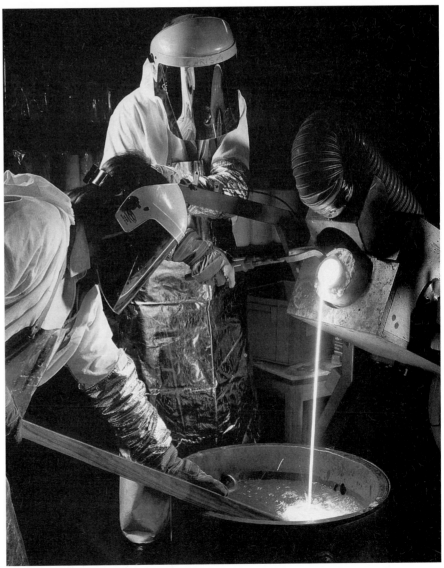

Foundry workers in protective clothing. Tek Image/ Science Photo Library.

three are the most significant. Obviously the accumulation of heat can be reduced by wearing less protective clothing, working less vigorously, and working for a shorter time. Thus those managing a work-force or a sporting event have a significant responsibility for the well-being of individuals who may be unaware of impending hyperthermia.

What should be done in extreme circumstances?

Some past human activities have left materials and situations now recognized as extremely hazardous and in which remedial workers would have to wear sophisticated protective clothing to obtain even partial protection. Stripping asbestos insulation off boilers and from fire barriers, decommissioning chemicals and munitions factories, making damaged nuclear reactors safe, and clearing landmines are examples. If protective clothing is only partially effective and itself causes heat stress, perhaps it is the wrong solution. The job should be done another way, or perhaps it should not be done at all. If for imperative reasons of public safety the job apparently has to be done, and has to be done by workers in close contact with the hazard, there will be injuries and possible deaths. Who should take the decisions balancing the level of the hazard, the risk of injury, the practicality of providing protective clothing, the cost of remote operation versus the cost of sending in people, and the benefit to society of the job being done compared with it being left undone?   RODERICK WOODS

See also COLD EXPOSURE; DIVING; ERGONOMICS; HEAT EXPOSURE; WORK AND THE BODY.

Proteins

The term 'protein' is derived from the Greek word *proteious*, meaning 'of the first rank'. Proteins are indeed 'of the first rank' of importance in all living creatures. Proteins consist of chains of AMINO ACIDS joined end to end by peptide bonds and are involved in all manner of biological processes and reactions. The majority of the chemical reactions in the body are controlled by ENZYMES, all of which are proteins. The carriage of OXYGEN in the blood from the lungs to the periphery is possible because a protein, HAEMOGLOBIN, forms a complex with oxygen, while in muscle another protein, myoglobin, acts as an oxygen transporter. Muscle contraction is dependent on two proteins, actin and myosin. Linear protein molecules, in the form of COLLAGEN, give tensile strength to tissues. Antibodies, produced as part of our body defence mechanisms, are proteins, as are the MEMBRANE RECEPTORS that respond to HORMONES and NEUROTRANSMITTERS. Some hormones, for example INSULIN, are also proteins. Membrane ION CHANNELS, as those activated during a nerve impulse, are proteins. A multitude of proteins are involved in growth and development. Thus it is obvious that proteins play a crucial role in living processes.

In spite of the variety and complexity of proteins they are composed of only twenty different amino acids. Nine of these are essential amino acids, that is they cannot be synthesized within the body but are derived from dietary sources. The amino acids in each protein occur in a unique sequence, from 100 to more than 1000, in accordance with the widely ranging size of protein molecules.

The amino acid sequence in a particular protein is determined by its gene. It is proteins and only proteins that are described by the genetic code. The most overarching, important rule in biology is that DNA (i.e. genes) makes RNA (messenger) that in turn makes protein. Thus it is essential that genes are accurately transcribed and that the messengers are accurately translated if the amino acid sequences in proteins are to be accurate. If the gene sequence is faulty because of an inherited mutation, then neither transcription or translation can correct the problem, and a faulty protein or no protein will be the result. Thus genetic disease that results when faulty genetic sequences are passed from parents to their offspring is a consequence of the loss of function due to faulty proteins.

Two conditions serve as examples. Human haemoglobin consists of four amino acid chains, combined with haem groups, namely two alpha and two beta chains. If glutamate is exchanged for valine in position 6 on the two beta chains, the resulting haemoglobin is faulty and *sickle cell disease* is the result. In the haemoglobin molecule there are 574 amino acids, and the replacement of just two glutamates by two valines leads to loss of normal function. In *cystic fibrosis* one tiny piece of the gene has been lost, resulting in the loss of a single amino acid, phenylalanine, from a protein containing 1480 amino acids; this small change produces a lethal genetic disease.

Although the sequences of amino acids in proteins are linear, the protein structures formed are rarely so, the chains being folded and linked together to give more globular structures. It is the amino acid sequence that determines the folding pattern, common motifs being the 'alpha helix' and the 'pleated beta sheet'. Disulphide bridges often form between sulphur-containing amino acids which become adjacent by folding, although they may be very distant in the linear sequence. Other sites on the folded molecules may become phosphorylated (phosphate groups added) or glycosylated (linked to sugar molecules), or may bind with non-protein groupings (e.g. haem in haemoglobin).

Digestion of proteins in the diet gives rise to amino acids that are absorbed into the bloodstream from the gastrointestinal tract. These amino acids can be used either as an energy source or in the synthesis of new proteins. In this way an individual amino acid may be part of many different protein molecules in many different species, including man, at different times.

The tertiary structure (the way the linear chain is folded) of many proteins is now known and this in turn has led to an understanding of their functions. Active centres and binding pockets have been revealed, into which substrates can fit — for example to bind a molecule which is to be cleaved, as in digestion, or to bind a molecule of neurotransmitter. The consequence for the protein is often a conformational change, which leads to the cleavage of the substrate, as in digestion, or the opening of an ion channel, as with some neurotransmitters. Loss by diffusion of the cleaved substrate or of the transmitter then allows the conformational change to reverse.

ALAN W. CUTHBERT

See also AMINO ACIDS; ENZYMES; GENETICS, HUMAN; MEMBRANE RECEPTORS.

Psychological disorders

The time is the late nineteenth century, the place a physician's clinic. A female patient complains of dramatic mood swings, paralysis on one side of her body, hallucinations, convulsive seizures, and religious delusions. Is she suffering from HYSTERIA, a nervous condition the Viennese neurologist Sigmund Freud believed to be treatable through an analytic discussion of the patient's dreams and memories of childhood? Or is she suffering from what German psychiatrist Emil Kraepelin called *dementia praecox*, the antecedent of today's schizophrenia? Or is she a victim of *syphilis*, once dubbed 'the great imitator' because of the mental disorder that it produces? Since her symptoms could fall into any of these three disease categories, what kind of disorder does she have? Is it psychological, that is, purely 'mental', or is it neurological, that is, caused by distinctly organic factors?

These questions all illustrate the complexity involved in defining the term 'psychological disorders'. It begins with the words 'psychological' and 'disorder'. A disorder can be described as a pathological condition of the organism, mental or physical. When the term is applied to PSYCHOLOGY — the study of the mind and behaviour — a disorder becomes a functional deviation from normal mental or behavioural conditions. As such, there is little to distinguish it from many psychiatric diseases, at least from a diagnostic point of view. Indeed, among psychiatrists the word 'disorder' is preferred to 'disease', as a glance at the American Psychiatric Association's *Diagnostic and Statistical Manual-IV (DSM-IV)* proves. In these terms, then, mental and psychological disorders are synonymous.

Captive to language

Nonetheless, psychiatrists remain dissatisfied with the use of the phrase 'psychological disorder' or its virtual equivalent, 'mental disorder'. To psychiatrists, both terms hark back to the French philosopher René Descartes (1596–1650), who argued that mind and body were utterly dissimilar. As the authors of the *DSM-IV* state: 'mental disorder unfortunately implies a distinction between "mental" disorders and "physical" disorders that is a reductionistic anachronism of [Cartesian] mind/body dualism. A compelling literature documents that there is much "physical" in "mental" disorders and much "mental" in "physical" disorders.' Probably because of their medical training as physicians, psychiatrists are loath to accept the notion that psychological disorders are purely mental. Hence, the *DSM-IV* concludes that there is no 'fundamental distinction between mental disorders and general medical conditions.' Mental disorders are in fact tied to 'physical and biological factors and processes', even if scientists are unable determine precisely what these processes are. Conversely, general medical conditions are often influenced by 'psychosocial factors or processes.'

In the eyes of modern psychiatrists, then, psychological disorders are biological phenomena just as much as certifiably medical diseases are. But in explaining how they arise, researchers must still use Cartesian terms of reference. To this point no new terminology to describe the natural reality of psychological disorders has been widely accepted, terminology that could transcend the ages-old concepts of mind and body. Psychiatry, so to speak, is captive to language that has not kept pace with the march of biomedical knowledge.

Challenges to classification

Psychiatrists and psychologists usually divide psychological disorders into three main classes: *mental handicap*, *personality disorders*, and *mental illness*. *Mental handicap*, also called mental retardation, is evident in the early years of individual development and is accompanied by abnormally low intelligence, though other psychological features might be affected. Severely mentally-handicapped people frequently have physical handicaps, such as difficulty in walking or controlling the bladder, but with help most can live fairly normal lives.

Personality disorders typically develop in teenage years, affecting all aspects of personality but not intelligence. One kind of personality disorder is the *psychopathic* personality disorder. Individuals with this disorder often combine superficial charm with serious inability to love, trust, respect, and care for other persons. Another is the *paranoid* type of personality disorder, featuring suspiciousness, secretiveness, insensitivity, and deception as salient personality traits.

Mental illnesses are divided into neuroses and psychoses. *Psychoses* are characterized by serious impairment of self-insight, inability to meet some ordinary demands of life, and loss of contact with reality. Although the terminology is still controversial (see PSYCHOSIS), three principal groups of psychoses are generally recognized: *schizophrenia*; the *affective disorders* (primarily mood disturbances); and the *organic psychoses*, which can be caused by things like brain tumours or toxic products in the bloodstream, and which sometimes culminate in dementia, or the severe loss of intellectual abilities. Schizophrenia and the affective disorders are usually called 'functional' psychoses, to denote the absence of a verifiable organic pathology.

The *neuroses*, or neurotic disorders, leave patients distressed, but there is no grave impairment of functioning or loss of self-insight, and contact with reality is maintained. Typical symptoms of the neuroses include obsessions and acute anxiety. Hysteria, often accompanied by symptoms of physical illness without physical causes, was once defined as a neurosis but is no longer recognized as a mental disorder by the American Psychiatric Association.

There is considerable MIND–BODY INTERACTION in psychological disorders. Delusions, phobias, HALLUCINATIONS, ANXIETY, and other mental dysfunctions can be caused by physical substances, particularly alcohol, amphetamines, CAFFEINE, NICOTINE, SEDATIVES, and COCAINE. The prolonged use of neuroleptic drugs (major tranquillizers) can produce movement disorders, including TREMORS, tics, and smacking of the lips. DEMENTIA can also be caused by HIV infection, head injuries, or the onset of Alzheimer's disease.

Then there is the class of disorders named *somatoform* or *psychosomatic*. This class generally refers to the condition labelled 'neurasthenic' by earlier generations of physicians. Today some of the best known of these conditions are *total allergy syndrome*, *chronic fatigue syndrome* (the 'Yuppie Flu'), and *anorexia nervosa* and *bulimia*. Symptoms vary from patient to patient, but nausea, lethargy, phobias, dyspepsia, malaise, and weight loss are often present, some at the same time. Until recently a widespread belief was that these disorders were due to a patient's unresolved mental conflict, possibly dating back to an earlier traumatic event, the awareness of which signalled a step towards cure. Other physicians prescribed rest and a medically-monitored regimen. However, with the rise of immunology since the 1960s numerous doctors and patients now believe that many of these symptoms can be traced to a viral origin.

The relationship between the body and another class of psychological disorders, the psychotic disorders like schizophrenia and the mood disorders like depression, is less evident. While an illness like postpartum depression patently corresponds to physical conditions, it is not clear what connections exist between the body and delusional disorders. The optimism surrounding the announcement, in the early 1990s, of the discovery of genes for schizophrenia and manic-depressive illness has subsided, though family histories still point to a hereditary dimension to these disorders. Recent research into brain biochemistry linking NEUROTRANSMITTERS to abnormal mood and thought functions has also sustained hope that more progress will gradually erode the ontological distinction between the mind and the CENTRAL NERVOUS SYSTEM.

One of the most troublesome obstacles to a proper classification of psychological disorders is the fact that patients can often suffer from more than one disorder; for example, personality disorder and mental illness. This and other problems have hamstrung psychiatrists' efforts throughout history to agree on a truly natural classification of mental disorders. Certain national communities of psychiatrists, like the French, have developed idiosyncratic classifications, based as much on chauvinism as clinical reality. Many have also argued that the entire classification enterprise is hopelessly relativistic, that mental disorders are wholly determined by cultural and socio-political environments. But much progress has been made in developing a valuable taxonomy, starting with the impressive efforts of Emil Kraepelin around the turn of the twentieth century. With the growing hegemony of the DSM there are hopes that a common vocabulary for recording mental symptoms is emerging in the early twenty-first century.

Therapeutic hopes

If diagnostic progress is a realistic expectation, optimism about therapeutic progress may even be more glowing. For much of its history psychiatry has swung back and forth between mainly psychological and physical approaches to treating mental disorders.

In the early nineteenth century, when numerous recognizably modern mental hospitals (or 'asylums') were built throughout the Western world, psychiatrists tended to emphasize what would later be called '*milieu therapy*' — that is, treatment based on the belief that an institutional environment exerted a huge influence on a patient's psychological state. But drug therapy never vanished from asylum medicine and in fact grew in popularity as the century wore on. With the emergence of Freudian psychoanalysis and similar theories of mental illness in the early twentieth century, there were renewed efforts to treat even severely psychotic patients with methods stressing non-physical therapies. At the same time psychiatrists and neurologists explored new and radical somatic treatments for long-term institutionalized patients, including electroshock, metrazol convulsion, malarial fever, insulin coma, and psychosurgical therapies. Many of these somatic treatments, however, died out when a series of new antipsychotic drugs were introduced, beginning with chlorpromazine in 1954. Despite studies that showed physical side effects of prolonged drug use, the pharmaceutical revolution of late-twentieth-century psychiatry shows few signs of being over. The controversy over the antidepressant *Prozac*, introduced in the early 1990s, underscores the fact that feelings run high on both sides of the debate.

Insanity and the arts

Psychological disorders have fascinated countless poets, novelists, painters, musicians, and playwrights throughout the ages, to say nothing of the public at large. Madness appears prominently in Shakespeare's plays, such as Hamlet and King Lear. James Boswell documented Samuel Johnson's melancholy. The madness of King George III attracted considerable attention and led to calls for more humane forms of treatment. The cultural profile of psychological disorders grew dramatically as the nineteenth century wore on. The Romantics in particular were deeply interested in madness, especially the mysterious boundaries between insanity and sanity and the curious combination of GENIUS and madness in certain individuals. The writer Emile Zola took a more naturalist approach when he vividly described abnormal mental states in his Rougons-Macquart series of novels. The Shakespearean character Ophelia was a favourite topic for Victorian artists and writers interested in the impact of madness on women. Indeed, the whole issue of women and their mental and nervous illnesses — especially hysteria — produced a literary avalanche in the late nineteenth century, centering on the well-publicized studies by the neurologist Jean Martin Charcot and the clinical theories of his former student Sigmund Freud.

In the twentieth century the romanticization of PSYCHOLOGICAL DISORDERS continued. The rise of psychoanalysis did much to validate the contents of mental symptoms, including delusions. To a lesser extent, the philosophy of phenomenology triggered subjective attempts by psychiatrists to study human behaviour and thought. Later in the 1960s the Scottish psychiatrist R. D. Laing argued that the mentally ill were actually saner than the apparently normal. Others like Michel Foucault and Thomas Szasz, though they never went as far as Laing, attributed malicious motives to the mental health care professions past and present, thereby running the risk of depicting the mentally ill as unwarranted victims of abuse and undermining their status as patients with bona fide diseases. Hollywood films like *Frances* and *One Flew Over the Cuckoo's Nest* reinforced this trend. But since the 1970s this view has gradually declined in the face of the theory that psychological disorders are indeed illnesses.   IAN DOWBIGGIN

Further reading
APA (1994). *Diagnostic and statistical manual of mental disorders* (4th edn) American Psychiatric Association, Washington, DC.

Berrios, G. E. (1996). *The history of mental symptoms: descriptive psychopathology since the nineteenth century.* Cambridge University Press.

See also MIND–BODY INTERACTION; PSYCHOSOMATIC ILLNESS.

Psychology
The word 'psychology', from the Greek *psyche*, meaning mind or soul, describes an academic and clinical subject concerned with reason and emotion, conscious and unconscious mental processes. It has become an umbrella term for such a wide variety of 'disciplines', paradigms, and cults that it is not clearly definable. The caring professions, especially for mental problems, are important activities under this rubric. Perhaps most intellectually respectable is *experimental psychology*, concerned especially with learning, memory, perception, attention, and emotions — with explicit links to physiological processes of the brain and body. These are of practical importance for understanding

the consequences of brain damage and mental illnesses such as schizophrenia.

Although the scientific aspects of psychology are increasingly seen as falling within the broad remit of NEUROSCIENCE, the conceptual association of physical brain to mental mind raises philosophical questions which remain controversial after thousands of years of debate. Current accounts of the mind, created by brain processes, generally refer to an analogy to the hardware–software distinction for computers. Computers, though physical, are 'cognitive' in that they carry symbols and meaning. But, so far as we know, computers are not conscious: the explanation of consciousness remains a great challenge for both psychology and brain science.

RICHARD L. GREGORY

Psychosis
The Greek *psyche* ('life' or 'soul') today can be translated as 'mind'. The suffix '-*osis*' means 'any illness of'.

The Oxford English Dictionary defines psychosis as:

> Any kind of mental affectation or derangement; especially one which cannot be ascribed to organic lesion or neurosis. In modern use, any mental illness or disorder that is accompanied by hallucinations, delusions or mental confusion and a loss of contact with external reality, whether attributable to an organic lesion or not.

The question of how far psychosis is an organic condition of the body or brain has fascinated psychiatrists ever since the term's origins a century and a half ago.

Origin of the term
The mid-nineteenth-century Austrian poet, politician, and psychiatrist, Feuchtersleben, introduced 'psychosis' to denote serious mental conditions affecting the personality; it was a subcategory of (Cullen's) neuroses. Psychosis soon comprised conditions besides the insanities and mental handicap, including minor psychological conditions and major organic disorders. Feuchtersleben coined the terms 'psychosis' and 'psychopathy' as identical terms because they were 'diseases of the personality' — and not of the body, nor of the soul or of the mind alone.

Psychosis-neurosis debate
Neurosis was already a popular term, and psychosis and neurosis were soon viewed in conjunction. Psychosis was seen as the psychological aspect of a neurosis — hence *psychoneurosis*. Thus the confusing picture arose whereby, in the late nineteenth century, there were three terms — psychosis, psychoneurosis, and psychopathy — for the same condition; by the late twentieth century by contrast these terms all referred to separate conditions. The development of this process of change over the course of the century will now be outlined, along with the different types of psychosis that were described.

At the end of the nineteenth century, attempts were made to find organic/cerebral causes for mental illnesses. The trend of 'organicization'

increased and culminated in the discovery in 1905 that general paralysis was caused by a physical agent (syphilis). However, there remained many mental disorders that had no known organic cause. The term 'functional' was applied to these psychoses in 1881 by the German psychiatrist Fuerstner. However, his compatriot, the anatomist Nissl, claimed that 'in all psychoses of whatever type there are always positive cortical findings' (i.e. anatomical evidence of pathology). A functional illness therefore meant one that was suspected of having a physical origin, which had not yet been discovered.

By the mid 1920s, in the absence of the discovery of physical causes for Kraepelin's dementia praecox (schizophrenia) or for manic–depressive insanity, Bumke, his successor as Professor of Psychiatry at the world famous Chair in Munich, unequivocally labelled these as functional as opposed to organic illnesses. An examination of the latter should be conducted in the BRAIN, while the study of the former had to be made in the mind, according to Bumke. The highly influential psychiatrist and philosopher Jaspers listed the functional psychoses as schizophrenia, manic–depressive insanity, and EPILEPSY.

Today, using computerised IMAGING TECHNIQUES, we know that functional psychoses are accompanied by organic changes in the brain. This has made the use of the term 'functional psychosis' unhelpful. In the nineteenth century, many mental disorders were considered to be due to DEGENERATION, that is 'being predisposed to a disorder which led to deterioration, either in that individual or in succeeding generations'. These disorders were termed 'endogenous', which could apply both to the psychoses and to disorders of personality (psychopathies).

In 1881 the German degenerationist psychiatrist, Schuele, began the process whereby psychoses were associated with the more serious, organic conditions — cerebropsychoses — and psychoneuroses with the less serious ones. Freud emphasized and popularized the 'psychoneuroses' at the turn of the century, and the successful treatment of otherwise healthy soldiers suffering from shellshock in World War I established the entity of the *neuroses*, as they were to become known.

By 1925 Bumke was writing that 'there has been no such thing as psychoneuroses for a long time. They have been reclassified into nervous reactions (neuroses), nervous constitutional states, psychopathies and functional psychoses.' The neuroses were further delineated from the psychoses by Jaspers because 'they do not wholly involve the individual himself, while those which seize upon the individual as a whole are called psychoses … [and] are generally thought to open up a gulf between sickness and health.'

In the early twentieth century, various terms were used for those conditions, which were deemed psychoses but which were not manic–depressive insanity or schizophrenia, but in the main these two remained the recognised 'mental illnesses'. Some have upheld the significance of atypical psychoses. The recent debate on these psychoses has also generated much renewed research in the unitary theory of mental illness.

Unitary psychosis

In the mid nineteenth century, the unitary psychosis theory referred to a continuum of mental conditions from health to disease and was based on the importance of symptoms. In the twentieth century, by contrast, the term 'unitary psychosis' was applied to the two psychoses, schizophrenia and manic–depressive insanity, with the atypical psychoses bridging these two. Contemporary British psychiatrists have split two ways in their views on this question. Some, who analysed symptoms and emphasized the genetic basis of these disorders, have favoured the concept of unitary psychosis. Others, on the basis of neuroimaging, have rejected the unitary theory in favour of three categories of psychosis: congenital dementia praecox with poor prognosis; an adult form of schizophrenia with good prognosis; and bipolar affective disorder.

'Psychosis' — useful or not

There are certain problems with the use of 'psychosis' in contemporary psychiatry. Firstly, its very definition is difficult because its defining criteria are not specific (*Oxford Textbook of Psychiatry*). 'Lack of insight' is difficult to define. If 'severity of illness' is used as a criterion, the problem then arises that conditions falling into the psychosis category can occur in mild as well as severe forms. Moreover, non-psychotic conditions such as obsessional–compulsive disorder can also be very severe. 'Impaired contact with reality, as evidenced by delusions and hallucinations' has been considered difficult to apply. Secondly, conditions to which the term refers appear to have little in common, especially from an aetiological viewpoint. For example, some psychoses can be caused by known organic factors, while others represent a severe depressive illness. Thirdly, it may be better to classify an individual condition like schizophrenia as such, rather than as a member of an umbrella term like psychosis. So, recent classifications have renamed *paranoid psychosis* as *paranoid disorder* and *affective psychosis* as *bipolar affective disorder*. Fourthly, the tenth International Classification of Diseases (ICD 10) no longer distinguishes between psychosis and neurosis.

The arguments for retaining the term are as follows. Firstly, the psychoses are recognizable — as the ICD 10 proposes — by the presence of delusions and hallucinations without the patient having insight into their morbid nature. Secondly, on a purely practical level, psychosis has carried with it less stigma than the alternative term of 'insanity'. Thirdly, it is very difficult always to use the term 'disorder' as an alternative for psychosis. For example, when it comes to the atypical psychoses the term 'atypical disorder' or 'atypical insanity' is unsatisfactory. Fourthly, the adjectival use of psychosis is a helpful shorthand term. This can be as in 'psychotic symptom'

(delusion or hallucination) or 'antipsychotic' medication. To use 'severe unipolar depression with delusions, hallucinations, and loss of insight' as a replacement for 'psychotic depression' is cumbersome.

The contemporary British professor of psychiatry, Tyrer, has written that 'classification stands or falls by its usefulness.' In the last two decades the psychiatric profession has made many improvements in the sphere of reliability, but it has been said that there has not been comparable progress in the validity of psychiatric diseases. Therefore, there is a continuing need for the 'umbrella' categories such as psychosis and neurosis. The danger with an unquestioning use, and one which does not take cognisance of its abuse and attempted reification as a disease concept earlier this century, is that the mistakes of the past are repeated and an overly organic approach is adopted at the expense of a careful consideration of other — for example psychosocial — factors.

In a clinical and pragmatic sense the combination of one of the definitions of psychosis as 'gross impairment in reality testing' and the evident possibility in clinical practice of differentiating psychosis from normality, make psychosis a term that is accessible and acceptable, and yet one which does not necessarily carry the longer term or immutable connotations of its fellow term 'insane'. Thus for the clinician and the man in the street, a psychotic person differs qualitatively from normal, while someone suffering an understandable neurotic or emotional disturbance usually only differs quantitatively from normal. The psychiatric profession should continue to use the term, but its conceptual limitations should not be overlooked.

M. DOMINIC BEER

Further reading

Berrios, G. E. and Beer, M. D. (1995). Unitary psychosis concept. In *A history of clinical psychiatry. The origin and history of psychiatric disorders*, (ed.) G. E. Berrios and R. Porter. Athlone Press, London.

See also PSYCHOLOGICAL DISORDERS; PSYCHOSOMATIC ILLNESS.

Psychosomatic illness

'Psychosomatic illness,' writes Edward Shorter, author of a comprehensive history of the subject, 'is any illness in which physical symptoms, produced by the action of the unconscious mind, are defined by the individual as evidence of organic disease and for which medical help is sought. But how, we may ask, do the actions of the unconscious mind produce these physical symptoms? 'Is it real, or just in your head?' is a most common turn of phrase, but does the juxtaposition bear scrutiny? Are symptoms any less 'real' if their origin lies in the mind, rather than in more tangible, organic sources? Should they be treated differently? What, in short, is the relationship between the mind and the body in the formation and expression of this type of ILLNESS?

Western thinkers have grappled endlessly with these issues, positing shifting and historically-contingent theories of the mind–body relationship for centuries. The dichotomy between mind and body, which traces back to Plato's distinctions between transient materiality and transcendent truths, was reinforced by the Christian belief in the supremacy of spirit over flesh, and found its modern expression in Descartes' philosophical dualism, which confirmed and celebrated the autonomy of consciousness.

Indeed, Western medical thinkers have long been aware of the mind's influence over the body. Nevertheless, the idea that illnesses originate — and can be cured — in the mind first entered modern medicine around the late eighteenth century. Before this period, madness — or what we now call mental illness — had been considered a thing of the body, originating in disturbances of HUMOURS (bodily fluids), physiological processes, or nerves. As the physician George Cheyne colourfully noted in his 1733 opus, *The English Malady*:

> I never saw a person labour under severe obstinate, and strong nervous complaints, but I always found at last, the stomach, guts, liver, spleen, mesentery, or some of the great and necessary organs or glands of the belly were obstructed, knotted, schirrous, spoiled or perhaps all these together.

A decisive turn from the body to the mind occurred just decades later. In 1789, the year of the Revolution in France, a British surgeon attributed insanity to the psyche, 'independent and exclusive of every corporal, sympathetic, direct, or indirect excitement, or irritation whatever.' This dictated a new focus on, in the words of the French alienist Esquirol, 'the ideas, thoughts, [and] projects of the lunatic. Accompanying this change was a shift in therapeutic tactics and the rise of the 'moral treatment', a non-coercive, semi-psychotherapeutic, and often highly theatrical doctor–patient encounter meant to reveal the delusion or moral (read 'mental') flaw at the core of the disorder. This approach was made most famous, perhaps, by the treatment of George III by the English physician Francis Willis.

But the path from the moral treatment to the therapist's couch was long and twisted. Mid-nineteenth-century doctors, seeking to elevate the status of the care of the insane, pinned their hopes on science and showed decreasing tolerance for these moral cures. By the end of the century, the new field of scientific psychiatry had established itself at the university, spawned numerous professional journals, and reverted, in a sense, from the mind to the brain. New research technologies and clinical facilities furthered attempts to localise behavioural anomalies in neuroanatomy, and new diagnostic systems subsumed mental illness to what the German neurologist Max Nonne called 'the narrow straight-jacket of exact science'. As a result, therapeutic success suffered; there was, according to an asylum doctor in Posen, 'an enormous blossoming of psychiatric literature alongside a low level of practical success. We know a lot and can do little.'

This late-nineteenth-century paradigm shift proved both incomplete and short-lived, collapsing under the weight of various medical and social forces. By the middle of World War I, a new, psychogenic view seemed to hold sway, as the tens of thousands of cases of 'shell-shock' — the tics, stuttering, shaking fits, and mutism so often observed among soldiers in the aftermath of explosions — were increasingly attributed to fear, ANXIETY, and MEMORY, rather than any somatic mechanism. The wishes and fears produced in modern war, noted Nonne, 'are of a previously unimaginable versatility.'

It was around this time that Freud and his followers first turned their attentions to mind–body disturbances. Freud had, of course, described the conversion of pathological ideas into hysterical symptoms already in the 1890s, but it was the 'wild analyst' Goerg Groddeck who first applied psychoanalysis to the treatment of specifically organic disorders. Groddeck's Baden-Baden sanatorium was soon supplemented by the clinic of the Berlin Psychoanalytic Institute under Max Eitingon and Ernst Simmel's Tegel sanatorium, all of which treated organic disturbances with psychoanalytic methods in the 1920s.

This brief sketch should suffice to show that today's belief in psychosomatic illness — a belief under siege by accumulating advances in genetics, biopsychiatry, and psychopharmacology — represents just one phase in a cyclical and fraught process. But even in its most 'psychological' phases, Western society seems to cling to distinctions between pain and suffering that is 'real' and maladies that lie 'just in the mind'.

PAUL LERNER

Further reading

Shorter, E. (1992). *From paralysis to fatigue: a history of psychosomatic illness in the modern era*. New York.

Porter, R. (1995). Psychosomatic disorders: historical perspectives. In *Treatment of functional somatic symptoms*, (ed. R. Mayou, C. Bass, and M. Sharpe). Oxford.

See also MIND-BODY INTERACTION; NERVOUSNESS.

Puberty marks the point in human development where both males and females gain the capability to procreate. Puberty occurs during ADOLESCENCE, which begins as early as age 10 and is usually completed by age 17. For girls, a rising level of OESTROGEN (female hormone) sets the process in motion. PELVIS and BREAST development are followed by a spurt in height and then the growth of underarm and pubic hair. Finally, MENARCHE, the beginning of the first MENSTRUAL CYCLE, occurs. Ovulation does not automatically coincide with menarche. It may take as many as forty cycles for ovulation to become a regular part of the menstrual cycle. Though they are uniform in order, the age of onset, pace, and duration of these changes vary widely from one individual to another. Since the beginning of the twentieth century, the average age of first menstruation has declined. In the US, it decreased from about 14 years old in 1900 to 12 years old in 1975. Scientists attribute this change to better living standards, particularly in regard to diet. In males a sharp increase in ANDROGEN (male hormone) and GROWTH HORMONE spawns skeletal development, followed by the lowering of the voice, the growth of facial hair, increase in sex organ size, height, spermatogenesis, and muscle development. The outward physical signs of puberty tend to occur earlier in girls than in boys, particularly the growth spurt.

While the physiological terrain of puberty is clearly mapped, psychological and cultural changes meander in a much less orderly direction. Adolescence, by definition, begins in childhood and ends with young adulthood. To negotiate successfully this stage of human development, girls and boys must develop conceptual powers, independence, a sense a their own identity, and a way to make moral or ethical decisions. All the while, they are grappling with their emerging SEXUALITY, marked by heightened sexual development and sexual interest.

The 'normal' routes through puberty vary according to cultural standards, socio-economic class, gender roles, and family structure. Some cultures and religions have clearly established rituals to mark puberty. The Jewish bar mitzvah, for example, celebrates a boy's entry into adolescence, and most of tribal Africa holds puberty rituals which may include dance, music, or seclusion.

According to John and Virginia Demos, adolescence is a rather modern invention which 'did not exist before the last two decades of the nineteenth century.' Its invention resulted from an increased focus on children among the middle classes, who no longer needed their children's labour for family survival and so re-defined childhood and puberty in more psychological and social terms. In addition, the nineteenth-century research of social scientists such as G. Stanley Hall and Sigmund Freud emphasized distinct categorizations for each stage of human development. The influential Hall defined adolescence as stressful, violent, and crisis-ridden.

MARGARET A. LOWE

Further reading

John and Virginia Demos (1973). Adolescence in historical perspective. In *The American Family in Social-Historical Perspective*. St Martin's Press, New York.

See also DEVELOPMENT AND GROWTH: SCHOOL AGE AND ADOLESCENCE; SEX HORMONES.

Pubic wigs The pubic wig, or *merkin*, as it was earlier known, made its debut in 1450. It was used as a device to cover syphilitic pustules and gonorrhoeal warts in the genital area. In its contemporary form, the merkin is used as a part of erotic play, and it has also crossed over the boundaries of intimate wear into some mainstream genres of dress. The chosen material the wig is made of — usually nylon, yak belly, or human hair — is woven onto a transparent mesh. This is then applied to the pre-shaved pubic area with spirit gum; alternatively the wig can be attached to a transparent G-string.

The wearing of a pubic wig is a sensory experience. The wig can allow the wearer a certain 'jouissance' (Roland Barthes, 1973) as it is made of a fibre/hair that has been selected by the wearer, and it is worn on an EROGENOUS ZONE. A fetish for the feel of silk, leather, fur, or hair against one's own skin, or that of others, is common, and can be incorporated into the design of a pubic wig to give heightened pleasure.

Bondage crossed over from erotic use into couture when it first glided down a Gianni Versace catwalk in 1992; and Vivian Westwood flirted with the pubic area, using tailored fig leaves to cover modesty under transparent fabrics. There has always been a *risqué* element to FASHION throughout the ages, whether it was baring ankles, knees, thighs, or breasts. The 'club scene' has taken fashion one step further. It has formulated its own look as pubic wigs are being worn under short 'baby doll' dresses in mainstream nightclubs, as well as being worn in private and fetish parties.

The pubic wig is a strong device for both the exhibitionist and the voyeur. Ideally the relationship between the two is best suited as a 'performer' and 'audience' scenario. The exhibitionist is allowed freedom of movement and a confidence in the unusual, and in doing so creates entertainment for the voyeur. In a professional and aesthetic capacity the wigs are frequently used by show girls.

The pubic wig has also become an essential piece of the serious drag queen's wardrobe, as it covers the genitalia that are otherwise the epitome of maleness. It is the finishing feminine touch and it is intrinsic to the pleasure of drag, as 'a little female finery' creates the sexual identity in the 'role play' of the subject.

Rick Stonell, a tonsorial expert in London, custom-makes pubic wigs or 'body furniture' designing them to suit the wearer and their moods. Two examples of his work are 'Heart' and 'Target'. The first is a pale pink, heart-shaped piece that is made from yak belly hair; the image it projects is one of virginal youth and subtleness. The colour and hair are soft and the shape is traditionally linked with love and romance. The overall look is of innocence, though ironically it is reminiscent of Eve's fig leaf! Alternatively he has created a piece that uses the shape of a target; this is made from red, white, and blue nylon. The strong design, colours, and fibre used in this wig carry a bold and sexual statement of availability. The wig has a phantasy element and gives the impression that it was designed with a superhero or heroine in mind. The range of pubic wigs in Rick Stonell's collection covers every aspect of SEXUALITY and PERSONALITY from 'whore' to 'madonna'.

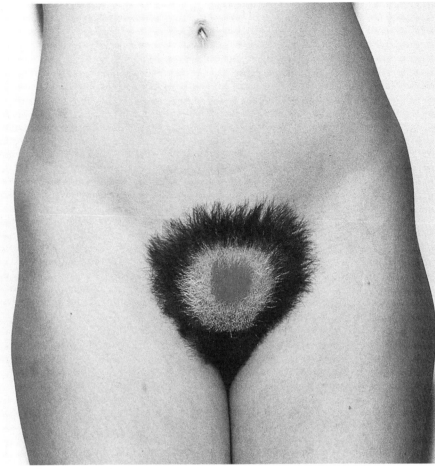

'Target' pubic wig designed by Rick Stonell, Archive Hairdressing, London. © Alpha, London.

The merkins of the past were made to cover the 'filthy running sores' of syphilis, a disease which:

> ... eroded the palate ... In some cases the lips, nose or eyes were eaten away, or on others the whole of the sexual organs.
>
> Arrizabalaya, p. 205.

Merkins were frequently connected with prostitutes. The women often worked while infected, because many of them were single mothers with no other form of income. Despite the horror of infection and the merkin's connections with it, amusing anecdotes have appeared in literature, such as A. Smith's:

> This put a strange whim in his head — which was to get the hairy circle of her merkin ... this he dried well and combed out, and then returned to the Cardinall, telling him he had brought St Peter's beard.
>
> The Oxford English Dictionary.

Fortunately, the merkin is no longer needed for its original function. The idea of the merkin has been displaced in time to be re-born into a different era as the pubic wig. It is now used as an accessory to alter the appearance of the pubic hair, which is usually, when left to its own devices, unruly, coarse, and shapeless. Body decoration is a primal and innate part of the human psyche, whichever way it chooses to express itself.

AMANDA BARROW

Further reading

Arrizabalaya, J. and French, R. (1997). *The French Disease in Renaissance Europe*. St Edmundsbury Press.

Brame, G. and Brame, W. D. (1997). *Different loving*. Century, London.

Freud, S. (1991). *Volume 9, Case Histories II*. Penguin Books Ltd., Harmondsworth.

Henning, J. L. (1995). *Rear view*. Souvenir Press, London.

Pulse Feeling the pulse is one of the hallmarks of the medical profession, and has been for many a century. As well as being informative, this action can give the doctor something physical to do while he takes time to think.

The pulse is most commonly felt where the radial artery lies near the surface on the thumb side of the wrist. It is made palpable by the 'pulse pressure wave' — initiated by each heart beat — reaching and expanding the artery. This wave is transmitted to the wrist at about 10 metres per second around forty times faster than the speed of the blood flow itself.

The information obtained from feeling the pulse is limited but important. The feel of the artery itself may suggest whether its wall has normal resilience, or is hardened and thickened by arteriosclerosis.

The pulse may feel, at one extreme, 'strong' and 'full' or, at the other, 'weak' or 'thready'. These are indirect indications of the stroke volume of the HEART. The impulse felt in the radial artery is related to the rise in arterial BLOOD PRESSURE generated by the heart at each beat — the *pulse pressure*. For any given stroke volume, this rise in pressure depends on the elasticity of the arteries: the more compliant they are the less the pressure rises; the stiffer they are with age and arteriosclerosis, the more sharply the pressure rises. These subtleties may be recognized by an experienced observer.

The *rate* may be faster or slower than normally expected in the circumstances. In healthy adults the rate at rest, although typically 60–70, can be anything from 40 per minute, say in an elite long-distance swimmer, to about 80 per minute. Even so the rate can, for example, be used to distinguish a simple faint (slow) from loss of consciousness caused by HAEMORRHAGE (fast).

The *rhythm* may be regular or irregular. In a person at rest an absolutely regular pulse is in fact unusual because of the phenomenon of *respiratory sinus arrhythmia* — an increase when breathing in and a decrease when breathing out. This is more marked in younger than in older people, and disappears at higher heart rates such as in EXERCISE or in FEVER. This is a 'regular irregularity' and the pattern is generated from the normal physiological PACEMAKER, the sino–atrial node. There are other, abnormal disturbances of rhythm which are 'irregular irregularities'; in this instance the rhythm is occasionally interrupted or persistently disorganized. Interruptions can either come in the form of extra heart beats, generated from a different part of the heart rather than from the sino–atrial node (*ectopic beats*), or else an occasional beat may be missed out entirely in mild forms of HEART BLOCK. 'My heart missed a beat' is not just poetic licence: the sensation of missing a beat, in healthy people, is usually because of a longer gap after a premature ectopic beat. A totally disorganized rhythm is felt at the pulse in the condition of *atrial fibrillation*.

An exaggerated sensation of the beating of the heart — *palpitation* — may or may not be associated with a faster than normal pulse rate; it is also a normal accompaniment of the increase in strength and rate of the heart-beat induced by strenuous exercise, or by the sympathetic nervous systems in stressful conditions, and can be a component of abnormal ANXIETY states.

Awareness of pulsation within ourselves, particularly when EMOTIONS are heightened — and even at the earliest in our mother's womb — may well be inextricably related to the creation and appreciation of MUSIC.

SHEILA JENNETT

See also HEART; MEDICINE; MUSIC; PACEMAKER.

Puppet A figure, usually human or animal, moved by human agency, used in a theatrical show. Puppets are thus to be distinguished from DOLLS, clockwork AUTOMATA, and other toys. They come in several varieties: glove or hand puppets are hollow bodies, usually made of cloth, into which the performer inserts a hand, with the fingers and thumb manipulating the usually wooden head and hands; marionettes are full-length figures moved from above by strings or wires; rod puppets are large, and manipulated by rods to the head and hands; shadow puppets, common in Java, Bali, and Thailand, are flat figures held between a light and a translucent screen. There are many other less familiar types, for instance living marionettes; bodies attached to the actual head of the performer, with either legs or arms manipulated by rods from behind; and 'held' puppets — figures carried about by one or several operators, like the characters in Japanese Bunraku theatre.

The origins of puppetry lie with ritual MAGIC. Puppet theatre has featured in almost all civilisations. In Europe there are written records of it from the fifth century BC, and puppets certainly figured in the repertoire of medieval *jongleurs*. In sixteenth-century Italy they were closely linked with the characters of the *commedia dell'arte*, though in England they played mainly folk stories and popular Old Testament stories. The introduction of Punch into England in the seventeenth century united these two traditions. Puppet theatre has customarily been a form of folk theatre, often featuring a comic character, such as Petroushka in Russia or Pulcinella in Naples.

Occasionally, however, puppet theatre has become a fashionable, élite entertainment. In the eighteenth century, various operas were composed for puppets; Alessandro Scarlatti wrote works for Cardinal Ottoboni's theatre in Rome, as did Joseph Haydn for Count Esterhazy. The puppet theatre occasionally provided a fine vehicle for parody, as in early Hanoverian England, when Powell's Covent Garden theatre attained celebrity by sending up the vogue for Italian opera, and Henry Fielding, Samuel Foote, and other comic writers presented puppet shows to burlesque contemporary fashions.

In the nineteenth century, various artists and writers sought to turn the puppet theatre into a serious medium. In Germany, an essay by Heinrich von Kleist, written in 1810, was a forerunner of this move; in France, George and Maurice Sand directed a home puppet theatre in the 1860s that inspired many imitators; in Belgium in the 1890s, Maurice Maeterlinck wrote symbolist plays to be performed by marionettes; in England in 1907, Gordon Craig hailed the *übermarionette* as the ideal actor. Alfred Jarry's *Ubu Roi* (1888), originally written for puppets, has been viewed as a precursor of the theatre of the absurd. In the 1920s the German Lotte Reiniger exploited film techniques to produce remarkable silhouette shows based on shadow figures. In Communist Eastern Europe, state subsidies led to work of great technical accomplishment and artistic sophistication. This highbrow interest, however, has been rather limited, and, for the public at large, puppets in modern culture have typically been regarded as children's entertainment — notably the Punch and Judy show.

Recent years have seen revived use of puppets for political satire, as in the British television show *Spitting Image*. Puppets have also served as an educational medium in the American TV programme *Sesame Street* and they are employed in child psychiatry as surrogate figures.

ROY PORTER

Further reading

Speaight, G. (1955). *The history of the English puppet theatre*. G. G. Harrap, London.

Baird, B. (1965). *The art of the puppet*. Macmillan, New York.

See also THEATRE.

Purdah literally means curtain or VEIL, and refers to the various modes of shielding women from the sight primarily of men (other than their husbands or men of their natal family) in the South Asian subcontinent. Purdah can refer to the veiling or covering of the entire body or of parts of the head and face through the manipulation of womens' attire. It can also refer to the practice of the seclusion of women inside their homes. In the sense of attire, purdah can denote the practice of completely covering a woman's body by wearing a loose, body-covering robe called the *burqa*. Among sari wearers, the end part of the sari called the *palla* is used to cover all or part of the head and face. In those parts of the subcontinent where women wear the *shalwar-kameez* (long, loose tunic worn over trousers) or long skirts (*lehenga/ghaghra*), a scarf (*dopatta*) is used to cover the upper part of the body as well as part of the head and face. Purdah in its many variations is still used by both Hindu and Muslim women, although the burqa is almost always exclusively associated with Muslim women.

Purdah, in the sense of seclusion, means restrictions on women's movements outside the home. Thus, a woman could be unveiled and yet observe purdah by remaining in seclusion within the home. Purdah has further connotations for living arrangements within the home in the sense of separate living spaces for men and women — a feature that is often manifest in the architecture of family residences. As Cora Vreede-De Stuers has pointed out, in its most extended sense purdah refers to approved norms of modest and circumspect feminine behaviour, as for instance in downcast eyes, the bowing of the head, the complete silence a woman observes in the presence of a man, or by the hasty gesture of veiling her head with a corner of her sari or *dupatta* if she is caught unawares. The degree and kind (the actual veiling or seclusion) of purdah observed by women has varied across time and place and from family to family and is also related to class status. Purdah in the form of seclusion is almost exclusively a characteristic feature of upper-class status, but one that is frequently emulated by lower-class aspirants to it.

The practice of purdah derives from a concern to control female SEXUALITY and to shield women from being the objects of the sexual desire of men other than their husbands. Secondly, in its association with circumspect feminine behaviour (which in turn was associated with female subordination), it is critical for preserving hierarchy within the patriarchal family. Thus, women observe purdah usually with male and often with senior female members of their husbands' families. Purdah is observed much more loosely and sometimes not at all by women when they are with their natal families.

The belief that the custom of purdah was introduced into the Indian subcontinent through Muslim conquests of northern India in about AD 1200 is of limited validity. The purdah, as veiling, was possibly influenced by Islamic custom, and the practice of covering the head and face is more prevalent in those parts of India believed to be more heavily influenced by Islam than others. But, in the sense of seclusion and the segregation of men and women, purdah predates the Islamic invasions of India. In the nineteenth century, the custom of purdah, specially in the sense of the seclusion of upper-class women, was increasingly viewed by British colonial rulers of India as an indication of the degraded condition of Indian women and, even more broadly, as a symptom of the overall primitiveness of Indian society. Indian social reformers in the nineteenth and early twentieth centuries attempted to eradicate purdah as part of a program to 'improve' the social conditions of women. The long-term results of this, as well as other factors, led to a reduction (but not elimination) in the observance of purdah in South Asia throughout the twentieth century. However, efforts to create Islamic theocratic states in certain parts of South Asia in recent times led to government directives ordering women to wear 'Islamic dress' — that is to observe purdah by covering their bodies with a garment (now called *chador*) and to cover their heads as well.

KUMKUM CHATTERJEE

Further reading

Mumtaz, K. and Shaheed, F. (ed.) (1987). *Women of Pakistan*. Zed Books, London and New Jersey.

Papanek, H. and Minault, G. (ed.) (1982). *Separate worlds. Studies of purdah in South Asia*. South Asia Books, Columbia, Missouri.

Vreede-De Stuers, C. (1968). *Purdah: a study of Muslim women's life in Northern India*. Humanities Press, New York.

See also HINDUISM AND THE BODY; ISLAM AND THE BODY; VEIL.

Purging Purgatives (or laxatives) are substances that encourage the bowels to move. They have probably always been some of the commonest drugs prescribed. They have been used as a form of medical treatment since at least the time of the ancient Egyptians. GALEN (c. AD 129–216), whose works were the basis of medical knowledge for the next 1500 years, was a strong advocate of purging and bleeding. The distinguished Thomas Sydenham (1624–89) said that the physician possessed two resources: to bleed and to purge.

The French philosopher Michel de Montaigne (1533–92) was sceptical. What was the evidence, he asked, that purgation did anyone any good? 'The violent struggles between the drug and the disease are always at our expense, since the combat is fought out within us.' He also noted how quickly doctors claimed success when the patient improved. There have been many such critics since and during the twentieth century: orthodox MEDICINE has come to doubt the wisdom of giving purgatives to all patients. In the 1950s a successful physician used to tell his students that the healthiest community he had ever looked after was a convent where the nuns opened their bowels once a week and the reverend mother once a month. True or not, he hoped to wean his students from the myth on which many of them had been raised, that failure to open the bowels at least once a day was likely to lead to serious illness and should be immediately remedied with purgatives.

Another famous critic was Molière (1622–73). In *Le Malade Imaginaire* all the patients, regardless of what is wrong with them, are treated with ENEMAS, bleeding, and purging. The physician of the time had little else in his repertoire that could produce a visible effect. William Buchan, addressing the general public in his *Domestic Medicine* (1800 edition), wrote, 'Persons who have regular recourse to medicines for preventing constiveness, seldom fail to ruin their constitution' — and he advised against the use of drugs.

Nevertheless, a century later many Victorians were taking a nightly dose of blue pill, aloes, colocynth, and castor and croton oils to purge their bowels. Enlightened doctors disapproved, but the practice continued into the twentieth century. It was still believed that CONSTIPATION was to be feared and avoided as the poisoner of the blood and the cause of many diseases. Many parents dosed their children regularly with purgatives, despite criticism of different kinds. 'Syrup of figs' diminished many English children's enjoyment of life. The Nobel Prize winner, Élie Metchnikoff, believed that toxic action in the bowel was the cause of ageing and death. He advocated sour milk and colectomy as purgatives instead of the usual stronger ones. Sir Arthur Hurst, a distinguished gastroenterologist, pointed out that regular use of purgatives caused them to be inactive. He wrote,

'If the fortunes made from purgative pills had been devoted to the hospitals which treat the victims of their abuse, the financial problems of the voluntary hospitals would have been solved.' He pointed out that bowel investigations were done with the patient *not* taking purgatives: 'It is interesting to observe how large a proportion of patients, who are supposed to be the victims of toxaemia from intestinal stasis, feel better whilst these examinations are being carried out. The fact is that symptoms result far more frequently from the artificial diarrhoea produced by purgatives than from intestinal stasis.'

Current thinking is that few people need laxatives unless they suffer from neurological disease such as multiple sclerosis, are old and very inactive, or need to avoid all strenuous activity, perhaps after a HEART ATTACK or STROKE. On the other hand the value of a high fibre diet for healthy bowel function is widely recognized and advocated. Still, many people, obsessed with their bowels, continue to swell the profits of pharmacists and pharmaceutical companies by consuming purgatives regularly, usually unknown to their doctor, often simply in the attempt to lose weight.

ANN DALLY

See also COLONIC IRRIGATION; CONSTIPATION.

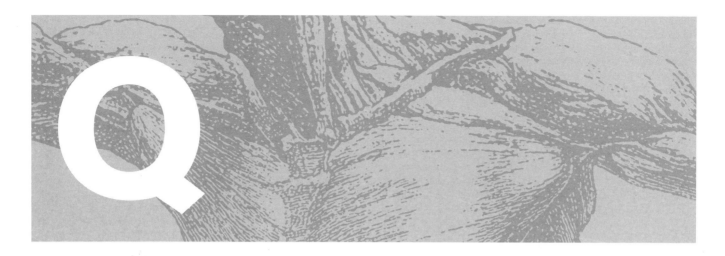

Q

Quadriceps The full name *quadriceps femoris*, or commonly 'quads', refers to the mass of muscle with four 'heads', partly surrounding the femur in the front of the thigh. This is the muscle that primarily extends the leg, straightening and stabilizing the KNEE by virtue of its strong attachments around the front and sides of the joint and to the tibia below it. Also, because part of it spans the front of the HIP joint, it assists other muscles around the hip in maintaining an erect POSTURE. The quads are thus essential simply for standing and for rising to standing, as well as for WALKING and running. The four components are partly distinct muscles with individual names: the *vastus lateralis*, the largest, lies mainly on the outer side, covering the deeper *vastus intermedius*; the *vastus medialis* lies on the inner side; the fourth muscle is attached to the pelvic bone above the hip and thence runs a straight course down the thigh — hence its name, *rectus femoris* — to end in a tendon that continues into the common quadriceps tendon in the front above the knee. The vastus muscles are attached above to the femur itself. Above the knee they curve in from the sides, accounting for the fleshy masses on either side just above the kneecap (*patella*), to be linked by fibrous sheets to the sides of the patella and to join the quadriceps tendon. This thick tendon is attached to the top of the patella, but also its strong fibrous extensions carry on downwards, embedding the patella within them, and linking up with the patellar tendon below it (the one that is tapped to elicit a knee-jerk REFLEX). This in turn is attached to the top of the tibia.

SHEILA JENNETT

See PLATE 5.

See also HIP; KNEE; POSTURE; REFLEXES; WALKING.

Quarantine All laws of quarantine have their origin and basis in the concept of disease transmission by contagion. Quarantine is a term which has been applied to many different systems of disease prevention, but it is generally used in two specific senses: first, it involves the segregation and isolation of individuals, suspected of being infected with a communicable disease, for at least the period of likely incubation; more generally, it refers to the maritime practice of forcibly detaining and segregating all vessels arriving in port, together with the people and things on board, when suspected of certain diseases, for specified periods, usually about forty days. The individuals quarantined may in each case be perfectly healthy, but the suspicion that they are harbouring disease provokes the application of quarantine procedures. The most notorious current practice of quarantine regards the entry of domestic pets and minor livestock into the UK.

The first known law of segregation on account of disease was enacted by the Emperor Justinian in AD 542. The earliest definite regulations against the spread of disease were, however, developed by Italian city states under the threat of bubonic plague in the fourteenth century. Venice, the great entrepôt of trade with the east, probably issued regulations as early as 1127, and was the first city to issue a complete quarantine code in 1448. This code provided the model for all subsequent regulations over the next four centuries. Initially these European quarantines were limited to the exclusion of goods and people from stricken localities, but as time went on they were increasingly extended to foreign places as well, especially in sea ports.

By the sixteenth century the practice of quarantine was well established across Europe, and British governments also began to adopt the policy. It was not until the eighteenth century, however, that comprehensive codes of practice were put into place in response to the last outbursts of plague on the European continent — in the Baltic states between 1709 and 1712, and at Marseilles in 1721. These early eighteenth-century regulations were apparently successful at staving off the menace of plague, and were repeatedly revised and renewed over the next hundred years.

The arrival of Asiatic cholera in Europe in 1830, against which quarantines proved singularly ineffective, heralded the demise of the system. In England, commercial and trade interests were already beginning to protest against the restrictions imposed by the system in the mid 1820s, and the experiences with cholera in 1832 and 1848 confirmed commercial opposition to the practice. Both England and France, as colonial trading powers with wide international interests, increasingly questioned the necessity of quarantine, and in 1851 an international congress was called to consider the issue. In following decades, opposition from countries like Spain, Portugal, Greece, and Sweden was gradually eroded at a series of international congresses, and by the successful development by the British of a rival system of surveillance and port supervision. Indeed, the development of the electric telegraph, which so greatly facilitated international communications, permitted the dissemination not only of information on local disease prevalences, but also on the route, condition, and expected arrival of individual ships. Technological developments, as much as commercial pressures, were critical in undermining the rationale for international quarantine systems. At the congresses of Venice and Dresden in 1892 and 1893, the international quarantine system was largely dismantled, to be replaced by supervision systems on the British model. For some years, however, quarantine remained an issue with regard to India, partly because of her reputation as the home of cholera and of plague, and partly because of the complications of the annual pilgrimages of Indian Muslims to Mecca and Medina.

Even into the twentieth century, quarantines were occasionally imposed under the threat of invading EPIDEMICS, as when Sydney was quarantined by other Australian states on the outbreak of plague there in 1900. On the smaller scale, too, informal domestic household quarantines continued to be adopted, until well into the twentieth century, for children and adults potentially incubating INFECTIOUS DISEASES such as measles and chicken-pox.

ANNE HARDY

See also INFECTIOUS DISEASES.

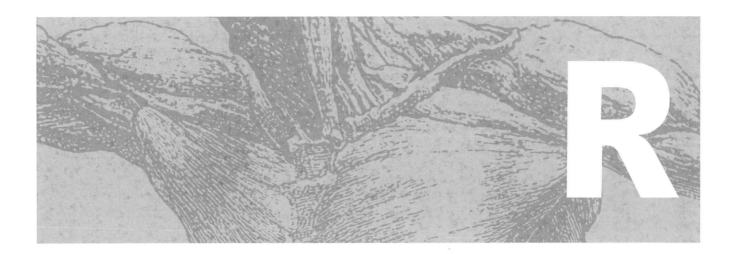

Race The origin of the term 'race' is obscure. It may have derived from the Arabic *râs*, meaning 'chief', 'head', and 'origin'. The word entered Europe between the fifteenth and sixteenth centuries. Initially 'race' was understood to signify descent of an aristocratic breed. In particular it referred to the lineages of the Frankish kings. Later, Europeans used 'race' as one of the possible translations of the Latin *natio* or *gens*; until the eighteenth century it was interchangeable with terms such as 'stock' or 'tribe'. All ethnicities, whether they were called 'peoples' or 'races' or 'tribes', were classified according to their political traditions, their geographical habitat, and climatic conditions. The European reference system of thought, being shaped by classical authors, was dominated by political paradigms and categories that paralleled natural and political phenomena. Only in the first decades of the nineteenth century did the term acquire its modern meaning. implying that original difference is biologically founded, the concept presupposes the genealogical continuity of 'racial' traits that supposedly remain the same irrespective of environmental influences, and it includes the idea that there are correlations between outward physiognomy and mental capacity.

The Greeks' emphasis on citizenship went hand in hand with the assumption that citizens were made, not born. From the Greeks onward, the state of government and civilization were seen to be the decisive characteristics of a people; some climates favoured the development of vigour of spirit and courage, instilling a war-like disposition, while others induced a phlegmatic attitude, laziness, and the tendency to succumb to tyranny. The roots of this view were laid down in Hippocrates' *Airs, Waters, Places*. It was only in respect to this sort of theorizing — dubbed 'environmentalism' at the end of the nineteenth century — that the notion of descent played any role. 'Blood', by contrast, had been invested since antiquity with mythical meaning, transcending the common sphere of everyday life. In heathen Greek theory, notably in the writings of Aristotle, notions of 'species', 'genus' and physiognomy

were closely linked to the concept of the 'essences', the basic elements of all matter. Therefore, Greek accounts of differing human physiognomies cannot be compared to modern-style theories of race or racism. The same applies *mutatis mutandis* to Roman theory.

Biblical anthropology

The Bible stipulated that mankind was derived from one common pair of ancestors. The concept of the 'chosen people' was integrated into Scriptural cosmogony; it resided in the idea that adherence to Moses' commandments qualified people for participation in the Abrahamitic covenant between God and the Jewish people. As for the cultural foundations of the Christian creed, the notion of the soul as the essential part of all humans prevented fixation on physiology alone as inherent in the concept of race. According to common Christian understanding, all converts to the faith, whatever their complexion might be, underwent what was evidently thought of as a spiritual 'white-washing'. Christian iconography abounds with depictions of this procedure in which the coloured convert was washed white. It was an allusion to Jeremiah 13:23 ('Can the Ethiopian change his skin, or the leopard his spots? Then may ye also do good, that are accustomed to do evil'). Christian doctrine confirmed that the curse of Ham could be removed. In another respect, too, Christian theory contradicted the Scriptural narrative. From the Jewish historian Flavius Josephus (AD 37–*c*.97) onwards, writers divided mankind into the posterity of Shem, Ham, and Japhet. The Japhetites were considered to inhabit Europe; the Shemites resided in the region of the Pacific Ocean and the Near East; the Hamites were to be found in Africa. The Catholic Church denounced this division, which threatened its claim to universality. Christian theory asserted that all mankind was one — though, of course, the ideal was remote from actual practice.

Until the eighteenth century, Judaeo-Christian traditions and classical theory dominated all philosophizing on mankind. Human nature was

discussed in terms of ideas about *polis* and *ecclesia*. The identity of a people was considered to depend on its faith, and on the fact that all citizens were subject to the same law. Philosophers had no concept of 'racial' traits, instead they discussed what they called 'national character'. Its shape was seen to depend on climate and geographical station — humoralism, the complex concept of an interplay between the outside world and human temperaments, lasted well into the nineteenth century. Until the middle of the eighteenth century it influenced all attempts to account for human diversity. On the whole, references in early modern literature to, say, the African or the Chinese 'race' do not imply the existence of a set of physical categories adding up to a system of human classification. And the notion of 'purity of blood' had no biological connotations.

During the sixteenth century the term 'race' had a socio-political rather than an anthropological meaning. It was part of the historiographical appreciation of the Frankish dynasties. The French historian François Hotman (1524–90) denied that the political institutions of Greece and Rome were the models of German and Frankish government. Distinguishing between the autocratic monarchies of antiquity and Franco-Germanic freedom, he supported the notion that different peoples were endowed with different spirits. As Europeans discovered foreign parts, the understanding of 'race' was increasingly extended to denote not only noble families, but entire peoples. However, the concept was still shaped by political concepts as opposed to biology.

As an ethnological category, 'race' is a modern idea. From the Renaissance onwards, study of the natural realm was increasingly distinguished from metaphysics. Francis Bacon, Thomas Hobbes, John Locke, Jean Bodin, and others relieved Aristotle's philosophy of its emphasis on the essences. The pursuit of evidence became the paramount scientific occupation; empirical observation of difference supplanted unifying philosophies. Classical learning gradually lost its grip on the European mind. As a result, 'racial' differences became independent of political discourse, and instead were investigated as natural phenomena.

Natural taxonomy, advanced by Carolus Linnaeus and the Comte de Buffon, was decisive in this development. In their panoramic views of nature, many naturalists arranged human tribes into a number of natural varieties. J. F. Blumenbach, a Professor of Anatomy at Göttingen University, proved especially influential. He distinguished five different human varieties: Caucasian, Mongol, Ethiopian, American, and Malay. Once some such divisions were made, it was only one step to a concept of race. That is not to accuse those thinkers who unwittingly prepared the ground — but it is difficult to imagine that history might have taken a different course.

The eighteenth century saw many methodical inquiries into the mechanisms of cross-breeding. Scientific travellers and other naturalists discovered that 'purity of blood' was anything but a guarantee of the excellence of stock. It was only in the nineteenth century that these insights would be applied to mankind.

Types of mankind

The eighteenth century also brought the heyday of the anatomists and pathologists who attempted to find bodily differences between different types of mankind. The German S. T. Soemmerring acquired dubious fame in 1784 by publishing a treatise on 'the physical differences between the Negro and the European'. He came very near to stating that there had been several creations of human kinds. Contemporary discussion turned to the question whether such a polygenist account of mankind could be true. The authority of the Scriptures was still great: the case for polygenism, put forward most famously by Henry Home, Lord Kames (1696–1782), met with widespread outrage. It was generally assumed that the differences between human varieties were due to differing physical and moral environments. As long as the Biblical story of creation was accepted doctrine, the notion of original difference was pure heresy. By the beginning of the nineteenth century, however, religion faced increasingly troubled times. It was then that the concept of race began to spread.

The established social hierarchy was overthrown in France and denied in America. The shock waves of the revolutions in the English colonies and in France were felt in the whole of Europe. While these developments may have induced some desire to erect biological hierarchies, where previously there had been social ones, simple observations gave an immediate boost to the idea of race: according to the environmentalist theories, under various climatic conditions any stock of people might transform into any other. Yet, as many writers noted, the progeny of black slaves in the northern hemisphere remained black, and white colonists who shunned intermarriage with the locals persisted in producing white offspring. Evidently the theory of climate was wrong. What

else, then, could account for physiognomical differences among the human species but a concept of race? Students of anthropology and its younger offshot, ethnology, began systematically to inquire into human physical and mental diversities. As early as 1824 the French doctor Julien-Joseph Virey advanced physiological arguments to support his opinion that mankind was originally divided into the white and the black 'species'. In the following years monogenism was increasingly undermined.

German romanticism has often been accused of having stimulated racialism. Johann Gottfried Herder (1744–1803) put forward the idea that the spirit of an age was determined by the prevailing culture, which in turn was represented not by outstanding individuals but by the people. He brought the cultural concept of the people to the fore. This notion suited racialist thinking, although not based on it. The Romantic movement was not only German but Europe-wide. Even France, nowadays officially proud of its traditions as a society based on the notion of citizenship, participated in the new emphasis on race.

While the Germans celebrated ancient Teutonic notions of freedom, similar ideas were thriving in England and France. In the early nineteenth century, the old British antagonism between Celts and Saxons was put on a biological footing. Explanations in terms of race came to be seen as the source of political struggles. In England, John Mitchell Kemble (1807–57) contended that the excellency of the English was due to their Germanic roots. Robert Knox (1791–1862), who, despite his intellectual shortcomings, became famous as Britain's first explicit racialist, juxtaposed noble Saxons to enfeebled Celts. In France, historians who opposed Bourbon rule argued that the Franks had been foreign invaders on French soil and therefore did not have the right to govern the original Gallic population. Before, racial thinking had turned around the blatant physiognomical differences between exotic peoples and the white man. Now European history itself was considered to be the result of racial struggle. Europe was made up of Celts and Gauls, Saxons and Germans — and minorities such as the Jews and Gypsies were increasingly seen as parasitical intruders. The concepts of 'Aryan' and 'Semitic' races were gradually transferred out of historical linguistics into ANTHROPOLOGY. The second half of the nineteenth century saw a host of antisemitic theories. It was only in the slave-holder society of America that racial theory continued to centre on the antinomy between blacks and whites.

From the 1820s anatomical investigations into race gained further momentum thanks to the activities of cerebral anatomists. PHRENOLOGY, the external examination of skulls, was first conceived to determine individual characters more reliably than earlier approaches to PHYSIOGNOMY. But very soon craniology was employed to classify human types, and the Swede Anders Retzius (1796–1860) gained

international acclaim with his 'cephalic index'. For several decades, SKULL measurements were seen as a key to a racial division of mankind and the various degrees of human intellect. When, in the 1890s, craniology went out of fashion, 'race' acquired a nominalist understanding, with the concept of racial 'types' superseding the idea of fixed races.

The notion of biologically grounded races had been developed at the expense of political discourse; once the biological 'laws' of race and racial mixture were established they were reintroduced into society. Increasingly, social problems were seen through the spectacles of racial theory. In 1845 Benjamin Disraeli famously spoke of the rich and the poor as being two 'races'. Herbert Spencer applied Darwin's theory of the survival of the fittest to the social sphere. Similar ideas were popularized in Germany and France. Darwin himself was not interested in race as a category. Yet, his theory of species differentiation continued to be exploited by Social Darwinists well into the twentieth century.

On another level the concept of purity of blood occupied the minds of cultural pessimists. Harking back to eighteenth-century theories, some accepted that cultural excellency required racial intermixture but warned that continuing hybridization would inevitably lead to degeneration. Others pleaded for purity of race, invoking the authority of Darwin; Houston Stewart Chamberlain denounced racial intermixture and supported racial inbreeding as the best means to perpetuate the qualities of a race. His *The Foundations of the Nineteenth Century* (published first in German in 1899), one of the most comprehensive accounts of the forces of race, was much appreciated — though not emulated — by the Nazis. Their racial doctrines, unlike Chamberlain's, were for the most part allusive in style. Hitler's *Mein Kampf* aptly linked ill-advised racial mixing to notions of sin and disease alike.

Class struggle by other means

Outside Germany, theoreticians of race were embroiled in the discussion of what came first: did social hierarchies, such as the caste system in India, have racial origins? Or were racial theories merely class struggles by other means? In 1950, after the experiences of World War II, the United Nations passed a *Statement of Race*, stipulating that national, cultural, religious, geographical, and linguistic groups had been wrongly considered as races. Some inveterate supporters of physical anthropology notwithstanding, this resolution remained until recently the last word on matters of race.

Since the 1980s there have been attempts to revivify theories of racial classification in the US and elsewhere. In this context, *The Bell Curve* by Charles Murray and Richard Herrnstein, investigating racial parameters of intelligence and based in part on sources already rejected by the scientific community, has gained notoriety. Latterly, an authoritative contribution to the problem of 'race' has been a publication under the guidance of the genetic historians L. Luca Cavalli-Sforza, Paolo Menozzi, and Alberto Piazza, whose team has investigated the genetic make-up of hundreds of individual populations (*The History and Geography of Human Genes*, 1994). The result is that the genetic programme shifts slightly but perceptibly from one tiny population to the other: 'By means of painstaking multivariate analysis, we can identify "clusters" of populations and order them in a hierarchy that we believe represents the history of fissions in the expansion to the whole world of anatomically modern humans. At no level can clusters be identified with races, since every level of clustering would determine a different partition and there is no biological reason to prefer a particular one.'

H. F. AUGSTEIN

Further reading

Augstein, H. F. (ed.) (1996). *Race: the origins of an idea, 1760–1850*. Thoemmes Press, Bristol.

Banton, M. (1987). *Racial Theories*. Cambridge University Press.

Barzun, J. (1965). *Race: a study in superstition*. Harper and Row, New York.

Hannaford, I. (1996). *Race. The history of an idea in the West*. Johns Hopkins University Press, Baltimore.

Poliakov, L. (1974). *The Aryan Myth: a history of racist and nationalist ideas in Europe*. Chatto and Heinemann, London.

See also ANTHROPOLOGY; RACISM.

Racism According to the *Oxford English Dictionary*, the term describes 'the theory that distinctive human characteristics and abilities are determined by race'. The word itself is rather recent, probably going back only to the 1930s. There are two attitudes towards the concept of racism: one says that 'racism' is usefully applied only where it is derived from a perception of race and the ensuing fixation on 'typical' racial traits. In this sense 'racism' describes the racialist attitudes of the nineteenth and twentieth centuries, deriving from the merger of physical ANTHRO-POLOGY und ethnography on the background of the idea of evolution. Another school has argued that racism consists in intentional practices and unintended processes or consequences of attitudes towards the ethnic 'other'. According to this line of thought, it is not necessary to possess a concept of 'race' to entertain prejudices towards other peoples.

As the term was coined in reaction to the rise of German Fascism and its antisemitic theory of race, 'racism' carries in itself the condemnation of what it means — it is true indeed that self-professed racists are very rare. Basically, racism lives in practice, not in theory; sociologists such as Michael Banton, therefore, have denied that the phenomenon of racism might be accessible to theory. Some theoreticians of imperialism have argued that only whites could be racists. Marxist thinking has tended to consider it as a corollary of the development of capitalist society.

The sociologist Robert Miles, by contrast, has pointed out that pre-capitalist societies, too, afford manifold opportunities to observe racism. Concentrating on racism under the conditions of colonialism and in societies with a large contingent of foreign immigrants, Miles has put forward the suggestion that it must be regarded as an 'ideology'. To rescue the concept of 'racism' from indiscriminate conflation with exclusionary practices, on the one hand, and from being tied up too closely with the nineteenth-century understanding of 'race', on the other hand, he has suggested that racism refers 'to a particular form of (evaluative) representation which is a specific instance of a wider (descriptive) process of racialisation'.

The psychological precondition of racism is ANXIETY. On a sociological level it may be said that mobile societies and those experiencing great social changes are especially prone to develop some or other sort of racism: contempt of the 'other' provides a reassuring feeling of identity. Philosophically speaking, racism is the result of a world view that does not leave any conceptual room for the strange, the unknown. The anthropologist Claude Lévi-Strauss has surprised his audience with his discovery that the Indians of Southern America possessed the very rare ability to accept the 'other'. According to Strauss, the cosmogony of these Indians included the idea that the world was complete thanks only to the existence of other beings different from themselves. When the conquistadores arrived they were initially taken for this complement to Indian identity.

Racism has many faces; its particular expressions are dependent on the socio-economic, religious, and cultural situation of any given society. This versatility notwithstanding, the moral overdetermination of SKIN COLOUR is one of its most conspicuous, ever-recurring elements. The Christian world has excelled at consigning dark complexion to the realms of the mysterious and the bad. In pagan antiquity, however, this was quite different: the stereotypes associated with black Africans were rather of a positive nature: blackness signified qualities such as wisdom, or the love of freedom and justice.

One of the earliest examples of what, in modern parlance, amounts to state-organized racism in European history was the persecution of the Jews in fifteenth-century Spain. In 1492 King Ferdinand succeeded in defeating the Arabs at Granada. Eight hundred years of Muslim rule in Southern Spain came to an end. In the wake of the victory, the Jews were expelled. Though converts to Christianity were allowed to remain, the enforced Jewish exodus signalled that the times were over when political rulers could tolerate the existence of the 'other' on their territory. This had been possible in the Roman Empire as well as in Greek city-states. Post-medieval, centrally governed countries, by contrast, had lost the will and the philosophical preconditions for putting up with foreign ethnic groups. Since the fifteenth century instances

of organized racism have accumulated. The holocaust happened in a cultural climate of which it has been said that it bore many resemblances to the atmosphere in Spain at the time of the expulsion of the Jews.

H. F. AUGSTEIN

Further reading

Benedict, R. (1983). *Race and racism*. Routeledge and Kegan Paul, London.

Miles, R. (1989). *Racism*. Routledge, London.

Banton, M. (1970). The concept of racism. In *Race and Racialism*, (ed. S. Zubaida). Tavistock Publications, London.

See also ANTHROPOLOGY; GENOCIDE; RACE.

Radiation, ionizing X-RAYS were discovered by Röntgen in Germany in November 1895. This caused tremendous public interest and very rapidly they started to be used for many medical diagnostic purposes. Within just a few years it was realized that high radiation doses from X-rays could cause severe skin burns, CANCER in exposed tissues, and even death. This resulted in steps being taken to reduce exposures, although in the early years after their discovery it was assumed that only high radiation doses from X-rays could cause cancer. By the late 1920s it had become apparent, from the studies of Müller on the fruit fly, *Drosophila*, that radiation damage from X-rays could cause effects in future generations, and through to the 1950s this was the principle cause for concern at lower radiation doses. By the early 1950s, however, follow-up studies of the A-bomb survivors in Japan and other exposed populations were showing that radiation-induced leukaemia and other cancers could arise even at low levels of exposure. The principle long-term effect of exposure to low doses of *ionizing* radiation is now considered to be the induction of cancer.

Ionizing radiations include X-rays, neutrons, cosmic rays, and radiation from radioactive materials, such as alpha particles, beta particles, and gamma rays. When ionizing radiations pass through matter, energy is deposited in the material concerned. Alpha and beta particles, being electrically charged, deposit energy through electrical interactions with electrons in the material. Gamma rays and X-rays lose energy in a variety of ways, but each involves liberating atomic electrons, which then deposit energy through interactions with other electrons. Neutrons also lose energy in various ways, an important means being through collisions with hydrogen nuclei, which are single protons. The protons are set in motion and, being charged, they again deposit energy through electrical interactions. So in all cases, these radiations ultimately produce electrical interactions in the material and this can give rise to ionizations when a neutral atom or molecule becomes charged as a result of a loss of an electron. Once removed from an atom, an electron may in turn ionize other atoms or molecules. When ionizing radiation passes through cellular tissue, it produces charged water molecules. These break up into entities called FREE RADICALS, such as the free hydroxyl radical (OH˙) composed of an oxygen atom and a hydrogen atom. These free radicals are highly reactive chemically and can themselves alter molecules in the cell. One molecule of particular importance in relation to radiation damage is *deoxyribonucleic acid* (DNA), found in the nucleus of the cell. Radiation may ionize a DNA molecule, leading directly to a chemical change, or the DNA may be changed indirectly when it interacts with a free radical produced in the water of the cell by radiation. In either case, the chemical change can cause a harmful biological effect, leading ultimately to the development of cancer or inherited genetic defects. The quantification of these effects has provided the basis for radiation protection standards.

The principal quantity used to assess exposure to radiation is the absorbed dose, with the unit of the gray, Gy (equivalent to a deposition of energy of 1 Joule/kg). The gray can be multiplied by a 'weighting factor' to take account of the effectiveness of different radiations in causing damage to tissues. Thus X-rays, gamma rays, and beta particles have a 'radiation' weighting factor of 1; for alpha particles it is 20. The unit of this weighted dose is the sievert, Sv, and it is termed the *equivalent dose*.

Exposure to ionizing radiation comes from a variety of sources. There are sources of natural origin, such as cosmic rays from the atmosphere, gamma rays from radioactive materials in the ground and in our own bodies, and inhalation of radon; we can be exposed as a result of medical diagnostic procedures and treatment; radiation is also present in the environment as a result of nuclear weapons testing and as a consequence of discharges from nuclear sites and from nuclear accidents. For most people the main source of radiation exposure is natural background, which, in the UK, gives a radiation dose of about 2.2 millisieverts (mSv) a year. There can be substantial differences between individuals, mainly reflecting differences in exposure to radon gas and its decay products.

Early radiation effects

The effects of ionizing radiation soon appear if a person receives a sufficient radiation dose. A very high radiation dose to the whole body can cause death within a matter of weeks. For example, an absorbed dose of 5 Gy (5000 mGy) or more received instantaneously by the whole body would probably be lethal unless treatment were given. Death would occur because of damage to the bone marrow and the gastrointestinal tract, both of which have rapidly-dividing and hence sensitive cell populations. If the same dose were instead restricted to a limited part of the body, it might not prove fatal but early effects could still occur. Thus an instantaneous absorbed dose of 5 Gy or more to the skin would probably cause erythema within a week or so. Higher doses would lead to more serious damage and break-down of the skin structure. Similar doses to the testes or ovaries might cause sterility. However, if the same radiation dose were to be received over a period of weeks or months, there would be the opportunity for body cells to repair some damage, with much less early sign of injury. Even in the absence of early signs, however, tissues could still have been damaged, with the effects becoming manifest only later in life, or perhaps in the irradiated person's descendants. The most important of these late effects is cancer, which is always serious and frequently fatal.

Radiation-induced cancer

Although the cause of most cancers remains unknown or poorly understood, exposures to a wide range of agents, such as tobacco smoke, asbestos, ultraviolet radiation, chemicals, and ionizing radiations, are all known to induce them. The development of cancer is a complex cellular process that occurs in several stages, usually taking many years. Radiation appears to act principally at the initiation stage by causing mutations in the DNA of normal cells in tissues. It is usually considered that damage is caused by double-strand breaks (DSBs) in DNA, which are not readily repaired. The production of DSBs can result in a cell entering a pathway of abnormal growth that can sometimes lead to development of a malignancy. In recent years, much has been learned about the processes by which radiation exposure leads to DNA damage, and also about the cellular systems that act to repair, or misrepair, such damage and the way mutations can arise. This information provides supporting evidence for the long-standing belief that, although the risk of cancer after low doses of radiation may be very small, there is no dose, no matter how low, at which we can completely discount the risk. For radiation protection purposes it is therefore assumed that the risk of cancer increases progressively with the dose, with no threshold.

Advances in knowledge also indicate that a person's genetic constitution influences the risk of cancer after irradiation. At present we can identify only rare families who may carry increased risk. In future, techniques may become available that allow the identification of more groups of individuals with increased sensitivity to irradiation. This is an important factor in medical exposures, as individuals treated medically — for example by radiotherapy — might have quite different responses to radiation exposure.

It is also known that tissues vary in their response to radiation-induced cancer, thus the lung and the gastrointestinal tract are particularly sensitive, whereas the brain and muscles are very insensitive. In assessing the risks of exposure to radiation we therefore have to allow for these differences in sensitivity.

How can we calculate the risk of cancer from exposure to radiation? Suppose we know the number of people in an irradiated group and the doses they have received. By observing the incidence of cancer in the group and analyzing it in relation to the size of the radiation dose and the number of cases expected, in another similar but unirradiated group, we can estimate the raised risk of cancer per unit radiation dose. This is commonly called a *risk factor*. It is most important to include data for large groups of people in these calculations so as to minimize the statistical uncertainties in the estimates and to take account of factors such as age and gender that can effect the spontaneous development of the disease. For this reason, the main source of information on risks of radiation-induced cancer comes from studies on nearly 100 000 survivors of the atomic bombs dropped at Hiroshima and Nagasaki in 1945. Other risk estimates for the exposure of various tissues and organs to X-rays and gamma rays can be obtained from studies of people exposed to external radiation for the treatment of non-malignant or malignant conditions or for diagnostic purposes, and also from people in the Marshall islands in the Pacific who were exposed to severe fallout from atmospheric nuclear weapons testing. Information on the effects of internally incorporated alpha-emitting radionuclides comes from miners exposed to radon and its decay products, from workers exposed to radium in luminous paint, from patients treated with radium for bone disease, and from other patients given an X-ray contrast medium containing thorium oxide, which tended to concentrate in the liver. Long-term follow-up studies on these groups of people have allowed both national and international bodies, such as the United Nations Scientific Committee on the Effects of Atomic Radiation (UNSCEAR) and the International Commission on Radiological Protection (ICRP), to estimate risks of radiation-induced cancer in various tissues as a function of time and age after exposure. A striking observation from these studies has been that whilst radiation-induced leukaemia starts to occur within a few years, and most have occurred by about thirty years following radiation exposure, in the case of most solid cancers the so-called latent period, before any induced cancers appear, may be five, ten, or even twenty years. Subsequently cancers may then occur over the remaining lifespan of the individual. For this reason, exposed groups must be followed for very many years to obtain accurate estimates of the total risk of cancer. In practice, as no populations have yet been followed for their entire lifespan, it is necessary to predict how many excess cancers will have been found by the time all the survivors have died. Various mathematical methods are used for this purpose, which inevitably introduces some uncertainty in the risk estimates.

Not all cancers are fatal. Mortality from radiation-induced thyroid cancer is about 10%, from breast cancer about 50%, and from skin cancer only about 1%. Overall, the risk of inducing any cancer by uniform irradiation of the whole body is about half as great again as the risk of inducing a fatal cancer. In radiological protection, the risk of fatal cancer is naturally of most concern.

The electromagnetic spectrum

Present estimates of the risk of radiation-induced fatal cancer provided by ICRP are 1 in 20 per Sv for exposure of a population of all ages and 1 in 25 per Sv for a working population. These values apply to a mixed population of all ages; there will be differences in sensitivity in males and females as well as between individuals of different ages.

Radiation-induced hereditary disease

Apart from cancer, the other main late effect of radiation is hereditary disease. As with cancer, the probability of hereditary disease, but not its severity, depends on the dose. Genetic damage arises from irradiation of the TESTES and OVARIES, which produce sperm cells in males and the egg cells in females. Ionizing radiation can induce mutations in these cells or in the stem cells that form them. Mutations occur as a result of structural changes to the DNA in single GERM CELLS, which subsequently carry the hereditary information in the DNA through to future generations. The hereditary diseases that may be caused vary in severity from early death and serious mental defects to relatively trivial diseases such as skeletal abnormalities and minor metabolic disorders.

ICRP has assessed the risk of severe hereditary disease in a general population of all ages exposed to low doses and dose rates. It estimated a risk factor of 1 in 100 per Sv for such diseases appearing at any time in all future generations. Mutations leading to diseases that are strictly heritable, such as haemophilia, make up about half of the total, with the remainder mainly coming from a group of so-called *multifactorial*

diseases, such as diabetes and asthma. Estimating the risk of multifactorial diseases is complex, as there is interplay of the genetic and environmental factors that influence the development of these disorders.

In genetic terms, irradiation of the testes and ovaries is potentially harmful only if it occurs before or during the reproductive period of life. For people who will not subsequently have children, there is, of course, no hereditary risk. Since the proportion of a working population that is likely to reproduce is lower than that in the general population, the risk factor for workers is smaller. ICRP estimates 1 in 170 per Sv for hereditary disease in all future generations.

Summary and conclusions

At high radiation doses, significant effects can occur in exposed individuals within a short time of exposure, and in severe cases this can lead to early death. At low radiation doses, the principal concern is the risk of radiation-induced cancer in exposed individuals and hereditary disease in their descendants. The risks of these late effects have been quantified and this provides the basis for recommendations on limits for exposure.

JOHN W. STATHER

See also CANCER; FREE RADICALS; RADIOACTIVITY; X-RAYS.

Radiation, non-ionizing
Electromagnetic fields and radiation have, perhaps through their historical associations with magnetic lodestones and electrical storms, been linked to forces of nature that are not readily understood. Early students of the effects of electromagnetic phenomena

on living organisms include the noted eighteenth-century Italian scientists Luigi Galvani and Count Alessandro Volta. The responsiveness of tissue to electrical stimulation described by these scientists no doubt provided some inspiration for Mary Shelley when writing the novel *Frankenstein*.

The foundation of modern electromagnetic theory, which accounts for the way in which electromagnetic radiation interacts with the human body, was laid down by the great Scottish scientist James Clerk Maxwell. His treatise on *Electricity and Magnetism*, published in 1873, was built on the experimental observations of another major British scientist, Michael Faraday, who, amongst other things, championed the concept of electric and magnetic 'lines of force'. It was Maxwell's theoretical understanding, however, that paved the way for Einstein's special theory of relativity, eventually leading to Max Plank's formulation of the quantum theory. The latter underpins our present understanding of the interaction between electromagnetic radiation and matter, and the subdivision of the electromagnetic spectrum into ionizing and non-ionizing regions.

The electromagnetic spectrum (see figure) extends from static (or DC) fields such as those generated by permanent magnets, through the extremely low-frequency electric and magnetic fields generated by the supply and distribution of mains electricity, to radiofrequencies used for radio and TV transmission and now for mobile phone communications. Higher frequencies extend to infra-red, visible, and ultraviolet optical radiations and to X-rays and gamma radiation. The quantum energies of these latter 2, highly energetic, short wavelength (<100 nm) radiations are sufficient to be able to eject electrons from an atom, and thus they comprise the ionizing part of the electromagnetic spectrum. Non-ionizing radiations are less energetic and are conventionally subdivided into electromagnetic fields and radiations and optical radiations.

Electromagnetic fields and radiations

Life originated in the static, geomagnetic field of the Earth. It is widely believed that migratory animals, which include species of birds, butterflies, and fish, can utilize this (and other) information for navigation. Surprisingly, however, human beings seem relatively unaffected by exposure even to the large static magnetic fields, some 20–40 000 times natural background levels, that are used in magnetic resonance imaging systems. This equipment is used to provide images of the soft tissues of the body, derived from radio signals emitted mostly by transiently excited hydrogen nuclei, for clinical diagnosis. Above these levels, the electrical potential generated across the aorta by the flow of blood in the static field becomes substantial. In addition, people working in such fields have occasionally reported feelings of vertigo and nausea, possibly because of electrical stimulation of the vestibular organs.

Static and power frequency electric fields, such as those encountered under overhead powerlines, generate an electrical charge on the surface of the body. Human volunteer studies, carried out at the Electrical Power Research Institute in Palo Alto, California and elsewhere, have shown that many people can perceive the hair vibration and other effects that result from exposure to electric fields typically greater than those likely to be encountered even under high voltage overhead powerlines. The time variation of the surface charge, in the case of power frequency electric fields, will induce the flow of small electrical currents; these are however tiny compared to the thresholds for nerve stimulation. In contrast, the most sensitive and well-documented response of the human body to extremely low frequency magnetic fields is the induction of flickering visual sensations — the *magnetic phosphenes* — which are thought to result from the interaction of induced eddy currents with cells in the retina. One early investigator, the English physiologist Sylvanus Thompson, described them thus: 'On inserting the head into the interior of the coil, in the dark, or with the eyes closed, there is perceived over the whole region of vision a faint flickering illumination, colourless, or of a slightly bluish tint.' However, such high magnetic flux densities are unlikely to be encountered except in very specialized situations.

Radiofrequency currents are not able to stimulate nerve and muscle tissue in the same way, as the reactance of CELL MEMBRANES renders them invisible to such high frequencies. The French physiologist, Arsène d'Arsonval, demonstrated around the turn of the century that the passage of a radiofrequency current through his colleagues sufficient to light a bulb resulted in a sensation of warmth, an observation that led to the development of short-wave and later microwave therapy for the treatment of injured tissue. Today, the most well-established effect of exposure to radiofrequency and microwave radiation from whatever source is that of heating through increased molecular kinetic energy, either heating of the whole body or localized heating of parts of the body, depending on various factors including the proximity of the exposed person to the transmitter. Much work on human physiological responses to radiofrequency and microwave radiation has been carried out by the American physiologist Eleanor Adair at the John B. Pierce Laboratory and at Yale University. Most people, however, encounter levels of radiofrequency and microwave radiation that are many orders of magnitude below those likely to induce measurable heating.

The pervasiveness of man-made electromagnetic fields and radiation, combined with some uncertainties about the possible existence of low level health effects, particularly in relation to childhood cancers, have generated much public concern over the past few decades. A large number of biological and epidemiological studies have now been carried out, centering mostly on the possible effects of exposure to power frequency magnetic fields. Generally speaking, however, there is at present no convincing evidence of any risk to health from such exposure; if there is a risk, most authorities agree that it is likely to be very small. The rapid expansion of mobile phone use has, however, led to some disquiet about the possible effects of exposure to the low levels of radiofrequency and microwave radiations emitted by these devices. Further biological and epidemiological research is being undertaken in order to address these concerns.

Optical radiations

The sun is the most important source of optical radiation, creating through its action on the environment the conditions necessary to sustain life. Light, which is only the visible part of the spectrum of optical radiation, drives photosynthetic processes in plants, generating food and oxygen, and enables our perception of the world through visual processes in the eye and associated parts of the brain. However, prolonged gazing at bright sources of light such as the sun can result in a loss of visual acuity through photochemical damage to the light-sensitive receptor cells in the retina. Such damage has been reported for example in anti-aircraft gunners and plane spotters during World War II, and in people viewing a partial eclipse of the sun.

Infra-red radiation, which is less energetic and of longer wavelengths than light, heats tissue through increasing molecular vibrational energies. It is mostly absorbed by the skin; we feel the warmth when we sit in bright sunlight or around a fire. With regard to the EYE, however, mid-wavelength infrared-B radiation is absorbed mostly by the crystalline lens; heat-induced opacities (cataracts) have historically been associated with work in industries handling hot materials. H. M. Chief Inspector of Factories, Thomas Legge, reported in 1907 that 'persons exposed to incandescent molten glass or to continual furnace glare in the flattening of glass suffer unduly, more than ten times as frequently as other people, from cataract.' 'Heat cataract' became a recognized industrial disease, although modern working practices, including the wearing of protective goggles, have virtually eliminated this risk.

Ultraviolet radiation is the most energetic of the non-ionizing electromagnetic radiations; the shortest, most energetic wavelengths are however attenuated by the atmosphere, particularly the ozone layer. Ultraviolet radiation is able to damage DNA and other biologically important molecules through direct absorption, and to generate highly reactive oxygen radicals, which can result in adverse health effects; tissues of the skin and eye are most at risk. In the absence of dietary supplements, however, we require some limited daily exposure to ultraviolet radiation in order to produce sufficient vitamin D. Short-term damaging effects resulting from acute over-exposure include sunburnt SKIN, which becomes painful and red, and may blister and peel, and inflammation of the cornea (*keratitis*) and conjunctiva (*conjunctivitis*) of the eye; the last two effects are also known collectively as 'snowblindness' or 'welder's eye'.

In the longer term, repeated exposure to excessively high levels of ultraviolet radiation may lead to photoageing of the skin and to an increased risk of cataract and skin cancer. Malignant skin tumours are the most severe health effect; their incidence has increased by about 50% over the last decade, possibly reflecting behavioural changes relating to sun exposure. Non-melanoma skin cancers are relatively common but rarely fatal; experimental studies carried out by Frank de Gruijl and his colleagues at Utrecht using mice have been invaluable in showing that both the mid-wavelength (UVB) and long-wavelength (UVA) regions are carcinogenic. Cutaneous malignant melanoma occurs much less frequently but accounts for the majority of skin cancer deaths. In contrast to the non-melanoma skin cancers, the aetiology of malignant melanoma is not clear; there are no good animal models. However, short-term, intermittent exposure to high levels of solar radiation, particularly during childhood, is thought to be a contributing causal factor.

RICHARD D. SAUNDERS

See also FREE RADICALS; MAGNETIC BRAIN STIMULATION; SUN AND THE BODY.

Radioactivity When Henri Becquerel established the existence of 'uranic rays' in March 1896, there was no way of appreciating the far-reaching implications of this discovery. Only 75 elements had been discovered by this time, two of which, uranium and thorium, were radioactive, although this was not known. The periodic table has since been expanded to 81 stable and 31 radioactive elements.

Radioactivity is the process of emission of radiation as a radioactive material changes form, often to a different element. To understand this process, we need to be familiar with a number of concepts and terms. Atoms of each element contain a different and defining number of protons and an equal number of electrons. The nucleus of the atom contains neutrons as well as protons and different numbers of neutrons are present in different *isotopes* of the same element. Isotopes of an element may be either stable, or unstable and radioactive — *radioisotopes*. Isotopes of all elements are referred to collectively as *nuclides*; those that are radioactive, as *radionuclides*. Radionuclides are specified by the elemental name and the mass number — the combined number of protons and neutrons — for example, carbon-14 (^{14}C), iodine-131 (^{131}I), plutonium-239 (^{239}Pu). Where an element is referred to as radioactive, as in the paragraph above, this is intended to mean that all isotopes of the element are radioactive. Radionuclides differ in their rate of decay as well as the radiation emitted. The rate of decay in a given mass of the radionuclide is measured in units called becquerels (Bq), where 1 Bq equals one transformation per second. *Alpha*-emitting radionuclides emit alpha particles, each consisting of 2 protons and 2 neutrons. *Beta*-emissions involve the loss of an electron from the nucleus as a beta particle during the conversion of a neutron into a proton. *Gamma* rays are high energy photons, often emitted together with beta or alpha radiations when the transformation has left the atom with excess energy. An important characteristic of a radionuclide, as well as the radiation emitted, is its *half-life* — the time taken for half the atoms present to decay to the daughter nuclide. Thus ^{131}I is a beta-emitter with a half-life of 8 days, while ^{239}Pu is an alpha-emitter with a half-life of 24 000 years.

We are exposed to radionuclides throughout our lives, mainly from natural sources. The greatest exposures are due to inhalation of radon-222 (^{222}Rn) gas, present in the atmosphere due to the decay of uranium-238 contained in rocks and soil. Artificial sources include the medical use of radiopharmaceuticals and small amounts released by the nuclear industry. There is, of course, the potential for greater exposures from nuclear installations if accidents occur, the most noteable example being the accident at Chernobyl in the former Soviet Union in 1986.

The health risk associated with exposure to a particular radionuclide will depend on the radiation emitted and its chemical behaviour. Beta and gamma radiations can penetrate through the skin and may pose an external radiation hazard, but the main concern generally is the entry of radionuclides into the body by inhalation and ingestion. Intake will lead to dose delivery to the respiratory and alimentary tracts, and absorption into the blood followed by entry into other organs and tissues. Depending on their chemical behaviour, some radionuclides concentrate in specific organs and tissues. For example, iodine-131 concentrates in the THYROID GLAND because iodine is an essential constituent of the hormone, thyroxine. Consequently, the dose to the thyroid is much greater than doses to other tissues, presenting a potential risk of thyroid cancer. Plutonium-239 is deposited mainly in the SKELETON and LIVER and presents a potential risk of liver and bone cancer and leukaemia. Doses are calculated for intakes of radionuclides, taking account of their distribution and retention in the body and the pattern of deposition of radiation energy in different tissues. These calculations are done primarily by the International Commission on Radiological Protection, and the calculated values of dose per unit intake (Sv per Bq) are used as a basis for restrictions on radionuclide exposure in legislation in Europe, the UK, and elsewhere.   JOHN D. HARRISON

See also IMAGING TECHNIQUES; RADIATION, IONIZING; RADIOLOGY; RADIOTHERAPY.

Radiology

This medical specialty originally involved the use of X-RAYS in the diagnosis and treatment of disease. Improved technology over the years with computer analysis of images has led to many sophisticated developments. *Computed tomography (CT scans)*, developed by Sir Godfrey Hounsfield in 1972, was probably the most spectacular advance in radiology, using X-rays to provide three-dimensional information. Along with a progressive increase in the use of X-rays in diagnosis, other methods such as those utilizing gamma rays from radioactive isotopes (*isotope scans*), and *positron emission tomography* (*PET scans*), became incorporated into the modern practice of radiology. More recently radiologists have become involved also in ULTRASOUND and MAGNETIC RESONANCE IMAGING (MRI) which do not involve ionising radiation. Further sophistication has led to *Doppler ultrasound, duplex scanning,* and *MRI angiography*. These diagnostic methods are all known as organ imaging or IMAGING TECHNIQUES and are described more fully elsewhere. They display in superb detail various organs or blood vessels and are very much a part of a modern radiologist's activities.

When one reflects that X-rays were only discovered in 1895, the developments have been quite staggering and expensive. Who could have foreseen, a hundred years ago, that putting patients inside magnets (MRI) could produce images? We are in the Golden Age of radiology with not enough gold to do all that is possible. Present day radiologists must be aware of the potential of these imaging methods, ensuring that optimal diagnostic pathways are followed. Radiologists now tend to subspecialize: neuroradiologists work solely within the nervous system, while others develop expertise in chest, bone, or gastrointestinal investigations.

Interventional radiology — dealing not with diagnosis but with treatment — is now a special field where various procedures are carried out using radiology for a visual display. Thus, under X-ray control, a catheter or needle may be positioned for various purposes; narrowed blood vessels in the leg or heart can be dilated (*angioplasty*); stents can be placed to widen arteries, bronchial airways, or ducts in the urinary or biliary tracts; tumours can be embolized (injected with material to block their blood vessels) to reduce their size; and abscesses can be drained.

J. K. DAVIDSON

See also IMAGING TECHNIQUES; MAGNETIC RESONANCE IMAGING; RADIOACTIVITY; RADIOTHERAPY; X-RAYS.

Radiotherapy

refers to the use of ionizing radiation in the treatment of disease — mainly CANCER.

Radiation — exposure to X-RAYS or gamma rays — can kill cells or stop their growth. It can be effective in the treatment of cancerous growths, because malignant cells are more sensitive than normal body cells: the radiation can be applied to a particular area, whilst the rest of the body is shielded from it.

Historically, radiotherapy dates back to the discovery of X-RAYS by Röntgen in 1895, and of the radioactivity of substances such as uranium by Becquerel in 1896, leading to that of radium, identified in 1898 by Marie and Pierre Curie.

The first use of X-rays as a treatment, for BREAST cancer, occurred in the USA within two to three months of their discovery. More followed within a year in Germany, France, and Austria. The loss of hair which followed exposure in these early cases alerted the medical profession to potentially harmful effects on normal tissues. The first report of successful treatment by X-ray was of a SKIN cancer in 1899. The use of radium in treatment was explored after Becquerel had been burnt by carrying a tube of radium in his pocket. The first accredited success, again for skin cancer, was in 1903. Radium tubes could be inserted, for example for treatment of uterine cancer (the standard method in the 1930s), or rays from a radium source could be directed at the lesion. Radium 'needles' were also inserted into tumours such as breast cancers. 'Teletherapy' — directing beams of radiation at the appropriate part — was thus a method applicable to either X-rays or radium. The two continued to be the mainstay of cancer treatment for the first half of the twentieth century.

Despite early realization of danger, protection of personnel involved in radiotherapy was not taken seriously before the mid 1930s nor implemented adequately until considerably later than that. In the late 1920s it was even recommended that the physician should use the redness produced on his own skin to determine the appropriate X-ray dose for a patient.

The discovery of plutonium-239 in 1941 led to the therapeutic use of artificially produced radioactive isotopes (as well as to nuclear weapons). The gamma rays which these emit can be directed at a tumour through a tube or needle. They are safer than X-rays both for patients and attendants; they have a much shorter half life than radium and emit gamma rays of lower energy. Thus cobalt-60 for example mainly supplanted radium for cancer of the uterus, and other radioisotopes, such as caesium-137 and iridium-192, have been developed for particular uses. These treatments, along with the diagnostic IMAGING TECHNIQUES which employ radioisotopes have become the province of the specialty of *nuclear medicine*.

X-rays, however, have not been supplanted. In recent years radiologists involved in radiotherapy have expanded their activities to include the use of radioisotopes and also the combination of radiotherapy with a variety of chemotherapeutic drugs or with hormones in the treatment of cancer. This specialty is now termed, 'radiation oncology'. J. K. DAVIDSON

See also CANCER; CHEMOTHERAPY; IMAGING TECHNIQUES; RADIATION, IONIZING; RADIOACTIVITY; RADIOLOGY; X-RAYS.

Rape has always been deemed a terrible crime. What has changed over time is the perception of what constitutes rape. Since the 1960s, rape is increasingly considered as sexual intercourse without consent. Not very long ago physical violence was taken to be intrinsic to the notion of rape; this is no longer so. It was also assumed that rape occurred predominantly between strangers. Now the idea of rape within MARRIAGE is no longer thought a contradiction in terms.

Defined as the unlawful carnal knowledge of a woman by force and against her will, rape was a capital crime already in early Anglo-Saxon times. It was deemed a crime even where legal codes said nothing of it. Thus the Chevalier de Jaucourt (1704–80 cited the argument which Cicero (106–43 BC) had made around 46 BC:

> [e]ven if there was no written law against rape at Rome in the reign of Lucius Tarquinius, we cannot say on that account that Sextus Tarquinius did not break that eternal Law by violating Lucretia, the daughter of Tricipitinus! For reason did exist, derived from the Nature of the universe, urging men to right conduct and diverting them from wrong-doing, and this reason did not first become Law when it was written down, but when it first came into existence; and it came into existence simultaneously with the divine mind.

Throughout the ages, political theorists warned princes of the consequences of rape. Machiavelli (1469–1527), for one, stressed the political danger it presented. 'Among the primary causes of the downfall of tyrants', he argued, 'Aristotle puts the injuries they do on account of women, whether by rape, violation or the breaking up of marriages . . . absolute princes and rulers of republics should not treat such matters as of small moment, but should bear in mind the disorders such events may occasion and look to the matter in good time, so that the remedy applied may not be accompanied by damage done to, or revolts against, their state or their republic.'

Amongst those who wrote about rape, some, like St Augustine (AD 354–430), stressed that the victim of rape was untainted by it. 'There will be no pollution, if the lust is another's; if there is pollution, the lust is not another's,' he contended, adding; 'While the mind's resolve endures, which gives the body its claim to chastity, the violence of another's lust cannot take away the chastity which is preserved by unwavering self-control.' Critical of Roman culture and the importance it gave to honour, St Augustine criticized Lucretia for taking her life following her rape by Tarquin. Christian women, St Augustine argued, 'did not take vengeance on themselves for another's crime.' The public gaze did not unduly concern them, for they knew themselves to be chaste in the sight of God. In the seventeenth century, the jurist, Samuel Pufendorf (1632–94), was one of the many authors who reiterated St Augustine's point, although he stressed that this did not impinge on the right of women to kill their aggressors in self defence. Jean Barbeyrac (1674–1744) drew attention to the fact that, under several ancient legal systems, seducers were actually thought worse than rapists, because they violated not only the body of their victims, but effectively their mind as well, and hence exercised power over their whole person and over their family.

To recognize that we are by no means the first to attend to the issue of rape, is not to presume, however, that rape is a timeless or universal feature of social existence. Women have not always lived in fear of rape, at least not to the extent to which they now do in some parts of the Western world. Anthropological and historical studies reveal some societies and ages to be far more 'rape-prone' than others. In 1887 Friedrich Nietzsche wrote: 'No act of violence, rape, exploitation, destruction, is intrinsically 'unjust', since life itself is violent, rapacious, exploitative, and destructive and cannot be conceived otherwise. Even more disturbingly, we have to admit that from the biological point of view legal conditions are necessarily exceptional conditions, since they limit the radical life-will bent on power and must subserve, as means, life's collective purpose, which is to create greater power constellations. To accept any legal system as sovereign and universal — to accept it, not merely as an instrument in the struggle of power complexes, but as a *weapon against struggle* (in the sense of Dühring's communist cliché that every will must regard every other will as its equal) — is an anti-vital principle which can only bring about man's utter demoralization and, indirectly, a reign of nothingness.'

Those who, like Cicero, endorse a natural rights theory, and who believe that natural law is the expression of God's will, have no difficulty in arguing what is wrong about rape. Nor should they face too much difficulty in making a case for a moral community which enforces certain ideals of conduct with respect to others and themselves. Those who don't ground their moral theories in a theocentric framework will have to

come to terms with the fact that liberty is not an empty ideal, a licence for anything, and that the liberty of women is conditional on the struggle against their being considered in any way men please. Or as Nietzsche contended, that wills cannot be regarded as equal. The law is indeed an instrument of struggle; it is one of the means by which society struggles against barbarism. Other means must be deployed to make for a culture in which sex is conceived not as something individuals have a right to, nor independent of personal relationships and the duties and responsibilities they entail. This will not be the reign of nothingness, it will be the assertion of the will of civilized women, and men. SYLVANA TOMASELLI

Further reading
Tomaselli, S. and Porter, R. (ed.) (1989). *Rape: an historical and social enquiry*. Blackwell, Oxford.

Rash A SKIN eruption: red spots or mottling of the skin, accompanying a variety of infectious illnesses, allergic reactions, chemical or heat irritation, or specific skin diseases. Rashes may be localized or body-wide and come in several descriptive categories; their distribution and character usually enable doctors to establish the cause. S.J.

See SKIN.

Reaction time Your hand accidentally touches the hot plate of an oven and is withdrawn immediately. A young child runs out in front of your car and you hammer on the brakes. A lottery ball falls into its position upside down and you have to shout out the correct number as fast as you can to a colleague who is checking off the numbers for your syndicate. All three examples of reaction time are the time it takes to make a movement in response to a sensory stimulus. However, even if we try to respond as fast as possible in each situation, the reaction time is quite different.

In this context, time is measured in milliseconds (ms) — thousandths of a second. It may take only 100 ms to withdraw our hand from the stove, 200 ms to stamp on the brakes, and 500 ms to read out the number on the ball. The difference occurs because of the different amount of time it takes for the CENTRAL NERVOUS SYSTEM (CNS) to process the sensory signals and to choose the appropriate course of action.

The quickest reaction times have the simplest neuronal circuitry. Tap the knee and the leg moves. This is the tendon jerk beloved of clinical neurologists. The tap excites receptors in the quadriceps muscle at the front of the thigh and these send signals back to the lumbar part of the SPINAL CORD. There, a direct connection is made to the MOTOR NEURONS that innervate the quadriceps muscle and cause it to contract, making the leg kick forwards. It takes a total of about 30 ms for this to happen. The receptors take 1–2 ms to respond, and another 1–2 ms is needed for the connections to operate in the spinal cord. The remaining 27 ms or so is taken up with the time it takes nerve impulses to travel from muscle to spine and back again. There is of course a price to pay for such a fast circuit. The circuit is so simple that the same thing happens every time the tendon is tapped; it is impossible to control what happens no matter how hard we try. Because of this we refer to this type of reaction as a reflex, and the time it takes as the reflex response time. In electronic jargon we can imagine that it is a hard-wired input–output circuit.

There are rather few examples where the circuit is so simple. The corneal reflex, which causes an eye blink when a speck of dust hits the cornea, is one of the few other familiar examples. Most other very rapid reactions turn out to be more complex. Withdrawal of a hand from a hot cooker is certainly automatic, but can, with great effort of will, be controlled. The neural circuit is more complex than that for the tendon jerk, and this gives it more adaptability at the expense of a longer response time. However, like the tendon jerk, this is a circuit that is innate, and ready for action from the moment we are born.

More complex reactions, like hitting the brakes to stop a car in an emergency, are neither innate nor hard-wired. After all, a person who had never been in a car before would have no idea how to stop the vehicle. They are learned responses that can be selected with remarkable speed in the correct conditions. In the simplest situation we may be asked to press a button as soon as possible after a light is illuminated. There is no ready-made circuit to do the job. Instead, the motor system prepares in advance the instructions for the response (move the arm), and all our attention is concentrated on the light. As soon as a change in illumination is detected, the instructions for movement are released and the button is pressed. In this situation the CNS narrows down the total possible number of movement options and sensory events to just one of each, and links them together with high security. Of the millions of possible connections between sensation and movement, one is highlighted by the preparation to respond in a particular manner. In the case of driving a car, there may be several circuits that have a particularly high probability of being called into action. One of them may link the operation to press the brakes hard with the unexpected arrival of an object in the path of the vehicle. Such very fast responses are sometimes referred to as *voluntary*, to indicate the necessary involvement of volition in preparing to respond in a particular way to what may well be an arbitrary event. The term 'voluntary', however, does not mean that we need consciously identify the sensory signal before issuing the instructions to move. Drivers will often volunteer that they pressed the brakes before knowing what it was that was in front of the car. They may well say that it was a 'reflex' response, presumably indicating that conscious appreciation of the action occurred only after the event.

There are some responses that require much more careful evaluation of the sensory input before an appropriate movement can be selected. These have longer reaction times, since the circuits cannot be prepared in advance with any certainty. Calling out upside-down numbers on lottery balls is probably in this category. First of all the visual field must be rotated mentally by 180 degrees, and even then, fifty possible responses are available, perhaps narrowed down to 10 if the colour of the ball is known. All of this takes the CNS a good deal of processing, and by the time the response (vocalization of the number) is selected, the sensory impression has probably reached consciousness.

In summary, reaction times span a spectrum of response types. At one end are very fast, predefined neural circuits such as the tendon jerk and the withdrawal reflex that always operate, but which can be modulated, depending on how complex their connections are, by volitional control. At the other end, sensations must first be evaluated and then assigned the correct motor response, which prolongs the response time by a factor of ten or more. In the middle, situations occur in which the CNS can accurately predict what to do when a certain simple sensation is received. In these circumstances, sensory and motor circuits are selected in advance and joined with high probability so that processing time is reduced to an absolute minimum.

J. C. ROTHWELL

See also REFLEXES.

Rectum The final part of the intestinal tract, 4–5 inches long, continuing from the COLON in the lower left part of the abdomen, and passing down through the pelvic cavity to the anus. It has a large tubular capacity for storing FAECES pending voiding, but is flattened and empty between times. Like the rest of the intestines it has a muscular wall and a mucus-secreting lining. Rectal examination can be medically informative: the other organs in the pelvis can be felt through its walls by a gloved finger, allowing recognition, for example, of enlargement of the PROSTATE gland or of the UTERUS. S.J.

See ALIMENTARY SYSTEM; DEFECATION.

PLATES 1 AND 8.

Reflexes The term 'reflex' was first used to describe an automatic, almost immediate movement in response to a stimulus, involving a nerve circuit that traverses the SPINAL CORD. It is now applied also to other types of automatic response to a stimulus, including those involving the BRAIN. A reflex requires SENSORY RECEPTORS that detect the stimulus, sensory nerve fibres that conduct the information to the CENTRAL NERVOUS SYSTEM (CNS), neurons in the CNS itself, nerve fibres conducting the command away from the CNS, and the *effector*. Sir Charles Sherrington (1857–1952) was the first to introduce the word 'reflex', taking the view that sensory information going into the cord was reflected out again along the motor nerve fibres, analogous to a beam of light being reflected by a mirror. Sherrington referred to the chain of structures — receptor, conductor, and effector — as a *reflex arc*.

The study by Sherrington and colleagues of the spinal reflex provided an understanding of the basis of the simplest neural circuits in the central nervous system, an understanding on which subsequent advances in neuroscience relied. Sherrington wished to remove the element of CONSCIOUSNESS and consciously-guided movement, so that he could study the nature of the behaviour repertoire of the spinal cord. The experimental results prompted Sherrington to define the term 'reflex' and, with this, the implicit assumption that a reflex response is independent of consciousness. Elimination of the effects of consciousness could be achieved in experimental animals by surgically interrupting influences from higher centres. This afforded the means of unravelling features of the activity of the cord that had hitherto escaped analysis.

Spinal reflexes

Although simple manifestations of activity of the central nervous system, spinal reflexes are meaningful, in that each reflex subserves an obvious function. For example, the reflex withdrawal of the hand from a noxious object minimizes the damage inflicted on the organism by the noxious agent.

One of the best-known reflexes is the *tendon jerk reflex* (see figure). When a tendon is tapped, the muscle to which it is attached gives a twitch. An example is the 'knee-jerk reflex'; a tap to the patellar tendon (just below the front of the knee) causes a reflex twitch in the quadriceps muscles (the muscle mass on the front of the thigh). This twitch may be sufficiently powerful to extend the lower leg at the knee. We now know that this reflex response is initiated from the class of sensory receptors called *muscle spindle receptors*. In animal experiments, Sherrington showed that the adequate stimulus for this reflex was a mere 0.01 mm elongation of the quadriceps muscle.

The tendon jerk reflex is the simplest reflex; within the central nervous system, the sensory nerve fibres form connections directly with the nerve cells that send out motor nerve fibres to innervate the effector muscle. The testing of these reflexes, together with a knowledge of the different levels of the spinal cord responsible for each of them, provides a clinical method of examining the integrity of a reflex arc involving particular peripheral nerves and segments of the spinal cord. Also, since tendon jerks are normally partly suppressed by nerve impulses descending from higher levels of the CNS, their exaggeration is a valuable sign of damage above the relevant spinal segments.

Transmission of information in the reflex arc

As with other cells in the body, each nerve cell is surrounded by its own thin lipid CELL MEMBRANE. This membrane has a high electrical resistance. Conduction of nerve impulses along nerve fibres is subserved by an electrical mechanism. The nerve fibre acts as a cable with a conducting core (the *cell sap*) surrounded by its insulating membrane. Nerve impulses can propagate in either direction along the nerve fibre.

The study of spinal reflexes allowed early workers to deduce properties of transmission of information from the sensory nerve fibres to the motor nerve cells within the spinal cord. In consultation with Classics colleagues in the University of Liverpool, in 1897 Sherrington introduced into our language the noun SYNAPSE to describe those areas of functional contact, between nerve cells, that are specialized for transmission of nerve impulses. He deduced that it was synaptic transmission that conferred the reflex with the property of directionality. In the reflex arc, information entered the cord along sensory nerve fibres to elicit activity leaving the cord in motor nerve fibres but, because of the special properties of the synapse, information could not flow in the opposite direction. Synaptic transmission was subsequently shown to be subserved by a chemical mechanism. Action potentials in the sensory nerve fibres cause the release of a NEUROTRANSMITTER chemical that diffuses to attach to specific recognition sites on the motor nerve cells. This attachment changes the electrical excitability of the nerve cells and may initiate nerve impulses in the motor nerve fibres. Synaptic transmission, the fundamental properties of which were initially revealed by the study of the spinal reflex, is the basis of the integrative activity of the nervous system. Modulation of synaptic transmission underlies the mechanism of action of most drugs, both therapeutic and drugs of abuse, that act on the brain.

Evolutionary aspects

In simple vertebrates the spinal cord and lower BRAIN STEM dominate, there being little or no developed forebrain. As higher centres have developed in the course of evolution, they have come to exert many of their effects by controlling and modifying the pre-existing spinal reflex mechanisms, not by replacing them. An example of modification of primitive cord activity by higher centres is afforded by another clinically useful test. When a firm stroke is applied to the sole of the foot, the primitive spinal reflex response, when influences from higher centres are absent, is withdrawal of the foot from the mildly noxious stimulus. The response of a normal human adult to this same stimulus, however, is a thrust, to push the stimulus away. This latter response is part of the complicated mechanism that allows us to stand; the pressure on the soles of our feet elicits a continuous muscular effort to keep the feet pushing against the ground to prevent us from falling. If a human adult suffers damage to the higher motor centres in the brain, the reflex reverts from its normal thrust to the more primitive withdrawal response. Doctors refer to the reflex as the *Babinski* response, named after the neurologist in Paris who first described its significance in 1896. It is a clinically useful indicator of the integrity of the higher motor centres together with the tracts projecting down from these centres to the motor nerve cells in the spinal cord. Normal new-born babies, in whom the higher central control of POSTURE has yet to develop, show the primitive withdrawal response. This reverses to the normal adult response at the age of about 6 months. This is the time in development at which the tracts from higher motor centres become functional.

For different reflexes, the reflex responses range from simple to complex. The tendon jerk reflex is relatively simple and involves a relatively small region of the spinal cord. This contrasts with complicated, repeated movements, such as those occurring in a limb of a dog showing a *scratch reflex* to dislodge an insect biting its flank. For these more complicated reflexes, extensive regions of the cord are involved and the reflex circuits are correspondingly elaborate. Whereas the tendon jerk reflex is executed by a direct connection in the cord between the sensory nerve fibres and motor nerve cells, a scratch reflex depends on long pathways involving multiple synaptic relays, and the triggering into action of a rhythm generator responsible for the frequency and vigour of the scratching movements.

Reflexes interact with each other. The reflex response to a stimulus which is severely threatening to the well-being, or even to the life, of an animal, will, whilst commanding its own response, simultaneously switch off any other interfering reflexes that are less important in survival and that utilize the same muscles.

Reflexes mediated by cranial nerves

The cranial nerves (the nerves that arise from the brain rather than the spinal nerves that arise from the cord) provide the pathways to and from the central nervous system for reflexes utilizing the muscles of the head, such as those controlling movements of the eyeball, face, and tongue. The nerve cells giving rise to the cranial motor nerve fibres lie in clusters (*nuclei*) in the brain stem; they represent an upward extension of the homologous groups of nerve cells in the spinal cord. Examples of reflexes involving the cranial nerves are the closure of the eyelids when the cornea is stimulated, or gagging when the back of the throat is irritated.

Autonomic reflexes

These reflexes produce effects such as: changing the rate or force of contraction of the heart; contraction or relaxation of smooth muscle; glandular secretion. The reflexes are mediated by the sympathetic or parasympathetic nerves of the AUTONOMIC NERVOUS SYSTEM, in response to information reaching the central nervous system from a variety of receptors in the organs and tissues. For example, when a light shines in the EYE, there is constriction of the pupil produced by contraction of the circular smooth muscle of the iris; when a person rises rapidly from bed or bath, the heart rate promptly increases in response to a fall in BLOOD PRESSURE; in response to the taste of a lemon, there is an outpouring of SALIVA.

In conclusion, the study of reflexes alone cannot solve the problems of higher neural function, of emotion, or of psychology. However, by providing a basis from which a study of higher functions could develop, the unravelling of the properties of reflexes was an historic, essential early step in the development of NEUROSCIENCE.

OLIVER HOLMES

See also CENTRAL NERVOUS SYSTEM; MOTOR NEURON; REACTION TIME; SYNAPSE.

Reflexology

is a form of complementary therapy that involves treating the body through the feet. It is based on the premise that there are reflex areas in the feet which relate to all the body parts and that therefore the whole body can be treated through the feet. The arrangement of these reflex areas is such that a map of the body is described on the foot, with the right foot corresponding to the right side of the body and the left foot to the left side of the body. (See figure.) A system of longitudinal energy zones is believed to provide the link between the reflex areas and the body parts. The body is divided into ten zones, with each zone linking the fingers up to the head and down the body to the toes; for example zone 1 is in line with the big toe and thumb on each side, zone 2 in line with the second toe and second finger, and zone 5 in line with the little toe and fifth finger. The zones were first described by an American, Dr William Fitzgerald, in the early 1900s. Fitzgerald had become interested in various pressure therapies whilst studying in Europe and described a method called Zone Therapy based on his findings from work dating back to the 1500s. It is probable that reflexology had been known for many years, originating in China, and there is evidence dating back to 2500 BC in Egypt, where a tomb drawing shows one man treating another man's foot by applying pressure with the thumb.

During a reflexology treatment, massage using the side and tip of the thumb will be used on each of the reflex areas. A firm but not heavy pressure is applied to the area, the pressure held for a moment or so and then, released. If the part of the body corresponding to the reflex area is out of balance then a degree of tenderness will be felt in the foot when pressure is applied. In some areas there may be a sharp feeling and in others a slight pain, but these feelings should never be very uncomfortable; in areas corresponding to parts of the body that are in balance, then just the feeling of pressure will occur.

Treatment to all of the reflex areas in both feet will take about one hour and during this time the patient will be sitting in a comfortable, reclining position with the feet raised.

Thus, an additional benefit of treatment is the relaxation effect. However, a wide range of disorders can be helped by reflexology, including problems such as migraines, sinus congestion, backache, digestive disorders, hormonal imbalances, and circulatory problems. Reflexology does not claim to be able to cure all disorders, but there are very many instances where treatment can be of great benefit.

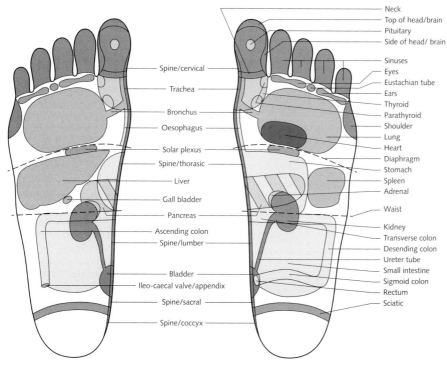

The reflex areas of the feet as described by reflexologists. Nicola M. Hall, The Bayly School of Reflexology, 1987.

If the correct technique and pressure are used, treatment will not do harm, and there are very few cases when reflexology treatment is not appropriate. Following treatment, it is possible in some instances for certain 'healing reactions' to occur, such as streaming nose (if there is sinus congestion) or increased bowel and bladder activity. These reactions will only be short term and will occur only after the first few treatments. After treatment, many people feel tired, though others may feel quite energized, and often people report how well they sleep.

For most conditions, a course of treatment is required — typically once a week for between three and six weeks. After three treatments, some response should be seen; in some cases there may already be a great improvement, whereas in others it may take longer. In many cases people have a course of treatment from which they benefit and then decide to continue at intervals of, for example, every four or six weeks in order to maintain good health and to try to prevent other problems from arising.

Reflexology treatment is suitable for people of both sexes and all ages. There are very few who do not feel benefit either on a physical or on an emotional level, with a general overall sense of well-being.

In recent years the popularity of reflexology has increased tremendously, helped by regular media coverage. The number of reflexology practitioners has also increased. Many training courses are available and a number of associations exist. In Great Britain it is estimated that there are about ten thousand practitioners. At the time of writing there is no set national

qualification for a practitioner in the UK but this is an area which is currently being addressed. In the US, practitioners in some States are required to hold a massage licence, but this is something which the reflexology associations are fighting, on the grounds that practitioners should receive thorough training and that their practice should be regulated by membership of a professional body.   NICOLA HALL

Further reading

Hall, N. M. (1991). *Reflexology: a way to better health*. Gateway Books, Bath.

Refractive errors Why, in our forties, does reading become progressively more difficult? People who have always enjoyed clear vision at any distance start to hold the book further away and employ brighter light for comfortable close work. The cornea and lens refract the incoming light rays to focus them on the retina at the back of the eye. In humans the cornea does some two-thirds and the lens one-third of this focusing. The power of the lens can be altered by changes in the shape of the lens — a process called ACCOMMODATION. This allows rapid changes in focus, according to how near or distant is the object of regard. Better light increases the contrast between print and page, the associated contraction of the pupil increasing the depth of field. Unfortunately, focusing for near objects gradually reduces with age (*presbyopia*) and has to be helped by converging or convex lenses.

The lens develops from the same layer of embryonic tissue that forms the skin (*ectoderm*). Both skin and the lens grow throughout our life.

Skin is slowly shed or rubbed away and replaced, but the lens is confined within the fixed volume of the eyeball. As it grows it becomes more compact and stiffer, less able to assume greater convexity for near vision. Further compaction causes opacities to develop within the lens — cataract formation. When this causes significant interference with vision it is extracted surgically and replaced by an artificial *intra-ocular lens* (IOL). However, the IOL cannot accommodate for near vision, and glasses are still needed for reading.

Light from a distant object is brought to a focus on the retina in a normal-sighted, or *emmetropic* eye. In *hypermetropia* the eyeball is too short, so that the image falls behind the retina (Fig. 1(a)). Most hypermetropes younger than 35 years can accommodate all the time for clear distance vision but, together with the extra effort still necessary for close work, they may suffer from headaches and other symptoms. Once an ageing hypermetrope has become presbyopic he cannot see clearly at any distance without refractive help (Fig. 1(b)).

Contrast this with *myopia*, where the eyeball is too long, and distant objects are focused in front of the retina (Fig. 2(a)). A diverging, concave lens can correct this (Fig. 2(c)). Note that diverging light rays from a near object can be accurately focused on the retina in myopia without correcting lenses (Fig. 2(b)). Because the myope can see clearly at short distances without glasses the term 'short-sighted' is often used. Hence my hypermetropic wife wearing her glasses can find my concave spectacles for me, but I can read the dials and shower safely without the risks of being scalded or frozen, or wetting my glasses.

Perfectly regular, spherical hypermetropia or myopia are not the commonest refractive errors. *Astigmatism* may be added to either condition, when the cornea has unequal curvature in different meridians, like the shape of an egg. Light rays from a single point are refracted to two separate focal lines at right angles to each other (Fig. 3). The astigmatic person does not know which focal line to look at, and 'hunting' between the two may cause eye-strain. Some people are much more susceptible to this than others and require correction of low levels of astigmatism, but the majority do not. Most astigmatism has its axes close to horizontal and vertical, with the curvature being less along the horizontal axis. Oblique astigmatism is usually more troublesome; even spectacle correction with cylindrical lenses is a compromise, but contact lenses may be much more effective.

Many surgical methods have been tried on the cornea in attempts to correct myopia. Radial cuts with a diamond knife to induce scarring, which changes corneal curvature, have been largely replaced by laser methods, in which the optical zone is re-profiled by removing tissue from the anterior corneal surface. In the latest method (LASIK) a thin corneal flap is cut, some of the underlying substance is removed by laser, and the flap is replaced.

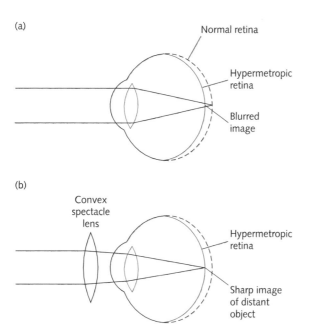

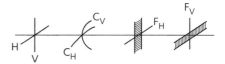

Fig 3 Astigmatism. Diagram of a cross with vertical (V) and horizontal (H) lines as focused by an astigmatic cornea with greater curvature vertically (C_V) than horizontally (C_H). The line H is sharply focused at F_H but the line V is still out of focus. Line V is sharply focused farther away at F_V. The retina can receive clear images only of either H or V: not both at the same time unless a correcting lens is used.

Fig 1 Hypermetropia. (a) parallel light rays from a distant object give a blurred image and (b) require a convex spectacle lens for a sharp image.

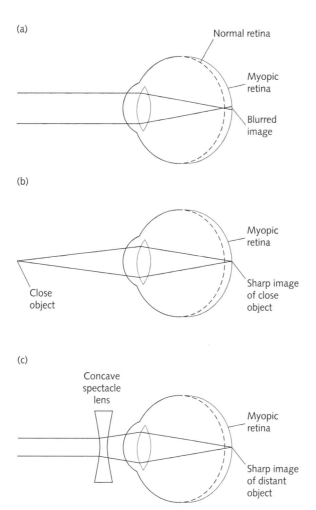

Fig 2 Myopia. (a) parallel light rays from a distant object give a blurred image. (b) Rays from a close object can be sharply focused without any spectacle lens. (c) Rays from a distant object require a concave lens for a sharp image.

The refractive power of a lens is measured in *dioptres* (the reciprocal of the focal length in metres). Refractive errors are expressed as the dioptres required for correction (positive or negative); thus hypermetropia requires additional refractive power to focus an image on the retina in the short eyeball (Fig. 1(b)), whilst myopia requires negative correction (Fig. 2(c)).

Measurements of refractive errors of large numbers of individuals, when plotted graphically to show their relative incidence, lie on a sharply-peaked curve, shown in Fig. 4 and compared with a theoretically derived 'normal' or 'Gaussian' distribution curve. Ninety-eight per cent of all refractions in one series of cases lay between +4 and −4 dioptres, and the number of emmetropes (normals) was greater than anticipated. Furthermore, the mean refractive level was at some +2 dioptres of hypermetropia in infants, moving towards +1 dioptre by 25 years of age, with a similar distribution of relative values at all ages. There appears to be a definite tendency towards normalization of refraction (*emmetropization*), which implies highly accurate and co-ordinated control of growth of the cornea, the lens, and the whole eyeball. Interestingly, when refractive errors are present they are often closely similar in the two eyes, even down to the degree and axes of any astigmatism. Occasionally there is a large difference between the focusing of the two eyes, making correction difficult and with profound implications for the development of normal binocular vision.

In the Western world some 15–20% of people are myopic and 40–50% hypermetropic, but in Japan and China 50–70% are myopic. The Jewish race has an excess of myopia, but Black African have more hypermetropia than average.

With vision being our principal sensory contact with the environment, it is not surprising that uncorrected focusing can have significant influences, so much so that separate myopic and hypermetropic personalities have been recognised. The myopic child can be introverted, studious, and solitary, with no interest in ball games or outdoor pursuits. 'Short-sighted' can be used as a derogatory term, implying an incomplete view, lacking in extent of intellectual outlook. As Disraeli put it, 'so short-sighted are politicians in power'. The distinctive style of Impressionist painters has been attributed to myopia, and

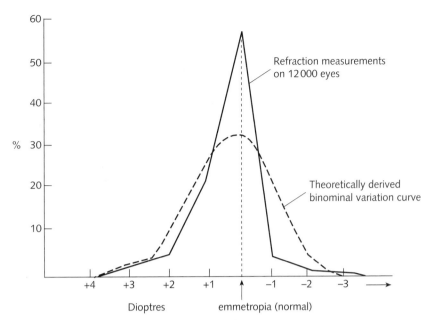

Fig 4 Relative incidence of refractive errors (after A. Franceschetti).

Cézanne, Degas, Pissarro, and Renoir were all known to be myopes. A survey of the teachers and pupils at the École des Beaux-Arts in Paris around the turn of the nineteenth century revealed 48% to be myopes, almost three times as many as in the general population.   PETER FELLS

Further reading

Donder, F. C. (1864). *On the anomalies of accommodation and refraction of the eye*. The New Syderham Society, London.

Duke-Elder, S. and Abrams, D. (1970). *System of ophthalmology*, Vol. 5. Published for Henry Kimpton by C. V. Mosby Company, USA.

Trevor-Roper, P. (1970). *The world through blunted sight*. Thames and Hudson Ltd., London.

See also ACCOMMODATION; CONTACT LENSES; EYES; OPTOMETRY; SQUINT.

Refractory period

Signals are transmitted around the nervous system, along the fibres (*axons*) of nerve cells, in the form of electrical impulses called ACTION POTENTIALS. After an action potential has swept along a single nerve fibre, a second nerve impulse cannot be initiated immediately. Instead a finite time, known as the *refractory period*, must elapse before another action potential can be generated in response to a further stimulus (such as an electric shock to the nerve). Neurophysiologists sometimes divide this interval into the *absolute refractory period*, during which a second action potential cannot be elicited, no matter how strong the stimulus, and the *relative refractory period*, during which a second action potential can be evoked, but only if the stimulus strength is increased.

The refractory period sets a limit on the frequency at which action potentials can be conducted along single nerve fibres. In mammals, the absolute refractory period is about 1 millisecond

and the maximum firing frequency is around 1000 impulses per second (although it is rare for fibres to fire naturally at rates above a few hundred per second). Some animals manage faster rates: the *Gymnotid* electric fish of South America, for example, can transmit impulses at rates of up to 1600 per second.

The refractory period is a consequence of the molecular processes that underlie the action potential. Action potentials are elicited when tiny pores in the nerve CELL MEMBRANE, known as sodium channels, open up in response to a stimulus. The sodium channels can exist in three different states: closed, open, and inactivated. At rest, the sodium channels are closed. In response to electrical stimulation, the sodium channels open, but they then pass into the inactivated state, in which the pore is closed but the channel is unable to open in response to a further stimulus. It takes some time for the sodium channels to recover from inactivation and return to the closed state, even after the action potential is over and the nerve cell membrane has returned to its resting state. During this time, the nerve is refractory to stimulation. The refractory period thus reflects the time it takes for the sodium channels to recover.   FRANCES M. ASHCROFT

Further reading

Hodgkin, A. L. (1963). *The conduction of the nervous impulse*. Liverpool University Press.

See also ACTION POTENTIAL.

Regurgitation

refers most commonly to stomach contents moving back up into the oesophagus or all the way to the mouth — but short of the full reflex drama of vomiting. Also applied to backflow of blood through a leaking heart valve.   S.J.

See HEART; INDIGESTION.

Rejuvenation

Resistance to the process of AGEING is a perennial preoccupation that refuses to die out. From legends of the Fountain of Youth, and the account of the rejuvenation of Aeson in *The Golden Fleece*, to the latest wonder drug, without fail science, magic, and medicine have pandered to the predominantly Western cult of youthfulness. More than merely camouflaging a pandemic fear of death, the desire for rejuvenation is primarily a rejection of the infirmities and diseases of old age and a desire to retain or regain the beauty and vitality of youth.

The most literal restorative was that devised by Hermippus Redivivus, who allegedly lived for 150 years and five days using the breath of young women. Pliny insisted that he would have lived even longer had he inhaled the breath of young men. Even less probable than Redivivus' longevity is the claim that he had in fact existed. It is likely that he was a product of the 1740s (invented by either John Henry Cohausen or John Campbell). The anarchistic philosopher, William Godwin was inspired by Campbell's history of Redivivus to write *St Leon* (1799), about an immortal, who drinks the legendary elixir of life. While Godwin drew upon the arcana of the Rosicrucian and Hermetic traditions for his novel, which was imitated by P. B. Shelley in *St Irvyne* (1801), his belief in prolongevity was grounded in Enlightenment rationalism. The laicization and secularizing of death stemming from the Scientific Revolution led to sublimation of the belief in a divine afterlife into the prospect of a sublunary life extension. Philosophers such as Descartes, Bacon, Franklin, and Condorcet embraced this secular eschatology. For Godwin, an improved intellect as part of the amelioration of the human race would lead to the prolongation of life.

Three years before the publication of *St Leon*, Christopher Hufeland, a disciple of the major exponent of longevity, Conaro, published *The Art of Prolonging Life*. Hufeland claimed that the human lifespan could be extended to 200 years if individuals kept within the limits of a macrobiotic lifestyle. This is in keeping with the commonly-held view that prolongevity is a consumerist rather than a cerebral matter. Plants, such as the mandrake, orchid, and sweet potato, have, as the history of folk medicine reveals, been credited with rejuvenating properties. Individuals deficient in MINERALS and VITAMINS could derive a sense of well-being or sense of rejuvenation after eating certain plants and herbs. Such may have been the case with the herb fenugreek, which is rich in vitamin A and D — although the trimethylamine it contains works as a sex hormone only in frogs.

APHRODISIACS have been used as an aid to rejuvenation, mainly because the diminution of sexual or reproductive powers has often been regarded as the least desirable effect of ageing. More aphrodisiac effects have been attributed to animal products than to plant remedies. The occultist Doctrine of Signatures and use of sympathetic magic, both of which are grounded in a science of cosmic correspondences, partly explain, for example, why an increase in male potency could be attributed to consuming powdered rhinoceros horn or the blood and internal organs of a snake. According to Nicholas Culpepper's *London Dispensatory* of 1679, the brains of sparrows were thought to increase lust. The most famous male aphrodisiac is the common blistering beetle or Spanish Fly, *Cantharis vesicatoria*, which is prepared using the soft part of the insect. John Quincy in *The Compleat English Dispensary* (1722) cites a case of a man who on taking a large dose so inflamed himself that he nearly killed his wife 'yet he continued even in distraction with fresh rage until he dy'd delirious.' The notorious trial of 1772 held at Marseilles involved the Marquise de Sade, who gave chocolates laced with Spanish Fly to prostitutes, causing them to suffer lumbar pain, cystourethritis, and vomiting.

The gendering of rejuvenation identifies increased sexual potency primarily with men. Even seminal fluid has been treated as a love philtre or prophylactic in WITCHCRAFT, and administered by Aborigines to dying or enfeebled members of their community. For women, the pressure to rejuvenate is greater, as ageing is socially constructed as 'defeminising' and undesirable in every sense. Cosmetics are often marketed not just as an enhancement of female beauty but also as containing rejuvenatory substances. The youth cult has been an effective way of undermining the power, sexual and otherwise, of post-menopausal women, and has been a potent weapon in the battle of the sexes.

Men and women were brought together in James Graham's Temple of Health and Hymen of 1780, where electric currents passed through his celestial bed, promising sexual rejuvenation for a nightly fee of fifty pounds. The high priest of health and prophet of prolongation also recommended earth bathing, which stipulated fasting and being buried up to one's neck in mud. Those unwilling to immerse themselves in the earth could strap to their chest a piece of Hampstead Hill turf in the hope of extending their lifespan far beyond a hundred years.

More familiar forms of bathing were popular with the Romans, who were predated by the Vedic physicians of the gods, whose knowledge of rejuvenation by water is recorded in Sanskrit literature. Spas and hydras flourished in Georgian England and nineteenth-century Germany, mainly due to Vincent Priessnitz, who made a fortune out of hydrotherapy.

Cashing in on life extension became a secular version of the medieval practice of buying plenary indulgences. Instead of sacred relics dispensed by a priest, the rejuvenating quack would supply potions and phials, while the Fountain of Youth and hydrotherapy served as a substitute for Holy Water. Hawkers of such chicanery have made claims that youth and restored body functions could be brought about through nerve tonics and elixirs of life. The twentieth-century 'Sanatogen', for instance, which was merely powdered casein (the protein of milk), was advertised in the *London Graphic* and endorsed by members of the establishment as 'The Life tonic and nerve tonic, Rejuvenates and Revitalises'. A more exotic product was El Zair. Advertised as having been harvested under specific phases of the moon, it was claimed that the ingredients could only be procured from 'almost inaccessible mountain ranges in Africa'. Not only was El Zair alleged to make hair grow on bald heads, but it could clear away the deeper-seated waste matter that was claimed to be responsible for old age. American medical scientists from Chicago found that they could reproduce the product a lot nearer home by dissolving $2\frac{1}{2}$ ounces of Epsom salt in a pint of distilled vinegar.

More sophisticated medical interventions have appeared since, which range from cellular therapy involving the injections of fresh cells, the Romanian practice of rejuvenation by novacaine, transplanting sex glands, monkey gland therapy, and forays into genetic engineering to produce the ultimate youth drug. The most effective route for prolongevity would still seem to be diet and lifestyle, while the cosmetic surgeon has become the modern guru of rejuvenation. Medical researchers and biochemists are still looking for the genetic key to slow down the countdown towards death. While the fascination with rejuvenation continues to span the centuries, maybe only when we can travel at the speed of light, and possibly then through time, will the ageing process be significantly slowed down.

MARIE MULVEY-ROBERTS

See also AGEING; APHRODISIAC; COSMETIC SURGERY; LIFESPAN.

Relaxation is that blissful state of being at peace with oneself and with the world. As Robert Browning put it about a hundred years ago, 'God's in his heaven/All's right with the world'. It is the consequence of an untroubled mind in a relaxed body — a body free from undue tension. It is something that we are all born knowing how to do, or rather to be — since relaxation is more a state of being, than an activity, although sometimes it becomes a skill that we have to relearn.

Relaxation creates measurable changes in the body, such as a reduction in oxygen consumption, heart and respiratory rate, blood pressure, blood cortisol levels, and muscle tension, and an increase in the production in the brain of SEROTONIN which leads to feelings of calmness and well-being. There is also a noticeable change in the pattern of our brain waves (ELECTROENCEPHALOGRAM) when we are deeply relaxed. Very deep relaxation and MEDITATION produce a pattern that combines the so-called alpha and theta rhythms, indicating a state of harmony. The collection of bodily changes that accompany relaxation is sometimes referred to as 'the relaxation response'.

The body and mind — or body/mind, since they are so intricately interconnected — is designed to cope with periods of effort interspersed with periods of rest and relaxation. Unless we allow the body/mind these respites, we become irritated, unhappy, stressed, and vulnerable to disease. Most of us instinctively know how to achieve relaxation, whether it is through LEISURE activities — taking walks, dancing, playing sports or games, knitting, reading, listening to music, watching television, having a drink, spending time with friends, laughing, making love — or simply doing nothing. Some forms of relaxation involve virtually no effort, other forms require effort as a means to achieve relaxation. Methods of relaxation that address both the physical and mental sides tend to be most effective. EXERCISE often works in this way. It gets us 'out of our heads' and into a greater awareness of our bodies. Thus, it distracts us from our worries. It also gives us a sense of accomplishment and 'satisfied tiredness', which may be related to the exercise-induced production of ENDORPHINS — the body's own morphine-like substances. Happy, healthy people tend to know what relaxes them and take time for it.

Problems arise when we fail to see relaxation as being important and continually prioritise getting through our 'to do' list. We get lost in the endless cycle of 'doing'. It became something of a feature of late-twentieth-century life to see constant busyness as the norm; to make oneself available for round-the-clock demands by means of mobile phones, laptop computers, faxes, and e-mails. The pace of modern life has speeded up to such an extent that we often feel that we simply cannot afford the time to relax because we have to run so hard to keep up.

Chronic STRESS can lead to significant physical and mental health problems — so a habitual stressed state requires serious attention. Firstly, we need to become aware that there may be a problem. Secondly, spending more time relaxing is half the battle. Nevertheless, we may feel dissatisfied with our usual repertoire and in need of new and more effective methods of relaxation.

Ancient Asian methods tend to be at the basis of most of what has been more recently learned about relaxation. YOGA and meditation are the most well-known methods. Starting to practise them may turn into a life-changing experience. Other relaxation methods, like 'cue-controlled relaxation' or 'progressive relaxation', have also blown over from the East. In essence, these Western adaptations have in common a way of regulating and slowing down the breathing, relaxing the muscles, and reducing mental activity. Progressive relaxation and cue-controlled relaxation differ in that the first requires the tensing of muscles before relaxing them, while the second addresses release of muscle tension directly: this may be preferred by a person who is already aware of how it feels to be tense.

The instructions are these (adapted by de Vries from Benson, 1975):

1. Sit down in a relaxed position and close your eyes. Make sure your position in the chair allows you to relax as many of your muscles as possible. Become aware of where you need tension for your posture.

2. Concentrate on your breathing, and slow it down. Breathe through your nose, making your exhalation longer. You will notice a little tension associated with inhalation. Concentrate on making exhalation feel pleasurable.

3. Pay attention to your position, and feel each part of you being supported by the chair so that you can relax your muscles further. Adjust your position if you wish to.

4. Begin searching your body for any signs of tension. Start at your feet and work your way up. If you find any tension, focus your attention on it, and, as you exhale, relax it away. Once you have reached your shoulders, work your way down your arms first and then finish with the neck and head. Pay extra attention to areas you know you find difficult to relax. Shoulders, neck, hands, and jaw are examples. Hands can be made to relax by 'instructing them' to feel 'soft'.

5. Keep breathing slowly through your nose, and begin to think or say the word 'one' to yourself. You don't need to produce sound as long as you make sure that you move your lips to say 'one'. Keep doing this for 5 to 10 minutes. If you get distracted, don't worry about it, simply go back to saying the word and continue repeating it. Because of its neutral content the word 'one' helps to take attention away from worrying thoughts.

6. When you are ready to end your relaxation training session, open your eyes and sit up slowly. Take one or two more deep, slow breaths. Notice that you are both relaxed and alert. This is one of the main reasons why you will want to practise relaxing, for example, just prior to beginning any performance before an audience.

This exercise can be used in many different circumstances. A comfortable chair is not even needed. In the beginning it may take about a quarter of an hour. After regular practice it may take only a couple of minutes to bring about the desired effect. Eventually, just sitting down and closing the eyes may automatically trigger the relaxation response. This makes it an excellent technique to use in preparation for exciting or stressful activities like hosting a party, making a speech, doing an exam, or going for an interview.

Relaxation is necessary for our health and sense of well-being. If we've forgotten how to do it, an exercise like cue-controlled relaxation may help — but essentially relaxation comes from a balanced lifestyle as reflected in this old Irish Prayer.

Take time to work
It is the price of success.
Take time to meditate
It is the source of power.
Take time to play
It is the secret of perpetual youth.
Take time to read
It is the way to knowledge.
Take time to be friendly
It is the road to happiness.

Take time to laugh
It is the music of the soul;
And take time to love and be loved.

ÁINE KENNEDY
JAN M. A. DE VRIES

Further reading

Ban Breathnach, S. (1995). *Simple abundance.* Bantam Books, London.

Benson, K. (1975, 1976). *The relaxation response.* Morrow Books, New York.

Davis, M., Robbins Eshelman, E., and McKay, M. (1995). *The relaxation and stress reduction workbook.* New Harbinger, Oakland, CA.

Gerzon, R. (1998). *Finding serenity in the Age of Anxiety.* Simon and Schuster, London.

Kirsta, A. (1986). *The book of stress survival.* Allen and Unwin, London.

See also BREATHING; ELECTROENCEPHALOGRAM; EXERCISE; LEISURE; MEDITATION; MIND–BODY INTERACTION; SEROTONIN; STRESS; YOGA.

Relics are material remains of SAINTS which are venerated as signs of their continued presence in the world. They are revered both as points of contact of this world with the divine, and as offering the promise of worldly intercession. The means by which relics gained devotional, theological, and liturgical value in the church were linked to the power and persona of a saint. Bodily fragments were venerated as representative of the worldly presence of a saint, the suffering that a martyr endured, as the miracles associated with the relics were testimonies of saintliness. The term literally refers to bodily remains, exhumed and moved to a church, but may include any object which was in contact with a saint. Either is venerated through pilgrimage, prayer, or worship since true relics are a site of the full presence of the saint, able to work miracles in the world.

The worship of saints' relics is closely tied to the growth of the Christian church. The reverence shown for relics has roots in the celebration of the Eucharist over the graves of the first Christian martyrs. Theological definition of the holiness of the relic is absent from both the Old or New Testament, but was perpetuated as Christianity grew, as a basis for seeking intercession, often in healing bodily ills. The reverence of early Christians for bodily remains of martyrs during the Age of Persecution (*c.* 200–313) mirrored the healing powers of the belongings of the Apostles in the New Testament, but the holiness of martyrs' bodies derives from their being seen as instruments of their faith. While other Christian traditions separated the body from the self, Church fathers assimilated remains of saints to the spiritual body of Christ. They described fragmentary parts of the body — an arm, a finger, or a head — as a synecdoche for the person of the saint after death, and as forecasting Christ's promise of eventual RESURRECTION. Encased in iron or under glass, such relics were especially esteemed for their power to reverse the

course of the body's eventual decay by effecting cures or allaying physical pain.

The cult of relics soon won a prominent place within the Church. If Jerome argued that the physical remains of martyrs were to be worshipped out of honour for Christ as records of individual faith, by Augustine's time (354–430) the cult of relics expanded to include objects associated with martyrdom or with the individual person. Early churches were built over the tombs of martyrs, and in 401 the Council of Carthage decreed that all churches not honouring the relics of saints should be destroyed. In the Eastern Church, worship of relics receded in the face of the growing cult of ICONS, but in 787 the second council of Nicaea required that relics be present in the altars of consecrated churches and gave a liturgical role to the salutation of relics after the celebration of the Mass. While the exhuming of bodies faced fewer restrictions in the East, the increased need for relics led prohibitions against the spoliation of graves to be relaxed. Relics were increasingly translated, or transported into, churches from sites of martyrdom, and as the basis for Christian burial *ad sanctos*. Their charismatic value played a prominent role in European conversion. The church distinguished primary relics, parts of bodies which had suffered TORTURE or martyrdom, from 'secondary' relics, objects valued for their contact with the body of a saint and as memories of a worldly presence. Secondary relics might be privately owned, and were believed to have power as protective charms.

Worship of saintly relics became a pressing theological concern in the high Middle Ages. The church emerged as a house of worship, as well as a place of the veneration of saints, at the same time as the number of relics in the West increased. Relics continued to be considered a treasure of towns and congregations, and as the papacy authorized translation of a large number of relics from the East during the Crusades, instruments of the passion, vials of Mary's milk, and relics of the apostles flooded Europe. Relics were treasured by towns and congregations, and the cult grew so rapidly that by 1274 the veneration of relics was forbidden without papal approval. The scholastic Thomas Aquinas emphasized the importance of relics as manifestations of the Godhead. He confirmed the doctrine of saintly intercession and also saw relics as confirming the promise of future resurrection. The combined emphasis on relics' divinity and physicality paralleled theologians' increased location of individuality in the human body.

The prominent place that relics came to occupy as material objects of veneration in medieval Christianity led reformers such as Jan Huss (d. 1415) and Martin Luther (d. 1546) to question their worth as points of access to the divine. In arguing that true faith was independent from the cults of saints, Luther condemned the worship of relics as a money-making invention of the worldly Church. In response, Catholic theologians argued for the importance of relics as signs of religious faith, reaffirming their role as illustrations of the continual presence of saints within the Church. Cults of relics regained a prominent role in counter-reformation religiosity. While earlier relics were associated with Christ, the Virgin, and the apostles, the Catholic reformers confirmed worship of existing relics and encouraged veneration of parts of the saintly body: arms, hearts, tongues, throats, hands, and blood of saints were prominently exhibited on altars. Pope Sixtus V responded to accusations about the worship of false relics when he gave juridical form to the authentication of sainthood and of relics in 1588. This preserved the doctrinal basis of relics in Catholicism, established uniform guidelines for reviewing claims to sanctity, and created norms for the exhibition of relics. New guidelines for the display of relics were drafted in the late nineteenth century, to ensure their accessibility to the individual believer.   DANIEL A. BROWNSTEIN

Further reading

Brown, P. (1981). *The cult of the saints: its rise and function in Latin Christianity*. University of Chicago Press, Chicago.

Geary, P. (1978). *Furta Sacra: thefts of relics in the central Middle Ages*. Princeton University Press, Princeton.

See also SAINTS.

Religion and the body

Across the ages, organized religions have always laid claim to the bodies of their adherents. The expression of religious belief through bodily conduct and comportment has served both to confirm knowledge of abstract creeds and to evoke expedient devotional attitudes. In the initiation ceremonies of the Araucanian shamanesses, for example, initiates were brought into a sacred circle of healers by having their bodies rubbed with canelo leaves and massaged repeatedly over breasts, bellies, and heads. When the celebrations reached their height, initiates climbed nine-foot trees that were barked and notched to form ladders. Ritualistically, they were ascending to the sky to acquire magical skills of HEALING, enacting physically their faith in the supernatural curing powers of the gods. In like manner, Chinese Buddhist practices of funereal feasting mirrored theological precepts. Through consumption of vegetarian dishes and the offering of food items to the world of the spirits, celebrants expressed filial piety and demonstrated concern for their ancestors' continued livelihood. In both ritual instances, human bodies were acting as depositories of deferred thoughts and values.

It is a quality characteristic of pre-literate societies that bodily rites and symbolic GESTURES have been used to articulate religious credo. Traditionally, the body has served as a living memory pad to reproduce abstract knowledge. In the absence, through most of humanity's religious experiences, of reading skills that might assist in retrieval of basic spiritual information and insight, knowledge has

survived in the memory, where it is recalled kinaesthetically through ritual gesture and orally through prayer. Bodily ritual helps reconstruct, often below the level of consciousness, the fundamental ordering of the cosmos in religion. Careful stagings, decorations, and scarifications of the body in liturgical ceremonies and theatrical productions are mimetic reproductions of complex oral and scriptural stories and ideas. It is in this manner that the Omaha Indians of North America paint and tattoo the skin of their young women with two significant symbols: a round disk representing the sun and a star standing for the night. Together, the two bodily signs are offered as a physical memorial to the power of day and of night to grant fecundity on all earthly things.

In many religions, theoretical ideas concerning the origins of the universe, the nature and power of divinities, and the fate of human souls are made visible in seemingly innocuous details of bearing and verbal manners. In Islamic prayer-habits, for example, the simple task of physical prostration before Allah demonstrates willed subservience to divine omnipotence. In similar ways, variable positioning of the body during Christian liturgy, with its initial acts of genuflection to complex patterns of standing, kneeling, sitting, and singing, involves the believer in a set of communal gymnastics that contributes to internal reflection on biblical messages. Like the mind, the body expresses itself in symbolic forms.

This 'incorporation' of abstract thought into bodily sign is in fact a key to the psychological formation of belief. Commitment to any symbolic order requires more than cognitive understanding. It includes as well, willed assent to moral regulations and emotional commitment to narrative mythologies. This order of identification with symbolic systems is most fully accomplished, as Pierre Bourdieu has said in *The Logic of Practice*, through 'bodily *hexis*', the realization or *em-bodiment* of abstract principles. Through many different styles of physical homage, symbolic systems are 'turned into a permanent disposition, a durable way of standing, speaking, walking, and thereby of feeling and thinking.'

Traditionally, among the three monotheistic religions of Judaism, Christianity, and Islam, each of which have set up strict ontological distinctions between the supernatural and the natural, or the SOUL and the FLESH, spiritual aspirations are made manifest through the body in characteristic ways. Although all three of these 'religions of the book', have their fundamental moral and theological precepts scribally recorded, they have nevertheless made extensive use of bodily resources. Internal devotional life has been maintained through external behavioural codes like dietary regimen, dress codes, and work and holiday schedules. These devotional habits have been structured to discipline the body according to cosmic principles of sacred and profane. Each one of them is designed to affirm

the theological notion of the superiority over the corporeal world of the transcendent realm of being in god. This is the reason for head-coverings, face-veilings, bowing, kneeling, genuflecting, and other signs of spiritual modesty. The body is daunted before the magnificent transcendence of the god of Light. Hierarchical distinctions in Jehova's religions between good and evil, and male and female, are likewise acclaimed through religious rituals such as these. The segregation of women in the back of synagogues, churches, and mosques, the 'purification' or 'churching' of women's bodies after childbirth, and the CIRCUMCISION of boys at INITIATION RITES into the covenant of Abraham, are all forms, as it has been said, of 'bodily *hexis*'. They articulate underlying theological notions concerning the inferiority of women in the deity's creation.

Judaism, Christianity, and Islam have also given account in their theologies of a distinctly positive role for the human body. As expressed in the foundational Hebrew myths of Genesis, the body is a creation of divine life; it is made in the image of the creator of the universe. The human sensory apparatus is designed, so these theisms affirm, to be an instrument through which the human soul apprehends supernatural truths. Nowhere was this acceptance of bodily existence more obvious than in the graphic works of Christian artists during the Renaissance. Donatello, LEONARDO DA VINCI, and Michelangelo were celebrating the divine content of the human form. Their attention to the beauty of bodily physique is still astounding to behold. This same affirmation of earthly existence in the body is apparent structurally in the pedagogical strategies of the various beliefs. Since ancient and medieval times, the main task of organized religions has been to instruct the moral person to pursue truth and piety through the natural abilities of mind and body. To study the sacred and traditional writings of the Torah, the Bible, and the Koran, making use of the body's temporal powers of reason, will, and memory, was expected to lead believers toward more complete and intimate understanding of eternal matters. Contemplation of created things, it was believed, deepens appreciation of god their creator. During spiritual services, sensitivity to the sacred order of things has been further heightened in many denominations by instrumental music, choral singing, psalm recitation, and hand-clapping. In some churches, the odour of incense and the sight of meaningful ICONOGRAPHY support the process of prayer and MEDITATION.

It is a matter of special interest to scholars of religion to determine how religious attention to corporal devotional strategies may have heightened awareness of the sentient nature of the human body. Corporal ritual calls for repeated reflection on some of the most intense sensory experiences, including hunger, sexual abstinence, sleep deprivation, and skin laceration. Across the centuries, holy men and women have engaged in heroic efforts to deny basic physiological drives and desires, and have consciously utilized their contrived situations of PAIN and FATIGUE to reflect upon the human condition. It may very well be true that religious efforts to regulate behaviour have contributed to the unprecedented consciousness among the human species of sensory experiences and bodily movements and passions. Centuries of monastic efforts to curb sexual impulses, for example, finally led among Christian ascetics of the high Middle Ages to the exoneration of sexual passion from charges of mortal sin and the creation of elaborate codes of amorous chivalry. It was indeed among the reflective body-chastening monks of several different religions in the past that 'crimes of passion' came to be identified and granted special status under the law. In this regard, religious attempts to design moral codes has led to continual re-investigation of the types of bodily desires that are conducive to willed control and the types that seem intransigent to reasoned opinion.   MAUREEN FLYNN

See also ASCETICISM; FLAGELLATION; MORALITY; MYTHIC THOUGHT.

Removing parts of the body
Removing surplus hair, nails, and skin is a convenience and part of normal life. Almost everywhere in the world removing other parts, or allowing a surgeon to remove them, is more unusual. Nevertheless, it has a long history.

'[I]t is no small presumption to Dismember the Image of God' wrote the military surgeon John Woodall in 1639, and he advised his colleagues to say their prayers before they did it. But this attitude did not last. From the late eighteenth century onwards there was a huge increase in surgical knowledge and practice, along with a much less holistic attitude to the parts of the body. It was also a period when many lost their faith in God and with it the idea that the human body was perfectly designed. Both surgeons and their patients developed an interest in removing parts of the body in order to improve human life and strive for bodily perfection. Some directed research towards discovering what parts the body could do without and how much of it could be removed without killing the patient. The arrival of safer SURGERY, with antisepsis and ANAESTHESIA, gave impetus to such procedures, particularly from the 1880s onwards.

Removing healthy parts of the body was not a new idea. For thousands of years young boys had been castrated to turn them into eunuchs, to avoid them becoming sexual rivals of their masters or so that their voices would not break. Many more young boys lost their foreskins for religious reasons. Since ancient times surgeons had removed diseased parts but now, in the pursuit of health and bodily perfection, this practice was extended to healthy tissues and to tissues that appeared to be healthy but which might, in accordance with new medical theories, be a concealed source of disease or ill-health. Healthy teeth were removed in huge numbers in case they

were a source of hidden infection. Tonsils and the foreskins of newborn boys were excised in their millions, often for social as much as prophylactic reasons (though 'medical' reasons were often constructed as rationalization). Wedges were taken from noses or behind ears to improve their shape or profile. 'Spare tyres' of fat were cut from abdomens. The uvula was removed for being too long, the frenum (the fold of membrane under the tongue) was divided to improve articulation, and part of the tongue was excised with the same intent. The thymus was removed (or irradiated to put it out of action) in babies, with the intention of guarding against sudden death. Colons were shortened to relieve constipation. Lengths of bone were even removed to shorten stature.

The idea of removing healthy parts of the body for the sake of improved appearance or health was supported by the evolutionary concept of 'vestigial organs' that were no longer required and, so it was argued, might cause trouble. Appendix, colon, tonsils, prostate, and coccyx were all at some time believed to come into this category. Darwin thought that these organs 'had to be those that once had been of some use but which now were degenerating because they served no purpose and were a waste of energy for the organism to produce.' The concept of declining organs was supported by nineteenth-century ideas of DEGENERATION.

Some people still develop desires to have normal parts of their bodies or their children's bodies removed. Even before the days of anaesthetics there were women who begged surgeons to remove their ovaries. The availability of anaesthesia made all forms of removal much easier. HYSTERECTOMY became popular even where the indications for doing it were doubtful. Transsexuals began to seek removal of their sexual organs. Parental pressure was the main reason that the practice of tonsillectomy on children without disease persisted. Infants are usually circumcised because their parents wish it. 'Nose jobs', face lifts, breast reductions, and other cosmetic operations are done because the patients want to have them done, or are persuaded by others that their lives will be transformed.

During the twentieth century we became even more obsessed with body image and appearance. Fay Weldon's novel, *The She-Devil*, is about a woman who had virtually her whole body removed and reconstructed. It is an appropriate satire on our times.   ANN DALLY

See also AMPUTATION; APPENDIX; CASTRATION; CIRCUMCISION; COSMETIC SURGERY; SURGERY.

Reproduction myths
provide many alternative accounts of procreation and birth in classical mythology. By challenging the need for contact between the two sexes, Greek myths of the fifth and fourth centuries BC express unease about the need for women as a means to continue the human race. While medical texts of the fourth century BC debated whether men simply planted their seed in the field which was the

female body, or whether women too contributed seed to the formation of an embryo, myth presented many far more imaginative variations on reproduction. The goddess Hera, angry at the repeated infidelities of her husband Zeus, conceived Hephaistos, the god of fire and metallurgy, not by being impregnated, but by eating lettuce: Zeus ate Metis (whose name means 'cunning intelligence'), so that the daughter she was carrying, Athena, was born fully-grown from the head of her father, thus being as free from female influence as possible. Hephaistos, the child of an all-female conception, was the only 'midwife' at this all-male reproductive event, by opening Zeus' head with his axe. Athena later rejected marriage for herself, remaining a virgin forever, and was represented in male armour. The nearest Athena came to motherhood was when Hephaistos tried to rape her. Because he was lame, he was unable to catch her, but instead ejaculated on her leg. Athena wiped off his semen, which fell on mother Earth who, in due course, produced a son, Erichthonios — thought to be the first king of Athens. Dionysos was born from his father's thigh. Greek mythology seems particularly concerned to deny the female. In the otherwise similar central African myth of Lianja, it is from his mother's thigh that the fully-grown and armed culture-hero emerges.

In the account of creation in Genesis, the first woman — Eve — is created from the *rib* of the first man, Adam. Graeco-Roman creation myths include the moulding of the first woman, Pandora, from earth and water by the gods, with each giving her a different gift. Hephaistos, whose attendance at abnormal births seems to be almost *de rigueur*, does the initial moulding of the raw materials. In the accounts of the creation of Pandora, the external appearance of the female body is seen as deceptive, with the adornments given to the first woman acting to conceal the reality within, in particular her possession of 'the mind of a bitch'.

An alternative Greek myth involves a first man, Deucalion, with his wife, Pyrrha, repopulating the earth after a flood by throwing stones over their shoulders. *Autochthony*, the belief in 'birth from the earth' which occurs in the Erichthonios story, was also found in the mythology of ancient Thebes, where the population emerged from the earth after the teeth of a dragon were sown there. An East Indonesian myth claims that Timor emerged from the sea in two pieces; a huge vagina opened up in the earth, and the first people climbed out of it.

HELEN KING

See also CREATION MYTHS; GREEKS; METAMORPHOSIS; MYTHOLOGY AND THE BODY.

Reproductive system
The gonads, which produce the GERM CELLS, and all associated organs and tissues in either sex that provide the mechanisms for fertilization and development of an embryo: in the male, the TESTES, vasa deferentia,

PROSTATE, seminal vesicles, and PENIS; in the female, the OVARIES, FALLOPIAN TUBES, UTERUS, VAGINA, and mammary glands (BREASTS). Also, in both sexes, the relevant SEX HORMONES and the tissues that produce them.   S.J.

See PLATE 8.

Respiration

Respiration is the absorption of OXYGEN and the output of CARBON DIOXIDE that take part in the metabolic processes in the body; it includes the burning of foodstuffs in the tissues, the transport of the gases in the blood and their exchange in the LUNGS. All but the smallest animals, for example single cells like amoeba, require specialized transport and exchange organs to provide sufficient supply and removal of the large quantities of gases involved. A vigorously exercising athletic human might take up as much as six litres of oxygen per minute, and excrete a similar amount or more of carbon dioxide.

It is usual to divide respiration into external and internal components, linked by the bloodstream that transports the gases but has little metabolism of its own. In mammals, external respiration — the VENTILATION of the lungs — is achieved by BREATHING, the mechanical basis of respiration: the terms are sometimes used synonymously. In fishes there is equivalent 'ventilation' of the gills with water. At rest an adult human inhales about 6–8 litres of air per minute, of which about two thirds gets to the alveoli and takes part in gas exchange, the rest remaining in the air passages. Fresh air contains 21% oxygen and almost no carbon dioxide. In the lungs, the entry of oxygen into the blood and the release of carbon dioxide results in exhaled gas having about 5% less oxygen and 5% more carbon dioxide. The gases pass in and out of the blood by passive diffusion, due to their relative pressures in the blood and in the alveolar gas, just as a fizzy drink will lose its gas and go flat when exposed to air. At rest an average-sized adult will take up about 250 ml of oxygen each minute, and exhale about 200 ml of carbon dioxide. In vigorous EXERCISE these values can increase over 20-fold in a trained athlete as a result of the increased metabolism in the muscles. The blood in the capillaries leaving the lungs, and therefore in the arteries carrying it round the body, have the same pressures of oxygen and carbon dioxide as those in the alveoli, at least in health. In some lung and heart disease, involving a problem of gas transfer, the arterial blood may have a lower oxygen and a higher carbon dioxide pressure than that in the alveoli, causing HYPOXIA and hypercapnia. In other types of lung disease these abnormalities in the blood result from inadequate breathing — failure to ventilate the alveoli with sufficient fresh air.

In the blood almost all the oxygen is carried combined with HAEMOGLOBIN in the red cells, while carbon dioxide is taken up in both plasma and red cells. Once the blood has reached the tissues, internal respiration takes over. Oxygen will diffuse from the capillaries into metabolizing cells, again passively following its pressure gradient. Vigorously contracting muscle cells use up almost all the available oxygen inside them, and strongly pull a fresh supply from the blood by diffusion. The oxygen combines with food materials, mainly SUGARS and FATS, to release heat and energy for contraction of muscle, with water and carbon dioxide as the main waste products. The water enters the general water pool of the body, while the carbon dioxide enters the blood and is carried to the lungs mainly as BICARBONATE but also in combination with hemoglobin and plasma proteins. An appreciable amount of carbon dioxide, unlike oxygen, is also free in solution in the plasma. Such aerobic METABOLISM occurs similarly in the great majority of body cells.

This understanding of the chemical basis of respiration was only developed in the eighteenth century, with the chemical identification of oxygen and carbon dioxide, mainly by Joseph Priestley (1733–1804) and Antoine-Laurent Lavoisier (1743–94). For two thousand years before then there were many speculations about the meaning of breathing, the main idea being that its function was to cool the blood by physically mixing air with it in the arteries and veins. The cooling function seemed proved by the fact that exhaled gas was usually warmer than inhaled air, and the mixing with blood was deduced from the fact that when arteries and veins were cut the blood flowing out was often frothy. (We now know that if large veins are cut they will suck air into the circulation, and it will pass through the heart and lungs and make the haemorrhaging blood bubbly.) In the second century AD GALEN wrote 'respiration is useful to animals for the sake of the heart, which to some extent requires the substance of the air and besides needs very greatly to be cooled because of its burning heat.' Even primitive men must have known that breathing was necessary for life; according to the Judaeo–Christian tradition, breath created it. 'And the Lord God formed man of the dust of the ground and breathed into his nostrils the breath of life; and man became a living soul' (Genesis 2:7). In the seventeenth century much experimental work established that one component of air was essential for life, and that another different fraction was exhaled. These were identified as oxygen and carbon dioxide a century later. There was much speculation about the 'respiration' of fetuses. Clearly they could not breathe air, since their lungs were full of liquid. Since the role of the blood circulation in gas exchange was not understood, the respiratory function of the PLACENTA, the 'external' respiratory organ of the fetus, was not apparent.

Sophisticated and accurate methods of analysing respiratory gases were developed in the twentieth century, and the mechanisms of external respiration are now well defined. At about the same time development of BIOCHEMISTRY and, later, of MOLECULAR BIOLOGY, led to an understanding of internal respiration. When oxygen combines with carbohydrates every molecule of oxygen creates one molecule of water and one in carbon dioxide. Thus the ratio of the exchange volumes of the two gases, the *respiratory quotient*, is 1; in practice this would only occur in someone living on a diet of, and metabolizing only CARBOHYDRATE — polished rice, for example. Fat and PROTEIN contain less oxygen than does carbohydrate, so more oxygen is needed for their consumption than the carbon dioxide that is produced. On an average diet in a developed country the ratio of carbon dioxide excreted to oxygen absorbed is about 0.8. However these values assume that there is enough oxygen for the metabolic needs of all the body — that we are at rest or in a state of *entirely* aerobic metabolism. 'Aerobic exercise' is exercise within this limit. If exercise is severe, not enough oxygen is available for the muscles, which pass an 'anaerobic threshold', and energy is provided additionally by the breakdown of carbohydrates without using oxygen and with the formation of lactic acid. This diffuses into the blood, causing a mild acidosis and acting on the bicarbonate to release carbon dioxide which is excreted in the lungs. (Lemon juice, put on self-raising flour, or bicarbonate of soda, will make it fizz as it releases carbon dioxide.) Thus in severe exercise we exhale more carbon dioxide than the oxygen we absorb. After the exercise we retain carbon dioxide in the body and most of the lactic acid is converted back into carbohydrate in the liver. Extra oxygen is needed for this, and the process is referred to as 'repaying the oxygen debt'.

JOHN WIDDICOMBE

See also BREATHING; BREATHING IN EXERCISE; CARBON DIOXIDE; HAEMOGLOBIN; LUNGS; METABOLISM; OXYGEN.

Resurrection

Resurrection from the Latin *resurgo* ('I rise'), refers to the belief that the dead will ultimately be raised and have their bodies restored to them. While this belief is found in Christianity, Judaism, and Islam, Christian belief in the resurrection and saving of the dead is shaped specifically by the resurrection of Christ who, according to the New Testament, on the third day after his death and burial rose again and appeared to his followers.

Several scriptural accounts of the resurrected Jesus stress the materiality of Jesus' body. For example, in Luke's gospel Jesus told his disciples to touch him, asking whether a ghost has hands and feet, as he has, and then proceeded to eat a fish in front of them. In John's gospel 'doubting' Thomas was invited by Jesus to put his finger on Jesus' hand where the nails had been, and put his hand in Jesus' side which had been pierced. In Matthew, Jesus met his disciples and they touched his feet. And yet, despite this stress on the material body of Jesus as 'proof' of his resurrected identity, on several occasions — on the beach at daybreak and on the Emmaus Road, for example — the men and women disciples did not recognise him; and in the account of the resurrected Jesus' appearance to Mary Magdalene, in John's Gospel, Jesus instructed Mary not to hold onto him because he had not yet ascended to the Father. This represents a tension, in the New Testament accounts, between the materiality and 'spiritual' nature of the resurrected Jesus.

From early on, Jesus' resurrection was an important part of Christian teaching as indicated in Acts and Paul's epistles. In 1 Corinthians, Paul wrote of Jesus being raised from the dead and appearing to Cephas, the twelve, some five hundred brothers and sisters, James and the rest of the Apostles, and finally to Paul himself. Thus Paul concluded that if Christ was resurrected, as his evidence attests, then the resurrection of the dead could not be denied. Paul expressed a variety of views about what that resurrection meant. Later in 1 Corinthians, Paul held that the resurrected body would be 'new' and spiritual, of a new order and raised above the limitations of the earthly body. In 2 Corinthians he suggested that the body will be discarded when we come to reside in heaven. But in Romans he expressed the notion that resurrection begins with baptism, suggesting, perhaps, that resurrection is the rebirth of the embodied person.

The Christian idea of the resurrection of the dead is found in the notion that at the Parousia or Second Coming of Christ, the dead will have their bodies restored to them and the saved will enter into heaven in this bodily form. Despite Paul's primary emphasis on the resurrected, 'spiritual' body, early Christian writers increasingly came to understand the resurrection of the dead as meaning the full reassemblage of bodily parts (and thus material continuity), as indicated by patristic debates about resurrection, from the second to fifth centuries. The apologist Justin Martyr defended the material continuity of the fleshly body at the resurrection against the criticism of pagan critics, such as Celsus, who asked why anyone would want to recover the body, given that corpses were revolting. Tertullian believed in the reassemblage of bodily bits, seeing all reality as corporeal and arguing that the whole person would be rewarded or punished, because the whole person — SOUL and body — had sinned or behaved virtuously. Such ideas were developed in the context of *Gnosticism* (which saw the resurrection as spiritual and an escape from the body) and *Docetism* (which saw Christ's body not as real but as metaphorical), and as Christians asked questions about what happened to the bodies of martyrs. Literal, physical resurrection was seen as victory over death after MARTYRDOM, for those Christians who had died voluntarily and sacrificially.

This idea of the resurrection of the literal body was continued into the Middle Ages, for example in the formulation of doctrines and creeds, in sermons, and in popular stories of miracles. Eschatology was seen in material terms, and there existed a strong sense of a self whose physical nature was linked to EMOTIONS, intellect, SENSATIONS, and reason, and thus to notions of salvation. Aquinas challenged these ideas, asserting that the soul accounts for a person's identity and therefore maintaining that the continuity of the fleshly stuff of the body was unnecessary. He

encountered considerable opposition to his ideas, especially between the 1270s and 1300, but the condemnations of his views were removed in 1325. This might be seen as a benchmark moment — when the idea that the soul was primary in the resurrection of the dead began to take precedence. Modern debate about bodily resurrection has tended to focus on the scientific plausibility of such a notion, although Stanley Spencer's painting, *The Resurrection, Cookham* (1927) is a modern rendering of the idea of bodily resurrection, as the fully embodied inhabitants of Cookham climb out of their tombs to enjoy eternal life.

In Judaism, belief in the resurrection of the body is found in some passages of the later Hebrew scriptures, and gradually became a central, if debated, tenet of Judaism, as found in parts of the Mishnah. It is the idea that body and soul are indivisible and will be resurrected together which is important in Judaism. In Islam, it is on the day of resurrection, *Yaum al-Oyama*, that all will die on the first blast of the trumpet, and, after an interval, and on the second blast of the trumpet, will be bodily resurrected to stand before Allah for judgment and division between heaven and hell. Hinduism has many notions of the return, reassemblage, and revival of the body — especially after it has been eaten or digested — if not any specific doctrine of resurrection.

JANE SHAW

Further reading
Bynum, C. W. (1995). *The Resurrection of the Body in Western Christendom*. Columbia University Press, New York.

See also CHRISTIANITY AND THE BODY; DEATH.

Resuscitation Normal function of the body requires an adequate delivery of OXYGEN to the tissues, and removal of CARBON DIOXIDE and other waste products of tissue metabolism. These items are carried by the bloodstream which must have sufficient flow and pressure to service all parts of the different tissues. The process requires both sufficient BREATHING and also adequate pumping by the HEART. The most important tissues are the vital organs — the BRAIN, heart, LIVER, and KIDNEYS. In particular, the brain requires a continuous supply of oxygen and glucose or the brain cells may die.

When a person loses consciousness it is often caused by the heart rate slowing down — as in a simple fainting attack. This leads to a reduced blood pressure, insufficient oxygen then reaches the brain. When the person falls and lies horizontally, the blood pressure is improved and recovery of consciousness occurs spontaneously. A patient who has 'passed out' for more serious reasons may require resuscitation when this process fails, and if breathing has stopped it is vital to apply ARTIFICIAL VENTILATION to ensure the delivery of oxygen. Similarly, when the heart has stopped, it is essential to provide cardiac massage to deliver oxygen-carrying blood to the vital organs.

The aim of resuscitation is to ensure that both the breathing and the blood flow functions of the body are maintained so that the brain and other vital organs receive a sufficient supply of oxygen and nutrients to maintain their functions, and that waste products of metabolism are removed. Brain damage can begin if the oxygen supply stops for more than a few minutes. The standard *aide memoire* for resuscitation is 'ABC': airway, breathing, and circulation.

Airway
The first essential of resuscitation is to make certain that the person's airway (the passage from the mouth via the larynx to the trachea) is clear. This may simply require the jaw to be pulled forward, to prevent the tongue falling backwards and blocking the airway; or there may be false teeth or vomit which must be removed before air can pass down into the patient's lungs. By placing the patient in the 'coma position', the tongue naturally falls forward and helps to maintain a clear airway. Where skilled assistance is available, as in a hospital, an anaesthetist may pass an *endotracheal tube* into the windpipe (trachea). This will guarantee the clear passage of air into the lungs.

Breathing
Once the airway is clear, the patient may begin to breathe spontaneously. If oxygen is available, this will be used to supplement the normal 21% oxygen present in the atmosphere. Pure oxygen may be used in extreme cases. Where spontaneous respiration does not begin, air must be forced into the patient's lungs either by mouth-to-mouth respiration or by using medical apparatus which can deliver air via a mouthpiece or by connecting it to an endotracheal tube.

Circulation: cardiac massage
Once the airway is clear and the patient can receive air or oxygen into the lungs, the blood flow to the tissues must be maintained. Following a faint, the heart usually returns to a normal rate and produces a normal flow. However, after an event such as a HEART ATTACK, the normal rhythm of the heart may be disturbed. The heart may stop beating or may vibrate at a very rapid rate which is too fast to move the blood forward (FIBRILLATION). In such cases, the patient will require urgent cardiac massage. This involves compressing the heart against the spine by pushing down rhythmically on the breast bone (sternum). Following several cardiac massages, a mouth-to-mouth breath is given if breathing has not started spontaneously. The sequence is repeated until pulse and breathing start or skilled help is obtained.

This form of cardiac massage can be very effective in maintaining the blood flow to the vital organs. Where the cause of CARDIAC ARREST is reversible, such as sudden cooling after falling through ice, the patient may make a complete recovery. However, where the underlying disease process has already produced

591

considerable damage to the heart, then cardiac massage may not be successful.

A DEFIBRILLATOR may be used if cardiac arrest occurs in a hospital or in some other places such as exercise laboratories which may be equipped with this apparatus and knowledge of its use. This may succeed in jolting the heart back into effective action.   GAVIN KENNY

See also DEFIBRILLATOR; DROWNING; FAINTING; FIBRILLATION; HEART ATTACK; HYPOTHERMIA.

Rigor mortis

Shortly after death all the muscles in the body become soft and flaccid. At a variable time later, they become firm and rigid. This is known as rigor mortis. Rigor commences in the smallest muscles such as those in the face and the hands, and then extends to the limb muscles. Rigor can be 'broken' by stretching the muscle, for example by moving the jaw or the elbow, and does not then return.

Rigor is brought about by a chemical change in the MUSCLE. The normal reaction between ADENOSINE TRIPHOSPHATE and adenosine diphosphate (ATP and ADP) within the muscle fibres, which supplies energy for their contraction during life, ceases and the ATP level in the muscle progressively diminishes. This is accompanied by accumulation of lactic acid and a fall of pH (increase in acidity), which leads to stiffening and firmness. Whether or not the muscle fibres actually shorten has not been established.

Temperature is an important factor in determining the time of onset of rigor. In normal circumstances and at room temperature rigor is complete in about three to six hours. If the temperature is higher the onset is more rapid — perhaps no more than an hour in tropical temperatures. Conversely, the onset of rigor is delayed at low temperatures. In cases of DROWNING in cold water, for example, rigor may not appear until the body has been removed from the water, even after several days of immersion. The onset of rigor is hastened if there has been intense physical activity shortly before death. Thus, in forensic medical practice, the presence of rigor is a poor determinant of the time of death. Once established, the duration of rigor ranges from 18 to 36 hours.

J. HUME ADAMS

See also CORPSE; DEATH.

Rites of passage

In all societies, major events in the life cycle are subject to ritualized forms of recognition. Across the world, such events are celebrated in diverse and sometimes elaborate ways, with different cultures singling out different stages of life for attention. Where ancestry is important, as in China or many of the societies of Africa, DEATH may be the subject of extended and intricate mortuary ceremonials, which act both to separate the living from the dead and to transform the dead from elder to ancestor. In others, death may be neglected and cultural salience given rather to MARRIAGE, to the installation of office holders, or to initiations into adulthood or into CULT groupings. In these cultural processes, actual biological events are subsumed and transformed, even negated in the various schemas of culture. Among the Kuria of Kenya and Tanzania, life for both men and women is said not to begin and end with their birth and death but rather to begin in early puberty when they are circumcized and to culminate in dramatic rituals of eldership, which celebrate the achievement of a full life course, of successful FERTILITY, and of wealth as evidenced in the growth of the homestead herd.

Despite the variety in the forms and meanings of such rituals, a certain unity has been given to the category by the work of the Belgian scholar, Arnold Van Gennep. His book, *Les Rites de Passage*, first published in 1909, has formed the backdrop to most anthropological work. Van Gennep envisioned life in society as a house with many rooms, in which the individual has to be conveyanced formally from one defined position to another. From this perspective, life is not a matter of gradual development and change but rather consists of a series of abrupt and ritualized transitions. Rites of passage, he argued, display common features — in particular, a definite three-phase structure, of *separation transition*, and *aggregation*. Initial rites of separation serve to remove the individual from normal social life, thus dissolving existing social ties and status. These rites are often mirrored in the opposing rites of aggregation, which end the ritual process and reinstate a normal social life when the individual is welcomed back into a new position in the community. In between these two contrasting phases are the rites of transition. This pattern, though discernible to some extent in all, tends to be most fully recognized in INTIATION RITES, where it may be given added force in the symbolism of death and rebirth.

Of particular interest has been Van Gennep's identification of the mid or transitional phase as one of *marginality* or *liminality* (from the Latin, *limen*, meaning threshold). It represents, he writes, the point of inertia for the novices between contrary ritual movements; they are regarded as being outside society — untouchable, dangerous, sacred as opposed to profane. Sharing with Van Gennep a similar concern with social classification and the cultural imposition of order on natural and social affairs, the British anthropologist, Mary Douglas, has argued that the idea of danger attaches to any situation or object that transgresses or cannot be placed within the dominant schema of social classification. Novices, betwixt-and-between defined social positions, are inherently anomalous and likely to be regarded as both polluted and polluting. Often this state is expressed in strict rules of seclusion, of physical as well as social invisibility, in which the neophyte's condition can be expressed only in terms of ambiguity and paradox. Outside and opposed to normal social life, liminality is also given ritual expression in licence, disorder, and role reversal.

For Van Gennep the theme of passage provides one clue to the diverse symbolic devices employed in such rites. The ritual passage may be represented in spatial terms, by exits and entrances, crossings and journeys, and in the general significance attached to crossroads, boundaries, and thresholds. By extension, too, the term may be used of other ritual events that, like life crisis rituals, are seen to share a concern with the social recognition of time — particularly communal rituals that serve to mark changes in the seasons or calendar, such as first fruits celebrations or those conducted to usher in the New Year. Other events that also imply a dramatic change in social life, such as going to war, or periods when the community prepares itself for major religious festivals, may also be subject to similar forms of ritualization.

Rites of passage, which disconnect ritual moments from the normal flow of life, break the passage of time, representing it as a constant replay of opposed movements. Rather than inexorable processes of growth and decay, the ritualization of the stages of life seems to speak to the discontinuity of personal experience and the oscillation of social life between contrasting moods and phases. These characteristics of rites of passage have been seen to make them most typical of traditional societies and repetitive social orders. In terms of the personal biography of individuals, this gives ritual the formative role, as the essential catalyst in major life changes and the key to the creation of identity and PERSONHOOD. To explore these aspects, one needs to abandon the simple metaphor of transition, bequeathed to us by Van Gennep, and focus instead on the idea of transformation. Thus life crisis rituals may not simply bestow or formally acknowledge changes in the life history, but in many societies have a truly transformational intent: the main and only means by which boys can be transformed into men, girls into women, elders into ancestors, the sick into spirit mediums, or princes into kings.   SUZETTE HEALD

Further reading

Van Gennep, A. (1960). *The rites of passage.* Routledge, London.

See also INITIATION RITES; FUNERAL PRACTICES; TABOOS.

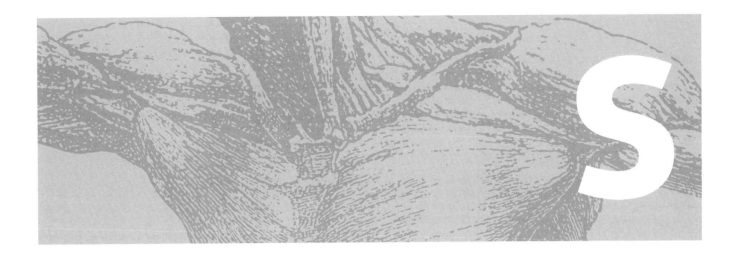

Sacrifice The Greek myth of the origin of sacrifice links it with the aftermath of Prometheus' attempt to trick Zeus by dividing the meat of an ox into two packages and trying to persuade Zeus to pick the one that had the tempting exterior, but that contained only the *bones* of the beast. In animal sacrifice, it was to be these bones which were burned on the altar as the divine share: the human sacrificers and onlookers then divided out the meat according to their degree of participation in the ritual. In the classical world, animal sacrifice was a daily necessity, reminding people of a lost past in which they had once shared food with the gods, but simultaneously acting to keep up communication between the human and the divine worlds. The Christian innovation of the 'one, true, pure, immortal sacrifice' of the son of God thus built on classical notions of the necessity of sacrifice, but also completely overthrew them by its insistence that no further animal sacrifices were necessary.

Not all sacrifice takes the form of animal sacrifice. Bloodless offerings of cakes, fruit, and bread were also common in antiquity. In all sacrifices fire was used to consume the parts which were being dedicated to the gods; a holocaust is a sacrifice in which the chosen offering is entirely consumed by the flames.

In the late nineteenth century, scholars of religion and sociologists tried to find a general theory of sacrifice. In his *Lectures on the Religion of the Semites* (1894), W. Robertson Smith proposed that *totemism* was the basic form of sacrifice, in which the clan shed the blood of its totem animal, then consumed it in a communal meal. The great French sociologist Émile Durkheim went further, arguing that sacrifice not only bonded the members of a social group, but acted to make the group aware of its common identity and thus, in a sense, to create the group. The anthropologist René Girard saw sacrificial violence as the basis of human culture; the classical scholar Walter Burkert links it to man the hunter who, by hedging around the slaughter of animals with the observation of strict ritual practices, attempted to allay his unease about whether the animal kingdom permitted him to take the lives of its members.

The problem with all such 'grand theories' of sacrifice is that they cannot always take account of individual societies' different myths and practices. However, a comparative approach can be illuminating; for example, the Greek myth of the *Bouphonia* (Ox-slaying) suggests that the beast to be sacrificed must agree to its role, and the story of the sacrifice of Christ also makes much of the need for the sacrificial victim to be aware of his role and willing to take it on. In classical Greek sacrificial ritual, the ox was even supposed to nod its head in consent, although this was often achieved by sprinkling water on its head to make it shiver.

Human sacrifice, like CANNIBALISM, tends to be an accusation levelled by a society against its most feared enemies, or a marginal group within it. The Romans accused the Carthaginians of sacrificing children; Christian communities from the Roman Empire onwards have accused Jewish communities of it, while Roman pagans accused the Christians of exactly the same offence. But, as the ultimate victims, human beings make perfect sense *in extremis*. In the biblical story, when God tested Abraham by asking him to sacrifice his only son Isaac, the command did not seem unreasonable, and the last-minute substitution of a ram became evidence that 'The Lord will provide'. In myth and drama, the Greek leader Agamemnon thought his daughter Iphigenia was an appropriate sacrifice to ensure a good wind for the fleet sailing to Troy; in many versions of the myth, the goddess Artemis substituted an animal for Iphigenia. In ancient Rome, the burial alive of two Gauls and two Greeks was performed when the city was believed to be in serious danger.   HELEN KING

Sadomasochism subsumes a whole array of practices whose practitioners may have very little in common. Sexologists have commonly included under this heading everything from love bites to lust-murder. What, if anything, conceptually unites the desire to receive mild pain, to give mild pain (and even these desires may take diverse forms), to be tied up or to bind one's partner, to participate in scenarios of humiliation or domination, or to receive severe pain or to inflict it? Perhaps the common factor in all these phenomena is some form of suffering, from the minor to the extreme, which has been given an erotic meaning by the actors involved. Whether, however, all forms of suffering have the same eroticized meaning is open to question.

The sadomasochistic practice with possibly the longest history of recognition as a sexual perversion, even before the development of the concept, must be FLAGELLATION. There have been numerous historical studies of corporal punishment, though it may be queried how far these illuminate one of the murkier areas of sexual diversity, or are merely a specialized form of PORNOGRAPHY masquerading as 'science'. Flagellation was long known to arouse sexual desire by stimulating nerves in regions adjacent to the genitals. It was employed, for example, in brothels, as a means of arousing the sluggish desires of the impotent or elderly. Sexual arousal tends to raise the threshold at which pain is experienced, and thus love bites, pinches, slaps, and other non-specifically arousing acts may feed back into the process of sexual arousal and enhance its intensity.

Theories

'Sadism' and 'masochism' as definitions emerged from the pre-existing writings of the French Marquis de Sade and the Austrian Leopold von Sacher-Masoch depicting sexualized forms of cruelty. The use of the word 'sadism' was already in vogue to describe the infliction of suffering when Richard von Krafft-Ebing commenced his massive study of *Psychopathia Sexualis* (first published in 1886), but 'masochism' was a coinage of his own. He claimed that the perversion described by Sacher-Masoch in novels such as *Venus in Furs* had previously been unknown to science, though he was able to cite a large number of cases. He classified the two phenomena as opposite perversions to some extent mirroring one another. He pointed out, however, that extremes of suffering, resulting in serious injury or death, were likely to be pursued by masochists only in fantasy, due to the instinct of self-preservation, whereas there were recorded cases of assault or MURDER committed by sadists for sexual motives. His conclusion may be contested in the light of cases where auto-erotic rituals have led, however inadvertently, to death.

Current thinking suggests that the division is not so clear-cut and that there may be something about ritualized scenarios of PAIN, bondage, domination, or humiliation which causes arousal quite separately from whether participation, real or fantasized, is as inflictor or sufferer. Individuals may switch roles, and indeed, there is some rather anecdotal evidence that within sadomasochistic subcultures preferences are predominantly masochistic, and good 'tops' or sadists are rare and much prized, so that 'bottoms' or masochists may perform the complementary role if required.

Practices

The aetiology of sadomasochism is, like that of much sexual behaviour, only partially understood. In the case of a desire for the infliction of certain kinds of pain, it may be that the individual has an innately high threshold of arousal and requires vigorous stimulation in order to become sexually aroused and potent. While sadomasochism may be seen as expressing innate human aggressiveness, any relationship is extremely complex. Aggression often interferes with satisfactory sexual interaction, as actual anger and hostility are likely to mute rather than enhance sexual responsiveness. While a certain degree of assertiveness may be necessary, aggression as such is likely to prove counter-productive. Submissive or sexually receptive behaviours are used by a variety of species, including other primates, to defuse offered aggression, but it is not clear whether this appeasement behaviour is sexually gratifying rather than strategic.

The influence of childhood experiences has been invoked to account for these preferences. Protests against the corporal punishment of children cited the dangers of premature sexual arousal (the most commonly quoted case was that of the Enlightenment philosopher, Jean-Jacques Rousseau, who described such an outcome in his *Autobiography*), and the deleterious effects upon the observers of public and ritualized floggings. Punishments might additionally involve the exposure of parts of the body normally concealed so that several factors could elicit sexual response to an event involving pain and humiliation. Given the decline of corporal punishment, however, there must be many sadomasochists who have never directly experienced or witnessed this as children: it cannot be the entire explanation.

Sadomasochism seems to be more evenly distributed between the sexes than some other sexual preferences, at least on the level of fantasy. Women report fantasies of RAPE or being forced

into sexual situations: however, there are major differences between such fantasies and 'real life'. It has been suggested that fantasies of being dominated and the abrogation of personal responsibility give permission for a sexual response which guilt would otherwise deny.

Active sadomasochistic subcultures, both heterosexual and homosexual, exist. It has been suggested that heterosexual subcultures, largely male, function as a support group — any women involved being prostitutes servicing this specialized clientele — whereas the homosexual subculture is a source of partners. However, there is some evidence, in particular from more recent surveys, that non-prostitute women are increasingly participating. One side-effect of the 'liberation' of women may be their exploration in person of practices which they perhaps used only to fantasize about, although women tend to have been introduced to sadomasochistic practices by a male partner. There is also a lesbian sadomasochistic subculture, which has aroused much feminist debate as to whether it constitutes a means of exploring the limits of SEXUALITY and of protesting against received ideas of female sexual apathy and passivity, or rather an internalized manifestation of the patriarchal sexual violence within society at large. Advocates for sadomasochism claim that it is a very safe form of sexual practice requiring participants to make their preferences clear from the outset. The 'bottom' is said to be the one actually in control, and a code of 'safe words' prevents situations going too far.

Sadism and masochism might be taken as extreme manifestations of the roles of the sexes as encoded by society and (in the view of many) by biology. Sexual dominance is associated with successful masculinity, while submissiveness and passivity are seen as appropriate feminine attributes. There has been a good deal of feminist debate around the contention that sadomasochism explicitly eroticizes this sexual dynamic. Such a view fails to account for the prevalence of male masochist preferences, which probably predominate over sadistic tendencies; however it could be argued that in a still male-dominated society, men have many opportunities outside the specifically sexual sphere to gratify impulses of sadism and the assertion of dominance. A sexual preference so contradictory to the expected social role was perceived as problematic from the earliest investigations of sexologists. Iwan Bloch, in *The Sexual Life of our Time* (first British edition 1909), drew attention to the remarkable prevalence of masochism among men holding power and influence within society, operating, he suggested, as 'a kind of liberation from conventional pressure and the professional mask.'

Only a minority of individuals ever deliberately seek out sadomasochistic partners and activities, though this may be more widespread than often assumed. Minor manifestations in sexual games and horseplay are probably common. On the evidence of prostitutes' advertisements, it is a commonly sought speciality in commercial sex

transactions. As a theme, it is widespread in many media; indeed, it is something of a truism that all sorts of acts of violence may be depicted, although there may be considerable restrictions on revealing the naked body and acts of normal coitus. But people who pursue sexual pleasure by this means are stigmatized, and in the recent notorious British case of 'Operation Spanner', a group of men practising consensual, though very extreme, sadomasochism received sentences which many regarded as disproportionately heavy, especially compared with the inconsistent penalties imposed for sexual assaults on women.

In a post-modernist age of sexual choices, where sadomasochism is presented as one more option among sexual activities, the once potent connection made between sexual repression and sadism or masochism has become somewhat occluded. This is a connection, however, which history tends to substantiate, because there have been perceptible associations in numerous societies between puritanical and repressive attitudes towards sexuality and a toleration, or even encouragement, of cruelty and violence, and vice-versa. It could be argued that those who are aware of their erotic response to pain and/or domination, and who orchestrate sadomasochistic scenarios for personal sexual gratification, are less socially dangerous than those who do not acknowledge the sexual component in their reactions to these phenomena and pursue them in less self-knowing and more oblique ways.

LESLEY A. HALL

See also FETISHISM; FLAGELLATION; RAPE; SEXUALITY.

Saints The terms 'saint' comes from the Latin *sanctus*, meaning sacred, inviolate, or holy. The term is used within Christianity to designate a holy person, one deemed to have lived a life of such great virtue and sanctity as to achieve special closeness to God. Such persons may be venerated in public cults after their deaths. This occurs not only through the commemoration of a saint's feast day and belief in the divine intercession of the saintly figure, but also through the veneration of RELICS, the physical remains of the holy person. These may include the intact body of the saint or portions of the body, as well as objects worn, used, or associated with him or her. Within medieval Christianity the cult of relics — those of Christ as well as of the martyrs and saints — was crucial to religious practice.

Historians of Western religion have expanded the category of saint to include holy and venerated persons within other religious traditions. The *hasid* in Judaism, the Islamic *wali*, the Buddhist *arahant* and *bodhisattva*, and Hindu gurus have been assimilated to this category for the purposes of cross-cultural comparison. Although questions remain about the appropriateness of using Western Christian categories to describe non-Christian practices and beliefs, careful attention to differences as well as similarities between various categories of venerated persons is itself informative.

First of all, not all traditions single out certain individuals as models for action and intercessors to be venerated by the community. Traditions in Africa, the Americas, and Australia tend to focus on established religious roles rather than individual sanctity. Classical rabbinic Judaism stresses the salvation of the community rather than that of the individual, although a certain reverence is granted to the rabbis themselves. Protestant Christianity rejects the cult of the saints so crucial to medieval and modern Catholic Christianity. Many Protestant groups return to early Christian usage, in which the redeemed are referred to as the community of saints.

Moreover, different religious traditions stress different poles of the twofold, sometime contradictory, nature of the saint. Whereas some religious traditions are most interested in identifying certain people as models for how all should act, others stress the wonder-working, miraculous, or even salvific nature of holy persons. Within many traditions, such as Christianity, the two functions exist uneasily side by side.

Even within those traditions that do single out certain individuals for (usually posthumous) veneration, what constitutes sanctity, and the methods of veneration, differ dramatically. Most crucially for our purposes, emphasis on the bodies of the saints and their miraculous powers is found most prominently in Christianity and Buddhism. Parallel practices can be found among the Sufi brotherhoods of Islam. Within Hinduism, on the other hand, the impurity of the dead prohibits development of a cult of relics. Living gurus, however, are often understood to be avatars of the divine, and venerated with incense and offerings in ways parallel to the treatment of divine images.

Christianity

Emphasis on the bodies of the saints began in early Christianity with the cult surrounding the Christian martyrs, put to death under the various Roman persecutions from the first to the fourth centuries. The bishop Polycarp's (second-century) executioners, for example, attempted to burn him at the stake, but the fire made a vault around his body, from which emanated a sweet aroma. The bodies of other martyrs were similarly spared suffering, suggesting their assimilation to the resurrected body of Christ. By the third century, believers commemorated the anniversary of martyrs' deaths and crowds flocked to the cemeteries where their remains were buried, a practice abhorrent to Roman sensibilities, as they regarded dead bodies as polluting. Christian enthusiasm for the often mutilated remains of their religious heros was so great, however, that religious leaders made altars of their tombs, claiming their patronage for local churches. At the tomb, people prayed for the cure of illnesses, the forgiveness of sins, and protections from enemies. Martyrs' bodily remains were sites of the divine on earth, possessed of miraculous and saving power.

Veneration of the relics of the saints increased throughout the medieval period, particularly with the spread and growth of Christianity. The Second Council of Nicaea in 787 CE made it obligatory for relics to be present for the consecration of a church. Although relics of Christ's Passion and the Virgin Mary were popular (these were of things associated with the Passion and the Virgin Mary, as Christ's and Mary's bodies were believed to have been assumed into heaven), those of the saints were key to the traffic in relics through which Christianity was disseminated and ecclesial power established. The bodies of those deemed to be saintly in life were often the subject of fierce disputes; many, like that of the well-known thirteenth-century theologian Thomas Aquinas, were divided and dispersed immediately after death. These body parts were not only institutionally and economically important, they also carried political power for ecclesiastics and secular leaders because of the religious powers vested in them by both lay people and churchmen. The thirteenth-century prelate James of Vitry tells readers, for example, that he wore the finger of his mentor Marie of Oignies around his neck and was, by this means, saved from a shipwreck.

Within both the early Christian and the medieval period, the bodies of the saints were depicted in hagiography and iconography as transformed into the resurrected body through their asceticism, suffering, and practice of prayer and virtue. At times, even stronger claims were made, associating saintly remains with the body of Christ. Hugh, bishop of Lincoln, for example, to the horror of those present, ate a piece of the arm of Mary Magdalen, arguing that if we eat the body of Christ we should also eat the bodies of his saints. The role of the body in sanctity was particularly strong in depictions of women saints, for whom bodily suffering, illness, and asceticism were the primary mode of attaining sanctity. These women's transformed bodies, like Marie of Oignies', were often depicted as healing the wounded or suffering bodies of men. Just as Christ's suffering body redeemed humanity on the cross, so these women's bodies were depicted as undergoing suffering to redeem their fellow Christians. Although there is evidence that some women pushed against these cultural prescriptions for female sanctity, such images pervade medieval hagiographies, in which women redeem sinners on earth, in purgatory, and even in hell through their prayerful suffering.

Martin Luther's revolt against many practices of the medieval church included a denunciation of the cult of the saints and of relics as superstition and idolatry. Although he recognized that certain saintly people were exemplars of virtue and good behaviour, he denied the intercessory power of the saints and claims to the miraculous and sanctifying power of their relics. In the face of the protests of Luther and other reformers, the Catholic Reformation systematized and reaffirmed these practices and beliefs for modern Catholicism.

Buddhism

There are two major divisions of Buddhism, each of which has its own understanding of sainthood. In Theravada Buddhism, based primarily in Sri Lanka and South East Asia, the *arahant* marks the pinnacle of human possibilities. The arahant achieves release from suffering, death, and rebirth through a rigorous pursuit of the monastic life and the 'three trainings' in higher morality, higher concentration, and higher wisdom. Through this the arahant destroys the *asavas*, the wrong mental states that bind one to *kamma* and rebirth. Although there have been few arahants since the time of the Buddha, their legends are found throughout the Pali canon.

The extraordinariness of the arahants' achievement make them figures of veneration rather than imitation. The arahant is connected to the community of believers through relics. By making offerings at pagodas containing relics of the saint, the householder purifies the mind and achieves merit. The action has a similar outcome to the care of monks, also undertaken by householders.

Mahayana Buddhism, which is found throughout East Asia, stresses the power of the saints to help ordinary lay people attain enlightenment. The saintly figure in this case, known as a *bodhisattva* or 'Buddha-to-be', is a person who puts his or her own enlightenment on hold in order to help others on the path. They emulate the compassion of the Buddha, who also delayed his enlightenment in order to teach the path of enlightenment. The *bodhisattva* ideal is available to men and women, but stories surrounding women *bodhisattvas* suggest that they must be sexually transformed in order to attain this state.

AMY HOLLYWOOD

Further reading

Brown, P. (1981). *The cult of saints*. University of Chicago Press, Chicago.

Kieckhefer, R. and Bond, G. (ed) (1988). *Sainthood: its manifestations in world religions*. University of California Press, Berkeley.

See also BUDDHISM AND THE BODY; CHRISTIANITY AND THE BODY; MARTYRDOM.

Saliva is a complex fluid secreted into the mouth by the various salivary glands. There are three pairs of major salivary glands: the parotid glands, situated behind the JAW in front of the ear, and the submandibular and sublingual glands that lie under the jaw and TONGUE. Also, there are many minor salivary glands, present throughout the mouth within the lips, cheeks, tongue, and PALATE. The parotid glands produce saliva with a watery (*serous*) consistency, whilst the sublingual and the minor salivary glands produce a more viscous (*mucous*) fluid. The submandibular glands produce a mixture of serous and mucous saliva.

Saliva contains 99% water, plus dissolved inorganic IONS and numerous organic substances. Most of the organic material in saliva is PROTEIN, some of which is glycoprotein or mucin, which contains both carbohydrate and protein components. The total daily flow of saliva from all the salivary glands is around 600 ml. Salivary flow rates are lowest during sleep and highest whilst EATING, when flow rates may reach 5 ml/min. Resting salivary flow averages around 0.3 ml/min. Salivary flow rates are reduced in dehydration and after significant blood loss. The resulting dry mouth is responsible for the accompanying sensation of thirst.

Although saliva is very useful for moistening postage stamps and cotton thread, its main roles are in feeding, and in protecting the oral tissues. When salivary flow is too low, dry mouth (xerostomia) may result. Here, normal oral functions such as chewing, SWALLOWING, and speaking can be uncomfortable and difficult to perform. Greatly reduced salivary flow may also result in increased incidence of dental disease (dental caries and periodontal disease), or disease of the oral mucosa — the lining of the mouth (stomatitis). Dry mouth may be due to salivary gland disorders, but it is also a prominent and undesirable side-effect of many commonly-used drugs.

Saliva coats the surfaces of the TEETH and oral mucosa with a thin film of mucins. This slippery film lubricates the oral tissues, making it easier to chew, swallow, and speak. Saliva assists feeding by moistening the ingested food morsels and helps to bind the chewed food particles into a compact mass (a bolus) suitable for swallowing.

ENZYMES in saliva begin the digestive process: an α-amylase breaks down starch molecules and a lipase digests fat. Saliva also contributes to taste by dissolving sapid substances in food and so making them accessible to the taste buds; a zinc-binding protein, gustin, is thought to contribute to the taste process.

The saliva also has defensive functions. 'Proline-rich proteins' coat the teeth with a thin layer — pellicle — that serves as a protective diffusion barrier on the tooth surface. Saliva is supersaturated with calcium and phosphate ions, which are effectively in balance with the minerals in the teeth. To a limited extent, calcium and phosphate ions in saliva can diffuse through the pellicle into the tooth and can reverse the very early stages of tooth decay, where acids have caused slight demineralization of the tooth surface, but before actual cavity formation occurs. This remineralization process is enhanced by fluoride ions, which may be present in toothpastes or other oral health products. While the high levels of calcium and phosphate in saliva may help remineralization of early carious lesions, they also increase the likelihood of spontaneous precipitation of calcium phosphates on the teeth as calculus (tartar). However, saliva also contains statherins and proline-rich proteins, which inhibit mineralization and so help to prevent precipitation of calcium and phosphate on intact tooth surfaces. Saliva contains all the ions usually present in body fluids,

and of these, BICARBONATE (hydrogen carbonate) ions play a major role in determining the pH and buffering capacity of saliva. Salivary bicarbonate can help protect teeth against attack from acids produced by bacteria in dental plaque. The bicarbonate concentration of saliva increases with flow rate, so buffering is improved during eating.

Salivary proteins prevent the oral mucosa from drying and provide a defensive barrier against bacteria, fungi, and viruses. Saliva contains growth factors which promote healing of the oral mucosa. Saliva contains various antimicrobial substances, including lysozyme, lactoferrin, sialoperoxidase, and histatins as well as more specific antibodies or immunoglobins. The main antibody in saliva is secretory immunoglobin A (sIgA), which binds to bacterial antigens and is of interest in view of its possible role in immunity to dental caries.

Salivary flow increases during eating. The physical action of chewing stimulates nerve endings in the periodontal tissues around the teeth. Sapid substances stimulate taste buds. Both of these stimuli are potent initiators of salivary flow. Olfactory (smell) stimuli have little effect in provoking salivary flow in humans, although irritants (such as spices) can increase salivary flow. Signals from nerve endings in the mouth evoke salivation by exciting the salivatory centres in the BRAINSTEM. Salivary secretion is controlled by the AUTONOMIC NERVOUS SYSTEM. The sympathetic and parasympathetic divisions of the autonomic nervous system often have antagonistic actions, but in the control of salivation they act in a complementary manner. Activation of the parasympathetic nerves elicits large volumes of a watery salivary secretion containing ions and enzymes; stimulation of the sympathetic nerves produces small amounts of saliva that is rich in proteins. The composition of saliva thus varies with the balance of activity in the autonomic nerves controlling salivary secretion.

Salivary responses to chewing and taste stimuli are innate. However, salivary flow may be elicited by events not necessarily associated with feeding. These are termed conditioned REFLEXES and are learned after a period of training or CONDITIONING during which a 'natural' stimulus (e.g. food) is presented at the same time as the 'artificial' or conditioning stimulus (e.g. light or sound). Eventually, the 'artificial' stimulus on its own will elicit salivary flow. The classical example of conditioned salivary secretion was originally observed in dogs by the Russian physiologist, Ivan PAVLOV, who was awarded a Nobel Prize in 1904 for his work on digestive secretions. Conditioned salivary secretion is also present in humans.   ROBIN ORCHARDSON

Further reading
Edgar, W. M. and O'Mullane, D. M. (ed.) (1996). Saliva and oral health, (2nd edn). British Dental Association, London.

See also ALIMENTARY SYSTEM; EATING; MOUTH.

Salt has always been an important commodity, especially in hot climates, where salt loss through the sweat can be considerable. Soldiers of the Roman legions were often paid part of their stipend in salt — the so-called salerium argentinium, giving us the word salary.

Salts in general are formed, together with water, when acids react with bases, but the common meaning of 'salt' refers in particular to sodium chloride, the same material that is found in salt cellars. Normal saline is a solution of salt in pure water containing 0.9 g of sodium chloride per 100 ml. This solution is often used for bathing and cleaning wounds, or given by intravenous infusion after excessive blood loss — but why is it called 'normal'? It is because the solution has the same tonicity as blood. Tonicity is a term related to osmotic strength, a property determined by the total number of molecules or IONS in a given volume of solution. If living CELLS are bathed in a hypertonic saline (with a greater tonicity than normal saline) then the cells shrink and cease to function properly, as water passes outwards from the cells into the concentrated solution. Conversely, if living cells are bathed in hypotonic saline (lower tonicity than normal saline) they swell, water passing from the dilute solution into the cells, and eventually the cells may burst. Thus fluids that exist in different body compartments must be of the same tonicity, to avoid any such shrinkage or swelling. Salt — that is, sodium chloride — is one of the most important salts used by the body to keep fluids at their correct osmotic strength.

In a 70 kg person, the extracellular fluid contains an amount of sodium ions equivalent to 125 g of salt, while in the intracellular fluid — the sum total inside all body cells — there is the equivalent of 25 g of salt. With an average urine output of 1 litre per day there is a loss of about 9 g of salt per day. The KIDNEYS filter off from the blood the equivalent of around 1500 g/day of salt, of which 99.5% is reabsorbed as the filtrate passes down the kidney tubules, so that only 0.5% ends up in the URINE. There are also small losses of salt in the saliva and faeces, and during strenuous exertion — particularly in a hot environment — there is significant salt loss through the sweat. Clearly the salt loss must be made up by dietary intake, but this alone is not sufficiently precise to keep the tonicity of body fluids constant. Therefore the body has control mechanisms to regulate salt levels, by either increasing or reducing its excretion. If the intake of salt is insufficient, keeping the concentration correct causes the extracellular fluid volume to decrease, with consequent dehydration.

As with most bodily control mechanisms, there is a system for dealing with deficiency as well as one for dealing with excess. They are, respectively, the renin-angiotensin system and atrial natriuretic peptide.

When the body is short of salt the extracellular fluid volume, including the circulating blood volume, decreases, and the BLOOD PRESSURE may fall; the sodium concentration falls and the potassium ion concentration may rise, especially in those eating a low sodium diet. All these changes act directly or indirectly as stimuli for the release of the enzyme *renin* in the kidneys, triggering a sequence of chemical events in the blood of which the end product is angiotensin II. This is a powerful constrictor of BLOOD VESSELS and therefore counteracts any fall in blood pressure. Many people with hypertension are treated with drugs which block the enzyme required for *angiotensin II* formation. (This same *converting enzyme* also breaks down *kinins*, which are powerful vasodilators, and therefore tend to lower the blood pressure. When kinins are preserved by inhibiting the converting enzyme, the decrease in blood pressure is probably due to both a lack of angiotensin II and also an excess of kinins.)

Angiotensin II also acts on the adrenal cortex to liberate *aldosterone*, which in turn causes the kidneys to increase the reabsorption of sodium ions from the filtered fluid.

When salt intake is excessive, the extracellular fluid volume and the blood pressure rise; stretching of the atria of the heart causes the release of stored granules that contain *atrial natriuretic peptide*. As the name implies (*natrium*, sodium: *ouron*, urine) this peptide causes natriuresis; that is, it acts on the kidneys to increase salt loss in the urine by reducing its reabsorption. More water is lost along with the salt, so the excess fluid volume is corrected.

In man excess salt intake has been considered to cause HYPERTENSION, but the supporting evidence is equivocal. Certainly there are salt-sensitive strains of laboratory animals that become hypertensive when fed salt, but other strains do not. In the animal kingdom low salt content of the diet is a problem. In seed-eating birds, like parrots, the seeds contain very little salt and an avid salt retaining mechanism has developed in the terminal part of the gut, the coprodaeum, so that little or no salt is lost in the faeces. Similarly, in frogs and toads, salt is avidly reabsorbed from the bladder, so that urine is free of salt. Darwin described how some primitive peoples would pick up a large toad (*Bufo marinus*), gently squeeze it, and be rewarded with several fluid ounces of almost pure water.

The old medical name, from the time when prescriptions were written in Latin to prevent patients knowing what they were getting, is *nat. mur.*, standing for *natrium of muriate*. Muriatic acid is hydrochloric acid, therefore nat. mur. is the chloride salt of natrium — that is, sodium. Many popular homeopathic remedies of today contain nat. mur. in infinitesimally low amounts. The reader may ponder how adding such miniscule amounts of salt to the very large quantities already present in the body can have any effect whatsoever.   ALAN W. CUTHBERT

See also BLOOD PRESSURE; BODY FLUIDS; KIDNEYS; SWEATING; WATER BALANCE.

Satiety Humans and many animals eat in discrete periods of time, that is, they eat meals. Before a meal begins the sensation of HUNGER rises, and this motivates food-seeking behaviour.

Once EATING starts, hunger declines, and people report that they start to feel full. The term 'satiation' describes the processes that bring a meal to an end. An interval of time will then elapse before eating begins again. 'Satiety' refers to the inhibition of eating following a meal, and it is measured both by the inter-meal interval and by the amount consumed when food is next offered.

Let us consider in more detail what happens during a meal. At the beginning, eating is rapid, with few pauses between bites. As the meal progresses, eating slows, there are more pauses between bites, and other behaviours such as fidgeting, grooming, or resting increase. A state of satiety is reached when the meal ends. This state is usually associated with a pleasant sensation of fullness or satisfaction. However, unpleasant sensations of nausea and bloating can be associated with satiety following excessive food intake. Of interest is that even when eating has stopped altogether, the introduction of a new food can restart eating. We call this satiety for one food but not for others 'sensory-specific satiety'. This specificity of satiety explains why, in a multi-course meal, dessert is eaten even when we feel full.

Satiation and satiety depend both on behavioural and physiological responses. The act of eating and our beliefs about what we are eating are important. As food is ingested, a number of physiological processes are sequentially activated. We chew food and it then moves down our throats and into our stomachs, thereby stimulating receptors which respond to the bulk of food and the nutrients it contains. Distension of the stomach and gut makes us feel full. The gut also releases HORMONES which affect satiety. All of these responses to food occur within minutes of eating, but the METABOLISM of food, that is, turning it into fuel several hours later, also affects satiety or when we will eat again.

Much recent research has explored how different types of foods affect the satisfaction and feelings of fullness that follow eating. While the calorie content of food can influence satiety, another important factor is the weight or volume of food consumed. Since FAT has more than twice the calories per gram as either CARBOHYDRATE or PROTEIN, a high-fat meal is smaller in size than a low-fat meal with the same number of calories. Imagine that before a meal you eat a first course of either tomato soup or an equivalent number of calories from cheese on crackers. The soup provides a greater bulk of food because it has a higher water content and little fat. You will feel fuller and hunger will be suppressed more following the soup than the cheese on crackers, thus you will eat less food during the main course. Understanding how different foods and nutrients affect satiety is leading to strategies to reduce energy intake and to control BODY WEIGHT. Eating a diet of low-fat, high-fibre, high volume foods such as fruits and vegetables is a healthy, natural way to increase satiety after a meal.   BARBARA ROLLS

Further reading

Rolls, B. J. (1986). Sensory-specific satiety. *Nutrition Reviews*, 44, 93–101.

See also EATING; HUNGER.

Savages have played an important conceptual role in the history of Western thought since its beginning. The idea of man living in a natural state, possibly even devoid of man-made laws or conventions, can be traced back to ancient times. It was, however, only with the rise of increasingly penetrating critiques of civilization that the notion of the savage came to be fully elaborated in the wholly positive sense it was to assume in the Enlightenment cult of the 'noble savage'.

A powerful influence on subsequent conceptions of savages is to be found in Michel de Montaigne's accounts of Amerindians in his *Essais* (1530). His depiction of their lives was not idealized as it often was later. But he endeavoured to challenge the moral and intellectual complacency of his contemporaries by subverting the notion of the *sauvage*: 'They are savages [*sauvages*] in the sense that we say fruits are wild [*sauvages*], which nature produces of herself and by her own ordinary progress; whereas in truth, we ought rather to call those wild, whose nature we have changed by our artifice, and which are diverted from the common order.' This idea was further exploited by Rousseau in his *Discours sur l'origine et les fondements de l'inégalité parmi les hommes* (1755). Natural man was healthy, robust, unreflective, and fearless, according to Rousseau; he was also indolent and had no cause to labour, as nature was bountiful and his needs were few and easily provided for. What is more, he was truly happy. His existence was mostly solitary. The chance encounters between men and women were very brief; women raised children single-handedly and children left their mothers, never to see them again, as soon as they could fend for themselves. Civilized man, by contrast, was dependent, weak, frail, enslaved to countless needs and desires, unhealthy and as profoundly unhappy as one might expect of a creature thoroughly alienated from his true nature. Not everyone agreed with this rendition of civilized existence. James Boswell reported that when he argued for the superior happiness of the savage life, Samuel Johnson was adamant: 'The savages have no bodily advantages beyond those of civilized men. They have no better health; and as to care or mental uneasiness, they are not above it, but below it, like bears.'

Most thinkers were agreed that the condition of women amongst savages was far from ideal. Even Diderot, who spoke favourably of the life of savage man, thought that civilized woman was far better off than her primitive counterpart, who was treated with unmitigated brutality by uncivilized males. However the idea of the savage was used in a negative manner by women writers who, like Mary Wollstonecraft, reflected on the contemporary condition of their sex: 'An immoderate fondness for dress, for pleasure, and for sway, are the passions of savages; the passions that occupy those uncivilized beings who have not yet extended the dominion of the mind, even learned to think with the energy necessary to concatenate that abstract train of thought which produces principles. And that women from their education and the present state of civilized life, are in the same condition, cannot, I think, be controverted.'

The debate over the merit or demerit of savage life continued throughout the nineteenth century and well into the twentieth. Likewise, the evolutionary view of the history of society and the family, like Lewis H. Morgan's *Ancient Society, or Researches in the Lines of Human Progress from Savagery through Barbarism to Civilization* (1877) exercised much influence, not least on Frederick Engels' *Origin of the Family, Private Property, and the State* (1884).

SYLVANA TOMASELLI

Further reading

Kierman, V. G. (1990). Noble and ignoble savages. In *Exoticism in the Enlightenment*, (ed. G. S. Rousseau and R. Porter). Manchester University Press, Manchester.

Scalping

The practice of removing the scalp, 'the haire skinne of the head', from a slain enemy as a trophy, originated in ancient headhunting. The English word 'scalp' is derived from the Danish *skalp* (shell, husk), which, like the Old Norse *skalpr* (sheathe), belongs to the Indo-European verb stem *skel-* (to cut), and is thus related to *skelo* (Danish: *skaal*, Swedish: *skål*), the Germanic term for 'drinking vessel'. According to Paulus Diaconus, *skelo* was originally applied only to vessels made from SKULLS, out of which the blood of vanquished foes was drunk both in Germanic and classical antiquity. Correspondingly, in Middle English scalp still meant 'skull', and only after the seventeenth century did the word take on the more common and specific meaning of the 'skin of the head'. From that point on the word 'scalping' was used to describe the 'peeling' of the skin from the head of dead and, on occasion, still living enemies, and above all to its practice among several Indian tribes of North and South America, where it served to satisfy a thirst for glory and honour or simply as a means of revenge.

Although American native peoples were all too often accused of being the sole practitioners of scalping, in reality they did nothing others had not done before. Herodotus found the practice among the Pontic Scythians, and, according to the Maccabees, the ancient Persians tore away the scalp of one of their prisoners. Orosius reports that Romans scalped during the battle on the Raudine plain. It is highly probable that Germanic tribes behaved similarly, for we know that they ascribed magical powers to a shock of human hair, regarding it as the symbol of the free man. In Germanic law, if a court demanded the guilty party's head to be shaved it was considered an especially grievous sentence — in very serious cases the court could decree that the hair be ripped out with the skin. The Vandals used this form of scalping (*decalvatio*) as a method of torture; several provisions of the *Sachsenspiegel*, the oldest and most influential legal code of medieval Germany, are tantamount to the same thing. The shaved, bald heads of prisoners in Nazi concentration camps, as well as those of *bochesses* (German-lovers) after the defeat of the *Wehrmacht* in the zones occupied by Germany during World War II, are horrible reminders of that dreadful tradition.

Outside Europe, tribes in western Siberia practiced scalping into recent times, as did the Naga peoples in the Indian state of Assam and various groups in the interior of Celebes. In 1845, the British traveller John Duncan watched the Apadomey regiment of the legendary black Amazonian army pass in parade before the king of Dahomey — bearing 700 scalps as trophies. Duncan's awe-struck description of the sight has been adapted many times, most recently in Richard Fleischer's *Conan the Destroyer*, where Grace Jones plays a warrior woman armed with a knife and draped, as it appears, with scalps. In the Caribbean, scalp hunts were organized by runaway slaves, especially the 'bushmen' of Surinam, who, following African custom, used scalps for ceremonial purposes inside their fortified asylums (*palenques*).

Among the native peoples of both Americas, scalping was originally not widespread and was practised only rarely and on a small scale. It was only after firearms and steel knives were introduced that the taking of scalps as booty became more frequent. Even then, scalping did not become extensive until the eighteenth century, when warring European groups adopted the custom of posting rewards for scalps in order to terrorize the foe of the moment. By that time, however, it was certainly no longer merely 'reds' scalping 'whites' and other 'reds', but also 'whites' scalping 'reds' and other 'whites'. In the Kansas — Nebraska War of the 1850s, 'damn'd abolitionists' were scalped, as were some political opponents during the 1856 presidential election campaign between Buchanan and Fremont.

PETER MARTIN

Further Reading

Friederici, G. (1906). *Skalpieren und ähnliche Kriegsgebräuche in Amerika*. Braunschweig.

Scan

The term used to describe a variety of IMAGING TECHNIQUES — ULTRASOUND, CT (computed tomography), MRI (magnetic resonance imaging), isotope, or PET (positron emission tomography) scans. 'Going for a scan' in pregnancy would mean an ultrasound scan of the unborn baby or of the mother's pelvis. Sometimes the term may be linked to the organ or part of the body being examined (e.g. brain scan, liver scan, bone scan) without defining the particular imaging technique, other times it may be qualified and more specific (e.g. CT brain scan, isotope bone scan). All types of scanners provide moving or consecutive pictures, focussed on an organ or region of the body, from which a two- or three-dimensional image can be built up and saved by computing techniques.   J. K. D.

See IMAGING TECHNIQUES; RADIOLOGY; X-RAYS.

Scars

Any disruption of the body surface, or of internal organs, will leave a scar, although the most skilful surgical repair can result in a scar which is virtually invisible. Permanent physical evidence of injury on or in the body is the end-product of a complex and highly effective system of repair. However skilful the mending of a tear in a man-made fabric, it does not achieve actual restoration of continuity between the interwoven threads: likewise for the SKIN and for internal tissues.

When injury — accidental or deliberate — or surgery breaks the skin, the normal WOUND HEALING processes result in restoration of continuity of the protective surface layer. Any gap is filled by a covering of EPITHELIUM, with an underlying layer of fibrous CONNECTIVE TISSUE, but this new 'skin' does not develop the full character of normal skin — there are no sweat glands, and no hairs. If the edges of a wound have been held close together during the healing process by stitching, or by careful dressing for smaller wounds, the gap — and therefore the final scar — is minimal. At the other extreme, a widely gaping wound will be covered over, but it may end up as an unsightly streak of 'keloid' tissue, or 'welts', lying proud and purplish above the surface of the adjacent normal skin.

Scarification, artistic marking of the body, practised around the world but especially in Africa, is used to indicate social status, progress through the cycle of life, or familial and dynastic affiliations. It is also employed to enhance bodily beauty and as medical treatment (cuts above the eyes are said to aid sight and those on the temples to relieve headaches). Among the Nubians, for example, one can read a woman's marital and fertility status in her skin. At puberty, Nubian women are marked by a pattern of scars on either side of their abdomens that join at the navel and continue into a point between the breasts. With menarche a second set of cuts are made in parallel rows under the breasts which continue around to the back and cover the entire upper body. After weaning her first child, a woman is marked with raised welts over her back, neck, arms, and buttocks to the knees. In Southern Egypt and Sudan these raised scars are made by a hooked thorn used to lift the skin, which is then cut with a small blade; ashes or indigo are often applied make the scars more prominent.

Scarring is common among both sexes. In men, the scars often indicate social standing or physical ordeals of individual valour. In the early part of the twentieth century, for instance, male students at German universities proudly bore duelling scars.

SHEILA JENNETT
LONDA SCHIEBINGER

Further reading

Brain, R. (1979). *The decorated body*. Harper and Row, New York.

See also BODY DECORATION; BODY MUTILATION AND MARKINGS; SKIN; WOUND HEALING.

Scrotum

To quote a 1940s edition of Gray's anatomy: 'The scrotum forms an admirable covering for the protection of the TESTES. These bodies, lying suspended and loose in the cavity of the scrotum … are capable of great mobility, and can therefore easily slip about within the scrotum, and thus avoid injuries from blows or squeezes.' Indeed so. Modern anatomical texts have lost a certain poetry.

The skin of the scrotum is exceptionally thin and 'beset with thinly scattered, crisp hairs …' but the whole pouch is thickened by an underlying sheet of involuntary muscle (*dartos*), closely linked to the skin, and responsible for its corrugated appearance. This muscle layer is continuous with a *septum*, which divides the scrotum into compartments for the two *testes* and their *spermatic cords*; it is 'separated from the subjacent parts by delicate areolar tissue upon which it glides with the greatest facility'. These subjacent parts are a *fibrous capsule*, and then a *serous* (fluid-secreting) *membrane*, which slides upon (and is continuous with) a membrane covering the testis. These membranes form a closed, fluid-lined sac, like a deflated balloon, that sometimes swells up to become a *hydrocele*. The *cremaster muscle* links the lowest part of the abdominal wall above the groin to these coverings of the testis, and can retract it upwards: this occurs reflexly when the inner thigh is stroked.

The contents of the scrotum have descended into it, usually before birth, from the abdominal cavity. The route was through the *inguinal canal* at the groin. Each testis dragged after it a string of elongating vessels and nerves and the *vas deferens*; these constitute the spermatic cords. Each cord maintains its connection with the abdominal cavity via the canal, whence the vas joins the urinary tract below the bladder. Because the inguinal canal breaches the muscular and fibrous integrity of the abdominal wall, it can become further weakened and expanded, allowing abdominal contents to extrude through it as an *inguinal hernia*. A large hernia can extend right down into the scrotum.

In the early weeks of fetal life, before gender differences are apparent, there is a *labioscrotal swelling* on each side; these swellings join up to develop into the scrotum when maleness is genetically ordained.   SHEILA JENNETT

See also GENITALIA; TESTES.

Sculpture

Breasts, bellies, and buttocks bulging, the female figurines of Paleolithic Europe are the earliest echoes of the human body in sculpture. Some 35 000 years old, such so-called 'Venuses' are an extraordinary breed. The 'Venus of Willendorf', for example, has a mere knob of a head, her face obscured by what has been interpreted as a cap of curls. Her puny appendages dangle below the swollen organs of an exaggerated fecundity, leading historians to make analogies, anachronistically, with the Greek goddess of love.

Numbers of these early carvings have been found, and most employ an already sophisticated symbolic play of miniaturization and metonymy. The body is constructed on an intimate scale, like most early sculpture (these figures are usually about 15 cm high), rendering these female forms both literally graspable and psychologically non-threatening. Yet the symmetrically-arranged limbs and organs are often significantly abstracted — visually bisected with deep lines between breasts and thighs (and even running down the midsection), so that the entire miniature body can be viewed as a slightly-larger-than-life-size equivalent for the female vulva. Whatever rituals they accompanied, and whatever practices gave them cultural meaning, have been lost. All that can be said with confidence of these first moments in cultic sculpture is that mimetic representation is far from the primary goal.

Authority figures

Sculpture of the body in the African continent participated in these wide Paleolithic trends, but more salient for art historians has been the enduring canonical tradition emerging with dynastic rule in Upper Egypt at the beginning of the third millennium BCE. As scholars have argued, the astonishing invariance of the dynastic Egyptian canon is a mark of its unremitting intentionality, as well as a sign of its social origins in systems that controlled representations and institutionalized their modes of transmission. Dynastic Egyptian sculpture of the body, based on an art of contour and shallow relief rather than sculpture in-the-round, presents different aspects of the human form as if each were seen from a different vantage point. Eye, shoulders, and one breast are shown as if viewed from the front; face, legs, feet, and the other breast are represented in profile. Junctures (such as the hip or neck) are non-anatomical transitions expressing sections of the contour.

The Egyptian canon was developed specifically to project a visual sign of one pre-eminent body, that of the ruler. The strong arm (its symbolic attributes fully preserved) is shown clenched, or in muscled extension (wielding a sceptre or other sign of authority); the (usually male) face is limned with its jaw jutting forward; the feet are stable on the ground line, yet one foot is shown striding forward in purposeful procession. Repeating this series of important attributes, the canon was a socially-enforced formula for achieving clarity in *delineating power*, not some 'way of seeing' or being-in-the-body that can be held to be innate in the distant Egyptian (or, for that matter, the ancient Mesopotamian or Mycenaean). As described by Whitney Davis, the canonized body of the Egyptian ruler stabilized only with the second period of pharaonic rule, 'symbolically [stating] certain social achievements that society had recently recognized as significant, potentially unstable, and problematic for its continued reproduction — namely, the stability and validation of a centralized state'.

When cultures in ancient Greece emerged to revise the Egyptian canon in specific and self-conscious ways, they built on local traditions of sculpture that manipulated patterns of nakedness and ritual. Greek sculpture of the body was intended primarily for ritual use; those being depicted are participants in religious practices or objects of devotion, not (or not only) articulating signs of statehood. Votive figures in the form of women (viewed as 'not-men') are shown draped; only men are naked. But, as Andrew Stewart argues, in an earlier (pre-Geometric) tradition, both men and women were shown naked, their basic forms marked by slits or penile protuberances that reveal a paramount goal of gender differentiation in which women were not merely partial or canceled men. In this pre-canonical period in Greece, the body was a differentiated sign for the human in general, but also for the self in particular. Clothing or other social implements were mere distractions from the true self, revealed by, and in, the body.

The shift from this early phase of nakedness to a bifurcation in Greek sculpture and vase-painting between the clothed female and the naked male, appears in the late eighth century BCE. Nakedness is the natural state of the human (male): clothing designates its socially-constructed (and female) state. Not coincidentally, this is also the period of consolidation for male rule in the *polis*, and the moment when running naked during the (male) Olympic Games becomes the rule. It also marks the inaugural moment for what would later come to be called 'classical' Greek art, a powerful conflation of ambitions, for mimesis and a new body ideal — twin goals that would haunt sculpture, and culture, for millenia.

The sculpted body in this highly mimetic phase of classical Greek art was preferentially bronze, a metal which carried all the connotations of Hesiod's descriptions of the race of strong men that preceded the classical age of heroes. (Fig. 1). The literally 'brazen' warrior stood poised for aggressive and immediate action — breath drawn into a barrel chest through slightly parted lips (made of copper, with gleaming silver teeth), nipples taut (and inlaid in contrasting copper), hands flexed around weapons, and inlaid eyes (with copper eyelashes) staring implacably at their prey. The polychrome realism of such works was lost by the later dominance of the Roman marble copies that were the primary means of transmitting classical forms. The bleached white headless and armless 'VENUS' came to represent the classical tradition for countless followers in later times — despite periodic archaeological revelations of the intense colours that once adorned Greek sculpture in marble *and* in bronze.

Corpus Christian

Tied as it was to pagan religions, the Greek mimetic model was devalued by the early Christians (and, for that matter, by the Judaic traditions on which they built). The play between illusion and the materiality of sculptural form was but one aspect of the devilment Christianity perceived in these body images. Medieval sculpture, then, was a sculpture of the body in dialectic — either dematerialized into architectural form or rendered abjectly material, ridden with the wormholes of corporeal death or dripping with the gore of the Passion. Arguably, the privileged Christian signifier of the cross is the ultimate sculptural abstraction of the body. As floorplan of the cathedral, icon above the altar, and punctuating votive on the rosary, the cross is both reminder of the body's dross mortality, and vehicle for its divine transcendence. Depicted medieval bodies (such as the curving apostles who adapt themselves to the portals of a Romanesque cathedral) are only part of the story, for the medieval body also moved, in worship, through the abstract sculptural void of the cruciform (body-formed) church.

Quattrocento Neoplatonists struggled to reclaim the naturalistic body as a signifier of the sacred. The triumph of High Renaissance sculpture marked the success of this project, but not without dramatic struggles, such as the iconoclastic burnings of 'pagan' art under the fierce eye of the preacher Savonarola. Buttressed by the support of powerful patrons and his own humanist ambitions, Michelangelo Buonarroti was but one of the most gifted Renaissance artists who restored sculpture to the profoundly mimetic status it had possessed in classical times (indeed, in one famous story the young Michelangelo buried one of his marble torsos, fooling fellow Tuscans into believing it was ancient when it was finally unearthed). Whether painting sculpted androgynes on the ceiling of the Sistine Chapel, hewing the colossal *David* from the quarries at Carrara, or achieving the dreamy torsion of the half-liberated *Slaves*, Michelangelo forced sculpted bodies (preferably nude and male) to the forefront of visual culture and public space, where they would remain until well into the twentieth century.

The apotheosis of the body in stone must surely be Gianlorenzo Bernini's (1598–1680) Cornaro Chapel altar depicting *The Ecstacy of Saint Teresa* (Rome, 1645–52). This well-known work instantiates the emotional intensity, drama, and erotic mysticism of the baroque (by one of the style's inventors). From a tangle of surging drapery, an upturned head, and a few exposed appendages, the sculptor convinces us of Teresa's sublime *jouissance*, amplified by gilded rays of light and a smiling angel (or Eros) looking on. Such extreme emotional states, and such twists and turns of the body, were tamed during the Enlightenment. Neo-classicism was reconfigured in terms of an archaic Greek ideal (the Egyptianizing *Kouros* rather than the explosive movement of Hellenistic Greece). Bodies aligned themselves in military phalanxes (Francois Rude's *Marseillaise*, 1833), or arranged themselves in tepid erotic displays (Antonio Canova's *Pauline Borghese as Venus*, 1808). Only the pressures of a restless, industrializing modernity would threaten the long reign of these classical echoes. Towards the end of the nineteenth century, twin emphases on specularity and an inner-directed abstraction (its seeming obverse) rendered figural sculpture increasingly irrelevant. Bridged by the accomplishments of French Impressionist sculptor Auguste Rodin (1840–1917), the tenure of the classical body ended, and the twentieth-century body emerged — fragmented, pocked by light, insistently unfinished, and usually cast in industrial scale foundries rather than carved 'by hand' (even if they had often been the hands of skilled *practiciens*).

Modern discipline

The multiple, serialized body characterized modern artists' production, with or without the artist's knowledge or consent. Rodin's sculptures still continue to be cast by the French government (with his blessing) and although Edgar Dega's *Little Dancer of 14 Years* (c. 1881) was made in a single wax original (dressed in gauze tutu and silk, with real hair whose ratty realism

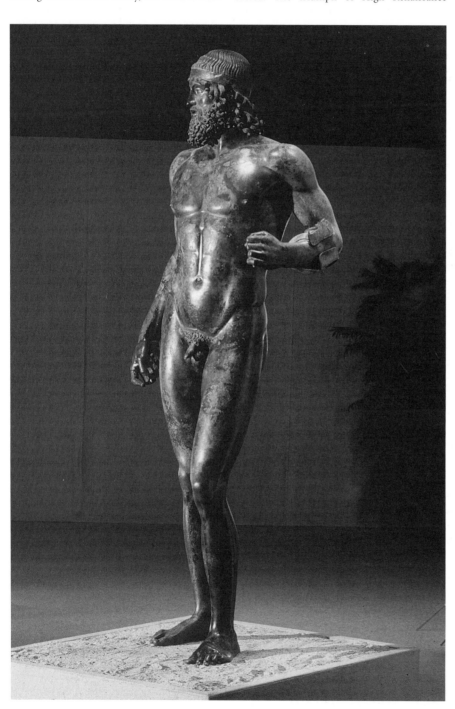

Fig 1 Bronze soldier retrieved from the sea at Riace, Sicily, c. 450 BCE. Museo Nazionale, Reggio Calabria, Italy/Bridgeman Art Library.

repulsed contemporary critics), market pressures resulted in its replication in bronze, with only the tutu in cloth. The possibilities presented by such industrial casting methods, and by the concept of serialization itself, became themes for later artists. Drawing from the vibrant vernacular tradition of African wood carving, Pablo Picasso's odd little Cubist abstraction *Glass of Absinthe* (1914) (Fig. 2) was cast in bronze and issued in a series of six, each painted differently to play with the object's anthropomorphic status as both cup and besotted drinker of the lethal drug.

The history of twentieth-century art is a history of the ebb and flow of abstraction; the projected and empathetic presence of the body *in* the sculpture shifted in mid-century to a dialectic between the body *and* the sculpture. Phenomenology codified this shift, focusing on the relationship of the perceiving body to forms in an experiential space. This was particularly important for the group of artists called the Minimalists (New York, 1960–8). Their central canonical form was the cube, although the rectangle and the paralleliped were contenders.

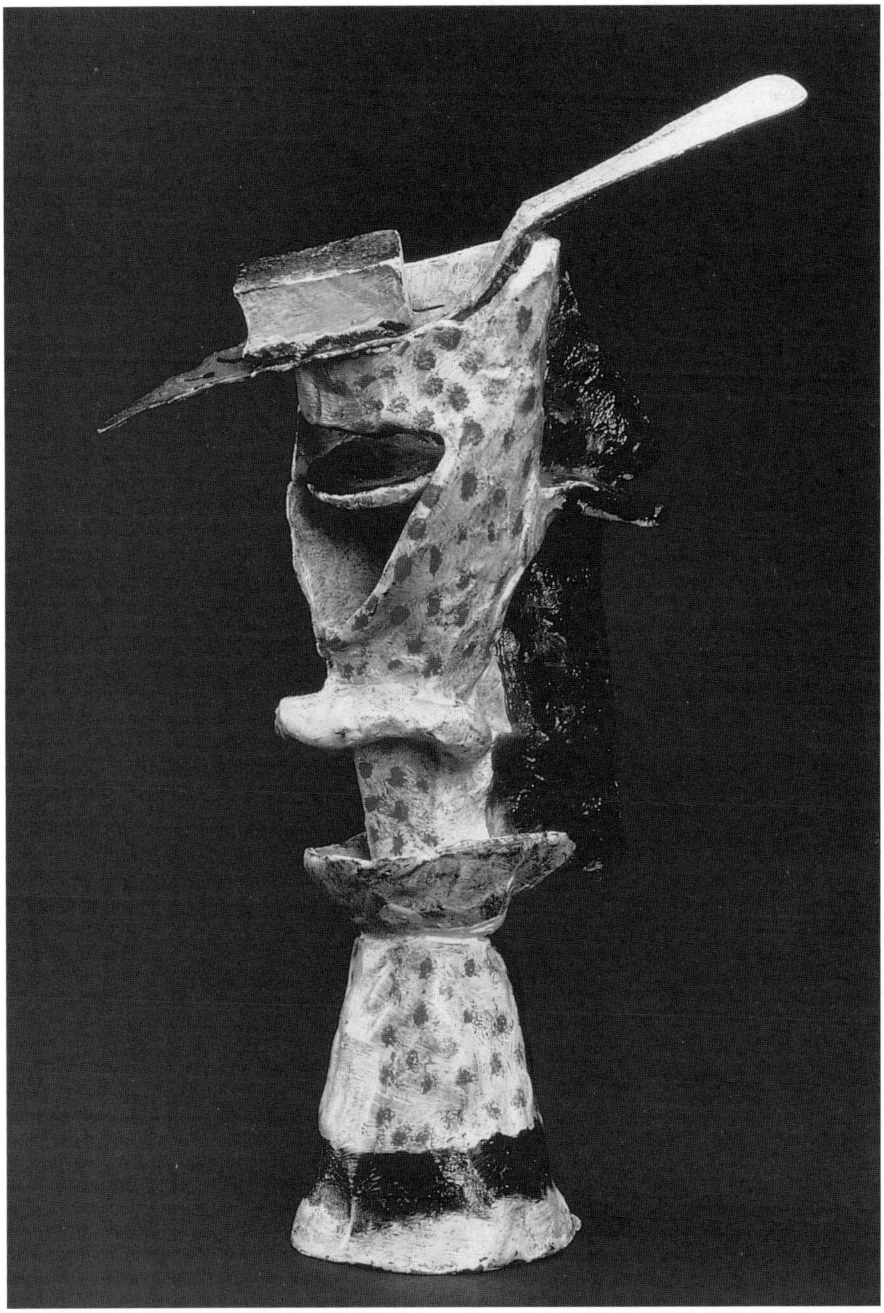

Fig 2 *Glass of Absinthe*, 1914 (mixed media) by Pablo Picasso (1881–1973). Private collection/Bridgeman Art Library. © Succession Picasso/DACS 2001.

Such basic geometric forms, many built to the scale of a standing man, were held to have 'presence', to command a response from the viewer of the type normally reserved for other human beings — to function, in other words, as another body, confronting, but not replicating, the viewer's own.

The reductive austerities of Minimalism were followed by a wide range of art movements that brought the body forcefully back into art — although not by the standard mimetic means. Art of the last decades of the twentieth century can no longer be contained within the genre called 'sculpture': body art, performance, and occasionally even installation art inserted the living body into the arena of display. Visual artists commanded theatrical stages, but they also worked in stadiums, seashores, sidewalks, subways, and conventional gallery interiors. Repetitive actions of bodies in Ann Hamilton's installations surfaced concerns with labour and ritual; Laurie Anderson's technologically-mediated performance art questioned the stability of gender; Adrian Piper's Explorations of the abject body strained the social fabric of public space in New York City; absent bodies, signalled by female-shaped depressions in the earth, were presented in Ana Mendieta's *Silueta Series*, performing the negativity so often ascribed to 'woman' in a binary economy of signs. The source of much of this fin-de-millenia energy lay in feminist and multicultural critiques of a prevailing Western tradition, seemingly not yet fully exhausted — that tradition in which living bodies are emptied and mapped onto the fetish known as sculpture.

CAROLINE A. JONES

Further reading

Davis, W. (1989). *The canonical tradition in ancient Egyptian art.* Cambridge University Press.

Stewart, A. (1997). *Art, desire, and the body in ancient Greece.* Cambridge University Press.

See also ART AND THE BODY.

Second wind The sensation of relief from breathlessness and FATIGUE that occurs at some point during sustained EXERCISE, even though the degree of muscular effort may be unchanged.

S.J.

See BREATHING DURING EXERCISE; FATIGUE.

Secretion describes the processes by which cells assemble materials and release them for action elsewhere. Commonly material is passed into a duct (*exocrine secretion*). For example, SALIVA, containing salts and ENZYMES, is assembled in the salivary gland cells, released into salivary ducts, and passed to the mouth to help with mastication and digestion. Other secretions are passed directly into the bloodstream (*endocrine secretion*). Generally the word is not used to describe how NEUROTRANSMITTERS or neurohormones are lost from cells; rather these are said to be released. Finally, secretion should not be confused with EXCRETION, which refers to the loss of waste products from the body. A.W.C.

Sedative Technically, a DRUG causing sedation. Useful for the treatment of patients with ANXIETY, and who are restless and agitated such that normal function is impaired. Sedatives are more properly called *anxiolytic* drugs. Anxiolytics should not be confused with *hypnotics*, which cause SLEEP — although sedation may often allow those with troubling anxieties to be able to sleep. Sedative drugs taken at higher doses can often act as hypnotics in those suffering from insomnia. Until twenty years ago the main group of sedative drugs were the *barbiturates*, now almost entirely replaced by the *benzodiazepines*. Miscellaneous other modern drugs, such as *glutethimide* and *meprobamate*, are also used as sedatives, as are some very old ones, such as *chloral hydrate*. The latter mixed with an alcoholic drink is known as a Mickey Finn, used, in detective literature at least, to knock out the 'goodies'.

A.W.C.

Semen consists of sperm from the TESTES, and seminal fluid secreted by the accessory glands of the male reproductive tract; these include the seminal vesicles, PROSTATE GLAND, and the bulbo-urethral glands (known as 'Cowper's glands after a seventeenth-century French anatomical plagiarist who was not in fact the first to describe them). The seminal fluid secreted by these glands provides a medium in which sperm can be carried to the female reproductive tract, and may provide nutritional and protective support, but we know that seminal fluid is not essential for fertilization, because sperm taken directly from the vas deferens is capable of fertilization in its absence.

Semen is produced during the complex genital reflexes which culminate in EJACULATION. Upon sexual stimulation, the muscular wall of each vas deferens contracts, pushing sperm towards its widened end, the ampulla, where it joins with the ducts from the seminal vesicles to form the ejaculatory duct. This duct then passes into the prostate gland, which lies below the exit of the BLADDER, and joins with the urethra — the final common tube for the excretion of urine and the passage of semen. The small, pea-sized bulbourethral glands lie on either side of the base of the prostate gland, and their ducts open into the urethra. As the sperm is pushed from the two vasa deferentia into the urethra during sexual stimulation (the emission phase), simultaneous contractions of the accessory glands add fluid to the sperm.

The bulk of seminal fluid is secreted by the seminal vesicles, which were previously thought to store sperm (storage is now known to be at the end of the long coiled tube of the epididymis in the testis). These two glands release a viscid, yellowish fluid into the ejaculatory duct. The seminal secretion from the prostate gland is a thin, milky fluid, which is responsible for the characteristic smell of semen, while the bulbo-urethral glands secrete mucus, which acts as a lubricant prior to ejaculation. In man the volume of semen produced at each ejaculation is about 3–4 ml,

containing about 300 million sperm. This is a very conservative volume compared with the wild boar which can produce up to half a litre (500 ml) of semen at ejaculation.

SAFFRON WHITEHEAD

See also COITUS, EJACULATION; SPERM; TESTES.

Senility can be defined as 'showing the feebleness of old age' and in this sense it is commonly used to imply feebleness of the mind. As Samuel Johnson has stated in his life of Boswell (1783), there is a wicked inclination in most people to suppose older people decayed in their intellects. He goes on to suggest that if younger or middle-aged men do not recollect where they have left their hats when leaving company it is nothing, whereas if the same happens with an old man then people will shrug up their shoulders and say 'His memory is going.' But are there such mental changes associated with normal AGEING or is the term 'senility' a generalization from the increasingly frequent DEMENTIAS which occur in old age?

Examining initially the gross changes which occur in the brain with ageing, it can be observed that the normal volume and weight of the adult brain begins to decrease from about 50 years of age. This is due to a reduction in the number of cells in a wide area of the brain: the CEREBRAL CORTEX, the hippocampus, the substantia nigra, and the CEREBELLUM. Depletion however does not necessarily result in impaired function because there is a generous reserve of cells. There is also a reduction in nerve cell size from the age of 85 years onwards in some areas of the brain.

A high resolution scanning technique, magnetic resonance imaging (MRI), has demonstrated increased white matter hyperintensities, and radioisotope scanning techniques such as single photon emission tomography (SPET) and photon emission tomography (PET) have shown a decrease in cerebral blood flow and metabolism, in normal people with advancing age.

At the microscopic level, we also know that old age is accompanied by the accumulation of certain substances in and around the brain cells. Abnormal structures known as 'neurofibrillary tangles' appear in some nerve cells of the cerebral cortex and 'senile plaques' containing the protein beta amyloid may be widespread. In a third of older people's brains amyloid deposits are also found in the thin membranous covering (leptomeninges) and in the walls of the blood vessels in the cerebral cortex. Some nerve cells show evidence of shortening or loss of dendrites (their multitudinous fine extensions through which incoming messages are received), whilst others have excessive branching dendrites. In addition to changes in the nerve cells, the intermingling glial cells, which normally form more than half of the brain's substance, spread themselves diffusely in some areas in a manner which resembles the way in which they would respond at any age to local damage.

But do all these changes result in an alteration in 'normal' brain function? Certainly there are neuropsychological changes associated with normal ageing and these can best be described as not inevitable and affecting different people at different ages to a variable extent. When population samples of different age groups are compared (cross-sectional studies), intellectual function appears to be at its peak at around 25 years of age, to remain static until the middle 50s and then to decline gradually. But consecutive assessments of large samples of people as they become older (longitudinal studies) demonstrate considerable individual differences, with 60–80% remaining stable or actually improving in some specific abilities. It appears that tests emphasising the need for speed are particularly prone to deterioration with age. Stored knowledge and its access is less susceptible to change than the more 'fluid' aspects of intelligence such as working memory. Thus older people can be viewed as demonstrating significantly faster forgetting of newly acquired information and having a smaller pool of processing resource available. This is evident for example in their difficulty in dealing with divided attention tasks. But at the same time age brings with it an enriched database and intellectual skills which have been accumulated during a lifetime.

The concept of senility may also be a generalization from the increasing number of older people who develop dementia. Dementia is a syndrome due to disease of the brain, usually of a progressive nature, where there is impairment of multiple higher cortical functions and deterioration in emotional control, social behaviour, and motivation, all occurring in clear consciousness. The commonest causes of dementia are Alzheimer's disease and those associated with arteriosclerotic changes in brain blood vessels. The prevalence of dementia in the population is 5% at 65 years and 20% at 80 years of age. The cognitive changes in dementia are widespread, affecting intellectual, language, and memory functioning and as with normal ageing, some functions may change more than others, indicating that there may be subgroups of patients with different cognitive impairments.

MARTIN BLANCHARD

See also AGEING; BRAIN; DEMENTIA; LIFESPAN.

Sensation A sensation is a subjective experience resulting from the stimulation of a SENSORY RECEPTOR (a specialized nerve cell that is excited by some physical or chemical stimulus). Sensations are presumed to arise as a result of nerve activity in certain areas of the CEREBRAL CORTEX, which receive incoming signals from the sensory receptors.

Aristotle recognized only five senses — *vision, hearing, taste, smell* and *touch*, each associated with a particular SENSE ORGAN (counting the skin as a sense organ). The term 'special sense' is still used for VISION, HEARING, TASTE AND SMELL. In reality, there are many more sensory systems, including those that mediate the sensations of PAIN and temperature, those of the positions of parts of the body (PROPRIOCEPTION), and those related to balance (conveyed by the vestibular apparatus). A more fundamental way of classifying sensory receptors is according to the types of physical stimuli to which they respond. It is remarkable that all the majesty of our sensory experiences depends only on sensitivity to light, and to mechanical, chemical, and thermal stimulation.

The experience of our own bodies, SOMATIC SENSATION (from the Greek 'soma' meaning body), conventionally includes sensations arising from nerve endings in skin, muscle, bones, and joints. A different term, VISCERAL SENSATION, is used to describe awareness (usually discomfort) arising from receptors in the internal organs (viscera). Such sensations are only vaguely localized compared to somatic sensations, and in some instances may be 'referred', that is, felt to be coming from a site quite different from where the excitation arises. For instance, the pain of angina, originating from sensory fibres in the muscle of the heart, is typically felt in the left shoulder and upper arm. Some visceral sensations, such as the feeling of a full bladder, are associated with normal functions; others signal abnormality, such as the pain of intestinal colic or a growing tumour.

Sensory experiences have distinct subjective qualities, such as colour, pitch, tickle, bitterness, and floral. These are sometimes referred to as 'modalities' or 'sub-modalities' of sensation, especially for sensations derived from the skin. Valiant, partially successful, attempts have been made to correlate each such mental property with a particular specialized type of sensory receptor, nerve pathway or region of the brain. In 1823, the British neurologist and anatomist, Sir Charles Bell, first described evidence for what subsequently became known as Müller's Law of 'Specific Nerve Energies' (after the German physiologist, Johannes Müller). Bell wrote: 'every nerve of sense is limited in its experience, and can minister to certain perceptions only'. He and Müller cited examples of false sensations, elicited by inappropriate stimulation of particular nerves. For instance, pressing on the side of the eyeball with a finger, which causes direct, mechanical stimulation of the retina, gives rise to a 'phosphene' — a visual sensation in the form of a curious blob in the part of the visual field corresponding to that region of the retina. Certainly, many modalities of sensation can be identified with particular specialization of the sensory receptors involved. Touch, vibration, warmth, and coldness are indubitably associated with particular, highly specialized nerve endings in the skin.

Sensory receptors provide information about the *quality* of the stimuli that they detect, giving rise to what philosophers call the *qualia* of conscious perceptual experience. We see colour and brightness, hear pitch and timbre, and taste sweetness and sourness: we can distinguish whether an object touching the skin is sharp or smooth, hot or cold. But stimulus quality is not the only kind of information that sense organs provide. They also transmit data on the intensity, duration, and location of the stimulus. Generally speaking (though there are exceptions), the quality of a sensation is determined by which type of specialized nerve ending or receptor cell is stimulated, but the perceptual intensity (brightness, loudness, etc.) depends on how strongly the receptor is stimulated.

However, there is not perfect congruence between particular individual sensory receptors and the qualia – the units of subjective experience. For example, our retina contains just three types of cone receptor cell which have slightly different but overlapping spectral absorption. The large number of different colours that we can distinguish are somehow derived by the brain from the relative strength of the signals from these three basic detectors.

PAIN is usually thought of as rather different from other modalities, in that it bears no simple relationship to the physical world. It is, most simply, a perception resulting from a noxious stimulus — one associated with actual or potential tissue damage. But pain may be caused by excessive stimulation of receptors ordinarily involved with other modalities: for example heat on the skin is felt as heat, but excessive heat is felt also as pain.

Although, strictly, sensation refers only to conscious feelings, it is clear that much of the massive, unremitting inflow of information from sensory nerves does not enter CONSCIOUSNESS. Even for the special senses, we are aware at any moment only of what we attend to, which is a tiny fraction of the information streaming in. Indeed, much sensory processing, essential for the regulation of the body, is entirely unconscious. The receptors in MUSCLES, JOINTS and TENDONS, some of which give rise to conscious proprioception, are involved in the constant, unconscious task of regulating posture and guiding movement. The HEART, LUNGS, and major BLOOD VESSELS have a variety of specialized sensory endings, conveying information to the brain about the pressure and composition of the blood, and about the stretching of the lungs. Within the brain itself, the HYPOTHALAMUS and parts of the medulla contain sensory nerve cells that are specialized to detect such properties as the acidity of the blood, its temperature and the concentration of glucose, salt and other constituents. These unconscious sensory systems play an essential part in HOMEOSTASIS — the maintenance of the internal environment of the body, by initiating reflex regulation of breathing, heart rate, blood vessel size, sweating and shivering, as well as in regulating essential behaviour such eating and drinking.

Psychologists and philosophers often draw a distinction between sensation (said to have a raw, unprocessed quality) and perception, the interpreted meaning of sensory activity. This view can be traced to Immanuel Kant's 'transcendental' philosophy, namely to the view that knowledge of the world arises from sensory experience, furnished by the mind with such 'archetypal' properties as space, time, relation, and causality.

The distinction between sensation and PERCEPTION is hard to defend on the basis of what we now know about how sensory receptors and their associated brain areas work. At each stage, even at the sensory receptors themselves, the particular, selective characteristics of the nerve cells impose expectation and order on sensory signals. The detection of stimuli and their cognitive interpretation, to provide knowledge of the world, are inextricably linked within our sensory systems. Effortless though our perceptions seem, they involve immense 'computational' tasks. More than half of the human cerebral cortex is devoted to analysing sensory signals.

'Common sense', meaning native intelligence, derives from the medieval term *sensus communis*. This described the place in the fluid-filled chambers of the brain at which signals from all the sense organs were supposed to mix together, to provide the ingredients of imagination and rational thought. The near-miraculous process that intervenes between the irritation of the membrane of a sensory receptor and our perception of the world is arguably the most intelligent thing that we do.   COLIN BLAKEMORE

See also CEREBRAL CORTEX; CEREBRAL VENTRICLES; HEARING; PAIN; PERCEPTION; PROPRIOCEPTION; SENSORY RECEPTORS; SOMATIC SENSATION; TASTE AND SMELL; VESTIBULAR SYSTEM; VISCERAL SENSATION; VISION

Sense organs Our sensory experiences, conscious and unconscious, derive from SENSORY RECEPTORS distributed throughout the body. But the five main senses — sight, hearing, taste (*gustation*), smell (*olfaction*), and touch — are associated with specialized structures known as sense organs (the skin being the 'organ' for the classical sense of touch). In addition, a sense organ in the inner ear known as the *vestibular apparatus* provides our sense of balance and equilibrium. It detects movement, and gravity (strictly speaking, angular and linear acceleration of the head).

The variety of specialized sensory experiences is very much greater than the classical five. The skin, as well as being sensitive to tactile contact, can also detect and distinguish warmth and cold, vibrations at various frequencies, and a whole range of different kinds of PAIN, itch, and TICKLE. Each of these definable 'sub-modalities' depends on the activation of a particular type of specialized nerve ending in the skin (or of more than one type of nerve ending). Visual and auditory senses also have a range of 'submodalities', each associated with a distinctly different sensory experience — for instance colour, movement, and brightness for VISION; loudness, pitch, and position in space for HEARING. These different aspects of sensory experience depend not only on receptor cells with different receptive characteristics in the eye and ear, but also on the way in which information from the sense organs is processed in the brain. Indeed, much of our sensory experience is determined not by the basic characteristics of our sense organs, but by the analysis of sensory messages in the brain, especially in the sensory areas of the CEREBRAL CORTEX. The perception of the distances of objects in space through stereoscopic vision is a good example. This depends on the detection of tiny differences in the two retinal images resulting from the fact that the two eyes are separated in the head and therefore view the world from slightly different angles. Obviously this striking aspect of our visual experience is not represented in the signals from either eye alone, and can be derived only in the brain, where the signals from both come together.

At the heart of all sense organs are sensory receptors — specialized nerve cells or the endings of nerve fibres, which detect particular physical or chemical events outside the cell membrane. Much of the variety of sensory experience depends on the physical characteristics of the tissues that make up the rest of the sense organs. For instance, receptors sensitive to mechanical stimulation (*mechanoreceptors*) have been put to an extraordinary range of tasks in the body. The hair cells in the cochlear of the inner ear are mechanoreceptors: they respond selectively to sound because the rest of the ear delivers sound energy directly to them and protects them from any other form of mechanical stimulation. The hair cells of the vestibular apparatus are very similar to those of the cochlea, but they respond to tilt or rotation of the head, not sound, because those are the physical forces to which they are exposed. All the receptors in the skin that respond to touch and vibrations, those in muscles, tendons, and joints that detect stretch and tension, and even various receptive endings in the heart, lungs, and blood vessels that signal changes in blood pressure and inflation of the chest, are basically mechanoreceptors. Their particular sensitivities are determined by where they are placed in the body.

The non-neural components of sense organs serve, then, to protect the sensory cells and also to deliver particular forms of stimulation to them. The nasal passages support the delicate olfactory epithelium and direct the airflow across it. Chewing, tongue movement, and swallowing force a flow of macerated food, dispersed in saliva, over the taste buds on the tongue. The cornea and lens of the eye ensure that the light rays are focused on the rods and cones of the retina. The eye is unique among sense organs in that it not only houses the receptor cells, forms an image on them, and directs them towards objects of interest (by means of eye movements), but it also contains a large number of other interconnected nerve cells, in the retina. These process and analyse signals from the rods and cones and then transmit processed messages to the brain, along the optic nerve.

Sense organs are our windows on the world. But, like windows, they restrict our perception to what passes through them. We blissfully imagine that, if our senses are normal, we know everything that there is to know of the world around us. But our environment is full of physical energy and chemicals that our sense organs cannot detect. Many other animals have sense organs that can detect stimuli beyond the confines of the human senses. Our wonderful vision is restricted to the narrow band of wavelength within the electromagnetic spectrum that our photopigments can catch, and our eyes are blind to the ultraviolet and infra-red wavelengths that lie just beyond this visible band of the spectrum. But the eyes of many invertebrates, fish, and birds can detect ultraviolet light — male and female blue tits distinguish each other by brilliant ultraviolet feathers whose 'colour' is invisible to our eyes. The family of snakes called pit vipers, which includes rattlesnakes, have a second set of 'eyes', in the form of pinhole cameras set in the cheeks, each consisting of a cavity lined with thousands of heat receptors. Like a thermal imaging camera, these 'pit organs' sense infra-red radiation, enabling the snake to detect the positions of warm-blooded prey in its vicinity. The ears of even a young child can detect frequencies only between about 50 and 20 000 cycles per second (Hz); but natural events, from thunderstorms to snapping twigs, generate much higher and lower frequencies. Whales and pigeons can hear frequencies of sound far below the capacity of the human ear. And many animals can detect sound frequencies up to 100 000 Hz: the vocal production and detection of such ultrasound is the basis of the radar-like echo location of bats.

Even more impressive (and more humbling to human beings) are sensory capacities found in many animals that differ from ours not just in degree but in kind. For instance, bees and many other insects can detect the plane of polarization of light (the axis of vibration of the light photons). This enables them to recognize the position of the sun, even when below the horizon or partially obscured by cloud, and hence it helps them to navigate. Pigeons (and probably many other animals) have magnetic sensory receptors through which they can detect the direction of the earth's magnetic field. A homing pigeon with a small bar magnet attached to the back of its head takes much longer to fly home! And certain fish have electroreceptive organs that are sensitive to weak electric fields in the water around them. Some emit electric pulses and use them to communicate. Others, such as sharks, use their electroreceptors when they attack other fish, sensing the minute electrical fields emitted by the gills of their prey.

FRANCES M. ASHCROFT
COLIN BLAKEMORE

See also EYES; HEARING; PROPRIOCEPTION; SENSORY RECEPTORS; SOMATIC SENSATION; TASTE AND SMELL; VESTIBULAR SYSTEM; VISION.

Senses, extension of

There are two, essentially different, ways in which human beings can extend their sensory powers (neither of which involves EXTRA-SENSORY PERCEPTION!). *Passive extensions* do not need extra power; *active extensions* require some source of energy.

The most obvious way in which we can escape from the physical limitations of our eyes is to employ a microscope, magnifying glass, or optical telescope to improve magnification and resolution. It is remarkable that such passive optical devices have no running costs. One seems to get something for nothing. But this is not quite right. Whatever the properties of the optical system within and in front of the EYE, its capacity to resolve patterns of light is ultimately limited by the spacing of the array of photoreceptors in the retina, which catch the light and initiate the signals that are sent to the brain. Consider the fact that coarse-grain film always produces grainy photographs, however excellent the camera in which it is used. Imagine an eye with only one photoreceptor: it would provide the BRAIN with no information about the *pattern* of light and dark in the image, whatever the quality of its optical system.

Although external magnification can be very useful for particular purposes, there is no gain of information. A magnifying glass enlarges things at the cost of reducing the total field of view: so, one sees more of less. This is valuable for close examination of small objects, but if the optics of our eye were designed to provide such magnification, vision would be perpetually limited to a small fraction of the normal field of view. EVOLUTION has generally provided animals with a wide field of VISION to warn them of danger from all sides. Hence the resolving power of their retinal photoreceptors is distributed across a wide region of space, sacrificing resolution for coverage. (The enormous blind region behind our heads is not, of course, evidence against Darwin! For animals that hunt or manipulate things with their hands, there are other advantages in having eyes that point forwards, with their fields of vision overlapping — not least the capacity to judge distance by stereoscopic vision.)

Try walking around while viewing the world through binoculars or a magnifying glass to see how inconvenient it would be to sacrifice the field of view for the sake of greater resolution. The rear-view mirror in a car does, however, provide the all-round view that evolution has failed to achieve — a very useful extension of vision. However, it does it by making use of part of the eye that would normally be viewing the world ahead. Using such a device requires a good deal of practice.

The sensitivity of the photoreceptors is so great that the best of them (the rods, which provide us with vision in dim light) attain the theoretical maximum: they respond to a single quantum of light. Why, then, does an astronomical telescope allow stars to be seen that are far too faint for unaided sight? The large lens (or even larger curved mirror) captures more quanta than the small pupil of the eye, and hence increases the chance that enough of them will be caught by photoreceptors for the brain to see the star. Also, the eye can be replaced with a camera that integrates quanta over minutes or hours, unlike eyes, which have to signal rapidly to the brain if their information is not to be too late to be useful for most behaviour. (Actually, when the eye adapts to dim conditions, it does integrate for a longer period, allowing it to detect fainter targets, but suffers the disadvantage of not being able to signal rapidly changing or moving objects reliably. This results in the dramatic *Pulfrich Illusion* — the apparent circular swinging motion of a pendulum when viewed with a dark glass over one eye.)

Devices have been invented to give new uses to our senses, extending them beyond the biological function for which they evolved. But for such a device to be valuable, it has to be *matched* to the normal use and situation of the sense it extends. And extension is always at some cost, though this may not matter for the particular, limited purpose of the instrument.

Active extensions can be unimaginably dramatic in their effects, providing entirely new kinds of information for everyday living, as well as for science and technology. The unaided eye is sensitive to just one octave out of the vast spectrum of electromagnetic radiation that exists in the universe. Radio and television (involving the transmission and reception of electromagnetic radiation for which we have no sense organs) gives communication undreamed of a century ago, opening our minds to entirely unexpected features of the universe. X-RAYS, discovered in 1895 by the Austrian physicist Wilhelm Röntgen, were immediately seen as valuable for medical imaging. Diffraction patterns of the short wavelength, high-energy X-rays pointed to the structure of DNA, and X-rays have revealed the hidden structure and dynamics of matter itself. Essentially such techniques extend human sensitivity to regions of the electromagnetic spectrum, outside the bounds of the tiny fraction of that spectrum that we can see.

Extensions of damaged senses are one class of PROSTHESES. Most common are SPECTACLES, which are passive, and HEARING AIDS. Electronic hearing aids are active, but their predecessors, ear trumpets, were passive. They worked by selecting the wanted source of sound, for example someone else speaking, while reducing surrounding auditory irrelevancies. This function is hard or impossible to achieve with inconspicuous, small electronic devices. Also, simple amplification can produce damage to the delicate hair cells of the cochlea. Vanity is the great obstacle to the design of hearing aids. The joke has it that the most effective aid is simply a piece of string dangling from the ear: this encourages others to speak more slowly and clearly — a psychologically active hearing aid!   RICHARD L. GREGORY

See also EAR, EXTERNAL; HEARING; HEARING AID; IMAGING TECHNIQUES; MICROSCOPY; VISION; X-RAYS.

Sensory integration Many of our perceptual and cognitive experiences involve the combination and interaction of different sensations. There are numerous ways in which our ability to recognize and localize events can be improved if we sample information from different sensory modalities that are present at the same time. One of the most compelling is the marked improvement of our ability to understand SPEECH if we can observe the speaker's lips moving. On the other hand, if the cues from different senses are discordant, perception can be distorted. For example, if you listen to a recording of a particular speech sound (say 'ba') while watching a silent video recording of the movement of someone's lips uttering a slightly different sound ('ga'), the sound that you actually perceive will change to something closer to that being produced by the lips (the *McGurk Effect*).

Many well-defined areas of the brain (such as the sensory areas of the CEREBRAL CORTEX) are each devoted to the analysis of signals from a particular sensory system. But if information from different sensory systems is to be integrated and co-ordinated, these signals must be combined within the CENTRAL NERVOUS SYSTEM. Indeed, nerve cells that receive converging sensory inputs are quite widespread in the brain. '*Multisensory convergence*' is occasionally found right at the level of the peripheral receptors: for instance, the smallest, naked nerve endings in the mammalian skin respond to damaging stimuli that may be mechanical, thermal, or chemical in nature, and many of them also respond to certain categories of non-damaging stimuli, such as gentle touch. However, neurons that combine different sensory inputs become more prevalent at higher levels of the central nervous system.

A simple example of interaction between sensory modalities is the way in which the sensation of PAIN from a cut or a blow to the skin can be reduced by rubbing the affected or surrounding area. This is thought to be due to interactions in the spinal cord: the large sensory fibres that respond to the rubbing exert an inhibitory influence on neurons that receive input from the smaller fibres that detect the noxious stimulus.

Nerve cells that have input from more than one sensory system are particularly abundant in specialized 'multisensory' regions or 'association fields' in the temporal, parietal, and frontal lobes of the mammalian cerebral cortex. But even areas of the cortex that appear to be devoted to a single sense may be influenced by other sensory modalities. Thus, recent studies involving the imaging of activity in the human brain have found that crossmodal influences on perception and attention can be associated with increased activity in the visual and auditory cortices.

Sensory integration plays an important role in a variety of neural functions. Neurons in the so-called 'reticular activating system', which extends through much of the BRAIN STEM, receive signals from more than one sense organ. They in turn modulate the activity of neurons in the midbrain, THALAMUS, and cortex, depending on the overall levels of incoming sensory stimulation, hence influencing the level of alertness and arousal.

The integration of gustatory, olfactory, and other sensory stimuli in areas of the LIMBIC SYSTEM plays an important role in EMOTION. Even neurons in those parts of the brain that are involved in the control of bodily posture can be modulated by different sensory cues. This allows motor commands to be modified to take account of the current position or motion of the eyes, head, or limbs.

Detecting the positions of objects in the environment (for instance, predators or prey) is of crucial importance to animals, and several of the sensory systems, especially VISION AND HEARING, are particularly specialized for this task. It is obvious that the various messages about the positions of stimuli must be co-ordinated for effective and accurate control of behaviour. One region of the brain that seems to be particularly important in this respect is the *superior colliculus* (*colliculus* means little hill) in the roof of the midbrain, which is concerned with the control of 'orienting' movements of the eyes, the head, and the rest of the body towards objects of interest. In mammals, this nucleus receives nerve fibres conveying signals from the eyes, the ears, and the body. Each sensory input is distributed across the superior colliculus to form a neural 'map' in a particular layer of the nucleus. The maps of the visual and auditory worlds and of the body surface are superimposed in such a way that, say, a visual stimulus and a sound at a particular point in space will excite cells at the same position in the superior colliculus. This registration of different sensory maps provides an efficient arrangement by which any stimulus, irrespective of its modality, can activate the pathways that control appropriate movements of the eyes or head towards the position of the stimulus in space. The specialization of this part of the brain for combining sensory information about spatial location is very widespread among vertebrates, even those with quite different sense organs from our own. For example, rattlesnakes have heat-detecting organs in their cheeks, which form an image of the infra-red radiation from warm objects (including potential warm-blooded prey). These infra-red 'eyes', like the real eyes, send signals to the superior colliculus and the two maps of space are superimposed.

Multisensory integration also provides a way in which one sensory system, most often visual, can 'calibrate' the neural representations of other modalities during development. There is evidence, for instance, that the projection from the eyes to form a visual map in the superior colliculus, which is itself probably largely genetically programmed, can, after birth, 'teach' the synapses formed by incoming fibres from the auditory pathway, enabling them to form a map of auditory space that is matched to the visual map.

Vision generally dominates human perception. When conflicts between the senses occur, vision tends to bias both auditory and tactile perception. For example, in ventriloquism, the visual cues (the movement of the puppet's mouth) can readily 'capture' the sound of the ventriloquist's voice. On the other hand, early blindness leads to substantial reorganization in the remaining senses. These changes include the heightened auditory and tactile sensitivity, and improved auditory localization of blind people. Recent studies of activity in the living human brain, using IMAGING TECHNIQUES, have shown that the regions of the cortex responding to auditory and especially tactile stimulation can expand enormously in people who have been blind from birth or childhood, even involving areas that would normally respond only to visual stimulation. This increase in the area of cortex occupied by the remaining senses may play a part in the improvement of sensitivity and discrimination. ANDREW J. KING

Further reading

King, A. J. and Hartline, P. H. (1999). Multisensory convergence. In *Encyclopedia of neuroscience*, (ed. G Adelman and B. H. Smith, 2nd edn.), Elsevier pp. 1236–40. Also available on CD-ROM.

Stein, B. E. and Meredith, M. A. (1993). *The merging of the senses*. MIT Press, Cambridge MA.

See also HEARING; SENSE ORGANS; SOMATIC SENSATION; SYNAESTHESIA; VISION.

Sensory receptors

Sensory receptors account for our ability to see, hear, taste, and smell, and to sense touch, pain, temperature, and body position. They also provide the unconscious ability of the body to detect changes in blood volume, blood pressure, and the levels of salts, gases, and nutrients in the blood.

These specialized cells are exquisitely adapted for the detection of particular physical or chemical events outside the cell. They are connected to nerve cells, or are themselves nerve cells. Many of them are enclosed in SENSE ORGANS. Others are the endings of nerve fibres that ramify within the SKIN, the MUSCLES, BONES, and JOINTS and the other organs of the body. Yet others are nerve cells within the brain that are sensitive temperature, to dissolved gases, salts, and other substances in the fluid around them.

In human beings there are just four basic types of sensory receptor — sensitive to mechanical stimulation, light, chemicals, and temperature — but they vary enormously in their form. The particular kind of stimulus to which they respond is largely determined by the structure of the sense organ around them or by their location in the body. Some animals have receptors sensitive to magnetic fields or to electrical fields.

All sensory receptors in the human body operate on the same general principles. Their membranes contain particular protein molecules that are activated and change their shape when the appropriate physical force or chemical substance comes into contact with them. For instance, light falling on the retina causes rotation of a small part of molecules called *photopigments*, which lie within the internal membranes of the rod and cone receptor cells. *Olfactory neurons* in the nose have fine hairs covered in a huge variety of protein molecules to which inhaled odorant molecules attach in a 'lock-and-key' fashion. Specialized proteins in the membranes of hair cells in the cochlea and the vestibular apparatus of the inner ear are sensitive to the mechanical forces caused by sound or movements of the head, respectively. Other types of *mechanoreceptive nerve endings* that detect touch and vibration of the skin, movements and stretch of muscles, tendons, and joints, and the pressure of blood in the blood vessels and heart, employ similar *stretch-sensitive proteins* in their membranes.

Activation of the specific protein receptors in the cell membrane is followed by a sequence of reactions, collectively called *transduction*, leading to the initiation of nerve impulses (ACTION POTENTIALS), which are transmitted along a fibre towards (or within) the central nervous system. The essential step, resulting directly or indirectly from the activation of the receptor molecules, is the opening or closing of tiny pores (ION CHANNELS) in the cell membrane. This causes a change in the movement of charged ions (usually sodium ions), which alters the voltage inside the receptor cell. The amplitude of this receptor potential varies with the intensity of the stimulus. This then leads to the firing of nerve impulses, either in the sensory cell itself or in an adjacent nerve cell. The sensory stimulus is thus translated into a train of impulses whose frequency varies with the stimulus strength.

The *sensitivity* of a sensory receptor usually depends on how much it has recently been stimulated. Hence, if a receptor (say a nerve fibre in the skin) is exposed to a constant stimulus (such as pressure on the skin) the rate of nerve impulses quickly falls to a much lower level, or even ceases altogether. This phenomenon, called *adaptation*, leads receptors to be more sensitive to *changing* than to steady stimulation. Hence they usually measure the stimulus as a percentage of its deviation from the background signal, rather than signalling its absolute intensity. This means that our sensory receptors are sensitive to small changes in signal strength but tune out constant signals. Everyone is familiar with this effect: it is the reason you cease to notice a constant background noise, quickly desensitize to strong smells, and are gradually able to see in a darkened room after leaving one that is brightly lit. It is one example of the way in which our sensory systems 'economize' in their use of nerve impulses.

FRANCES M. ASHCROFT
COLIN BLAKEMORE

See also BARORECEPTORS; CHEMORECEPTORS; EYES; HEARING; SENSE ORGANS; SOMATIC SENSATION; TASTE AND SMELL; VESTIBULAR SYSTEM; VISION.

Septic

Septic From the Greek *sepsis* meaning putrefaction. 'Septic' may describe any INFECTION usually bacterial infection of a wound, which causes both damage to tissues and also the defensive accumulation of white blood cells; the debris of the battleground leads to the accumulation of the thick yellow fluid *pus*. If this is confined beneath the skin or in any enclosed space (root of a tooth, breast, brain, middle ear, for example) it needs to be released before healing can occur — either by spontaneous bursting or with surgical assistance, for example by the traditional 'lancing' of an abscess, now referred to as incision and drainage. The derived term *septicaemia* means infection which has spread into the bloodstream (the ending *-aemia* always refers to the circulating blood). S.J.

See IMMUNE SYSTEM; INFECTION; INFLAMMATION.

Serotonin

Serotonin After blood is allowed to clot a substance can be extracted from the fluid serum which, when injected, causes an increase in blood vessel 'tone' (the vessels' state of contraction). This serum-derived substance was therefore called *serotonin* or *vasotonin*. Similarly, extraction of animal intestines yielded a material with similar actions termed *enteramine* — the name being derived from the term *enteron* (gut). Serotonin, vasotonin, and enteramine were found to be identical. Chemically the vasoactive agent was *5-hydroxytryptamine (5HT)*. This is an endogenous autacoid (a substance made by body cells, which has some action on other cells) and is derived from the amino acid tryptophan, obtained from protein in the diet.

It is now known that 5HT is widely distributed throughout the body, with a multitude of actions. Ninety per cent of the total body content of 5HT is found in the *enterochromaffin cells* in the wall of the intestine. Most of the rest is found in blood platelets, and released from these when blood clots. A small amount is also found in the brain, especially the mid-brain, where it acts as a NEUROTRANSMITTER.

5HT can act on a cell only if the cell membrane has specific 5HT receptors, and there are sub-types of these receptors on different cells, associated with different actions of 5HT upon them. 5HT causes many SMOOTH MUSCLES (involuntary muscles) to contract, such that gut motility and peristalsis are increased and contraction of the smooth muscle of blood vessels causes the BLOOD PRESSURE to rise. The smallest arterioles, however, are dilated, resulting in increased capillary pressure and capillary permeability, causing an increase in the rate of formation of tissue fluid. But 5HT also reduces the release of NORADRENALINE from sympathetic nerves, by acting on $5HT_1$ receptors on the nerve terminals, which tends to reduce blood pressure. The vasoconstrictor response on the larger blood vessels is mediated by $5HT_2$ receptors. Consequently, in the presence of a $5HT_2$ antagonist, when 5HT can act only on the $5HT_1$ receptors, it causes a fall rather than a rise in blood pressure.

5HT exerts many of its actions indirectly by either stimulating or inhibiting the release of other neurotransmitters. An example of inhibition of neurotransmitter release is given above, whereas in the gut it is stimulation of ACETYLCHOLINE release from neurons of the *myenteric plexus* in the gut wall that increases contractions and secretions. 5HT can also stimulate sensory nerve endings directly, causing a PAIN sensation — well known to those who have suffered nettle stings, which contain 5HT.

Although only 1% of the body's total 5HT occurs in the brain it is here that the actions of this substance are the most profound. The neurons containing 5HT are concentrated in the *raphe nuclei* in the mid-brain and their fibres project in a diffuse way to the CEREBRAL CORTEX, hippocampus, LIMBIC SYSTEM, and HYPOTHALAMUS as well as down the spinal cord — a distribution not dissimilar to that of noradrenergic fibres.

Modern molecular biological studies have shown that there are many different types of receptors for 5HT — perhaps as many as ten — whose precise functional responsibilities are not yet clear. There is clear evidence that 5HT is involved in SLEEP, wakefulness, and mood. Descending 5HT pathways (from the brain down the spinal cord) affect the excitability of spinal MOTORNEURONS, activating those involved in simple reflexes and inhibiting more complex reflexes. Animals deprived of 5HT (by giving agents that prevent its synthesis) show exaggerated responses to many types of sensory stimulus, indicating that 5HT normally exerts a modifying effect, allowing irrelevant stimuli to be ignored and the response to pain palliated. 5HT is also involved at the level of the hypothalamus in temperature regulation and in the control of factors which release hormones from the anterior PITUITARY GLAND; also in the central control of vomiting.

There is much evidence to suggest that major changes in the blood vessels on the surface of the brain, which underlie MIGRAINE, are caused by release of 5HT. After an initial vasoconstrictor phase has passed the brain vessels dilate, and it is thought this is responsible for the pain. Drugs used to treat this condition, such as Sumatriptan, are antagonists at the receptor sub-type $5HT_{1d}$.

Lysergic acid diethylamide (LSD) is one of the most notorious mood-altering (psychomimetic/hallucinogenic) drugs, producing bizarre visual experiences together with marked motor unrest and vocalisation of extraordinary utterances. Mental function is altered so that perception of all sensory input — visual, auditory, tactile or olfactory — is distorted. In the brain LSD is able to activate 5HT receptors although elsewhere LSD is an antagonist. The psychomimetic effects of LSD certainly involve interference with the multiple actions of 5HT in the brain. Users of LSD describe both good and bad 'trips', which may mean that the response to LSD is dependent on the state of the 5HT system when the drug is taken. With 5HT, as with many neurotransmitters, the body economises by using reuptake mechanisms: after a neurotransmitter has been released and has acted on post synaptic receptors the transmitter in the vicinity of the nerve terminal is taken up, stored, and recycled when the next nerve impulse arrives. In recent years drugs have been developed which specifically block the reuptake of 5HT. Clearly this is useful if reduction in the effectiveness of 5HT transmission in the brain has led to depression. Selective *serotonin reuptake inhibitors* (SSRIs) have proved useful mood-improving drugs; the best known is *fluoxetine* (Prozac), although there have been adverse criticisms of its use as many patients are reluctant to give it up, even when the condition precipitating the depression has passed.

ALAN W. CUTHBERT

See also NEUROTRANSMITTERS; MEMBRANE RECEPTORS.

Sex is a short word, but an immense concept, and many of us spend a lot of time thinking about it. Sex is the engine that drives creation, ensuring propagation of the race and ultimate survival of the species. The imperfection of biological machines means that after a certain period of time they become dysfunctional and obsolescent, and it becomes more economic and energy-efficient to replace them completely than to continue to renew the old ones.

So how can selfish organisms, intent only on their own survival, be persuaded to reproduce and hand on their heritage and their living space to an utterly new individual?

There are a number of instruments, such as the selfish gene theory and the maternal instinct but the chief contrivance is sex, and Mother Nature has been capriciously kind in allowing us this delightful inducement to procreation.

Apart from being great fun, sex allows the mixing of genetic material with its consequent crucial increase in adaptability; no two progeny are exactly alike, as the cocktail of genes will never mix in exactly the same way. This genetic diversity permits adjustment to any environmental changes, as any advantageous characteristics will promote survival and increase their chances of being further propagated. For example, if the weather gets colder, people with a tendency to wear warm pyjamas will be more likely to survive and pass on their cuddly proclivities; thus the human race will tend to become more huggable, and I say go for it.

The act of sex is also of immense symbolic significance, a gesture of trust and vulnerability. The woman lies on her back (usually) exposing herself without guard or guile to the frenzied thrusting of the man.

The man is also uniquely vulnerable at this time; at the point of ejaculation his back arches, his eyes close in rapture, and he is oblivious to all ordinary sensations. This vulnerability is exploited more cold-bloodedly in other species; the male spider and praying mantis pay the ultimate price for sex, for that gasping moment of desire, for the chance to perpetuate their genes; they form a tasty little post-coital snack for their partner.

And one of the consequences of the desire for sex is that sublimation of that desire has led to that finest of human emotions: romantic love, the passionate unconditional constant devotion to another person, the inspiration for great art, great literature, great poetry, great food, and great, great pop songs. Some authors, however, have argued that it is implausible to suggest that this remarkable harmony between the interests of the species and the ecstasy of the individual came about solely though evolutionary pressure; that the sheer joy of sexual love is far greater than can be explained by reference to biological utility or Freudian psychology — as Tina Turner rasped, 'What's love got to do with it?'

As one of our great primal drives, cultures and religions have naturally developed many different ways to depict and control sex. For example, many traditional religions consider the act of sex without procreation to be sinful, whereas contemporary Western social mores and wider environmental concerns about over-population take the opposing view. In Western society, most forms of sex are now acceptable, so long as they involve consenting adults, and these increasingly bizarre forms of non-procreational sex may be a species response to overcrowding and an inherent, if unconscious, awareness of the dangers of over-population; they might be considered analogous to the legendary mass migrations and suicides undertaken by lemmings when their numbers become too great to support their food supply, though thankfully outre sex is much more diverting both to partake in and to watch.

So the bottom line, so to speak, is that sex represents a ferociously potent device for ensuring that our species continues to adapt and survive (and have great parties on the way).

LIAM FARRELL

See also COITUS; ORGASM; SEXUALITY; SEXUAL ORIENTATION.

Sex change In humans, sex change normally refers to the surgical and legal conversion of a man to a woman or a woman to a man; these individuals are known as male and female transsexuals, respectively.

The term 'transsexual' was first coined — to describe the case of a woman who wanted to be a man — by Cauldwell, an American sexologist, in 1949, although transsexualism is known to have existed since antiquity. The first scientifically documented case of sex change surgery was that of Lili Elbe in the UK in 1930. However, public interest in sex change surgery was first aroused by the sensationalism of Christine Jorgenson's case in Denmark in 1953. Born as a male, it was she who popularized the notion that a man who felt like a woman could change sex. Although the first sex change operation was carried out that long ago, the controversy and emotion stirred up by the use of the procedures in the management of transsexualism are unmatched by most other psychosexual issues today.

According to Dr Harry Benjamin, the esteemed American pioneer in the field of gender disorders since the 1950s, transsexualism is generally accepted to occur independently of other mental disorders and in individuals of varying personality types. He defines transsexualism as a disturbance of GENDER identity in which persons anatomically of one sex have an intense and persistent desire for medical, surgical, and legal 'change' of sex so that they may live as members of the opposite gender. Overtly they may appear to be homosexual, a label which they vehemently deny, although their sexual attentions from the time of puberty have been directed to members of the same sex. They consider their genitalia as foreign, and their one obsession in life is to get rid of them. For these patients, surgery is the finishing touch, rather than a sudden leap into either femaleness for male transsexuals, or maleness for female transsexuals.

Transsexualism has been described as the most extreme form of gender reversal. To alter their body to match their inner self is an intense desire in every transsexual's life. Gender confusion is a dominant feature present in all transsexuals. However, gender confusion is not restricted to transsexuals alone; it may accompany patients suffering from other psychosexual disorders. It is common during the course of almost every child's development to experience some degree of gender confusion. For most, this gender confusion dissolves with the passage of time and growth. Therefore, all transsexuals suffer from gender confusion, but not all who suffer from gender confusion are true transsexuals.

Because of the nature of transsexualism and the apparent similarities it has with other psychosexual disorders, transsexuals are often confused with homosexuals, lesbians, and transvestites. The lack of definitive and easy diagnostic criteria for transsexualism has resulted in many patients with other psychosexual disorders being wrongly diagnosed as transsexuals. The ability to make a clear differential diagnosis, distinguishing patients with various psychosexual disorders from transsexuals is, therefore, an important management requisite.

Advancement of surgical techniques and plastic surgery have made sex change surgery available to both male and female transsexuals. Surgical outcomes have become more predictable, and cosmetically and functionally acceptable to patients. This has resulted in an increasing number of patients seeking sex change surgery. This increase is further enhanced by media exposure, and the establishment of gender identity clinics all over the world.

Despite more openness in discussing the subject of transsexualism and more autobiographies written by transsexuals themselves, the pain and confusion experienced by an average transsexual is not understood by the public at large. Historically, there has been much stereotyping of such patients. Many have viewed them with disdain, others have made them the butt of their jokes, and still others have seen them as sexual objects: in all, making such people feel they are the accursed minority.

Transsexualism is an emotionally crippling disease that impinges on all developmental stages. While sex change surgery has definite medical, surgical, and psychological limitations, there is strong evidence suggesting that true transsexuals have benefited from it, and it remains the treatment of choice for them. The problem is how to identify these patients. Instead of ruthless exclusion of doubtful cases and prolonged pre-surgery observation, thorough screening has led to successful results with excellent individual, social, and sexual adjustment.

The lack of a simple 'litmus test' to predict which patients will benefit from sex change surgery has created a tremendous ethical unease among professionals managing transsexuals. To provide guidance for this particularly difficult area of patient management, the Harry Benjamin International Gender Dysphoria Association has developed 'standards' that set minimal requirements of care. A team approach is recommended. The 'standards' require that a patient should have the gender disorder for at least two years, and that a person with this condition be known to a clinical behavioural scientist, and be his or her patient, for at least three months. Hormone therapy should be initiated only upon the recommendation of the clinical behavioural scientist. The endocrinologist of the team should be aware of the risk factors or side-effects of the hormone therapy. He needs to appraise the patient in the light of those risks. Regular monitoring of relevant blood chemistries and routine physical examinations must be included.

The management strategy can therefore be divided into six stages:

(i)   Initial evaluation by the psychiatrist/psychologist to diagnose the underlying cause of the patient's gender confusion and to identify true transsexuals from 'wish-to-be' transsexuals.

(ii) To attempt psychotherapy to reverse the patient's desire for the sex change operation. To help patients with other compounding problems that may confuse them as to their real motives behind the desire for a sex change.

(iii) Cross-gender hormone therapy to initiate reversible 'changes' of sex. To explain to patients the reasons, strategy, and possible side-effects of the hormone therapy. Female transsexuals are usually given testosterone-esters as a monthly or bi-weekly depot injection, while male transsexuals are given a combination of oestrogen/progestagen or oestrogen alone. Hormone therapy will bring about physical and perhaps psychogenic changes. A subsequent change of mind can be helped as most of the changes brought about by hormone therapy are reversible.

(iv) On top of cross-gender hormone therapy, patients next go through a stage of total cross-dressing. This will provide a real-life test of the patient's intention and ability to adjust and cope in society.

(v)   When the patient is adequately prepared and ready, the sex change surgery is carried out.

(vi) Post-surgery management includes monitoring of cross-gender hormone therapy, adjustment of hormone therapy according to the individual patient's response, and continuing to provide counselling to patients.

The sex change surgery may be classed into two types, namely, genital and non-genital. Non-genital surgery includes plastic reconstruction of the nose, chin surgery, revision of thyroid cartilage, breast surgery, and revision of the buttocks. These surgical procedures are not exclusive to transsexuals seeking sex change surgery. Many females not suffering from gender confusion do seek these kinds of plastic surgery to improve their body image. For example, women who are bothered by large, pendulous and heavy breasts may seek reduction in breast size. All female transsexuals will ask for breast reduction surgery, while most male transsexuals will seek breast augmentation mammoplasty.

The sex change genital surgery for male transsexuals differs greatly from that for female transsexuals. Currently, it is performed as a one-stage procedure. The major steps include: (i) bilateral orchidectomy (castration); (iii) penectomy (amputation of the penile shaft); (iii) creation and lining of the neovagina; (iv) shifting of the urethra and; (v) fashioning of the labia.

The genital surgery for female transsexuals is carried out over several stages and it includes: (i) total radical hysterectomy (removal of womb, fallopian tubes, and ovaries); (ii) construction of an artificial penis (penoplasty); and (iii) closure of the vagina. Future advancement in the surgical procedures may include the fashioning of a scrotum to house artificial testes.   S. S. RATNAM
VICTOR GOH HNG HANG

See also GENDER; SEXUAL ORIENTATION.

Sex determination

Theories and myths about what might cause a child to be boy or girl, and what action might be taken to select one or the other, have no doubt been part of all human cultures. Of those that are recorded, we know that it was a common Hippocratic view, believed by GALEN, that the right testicle and the right side of the womb produced male children, and the left counterparts, female. This was disputed by Aristotle, who contended that the male determined the sex of the offspring. And he proved to be correct: the sex of a child is determined by the father's SPERM.

The germinal cell from which the sperm was formed contained, like all other cells in the man's body, 22 pairs of chromosomes plus another dissimilar pair of sex chromosomes — an X and a Y. The split that resulted in sperms meant that each sperm carried one of these two alternative chromosomes: either an X or a Y, and one copy of each of the other 22 chromosomes. The mother's germinal cells had 22 pairs plus paired X chromosomes, so that every ovum had an X. Fertilization may therefore result in an embryo carrying either two X chromosomes (one from the father, one from the mother), when development will be female (XX), or an X chromosome from the mother and a Y from the father chromosome, when development will be male (XY).

How does this happen? Sometimes the inheritance of the *sex chromosomes* is disturbed, and this provides clues to the normal mechanism. A person with only one X chromosome and no Y chromosome (XO) develops as a female, whereas an individual with one or more X chromosomes but also at least one Y chromosome develops as a male. An experiment by the French physiologist Jost provided the basis of our understanding of the processes underlying male or female development. He operated on fetal rabbits to remove their gonads at a stage before they had developed in either a male or female direction. All fetuses from whom the testis rudiment had been removed developed as though they were female, as also did those from whom the developing ovary was removed. Thus female development is the default. It is the presence of a testis which causes male development. The testis itself develops as a result of the presence of a Y chromosome. Thus the Y chromosome determines male development by the possession of some *testis determining factor* (TDF).

Analysis of individual people who have either inherited an altered Y chromosome and are still female, or who apparently have 2 XX chromosomes but are male, revealed that it was only a small region of the Y chromosome which was responsible as TDF. Pieces of the Y chromosome were either missing or located in another place, and it was therefore possible to identify the gene responsible, by a positional cloning approach. At the same time as this work was progressing a mouse was discovered with a Y chromosome with a mutation that made its TDF non-functional.

Other workers isolated a candidate human gene that fulfilled all the criteria for the TDF. The scientist who had isolated the mutant mice was able to show that the equivalent gene was mutated and that its normal expression was at a critical early stage of testis development. The final proof that this was the gene responsible for sex determination came when the two groups collaborated to make mice carrying an extra copy of the human gene. These mice developed as males.

This is therefore an example of a gene which causes a switch in developmental direction. We now need to know how this gene function is turned on at the critical point of gonad development and what downstream functions it itself controls to cause male development.

MARTIN EVANS

See also GENETICS, HUMAN; GERM CELLS; GONADS; HEREDITY.

Sex hormones Reproduction in both sexes is ultimately controlled by a hierarchy of hormonal secretions form three sites: the HYPOTHALAMUS (in the brain), the PITUITARY GLAND, and the GONADS (the testes or ovaries). The gonads require HORMONES from 'higher' sites to initiate and maintain their activity, and these are known as gonadotrophins. (*Trophin*, from the Greek, means something that nourishes — not strictly appropriate, except in the broad sense of maintaining the healthy function of the gonads.)

The sequence is this: neurons in the hypothalamus secrete gonadotrophin-releasing hormone (GnRH), which is transported through local blood capillaries to the nearby anterior lobe of the pituitary gland. Here GnRH stimulates the cells which synthesize and release the pituitary gonadotrophins — *luteinizing hormone* (LH) and *follicle stimulating hormone* (FSH). LH and FSH are secreted into the circulating blood and transported to the ovaries or testes, where they stimulate the production of the STEROID hormones specific to each sex — oestrogen and progesterone, or testosterone. The gonadotrophic hormones and the gonads' own steroid hormones act together to maintain the prime function of the gonads: the production of mature eggs (OVA) or SPERM. The whole cascade of hormone secretions, from the hypothalamus to the anterior pituitary gland to the gonads, is tightly controlled by feedback effects of the gonadal steroids, which in turn act on both the hypothalamus and the pituitary gland to regulate the secretion of GnRH and of gonadotrophins. In the male these feedback effects are always negative. This means that when secretion of the male hormone, *testosterone*, increases, the release of GnRH and LH will decrease — inhibited by the rising level of testosterone in the blood. Conversely, when testosterone secretion declines,

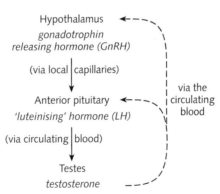

Fig 1 Diagram of the interaction among hypothalamic, anterior pituitary, and testicular hormones: negative feedback loops illustrated in terms of luteinizing hormone (LH) (sometimes known in the male as interstitial cell stimulating hormone). Solid arrows: an increase in secretion of the hormone causes an increase in secretion of the next hormone down the 'cascade' (or a decrease causes a decrease). Dotted arrows: an increase in secretion of the hormone (testosterone) causes a decrease in secretion of the hormones higher in the cascade (GnRH and LH) (or a decrease causes an increase).

the hypothalamic and pituitary secretions increase (Fig. 1). Similar negative feedback effects are seen with the female hormones, *oestrogen* and *progesterone*. However, in females a unique event in the control of hormone secretions occurs just before ovulation. In the ovary, oestrogen production by the cells surrounding the maturing eggs reaches a peak, and the rise of oestrogen level in the blood exerts a *positive* feedback effect: there is an *increase* in both the release of GnRH and the responsiveness of the pituitary gland to GnRH. The result is a huge surge of LH secretion, and a smaller surge of FSH secretion from the pituitary gland; a few hours later the egg bursts from a mature ovarian follicle — the phenomenon of ovulation.

GnRH and the pituitary gonadotrophins are the same in both males and females. (The names used for the gonadotrophins (LH and FSH) refer to the female: 'luteinising' and 'follicle stimulating' are their actions in the ovary. Identical hormones were found to exist also in the male, but the names have persisted.) It is the different steroid hormones secreted by the gonads themselves which are important not only in controlling their own function but also for the development and maintenance of sexual characteristics in the rest of the body.

The major hormone secretions of the ovaries and testes are *steroid hormones*, which are all synthesized from the same precursor — CHOLESTEROL. Cholesterol is derived from animal fats in the diet, and reaches the gonads in the circulating blood, where it is bound to low density lipoproteins (LDLs). The LDL-cholesterol complexes are taken up by the gonads and broken down there to release free cholesterol. Alternatively, cholesterol can be synthesized within the gonads themselves from its percursor molecule, acetate; this is the preferred pathway for generating cholesterol in the testis, but not in the ovary. The synthesis of steroid hormones involves many chemical steps from cholesterol to finished product. In both sexes, molecules related to progesterone (*progestogens*) are formed first; *androgens* — male-type steroids — follow, and these give rise to testosterone and also to the oestrogens. The production of the appropriate end products depends on the presence of different enzymes in the respective gonads (Fig. 2). So there is a common chemical pathway through which both male hormones (androgens) and female hormones (progestogens and oestrogens) are synthesized, but the relative proportions of these different 'male' and 'female' hormones produced within the gonads depend on whether the process is occuring in a testis or an ovary. Testosterone is the major steroid synthesized in the testis, with much smaller amounts of oestrogens, while oestrogen and progesterone predominate in the ovary with lesser amounts of androgens.

In the testes

Testosterone is synthesized by the *interstitial*, or *Leydig*, cells, which lie between the seminiferous tubules, under the stimulating influence of LH. In adults testosterone diffuses into the tubules and, together with FSH, helps to maintain spermatogenesis; also, via the circulating blood, it exerts negative feedback effects on the hypothalamus and pituitary gland, inhibiting gonadotrophin release — signalling that stimulation of more testosterone production is unecessary. In the fetal testis, testosterone production is responsible for the virilization of the male reproductive tract. At puberty an increase in testosterone secretion stimulates the changes associated with sexual maturation, including growth, pubic hair development, genital enlargement, and the breaking voice. For these generalized effects to take place, it is necessary for the 'target' cells, to which the circulating hormone attaches, to possess a particular enzyme which converts testosterone itself into a closely related, but crucially different steroid molecule — *DHT* (5α-dihydrotestosterone). When this enzyme is missing, a rare condition known as testicular feminization occurs: a male has the external appearance of a female.

In the ovaries

Steroid synthesis here is more complicated. Whereas the testis requires only LH stimulation the ovary requires the actions of both LH and FSH for the production of progesterone and oestrogen. The two gonadotrophins act on two different cell types (the thecal and the granulosa cells of the developing ovum-containing follicles). Once follicles becomes sensitive to the gonadotrophins, the outer thecal cells respond to LH and synthesize progesterone and androgens. The androgens then diffuse into the inner granulosa cell layer and here, under the influence of FSH, they are converted to oestrogens. Then, at mid-cycle, the single dominant follicle that is destined to release a mature egg develops receptors for LH in the granulosa cell layer, and the action of LH (in its 'surge' of secretion described above) precipitates ovulation. After ovulation the empty follicle is 'luteinized' — turns yellowish — it becomes a *corpus luteum*, secreting predominantly progesterone and some oestrogen under the influence of the gonadotrophins, until the next menstrual cycle begins.

Like testosterone secreted by the testes, the oestrogen and progesterone which the ovaries secrete not only act within the ovaries themselves to stimulate their function, but also enter the circulation to exert feedback effects on the hypothalamus and pituitary gland and to act on other target organs including the UTERUS, VAGINA, and BREASTS. However, unlike testosterone, which plays such a crucial role in the fetal development of the male reproductive system, the ovarian hormones have little if any effect on the fetal differentiation of the female reproductive system: this simply occurs in the absence of the male hormone. The female sex hormones do, however, become important later during puberty for growth of the breasts, changes in body shape and composition, and other characteristic

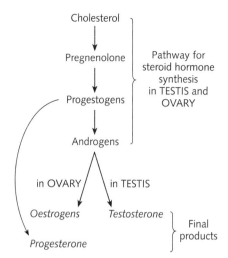

Fig 2 Outline of the derivation of the major steroid sex hormones from the precursor, cholesterol.

physical changes. After the MENOPAUSE the ovaries no longer produce sex hormones, although the cortex of the adrenal gland does produce small amounts of androgens. These can be converted to oestrogens, and are thus an important source of oestrogens in postmenopausal women, but they are not produced in sufficient amounts to replace the loss of oestrogen secretions from the ovary.

It is becoming clear that oestrogens, and to a lesser extent progestogens, have important effects on a variety of body functions apparently unrelated to reproduction. Thus, changes in the secretion of oestrogens and progestogens (occurring during the MENSTRUAL CYCLE, during PREGNANCY, and after the menopause) can, for example, influence mood, metabolism, bone structure, and cardiovascular and immune function, and can cause water retention and breast tenderness.

Aside from the steroid hormones, the gonads also produce a wide range of protein and peptide hormones, which may simply act as local regulatory hormones, such as growth factors, within the gonads themselves or may circulate in the blood and influence pituitary gonadotrophin secretion; one such is 'inhibin', from the testis, which can depress FSH secretion.

Synthetic sex hormones are widely used for CONTRACEPTION and HORMONE REPLACEMENT THERAPY. Oestrogens may also be prescribed to suppress lactation and as a palliative measure in cancer of the breast or prostate, and progestogens for menstrual problems and for habitual abortion.   SAFFRON WHITEHEAD

See also STEROIDS.

Sexuality
This word initially denoted organisms capable of reproducing sexually (thus plants had sexuality), and was applied to things rather than people (humans had sex, a man's spermatozoa had sexuality). Then, early in the nineteenth century, it began to be used to denote

a whole nexus of concepts around sexual expression, sexual activity, and sexual powers, detached from the original connotation. In spite of this, it took some time to develop as a concept: for example, the pioneer British sexologist Havelock Ellis entitled his series of investigations *Studies in the Psychology of Sex* (1897–1928), rather than *Studies in Sexuality*, which might now seem a more appropriate title.

Freud and Foucault

It was perhaps Freud who gave it its particular modern meaning as a term describing not only the sexual drive as such but the direction which it takes in a particular individual. He distinguished the sexual instinct from the sexual object, arguing that the very numerous instances in which the instinct was not attached to something appropriate — a suitable member of the opposite sex — suggested that the instinct was initially independent of any object. The sexual instinct permitted much variation in the choice of objects it was directed towards, and often also, he pointed out, a considerable lack of discrimination — he cited bestiality as an example. These vagaries, however, were not to be confused with insanity. Sexuality was thus not coterminous with the sexual instinct. Freud was accused of making sexuality too important, allocating it a central place in human motivation and extending its ramifications into areas that many had not previously thought to be sexual. It could, conversely, be argued that he was making explicit an obsession with the importance of sex that characterized his times.

Michel Foucault has famously described sexuality, in *A History of Sexuality; Volume I, Introduction* (1976), as a system of discourses rather than a 'given', that came into existence during the nineteenth century — created, he argued, by the desire to regulate sex, and to define and prohibit certain kinds of behaviour. While Foucault's conclusions are supported by perhaps over-broad and sometimes unsubstantiated generalizations, and the establishment of elegant antitheses with which one might want to contend, he has certainly drawn our attention to the rise of a particular way of looking at and defining sexual matters. Sexuality, in the sense of a personal and idiosyncratic amalgam of drive and direction, central to a person's individuality, was generated out of a perception of sex as a problem, or a series of problems.

Foucault has also forced us to think differently about existing naïve concepts of what sexuality is and does. It is not a force of nature which was repressed during the course of the nineteenth century and then liberated through the breaching of the taboo of silence which had prevented it being spoken about. Rather, it is a nexus of concepts and relationships brought into being through a complex process of naming the forbidden, in order to control and regulate it. And through that process, forbidden desire and behaviours were given names by which they could be discussed and spoken. In fact it was a product of the great nineteenth-century urge to catalogue and classify, mediated by a sense that there was something peculiar, slippery, elusive, and dangerous about the subject. The 'hydraulic' view of sexuality as something that can either be dammed up, liberated, or channelled, is thus seen to be just one way of looking at the phenomenon of sex, and one which is, moreover (though Foucault does not make this point) open to the criticism of being heavily dependent upon a male model of sexual functioning.

Towards a plurality of sexualities

With this delineation of 'sexuality', as a particular way of looking at or talking about sex created by a particular kind of society during a particular historical epoch, often goes an assumption that previously there was no such thing as 'sexuality'. There was the sexual instinct, there was lust, there was sin or crime or insanity, but there was not 'sexuality' in the sense of the individual's personal and centrally-defining blend of drive and desire. This assumption has been much contested, in particular the corollary that prior to the definition of the homosexual as an individual of innately inverted sexuality, in the late nineteenth century, there was no such thing as the 'homosexual' but merely individuals convicted of acts which were defined by the law as sodomy. Historians had demonstrated a strong case for the emergence of something like a 'homosexual identity' well before the writings of the sexologists created the category, and in fact these writers based their conclusions on contacts with individuals who already had the sense of their own difference from a norm.

With the rise of FEMINISM and feminist analyses of sex in society, and with the contemporaneous rise of gay studies and theory, the idea of 'sexuality' meaning a particular association of sexual desire and its object (hetero or homo) is itself seen as too coarse a definition; it tends to conflate very different kinds of preference and behaviour. Recent feminist, gay, and 'queer theory' writers have preferred to talk about 'sexualities' rather than sexuality as such. These sexualities may be defined as constructed partly through social means (the provision of roles or scripts for sexual identity and behaviour) and partly on the basis of personal psychological factors.

It thus follows that the notion of some biological basis for 'sexuality' is an over-simplistic concept. While there may be (as a current example) some predisposition in biochemistry or brain structure to same-sex attraction, it will be manifested in various ways because of the ways society defines 'sexuality'. The same predisposing factor at different times and in different cultures, and according to other elements of personal psychology, will be expressed in very different ways — a furtive (married) cottager, a drag queen, an AIDs activist. 'Sexuality' is a bundle or a container rather than a reified thing in itself.

LESLEY A. HALL

Sexually transmitted diseases were previously called 'venereal diseases', of which there were three: syphilis, gonorrhoea, and chancroid. Over time, but particularly during the second half of the twentieth century, the range of diseases spread by sexual contact have increased considerably, and include infection by a variety of organisms, particularly BACTERIA and VIRUSES, of which the newest is the Human Immunodeficiency Virus, causing AIDS (see table).

Currently, the geographical distribution of the sexually transmitted diseases (STDs) varies in number and type of condition. The World Health Organisation (WHO) estimates 333 million new infections per year (excluding HIV/AIDS). The major focus is South and South-East Asia, with an estimated 150 million new cases in 1995, and sub-Saharan Africa, with 65 million. In the developing world, the commonest diseases are gonorrhoea, syphilis, chancroid, and HIV infection, whereas in developed countries they are chlamydial infections, non-specific urethritis, genital warts, and herpes.

The STDs are important because of their complications and social stigma. The most serious sequelae occur in women, and are pelvic inflammatory disease (infection in the fallopian tubes) and ECTOPIC PREGNANCY (pregnancy in the tubes), but the infections also increase the risk of stillbirth and prematurity, and can affect the new-born baby. In sub-Saharan Africa, 50% of cases of INFERTILITY can be attributed to prior tubal infection, usually with gonorrhoea or chlamydia.

The risk of acquiring a sexually transmitted infection is related to a number of factors, which include demography, partner change, poverty, urbanization and migration, social unrest, and war, as well as lack of diagnostic and treatment facilities.

The diseases and their features

The three most common presenting symptoms of STDs are urethral discharge, genital ulceration, and vaginal discharge. Whereas the first two are usually due to an STD, vaginal discharge is not. Most women have a physiological vaginal discharge, which can vary from day to day, and can also be related to their MENSTRUAL CYCLE. It can be due to other infections, such as candida (thrush), which are not usually sexually transmitted. Pointers to the possibility that a vaginal discharge is due to an STD are development of symptoms after a recent partner change, recent multiple sexual contacts, symptoms that are recurrent or persistent, and symptoms in the woman's partner. Finally, there may be general symptoms such as abdominal pain, menstrual problems, or pain on intercourse.

Gonorrhoea, non-specific genital infection, and chlamydia In heterosexual men, these conditions give rise to discharge from the penis, 3–14 days after exposure. In homosexual men, the rectum can be infected, but in many incidences the patient is unaware of this unless they attend a clinic for a routine check-up, or at the request of a partner who develops symptoms. In women, these three conditions can often be without specific symptoms, especially since vaginal discharge is common. These infections are particularly important in women because of the complication of pelvic inflammatory disease; if this arises, it usually causes abdominal pain, perhaps with menstrual disturbances, and pain on intercourse. Women may only become aware of their infection when their male partner develops problems. Gonorrhoea can be treated with penicillin, and non-specific genital infection and chlamydia with tetracycline.

Genital warts — small lumps around the genital regions — have become increasingly common. They have a very long incubation period after exposure (anything up to 6 months). Treatment is straightforward, by freezing or applying acidic substances such as podophyllin. Warts tend to recur. It is important that they are treated, particularly in women, where there is a possible association between some types of warts and the later development of carcinoma of the cervix. All women with genital warts should have regular CERVICAL SMEARS.

Genital herpes is a viral condition with a short incubation period of approximately 3–7 days. If it is a first attack, the symptoms can be particularly severe, with pain, and blisters breaking down into sores, which sometimes can be extensive. Occasionally patients may have a temperature

Microorganisms that can be sexually transmitted	
Bacteria	*Chlamydia trachomatis*
	Neisseria gonorrhoeae
	Gardenerella vaginalis
	Treponema pallidum
	Group B Haemolytic streptococcus
	Haemophilius ducreyi
	Calymmatobacterium granulomatis
	Shigella species
Viruses	Herpes simplex virus types 1 and 2
	Wart virus (papillomavirus)
	Molluscum contagiosum virus (poxvirus)
	Hepatitis A, B, and C virus
	Cytomegalovirus
	Human immunodeficiency virus 1 and 2
Mycoplasmas	*Ureaplasma urealyticum*
	Mycoplasma hominis
Parasites	*Sarcoptes scabiei*
	Phthirus pubis
Protozoa	*Entamoeba histolytica*
	Giardia lamblia
	Trichomonas vaginalis
Fungi	*Candida albicans*

and headache, and feel generally unwell. There are two types of herpes simplex virus. Herpes type 1 normally causes cold sores, but oral–genital contact can transmit this from the lips to the genital area, therefore one should avoid this type of contact with people during the time that they have cold sores. There is no cure for this condition, and it tends to recur, but with unpredictable frequency from patient to patient. Pregnant women can pass herpes on to the baby at the time of delivery, so they should be under specialist care.

Syphilis is now very uncommon in the UK. *Primary syphilis* occurs after an incubation period of about 9–90 days. Usually a solitary, painless ulcer appears at the site of exposure (penis, vulva, rectum, etc.). This will heal without treatment. *Secondary syphilis* appears 4–8 weeks later, in the form of a widespread rash, mainly on the shoulders, chest, back, abdomen, and arms. *Tertiary syphilis* occurs any time from 3–20 years after exposure, with complications affecting the CENTRAL NERVOUS SYSTEM and HEART.

Candidiasis, trichomonas, and bacterial vaginosis cause vaginal discharge, and are not usually sexually transmitted.

Genital ulcers are not necessarily due to STD. In Britain the commonest causes are genital herpes and syphilis, but in tropical countries there are other conditions commonly causing genital ulceration.

HIV and AIDS Even though North America and Europe experienced the first impact of the AIDS epidemic, infections with HIV are now seen throughout the world, with the focus having switched to developing/resource-poor countries. WHO estimate that, by the end of 2000, 36.1 million people were living with HIV/AIDS, and that 5.3 million new infections occurred during that year. At the time of writing, 90% of all infections occur in developing countries and continents, with the major brunt of the epidemic in sub-Saharan Africa (22.5 million cases), and south and south-east Asia (6.7 million cases).

It is now realized that cases of AIDS were first seen in central Africa in the 1970s, even though at that time it was not recognized as such. Current surveys from some African countries show that the level of infection is high amongst certain groups: in 50–90% of prostitutes and 30% of those attending departments for STDs and antenatal clinics. The advent and increase of HIV infection since the 1980s has highlighted the importance of infections spread by the sexual route. It has also been recognized that the presence of a sexually transmitted disease, particularly (a) genital ulcer(s) and/or a vaginal/urethral discharge, can enhance both the acquisition and transmission of HIV by increased shedding of the virus within and from the genital tract.

The most common mode of transmission of this virus throughout the world is by sexual intercourse, vaginal or anal. Other methods of transmission are through the receipt of infected blood or blood products, semen, or donated organs; and through the sharing or re-use of contaminated needles by injecting drug users, or for therapeutic procedures. Also, transmission from mother to child can occur, in the womb, possibly at birth, or through breast milk.

Acute infection with HIV usually passes unnoticed, although there may sometimes be fever, swollen lymph nodes, muscular pain, and a rash. Most patients are unaware of their infection unless they are tested. The antibody test carried out on blood can take approximately three months to become positive (the window period). In view of this, patients are encouraged to delay being tested after possible exposure. Chronic infection follows and again the patient may not be aware that they are infected — or they may have non-specific symptoms such as fever, night sweats, diarrhoea, and weight loss. The time between infection with HIV and developing AIDS can be very long: on average about 8–9 years. Once a patient develops AIDS, they can have tumours and/or infections in various parts of the body. There is no cure for AIDS, but the infections can be treated, and new antiviral agents against HIV are now more powerful, and may alter the medical history and life expectancy of those infected.

Control of sexually transmitted diseases is served in the UK by a network of specialist clinics: departments of Sexually Transmitted Diseases or Genitourinary Medicine clinics. The image of such clinics has changed considerably; they have become more friendly, with far less associated stigma. Most people attend without medical referral, and because the remit of these clinics has extended in recent decades, many use them for check-ups, screening for HIV, and for gynaecological problems or contraceptive advice. In developing countries, such specialist services do not usually exist, and sexually transmitted diseases are normally managed in non-specialist services, usually in rural primary health centres by non-medical staff.

Prevention of STDs involves primary and secondary approaches. Primary prevention aims to educate individuals about the advantages of discriminate and safe sex (prevention by the use of CONDOMS), about the symptoms of the common sexually transmitted diseases, and about how to seek care for them. It is also important to point out that some conditions may cause no symptoms, so that regular check-ups are advised for those who often change their partners.

Secondary prevention aims to encourage people to seek care without delay once the symptoms of a disease are recognized, to stop sexual intercourse until medical advice has been sought, and to adhere to the advice and treatment given. The final aspect of control is the tracing of the sexual contacts of the infected patient, who may have infection without being aware of it.   M. W. ADLER

Further reading

Adler, M. W. (1980). The terrible peril — a historical perspective on the venereal diseases. *British Medical Journal*, **281**, 206–11.

Adler, M. W. (1997). *The ABC of AIDS*, (4th edn). BMJ Publications, London.

Adler, M. W. (1999). *The ABC of sexually transmitted diseases*, (4th edn). BMJ Publications, London

Sexually transmitted diseases: a brief history

Sexually transmitted diseases (STDs) have been known since antiquity: gonorrhoea was certainly described by the ancient Egyptians, and was recognized by Greek and Roman medical writers. The prevalence and spread of these diseases was exacerbated by war or other travel, and the rise of city dwelling, with the concomitant increase of people living in close proximity to each other. By the Middle Ages both gonorrhoea and syphilis were widespread. One view, by no means unchallenged, was that syphilis was brought to Europe by Christopher Columbus' sailors on their return from the New World. The differentiation of the 2 diseases from each other was often a matter of medical debate, from the sixteenth up until the nineteenth century, many authors believing that the symptoms of gonorrhoea (clap or gleet) were the early stages of syphilis (the pox). This view was substantiated by the British surgeon John Hunter (1728–93), who undertook heroic self-experimentation by injecting his own penis with material taken from a patient with gonorrhoea. On developing the signs of syphilis he concluded the two infections were the same — little realising that his patient, like many others, actually suffered from both infections at the same time.

The main orthodox treatment for syphilis from the Middle Ages until the early years of the twentieth century consisted of the application of a mercury ointment, a favourite treatment for skin lesions. But sufferers from the disease were particularly susceptible to the blandishments of quacks and charlatans, and many successful businesses profited during the seventeenth through to the twentieth centuries from selling useless remedies.

In the middle of the nineteenth century a French physician, Philippe Ricord (1799–1889), convincingly demonstrated the differentiation of the two main STDs and determined the three stages — primary, secondary, and tertiary — of syphilis. Shortly afterwards Rudolph Virchow (1821–1902) established that syphilis was spread through the body by the blood, explaining the known cardiovascular, muscular, and psychiatric complications. At the turn of the twentieth century up to a third of inmates in mental asylums were reckoned to be suffering form tertiary syphilis.

During the nineteenth century an increasing number of public health measures, usually aimed at prostitutes, were taken to prevent or control the spread of STDs. The Contagious Disease Acts of Great Britain clearly tolerated prostitution, as they permitted, amongst other regulations, the compulsory examination and incarceration of infected women, often in the so-called Lock hospitals. A vociferous campaign was mounted by women's groups, civil rights activists, and members of the medical profession, and the Acts were repealed in 1886.

Advances against the diseases were notably improved by the discovery of their causative microorganisms. That of gonorrhoea was found in 1879 and that of syphilis in 1905. Shortly after this the German bacteriologist Paul Ehrlich (1854–1915) announced the efficacy of Salvarsan, an arsenic-based treatment for syphilis. Also a diagnostic test was devised, which was enormously important as it allowed the disease to be detected in sufferers not yet displaying the symptoms; they could then be advised on how to prevent or minimize passing on the infection. The development of the sulpha drugs and more potent antibiotics provided a wider range of effective drugs against these diseases. However, it rapidly became apparent that the provision of appropriate treatments did not eradicate these diseases, and that public health advice and personal hygiene education were also necessary. The appearance and world-wide spread of AIDS (Acquired Immune Deficiency Syndrome), for which an effective treatment is still unavailable, during the 1980s, has emphasized the complex nature of these diseases.   E. M. TANSEY

Further reading

Brandt, A. M. (1993). Sexually transmitted diseases. In *Companion encyclopaedia of the history of medicine*, (ed. W. F. Bynum and R. Porter), Vol. 1. Routledge, London.

Sexual orientation

Assumptions about the exceptions

The idea of an innate and idiosyncratic direction to the sexual drive of the individual — like so many ideas around sex — largely originated in the efforts of late-nineteenth-century sexologists to classify the vagaries of human sexual behaviour. Influenced by evolutionary science and developments in psychology, authorities such as Krafft-Ebing or Havelock Ellis wished to remove the stigma of sin or wanton debauchery from those whose sexual conduct diverged from the received model of heterosexual MARRIAGE for reproductive purposes. They endeavoured to suggest that those who did not conform, or conformed only with difficulty, to this model, were not necessarily lascivious sinners committing perverse acts for a corrupt thrill, but individuals who could not help themselves — individuals for whom, in fact, behaviour which might seem bizarre to the majority felt 'normal'.

However, while the late nineteenth century saw the codification and elaboration of the idea of sexual orientation, the idea that there were certain kinds of people with certain kinds of drives which set them apart from their neighbours did have a less formal and scientific existence before that. It has been plausibly argued that, as a result of increasing urbanisation facilitating meeting with individuals of like desires and the formation of subcultures, and additionally in response to legal penalisation, a sense of homosexual identity was emerging from the early eighteenth century. 'Sodomites' began to perceive themselves not as men who might from time to time commit acts defined by the law as sodomy, but as men with a particular sexual identity, forming part of a community of similar men.

Initially, sexual orientation was very much about desires which did not fit into a simple model of a biological drive intended for the reproduction of the species. Being attracted to members of the same sex, aroused by pain or domination, or sexually stimulated by wellington boots, had no apparent biological purpose and could become completely detached from sexual activity with another person. The notion that being heterosexual and becoming a parent were possibly equally problematic was seldom registered: few scholars of sex took Freud's ruthlessly logical line in the *Three Lectures on the History of Sexuality* (first published in German in 1905), that 'the sexual instinct and the sexual object are merely soldered together' and therefore the development of a heterosexual preference also required explanation and was by no means a given.

Those who are aware that their sexual preferences are such as to preclude them from living the kind of life society designates as normal are conscious of those preferences and the difficulties they bring with them, and may also present problems to society at large, if only by complicating categories which are assumed to be clear cut. Those who have never had to question the path set out for them are unlikely to have as clear a sense of their own desires and preferences as being distinct from what society deems appropriate. They may be dissatisfied with their lot in a greater or lesser degree without ever querying whether society's prescriptions meet their needs. As Freud noted in *Civilised Sexual Morality and Modern Nervous Illness* (1908), 'what a degree of renunciation, often on both sides, is entailed by marriage, and to what narrow limits married life … is narrowed down.'

Coping with it

Some cultures deal with same-sex-preference, the form of diverse sexual orientation that is perhaps most obvious, by assimilating the anomaly of sexual object-choice into an anomaly of gender. This may place the individual who prefers his or her same gender as an intermediate 'third sex', or situate the male homosexual as effeminate and the female homosexual as masculinized. In some cases these are recognized social roles associated with specific sexual practices, but in many societies although the roles exist as categories they are stigmatized and marginalized to various degrees, from being subjected to mild social disapproval and mockery to being penalized by death. Another way of integrating homosexual orientation into society has been through the structuring of male homosexual relationships into older man–younger man (or adolescent boy), in which the senior man is supposed to have a tutelary function in inducting the younger into full adult manhood. Behaviour which does not fit into these categories may be stigmatized, or else invisible. The macho male who took the insertive, 'masculine' role with an effeminate male, or the female partner of the crossed-dressed 'passing' woman, created problems for theorists. The first was often seen as hypermasculine with an excessive sexual drive, 'perverted' in his search for sensation rather than 'inverted' in his desires, the second was assumed to have been deceived by her partner or to be a shy, passive creature more scared of men than actively attracted to women.

While these may be the most obvious (and to many, the most disturbing) examples of sexual orientation, few individuals are completely free from some form of preference as to their sexual partner or type of activity. When someone is attracted to persons of the opposite gender, there may be quite a narrow range of actual individuals who are found attractive within that larger category. Again, those preferences which coincide with societal norms may go unremarked: a man who seeks out female partners younger than himself and physically smaller is not going to arouse much comment, whereas a man who manifests desire for women older or larger than himself is more likely to be conscious of a potentially embarrassing personal idiosyncrasy. Awareness of a particular orientation may also arise when an individual finds features attractive which are not currently fashionable: for example, plumpness in women when the trend is for supermodel slenderness. Individuals may also have specific situations in which their desires are most acutely stimulated: this is perhaps most noticeable in the case of people who invariably fall for unattainable others, or for partners who treat them badly in some way. Particular forms of sexual stimulation may also be desired, which may present problems unless the partner's desires are complementary.

Attempts at explanation

The reasons for such preferences are extremely hard to account for. There are many elements within sexual preference which it is exceedingly difficult to interpret as innate and part of the biological make-up. While identical twins are more likely than non-identical both to be homosexual, the likelihood only runs at about 50%: Bancroft, in *Human Sexuality and its Problems* (1989), hypothesizes a genetically-determined predisposition to react in similar ways to environmental influences. Though there may, debatably, be some innate predilection to become homosexual, the ways in which homosexual identity may be expressed are manifold and subject to a large degree of structuring by particular societies. In differing individuals in different societies such a predisposition might result in bisexual behaviour, in CELIBACY, or in becoming a drag queen or an activist for gay rights.

There are also individuals who may indulge in a particular type of sexual behaviour without its impinging on their sense of preferred identity. For example, homosexual behaviour is relatively common in single-sex institutions but does not necessarily lead to self-identification as homosexual or to similar activity outside the institution. Conversely, homosexual men and women may marry or have sexual intercourse with members of the opposite sex, without losing the belief that their 'innate' sexual leanings are entirely different. Furthermore, individuals have been known to undergo radical changes in their sexual preferences over the course of a lifetime.

Animal studies are not particularly illuminating. In some birds, imprinting takes place at an early age, and exposure to something seen at the critical stage of development is crucial for later object choice. However, such a mechanism does not seem to operate to anything like the same extent in mammals. Various forms of same-sex contact have been observed in different mammalian species, but these often serve the purpose of establishing dominance or submission for social purposes between individual animals or within the group, and to have a dubious relationship to sexual gratification as such. There are also cases in which animals in single-sex groups will mount one another, often at the dictates of a hormonal cycle: cows and heifers mounting one another is taken as a reliable sign that they are ready for breeding. There is little evidence, however, that homosexual relationships in any species are formed when opposite-sex partners are available and receptive.

Childhood influences of various kinds play an important role in the evolution of adult sexual orientation in the individual — for example, certain experiences can become associated with sexual arousal. Emotional experiences, in particular relationships with parents, can form patterns which are reiterated in the sexual sphere in later life. The reasons why similar influences (for example, among different members of the same family, with both heredity and environment in common) may result in different outcomes is, however, still obscure. Complex factors, involving idiosyncrasies of biological make-up, the individual's personal experiences, and the wider social environment, are probably all involved in the evolution of a person's sexual orientation.

LESLEY A. HALL

See also GENDER.

Shamans

Ethnologists since the nineteenth century have sometimes used the terms 'shaman', 'medicine man', 'sorceror', and 'magician' interchangeably to designate individuals, found in all 'primitive' societies, who possess magico–religious powers. 'Shamanism' has been used to describe a wide variety of practices and beliefs observable in many geographic areas, such as North and Central Asia, the Americas, Indonesia, and Oceania. By extension, the same term is applied in studying the religious history of 'civilized' societies such as the Indian, Germanic, and Chinese, all of which have 'mystical' or 'magical' elements. Yet it is misleading to identify shamanism simply with the 'primitive elements'

within a religion, for it is a clearly defined and symbolically sophisticated religious phenomenon in itself.

In the strict sense, shamanism is a religious phenomenon of Siberia and Central Asia, where the religious life of society centred on this figure. The word comes to us through Russian, from the Tungusic *saman*. Shamanism can best be defined as a technique of ecstasy, in which the soul of the shaman leaves the body and journeys through the spirit world. In their trances, shamans are able to communicate with the dead, and with demons, nature spirits, and the elements, without becoming subject to them. They speak secret or otherworldly languages, and, in the soul's 'magical flight', they can travel immense distances, ascend to the sky or descend to the underworld. Shamans cure illnesses, accompany the dead to the next world, and serve as mediators between people and the gods. They form a small mystical elite which directs the community's religious life and guards its 'soul'.

Shamans are of the elect, and have access to a region of the sacred inaccessible to other members of the community. They are persons who stand out in their respective societies by virtue of characteristics that, in modern Europe, represent the signs of a vocation or a religious crisis. They are recruited either by hereditary transmission of shamanic profession, or by spontaneous vocation ('calling' or 'election'). They are taught by ecstatic means, through dreams or trances, or by masters who instruct them in shamanic techniques, mythology, genealogy, secret languages, and the names and functions of spirits.

Initiation may take the form of a public ritual or a private dream or experience. One of the commonest forms of election is when the shaman encounters a divine or semidivine being who appears in a dream, sickness or other circumstance, tells him that he has been 'chosen', and incites him to follow a new rule of life. Sometimes the shaman's relation to the initiatory spirit is sexual, and the spirit becomes the shaman's celestial spouse. The spirits associated with a shaman vary in relation and familiarity to him: some are 'helpers' or 'familiars', whom he controls; others are 'tutelary', and teach him; still others are the divine or semidivine beings he conjures during seances.

The secret languages of a shaman are used to communicate with spirits and animal spirits: they are learned from a teacher or through his own efforts, i.e. directly from the spirits. A language often originates in animal or bird cries. The shaman's costume varies widely, and often incorporates animal symbolism (e.g. the feathers of birds, essential for the flight of the soul). The shamanic experience does not take place while shaman is in his everyday, profane dress, but only when he dons his sacred wardrobe.

The shaman is indispensable in any ceremony concerning the experiences of the human soul (which is, for example, inclined to forsake the body in ILLNESS). This is why, all through Asia and North America and elsewhere as well (e.g. in

Indonesia), the shaman performs the function of doctor and healer. Disease is generally attributed to the soul's having strayed away or been stolen (by the spirits of recently dead people), and treatment consists principally of finding it, capturing it, and forcing it to return to the patient's body. It is the shaman who announces the diagnosis, searches for and finds the patient's fugitive soul, and makes it return to animate the body.

The origin of sickness can also be the intrusion of a magical object into the patient's body or his 'possession' by evil spirits: the cure then consists of extracting the harmful object or expelling the demons. This may be accomplished by the shaman 'sucking' or seeming to pull out the object, such as a stone or an animal bone, from the afflicted part of the patient, thus removing the cause of the illness.

Shamans are known to possess unusual physical endurance, demonstrated in heavy masturbation, and insensitivity to fire and to knife cuts, and they also perform bodily feats such as escaping from tied ropes. Yet their principal gifts are those of the spirit, which include divination and clairvoyance. The shaman is a healer and a seer because he commands the techniques of ecstasy: his soul can safely abandon his body and roam vast distances before returning to his body, ascend to the sky and descend to the underworld. He knows the roads of extraterrestrial regions: sanctified by initiation, instructed by tutelary spirits, and protected by guardian spirits, he is the only human being able to challenge the dangers of these regions, and venture into a mystical geography.

Certain currents in modern medicine have initiated a renewal of focus on the powers of the imagination to heal the ailments of the body. Traditional shamans are thought to perform cures 'through the mind', by various ritualized, symbolic actions designed to dispel sickness by mimetic means. Thus, techniques and phenomona in contemporary medicine such as HYPNOSIS, autogenics, placebo response, and imaging, which stress the effects of mental or emotional states on physical illness or wellbeing, are occasionally referred to as a twentieth-century Western form of 'shamanism'.

NATSU HATTORI

Further reading
Achterberg, J. (1985). *Imagery in healing: shamanism and modern medicine.* New Science Library, Boston.

Eliade, M. (1964). *Shamanism: archaic techniques of ecstasy.* (trans. W. R. Trask). Routledge and Kegan Paul, London.

See also HEALING; MAGIC; POSSESSION.

Shame

In the beginning, there was no shame. *Genesis* tells us that Adam and Eve 'were both naked, the man and his wife, and were not ashamed.' Having eaten the forbidden fruit, however, they knew of their nakedness and sought to hide it. Shame thus came into existence, along with mortality, physical toil, and the pains of childbirth. In the Bible, shame is intrinsically connected with both the body and wrongdoing, or more precisely with self-consciousness of one's body and awareness of wrongdoing. Once they had disobeyed God, Adam and Eve became ashamed of their nakedness and took cover.

Similarly, in the ancient Greek world, shame was linked to the body etymologically and in Homer's tales also to nakedness and sexuality. The dread of being seen naked or making love, or being seen to witness love-making, to use examples from the *Odyssey*, might indicate that the idea of shame is tied to that of physical vulnerability. It also suggests that it is a fear of appearing other than one might like to in the eyes of others, mortal or divine. In a heroic culture, in which men like Odysseus and his son, Telemachus, are repeatedly referred to as 'god-like', this is more likely to be a fear of seeming base, stripped of dignity, and lacking in the requisite virtues of courage, wisdom, temperance, and so forth. It is the fear of revealing oneself as being closer to an animal than a god, of being no more than flesh and ruled by it, concomitant with the ignominious need to conceal oneself and crouch, rather than to be able to stand or walk tall — images associated by contrast with honour and pride.

In moral philosophy, feeling shame has generally been considered a natural disposition or sensation, and the fear of incurring it an universal motive for action or forbearance from antiquity onwards. It has also been taken as crucial evidence of the existence of an innate moral sense, most notably by Francis Hutcheson (1694–1746) and the Scottish school of moral philosophy.

Its management and careful manipulation has been deemed crucial in pedagogical practice and theory, especially in times when physical punishment was thought inefficacious or aberrant. In one of the most influential pedagogical treatises of all time, *Some Thoughts Concerning Education* (1693), John Locke urged parents to desist from beating their children and encouraged them to use the softer, but more effective, ways of shame and its counterpart, commendation.

Following World War II, especially in the context of understanding Japanese society from a Western point of view, much was made of the distinction between so-called 'shame' and 'guilt' cultures, a distinction introduced by Ruth Benedict (*The Chrysanthemum and the Sword*, 1946). The former rely on 'external sanctions for good behaviour', the latter on 'an internalized conviction of sin'. Although there seems to be a psychological difference between shame and guilt, to contrast cultures on that basis is at best misleading. Thus, while feelings of guilt tend to imply that someone other than oneself has been wronged in some way, one could feel ashamed of an action which did not involve anyone else. Beyond this, however, the two concepts and the feelings which they identify overlap to a large extent and are too complex to admit of a sharp contrast. At the cultural level, the matter is, if anything, more complex still; it is difficult to

imagine a society in which fear of shame was a significant or leading motive for action or forbearance, without 'an internalized conviction' of wrongdoing and of breach of a socially accepted code of behaviour. SYLVANA TOMASELLI

Further reading
Williams, B. (1993). *Shame and necessity*. University of California Press, Berkeley.

Shinto Dictionaries, both English and Japanese, commonly present 'Shintoism' or 'Shinto' (the more common term), as a system of ancestor and nature worship native to Japan. Shinto as a systematic, unified religion is as much a creation of modern Japan's Meiji state (1867–1912) as it is something that has existed throughout Japan's history. The basic meaning of the word 'Shinto' until the nineteenth century was local religion in general, and although Shinto usually referred to Japanese religion, it did not necessarily have to (e.g. the 1605 anthropological work *Ryūkyū shintō-ki*, or *Account of Local Religion [Shinto] in Ryukyu*, the Kingdom of Ryukyu then being a separate country from Japan). Viewed historically, we may identify three related yet distinct varieties of 'Shinto': (i) local religious practices and beliefs that originated before Buddhist influence; (ii) certain of these local practices and beliefs that Buddhism later subsumed, systematized, and modified, from the ninth to the eighteenth centuries; and (iii) Japan's 'national religion', with varying degrees of connection to the state, in the nineteenth and twentieth centuries. Shinto never articulated an overall theory of the body, but the first variety of Shinto closely linked the sexual body with agriculture and the forces of nature.

Important artifacts from the middle Jōmon period (*c.* 3500–2400 BCE) and later, include phallic stones (*sekibō*), ranging in height from 2 m to 50 cm, and clay female figures with prominent breasts and hips (*dogū*), sometimes appearing pregnant, most approximately 30 cm in height. Although there is disagreement over the details, most scholars agree that ancient inhabitants of Japan connected these objects with magico-religious rites to promote bountiful harvests. Prehistoric residents of the Japanese islands probably connected the mystery of human reproduction with agricultural productivity, and the female figures symbolized both mother and earth as locus of mysterious power.

The notion of mysterious power gradually developed into the Shinto concept of *kami*, often translated as 'deity'. The most basic meaning of the term is: that which is above other things like it — in other words, that which is distinctive. An unusually large tree, an outcropping of rock, a waterfall, certain animals, and even certain people are examples of things that have qualified as *kami* owing to some distinctive attribute the local people regarded as significant. Though part of a world of spirits, *kami* were not transcendent. They linked the visible world with the realms beyond direct sensory apprehension.

According to ancient mythology, the Japanese islands themselves were created by the sexual activities of anthropomorphic *kami*. For example, in *Chronicles of Japan*, two creation deities, Izanagi and Izanami, stand on the Floating Bridge of Heaven and say 'Is there no country beneath?' They then thrust down a heavenly jewelled spear, repeatedly, until they found the vast ocean beneath. Brine dripped from the point of the spear, coagulated, and became an island on which the two deities dwelt. They continued the creation process after the female deity explained that her body has a place that is the source of femininity and the male deity explained that his had a place that is the source of masculinity. They united these two places to form numerous other islands. In these myths the deities' sexuality was the creative power of nature.

Shinto typically associated disease and death with pollution and, accordingly, developed purification rites. It celebrated health, prosperity, and life, which it associated with the creative forces of nature. A common metaphor for nature's generative forces was the sexual body. Phallic stones, poles, and etchings along roadsides, for example, functioned to protect against nature's polluting forces. Ancient agricultural deities often existed as a male and female pair, sometimes depicted embracing each other. Wooden or stone representations of male or female genitalia, or a pair of such objects, became the *kami*-body in shrines throughout many parts of the Japanese islands (the *kami*-body is an object in which the spirit of a deity was thought to reside). Even today, representations of sexual organs occasionally serve as the *kami* in Japanese shrines and can be seen in public festivals celebrating the shrine's *kami*.

During the late nineteenth century, Japan's Meiji state sought to revamp Shinto to enhance the process of nation-building (i.e. of Japanese thinking of themselves as Japanese). As part of a general policy of policing morality, the leaders of modern Japan sought to suppress the overtly sexual symbolism of Shinto. Instead of the sexual body, modern Japan's state Shinto stressed *kokutai*, the 'national body' (often translated 'national polity') — a vague but potent concept of Japanese essence embodied in an allegedly unbroken lineage of emperors descending from the solar deity (Amaterasu). What began in ancient Japan as worship of the sexual body, ended in modern Japan (until 1946) as worship of the national body. Neither 'body' plays a major role in today's Shinto, but vestiges of each remain. G. SMITS

See also CREATION MYTHS.

Shivering A common experience; the explanation is a stimulus to rapid muscular contractions, set off from the temperature-regulating centre in the HYPOTHALAMUS, in response to cooling of the skin and the blood. The contractions generate heat, helping to maintain deep body temperature despite increased heat loss during COLD EXPOSURE. Shivering occurs in

FEVER when there is effectively a re-setting of the hypothalamic 'thermostat'.   S.J.

See FEVER; TEMPERATURE REGULATION.

Shock has many meanings in common usage.

Most often it refers to a sudden mental or emotional experience ranging from a trivial unpleasant surprise to the deep disturbance of personal disaster or bereavement; 'shell-shock' refers to distress and disturbed behaviour in the aftermath of battle. When the media report someone as 'suffering from shock' this may vaguely imply 'only' shock, without physical INJURY, whereas a clinician will use the term for a potentially dangerous condition with quite specific physical features. This last will be the main topic under this heading.

In medical terms, shock occurs when the blood supply to the tissues is inadequate to meet the requirements of the body. It is a sudden, or acute, failure of the circulation.

Causes of shock

The simplest and most frequent example of acute failure of the circulation is FAINTING. The cause may be a sudden emotional or painful experience — a physical reaction, linked to a mental 'shock' via the AUTONOMIC NERVOUS SYSTEM, which causes slowing of the heart rate. When the heart slows excessively, it does not pump out enough blood and the BLOOD PRESSURE decreases. The person may say that they 'feel faint' because they experience dizziness due to the decreased blood pressure and the resulting inadequate blood flow to the brain. If the blood pressure is not restored by, for example, lying down or sitting with the head between the knees, they may lose consciousness. Generally, the heart rate will quickly return to normal and the person awakens with an anxious crowd looking down at them.

Fainting may result also from standing still particularly in very hot conditions. This can cause the blood to collect or 'pool' in the lower limbs. Less blood reaches the heart and so less can be pumped out. If the blood pressure decreases excessively, then the patient may faint. Fighter pilots can encounter a similar effect when they make their aircraft turn very tightly at high speed. The high 'G' forces cause blood to drain into their lower limbs. They may experience a 'grey out 'and then a 'black out' before losing consciousness as the blood pressure gradually decreases. An anti-gravity suit is designed to maintain pressure on the blood vessels in the lower limbs and so prevent pooling of the blood with the resulting reduction in blood pressure.

A simple faint can be treated by laying the person flat. This will help to restore the blood pressure to normal; consciousness will then return within a short time. More serious causes of shock require appropriate medical treatment.

The clinical picture of shock which is more than a transient faint includes the signs and symptoms of both inadequate circulation and the body's attempt to compensate for this circulatory failure. Reflex responses to reductions in blood pressure act to prevent or minimize the decrease. The heart rate will increase in an attempt to pump out more blood and this can be felt as a rapid pulse rate (although in a simple faint it is *initially* slow). The blood vessels to the non-vital organs may constrict in an attempt to move blood away from these tissues towards the vital organs. This can be seen as extreme pallor of the skin and may be one of the first signs that a person is about to faint. The pulse is not only rapid but is described as 'thin' or 'thready'. Hormones, such as ADRENALINE, are released into the blood stream, and SWEATING, due to autonomic nervous activity can make the patient's skin feel moist to the touch.

Types of shock and their treatment

Hypovolaemic shock follows major blood loss which may be caused by trauma or during surgery. The blood loss can be visible and obvious or may be hidden as occurs in some types of fractures of leg bones or in internal bleeding from abdominal organs. The signs are similar to those in a patient who has fainted, with a low volume pulse and a pale, moist skin. However, the pulse rate will always be rapid in a patient suffering from hypovolaemic shock as the heart attempts to compensate for the low blood pressure.

RESUSCITATION from haemorrhagic shock following blood loss or a major burn requires rapid BLOOD TRANSFUSION and/or administration of other intravenous fluids to replace the circulating volume and to ensure the circulation of well oxygenated blood from the lungs to the brain and other vital organs. An intravenous cannula is inserted and fluids are administered directly into the circulation. As well as whole blood, fluid replacement may involve administration of salt fluids, plasma, or artificial substitutes, and concentrated red blood cells. Blood contains many different components including antibodies which require the blood to be 'cross-matched' before administration to the patient. There is considerable research directed at producing artificial blood substitutes which can be used without the need for cross-matching. These are designed to be able to transport oxygen efficiently to the tissues with less risk of producing a transfusion reaction and of transferring infection from the donor to the recipient.

Cardiogenic shock A HEART ATTACK (myocardial infarction) is usually the result of a blockage of one of the coronary arteries which supply the heart muscle. If the artery is relatively large or supplies a particularly vital part of the heart, the damaged tissue may reduce the ability of the heart to pump blood around the body. If blood supply to the tissues is decreased because of the reduced output from the heart, then the patient may be in cardiogenic shock.

Cardiogenic shock is usually treated in a specialist intensive care unit where the patient's condition can be monitored closely and the appropriate drugs administered. Anaphylactic shock also requires rapid and skilled medical treatment using intravenous fluids and powerful drugs to restore the circulation to normal. Drugs which cause constriction of the blood vessels may be required. However, the major complication of this therapy is that these drugs produce an increase in the work performed by the heart and an increase in the heart's oxygen consumption, with the result that any primary heart disease may be worsened.

Anaphylactic shock can develop as a result of a serious ALLERGY. The allergen causes the release of chemicals within the body which act to make the small arterial blood vessels dilate and to leak fluid from the capillaries into the surrounding tissues. The dilation of the blood vessels has the effect of expanding the capacity of the circulation, whilst leakage of fluid into the tissues reduces the volume of the blood. The net effect is that there is insufficient filling of the circulation and the blood pressure falls. This can cause a major decrease of blood pressure but the person's skin may be flushed and reddened rather than pale. Leakage of fluid into the tissues may cause swelling which may be seen most clearly around the face. Swelling of the vocal cords can reduce or completely block the patient's airway and so prevent them breathing. In a severe case, the condition can be life threatening and immediate medical treatment is required to combat the allergic response and to assist breathing.

Septic shock Some types of very severe INFECTIONS (sepsis), can release toxins which also cause the small blood vessels to dilate and to leak fluid into the tissues. This septic shock has the same effect as an anaphylactic shock but is preceded by signs of a severe infection and develops much more gradually. The lungs may be badly affected and the leakage of fluid into the lungs can greatly reduce the ability to transfer oxygen into the blood stream.

The mainstay of therapy for any infection and particularly for septic shock is eradication of the infection. Powerful ANTIBIOTICS are administered according to the specific clinical situation, and any focus of infection or abscess must be drained surgically.

Consequences of severe shock of any type

When the patient's blood pressure decreases, sensors in the blood vessels (baroreceptors) send signals which lead to an increase in heart rate, more powerful beating of the heart, and constriction of the blood vessels supplying the less vital organs. Breathing becomes less effective **because** blood **flow** to parts of the LUNG, and therefore the uptake of oxygen is inadequate, and the patient may be seen to breathe more heavily. Fluid begins to move into the circulation from the tissues to restore the balance, but this is a relatively slow process.

Some tissues are particularly sensitive to severe shock if it is prolonged. The KIDNEYS can be damaged by insufficient blood flow and the patient may develop acute kidney failure. This can require treatment with an artificial kidney until normal function recovers.

After major shock, respiratory failure can occur and this may require the patient to receive ARTIFICIAL VENTILATION to maintain sufficient delivery of oxygen to the tissues.

A *shock liver* syndrome can occur in patients in whom marked reduction in blood pressure has persisted for some hours. This can lead to many complications. For example, the LIVER is responsible for making components necessary for clotting of the blood and lack of these components causes bleeding spontaneously or from relatively minor injury.

Shock, defined as a failure of the circulation, can therefore range from a simple faint which requires minimal treatment to more serious conditions which require skilled medical and nursing care to treat successfully. The essential feature of shock is an inadequate blood supply to the tissues to meet the requirements for oxygen supply and the removal of waste products of metabolism. Treatment must be rapid to protect organs such as the kidneys, lungs, and liver from damage. The challenge for medical staff is to prevent death from irreversible shock by perfecting in-hospital treatment of the seriously ill. Such optimum care will give these patients a chance to return to functional life. GAVIN KENNY

See also ALLERGY; AUTONOMIC NERVOUS SYTEM; BLOOD PRESSURE; BLOOD CIRCULATION; FAINTING; G AND G SUITS; HAEMORRHAGE; INJURY; STRESS.

Shoes

Shoes may be divided into two categories: open shoes, such as the sandal or Japanese *geta*, and closed shoes, including ankle boots and high shoes. No doubt the first shoes were simple protective wraps. Until the seventeenth century, men and women wore similar styles of shoes.

The thirteenth to fifteenth centuries witnessed the popularity in Europe of the long, pointed *poulaine* or *cracowe*, with the point often stiffened and curled up to facilitate walking. Clearly phallic, the poulaine received condemnation in a Papal bull of 1468 (see figure). Another extreme style, the *chopine*, with a very thick sole of wood or cork, was popular in the fifteenth and sixteenth centuries and was unsuccessfully outlawed by the Venetian Republic in 1430.

From antiquity, shoes constructed of costly materials, including gems or gold embroidery, revealed wealth and social class. Beginning in the last quarter of the fourteenth century, shoes were worn with *pattens* — carved wooden supports with pedestals under the heel and ball — to protect the shoes. In the sixteenth century the high heel appeared, worn by both men and women. These, too, were worn inside another shoe, or *pantofle*, to protect them. Prominent persons sometimes wore shoes to increase their height. Louis XIV, who was only 5 feet 5 inches tall, wore shoes with 5-inch heels covered in red leather, setting off a fashion trend among courtiers.

By the end of the seventeenth century, only women wore the high heel, which accentuates the

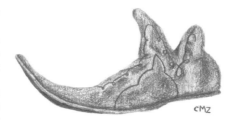

A fifteenth century poulaine. Drawing by Caitlin Marie Zacharias.

curvature of the spine, thrusts out the posterior and breasts, and creates a gait in which the hips sway from side to side. Good deportment called for learning how to walk properly in fashionable shoes. Toward the end of the eighteenth century, Petrus Camper, a professor of anatomy, wrote a little book detailing the ill effects of high heels on women's health, particularly during pregnancy.

Tiny feet in women have been admired in different cultures. The practice of foot binding in China produced the lotus-foot, which fitted into a tiny, pointed shoe. In the fairy tale, the glass slipper could fit only the tiny foot of Cinderella, who became the bride of the prince. Historically, some women purposely wore shoes too small to make their feet look smaller.

Shoes are involved in a number of customs. An Anglo-Saxon father gave one of his daughter's shoes to her bridegroom. During the Middle Ages, it was customary to kiss the Pope's shoe. In an old Flemish custom, Christmas gifts were brought in *sabots*, or wooden shoes.

Shoes, including the lotus-shoe, modern stiletto, and extremely high heels, have been the object of shoe fetishism. The eighteenth-century novelist Nicolas-Edme Restif de la Bretonne imagined a story in which the narrator steals some rose-coloured shoes from his employer's wife and kisses one shoe while he ejaculates into the other. The male shoe fetishist is often a masochist who imagines himself being impaled by the high heel. Fetish-style shoes have been brought out into the open by members of heavy metal bands, such as KISS, who wear high-heeled platform shoes during performances.

KRISTEN L. ZACHARIAS

See also FEET.

Shoulder

Shoulder Like the HIP, this is an example of the 'ball and socket' (or *multiaxial*) type of joint, with the head of the long bone of the upper arm (*humerus*) articulating with a hollow in the shoulder blade (*scapula*). The collar bone (*clavicle*) also plays a role in maintaining the stability of the shoulder joint, as it acts like a strut, holding the joint and the upper arm away from the chest and thus allowing the upper limb to swing freely. Because it is relatively thin and in a vulnerable position, the clavicle is broken more often than any other bone. The clavicle and scapula together form the shoulder (*pectoral*) girdle. Movement occurs in three planes: forwards (*extension*) and backwards (*flexion*); outwards (*abduction*) and inwards (*adduction*); twist in (*internal rotation*) and twist out (*outward rotation*). Combinations of these movements also give rise to 'circumduction', as at the hip. The shoulder has a greater degree of mobility than the hip, but is less stable, and therefore is more likely to be dislocated by injury. This is

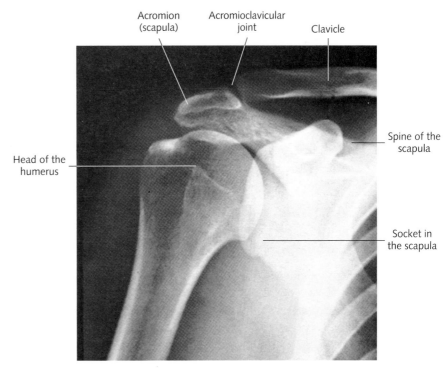

X-ray of adult shoulder. Reproduced, with permission, from *Cunningham's textbook of anatomy*, (12th edn), OUP.

partly due to the fact that the shoulder 'socket' (*glenoid fossa*) is much shallower than the socket of the hip (*acetabulum*). In addition, the capsule is less strong than in the hip and the muscles acting at the shoulder, are less powerful. This vulnerability is the trade-off for the greater mobility of the shoulder joint, which is essential for even simple activities such as combing the hair. Inflammation of the tendons of the muscles surrounding the shoulder joint (*rotator cuff muscles*) can give rise to pain on lifting the arm (*frozen shoulder*). WILLIAM R. FERRELL

See also JOINTS; SKELETON.

Siamese twins

Conjoined twins result when there is incomplete cleavage and separation of *monozygotic* (single egg) twins. The twins may be joined at the head end (*craniopagus*) or tail end (*ischiopagus* and *pyopagus*), but the majority who survive are joined ventrally with varying degrees of coalescence (*thoracopagus* and *omphalopagus*). They may share heart, blood vessels, liver, and gut. Successful surgical separation will depend upon the degree of coalescence of major organs.

Throughout recorded history there are many references to surviving conjoined twins. One of the earliest reports concern Mary and Eliza Chalkhurst, born at Biddenden, Kent, England in the year 1100. They died in 1134 within six hours of each other. They bequeathed 20 acres of land to the church wardens from which a yearly income was used to provide, for the poor, cakes with the imprint of their effigies 'in their habit as they

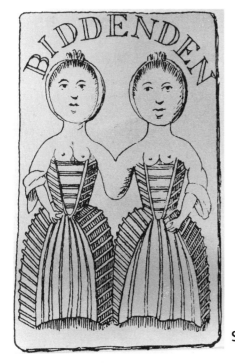

'The Biddenden Maid biscuits' — reproduction of an imprinted cake. From Ballantyne, J. W. (1904), *Manual of antenatal pathology and hygiene*. Wm. Green, Edinburgh.

lived' together with bread and cheese. For many years this ceremony took place on Easter Monday at their birthplace. As late as 1874 an observer noted that the Biddenden Maids cakes are 'simple flour and water, are four inches long by two inches wide and are much sought after'. They bear the date 1100 and also their age at death.

The most notable were the Siamese twins, Eng and Chang, who were born in Siam in 1811, the fourth pregnancy of a Chinese father and a half-Siamese/Chinese mother. They were joined at the chest and upper abdomen. They were 'discovered' in 1829 by a Scottish trader, Andrew Hunter who realized their commercial potential and took them to England in 1830, where he exhibited them as 'The Siamese Double Boys' for five years. Chang, Eng, and Hunter then embarked on a tour of America, where Phineas T. Barnum 'acquired' them in 1835 as exhibits in 'The Greatest Show on Earth'. By 1840 they had earned enough money to retire and became gentlemen farmers in North Carolina. In 1844 they married Addie and Sally Yates, daughters of a nearby farmer, and during the next 20 years had 21 children between them, 10 to Addie, who was married to Chang, and 11 to Sally.

With the advent of the Civil War in 1861 Chang and Eng were forced to move north with their families, and in New York they rejoined Barnum and recouped their lost fortunes. During their travels on show they were seen by many famous surgeons, who considered their separation. Sir James Young Simpson, Professor of Medicine and Midwifery in the University of Edinburgh, gives full details of his examination of them in the *British Medical Journal* of February 13, 1869.

Whilst on a voyage from Liverpool to New York in 1872, Chang had a paralytic stroke and was partially dragged about by Eng for some months thereafter. Fortunately they had by this time amassed sufficient money to return to the South and rebuild their mansions. At the age of 63, Chang, who was the more argumentative and aggressive of the brothers, and who drank to excess, developed a chest infection. It had been the custom for many years for the families to spend two weeks in alternate mansions. Chang's 'bronchitis' developed on Monday 12 January, 1874, and in spite of being unwell he moved to Eng's house on the Thursday of that week. He died on the Saturday morning whilst sleeping on a couch in front of the fire. Eng wakened and discovered his dead brother but died a little more than two hours later. Postmortem examinations showed that they shared muscle and liver tissue, and they were buried, still joined, in a single grave in North Carolina. JIM NIELSON

FORRESTER COCKBURN

Sighing

is commonly interpreted as an expressive, though usually involuntary, 'gesture', perhaps of boredom or despair, or sometimes of relief. But there is more to it than that — it is of interest both for its reflex mechanism and for its physiological significance

A sigh, defined as a breath larger than 3 times the average breath volume, is a normal phenomenon occurring in healthy adults, when they are relaxed in a semi-recumbent position, at an average rate of 9–10 per hour. There are two types of sigh, according to the exact point at which they interrupt the regular BREATHING cycle. Fifty per cent of sighs 'take off' from the early expiratory phase following a normal intake of breath (Type I), while the rest 'take off' from the end of the expiratory phase (Type II). The new-born human infant, asleep, typically has Type II sighs (2 × average breath volume) at a frequency of 18–70 per hour in the first 24 hours of life; by 5 days the frequency is down to 6–36 per hour. Studies in anaesthetized cats and rabbits, who also sigh, have demonstrated the presence of an inspiratory-augmenting reflex, mediated by VAGUS NERVE receptors within the lung airway, and this mechanism may be responsible, in part, for the sighing. The reflex is particularly sensitive to excitation after short periods of airway occlusion resulting in patchy lung collapse with increasing lung stiffness and hypoxia. With a sigh, collapsed areas of lung open up, removing the stimulus to sigh and at the same time restoring lung stiffness to its normal range. Moreover, we now know that a large breath will stimulate production, by some cells in the lung airspaces, of a surface-active material that minimizes the surface tension in the fluid lining the airspaces. This surface tension would otherwise tend to close the airspaces, particularly when they are small. Quiet breathing, whether spontaneous or on a ventilator, in adult humans at rest is associated over time with an increase in lung stiffness; this is completely reversed by 1–2 sighs, which may explain the sense of satisfaction and well-being produced by the sigh.

During the 1930s, sighing became a symptom of a 'respiratory neurosis'. It was a particular feature of soldiers who had served in the 1914–18 War and developed 'effort syndrome'. This was first thought to be a 'cardiac neurosis', particularly because of the frequency of left submammary pain and the complaints of 'breathlessness at rest' together with 'inability to get enough air into the lungs'. Objectively, all that was found was an irregularity of respiratory depth and rate together with frequent (Type I) sighing; the heart and lungs were normal. Breathing became abnormal with the slightest emotional stimuli. Extreme yawning often accompanied the sighing, and this commonly caused temporary relief of the sense of respiratory oppression. Nowadays, we would consider these patients as having a *chronic anxiety state*, with or without *panic*, with a predisposition to overbreathe in response to stress. Sighing (Type I) may occur at rates of up to 25/min! We have no clear-cut neurophysiogical basis for this breathing behaviour, now called a 'HYPERVENTILATION disorder'. However, we do know that breathing can be 'driven' by activation of the amygdaloid nucleus within the limbic system — a complex brain area concerned with feeling and emotions. Common experience confirms the reality of this link, no better documented than by W. Shakespeare in Jacques' soliloquy in *As You Like It*, Act II, Scene 5 — 'All the world's a stage ... And then the lover, Sighing like a furnace, with a woeful ballad, Made to his mistress' eyebrow.' ABE GUZ

Further reading

Baker, D. M. (1934). Sighing respiration as a symptom. *The Lancet*, **Jan 27th**, 174–6.

Bendixen, H. H., Smith, G. M., and Mead, J. (1964). Pattern of ventilation in young adults. *Journal of Applied Physiology*, **19**(2), 195–8.

Thach, B. T. and Taeusch, H. W. Jr. (1976). Sighing in newborn human infants: role of inflation-augmenting reflex. *Journal of Applied Physiology*, **41**(4), 502–7.

See also HYPERVENTILATION; LUNGS; SURFACTANT.

Singing

One definition of singing is 'the utterance of words or sounds in tuneful succession'. Another is 'to make musical sounds with the voice'. But the oldest musical 'instrument' is the human voice, so tautology leads us to *musiche*, the Greek word signifying the 'art of the Muses'. Such chanting, together with that derived from Jewish traditions, evolved into Gregorian Chant, the sacred music of the Catholic Church, taught at the Schola Cantorum in Rome (founded in 590 by Gregory the Great).

Evolution of song

Save for early manuscripts and the sacred music still sung in synagogue and church, little can be known about the origins of song. In his brilliant survey of the evolution of SPEECH in relation to LANGUAGE and human brain development (1996), the neuroscientist Deacon has observed that there are no extant 'simple' languages, only the present complex ones. These comprise different linguistic forms of grammar and syntax, moulded by cultural idiosyncrasies, mutual interaction, and, above all, the specific influence that the language potential of early hominids had on brain evolution through natural selection. This surely would also have been the case for song's prehistory, which of course is also unknown. However, its nature may perhaps be surmised from the first linguistic communication between mother and infant which, if not in the womb itself through transmitted sound, is in the instinctive, inherently tuneful, and innately beautiful sound of the lullaby, whether sung or simply hummed. Musicologists recognize that Jewish and Greek sacred chant, plainsong, psalmody, and motet, both liturgical and secular, and their parallels in folksong, the lyric poetry of the troubadours' song and the madrigal, were all formative in the subsequent development of opera as an important aspect of the Renaissance. All of these, together with the later development of *lieder*, that distinctive German song style for the accompanied solo voice, which joins music, poetry, and its interpretation into a singular whole, have contributed to sung music — both classical and in the multitude of forms today.

As a musical instrument the singing voice has wide tonal compass and uniquely variable pitch, intensity, and stress. These and other prosodic features can fill even simple tones with emotional charge, as in psalmody. Here, in the solemn context of the mass and of the expectations of those hearing it, agony and love are portrayed as spiritual and reverential, appropriate to sacred music; intensely beautiful in its own way but, through religious observance, containing, not freeing, the spirit. When it encompasses all emotions, beautiful singing is epitomized by the ideals sought in the Italianate *Bel Canto* tradition, which came to perfection through the development of the operatic form. Its essence and secular appeal rested then, and to this day, on the emotional response of the listener to the production particularly of perfectly sung vowels in the arias for the solo voice, now in harmony with orchestra and chorus. Indeed, such emphasis on the quality of the open vowels, achieved by years of assiduous practice, was also at the heart of Gregorian chant, in which voices of different *tessitura* (the natural centre and tonal surround of each voice) would sing the tenor or falsetto parts. Then, the 'tenor' voice was the 'lower' voice, 'holding' the plainsong melody in long, drawn out notes, progressing smoothly from one note to the next in 'legato', sung either solo or by one half of the chorus. The upper (falsetto) voices responded in Amens or *antiphons* (short refrains). These, as well as other exclamatory additions, such as the *Kyrie* and *Gloria in excelsis*, allowed a more florid style of singing, but constrained nevertheless, so that emotion was subservient to the awe and solemnity appropriate to the Mass. But not so in opera, where legato in a favourite aria can still an audience and then climactically bring it to its feet over the full spectrum of human emotions, from love to hate, from grief to happiness. It can reveal evil or good intent as in Iago's scheming, or display the ambivalence of Carmen's love.

And so on to the German *lieder*, epitomized by Schubert's extraordinary genius in creating songs and song cycles. These were no longer constructed so that each repeating verse had the same musical form; instead, based on the poetry of Goethe, Schiller, and their successors, sonority and melody now captured and enhanced the dramatic content of their lyric poetry, for each consonant, word, and line.

Beautiful singing, then, perhaps even more than speech itself, proclaims the emotional state of mind of the singer and hence, through the linguistic and emotional content of the words and the quality of the composed music, recapitulates a similar state in the minds of listeners, magically uniting composer, performer, and audience. The commonality of such a collective experience thus reveals the full extent of the communicative power of the highly evolved, culturally moulded gift (but from whom?) of human language, expressed in song as well as speech.

Sound generation

The terms 'tenor' and 'falsetto' refer to the early recognition that in the singing of notes of ascending or descending pitch within the great scale, individual voices show a 'break', requiring a distinct readjustment of voice production. The lower range was called *voce di piena* or *voce di petto*, meaning 'full voice' or 'voice of the chest'; the upper one, *voce finte*, or 'head voice'. These descriptions reveal the early recognition of the two principal voice 'registers' by relating them to the perceived placement or apparent source of the voice. In either case there is in fact only one sound source, that of the 'phonating' glottis (the aperture between the vocal cords). It is this sound which is modulated by the articulatory movements of the jaw, tongue, lips, and palate to add syllable, fricative, and other phonetically-distinct components to shape the natural sound or timbre of the individual voice. The willed intention to sing or speak, or for that matter the occurrence of an involuntary gasp or groan, depends on two sets of movements due to muscular activity; those of the thorax leading to expiratory airflow (see BREATHING), and those of the laryngeal cartilages in the voice box. In the latter case the vocal cords are brought together (*adduction*), interrupting the airflow. This process is not itself directly perceived, only the sense of vocal effort in generating the intensity of the intended sound, which through lifelong learning is inextricably bound to the sound heard 'in one's head'. In common usage it is said that the vocal cords 'vibrate', but this is not actually correct in physical terms. Instead, the sound is generated secondarily to the sudden interruption of the expiratory airflow by cord adduction; the driving pressure in the airway below the cords (*subglottal pressure*) then forces the cords apart and a spring-like action closes them again. This cycle repeats in oscillatory fashion until the singing breath is exhausted or the 'voicing' ceased through voluntary action, by the moving apart (*abduction*) of the vocal cords. Such 'valving' of the airflow occurs at a frequency governed by the endowed mass and thickness of the vocal cords, and most importantly by the tension within them; this latter, a function of their length, is determined by the position of the different laryngeal cartilages, which is governed by activity in the extrinsic laryngeal muscles, supported by the intrisic 'vocalis' muscle. The actual sound is generated by the repeated compression and decompression of the gas particles immediately above the glottis, this process being acoustically magnified and harmonically enriched by the resonance and filtering properties of the vocal tract above. But control over the harmonic balance, and hence over the timbre of the voice, can only occur within the harmonic range determined by the overall frequency content of sound emission from the cords themselves.

These scientific facts only complement that which those versed in the Gregorian and *Bel Canto* traditions already knew, and which is still emphasized: that the aesthetic goal of perfectly sung vowels can only be met, with few exceptions, by years of diligent practice. The trained singer learns to control these properties, not through proprioception, as with the learning of limb motor skills, but through the acoustic goal of the quality of the sounds produced. Interestingly — save perhaps for the low frequency (6–8 Hz) intensity modulation of tones that occurs in *vibrato* — the frequency of sung notes is not directly represented in the frequency of the neural commands to the laryngeal muscles; rather, the frequency of action potentials in the motor nerves is simply that which is necessary to generate the muscle tensions for the intended note. Thus a larynx removed from a cadaver will generate rich, pure tones if the vocal cords are manually adducted in the presence of a supplied flow of air: a macabre scientific fact about the production of human sound in stark contrast to aesthetic considerations!

Musical prosody

Simulation however could never match the human skills used in singing, the way the physical attributes of intensity, pitch, and harmonic content are used serially to create stress and intonation. These, together with tempo and rhythm, link the unitary phonetic events (*phonemes*) of consonant, syllable, and fricative into the linguistically-complete words which symbolically represent, through verb and noun, both the world of action and things about us, and also our emotions ('affect') generated within.

The fundamental importance of prosody in relation to human speech and song, where the timing of stress within a word can determine its linguistic function as noun or verb, is well expressed in 'office psalmody'. There each syllable is represented by a single or sustained note as in *Dom in nus vo bis cum*, and it is only the entire tonal progression of notes and intervals within this simple vocal line which conjoins the phonemes into linguistically meaningful words. The control over sound intensity needed to produce a beautiful, sustained tone at constant or smoothly-changing pitch and intensity in legato, or needed for stress, as in vocal attack, is wholly dependent on the dynamics of the pressure (*subglottal pressure*) that drives the expiratory airflow and that can be said to 'power' vocalization. The release of this pressure for the normal, vocally 'clear' attack (*coup de glotte*), or the *mezza voce* or 'breath' attack, requires precise timing of respiratory and laryngeal movements. If this timing fails, tones are slurred; if the vocal cords do not fully oppose a 'breathy' sound is produced. It is the timing of such skilled movements that is probably disrupted in the particular disturbance of vocalization (*dysarthria*) associated with lesions of the cerebellum, a structure intimately involved in motor 'learning' and now shown by imaging techniques to be active during vocalization. These and related topics, including the mechanical characteristics of breathing, bear also on the usually contentious matter of breath control in singing.

One surprising feature of the scientific analysis of breathing movements in singing is the finding that, except at high lung volume and at the onset of high notes at low intensity, the diaphragm is not actively involved, contrary to the emphasis given to the diaphragm's importance by voice teachers. Pressure measurements have shown that the diaphragm is mainly in a passive state, not undergoing active contraction through nervous control, so that it does not directly power sound production. However, it does serve mechanically to couple abdominal and ribcage motions, in which case abdominal muscle activity would relieve the ribcage from gravitational effects due to the mass of visceral organs. This frees the ribcage to contribute to the dynamics of subglottal pressure changes used in vocal stress. Nevertheless, the sensations generated in the chest wall during singing have traditionally been referred to the diaphragm, and this practice will doubtless continue.

When, through lifetime learning, habit, and experience, our movements become more and more automatic, the total sensory experience associated with them reduces to one of 'effortless' action that barely intrudes into consciousness. Breath and laryngeal control during speech and singing epitomize this state and when achieved set the cornerstone of supreme vocal performance, freeing the mind to dwell solely on artistic matters of interpretation — and it is these which eventually unite singer and audience.   TOM SEARS

Further reading

Crocker, R. L. (1966). *A history of musical style.* Mcgraw-Hill, New York.

Deacon, T. (1997). *The symbolic species.* The Penguin Press, Allen Lane.

Sears, T. A. (1977). Some neural and mechanical aspects of singing. In *Music and the brain*, (ed. M. Critchley and R. A. Henson), pp. 78–94. Heineman, London.

See also LARYNX; MUSIC AND THE BODY; VOICE.

Sinus From the Latin, meaning a cavity, channel, or hollow. In the body there are several types of sinus, matching these definitions. The air-containing *cavities* so-named are within the SKULL bones, enclosed except for openings into the nasal cavity; these are the frontal sinuses (in each side of the forehead), and the maxillary sinuses (in the cheek bones). Their lining can become acutely or chronically infected (sinusitis), causing pain and muco-purulent nasal discharge (catarrh). The *channels* known as sinuses are blood-containing spaces such as those in the SPLEEN, LIVER, and bone marrow; they are not shut off from the circulating blood, but their width allows greater stagnation than capillary BLOOD VESSELS, for specific functions such as the addition and the removal of blood cells and other constituents. The venous drainage channels of the BRAIN, inside the skull, and that of the HEART MUSCLE, also go by this name; likewise dilated regions of some blood vessels, notably the

carotid sinuses in the neck, which have stretch receptors important in the regulation of the arterial BLOOD PRESSURE; also dilated parts of lymphatic channels, and of milk channels behind the NIPPLES. The *hollows* so named are more often like dead-end channels or pits–abnormal connections to the surface of the skin from deeper areas of infection.   S.J.

Skeletal muscle moves the SKELETON and is responsible for all our *voluntary* movements, as well as for the *automatic* movements required, for example, to stand, to hold up our head, and to breathe. (Other involuntary functions involve SMOOTH MUSCLE and CARDIAC MUSCLE.)

As well as being the 'motors' of the body, muscles are also the brakes and shock absorbers. They can be used as heaters (when shivering) and also function as a store of protein if we should face malnutrition.

Individual muscles, such as the biceps in the arm, are made up of large numbers (about 100 000 in biceps) of giant cells, known as *muscle fibres*. Each fibre is formed from fusion of many precursor cells and therefore has many nuclei. The fibres are each as thick as a fine hair (50 μm in diameter) and 10–100 mm long. They are arranged in bundles, separated by sheets of connective tissue containing COLLAGEN. These bundles rarely run straight along the axis of the muscle, more usually at an angle, called the *angle of pennation* because many muscles show a pennate (featherlike) pattern of fibre bundles.

Each muscle fibre is surrounded by a CELL MEMBRANE, which allows the contents of the fibres to be quite different from that of the body fluids outside them. Inside the fibre are the

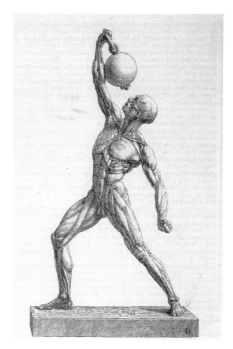

Muscles of the human body in movement (nineteenth century). Christian Roth. Mary Evans Picture Library.

myofibrils, which constitute the contractile apparatus, and a system for controlling the myofibrils through changes in calcium concentration. This system, the *sarcoplasmic reticulum* (SR), is a closed set of tubes containing a high concentration of calcium. Each myofibril runs the whole length of the muscle fibre with a variable number of segments, the *sarcomeres*; it is only one or two micrometres in diameter, and is surrounded by the SR network. The myofibril consists of many much thinner and shorter protein rods, which are the *myofilaments*. These are of two kinds: thick filaments, which are made predominantly from a single protein, *myosin*, and thin filaments, which contain the protein *actin*. The actual contraction takes place by an interaction of the actin with projections on the myosin molecules (*crossbridges*). Each of the crossbridges can develop force (about 5×10^{-12} Newtons) and can pull the thin filament along past the thick filament by about 10×10^{-9} metres (10 millionths of a mm). The net effect of many of these small movements and small forces is to shorten the myofibrils, and thus the whole muscle; hence some part of the skeleton is moved, by means of the attachment of the muscle at each end to bone, directly or via TENDONS.

When a person initiates a movement, events in the BRAIN and the SPINAL CORD generate action potentials in the axons of the MOTOR NEURONS. Each of these axons branches to send ACTION POTENTIALS to many muscle fibres. (A *motor unit* is this collection of perhaps several hundred muscle fibres controlled by one axon.) At the nerve terminals of each axon branch (NEURO-MUSCULAR JUNCTION) ACETYLCHOLINE is liberated by the arriving action potential, and this combines with receptors on the membrane of the muscle fibre, causing it, in turn, to generate an action potential. This action potential spreads over the whole surface of the fibre and also down an extensive network of fine tubes (*T-tubules*), which conduct it into the interior. Here a message, the nature of which is uncertain, passes from the T-tubule to the sarcoplasmic reticulum, causing it to allow some of the calcium it contains to leak out into the interior of the muscle fibre. The thin filaments in the myofibrils contain, as well as actin, two proteins, *troponin* and *tropomyosin*; the calcium which leaks from the SR is able, for a brief period, to interact with the troponin molecule of the thin filament; this, through movements of the tropomyosin molecules, alters the thin filament

so that the actin molecules are available to be joined by the crossbridges, starting the process of contraction. As soon as calcium escapes from the SR the process starts of mopping it up again. There are *calcium pumps* in the membranes of the SR, which are able to move the calcium back inside, thus bringing to an end the short period of muscle activity (a *muscle twitch*). More sustained periods of activity are the norm in the movements we make; they require a sequence of action potentials to be sent to the muscle, at perhaps 30 per second. The contractions produced in this way are stronger than a twitch.

Muscle contraction requires energy to drive the crossbridges through their cyclic interactions with actin: in each cycle the myosin molecule does work in moving the thin filament. Also, energy is used for the process of calcium pumping by the SR. Energy consumption is highest when muscles are used to do external work — for example in climbing stairs, when the body weight has to be lifted. However energy is also used when a weight is held up without doing work on it (*isometric contraction*). Least energy is used when muscles are used to lower weight, as when descending stairs.

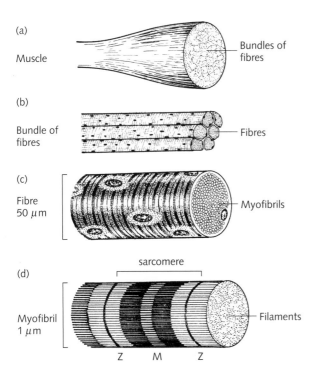

Skeletal muscle at increasing magnification: (a) the whole muscle; (b) bundle of muscle *fibres*; (c) a single muscle fibre, composed of *myofibrils*, showing nuclei and striations; (d) a single myofibril, composed of *myofilaments*. A single *sarcomere* extends between two 'Z discs'. The darker bands are where actin and myosin filaments overlap.
The regular alignment of the light and dark bands of the sarcomeres across the whole muscle fibre accounts for the striped or 'striated' microscopic appearance. (*See also* figure under GLYCOGEN.) (Adapted from Jennett, S. (1989). *Human physiology*. Churchill Livingstone, Edinburgh.)

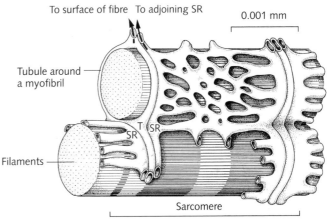

Section of myofibrils with sarcoplasmic reticulum (SR) and T-tubules (T).

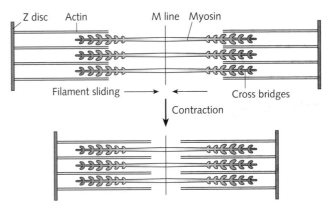

Schematic diagram of a single sarcomere: (above) in relaxation; (below) shortened during contraction.

The energy for muscle contraction comes from the splitting of ADENOSINE TRIPHOSPHATE (ATP) to adenosine diphosphate (ADP) and phosphate. The muscle contains enough ATP to power it at maximum output for only a couple of seconds. ATP can be regenerated in muscle rapidly from *phosphocreatine* (PCr), and there is enough of this substance in the muscle to last perhaps 10 to 20 seconds of maximum activity. The fact that we can sustain strenuous activity beyond 10 seconds is due to the utilization of carbohydrate in the muscles, where it is stored as GLYCOGEN. This can be used to regenerate the ATP supply in two ways. If oxygen is available, glucose can be oxidized to water and carbon dioxide, with two-thirds of the energy released used to rebuild the ATP supply. If oxygen is not available, the process stops with glucose converted to lactic acid and only about 6% of the energy used for building ATP. The lactic acid leaves the muscle cells and can accumulate in the blood. In addition to carbohydrate, muscles use fat, in the form of FATTY ACIDS taken up from the blood, as a substrate for oxidation; this is important for prolonged activity, since the body's energy stored as fat is much greater than that stored as carbohydrate. The availability of oxygen depends on its delivery by the blood; when muscle becomes active, the products of its metabolism cause the vessels to dilate, and this enables a rapid increase in the blood flow.

Muscle FATIGUE is the effect of a set of mechanisms which ensure that muscle is not made active when there is not enough energy available for the activity. If that were to happen, theoretically the muscle could go into RIGOR MORTIS, and could fail to retain the large amount of potassium it contains, with dire consequences for the body as a whole.

The body contains several different varieties of skeletal muscle fibre, which can be seen as specialized for different purposes. The 'slower' muscles are more economical at holding up loads, such as maintaining POSTURE of the body itself, and probably also more efficient at producing external work. Related to their lower energy use they are less easily fatigued. Faster muscle fibres, however, can produce faster movements and higher power outputs, and are essential for such tasks as jumping or throwing. The way different muscles are constructed also allows for specialization of function: muscles with shorter fibres hold forces more economically, muscle with longer fibres can produce faster movements. A pennate arrangement allows muscles to be built with many short fibres, increasing the force they can exert, whereas long fibres, running almost parallel to the axis of the muscle, give the fastest movements.

Some people have more muscular strength than others; they can exert larger forces, do external work more rapidly, or move faster. To a large extent this is because the stronger individuals have larger muscles, but there seem to be other factors at work as well. Training can change the properties of muscle. STRENGTH TRAINING consists in using the muscles to make just a few very strong contractions each day. Over months and years this leads to an increase in the force that can be exerted and in increase in the size of the muscles. Force increase often precedes size increase. *Endurance training* consists of using the muscles less intensely but for longer periods. Again, over months of training the ability of the muscles to get energy through the oxidation of carbohydrate and fat is raised. The supply of blood to the muscle is also increased through changes in the blood vessels and also in the heart. Training can also lead to changes in the fatigue resistance of muscle fibres, and perhaps cause them to change into a slower type of fibre.

ROGER WOLEDGE

See PLATE 5.

See also EXERCISE; FATIGUE; GLYCOGEN; METABOLISM; MOVEMENT, CONTROL OF; MUSCLE TONE; SPORT; STRENGTH TRAINING.

Skeleton The human skeleton has been somewhat nebulously defined as 'a man with his insides out and his outsides off'. It is probably the most durable reminder of man's mortal existence and has intrigued, challenged, and stimulated morbid, mystical, and scientific minds from at least biblical times and probably before. To appreciate the public interest in this subject, one need only observe the media frenzy that ensues when a human skeleton is discovered. Paradoxically, the level of media interest seems to be almost inversely proportional to the academic value of a find. Remains that date from fossil times can have a monumental influence on our understanding of the EVOLUTION of our species but often attract less attention than more recent remains, especially if there is some hint of criminal involvement. It is the inseparable and inextricable nature of the bond between the skeleton and DEATH which ensures that human bones are often perceived in a supernatural light that passes beyond common sense. Hopefully any sane anatomist will tell you that the bones in the dissecting room never rattle ominously and any sober gravedigger will assure you that they do not rise from their coffins and dance around the tombstones at midnight.

There are essentially five basic functions attributed to the skeleton. Each is arguably as important as the other, but given the evolutionary evidence for bone development, the primary function is probably to provide a stable framework that gives support and structure to the soft tissues. Various clinical conditions such as *osteomalacia, osteoporosis,* and *osteogenesis imperfecta* bear witness to the inadequacies of poorly formed bone in fulfilling the role of support to the human body. The skeleton also plays a protective role and this is most clearly seen in the region of the SKULL, which not only forms a box around the delicate tissues of the brain, but also serves to protect the special senses of sight, smell, and hearing. It is said that the thorax protects the heart and lungs, but this theory has little merit when one considers that equally delicate structures in the abdomen are not guarded in this way. It is more likely that the bones of the thorax are involved in the third function of the skeleton, which is to provide a rigid framework for the attachment of muscles and, in the case of the thorax, thereby facilitate BREATHING. For efficient movement to occur, each muscle must originate on the surface of one bone, pass across a joint and insert onto the surface of another bone. In this way one can accurately predict the movement produced by the contraction of each individual muscle or muscle group. The fourth function of the skeleton is to house sites of *haemopoetic* (blood-making) activity within the red marrow that occupies the cancellous spaces of many bones. In bone marrow transplantation, the blood-forming cells are aspirated from sites rich in red marrow, such as the iliac blade of the pelvic bone and the sternum. The final function of the skeleton is to provide a reservoir of MINERALS (calcium, phosphates, potassium, and many other trace elements), which the body can call upon to replenish depleted levels.

There is a myth that BONE is an inactive, dry, and dusty material. This is reflected in the origin of the term 'skeleton', which is derived from the Greek word *skeletos* meaning 'dried up'. However quite the opposite is true in life, as bone is

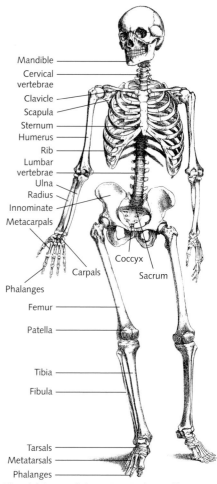

Mandible
Cervical vertebrae
Clavicle
Scapula
Sternum
Humerus
Rib
Lumbar vertebrae
Ulna
Radius
Innominate
Metacarpals
Phalanges
Carpals
Coccyx
Sacrum
Femur
Patella
Tibia
Fibula
Tarsals
Metatarsals
Phalanges

The adult human skeleton. From Luther Holden (1882) *Human Osteology: a description of the bones.* J. T. A. Churchill, London.

unquestionably a dynamic tissue that will bleed if it is cut, hurt if it is damaged, and mend itself if it is broken. Furthermore, it will be resorbed if it is not needed and conversely will develop where it is required.

The official statement, although a virtually meaningless concept, concludes that there are 206 individual bones in the adult skeleton. However, when one considers that over forty inconstant accessory bones have been described in the foot alone, it is clear that, whilst of some value in a trivia quiz, the statement is essentially meaningless. Bones are classified according to either their location within the body or their shape. The latter should be avoided where possible, as the wide variety of bone shapes almost seems to defy useful classification. Whilst the skeleton is bilaterally symmetrical, those structures that lie on the midline do not have a corresponding partner and therefore form the axis, and hence the 'axial' skeleton (see Figure). This comprises the skull, the vertebral column (24 presacral, cervical, thoracic, and lumbar vertebrae; the sacrum; and the coccyx), and the sternum. The limbs and their attachments to the axial skeleton (*girdles*) belong to the 'appendicular' skeleton and are all paired. The *pectoral girdle* (scapula and clavicle) attaches the upper limb to the axial skeleton whilst the *pelvic girdle* (innominate bone) attaches the lower limb to the axial elements. In addition, the rib cage attaches the sternum in front to the vertebral column behind.

Each bone displays an intimate correlation between form and function. This relationship is fundamentally governed by a variety of factors including genetics, mechanics, and metabolism. It is clear however that the human skeleton is unlike that of any other animal and this uniqueness is exploited in the science of *osteology*, where recognition of 'human' plays a vital role. The human skeleton is different for many reasons, including the fact that we are the only habitual biped with upper limbs that are solely dedicated to manipulation and not involved in locomotion. Relatively speaking, we also have the largest brain and give birth to babies with relatively large heads. All of these factors, plus many others, lead to levels of specialization in our skeleton that allow anthropologists (both archaeological and forensic) to persuade our bones to give up many secrets regarding our identity and way of life. One of the first steps in the analysis of human skeletal remains is to establish whether or not they are human, since a murder investigation initiated on the misidentification of some sheep bones is unlikely to be successful. The second question is often an attempt to establish how long the person has been deceased. If more than 70 years have elapsed since death then the remains are classified as archaeological, but if they are more recent then it is a forensic problem. Biological identity is one of the first things to be established and this includes sex, age at death, stature, and race. Beyond that, information regarding individual identity may be established through recognition of personal idiosyncrasies (previous fractures,

dental treatment, previous diseases, congenital anomalies, etc.), all of which might lead to a positive identification of the deceased in a forensic situation. Given an intact skeleton, sex can be determined with up to 95% accuracy, and whilst this is relies heavily on differences in the PELVIS, every bone displays some degree of sexual dimorphism. The determination of age at death is accurate if the individual was younger than 25 years of age but becomes more difficult with advancing age as there are degenerative changes which occur at different rates in different individuals. Stature is relatively easy to determine as it involves measuring the lengths of the limb bones and inserting the values into previously computed regression equations. The ethnic affinity of skeletal remains is very difficult to assess and normally requires the skull to be intact and to show characteristic racial traits. In cases of trauma-related deaths, evidence of the cause of death may remain on the skeleton, such as bullet entry and exit wounds, fractures caused by implements such as hammers or crow bars and also, in cases of stabbing, blades may penetrate and leave marks on the underlying bone. It is probably true that the most important evidence left behind at the scene of a homicide is the body, and this holds true even if it is not discovered for a very long time and only the skeleton remains.　　　　　　　　　　SUE M. BLACK

Further reading

Brothwell, D. R. (1981). *Digging up bones. The excavation, treatment and study of human skeletal remains.* Oxford University Press, Oxford.

Reichs, K. J. (1998). *Forensic osteology: advances in the identification of human remains*, (2nd edn). CC Thomas, Illinois.

See also ANTHROPOLOGY; BONE; JOINTS; PELVIS; SKULL.

Skin The skin is the largest organ of the human body, exceeding two square metres in area in the average adult. Whilst it is rarely more than 2 mm in thickness, the skin plus subcutaneous fat may weigh 9 kg — approximately 14% of the body weight. The primary function of skin is to act as a physical barrier between the organism and its external environment, preventing water loss in dry conditions, hydration in humid or aquatic environments, and access to the body by microbes, and screening the harmful effects of ultraviolet rays of the sun. The skin also plays an important role in transmitting signals from the external environment and in regulating body temperature. The structure of skin confers mechanical strength, enabling it to withstand considerable physical insults, and when it is breached, it exhibits an amazing power of regeneration and repair.

The epidermis, the outer layer of the skin, is a multi-layered epithelium approximately 0.1 mm thick, although there are great variations, such as on the palms and soles, where it may reach 1.4 mm. (The underlying dermis is about 3 mm

thick.) The major cell type of the epidermis is the keratinocyte, so named because of the protein keratin, which it synthesizes in abundance. The epidermis is in a state of constant turnover, with keratinocytes being generated by mitosis (cell division) in a basal layer adjacent to the underlying dermis, and daughter cells passing outward toward the skin surface through successive stages of differentiation, characterized by dramatic changes in shape and size (see figure). After leaving the basal layer, the cells become large and polyhedral (spinous), and are joined to adjacent cells by complex structures called 'desmosomes', which are like spot welds. This spinous layer may be several cells thick, with the cells becoming increasingly flattened before they form the granular layer and then ultimately the cornified horny outer layer, in which the cells lose most of their internal structures including their nuclei and essentially become dead packages of compacted keratin coated with lipid. Cell-to-cell adhesive processes degenerate and the dead cells are eventually shed from the skin surface. It takes 26–42 days for a cell to transit from the basal layer to the outer horny layer, and a further 14 days before being shed, so the epidermis can completely replace itself within two months. The rate of epidermal cell turnover is normally strictly controlled, but a number of diseases are characterized by epidermal hyperproliferation. In psoriasis, for example, the rate may be increased twenty-fold.

The keratin proteins within the keratinocytes are fundamental to the protective functioning and integrity of the skin. The mixture of compacted fibrous keratins in the outer horny layer (the word, 'keratin' is derived from the Greek *keratos*, meaning horn) is highly stable, inert, hard, waterproof, and resistant to physical insult, and therefore is ideally suited to act as a protective layer. The dehydrated nature of the horny surface layer together with an acidic environment due to various secretions, makes it an inhospitable environment for MICROORGANISMS. That this outer surface of dead, keratin-rich cell layers is important in regulating water loss or skin saturation in humid conditions and infection can be demonstrated by removal of the outer layers by successive stripping with sellotape. The resulting denuded skin surface is highly permeable to water and susceptible to infection by a number of microorganisms. Defects in keratins have now been identified as having a causal role in a number of skin disorders.

Other cell types within the epidermis include melanocytes, Langerhan cells, and Merkel cells. The melanocytes are confined to the basal cell layer, are highly dendritic (i.e. they have many branching extensions, like nerve cells), and synthesize the pigment melanin, which moves into surrounding keratinocytes, via the dendritic processes, in small packages termed melanosomes. The Langerhan cells appear to be involved in immunological monitoring of the skin, while the Merkel cells are associated with sensory perception.

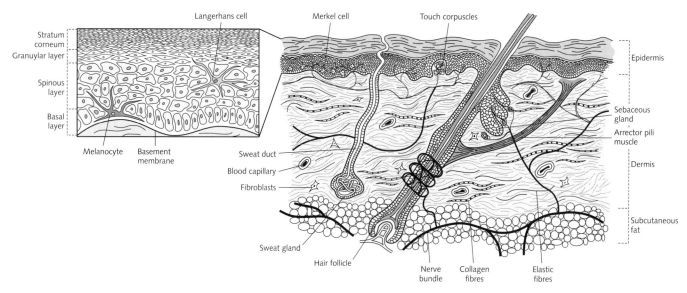

The layers and components of the skin. Right: the full thickness; left, the epidermis only.

The dermis is a dense fibroelastic tissue, of which the major constituents are COLLAGEN, forming a fibrous rope-like network predominantly in a plane parallel to the epidermis, and elastic fibres, which form a fine network in all directions. The collagen fibres confer tensile strength to the tissue, while elastic fibres allow restoration of the normal skin architecture following deformation by external mechanical forces. The space between this fibrillar network is filled with glycosaminoglycans, which are large polysaccharides, and, although they are present in small amounts, they bind vast amounts of water, forming a gel-like matrix which controls the tone and turgor of the tissue and helps to resist compressive forces. The outer region of the dermis is highly uneven, with numerous projections called papillae, which conform tightly to the contours of the epidermis, imparting a resistance to sheer forces upon it. The boundary between the epidermis and dermis is demarcated by a thin membrane and by complex structures which ensure tight anchorage of each to the other. Defects in some of these junctional complexes are associated with certain blistering diseases, such as epidermolysis bullosa, where there there is an abnormality of anchoring fibrils. The dermis contains a number of structures which are derived during development from the epidermal layer, notably sweat and sebaceous glands and HAIR follicles.

The dermis has a copious blood supply, with capillaries extending right up into the dermal papillae projections; these are the nearest vessels to the epidermis, which is itself avascular. Constriction or dilation of the blood vessels alters the temperature of the skin, plays an important role in whole body TEMPERATURE REGULATION, and may be observed as pallor or flushing. The skin also has a rich sensory nerve supply, particularly abundant on the face, hands,

and genitalia. Some nerve endings lie in the epidermis adjacent to Merkel cells, where they can detect pain, temperature changes, and itch. Nerves of the sympathetic system are associated with blood vessels, sweat glands, and the arrector pili muscles of hairs, which allow hairs to 'stand on end'.

Hair While in most animals hair and fur plays an important role in heat conservation, in humans its primary function is in sexual attraction. The keratinous hairs cover the whole body surface except the palms and soles, and are present as either 'terminal' hair characterized by that of the scalp, or 'vellus' hair such as the very fine short body hairs. Hair fibres arise as a result of cell division within the hair follicles, which go through a cyclical pattern of active growth, regression, and a resting phase. The rate of hair growth varies depending upon body site: eyebrow hair, for example, grows much faster than the scalp hair rate of about 0.33 mm per day. Loss of hair in males (*male pattern* BALDNESS) is essentially inherited and androgen-dependent: from the second decade, following multiple growth cycles, the terminal hairs gradually convert to fine vellus hairs. Other types of baldness (*alopecia*) may occur due to infection or immunological disorders.

Sebaceous glands are sac-like structures that arise from an epithelial outgrowth of the hair follicle outer root sheath, and are composed of a single cell type, the sebocyte. The gland produces an oily 'sebum' secretion, of unknown function. The glands remain immature until puberty, and it is the secretion of sebum that is associated with pubertal acne. This is a chronic inflammation of the hair follicle and sebaceous gland (*pilosebaceous unit*) characterized by pustules, comedones (blackheads), cysts, and scars, and it affects most adolescents. Treatments may include anti-androgens, retinoids, or antibiotics.

Sweat glands are of two types. *Eccrine* sweat glands are distributed over almost all of the body surface (2–4 million in total), but they are particularly numerous on the palms, soles, axillae, and forehead. The eccrine sweat gland is a simple unbranched tube which runs from the epidermal surface deep into the dermis, where it develops into a coiled structure. These glands are responsible for the secretion of large amounts of sweat, particularly during strenuous exercise or heat stress, when up to 10 litres a day may be produced; evaporation of the sweat cools the body. Elevated sweat production may also be stimulated by emotion or the consumption of spicy food. *Apocrine* sweat glands differ from the eccrine in that the gland ducts discharge into the lumen of a hair follicle; also they are confined mainly to the underarms, and the genital area in women. Their secretion is probably of limited functional significance, but as a result of bacterial action it is responsible for body odour.

Wound healing

Skin has an amazing ability to heal wounds, but the rate of healing is dependent upon the severity of the wound. Superficial wounds may be repaired rapidly by simple migration of keratinocytes over the defect. Deeper wounds involve blood coagulation, inflammation, re-epithelialization, wound contraction, and new tissue synthesis and remodelling. These processes have been optimized for rapid wound closure, thus preventing fluid loss and infection, but usually at the expense of subsequent function and cosmetic appearance by the formation of SCAR tissue. Some large wounds, such as severe burns, may be assisted in their healing response by grafts, or by the use of keratinocyte sheets — grown in the laboratory from keratinocytes derived from biopsies of the patient's own skin. Much research effort is currently devoted to accelerating WOUND HEALING and reducing scar formation.

Sun exposure

Exposure of the skin to non-ionizing ultraviolet emissions of the sun is unavoidable, but the effect of such exposure is dependent upon both skin type and the length of exposure. Skin is classified as a certain type depending upon its susceptibility to burn, ranging from type I for very fair skin which burns easily and never tans, to type VI-black negroid skin. Within the spectrum of sunlight, ultraviolet B (UVB, 290–320 nm wavelength) causes sunburn, while both UVB and UVA (320–400 nm) will induce pigmentation. UVB is predominantly absorbed by the outer horny layer, allowing only about 10% to reach the dermis, while all UVA penetrates the epidermis to reach the dermis. Exposure to UVA (the predominant wavelength used in sunbeds) is therefore likely to be a major contributor to connective tissue damage in the dermis, resulting in the features of aged, wrinkled skin. More seriously, sun exposure is a major cause of skin cancer (see below).

Sun exposure does have some benefits, such as promoting the synthesis of vitamin D3 from its precursor in the skin, while stimulation of tanning has a protective effect from subsequent sun exposure. Many psoriasis patients also exhibit a marked improvement in their disease following sun exposure.

Ageing

Aged sun-protected skin is characterized by a general laxity, thinning, and the presence of numerous fine wrinkles. The skin becomes less elastic, is greatly reduced in its tensile strength, and exhibits a diminished ability to resist various insults such as injury, infection, and irritants. Chronic sun exposure induces substantial photoageing characterized by a coarse leathery texture, loss of elasticity, deep wrinkles, yellowish colouration, and the presence of numerous irregular pigmented lesions including actinic keratoses. While the youth of today may regard a deep tan as attractive, in their later years they will undoubtedly suffer the consequences of their actions. A more sinister consequence of prolonged sun exposure is the greatly increased incidence of both benign and malignant tumours.

Skin diseases

In the UK, skin diseases account for approximately 10% of patient visits to general practitioners and 6% of hospital outpatient referrals, and this, combined with the fact that they are the most prevalent cause of occupational absence, has substantial economic implications. In addition, many skin diseases, such as those that are debilitating or particularly apparent and extensive, can have serious psychological effects. Some of the more common skin complaints include urticaria (an eruption characterized by usually itchy weals and swelling), acne, viral warts, infections (bacterial, viral or fungal such as ringworm and athlete's, foot), eczema/dermatitis, rashes, and psoriasis. Psoriasis affects approximately 2% of the population in Europe and North America, and is characterized by well demarcated, inflammatory red plaques topped by silvery scales; it is a major medical problem, causing anxiety and distress, and can be debilitating in severe cases. Although our knowledge of the disease has progressed greatly in recent years, the primary cause of the excessive epidermal proliferation which underlies psoriasis has eluded major worldwide research efforts.

Tumours

Tumours of the skin may be benign or malignant. Benign epidermal tumours such as 'seborrheic keratoses' are extremely common. Malignant skin tumours are much the commonest type of cancer overall. Excess exposure, particularly of pale Caucasian skin to ultraviolet irradiation in the form of sunlight, is currently recognized as the major cause of skin cancers, of which the most frequent are basal cell carcinomas (rodent ulcers), squamous cell carcinomas, and malignant melanoma. Basal cell carcinomas are most frequently found on the faces of middle-aged or elderly patients and do not spread to other parts of the body, whereas squamous cell carcinomas may spread. Both of these tumour types are derived from keratinocytes, and are usually treated by simple excision. Malignant melanomas are derived from epidermal melanocytes, and frequently arise from pre-existing pigmented lesions such as moles. The incidence has increased dramatically over the last two decades and this is the most lethal of all skin cancers, spreading rapidly to other organs. If caught at an early stage, however, the prognosis is good, and, due to public education campaigns, the use of sun screens has become more prevalent, and patients are presenting at the clinic much earlier.

Cosmetics

Cosmetics play an important role in skin protection, either as moisturisers or sunscreens, but many are simply used to promote attractiveness, to mask unwanted smells, or to impart pleasant smells and camouflage skin defects. Many contain so-called active ingredients which may alleviate the damage inflicted by sun exposure such as anti-wrinkle creams, or skin lightening creams, or artificial tanning creams. However, a number of cosmetic preparations may elicit a reaction in some people resulting in either irritant dermatitis or allergic sensitivity and contact urticaria.

MIKE EDWARD
RONA MACKIE

Further reading

MacKie, R. M. (1997). *Healthy skin — the facts.* Oxford University Press, Oxford.

MacKie, R. M. (1996). *Clinical dermatology*, 4th ed Oxford University Press, Oxford.

See also BODY DECORATION, BODY ODOURS, HAIR, SUN AND THE BODY, SWEATING; TEMPERATURE REGULATION.

Skin colour The various shades of colour in human skin are due primarily to the presence of melanin, a pigment that protects the skin from ultraviolet radiation, but fat content and thickness of the skin likewise play their roles, as do BLOOD CIRCULATION and varying levels of carotene. Pigments are found mainly in the inner region of the many-layered *epidermis* (the outer skin). Over 300 years ago, the Italian anatomist Marcello Malpighi localized the black colour of 'Negroid skin' in this 'intermediate layer'; 'for when it is washed and kept for a long time in lukewarm water, its colour does not change, but remains black, whereas the true skin (*cutis*), and the epidermis appear almost as white as those of other persons. Today we know that the cells responsible for producing PIGMENTATION, the *melanocytes*, are located here and that their variable and genetically determined activity is the sole determinant for individual skin tone and classification according to 'racial type'.

Even in ancient times human beings were aware of varying shades of colour in individuals and groups in the world around them. For people living on the shores of the Mediterranean — who themselves were usually well tanned — both the 'black' skin of Africans to the extreme south and the pallid 'whiteness' of peoples in the far north seemed remarkable; Homer and Xenophanes made mention of it, as did, above all, Herodotus and a majority of his fellow geographers in the Greco-Roman world. Early on the Greeks and their students raised the question about the origin and nature of 'coloured' skin, which also contained hidden within it the question about the relationship of various peoples to one another. They traced the 'blackness' of Africans and the 'pallor' of 'Northmen' to their extreme and inhospitable environments (blazing sun and gloomy cold), and were the first to associate 'coloured people' with what they viewed as the uncivilized outer limits of their world and a 'barbaric' way of life.

In much the same way that, in Greco-Roman antiquity, 'barbarians' were found far from the civilized centre of human life, for later Christian missionaries coloured 'heathens' lived at a geographical and spiritual distance from God. Christians at first showed little concern for the origin and nature of skin colour and were more interested in the 'eternal soul' than in the composition of its mortal shell. But working to the detriment of 'coloureds' was the age-old Christian symbolism by which 'white' and 'black' were opposites associated with light and darkness, beauty and ugliness, innocence and sin, good and evil, God and Satan. Whereas 'white' was held to be more or less ennobling, a person was discredited by dark skin, which was interpreted as a token of, or sometimes even as the result of, a challenge to Christian norms. Despite the fundamental equality before God postulated by the Church, a converted 'heathen' could not be washed 'white' even by baptism and so in fact remained generally (and even disconcertingly) a Christian of second rank.

Since the sixteenth century, Europeans have seen 'coloured' peoples not only as being far from civilization and God, but also and above all as distant from the centres of capital. In the same way as the Church dealt with 'heathens', now 'coloureds', who previously had been of no 'economic use', were integrated into the global economy — treated not as equals among equals as in the Christian community, but rather subjected simply on the basis of a different skin colour and as a matter of principle, to political, economic, and social discrimination. In a differentiated colour spectrum, 'white' now stood for the functions of management and planning, whereas 'black', for instance, meant 'common' (manual) labour and 'red' meant something to be excluded as worthless.

Against this background, it should be emphasized that during the era of colonialism numerous theories concerning the origin and nature of skin colour asserted, almost without exception, the 'natural' inferiority of 'coloureds'. Some scholars thus called into question the Church's dogma of a single origin for all humankind (so-called 'monogenism'), and resolved the discrepancy with a second creation. For the physician Philippus Paracelsus (1491–1541), the philosopher Giordano Bruno (1548–1600), the biblical scholar and philosopher Isaak la Peyrère (1594–1676), and even Voltaire and Goethe, certain groups like the indigenous inhabitants of the 'American islands' were 'lower' creatures, so-called 'pre-Adamites', created simultaneously with the animals on the sixth day of creation. Other theorists, remaining faithful to the Church's worldview, rejected such 'heretical' ideas and defended the theory of a single Adam, a belief deeply rooted in the Christian faith. In his *Mémoire sur l'origine des Nègres et des Américains* (1733), the Jesuit priest August Malfert retained the theory of monogenism by applying moral theology and interpreting the black colour of Africans as a kind of mark of Cain — which did not do 'coloureds' much good, since it thereby turned the individual stigmatization of a single evil-doer into the collective punishment of a whole 'race'. Finally, a secularized version of such explanatory attempts was provided by a third group of protoscientific theories, in which climate, the chemical environment, or illness assumed the role of a just and vengeful God. The American physician Benjamin Rush (1745–1813), for example, having observed that black children are significantly lighter in the first days after birth than they will be, relatively, as adults, explained the colour of blacks as the hereditary consequence of illness, in this case of leprosy. For Rush 'Negroes' were therefore not the product of a second creation, but simply ill; their blackness was to be understood as a deviation from a healthy condition and in need of rectification. In other words, the doctor wanted to combat racial discrimination with medicine and even appealed to the work of the English chemist Thomas Beddoes (1760–1808), who had already used 'oxygenated muriatic acid to almost bleach' the hand of an African — prompting one wag to suggest that 'bleaching societies' be sent to Africa along with missionaries.

A major division of modern physical ANTHROPOLOGY now concerns itself, for the first time since antiquity, with the question of the origin and nature of skin colour but *without* regard to any social or cosmological notions of rank — since these lie outside the limits of scientific inquiry. Yet, because the residue of a long series of traditional theories on skin colour, which were influenced by such cosmology, continues to determine public perception even today, and because the influence of such a mindset is not always adequately taken into account in the formation of scientific theory, such notions are occasionally incorporated into particular theories. One cannot therefore rule out the possibility that 'coloureds' will continue to be marginalized and discriminated against — even in cellular or genetic research. The extent to which researchers are successful in overriding such discrimination remains to be seen.   PETER MARTIN

See also ALBINO; PIGMENTATION; SKIN.

Skull The human skull has been rich in symbolism over the course of Western history. The skull as an emblem of DEATH appeared as a result of the casualties brought on by the bubonic plague or the Black Death that ravaged the inhabitants of Europe throughout the fourteenth and fifteenth centuries. The *Dance of Death*, which portrayed men and women of all classes dancing with a SKELETON, became a popular artistic motif.

The skull as an intimation of death was also an obvious aspect of sixteenth-century century fashion and art. In the early decades of the century, portraits had skulls printed on the back in order to symbolize the inevitable demise of the sitter. Men and women of the upper classes wore medallions engraved with skulls and ivory heads as jewelry. These objects normally portrayed a living face on one side and the human skull on the other side. The mementos were to remind both the wearer and the onlooker of death and their obligation to lead moral lives. The keepsakes also revealed the tension experienced by members of the upper classes who desired to display their wealth while appearing to obey the dictates of Christian piety.

In the eighteenth century, Caribbean pirates flew flags that featured the human skull and crossbones. The symbol, known as the *Jolly Roger*, may have been a corruption of *joli rouge* (pretty red), the original colour of the flag. The phrase also may have referred to a pirate known as 'Ali Raja' or simply have designated the British term for devil, vagabond, and rogue. The eighteenth-century French pirate Emanuel Wynne was the first to use the skull and crossbones. Wynne also displayed an hourglass on his flag to indicate that time was running out for his intended victims.

In the twentieth century, the Nazi SS adopted the human skull and crossbones, called *Death's Head*, as the badge of their organization. The *Totenkopfverbande*, or 'Death's Head units', were among the most élite and most feared members of the SS. Taking their name from the death's head symbol they wore on the right collar of their uniform, the Totenkopfverbande initially guarded concentration camps, but their role was expanded to include military service, most prominently in Poland and the Soviet Union, where they were responsible for killing Jews, soldiers, and civilians.

The human skull and crossbones have not simply been the mark of infamous men and women; more significantly, they have warned young and old alike of the dangers posed by poisons, toxins, and other hazardous materials. The poison symbol is successful because it is easily identifiable and can be understood by those who are unable to read.

Finally, the human skull figured in nineteenth-century scientific debates, especially those that concerned the attributes of the various races. Practitioners of CRANIOMETRY, or the science of measuring skulls, maintained that they possessed empirical evidence that showed the superiority of Caucasians over other races. Nineteenth-century criminal anthropologist Cesare Lombroso employed craniometry to bolster his claim that

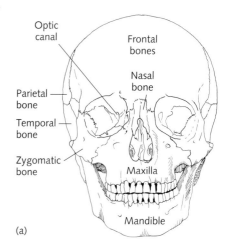

(a)

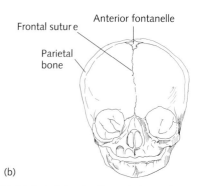

(b)

(a) Adult skull showing the main bones that can be seen from the front.
(For side view see CRANIOMETRY.)
(b) The skull at birth. Note the relatively large size of the neurocranium. Most of the enlargement of the skull occurs in early childhood: the greatest increase in size (about two-thirds) occurs in the first two years.

CRIMINALS possessed an innate predilection to commit crimes. Lombroso said large jaws, low and narrow foreheads, and smaller cranial capacity were characteristics of natural-born criminals.

Like craniometry, PHRENOLOGY flourished in the nineteenth century in the US and Europe as a way to determine the future successes and setbacks of men and women. The phrenologist professed that by studying the shape of a subject's skull he or she could determine the person's unique attributes and abilities. The size and form of the cranium revealed the character of the phrenologist's client.

Structure and evolution

Anatomically, the adult cranium is an extremely complex region of the skeleton. It comprises some 27 bones, forming two components, — the *neurocranium* (brainbox) and the *splanchnocranium* (face). The neurocranium consists of a base and vault whose side walls and roof complete the protective encasing around the delicate brain. The splanchnocranium houses and protects many of the organs of special sense — sight, smell, and taste — as well as accommodating the first part of both the respiratory and alimentary tracts. The upper part of this face-skeleton forms the orbits and nose, whilst the lower part, together with the mandible, forms the JAWS. The FACE is probably the most expressive aspect of human anatomy and this is made possible by more than 50 muscles that attach to the underlying skull. Despite the mobility which these provide, with the exception of the small bones of the middle ear there are only two moving joints in the entire face region, and even they cannot move independently, as the two sides must work in unison. The free movement of the jaw at these *temporomandibular joints* is critical to the success of both *phonation* (SPEECH) and *mastication* (chewing). In historical times, infection of the joint could lead to *ankylosis* (fusion), which was obviously not compatible with sustained life.

The skull is probably the region of the human body that is most avidly studied with respect to human EVOLUTION. The size of the neurocranium and its size relative to the splanchnocranium have been critical to the definition of the hominid lineage. The apes tend to possess a relatively smaller neurocranium and larger face than modern man and his immediate ancestors. The modern human face is suspended under the BRAIN, having rotated backwards and downwards underneath the neurocranium, whilst the brain has extended above and over the top of the face, giving modern man his characteristically high FOREHEAD that protects the frontal lobes of the brain.

Development and growth

In the child, the neurocranium develops in parallel with the early maturation of the CENTRAL NERVOUS SYSTEM, whilst the splanchnocranium lags behind and is more closely linked to the development of the TEETH. Hence the 'cutesy' and non-threatening appeal of baby cartoon characters with big eyes, a big head, and a small face. This early development of the brain along with its protective case has enormous implications with regard to the evolution of man and encephalization in particular. This is the study of the degree to which the nervous system of the human fetus matures *in utero*. Compared with all other animals, including other primates, human babies are born with relatively big heads that house a large brain. During the early part of this century, before CAESAREAN SECTIONS were commonplace or indeed safe, *pelvimetry* (measurements of the maternal PELVIS) was frequently employed in an attempt to predict the outcome of labour. *Cephalopelvic disproportion* — when the baby's head was too large to pass successfully through the birth canal — was a serious clinical concern, as it led to high levels of fetomaternal mortality. However, to overcome this transitory problem, the fetal skull retains considerable flexibility, as the bones are not fully formed and so can ride over each other as the head passes down through the birth canal. It is whimsical to suppose that perhaps new-born babies cry because they start life with a blinding headache!

Forensic applications

In physical and forensic ANTHROPOLOGY, the skull is extremely informative with regard to the identification of sex, age at death, and racial assignation. It also plays a pivotal role in establishing the identity of the deceased — it has been described as the 'bony core of the fleshy head and face'. There are various techniques available to the forensic investigator in this context. To confirm or reject a proposed identity, the skull of the deceased can be compared with a portrait or photograph of the person during life; the image of the skull, live on camera, is superimposed on the static photograph until the correct sizing and orientation are achieved. Then, using specific anatomical landmarks, the 'degree of fit' of the two images can be assessed. When the identity is entirely unknown, facial reconstruction is employed. This can be achieved either by computerized methods, where a standard face is wrapped around the scanned image of the skull, or alternatively by clay modelling. The latter approach requires a considerable degree of skill and generally leads to a more realistic image of the deceased. The function of facial reconstruction is not necessarily to produce a near-photographic image of the deceased, but more realistically to strike a chord with family or friends of a missing person. Such was the case of a young man who was found on the top of a Scottish mountain. He had been dead for nearly two years when he was found accidentally by two climbers. Investigations by the local police did not lead to any success in his identification and so it was decided to reconstruct his face. The outcome was shown on the television programme *Crimewatch* and was picked up by its French television counterpart. It was recognised by a French family who knew that their son had gone walking in Scotland before he went missing, but whose own investigations had been unsuccessful. A simple DNA test confirmed his identity. Such is the way, in osteology, that the dry bones have, of coming back to life to tell their own story.

KAROL K. WEAVER

SUE M. BLACK

Further reading

Aiello, L. and Dean, C. D. (1990). *An introduction to human evolutionary anatomy*. Academic Press, London.

Cohen, K. (1973). *Metamorphosis of a death symbol: the transi tomb in the late Middle Ages and the Renaissance*. University of California Press, Berkeley.

Davies, J. D. (1955). *Phrenology fad and science: a nineteenth-century American crusade*. Yale University Press, New Haven.

Reichs, K. J. (1998). *Forensic osteology: advances in the identification of human remains*, (2nd edn). CC Thomas, Springfield, Illinois.

Scheuer, J. L. and Black, S. M. (2000). *Developmental juvenile osteology*. Academic Press.

See also ANTHROPOLOGY; CRANIOMETRY; EVOLUTION; PHRENOLOGY; SKELETON; SKULL-SHAPING.

Skull shaping In late eighteenth-century Europe skull shape and size became the measure *sine qua non* of intelligence. It seems most remarkable, then, that mothers and midwives should have been seen as a crucial force giving shape to this particular part of the body. Germans had especially broad heads, it was said, because German mothers always slept their babies on their backs. Belgians had oblong heads because Belgian mothers wrapped their infants in swaddling clothes and slept them as much as possible on their sides and temples. Greeks had nearly spherical heads through the special care of midwives. As Jean-Jacques Rousseau remarked, if the way in which God has shaped our heads does not suit us, we have them modelled from without by midwives, and modelled from within by philosophers.

Skulls were only one bodily feature that supposedly lay within mothers' manipulative powers. Noses, especially the noses of African infants, were said to be flattened by the rhythm of their mothers' daily work while they were carried on their mothers' backs. SKIN COLOUR was also said to depend on the vivacity of women's imaginations during conception or pregnancy (Lot's daughters, who saw smoke as they fled burning Sodom, fixed that colour upon their children through the unconscious workings of their imaginations). Mothers among the Khoikhoi in southern Africa were deemed 'villainous' for excising the left testicle of newly born males to make them faster runners and better hunters. The notion that mothers wielded such power derived from the eighteenth-century theory of environmentalism, the notion that bodily characteristics — the shape of noses and lips, the colour of skin, the texture of hair, and the shape of skulls — were fluid, formed over a number of years by external forces working on the body. These forces included climate, diet, and customs; the vagaries of EPIDEMICS or disease; the crossing of different races; and the manipulative hands of women. In the idiom of Buffon, mothers and midwives took the homogeneous stuff of humanity and carved from it the peculiarities of national types. As late as the 1930s, adherents of Hitler strove to transform unsightly round heads into long, dolichocephalic ones.

While some of these notions are mythical, the skulls of very young children do respond to consistent pressure. The bones which will later fuse together around their edges are linked by soft membranes in the infant. This provides some pliability during descent through the birth canal and allows the 'moulding' which can change the shape of the skull considerably, though temporarily, if LABOUR is long and the head is large; babies born by CAESAREAN SECTION start off with rounder heads. Skull-shaping has also been popular outside Europe. Hindus of Baluchistan form a round head and broad forehead by wrapping the baby's head in bandages and keeping it immobile for some time on a cushion. The broad head marks their superior caste standing. The Chinook of the northwest coast of North America flatten infants' heads by pressing a baby's forehead between two pieces of wood tied together by leather thongs, making their faces appear remarkably broad. Only the free-born among them enjoy these carefully crafted heads; slaves are recognized by their 'ugly' round heads. The Caribs of the lesser Antilles, by contrast, formed flat foreheads but peaked crowns by banding their young children's heads. Various peoples of Africa prefer elegantly elongated skulls. For ancient Egyptians, this was a mark of royalty. In northeastern Zaire, still today, Mangebetu women bind their children's heads to produce elongated skulls.

LONDA SCHIEBINGER

Further reading

Brain, R. (1975a). *The decorated body*. Harper and Row, New York.

Schiebinger, L. (1993). *Nature's body*. Beacon Press, Boston.

Sleep is a complex behaviour that is an integral part of the body's strategic adaptation to daily changes in light and temperature. Because we lose CONSCIOUSNESS so dramatically when we fall asleep, it was erroneously assumed that brain activity ceased in sleep. The presence of vivid dreams made such a simplistic theory unlikely and, during the past fifty years, scientific research on the BRAIN and body has shown sleep to be richly variegated, exquisitely controlled, and essential to life. It is now also clear that sleep is not always benign but has its own built-in propensity for disorder and disease.

The rich variegation of sleep phenomena can already be appreciated in its definition as a behaviour characterized by postural immobility (but with periodic changes in body position and muscle tone), by decreased response to external stimuli (but with marked fluctuations in threshold to response), by selective sensitivity to some stimuli, and by an orderly sequence of electrical and chemical changes in the brain that affect the entire body and greatly alter the mind. Clearly, sleep is an active, global, organismic state requiring central control by the brain and affording the brain and body a wide variety of functional opportunities.

Subjective experience was not the only obstacle to appreciation of the manifold complexity of sleep. Because of our MODESTY, we do not normally welcome the observation of our sleep. And because we all tend to sleep at the same time, there is no one to watch over those few who are willing to be observed. The development of sleep laboratories in the last half century has begun to counter these trends and to create the detailed picture we have today, but naturalistic studies of sleep are still woefully inadequate.

Sleep laboratory studies

Most sleep laboratories consist of two rooms; one with a bed for the subject, connected via a one-way window and by cables to the other, an instrument room where a technician monitors the sleeping subject (sometimes also by video). Recordings are made of electrical signs from the brain (ELECTROENCEPHALOGRAM or EEG); from the eye (electro-oculogram or EOG); and from the muscles (electromyogram or EMG). *A polygraph* is used to keep track (graph) of the several (poly) signals simultaneously. Other important bodily functions, like body temperature, breathing, heart rate, blood pressure, and even sex organ volume, can also be recorded.

A typical night of sleep in an adult human is divided into four or five distinct cycles of body and brain activity. Each cycle begins with a *relaxation phase*, showing declines in brain wave (EEG) activation, muscle tone (EMG), eye movement (EOG), heart rate, breathing rate, and blood pressure, all of which typically reach a nadir after 45–60 minutes. This relaxation phase then gradually gives way to an *activation phase*, in which many of the brain and bodily functions resume the high levels of the awake state. In the face of this activation, sleep is maintained by the active suppression of sensory (input) signals and motor (output) commands.

Over the course of the night the length and depth of the relaxation phase (which is called *quiet*, NREM (non-rapid eye movement), or *EEG slow-wave* sleep) declines as the duration and intensity of the activation phase (called *active, REM* or *EEG fast-wave* sleep) increases. About 70–80% of an average sleep bout of 6.5–8.0 hours consists of NREM sleep, while 20–30% is REM. Other bodily functions which are associated with NREM sleep include the secretion of the HORMONES regulating growth and sexual maturation. REM sleep is associated with profound muscle relaxation and with sex organ distension, including full ERECTION (and is therefore a built-in test of physiological potency), and a loss of the capacity for internal TEMPERATURE REGULATION. The rapid eye movements that give REM sleep its name are not continuous but occur in flurries or clusters, each of which is associated with (sometimes dramatic) increases in the rate, or with irregularity, of heartbeat and BREATHING. Awakenings which follow these REM clusters are very likely to yield long and detailed reports of dreaming.

Variations in sleep

Sleep varies markedly over the life cycle as well as overnight. New-born infants lack the capacity for long, deep NREM sleep. This only develops, with brain maturation, during childhood and adolescence. But babies have an exaggerated propensity for REM sleep, often entering it directly from waking (so it can easily be observed by curious carers). Since sleep duration is about twice as long in neonates (16 vs. 8 hours) and REM is twice as common (50% vs. 25%), the new-born spends four times longer in REM than does the adult (8 vs. 2 hours). REM sleep declines dramatically as sleep depth increases with brain maturation and the emergence of the adult pattern.

But this is not the end of the dynamism of sleep development. The capacity for deep NREM sleep falls precipitately between ages 30 and 40. This leads to a normal decline in the ability to sustain sleep and to feel deeply rested by it. REM sleep remains relatively stable, but its decline may cause further deterioration of sleep quality after age 60, especially as other medical problems interfere with sleep.

Individuals also show marked differences in sleep behaviour. Most of us lie between two extreme ends of a bell-shaped curve of sleep length and efficiency. At one end are the short-sleepers, who need as few as 3–5 hours, and at the other are long-sleepers, who need 8–11 hours to feel rested and refreshed by sleep. Short-sleepers tend to be energetic, active, and productive, while long-sleepers tend to be lethargic, sedentary, and reflective. Society, with its interest in tight schedules and productivity, is kind to short but merciless to long-sleepers. Long-sleepers are ill-advised to seek professions, like medicine, which greatly curtail sleep.

Even within individuals of a given sleep need and age, sleep varies from night to night, and poor or lost sleep tends to be rapidly compensated. This reciprocal dynamic is dramatically revealed by studies in which one or another sleep phase or time is deliberately altered and the recovery process is monitored.

Much has been learned about sleep from laboratory studies of non-human animals. For example, the diversity of sleep behaviour increases as the brain becomes more and more specialized during EVOLUTION. Below the level of the reptiles (who have clear-cut NREM sleep but not REM), it is difficult to distinguish sleep from simple inactivity. REM sleep first appears in birds and then only fleetingly, because while hatchlings have it in abundance, adults have little or none. REM sleep is first clearly and enduringly seen in mammals, suggesting a relationship to the two features which distinguish that class of animal: large, highly developed brains and the capacity for strong internal temperature control.

Brain mechanisms of sleep

There is exquisite control of sleep by the brain. In mammals, sleep is one of the key bodily functions controlled by the body clock in the hypothalamus. By these means it is also tied to the rhythm of body temperature, such that sleep occurs as body temperature falls and waking occurs when body temperature is highest. For most animals, including humans, these peaks in alertness and energy availability occur during the daylight hours, but animals (like rats) that rely more on smell than on vision are active at night and sleep in the daytime. In very hot climates humans may also shift their activity into the darker, cooler night and have a siesta during the forbiddingly hot period of the early afternoon.

The BODY CLOCK times the occurrence of sleep via its direct nervous connection between the hypothalamus and other subcortical structures in the lower brain. Of particular importance are those collections of brain cells in the brain stem which manufacture and liberate from their endings two brain chemicals, NORADRENALINE (norepinephrine) and SEROTONIN, which appear to have energizing effects needed for the waking functions of the brain and the body. In order for sleep to occur the activity of these brain cells must be quelled by the mechanism of inhibition. As their activity is more and more completely diminished, another group of cells becomes increasingly active and liberates more and more molecules of another chemical (*acetylcholine*), which appears to mediate restorative functions throughout the body and the brain. It is the reciprocal interaction of the two cell groups that appears to provide the basis of the cyclic alternation of NREM and REM sleep and their functional differentiation.

Functions of sleep

Sleep is vitally necessary. Recent experiments on the effects of prolonged sleep deprivation give hints as to why even short-term sleep loss is so disabling and why it is so vigorously compensated by the brain. If sleep deprivation is extended beyond two weeks, rats develop a distinctive group of signs that inevitably leads to their demise. Their skin breaks down and they show an increasing craving for food but cannot maintain their body weight no matter how much they eat. At the same time they develop more and more determined heat-seeking behaviour, as they cannot control their body temperatures when exposed to normal variation in environmental temperature. Short of these extreme effects, more modest sleep deprivation has been shown to create a wide variety of difficulties. Taken together these suggest that sleep may normally play an important role in the maintenance of such important bodily functions as the immune response and metabolic balance, as well

as such critical mental functions as attentiveness, learning and memory, and emotional equilibrium. Shakespeare may have been correct when he said that sleep 'knits up the raveled sleeve of care', but he was underestimating the more active developmental and survival functions of sleep.

J. ALLAN HOBSON

See also DREAMING; ELECTROENCEPHALOGRAM; SLEEP DISORDERS; SNORING.

Sleep disorders

The ability to fall asleep, stay asleep, and wake up are all considered inalienable rights. We should neither stuporously wander about our houses nor suddenly decide to jump off our beds into imaginary swimming pools. The child's prayer, 'Now I lay me down to sleep', epitomizes the fond hope that sleep is a safe passage across a sea of unconsciousness undisturbed by life-threatening deficits in vital physiological processes. Still, it should have come as no surprise that a system as complicated and differentiated as the brain mechanisms underlying sleep and dreaming would have its own intrinsic propensity for dysfunction and disorder as well as its amazing capacity as a health-conveying operation. And the normal variation in sleep propensity, sleep depth, sleep length, and sleep stage distribution is already proof that such mundane events as excessive daytime sleepiness, or its converse, excessive night-time wakefulness (*insomnia*) should be viewed at least in part as expressions of extremes of normal physiology.

Yet even the most sophisticated and perspicacious sleep scientists were unprepared for the discovery that breathing sometimes stopped or was blocked in sleep (as it is in *sleep apnea*) or the recognition that all of the symptoms of the compelling need to sleep (as seen in *narcolepsy*) could be explained as abnormalities of sleep neurophysiology. More surprising still were the twin discoveries that sleepwalking, sleep-talking, and bedwetting had little to do with dreaming but that a previously unrecognized process, the *REM sleep behaviour disorder*, was not only dream enactment but the harbinger of degenerative disease of brain motor control systems!

There are three major kinds of sleep problems and each can be understood through sleep physiology:

1. Difficulty falling asleep (which is caused by excessively strong or inadequately suppressed brain drives toward waking) — the classic example is *insomnia*.

2. Difficulty staying awake (caused by excessively strong or inadequately suppressed brain drives toward sleep). The classic example is *narcolepsy*.

3. Abnormal movements that occur as the depth of sleep varies over the course of the night. For example, the movement-generating centres of the brain can sometimes become active without the brain's consciousness-generating arousal systems becoming simultaneously activated to waking levels. The classic example is *sleepwalking*.

The *sleep apnea syndromes* are an ambiguous but critically important class of sleep disorder with characteristics of all three categories. Victims of this life-threatening tendency to stop breathing when they fall asleep — and then to choke when they make compensatory efforts to wake up and breathe again — may be insomniac (because their bodies will literally not allow them to go to sleep); they may have excessive sleepiness by day (because they are chronically sleep deprived); and their laboured efforts to breathe while asleep can be seen as a form of chronic abnormal sleep movement, which, in the long term, may prove to be much more physiologically harmful than other sorts of abnormal sleep movements such as sleepwalking.

Sleep apnea sufferers are usually overweight (which makes breathing more difficult as the airway closes normally — causing snoring — at sleep onset) and male (which deprives them of the unexplained protection of sleep breathing afforded by female sex hormones). But they also just exaggerate the surprising normal tendency of men to have long pauses in their breathing efforts, especially during NREM sleep but also in REM. As their oxygen hunger increases and their brain alarm clock arouses them, they make a gasping effort to gulp air, at which point their flaccid, fat-compressed airway closes and they move even closer to self-strangulation. Because treatment is now quite effective it is crucial that any person suspected of having sleep apnea consult a physician or a sleep disorders centre.

Narcolepsy is a rare but instructive illness with four defining attributes: (i) excessive daytime sleepiness and irresistible attacks of sleep; (ii) the sudden loss of postural muscle tone (called *cataplexy*, often leading to total collapse; (iii) the occurrence of frightening dream hallucinations at sleep onset and upon awakening; and (iv) the persistence of REM sleep motor paralysis, also on arousal from sleep.

All of these symptoms are manifestations of a genetically-determined failure to inhibit REM sleep physiology, which most of us can do quite easily, especially during waking. Like new-borns, many adult narcoleptic patients have prolonged REM sleep bouts at sleep onset. Effective treatment is achieved using drugs that potentiate the brain chemicals responsible for effective waking, and/or suppression of the brain chemicals responsible for REM sleep.

Insomnia is by far the most prevalent disorder of sleep. It is also the most problematic to manage, because none of the myriad sedative drugs available for its relief is a physiological sleep inducer or enhancer. For this reason all of the effective sedatives have one or more defects: undesirable side-effects, diminished efficacy with prolonged use, or a worsening of symptoms upon withdrawal.

Because so much insomnia is psychologically and behaviourally driven, effective treatment should always include attention to such factors as (i) regular, early times of retirement; (ii) elimination of the commonly abused anti-sleep ingestants tobacco and alcohol; (iii) a review of daytime work and interpersonal concerns with special attention to identifying and eliminating the sources of nocturnal rumination and anxiety; (iv) the prescription of sleep-enhancing aerobic exercise; and (v) instruction in systematic body relaxation techniques.

This naturalistic approach to insomnia does not deny its sometimes strong physiological basis, which may demand pharmacological adjuncts, but it is cautious and conservative in warning against the undue expectation and the unacceptable risks of uncritical sedative treatment.

The *REM sleep behaviour disorder* is easily distinguished from ordinary sleepwalking. Sleepwalking is a self-limited and usually harmless problem of adolescence and early adulthood that occurs in NREM sleep and disappears when that sleep stage declines in the fourth decade. By contrast, the REM sleep behaviour disorder usually begins at that age or later, and reflects the dangerous and prognostically grave failure to inhibit the motor commands of REM sleep that are normally experienced as only the illusion of movement during dreaming.

Early degeneration of the brain (and especially Parkinson's disease) is heralded by REM sleep behaviour disorder, but it has also recently been reported to arise in younger subjects who have been treated for depression with drugs that specifically potentiate serotonin, one of the chemicals that the brain uses to energize itself in waking and to influence the excitability of the motor system in all of its states.

The study of sleep disorders is still a young, rapidly-developing field at the interface of neurology, psychiatry, and internal medicine. Its inventory of disorders, its methods of investigation, and its approaches to treatment can all be expected to change rapidly in the next few decades.　　　　　　　　　　J. ALLAN HOBSON

See also BODY CLOCK; SLEEP; SNORING.

Slipped disc
This applies to an abnormality of an intervertebral disc in the spine. These discs are cushions of CARTILAGE acting as shock absorbers between the bodies of the vertebrae that comprise the SPINAL COLUMN. They are therefore subject to considerable pressure, especially those in the lumbar spine, and these pressures are increased when a person lifts heavy weights. The discs are firmly fused to the vertebral bodies above and below, and the popular term is misleading — in suggesting that they are mobile structures that could slip out of place, and by implication could be 'put back' by manipulation or surgery. Rather, the discs can degenerate, a process that can be accelerated by repeated strains. Degenerated discs protrude and can press on spinal nerve roots or on the spinal cord, causing pain, with associated muscular spasm and sometimes weakness of the muscles of the arm, or of the leg, according to whether cervical or lumbar discs are affected. Such protrusions may require surgical removal. Only occasionally does acute injury tear part of an abnormal disc

and release a loose fragment; this also may compress nervous structures and need to be removed.　　　　　　　　　　BRYAN JENNETT

See also SPINAL COLUMN.

Small intestine
The part of the gut between the stomach and the large intestine, comprising consecutively the duodenum, jejunum, and ileum. 'Small' because it is a narrower tube, though at about twenty feet a much longer one, than the 'large' intestine. It is covered by a membrane of peritoneum, and receives its blood vessels and nerves via the mesentery — a flat but fatty double membrane which fans out from the back of the abdomen to the loops of the small intestine. Digestion (started in the stomach) continues here, and absorption begins of the resulting simple nutrient molecules, and of water and minerals. The lining has many folds and protrusions (villi), and secretes mucus and ENZYMES.　　　　　　　　　　　　　S.J.

See ALIMENTARY SYSTEM.

Smiling
The French neurologist, Duchenne du Boulogne, writing in the nineteenth century, made a fundamental discovery about the nature of smiling, a discovery that was forgotten for a hundred years. Duchenne electrically stimulated different positions on the face of a patient who had no pain sensation, and photographed the resulting expressions. By this means he learned how the different facial muscles produced different expressions. He showed that the *zygomatic major* muscle, which runs from the cheek bone down to the lip corners, pulls those lip corners upwards into a smiling shape (Fig. 1). Importantly, Duchenne noted that the man in this picture did not really look happy. He told him a joke, and noted that, when the man smiled spontaneously, it involved not just the *zygomatic major*, but part of a second muscle, the *orbicularis oculi*, which encircles the eye (Fig. 2). Duchenne noted that this is a muscle that most people cannot contract voluntarily, and so it 'unmasks the false friend'.

Although Charles Darwin, in his book on expression, published this photograph and described Duchenne's finding, it was ignored until very recently. In 1982, Paul Ekman resurrected Duchenne's distinction to explain why people often smile when they are not happy. As Duchenne had noted, Ekman found that people who smile when they are not feeling enjoyment do not show activity of the muscle around the eyes, just the lip muscle. Many studies now support Duchenne's distinction between these two types of smiling — what scientists now call, in honour of Duchenne, Duchenne smiles, or D-smiles for short (*zygomatic major* outer part, and *orbicularis oculi*) and non D-smiles (*zygomatic major* only). For example, 5-month-old infants show D-smiles when approached by their mother, non D-smile when approached by a stranger. In adults the D-smile is accompanied by the pattern of brain activity found with enjoyment, but that brain activity pattern is not found

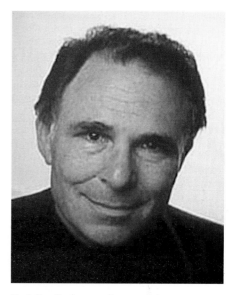

Fig 1 Non-Duchenne smile.

when the non D-smile is shown. Happily married couples show D-smiles when they meet at the end of the day, while unhappily married couples show non D-smiles.

It is not always easy to distinguish these two types of smiles. If the lips are pulled only slightly or moderately by the *zygomatic major* muscle, it is easy to see whether the eye muscle is involved, for it will produce crow's feet wrinkles and bagging of the skin under the eyes. Those signs are absent in a slight to moderate non D-smile. However, when the smile is very broad, the lip pulling itself will produce those changes in the face and it is necessary to look elsewhere. Only in the D-Smile will the eyebrows move down ever so slightly.

Instead of signalling genuine enjoyment, non D-smiles serve many different social functions. They may indicate agreement, they show a person is willing to go along with something, even

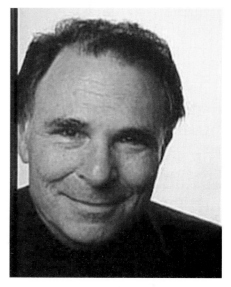

Fig 2 Duchenne smile.

something unpleasant (grin and bear it), and they may also be used to send a false message of enjoyment when none is felt. Research has shown that most people do not notice the difference between D-smiles and non D-smiles, and it is hard not to reciprocate a smile, even a non-D smile.

There is as yet no clear answer to the question, 'Why do the lip corners go up rather than down with enjoyment?' Research has found that the smile is a very powerful signal that stands out from all the negative emotional expressions. If the expression is broad, it can be accurately recognized (although not, of course, the distinction between D- and non D-smiles), at about 100 m — the maximum distance of a javelin throw.

PAUL EKMAN

See also FACE; FACIAL EXPRESSION.

Smoking Tobacco is believed to have been grown in the Americas for many thousands of years, and native Americans are thought to have discovered ways of using the plant, including smoking the leaves, a thousand years before Christ. A pottery vessel, found in Guatemala, dated earlier than the eleventh century, depicts a Mayan smoking a roll of tobacco leaves tied with string. Landing at San Salvador in 1492, Columbus was presented with dried fragrant leaves, but threw them away, not realizing the value placed on them by the natives. Rodrigo de Jerez was probably the first European smoker, learning of the practice from Cubans in the 1490s and taking the habit back to Spain. He was imprisoned by the Holy Inquisitors for seven years, but the practice was common by the time he was released. By the middle of the sixteenth century, smoking of tobacco was known in Mexico, Santo Domingo, Cuba, Brazil, Canada (in Montreal), France, Holland, Portugal, Spain, Germany, and Britain. It spread eastwards to Turkey and Poland by the 1580s, and in 1586 the first cautionary remarks about its use were made in Germany, where it was described as the 'violent herb'. The smoking habit was spread largely by sailors, who both experienced it on their journeys and brought back supplies for continuing use at home. Certainly the naval explorers Sir John Hawkins and Sir Francis Drake, or at least their crews, brought back supplies and made use of the leaves. It was Sir Francis Drake who introduced tobacco to Sir Walter Raleigh in 1585, and, as the story goes, a servant finding Raleigh smoking thought he was on fire and drenched him with beer. Tobacco was smoked in various ways — rolled into a cigar, as cigarettes made with reed stems, and in pipes. Raleigh, while not the originator of smoking in England, did much to improve the method of curing the leaf, and popularized it amongst the courtiers of his day. The rich would smoke the leaf in silver pipes, while in the taverns clay pipes filled with smouldering tobacco would be passed from hand to hand. The poor man made do with a walnut shell and a straw stem. The price of tobacco was high, the purchaser getting

enough leaf to balance the silver coins placed on the other pan of the scales. Numerous claims were made for the benefits of tobacco, such as prevention of toothache, falling fingernails, worms, hallitosis, lockjaw, and cancer. In 1566, Catherine de Medici, Queen of France, received snuff (powdered tobacco) to treat her migraine, and later decreed it *Herba Regina*.

The impact of tobacco, particularly in Europe, was considerable, and often contradictory. For example, importation of tobacco from the colonies prompted governments to impose a heavy duty, which in turn encouraged smuggling, bootlegging, and attempts to grow tobacco at home. In 1604, James I published a 'counterblaste' against tobacco, concluding that smoking was

'a custom lothsome to the eye, hateful to the nose, harmefull to the braine, daungerous to the lungs, and in the blacke stinking fume thereof, nearest resembling the horrible Stigian smoke of the pit that is bottomelesse'.

In the colonies it was realised that the Spanish leaf (*Nicotiana tabacum*) was superior to the indifferent leaf found in the colonies (*Nicotiana rustic*), and English colonials were very influential in setting up the tobacco growing industry in Virginia and Maryland, to the obvious advantage to trade. Indeed, an article in the Washington Post in 1997, by Susan de Ford, was entitled 'Tobacco: the noxious weed that built a nation' — referring here, of course, to the US. In the Americas a special tax levied in 1693 helped establish the college of William and Mary at Williamsburg, and in the nineteenth century Duke University in North Carolina was founded on tobacco. Spenser's *Fairy Queen*, published in 1590, contains the earliest poetical allusion to tobacco. Six years later Ben Jonson's *Every Man is his humor* has a scene in which an argument about tobacco is played out. By 1614 there were 7000 tobacconists' shops in London alone. Cigarettes became the most popular form of tobacco, use by the 1880s, made by huge corporations, particularly in the US, supplying the worlds' smoking needs: pipes were in decline. The taking of snuff and the use of chewing tobacco are now almost extinct, although dedicated pipe smokers and cigar devotees are still to be found.

Over the years increasing statistical evidence related smoking to cardiovascular and LUNG disease, especially bronchitis, emphysema, and CANCER. It is undoubtedly true that the pleasures of smoking are derived from the actions of nicotine on the CENTRAL NERVOUS SYSTEM. Nicotine is rapidly absorbed from the mucosal membrane of the mouth and from the lungs, and readily penetrates the nervous system. It also has peripheral actions, tending to increase BLOOD PRESSURE and heart rate. The Surgeon-General's Report in the US in 1964 was the real start of the campaign to prevent or abolish smoking. Vested interests in the tobacco companies promoted ideas to reduce the harmful effects by the introduction of filters and creation

of low tar cigarettes. It is the carcinogenic compounds in the tar which are the serious hazard to health, and some, but not all, of these compounds are removed by the filters. People changing to cigarettes with low nicotine content tend to smoke more and draw more deeply. Artificial smoking materials have been developed, consisting of pure cellulose-based material impregnated with nicotine. However, combustion of all plant material, and of pure cellulose, seems to produce some carcinogenic agents. The ultimate in the safe cigarette consists of a hollow tube which is not ignited but releases nicotine as the 'smoker' draws air through. Nicotine chewing gum and nicotine patches, which release the alkaloid when applied to the skin, have also been produced as substitutes, largely for those who are breaking the habit.

The taking of nicotine is habit forming, indeed it can be described as addictive. The balance of psychological to physical dependence is generally more towards the former, as physical withdrawal symptoms are less severe than with drugs such as heroin. However, individual tobacco addicts vary enormously in their level of dependence. Some of the pleasures of smoking are due to ritual — particularly so in pipe smokers, who carry a variety of equipment for preparing for a satisfying smoke. Many smokers never do so in the dark, for the curl of the smoke from the pipe or cigarette end is part of the ritualistic satisfaction. Many psychological tests have shown that mental activity and performance is enhanced by smoking, particularly when fatigued — but the young often take up smoking to imitate their peers or idols. Serious programmes to stop people smoking or to prevent the young from starting are now being offered, particularly in the Western world, and the number of public places in which smoking is acceptable has greatly reduced.

To understand why smoking is still so common, despite all that is known about its effects, it is necessary to appeal to experiments made in model systems. In the brain a tract of nerve fibres run from the *ventral tegmental area* (VTA) of the *mesolimbic dopamine system* to the *nucleus accumbens* (NA). When this tract of nerve fibres is activated, DOPAMINE is released in the NA. Application of nicotine to the VTA also causes dopamine release in the NA. Experimental animals which have been trained to self-administer nicotine by lever pressing fail to do so if the mesolimbic pathway from the VTA to the NA is cut. Thus, in this experimental paradigm, release of dopamine in the NA seems to be part of a reward response which reinforces administration. More importantly, other addictive drugs, such as amphetamine, COCAINE, or morphine, also cause dopamine release in the NA. Most drugs when administered repeatedly result in *desensitisation* — the CELL MEMBRANE RECEPTORS upon which the drug acts fail to respond or they 'down regulate', meaning that the number of receptors decreases, thus limiting the response. This is the basis of tolerance. In the case of nicotine receptors in the brain, the numbers *increase* with continued and repeated administration of the drug, though not uniformly in all areas of the brain. How this increased number of receptors is related to tolerance is unknown. Tolerance to nicotine does exist, for obviously smokers are used to low levels of nicotine for much of their waking hours and have increased numbers of nicotinic receptors. Yet the non-smoker who for one reason or another takes a cigarette or cigar often shows profound effects not only in the psyche but in the periphery as well, often vomiting and feeling very unwell. Stories of fathers making their children smoke a cigar if caught trying to smoke have claimed life-long cures by this ruse. Finally, nicotinic receptors are so called because they can be activated by nicotine, as well as by the natural transmitter ACETYLCHOLINE. Activation of the dopaminergic mesolimbic system by release of acetylcholine in the VTA is presumably involved with pleasurable feelings, even in non smokers.

ALAN W. CUTHBERT

See also ADDICTION.

Smooth muscle

The cardiovascular, gastrointestinal, genitourinary, and respiratory systems are composed mostly of hollow organs (tubular or sacular), which transport and/or store fluids (either liquids or gases) within the body. The walls of these organs contain smooth muscle, a type of tissue which enables them to constrict or dilate, in this way retarding or facilitating fluid movement as required. This is accomplished by the shortening or lengthening of the individual smooth muscle cells, which occurs in a co-ordinated fashion because the cells are electrically coupled by intercellular connections, known as *gap junctions*. Other structures in the body that contain smooth muscle include the *myometrium* — the muscular wall of the uterus — which is responsible for the rhythmic contractions of LABOUR; the *piloerector* muscles, which cause skin hair to stand up; and the *irises*, which control the diameter of the pupils.

Smooth muscle thus subserves all internal, involuntary functions, except the movements of BREATHING and the beating of the HEART. Many directly acting chemical agents affect its contraction, but most smooth muscle is also under the control of the AUTONOMIC NERVOUS SYSTEM; in some sites (notably most BLOOD VESSELS) it is influenced only by the sympathetic component, and at others (for example in the gut and the iris) by dual, and sometimes opposite, effects of sympathetic and parasympathetic nerves.

As befits its many functions, smooth muscle at different sites is much more heterogeneous than skeletal or cardiac muscle. By creating diverse structural arrangements of smooth muscle and other associated cells, and at the same time varying the mechanisms that control contraction, evolution has achieved a remarkable diversity of smooth muscle-containing organs, each of which is designed to fill a unique functional niche.

Calcium and contraction

On a cellular level, however, all smooth muscles share many characteristics. When relaxed, the cells assume the shape of long, narrow spindles or worms. The cells are termed 'smooth' because they lack the regular bands or *striations* which are prominent in SKELETAL MUSCLE fibres and CARDIAC MUSCLE cells. Smooth muscle cells are capable of contracting dramatically, to half or less of their relaxed length. Contraction may be sustained, as in the smooth muscle cells present in the blood vessels or airways, or rhythmic, as in the cells of the myometrium and gastrointestinal tract. The main stimulus for contraction is a rise in the cellular concentration of CALCIUM. This can be triggered by an impressive array of chemical signals, that differ depending on the type of smooth muscle involved, including a variety of NEUROTRANSMITTERS released at autonomic nerve endings.

As in striated muscles, contraction occurs because the rise in cellular calcium causes an interaction between cellular action and myosin filaments, although the arrangement of these filaments within the cells is not of a similar consistent pattern. Also, the mechanism whereby calcium stimulates this interaction in smooth muscle differs from that in striated muscle, in that it involves activation of a different signalling protein (*calmodulin* rather than *troponin*). Another important difference between smooth and striated muscle is that smooth muscle never becomes fatigued, because it uses metabolic energy much more efficiently than does striated muscle.

In common experience, some obvious manifestations of altered smooth muscle activity are the widening of the pupils in the dark when the radially arranged muscle of the iris contracts; asthmatic wheezing, when the smooth muscle in the walls of the bronchioles impedes airflow; and the phenomenon of erection, when blood vessel relaxation allows engorgement.

Self-regulating pipes

The functioning of each type of smooth muscle is intimately tied up with the organ or system of which it is a part, so that this type of tissue is perhaps best appreciated if one abandons the attempt to generalize and considers, for example, the blood vessels.

The arteries and veins are not merely conduits designed to convey blood passively to and from the capillaries. Rather, they exist in a dynamic state of partial constriction, regulated by the smooth muscle cells which form much of the vascular wall, where they are arranged in multiple layers embedded in a tough and elastic matrix of connective tissue. The cells wrap around the vessel in a low-pitch spiral, so that, when they shorten, the vascular lumen is constricted. The layers of smooth muscle cells are separated from the blood by a monolayer of flat, polygonal *endothelial cells*. These remarkable cells carry out multiple vital tasks, which include controlling the clotting of blood and releasing substances which influence the contraction and also the growth of the smooth muscle cells. The most important of these substances, NITRIC OXIDE, is a short-lived gas which reacts with the protein *guanylyl cyclase* in the smooth muscle cells, causing them to relax and lengthen. Nitric oxide release is controlled by many factors, including the friction exerted by the flowing blood, and also by HORMONES and other messenger molecules present in the blood.

The outer layer of blood vessels contains nerves of the sympathetic component of the autonomic nervous system, the activity of which is controlled by the brain. The sympathetic nerve endings are constantly releasing minute quantities of *norepinephrine* (also called 'NOR-ADRENALINE'), a neurotransmitter which stimulates the smooth muscle cells to shorten. The length of the smooth muscle cells, and therefore the diameter of the blood vessel, is largely determined by the ongoing balance between the opposing influences on constriction of nitric oxide and norepinephrine.

These factors account for the dynamic state of partial constriction of the blood vessels, of which the overall effect is to impose a net resistance to the flow of blood from the heart; along with cardiac output, this is an important determinant of blood pressure. This resistance can be varied by alterations in the levels of norepinephrine release and nitric oxide production; by a myriad of other factors such as local tissue acidity, the oxygen concentration in the blood, temperature; and also by other hormones which can stimulate or inhibit smooth muscle cell shortening.

Apart from variation in the overall net resistance to blood flow, the degree of constriction or relaxation varies from region to region in different physiological circumstances. For example, although during strenuous EXERCISE the heart may increase its pumping rate by about five times, the rate of delivery blood to each organ does not increase by this amount. Instead, the combined effects of activation of the sympathetic nervous system, and the release of substances generated in the heart and working muscles, causes the arteries in the heart and muscles to dilate dramatically, while the arteries in the non-working muscle and the digestive organs constrict. In this way, the flow of blood and therefore of oxygen to the muscles and to the heart may increase by twenty- and five-fold respectively, while the flow of blood to the rest of the body, excepting the brain, actually falls. Conversely, at rest after a meal, it is the vessels of the digestive organs which dilate.

The humble workhorse

In the gut, the smooth muscle is responsible for the many types of motility — *peristalsis*, which moves the contents along; *relaxation*, which accommodates a meal in the stomach; various *churning* and *mixing* movements; and finally *expulsion* of faeces — assisted by voluntary action.

Analogous changes in the functioning of the smooth muscles embedded in other organs are needed to support an enormous variety of involuntary activities, ranging from childbirth and ejaculation to urination, digestion, and visual adjustment to darkness and light. Indeed, as it faithfully performs its various automatically controlled tasks, this humble cousin of the heart and voluntary muscles plays many vital but unheralded roles in shaping both the most dramatic and the most routine events of our lives.

PHILIP AARONSON

See also ALIMENTARY SYSTEM; AUTONOMIC NERVOUS SYSTEM; BLOOD VESSELS; LUNGS.

Snoring
'Laugh and the world laughs with you, snore, and you snore alone' — from Anthony Burgess's *Inside Mr Enderby* (1963). It is a misquote of the original 'Laugh and the world laughs with you, weep, and you weep alone', from Ella Wheeler Wilcox (1855–1919).

Snoring has been a source of material for music hall mirth and general humour for centuries. Its association with obesity and alcohol has offered further scope for the stand-up comedian. Until relatively recently snoring was not considered a significant problem, except by the long-suffering partner behind closed bedroom doors, and those musing on the possible evolutionary advantage of snoring — the most entertaining suggestion from the latter being that snoring is a signal during the dark hours to potential marauders that there are large men about, so attack at your peril!

All this has changed since about 1965, when it was first reported that the PHARYNX, more specifically the airway behind the TONGUE, could collapse repeatedly during SLEEP, thus recurrently asphyxiating the sufferer, over and over again, hundreds of times a night. This condition is generally called *obstructive sleep apnoea*. This incompetence of the pharynx and failure to remain adequately patent only occurs during sleep, when muscle tone is at its lowest. It is always accompanied by loud snoring, which develops when the pharyngeal walls are close enough together to vibrate, a half-way house to complete obstruction. This condition of obstructive sleep apnoea is not just a physiological curiosity, but has been shown to lead to profound sleep fragmentation and excessive sleepiness. More recently, this excessive sleepiness has been shown to increase substantially the risk of driving accidents.

Both snoring and sleep apnoea are common; about a quarter of men snore regularly and about 1% have sleep apnoea sufficient to cause some degree of excessive daytime sleepiness. Why should this be the case? To some extent the pharynx represents an area of 'compromise engineering'. Because we must both eat and breathe through the pharynx, sometimes it has to be held open by muscles to allow air to pass unheeded, and sometimes it must collapse and propel food on its way into the *oesophagus* (gullet). Thus it is essentially a floppy tube, which requires muscle action to hold it open when required for breathing. The main factor that

encourages narrowing and collapse is OBESITY, which crowds the pharyngeal airway and can overwhelm the dilator muscle action during sleep. For example, collar size is one of the best predictors of whether someone snores. In addition, if the pharynx is small to start with — for example if the lower face is relatively set back — or occupied by large tonsils, then it takes little further narrowing to obstruct airflow. It would have been so much better if nature had provided us with separate routes through which to eat and breathe!

Other factors that encourage snoring and sleep apnoea are the muscle relaxation brought about by alcohol, and a blocked nose (which encourages further collapse of the pharynx during inspiration).

What does all this mean to the health of the human body? There is little evidence that occasional light snoring does any harm at all. As the amount of obstruction in the pharynx gets more, and the snoring gets louder, then this indicates a compromised airway and increasingly obstructed breathing. This in turn produces poor, fragmented sleep and daytime sleepiness. Thus a snorer with daytime sleepiness should be encouraged to seek help. There is also increasing evidence that heavy snoring and sleep apnoea may contribute to a raised BLOOD PRESSURE, with secondary consequences such as STROKE and HEART ATTACKS. However, this effect is likely to be small when compared with other known risk factors such as SMOKING.

The sound of snoring alone causes much misery to partners, and for this reason many remedies are peddled. Few have robust scientific support, although weight loss, alcohol reduction, and sleeping semi-propped up are usually the simplest first approaches. Small intra-oral devices worn in the mouth at night to hold the lower jaw forward are increasingly popular. Surgery should be viewed as a last resort for the desperate, as it is of only limited efficacy. At the more severe end of the spectrum, for obstructive sleep apnoea, *nasal continuous positive airway pressure* treatment is highly effective. This requires wearing, during sleep, a mask over the nose that gently pressurizes the upper airway and splints it open, preventing the narrowing and collapse. However, this is difficult to get used to, and is only tolerated by individuals suffering from incapacitating daytime sleepiness — which this treatment abolishes, leading to spectacular improvement in quality of life.   J. STRADLING

See also SLEEP; SLEEP DISORDERS.

Sociobiology
Some animals lead very solitary lives, but others, including humans, live in complex social groups. Sociobiology is the branch of biology that deals with the behaviour of these social animals. The term was coined by the Harvard entomologist, Edward O. Wilson, whose book of the same name brought to a wider public several important developments in theoretical biology that had been made during the 1960s and 1970s.

These developments addressed the phenomenon of altruism, which had long been seen as a problem in evolutionary biology (see EVOLUTION). Altruism is defined by biologists as any act that makes the recipient more likely to survive and reproduce while reducing the donor's own reproductive success. Since natural selection cares only about reproductive success, it seemed that altruism could not have evolved by such a process. And yet it was everywhere visible, from the parental care exhibited by mammals and birds to the selfless devotion of worker ants to their nest.

In the 1960s and 1970s, two solutions were proposed to this problem. The first of these was the theory of kin selection, which was first proposed by W. D. Hamilton in 1964. Hamilton argued that the spread of a gene did not depend only on its effects on the reproductive success of the body in which it sat, but also on its effects on the reproductive success of close kin, because they are likely to carry the same gene. A gene that caused its owner to risk his or her life to save several siblings, each of whom has a 50% chance of having the same gene, would spread quickly through the population, even if it often caused its owner to die childless. As Richard Dawkins put it graphically in *The Selfish Gene* (1976), the theory of kin selection showed that genes could proliferate by helping copies of themselves in other bodies.

Hamilton's theory of kin selection explains altruism between closely related individuals, but what about altruism between unrelated organisms? This is where the second solution to the problem of altruism comes in. In 1971, Robert Trivers argued that altruism may often be merely apparent, since it will turn out on a closer analysis to be a reciprocal exchange of favours. Trivers dubbed the phenomenon 'reciprocal altruism', and argued that the appearance of altruism is generated by the fact that the reciprocation may not be immediate. For example, a vampire bat may give up some of its food to a hungry companion one day without any immediate reward, but only because it expects that the favour will be returned in the future. In the years following Trivers' initial paper many biologists thought that reciprocal altruism was widespread in the animal kingdom. More recently, however, considerable doubt has been cast on this assumption.

The theories of kin selection and reciprocal altruism have led to much productive research in animal behaviour. When applied to human behaviour, however, they have generated much more controversy. Wilson's *Sociobiology*, for example, unleashed a torrent of criticism when it was published in 1975. Although he dedicated only a short final chapter of the book to human behaviour, the ensuing debate focused almost entirely on the possibility of applying sociobiological tools to humans. Social scientists, in particular, objected to such biological explanations on the grounds that they did not do justice to the rich cultural variability of human behaviour (see INSTINCT).

After the initial backlash against sociobiology in the late 1970s, attempts to apply theories such as those of Hamilton and Trivers to human behaviour regained popularity during the 1990s. The second generation of sociobiologists, who are much more circumspect in avoiding some of the brash pronouncements of the 1970s, go under the name of 'evolutionary psychologists'. Evolutionary psychology, while in many ways the heir of sociobiology, differs in stressing the importance of the mental mechanisms that mediate selective pressures and behaviour. It is thus more mentalist than sociobiology, and draws on the explanatory tools of cognitive science, such as the use of the language of information processing to describe the mind.

However, unlike cognitive scientists of a more classical bent, evolutionary psychologists reject the idea of a central 'executive' within the mind, arguing instead that co-ordinated behaviour emerges from a collection of psychological mechanisms, none of which is 'in control'. These 'mental modules' are thought to be designed by natural selection to solve adaptive problems that were recurrently faced by our ancestors. For example, it is has been hypothesized that there is a module for detecting cheats, another for recognizing faces, and so on.

Like sociobiology, evolutionary psychology has attracted more than its fair share of critics. Some of these attack evolutionary psychology for allegedly excessive speculation, while others have ethical and political objections. Evolutionary psychologists reject both kinds of criticism. The debate goes on. DYLAN EVANS

Further reading
Pinker, S. (1997). *How the mind works.* Penguin, Harmondsworth.

Wilson, E. O. (1975). *Sociobiology: the new synthesis.* Harvard University Press, Cambridge, MA.

See also EVOLUTION, HUMAN; GENETICS, HUMAN.

Sociology
The human body has always been central to sociology because sociology is about the organisation of collections of human bodies into forms of social life. Sociologists have also always been concerned with the question of the boundary between the biological and the social in the formation of human identity; the so-called *nature/nurture* controversy. But until the late 1970s the body as the physical expression or embodiment of human identity, personal experience, and action was largely ignored by sociologists, who concentrated on the structuring of groups and societies. Against this background it is generally agreed that the recent specific interest in the sociology of the body has developed for three main reasons.

Modernity and the body
Firstly, there is the series of complex social and cultural changes associated with the rise of modernity. Modernity has a long history, but amongst the most significant social processes identified with rapid socio-economic and technical change since the nineteenth century, is the emergence of consumer culture. The marketing and consumption of mass-produced consumer goods involves an unprecedented exploitation of visual images of the body, ranging from photography and the cinema to computer-mediated forms of communication. Linked with innovations in processes of mass communication, consumer culture encourages the cultivation of individualized lifestyles in which bodily and self-display play a prominent part. An easy test of the extent of this influence on everyday life is to make a rough count of the images of human bodies in various states of dress encountered during the course of an ordinary day and then add to these the number of mirrors and other surfaces reflecting one's own face and physical appearance. This account can then be compared with an estimate of such images one would have been likely to see before the end of the nineteenth century, especially images of one's own face and body.

The proliferation of images of the body is a significant aspect of the growth of individualism — the high value given to the private individual or person — which is regarded by sociologists as a key feature of modernity. Modernity has been equated with the shift from the social to the individual person who spends increasing amounts of time cultivating personal identity through the cultivation of the body. A good example is the growth in regimes for body modification, including gymnasia, LEISURE and keep fit centres, and health farms; also the expanding selection of magazines, newspaper articles, and TV programmes designed to encourage body-consciousness and self-expression. It is argued that a key reason underlying this change is the transition from traditional to modern forms of human association, where the links between human beings are no longer established by the rules of traditional community life. Rather, they have been replaced with those based upon agreements and contracts made between people who regard themselves as private individuals operating in a free market. In this situation the individuals are dependent upon their own resources, including those of the body; the competent self requires a functioning body which is capable of sustained activity and of responding to the demands of rapid and risky social change. The move from traditional forms of social and economic organization to 'late modern' societies is therefore seen as one requiring a flexible embodied self whose identity is much less stable than perhaps was the case in the past. The result is an increasing tendency to regard the nature of the body not as fixed, but as highly flexible and open to social construction/reconstruction through various techniques of body- and therefore self-modification. Another good example is the rising demand for COSMETIC SURGERY, a reflection of the current value placed upon the interdependence of body and self, and of the importance of embodied self-expression in an individualized social world.

Feminism and the body
The second major influence on the emergence of sociological interest in the body is the feminist movement. From the 1970s feminist scholarship has played an important part in bringing the body back into sociology. The traditional concern of feminists with the exclusion of women from the public sphere is expressed in sociology as a major critical attack on their neglect by male sociologists, who have taken 'man', and especially 'public man', as the model for the whole of 'humanity'. Feminists argue that the equation *'man' = society* stems from a neglect of the personal and social lives of women. This arises from assumptions about the nature of biological differences between the bodies of men and women and their influence on the roles they should play in society. At the heart of this issue is the recurring question of biology and society: to what extent are the differences between male and female bodies biologically determined, or socially and culturally constructed? Whilst biological differences in the reproductive functions of men and women are clearly evident the question remains of the social interpretations placed upon this difference and the ways in which perceptions of these differences influence forms of social discrimination between the genders.

One typical area is the matter of GENDER differences in the AGEING process. Because their bodies are biologically programmed for conception and childbirth, women undergo a number of changes called the MENOPAUSE, with the cessation of the ability to produce children. With the apparent exception of a few unusual cases, this process of biological change is unknown in men. That much is generally agreed but, as feminist scholars argue, the fact of this bodily change is no justification for the elaborate construction of personal and social distinctions between middle-aged men and women which characterize social stereotypes of 'menopausal women'. In fact menopausal changes are highly variable and there are good reasons to believe that the severity of these physical effects is widely exaggerated. Yet the menopause is also widely stereotyped as a troublesome period for women.

The major contribution of feminists to the sociology of the body has been to challenge the belief that the biology of the body is the bottom line and to show how the meanings given to the body are socially constructed by those who are in a position to create ideas about the body and put them into practice. In this area many sociologists have been influenced by the work of Michel Foucault, who regards the body as the subject of power and discipline, especially the power and disciplined knowledge of the expert. Partly because power and the exercise of power has always been a central concern for sociologists, Foucault's theoretical and historical analyses of body discipline have formed the basis for much contemporary empirical research on the body, including SEXUALITY, health education, doctor–patient relationships, mental illness, the social organization of hospitals, DENTISTRY, geriatric medicine, and crime and punishment. In this work sociologists are principally concerned to show how experts such as medical investigators do not simply discover the biological secrets of the body, which are somehow waiting there to be observed, but also actively construct ways of perceiving the body and giving meaning to it; observations of the body, even using the most advanced technology, are influenced by the ideas and beliefs of the day. According to Foucault, experts in sexology during the nineteenth century were instrumental in creating a whole new range of sexual experiences and behaviour through their prescriptions of what could be defined as 'normal' sexual practice. Their 'discoveries' of new sexual deviations and 'PERVERSIONS' had the unintended effect of extending the repertoire of sexual behaviour and producing new forms of social problems for experts to resolve. Similarly, geriatric medicine, also an invention of the nineteenth century, can be seen sociologically as an attempt to determine the nature of the ageing body by constructing categories of distinction between 'normal' and 'pathological' ageing processes. This development is a crucial part of the process whereby members of the medical profession lay claims to certain forms of expertise and therefore the power to discriminate between older people. The point is not that there is no such thing as biological sex or the biologically ageing body but that our perceptions and understanding of them are shaped by the practical social activities of those who wish to set themselves up as experts working within specific professional fields.

The civilizing process and the body

In the sociology of the body all roads ultimately lead to contemporary versions of the old nature/nurture debate — the question of the boundaries between the biological, the social, and the psychological. Another key influence here is the German sociologist Norbert Elias (1897–1990), for whom it is a waste of time and intellectual effort to assess the relative contributions of biology, society, and psychology to the causes of any human behaviour. His argument, based on detailed studies of the history of human VIOLENCE, bodily functions (sexual activity, eating habits, excretion), and the EMOTIONS, is that over a long period of time these three have become indivisible. Although human behaviour is inevitably grounded in biology and we cannot escape the material limitations of our bodies, this basic physical potential is overlaid by the long-term cultural transformations that Elias calls 'the civilizing process'.

The civilizing process is characterized by the gradual domination of learned over instinctual experience, a process he describes as 'symbol emancipation'. Through the long history of the species, human beings have gradually become distanced, by the accumulation of a vast cultural heritage, from their basic instinctual drives and biological urges: human beings survive because of their innate capacity for learned behaviour. Whilst therefore human societies are composed of bodies these are collections of the bodies of individuals who have learned from a vast inherited cultural repertoire the importance of exercising control over their bodies and who are subject to the often self-imposed restraints of guilt, shame, and embarrassment. One consequence of this long-term process is the emergence of the disciplined individual, who through self and bodily discipline is able to establish collaborative relationships with other people, many of whom, in the modern world, will be strangers. The civilized individual is slow to anger and emotionally calculating, exercising a high degree of discipline over bodily functions such as eating, excretion, and sexual activity. The civilized individual has a strong sense of the boundaries prescribed by good manners and etiquette between one human body and another and the subtle distinctions between public and private space. The civilized individual is the citizen of the modern world.

Body and self

If at the present moment a generalization about the sociological analysis of the human body can be made, it is that recent work is marked by an increasingly sophisticated and theoretically complex rejection of crude attempts to reduce the body to a biological mechanism. In particular, the dualistic or binary approach — inherited from Descartes, who separated the mind from the body — is regarded at worst as totally unacceptable and at best as an issue for further enquiry and research. The idea of the self (or SOUL) having a separate existence within the body is seen by many sociologists to be indefensible at a time when science and technology are transforming human beings into part biology and part machine. The emergence of 'cyborg culture' raises urgent questions about what it is to be a human body, when increasingly our bodies are invaded by surgical techniques, and deficient organs are replaced or given mechanical substitutes. One hope for those who regard the ageing of the population as a major social problem is in the prospect of advances in 'young' laboratory-grown replacement tissues and organs to replace the 'aged' in the bodies of older people. Similarly developments in genetic science hold out hope for the discovery of the ageing gene and the abolition of old age.

Technology as culture frees the body from biology, because it enables humans to modify their bodies, both in their external appearance and in their inner structures and functions. A concern with modern identities has resulted in much closer enquiry into the emergence of individuality and self-consciousness in late modern forms of social organization, where technology and consumer culture have produced a significant change in the relationship between the social, the cultural, and the biological. Yet at the same time, as many sociologists indicate, the spectre of the death of the body continues to haunt the modern world. The ageing of the population on a global scale is, therefore, a final reason for the increasing interest in the sociology of the body. In modern societies old age takes us to the limits of the increasingly blurring boundary between the biological and the social: old age becomes in a very real sense the final problem. For another twentieth-century German sociologist, Zigmunt Bauman, modern societies conceal death because death conflicts with the continual process of making and re-making the self, which is central to modernity. Selfhood is grounded in consciousness of one's own bodily processes and the belief in science, yet the desire of human beings for complete control over their lives and destinies exists uneasily alongside an increasing awareness of the limitations of scientific knowledge and of the risks it entails.

If the self and the body form a culturally integrated whole and the self is essentially embodied — has no existence outside the body — then problems arise when the body begins to decline or is disabled. For some sociologists the future lies in the disembodied world of 'cyberspace', where the electronic media liberate individuals from the encumbrance of the body, a development which is seen as potentially beneficial for those excluded from normal social interaction through bodily impairment and disability. But the reference point of individual identity, even in cyberspace, is still the human body, and in the last analysis images have to be related to embodiment as it is experienced, if they are to influence practical human relationships and shape the quality of the experience of everyday life.

MIKE HEPWORTH

Further reading
Shilling, C. (1993). *The body and social theory.* Sage, London.

Turner, B. S. (1996). *The body and society,* (2nd edn). London.

See also AGEING; FEMINISM; LEISURE; PHILOSOPHY AND THE BODY; WORK AND THE BODY.

Solar plexus
Plexus (from the Latin for 'braid') is the name used to describe a network of nerves; a 'spaghetti junction' which many nerves pass through and where their branches split off to merge with those of others. A plexus such as this one, where most of the nerves belong to the AUTONOMIC NERVOUS SYSTEM, also embeds relay stations — the *ganglia* where sympathetic nerve fibres coming from the SPINAL CORD relay at synapses with the *post-ganglionic* nerves that then proceed to their destination on smooth muscles or glands.

Solar is the more colourful adjective for the plexus, otherwise known as *coeliac* (derived from the Greek for 'belly'). Its widely-radiating incoming and outgoing nerves, linking the two coeliac ganglia, are fancifully likened to the sun's rays. It lies mainly on the front of the aorta, where this main artery enters the abdomen by passing down through the DIAPHRAGM — at the 'pit of the stomach', and behind the stomach itself. The sympathetic nerves to the abdominal organs, glands, and blood vessels relay here, or pass through in branches to other satellite plexuses and relay there. Since these nerves originate from the lower thoracic segments of the spinal cord, they reach the plexus by passing down from the thoracic cavity. The ADRENAL GLANDS are among the organs innervated via the plexus, which therefore incorporates the nerve pathway for switching on the release of adrenaline into the bloodstream from the adrenal medulla. In addition to the sympathetic components, branches from the VAGUS NERVES also pass this way, to be distributed to the abdominal organs. They carry parasympathetic nerve fibres descending from the BRAIN STEM, which activate the muscle and glands of the gut, and ascending fibres serving VISCERAL SENSATION. Injections that block nerve transmission in the plexus may be helpful in the treatment of intractable abdominal PAIN, such as in cancer of the pancreas. A *coeliac plexus reflex* is described, consisting of a fall in BLOOD PRESSURE when the upper abdominal organs are handled during a surgical operation. A reflex as well as a mechanical effect may also be involved in the sensation of being 'winded' by a blow in this region.   SHEILA JENNETT

See also AUTONOMIC NERVOUS SYSTEM; VAGUS NERVES; VISCERAL SENSATION.

Somatic sensation
Sensations arising from the SKIN — such as touch, pressure, cold, warmth, and pain — and from the MUSCLES, TENDONS, and JOINTS — such as the position of the limbs and pain — are known as somatic sensations. *Soma*, the Greek word for body, refers to the whole of the body structure, apart from the GERM CELLS (eggs and sperm). Sensations arising from the internal organs (the viscera), such as pain or the sense of fullness of the stomach or bladder, may therefore be included, although they are usually considered separately as VISCERAL SENSATIONS. Pain arising from the viscera is often felt as though it comes from some part of the body surface or underlying tissue (referred pain).

All somatic sensations start with the excitation of SENSORY RECEPTORS located in the appropriate tissue — skin, muscle, joints etc. But we are not passive recipients of stimuli, and indeed the amount of information received in a passive way is severely limited. We, and other animals, actively explore objects to obtain information about them. Somatic sensation is intimately associated with movement (and also with resistance to movement). We use our fingers and also our tongue and lips to explore objects in order to identify their structure and form. Good examples of such 'active touch' include reading of Braille characters and the sorting and selecting of objects in a pocket, out of sight. Coins can be selected on the basis of size, shape, weight, and other distinguishing characteristics, such as the presence of a milled edge. Metal objects may be differentiated from non-metal ones on the basis of perceived temperature differences due to their different heat conducting properties, or by their weight relative to their size.

Modern experimental research on the mechanisms underlying somatic sensation (somatosensory mechanisms) began in the nineteenth century with psychophysical experiments on humans, supported by studies of the structure of sense organs in both human and animal tissues. Then, with the advent of electronic amplifiers, in the 1920s and 1930s the emphasis switched to animal experiments, where it continues to the present: electrical recordings of neural activity evoked by the stimulation of sensory receptors have been made from all parts of the nervous system concerned with somatic sensation. In the past thirty years, electrical recordings have also been made from peripheral nerves in conscious human subjects, and these important experiments have added enormously to our understanding. Most recently, advanced IMAGING TECHNIQUES have been used to examine which parts of the brain are active during particular tactual tasks in awake humans.

The sensory receptors in the different tissues and organs are highly selective (or specific). Each type responds only to a particular stimulus, such as mechanical displacement, or cooling, or warming, or harmful stimuli, and not to more than one such kind of stimulus. These receptors, in turn, are connected through chains of nerve cells (neurons) to the somatosensory areas of the brain's CEREBRAL CORTEX in such a way that the specificity of the information is maintained — the ascending information travels along parallel pathways that may be considered as 'pure lines'.

The idea that SENSE ORGANS are specific for particular stimuli and that their excitation leads to specific sensations was first clearly stated in 1811 by the Edinburgh anatomist Sir Charles Bell, but is more commonly attributed to Johannes Müller, who elaborated his Law of Specific Nerve Energies in 1826. Müller did not distinguish between the various sensations that can be elicited from the body, being more concerned with the special senses such as VISION. Various workers established that *cutaneous sensation* (that arising from the skin) is punctate (spotty) in character, and attempts were made to identify particular structures (sensory receptors) at the sites of the sensory spots. These attempts were, at best, only partially successful, although the classical theory of von Frey (1852–1932) allots a particular type of receptor to each of the main cutaneous sensations (touch, cold, warmth, and pain). It was not until careful animal experiments were carried out that the situation clarified. A most important step forward was made by E. D. (later Lord) Adrian, the Cambridge physiologist who, in the 1920s, showed that there are specific sensory receptors in skin and muscle responding only to particular stimuli, and that these receptors transform the stimuli into trains of nerve impulses which are conducted into the CENTRAL NERVOUS SYSTEM along peripheral nerve fibres. The analysis of the quality of a stimulus is therefore carried out by specific receptors, while information about stimulus intensity is carried

by the frequency of the nerve impulses in the sensory nerve fibres. We now know that all mammalian species, including humans, have the same types of sensory receptors in skin, muscle, tendon, and joints. Remarkable experiments initiated by the Swedish neurophysiologists, K.-E. Hagbarth and Å. B. Vallbo, in the late 1960s, in which electrical recordings were made from single peripheral nerve fibres in conscious human subjects, have confirmed that humans have the same sensory receptors as animals such as the cat. In addition, by electrically stimulating the individual nerve fibres from which recordings were made, they were able to determine the *conscious experience* (sensation) which results from activation of a particular receptor type. Thus, in the skin there are separate receptors responding to touch, light pressure, hair movement, vibration, cooling, warming, and harmful (painful) stimuli. In muscle and tendon there are receptors responding to muscle length, muscle tension, and harmful stimuli, and in the joint capsule there are receptors monitoring joint position and also responding to harmful events, these latter being exaggerated in inflammatory conditions, mimicking arthritic disease.

The peripheral sensory apparatus, consisting of the sensory receptors and the nerve fibres which connect them to the central nervous system, is therefore responsible for establishing which kinds of stimuli we can respond to, for setting the sensitivity of the system, and for determining the intensity of stimulation. Furthermore, it is also largely responsible for sensory acuity of the different parts of the body, because certain parts contain a higher density of receptors than others. There are very high densities of cutaneous receptors on the tips of the fingers, the lips, and the TONGUE: the parts of the body surface at which the greatest spatial resolution of sensation can be made, and the parts which are actively used to explore objects.

The information carried by the peripheral nerve fibres enters the central nervous system either at the SPINAL CORD or, for information from the head, at the BRAIN STEM. Here the various inputs from different receptors are distributed into separate sets of ascending channels (pathways or components of pathways) and passed on to the cerebral cortex. Because of the selective channelling of information from different receptor types into different ascending neuronal pathways, it is possible for damage to a particular pathway to produce a selective loss of sensations. For example, damage to part of the spinal cord (*posterior* or *dorsal columns*) leads to loss of vibration sense, whereas damage to another part (*anterolateral columns*) may lead to loss of temperature sense.

As the sensory information ascends to the cerebral cortex, considerable neuronal processing occurs at places where one set of nerve fibres connects with the next set of nerve cells in the chain, usually in clearly-defined parts of the nervous system called 'nuclei'. The processing extracts information from the input and performs analyses on it, such as the enhancement of contrasts (e.g. detection of edges), the orientation of linear stimuli, and the direction of movement of moving stimuli. At each processing station there is the opportunity for certain parts of the information to be suppressed, as would be necessary for selective attention. The *nociceptive* information — information concerning harmful events — that ultimately gives rise to the sensation of *pain* is commonly suppressed, especially during activities that are highly charged with emotion, such as during sports activities or in battle.

Each of the central processing stations, including those in the cerebral cortex itself (*cortical somatosensory areas*), are organized such that they contain a map of the body which can be revealed by recording from the nerve cells. Adjacent nerve cells are excited from adjacent parts of the body. In this way the nervous system locates the position at which a stimulus is acting on the body. Damage to part of one of these sensory maps, for example in the cerebral cortex, will produce sensory changes (a loss or reduction in a particular sensation or group of sensations) localized to a particular part of the body. It is therefore possible for a clinician to determine where brain damage might be located, by testing sensation. Similarly, with special averaging techniques it is possible to record, from the human scalp, the electrical and, more recently, the magnetic activity evoked in localized areas of the brain following localized stimulation of the body surface.

Initial processing in the cerebral cortex takes place in the somatosensory cortical areas. In order to allow for more subtle analysis by the brain, the information is then passed on to motor areas (since active motion is important in active touch) and also to other parts of the cortex (*parietal cortex*), where higher-order analysis takes place and where information from other senses is received as well. Here, the analysis of spatial relations is important, as is the co-ordination of eye and hand movements. Damage to the parietal cortex, especially on the side of the brain not concerned with *language*, leads to impairment in the ability to deal with extrapersonal space, and the patient may even deny that the opposite side of his body exists. Conversely, phantom sensations of movement may occur following amputations.   ALAN G. BROWN

See also SENSORY RECEPTORS; VISCERAL SENSATION.

Sonogram
An image of the body's interior produced by sound waves — or, rather, by ULTRASOUND, because the waves are of much higher frequency than those which can be heard. Sound imaging originally helped military personnel locate enemy aircraft and submarines in World War II. After the war, medical researchers began to apply this technology to the human body. Doctors first employed ultrasound to look at the brain, to diagnose heart disease, and to detect tumours. Obstetricians also started to utilize the diagnostic technique because of the

dangers associated with X-raying fetuses, a practice that resulted in deaths from cancer in children under the age of 10. Sonograms have become an established part of prenatal care in the First World because the equipment used to produce these images is affordable and can be used in the doctor's office. Ultrasound is ordered routinely — although one study in 1993 concluded that sonograms provide no substantial health benefit for the mother or the fetus. Many physicians, however, disagree with this assessment and argue that sonograms furnish important information about the development, health, and age of fetuses. Sonograms confirm pregnancies, ensure that fetuses are developing normally, determine age, and indicate delivery dates more accurately. Ultrasound technology also represents a non-invasive form of medical diagnosis that can take the place of exploratory surgery.

The ability to 'see' inside the human body has had effects far outside medicine. Mothers and fathers proudly display sonograms in baby albums and on refrigerators. The sonogram itself is an expected element of modern pregnancy. Pro-choice defenders argue that the fetus, not the pregnant woman, has become the major actor in this biological and cultural drama. Pro-life proponents, by contrast, embrace the fetus as the symbol of their struggle. They have employed ultrasound technology in the film *The Silent Scream* in order to highlight the PERSONHOOD of the fetus and they use fetal imagery in their advertising campaigns.   KAROL K. WEAVER

Further reading
Busch, A. (1995). Ethical fervor and the graphics of choice. *Print*, **49**, 52–6.

Duden, B. (1993). *Disembodying women: perspectives on pregnancy and the unborn*, Hoinacki. Harvard University Press, Cambridge, MA.

Kevles, B. H. (1997). *Naked to the bone: medical imaging in the twentieth century*. Addison Wesley, Reading, MA.

See also IMAGING TECHNIQUES; ULTRASOUND.

Soul
In the Hebrew scriptures, the human being is a single and undivided entity: the soul and body are not clearly distinguished from one another. Thus any discussion of life after death points to the resurrection of the body rather than the immortality of the soul (Isaiah 26: 19 and Daniel 12: 2). Jewish and Old Testament scholars have debated whether the authors of the Hebrew scriptures ever thought of the body and soul as distinct entities; certainly, later Jewish writers have interpreted passages such as Ecclesiastes 12: 7 — 'Then shall the dust return to the earth as it was; and the spirit shall return unto God who gave it' — to mean that at the death of the body the soul returns to reside with God forever.

The Greek, especially the Platonic, tradition saw the soul and body as utterly distinct and separate entities. For the Platonists, the soul is the human being; the intellect is eternal, and pre-exists and survives the body. In this earthly life, the soul makes use of the body and its instincts

which, while not seen as evil, must be kept under control. While Aristotle modified this Platonic teaching, the Neoplatonist, Plotinus, developed it such that his biographer, Porphyry, recorded that Plotinus would tell no one his birth date, as the day of his soul's entry into his body was cause for mourning, not celebration.

This Greek tradition affected Judaism. The Greek-speaking community in Alexandria, of whom the foremost member was the philosopher Philo, began to understand the body and soul as completely distinct from one another, and Philo taught the immortality of the soul. The distinction between body and soul exists everywhere in the Rabbinical/Talmudic literature, and medieval Jewish thinkers understood the body and soul as being in struggle, and therefore promoted a denial of bodily pleasures; Maimonides saw the building up of the body as occurring at the expense of the destruction of the soul. The Kabbalists believed that the soul was a divine entity which had to descend into the body.

The Christian tradition took on both the Hebrew and Greek traditions in its thinking about the soul. The Incarnation — the Word made flesh — emphasized the Hebrew notion of the unity of body and soul: Jesus was born of a woman, and thus God took human form, with a body and soul. However, in the Hellenistic world in which much of Christianity spread, Platonic notions of the soul as temporarily imprisoned in the body took hold, so that Origen, for example, believed that humans were originally created as intellects without a body, and taught that the pre-existing soul entered the body after it had fallen into sin, and was bound to the body as a punishment. However, he also taught that the soul uses the body for healing and restoration: the body itself is not evil, but rather our misuse of free will is the root of our evil (Origen's teaching on the soul was condemned, after his death, at the fifth ecumenical council in Constantinople, in 553). By contrast, Clement, another Platonist, did not understand the soul as pre-existing and saw the body in a more positive way, as the 'soul's consort and ally'.

Ideas about the soul were linked to notions of RESURRECTION of the body, and from the third century to the late Middle Ages many theologians emphasized the full and literal resurrection of the body after death. Tertullian, for example, following a stoic metaphysics, not only believed that resurrection meant the full reassemblage of the body but also that all reality is corporeal, and therefore even the soul is composed of fine material particles. Irenaeus held a similar view. However, such ideas gradually declined, and by the later Middle Ages Aquinas' view that the soul is an individual spiritual substance was becoming predominant (though it did not go unchallenged) and eventually received wide acceptance amongst many branches of Christianity. For Aquinas, influenced by Aristotle, body and soul together form the human unity, though the soul can be separated from the fleshly body, as happens at death, and continue to exist. It is believed, in this scholastic tradition, that each soul is made by God individually for each human body (*Creationism*, as opposed to *Traducianism*, a belief in which the soul is the product of the generative, material power of human beings, a view that was to be held by many Lutherans and Calvinists).

In some other religious systems and philosophies, body and soul are not as sharply opposed as they often have been in Christianity. In Taoism, the religious philosophy developed in China, the soul is essential to the body's wholeness and healing. Central to Taoism is a system of meditation and prayer in which the soul relates to the inner body and the external world. The 'shen', meaning soul or spirit, resides in the heart. When *ch'i* (mind energy), *shen* (soul), and *ching* (intuition and physical powers) are in harmony, the body is healthy, works in concert with nature and the person lives a long time. However, a person dies when the *ch'i* and *ching* are exhausted and at that point the soul leaves the body. In Zoroastrianism, the world's oldest prophetic religion, which originated in Iran, body and soul are seen as distinct from each other, but not necessarily opposed in a dualistic manner; indeed, bodily sickness is said to indicate the soul's sickness, while bodily HEALTH, FERTILITY, and maturity indicate spiritual health. The body is to be treated with respect and is seen as a part of the human being's ultimate nature, not a means to an incorporeal nature.   JANE SHAW

See also MIND–BODY PROBLEM; RELIGION AND THE BODY.

Sounds of the body
The healthy functioning of the human body produces a variety of sounds. We can readily hear the movement of air through the MOUTH and NOSE, and in and out of the bronchi and the LUNGS; the sounds which come from the beating HEART as its valves close in sequence; blood pulsating along the arteries; and the rumblings of gas in the alimentary canal. Coughing serves to clear fluid from the airways; hiccuping has no known function. Not so long ago, aural detection of the fetal heartbeat within a swollen female abdomen was the only totally unequivocal clinical indication of PREGNANCY.

All of the body's normal sounds may become modified in disease. The rhythms of BREATHING may change, becoming laboured or irregular. The note of the COUGH alters. Bronchi, inflamed or otherwise constricted, wheeze. The lungs and their membranes may begin to creak, rasp, or hiss, to transmit the voice more clearly or the breath sounds less so. Narrowing of the arteries and valvular disease of the heart both replace the relative quiet of smooth blood flow with the gurgles of turbulence.

Pathological processes may also reveal themselves by the production of sounds unheard in health, such as the creaking of arthritic JOINTS; the crepitus of broken bones; and slopping of abnormal accumulation of fluid in the abdomen. A tinkling sound in the flesh around an infected wound is a dreadful sign, indicative of gas gangrene. The absence of sound may be equally

ominous. A blocked artery is quiet downstream of the occlusion. Silence in the bowel demands urgent investigation.

The physicians of ancient Greece knew of the diagnostic value of applying the ear to the chest wall in order to listen to the sounds of the lungs. Sometimes they would shake their patients in an attempt to elicit splashing noises in the thoracic cavity. In the eighteenth century, Leonard Auenbrugger invented the technique of percussion; tapping the thorax with the finger. Regions of the chest that were filled with air resonated; solid or fluid-filled regions did not. The character of the sound elicited by tapping was, thus, indicative of the state of health of the underlying tissues.

The invention of the STETHOSCOPE, in 1816, made the clinical study of both normal and pathological sounds much easier, but it was only after considerable research and controversy that the cause and meaning of many of the pathological sounds, and even some of the normal ones, were fully clarified. In the nineteenth century, more than thirty-five different theories were suggested to account for the two principal cardiac sounds. The study of pathological noises was hampered both by deficiencies in the understanding of the physics of sound and by an unduly slavish allegiance to the idea that particular sounds were the characteristic signatures of particular diseases. It only gradually became appreciated that an abnormal sound signifies not necessarily a specific disease but rather a specific alteration of bodily structure.

MALCOLM NICOLSON

See also AUSCULTATION; DIAGNOSIS.

Space travel
Manned space flight commenced with the orbital flight by Gagarin in April 1961. By 1996 over six hundred human beings had flown in space for periods of time varying between a few hours and 438 days. Space travel is set to become more frequent in the twenty-first century, although the financial cost of the vehicles and their propulsion systems will limit the number of individuals who will experience the excitements and wonders of space flight. Flight in space is characterized by the absence of gravity, the absence of the Earth's atmosphere with the associated absence of protection against solar and cosmic radiation, and the vast distances which have to be traversed to reach other planets.

A spacecraft must be accelerated to a velocity of 8 km per second (17 900 mph) to enter into orbital flight around the Earth and to a velocity of 11.6 km per second (25 900 mph) to escape Earth's gravitational field and travel into outer space. Similar changes in velocity are required to return safely to the surface of the Earth. The velocity required to enter orbital flight can be attained by suitable combinations of acceleration (G) and time (828 G seconds are required to reach orbital velocity). In practice, the pattern of acceleration is determined by the design of the rocket motors. Development of the latter has

resulted in a progressive reduction in the maximum acceleration from 5–7 G in early flights to 3 G in the Space Shuttle. The effects of the G on the circulation are minimized by placing the long axis of the body of the astronaut at right angles to the direction of travel of the space vehicle. The accelerative forces associated with returning to the Earth from orbital flight are about half those of launch into orbit, and the physiological effects are minimized by appropriate orientation of the spacecraft.

An artificial gaseous environment must be produced with the spacecraft, and its cabin must be sealed to a very high standard to avoid the loss of gases to the vacuum of space. Although 100% OXYGEN at a pressure of 1/3 atmosphere was employed in early American space vehicles, air at 1 atmosphere is the environment of choice in order to avoid the deleterious physiological effects of prolonged exposure to 100% oxygen and the high risk of fire associated with an oxygen atmosphere. Air at a pressure of 1 atmosphere does, however, have the disadvantage that, with present designs of space suits, 100% oxygen must be breathed for several hours before undertaking extra-vehicular activity in order to avoid DECOMPRESSION SICKNESS. The atmosphere of the sealed cabin must be conditioned continuously by the removal of carbon dioxide and the addition of oxygen. The heat generated by occupants and some of the equipment within the cabin is removed by cooling the air and removing water vapour. The environmental control required in the cabin of a spacecraft has also to be provided in individual space suits. Inflation of a space suit to a pressure of 1 atmosphere is associated with an unacceptable loss of mobility due to the 'stiffness' of the suit. Suit pressures of the order of 0.3 to 0.5 atmosphere are generally employed, with an internal suit atmosphere of 100% oxygen. Heat produced by the body and by incident solar radiation is removed by means of a liquid conditioning garment worn beneath the suit. The heat gained by the fluid circulating through the garment is rejected to space by evaporation of a suitable refrigerant.

Microgravity

The principal effects of the *microgravity* (also termed WEIGHTLESSNESS) of space travel arise in the vestibular, cardiovascular, and musculoskeletal systems. Space sickness, which comprises nausea, a general feeling of malaise, and often actual vomiting, occurs early in a flight and is greatly aggravated by rapid movements of the head. Adaptation occurs over the first few days of flight and the condition seldom persists for longer than 5–6 days. Like other forms of MOTION SICKNESS, space sickness is due to a conflict of sensory information from the VESTIBULAR SYSTEM and eyes to the CENTRAL NERVOUS SYSTEM. The abnormal sensory input in space sickness is the absence of signals from the *otolith* organs. The incidence and severity of the condition is reduced by avoiding head movements, especially rapid ones. The use of anti motion-sickness drugs during the first few days of flight is of considerable value.

In contrast to the effects of +G$_z$ (see G AND G-SUITS), microgravity abolishes all the hydrostatic pressure gradients within the circulation so that blood and tissue fluids move from the lower parts of the body to the head and chest. It is estimated that the volume of blood and tissue fluid in the lower limbs is reduced by 1.0–1.5 litres within the first 24 hours of exposure to microgravity. The veins of the head and neck are distended, and there is puffiness of the face and congestion of the nasal passages. The distension of the heart caused by the central movement of blood stimulates an increase in the excretion of urine, which in turn produces a reduction in the total volume of blood in the body. The circulation is well maintained whilst in microgravity. The most important effect of the circulatory changes induced by microgravity, is, however, a reduced tolerance to the shift of blood to the feet which occurs on return to the 1 G environment on the surface of the earth. The astronaut may feel faint and indeed a few have fainted on standing upright after landing.

The muscular effort required to maintain posture and to carry out physical tasks is reduced in microgravity. This reduction in muscle activity gives rise to a progressive loss of muscular strength and wasting (atrophy) of muscles over days and weeks in much the same manner as a long period of rest in bed. These effects of microgravity can be reduced by special regimes which exercise the muscles, especially those of the trunk and lower limbs. Cycling on an ergometer has been widely used during prolonged space flights.

Of even greater concern in long duration spaceflight is the loss of MINERALS from BONE produced by microgravity. The maintenance of normal bone structure and calcification of bone depend upon the physical stresses which living and working in a 1 G environment impose upon the bones. The greatly reduced forces in microgravity lead to *demineralization* of the bones. There is an increase in the loss of CALCIUM from the body and a decrease in the absorption of calcium from food. Studies conducted to date suggest that the loss of calcium, bone structure, and bone strength continue for as long as the individual is exposed to microgravity. The concern is the risk of fracture of bones on return to normal gravity, or even in spaceflight when the duration of the flight extends into many months. Although exercises which place high stresses on bones may retard the demineralization process, the effect of microgravity upon bone is probably an important determinant of the time which an individual may spend in space.

Cosmic radiation

Very little of the ionizing radiation present in space reaches the surface of the Earth, owing to the shield provided by the atmosphere and the magnetic field of the Earth. Once outside this protection a space vehicle is exposed to galactic radiation and to radiation from the sun. Furthermore, the Van Allen belts of high energy particles which lie between 250 and 44 000 km above the surface of the Earth form a potential hazard on missions deep into space. Most manned space flights to date have occurred at altitudes well below the inner Van Allan belt. The damaging effect which ionizing radiation has upon living matter varies with the nature and dose of the radiation, from damage to blood-forming organs to prolonged vomiting and nausea, to incapacitation and death within a few hours. At present the cumulative dose of radiation to which astronauts can be exposed over their total career in space is limited by considerations of damage to the most sensitive tissues such as the bone marrow, the lens of the eye, and the skin. The dose of radiation received by individual astronauts is monitored routinely in space flights. The effect of cosmic radiation is probably the principal hazard for prolonged interplanetary space flight. There is a limit to the protection which can be afforded by either passive or active shielding against the ionizing radiation of space.

JOHN ERNSTING

Further reading

Ernsting, J. and King, P. (1988). *Aviation medicine*, (2nd edn). Butterworth-Heinemann, Oxford.

Nicogossian, A. E., Leach Huntoon, C., and Pool, S. L. (1993). *Space physiology and medicine*, (3rd edn). Lea and Febiger, Malvern, Pennsylvania.

See also G AND G SUITS; RADIATION, IONIZING.

Spasticity is an abnormal physiological state of increased MUSCLE TONE with exaggeration of the tendon jerks or REFLEXES. The definition implies comparison with normal muscle tone, and therein lies the importance of clinical experience. Physicians use their own 'proprioceptive' sense to assess whether muscular tone is normal, by slowly moving the patient's limbs at the knee, ankle, and wrist joints so as to stretch the muscles acting on them — the quadriceps at the knee for example, and the biceps at the elbow. The slight resistance to movement in a normal subject is attributable to the intrinsic, passive mechanical properties of the muscles, tendons, joints, and ligaments, because in a resting and, equally important, relaxed subject, there is no muscle activity to generate an opposing force. However, in a spastic limb, for all but the very slowest of joint movements the physician perceives an opposing resistance to movement, the immediate cause of which is an exaggerated 'stretch' reflex. This spinal reflex, which arises in muscle receptors exquisitely sensitive to muscle stretch, is notable for the fact that the relevant afferent fibres pass directly to the motor neurons innervating the same and closely related (*agonist*) muscles. Thus, when muscle tone is enhanced, so also are the tendon jerks; if the patellar or other tendons are tapped, which applies a brief stretch to the muscles, the reflex jerk is larger or more 'brisk' than usual. Indeed, brisk jerks may be the earliest indication of a developing spasticity.

Spasticity results from loss of the control of the spinal reflex centres that normally descends from higher parts of the CENTRAL NERVOUS SYSTEM, via several different nerve pathways. Thus, for example, a STROKE can interrupt the pathway descending from the CEREBRAL CORTEX, resulting in spasticity of the limbs on the affected side of the body; or a complete transection of the SPINAL CORD can leave the reflex centres for both legs uncontrolled, so that they become spastic (after recovery from an initial period of 'SPINAL SHOCK'). The importance of such descending control over the reflex pathways within the spinal cord has been known for many years. However, the fine detail concerning the many different types of interneuron that subserve such control has only been established over the last 20–30 years through experiments on anaesthetized animals. From these, new concepts have emerged which in turn have led to the development of sophisticated, electrophysiolgical measurements for use in man. These will be important in establishing the usefulness of the concepts in the search for symptomatic therapies that might ease the mobility problems resulting from spasticity. Meanwhile, direct recording in man of the electrical activity of the muscle receptors, using the technique of *microneuronography*, in which ultra-fine electrodes are inserted into the relevant peripheral nerves, has proved to be a valuable technique. It has been established, with respect to the muscle nerves so far examined, that spasticity is not due to an exaggerated sensitivity of the muscle receptors ('spindles') to stretch. This factor had preoccupied much of the thinking about the cause of spasticity since the early 1950s, following the discovery that the sensitivity of muscle spindles depends on central nervous system control over the 'gamma' motor neurons that innervate the special types of muscle fibre within the muscle spindles.

TOM SEARS

See also CEREBRAL PALSY; MUSCLE TONE; PARALYSIS; REFLEXES; STROKE.

Spectacles Many claims have been made with regard to where spectacles originated. Both China and India have their advocates, but the best evidence is that they reached these countries from Europe via circuitous routes. The Romans considered myopia ('short-sightedness') a permanent defect that reduced the market value of a slave. However, ageing patrician Romans appreciated that the only way to counteract *presbyopia* (the refractive error of AGEING) was to be read aloud to by a younger slave. Pliny wrote of Nero viewing gladiatorial events *zmaragdo*, that is, through beryl, one of a family of transparent green precious stones of which emerald is another. Nicolaus Cusanus first wrote of using concave lenses for myopia in his book *De Beryllo* in 1441. The word beryl has lived on as *beryllia* (Venice) and as *Brille* (German), meaning 'spectacles' — a word which itself comes from *perspectare* (Latin), 'to look all about'.

A glass bowl full of water had been used as a magnifier and burning glass in antiquity. Roger Bacon (thirteenth century) wrote of looking through the 'lesser segment of a sphere, with the convex side towards the eye' to make letters and minute objects appear larger. Even today a simple magnifying lens — the monocle — is occasionally used as a temporary aid to reading, hand-held or kept in place over the eye by contraction of the orbicularis muscle that encircles it.

It was in Venice, the centre of glass making, that the first pair of spectacles appeared, around 1280. Two convex lenses mounted in a frame were used for presbyopia. Brother Giordano da Rivolto of Pisa, in a sermon in 1305, said, 'It is not yet twenty years that the art of making glasses was invented; this enables good sight and is one of the best as well as the most useful of arts that the world possesses.' Contrast this with the comments of Mr Cross, Vicar of Chew Magna in Somersetshire, who declared: 'The newly invented optick glasses are immoral, since they pervert the natural sight and make things appear in an unnatural and a false light.'

The spectacles worn by Hugues de St Cher may be the first ever painted and are to be seen in the fresco by Tomaso da Modena in the Dominican chapter house of San Nicolo, Treviso, Italy, dated 1352. The earliest myopic glasses were painted by Jan van Eyck in the early fourteenth century. The Medici family provide a pedigree of myopia but Pope Leo X is the only member known to have used glasses. Raphael's painting of 1518 shows Pope Leo X holding his concave lens.

Reading corrections

The strength of reading glasses was originally based on the patient's age. For a man of 30–40 years lenses of 2 degrees were used, for 70–80 years, lenses of 4 degrees. Even as late as the second half of the nineteenth century, glasses were provided by itinerant pedlars. It is remarkable that in our present scientific age, when the appropriate corrective lenses can be prescribed on the basis of precise measurement of refractive errors, some people still choose their own reading glasses at the chemist's shop. Astigmatic correction was not generally available until late in the nineteenth century, despite Airy's cylindrical correcting lens (1827) and Donders' comprehensive book on refraction (1864). Benjamin Franklin devised bifocal lenses, originally for himself, around 1775, by cutting each lens horizontally from his distance and reading glasses, and then binding half from the distance pair with half from the reading pair into the same frame, with the stronger lens lower, i.e. in the reading position. Hawkins introduced trifocal lenses in 1826. Successful multifocal lenses, which have smoothly increasing power over the lower half of the lens, with no visible segment line, were brought in during the 1960s. Unfortunately, these lenses are such a compromise in optical terms, and the field of clear vision in the reading area is so small that, for even the short lines of print when it is in double columns, the reader is obliged to turn his head slightly to follow along each line. Multifocal lenses have their best chance of acceptance if introduced when presbyopia first appears as then the necessary increases in strength with age are more readily tolerated.

Optical defects

Spectacle lenses have inherent optical defects, such as chromatic and spherical aberration, some of which are correctable. It was early apparent that a fixed lens in front of a mobile eye could only be optimally focused in the straight ahead position. Side vision is distorted and oblique rays of light passing through a spherical lens produce astigmatism. Instead of having a spherical front surface with a flat (*plano*) back, a lens with a more strongly convex front surface and less convex back was devised. Similar double curvatures were used for concave lenses, and even more complicated corrections for astigmatism.

Special lenses

Originally made of glass, with the dangers of breakage and eye injury, most spectacle lenses are now made of plastic — they have to be by law if they are for children or for adults with dangerous occupations. Lenses can be specially formulated to protect against radiation — principally ultraviolet light, but also against infra-red light. *Photochromic* lenses, which darken in sunlight and become lighter in the shade, now change colour at acceptable speed for most purposes. Another way of reducing glare is by 'Polaroid' lenses, which cut out much of the reflected light that has been partially polarized by reflection from water or from glass surfaces. Reflecting glasses, with an extremely thin metallic layer to reject harmful rays, render the wearer's eyes totally invisible behind the silver surface in a most disconcerting manner.

The author currently wears spectacles made of plastic, photochromic lenses with multifocal capabilities in a 'rimless' frame to be as light in weight as possible. But the definitive, all-purpose lens has yet to be devised. The huge choice of frames, of colours, and of lenses allows spectacles to make a fashion statement even if their physiological necessity is questionable. Finally, very dark or reflecting glasses may be used not only for purposes of anonymity but as a shield for an inadequate personality.   PETER FELLS

Further reading

Sorsby, A. (1948). *A short history of ophthalmology*, (2nd edn). Staples Press Ltd., London.

See also CONTACT LENSES; EYE; REFRACTIVE ERRORS.

Spectator John Berger opened his well-known BBC television series *Ways of Seeing* (1972) by noting that 'it is seeing which establishes our place in the surrounding world.' His comment stresses the most important presupposition about the activity of spectators: spectating creates and reinforces our social, political, and even bodily place in the world. In the late nineteenth century new media technologies, especially the cinema, called attention to the role of the audience in creating meaning — not merely understanding messages. As Walter Benjamin expressed it in the 1920s, 'Then came film and burst this prison-world asunder by the dynamite of the tenth of a second, so that now, in the midst of its far-flung ruins and debris, we calmly and adventurously go travelling.' The cinema expressed the spectators' desires to see more and go farther.

This conception of the spectator is a relatively recent invention, because before the late nineteenth century most analyses focused on the aesthetic object rather than the specific mechanisms of reception within each individual spectator. For example, to modern readers Aristotle's discussion about catharsis might seem to focus on spectators, but his interest was in particular dramatic strategies rather than in the importance of seeing *per se*. Likewise, Bacon and Locke opened the Enlightenment's interest in spectating by arguing for a visual accounting of the world, but the Enlightenment movement sought edification from objects in the world — not by studying *how* people view the world.

In the twentieth century, the new interest in how spectators understand was epitomized in research for the US Pentagon during World War II. The army commissioned behavioural studies of how well soldiers understood and accepted military propaganda. In those studies, researchers showed propaganda films (like the 'Why We Fight' series directed by Frank Capra) to new US Army inductees, to determine what effect the films had on the new soldiers. The studies initiated 'media effects' research. The films sought to convince soldiers that this was indeed a 'good cause' in spite of enormous opposition to entering the war and significant pro-German sentiment. The studies concluded that the soldiers did not understand the films and were left bemused. The films contained too much historical contextualization for the audiences to understand, and the researchers argued that the messages needed to be simplified. Before these studies, the role a spectator played in the creation of meaning was considered secondary to the actual message. After these studies, the role and experience of spectators became a major concern of social scientists and of many humanities disciplines as well. Scholars, like John Fiske, now investigate precisely how particular audiences get the 'wrong' message, but a message that is particularly useful for local socio-political needs. The spectator is seen as having an active role in creating meaning, rather than functioning merely as a passive viewer.

Examining popular notions of the spectator's role throughout the twentieth century, we can see a shift from a bodily, social experience to an isolated visual experience. One of the earliest examples of the earlier type of bodily spectating was Hale's Tours, which appeared in the late nineteenth century. Hale was an American fireman turned impresario; his spectacles and tours began as part of exhibitions and World's

Fairs. In his Tours, the spectators would enter a pavilion and buy a train ticket; they then entered a railroad car which was open on one side. The train moved back and forth on uneven tracks in a dark tunnel. The wall facing towards the open side was a continuous screen. As the train began to shake, the films showed the countryside or city streets. Often a tour guide would lecture during the adventure. The unevenly laid tracks heightened the illusion, which was so overwhelming that frequently passengers would yell at pedestrians to get out of the way. One passenger who went to the same show week after week was quoted as saying that he was waiting to see if the conductor would make a mistake so he could see a train wreck. Strangely, the films were shot both from the cowcatchers and from other locations on the train; these different views were then edited together without regard for a continuous point of view. The visual films taken alone make no sense, but in the context of the entire bodily experience, the spectators did not notice the cinematic discontinuities.

Although cinema heightened the awareness of the spectator's activities, it also effaced previous spectacles that involved more synaesthetic and bodily experiences, though theatre-going was still a social, group experience. As television became the dominant medium, the popular concern was that the spectator had become more passive and isolated. In the last decade of the twentieth century, with new technologies that stress 'virtual realities', interactivity, and connections through telecommunication, our view of the spectator's role is again undergoing a shift to a more bodily, social, active role.

While the twentieth century saw the rise in the importance of the spectator, the present century will introduce new formations of spectating that go beyond ways of seeing immersive bodily interactions. The sense of sight will no longer be synonymous with spectating, and socio-political control through participation will become much more specific to individuals and particular demographics. The notion of 'the' spectator may be superseded by 'a' spectating situation, and the emphasis on a singular response to a mass media visual spectacle will appear anachronistic.

CRAIG SAPER

Further reading

Staiger, J. (2000) *Perverse Spectators: the practices of film reception.* New York University Press, Chicago.

Taylor, M. C. (with a forward by Jack Miles) (1997) *Hiding.* Univeristy of Chicago Press, Chicago.

See also CINEMATOGRAPHY; ILLUSIONS; VIRTUAL REALITY.

Speech involves voluntary initiation and involvement of a complex set of muscles around the LARYNX, throat, and MOUTH, together with interruption of the rhythm of BREATHING and utilization of the muscles of expiration. Like other patterns of voluntary movement, speech originates in the CEREBRAL CORTEX. Several other parts of the brain (notably the CEREBELLUM), together with sensory feedback, modify and regulate the outgoing nerve impulses to the MOTOR NEURONS whose axons activate the relevant muscles. In this instance, the motor neurons concerned are in the brain stem, and their axons travel in the lowermost cranial nerves to the muscles of the vocal apparatus. Effective speech depends also on the motor neurons in the cervical and thoracic parts of the spinal cord that serve the muscles of breathing.

The process of speech production, speech transmission, and speech perception is often referred to as the *speech chain*. It is the configuration of the human vocal tract that gives rise to the *acoustic properties* of speech. The major speech articulators are the lips, JAW, the body, tip and velum of the TONGUE, and the hyoid bone position (which sets larynx height and pharynx width). The configuration of the speech articulators and their co-ordinated movement generate the acoustic consequences that we perceive as the sounds of our LANGUAGE. These *phonemes* (the consonant and vowel units of language) are not produced in a sequential and isolated manner but rather are co-articulated, and they coalesce to form a complex sound stream. The speech production system may be thought of as a set of *physical acoustic sources* (e.g. larynx) and *physiologically-determined filters* (e.g. lips) that are combined. The human speech system is particularly well suited for the rapid transfer of information.

There are a variety of ways to produce speech sounds. One method involves using the air pressure provided by the lungs to cause the vocal folds of the larynx to vibrate. The resulting sound can be altered by a variety of constrictions or closures in parts of the upper vocal tract. The modern study of the physiology of speech production began in 1928 with Stetson, who measured the speed and force of articulators. The development of X-ray photography led to the dynamic visualization of the vocal tract during speech production. The *sound spectrograph* (developed by Koenig in the 1940s) made it possible to study speech acoustic events in greater detail and revealed phoneme-specific information in the acoustic patterns. In particular, vowel formants and consonant-dependent formant transitions were recognized as key components to phoneme identity, leading to the initial attempts at computer speech synthesis.

The acoustic properties vary among different speakers producing the same sound and, more crucially, each utterance produced by an individual is unique. The mapping between the variable acoustic characteristics of speech production and the successful and stable identification of linguistically meaningful units in speech production is a major paradox. Recent research suggests that visual information is used to resolve acoustic difficulties in speech perception.

MARJORIE LORCH

See also JAW; LANGUAGE; LARYNX; LIP-READING; TONGUE; VOICE.

Sperm A mature sperm (*spermatozoon*) is a complex and highly specialized cell, genetically programmed, and unique in both function and shape. Its production — *spermatogenesis* — involves cell divisions and reorganisation of chromosomal material, which generates genetic diversity. After extensive cell modelling it eventually becomes mobile and capable of penetrating and fertilizing an egg.

Spermatogenesis occurs in the hundreds of *seminiferous tubules* of the TESTES, and is dependent on the actions of *testosterone* produced from cells which lie among these tubules (*Leydig cells*) and of the gonadotrophic hormones from the PITUITARY GLAND. It begins at puberty when the germ cells (*spermatogonia*), which have been in the testes since fetal life, start dividing by *mitosis* to produce a small clone of daughter cells with the normal 23 pairs of chromosomes (*diploid cells*). One of these pairs constitutes the sex chromosomes: in males an X chromosome and a smaller Y chromosome, which carries the male-determining gene. The majority of these cells (now termed primary *spermatocytes*) push their

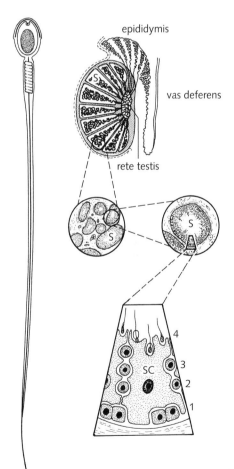

A mature sperm and sections of the testis and seminiferous tubules (S). 1,2,3,4, represent stages of development of spermatogonia to spermatocytes, to spermatids, beside the Sertoli cells (SC). Adapted from Jennett, S. (1989). *Human Physiology*. Churchill Livingstone, Edinburgh.

way through the junctions between the large protective and nourishing cells (*Sertoli cells*) which lie between them and the lumen of the tubule. In their new environment, created by secretions of the adjacent Sertoli cells, they undergo divisions which halve their number of chromosomes. In the first *meiotic* division the pairs of chromosomes come together and strands of DNA are swapped between them (*crossing over*), thus changing the genetic code carried by each chromosome. Eventually the pairs separate and two *haploid* cells, each containing a single set of 23 chromosomes, are formed. Thus one of these 'secondary spermaocytes' contains an X chromosome and the other a Y chromosome. Almost immediately after this first meiotic division a second meiotic division takes place. This involves the separation of the two halves of each single chromosome. These haploid cells — now called *spermatids* — thus contain 23 single half chromosomes. By this stage the important genetic events have taken place, but these spermatids are still simple round cells and must now undergo extensive remodelling (*spermiogenesis*) before they are capable of performing their function.

The first stage is the formation of the *acrosome*, which is an ENZYME-rich structure covering the head of the sperm. This is essential for fertilization. Then a tail develops for forward propulsion and mitochondria (energy generators for the cell) form in the midpiece of the sperm. By now, the work of the Sertoli cells in nurturing the primary spermatocytes through the process of spermatogenesis is complete. As these processes have occurred the developing cells have moved closer and closer to the lumen of the seminiferous tubule. Finally they are extruded and released into the tubule (*see figure*). In humans this whole process of spermatogenesis takes 64 days.

Once in the lumen of the tubule, the sperm are washed away by secretions from the Sertoli cells, and eventually reach the confluence of all the tubules in the single, highly-convoluted tube of the *epididymis*, which eventually drains into the vas deferens. The passage of sperm from the seminiferous tubules of the testis to the vas deferens takes about 12 days. During this time the sperm are subjected to major environmental changes due to testosterone-dependent secretions within these tubes. As a result, sperm not only acquire the ability to swim (on leaving the testis they are only capable of an infrequent twitch), but they also change in the way they utilize and break down energy substrates, and finally reach full fertilizing capacity. Sperm obtained before their passage through the epididymis are incapable of fertilizing an egg even if implanted directly.

By the time sperm reach the vas deferens they are fully mature and mobile and, due to fluid absorption in the epididymis, they are now densely packed. In fact 1 ml of fluid in the vas deferens contains about 5000 million sperm. Sperm can be stored for as long as five weeks in the tail of the epididyms and the vas deferens until they are released at ejaculation. In the absence of ejaculation sperm dribble into the urethra and are washed away in the urine. In men who have undergone a vasectomy, sperm build up behind the ligation, and are then removed by phagocytes in the epididymis.

Each sperm produced by the testis is only a few thousandths of a millimetre in length and must travel through some 30–40 cm (100 000 times its own length) in the male and then in the female reproductive tract before it reaches the FALLOPIAN TUBES and can perform the function for which it was intended. Needless to say, many fewer than 1 in a million ever complete this hazardous journey.   SAFFRON WHITEHEAD

See PLATE 8.

See also EJACULATION; SEMEN; TESTES.

Sphincter A band of muscle encircling one of the body's 'tubes', and so able to alter the 'bore' by contracting/relaxing. In the alimentary tract there are sphincters at the exit from the STOMACH, between the small and large INTESTINE, and at the anus; another regulates the flow of BILE and pancreatic juice into the DUODENUM. In the urogenital tract, there are sphincters at the exit from the BLADDER. They occur also in the walls of small arterial BLOOD VESSELS, regulating the flow into the capillaries beyond, according to local requirements. Those which assist retention of the excreta are partly under voluntary control; all the others, formed only of SMOOTH MUSCLE, are regulated by the AUTONOMIC NERVOUS SYSTEM; in general, sympathetic nerves constrict them; in the gut, parasympathetic nerves relax them. The thin sheet of circular muscle of the iris which constricts the pupil of the EYE is also known as a sphincter — it is stimulated by parasympathetic nerves, in response to light and as part of ACCOMMODATION for near vision.

S.J.

See ALIMENTARY SYSTEM; AUTONOMIC NERVOUS SYSTEM; BLADDER.

Spinal column The terms 'spine', 'spinal column', and 'vertebral column' all refer to the series of bones — 24 separate vertebrae plus the sacrum and the coccyx — that extend from neck to tail. They represent the segmental architecture of our phylogenetic ancestors. The topmost vertebra is known as the 'atlas' because it supports the skull at joints with the occipital bone, as the Titan of Greek mythology supported the earth. For descriptive convenience the bones are described as 7 cervical, 12 thoracic, and 5 lumbar vertebrae. The lowest lumbar vertebra articulates with the sacrum, and this in turn with the coccyx. The sacrum itself represents 5 fused bones, and the coccyx another vestigial 2–3 or more — the remains of the ancestral tail. Each of the vertebrae is a bony ring, and they are aligned to form a continuous tunnel, the *vertebral canal*, down the whole column to the end of the sacrum. This encloses the SPINAL CORD and the spinal nerve roots that enter and leave it, together with their surrounding membranes. The thick 'bodies' of the vertebrae are in the front of the canal, and their arches form the sides and back. The flat upper and lower surfaces of the vertebral bodies are linked, each to the next, by an adherent, cartilaginous *intervertebral disc*; each disc is fibrous and strong where it adheres to bone and around its circumference, but encloses a softer centre that allows some angulation of one vertebral surface relative to the next; thus there is a degree of flexibility — greater at some levels of the spine than others. The vertebral arches each have seven bony projections, including the midline 'spines' that can be felt through the skin of the back. The other pairs form joints with those of adjoining vertebrae and provide attachment for muscles and ligaments. The arrangement of the projections and joints is such as to allow some rotation in parts of the spine above the lumbar region. Nerve roots pass to and from the spinal cord through gaps between the arches of adjacent vertebrae, linking the cord with the peripheral nerves. The thinnest, flat parts of the arches — the *laminae* — provide surgical access to the spinal cord within the canal: hence the term *laminectomy* for making an opening into the spinal canal. The gaps between the arches of adjacent lumbar vertebrae, when the spine is flexed, allow the insertion of a needle for sampling CEREBROSPINAL FLUID in a *spinal tap* or *lumbar puncture*.   SHEILA JENNETT

See also BIPEDALISM; EVOLUTION, HUMAN; SKELETON; SLIPPED DISC.

Spinal cord The spinal cord extends down from the BRAIN STEM at the base of the SKULL, enclosed in the vertebral canal; brain and spinal cord in continuity comprise the CENTRAL NERVOUS SYSTEM. Like the brain, the cord is ensheathed by membranes (MENINGES), and bathed by CEREBROSPINAL FLUID. In the spinal cord are tracts of WHITE MATTER, nerve fibres carrying information to and from the brain as well as between different levels of the cord itself; and a core of GREY MATTER, containing nerve cells and SYNAPSES that mediate motor, sensory, and reflex functions. The substance of the cord is continuous, but functional segments are marked by the series of nerve roots at intervals down its length. At each level, two nerve roots (*dorsal* or *posterior* carrying ingoing nerve impulses; *ventral* or *anterior* carrying outgoing impulses) join to form a spinal nerve on each side. The uppermost emerges between the skull and the uppermost cervical vertebra; the rest emerge between two adjacent vertebrae, and between the segments of the sacrum. There are 8 cervical nerves, and below this the nerves are named according to the vertebra above their point of exit: thus there are 12 thoracic, 5 lumbar, 5 sacral, and 1 coccygeal nerve. The spinal canal is longer, however, than the spinal cord, which ends in the lumbar part of the canal. Therefore the distance that a spinal nerve must travel to reach its point of exit increases from above downwards, from zero for the first cervical nerve to about 20 cm for the lowest sacral and coccygeal. In the canal below the

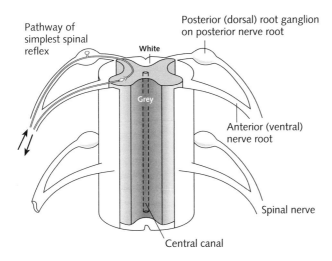

Diagram of part of the spinal cord, with the anterior white matter cut way, and two sets of segmental nerve roots.

[Labels on diagram:]
Pathway of simplest spinal reflex
White
Posterior (dorsal) root ganglion on posterior nerve root
Grey
Anterior (ventral) nerve root
Spinal nerve
Central canal

end of the cord, there is therefore a sheaf of descending spinal nerves that becomes progressively smaller as the nerves leave; this is known as the horse's tail — the *cauda equina*. This arrangement has consequences for the effects of spinal injury at different vertebral levels. Anywhere above the second lumbar vertebra, it is the spinal cord that is damaged; below this, it is spinal nerves. Spinal cord damage leaves uncontrolled MOTOR NEURONS below the level of the lesion; voluntary movement is lost, but after recovery from an initial period of SPINAL SHOCK, the muscles can and do contract, spontaneously and reflexly: a spastic PARALYSIS. Damage to the spinal nerves in the cauda equina, by contrast, separates the affected muscles from their spinal motor neurons; voluntary movement is lost and the muscles remain relaxed: a flaccid paralysis followed by wasting. In either case paralysis is accompanied by loss of sensation.

SHEILA JENNETT

See PLATE 6.

See also CENTRAL NERVOUS SYSTEM; MENINGES; MOTOR NEURONS; PARALYSIS; REFLEXES; SPINAL SHOCK.

Spinal shock The term 'spinal shock' refers to the fact that transection of the SPINAL CORD produces an initially complete but temporary absence of spinal REFLEXES in body parts whose innervation arises from levels of the spinal cord below the level of transection. In current clinical usage, the state of spinal shock would never be considered in isolation, but together with the absence of voluntary movement in, and the loss of sensation from, corresponding regions of the body, it forms the basis of the clinical diagnosis of a functionally-complete transection of the spinal cord. This distinction between current and past usage is not without academic interest, as, historically and conceptually, spinal shock could not be understood until the 'spinal reflex' itself was fully defined and its nature investigated by experiment. Thus, although the phenomena of

spinal shock were first described and investigated by the physician Whytt in 1750, its naming as such, by the physician and physiologist Marshall Hall, did not occur until a hundred years later. That naming was the outcome of animal experiments in which he clearly defined *spinal reflex* for the first time and later their counterpart *cranial reflexes*, such as the blink reflex. Whytt had recognized that mechanical stimulation of the foot in a decapitated frog resulted in withdrawal of the hindlimb. He termed such movements 'vital motions' and recognized that they depended on the spinal cord. However, in accord with lingering ideas of 'vitalism' (for which 'soul' corresponds to the contemporary usage of 'consciousness'), he deemed the spinal cord to contain a *sentient* principle or 'SOUL'. Hall, who can be regarded as the first professional physiologist, and wedded therefore to functional explanations, conceived a distinct class of 'involuntary motions', the spinal reflexes, that depended on ingoing influences to the spinal cord on the spinal cord itself, and on outgoing influences to the muscles (and glands); such 'reflected' actions were purposive in nature, but not dependent on sensory experience and hence not involving consciousness, which he attributed to the BRAIN alone. Indeed, these and related experiments and philosophical enquiry all contributed to the then current debate as to whether movements induced by touching a part of the body (e.g. the tail) which, together with the spinal cord, had been surgically isolated from the rest of the body, were the result of a sensory experience, i.e. whether they concerned the 'soul'. In contrast, Hall believed reflex action to be a manifestation of sensitivity to the stimulus but without sensibility; for him the 'soul' could not be so divided between brain and spinal cord.

As evident from the early experiments on the frog, spinal shock can be very transitory, lasting only for a few minutes, but it is of increasing duration according to cerebral dominance, lasting weeks in monkeys and still longer in apes and

humans. In man the effect of injury of the spinal cord depends on whether it is completely or incompletely divided and on the level of the spinal cord that is affected. For example, with transection at the third cervical level or above, functions depending on the cranial nerves, such as swallowing and facial movements, persist, but all BREATHING movements cease and life support by ARTIFICIAL VENTILATION is necessary. Speech remains possible, so long as a source of air pressure is provided below the vocal cords, to energize their oscillation when they are brought together (through activity of the still intact cranial nerves serving the LARYNX) as the patient attempts to speak. With transection a little lower, below the fourth cervical level, speech and also breathing are now independent because the BRAIN STEM motor control of the diaphragm remains mainly intact, via the phrenic nerve, whose motor neurons leave the cord mainly above this level; however all active expiratory-dependent activities, such as coughing, straining in defecation, and vocal power, remain absent, because the motor innervation of the relevant muscles lies below the transection. Even one segmental level can make a remarkable difference in the person's dependence on others or independence. A lesion at the seventh thoracic segment would leave the person independent for much of his personal needs, but standing unassisted and walking would be impossible, as would normal control of DEFECATION and micturition. The 'tendon jerk' is important to the assessment of spinal transection, because normally it would be present in a range of muscles in the arms and legs. This allows the level of transection to be identified, along with other features, based on knowledge of the spinal segmental motor nerve supply to the individual muscles. Furthermore, extensive anatomical and physiological research has clearly established that the reflex pathway of the tendon jerk is *monosynaptic*. This means that when the muscle receptors are briefly stretched by the tap, the nerve impulses in the afferent pathway travel directly to the motor neurons and excite them reflexly to cause the normally visible muscle twitch. Thus the complete absence of this particular class of spinal reflex activity, in the initial phase of spinal shock that follows spinal transection, indicates how strongly in man motor neuron excitability is dependent on impulses descending from the brain stem and above.

However, not all the pathways are necessarily excitatory. The spinal neural circuitry is itself extremely complex, and some descending pathways may equally normally inhibit 'inhibitory' interneurons whose activity is then 'released' by the loss of the descending inhibitory control, causing the motor neurons to be inhibited. It is not surprising, therefore, that the basis of spinal shock remains an enigma; its unravelling would undoubtedly contribute to future attempts to restore — prosthetically, or biologically by cell transplantation, for example — useful function to spinal man. But until more research is done, any such interventions when first undertaken would be unlikely to be introduced at the time of 'spinal shock', because at that stage the final clinical outcome would remain uncertain if not unknown.

With regard to the reflexes, spinal shock is not permanent and spinal reflex activity is restored; this is a gradual process starting some weeks following the lesion. It is not simply as before but has a distinct bias in which increasingly the flexor muscles are readily thrown into reflex contraction by cutaneous stimulation or muscle stretch, the process commonly being first seen in the big toe (*Babinski's sign*) and ankle, and later in the knee and hip. Still later, reflexes return in the extensor muscles. Another aspect of this functional recovery is the enlargement of the *receptive field* of the cutaneous reflexes so that they can be elicited by minimal stimulation from a progressively wider area of skin. Spinal reflexes involving micturition and defecation are also affected during spinal shock. In particular the BLADDER is completely without its normal 'tone' and the immediate loss of the 'voiding' reflex, whose reflex pathway normally involves the brain stem, can result in overfilling of the bladder, with urination only by overflow if not managed clinically. Eventually, as spinal shock diminishes, a wholly spinal reflex emerges to create an 'automatic bladder,' which the patient can learn to empty by manual stimulation in the groin.

The study of spinal shock indicates the extraordinary capacity of the nervous system to reorganize after a lesion, and raises many important questions and theoretical concepts about the way the CENTRAL NERVOUS SYSTEM functions. The International Spinal Research Trust (now usually known as 'Spinal Research') funds the majority of research in spinal cord injury and for further information readers are referred to this Trust.   L. S. ILLIS

Further reading

Manuel, D. E. (1980). Marshall Hall, F. R. S. (1700–1857): a conspectus of his life and work. *The Royal Society Notes and Records*, **35**, 135–65.

International Spinal Research Trust, Station Road, Bramley, Surrey, GU5 0AZ, UK. e-mail: isrt@spinal-research.org

See also BREATHING; CENTRAL NERVOUS SYSTEM; PARALYSIS; REFLEXES; SPINAL CORD.

Spirit possession

Spirit possession, simply defined, is the seizure of a human being by the divine, or by external spirit(s). It refers to the ways in which a person is changed in terms of both identity and bodily manifestations through the presence within him or her of a spirit entity or power. Thus spirit possession is interpreted as a transcendental experience which has material, bodily manifestations. The spirit(s) might be good or bad. It is a phenomenon found across different cultures and religions.

Amongst the bodily, that is physiological, manifestations of spirit possession are: trance, muscle rigidity and/or loss of motor control, jerky movements, uncontrollable shaking, falling (often accompanied by difficulty in rising); and even various forms of sickness. Ritual possession may end abruptly when the possessed person becomes limp or falls with exhaustion. Those who have experienced spirit possession often describe this exhaustion as pleasurable, peaceful, joyful, and even euphoric. The spirit-possessed person may also speak in the 'voice' of the spirits: through *glossolalia*, or speaking in tongues — described, in the Christian tradition, in the Pentecost event (Acts 2: 1–4), and by Paul in 1 Corinthians 14: 18; in shouts, barks, or other inarticulate sounds; by babbling; and by acting as a medium for a spirit, conveying messages to living human beings, as for example in a seance. Some might include prophecy as an example of spirit possession.

These bodily manifestations often make the rituals of spirit possession dramatic and theatrical. For in so far as the spirits are embodied, they rely both on the 'host', that is the possessed, and the various elements of the performance. Thus the 'embodiment' of the spirit(s) lies in the discrepancy between the usual behaviour of the person who is possessed (that is, the behaviour displayed by that person when in their usual state of CONSCIOUSNESS and as a recognized member of the community) and the transformation that occurs in their behaviour when they are possessed by the spirit(s). Thus the 'embodiment' of spirits impinges on the possessed person's selfhood, and raises interesting psychoanalytical questions about dissociation, and how the dissociated parts of the self might be linked in a larger whole.

Possession is a central feature of some religious traditions, as, for example, in Voodoo — in Haiti and parts of the US, and Santeria — in Cuba, Puerto Rica, and parts of the US. In these religions, possession is the means by which the deities interact with humankind, entering the human world to punish or reward human beings, to treat their ills or problems. This may suggest that all human beings have the psychobiological capacity to enter possession states, but that cultural expectations and social context determine whether that occurs or not. For spirit possession usually occurs in social — that is, community — contexts: people do not usually become possessed by spirit(s) when on their own, though the example of well-known mystics such as Teresa of Avila may stand as an exception, depending on whether we categorize mystical experiences as forms of spirit possession or not (see MYSTICISM).

It has been observed by some anthropologists and historians that those most frequently possessed by spirits are those marginalized in society, such as women. Thus spirit possession can be seen to have social uses, allowing the expression of discontent and acting as a safety valve in certain societies; or creating a situation in which those without a public voice can speak publicly, all the while abdicating any responsibility for their transgressive speech, for they can claim it is the spirits who are speaking. For example, wives might be able to express demands to husbands through spirits in situations where they would not be able to express those demands directly. In those cultures where women are seen as 'naturally' weak or vulnerable, they might be seen as more prone to spirit possession. In Victorian Spiritualism, for example, women were seen as making the best mediums because, being seen as 'naturally' passive, they were thought to make good repositories or vessels for the spirits, able to renounce self and thereby become good channels for divine communication. A number of nineteenth-century working-class women became star mediums, acquiring fame and the ability to speak and act publicly — at least in the context of the seance: they exemplify the ways in which the spirit-possessed, often from a marginalised position in society, can enjoy an elevated social status, at least for the time while they are possessed.

JANE SHAW

Further reading

Lewis, I. M. (1971: new edition 1989). *Ecstatic religion. A study of shamanism and spirit possession.* Routledge, London.

See also EPILEPSY; MYSTICISM.

Spleen

Spleen The spleen was linked in past centuries to a variety of EMOTIONS, characteristics, or behaviours — usually spitefulness, bad temper, or melancholy, but also sometimes to general liveliness and explosive wit. In the seventeenth century Shakespeare provided many a quote, including the tag 'spleeny Lutheran'. In the eighteenth century we have Addison's 'touchy testy pleasant fellow' with 'so much Wit and Mirth and Spleen', whilst less positively a 'touch of the spleen' was what we would now call PSYCHOSOMATIC illness. In the late nineteenth century the concept still survived in such whimsies as Gilbert's in *Patience*: '… a sentimental passion of a vegetable fashion must excite your languid spleen'. And 'venting one's spleen' has traditionally described a vituperative outburst.

There seems no good reason why the spleen should have deserved these associations — unlike, say, the HEART which manifests its link with love by an increase in beating rate with excitement. The spleen is physiologically and anatomically unobtrusive. It is in fact — unusually in the body for an unpaired organ — dispensible. We can live without it because its functions can be taken over elsewhere. It is a small spongy purple mass in a fibrous capsule, tucked under the left side of the diaphragm (smaller than the liver which is tucked under the right side).

The spleen is in a way a poor relation among organs in that it is rarely in the public eye — not even on the butcher's counter. It is not susceptible to dramatic televisual imaging and it does not invite TRANSPLANTATION. It does however sometimes need to be removed: it can suffer hidden injury, for example in crushing or road traffic accidents, when its rupture can cause internal bleeding; other causes for *splenectomy* include some BLOOD diseases.

Although we can do without it if necessary, the spleen does normally have important functions. In fetal life it is the site of red blood cell formation, until this is taken over by the bone marrow. It contributes to the IMMUNE SYSTEM, forming antibodies and producing and storing masses of lymphocytes. It contains extensive channels and spaces (sinuses) where the blood flows slowly and where senescent red blood cells break down and are removed from the circulation. It therefore becomes enlarged in some infective, parasitic, and blood diseases.

The spleen acts to some extent as a blood reservoir, although this mechanism for increasing circulating blood volume is relatively minor and unimportant in humans compared with some other animals. The smooth muscle in its capsule is activated by the AUTONOMIC NERVOUS SYSTEM in conditions of 'fight or flight' or after blood loss, squirting a little extra blood into the circulation — which is perhaps the nearest physiological equivalent to the metaphoric 'venting'.

SHEILA JENNETT

See PLATE 4.

See also BLOOD; HUMOURS; IMMUNE SYSTEM.

Split brain

In the 1940s, it was discovered that surgical disconnection of the two cerebral hemispheres, by dividing the *corpus callosum*, the bridge of nerve fibres that connects them, effectively reduced seizures in patients with intractable EPILEPSY. When behavioural studies with these patients were first carried out, it appeared that sectioning the callosum led to no major breakdown in interhemispheric processing. A simple test, however, can reveal that there are in fact dramatic effects of this disconnection, known as the split-brain syndrome.

If such a patient's hands are obscured from his view and an object is placed in the right hand, he can name it easily. Conversely, if it is placed in the left hand, the patient is unable to identify it verbally. Given an array of items to choose from, however, the left hand is immediately able to pick out this same item. Since initiation of left-hand movement occurs in the right hemisphere, this indicates that the right hemisphere has knowledge about the object but is unable to name it.

Over the years, more sophisticated testing procedures have taken advantage of the contralateral organization of various perceptual systems, such as the visual system, to explore the specialized functions of the two hemispheres. These studies have resulted in remarkable insights into the specialized capacities of each disconnected hemisphere. They have also revealed how the two hemispheres work in concert in the normal brain to provide seamless integration of sensory, motor, and cognitive functions.

Split-brain patients behave in ways that were to a large extent predicted by classical neurology. For example, the most striking aspect of the split-brain syndrome is that the left hemisphere has access to SPEECH and the right hemisphere does not. The left hemisphere's specialization for LANGUAGE was already long established, based on data from patients with unilateral brain damage. Although the effects of disconnection on language were therefore not unexpected, it was surprising to discover the extent to which the left hemisphere was specialized for problem-solving of all kinds. Indeed, not only could it, and it alone, solve a wide range of cognitive problems, it also possessed a special device that has been called the 'interpreter'. In brief, this was revealed by presenting two pictures, one to each half brain. For example, a picture of a snow scene was presented (from the left field of vision) to the right hemisphere of a split-brain patient. The non-talking right hemisphere had four cards to choose from, one of which was a shovel. At the same time the left hemisphere was shown a chicken claw and its four choices included a picture of a chicken. Following presentation of these pictures the patient was allowed to choose between the eight possible pictures. The left hand, governed by the right hemisphere, chose the shovel and the right hand, governed by the left hemisphere, chose the chicken. When asked by the experimenter why he had responded in that manner, the speaking left hemisphere said, 'Oh, the chicken claw goes with the chicken, and you need a shovel to clean out the chicken shed.' The left hemisphere in fact did not know why the left hand chose the shovel. The left brain observed what the right hand was doing and came up with a theory that explained away an action.

The right hemisphere appears to lack the interpretive capacities of the left and consequently is markedly impoverished in problem solving. Nevertheless, the right brain has it own specializations. The right hemisphere is superior to the left in a wide range of perceptual skills, such as grouping of visual elements into a whole picture. Early demonstrations of this involved copying drawings with each hand separately. With their hands obscured from view, right-handed split-brain patients were able to produce reasonable copies with their left hands but not with their right. The drawings made by the right hand contained details of the original pictures but had little or no spatial coherence. More recent research has revealed the right hemisphere's superiority in making orientation judgments, remembering unknown, upright faces, and a host of other visual tasks.

Investigations into the realms of language and PERCEPTION clearly reveal the functional differences between the two hemispheres. Studies on memory and attention, however, provide insights into the ways in which the two hemispheres work together in an intact brain. MEMORY research with split-brain patients suggests that the two hemispheres each provide a unique input into storing information and later retrieving it. The left hemisphere interpreter is thought to be continually generating theories to explain the information it is currently processing. As a result, this hemisphere is particularly suited to getting the 'gist' of an event. This interpretive function, however, means that the left hemisphere often makes errors in recalling details of an event. The more literal right hemisphere does not make inferences and generalizations about incoming information, so this hemisphere is much less likely to make factual errors. The two hemispheres therefore work together to provide a system which is capable of accurately recalling details while still allowing for elaboration and inferences about the world.

Attention is something else that involves interaction between the two hemispheres. Both hemispheres are able to orient reflexively to external stimuli, and this focusing of attention occurs independently in each hemisphere. Voluntary orienting, however, appears to involve a single shared resource. This is illustrated by experiments that require each hemisphere to be performing a task independently of the other; then, when one hemisphere has a difficult task, the performance of the other hemisphere on a separate task is impaired. If the task of the first hemisphere becomes relatively easy, however, the performance of the other hemisphere improves markedly. Thus although the two hemispheres co-operate in many aspects of neural functioning, in the realm of voluntary control of attention the two hemispheres appear to compete. Studies that demand this kind of hemispheric competition have revealed that control over voluntary attention seems to be preferentially lateralized to the left hemisphere.

In summary, studies with split-brain patients have provided invaluable insights into the specialized functions of the two hemispheres and the ways in which they interact to enable myriad perceptual and cognitive functions.

MICHAEL GAZZANIGA
PAUL M. CORBALLIS

See also BRAIN; LANGUAGE AND THE BRAIN.

Spontaneous human combustion

On the morning of 2 July 1951, Mary Reeser, of St Petersburg, Florida, was found dead. Her landlady had attempted to deliver a telegram but the doorknob was too hot to touch. When rescuers entered the smoke-filled apartment, they found a pile of ashes and fragments of bone, along with one blackened foot encased in a satin slipper — the remains of Mrs Reeser. Dubbed by the newspapers 'the cinder woman mystery', this was one of several dozen grisly cases, recorded over the past three centuries, of spontaneous human combustion (*SHC*).

What happened in this case and others like it? In some mysterious way, solitary human beings have burned up almost entirely, without setting fire to their surroundings, and with no apparent outside cause. Even James Randi, the famous hoax-breaking sceptic, has described SHC as a 'not-too-well-explained phenomenon'.

The great period in this form of auto-incineration, SHC's Elizabethan period, so to speak, was in the mid nineteenth century. No man did more to draw attention to the phenomenon and its dramatic possibilities than Charles Dickens. In the December 1852 instalment of *Bleak House* he did away with the repugnant junk-dealer Krook in spectacular fashion, by turning him into soot, smoke, and what the novelist describes as 'a dark greasy coating on the walls and ceiling'. Although other novelists had lit the way — Herman Melville in *Redburn* (1842), Captain Marryat in *Jacob Faithful* (1834), and Nikolai Gogol in *Dead Souls* (1849) had recently turned their villains into human tapers — Dickens' was the most detailed and repulsive account. It was also the most believable, which Dickens ensured by citing in his book corroborating testimony from the *Philosophical Transactions* of the Royal Society, works of jurisprudence, and the medical literature. Bodies — especially vile bodies — burned.

In an immediate and caustic reaction, the journalist, positivist philosopher, and physiologist G. H. Lewes denounced Dickens' credulity in the pages of *The Leader*, labelling Krook's demise a 'vulgar error' whose endorsement by novelists could only perpetuate ignorance and superstition. To support his attack, Lewes cited the damning evidence of the brilliant German chemist, Justus von Liebig, who had recently completed a series of experiments showing that beyond any shadow of a doubt SHC was an impossibility. Liebig had tried to set alight bones and flesh, dried and wetted, all without being able to reduce them to ashes. Bodies did not burn.

Liebig ought to have settled the matter, but did not, and for two reasons. In the first place, he was a chemist, using new-fangled (and foreign) experimental procedures to explore what was judged at the time to be a matter of and for medicine. Doctors who had come on the scene soon after a death by SHC had no reason to doubt the evidence of their eyes. At a time when experimental chemistry and medicine were making great efforts to establish themselves as credible and reliable, there was a veritable tussle over the rights to pronounce on causes of death, and over who had disciplinary ownership over corpses (the matter was settled by the formation of forensic science in the late 1800s).

Apart from disciplinary tussles over the credibility of on-the-scene and laboratory evidence, the conflict between sceptics and believers was, and remains, one between those who concern themselves with causes and those who deal with effects. With most of the human body a mystery, lying seemingly beyond medicine, many doctors were happy enough 150 years ago to treat effects, and to accept as real many phenomena (including most diseases, in fact) for which they had no explanation. Scientists, however, were reluctant to credit any effects for which causes could not be discovered, and steadfast in discrediting any whose conceivable causes violated known laws.

As the scientific and medical controversy continued, many commentators found that SHC, if not scientifically credible, was morally proper. Almost without exception, those who went up in a puff of smoke were the lazy, the corpulent, the solitary, the aged, and the drunk. What better way to eliminate a degraded character, like the unfortunate but deserving victim in Emile Zola's *Doctor Pascal* (1893)? In any event, it was a death

too good for scandal sheets to give up. Are we to sense trouble on the horizon when, early in Fyodor Dostoevsky's *Crime and Punishment* (1866), Raskolnikov enjoys a lurid newspaper account of SHC?

While believers have documented the characteristics of SHC victims, sceptics have used precisely these characteristics to explain away the phenomenon. In a recent re-evaluation of over twenty-five deaths attributed to SHC, Joe Nickell and John Fischer have found that simple explanations account for each case. In some cases, an alcoholic's carelessly-dropped cigarette sets the victim ablaze. In others, an oil-heater or a spark from the coal fire have done the job. Meanwhile, those reluctant to discount the reality of SHC have supposed that a perfectly natural 'candle effect' may be responsible: the result of human fat dripping out of the body, permeating the clothing, and then burning like a giant human candle wick.

Thousands each year revisit the death of Krook, and are horrified by Dickens' ability to portray 'the romantic side of familiar things'. Thousands devour lurid reports, often illustrated, of recent deaths by SHC and, like that famous connoisseur and collector of impossible facts, Charles Fort, ask 'why not?' For a large segment of the population — those alienated, or at least not persuaded, by scientific authority — SHC is a fact, whether explained by recourse to people's 'electrodynamic potential' or the Earth's 'geomagnetic fluctuations', or not explained at all. Reporting the freakish fate of Mrs Reeser, a Florida newspaper ran the story under the wry headline, 'How Woman Was Incinerated Stumps All But Amateurs'. While physicians and scientists denounce the credulity of the general public, thousands of amateurs have ready answers to this particular mystery of death.

MICHAEL SHORTLAND

Further reading
Harrison, M. (1976). *Fire from heaven: a study of spontaneous combustion in human beings.* Sidgwick and Jackson, London.

Sport has been defined by a UNESCO Committee as: 'Any physical activity which has the character of play and which involves a struggle with oneself or with others, or a confrontation with natural elements'. They added 'If this activity involves competition, it must then always be performed in a spirit of sportsmanship. There can be no true sports without the idea of fair play.' The UK Sports Council in 1992 stated; 'We know that sport can make a positive contribution to national morale, health and the economy. We believe that it can enhance community spirit, equality of opportunity, personal development and social integration.' Over 150 activities are recognised by the Sports Council as sports, and a line has been drawn to the exclusion of chess, as a game, not a sport.

The origins of sport in general lie in their practice for combat and war. *Fencing* is depicted

on Egyptian murals from the time of the pyramids; appropriately, sabre and foil are two of only fifteen disciplines included in every modern Olympic Games since 1896.

Robert Dover codified English country sports into his celebrated *Dover's Cotswold Olimpicks*, in 1612, almost certainly attended by Shakespeare, which continued until 1853. Baron de Coubertin had his idea to found a modern Olympics partly from his attendance at the similar Much Wenlock Olympics in Shropshire. Both these festivals run today. The equivalent sports festivals in Scotland are the Highland Games. In both countries from the seventeenth to the nineteenth centuries local girls and women of all ages ran footraces at country fairs for holland smocks, or shifts — the 'smock races'. In Scotland also, during nearly 200 years from the Peace of Glasgow in 1502 to the Revolution of 1688, every reigning monarch of the Stuart line, including Mary Queen of Scots, played golf — a sport which has been played on the moon.

The ancient *Olympic Games* were religious festivals which commenced with a procession along the sacred way, the Pompike Othos, followed by sacrifice and oath-taking. The athletes were all men and competed naked, and only one woman was permitted to spectate, a priestess of Demeter, the Goddess of earth and harvests. The Komos was the ceremonial crowning of the victors with olive leaves on the fifth day, after which they returned in triumph to greater wealth and status in their city states. The Olympic Games were primarily occasions to honour Zeus, but their origins are to be found long before the GREEKS came to the Mediterranean. Although the first Games are reputed to have been held in 776 BC, the site was occupied a thousand years earlier. After 293 celebrations, Emperor Theodosius banned them in AD 393, ostensibly for corruption and professionalism, but essentially because as a converted Christian he disapproved of their pagan associations. An idea of such festivals may be gained in the Duveen gallery of the British Museum, from the frieze which originally decorated the Parthenon. The modern Games, and many other major sports festivals, follow a similar format.

The major change in modern sport (apart from the expansion of women's participation) is the massive impact of money and professionalism. It is reported that the American television network NBC has paid $3.4 billion for certain future Olympic rights, and on a lesser scale this is happening throughout particular sports, aided by lottery and other funding. This is not entirely new: many of the ancient Greek Olympians had their training expenses paid and subsistence provided, and although there were no money prizes at the Games, nevertheless, the champions could look forward to major material rewards back in their city states. The concept of *amateurism* in Britain arose as a means of preventing the working classes from competing against the aristocracy. As late as the 1930s physical education teachers were considered professional athletes and thus ineligible for the Olympics. An important change in Britain has been much better subsistance finance (mainly lotttery funding) for full-time training for selected athletes. At the Sydney Olympics 28 medals (and ten 4th places) vindicated this policy.

Rules of the games

It is axiomatic that sport is played to rules, which are formed to establish equality. Sports sociologist Alan Tomlinson has commented: 'Sports … are contested in theoretically equal terms: they are increasingly specialized; they are based upon officially drawn-up rules and extraordinarily sophisticated approaches to them; they are run by organisational personnel; they are measured in unprecedentedly detailed ways; and they stress the unsurpassable, the far horizon, the stretching of limits.' Regarding the measurement of such limits, when Said Aouita officially beat David Moorcroft's 5000 metres world record of 13.00.41 by 0.01 seconds — or 0.0013%, the current author wondered if the track itself was measured with comparable accuracy. By contrast, 0.01 of a second would be an acceptable 0.01% of the 100 metre world record time of 9.79. But beyond the rules there are also meta-rules, unwritten systems of conventions which embed the rules in a value system, signalled by victory award ceremonies or football team celebrations. A bowler, bowling a grubber to prevent a winning run being scored, defies the *conventions* of cricket, but not its *rules*. When Oliver McCall refused to fight Lennox Lewis in the BOXING ring in Las Vegas in 1997, he defied not the rules, but the conventions. And sport is often powerless against those who defy its conventions.

The requirements of modern sport

The requirements of modern sport can be considered in terms of the total expert input into a National Team or *Olympic Squad* (although a much scaled down version is applicable to the preparation of a Saturday primary school team). Many areas of expertise are needed:

Specialist equipment advances continually. The 'shovel blade' in rowing, and the 'wing paddle' in canoeing, both gave significant advantages when first introduced. It was noted that a marathoner running at 322 metres per minute (around 2 hours 10 minutes) needed 62 ml of OXYGEN per kg per minute with a then conventional shoe, but only 60.8 ml at the same speed with an air-soled shoe. An aerodynamic, low profile, smaller wheeled, helium-tyred, lighter bicycle (5.9 kg compared to conventional 8.1 kg) reduces drag by about 7%, giving a 5 second advantage over 4000 metres at 50 kph. From 1940–60 the pole vault world record improved by 23.5 cm, but in the next twenty years it improved by over 100 cm — mainly by improvements in the pole itself. Modern rackets in tennis and squash have increased ball speed. The Formula 1 Grand Prix car has changed out of all recognition in the past thirty years — and so on.

Technical and motor skills have also vastly improved, due to education of coaches regarding motor skill learning and also to detailed biomechnical analysis, in sports ranging from gymnastics to the football free kick. As a *biomechanist*, Dick Fosbury won Olympic gold and set a high jump record by realizing that, as the centre of gravity of the body is nearer the back than the front, it made more sense to go over the high jump bar on his back, thus not needing to lift the centre of gravity quite as high, for the same height of jump. Hence the 'Fosbury Flop' — although it needed the technology of the raised foam landing area. Not all technical improvements are feasible; for example a new javelin technique was perfected whereby the thrower greased the javelin tail, held it initially in the middle, and span like a discus thrower before release. Use of the technique immediately led to throws beyond the then world record, but the accuracy was too uncertain for use in stadia.

Tactical innovations and identification of weaknesses in the opposition have been assisted by videotaping and *notational analyses* especially of the 'invasion' team games, from rugby to camogie, and of the racket sports.

Sports psychology plays a major part in most modern competition at high level, in a variety of ways, ranging from STRESS handling and motivation, to acceptance of defeat and of injury.

Sports nutrition and biochemistry are vitally important, with techniques such as carbohydrate loading for muscle GLYCOGEN boosting now standard, the importance of maintaining fluid balance being recognized in a wide variety of sports, the use of creatine supplements benefitting short term anaerobic work, and promising innovations being made regarding AMINO ACID supplementation.

Sports medicine (including physiotherapy and podiatry) is, of course, vital, not just to help treat or even prevent injury, but also in areas such as *sports amenorrhoea*, due to too high volume training, which may lead into, or already be part of, the deadly triad of amenorrhoea, OSTEOPOROSIS (with its sports risk of stress fractures), and EATING DISORDERS.

Team selection is obviously of major importance and *team management* is no longer a perk for a long-serving official, but a full-time high profile job demanding a broad range of managerial, organizational, and personal skills.

Physical fitness which falls into six components:
(i) *aerobic (cardiorespiratory) fitness* — or 'stamina', dependent on maximal oxygen uptake, and what percentage of that maximum may be sustained during the sport, as assessed by techniques of 'anaerobic threshold', 'critical power', or the more recent 'lactate minimum' analysis;
(ii) *local muscle endurance* (often, somewhat inaccurately, called anaerobic fitness), assessed in terms of peak power output (in watts), time to peak power, rate of fatigue, total work done (in kJ), and rate of recovery;

(iii) *muscle strength* (increasingly measured on isokinetic dynamometers, to assess the force output at the contraction velocity required in the sport);
(iv) *muscle speed* itself — often combined with muscle force to provide a measure of power;
(v) *flexibility*; and
(vi) *body composition*, in terms of the percentage of body fat.

Some sports, such as marathon running or sea SWIMMING, require very high levels of fitness in just one or two areas; others, such as GYMNASTICS, DANCE, and some MARTIAL ARTS, require high levels in almost all of them. Each sport requires an individual fitness profile and, as each competitor is different, this usually requires subtly different emphases within the training cycles. Analysis of the fitness components must always be the basis of training advice to coach and to competitor.

Sports science is now a major feature of competition. Yet the author competed in athletics in the late 1940s and 50s, and in those days of no tracksuits, we ran in winter with newspaper down the front of our vests, and had a squirt of methylated spirits onto the back of our pharynx at the end of the training run; we changed in a 'steamie' attached to a public baths, and washed ourselves in its iron tubs — always with a 'rub-down' from an old trainer. A club member vulcanized pieces of car tyre treads onto our ex-army 30p thin-soled black plimsoles; yet on this regime, the club, from inner-city Glasgow, won the English National Senior Cross-Country Championship and provided a string of international and Olympic team members.

Sport and health

A very large number of people engage in sport, or EXERCISE, for the benefits of 'health-related fitness', with a major rise in recent years of jogging and aerobics. Sir Phillip Sydney Smith in the seventeenth century said 'You will never live to my age except you retain your breath through exercise and your heart through joyfulness', and famous exercise epidemiologists, Jerry Morris and Ralph Paffenbarger, have provided a very firm modern foundation for the belief that exercise is a major factor in the prevention of coronary heart disease. *Aristotle* (384–22 BC) pertinently observed that 'Men may fall into ill-health as a result of hypo-activity.' On the other hand, *Hippocrates* (469–399 BC) observed that 'Health is at risk when exercise is at very high levels', and indeed, 'Sport for All' implies sports injuries for all. This has long been recognized: the Scottish Maitland Folio Manuscript of 1582 (transcribed into modern English) has:

Bruised muscles and broken bones
Strife, discord and spoiled bairns
Twisted in age and lame withall,
These are the beauties of football.

Sport and age

The *oldest Olympic medallist* was Swedish shooter, Oscar Swahn winning silver in 1920 aged 72. The oldest woman Olympian was 70-year-old Hilda Johnstone at Munich. Youngest known competitor was a 10-year-old Greek gymnast in 1896, and youngest individual medallist was Danish woman breast-stroker Inge Sorensen in 1936, at just 14. Of course, many sports now have Master's national and even world championships. In athelics, for example, these have categories extending into the 1990s. Norwegian Herman Smith-Johannsen was still skiing Nordic style into his eleventh decade, and George Stelback of USA was still golfing at 106. A recent Himalayan expedition had an average age of over 70, and in the final of the 1996 world indoor athletics championsips, Yekaterina Podopayeva, aged 42, just beat Mary Decker-Slaney, 38, in a thrilling 1500 metres final. Sandy Neilson swam 100 m freestyle in 58.59 s to win Olympic Gold at 17, 22 years later she swam the distance in 58.87 s, and just failed to make the USA Atlanta team.

Ergogenic aids and doping

A cynic has suggested that the difference between *ergogenic* work-producing aids, and doping, is that doping works. Perhaps the most bizarre such aid was the East German experimentation with rectal insufflations of air to optimize the buoyancy of swimmers; and among the most controversial — and most popular — is the use of altitude as an ergogenic aid to training. Doping itself is not new, e.g. the 1904 marathon winner Thomas Hicks was given multiple doses of strychnine and brandy *while* he was running! Just before the men's 100 metres in 1920, the US coach gave his men a mixture of sherry and raw eggs. Aids like that are harmless enough, but in 1960 the Danish cyclist Knut Jensen died during the Olympic road race, having taken amphetamines (which interfere with heat dissipation) and nicotinyl tartrate. Full scale Olympic doping control started in 1972, and rule 29 of the Olympic Charter states, simply, 'Doping is forbidden.' Hence, doping is cheating. Dr Robert Kerr, in practice in San Gabriel, was quoted as saying: … 'in 1983 I was seeing 2000 patients for steroids alone … There were seven physicians who prescribed steroids right here in San Gabriel, and at least seventy of them in the Los Angeles area. Nationwide thousands of doctors were involved.' The drugs causing most current concern are erythropoietin (in the aerobic endurance sports), insulin-like growth factor-1, INSULIN itself and nandrolone (in the strength-power sports).

A major problem facing governing bodies and national associations who ban competitors for doping is that they may be taken to court by professional athletes in terms of 'unlawful restriction of earnings', and the association may find itself on the end of an expensive lawsuit. There is now a whole legal area connected with sport, from arranging the contracts to taking up cases such as that of 11-year-old Teresa Bennett, who took the FA to court because their rules denied her playing in her school football (boys') team, in which she was the best player. Another case was the attempt before the Lillehamer winter Olympics of 1994, by the husband of American skater Tanya Harding, deliberately to cripple her main rival, Nancy Kerrigan, by hitting her knee with an iron bar. Fortunately Kerrigan recovered, and went on to win a medal.

Sport and religion

Sport has long been seen, rightly or wrongly, as a very useful means of education, of social control, and even as a means of evangelizing. An increasing number of Christian athletes, for example Jonathan Edwards, the current triple-jump Olympic champion and world record holder, are following the example set by 1924 400 metres champion Eric Liddell, who in 1925 went as a missionary to China. But even he was just the latest in a long line of 'Muscular Christians.' Jean Jacques Rousseau's Emile, in 1762, was the inspiration for famous physical educators such as J. F. G. Salzmann. But Charles Kingsley and Tom Hughes are generally credited with being the pioneers of *Muscular Christianity* — title of a chapter in 'Tom Brown at Oxford' (1861) which contains: 'The least of the muscular Christians has got hold of the old chivalrous and Christian belief that a man's body is given him to be trained … then used for the protection of the weak, the advancement of righteous causes. He does not hold that mere strength or activity are in themselves worthy of any respect or worship.' As one of the founders (later principal) of the Working Men's College in London, Hughes launched an athletic programme there in 1854, with a cricket team and a fully equipped gymnasium. He also taught boxing in the basement. Elspeth Huxley's 1973 biography *The Kingsleys* noted: 'In Amyas Leigh he created the quintessentially muscular Christian, transparent, honest, brave, strong, chivalrous, none too bright but resourceful in emergencies, chaste, loyal to God, Queen, Devon and his mother.'

Sport and nationalism

There is a powerful nationalist element behind all international sport — as those who witnessed the extreme partiality of the American crowds in the Atlanta Games will testify although Sydney 2000 was very fair. Within the UK, Wales and Scotland advertise the fact that they exist as a countries through sporting success, hence their extreme fondness for rugby and football, respectively. The Republic of Ireland gained huge recognition with Michelle Smith's three swimming 1996 Olympic gold medals. Yet among the athletes, as the current author witnessed in Munich after the terrorist attack which killed eleven members of the Israeli team, there is a very strong feeling to require future Olympic teams to march into the arena, not by country, but by event. (The competitors in each event tend to know each other very well, while hardly knowing at all the majority of their own country's team members, so it makes social sense.) Also, many felt they would prefer the Olympic flag to be raised, and an Olympic anthem to be played at medal presentations. This will not happen. The television companies have a massive incentive in playing the nationalist card to augment their viewing figures.

The sociology of sport

Finally, the whole sociology of sport, in terms of race, class, gender, local history, professionalism, empowerment, — inter multa alia — is being increasingly analysed by sports sociologists, such as Professor Jennifer Hargreaves with, for example, her widely acclaimed texts 'Sporting Females' and 'Heroines of Sport: The Politics of Difference and Identity', and Professor Grant Jarvie, who focusses deeply into local community sport (eg *Highland Games and shinty*). In addition, sport provides a very large employment outlet, being economically of major importance in the leisure and tourism, and sports equipment, clothing and shoe industries. Think of football, golf, fishing, skiing and horse-racing — and leisure sports wear. In Ireland, for example, sport is one of the country's major employers.

Sport and the arts

Don Masterton, a commentator on the arts and sport, noted that 'If sport does have a relationship with the arts, then drama is its closest kin', and dance indeed would seem to have a foot in both camps. Robert Frost thought that 'writing poetry without rhyme, is like playing tennis without a net.' Lillian Morrison wrote. 'There is an affinity between sport and poetry. Each has power to lift us out of ourselves. They go naturally together wherever there is a zest for life.' While we may think it the province only of poets and artists to seek beauty, consider Robert Francis' description of 'The Skier':

> He swings down like the flourish of a pen
> Signing a signature of white on white

or of gymnasts:

> Competing not so much with one another
> As with perfection,
> They follow follow as voices in a fugue,
> A severe music.

Sport and war

George Orwell held that 'International sport is bound up with hatred, jeolousy, boastfulness, disregard for all rules and sadistic pleasure in witnessing violence — in other words it is war minus the shooting' Conrad Lorenz took a different view: 'A simple and effective way of discharging agggression in an innocuous manner is to redirect it into sport.' In war, men fight to support comrades, not to dominate the enemy, and Jean Rostrand noted: 'In *war*, man is much more sheep than wolf; he follows, he obeys. War is servility, rather a certain fanaticism and credulity, but not aggression.' Yet especially in the First World War, the boundaries with sport seem blurred, as a contemporary account shows: '7.30 am 1 July 1916. As the gunfire died away I saw an infantry man climb onto the parapet into No-Man's land, beckoning others to follow. As he did so, he kicked a football; a good kick, the ball rose and travelled towards the German line. That seemd to be the signal to advance.' Thus began the blackest day in the entire history of the British Army.

On through he heat of laughter
Where gallant comrades fall
Where blood is poured like water
They drive the trickling ball

Anon.

There is a hill in England
Green fields and a school I now
Where the balls fly fast in summer
and the whspering Elm trees grow
There is a hil in Flanders
Heaped with a thousand slain
Where the shells fly at night and noontide,
And the ghosts that died in vain.

Everard Owen *Three hills and other poems.*

Again: '… on Christmas Eve, along several stretches of the Flanders front, curious festive scenes took place, including some of he most incredible sporting scenes in the war — in at least two places along the front, footballs were produced and impromptu matches were started between German and British soldiers.'

These happy boys who left the football field,
The hockey ground, th river, the eleven,
In a far grimmer game, with high elated souls,
To score their goals

W. M. Letts *Golden Boys*

In 1884, headmaster Haslam of Rippon school emphasized the values in his Speech Day sermon: 'Wellington said that the *playfields of Eton* won the battle of Waterloo, and there was no doubt that the training of English boys in the cricket and football field enabled them … to undergo fatiguing marches in Egypt … to stand up to work, and how to give and take a blow.' this aspect of sport is still subject to contemporary debate   CRAIG SHARP

See also EXERCISE; FITNESS; MARTIAL ARTS; WAR AND THE BODY.

Sports science

Two approaches

'Doing science in the context of sport' is one definition of sports science. Arguably the greatest scientist seriously to study sport, Nobel Laureate A. V. Hill, did so in this vein — 'The complaint has been made to me — "why investigate athletics, why not study the processes of industry or disease?" The answer is twofold. (1) The processes of athletics are simple and measurable, and carried out to the utmost of a man's powers: those of industry are not; and (2) athletes themselves, being in a state of health and dynamic equilibrium, can be experimented upon without danger and can repeat their performances again and again' (1927). Only a minority of top-class athletes are prepared to offer themselves as subjects for experiment in the way which Hill implies, but they are an invaluable minority. With their help, much has been learnt about the human body performing at its limits.

However, this is not the approach which would be favoured by Sports Councils, governing bodies of particular sports, or the majority of top-class sportspeople. The organisations which fund most sports science research are seeking support and service to their ongoing training programmes. This approach to sports science is much less likely to produce results which are fundamentally illuminating, but obviously it serves substantially better the purpose for which it is designed.

Four main streams

The two approaches just noted represent differences of purpose, but they say nothing about the content of the science involved. Yet sports performance involves the whole person, and its complete study must take account not only of the body but also of the mind of the sportsperson, and the societal aspects of the sport itself. Thus sports science is an envelope term, embracing at least the following disciplines: (i) Physiology of sports performance; (ii) Biomechanics of Sporting Movement; (iii) Sports Psychology; (iv) Sociology of Sport.

Furthermore, between and derivative from these four main streams are sub-disciplines, many of which have great practical importance. Thus, sports nutrition combines relevant aspects of both physiology and psychology; skill learning is studied by combining techniques from psychology, biomechanics, and neuromuscular physiology; while sports PHYSIOTHERAPY and podiatry (the therapeutic study of FEET and GAIT) are examples of disciplines allied to medicine which draw heavily upon the various aspects of sports science. Another such area of important study, bridging medicine and science, concerns the influences of drugs on performance — whether or not they were deliberately taken to try and enhance it: this could be termed 'sports pharmacology', though in fact that term is rarely used. A final mention, with very different emphasis, should be of match analysis; this is the detailed recording of movements and events in a contest, to aid the evaluation of tactics or physical demand.

Relation to sports medicine

The range of these examples will indicate that the division between sports science (particularly in its service role) and sports medicine is not sharp. The American College of Sports Medicine, indeed, is that country's leading sports science forum also. In Britain the two disciplines have separate professional associations, yet with considerable overlap of membership; and this pattern is repeated in many countries. The two books suggested below for further reading embody just this feature: each, despite its title, devotes more than half its space to what would normally be regarded as sports science.

Representative questions

As to the mainstream sports science disciplines listed above, some examples will help clarify their coverage. Sports physiologists address such questions as:

(i) What distinguishes a sprinter from a marathon runner — and each from the ungifted struggler?

(ii) Why are the effects of training so specific to the particular programme undertaken?

(iii) What are the optimum proportions of glucose, salt, and water in a drink to be taken during competition?

A sports biomechanist might study:

(i) The effects of shoe design on the shock waves caused by foot–ground impact.

(ii) The kinematics of a high diver's multi-axial rotations.

(iii) The optimum techniques of fast bowling, rowing or putting the shot.

Some representative topics of sports psychology are:

(i) The function of a performer's mental images during a gymnastic routine.

(ii) The effects of concentration on reaction time.

(iii) Maintaining the right amount of aggression — not too little, not too much!

And sports sociologists study matters like:

(i) Class, race, gender, and social expectation.

(ii) Sportspeople as role models.

(iii) Politics and the funding of sport.

Future theme?

It is tempting to ask whether a common theme is likely to crystallise out of the interactions of these disciplines as the new millennium gets under way — a theme, that is, at subtler level than the perpetual quest to improve performance by minute particular developments. If there is such a theme, it seems permissible to suggest that it will centre round the interactions of genetic and social inheritance, environment, nutrition, and personal training in the individual's sports performance
NEIL SPURWAY

Further reading

Kent, M. (1994). *The Oxford dictionary of sports science and medicine.* Oxford University Press.

Dirix, K. *et al.* (1988). *The Olympic book of sports medicine.* Blackwell, Oxford.

See also EXERCISE; SPORT.

Sprain A term used loosely for an injury involving JOINTS and MUSCLES: a 'soft tissue injury' which does not damage bone. Since a 'sprain' is characterized chiefly by subjective symptoms (though there may be swelling) and reveals no abnormality on X-ray, the precise site and nature of damage can only be guessed from the description of the type and direction of the strain suffered and the location of pain and tenderness. Sprains are probably mainly due to small tears in LIGAMENTS or muscles.   S.J.

Squint Eye contact is essential for effective social intercourse. This ranges from the parental insistence that an erring child should 'Look at me when I'm talking to you' to the speaker who must look at his audience, even if it is via a TV camera, to keep their attention. Avoiding eye contact can be equally important in ignoring importuning beggars, canvassers, and touts. The evasive glance of the liar is sometimes replaced by an over-emphatic, frank stare in an attempt to establish veracity — a sort of double bluff.

Types of squint

Binocular single vision (BSV) is the simultaneous use of the two eyes to give a single mental impression under normal conditions of seeing. Anyone who has a squint or cast of the eye, such that the two eyes are not pointing towards the object of regard, is seriously disadvantaged, both socially and physiologically. Squinting eyes are most commonly convergent, but divergent squint and vertical squint — with one eye looking higher or lower than the fixing eye — occur as well. Where the squint is constant, the vision in the deviating eye is ignored or suppressed, resulting in reduced acuity. When this defective visual acuity persists after correction of any refractive error it is called *amblyopia* (literally 'blunt vision').

Consequences of squinting

Squints may be constant, intermittent, or latent. An *intermittent*, divergent squint on distant viewing may disappear on looking at near targets, with recovery of BSV. There can be *latent* squint when a tendency to squint is controlled by the individual's quality of BSV. Depending upon the angle of a *constant* squint, the patient may have some low quality or degraded BSV, or even none at all. Here the lack of depth perception can reduce the ability to do detailed close work or to pour liquids accurately, and can make driving even more hazardous than it is already. These problems assume a lesser degree of importance when the faculty of BSV has never developed than in the case of a normal-sighted adult who suddenly loses the ability to fuse the images from the two eyes and is afflicted with double vision (*diplopia*).

Application of animal studies

The infant visual system, comprising eyes, optic pathways, relay stations, and visual cortex, is partly pre-programmed, and the remaining development is governed by the visual environment. Important experimental work with kittens and cats, by Hubel and Wiesel at Harvard in the early 1960s, and later by Blakemore (Professor of Physiology at Oxford), established how columns of nerve cells in the visual cortex could be tuned to respond to the length, orientation, and direction of movement of lines in their field of vision. Amblyopia was produced by unilateral lid suturing, by unilateral squint (induced by surgery or prisms), by defocusing the image optically, or by using ATROPINE. Amblyopia caused a decrease in the number of cortical cells receiving input from the deprived eye, with corresponding cell shrinkage in the layers of the relay station. The number of binocularly-driven visual cortical cells fell from 80% to less than 20%, with a shift in cortical dominance to the side of the non-deprived eye. Some of the changes could be rectified by reverse lid suturing — that is, opening the sutured lids of the visually-deprived eye and suturing the lids of the fellow eye. Similar processes were demonstrated in immature monkey visual systems by von Noorden, at Baylor, Texas. Animal experiments showed that there was a sensitive period of limited duration when cortical cell responses could be reversed and, by analogy with results from occluding the preferred eye in amblyopic children, there is a sensitive period in humans, although its extent cannot be determined so precisely. Certainly this work has led to modifications in the management of childhood amblyopia — for example, part-time occlusion instead of total occlusion or atropinization of the preferred eye. Surgical straightening of congenital convergent squint has only rarely been done as early as 4 months of age, but many surgeons will operate by 9–12 months of age. However, there are many different types of squint, in some of which treatment at four to five years of age can be successful.

Refractive correction

Donders, Professor of Ophthalmology in Utrecht, as long ago as 1864, laid the foundations of the importance of correcting REFRACTIVE ERRORS in squinting children. In particular, if a child has to exert marked accommodation to overcome *hypermetropia* (long-sightedness) for clear sight, the normal close link is broken between focusing the eyes and attaining just the right amount of convergence. The excessive focusing power produces over-convergence, which drives one eye too far inwards. If corrective spectacles are not worn this convergent squint may become permanent.

In some children, the focusing of the two eyes is widely different, usually with one being much more hypermetropic than the other. The more hypermetropic eye never receives a clear image, so visual cortical cells fail to be properly stimulated. Full spectacle correction may not be tolerated because of the large difference in image size on each retina. Instead, contact lenses can be used, as they cause a much smaller difference in image size between the two eyes, thus allowing central fusion.

Early detection

Because of the importance of early correction of obstacles to binocular vision, enthusiastic programmes to visually screen all children by 3–4 years of age have been undertaken, but this is a doctrine of perfection. Their cost-effectiveness — in terms of eventual outcome versus the time and effort expended by orthoptists — has been challenged.

Both parents and family doctors must be educated about the importance of early detection of squints. Any child in a family where either parent or a sibling is hypermetropic or has a history of squint should be screened by an orthoptist. If the results are clearly positive, or equivocal, the child must be referred on to the consultant ophthalmologist, for detailed examination of the eyes, their refractive errors, and their movements. Appropriate therapy, if indicated, can then be started and supervision continued by the orthoptist. Once best visual acuities have been achieved, with glasses if needed, any residual squint is treated by surgical realignment of the eyes under general anaesthesia. This involves moving ocular muscle attachments to new positions in the eyeball and shortening their antagonist muscles. Ideally, fusion of the images of the two eyes can be (re)established, but a more usual result is significant improvement in appearance, with good acuity bilaterally but no or only low-grade fusion.

Double vision in adult squints

In the adult, or visually-mature child of 8 years or older, 'paralytic' squint may develop suddenly as the result of injury or illness. Road traffic accidents are a continual cause of head injury, despite seat belts, as are other means of personal transport — such as cycling, roller blades, and skiing — and also body contact sports. Damage to the CRANIAL NERVES which control the eye muscles, or direct orbital injury to the muscles and their connective tissues, causes uncoordinated eye movements with diplopia. This is a dramatic symptom, demanding medical help urgently. Illnesses capable of such devastating visual results include diabetes, high blood pressure, multiple sclerosis, cerebral aneurysms, and tumours.

In the early stages of paralytic squint, very thin, plastic Fresnel prisms can be pressed onto spectacle lenses to restore fusion. Fresnel, a French physicist, used racks of glass prisms to direct the beam from a lighthouse. Plastic spectacle prisms, based on the same principle, are invaluable orthoptic aids to therapy. Later, in adult patients, surgical repositioning of ocular muscles using adjustable sutures under local anaesthesia gives the best results. *Botulinum toxin* (Botox) (in minute doses, as this is one of the most powerful poisons known) may be injected directly into the antagonist of a weakened ocular muscle to let the eye move into a more central position. For example, in damage to the sixth cranial nerve, which paralyses outward movement, causing horizontal diplopia, this treatment may allow useful binocular vision with a compensatory head posture, and it may even hasten recovery. Botox can be used to create cosmetically straighter eyes in patients embarrassed by noticeable squint. The improvement may only last a matter of months, but a significant number of such patients prefer repeated top-up injections of Botox to a series of squint operations.

PETER FELLS

Further reading

Donders, F. C. (1864). *On the anomalies of accommodation and refraction of the eye.* The New Sydenham Society, London.

Mein, J. and Harcourt, B. (1986). *Diagnosis and management of ocular motility disorders.* Blackwell Scientific Publications, Oxford.

See also EYE MOVEMENTS; GAZE; ORTHOPTICS.

Starvation

Starvation The sight of the ravages of starvation in far too many parts of the modern world is all too familiar on the television screens of

Western society. In our 'developed' countries starvation is encountered only occasionally: self-inflicted as an ultimate political statement by the hunger striker, or in the effort to lose weight, whether reasonably in the obese, or unreasonably by sufferers from EATING DISORDERS; or even more rarely in prolonged SURVIVAL AT SEA or other circumstances of accidental isolation.

In normal circumstances, with an adequate and balanced diet, all tissues take up the required amounts of nutrients from the passing blood, in the form of simple SUGARS (mainly glucose), FATTY ACIDS, and AMINO ACIDS. Tissues differ in the ratio of different fuels used: the BRAIN and SPINAL CORD, and also the red blood cells, can normally utilize only glucose. Excesses from the diet are converted to storage forms, mainly as lipid in fatty tissue and as GLYCOGEN in the LIVER.

Adults can survive for many weeks without FOOD, provided they have water. For just how long depends partly on the extent of their body stores of nutrients, mainly fat. But unfortunately it is not only the fat which is broken down to simpler substances to be used for metabolic energy production and for essential repair and maintenance of the body's tissues. As soon as carbohydrate stores have run out, proteins are mobilized from muscles for the manufacture of sugars by the liver, causing progressive physical weakness.

The physiological priorities in the face of zero food intake no doubt evolved in early millenia when hunting and gathering was an unpredictable and variable source of food. The first priority is to provide the brain with glucose, which is its staple diet, and this requires a certain level of glucose in the circulating blood. The carbohydrate store in the form of liver glycogen is used first to provide this glucose but is used up in the first day or two. Then glucose has to be made from lactic acid and from amino acids derived from muscle protein, released into the blood and taken up in the liver.

But how do the various parts of the body involved 'know' that there is a state of starvation and 'act' accordingly? A fall in blood glucose directly affects the endocrine part of the PANCREAS to change the balance of its hormonal secretions, suppressing *insulin* and enhancing *glucagon* synthesis and release. A fall in blood glucose is sensed also in the HYPOTHALAMUS in the brain, which is the co-ordinating centre for homeostatic processes — those which tend to maintain the body's status quo. This orchestrates a complex hormonal response and also switches on autonomic nervous mechanisms, which stimulate the release or synthesis of glucose in the liver; adrenaline secretion is increased from the adrenal medulla; and the anterior PITUITARY GLAND is brought into action, releasing GROWTH HORMONE, and ACTH which in turn stimulates the release of cortisol from the adrenal cortex.

Glucagon promotes all the processes which tend to raise blood glucose — first its release from liver glycogen, then its synthesis from

amino acids. Adrenaline, growth hormone and cortisol all promote mobilization of lipid from adipose tissue (fat stores) and the use of the resulting circulating fatty acids as metabolic fuel in preference to glucose — everywhere except the brain and the red blood cells, which do not have the necessary chemical apparatus to use them. In the liver, the predominant metabolic use of fatty acids produces the 'ketone bodies', acetoacetate and β-hydroxybutyrate, which circulate in the blood and can be used by other tissues for energy production. If starvation is prolonged even the brain is able to utilize these when glucose is seriously depleted. Some of the acetoacetate is converted to *acetone* — another 'ketone body' — mainly in the lungs, and this becomes noticeable on the breath. The blood becomes progressively more acidic.

In the end, of course, there can be no hope of maintaining life in the absence of food intake. Some of the defence mechanisms become counter-productive. Thus the necessary production of extra acid as a by-product of altered metabolism puts an additional load on the KIDNEYS to deal with H⁺ excretion; the acidity also stimulates breathing, helpfully counteracting acidity by the excretion of more CARBON DIOXIDE, but imposing extra breathing work on a weakening body. Muscles waste away; oedema and accumulation of fluid in body cavities follows depletion of plasma proteins. Ultimately there is multi-organ failure from lack of fuel and loss of vital enzyme activity. Shortages of MINERALS and VITAMINS will also take their toll if starvation is not total, and hence attenuated enough for these deficiencies to take effect, but in terms of aid to starving communities, the urgent requirements are for the basic nutrients.

SHEILA JENNETT

See also ACID BASE HOMEOSTASIS; BLOOD SUGAR; FASTING; HORMONES; HUNGER.

Stem cells

are 'uncommitted' cells, capable of dividing to make more stem cells, or, under appropriate conditions, to produce the kinds of specialized cells that make up the tissues and organs of the body.

A newly fertilized egg is the ultimate stem cell. It is *totipotent* – capable of generating all the different types of cells found in the body, and also the fetal part of the placenta and supporting tissues. The fertilized egg splits into two, and those into four, and so on. For the first few divisions, up to at least the 8-cell stage, all the cells of the tiny embryo are totipotent stem cells. Indeed, if these early cells separate, they can each continue to develop, making identical twins, triplets, quadruplets, etc.

About four days after fertilization, the route to commitment starts. Some cells form an outer layer, which becomes part of the placenta, while others make the inner mass, which is the beginning of the true embryo. Initially this consists entirely of *pluripotent* stem cells, which cannot give rise to placental tissue but can make any component of the fetus itself. As the embryo

grows, and the parts of the body start to emerge, the individual stem cells within each future organ or tissue become further specialized so as to be capable of producing only a certain range of possible final cell types. These stem cells are then called *multipotent*. At a certain stage in the development of each 'family tree' of cells, one or both of the daughter cells produced by the division of a stem cell becomes 'committed', that is, incapable of further division. These committed daughters continue to *differentiate* and become the normal functional cells of the heart, skin, brain, kidney, and other organs.

Adult animals still have some multipotent stem cells, especially in tissues such as skin and blood, in which cells last only a short time and have to be replaced. Indeed, even in the adult brain, previously thought to be incapable of making new nerve cells, there are populations of stem cells, which are constantly producing relatively small numbers of new neurons.

We now stand at the threshold of a potential revolution in medical treatment for diseases and disorders in which organs stop working properly. At present, some such conditions, such as heart, kidney and liver disease, can be treated by transplantation of a replacement organ from another person. But demand for donor organs is far outstripping supply, and the failure rate of such surgery is quite high, mainly because of the problem of rejection. Many other disorders, such as stroke, diabetes and Alzheimer's disease, cannot presently be treated by transplantation. The great hope is that suitable stem cells, produced in large quantities through cell culture methods and injected into failing tissues and organs, will produce fresh, replacement cells to take over from lost or damaged ones.

Stem cells for such replacement therapy could be produced in a number of different ways. Ultimately, it might be possible to make them with the kind of methods used to produce the first cloned mammal, *Dolly* the sheep. An ordinary specialized adult cell from the patient could be used to produce a totipotent stem cell by removing the nucleus (with the DNA-containing chromosomes), and inserting it into a human egg from which the nucleus has been removed. But there are many problems with this approach, not least the fact that adult cells may have accumulated genetic errors, which will be transmitted to the stem cells produced. Everyone agrees that formidable technical obstacles must be overcome before the cloning of stem cells from adult cells becomes safe. There is also concern that the development of methods for *therapeutic cloning* would inevitably lead to the production of whole human beings, who, like *Dolly*, are genetic replicas of an adult. At present, the vast majority of scientists and clinicians, not to mention ethicists and politicians, are opposed to such *reproductive cloning*, but it must be said that resistance may decrease if the techniques involved can be made more reliable.

In principle, some of the patient's own stem cells could be harvested (most likely from bone marrow or certain parts of the brain), multi-plied in culture and injected into a diseased or damaged region to produce new cells. Stem cells derived from the patient's own body would have the great advantage that they would not be rejected. This approach has already been successful in experimental animals, with stem cells from bone marrow used to replace damaged heart muscle. It may soon be used in humans to treat heart disease, diabetes, and other such diseases. However, it would not be appropriate for the replacement of tissues that are diseased because of a genetic disorder (such as Huntington's disease or cystic fibrosis), since stem cells from the patient would have the same genetic mistake in their DNA. This strategy would also be inappropriate in acute conditions, demanding immediate treatment, because of the time needed for stem cells to multiply in culture.

The most immediately promising strategy is to isolate pluripotent stem cells from human embryos just a few days after fertilization, to culture them, and to inject them into the patient's diseased or damaged organ. Since such cells carry different DNA from that of the patient, they could be used to treat genetic disorders. On the other hand, this means that precautions would have to be taken to avoid rejection.

Transplantation of immature nerve cells and stem cells from the brains of aborted human embryos has been used for several years to treat the degenerative brain condition, Parkinson's disease, with reasonably encouraging results. Such treatment has not greatly alleviated the characteristic tremor of the hands, and some patients have developed disturbing unintended movements. But most have regained the ability to initiate and control their actions. It is probable that embryonic stem cell injection will soon be used in efforts to treat the degenerative diseases Huntington's disease and Alzheimer's, and even STROKE, in which parts of the brain are destroyed becomes of interruption of the blood supply.

There is wide agreement among medical scientists that research on human embryonic stem cells is an important first step towards stem cell therapy, even though it may eventually be possible to use adult stem cells. Yet the prospect of harvesting cells from living human embryos smacks of *Frankenstein* or *Brave New World*, and 'pro-life' religious groups have mounted stout moral opposition. However, it would not be necessary to fertilize additional human eggs specifically for such research. Present methods for the production of 'test-tube babies' involve the production and storage (by freezing) of several fertilized eggs, the unwanted ones simply being destroyed or permanently stored. These surplus eggs could, with parental agreement, provide a ready source of embryos for stem cell collection. Moreover, as long as there are strict limits on the time for which the embryo is allowed to develop, it will have no nervous system or other organs, no possibility of feelings, and nothing approaching an independent life. Also, the indubitable suffering of the many people who might be helped by stem cell therapy

ought to weigh heavily in the complex moral equation.

In 2001, the British government authorized stem cell research on human embryos up to 14 days post-conceptual age. Given the huge potential benefits of stem cell therapy, it is likely that other nations will follow suit.

COLIN BLAKEMORE

Further reading:

Thomson, J. *et al.* (1998) Embryonic stem cell lines derived from human blastocysts. *Science* 282: 1145–1147.

US National Institutes of Health website. Stem cells: a primer.
www.nih.gov/news/stemcell/primer.htm

See also: ANTENATAL DEVELOPMENT; ASSISTED REPRODUCTION; CLONING; DISEASE; GENE THERAPY; GENETICS, HUMAN; ORGAN DONATION; PREGNANCY; TRANSPLANTATION.

Sterilization

Voluntary sterilization: the clinical possibilities

Sterilization refers to the procedure performed to stop FERTILITY permanently, in either the male or the female. It is the most reliable type of CONTRACEPTION; consequently it is the most common form of contraception in couples over the age of 35 in the UK who have completed their families.

Fertilization occurs when a man's SPERM reaches and joins an egg released from the OVARY of a woman. The released egg is picked up by one of the two Fallopian tubes, which transports it to the UTERUS. Fertilization usually occurs in the Fallopian tube; if fertilized, the egg then implants into the wall of the uterus to establish a PREGNANCY. Sterilization interrupts this process permanently, either by preventing the release of sperm or by stopping fertilization by blocking the Fallopian tube.

Female sterilization may be achieved by a number of techniques, over a hundred having been described since Lungren performed what is thought to be the first tubal sterilization in 1880. Operations on women are commonly called *tubal ligation*, as the procedures aim to occlude or 'ligate' (tie) the Fallopian tubes. The majority of operations described involved cutting the Fallopian tube and oversewing the cut end so that it was hidden. These operations required an incision either on the abdominal wall or through the top of the VAGINA to gain access to the tubes. The early operations are thought to have had a failure rate of around 1 in 200.

Sterilization can be performed at the time of CAESAREAN SECTION, which allows easy access to the Fallopian tubes. This is seldom done now, as the failure rate is higher than with other techniques applied after the womb has returned to its non-pregnant state.

Modern surgical techniques have been developed and now include *laparoscopic* (telescopic) procedures to occlude the Fallopian tubes. These may use *diathermy* (burning) of the tubes to

damage them and seal them. Alternatively, one of two common types of device are used to block the tubes. The first type involves placing small rubber bands over a pinched-up portion of each tube. The second type involves placing a crushing clip across them.

If a sterilization procedure fails there is an increased risk of the pregnancy implanting outside the womb. This is known as an ectopic pregnancy, which most commonly occurs in the Fallopian tube and can sometimes, if the pregnancy grows, result in the tube rupturing and causing internal bleeding.

Male sterilization is achieved by the operation of *vasectomy*: cutting or ligating, on both sides, the vas deferens, which transports sperm from the testicles to the penis. The major advantage to a couple of a vasectomy is that it is a much simpler operation than female sterilization, due to the easy access to the vas within the scrotum. Vasectomy can easily be performed as an outpatient operation under local anaesthetic. After the operation the man must wait for around twelve weeks before the sperm count falls to sterile levels. Normally doctors ask for two sperm samples to check the operation has worked before alternative contraception can be abandoned.

Men and women requesting sterilization are usually seen at least twice by doctors prior to being sterilized, as the operation is designed to be permanent. Although reversal may be possible, sterilization should not be performed if either of the partners is unsure. It is also important that the doctor excludes any medical reason why the operation should not be performed. Women who have been taking the contraceptive pill because of painful periods are warned that these may recur if the Pill is stopped.

Current research is investigating reversible forms of contraception such as foam plugs for the Fallopian tubes or for the vas deferens.

Eugenical sterilization as a solution to social problems

Eugenicists in the US were particularly active in lobbying for the passage of state eugenical sterilization laws in the 1920s and 30s. Similar movements occurred in Canada, Britain, and Germany, but no laws were passed. Scandinavian countries — Denmark, Norway, Sweden, and Finland — passed laws in the 1930s. In the US, Harry H. Laughlin, of the Eugenics Record Office in Cold Spring Harbor, had drawn up a 'Model Sterilization Law' that served as a prototype for local use at home or abroad. Although the earliest such laws had been passed before World War I, the majority were established in the inter-war period. Eugenical sterilization laws were considered quite different from the punitive sterilization laws that existed in many states and countries in the nineteenth century. Although both types were compulsory, eugenical sterilization was aimed at prevention of future problems rather than serving as a punishment for past ones.

Eugenical sterilization was always couched in medical and scientific terms, and was justified as a means of saving the taxpayer money. In most countries it was aimed specifically at those individuals in mental or penal institutions who, from family pedigree analysis, were considered likely to give birth to socially defective offspring. In the US, sterilization could be ordered only after a patient had been examined by a eugenics committee, usually composed of a lawyer or family member representing the individual; a judge; and a doctor or other eugenic 'expert'. Lobbyists often included members of the local state American Eugenics Society and a network of progressive enthusiasts who thought this was the way to cure social problems at their roots — it was the prime example of 'social efficiency'.

Between 1907 (when the first law was passed, in Indiana) and 1941, over 38 000 eugenical sterilizations were performed in the US, with California in the lead. By the early 1960s the number had risen to over 60 000. The most famous sterilization case was that of Carrie Buck in Virginia, where a test case was set up to determine whether the law which had been passed was constitutional. Buck v. Bell was tried in 1925 in the Virginia Circuit Court. When the lower court ruled in favour of the law, an appeal was sent to the Supreme Court of the US, where Justice Oliver Wendell Holmes wrote the majority report. In upholding the lower court ruling Holmes made his oft-repeated assertion: 'Three generations of imbeciles are enough.' More to the legal point, Holmes claimed that 'The principle that sustains compulsory vaccination is broad enough to cover cutting the Fallopian tubes.'

Laughlin's model law served also as a basis for a similar law in Germany, passed by the National Socialist government in 1933. For this effort, as well as for his enthusiastic support of Nazi eugenics programmes, Laughlin was awarded an honorary doctorate from Heidelberg University in 1936 — three years after the Nazis had come to power, and two years after their sweeping sterilization act had gone into effect.

While it would not be historically accurate to claim that state sterilization laws were repealed *en masse* after World War II and the disclosure of Nazi eugenic excesses, the general trend in 1945–55 was a decline in their application, increasing challenges to their constitutionality, and repeal of laws in some states — but it was not, for example, until 1977 that New Jersey outlawed the compulsory sterilization of the 'developmentally disabled'. More telling, perhaps, than legislative changes, is the history of the actual application of sterilization laws in the post-war era — where they were not repealed, there was a dramatic decrease in the number of sterilizations reported. This decline was partly due to changing attitudes about the actual genetic effectiveness of sterilization — the acceptance that feeblemindedness might not have such a hereditary basis as had been supposed.

Influenced by their proximity to the Nazi experience, the Scandinavian countries repealed their laws after World War II. However, related issues of sterilization and control of reproduction in other guises continued, and gained considerable momentum after 1950, with respect to world population growth. Funded by the Rockefeller Foundation, pilot population control programmes were initiated in India, Puerto Rico, and other Third World countries; by 1960 these had been taken over and expanded by the US government funded bodies. Some post-war proponents of population control had been involved in eugenics in the 30s and 40s, and they used comparable arguments to those advanced earlier for eugenical sterilization — the differential birthrate of non-Western, non-European/American peoples. Now on a global scale, population control was, in the words of historian and critic Allan Chase 'aimed at the gonads of the poor'.
LINDA CARDOZO
PHILIP TOOZS-HOBSON
GARLAND E. ALLEN

Further reading

Allen, G. E. 1986. The eugenics record office at Cold Spring Harbor: an essay in institutional history. *Osiris 2* (**2nd Series**), 224–64.

Chase, A. 1977. *The legacy of Malthus*. Alfred A. Knopf, New York.

Reilly, P. 1992. *The surgical solution: a history of involuntary sterilization in the United States*. Johns Hopkins University Press, Baltimore.

See also CASTRATION; EUGENICS; VASECTOMY.

Steroids comprise a large group of substances that mediate a very varied set of biological responses. The most widespread in the body is CHOLESTEROL, an essential component of CELL MEMBRANES, and the starting point for the synthesis of other steroids — the SEX HORMONES, adrenal cortical hormones, and the BILE salts.

The steroids are grouped together because their chemical structures are all very similar. The steroid chemical nucleus consists of four carbon rings, three 6-sided and one 5-sided, joined together by their edges. The specificity of their different biological actions is due to the various groups attached to a common nucleus. When alcohol groups (OH) are attached, steroids should properly be called *sterols* (such as *cortisol*), whereas ketone groups (C=O) make them *sterones* (such as *aldosterone*).

Different steroids react with different MEMBRANE RECEPTORS in cells, and a precise fit between the steroid and the receptor is required. Therefore a single steroid can be expected to have a specific effect.

Steroids have major responsibilities as hormones, controlling METABOLISM, salt balance, and the development and function of the sexual organs as well as other bodily differences between the sexes. Steroids in the form of bile salts assist in digestive processes, while another steroid is a vitamin that takes part in CALCIUM control.

Steroid hormones

Steroid hormones are made and secreted into the circulating blood by the cortex of the ADRENAL GLANDS and the gonads (testes or ovaries). Mostly, their secretion is regulated by hormones from the PITUITARY GLAND, and those in turn by chemical messages from the HYPOTHALAMUS.

Two types of steroids are released from the adrenal cortex, the *glucocorticoids*, mainly cortisol (hydrocortisone) and the *mineralocorticoids*, mainly aldosterone. Both types of hormone are important in stress situations such as disease or INJURY.

Glucocorticoids mobilize glucose, which is particularly important in fasting conditions. They do so by promoting glucose formation from non carbohydrate sources in the liver, increasing GLYCOGEN levels, and raising the blood glucose concentration. Liberation of glucocorticoids from the adrenal cortex is caused by *adrenocorticotrophic hormone* (ACTH), released from the pituitary gland. When the glucocorticoid level in the blood is low, ACTH is released, but when it is high the release of ACTH is suppressed. This is a good example, one of many that occur in the body, of a feedback system. Large doses of glucocorticoids are anti-inflammatory and at one time it was thought they would provide suitable treatment for inflammatory conditions such as rheumatoid arthritis. However, the excessive breakdown of proteins, mobilized to form glucose in the liver, leads to muscle weakness and osteoporosis and there is also 'moon face' and OBESITY. This describes exactly the features of *Cushing's syndrome*, a condition caused by excess secretion of corticosteroids. Furthermore, if therapy with glucocorticoids is withdrawn rapidly the pituitary system is so suppressed that the body's own system takes a while to trip in, leading to an 'Addisonian crisis', mimicking Addison's disease in which there is a deficiency in glucocorticoid production. With due precautions, however, corticosteroids remain a useful treatment in some severe allergic and inflammatory conditions.

The mineralocorticoid aldosterone is released at an increased rate from the adrenal glands if the body is salt depleted; this is stimulated by a complex detecting system in the KIDNEYS, resulting in an increase in circulating *angiotensin*, which acts in turn on the adrenal glands. Aldosterone promotes sodium reabsorption by the kidneys, so that there is less salt in the urine, thus correcting the deficiency. It acts on sweat glands similarly, diminishing salt loss in sweat.

Male steroid sex hormones, *androgens*, are produced in the testes. Testosterone is the most important of the androgens and is responsible for controlling the production and maturation of sperm, as well as male characteristics, such as the distribution of body hair. *Anabolic steroids* are derivatives of testosterone and act on androgenic receptors. They build up muscle mass and cause virilization — features of masculinity. They are useful in the treatment of debilitated patients to help restore their physique. Unfortunately these substances have been taken illicitly by athletes for

BODY-BUILDING. Their use carries considerable risk, as sudden withdrawal will leave the body's natural processes suppressed, by interference with the feedback system as described above. Detection of the use of anabolic steroids has become difficult as it appears that one that is commonly used, namely *nandrolone*, can be synthesized by the body itself in small quantities, especially when under physical stress. Female steroid sex hormones are of two types, *oestrogens* and *progestins*, both from the ovaries. Again under pituitary hormone regulation, their relative secretion varies within the menstrual cycle. Oestrogens promote the growth of the lining of the uterus in preparation for implantation of a fertilized egg. Once the egg has been shed from the ovary, the *corpus luteum* (yellow body), which develops in the cavity left behind, secretes progesterone; this promotes further development of the uterine lining and, if implantation of an embryo occurs, maintains changes here and elsewhere for the duration of pregnancy.

The understanding of these processes is the basis of the contraceptive pill. Synthetic steroids were devised for this purpose, as natural steroids are metabolized by the liver if taken by mouth. As with the other steroid hormones, there are feedback systems involving the pituitary gland. Taking oestrogens inhibits the release from the pituitary of the *follicular stimulating hormone* that would normally cause maturation of eggs in the ovary: so, no ovulation, no conception. Contraceptive pills usually contain both oestrogens and progestins, which are taken concurrently or sequentially during the 4 week course, menstruation following when the course ceases. A large dose of both an oestrogen and progestin promotes uterine bleeding within a few hours and is the basis of the 'morning after' pill.

Steroids and bile

Cholesterol, taken up from the blood into the liver or synthesized there, can be oxidized in the liver to cholic acid. Conjugation of this with taurine or glycine gives the bile salts, *taurocholate* and *glycocholate*. These bile salts pass into the small intestine and have important actions in aiding the digestion and absorption of fats. Cholesterol itself is excreted in the bile.

The steroid vitamin

Exposure to ultraviolet light converts a steroid, *dehydrocholesterol*, in the skin to vitamin D. This is what happens when you sunbathe, but in climes where exposure to the sun is limited it is necessary to supplement the diet with the vitamin. Fish oils are rich in vitamin D and the Eskimo diet ensures that they get a sufficient supply. The vitamin primarily promotes calcium absorption from the gut. Calcium is essential for bone growth and maintenance, muscle contraction, and many signalling processes in the body.

While steroids have many different actions on the body, their mechanism of action is similar in all instances. The receptors for steroids are inside cells (unlike those for many other substances, which are on the cell membrane). The complex formed by combination of the steroid with its specific receptor enters the nucleus and switches on or off the appropriate genes, which then gives rise to the characteristic effect. Their actions are not therefore immediate as with, for example, NEUROTRANSMITTERS, nor are they as rapid as those of the peptide hormones; several hours elapse before the effect appears. To give one example, the receptors for aldosterone are located in the end part of the kidney tubules. Here genes are switched on which lead to the synthesis of the molecules that actually handle the reabsorption of sodium ions from the urine back into the blood. The process becomes more efficient because there are a larger number of molecular entities dedicated to the task.

ALAN W. CUTHBERT

See also BILE; BODY BUILDING; HORMONES; MENSTRUAL CYCLE; SEX HORMONES.

Stethoscope
The stethoscope is an instrument for listening to sounds originating within the body. It was invented in 1816 by the French physician, Rene Laennec. The older diagnostic method of direct AUSCULTATION — applying the ear to the chest wall — was known to the ancient Greeks, but had fallen out of general use. It was, however, experimented with by Jean-Nicolas Corvisart, at the end of the eighteenth century. Laennec, who had been Corvisart's student, took a special interest in chest disorders. One day, he was consulted by a young woman with the symptoms of heart disease. Still a young man, Laennec felt too embarrassed to press his head against his patient's bosom. Remembering a children's game, he picked up a sheet of paper, rolled it into a tube, and placed one end upon the woman's chest. He was able to hear the sounds of her HEART and her BREATHING quite distinctly. The stethoscope had been invented.

Leannec experimented with various materials and shapes for his new instrument, finalizing upon a simple hollow wooden cylinder, about 25 cm long. With this tool, Laennec undertook a comprehensive investigation of the sounds emanating from the heart and LUNGS, correlating his findings with post-mortem results. His treatise on the subject is the basis of our modern understanding of the pathology of the lung.

While there was some early opposition, Laennec's innovation came into general use quite quickly. The development of clinical teaching in the hospitals provided students with the necessary supply of patients upon whom to practice. By the 1850s, the stethoscope had become virtually the indispensable badge of office of the medical practitioner. Its widespread adoption encouraged the development of other methods of physical diagnosis.

However, despite Laennec's claims, the stethoscope possessed only a few technical advantages over direct auscultation. In most circumstances, the instrument did not enable one to hear the thoracic sounds any more clearly than one could with the unaided ear. What it did do was enable the physician to examine the patient's chest more conveniently, more hygienically, and less intrusively. In 1828, N. P. Comins, in Edinburgh, designed a stethoscope with a hinge in the middle of its barrel, to facilitate bedside application. Comins also suggested that a binaural stethoscope might be clinically useful, and in 1851 Arthur Leared designed an instrument with two flexible rubber tubes. This was the basis of the modern stethoscope, equipped with either an open bell or a diaphragm at the chestpiece, but it did not come into common use until the 1890s. Throughout the nineteenth century, many other modifications were suggested to improve the acoustics or the ease of use of the instrument, and methods for amplifying the heart and lung sounds were investigated.

While now superseded, to a large extent, in the diagnosis of lung disorders by the X-RAY machine and other IMAGING TECHNIQUES, and of heart disorders by investigative techniques ranging from the electrocardiogram to the ultrasonic scanner, the stethoscope remains indispensible in the initial detection of abnormalities in both hospital and general practice. Numerous applications have been found outside the thoracic region, such as in the monitoring of bowel function and of pregnancy, and in the measurement of BLOOD PRESSURE.

MALCOLM NICOLSON

See also SOUNDS OF THE BODY.

Stigmata
are the wounds of Christ as reproduced in a human body. Visible stigmata are frequently located in both hands and both feet, and on the right side of the chest, replicating the sites of Christ's wounds, which he showed to the disciples in his post-resurrection appearances (Luke 24: 36–40 and John 20: 19–29). The most famous of the stigmatics, St Francis of Assisi, received the stigmata in these places. Occasionally wounds on the head, in the shape of a crown (copying the crown of thorns), and marks on either shoulder (representing the carrying of the cross and scourging) are evidence of stigmata too. Stigmata might also be invisible, marked by the pain of wounds in the classic places, or alternately invisible and visible. St Catherine of Sienna received the stigmata of the five wounds in a vision but asked God to make them disappear, after which she experienced only the pain of the wounds.

The appearance of stigmata varies greatly. Stigmata have ranged from the nail imprints of St Francis' wounds — for which Francis consequently required bandages to cover the protruding nail shapes so that he might use his hands and feet (though he had no bandages from Thursday evening to Saturday morning in order that he might share Christ's Good Friday suffering) — to cuts of varying length and depth, blisters, and scabs of dried blood. Bleeding or manifestation of the stigmata might in some cases be continual while in other cases occur only periodically — for example, in Lent and Holy Week, or on particular days of the week, especially Fridays or Good Friday. In the case of Padre Pio, the twentieth-century stigmatic, his hands bled lightly but almost continually, soaking the gloves he wore, and the wound in his chest produced a cup of blood each day.

Stigmata are often accompanied by other bodily phenomena such as pain, blood, sweats, levitations, or even lameness or blindness, and they quite often occur in people who are already ill or are voluntarily abstaining from food for religious reasons. Many of the women nuns and saints who fasted and/or existed on the host alone, in late medieval and early modern Europe, received the stigmata, such as St Catherine of Sienna, who fasted — except for eating the blessed host — for eight years. Stigmatics often receive religious visions or ecstasies, having visions of Christ and various saints, and also 're-living' or seeing parts of Christ's passion and sharing in his suffering.

Stigmata seem to have begun to appear only in the thirteenth century, with the growing popularity of the imitation of Christ, especially the suffering Christ, in patterns of piety and devotional life. Of some 330 recorded cases of persons receiving the stigmata, only about 60 of those have been made saints. The official Roman Catholic position towards stigmata has always been rather guarded.

It seems that the vast majority of stigmatics have been women. In the case of the late medieval and early modern female religious, their receiving the stigmata has been interpreted as one of a number of experiences or phenomena, including fasting and other forms of asceticism, by which women participated in the imitation of Christ. Through their bodies they could share in the suffering of Christ, who in his body suffered to save humankind, and by the signs of their suffering, such as the stigmata, they gained access to power and authority, not by virtue of office (which was denied them) but through experience. In the modern period, female stigmatics have been consistently subjected to medical testing, in the quest for authenticity, and there is an abundance of medical evidence for stigmatics, such as Catherine Emmerich (1774–1824), Louise Lateau (1850–83), and the early twentieth-century Teresa Neumann. In nineteenth-century France especially, this kind of medical testing of female bodies by male doctors bears some comparison with Charcot's study of hysteria, especially as stigmatics and hysterics were seen to share some of the same pathologies or symptoms. In both cases the body was seen to hold the 'truth'. A medical doctor, Imbert-Gourbeyre, visited and examined as many of the nineteenth-century stigmatics as he could, as well as examining and compiling evidence about other unusual religious phenomena such as the miracles reported at Lourdes, and his medical study of 1894, *La Stigmatisation, l'extase divine, les miracles de Lourdes*, illustrates very well this sort of approach. JANE SHAW

See also BODY MUTILATION AND MARKINGS; SAINTS.

Stimulants A stimulant is a rather imprecise term used for a variety of different kinds of drug, some with medical uses and others with only recreational use. *Psychomotor stimulants* produce *locomotor activity* (the subject becomes hyperactive), *euphoria*, (often expressed by excessive talking and garrulous behaviour), and *anorexia*. The *amphetamines* are the best known drugs in this category, the actions in the central nervous system depending on the release of NORADRENALINE, DOPAMINE, and possibly 5HT. Many tests show that the amphetamines reduce physical and mental fatigue, but the accuracy of mental deliberations is likely to be reduced also. Nevertheless, the amphetamines once enjoyed a reputation among students for improving performance at examinations. Excessive use leads to insomnia and repeated use leads to a level of dependence. Amphetamines also have actions outside the nervous system, causing hypertension.

COCAINE is also a psychomotor stimulant and users are typically extroverted, party-loving individuals. Cocaine blocks the re-uptake of noradrenaline at SYNAPSES within the brain and elsewhere, with effects similar to the amphetamines. Cocaine is produced by bushy plants growing in Bolivia and Peru, and hardworking peasants chew the leaves to reduce the FATIGUE they feel from their toiling, but also to reduce hunger. The dependence which develops with cocaine presents a serious problem in the developed world.

CAFFEINE and *theophylline*, both *methylxanthines*, found in tea, coffee, and some soft drinks, are mild psychomotor stimulants. They reduce mental and physical fatigue, without affecting locomotor activity or producing euphoria. It is doubtful whether caffeine and theophylline can produce true dependence. Methylxanthines have some other actions, causing increased urine production and stimulation of heart muscle.

Drugs of another type are used as *respiratory stimulants* in deeply comatose patients or those with respiratory failure. These are more properly described as *analeptics* (meaning restorative); *nikethamide* is an example. Some purgatives, such as *cascara* and *senna*, are described as *stimulant purgatives* and work in the gut, releasing substances which cause peristaltic movements and lead to a temporary diarrhoea.

ALAN W. CUTHBERT

Stoicism Stoic philosophy was developed in Athens in the third century BC, and reached the peak of its popularity among the upper classes of Rome during the first century BC and the first century AD. The Stoic view of knowledge is empirical; knowledge comes to us from the world through 'appearances', which are impressed on our minds. Reason, seen as the quintessentially human characteristic, enables us to understand the world; it is possible to form a community of those who use reason, which will be superior to any secular community. While in pursuit of this ideal, Stoics did not always withdraw from participation in political life; the Roman Stoic Seneca served in the Roman senate and influenced the emperor Nero, although in later life he moved away from Rome to concentrate on writing.

Stoicism denied the importance of all bodily conditions, and EMOTIONS were always regarded as bad. The only factor seen as essential to human happiness was virtue, all else in life having significance only as an opportunity to demonstrate that one possesses virtue. Seneca claimed that one could demonstrate virtue equally well through PLEASURE or through PAIN, whether enjoying a banquet or submitting to TORTURE. Since all bodily experience equally provided an opportunity to show virtue, no experience was to be deliberately sought out over another. This contrasted with other philosophical approaches; for example, Epicureanism, which regarded pleasure as the goal of life. For the Stoic, poverty and detachment from the world were not seen as essential for the achievement of the good life, nor need worldly wealth be abandoned in the quest for virtue.

In the treatise *De Officiis* (On Duties), written after the assassination of Julius Caesar in 44 BC, the Roman politician and philosopher Cicero gave a Stoic account of the correct use of the body as part of his advice to his son — and to the Roman governing classes in general — on how to make moral decisions and to live in the best way possible. As a manual for the upper classes, this text was highly influential in Western political and social thought. Cicero says that both the mind and the body should be trained from childhood into moderate and appropriate behaviour, and this should be expressed through every action — there being a seemly way to stand, walk, or sit. Nature, Cicero argues, has constructed the body so that the most honourable parts are the most visible. Sane people mirror Nature's wisdom in keeping out of sight the parts Nature has hidden away, and in performing bodily functions in private. Moving too slowly is seen as effeminate: hurrying around makes someone out of breath, thus distorting the face. Anger, pleasure, and fear equally transform the faces, voices, and GESTURES of those experiencing them: the ideal is to control the body, avoid excessive gestures, and follow a moderate way of life. While recommending following 'Nature', Cicero also recommends training the body in such a way that one's natural faults are played down; presentation of self can thus be achieved in a way which deceives the onlooker. HELEN KING

Stomach The part of the alimentary tract into which the oesophagus (gullet) opens immediately below the diaphragm. A term often used colloquially for belly or abdomen, which it is not; so-called 'stomach-ache' arises most commonly from the intestine and is felt near the umbilicus. Pain from the stomach itself is higher — just below the breast bone. The stomach expands to receive a meal, holds it for up to four hours depending on the amount of food, churning it to a pulp and initiating digestion, then passes it on by degrees into the duodenum. These functions depend on its muscular wall and the acid- and enzyme-secreting glands in its lining, all of which are under the control of autonomic nerves.   s.j.

See ALIMENTARY SYSTEM; PLATE 1.

Strength training

Specificity of training

The adaptation of MUSCLES, and indeed body systems generally, to tasks with which they are repeatedly challenged, is highly specific. Thus training for endurance, for flexibility, or for speed are all very different; and training for strength has little in common with any of them. One must 'overload' (in the physical educator's sense of 'load beyond the ordinary', not the engineer's sense of 'break') the ability of muscles to produce extreme force, not their ability to produce lesser forces very often or very fast, if strength is to be increased.

Resistance

Strength is increased by work against high resistance — 'strength training' and 'resistance training' are synonymous. After warming up against lesser loads, strength athletes during a high-intensity phase of training will perform, in a weight-room session, no more than perhaps ten efforts against loads almost as great as they can possibly manage. Strength trainers characterize loads in terms of the individual's 'repetition maximum' (RM). A 1 RM load can be managed just once in a session, a 10 RM load can be tackled 10 times within a period measured in minutes. Working against loads less than 60% of 1 RM is not considered capable of increasing strength at all.

(By contrast, in endurance training, any one stride or stroke or pedal-turn probably involves only 10–15% of the maximum force the limb can produce; however, not 10 but at least 10 000 such actions are performed in the course of an endurance training session.)

Phases of training

In someone whose genetic makeup allows a good response to strength training, the maximum load which can be handled may increase by 50–100% in the first 6–12 months. The improvement, however, is not all of one kind, but falls into two phases.

The first phase, lasting probably 8–12 weeks, is termed the 'neural phase' of strength training. Muscle bulk does not increase, though strength does. Electrical recordings show that more of the muscle fibres are being called into action simultaneously at the end of this phase than at the beginning. It is as if the nervous system has been teaching itself how to get the most force out of the muscle bulk it already has available to it. (The inability to do this without training should not be thought of as poor evolutionary design; it may well have protective benefits, while TENDONS, JOINTS, and other parts of the system are also not adapted to the high loads being tackled.)

After this period, muscle bulk does increase. In high responders this 'hypertrophic' (enlargement) phase may continue for years, though the rates of increase of bulk and strength slow down markedly after 8–12 months. The hypertrophy is expressed at the individual fibre level: strength-trained muscles have bigger fibres, not more fibres.

Real programmes

The above account is a simplification. Within an actual session, lifts are grouped into 'sets' with rests between them, and repeated say 2–10 times in a set. Not all exercises are done each training day; they may recur only twice a week. Finally, over a year, the established strength athlete will probably alternate two periods of 'volume' training with two of high intensity.   NEIL SPURWAY

Further reading

Komi, P. V. (1991). *Strength and Power in Sport.* Blackwell, Oxford.

See also BODY-BUILDING; EXERCISE.

Stress is a word derived from the Latin word *stringere*, meaning to draw tight, and was used in the seventeenth century to describe hardship and affliction. During the late eighteenth century (as Hinkle records), stress denoted 'force, pressure, *strain*, or strong effort', referring primarily to an individual, or to the individual's organs or mental powers.

Definitions of strain and load used in physics and engineering eventually began to influence our understanding of how stress affects individuals and their HEALTH. Under this concept, external forces (load) are seen as exerting pressure upon an individual, producing strain. Proponents of this view felt that they could measure the stress to which an individual is subjected, in the same way we can measure physical strain on a machine. While this concept looks at stress as an outside stimulus, an alternative concept defines stress as a person's response to a disturbance. As early as 1910, Sir William Osler explored the idea of stress and strain causing 'disease', when he saw a relationship between chest pains (angina pectoris) and a hectic pace of life. The idea that environmental forces could actually cause disease rather than just short-term ill health effects, and that people have a natural tendency to resist such forces, was seen in the work of Walter B. Cannon in the 1930s. Cannon studied the effects of stress in animals and people, and in particular studied the 'fight or flight' reaction. Through this reaction, people, as well as animals, will choose whether to stay and fight or try to escape when confronting extreme danger. Cannon observed that when his subjects experienced situations of cold, lack of oxygen, or excitement, he could detect physiological changes such as emergency adrenaline secretions. Cannon described these individuals as being 'under stress'.

One of the first scientific attempts to explain the process of stress-related illness was made in 1946 by physician Hans Selye, who described three stages an individual encounters in stressful situations: (i) *alarm reaction*, in which an initial phase of lowered resistance is followed by countershock, during which the individual's defence mechanisms become active; (ii) *resistance*, the stage of maximum adaption and, hopefully, successful return to equilibrium for the individual. If, however, the stress agent continues or the defence mechanism does not work, he will move on to a third stage; (iii)*exhaustion*, when adaptive mechanisms collapse.

Critics of Selye's work say it ignores both the psychological impact of stress on an individual, and the individual's ability to recognize stress and act in various ways to change his or her situation.

Newer and more comprehensive theories of stress emphasize the interaction between a person and his or her environment, describing it as a response to internal or external pressures which reach levels that strain physical and psychological systems beyond their coping capacities.

In the 1970s Richard S. Lazarus suggested that an individual's stress reaction 'depends on how the person interprets or appraises (consciously or unconsciously) the significance of a harmful, threatening, or challenging event.' Lazarus' work disagrees with those who see stress simply as environmental pressure. Instead, the intensity of the stress experience is determined significantly by how well people feel they can cope with an identified threat. Any person who is unsure of his or her coping abilities, or is likely to feel helpless and overwhelmed.

Similarly, Tom Cox and colleagues in the late 1970s rejected the idea of looking at stress as simply either environmental pressures or physiological responses; they suggest that it can best be understood as 'part of a complex and dynamic system of transaction between the person and his environment' and criticize the mechanical model of stress: 'Men and their organizations are not machines … Stress has to be perceived or recognized by man. A machine, however, does not have to recognize the load or stress placed upon it.'

By looking at stress as resulting from a misfit between an individual and his/her particular environment, we can begin to understand why one person seems to flourish in a certain setting, while another suffers. Tom Cummings and Cary Cooper in 1979 explored the stress process in a cybernetic framework as follows:

(i)   Individuals, for the most part, try to keep their thoughts, emotions, and relationships with the world in a 'steady state'.

(ii)   Each factor of a person's emotional and physical state has a 'range of stability', in which that person feels comfortable. On the other hand, when forces disrupt one of these factors beyond the range of stability, the individual must act or cope to restore a feeling of comfort.

(iii)   An individual's behaviour aimed at maintaining a steady state makes up his or her 'adjustment process', or coping strategies.

Accordingly, a stress is any force that puts a psychological or physical factor beyond its range of stability, producing a strain within the individual. Knowledge that a stress is likely to occur constitutes a threat to the individual. A threat can cause a strain because of what it signifies to the person.

Stress certainly involves a range of bodily reactions. Man is the product of many thousands of years of evolution, and to survive required a quick physical response to dangers. The body developed the ability to 'rev-up' for a short time. Cannon described this mobilization of forces as the 'fight or flight' reaction mentioned earlier. Primitive man expended this burst of energy and strength in physical activity, such as a life and death struggle or a quick dash to safety.

Modern man has retained his hormonal and chemical defence mechanisms through the millenia. But for the most part, the lifestyle in the Western world today does not allow physical reaction to the stress agents we face. As Albrecht pointed out, attacking the boss, hitting an insolent customer, or smashing an empty automatic cash dispenser are not solutions allowed by contemporary society. Even the non-aggressive 'flight' reaction would hardly be judged appropriate in most situations. The executive who flees from a tense meeting, and the assembly worker who dashes out in the middle of a shift, will likely suffer the consequences of their actions. Our long-evolved defence mechanisms prepare us for dramatic and rapid action, but find little outlet. The body's strong chemical and hormonal responses are then like frustrated politicians: all dressed up with nowhere to go, as Melhuish describes it.

It is this waste of our natural response to stress which may actually harm us. Although scientists do not fully understand this process, our thought patterns regarding ourselves and the situations we are in can trigger widespread physiological changes, acting through the HYPOTHALAMUS — the part of the brain which co-ordinates a complexity of neural and hormonal mechanisms for taking care of bodily functions. In a situation of challenge, tension, or pressure, the hypothalamus activates both the sympathetic branch of the AUTONOMIC NERVOUS SYSTEM and certain hormone secretions from the PITUITARY GLAND. The resulting release of ADRENALINE and other hormones, together with other actions of sympathetic nerves, enhances the level of arousal and stimulates the cognitive, neural, cardiovascular, and muscular systems, whilst also mobilizing metabolic fuels to provide energy for an increase in muscular activity. These physiological changes are designed to improve the individual's performance: the HEART speeds up and beats more strongly; this and widening of muscle BLOOD VESSELS increase the blood supply of the muscles; BREATHING rate and depth increase. BLOOD PRESSURE rises, and less blood flows to the stomach and the intestines, as well as the SKIN, resulting in the cold hands and feet often associated with a nervous disposition.

All of the body's 'rev-up' activity is designed to improve performance. But if the stress which launches this activity continues unabated, researchers believe, the human body begins to weaken as it is bombarded by stimulation and stress-related chemicals. As stress begins to take its toll on the body and mind, a variety of symptoms can result. We have identified physical and behavioural symptoms of stress occurring before the onset of serious stress-related illnesses; these include: insomnia, eating difficulties, breathlessness without exertion, a tendency to sweat with no good reason, frequent intestinal difficulties, loss of sense of humour, constant irritability with people, difficulty with making decisions, suppressed anger, difficulty in concentrating, the inability to finish one task before rushing on to the next, and so on. Many of these symptoms are the prelude to more serious illnesses, in which stress is one of the risk factors. Recent research has shown that the psycho–social or stress risk factors can be found in hypertension, chronic fatigue syndrome, coronary artery disease, mental disorders, and a range of other illnesses; also suppression of immune responses by the stress-related hormones may provide chemical explanations of links between environmental and emotional pressures and susceptibility to diseases.

CARY L. COOPER

Further reading

Albrecht, K. (1979). *Stress and the manager. Making it work for you.* Prentice-Hall, New Jersey.

Cooper, C. (ed.) (1996). *Handbook of stress, medicine and health.* CRC Press, Boca Raton, Florida.

Hinkle, L. E. (1973). The concept of stress in the biological social sciences. *Stress medicine and man* 1, 31–48.

Lazarus, R. E. (1976). *Patterns of adjustment.* McGraw-Hill, New York.

Melhuish, A. (1978). *Executive health.* Business Books, London.

See also AUTONOMIC NERVOUS SYSTEM.

Stretch marks SCARS on the skin, most commonly developing on the abdominal wall in the later stages of PREGNANCY, and remaining thereafter. They may also appear when the skin is overly stretched by OBESITY. They accompany the weight gain in 'Cushing's syndrome' —overaction of the PITUITARY GLANDS causing an excess of corticosteroid secretion from the ADRENAL GLANDS, or in the equivalent condition caused by an excess of medicinal STEROID hormone.

S.J.

Stroke Apoplexy or stroke has been recognized at least since the beginning of Western medicine, in ancient Greece. Stroke arises from injury to the brain caused by interruption of the blood supply, rather like a heart attack: in fact stroke is now sometimes called a 'brain attack'. Over 250 000 people suffer some type of stroke in the UK each year. Stroke now is the third leading cause of death and the most common cause of adult DISABILITY.

The most typical manifestations include sudden weakness of the face, arm, or leg, and altered sensation or numbness on the side of the body opposite the stroke. LANGUAGE expression and comprehension can be impaired, usually for strokes in the left cerebral hemisphere. A stroke in the occipital lobe, at the back of the hemisphere, can cause BLINDNESS in the opposite half of the visual field. Sometimes a stroke in the parietal lobe of the right hemisphere renders the patient unable to attend to the left hand side of objects or even without awareness of the left side of their own body (the so-called *neglect syndrome*). Most bizarre of all, damage to the right hemisphere can produce *anosagnosia* — denial by the patient of any deficit at all, despite virtual PARALYSIS of the left arm and leg.

The brain — especially the CEREBRAL CORTEX, a frequent target of strokes — is divided into distinct regions, functionally specialized for one sense or another, for the control of movement, for aspects of language, etc. The sensory, motor, linguistic, and cognitive deficits caused by small strokes can therefore be extraordinarily specific, and their interpretation by neuropsychologists has been a major source of evidence about the organization of the human brain. But major strokes can have devastating effects, sometimes eliminating CONSCIOUSNESS completely, or, perhaps even worse, leaving a conscious mind in a useless body. The French writer Jean-Dominique Bauby gives a unique view of this state in his autobiography — paralysed except for the capacity to blink an eye, he described himself as a 'butterfly' trapped inside a 'diving bell'.

In 1761, Battista Morgagni, Professor of Anatomy in Padua, first clearly attributed strokes to limitation of blood flow to the brain. In 85% of cases this comes from blockage of a blood vessel giving a so-called *ischaemic stroke*. Most of the remaining 15% are due to sudden bleeding into the substance of the brain to create a *haemorrhagic stroke*. A small percentage are due to rupture of an artery in the surface of the brain — a *subarachnoid haemorrhage*.

The brain is metabolically highly active. Although it accounts for only about 2% of the body weight, it uses 20% of the total OXYGEN intake and has a high demand for the BLOOD SUGAR, glucose. At least 15% of the blood output from the heart is needed to supply this amount of oxygen and glucose. If this blood flow is interrupted, even for minutes, then brain cells die. The pattern of clinical deficits after strokes (other than subarachnoid haemorrhage) is determined by the particular blood vessel that is primarily affected. Interruption of flow in the left middle cerebral artery, for example, typically leads to specific impairments of language or calculation, while occlusion of the right middle cerebral artery may disturb visual–spatial skills. Subarachnoid haemorrhages lead to changes in pressure on the brain and chemical effects that cause more general deficits.

The most common cause of ischaemic strokes is blocking of a vessel by a so-called *embolus,* which forms on a pathologically abnormal wall of a larger vessel and then detaches and circulates in the blood. The wall of the larger vessel, particularly in areas of high-flow turbulence and around major bifurcations (e.g. the point at which the internal carotid artery branches off from the aorta), may become thickened and irregular, and calcified atherosclerotic plaques may form.

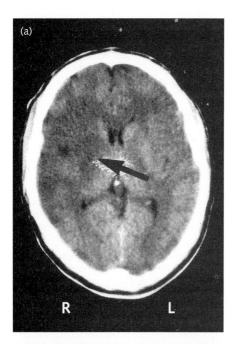

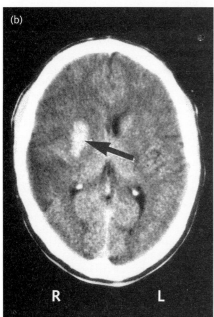

(a) CT brain scan within 24 hours of an ischaemic stroke due to blockage in large middle cerebral artery (arrow). (b) The next day the CT scan shows a transformed area (arrow). Without knowledge of (a) it would be very difficult to distinguish this area of change from intra-cerebral haemorrhage. (Donaghy, T. (2001). *Brain's diseases of the nervous system*, 11th edn, Oxford University Press, Oxford.)

Rupture of these plaques can form a blood clot, fragments of which can be carried along the course of flowing blood to block smaller vessels. Alternatively, platelets that aggregate on the abnormal surface of a plaque, or fragments of the plaque, can themselves act as emboli. Emboli also can be formed in the heart, or, more rarely, can come from elsewhere in the body.

The risk of stroke is determined by both genetic and environmental influences. A number of specific risk factors include: a family history of stroke in first-degree relatives; older age; male sex; hypertension; SMOKING; DIABETES; and heart disease.

Control of risk factors (e.g. giving up smoking, control of hypertension or diabetes, treatment of heart disease) can reduce the risk of stroke in affected individuals. The importance of hypertension has been recognized in a practical way since the time of GALEN (*c.* AD 130–210), who advocated treatment of APOPLEXY with vigorous BLOOD-LETTING.

Perhaps half or more of strokes are preceded by neurological symptoms (such as difficulty with SPEECH or with movement of one hand) that last less than 12 hours and reverse completely. However, the risk of a full-blown stroke following these transient ischaemic attacks (TIAs) is similar to the risk that a stroke leaving persistent deficits will be followed by another (approximately 12% overall risk over 12 months). The precise risks vary substantially, however, depending on the underlying cause and the particular blood vessel involved.

Acute treatment of smaller ischaemic strokes is generally based on use of drugs that limit platelet aggregation, such as ASPIRIN. Patients with occlusion of relatively large vessels, who reach medical care within the first few hours after the onset of deficits, may benefit from infusion of *thrombolytic agents* (clot-busters) such as tissue plasminogen activator (tPA) that can dissolve emboli and restore blood flow in the ischaemic area. This may benefit particularly the tissue at the outside of the core of the damage, in the so-called *ischaemic penumbra*, where the function of brain tissue is not irreversibly impaired.

Patients who survive their strokes without massive neurological deficits always show significant functional improvement. This occurs most rapidly over the first month after the stroke, but can continue for two years or more. The degree of recovery depends not only on the size of a stroke but also on its location. For example, small ischaemic strokes in the BASAL GANGLIA — nuclei deep in the cerebral hemispheres, involved in the control of movement — have a much better prognosis than strokes in the posterior limb of the internal capsule (see BRAIN), which contains major nerve fibres running between the cerebral cortex and the rest of the brain.

Recovery is often complicated by less well-understood consequences of stroke, which illustrate the complex interconnectedness of brain functions. Alfred Brodal, the famous

Danish neuroanatomist, observed in 1973 after his own small, 'pure motor' stroke that, in addition to difficulties moving one half of his body, he suffered from a 'loss of powers of concentration, reduced short-term memory, increased fatigue, reduced initiative, [and] incontinence of movements of emotional expression'. Depression can also be a major problem. In part this is a consequence of the patient's perception of the new disability. Sir Peter Medawar, Nobel Laureate in Medicine, describes this well in personal reflections on his own stroke entitled *Memoirs of a Thinking Radish* (1986). Strokes can have direct effects on the balance of NEUROTRANSMITTERS in the brain that are responsible for mood.

Current experimental strategies for treatment in stroke are focusing simultaneously on several areas: safer and more effective ways of delivering thrombolytic therapy to patients, with particular attention to the possibility of rapid, on-the-spot treatment; neuroprotective agents, designed to guard the surrounding area of brain from the effects of neurotransmitters released by dying neurons following the initial damage of the stroke; and other experimental drugs, directed at limiting damage from the breakdown of nerve cell membranes and highly reactive oxygen radicals that are generated in the damaged tissue.

An intriguing possibility is that cells derived from bone marrow (*stem cells*) could be implanted surgically into areas of brain damaged by stroke, where they may be able to differentiate into new neurons that could take over functions of those that have been damaged.

PAUL M. MATTHEWS

Further reading

Bauby, J.-D. (1998). *The diving-bell and the butterfly*. Fourth Estate, London.

Kapur, N. (1997). *Injured brains of medical minds*. Oxford University Press.

Porter, R. (1999). *The greatest benefit to mankind*. Fontain Press, London.

See also APOPLEXY; BRAIN; LANGUAGE AND THE BRAIN; PARALYSIS.

Stunts Stunts are actual or simulated dangerous physical activities, undertaken during movie production or sometimes performed live, for public entertainment.

The once private world of stunt work is increasingly in the news, with the growing media interest in the technology of film-making. In the early, golden years of the movies, stars cultivated the myth that they were, in real life, the kinds of characters that they portrayed on the screen, and they were usually unwilling to disclose that others stood in for them in risky or highly skilled sequences. Nowadays, most film actors openly admit that they have stunt doubles and these professionals are acknowledged in their own right.

Stunts were first recognized by silent-movie production companies in the early 1900s, in newly-discovered Hollywood. With genuine cowboy farming dying out, but cowboy movies becoming popular, it was no surprise that production companies recruited former or out-of-work cowboys to recreate their rough-and-tumble skills on film, largely for the entertainment of city dwellers. It was a natural progression for these strong, skilful, and fearless characters to be employed to perform risky sequences in a whole range of other early movies, notably the amusing but dangerous scenes in comedies, such as the Keystone Cops. Yakima Canutt was one of the founders of this profession. He progressed from being a real cowboy, and world champion rodeo rider, to working as a stuntman in silent movies. He became recognized as a 'stunt co-ordinator' and worked on stunts until the late 1960s, serving as '2nd unit' director on some of the greatest movies ever made, including *Stagecoach*, *Gone with the Wind*, and *Ben Hur*. A stunt co-ordinator is a person who works out the mechanics and rigging needed to execute stunts, and a so-called '2nd unit' films most of the stunt sequences.

Some stuntmen became recognized actors in silent movies, and this trend has been repeated in recent years. Ben Johnson, for example, graduated from being a stuntman in many John Wayne movies to being a very accomplished actor.

A movie stunt, as it is known these days, is usually a section during an action sequence when an actor/character appears to carry out a spectacular leap, jump, fall, punch, or something similar. It is for this kind of sequence that a stuntman (or stuntwoman), called a 'stunt double', usually stands in for the actor. Even when an actor is physically capable of performing a stunt, studios usually prefer to use a stunt person (especially if the scene can easily be filmed so that the person cannot be identified), because of the insurance risk and the huge cost that would result if the production were to be delayed, or cancelled because of an injury to a star. In the movie *Indiana Jones and the Last Crusade*, the character 'Indy' (played by Harrison Ford) had to jump off a rock, falling about five metres, onto

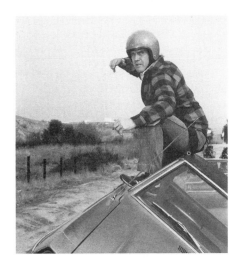

Lee Majors in *The Fall Guy*. The Kobal Collection.

the back of a passing horse, knocking off the rider and throwing the (trained) horse to the ground, and then stay mounted as the horse stood up and galloped away. Harrison Ford, paramount professional that he is, desperately wanted to perform this stunt himself, and he was certainly capable of doing so. But the risk of breaking a leg or getting a black eye or a tooth knocked out were simply too high. I (Vic Armstrong) as stunt co-ordinator had also been engaged to perform the stunt, but managed to persuade Harrison Ford to let me do it only by appealing to his good nature. I told him that he would deprive me of a small fortune in lost 'stunt adjustment' (the fee for a particular stunt, paid over and above the stuntman's salary) if he did the stunt himself, and he actually apologized and let me do it!

Other types of stunts are undertaken as public spectacles. These include motor cycle jumps performed as part of a stadium-type show or other public event. The famous American stuntman Evel Knievel brought this type of stunt to Europe. He was subsequently upstaged by the English super stuntman Eddie Kidd, who, sadly, paid the price of his profession and was seriously injured during one of his spectacular jumps. There are many other categories of public stunt, including jousting (based on the medieval sport of fighting from horseback), high-diving into small tanks of water, and crashing cars purely for the spectacle and the amusement of an audience. In the early 1930s and 1940s 'barnstorming' was very popular: intrepid aviators deliberately crashed their aircraft to amuse spectators! Such public spectacles have a long history, predating the movies. They can be traced back at least a thousand years, to the amusing or gymnastic feats performed by jesters and tumblers to entertain the court or other audiences.

Movie stunts, which started as an invisible yet integral part of film-making, have become so popular that they have spawned their own movies, notably *Hooper*, written and directed by the famous modern-day stuntman Hal Needham, and the television show *Fall Guy*, for which I wrote the first treatment.

Modern technology and new materials have contributed enormously to the stunt business. In the early days, stuntmen would perform high falls onto hay, but this was replaced by the miracle of empty cardboard boxes, which, when stacked correctly, would collapse and break the fall. As they say: 'it isn't the fall that hurts but the stopping'! Cardboard boxes have since been superseded by the airbag, with multiple chambers to stop it collapsing if it develops a tear. The multi-chamber airbag has enabled stuntmen to fall more safely from much greater heights.

A device called a 'fan descender', which I invented in the early 1980s for a movie called *Green Ice*, enables a stunt person to fall from great heights at a controlled speed. It has been used all over the world, on such movies as the *Indiana Jones* trilogy, through to *Titanic*, and

recently earned an award from the Academy of Motion Pictures Arts and Sciences.

Stunts involving vehicles have been popular since at least the days of the Keystone Cops. A few years ago, a cannon, detonated by black explosive powder, was developed to flip cars over for such stunts, and this has recently been replaced by the less dangerous air cannon. Both systems were devised by Hal Needham. Rolling-over of vehicles used to be achieved by running the wheels onto a ramp. But nowadays, compression of the suspension caused by wheel ramps is avoided by the use of the more accurate and safer 'pipe ramp' — a long metal pipe set at an angle of approximately 45 degrees to the ground, on to which the vehicle is driven, lengthways, so that it slides along the under carriage, lifting the vehicle and rolling it over. With the advent of better metal materials for the roll cages that strengthen cars, and better welding techniques to fix them in place, car-crash stunts have become safer. Fire retardants and fireproof clothing, along with miniature breathing apparatus, have greatly improved the chances of survival during fire stunts.

With all these advances in technology the stunt person has had to modernize as well. In Great Britain there is now a system of qualification. Aspiring stuntmen and women have to attain advanced proficiency in several disciplines, such as horse riding, sword-fencing, MARTIAL ARTS, DIVING, GYMNASTICS, SWIMMING, etc. Applicants must also be members of the actors' union Equity, in recognition of the professional performing skills of the modern stunt person. Even after joining the Stunt Register (the governing body for stunt work in the UK), stunt persons still have to go through a long apprenticeship, during which they must be supervised by a qualified stunt co-ordinator.

The British stunt business really got off the ground in the late 1940s and 1950s, led by such icons as Joe Powell, Jock Easton, George Leech, Paddy Ryan, and Ken Buckle. They were the real groundbreakers, pooling their own money to drive to such places as Almeria in Spain, to try to find work on American epics that were being made in Europe because of lower wage costs. Nowadays, stuntmen travel first-class and command top wages. Britain also produces world-class stuntwomen, including Wendy Leech, who doubled the heroines in the *Indiana Jones* trilogy, *Superman*, and several James Bond movies. British stunt people are now considered the most proficient in the world.   VIC ARMSTRONG

Stuttering Stuttering (or *stammering*, as it is often called in Britain) is probably the best known and most researched SPEECH disorder, but perhaps the most difficult to define, to explain, and to treat, especially in adults. Both names are onomatopoeic: the essential features of stuttering are frequent repetitions and prolongations of sound or syllables. Other problems of fluency may also characterize stuttering, including blocking of sounds or interjection of words or sounds. However, the sudden sensation of a loss of control over the ability to produce an utterance distinguishes stuttering from other forms of unfluent speech. Another characteristic of stutterers, especially adults, is their avoidance of anticipated problem words and situations, in order to cope with the problem.

Chronic stuttering usually begins in early childhood (*development stuttering*), although occasionally the disorder starts in adulthood (*acquired stuttering*), usually as a result of brain damage. Stuttering seems to occur in all nationalities with a prevalence of approximately 1% and an incidence of 4% to 5%. Approximately 40% to 80% of children with the disorder recover, for various reasons, by the time they reach adolescence or adulthood. More males than females stutter: the ratio of males to female stutterers ranges from 2–3:1 in childhood, up to 4–5:1 by adulthood. The incidence of the disorder is much higher among other members of the family of a stutterer than in the general population: in other words, there is probably a genetic factor in this condition.

Stuttering may vary greatly in its frequency and severity in different situations. It is, for instance, dramatically reduced when speaking alone or reading aloud in chorus with an accompanist. Wearing headphones that alter the feedback of one's own voice can also reduce stuttering, and so too can the use of certain regular speech patterns (e.g. singing, unusual accents, speaking in rhythm). The reliability with which such techniques for inducing fluency can reduce or even abolish stuttering is considered a key to understanding the disorder — they also form the basis of some treatments.

The social and vocational effects of chronic stuttering may be quite devastating, perhaps because of the suspicion that it is the outward sign of a PERSONALITY disorder. However, there is remarkably little evidence that stuttering is related to any unusual personality characteristics or neuroses; and there is little support for the claim that stuttering is associated with anxiety. Many prominent individuals, including well-known actors and politicians, have managed to control their stuttering and achieve successful careers. Nevertheless, the handicapping effects of the disorder in children and adults are undeniable.

There is currently no accepted theory that offers a satisfactory explanation for all the features of stuttering. At different times, psychoanalytic or organic theories have held sway over research and/or therapy. Traditional, formal learning has been blamed; so too have errors in control systems in the brain. Most current researchers consider developmental stuttering to be a disorder of motor control, with strong genetic underpinnings, influenced by environmental factors. This position has gained support with evidence that signs of severe stuttering may appear almost as soon as a child starts to produce connected speech.

Recent studies of right-handed adult stutterers, using techniques for imaging activity in the brain, have revealed unusual patterns of activation and inhibition during stuttered speech, particularly in parts of the right hemisphere involved in hearing and the control of movement, and especially exaggerated in the CEREBELLUM. The unusual activity in these regions, which appears to occur only during speech, is very different when stuttering is reduced or absent as a result of strategies for improving fluency. These findings have intensified the search for a neurological system or systems that might be specifically related to stuttering.

The treatment of stuttering is an area of controversy. There is no evidence that any drug treatment is effective in removing stuttering in children or adults. The most convincing effects have been reported for behavioural treatments, although there is much debate about the evaluation of such therapy. Other forms of treatment emphasize learning to adjust to the disorder rather than removing the problematic behaviour.

Probably the most dramatic change to therapy for stuttering in the last decade is the use of mild verbal corrections for each occasion of stuttering, and verbal praise for periods of fluency, which has beneficial effects in treating young children. Recovery commonly occurs without treatment in the first year after onset, but this becomes less likely without intervention if the disorder persists. Indeed, there is an urgent need to correct the widely-held belief that children will recover from stuttering if their problem is merely ignored. Currently, the preferred therapies for older stutterers involve a combination of behavioural techniques and methods for training speech–motor strategies. However, there is no convincing evidence that these therapies result in complete recovery.

The most successful therapeutic approaches for adults and children involve three general features: first, a method that *establishes* reduced stuttering or stutter-free speech under relatively controlled conditions; then a procedure for *transferring* that improvement beyond the treatment setting; and finally, strategies for *maintaining* that improvement. The most favoured techniques for establishing control over stuttering fall into three categories: behavioural methods based on rewarding performance; teaching stutterers to prolong their speech; and mechanical aids. These techniques are also often used in conjunction with control of the rate of speaking. Once improvement has been produced in the controlled conditions, 'transfer' procedures are used, which systematically introduce increasingly demanding speaking situations. The most successful maintenance procedures require intermittent management over periods lasting up to two or three years. Given the variability of stuttering across situations, over time, and with relatively slight alterations to the manner of speech production, stuttering therapy evaluation presents considerable challenges, which are now occupying the attention of clinical researchers.

ROGER J. INGHAM

Further reading

Bloodstein, O. (1995). *A handbook on stuttering*. Singular, San Diego, CA.

Fox, P. T., Ingham, R. J., Ingham, J. C., *et al.* (1996). A PET study of the neural systems of stuttering. *Nature*, 382, 158–62.

Suffocation is a general term denoting a death brought about by a reduction of the OXYGEN content in inspired air. It is one cause of HYPOXIA. Smothering is often classified as a type of suffocation, in which air, and therefore oxygen, are prevented from reaching the lungs by obstructing the nose and the mouth.

The oxygen in the atmosphere can be displaced by other gases, for example in industrial and domestic fires. In such circumstances toxic gases such as CARBON MONOXIDE or cyanide produced by burning plastics may be liberated and accelerate the process of suffocation. Another example is the replacement of oxygen in the atmosphere by CARBON DIOXIDE, which may build up in grain silos when some technical fault develops. There may also be a greatly reduced oxygen content in the air at the bottom of deep wells.

Suffocation may also be the cause of death when oxygen is being used up and there is no fresh air supply. In ships' tanks nitrogen can replace oxygen as a result of the damp inner linings using up oxygen as rust is formed: entry into such an atmosphere can result in almost instantaneous death — usually this means someone has ignored health and safety regulations. Another cause is when a defective heating apparatus in an inadequately ventilated room has removed oxygen from the atmosphere — in such circumstances suffocation may be compounded by the apparatus producing carbon monoxide, which displaces oxygen from the blood. Or the oxygen may be used up by the victim, when someone — often a child — has inadvertently been confined in an enclosed space such as a cupboard or a discarded refrigerator or deep freeze. Another example is plastic bag suffocation which may be accidental, suicidal, or homicidal and results from the bag being placed over the head down to neck level. Death can again be very rapid. This is of relatively recent occurrence — and has led to the familiar warnings on all plastic packaging.

Smothering is the usual term for external obstruction to breathing — perhaps by a hand, a pillow, a gag, or a sheet of plastic — which prevents air, and therefore *oxygen*, reaching *the lungs*. Smothering by 'overlaying' of an infant in the parental bed was in the past assumed to be the cause of what would now be called COT DEATH.   J. HUME ADAMS

See also BREATHING; CARBON MONOXIDE; COT DEATH; HYPOXIA.

Sugars CARBOHYDRATES, along with FATS and PROTEINS, water, some MINERALS, and VITAMINS, constitute the diet. Thus what the body is made of, plus what is needed to keep it functioning, must be derived from these elements. The building blocks of carbohydrates are the sugars. The general formula for sugars is $(CH_2O)_n$ — that is, carbon combined with water multiplied n times — indicating the derivation of the word 'carbohydrate'. The value of 'n' can be from 3 to 7, in trioses, tetroses, pentoses, hexoses, and heptoses respectively. These are all *monosaccharides*.

The common sugars that form part of the diet are sucrose, lactose (milk sugar), and maltose. They are all *disaccharides* and are split into monosaccharides during digestion; sucrose to glucose and fructose, lactose to galactose and glucose, and maltose into two glucose molecules. All three monosaccharides — glucose, galactose and fructose — can be metabolized by the body and used as a source of energy, although glucose is by far the most important, and is normally maintained within a narrow range of concentration in the blood. Fructose is also a dietary component in fruit. Some people congenitally lack lactase, the ENZYME which splits the lactose molecule in the intestine, and consequently suffer abdominal discomfort and DIARRHOEA after ingesting lactose. Lactose is present in milk and while few Europeans suffer lactase deficiency, some 97% of Thais, for example, are without this enzyme; in most instances this is likely to be the consequence rather than the cause of the rarity of milk-drinking and cheese-eating in this and Eastern communities, since their infants have no problem. Starch (a *polyglucose*) is broken down during digestion into maltose and then into glucose.

Sugars have multiple functions within the body and are used as a primary source of energy, through the synthesis of ATP, and for energy storage. When the body stores glucose it does so as GLYCOGEN (body starch). Glycogen stores in muscle provide readily available glucose for EXERCISE; glycogen stores in the liver are crucially involved in the maintenance of BLOOD SUGAR — the concentration of glucose in the blood. This in turn is vital as a nutrient supply to the brain, which normally utilizes only glucose for energy production.

Five-carbon sugars (*pentoses*) also have a crucial significance in the body. For example, ribose and deoxyribose are essential for the formation of the backbone of RNA and DNA. As well as forming part of the molecules determining inheritance and phenotype, sugars are linked to PROTEINS and LIPIDS, to form glycoproteins and glycolipids. Glycoproteins include antibodies and clotting factors. Other proteins and lipids expressed in the membranes of cells and linked to sugars are responsible for cell-to-cell recognition and adhesion, and are involved in the processing of messages brought by HORMONES and NEUROTRANSMITTERS and, in cells in the spleen and elsewhere, in recognizing old circulating red cells and removing them.

ALAN W. CUTHBERT

See also BLOOD SUGAR; CARBOHYDRATES; INSULIN; METABOLISM.

Suicide Current attitudes toward suicide derive from the debates of centuries long past. Aristotle condemned suicide on political grounds, arguing that the allegiance individuals owe to the state precludes them from taking their lives. Plato had likened the state to a parent in the *Crito*, a position which might seem to support a similar restriction of the individual's right to commit suicide. But Plato actually objected to self-destruction on religious grounds, claiming that human beings are the gods' possessions and risk punishment for daring to decide when to die. Nevertheless, a precedent for the right-to-die position may be found in the *Phaedo*, where Socrates argues against prolonging life at any cost.

The death of Socrates seemed to embody both reason and self control, qualities prized by the early Stoics, and EUTHANASIA was practised among elderly members of the school. In theory, suicide was an option available to the Stoic at any time. In practice, however, only the first century statesman and philosopher Seneca glorified death to the point of advocating self-destruction as an end in itself. His own death at the command of the emperor Nero was entirely consistent with the principles he espoused. Witnesses described how he managed to stretch the event over the course of a full day, drinking wine and conversing with his friends while periodically opening his veins until he eventually bled to death. Seneca's willingness to end his career in cold blood earned the admiration of his contemporaries — and his was but one of the many heroic suicides that have come down to us from Roman antiquity. The legends of Lucretia, Cato, Brutus, Portia, Antony, and Cleopatra became models for the suicide of honour. To die for some higher ideal, for the sake of virtue, patriotism, or faith, as would become the case with the early Christians, was to make death a cause for celebration.

The Christian case against suicide was formally stated by St Augustine, who prohibited the act as a violation of the sixth commandment, 'Thou shalt not kill'. But Augustine was actually ambivalent on the question of suicide, permitting it in instances where individuals behaved with divine sanction in ending their lives. This exception was necessary to allow for the voluntary sacrifice of Jesus, who freely chose to die on the cross for humanity's sins. In subsequent centuries the escape clause was widened to admit the martyrs of the early Church, whose sacrifices were essential to the mythology of medieval Christianity.

The Church policy regarding suicide that emerged during the Middle Ages was loosely based on Roman law. Picking up on ancient Greek traditions, the Romans had punished self- destruction, but only under certain conditions: when an individual killed himself to escape legal prosecution or in the case of a soldier or a slave. The act of suicide was not itself considered blameworthy. Rather, the suicide's civil status, combined with his presumed motivations — the cowardliness of the accused man

who sought to pre-empt the law, the disobedience of the soldier or the audacity of the slave who disposed of a life that was not truly his — determined whether the act should be punished. (The legal status of Roman women was akin to that of the slave. An unmarried female was treated as her father's dependent; the *pater familias* held absolute power over his daughter's life. With marriage, this power was transferred to her husband.)

The Christian position was different. What made suicide a sin was its voluntary nature. Self-destruction was prohibited because it represented an individual's choice to do wrong, a deliberate challenge to divine authority. Following the publication of the *Summa Theologiae* of Thomas Aquinas, suicide came to be seen as a crime against society as well. Aquinas revived Aristotle's view of suicide as an act of political insubordination and also condemned self-destruction on the grounds that it went against the natural instinct for self-preservation. To the traditional religious objection, which served to deny the sinner a Christian burial, Aquinas thus added a provision which could be used to support the implementation of civil penalties against people who killed themselves. During the high Middle Ages, civil legislation against self-murder was enacted in the majority of Western European states. Under no circumstances were men or women permitted to sacrifice themselves without divine sanction or to place their needs above the needs of the community to which they belonged.

The Enlightenment brought into question the moral implications of self-destruction. For the eighteenth-century *philosophes*, the issue proved to be an effective weapon in their crusade against absolutism and the Christian religion. Voltaire and others revitalized the classical tradition in the name of rationalism and freedom, portraying Lucretius, Cicero, and Seneca — all advocates of the right to die — as early upholders of the secular cause. The Romantics turned self-destruction into a literary convention, further weakening the stigma attached to the act. Driven to despair by the death of their beloved or, worse still, loving and being loved by someone who belonged to another, countless characters in nineteenth-century fiction actively courted the solace which death alone could provide.

Suicide was decriminalized during the French Revolution, and neither Napoleon nor his monarchist successors reinstated the laws against it. And with the emergence of the psychiatric profession in the nineteenth century, the tendency to interpret the act as the inadvertent consequence of psychological problems, which could be diagnosed, treated, and cured, displaced the religious impulse to judge it in moral terms. Thus, while the Catholic Church continues to regard suicide as a sin, the modern inclination to attribute it to depression makes the deprivation of a religious funeral rare.

The greatest controversy today is over the question of assisted suicide. It is a felony to help someone commit suicide in Great Britain and in twenty-eight American states, but in neither country is it illegal to kill oneself. In effect, this means that only healthy people are allowed by the law to take their lives, since people who are seriously ill are often unable to kill themselves without assistance. Supporters of euthanasia aim to do nothing more than to decriminalize assisted suicide for the terminally ill, as has been done in the Netherlands. Opponents of the right to die range from Christian activists who invoke religious arguments against the taking of human life to physicians who think the need for assisted suicide would vanish with more effective strategies for pain management in the last months of life. On a policy level, some argue in favour of allocating limited health care resources toward people whose lives can be saved instead of prolonging the existence of someone already near death, particularly when that person no longer wishes to live. This line of argument has been criticized by those who envision the day when sick people will be hurried to their deaths for reasons of economic expediency.

Current thinking on suicide also owes much to the development of the social sciences, and to the work of Durkheim in particular. What distinguishes the sociological approach from the psychological is that it diminishes the importance of individual intentions in assessing the causes of suicide. Even the most private of human activities, the decision to end one's own life, turns out to be socially determined. Like other forms of collective behaviour, its incidence is governed by regular laws. To isolate the social factors conducive to high rates of self-destruction is the object of suicide prevention programmes today.

LISA LIEBERMAN

Further reading

Kushner, H. I. (1989) *Self-destruction in the Promised Land*. Rutgers University Press, New Brunswick and London.

Lieberman, L. (2003) *Leaving You: the cultural meaning of suicide*. Ivan R. Dee, Chicago.

See also EUTHANASIA.

Sun and the body
The sun has exercised a powerful influence on the physical and mental lives of human beings. The sun emits *visible light, heat, ultraviolet rays, radio waves,* and *X-rays.* Ultraviolet light affects the human body in a number of ways. One of the greatest health benefits of ultraviolet light is the production of vitamin D, which is essential to CALCIUM metabolism and the formation of BONE. High energy ultraviolet light enters the skin and causes the photochemical conversion of *7-dehydrocholesterol* to previtamin D_3, which at body temperature undergoes isomerization to vitamin D_3. When the skin is exposed to excessive sunlight, previtamin D_3 is changed into two biologically inert substances, *lumisterol* and *tachysterol,* which prevent the synthesis of excessive amounts of D_3. The production of vitamin D is affected by time of day, season, and latitude. A century ago, the lack of sunlight in industrial cities, and

hence, of vitamin D, caused widespread *rickets,* characterized by bowleggedness. There is evidence that breast-fed babies require exposure to ultraviolet light — perhaps only 30 minutes a week — in order to acquire adequate vitamin D. Studies also reveal that mobility-impaired geriatric patients have only about one-quarter of the serum vitamin D of healthy middle-aged persons. Dietary changes and increased sunlight may help solve this problem. Vitamin D can also be taken in various vitamin supplements.

Ultraviolet light has several therapeutic effects. In combination with drug therapies, it is useful in treating skin diseases, such as psoriasis, herpes, and eczema. 'Phototherapy' — exposure not to ultraviolet but to light from the blue end of the spectrum — is used for JAUNDICE in newborn babies, caused by the immature liver's inability to rid the body of bilirubin, which, if it accumulates excessively, can cause brain damage.

Another positive effect of the sun is psychological. In the early 1980s a report appeared of a woman whose depression increased when she went north in the winter and disappeared when she visited Jamaica. Her condition later acquired the name *Seasonal Affective Disorder* (SAD). An accepted treatment for this condition is exposure to a full-spectrum light of at least 2500 lux — 5–10 times as strong as standard indoor lighting. By comparison, sunlight gives 10 000 lux on a cloudy day, and 80 000 lux (at the Equator) on a sunny day.

The human body apparently evolved a daily rhythm in response to the length of daylight. Sunlight suppresses the secretion of *prolactin,* which aids in rest; *melatonin,* which affects mood and subjective energy levels; and GROWTH HORMONE, which is needed for bodily construction and repair. When male subjects were put on a 10-hour photoperiod, they typically experienced a 2-hour period of non-anxious wakefulness in the middle of their sleeping period, and prolactin was found to be elevated for 14 hours. Those on a 16-hour, modern period, experienced less melatonin secretion than other test subjects, while growth hormone levels doubled. Women seem to be more sensitive to seasonal changes in length of day, perhaps explaining why they are more susceptible to SAD. *Photoperiodism* also seems to be involved in the production of the neurotransmitter, SEROTONIN, which controls the appetite for carbohydrates. People affected by SAD crave carbohydrates during the winter.

Sunlight can also harm the human body. Excessive exposure of the unprotected skin results in *erythema* (sunburn). With one *Minimum Erythemal Dose* (MED) the skin turns pink and starts to produce melanin. With 5–10 MED an excruciating sunburn results after 4–14 hours. Certain medications, including *tetracyclines* and *estrogens,* increase the skin's susceptibility to sunburn. The body has ways to protect itself from skin damage from sunlight. Repeated exposure to the sun creates a tan, as melanin accumulates close to the surface of the skin. A deep tan can filter out 95% of the sun's rays. However, after

only 2–3 minutes of exposure to the sun, skin damage begins. Two main structural proteins of the skin, *collagen* and *elastin,* begin to break down, ultimately resulting in WRINKLES. The skin has the ability to repair itself, but repeated and prolonged exposure to the sun damages the skin permanently. Prolonged exposure to the hot sun or any other heat source may cause *heat exhaustion* or the more serious *heatstroke* or *sunstroke.*

By far the most serious ill effect of the sun is *skin cancer.* Skin exposed chronically to the ultraviolet light of the sun shows a tenfold increase in mutations of a gene called P53. Sunlight further causes the cells containing the mutated cells to spread, where they copy themselves. This mutated gene has been linked with *basal cell* and *squamous cell skin cancers.* The most serious form of skin cancer, *melanoma,* has also been linked with exposure to the sun. Even one or two blistering sunburns in childhood have been associated with an increase in the incidence of melanoma.

The sun has profoundly influenced human intellect and custom. To the pre-technical mind, it ordered the world and set the rhythm of daily life. For many early peoples, solar observations formed the bases of their agricultural, religious, and ceremonial lives. The power of the Egyptian Pharaoh is underlined by the belief that he was the son of the sun god *Ra.* Images and designs found world-wide depict the sun. The sun governed conceptions of *time*; ancient *observatories* measured the time in terms of seasons, while, at least in antiquity, only *the sundial* existed to measure the time during a single day. The ancient GREEKS considered the sun to be unchangeable and divine, and *Plato* likened the highest form of human understanding, the understanding of unchanging truths, to the sun. In many cultures, particularly more northern ones, the end of winter is marked by celebrations. Even the *Copernican revolution* played a role in the conception of the central power of the sun, as the gravity of the sun became the literal controller of the solar system, displacing the changeable and corruptible earth from the centre position. It is little wonder, then, that the absolute monarch *Louis XIV* assumed the title of *Sun King.*

KRISTEN L. ZACHARIAS

Further reading

Smithsonian Institution (1981). *Fire of life. The Smithsonian book of the sun.* W. W. Norton and Company, New York and London.

See also AGEING; BIOLOGICAL RHYTHMS; SKIN.

Surfactant
is a chemical that sounds like a detergent — which it is. If you could get enough you could try it in a dishwasher, although it would froth too much: the word is from 'surf' or sea-froth.

The most important site of surfactant is the lining of the alveoli of the LUNGS. Here it reduces the force needed to inflate the lungs and allows comfortable, quiet BREATHING. If you compare blowing up a bubble of a soap film with a party balloon, much more force is needed for the latter. This is because the molecules of the balloon stick together far more tightly than do those of soap solution; they are said to have a higher surface tension. In the 1920s it was shown that something in the alveoli must be reducing the surface tension of of the lining liquid, and this was subsequently shown to be surfactant. It is a mixture of fatty substances linked to proteins, the main ingredient being dipalmitoyl lecithin. It is made in one of the types of cell in the alveolar walls (type II cells), where it can be seen under the electron microscope as onion-like granules. Released into the airspace it spreads out and lines the alveolar surface.

In fetal life, surfactant first appears at about 20 weeks' gestation, and is being fully secreted by 30 weeks, 10 weeks before birth normally takes place. If it is absent the lungs are not only immature, but they can only be inflated with pressures 5–10 times greater than normal. Even if the baby can achieve this, it will rapidly lead to exhaustion. The condition is called Respiratory Distress Syndrome of the Infant (RDSI). Between 20 and 30 weeks' gestation more and more surfactant appears and the premature baby is progressively better able to overcome the defect in its lungs if born during this period. Surfactant production can be encouraged by giving the mother steroids (e.g. cortisol) before delivery, but nowadays these are combined with attempts to put surfactant directly into the infant's lungs. This was first attempted in 1964, but it was twenty to thirty years before the treatment became widespread and successful for premature babies. Either surfactant extracted from animal lungs or a synthetic version is used, and it can be administered directly into the airways or as an aerosol.

Adults can suffer a rather similar condition to RDSI, called ARDS (A=adult). With major traumatic injuries, or in some cases of severe septic shock or tissue destruction, the lining of the alveoli is damaged and the surfactant is ineffective. This leads to serious respiratory difficulties, which can be treated by surfactant replacement.

Surfactants are found in many other sites in the body, as well as in the lungs. For example, in the stomach surfactants may act as a barrier on the surface of the mucosa, which may explain in part why our stomachs are not digested by their own gastric juice. In the airways surfactants probably act as lubricants, allowing mucus and other materials to be cleared easily from the lungs by coughing or by ciliary transport.

JOHN WIDDICOMBE

See also ANTENATAL DEVELOPMENT; BREATHING; INFANCY; LUNGS.

Surgery
The word 'surgery' comes from the Greek *cheirourgen*, made up of *cheir* — hand and *ergo* — to work. Literally the term means 'to work with the hand'. Surgery can therefore be defined as those manual procedures used in the management of injuries and disease.

Throughout his existence, man has been an aggressive animal and has always been the subject of VIOLENCE; contusions, fractures, dislocations, impalements, eviscerations, and so on. The earliest surgeons were no doubt those men and women who showed particular interest and skill in dealing with the injuries. Long before written records existed, we have to rely on the only available evidence, obtained from ancient SKELETONS, to learn something of the diseases which afflicted primitive man and of the earliest surgical endeavours. Archaeologists have unearthed evidence of arthritis, bone infections, and bone tumours from the earliest times. Fractures, of course, are obvious, and splints of wood and of bark recovered from excavations from tombs of the Fifth Dynasty in Egypt have been dated at approximately 2450 BC. However — remarkably and inexplicably — the earliest major surgery of which we have undoubted evidence is trephination of the SKULL, which dates back to at least 5000 BC in the Stone Age period. Not only did these primitive surgeons, using no more than crude flint or stone instruments, actually bore holes through the skull, but undoubtedly a proportion at least of their patients survived. We know this because about half of the skulls that have been excavated show evidence of healing around the edges of the bone defect. Others show that repeated operations had been performed. Moreover, this procedure was performed in widely different areas of the world. Trephined skulls have been excavated in Western Europe (including England), North Africa, Asia, the East Indies, and New Zealand. In the New World, evidence has been found of the operation in Alaska and down through the Americas to Peru.

There are many unanswered questions about this remarkable operation. There might be a single trephine defect or up to seven in number. Size could vary from a tiny hole to two or more inches in diameter. The operation was performed on men, women, and children. Did this operation, which is today regarded as a sophisticated procedure to be done by an expert neurosurgeon, arise spontaneously in numerous centres throughout the world, or did knowledge of the operation spread gradually from centre to centre? Why was the operation performed? In many cases it was undoubtedly carried out because of injury to the skull. This is particularly so in Peruvian skulls, where fractures in the region of the trephine were commonly found. Among the ancient Peruvians large clubs of wood and stone, and also hatchets have been excavated — reason enough for the production of serious skull injuries. In many other examples, however, there is no evidence of skull injury, and evidence that the operation was repeated at intervals of time. We can only guess that it might have been performed in patients who suffered from mental illness, intractable HEADACHE, or EPILEPSY in order to let out the demon which had possessed the patient — belief in such demons is still held in some primitive races.

To perform safe and effective surgical operations, four major hurdles had to be overcome:

(i) The surgeon has to have an effective knowledge of the ANATOMY of the body.
(ii) He must be able to control HAEMORRHAGE effectively, whether this is the result of trauma or follows his own surgical incision.
(iii) Effective PAIN relief is necessary in order to spare the patient the agonies of the knife: the development of anaesthesia. Without this, the patient will only submit to the surgeon when his symptoms are intolerable, and then will only allow the shortest and quickest procedure to be carried out.
(iv) There must be effective control of INFECTION of the wound, both by the prevention of the access of bacteria (antiseptic and aseptic surgery) and by having the means of killing bacteria which have already invaded the tissues (antibiotics).

These four barriers were successfully overcome over a period of many centuries.

Appreciation of the body's anatomy
In the centuries before an understanding of human anatomy, surgical procedures were necessarily both limited and crude. The major advance was the introduction of human DISSECTION in the European medical schools in the sixteenth century. An important landmark was the publication of the first comprehensive and fully illustrated textbook of human anatomy by Andreas Vesalius in 1543. Surgeons were now at least familiar with the location and relationships of anatomical structures, which enabled them, for example, to expose injured BLOOD VESSELS and to appreciate what structures might be injured in deep body wounds. Of course, the scope of their endeavours was still seriously limited by the other three problems listed above.

Control of haemorrhage
For centuries, major haemorrhage from injured blood vessels was controlled by pressure or by the application of the cautery iron — what amounts to a red-hot poker. Not only was this inefficient but, of course, it was also horrifyingly painful. The alternative of tying the damaged vessel with a ligature had been employed by various surgeons dating back to Celsus, a Roman medical author in the first century AD. A great advance was made by the French surgeon Ambroise Paré (1510–90) — a contemporary of Vesalius, and who actually met him once in consultation; he taught that ligation of blood vessels was safer and far kinder in major operations, especially in AMPUTATIONS. From then on, the control of haemorrhage became a safer and more accurate procedure.

Relief of pain
The agonising pain of surgical procedures, whether to deal with a major wound, a fractured bone, an AMPUTATION, or removal of a tumour, was a major obstacle to the development of

surgery. Surgeons would attempt to stupefy the patient with alcohol, opium, or morphia, but with little effect. It was the discovery of the anaesthetic properties of ether by William Morton (1811–68), a dentist in Boston, in 1846, and of chloroform by Sir James Young Simpson (1811–70) of Edinburgh, in the following year, that at last allowed the surgeon to carry out his procedures painlessly and in an unhurried manner under general anaesthesia.

Control of infection

Infection, the fourth in our list of problems, was the greatest impediment to surgical progress and the last to be conquered. Over the centuries, the wounds which surgeons were tending, either as a result of injury or inflicted by themselves on their patients, would swell, redden, and suppurate with the discharge of pus. Indeed, this was regarded as the normal process of WOUND HEALING. The patient often became severely ill from the general manifestations of infection — FEVER, rigors, and toxaemia — and was very likely to die when this occurred. Nowadays, of course, we know that both the local and the general effects of infection are due to bacterial contamination of the wound. It was Louis Pasteur (1822–95) who proved conclusively that putrefaction of milk, urine, meat, and wine was due to bacteria and not merely to exposure to the air. It was the genius of Joseph Lister (1827–1919), the professor of surgery in Glasgow, to realize that it was these BACTERIA, carried into the wound, which resulted in the suppuration, pus, gangrene, and other dreaded complications which plagued the surgical wards of those days. It was obviously impossible to kill microbes in the wound by means of heat as Pasteur had shown in his experiments, so Lister developed chemical methods to destroy the bacteria, initially carbolic acid. Lister's first operation using this antiseptic method was in 1865, and he was soon able to show that major surgery could be performed with what had virtually never been seen before: healing without infection. The next stage was to progress beyond killing the bacteria that reached the wound to the prevention of contamination by eliminating bacteria from the operating theatre — aseptic surgery, with steam sterilization of instruments, dressings, and gowns, and the other rituals of the modern operating theatre.

Since the days of Lister, the dream had been to discover an agent that would kill the bacteria that spread through the body, without damaging the patient, as well as dealing with local contamination of the wound. It was Howard Florey, Ernst Chain, and their team in Oxford who succeeded in extracting penicillin in 1941. Its effects in both the prevention and the treatment of wound sepsis were dramatic and heralded the onset of today's 'antibiotic era'.

The conquest of pain, haemorrhage, and infection, together with today's detailed knowledge of the anatomy and physiology of the human body and its derangements under pathological conditions, has opened the way to the

extraordinary burgeoning of surgery in the past century or so, with advances being made in the past decades in what seems like geometrical progression. Only some aspects of this vast subject can be chosen here to illustrate this theme.

Abdominal surgery

Abdominal cancers are common and serious problems, and were among the first conditions to be dealt with in the post-Lister period. In 1881, Theodor Billroth (1829–94) carried out the first successful resection of a carcinoma of the stomach, soon to be followed by successes in dealing with CANCERS of the large bowel, kidney, and other structures. Abdominal emergencies, previously almost invariably fatal, were soon shown to be curable by surgery. Removal of the APPENDIX for acute appendicitis, repair of perforated peptic ulcers, and removal of the ruptured SPLEEN after trauma all became routine procedures.

Cardiac surgery

It was long thought that even touching the HEART would be fatal, and it was not until 1897 that Ludwig Rehn (1849–1930) performed the first successful repair of a wound of the heart. Henry Souttar (1875–1964) made a considerable advance in 1925 when he passed his finger through the wall of the heart to dilate a stenosed mitral valve, an operation that was popularized by Harken in 1948. However, to perform careful procedures on the open heart itself under direct vision, the heart must be put out of circulation and stopped. This required the development of an effective pump oxygenator, which was developed successfully by Gibbon in the US and Melrose in London, allowing the first successful operation with this technique to be carried out by Lillehei in 1956. It was now possible to repair complicated congenital anomalies of the heart, replace diseased and defective valves (either with artificial valves or using pig or human cadaver valves preserved by freeze-drying), and, most commonly of all, to perform bypass operations on occluded coronary arteries, using either a superficial vein taken from the leg or an artery from the front of the ribs. This procedure, the CORONARY ARTERY BYPASS graft, is now performed in tens of thousands of patients each year.

Minimal access surgery

Refinement in fibreoptic technology and engineering have produced instruments which are used for so-called 'keyhole' surgery. Fine tools can be passed into the abdominal and chest cavities so that many operations which previously required major incisions can now be performed through quite small puncture wounds. This is particularly well established in gynaecological surgery and in operations upon the gall bladder, and techniques are being devised for similar operations on other organs. This technology also involves the development of instruments to pass along every tube in the body, for example to remove obstructions in the oesophagus, bile

ducts, bowel, prostate, and major blood vessels. Many procedures on JOINTS — for example, removal of a torn cartilage from the KNEE — can now be performed safely, using these minimal access techniques. HAROLD ELLIS

See also ANAESTHESIA, GENERAL; ANATOMY; DISSECTION.

Survival at sea has been a problem confronting man ever since he took to the sea in boats. An emergency can result in survivors finding themselves: (i) immersed in water; or (ii) aboard some type of life-saving craft such as a lifeboat or life-raft.

Immersion in cold water

Represents one of the greatest stresses to which the human body can be exposed and has been recognised as such since the beginning of recorded history. Around 450 BC, Herodotus described the ill-fated seaborne expedition by the Persian General Mardonius; he wrote: 'those who could not swim perished from that cause, others from the cold.' Thus, Herodotus clearly distinguished between the inability to swim and cold, a distinction which remained forgotten for over two centuries, despite evidence from countless shipwrecks that airway protection alone did not guarantee survival. The most notable of these was the tragic loss of the *Titanic* on 14 April 1912. The 712 people who boarded lifeboats survived, while all of the 1489 who entered the water died in less than two hours. The sea they entered was calm but icy cold, all were wearing life-jackets, yet evidence was provided at the subsequent enquiry that all cries for help from those in the water quickly waned, and disappeared completely in under an hour. The circumstantial evidence all pointed towards cold as the precursor to death, but despite this the official inquiry gave DROWNING as the cause of death in every case. Again the opportunity to identify the importance of protection against *cold* for survivors at sea was missed.

It was not until the height of World War II that the threat of cold and the inadequacies of the lifesaving equipment being provided were correctly identified. Post-war work by Molnar in the in the US, and groups such as the Royal Navy Personnel Research Committee in the UK, consolidated this thinking. Currently, predicted 50% immersion survival times for normally clothed individuals are in the order of 6 hours at 15°C, 2 hours at 10°C, and 1 hour at 5°C.

Up until recently, the primary threat associated with immersion in cold water was thought to be HYPOTHERMIA. This belief is still perpetuated by the press, manufacturers, in standards and specification, and in the findings of fatal accident inquiries. However, later research has further refined thinking, and there is now a significant body of evidence to implicate other physiological responses as the precursors to death in many immersion incidents. In 1981 Golden and Hervey identified four stages of immersion associated with particular risk; these are:

(i) Initial immersion (first 2 minutes): a large percentage of those who die on immersion do so within three metres of a safe refuge, and many are regarded as 'good swimmers'. Such statistics suggest much quicker incapacitation than can occur with the protracted period of cooling necessary to produce hypothermia. We now know that rapid cooling of the skin on immersion in cold water initiates a set of undesirable respiratory and cardiac responses given the generic title of 'cold shock'. The responses include a 'gasp' response, uncontrollable rapid breathing, an increase both in blood pressure and with work required of the heart. The inability to control respiration can result in drowning, and the cardiac responses can result in a STROKE or HEART ATTACK in susceptible individuals. The magnitude of the response can be reduced by entering the water slowly, or by keeping as much of the body surface as dry and warm as possible. It also shows a high degree of HABITUATION, being reduced by as much as 45% following just six 3-minute, immersions in cold water. This habituation appears to occur in the central nervous system and lasts for at least 7 months.

(ii) Short-term immersion (2–30 minutes): cooling in water results in a rapid loss of neuro-muscular function, which can produce significant decrements in muscular strength, dexterity, proprioception, and co-ordination. These alterations can impair swimming performance and other actions essential to survival during the early minutes of an immersion. Survival may therefore depend on the immersion casualty understanding this and undertaking essential survival actions as soon as possible following immersion or on boarding a life-raft. Legislators and designers of survival equipment should recognize these limitations in their safety standards and design criteria.

(iii) Long-term immersion (30 minutes plus): for the first time, falling deep body temperature becomes the primary hazard. Progressive hypothermia can cause: confusion, disorientation, introversion (35°C), amnesia (34°C), cardiac arrhythmias (33°C), clouding of consciousness (33–30°C), loss of consciousness (30°C), ventricular fibrillation (28°C), and death (25°C). The figures in parenthesis represent deep body temperatures, and should be regarded as only a very rough guide, as great variation exists between individuals. Depending on conditions, consciousnes can be lost some time before death; this emphasizes the importance of wearing a good life-jacket, which will support the airway clear of the water and prevent death by drowning at an early stage. Protection against hypothermia is provided primarily by immersion suits and liferafts. People cool 4–5 times faster in water than in air at the same temperature and, therefore, should get out of the water whenever possible.

(iv) Post-immersion: approximately 17% of immersion deaths occur during, or immediately following, rescue. Originally it was thought that the continued fall in deep body (rectal) temperature seen following immersion, the *after drop*, was responsible for these deaths. More recent work has suggested that they are more probably caused by the collapse of blood pressure when hypothermic casualties are removed from the water and re-exposed to the full effects of gravity. One practical way of reducing this effect is to remove casualties from the water in a horizontal rather than vertical posture; this helps to maintain venous return and cardiac output. These considerations apply equally to the rescue of survivors who have been adrift in life-saving craft for some time.

Survival in a life-saving craft

Accounts of epic survival voyages are newsworthy and tend to be recounted in folklore or make media headlines, with descriptions ranging from heroic selfless behaviour to CANNIBALISM. However, such accounts, involving dehydration and starvation, tend to obscure the more serious immediate thermal threat, which is frequently the major problem confronting survivors in such craft even in temperate waters. In thermoregulatory terms man is a tropical animal and, in order to survive outside a tropical environment, he must use clothing and shelter to prevent body cooling. In a survival at sea situation these are usually unavailable; the survivor is then at the mercy of the elements. As a result, in temperate and subarctic environments, death from a fall in body temperature (hypothermia) usually occurs long before dehydration or STARVATION come into consideration.

Longer-term non-thermal problems manifest themselves with time adrift. These include: MOTION SICKNESS; dehydration; starvation; sunburn; salt-water ulcers. Of these, dehydration and starvation are worthy of special mention here, along with the importance of refraining from drinking sea water or eating protein (fish/seabirds) when drinking water is not freely available. The concentration of SALT in body fluids is normally maintained at 0.9%. Any excess salt ingested is excreted by the kidneys in urine, and the maximum urinary salt concentration achievable is in the region of 2%. Sea water contains about 3.5% salt and, in the absence of copious amounts of fresh drinking water, the extra salt ingested can be excreted only at the expense of body fluids, thereby accelerating the onset of the deleterious effects of dehydration.

When starvation is present in a survival at sea situation, the body will catabolize its own muscle PROTEIN. The end product of this process is urea; a toxic substance which is excreted in urine by the kidneys. In the absence of drinking water, the excretion of urea can only be achieved at the expense of body water, thereby increasing dehydration. It follows that when water is scarce, protein consumption (fish/sea birds) will hasten death by dehydration. Survival rations of CARBOHYDRATES (sweets), or a mixture of carbohydrate and FAT in fudge-like compounds, not only reduce this catabolism, but also provide additional water to the body as an end-product of their METABOLISM.

It is concluded that the four essential biological ingredients for survival in any environment are, in order of priority: (i) an adequate supply of breathable air; (ii) a tolerable ambient temperature; (iii) the provision of potable water; (iv) sufficient edible food.

In terms of survival at sea, these can be translated into: (i) protection against drowning; (ii) protection from temperature extremes, both in and out of water; (iii) protection from dehydration; (iv) amelioration of the longer effects of starvation.

When planning for surviving at sea one must identify, in order of priority, the physiological threats which are likely to be encountered, and the appropriate protective measures. The thermal threat must be given a high priority.

MICHAEL J. TIPTON
FRANK ST. C. GOLDEN

Further reading

Adam, J. M. (1981). *Hypothermia ashore and afloat.* Proceedings of the Third International Action for Disaster Conference. Aberdeen University Press, Aberdeen.

Keatinge, W. R. (1978). *Survival in cold water,* (reprinted). Blackwell Scientific Publications.

Tipton, M. J. and Golden, M. J. (1994). Immersion in cold water: effects on performance and safety. Chapter in *Oxford Textbook of Sports Medicine* (ed. M. Harries, C. Williams, W. D. Stanish, and L. J. Micheli). Oxford Medical Publications, Oxford.

See also COLD EXPOSURE; DROWNING; HYPOTHERMIA; NEAR-DROWNING; PROTECTIVE CLOTHING; STARVATION; WATER BALANCE.

Swallowing

In preparation for swallowing, a softened or liquid *food bolus* is moved through the MOUTH by the action of the TONGUE. The bolus lies in a longitudinal midline furrow on the tongue, and the floor of this furrow is progressively raised from before backwards, squeezing the bolus back against the hard PALATE. The kinetic energy imparted to the bolus then moves it into and through the pharynx, the cavity of which continues on from the mouth. In the pharynx, contractions of circularly-arranged muscles complete the movement of the bolus down into the oesophagus and thence to the stomach.

The whole process is complicated by the fact that, in the adult human, the pharynx also forms part of the airway leading from the NOSE to the LARYNX. The opening into the larynx (the *glottis*) is sited about halfway down the front of the pharynx. As a consequence, swallowing and BREATHING cannot safely occur at the same time. In contrast, in the human new-born and generally in other mammals (both infant and adult), the larynx occupies a higher position relative to the pharynx so that its opening is usually above the soft palate, which extends around it. In this situation there is a degree of anatomical separation of the respiratory tract and the alimentary tract (and in many animals the high larynx divides the pharynx into two passages, which pass laterally either side of the larynx and then rejoin lower down in the pharynx). The timed separation of swallowing and breathing is consequently less critical in this situation than it is in adult man.

The anatomical differences also produce differences in the way that the swallow is executed. The important point with the high larynx is that if the larynx, with the *epiglottis* that protects its opening, contacts the posterior edge of the soft palate, a space is formed, which is bounded above by the soft palate, behind by the anterior surface of the larynx, and in front and below by the top of the tongue. This space temporarily accumulates food, prior to its onward passage via pharynx and oesophagus. This storage area includes the *valleculae* (pockets formed between the larynx and the surface of the back of the tongue) and will be referred to as the *vallecular space*.

Growth in length of the human pharynx (starting a few months after birth) is associated with a descent of the larynx so that its contact with the soft palate is lost. There is consequently no longer an enclosed space in which food can be stored or accumulated, and the airway is no longer anatomically separated from the food passage. A variety of measures operate to protect the airway during swallowing in this situation. They include interruption of breathing, closure of the glottis, tipping the larynx forward so that the back of the tongue bulges over it during swallowing, plus bending of the epiglottis back and down over the laryngeal opening. Because of the low position of the glottis, the pattern of swallowing in the mature human is the exception to the general pattern in mammals. All the early studies of swallowing were carried out on human adults so that the traditional ideas and terminology of swallowing all reflect that origin. Thus swallowing of food is described as being divided into three phases (usually oral, pharyngeal, and oesophageal). In man, approximately 600 swallows occur every 24 hours, but only about 150 of these are concerned with food and drink; the rest simply clear SALIVA from the mouth.

When cineradiographs of mammalian (non-human) feeding are examined, it becomes clear that there are two separate processes that first fill, and then periodically empty the vallecular space so that the contents pass directly down the oesophagus. Adequate filling of the space appears to be the trigger for emptying. Unless one includes all of the tongue and jaw movements involved in suckling, lapping, or chewing, the true swallow consists only of emptying the vallecular space and the subsequent movement of the bolus down the oesophagus. In contrast, in the human adult, only one transport cycle occurs as the two processes of vallecular filling and of vallecular emptying coalesce within a single cycle of jaw and tongue movement. This

occurs because emptying is usually initiated immediately the first trace of food material enters the vallecular region. The question then becomes one of how vallecular emptying is triggered so readily in the adult human, when (unlike other mammals) only a trace of food or liquid may have reached the region. In adult man, unlike other mammals, the movement of a bolus backwards within the mouth (*intra-oral transport*) is consequently described as the first phase of a swallow, because of its continuity with vallecular emptying.

The neural mechanisms involved in swallowing involve a number of nerves supplying the mucous membrane that lines the structures forming the vallecular space. The most important are the ninth and tenth pairs of CRANIAL NERVES (*glossopharyngeal* and *vagus*). A branch of the vagus nerve carries important sensory input from the larynx, the epiglottis, and particularly from the vallecular storage area that is present in infants and in all other non-human mammals, i.e. in all those with a high glottis. In these cases, swallowing can be elicited reflexly by fluid in the vallecular space even when there are no connections from higher parts of the brain

above the BRAINSTEM (e.g. in decerebrate animals and in infants with anencephaly, where the cerebral hemispheres are congenitally absent). It can therefore be assumed that all the necessary neural components for swallowing are present below the level of the midbrain and that sensory input from the surface of the palate, epiglottis, and tongue (the walls of the vallecular space) is alone sufficient to provide the activation necessary to elicit a swallow.

The same argument applies to swallowing in the fetus and in the new-born human with an immature central nervous system. However, in the adult human there is no longer an enclosed vallecular space. Consequently, the level of sensory input must be less than that which would arise when all the mucosal surfaces surrounding that space were stimulated by its filling.

The generally accepted view is that the sensory input from the back of the mouth activates a set of neural circuits within the brain stem that collectively produce the pattern of motor activity constituting a swallow. These circuits constitute a *pattern generator* for the activity involving the thirty or so muscles that take part in a swallow. The relevant network of brain stem neurons

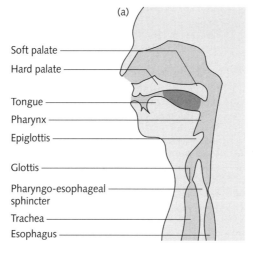
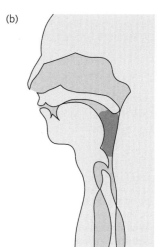
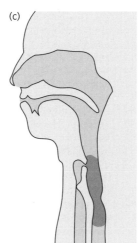
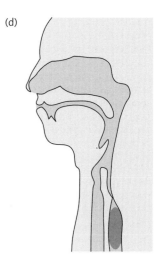

Soft palate
Hard palate
Tongue
Pharynx
Epiglottis
Glottis
Pharyngo-esophageal sphincter
Trachea
Esophagus

(a) (b) (c) (d)

Movement of food bolus (black) during swallowing.

receives sensory input from nerves innervating the mouth, and it also receives excitatory fibres descending from the CEREBRAL CORTEX.

To explain the situation in adult man, it is proposed that the activity in the nerve fibres descending from the cortex is sufficient to lower the threshold for reflex emptying of the valleculae so that only a trace of material has to reach this region to elicit emptying. A conscious swallow therefore seems to differ from other voluntary movements. One can test this oneself by repeatedly swallowing to eliminate saliva from the mouth; swallowing becomes progressively more difficult to perform and it eventually becomes impossible even to initiate the movement; i.e. there is nothing left to elicit the reflex. The corollary is that, in the presence of excitation from the cortex (a conscious desire to swallow), sensory inputs can elicit vallecular emptying very easily, even though only a trace of material has entered the vallecular region. Vallecular emptying and pharyngeal transit are then followed immediately by *oesophageal peristalsis* (a moving wave of contraction), so that these events follow seamlessly upon the first phase of intra-oral transport, giving rise to the classical appearance of the three-stage human swallow. It is also necessary to relax the *sphincters* (rings of muscle fibres) at the top and the bottom of the oesophagus so as to allow the passage of the bolus into the oesophagus and then into the stomach respectively.

'*Dysphagia*' is a word used to describe difficulty or discomfort in swallowing. Clearly a cyst or tumour restricting the width of the pharynx or oesophagus could give rise to such a state. A number of other types of disorder affect swallowing. These include muscle weakness, inability to relax a sphincter, peripheral nerve lesions, and central nervous system damage: a lesion in the medulla can directly damage the neurons making up the swallowing centre. More commonly, swallowing becomes disordered when the motor nerve fibres descending from the cerebral cortex are interrupted, as in a STROKE. The malfunction occurs presumably because an important source of excitation to the relevant cells in the medulla is removed, so raising the threshold for reflex emptying of the valleculae. Failure to maintain a competent sphincter at the lower end of the oesophagus (which can occur in *diaphragmatic hernia*, when part of the stomach protrudes upwards through the diaphragm into the chest) permits regurgitation of the acid contents of the stomach; this can cause discomfort when swallowing and is sometimes loosely classified as dysphagia.　　　ALLAN THEXTON

Further reading

Thexton, A. J. and Crompton, A. W. (1999). 'Control of Swallowing' in *Scientific Basis of Eating* (Frontiers of Oral Biology. Vol 9) Ed. R.W.A. Linden, Karger, Basel, p. 168–222.

See PLATE 1.
See also EPIGLOTTIS; LARYNX; PHARYNX; TONGUE.

Sweating Sweat is secreted by glands in the SKIN when it is necessary to lose excess heat from the body. They are stimulated to do so by sympathetic nerves of the AUTONOMIC NERVOUS SYSTEM when sensors in the HYPOTHALAMUS are activated by blood reaching it at a higher than normal temperature. There are also other contexts in which sweating occurs which have a less obvious physiological role — the 'cold sweat' of fear, of HAEMORRHAGE, and of SHOCK.

There are sweat glands all over the skin, but more densely distributed in some sites than others, and there are also two types, according to the way in which their cells produce secretions.

The secretion of the *apocrine* sweat glands includes cast-off parts of the sweat-generating cells themselves (the secretion of milk by the glandular tissue of the breasts is similarly apocrine). They are to be found in relatively few places (armpit, groin) and these are the ones responsible for the characteristic odour which nowadays in Western society triggers the application of deodorants rather attracting the attention of the nose — thus perhaps dispensing with a more primitive role in sexual attraction.

The *epicrine* sweat glands produce secretions by the more general method of extruding liquid from the glandular cells in their depths into the spiral ducts which discharge on the skin surface. They are present over the whole body surface, though more concentrated in some areas, such as the palms of the hands and the soles of the feet. They have an essential function in TEMPERATURE REGULATION.

Any moisture on the surface of the skin will evaporate unless the environment is highly humid, and by the laws of physics, evaporation causes cooling. Cooling of the skin in turn causes cooling of the venous blood flowing away from it, and hence cooling of the whole circulating blood. Since body tissues are moist and the skin is not entirely waterproof, some evaporation inevitably takes place all the time, without active stimulation of sweating; this is 'insensible perspiration'. In contrast to colloquial usage therefore, perspiring is not the same as sweating. Sweat provides additional water for evaporation — and to be effective as a body cooler, sweat must not be wiped away, since that defeats the purpose.

Sweat is not just water. It is well known that sweat, or the residue on the skin after evaporation, tastes salty. It is formed by movement of water and inorganic solutes out of the blood plasma into the cells of the sweat gland and thence out into its duct. Since sodium chloride is the main salt in the plasma, it is a major constituent of sweat. The ducts of the sweat glands are not just passive conduits: they reabsorb some of the salt from the fluid on its way to the surface, thus conserving it for the body fluids, although as the flow of sweat increases, a smaller proportion of the salt is reabsorbed. During work or exercise in a hot environment, loss of water could reach between 1 and 2 litres in an hour. This comes initially from the body's extracellular fluid volume (blood and interstitial fluid).

If too much fluid is lost blood volume becomes depleted, with potentially harmful consequences for cardiac output and BLOOD PRESSURE. Proportionally more water is lost than salt, so the body fluids also tend to become over-concentrated. Unless enough water is drunk to correct this, water moves by osmosis out of cells, causing generalized dehydration of the tissues. Thirst promotes intake of replacement fluid and there is also a physiological mechanism which helps to conserve water. When body fluids become concentrated, more antidiuretic hormone is released from the posterior lobe of the PITUITARY GLAND, and acts in the KIDNEYS to promote retention of water.

Acclimatization has important effects on sweating. Going to a hot climate and indulging in heavy work or exercise will lead over a period of weeks to an increased maximal sweating rate, assisting temperature control, and accompanied by an increase in the reabsorption of salt. This latter may seem unhelpful, since it tends to exaggerate the disproportionate loss of water relative to salt, and hence the concentration of the extracellular fluid and generalized dehydration. But it enhances thirst, and all is well if water is available. The conservation of salt can be important. Although in a modern Western diet salt is plentiful — sometimes harmfully superfluous — its normal concentration in the body fluids is essential to the maintenance of a normal blood volume, and hence of an effective circulation. In man the hunter, sweating in a hot climate, in regions where salt is scanty in the diet, it is a precious commodity, and the physiological mechanism evolved to conserve it can cut its loss in urine and in sweat to virtually nil. When sweating starts to deplete blood volume, the ADRENAL GLANDS receive signals to increase the output of the hormone ALDOSTERONE; this acts both on kidney tubule cells and on sweat duct cells, causing them to retrieve more salt from the escaping fluid.

SHEILA JENNETT

Further reading

Bursztyn, P. G. (1990) *Physiology for sportspeople — a serious user's guide to the body*. Manchester University Press. Manchester and New York.

See also ADRENAL GLANDS; BODY FLUIDS; SKIN; TEMPERATURE REGULATION.

Swimming is one of the most popular recreational sports that can be enjoyed by all ages. The ability to swim enables people to participate in a wide variety of water sports such as snorkelling, water skiing, jet skiing, wind surfing, sailing, boating, fishing, rowing, and canoeing, without the fear of getting into trouble, and reduces the risk of drowning. Fear of water, particularly if a person suddenly gets out of their depth, prevents a lot of people going into a swimming pool or enjoying beach holidays. Many of the newer watersports require expertise in handling a craft as well as swimming proficiency.

Water is a very dangerous place for non swimmers, particularly if it is cold and an excessive amount of alcohol has been drunk. Unfamiliar surroundings, and no knowledge of local tides, can be lethal to careless individuals. Water-related fatalities are the second leading cause of accidental death in the UK and Australia, and the third in the US. The risk of drowning is 2.5 deaths per 100 000 in USA and 1 per 100 000 in the UK.

Babies are taught to swim at a very young age in some countries; this enables them to learn to swim without fear of the water. They should have had their first two combined immunizations, unless they are being breast-fed. The water temperature should be higher than normal, a minimum of 86°F or 27°C. The time spent in the water should be carefully monitored; this can vary from 10 minutes to 30 minutes but babies should not stay too long in the water as they lose heat rapidly.

Swimmers are usually taught the four swimming strokes used for competitions; the front crawl, backstroke, breaststroke and butterfly, which are swum either as a single stroke or in combination over various distances.

There are four phases of each stroke; the reach, catch, pull, and recovery. The arm action during the pull phase provides 75% of the propulsion in all strokes except the breast-stroke, where the contributions from the upper and lower limbs are equal. During reach or entry the arm reaches forwards to enter the water. In backstroke the arm entry occurs with the shoulder in the fully elevated position. Catch is similar in all competitive strokes except backstroke; the elbow flexes, the arm extends forwards at the shoulder and moves outwards in the horizontal plane whilst rotating towards the body. The pull is the propulsion phase and can vary; the swimmer either sculls or pushes the water. The arm action starts at maximum elevation and ends in extension except in breast-stroke. Recovery is the out of water phase (except breast-stroke), and the arm then returns to start position.

In breast-stroke the arms move together in pull and recovery phase and the arms do not pull below the waistline.

Swimming is a sport that attracts participants of all ages although it is largely a young sport. Competitions are organized by clubs, schools, and national associations. Short course competitions take place in a 25-metre pool, long course in a 50-metre pool. Olympic swimming competitions are over a variety of distances and strokes, and they take place in 50-metre pools. Synchronized swimming, waterpolo, and diving are also included in the Olympic programme. Swimming in the sea may be part of a triathlon race, and open sea races, including Channel swims, are also held. 'Masters' swimming competitions are held for those over 24 years of age whereas 'veteran' sports competitions in athletics are for the over 40s. Competitions for different age groups are held in most countries, and world championships also take place.

Competitive swimming is a high-intensity training and performance sport. During the school year swimming training is divided into two sessions: the first session is in the early morning before school and the second session after school. The competitive swimmer usually does an average of 12 000–18 000 metres per day. The competition programme for the season should be planned well in advance so that the swimmer can peak for a specific competition, i.e. the swimmer reduces the amount of training to get the best result.

Swimming is a relatively injury-free sport and was found to be the safest of eleven sports surveyed by Weightman and Brown in 1975. It is non-load-bearing and does not involve antigravity work, resulting in fewer injuries. The injuries that do occur are usually due to overuse, doing too much too quickly, or breaking the rules.

To ignore warning signs of strong currents, king waves or rip tides may have lethal consequences. Diving into the shallow end of a pool or into a wave or sea where rocks are submerged may result in severe injuries. Pools should have the depth clearly marked so that swimmers do not dive into shallow water. Pools used for competition should be marked 2 metres from the wall at each end to judge when to turn. Flags are placed above the pool 5 metres from the end of the pool for the backstroke turn. There are rules against running around the pool. Pool discipline should be maintained, particularly out of the pool to prevent people slipping or jumping into the pool on top of other swimmers. There should also be strict discipline in the pool when swimming lengths. HYPERVENTILATION before trying to swim a long distance under water should be forbidden, as it increases the risk of HYPOXIA (lack of oxygen), and may result in loss of consciousness and death by drowning. The hyperventilation removes carbon dioxide and hence delays the stimulus to breathe when breathholding.

Swimming programmes are helpful for both the mentally and the physically handicapped as they weigh less in water, and this makes it easier for them to move their muscles, enabling them to improve muscle tone and co-ordination of movement. Pregnant women can swim during their pregnancy while many other sports are not suitable. Swimming is also useful in rehabilitation of injured athletes. Patients with rheumatoid arthritis can improve their aerobic capacity by swimming in warm water. Asthmatics should be encouraged to swim, as swimming is the sport that is least likely to precipitate an asthmatic attack, and the fitter they are the fewer attacks they have; swimming improves their breathing. Asthma is not a handicap in achieving excellence in sport as shown by the number of Olympic gold medal swimmers who were asthmatics.

Water aerobics is becoming a popular method of keeping fit, with less potential for injury than high impact aerobics. Running in the water is a useful method for athletes to keep fit, if they are injured and unable to cope with full weight-bearing on hard surfaces. Hydrotherapy is also an effective rehabilitation after injury. Swimming is thus a sport that can be enjoyed by many different groups.   MOIRA O'BRIEN

See also COLD EXPOSURE; DROWNING; EXERCISE; SPORT.

Symmetry and asymmetry

Exhibiting external bilateral symmetry about a vertical midline, the human body consists of two *enantiomorphs* — the right and left sides. The overwhelming preponderance of bilateral symmetry in the animal kingdom suggests that it provides an enormous evolutionary advantage. A close inspection of many individuals, however, reveals that small differences between left and right structures exist. These variations are called *fluctuating asymmetries* because neither side differs in a consistent manner when compared to the other.

What is the origin of bilateral symmetry? In the *Symposium* (190–1), Plato had Aristophanes explain that the original human beings were globular wholes with two faces on a single head, eight limbs, and double of every other structure; to punish them for their insolence and power, Zeus bisected each spherical human, and Apollo rotated each face toward the cut edge, pulled skin over the gash and tied it into a tight bundle at the navel.

Wilhelm Ludwig (1816–95) believed that bilateral symmetry was the basic body plan of all vertebrates, and that all asymmetries were superimposed upon the ground plan consequent to the lengthening and folding of the intestinal tract during evolution. Jacques Monod (1910–76) took a stance opposite to Ludwig's and, because the fundamental molecules — proteins and nucleic acids — responsible for organic structure are not symmetrical, considered asymmetry to represent the true order of living beings and symmetry to be a superficial phenomenon acquired during evolution.

Bilateral symmetry appears mainly in structures such as the BRAIN, NERVOUS SYSTEM, SKIN, HAIR, and NAILS, and in parts of the eye and ear — all of which arise from the *ectoderm* (outer germ layer) of the embryo — and in some structures, including the SKELETON and SKELETAL MUSCLES, tendons, glands, and reproductive organs, which develop from the *mesoderm* (middle germ layer). The HEART, originating in the mesoderm, and the LIVER, STOMACH, PANCREAS, and INTESTINES, which arise from *endoderm* (the inner germ layer) appear singly to one side of the midline.

Struck by the general doubling of organs, Aristotle rescued symmetry by asserting that the SPLEEN was a bastard liver and by pointing out that the heart has two halves. The bilateral symmetry of ectodermal and some mesodermal structures appears to have resulted from the interactions of the organism with its environment where left–right bias does not exist. Directional locomotion almost always requires bilateral symmetry and precludes the front — rear symmetry of Dr Dolittle's pushmi-pullyu (and Plato's original spherical human). The development of limbs for locomotion requires concomitant development of symmetry in the SENSE ORGANS and in the CENTRAL NERVOUS SYSTEM.

Certain anatomically symmetrical structures, notably the human hands and brain, do not exhibit functional symmetry. The evolution of bipedalism freed the hands from participation in locomotion and allowed them to evolve new functions, such as feeding, food gathering, tool using, and manipulating rather than simply reacting to the environment. The hands came to perform different functions, for example, in tool-making, for which one hand holds the material while the dominant hand shapes it. The bias of right-handedness in 88–90% of humans seems to be unique among animals. Some stone-flake evidence suggests that even the earliest human ancestors, the *Australopithecines*, were predominantly right-handed. As the human hand adapted, the mouth, freed from grasping functions, could specialize partly for communication, controlled by the brain.

Functions such as SPEECH, reading and facial recognition are asymmetrically located in the brain. During the evolution of handedness, duplication of functions in the brain might have wasted precious space and caused cognitive confusion. Such asymmetry of function correlates with the necessity of the association of the control of linked bodily movements and sensations. Some controversial evidence suggests that asymmetry of brain function may be more pronounced in males than in females, though it is an open question whether such differences are innate or environmentally determined.

External symmetry is a measure of health and provides a criterion of reproductive fitness in many species. Some research provides evidence that body symmetry also enhances human reproductive success. One study found that college males exhibiting greater body symmetry, as determined by measurements of ankles, feet width, wrists, hand, elbows, and ears, begin sexual intercourse several years earlier and have women partners who achieve orgasm more frequently. Another study indicates that slight asymmetries in women's fingers, ears, and breasts tend to diminish around ovulation, when women are fertile.

Critics of this research point out that much of the evidence linking symmetry with reproductive success rests on studies of non-humans and that the asymmetries discussed require fine calipers for detection. Furthermore, there is an alternate explanation for the greater approval of symmetry. A Swedish study suggests that the preference for symmetrical mates may be a by-product of a general preference for symmetry that evolved because it facilitated recognition of signals and objects varying in position and orientation in the field of vision.

Whatever the cause, it is certain that humans, including infants, find the symmetrical face — and body — more beautiful. In early representations, such as Mesopotamian and Etruscan

sculpture, the human body was rigidly symmetrical. The Roman architect Vitruvius (first century BCE) wrote that sacred buildings should be scaled according to human proportions because the human body, with legs and arms extended, fits into both the circle and the square. The 1480 drawing of a Vetruvian man by LEONARDO DA VINCI (1452–1519) illustrates how mathematical proportion became the foundation of an aesthetic philosophy in the Renaissance. Dürer (1471–1528) also applied Vetruvius' measurement to the human form, which he represented in numerous studies of the male and female figures, many of which were bisected vertically, with numerous horizontal lines to assure perfect symmetry and proportion. Varying from slender to obese, many of these figures are unattractive. The conscious artistic preference for symmetry tends to resurface, as suggested by a German physician's assessment that the *Venus de Milo*, discovered in 1820, had too many flaws and asymmetries to be considered beautiful. He lived too early to see works such as Picasso's *Guernica* (1937).   KRISTEN L. ZACHARIAS

Further reading

Corballis, M. C. (1991). *The lopsided ape. Evolution of the generative mind.* Oxford University Press, New York.

Weyl, H. (1952). *Symmetry.* Princeton University Press, Princeton, New Jersey.

See also BEAUTY; HANDEDNESS; LANGUAGE AND THE BRAIN.

Synaesthesia literally, 'joining the senses'. People who experience synaesthesia (*synaesthetes*) inhabit a world slightly, but magically different from that of most people — a world of extra colours, shapes, and sensations. 'Mine is a universe of black "Is" and pink "Wednesdays", numbers that climb skywards and a roller-coaster shaped year' is one description, reported by Motluk (1997). For synaesthetes, the experience of a single sense is accompanied by sensations in other sensory modalities.

Coloured-hearing is the most common form of synaesthesia, in which hearing a word elicits the perception of colour. The colour sensation elicited by a word is often determined by the letters in the word, with the first letter being the most influential. 'For me "run", "right", and "religion" are all black … because the letter R is so strikingly black. … Even the word "red" … is a black word, while the "black" is, because of its B, blue', said one synaesthete. The experience that words have particular colours can be helpful. Miss Stone, reported by Francis Galton in 1883, said 'I have always associated the same colours with the same letters, and no effort will change the colour of one letter … Occasionally, when uncertain how a word should be spelt, I have considered what colour it ought to be, and have decided in that way. I believe this has often been a great help to me in spelling, both in English and foreign languages.' Some composers report experiencing colours in response to chords or notes. For

example, Olivier Messiaen stated; 'I see colours which move with the music, and I sense these colours in an extremely vivid manner.' Other forms of synaesthesia combine many of the senses. An extreme example was experienced by the patient 'S' who was intensively studied by the Russian neuropsychologist, Alexander Luria. Presented with a tone of 2000 Hz at 113 decibels, S said, 'It looks something like fireworks tinged with a pink-red hue. The strip of colour feels rough and unpleasant and it has an ugly taste — rather like that of a briny pickle.' In this example a sound is eliciting experiences of colour, touch, and taste.

Synaesthetes are not simply using metaphorical language to describe sensations that are, in reality, no different from those of other people, nor have they simply learned peculiar associations between different senses. The synaesthetic experience is an automatic and involuntary response to certain stimuli. The experience is vivid and consistent: true synaesthetes give precisely the same descriptions of their experiences even when these are separated by months or years. In support of an organic basis, synaesthetes seem to have had their experiences from earliest childhood and certainly before the age of four, and the syndrome seems to run in families. A transient experience of synaesthesia can be induced in non-synaesthetes by drugs such as *hashish* and *mescaline*. All these observations suggest that an explanation of synaesthesia needs to be sought at the level of brain function.

The techniques of functional brain imaging (positron emission tomography and functional magnetic resonance imaging) have been used to observe brain activity associated with a synaesthetic experience. As yet, only one fully-controlled study has been reported, by Frith and Paulesu (1997). Volunteers were scanned who experienced colours when they heard words. In comparison to people who did not have such experiences, extra areas of brain activity were identified in the synaesthetes when they were hearing words. This extra activity occurred in regions of the brain normally activated when naming the colours of objects, e.g. reporting 'yellow' in response to 'banana'. Activity was not detected in regions of the visual cortex concerned with earlier stages of colour processing. This study confirms that the experiences reported by synaesthetes are associated with characteristic patterns of brain activity. The same regions are activated in non-synaesthetes when they are having experiences which are, to some extent, qualitatively similar. We remain, however, far from an understanding of the physiological basis of synaesthesia.

The problem is to explain how activity occurs in brain regions concerned with aspects of one kind of sense when the incoming stimulation derives from some other sense. There are essentially two possibilities (though very speculative), both of which involve some kind of 'miswiring' in the brain. The *crosstalk* theory suggests that information within the processing stream of one sensation crosses to another stream, leading to anomalous sensations. The *feedback* theory proposes that information from one sensory stream reaches a central region (e.g. a region concerned with object identity) and is then fed back towards the periphery, activating regions concerned with another sensory modality. Both ideas imply that, for a synaesthetic experience to occur, neural connections exist, that are not present, or not activated, in the more usual, non-synaesthetic individual. One suggestion is that the brain of an infant is naturally synaesthetic, such that information from any modality activates all sensory regions; activity in the cerebral cortex simply reflecting the amount of sensation, whatever its source. During maturation, responses to different modalities become localized in distinct brain regions. This differentiation may be achieved by the selective death of nerve cells, which is known to occur during infancy. Synaesthesia lasting into adulthood could be the consequence of partial failure of this mechanism.

Although synaesthesia is a relatively rare phenomenon (estimated to be 1 in 2000), understanding its physiological basis is of considerable importance to neuroscience. If we can understand synaesthesia then we might also understand the general mechanism by which neural activity is translated into conscious sensory experience. The main philosophical interest of synaesthesia, however, is the vivid example that it provides of how subjective our perceptions really are.   CHRIS FRITH

Further reading

Baron-Cohen, S. and Harrison, J. E. (1997). *Synaesthesia: classic and contemporary readings.* Blackwell, Oxford.

See also PERCEPTION; SENSATION; SENSORY INTEGRATION.

Synapse A specialized junction where transmission of information takes place between a nerve fibre and another nerve cell, or between a nerve fibre and a muscle or gland cell. The term was introduced at the end of the nineteenth century by the British neurophysiologist Charles Sherrington, who argued, on the basis of his own observations of reflex responses and the studies of the great Spanish anatomist, Ramón y Cajal, that a special form of transmission takes place at the contact between one cell and the next.

Synapses serve as one-way communication devices, transmitting information in one direction only, from the fibre ending to the next cell. They come in two varieties, known as chemical and electrical, according to the mechanism by which the signal is transmitted from the presynaptic to the postsynaptic cell. At *electrical synapses*, which are relatively rare in vertebrates, the membranes of the two cells are in tight contact, producing electrical coupling, which enables a nerve impulse (or ACTION POTENTIAL) arriving at the presynaptic nerve ending to pass swiftly and reliably to the next cell. *Chemical synapses* are more complex, because the pre-

synaptic and postsynaptic cells are physically separated by a minute gap (the *synaptic cleft*), which prevents simple electrical transmission of the action potential to the postsynaptic cell. Instead, transmission is accomplished by the release of a chemical NEUROTRANSMITTER substance from the presynaptic fibre.

The cytoplasm of the presynaptic nerve terminal (in a chemical synapse) is packed full of small vesicles, each containing a few thousand molecules of neurotransmitter. When an action potential arrives in the terminal it stimulates the opening of calcium channels in the terminal membrane. As a consequence, calcium ions flood into the cell and cause the synaptic vesicles to release their contents into the synaptic cleft. The neurotransmitter molecules that are liberated diffuse across the cleft and interact with specialized protein receptor molecules in the postsynaptic CELL MEMBRANE. The molecular structure of the neurotransmitter and its receptor are matched, so that they fit one another like a lock and key. At nerve–muscle synapses, and in many nerve–nerve synapses, the receptors have a double function, since they also serve as ION

CHANNELS. Binding of a neurotransmitter molecule produces a change in the three-dimensional shape of the receptor that opens a tiny intrinsic pore in the protein. In the case of neurotransmitters that excite the postsynaptic membrane, the pore permits positively-charged sodium ions to move into the cell, making the potential across its membrane less negative. This local depolarization is known as an *excitatory synaptic potential*, and its amplitude is determined by the number of vesicles released from the presynaptic cell. If it is sufficiently large, the synaptic potential initiates an action potential in the cell. If the target cell is a neuron, the action potential sweeps along its fibre. If it is a muscle, it also propagates over the surface of the muscle cell and causes it to contract.

Not all synaptic transmission is excitatory. *Inhibitory transmitters* also exist which render the post-synaptic cell less excitable and thus less likely to generate an action potential. They often act on receptors that act as channels for chloride ions, and generally make the interior of the postsynaptic cell even more negative (*hyperpolarization*). ACETYLCHOLINE is the excitatory

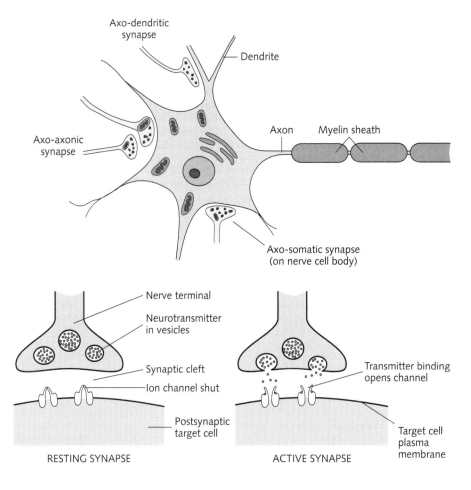

The main types of synapse and the structure of a typical chemical synapse simplified from electron micrographs.

transmitter at nerve–muscle synapses, and *glutamate* is the main excitatory transmitter in the CENTRAL NERVOUS SYSTEM. Examples of inhibitory neurotransmitters include *glycine* and *gamma aminobutyric acid* (GABA).

The action of 'fast' neurotransmitters is brief, because they unbind quickly from their receptors and are then rapidly cleared from the synaptic cleft, usually by breakdown into inactive substances or reuptake into the cell. Because the receptor channels remain open only as long as neurotransmitter is bound, and because binding is only transient, the synaptic potential is also brief and the membrane potential returns rapidly to its resting level. Many other transmitters, sometimes called *modulators* (including SEROTONIN, DOPAMINE, NORADRENALINE, and many small peptide molecules), act more slowly and for much longer periods of time. In general, their receptors do not act as channels but instead activate messenger molecules inside the cell, which can initiate a variety of responses, even including the switching-on of genes in the chromosomes. It used to be thought that each nerve fibre releases only one neurotransmitter ('*Dale's principle*', after the British pharmacologist, Henry Dale), but it is now known that two or more transmitters and/or modulators can be produced by individual nerve terminals.

Each SKELETAL MUSCLE fibre is innervated by a single excitatory nerve fibre, which discharges 100–300 vesicles for each arriving nerve impulse (enough to produce an action potential in the muscle cell). In contrast, a single nerve cell may have tens, or hundreds, of thousands of synapses. These are not only inhibitory as well as excitatory, but may involve many different type of transmitters and post-synaptic receptors (it is thought there may be more than 100 different neurotransmitters). Each pre-synaptic input may release just a few vesicles in response to a nerve impulse, so that the synaptic potential may be far smaller than that of a muscle fibre and many simultaneous or closely-successive inputs are needed to elicit one action potential. The output of the post-synaptic neuron will therefore be an integrated response to all of its many different inputs.

Most DRUGS that work on the brain, as well as drugs of abuse, act on synapses. One of the best known is NICOTINE, which activates acetylcholine receptors (its effect is mediated primarily at neuronal synapses in the brain). CURARE, traditionally used by South American Indians as an arrow poison, paralysed the prey because it is an antagonist of the acetylcholine receptor and therefore blocks neuromuscular transmission. *Morphine* and HEROIN act on opiate receptors, and *cannabis* (unsurprisingly) on cannabinoid receptors. COCAINE works differently. It blocks the uptake system that clears the neurotransmitter dopamine from the synaptic cleft: consequently, dopamine hangs around for longer, which explains why cocaine acts as a stimulant. Some *nerve gas* POISONS work in a similar fashion, by blocking the removal of the transmitter acetylcholine at nerve–muscle synapses.

A range of human diseases result from disorders of synaptic function. For instance, the inherited neuromuscular disorder, *myasthenia gravis*, occurs when the body produces antibodies to the acetylcholine receptors on muscle fibres. This causes them to be taken in by the cell, and the reduced number at the cell surface means that neurotransmission is compromised. Consequently, the patient is easily fatigued. Other myasthenias may result from a deficiency of the enzyme that breaks down acetylcholine, from presynaptic abnormalities that influence the amount of transmitter released, or from postsynaptic abnormalities associated with a reduction in the number or function of the acetylcholine receptors. EPILEPSY is sometimes due to a decrease in the efficiency of inhibitory transmission in the brain, leading to over-excitability of networks of neurons. There is some evidence that the major psychiatric conditions, *depression* and *schizophrenia*, involve disorders of synapses in which serotonin and dopamine, respectively, act as neurotransmitters.

FRANCES M. ASHCROFT

See also ACTION POTENTIALS; MOTOR NEURONS; NERVES; NERVOUS SYSTEM; NEUROMUSCULAR JUNCTION; NEUROTRANSMITTERS.

Syncope The technical term for FAINTING. The immediate cause of loss of CONSCIOUSNESS is failure of OXYGEN supply to the brain, because of failure of adequate blood flow, due in turn to a severe fall in BLOOD PRESSURE. Syncope usually refers to a 'vaso–vagal' episode, in which the heart is slowed by parasympathetic stimulation (via the VAGUS NERVES), perhaps as a result of fear or disgust, and the blood pressure falls, causing first faintness and then loss of consciousness. Standing or sitting still for a long time can also contribute — gravity tends to 'pool' blood in the legs, causing inadequate return to the heart. In quite different circumstances, a person may 'pass out' due to blood loss, again because of a fall in blood pressure, but in this instance the heart rate is fast. Fainting, with a slow heart rate, occurs also with HEART BLOCK. S.J.

See FAINTING; SHOCK.

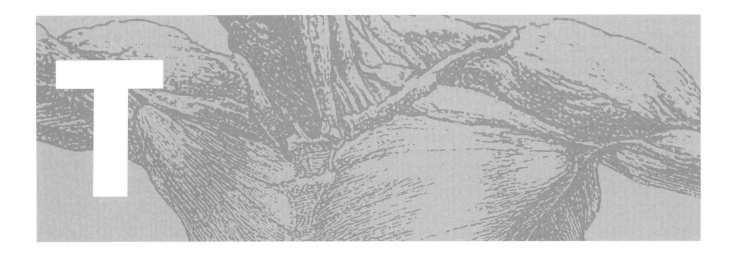

Taboos

Taboos The word 'taboo' passed into English from its Polynesian origin with remarkable rapidity. It was barely seven years from Captain Cook recording it in his journal of the South Seas to its being included in the New English Dictionary of 1791, with the simple meaning of 'forbidden'. The Polynesian concept is more complex. It is said to be derived from the two roots, *ta*, to mark and *pu*, an adverb of intensity — something marked thoroughly, as opposed to *noa*, things not so singled out. In these stratified societies, the persons of chiefs and priests were marked out by their being taboo. They were thus to be avoided by those of lower rank, and must subject themselves to numerous personal restrictions. A measure of their rank and power was also given in their ability to impose taboos on other persons, places, and objects, restricting access to them and making them also into a source of dangerous power. Yet, such 'marked out' things applied not only to the elevated and auspicious but also to the unpropitious and unclean, such as corpses and the new-born.

At one level, taboos shade into other rules of law, custom, or morality; they indicate membership of a given community, just as they support the dominant social system. In Polynesia, infractions of taboo were subject to punishment by the chiefly and priestly hierarchies. But one aspect often considered characteristic of taboo rules is that punishment is automatic, triggered by the infraction itself without further intervention by earthly authorities. Often this takes the form of a disease. Nineteenth-century scholars were perplexed by the combination of ideas involved. Interested in the odd 'dos', they were equally fascinated by the odder 'do nots' of what they took to be primitive religion. Why, for example, should the person of the mother-in-law in many African societies be so utterly revered by a man that he must scrupulously avoid all contact, even sight, of her? And why should even inadvertent breaking of such distance plunge both parties into a state of pollution, contaminating to other persons and bringing in train the threat of direct mystical retribution unless and until the pollution be cleansed? The apparent lack of ethical content, the contagious nature of the fear, the apparent confusion of holy with unclean, could all be seen as the mark of primitive.

It was not until the 1960s, with Mary Douglas's justly famed book, *Purity and danger*, that a new and decisive mode of interpretation was brought to bear on the subject. Adamant that primitive and modern are subject to similar forms of understanding, she begins with our own attitudes to dirt and HYGIENE, arguing that pollution beliefs are a by-product of the way people strive to create order in their lives. Dirt, she argues, taking a clue from Lord Chesterfield, is matter out-of-place. Thus, the concept is always relative to a system of classification; shoes are not dirty in themselves, but only when placed on the dining room table. It follows from this that ideas of dirt or pollution cling to things or behaviour which transgress the dominant schemas of society. From this perspective, dirt appears as a residual category, clinging to the margins and boundaries of things. However, she goes further, in arguing that, far from being solely unfortunate by-products of a system of classification, ideas about pollution are absolutely essential to it. Any system of classification is arbitrary and thus frail, subject to the contradictions of experience. Thus the categories we erect are all-important, because it is only by exaggerating the differences — above/below, inside/outside, male/female, marriageable/unmarriageable — that any semblance of order is created at all. It is here that taboos play their part, for the ambiguity which is perceived at the boundaries of categories can by its very nature be used as a means for demarcating and giving them added force.

With ideas as to the conceptual function of hygienic precepts, she turns to an examination of the abominations of Leviticus, pouring scorn on those who have seen Moses as an enlightened public health administrator, protecting the ancient Israelis against the dangers of eating pork or shellfish. A more literal reading relates us directly to the pattern of the cosmos, with its insistence on the separation of categories. Thus, she argues that pork is forbidden for exactly the reasons given in the dietary laws, which recognize as meat only those animals, like the sheep and cattle of their herds, which chew the cud and are cloven-footed. The pig, which is hoofed but does not chew the cud, is anomalous in this classification and is thus regarded as inedible. So also are other animals such as the camel, hare, and rock badger, because they chew the cud but do not part the hoof. In all such cases, materialist interpretations give way to conceptual ones, to the variable way in which the cosmos is structured.

With this approach, some unity is given to the subject of taboos. The frequency of taboo attitudes surrounding FOOD and things ingested becomes immediately interpretable; as do those concerning bodily waste products such as faeces, urine, sexual emissions, spittle, sweat, hair, and nail clippings. All can be seen to threaten the inviolability of the body's boundaries, the divide between self and not-self.

Again, life passages, such as BIRTH, DEATH, and initiations, which involve the negotiation of social and physical boundaries, are prime sites for such danger beliefs. To take another example, separation is a key idea in Rom Gypsy cosmology, where male and female, upper and lower body, inside and outside, things ingested (through the upper body) and things excreted (from the lower body) must be held rigidly apart. Thus, in Rom communities, the household washing is strictly divided into male and female items, and these in turn divided into those belonging to the top half of the body and those belonging to the bottom. Ideally, these should all be washed in different bowls, and a further bowl is required for food preparation and for washing kitchen utensils. Any breakdown in these prescriptions risks serious pollution, bringing danger to those affected and outcast status to the perpetrator.

Yet the subject in a sense only begins here, for Douglas also wants to explain the culturally variable way in which societies recognize taboos. For Douglas, pollution ideas work at two levels in society: in the first place they carry a symbolic load, making taxonomic schemas that relate to animals and the natural world as well as those that relate to the body metaphors for society. If these operate as part of the tacit, taken-for-granted assumptions of a social world, the second aspect relates them to current and manifest social concerns. Concepts become tactics; metaphysical and practical issues run together as people call down the powers of the cosmos in debates about membership and accountability for misfortune. Insofar as pollution beliefs guard social definitions and distinctions, she suggests they are likely to be strongest in societies in which these are most valued and subject to threat. For example, among the Gypsy, the rules of purity reinforce not only divisions within Rom society itself but also its divide from the wider world of which it forms a part. The fear of wrong-mixing metaphorically reflects the problems experienced by the Rom in maintaining a moral divide between themselves and non-Gypsy outsiders, with whom they must engage on a daily basis for survival.

Yet cultural attitudes to the anomalous and unclassifiable are not always so rejecting. Not only do cultures vary in the strictness of their purity rules, but she suggests that there are limits to the search for purity. This is often apparent in religious contexts, when the normally unclean is transformed into a positive source of potency and power. Liminal phases of rites of passage, carnivals, and fetes are often pervaded by images of chaos and misrule. Through displays of sacrilege and sedition, incest, or cannibalism, the normally abhorred becomes a source for world renewal. Again, in the ascetic traditions of both Christianity and Hinduism, defiling contact with the unclean on the part of its saints and sadhus is seen as a mark of holiness, a sign of freedom from the constraints of this world. In such situations, the arbitrary structuring of the social world, in its cosmological as well as social forms, is recognized and confronted.

SUZETTE HEALD

Further reading
Douglas, M. (1966). *Purity and danger*. Routledge, London.

See also BODY CONTACT; INITIATION RITES; RITES OF PASSAGE.

Tachycardia A rapid heart beat. This happens as a normal response to physical work and exercise, up to a maximum of about 200 beats per minute in a young adult, decreasing with age to about 150 at age 70. This is *sinus tachycardia* and it is brought about by the increased discharge rate of the heart's built-in PACEMAKER, the sino–atrial node, under the influence of the sympathetic nervous system. Likewise heart rate increases in response to excitement or anxiety or to blood loss. *Paroxysmal tachycardia* — disturbing attacks of palpitation — can occur for no apparent reason and often with no evidence of cardiac abnormality. *Ventricular tachycardia* is

more ominous: driven from an abnormal focus of electrical activity in the ventricles themselves.

S.J.

See HEART.

Taste and smell When we eat or drink we perceive a SENSATION that most people call 'taste'. However, we all know that when the nose is blocked, for instance when one has a common cold, the sensation is considerably reduced. This is because it results from a combination of stimulation of chemical receptors (chemoreceptors) in the nose as well as the MOUTH. The chemoreceptors in the mouth are called *gustatory receptors* and those in the nose are *olfactory receptors*. The sensations that result from individual stimulation of these two types of chemoreceptors are respectively taste and smell. Chemoreceptors are not, however, the only SENSORY RECEPTORS involved in the appreciation and discrimination of food and drink. At least two other modalities of sensation affect the overall experience. The smoothness, texture and crunchiness of food are conveyed by mechanoreceptors on the tongue, and throughout the rest of the mouth, including the teeth, and in the pharynx. Thermoreceptors in the mouth also detect the temperature of solids and liquids. Just think of the combination of experiences – touch, fizziness, coolness, acidity and exquisite smells – that make up the experience of drinking champagne. Those who like spices in their food even derive pleasure from the stimulation of receptors normally involved in the sensation of pain (nociception). These nociceptors in the mouth are stimulated by chemicals found in common spices, such as Chilli peppers, and the resulting sensation is referred to as the *common chemical sense.*

The taste/smell system fulfils two separate physiological roles. Not only does it help us to identify 'good' food, containing essential nutrients (salts, carbohydrates, proteins and fats), but it also provides a warning of the unsuitability of harmful and potentially toxic substances by detecting them before they are ingested.

Gustatory receptors
The receptors involved in gustation are found in specialised 'end-organs' called *taste buds*, embedded in the EPITHELIUM that covers the surface of the TONGUE, soft PALATE, PHARYNX, LARYNX and EPIGLOTTIS. However, they are not uniformly distributed in these regions. The taste buds on the tongue are associated with characteristic 'papillae' (from the Latin for pimples), whereas those in the other regions are found on the smooth epithelial surface. In humans, the number of taste buds varies considerably from person to person, with the majority having 2000 to 5000, distributed over the various regions. However, the number can be as low as 500 and as high as 20 000 in some individuals.

The papillae in different regions of the tongue have distinctive shapes and characteristic numbers of taste buds associated with them. Scattered over the main body of the tongue are approximately 200, small, mushroom-shaped (*fungiform*) papillae, which have, on average, only three taste buds each. Larger (*foliate*) papillae are found at the back and sides of the tongue. They consist of up to nine folds of epithelium and have as many as 600 taste buds each. Eight to 12 larger mushroom shaped (*circumvallate*) papillae, each surrounded by a circular trough, lie at the back of the tongue in a V-shaped formation; these have on average 250 taste buds each. Scattered taste buds are also found in the epithelium of the soft palate, pharynx, larynx and epiglottis.

Each taste bud is contacted, at its base, by the terminals of sensory nerve fibres. These taste fibres belong to three different CRANIAL NERVES, connected to the brain. The nerve supply for most of the taste buds on the soft palate and

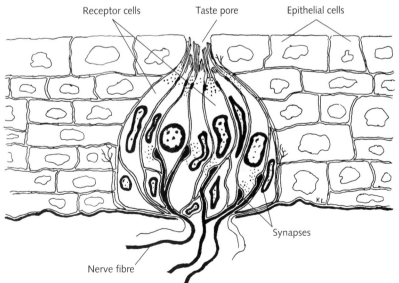

A taste bud, embedded in the epithelium of the tongue. After Linden, R.W.A. (1993) Taste. *British Dental Journal* **175**, 243–53.

towards the front of the tongue come from a division of the VIIth (facial) cranial nerve, called the *chorda tympani*, because its route to the brainstem passes close to the tympanic membrane in the ear. The IXth (glossopharyngeal) and Xth (VAGUS) nerves innervate taste buds in the back of the mouth and the pharynx respectively.

Each taste bud contains 50-150 neuroepithelial receptor cells arranged, like segments of an orange, to form a compact, pear-shaped structure, about 70 μm high and 40 μm in diameter. There is a small 2-10 μm opening in the epithelial surface called the taste pore, which allows direct contact between chemicals dissolved in the SALIVA and the tips of the receptor cells. These exposed parts of the receptor cells are made up of many long corrugated folds in the membrane called *microvilli*, which provide a greater surface area for contact with the saliva. It is difficult to taste food with a dry mouth. Saliva is essential for normal taste because it acts as both a solvent for the chemicals as well as a transport medium for those chemicals to reach the receptors. A layer of saliva extends into the taste pores and constantly bathes the receptors. The dissolved chemicals diffuse through this thin layer of saliva to reach the microvilli. Reflex secretion of saliva from the salivary glands under the tongue and in the cheeks is stimulated by chewing, taste and smell, to varying degrees. And, as Ivan PAVLOV demonstrated in his classical experiments on dogs, the simple form of unconscious learning known as CONDITIONING couples the reflex secretion of saliva to the familiar signs of an impending meal – the sound of a dinner bell, the clatter of crockery, the sight of the food.

The taste bud complex is a dynamic system in which the receptor cells are rapidly turning over. The life-span of an individual receptor cell is about 10 days: cells are continually being born (through the division of epithelial STEM CELLS within the bud), maturing, performing their gustatory function and eventually dying. Even though the receptor cell does not itself have an axon or fibre, the base of the cell has specialised regions that look like the terminals of nerve fibres. The cytoplasm in these regions is packed with tiny spherical vesicles, filled with a chemical transmitter substance, which is released when the potential inside the receptor cell becomes more positive (depolarisation). In close association with these regions are the endings of the sensory nerve fibres, making an assembly like a SYNAPSE. Each taste bud is innervated by more than one nerve fibre and each single nerve fibre can connect to a number of receptor cells, taste buds and even papillae. This suggests a high degree of convergence of input from taste buds on to the sensory nerve fibres. Because of the rapid turnover of receptor cells, the connections between cells and nerve fibres is constantly changing. The nerves are continuously sprouting new processes, forming new synapses with young cells and retracting synaptic connections with dying cells. At any one time less than a third of the cells in the taste bud are innervated.

An intact nerve supply is necessary for the normal function of taste buds. If the nerves are damaged the taste buds degenerate and slough off, and following regeneration of the nerves, the taste buds reappear.

Since the time of Aristotle (384-322 BC) there have been attempts to categorize taste into primary or basic tastes. Although many hundreds of different chemicals can stimulate activity in taste receptor cells, the four basic taste qualities of salt, sour, sweet and bitter have stood the test of time. However, there is still controversy as to whether combination of these four primary tastes adequately describes all gustatory experiences. Metallic and astringent tastes have, in the past, been suggested as primaries, and more recently Japanese researchers have proposed that the characteristic taste of monosodium glutamate (used as a taste enhancer by the food industry) is also a basic taste, with its own receptive mechanism. They have called it "*umami*" meaning "delicious taste".

Because of the dual role of gustatory receptor cells, detecting both nutrients and toxins, they must be able to respond, either individually or collectively, to a wide variety of chemicals. These chemicals range from simple ions such as sodium (salt) and hydrogen (sour) to the more complex compounds that give the sensations of sweet (e.g. sugar) and bitter (e.g. quinine). The mechanisms by which the chemical stimuli are translated into electrical events in the receptor cell (*transduction*) are numerous, varied and complex. The essential process depends on specific interactions between taste substances and specialized protein receptor molecules embedded in the membrane of the receptor cell, which trigger a series of chemical reactions, leading to a change in the flow of ions through pores in the membrane, and hence a change in the electrical potential inside the cell. However, there does not appear to be a unique mechanism for each of the basic tastes: each seems to use several different mechanisms. There may even be similarities of mechanism for different basic tastes. The way in which we can perceive many subtle tastes and distinguish between different compounds of the same basic taste category might be explained by the multiplicity and specificity of these mechanisms.

The evidence for a particular receptor mechanism is best for sweet sensation. First, certain drugs have specific effects on the detection of sweetness. For instance, after eating a West African fruit called *miracle fruit*, even quite acidic substances (such as lemon juice), which would normally be sour, taste extraordinarily sweet. Miracle fruit contains a substance that is thought to attach to the protein receptor molecules that detect sweet-tasting substances. A subsequent increase in acidity in the saliva is thought to alter the binding of this substance with the sweet receptor protein such that it stimulates the receptor, like a genuine sweet substance. In contrast, gymnemic acid, found in an Indian plant, *Gymnema sylvestre*, blocks the sweet receptor in

some manner, and abolishes the sensation of sweetness for half an hour or so. Very recently, a gene called T1r2 has been identified in mice, which is selectively switched on in taste bud receptor cells. It turns out that strains of mice that lack sweet taste (they don't prefer sweet food to non-sweet) have a mutation of this gene. There is a very similar gene in human beings.

Researchers have recorded with tiny electrodes from individual nerve fibres innervating the taste buds, in anaesthetised animals. One might have expected that each fibre would respond, with a burst of impulses, when a solution of just one of the primary taste substances was dripped on to the appropriate taste bud or buds. Such selectivity of response is, in fact, very rare. Most nerve fibres respond to two or more of the basic taste stimuli, the magnitude of the response varying from one taste substance to another. In other words, the activity of such a fibre does not provide unambiguous information to the brain about the nature of the stimulus. At some point the brain must perform a comparison between the activity in several different nerve fibres in order to decide what the taste actually is.

The signals from the taste buds are relayed, via a chain of nerve cells and fibres, at various cell stations in the BRAINSTEM and THALAMUS, up to the cerebral cortex. Some experiments in monkeys suggest that nerve cells at higher levels in the taste pathway respond more selectively, with a larger proportion of them essentially responding to only one basic taste. At the first relay in the brainstem almost no neurons respond to one taste, yet in the taste area of the cortex, about 75% of neurons respond to a single taste.

The 'common chemical sense' is the sensation caused by the stimulation of free nerve endings by potentially harmful chemicals. The evidence suggests that the free nerve endings are 'polymodal' nociceptors (receptive nerve endings that respond to mechanical, thermal and noxious stimulation). Amongst the chemicals that are known to stimulate these receptors, besides noxious, damaging chemicals, are alcohol, menthol, peppermint and capsaicin (chilli pepper).

Olfactory receptors

The human olfactory organ, the olfactory epithelium or mucosa, is a sheet of cells 100 –200 μm thick, situated high in the back of the nose cavity and on the thin bony partition (the central septum) of the nasal passage. The olfactory system responds to airborne, volatile molecules that gain access to the olfactory epithelium with the in-and-out airflow through and behind the nose. The odour molecules are distributed over the receptor sheet in an irregular pattern by the turbulence of the airflow set up by the turbinate bones in the side walls of the nose. The molecules diffuse through the surface layer of mucus and stimulate the olfactory receptors. Hydrophilic (water-soluble) molecules dissolve readily in the mucus, but the diffusion of less soluble molecules is assisted by 'odour binding proteins' in the mucus. These odour binding proteins are also thought to assist in removing odour molecules from the receptor cells. The mucus layer moves across the surface of the olfactory mucosa at 10 to 60 mm per minute toward the nasopharynx (the continuous of the nasal cavity backwards and downwards to link to the pharynx. This flow of mucus (which is increased and becomes more watery in such conditions as infection of the nasal cavity and hay fever), also assists in the removal of odours after they have been sensed.

The olfactory epithelium contains specialized, elongated nerve cells (olfactory receptors). These cells have very thin fibres that run upwards in bundles through perforations in the skull (the *cribriform plate*) above the roof of the nasal cavity, below the frontal lobes of the BRAIN. These bundles of nerves constitute the Ist cranial nerve, the olfactory nerve. They extend only a very short distance, ending in the olfactory bulbs, which are a pair of swellings underneath the frontal lobes.

The other end of each olfactory receptor, pointing down into the nasal cavity, is extended into a long process, ending in a knob carrying several hairs (cilia) between 20 and 200 μm in length. These cilia are bathed in a thin (35 μm-thick) layer of mucus, secreted by specialized cells in the olfactory epithelium, in which the molecules of odorous substances dissolve. In the membrane of the cilia are olfactory receptor proteins, which interact with the smelly molecules, and initiate a cascade reaction inside the cell that leads to a change in the rate of impulses (ACTION POTENTIALS) passing along the nerve fibre.

Human beings are able to distinguish 10 000 or more different odours. There have been valiant attempts to classify these into a smaller number (usually 10-20) basic or primary smells, comparable to the four or so primary tastes, but no scheme is universally accepted. The human nose (not to mention that of a sniffer dog) can be incredibly sensitive to very low concentrations of odorous substances. Certain male moths use similar receptor cells on their antennae to detect even single molecules of a PHEROMONE secreted by female moths.

Individual olfactory receptor neurons fire off spontaneously at between 3 and 60 impulses per second. When stimulated with particular odours they increase their firing frequency. Each receptor cell responds, but not equally, to many different types of odour. As in the gustatory system, the successive nerve cells in the pathway become more selective, each responding to fewer odours. Interestingly, despite the poor selectivity of individual receptor cells, different regions of the olfactory sheet (consisting of hundred or thousands of receptor cells) are maximally responsive to particular odours. The overall pattern of activity in the olfactory epithelium can be mapped with electrical recording methods (electro-olfactogram) or other techniques for detecting active regions. Each distinctive odour produces its own 'fingerprint' of activity across the epithelium. This mapping is thought to reflect the patterns of expression (activation) of genes that make the receptor proteins in the receptor cell membranes. A huge family of odour receptor genes exists in the mouse, perhaps as many as 5% of all the genes.

The spatial coding of odour quality is transmitted to the first relay of the olfactory pathway, the olfactory bulb. There is a loose topographical projection from the receptor sheet to the bulb, where the axons form synapses with neurons called *mitral cells*. The olfactory bulb contains a complex network of nerve cells and is responsible for a considerable amount of sensory processing. Hence, neurons in the olfactory bulb respond with one distinct temporal pattern of impulses to one odour and different patterns to another smells. The mitral cells send their fibres into the olfactory tracts, which run backwards. Some end in the THALAMUS, which in turn sends fibres up to the olfactory cortex. The neurons of the olfactory cortex are still not highly specific for particular odours. Other fibres of the olfactory tract have direct connections to areas of the limbic system around the region of the hypothalamus. Since the LIMBIC SYSTEM is thought to be responsible for regulating emotions, this might explain the fact that smells can evoke strong feelings of enjoyment or aversion (the hedonic component of sensation).

Unlike other stimuli, olfactory stimuli are not very time-dependent. The effects of visual, tactile and auditory stimulation follow the stimulus immediately, whereas some olfactory stimuli, such as those left by animals when marking their territory, remain when the animal is long gone. In this way olfactory stimuli, and their behavioural and social effects, can have more lasting consequences.

The olfactory system occupies a smaller fraction of the brain in humans than in many other species, and this is part of the evidence for the commonly-held belief that people are generally inferior in their sense of smell. Studies in other animals, from insects to hamsters to monkeys, have revealed the importance of olfaction for many aspects of behaviour, especially reproduction. For example, male rhesus monkeys use smell to sense the hormonal status of females (ovulating or not), with a marked effect on their level of sexual activity. But even in humans, there is growing evidence that olfaction (mainly unconscious) is important in such functions as sexual preference, and recognition of other people.   R.W.A. LINDEN

See also BRAIN; CEREBRAL CORTEX; LIMBIC SYSTEM; NOSE; PHEROMONES; SENSATION; SENSORY RECEPTORS; TONGUE.

Tattooing The tattoo — an indelible coloured image on the skin, is historically the most commonly practised form of permanent BODY DECORATION. Tattooing is thought to have diffused from Egypt about four thousand years ago; it has been found since then in most cultures of the world, though among dark-skinned peoples incised decoration (scarification, cicatrization) is a more common form of permanent alteration. Carved figures suggestive of tattooing survive in Egypt from 6000 BCE but the physical evidence of mummified bodies dates from Middle Kingdom Egypt (*c.* 2000 BCE). Widespread archaeological and literary evidence of tattooing since the seventh century BCE exists for many parts of Eurasia, and ethnographic evidence for these and other parts of the world, including the Americas, Africa, Polynesia, and New Zealand, has been collected since the sixteenth century.

The technique involves puncturing the dermis with a needle or other sharp instrument to a depth of 0.25–0.5 cm and simultaneously applying a dark pigment. The pigment rests in linear strata in the dermis; the fading and blurring of older tattoos is due to local dispersal of pigment through the lymphatic system. Small-scale needle tattoos are relatively painless, unless on sensitive areas of the body, but elaborate or semi-incised designs are a more severe ordeal. Temporary local inflammation may occur; more serious medical complications may develop where hygienic standards are poor (for example, from cross-infections through contaminated needles, or from use of harmful pigments), though more rarely than might be expected. Tattoos can be removed by various means, including dermabrasion, excision and suturing, and laser surgery, though usually with some residual scarring.

In pre-literate societies where tattooing is culturally embedded, the practice is normally highly ritualized, and alongside its decorative value it carries information about status and identity, as well as religious, therapeutic, or prophylactic significance. Designs are enormously varied in imagery and location, from the elaborate geometrical designs across arms, legs, and abdomen of Burma or the Marquesas; to the miniature stylized images of Gujarati tattooing; the elaborate curvilinear form of New Zealand *moko* tattooing on men, which combined incision and pigmentation to produce individually unique facial designs; or the vivid figurative images of Japanese *irezumi*, derived from eighteenth-century wood-block illustrations and patterned onto the body like ornate clothing. The English term 'tattoo' (from the Polynesian *tatu/tatau* — mark, strike), versions of which were adopted into other European languages, testifies to the profound significance of the eighteenth-century encounter with the Pacific cultures for the spread of tattooing in modern Europe. Alternative and older European words, carrying connotations of marking or piercing (e.g. English 'pounce', Dutch 'prickschilderen', French 'piqûre'), suggest that tattooing must have been known in Europe before its eighteenth-century reimportation and renaming, but the extent of its survival from the Scythian, Celtic, and Germanic customs documented in classical sources (e.g. Herodotus, Tacitus) is unclear. Greeks and Romans disdained the practice as barbarian; in the Roman empire it was used only on criminals, slaves/

indentured labourers, and soldiers. This outcast association was strengthened when the medieval western Church picked up and repeated the biblical proscription of body-marking (cf. Lev. 19:28). There is thus little reference to tattooing in medieval and early modern Europe — but there is scattered evidence of its popular survival within Europe or on its margins. Tattoos were certainly acquired by European crusaders and pilgrims in Jerusalem, as also by pilgrims to the medieval Italian shrine of Loreto and by Coptic Christians and Bosnian Catholics. However, decorative tattooing was largely effaced from European cultural memory before the eighteenth century, and its recurrence was marked by the absorption of a new and diverse repertoire of secular images from popular culture, many of which remain familiar today. (A similar process of cultural forgetting and marginalization seems to have occurred in Japan, where a revival of highly skilled tattoo artistry coexisted with more strenuous official attempts to suppress it in the nineteenth century.)

Even after its eighteenth-century reimportation, via European sailors, from Polynesia and New Zealand, and a brief period as an exotic novelty, tattooing retained its association with disreputability, though to differing degrees. In continental Europe, it was regarded as the habit of common soldiers, sailors, labourers, and criminals, or was displayed by fairground and freak-show entertainers. In Britain, by contrast, tattoo images were widely sported by naval and military officers, despite the fact that tattoos were also used as penal marks in the army until the 1870s; little social stigma attached to the practice, and its adoption by aristocrats and royalty helped spark a tattooing craze around the turn of the century that spread throughout Europe and the US. Britain and the US also saw the first professionalization of tattooing, the invention (1891) of an electrical tattooing machine, and the improvement of techniques and inks. This period of popularity was short-lived, however, and the 1920s–50s saw the social and aesthetic decline of tattooing in Western culture. However, since the 1960s successive periods of reinvention and expansion have given it an unprecedented prominence and visibility, and women have entered this previously largely male domain. The tattoo is currently enjoying a cultural renaissance, alongside and perhaps by contrast with other body-altering practices of scarifying, branding, and extensive piercing, which have entered modern Western culture for the first time.

Medical interest in the tattoo since the nineteenth century has included research into its anatomy and pathology, its applications in COSMETIC SURGERY, and means of its removal. In modern scholarship, tattooing has been the province of ANTHROPOLOGY for pre-literate societies, and of criminology, sociology, and psychology for non-tribal societies. Thus in the West it has been largely pathologized as the expression of a marginal subculture of resistance, associated

especially with communities of male confinement and group identification. Only recently has this perspective shifted, and the history, ethnography, and aesthetics of tattooing in the West become more serious subjects of study.

JANE CAPLAN

Further reading

Caplan, J. (ed.) (2000). *Written on the Body. The Tattoo in European and American History.* Reaktion Books, London and Princeton University Press, Princeton, NJ.

DeMello, M. (2000). *A Cultural History of the Modern Tattoo Community.* Duke University Press, Durham and London.

Gell, A. (1993). *Wrapping in images. Tattooing in Polynesia.* Clarendon Press, Oxford.

Rubin, A. (ed.) (1988). *Marks of civilization. Artistic transformations of the human body.* Museum of Cultural History, Los Angeles.

See also BODY DECORATION; BODY MUTILATIONS AND MARKINGS.

Teeth have a distinctive anatomy and physiology that is different to the biology of the SKELETON. The great eighteenth-century zoologist and anatomist Baron Georges Cuvier was once quoted as saying, 'show me your teeth and I will tell you who you are.'

Our teeth tell us something about our ancestry, ethnic background, and age, our environment and our health. Teeth are one of the hardest tissues in our body and a valuable source of evidence in understanding the biology of ancient communities throughout the evolution of mankind. Teeth can be used as part of our repertoire of behaviour, by showing or 'baring' one's teeth as a means of aggression, or by adding them to a perfect smile. The movement of teeth during eating can stimulate reflex salivation or can limit damage if excessive force is applied. Teeth can therefore serve a variety of functions in our lives from the time that the first deciduous (milk or primary) teeth appear, a process commonly known as teething. By the age of 3 the deciduous teeth are fully formed and by the age of 6 the first permanent teeth appear by displacing their predecessors. A complete permanent *dentition* (set of teeth) is present at or around the age of 18 years. In the complete deciduous dentition there are 20 teeth, 10 in each jaw. In the complete permanent dentition there are 32 teeth, 16 in each jaw. There are different classes of teeth each with a particular role in eating; incisors (Latin *dentes incisivi*; cutting teeth), canines (Latin *dentes canini*; dog teeth), premolars, and molars (Latin *dentes molars*; grinding teeth).

Each tooth is divided into a crown that projects into the mouth and a root that is embedded into the jaws. The crown is coated with heavily mineralized *enamel* and the root with a thin layer of cement. The visible crown surface is usually smooth, translucent, and white but may show defects in thickness, mineralization, and colour. During development these defects can be attributed to an interruption of the normal growth

processes due to malnutrition or diseases (such as rickets and measles) or to high levels of fluoride in drinking water. Betel nut chewing and smoking can also lead to discolouration.

The bulk of the tooth consists of the bony substance dentine, surrounding the soft inner pulp that contains blood vessels and nerves. In the crown, the pulp has small conical extensions (pulp horns) into the cusps of the tooth, and in the root it extends along one or more canals to the tooth apex, where the nerves and blood vessels enter. The density of nerve fibres in dental pulp is very high; in the mid crown of the average tooth there may be as many as 3000 axon branches with approximately 2000 nerve endings per mm^2, the highest density in the body. The role these nerve fibres play in the normal sensations from teeth has been a point of conjecture for dentists for over a century, but whatever the stimulus it invariably leads to the pain usually described as toothache which, according to Robert Burns was, 'the hell o' a' disease'.

Sufferers are well aware that a tooth can become acutely sensitive. Yet there are no nerve endings on the exposed surface. The mystery of the process that activates the nerve endings inside the teeth has only recently been solved. The dentine contains a honeycomb of dentinal tubules that radiate out from the pulp chamber, tapering along their length and increasing in spacing. At the pulp end of dentinal tubules is a layer of cells called *odontoblasts*. These cells secrete the initial *predentine matrix* and mineralize it to produce mature dentine. At the dentinal surface of each odontoblast is a process arising from the cell, which tapers as it penetrates up to half the thickness of the dentine. Some of the dentinal tubules containing odontoblast processes also have nerve fibres and most, if not all, also contain dentinal fluid that is formed from the blood capillaries in the pulp. Under normal circumstances the whole system is in equilibrium, with little movement of dentinal fluid, and the tooth is relatively insensitive. Only when the dentinal tubules are open to the atmosphere through damage, disease such as caries, or wear of the enamel (through the excessive use of a toothbrush or acidic drinks) can the dentinal fluid flow out through the tubules into the mouth (see figure of exposed dentine, showing movement of dentinal fluid). Despite the lack of nerve endings at the exposed surface, the area is now acutely sensitive to thermal, mechanical, and osmotic stimuli. An explanation for this apparent paradox involves the nerve fibres at the pulpal end of the dentinal tubules, and the dentinal fluid, which forms a hydraulic bridge. Most investigators now agree that the movement of fluid due to changes in pressure or in surface tension at the open end of exposed dentinal tubules is transferred through the odontoblast process to nerve endings at the base of the tubules. The dentinal fluid in the tubules can now move when a stimulus is applied, and it is this movement that is picked up by the nerve endings — the sensory receptors. All manner of stimuli would then

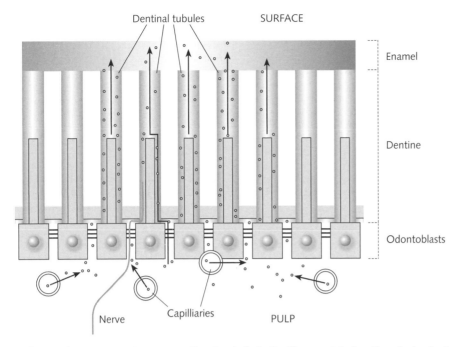

Dentinal tubules

SURFACE

Enamel

Dentine

Odontoblasts

Nerve

Capilliaries

PULP

A schematic diagram representing a cross section of part of a tooth with exposed dentine. The pulp chamber is richly supplied by nerve fibres and blood vessels. Exposing the dentine allows the fluid content of the dentinal tubules to move, thus exciting the sensory nerve endings at their base; this eventually gives rise to dental pain.

cause fluid movement; *temperature* — heat greater than 45°C, cold less than 27°C; *mechanical* — use of a dental bur, a probe, or a toothbrush; *removal of fluid* by an air stream, absorbent materials, or hyperosmotic solutions such as strong sugar solutions. Blocking the dentinal tubules using dental resins restores the equilibrium and the tooth will once again become relatively insensitive. Thus the hydraulic or *hydrodynamic* theory of movement of fluid through the dentinal tubules goes some way to explaining this exquisitely sensitive and unique system of receptors that occasionally gives rise to the 'sensitivity' of teeth.

DUNCAN BANKS

Further reading
Bradley, R. M. (1995). *Essentials of oral physiology.* Mosby, St Louis.

See also DENTISTRY.

Temperament From at least classical times, temperament has referred to an individual's or a group's consistent and stable pattern of behaviour or reaction, one that persists across time, activity, and space. The roots of the theory of temperament lie in classical Greek medicine and astronomy. A central component of the humoral theory of the body, temperament ('*crasis*' in Greek) denoted the particular balance of the four primary qualities — hot, wet, cold, and dry — characteristic of a given individual in a healthy condition. The mixture was fixed at birth, largely through astrological influences, though modifications could occur with ageing, changes in environment, disease, geography, etc. Although each person was deemed to have

his or her own individual temperament, they were generally described as variations on four basic types: choleric, melancholic, sanguine, and phlegmatic. These states were at once physiological and psychological, denoting both the organization of the internal body and what might be called an attitude toward life. Galen's *On Complexions*, drawing on Hippocratic sources and the ideas of the Pneumatics, presents an elaborated account of the theory of temperaments (*complexio* in Latin), one that had much influence on medieval medical authors. According to ancient and medieval medical theory, most internal illnesses could be explained as the result of complexional imbalances, and therapy consisted of various interventions designed to restore the proper mixture of the four elements. Because temperament was understood to be something individual, however, remedies had to be patient-specific, tailored to the unique complexion of the particular sufferer.

The medical theory of temperament began to lose favour in the early modern period. As a characterization of a person's psychological state, however, temperament continued to be employed by both psychologists and the lay public well into the twentieth century. In general, the concept has continued to refer to something both physiological and innate, although there is much dispute in the literature over whether temperaments are inborn or develop early in life through an interaction of genetic and environmental factors. Whatever their origin, it is widely accepted that temperaments both help to shape, and are themselves shaped by, the social environments in which an individual develops and lives, and that they represent

styles of thought and behaviour that are both personal and consistent. As an individual develops, it is his or her temperament that helps to orient that development, influencing the growth of both intellect and character along particular lines.

While the possible varieties of temperament are almost limitless, psychologists have identified a number of dimensions — including relative ego strength, radicalism–conservatism, dominance–submissiveness, and extroversion– interoversion — that they believe characterize important aspects of an individual's temperament. Research on temperaments has generally been oriented toward determining whether a functional unity exists within a given constellation of behaviours, so that it can be demonstrated that a recognizable style of action persists from one domain to another. Since the 1950s to 1960s, psychoanalytic ego psychology, personality psychology, and cognitive psychology have all become more interested in the phenomena associated with temperament, seeking to identify and understand individual differences or cognitive styles that are consistent across settings. It remains the case, however, that the term itself has fallen largely into disuse, especially within professional circles.

JOHN CARSON

See also PERSONALITY.

Temperature regulation The human body is a heat-generating object. Even at complete rest at a comfortable temperature, the vital functions of the body generate heat. When it is at a minimum this is called basal metabolic heat. Heat production rises with activity: the more vigorous the activity the greater the quantity of heat produced. Excess heat has to be lost. Considering this variation in internal heat production, together with the wide variety of thermal environments inhabited by humans, it is remarkable that, except during exercise or fever, the body temperature can be kept within such narrow limits. This is achieved partly by the physiological mechanisms that control the rate of heat loss and heat production to achieve a balance. If the rate of heat loss exceeds the rate of heat production, the body temperature will fall, leading ultimately to hypothermia. Conversely, if the rate of heat loss is less than the rate of heat production, or is defected by external heating the body temperature will rise, leading eventually to heatstroke. Death may be the end result of either.

Body temperature is controlled through a central mechanism in the BRAIN which, while it acts in a manner similar to a thermostat, is not a simple on/off device but is more akin to a 'black box' with a complex system of neurons cross-linking the sensory input and the effector output. The thermostat is activated by impulses from central receptors, which detect changes in the temperature of the BLOOD, and from peripheral receptors mainly in the SKIN. The thermostat regulates the temperature of the body by adjusting heat production and heat loss, but the setting of the thermostat itself may be altered. During SLEEP the cerebral thermostat is reset to a new low level, skin BLOOD VESSELS relax, causing an immediate rise in skin temperature and heat loss, and the metabolic rate is reduced.

There are racial variations in the response to heat and cold, and at the extremes of age there is an increased risk of HYPOTHERMIA and heatstroke. Many medical disorders and a range of drugs predispose to temperature disorders.

Heat is lost, and gained, through convection, radiation, and conduction, while evaporation contributes only to heat loss. Even for humans, the standard thermodynamic laws of physics apply. The rate at which the body loses heat depends on the temperature difference between the skin and the environment. In the cold, therefore, the aim is to reduce the skin temperature as much as possible, whereas in the heat the skin temperature should be as high as possible.

Conductive heat transfer depends on the surface area in contact with a substance, the temperature of the substance, and its thermal conductivity. Air is a poor conductor of heat, and therefore most insulating systems, including clothing, act by trapping air. Conductive transfer is high in water. Wet clothing not only has decreased insulating properties, but it rapidly conducts heat from the body to the colder surface of the clothing. In an emergency in the cold, conductive heat loss may be forgotten, with the casualty being well covered with blankets but continuing to lie with nothing between him and the ground.

Convective heat loss is increased by wind, hence the 'wind chill' index, which gives the total heat loss under any particular combination of cold and wind speed, and relates it to the still air temperature which would produce the same rate of heat loss. The rate of heat loss at −10°C in still air is almost exactly the same as that at +10°C with a 10 mph wind. Convective heat loss is also increased by movement, not only by the person physically moving forward but also through the 'pendulum' movement of the limbs, and through the clothing producing a bellows effect and blowing warm air out to be replaced by cold air, or water, at the next movement. Increasing convective loss is dangerous in the cold but beneficial in the heat.

Radiant heat exchange is often overlooked. Standing near a glacier causes a feeling of chill even though there is no contact and no wind. Similarly, people may gain heat radiating from hot walls, concrete, or sand in a hot environment, as well as from fires or central heating radiators in the cold.

Evaporation is an effective way of losing heat because of the high latent heat of evaporation. However, the rate of evaporation depends on the surface area of fluid and its vapour pressure immediately above the surface. Evaporative heat loss is greatest when the air is dry and the moisture vapour is constantly being removed from the body surface, and least when there is high humidity and no air movement. Any factor which increases convective heat loss also increases

evaporative heat loss. In man evaporative heat loss occurs through sweating and when clothing is wet. Wet clothing is used to reduce the temperature in heatstroke.

In animals with LUNGS, heat is also lost by warming and humidifying the inspired air during breathing, with the greater proportion being through humidification. Even in a mist in winter, with an ambient relative humidity of 100%, when the inspired air is warmed to core body temperature the relative humidity falls and the body expends heat in raising the relative humidity to 100% before it reaches the alveolar surfaces of the lung. Although some of the heat and moisture is retrieved from the air on its way out again, in temperate conditions 10–15% of the total heat loss from the body is from the respiratory tract, and the proportion increases in colder or drier air.

In the cold

The body responds by constriction of the superficial blood vessels, mainly via the sympathetic nervous system but also through direct action of cold on the blood vessels. Vasoconstriction is very effective in reducing heat loss by limiting blood flow to the periphery, thus increasing the depth of 'shell' insulation and reducing the temperature differential between the skin and the environment (see Figure). In fact vasoconstriction can result in the outermost inch of the body having a thermal conductivity equivalent to that of cork. To reduce the surface area exposed to cold the person may adopt a ball-like fetal position. There is also a counter-current exchange of heat between the arteries and veins in the distal half of the limbs. Below a limb temperature of 10–12°C the peripheral vasoconstriction fails and alternating vasodilatation and vasoconstriction occurs, though there may actually be very little increase in the volume of blood circulating in the skin during the vasodilatation, which would preserve the insulating effect of the vasoconstriction. Though there is some vasoconstriction in the face, it is minimal in the scalp, and this plus the lack of tissue depth makes the regulation of heat loss from the head inefficient; the rate of heat loss by this route increases in a linear manner between ambient temperatures of +32°C and −20°C, and indeed may be equal to half the total body heat production at rest at −4°C. Mental stress even of as mild a degree as mental arithmetic increases this heat loss, as also do nausea, vomiting, fainting, trauma, and haemorrhage.

Heat production rises with muscle activity, either deliberate activity (10–15-fold during hard physical exercise) or shivering. In severe cold stress CATECHOLAMINE secretion increases and stimulates increased heat production. The less fit a person is, the less the degree of cold stress at which the catecholamine 'overdrive' occurs. Any increase in heat production is always accompanied by a rise in OXYGEN consumption: in shivering it may double or treble. Activity and shivering are not economical in thermo-

regulation, because they are accompanied by an increased blood supply to the muscles and this in turn raises the surface temperature and increases heat loss. In fact only 48% of the extra heat generated is retained in the body.

The greatest rate of heat production which an individual can achieve depends on his maximal ability for muscular work, linked to his maximal rate of oxygen usage. This in turn depends on the supply of oxygen and therefore on the greatest rate at which the heart can pump blood around the body, and on the efficiency with which the muscles can utilize the oxygen. These all increase with improving fitness. For any level of exercise the oxygen consumption and cardiac output need to be higher in a cold environment than in a warm one; this explains, for example, why angina may develop during a particular level of activity in the cold but not at normal temperatures. Also, during sleep in the cold, unfit people are repeatedly awakened by shivering, whereas the greater heat generating ability of 'fit' muscles allows sleep undisturbed by shivering.

In conditions of very severe cold, if the person has to undertake very vigorous exercise, the maximal oxygen uptake may be insufficient to provide for the high demand of both the exercise and the severe cold stress, and a person can develop unexpected and unsuspected hypothermia despite vigorous muscular activity. If hypoxia is also present, as at high altitude, this decreases the total possible oxygen uptake, and therefore heat production and shivering may be inhibited. Finally, if the person is exhausted or suffering from malnutrition he cannot increase heat production because of the lack of substrate (fuel) for metabolism.

Alcohol produces a number of effects which increase the risk of hypothermia; the greatest danger is decreasing the awareness of cold and increasing bravado, while impairing the ability to assess risks.

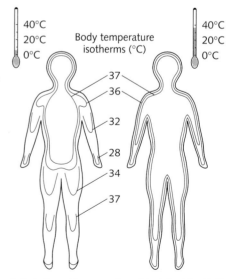

Left: In the cold: conservation of body heat by 'shell' insulation. Right: In the heat: increasing heat loss by warming the skin.

In the heat

The skin and superficial blood vessels open up and the skin temperature rises, thus increasing the possibility of heat loss. Sweating increases and, in a dry, hot environment, evaporation can become the major means of losing heat. Unfortunately in a hot and humid environment there is less scope for evaporation, and sweating becomes less effective. The person tends to adopt an 'open' posture e.g. lying spread-eagled to maximize the surface area available. This is usually done for suntanning but also works for heat loss. By contrast with the cold, there is little scope for adjusting the production of heat except by reducing activity.

In fever the thermostat in the brain is set at a higher level. Therefore the person shivers to raise the temperature to the new, higher setting, and, when the fever breaks and the thermostat setting drops back to normal, the person sweats to dispose of the (now) excess heat.

Clothing and shelter

Clothes are the obvious protection from the cold, especially those that trap air. It is more efficient to have several thin layers than one thick. Cold weather clothing effectively reduces the temperature of the outermost surface and therefore reduces heat loss. A windproof layer stops or reduces convective loss. In the heat, clothing should be thin and loose to cause the least barrier to heat loss by conduction and convection. White or light-coloured clothing reduces the heat load by reflecting radiant heat.

Shelter may take many forms, from simply sheltering behind a boulder or digging a snow hole to the high technology of modern housing. In cold climates houses tend to have wooden floors with carpets, fires or central heating, attic insulation, and double glazing, and everything is done to reduce draughts. In a hot climate many houses have stone floors, the windows and doors are placed opposite each other to encourage through draughts, and the buildings are often painted white to reflect radiant heat from the sun.

Comfort

Humans are very sensitive to differences and changes in temperature, especially changes downwards. The sensation of cold is related to the lowered average skin temperature, and the sensation of local cold becomes more intense with increasing duration of exposure. A hot or cold stimulus is considered pleasant when it tends to restore temperature towards normal, and unpleasant if it has the reverse tendency. Thus cold applied to the skin is pleasant if the core temperature is raised but unpleasant if the core temperature is lowered. A person may feel warm on moving from the cold into the warmth, even if the body temperature is still low; this suggests that the discomfort caused by cold may be the result of the superficial vasoconstriction. Subjective discomfort is greater if certain areas, such as the forehead or feet, are cold, and the discomfort is increased by shivering. Because cold is a common human experience, the fact that it can cause injury, illness, and death is often overlooked.

Symptomless cooling

The central thermostat responds to the rate of firing of temperature-sensitive neurons, and the rate of firing is partially dependent on the rate of change of the stimulus. If the peripheral and central temperatures change slowly enough, the body may fail to activate the mechanisms for reducing heat loss and increasing heat production. During experimental cooling (in a water bath) it is possible to abolish shivering and the sensation of cold without interrupting the progressive reduction in body temperature, by slightly raising the temperature of the water, and therefore of the skin, at the onset of shivering; the perceived warmth is increased although the water temperature remains cold enough to cause continued cooling.

Perceived warmth has practical and clinical implications:

(i) Deep divers have hot water flowing over the surface of the body, which gives a sensation of warmth whilst it may not be enough to balance the large quantities of heat they lose through breathing cold oxyhelium. They may therefore become hypothermic while feeling warm.

(ii) Coming out of a refrigerated room at −30°C into a cold room at 0°C gives a feeling of warmth and comfort but the risk of hypothermia is still present, especially if the person is moving frequently between the two chambers.

(iii) For the elderly a single bar fire in a large cold room gives a sensation of warmth which prevents vasoconstriction and therefore allows an increased heat loss for which the heat from the small fire cannot compensate; so they can become hypothermic without being aware of discomfort. Inadequate heating may therefore be more dangerous than no heating.

It is salutary to realize that humans can live in and explore very hostile areas of the world, not because of the physiology of thermoregulation, but because of man's technological ability to manipulate his thermal environment by the use of clothing, heating, and shelter. The proof of this is the fact that the temperature of the skin of the abdominal wall is the same in the Arctic as in the tropics.

EVAN L. LLOYD

Further reading

Lloyd, E. L. (1986). *Hypothermia and cold stress.* Croom Helm, London.

Maclean, D. and Emslie-Smith, D. (1977). *Accidental hypothermia.* Blackwell, Oxford.

See also COLD EXPOSURE; HEAT EXPOSURE; HYPOTHERMIA; SWEATING.

Tendons

are the tough extensions of muscles that attach them to BONES, usually focusing the pull of the muscle on a relatively small area. They also allow MUSCLES to act at a distance. For example, the fleshy bulk of the forearm muscles is well out of the way of the hand and finger movements that they control, whilst their tendons reach as far as the bone of the fingertip. Tendons come in many shapes and sizes. There are the long, narrow, flattened tendons (sinews) at the wrist and ankle, and those visible on the back of the hand. The broad and thick 'Achilles' tendon links the calf muscles to the foot. The patellar tendon links the quadriceps to the tibia via attachments to the knee cap. The rounded hamstring tendons are readily felt behind the knee. Whilst some tendons are attached to the end of a muscle, others are attached along the side or down the centre. Tendinous sheets or strips attach the edges of flatter trunk muscles to bony ridges, such as the ridge on the shoulder blade or the upper rim of the pelvic bone. Other sheets of tendon link muscles to each other or blend with the outer capsules of joints.

Tendons consist almost entirely of parallel collagen fibres, with elongated cells scattered among them. At the junction with muscle there are strengthened connections to infoldings of the muscle fibre membrane; at the junction with bone there are strong links to the fibrous covering (*periosteum*) adherent to it. To cause movement in exact proportion to the shortening of the muscle, a tendon would need to be inextensible; there is, however, a small degree of elasticity. Tearing of tendons is rare, because their breaking strength is high, but the Achilles tendon for example is sometimes the victim of sports injury. The solid structure, with few blood vessels, is then a disadvantage, making healing tediously slow.

At any site where a tendon lies in a tunnel or groove, it is surrounded by a smooth, double-layered, fluid-containing (*synovial*) sheath, facilitating mobility with minimal friction. Inflammation in such a sheath, for example at the wrist, is the painful condition of *tenosynovitis*.

Tendons are furnished with SENSORY RECEPTORS (*Golgi tendon organs*) that detect the tension within them and therefore the extent to which the attached muscle is exerting force upon them. Excessive nerve impulses generated by them cause reflex inhibition of the muscle contraction via the SPINAL CORD. This provides defence against overstretching and potential tearing.

SHEILA JENNETT

See PLATE 5.

See also SKELETAL MUSCLE.

Testes

Each testis (*synonym*: testicle), enclosed in its fibrous capsule, moves freely within its scrotal sac. Above and behind its oval 'ball' is the *epididymis* — a complex of coiled tubes which convey SPERM from their origin in the testis to the vas deferens. The testes have two major functions; to produce sperm and to produce male SEX HORMONES.

Spermatogenesis

The testis is divided into 200–300 lobes, made up mainly of seminiferous tubules where sperm are generated. By the time of puberty there are some 700 coiled tubules, each as long as an arm and as thin as a hair. These tubules are formed from two cell types, the cells which are developing into sperm and the *Sertoli cells* — named after the

Italian physiologist who described them in 1865. Each Sertoli cell spans the thickness of the tubule wall, and all the germinal cell types, in different stages of maturation, lie in between these Sertoli cells. The role of the Sertoli cells is to nourish the developing and maturing germinal cells which are eventually released into the lumen of the tubule as spermatozoa. Each Sertoli cell is closely attached to the adjacent ones near its base. This attachment forms a barrier which protects the maturing sperm cells from potentially harmful substances circulating in the blood (see SPERM).

The primitive germinal cells are the *spermatogonia*, which lie peripherally in the tubule wall, outside the barrier of Sertoli cell junctions. After they have divided and formed primary spermatocytes with the normal complement of 46 chromosomes, these push their way through the barrier. Lying between, and nurtured by, the Sertoli cells, the primary spermatocytes undergo two meiotic divisions (reducing to 23 chromosomes) and cellular remodelling to produce mature sperm.

The production of mature sperm from spermatogonia takes about 10 days and, during this process of development and maturation, the germinal cells move closer and closer to the lumen of the seminiferous tubules. Eventually they are released from the protection of the Sertoli cells. With little motility of their own at this stage, they are helped by fluid secretions to move into the epididymis; traversing the coils of this final tube takes about two weeks and the sperm become fully fertile and mobile along the way. This process of spermatogenesis is normally achieved by the age of 16 in most males. A fully-functioning testis has the capacity to produce 200 million sperm each day.

Hormone secretion

Lying between the seminiferous tubules are the interstitial cells, commonly referred to as Leydig cells after the German histologist who described them in 1850. These are the cells which produce the male sex hormones, the androgens. Testosterone is the major product and is the most potent of the androgens. It diffuses into the seminiferous tubules where it is essential for spermatogenesis. It also diffuses into the general circulation and is thus carried to its target tissues, where it is responsible not only for the development of male characteristics, both in fetal life and at puberty, but also in maintaining them after puberty.

The functions of the testis are primarily controlled by two hormones secreted by the pituitary gland. *Follicle stimulating hormone* (FSH) acts on the Sertoli cells to maintain their nursemaid function in spermatogenesis, whereas *luteinizing hormone* (LH) stimulates the Leydig cells to produce testosterone. (Both hormones rather oddly retain the names which originally referred to their actions in the ovary in the female.) If the testes are not maintained at a temperature about 2 °C lower than body temperature the process of spermatogenesis is arrested, although male hormone secretion is unaffected. Thus in normal

development the testes descend into the scrotal sac between the seventh and eighth months of fetal life, and remain outside the body at a cooler temperature throughout life. Failure of the testes to descend is known as *cryptochordism*.

Inflammation of the testis is orchitis, and its removal, orchidectomy — from its Greek name, *orchis*. SAFFRON WHITEHEAD

See PLATE 8.

See also SEX HORMONES; SPERM.

Testosterone The most potent of the male steroid SEX HORMONES, which are collectively known as androgens. It is produced by the interstitial (*Leydig*) cells of the testis, and acts locally to stimulate development of SPERM, and via the circulating blood to promote male characteristics. However, in many target tissues testosterone must first be converted to 5α-dihydrotestosterone (DHT) before it is active. S.A.W.

See SEX HORMONES.

Tetanus is perhaps better known through its more dramatic description 'lockjaw'. This potentially life-threatening condition is characterized by uncontrollable muscular contractions, which can be continuous or spasmodic. The immediate cause of this presentation of a disease state is the presence of a circulating poison (toxin) produced at the site of a wound by spores of the bacterium *Clostridium tetani*. This bacterium resides normally in human and animal intestines without causing disease, but contact with heavily manured soil or other material containing the spores, which are extremely resistant to heat and other agents, will readily infect those not immunized against such infection. Active IMMUNIZATION by vaccination with tetanus toxoid (an inactivated form of the toxin) is now usual in childhood, along with diphtheria and whooping cough vaccines. Also immediate passive immunization is available for anyone with a wound which could be contaminated, by injection of human immunoglobulin prepared from the plasma of blood donors; this has taken over from the earlier use of antitetanus serum from horses, which sometimes caused adverse reactions.

Insight as to the mode of action of this toxin at the cellular level has interestingly first been gained from research on muscles of the crayfish. In contrast to the single excitatory innervation by motor axons in mammalian SKELETAL MUSCLE, these invertebrate muscles have a twin innervation, one type of nerve fibre exciting, and the other inhibiting transmission at the NEUROMUSCULAR JUNCTION. This inhibition does not occur through a process directly affecting the muscle fibre or indeed the 'motor endplate' of the neuromuscular junction. Instead, it depends on the release of a chemical transmitter 'GABA' which acts on the excitatory motor nerve terminals by opening a chemically-gated chloride channel; the effect of this is to reduce the amplitude of the ACTION POTENTIAL that reaches the terminal, thereby reducing the amount of

excitatory transmitter (ACETYLCHOLINE) released. As human and mammalian muscles lack such a mixed dual action, the muscular contractions must arise centrally in the axons or motor neuron cell bodies within the SPINAL CORD or BRAIN STEM. Experiments show that tetanus toxin actually inhibits the release of GABA in the central nervous system. GABA normally damps downs the excitation of motor neurons; the effect of tetanus toxin is therefore to allow a now unchecked excitatory barrage to cause a sustained and uncontrollable discharge of motor neurons; this accounts in turn for the muscular contractions.

Because the muscle spasms may cause airway obstruction, such as by closing the jaw and the larynx, or may render the respiratory muscles functionally useless because contractions are sustained instead of rhythmic, tetanus is potentially fatal, but it can be treated successfully by antibiotic drugs. Meanwhile the patient may need to be sedated or, in more severe intoxication, to be paralysed by muscle relaxant drugs and artificially ventilated. TOM SEARS

See also IMMUNIZATION; INFECTIOUS DISEASES.

Tetany refers to a state of increased excitability of nerve and muscle, characterized by muscle spasms. At one end of the spectrum, tetany can occur in otherwise healthy people as a consequence of sustained HYPERVENTILATION or following excessive VOMITING. At the other extreme, tetany signifies a pathological state, arising most often from an endocrine disorder.

Whatever its cause, the common denominator appears to be a reduced level of ionized CALCIUM in the plasma of the circulating blood. Although present in the relatively low concentration of approximately 0.1 g/litre (2.5 mmol/litre), with only about half of this normally ionized or 'free', calcium nevertheless plays a crucial role in controlling the electrical excitability in nerve and muscle membranes, including those of the HEART. Hormonal mechanisms normally maintain a near-constant concentration of free calcium, but the constancy depends also on that of the pH (relative acidity/alkalinity) of the blood.

The prevailing pH determines the ratio of the calcium bound to plasma proteins (calcium proteinates) and the calcium in its electrically charged 'cationic' form of calcium ions ($[Ca^{++}]$). The more acid — the higher the concentration of hydrogen ions ($[H^+]$) — the more $[Ca^{++}]$ is 'freed' from the proteins, and vice versa. This is important because it is the free $[Ca^{++}]$ which crosses capillary walls and determines the concentration in the tissue fluids; this in turn influences the electrical excitability of nerve and muscle membranes. Experiments show that low $[Ca^{++}]$ increases excitability and high $[Ca^{++}]$ diminishes it.

Hyperventilation (overbreathing), whether deliberate or as an aspect of an anxiety state, removes too much carbon dioxide from the body, resulting in respiratory alkalosis (lower $[H^+]$, increased pH); this in turn increases the calcium proteinate and lowers free [Ca^{++}]. The increased excitability causes spontaneous tingling in lips and fingers and, through analogous effects on motor nerve fibres, characteristic muscular 'carpo-pedal' spasms, mainly affecting the wrists, hands, and feet. Short of full-blown tetany, in medical conditions with a low blood calcium (*hypocalcaemia*) the motor axons in the peripheral nerves may show an increased sensitivity to mechanical stimulation. The physician can make diagnostic use of this by tapping the facial nerve near the jaw joint in front of the ear, and looking for a twitch in the facial muscles — the so-called '*Chvostek's sign*', named after the Austrian physician who first described it. The detection of a low calcium is clinically important, because tetany can be fatal should it be severe and involve laryngeal or pharyngeal muscles causing upper airway obstruction. The hormone *parathormone*, from the PARATHYROID GLANDS, is the main regulator of blood [Ca^{++}], so tetany is a major sign of the condition of *hypoparathyroidism*. This rare condition occurs most often from autoimmune destruction of the cells that secrete the hormone; it can also result from the inadvertant or inevitable removal of the parathyroids when the THYROID gland, with which they are intimately associated, is surgically removed for independent medical reasons.

TOM SEARS

See also ACID-BASE HOMEOSTASIS; CALCIUM.

Thalamus

The *cerebral hemispheres* of the BRAIN consist of an outer layer of GREY MATTER called CEREBRAL CORTEX, with a core of WHITE MATTER, surrounding masses of GREY MATTER. The thalamus (of which there is one on each side) is a large and important mass of nerve cells or *neurons*. All sensory pathways (from eyes, ears, skin, etc.), except some of those concerned with the sense of smell, pass through the thalamus on their way to the cerebral cortex. The incoming fibres from each sensory system terminate on a dense clump of nerve cells called a *nucleus*, or on a set of such nuclei. In turn, the fibres of the cells in each thalamic nucleus run up to a particular area (or areas) of the CEREBRAL CORTEX. Important pathways concerned with the control of movement, from the cerebellum and from motor nuclei called the BASAL GANGLIA, also pass through the thalamus. But the thalamus is more than merely a relay station.

Each thalamus is a large, bullet-shaped mass, consisting of a number of closely-packed nuclei. The two lie side by side, roughly in the middle of the entire brain, forming the walls of the central fluid-filled CEREBRAL VENTRICLE called the third ventricle. And above each thalamus is the lateral ventricle, within the cerebral hemisphere. In some individuals they are joined by a bridge of grey matter, the *massa intermedia*, stretching across the third ventricle. Below and in front of each thalamus is the HYPOTHALAMUS, and to the side of each is the *internal capsule* – the important band of WHITE MATTER containing the fibres of thalamic nerve cells, passing to the cerebral cortex above,

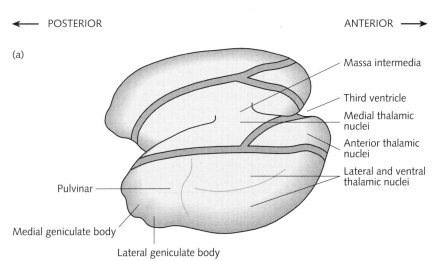

(a)

Massa intermedia

Third ventricle

Medial thalamic nuclei

Anterior thalamic nuclei

Lateral and ventral thalamic nuclei

Pulvinar

Medial geniculate body

Lateral geniculate body

The left thalamus and right thalamus (partly obscured), linked by the massa intermedia, viewed from above, left.

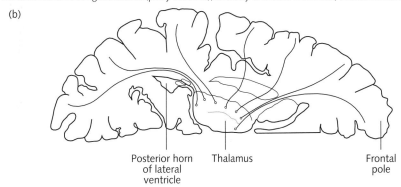

(b)

Posterior horn of lateral ventricle

Thalamus

Frontal pole

This horizontal section through the left hemisphere shows nerve fibres radiating out to different regions of the cerebral cortex.

together with fibres from the cortex running down. The thalamus is split into three major parts, *lateral*, *medial* and *anterior*, by a thin, Y-shaped fibrous sheet (see figure), containing so-called 'non-specific' nuclei (see below).

'Specific' thalamic nuclei

The lower part of the lateral thalamus contains large and very important nuclei, called *specific* nuclei, which relay sensory information to primary areas of the cerebral cortex. For instance, the *ventral posterior nucleus* (*VP*) is the main relay for information from the skin and deep tissues of the body, passing it up to the somatic sensory area of the cortex. The *ventral anterior* and *ventral lateral nuclei* receive fibres from, respectively, the *corpus striatum* (part of the basal ganglia) and the *cerebellum*, and they send fibres to parts of the frontal lobe of the cortex that are concerned with motor control. At the rear end of the thalamus are the smaller *medial* and *lateral geniculate nuclei*, relaying auditory and visual pathways, respectively, to the auditory and visual areas of the cortex.

In the major sensory nuclei of the thalamus, incoming fibres are generally distributed in strict topographic order and they therefore form 'maps' of the array of sensory receptors from which they derive. For instance, the opposite half

of the body is represented within each VP. Fibres ascending from the spinal cord reach the lateral part, carrying signals from the main part of body, while the medial part receives input from the face and head via the fifth cranial nerve, the *trigeminal nerve*. This spatial arrangement is conserved as the fibres of cells in the VP run up, so that the input from the whole body is draped, upside down, over the somatic sensory cortex (which occupies a strip running vertically down the middle of the side of each hemisphere).

The nuclei of the upper part of the lateral thalamus send their fibres to regions of the cortex other than the primary sensory and motor areas. The *lateral posterior nucleus* and *pulvinar* are large structures, which send fibres to regions of the *parietal* and *occipital* lobes that are concerned with visual understanding and the integration of sensory information. The *lateral dorsal nucleus* receives fibres from the *hippocampus* and sends its axons to regions of *limbic cortex* on the inner surface of the hemisphere.

The medial thalamus consists essentially of the *mediodorsal nucleus,* which relays signals from HYPOTHALAMUS and *amygdala* to the frontal lobe and also to the corpus striatum.

The anterior thalamus contains the *anterior nucleus,* which receives input from the *mamillary body* of the HYPOTHALAMUS and sends fibres to a region called the *cingulate cortex*, on the midline surface of the hemisphere. All these structures are parts of the LIMBIC SYSTEM, which is concerned with the regulation of vital rhythms, emotions, appetites, and memory.

The cerebral cortex and the thalamus have evolved in parallel during mammalian EVOLUTION, and they constitute an intimately related functional system. Perhaps the most intriguing and least-understood feature of the thalamus is the fact that each specific nucleus receives at least as many fibres from its region of cerebral cortex as it sends fibres to that region. Thus thalamus and cortex are reciprocally interconnected, with some sort of recursive interplay occurring between them. Some argue that the thalamus acts not just to relay signals to the cerebral cortex, but as a dynamic conduit of information between one cortical area and another, regulating the flow of information according to attention and intention.

'Non-specific' thalamic nuclei

In between the specific sensory and motor relay nuclei of the thalamus is a system of smaller, more diffuse 'non-specific' nuclei, which are organised quite differently. They receive ascending fibres from the reticular formation, which stretches through the core of the brainstem and itself receives and integrates input from the sensory pathways. In turn, the non-specific nuclei of the thalamus send their fibres diffusely over the cerebral hemispheres, rather than to distinct areas. This pathway, from reticular formation to non-specific nuclei to the cortex, which is called the *ascending reticular activating system,* is thought to be involved in regulating the state of 'arousal' of the cortex during the cycle of sleeping and waking.

LAURENCE J. GAREY
COLIN BLAKEMORE

See also BRAIN; CEREBRAL CORTEX; HEARING; SOMATIC SENSATION; SLEEP; VISION.

Thalidomide

Thalidomide and the thalidomide disaster are firmly riveted together in the minds of the population, and it is worth considering how such a tragedy could occur and whether a similar occurrence might be repeated with another new and promising drug. Thalidomide was introduced around 1957 as a safe hypnotic and SEDATIVE. In an immediate sense it was safe, massive doses producing no acute toxicity in animals. It was considered that the drug was far safer than the barbiturates, which were at that time the commonly used hypnotic, and often used by people committing SUICIDE. It was impossible to commit suicide using thalidomide.

The drug became popular in Germany and because of the lack of acute toxicity it became available over the counter without prescription. Around 1960 a number of cases of *phocomelia* (meaning 'seal-like limbs'), in which long limb bones failed to develop, appeared in new-born babies both in Germany and Australia. It took a long time before the connection was made

between thalidomide and birth defects. The reasons for this are clear in retrospect. First, only a small proportion of the population taking the drug were pregnant, and even women who were pregnant needed to take the drug between the thirty-seventh and fifty-fourth day following the last menstruation for the *teratogenic* effects (drug-induced fetal abnormalities) to be manifest. Finally, not all women who took the drug during the crucial period produced babies with teratogenic abnormalities. Other candidates considered to be responsible were radioactive fallout from atomic testing, X-rays, hormones, food additives, and contraceptive pills. The correlation between those taking thalidomide in the crucial period and the incidence of phocomelia became more evident, and the drug was withdrawn in 1961. It must be noted that correlation and causation are not the same, although there can now be no doubt that thalidomide was the cause.

At the time questions were asked why tests for teratogenic potential of the drug had not been made before it was released. First, the effects produced by thalidomide in pregnant women had not occurred before with other drugs and secondly, it was not easy to replicate the effects seen in humans in animal species. Altogether there were some 10 000 cases of babies with phocomelia, mostly in Europe, with some in Australia and a few in the US, of whom about 50% survived with deformed limbs, eyes, hearts, alimentary, and urinary tracts. All of these have required long term care and treatment, only partially ameliorated by the settlement made by the manufacturer. Another question asked was why there were so many cases before the cause of the teratogenic effects was identified. It was unlikely that any medical practitioner would have seen more than one case, and while the incidence of fetal abnormalities of the thalidomide type in normal pregnancy are very rare, the incidence is not zero. It was a German paediatrician who had encountered more than one case, and noted that thalidomide had been taken in all instances, who suggested the connection which was eventually verified.

While the human misery that resulted from the introduction of this seemingly harmless drug is incalculable, an important new development was introduced. To make it less likely that other, yet unknown, bizarre effects from the introduction of new drugs can ever occur on the same scale, most countries have introduced a monitoring system. In the UK, practitioners record any effect a patient reports, or signs which become obvious upon examination, together with the drugs prescribed. This data is entered immediately onto a national database. Of course, most of the reported effects will be nothing at all to do with drug treatment, but as the data will come from an entire country, or group of countries, correlations of effects with drug usage will be quickly spotted and sound the alarm before thousands of people are affected. The thalidomide story also illustrates another problem in

regard to the introduction of new drugs: the public demand the unattainable — that all drugs should be perfectly safe under all conditions — but ultimate answers can be provided only by the consequences of general release.

ALAN W. CUTHBERT

See also CONGENITAL ABNORMALITIES; DRUG.

Theatre

Theatre In Peter Brook's famous description of the essential ingredients for theatre as simply 'the audience and the message', the physical presence of actors is not judged strictly necessary. Yet the history of theatre worldwide makes clear that the first requirement of spectacle or drama is the performer's body. As the mime, Etienne Decroux, ironically put it: 'When the actor ceases to appear on the stage with his body, he will be justified in disregarding the art of the body.' Decroux condemned the use of elaborate scenery, lighting, costume, and properties (characteristic of the naturalistic or 'fourth wall' style of drama prevalent since the nineteenth century) — all of which, he held, obscured the bodily art of acting itself. Contemporary mime stripped the art to its essentials: to act naked on a naked stage, dispensing with all visual or musical support or accompaniment, and thus proving that the gesture can be self-sufficient. A mime, Jean Dorcy claimed, could portray the universe in two square feet.

Older theatre traditions such as classical Greek drama, the *commedia dell'arte*, and the Japanese Noh theatre, all influenced the development of contemporary mime. Whereas the Classical Greek tragic actor's physical movements were restricted both by his heavy costume and by the transcendant dignity of his roles, and he relied for expression on his voice, the actor in Greek comedy was expected to be something of an acrobat, displaying physical agility and skill in a primarily bodily form of theatre. The Japanese Noh was a drama of soliloquy and reminiscence, rather than one of conflict, in which the actor's stylized movements and stamping provided a rhythmic accompaniment to his narrative, with subjects taken from myth and legend. The *commedia dell'arte* was a mainly improvisatory form of theatre developed in sixteenth-century Italy: its influence has extended to the present in the stock characters its actors created — most famously Pantalone and Arlecchino — and the comic stunts and routines which evolved around them.

Contrary to the practice of Decroux and other mimes, these forms of drama do make use of spoken dialogue, costume, stage settings, and music. However, the feature these share in common with mime, and which epitomizes the non-naturalistic and body-based nature of these traditions, is the concealment or disguising of the face, by the use of a mask, or heavy stylized makeup which obscures the natural expression of the actor.

The purpose of this is to turn the eyes away from the face and towards the body of the actor. Dorcy once wrote of acting that 'one cannot simultaneously and fully use the body and the face as means of expression without one of these two being overshadowed by the other.' Perhaps it is appropriate, for a proponent of unspoken theatre, that the third instrument of the actor, the voice, is missing from the this statement. Indeed, practitioners of mime often claim a conflict between bodily movement, gesture, and attitude, and the spoken text, in holding the attention of the spectator. (This word is preferred by Dorcy and others over the word 'audience', for prioritizing the visual over the aural dimensions of theatre.)

Once the face is concealed, the spectator loses sight of what is commonly thought to be the most expressive part of the human frame. Attention is focused instead on the body, which becomes the sole vehicle of expression. Bodily movement, gesture, attitude are heightened and intensified in order to emphasize contrasts, and to eliminate superfluous movements and amplify or exaggerate the remaining motions.

The movement of the actor's body is inseparable from theatre, according to Dorcy: 'The stage is a place where space changes nature, size and architecture according to the body occupying it; without a body in motion, the stage would be a desert.' In such physical acting, each image created by the body, viewed separately, will reveal distinct emotions and circumstances. The gesture of the mime can conjure up absent objects; sometimes it serves as an interjection and expresses the psychological content of the moment: hesitation, joy, fear, etc. A successful attitude is like a condensed drama; perfect, complete, it is an image epitomizing identity, origin, destination, and intent.

The ideal intensity of bodily expression on the stage is summarized by Jean-Louis Barrault, who wrote that 'As soon as I found myself . . . I was put to death. My life is an execution. My conduct will therefore be a struggle against death, against the clock, against time. A single watchword must be issued in this inner world of the body: to delay the hour of surrender, to delay the "moment of truth". Accordingly, from head to toe, every part of this body is placed in a state of alert.' Its enactment of the absurd and tragic collision between the inner world of the self and the outer world of destiny links mime to the plays of Beckett and Ionesco, in the Theatre of the Absurd. Its dictates, based on Jarry's 1896 play, *Ubu Roi*, held that human life was so illogical and language so inadequate as a means of communication that one was thrown back onto the body as the sole vehicle of expression, whether laughter, pain, or bewilderment.

Bodily confrontation is emphasized in the later Theatre of Cruelty movement, begun in the 1960s. Inspired by the writings of Antonin Artaud, it sought to free humans from the restraints of morality and reason, returning to a state of unfettered expression of power and desire. This was a precursor to the recent resurgence of 'new melodrama', which employs non-naturalistic, expressionistic styles of acting, and physical theatre, with its emphasis on extreme bodily states and forms of expression.

NATSU HATTORI

Further reading

Cheney, S. W. (1972). *The theatre. Three thousand years of drama, acting and stagecraft*. McKay, New York.

Dorcy, J. (1961). *The mime*, (trans. R. Speller and P. de Fontnouvelle). (5 vols.) McGraw-Hill New York.

Hochman, S. (1984). *Encyclopaedia of world drama*. Robert Speller & Sons, New York.

Theory of mind 'Theory of mind' is a catch-phrase in contemporary psychology, referring to a universal human tendency to attribute mental states (feelings, beliefs, intentions, attitudes) to oneself and to others. 'Mentalizing' has much the same meaning. Mental states are used to explain and predict other people's behaviour intuitively — as if guided by a theory about the nature of mind.

Imagine you are watching a movie. 'Why did the detective duck into the doorway? Because he thought he was being followed.' This explanation holds even if the detective was not actually followed by anybody. What counts is that he believed he was being followed, and this determined his behaviour. Belief is more significant than reality. It is vitally important not to confuse mental states and physical states. To achieve this, the human brain is equipped with a mechanism that represents mental states in a special way. The underlying mechanism is likely to have an innate basis, which explains why social learning early in life is both rapid and universal. One early function of the mechanism may be to direct infants' attention to other human agents, who are likely to affect their lives.

There is increasing interest in the biological basis of mentalizing among neuroscientists and primatologists. It is uncertain whether any non-human primates possess the mechanism, but if so, it is probably limited to apes (gorillas and chimpanzees). Monkeys are thought not to possess it at all. Clues to the physiological basis of mentalizing come from *autism*, a developmental disorder, which is characterized by severe impairments of social communication. These impairments can be explained by a deficit in the ability to attribute mental states to self and others, suggesting a failure of the mentalizing mechanism. In contrast to children with autism, normally-developing children show evidence of mentalizing during the first year of life. For example, from about 8–12 months of age they spontaneously establish 'joint attention' with adults. They follow with their gaze to where an adult looks or points and begin themselves to point at things to show objects of interest to others. This is not so as to obtain things there and then, but to share mental states and to build communicative relationships to other people in the long term. Some time in the second year, children begin to understand pretend play, which relies on the ability to represent mental states and not to confuse them with reality. From the age of 4 or 5, children in all cultures show a reliable and explicit appreciation that mental states may differ from reality, and that one person may think something different from another, and different from what they know to be the truth.

A standard test to demonstrate mentalizing ability requires the child to track a character's *false belief*. This test can be done using stories, cartoons, people, or, as illustrated in the figure, a puppet play, which the child watches. In this play, one puppet, called Sally, leaves her ball in her basket, then goes out to play. While she is out, naughty Anne moves the ball to her own box. Sally returns and wants to play with her ball. The child watching the puppet play is asked where Sally will look for her ball (where does Sally think it is?). Young children aged around 4 and above recognize that Sally will look in the basket, where she (wrongly) *thinks* the ball is.

Mentalizing is pervasive in everyday life, in communication and co-operation, in pedagogy, in play-acting, but also in deceiving, cheating, and outwitting.

Autism — a specific disorder of mentalizing

Autism is a life-long developmental disorder that affects 0.1–0.5% of the population. It is characterized by qualitative impairments in social interaction and communication and the presence of restricted and repetitive interests and activities. Autism is associated with EPILEPSY (one in three cases) and mental retardation (three in four), and affects at least three times as

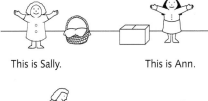

This is Sally.   This is Ann.

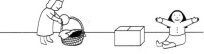

Sally has a ball. She puts it into her basket.

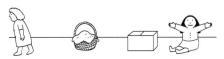

Sally goes out for a walk.
Ann takes the ball out of the basket.

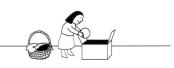

Ann then puts the ball in the box.

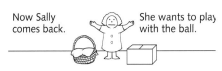

Now Sally comes back.   She wants to play with the ball.

Where will Sally look for the ball?

many males as females. Studies of families and of identical TWINS suggest a major genetic contribution to autism. Various types of brain abnormality have been found, although the specific and defining features of autistic brains have not yet been identified. This is in part because of the heterogeneity of the condition, which makes it problematic to correlate behavioural observations and physiological data. Autism is now conceptualized as a spectrum of clinical signs — a range of manifestations varying with age and ability, but showing core impairments in social, communicative, and imaginative abilities. One extreme of the spectrum is the severely impaired child of low IQ, who may be silent, aloof, and locked into repetitive motor behaviour (*stereotypy*). But at the other extreme is the high-functioning individual, who may be pedantic and verbose, active but odd in social approach, with an obsessive pursuit of narrow interests (e.g. collecting registration numbers on lamp posts). This latter picture conforms to the new diagnostic category of *Asperger syndrome*.

Among the first reliable signs of autism in the young child is an absence of joint attention activities, e.g. a lack of spontaneous pointing or pretend play. These early difficulties signal a failure to attend to other minds, which is later manifest in failure on simple false-belief tests, such as the Sally–Anne task (see figure). Children with autism, even high-functioning ones, seem to be unable to pass this test at the appropriate mental and chronological age. This is in contrast to other children with LEARNING DISABILITIES, such as those with Down syndrome or Williams syndrome. Furthermore, this result holds when alternative reasons for task failure, such as problems of motivation, language, or memory, have been ruled out through the use of closely matched control tests.

A deficit in mentalizing explains the particular social communication difficulties that are typical of children and adults with autism, who nevertheless display a range of other apparently normal social and emotional behaviours. For instance, children with autism are able to use 'instrumental' gestures (to affect behaviour directly) much better than expressive gestures (to affect inner states). They are able to understand and engage in sabotage (affecting behaviour directly) better than in deception (to alter somene's belief). They are able to remember messages verbatim, to give factual and honest answers to questions, and to deliver speeches. But they are curiously unable to respond to hints, to engage in gossip, to keep secrets, and to make confidences.

In individuals with Asperger syndrome, verbal ability and social adaptation tend to be higher than in autism. Thus, compensatory learning of social communication skills can occur even in the absence of a start-up mechanism early in life. A proportion of sufferers do gradually acquire mentalizing abilities with practice, and through the application of logical inference. And in some, mentalizing may be merely delayed. However, late-acquired mentalizing appears to lack an intuitive basis, and tends to be fragile and effortful.

What is the neural substrate of 'theory of mind'? To date there are only a handful of relevant studies, but the new IMAGING TECHNIQUES, which allow activity to be detected in the living human brain, are producing interesting results. In such experiments, the brains of volunteers are scanned while they perform tasks in which they must make inferences about mental states in contrast to physical states. During mentalizing, a number of brain areas become active, most notably a region called the *anterior cingulate cortex* (lying on the medial surface of the frontal lobe, hidden from view in the split between the two hemispheres), a region at the junction of the temporal and parietal lobes, and part of the LIMBIC SYSTEM called the *amygdala*. Each of these areas of the CEREBRAL CORTEX appear to have analogous regions in the brains of non-human primates, and even non-primate mammals. For example, some nerve cells in the equivalent of temporo-parietal region in monkeys become active when the monkey watches humans or other monkeys walking. In the same general area are found nerve cells that are similar to the 'mirror neurons' described sby the Italian neurophysiologist, Giacomo Rizzolatti, in a part of the monkey's frontal lobe. These cells respond when the monkey looks at particular actions (e.g. grasping) being carried out either with his own hands or by the hands of another monkey. The other main component of the mentalizing system, the *anterior cingulate cortex*, is involved in the 'monitoring' of action. In humans it is particularly active when we monitor our own thoughts and feelings.

To speculate, the brain's mentalizing system might have evolved from a system concerned with analysing the movements of other creatures and from a system that processes information about our own inner states. UTA FRITH

Further reading

Baron-Cohen, S., Tager-Flusberg, H., and Cohen, D. (ed.) (2000). *Understanding other minds: perspectives from developmental neuroscience*, (2nd edn). Oxford University Press.

Happé, F. and Frith, U. (1996). The neuropsychology of autism. *Brain*, **119**, 1377–400.

See also LEARNING DISABILITIES.

Third eye

A number of yogic traditions from around the world have developed the metaphor of the so-called 'third eye'. This eye is not usually conceived of as a physical organ, although most forms of YOGA will emphasize that all mental and spiritual realities have some kind of physical counterpart. The image is used particularly to refer to certain meditative techniques of self-reflection. The third eye is understood as a spiritual eye which perceives spiritual realities, a seat of *intuition*. Practically speaking, it can also serve as a metaphor for the relationship between *concentration* and MEDITATION. The ability to concentrate is often likened to the ability of the eye to stare at a single object for long periods of time. Just as the muscles of the eye can be strengthened through exercise to facilitate vision, so too the capabilities of the third eye can be cultivated and thus its sensitivity and range of perception can be deepened, increased, and augmented. Meditation subsequently involves this strengthened eye watching itself watch itself watch itself, in order to stop identifying with the ego and to identify properly with the true, essential reality of the Self, according to tradition.

Although many attempts have been made over the years, and particularly upon the reception of yoga by the West, to find physical organs corresponding to the spiritual organs of Asian psychospiritual systems, no such discoveries have been made with any degree of certitude. The third eye is sometimes associated with either the PINEAL GLAND or the HYPOTHALAMUS, which themselves have been considered the seat of the soul by a number of Western traditions.

ALAN FOX

See also PINEAL GLAND; YOGA.

Thumb-sucking

Between 75% and 95% of all infants suck their thumb, making thumb-sucking the most prevalent kind of nonnutritive oral activity in infants and young children. Thumb-sucking continues in approximately 45% of American pre-school children, but in only 30% of Swedish children of the same age. In a significant percentage of American 7–11-year-olds, thumb-sucking persists. Among Inuit, American Indian, and African children thumb-sucking is rare.

Thumb-sucking may begin before birth. The thumb has been observed in the mouths of fetuses as young as 18 weeks of gestational age, and true sucking movements and protrusion of the lips may occur by 24 weeks. New-borns often have blisters on their hands and arms, indicating the probable occurrence of sucking before birth. After birth, infants have a strong *rooting reflex*: they turn their head toward an object touching the cheek. This reflex allows them to find the nipple. Around the age of 3 months, an infant may accidentally discover its thumb or another digit and suck on it. Thumb-sucking is usually established before the first birthday.

A number of theories have been advanced concerning the origins and import of thumb-sucking. Freud believed that thumb-sucking is an instinctual activity. Following S. Lindner's 1879 argument that thumb-sucking is sexual in nature, Freud found that it fulfilled all the criteria to be considered the model of *infantile sexuality*. It relies on a physical function — the need for nourishment and the PLEASURE derived from it; it is autoerotic, or directed toward self-gratification; and it is controlled by an EROGENOUS ZONE, the lips, which first experience the pleasure of sucking. Freud believed that thumb-sucking (or sucking another part of the body) arises when the gratification of the erogenous zone becomes separated from the desire to take nourishment. During thumb-sucking an infant desires to grasp something, such as its own or another's ear, and pull it rhythmically. Since this activity is very pleasurable and may become associated also with rubbing sensitive parts of the body, such as the breast or genitals, Freud believed that thumb-sucking led to MASTURBATION.

The behaviourist John B. Watson rejected instinct as an explanation for human behaviour. In *The Psychological Care of the Infant and Child* (1928), he promoted child-rearing practices based on his belief that children are made, not born, and that almost all behaviours result from CONDITIONING. An implication of this view was that thumb-sucking, a bad habit, resulted from a conditioned response associated with eating, and must be cured within the first few days after birth. Charles Anderson Aldrich and Mary Aldrich, the authors of *Babies are Human Beings* (1938), by contrast, viewed thumb-sucking as a prenatal sport designed to exercise the facial muscles, and assured their readers that a child would stop it as soon as he developed other interests.

Other explanations for the origin and significance of thumb-sucking abound. Some consider it a natural stage of development that usually ceases by the end of the third year, though it may become a habit. Still others characterize it as a means by which infants comfort themselves. In contrast to these explanations, one study finds that thumb-sucking seems to improve respiratory function in babies with an immobile tongue (*ankyloglossia*) and a deviated epiglottis and larynx. Another group of theories links the development of thumb-sucking with inadequate sucking during breast-feeding or with bottle feeding, which takes less time. Some children suck their thumb only while falling asleep or sleeping. In older children thumb-sucking occurs in stressful situations, such as fatigue, boredom, hunger, insecurity, parental deprivation, or frustration.

Thumb-sucking may entail certain risks to physical health. It pushes the upper incisors out and the lower incisors in. Such *malocclusions* resolve spontaneously if thumb-sucking stops before the permanent teeth erupt. Other undesirable effects can include problems with jaw movements, narrowing of the cheek bones due to the contractions of the cheek muscles, ulcerations beneath the tongue, and root resorption. More commonly, the thumb may develop calluses or an irritant eczema, and the digit itself may become deformed.

Parental and expert responses to thumb-sucking underwent significant changes during the twentieth century. Before the end of the nineteenth century, little was said or written about it. In the final decades of the century, however, it became a cause for concern. Freud noted disapprovingly that, in the nursery, thumb-sucking was treated like any other 'sexual naughtiness'. It was recognized that thumb-sucking could also lead to a misshapen mouth. Luther Holt recommended mittens or a splint to the elbow to prevent it. In 1922 Charis Barlow warned that thumb-sucking introduced dirt and germs into the mouth, caused adenoid inflammation, weakened the digestion, and spoiled the mouth and thumb shape. To prevent thumb-sucking, she recommended pinning the sleeves shut or wrapping the baby in a shawl to sleep, while Watson advised sewing mitts onto pajama sleeves. In the first edition of the *Common Sense Book of Baby and Child Care* (1945), Dr Benjamin Spock recommended increasing the time taken in breast- or bottle-feeding in young infants to discourage thumb-sucking, but cautioned parents against using restraints such as aluminum mittens for older children, as such devices frustrate the child.

Pediatricians now recommend that no action against thumb-sucking be initiated during the first two or three years. In the older child, an environmental cause for thumb-sucking should be sought and eliminated; for cases where thumb-sucking is an empty habit, parents are urged to remind the child gently only if the child wants to quit. Other cures involve bitter tasting liquids applied to the thumb, and palatal bars. In all cases children require emotional support.

KRISTEN L. ZACHARIAS

Further reading

Hardyment, C. (1983). *Dream babies. Three centuries of good advice on child care*. Harper and Row, New York.

Leung, A. K. C. and Robson, W. L. M. (1991). Thumb sucking. *American Family Physician*, **44**, 1724–8.

Thymus The thymus has had a varied history in terms of attribution of function, from at least the time of GALEN, who named it the seat of the soul.

It is a relatively large organ at birth, centrally placed in the upper chest behind the sternum, and extending into the neck. It grows with the child until puberty, then regresses to almost nothing in adulthood. It consists mostly of lymphocytes. Up until the early twentieth century, an excessively large thymus was from time to time held responsible for some unexplained infant deaths, as part of so-called *status lymphaticus* believed to be a generalized superfluity of lymphatic tissue. This theory was discredited in the 1930s. Since then, the role of the thymus as part of the LYMPHATIC SYSTEM has become better understood, along with the study of the mechanisms of immunity, of AUTOIMMUNE DISEASE, and of factors causing rejection of transplants.

The thymus is now known to be involved in processing lymphocytes, which are crucial for the 'cellular component' of the immune response and also assist the provision of the 'humoral component' — the antibodies in the blood. It is a highly active organ in the young body, and the unique site for the selection of lymphocytes that will be 'competent' for this role in the immune response and for the maturation that prepares them for it.

Some of the lymphocytes that originate in the bone marrow move early in life to the thymus. These are the candidates for giving rise to *T-lymphocytes*, if their progeny emerge as the few survivors of a rigorous selection process, according to the appropriateness of the cell membrane receptors that result from random rearrangement of their genes. This process takes place in the outer layer, the 'cortex', of the young thymus, where lymphocytes are densely packed and actively dividing. Those that develop receptors that are able to bind the right sort of peptides proliferate; the others die. The 'good' ones proceed to the central 'medulla' and are further weeded out, until only those that have 'learnt' to bind 'non-self' peptides remain; rejects at this stage are those which could bind the body's own 'self' peptides, and would therefore be liable to cause autoimmune diseases.

The T-lymphocytes that leave the thymus enter the circulation, and some settle in lymphoid tissue, including the lymph nodes and the spleen. Their further story is that of the immune response: subsets of T-cells take part in several different ways, including the activation of phagocytic cells, killing specific antigen-producing cells, and regulating the production of antibodies by the *B-lymphocytes* (those which have not been processed by the thymus).

The thymus has sometimes been surgically removed in the treatment of *myasthenia gravis*, in which antibodies are formed to the body's own acetylcholine receptors in skeletal muscle, but in most instances there are other, more appropriate treatments. SHEILA JENNETT

See PLATE 4.

See also AUTOIMMUNE DISEASE; IMMUNE SYSTEM; LYMPHATIC SYSTEM.

Thyroid gland The thyroid gland secretes HORMONES which are necessary for normal growth and development from fetal life onwards, and for maintenance of normal METABOLISM in the adult body.

The gland is located just below the LARYNX and attached to the front of the trachea. The adult gland weighs 10–20 g and consists of two relatively flat oval lobes linked by an isthmus. It is so named because of its resemblance to the classical shield (*thureos*) used by the ancient Greeks. However, unlike the shield, in any one individual the thyroid is generally asymmetric, with the right lobe being significantly larger than the left. The gland is usually larger in women than in men and it increases slightly in size during pregnancy. This is exploited as an early pregnancy test in some African communities: the neck of a bride is adorned with a tight necklace and pregnancy is indicated when in due course the necklace is broken by the swelling thyroid gland.

The embryonic thyroid originated in the floor of the PHARYNX and it can be detected as a midline thickening, as early as day 24. By weeks 6–7 the characteristic bilobed structure can be distinguished. At about this time, the gland becomes detached from the pharynx and the developing tissue mass descends into the neck. The two lobes finally come to rest on either side of the trachea with the joining isthmus lying across the front of it. Occasionally the thyroid fails to descend, or may descend too far; the fully developed gland is then found below the root of the tongue or within the thorax. Such developmental abnormalities do not necessarily affect thyroid function.

During its descent down the neck the developing thyroid incorporates 'C-cells' into its tissue mass; also two pairs of discrete PARATHYROID GLANDS become attached to the back surface of the thyroid gland itself. These secrete hormones which regulate the concentration of calcium in the blood: the C-cells secrete the protein calcitonin, and the parathyroids the protein parathyroid hormone. Neither of these are regarded as thyroid hormones since they are not produced by the main mass of thyroid tissue; the latter consists of spherical follicles where the thyroid hormones are synthesized and stored.

The major functional and structural unit of the thyroid is the thyroid follicle. There are many thousands of follicles, and their individual sizes vary considerably, ranging in diameter from 20 to 100 μm (2/100–1/10 mm). A rich network of fenestrated capillary blood vessels surrounds small groups of follicles and there is an impressively high rate of blood flow through the gland as a whole (per unit mass, the flow is twice the flow through the kidneys, which themselves have a much greater blood supply than other organs relative to their size). The even greater flow through an overactive thyroid produces a 'bruit' which can be heard when a stethoscope is placed over the gland. The high blood flow ensures an adequate supply of blood-borne nutrients to the follicles — in particular the delivery of iodide derived from the diet — as well as uptake of the thyroid hormones into the bloodstream.

The unique biochemical characteristic of thyroid follicular cells is their ability to concentrate and to utilize dietary iodide. The cell possesses an iodide 'pump' which enables it to accumulate iodide internally, so that it can achieve a concentration twenty- to a hundred-fold higher than that in the circulating blood. Two other tissues which share a closely related embryonic origin with the thyroid (some cells of the stomach lining and the salivary glands) also possess this pumping mechanism, but the thyroid is unique in its ability to retain and utilize the iodide for the biosynthesis of its hormones. These hormones are small molecules derived from the amino acid tyrosine and they have iodine incorporated into their structures. There are two thyroid hormones, which have either 3 or 4 atoms of iodine per molecule; they are known respectively as T_3 (tri-iodothyronine) and T_4 (thyroxine). Both are synthesized within the thyroid follicles and secreted into the bloodstream when the cells are stimulated to extrude them by the thyroid stimulation hormone (TSH) from the PITUITARY GLAND. The thyroid hormones in the circulation in turn regulate the production of TSH by the pituitary, switching off TSH production when the appropriate level of T_3/T_4 is attained in the blood. Thus the 'pituitary–thyroid axis' is a classical example of a negative feedback system.

Following the accumulation of iodine in the follicular cells, the T_3 and T_4 are first synthesized separately and are then incorporated into a much larger molecule known as thyroglobulin. This large glycoprotein, which is sometimes referred to as 'colloid' is stored in the hollow interior of each follicle. If a thyroid gland which has been removed is cut across and gently squeezed, the colloid can be observed leaking from the transected follicles as a glistening yellowish fluid. TSH stimulates the release of the T_3 and T_4 from the thyroglobulin so that the hormones can be secreted from the cells into the bloodstream in a regulated fashion. This hormone storage system is unique in endocrine physiology; it ensures that there is a two-month supply of thyroid hormones in the event that a person encounters an iodine deficient environment. This occurs in many parts of the world, such as some mountainous regions in China and India. However, this capacity to store thyroid hormones within the follicles as thyroglobulin becomes disadvantageous if an individual inadvertently ingests radioactive iodine. This occurred after the huge release into the atmosphere of radioactive isotopes, including radioiodine, during the week following the Chernobyl accident on 26 April 1986. The natural storage of the radioiodine in the follicles delays clearance of the ingested radionuclide and concentrates the damaging radiation on the thyroid. In Belarus and the Ukraine this resulted in a major increase in the incidence of thyroid cancer in the 1990s amongst children born before the accident.

Thyroid hormones circulate in the blood in minute concentrations (nanomolar — of the order of $10^{-9} \times$ molecular weight per litre). Although this is very low compared with many blood constituents such as glucose or sodium ions, which circulate at millimolar concentrations (a million times greater), it is high relative to hormones in general. The blood concentrations of the thyroid hormones are tightly regulated by TSH and remain very stable in a healthy individual over prolonged periods. Thyroid hormones are relatively insoluble in water and this has two important consequences. Firstly, in the circulation more than 99% of them are linked to specific 'binding proteins'; this prolongs their half-life in blood, and since the binding is reversible, maintains a biologically active 'reservoir' in the circulation. Secondly, on arrival at a target cell, the hormones, being relatively soluble in lipid, are able to cross the plasma membrane of the cell and then bind to specific receptors associated with gene regulation in the nucleus of the cell.

Thyroid hormones regulate the activities of almost all cells in the body. They exert three main classes of action. Firstly they control the basal metabolic rate (BMR). Secondly they influence cell differentiation and growth. Thirdly they may modify the action of other hormones, extending their importance still more widely. Thus a lack of thyroid hormones is manifested in diverse ways. In the developing fetus an inadequate supply

leads to impaired brain development with the danger of the infant being borne a cretin. In an adult there is a depressed BMR with attendant lethargy. By contrast, excess thyroid hormones raise the BMR and may lead to cardiac problems due to potentiation by thyroid hormone of the effects of ADRENALINE.

T_3, the form of thyroid hormone which contains only 3 atoms of iodine per molecule, is now considered to be the physiologically active hormone, and T_4 to be a precursor of T_3, which can be converted to T_3 by specific enzymes within the target cells. Since T_4 circulates at a concentration about a hundred-fold higher than that of T_3, it can therefore be considered to be a storage form of the active hormone. Thus the thyroid system as a whole is designed to buffer any possibility of a reduction in the adequate supply of T_3 to target cells: large reserves are maintained in the thyroglobulin stored in the follicles, in the T_3 and T_4 attached to the circulating binding proteins, and in T_4 itself.

N. J. MARSHALL

See PLATE 7.

See also GOITRE; HORMONES; HYPERTHYROIDISM; HYPOTHYROIDISM.

Tickling is a common, perhaps universal, human experience. Depictions of people engaged in some kind of tickling activity, whether between siblings, parents and children, or lovers, can be found in the art of many countries and cultures. Tickling someone often causes them to smile and laugh in a way that is indistinguishable from the reaction to other forms of PLEASURE or even intense amusement. However, tickling is a curious, paradoxical phenomenon. Particularly 'ticklish' individuals wriggle and writhe in apparent agony, as well as laughing hysterically, when being tickled. Francis Bacon in 1677 commented that: '[when tickled] men even in a grieved state of mind . . . cannot sometimes forbear laughing.'

Tickling usually occurs only between people who know each other well: children are likely to be tickled by their parents and siblings, adults may be tickled by their lovers. Normally the tickler is someone who desires to express intimacy, emotion, and affection through their tickling — in other words the tickle is intended as a friendly gesture. The degree of 'ticklishness' increases if the 'ticklee' feels that he or she cannot escape from the tickler. Although there is often such inequality of power during tickling, it normally occurs in situations that are entirely non-threatening. Charles Darwin in 1872 claimed that if a stranger tried to tickle a child the child would scream with fear rather than squeal with laughter.

But tickling is a pleasure that 'cannot be reproduced in the absence of another' as Adam Phillips wrote. The inability to tickle oneself seems to be hard-wired in the CENTRAL NERVOUS SYSTEM: the BRAIN reacts differently when people tickle themselves compared with when someone else does the tickling. The areas of the CEREBRAL CORTEX associated with the sensation

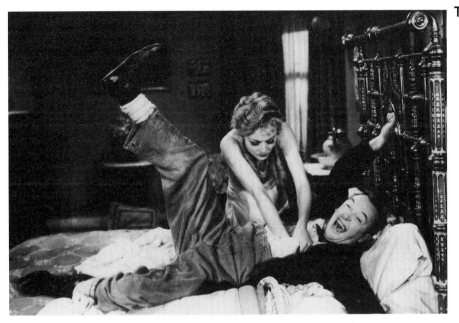

A serious exploration of tickling From Laurel and Hardy's *Way Out West*. The Kobal Collection.

of touch (the *somatosensory cortex*) and pleasure (the *anterior cingulate cortex*) react much more strongly to a tickling stimulus delivered by an external agent than to a self-tickle. This hard-wired mechanism suggests that tickling is useful in social bonding — there is little point in social bonding with oneself.

This view was argued by Charles Darwin over a century ago. He wrote that tickling is an important aspect of social and sexual bonding, and prominent in the development of communication between mothers and babies. Tickle-induced LAUGHTER, he argued, is socially stimulated and results from close physical contact with another person. An alternative claim is that the laughter is purely reflexive — something that happens without our voluntary control, similar to the reflex muscle contraction induced when a doctor taps the tendon of your knee. Just as people laugh when they read an amusing story on their own, so they will laugh out loud when they are being tickled by a robotic hand, even when no other person is around to hear them.

Some animals seem to be ticklish. Great apes (chimpanzees and gorillas) react with what is believed to be an analog of laughter — a panting sound — when tickled. Recent research shows that even baby rats squeal with apparent pleasure when tickled, although you need an ultrasound detector to hear the sounds because they are at frequencies too high for human ears to detect. They are interpreted as sounds of joy because they differ markedly from distress calls, being similar to the sounds made by a male rat while courting a female. The possibility that tickling behaviour is widespread among mammals suggests that it may lie at the heart of the evolution of complex social behaviour.

Why then do we laugh when tickled? Laughing might not simply be a social expression of happiness. Some have suggested that the components of laughter — convulsion of the abdomen, production of sniggering noises, tears streaming from the eyes — all serve the general purpose of releasing tension in a social situation. Nervous laughter often occurs during tense situations, and there are striking similarities between laughing and crying hysterically. Being tickled certainly causes the body to become tense, through increased muscle tone.

An alternative view is that of Vilayanur Ramachandran of the University of California, San Diego, who claims that we laugh to tell other people that a potentially threatening situation is not serious. 'You approach a child, hand stretched out menacingly . . . But no, your fingers make light, intermittent contact with her belly,' he writes. As a result of being tickled the child laughs, as if to inform other children, 'He doesn't mean harm. He's only playing.' Some psychologists have suggested that the sense of humour evolves during individual development, starting with the baby's giggling in response to being tickled, later maturing into a tendency to laugh at unusual faces and situations, and finally maturing into an appreciation of jokes, subtle wit, and irony.

It all starts, though, with that first tickle. Without tickling, some suggest, there might be no humour at all.   SARAH-JAYNE BLAKEMORE

Further reading

Darwin, C. (1872). *The expressions of the emotions in man and animals*. John Murray, London.
Ramachandran, V. S. (1998). *Phantoms in the brain*. Fourth Estate, London.

See also LAUGHTER AND HUMOUR; PLEASURE.

Tinnitus refers to the sensation of sound, most often a high-pitched, noisy whistle, in one or both ears in the absence of external stimulation. Like pain, tinnitus is a very subjective phenomenon, and descriptions by sufferers tend to be in terms of a familiar sound such as the roar of the ocean or the ringing of bells. Nearly everyone experiences a mild and transient form of tinnitus. Estimates of the incidence of more severe forms vary, but around 10–14% of adults complain of tinnitus that is either prolonged or present for much of the time, and 0.5% are so affected as to have difficulty in leading a normal life.

The first written record of tinnitus appears to date back to ancient Egyptian medical documents. There are several references in Babylonian medicine to the 'singing ear' or the 'whispering ear', for which incantation of charms was advocated. Descriptions of noises in the ear and their possible causes were placed on a more scientific footing through the works of the Greek scholar Hippocrates in the fourth and fifth centuries BC and the term tinnitus originates from ancient Rome. Over the subsequent centuries, different types of tinnitus were recognized and described more completely. However, tinnitus remains one of the least understood HEARING conditions, for which there is still, in many cases, no specific cure.

Many sounds are generated within the head as a result of muscular activity and by blood rushing through the cranial vessels. However, we are rarely aware of these sounds because the cochlea is shielded by the hard temporal bone. Although people with apparently normal hearing do experience tinnitus, it usually accompanies some form of hearing loss. Indeed, most people who complain to their general practitioners of deafness will also have tinnitus. Although it is often associated with disorders of the ear itself, including blockage of the ear canal by wax, otosclerosis, and Menière's disease, it is now apparent that neural activity within the BRAIN may be a more important factor. The discovery in the late 1970s that the ear produces sounds that can be detected in the ear canal suggested a possible link between tinnitus and the activity of outer hair cells in the cochlea. However, because drugs such as ASPIRIN both eliminate these emissions and induce tinnitus, this seems to provide an explanation in only a few cases. Moreover, tinnitus is often found in people with severe sensorineural hearing loss or following physical damage to the inner ear, which would argue against a cochlear origin for the condition.

Because of its subjective nature and the paucity of external signs associated with tinnitus, the development of animal models has been problematic. Nevertheless, studies in animals have shown that high doses of aspirin give rise to increased spontaneous activity both in the auditory nerve fibres that leave the inner ear and in the auditory midbrain. We do not yet know the mechanisms underlying central tinnitus or even which areas of the auditory pathway are responsible, but it is possible that a change in the level of inhibitory activity may be involved.

Early remedies for tinnitus usually involved the administration, either orally or into the ear canal, of a variety of substances ranging from oils to ox urine. It was observed in ancient Greece that external noise could mask buzzing in the ears and this was used therapeutically in the nineteenth century. Unless the patient is completely deaf, noise generators are still useful today as a means of providing temporary relief. By amplifying speech or environmental noise, hearing aids can also be effective in many cases. It was claimed at the beginning of the nineteenth century that electrical stimulation of the ear could be used to treat tinnitus. In a similar vein, tinnitus is often reduced after profoundly deaf patients are fitted with a cochlear implant in which sounds are transduced into electrical signals that are delivered to electrodes inserted into the cochlea of the inner ear.

In a small minority of cases tinnitus may be alleviated if the cause of the hearing loss can be treated by surgical or medical means. Because tinnitus is aggravated by STRESS or FATIGUE, the most successful treatment involves psychological counselling or some form of RELAXATION therapy, often in conjunction with devices that use external noise to mask the sounds that are generated within the head.   ANDREW J. KING

Further reading
Shulman, A., Aran, J.-M., Feldmann, H., Tonndorf, J., and Vernon, J. A. (1991). *Tinnitus: diagnosis/treatment*. Lea and Febiger, Philadelphia.

Vesterager, V. (1997). Tinnitus — investigation and management. *British Medical Journal*, **314**, 728–31.

See also DEAFNESS; HEARING; HEARING AID.

Tissue (singular): the term used to describe an aggregation of body cells with specialized structure and function (muscle, nerve, glandular, adipose, connective tissue and so on). Within each category there is usually more than one cell type — usually the main cells with a special function, plus connective tissue cells. Tissues (plural) refers in general to the whole fabric of the body — as in the statement 'the blood transports oxygen and nutrients to all body tissues', or sometimes '. . . to all organs and tissues', using the word to cover everything which is not a discrete organ.   S.J.

Titans The twelve Titans, children of Uranus (Heaven) and Gê (Earth), were the group of gods immediately preceding the Olympian gods in Greek mythology. The Olympians defeated the Titans in a battle — the *Titanomachy*. The word 'titanic' refers to the great size and power of the Titans, attributes necessary to make their defeat by their children, the Olympians, more impressive. In appearance, they are thus much like the Giants, and in classical and later art it is often difficult to tell whether Titans or Giants are represented. In addition to the Titans, Uranus and Gê produced monstrous offspring: three beings

each with a hundred hands, and three one-eyed giants (the *Cyclopes*).

The youngest Titan was Kronos, who castrated his father with a sickle given to him by his sister Rhea, and threw his genitalia into the sea; the Giants sprang to life from Kronos' blood, which fell on the earth, while Aphrodite was born from the foam of the sea. Kronos took his father's throne, then married Rhea; but he proceeded to swallow every child born to her, from fear that a child would copy his example and take control of the world. But one child, Zeus, was smuggled away to be brought up in Crete; instead Rhea passed a stone wrapped in a cloth to Kronos to swallow. When Zeus reached adulthood, he gave an emetic to Kronos that made him vomit up Zeus' long-lost brothers and sisters, the Olympian deities. These fought the Titans for ten years, and after the eventual Olympian victory the Titans were banished to Tartarus, a place below the underworld. Despite the cruelty and violence of these stories, the time when Kronos ruled was nevertheless also regarded as a Golden Age by the GREEKS, and in some myths he now rules the Isles of the Blessed, where some of the dead are privileged to dwell.

A variant from of Greek mythology given in Orphic theology, known from Neoplatonist sources, told an alternative version of the Titan myth, which also involves the separation of body parts but suggests a dual nature for human beings. In this variant, it is said that the young god Dionysos was dismembered, cooked, and eaten by the Titans, acts for which Zeus subsequently punished them by destroying them with a thunderbolt. Human beings were then created out of the ashes of the Titans; this suggests that, as part of our identity as humans, we have not only a tendency towards violent criminal acts, from the Titans, but also something good, from the parts of Dionysos they had consumed before their own destruction. Dionysos himself was reborn from the one remaining part of his body, the heart, which the goddess Athena preserved. The Orphic literature influenced many Bacchic mystery groups in antiquity; initiates seem to have regarded the body as a 'prison', and believed that they must liberate the divine 'Dionysiac' part of humanity from the evil 'Titanic' part.

At least one of the offspring of the Titans took on an important role in the period of the rule of Zeus in which the classical Greeks believed themselves to be living. Prometheus, son of the Titan Iapetus, was the major culture-bearer in Greek thought, responsible for many of the arts, crafts, and sciences. In some myths he creates men from clay. A friend to humankind, he stole fire from Zeus to bring to earth, making possible not only the cooking of food, thought to separate humans from beasts, but also sacrificial practice, which allows humans to communicate with the gods. However, Prometheus' cunning tricks annoyed Zeus, causing him to send the first woman, Pandora, as an unsolicited gift to humans; made by the gods to be a seductive snare, attractive on the outside, but containing an evil mind and an

endless hunger for all the food a man can work to produce, Pandora went on to open the forbidden jar containing all the evils of the present age. Prometheus himself was punished by being tied to a pillar, with an eagle visiting him daily to consume his liver. Overnight, his liver regenerated, making his punishment unending until Heracles (Hercules) came to set him free.   HELEN KING

See also BACCHUS; GREEKS; HERCULES; MYTHOLOGY AND THE BODY; SACRIFICE.

Toilet practices In contemporary Western society going to the toilet is generally viewed as a somewhat shameful necessity. A whole series of euphemisms exists covering both the technology and architecture of sanitation as well as the process and products. We talk of the 'smallest room', the 'loo', 'spending a penny', 'number ones', and 'number twos'. Obscenity is the reverse of the scatological medal, the corollary of the power associated with these functions and products. Like SEX, the excretory bodily functions provide us with some of our most basic symbolic language; when wishing to express ourselves strongly it is to words like 'shit' and 'piss' which we resort.

It seems that in modern Western societies URINE and FAECES are simply shameful waste matter — pollutants to be flushed from our bodies and our homes as swiftly as possible — but this has not always been the case. In Europe a more practical attitude to body products existed for many centuries. Human as well as animal dung has been an important form of fertilizer probably since the beginning of agriculture. With the development of towns a symbiotic relationship developed — the countryside produced food for the townspeople, who gratefully sent their soil-enriching waste products out in return. In the nineteenth century a global dung trade developed, as English farmers began to import guano from Argentina. Alongside its use as fertilizer, dung has been valued as a form of fuel in many peasant economies. William Buchan, the eighteenth-century Scottish physician, praised the folk tradition of using cow dung as a poultice.

Urine too has had a number of practical applications. Stale urine contains ammonia; in ancient Rome fullers used it in the cleaning and dyeing of clothes; in Britain it was known as lye and was the choice of poor housewives well into the nineteenth century. In Scotland it was called 'strang' and kept in buckets for use in a variety of herbal remedies — even in the twentieth century rural GPs have reported its use by farm labourers to treat burns.

In a period before the advent of X-rays and stethoscopes, faeces and urine offered a rare insight into what was going on inside the body. Excreta thus have a long history as diagnostic tools; indeed, during the medieval period the mantula, or urine flask, was the trademark of the medical profession. However, in the sixteenth century the Royal College of Physicians discouraged the use of uroscopy as a sole diagnostic technique, and by the eighteenth century the 'pisse-prophet' was a marginal figure, attacked by regular practitioners as a quack. Urine and stool samples still remain important in DIAGNOSIS of many conditions, but they are now more likely to be subject to chemical analysis — for the twentieth-century doctor smelling and tasting urine was no longer a routine.

However, orthodox medicine's interest in excreta has been more than diagnostic. In the eighteenth century, the physician George Cheyne exemplified contemporary attitudes when he advised one patient on the importance of bowel movements: 'Nothing will do but to keep your body open.' Since at least the days of Hippocratic hygiene, and until at least the mid nineteenth century, the Western medical profession urged the regular prophylactic use of emetics and clysters. Regardless of the particular medical theory invoked it was generally believed to be essential to purge regularly. Similar concerns have been present in Asian and African medical systems. Whilst gastroenterologists may bemoan an obsession with laxatives, the historical fascination with autointoxication and 'staying regular' has persisted to the present day. In Britain COLONIC IRRIGATION has gained publicity if not popularity from royal patronage, although proper contemporary concern focuses on the positive effects of a high-fibre diet, which has been linked to a decreased incidence of colon cancer.

In the eighteenth century the emphasis on regularity led the philosopher John Locke to advocate a strict regime of early POTTY TRAINING. In the first few months babies were to be encouraged to evacuate each morning. This kind of regime found increasing favour in the nineteenth century and by the 1920s a highly regimented approach to infant care was being mass-marketed by figures like Frederick Truby King. Under such systems cleanliness took precedence over affection, and all aspects of child-rearing, including potty-training, were subject to strict timetables. Potty-training was to begin at around 2 months and the baby was encouraged to perform regular bowel evacuations at the same time each day, aided by a salt-water enema if necessary. However, by the 1940s a more relaxed, child-centred approach was finding favour, epitomized by the work of Benjamin Spock. In his early work Spock advocated that the child rather than the parent was to initiate training but by the 1960s he was more prescriptive and recommended that training should commence at 18 months.

A cross-cultural study of child training in the 1950s showed a wide divergence of attitudes and approaches. The Tanala of Madagascar, where babies did not wear nappies, would slap their infants for wetting the mother as early as 6 months, whereas the Siriono of South America only began toilet training when the child was old enough to walk and would not expect full independence in toilet practices until around the age of 6. Amongst the Kwoma people of New Guinea the process did not commence until the child possessed verbal communication skills strong enough to make the process relatively straight-forward: 'You just tell the child what to do and he does it,' reported one villager.

For some young children bladder control is more difficult to achieve at night — *enuresis*, commonly known as bed-wetting, has been discussed by physicians since the days of Galen and Hippocrates. The ancient physicians generally blamed the problem on defects in the kidneys, bladder, or testicles, their remedies, involving extracts from the same organs in animals, persisted until the eighteenth century. By the late eighteenth century William Heberden was recommending cold baths and blisters 'applied to the loins' and belladonna was later used as a cure. Folk wisdom has ascribed the problem to children sleeping too deeply, and children were therefore forced to sleep on hard beds, but now technology has taken over in the shape of the enuresis alarm — two detector mats on a bed connected to a buzzer, which wakes the child when wetting occurs. Nowadays some doctors prescribe drugs, but behavioural training is the most common treatment.

The shame and anxiety aroused in both parents and children by potty training and bed-wetting demonstrates the importance attached to mastery of bodily functions. Since Freud we have seen toilet training as a battle between infant and mother fraught with danger — the anal personality, characterized by orderliness, obstinacy, and parsimony, stemmed from this confrontation. The development of excremental taboos seems to be fundamental to socialization in modern Western society. It may not always have been thus. Until recently, European society appears to have had a more robust attitude to waste products.

In early modern Europe the ritual power of body products was displayed during carnivals. In the mock mass, incense was replaced by excrement, whilst in processions the festive clergy were paraded in carts filled with dung, which they threw at onlookers. In Georgian London it was an accepted dinner-party custom that once the ladies had retired the men would be free to relieve themselves in chamberpots. 'The operation is performed very deliberately and undisguisedly . . . and occasions no interruption of conversation,' observed a visitor in 1810. In the same period people commonly relieved themselves publicly on the city streets. In art and literature too, scatology was an important and widely accepted form of humour. Eighteenth-century satirists like Swift raised the tradition to new literary heights.

This more open attitude partly reflected the technology of the period. As long as they relied on domestic servants to empty their chamberpots it was difficult for the upper and middle classes to deny faecal reality. Even privies were not necessarily private — many had more than one seat. The modern water-closet had its precedents in ancient civilisations, but for many centuries Europe lacked the kind of water supply systems needed for the easy use of such technology. Wastes were either collected above ground in dung-heaps and then periodically removed by street-cleaners, or collected underground in cesspits, which were periodically emptied by night-soil-men (so-called from the hours when they were permitted to perform their duties). Ironically, when the water-closet was popularized in the late eighteenth century it made cities dirtier rather than cleaner — connected to sewers built only for draining storm water from the streets, human wastes flowed into rivers which were often major supplies of drinking water.

However, the evidence of etiquette manuals dating back to the Renaissance suggests that this easygoing attitude was challenged. Bodily behaviour, from spitting to nose-blowing, was subject to increasing restraint. Historians may now have exonerated the Victorians of the charge of sexual prudery, but in the nineteenth century excremental taboos flourished. The water-closet encouraged the privacy: kept in a room of its own and with only one seat, solitude was guaranteed, and you disposed of the waste yourself — a pull on a chain now summoned the flushing water rather than a maid to empty your pot. The great sewer systems built by sanitary reformers thus represented much more than simply a response to the period's deadly cholera EPIDEMICS: the water-closet became not only convenient and hygienic but also a weapon of moral reform. Sanitation had become a fundamental aspect of Western civilization. As Somerset Maugham suggested: 'the cesspool is more necessary to democracy than parliamentary institutions.' S. HOGARTH

See also BODY CONTACT; HYGEINE.

Tongue The tongue plays an essential part in three main processes: in moving food around in the MOUTH — towards the TEETH for mastication, and towards the throat for SWALLOWING; in the special sense of TASTE; and in normal SPEECH production. It is covered by a mucous membrane that is continuous with the lining of the rest of the mouth and the throat; this is kept moist by the mucous SALIVA secreted from small glands in its own surface as well as from the main salivary glands. The characteristic roughness of the healthy tongue is due to four types of *papillae* that cover the top and sides of the front two-thirds. These are outgrowths of the epithelium — the covering layer — and are of various shapes and sizes. Three types of papillae contain taste buds; the largest but least numerous of the papillae, found towards the back of the tongue, have taste buds arrayed in grooves that surround them.

The bulk of the tongue is made up of a set of muscles attached at one end to hard tissues external to the tongue and inserted at the other end into the fibrous tissue of the tongue itself; these are the extrinsic muscles. There are, in addition, vertical and transverse intrinsic muscle fibres that are attached at both ends to fibrous tissue within the tongue; their prime function is to alter the shape of the tongue. The tongue musculature is largely contained within a fibrous sac, so the whole maintains a constant volume irrespective of its shape.

There are three main paired extrinsic muscles on each side; their attachments allow the production of the three main components of tongue movement:

The *genioglossus* muscles take origin from the middle of the back of the lower jaw and have a fan-like insertion into each side of the midline of the tongue. Their contraction protrudes the tongue.

The *hyoglossus* muscles take origin from each side of the horseshoe-shaped hyoid bone. (This lies below the tongue and is suspended by a sling of muscles from the jaw and the skull.) They extend forward into the tongue at the sides of the genioglossus muscles. Their contraction shortens the tongue towards its base on the hyoid.

The *styloglossus* muscles take origin from the styloid process on the base of the skull and pass downwards and forwards into side edges of the tongue. Their contraction elevates the sides of the tongue, forming a gutter in the middle.

During feeding, contraction of the styloglossus muscle of one side causes that side of the tongue to tilt upwards. Consequently, solid food is moved to the opposite side of the mouth, placing it between the occluding surfaces of the teeth for chewing. In contrast, all movements involved in the intra-oral transport of food, and in swallowing, are bilaterally symmetrical, so that the bolus moves in the midline.

During mastication, the *mechanosensory function* of the tongue is essential for the ability to sort the broken particles of food so that the largest remaining particles are always preferentially selected for placement between the occluding teeth. The mechanosensory receptors in the mucosa have an additional role because the control of tongue posture depends mainly upon information supplied by them. The nerves that carry the information to the BRAIN STEM for this and for the sense of taste are the CRANIAL NERVES V, VII (taste), and IX (the trigeminal, facial, and glossopharyngeal nerves). The motor nerve from the brain stem to most of the tongue muscles is the hypoglossal (XII).

During speech, movements of the tongue take part, along with those of the jaw, the lips, and the cheeks, in the complex configurations of this part of the 'vocal tract' that are necessary for articulation.

Looking at the tongue is a diagnostic tradition. It can become coated, glossy, or smoothed in a variety of systemic illnesses, but most changes are non-specific. Because the tongue is essentially a bag of muscles, a drop in the activity of those muscles makes the bag floppy so that its posture is governed primarily by gravity. Failure to maintain the tongue in a forward position, by maintaining contraction of the genioglossus muscles, may therefore restrict or block the airway, especially if a person is lying on their back. Such a blockage can occur in someone who is unconscious from any cause — from fainting to brain damage. Under normal circumstances the converse also applies: a restriction of airflow causes a reflex increase in genioglossus activity.

ALLAN THEXTON

See PLATE 1.

See also JAW; MOUTH; SPEECH; SWALLOWING; TASTE.

Torture In a broad sense, torture might be regarded as any instance in which pain is inflicted by one human being on another, either for personal gratification or to demonstrate power. But historically torture has most often been defined more narrowly, as an aspect of legal systems or of state repression. The third century Roman jurist, Ulpian, noted that by torture 'we are to understand the torment and suffering of the body in order to elicit the truth', and much the same definition was offered by Article 1 of the Declaration against Torture adopted by the General Assembly of the United Nations in December 1975: 'torture means any act by which severe pain or suffering, whether physical or mental, is intentionally inflicted by or at the instigation of a public official on a person for such purposes of obtaining from him or a third person information or confession, punishing him for an act he committed, or intimidating him or other persons.'

Viewed in this way, torture has a long history. It was part of the judicial practice in a number of ancient cultures, notably among the Egyptians, Persians, Greeks, and Romans. Among the Romans it was reserved mainly for the investigation of treason or of criminal acts perpetrated by slaves or other persons of low status. What has been termed judicial torture probably fell into at least partial disuse after the fall of the Roman Empire, but it returned in Western and Central Europe when interest in Roman Law revived during the 'judicial revolution' of the twelfth century. More specifically, a papal ruling of 1215 which denied the validity of the ordeal as a means of establishing proof in criminal trials left those running Europe's legal systems with the problem of how to prove that suspects were guilty. Most states adopted the notion that a confession was the best form of proof, and adopted torture as a means of gaining confessions as well as information which might implicate other persons. Torture also became part of the judicial repertoire of the Inquisition. In theory, and frequently in practice, the application of torture was subjected to set rules aimed at avoiding the infliction of excessive suffering. More specifically, torture was only to be used against persons against whom there were already strong presumptions of guilt; it was not to be used against children, pregnant women, or the aged and infirm; examining judges were not meant to shape confessions through leading questions; and, of course, in the Christian West torturing was did not take place on Sundays. Preferred forms of judicial torture were the rack, the strappado (which involved binding the arms together behind the suspect's back, and then lifting him by a rope secured to his hands and slung over a beam), thumbscrews, and irons designed to crush the legs.

Cross-cultural studies reveal that torture was used in a number of extra-European states. In Japan, for example, torture was used from a very early date to extract confessions, and from the beginning of the Tokugawa period in the seventeenth century the Japanese seem to have used something very like the strappado. Some legal systems were opposed to judicial torture. Islamic law rejected the use of coercion to gain confession, although the authorities in the Ottoman Empire frequently ignored this.

The abolition of torture as a part of criminal trial process occurred over most of Europe in the second half of the eighteenth century, and has usually been regarded as a symbol of the arrival of Enlightenment values. More recent scholarship has suggested that the emergence of forms of secondary punishment which made the former stress on the confession redundant may also have been at play, along with other changes in criminal process. Yet it is certainly true that nineteenth-century liberals regarded the abolition of torture as one of the major achievements of European culture, something which distinguished their rational and progressive world from the brutal past. Thus the entry on torture in the famous eleventh edition of the *Encyclopaedia Britannica*, published in 1911, could congratulate itself that 'the whole subject is now one of only historical interest as far as Europe is concerned'.

Sadly, twentieth-century developments shattered such complacency. Both Stalin's Russia and Hitler's Germany experienced a massive upsurge in torture, with the greater morality of the need to defend the Revolution or the State relegating other forms of morality to a secondary position. Since 1945 torture has been widely used in many parts of the world, notably in such South American States as Uruguay, Brazil, Argentina, and, under General Pinochet, in Chile, along with South Africa and Turkey. In such areas, torture has become one of the standard methods by which regimes have supported themselves, usually with a lack of control or supervision which would have been unthinkable in medieval Europe. The rack and the strappado have been rendered obsolete by electric shocks to the genitals, the use of electric cattle prods, regular beatings, cigarette burns, the insertion of police truncheons and similar objects in the anus or vulva, threat of RAPE or rape itself, and sophisticated psychological torments, applied to persons suspected of political deviance in a large number of states. Amnesty International has estimated that a third of the political regimes currently in existence use torture on a regular basis. The preface of that organization's 1973 *Report on Torture* commented that 'torture has virtually become a worldwide phenomenon and that the torturing of citizens regardless of sex, age, or state of health in an effort to retain political power is a practice encouraged by some governments and tolerated by others in an increasingly large number of countries.'

As an historical phenomenon, torture, apart from those occasions when it has simply been treated as a symbol of past brutality, has been most studied in its legal aspects, and there has been little attempt to integrate it into the history of the body. Obviously, however, it does raise questions about how physical pain and suffering were regarded, and hence how one human being might regard the body of another. At least initially, medieval codes regulating torture held that persons who refused to confess under torture had removed the presumptions of guilt against them, and long before the eighteenth century European critics of judicial torture were arguing that torture was more likely to reveal individual tolerance of pain rather than encourage accurate confessions. Thus the English legal writer Sir John Fortescue, in *De Laudibus Legum Anglie*, a treatise probably composed around 1470, asked 'who is so hardy that, having once passed through this atrocious torment, would not rather, though innocent, confess to every kind of crime, than submit again to the agony of torture?' (The English common law, which Fortescue was praising, did not use torture as a part of normal criminal process.)

This theme was taken up in the mid eighteenth century, with the arrival of the Enlightenment. The most noted Enlightenment writer on crime and punishment was the Italian Cesare Beccaria, who published his influential *Dei Delitti e delle Pene* (*On Crimes and Punishments*) in 1764. Beccaria discussed torture at length, giving a number of reasons why it should be abolished, some humanitarian, others returning to a discussion of what torture was actually testing. Using contemporary notions about sensitivity to pain, Beccaria argued that 'the impression of pain may become so great that, filling the entire sensory capacity of the tortured person, it leaves him free only to choose what for the moment is the shortest way to escape from pain . . . the sensitive innocent man will then confess himself guilty when he believes that, by so doing, he can put an end to his torment.' Conversely, argued Beccaria, 'robust scoundrels', although guilty, would not crack under torture. This line of argument became axiomatic in Enlightenment critiques of judicial torture.

There is currently a growing corpus of studies of the effects of torture, both physical and psychological, upon those who have suffered it in the modern world, and such studies might offer perspectives on how a wider history of torture might be written. What is perhaps most needed, however, is some sort of insight into how torturers regarded those upon whom they were inflicting pain. It seems likely that in many cases the torturer would regard torture as a necessary evil, vital in either defending a regime or expediting a criminal process, or might regard the person being tortured as a creature so deviant as not to merit consideration as a fellow human. Yet it remains clear that the practice of torture does hold some clues, as yet largely uninvestigated, to past attitudes towards the human body.

J. A. SHARPE

Further reading
Peters, E. (1985). *Torture*. Blackwell, Oxford and New York.

See also MARTYRDOM; VIOLENCE; WAR AND THE BODY.

Toxicology is essentially the science of POISONS. It was recognized long ago that the toxicity of any substance is related to dose. The sixteenth-century iconoclast Paracelsus is credited with the statement: 'All substances are poisons, there is none which is not a poison. The right dose differentiates a poison from a remedy.' Toxicology had its origins in medicine and therapeutics, and to this day one of the key steps in the development of new drugs is the evaluation of the 'therapeutic window'. This window corresponds to the range of doses where a beneficial effect is obtained but below the dose which causes unacceptable side-effects.

Throughout history the substances that have been used for medicine — as well as the poisons used to eliminate political rivals, as practised from classical times through to the Renaissance — have been almost exclusively derived from natural sources. Despite a recent emphasis on the toxicity of synthetic chemicals, arising in part from the influential writings of Rachel Carson, it is interesting to note that Nature has been endlessly inventive in its production of toxic agents. Such natural toxic substances are sometimes used as part of defence mechanisms as, for example, in the case of snake venoms. However, sometimes the toxic substances are by-products of normal metabolism by many different species. Several varieties of the mould *Aspergillus* produce a group of carcinogens called *aflatoxins*, which cause LIVER injury and CANCER. A proper understanding of the occurrence and actions of natural toxins is vital to the maintenance of a healthy lifestyle. In a number of countries cassava is a major source of carbohydrate, but if it is not properly treated ingestion of the naturally occurring *cyanogenic* (cyanide-forming) glycosides can be fatal.

From the mid nineteenth century onwards the increasing use of pure chemicals as DRUGS paved the way for the development of toxicology as a more exact science which aimed to unravel the mechanisms of action of toxic substances. Very few drugs or toxic agents are active without some sort of metabolic activation; a chemical or physical change brought about in the body. Usually the effect of these changes is to render the substance more water soluble so that it may be excreted as rapidly as possible. In some instances metabolism results in the formation of a reactive chemical species, which binds to cellular macromolecules such as DNA or PROTEINS. Such modifications can then lead to biological consequences, which are manifested as a frank toxic effect. However, there are protective mechanisms for dealing with such reactive species within cells; many are converted into substances that are ultimately excreted in urine.

In some cases unfortunate toxicological incidents can have beneficial consequences in the long term. For example, it was noted that soldiers returning from World War I who had been exposed to sulphur mustard had very depressed white blood cell counts. Ultimately, this observation led to the development of nitrogen mustards which, soon after World War II, began to be widely used in the treatment of cancers such as leukaemia. A rather different story relates to the discovery of a class of potent carcinogens, the *nitrosamines*. Several poisoning incidents in the textile industry, starting in the late 1930s, were associated with the use of *dimethylnitrosamine* (DMN) as a solvent for rayon. It was shown in animal models that acute administration of DMN produced a characteristic type of liver damage similar to that seen in workers. However, chronic administration of low doses of DMN produced liver tumours. It was subsequently found that many other nitrosocompounds produced tumours in different organs in many species of animals. Paradoxically, some nitrosocompounds were found to have antitumour activity and, like the nitrogen mustards described above, probably act by damaging the DNA in tumours in such a way that the cells cannot repair the damage and die.

There are sometimes great differences between species and between individuals with regard to the toxicity of a particular substance. A famous example is penicillin, which was tested for toxicity in rats before being given to humans. As rats tolerated large doses of penicillin with no ill effect, the drug was considered safe enough to be administered to humans, and the age of antibiotics was born. It was subsequently found that guinea pigs are very susceptible to toxicity from penicillin — history might have been very different if guinea pigs had been the test animal of choice. For many drugs which require metabolism to be active, or, in some cases, for toxicity to be apparent, *polymorphism* (occurrence in more than one form) of key metabolic enzymes can lead to spectacular differences in individual susceptibility. *Debrisoquine*, a drug used in the treatment of high blood pressure, was found to be very slowly metabolised by 1 in 10 Caucasian people, due to a genetic polymorphism for a particular enzyme. In affected individuals, administration of the drug caused a dramatic fall in blood pressure due to the persistence of the active drug in the circulation.

Despite much current public concern about health effects from environmental chemicals, there is little or no evidence of large numbers of cases of any disease being due to exposure to such agents. It is not that chemicals are any more or less toxic than those to which earlier generations were exposed — it is rather that contemporary exposure levels have been progressively reduced to such an extent that effects are almost undetectable. As our understanding of the mechanisms of toxicity of chemicals has improved, it is less likely that highly dangerous industrial chemicals will be present in the environment. However, as indicated above, our exposure to natural toxic agents remains a major source of concern.

Over much of its history the study of toxicology has relied upon the manifestation of some adverse health effect, in either humans or experimental animals, as an indication of the toxic effects of any particular substance. As the Human Genome Project attains one of its first goals of obtaining the complete sequence of the human genome (and as the complete sequences of the genomes of many other species have either already been, or will shortly be, completed), it is likely that approaches to toxicological questions will be quite different in the near future. Many pharmaceutical companies have led the way in the exploitation of this technology for rapid and comprehensive screening of adverse side effects of the increasing numbers of novel substances that are being examined for beneficial effects.

DAVID SHUKER

Further reading

Klassen, C. D. (1996). *Casarett and Doull's Toxicology: the basic science of poisons*. McGraw Hill, New York.

Timbrell, J. A. (1991). *Principles of biochemical toxicology*, (2nd edn). Taylor and Francis, London.

See also DRUG; ENVIRONMENTAL TOXICOLOGY; POISONING.

Toxins A term applied to POISONS which are toxic to the human body. Many come from microorganisms — for example, cholera toxin and TETANUS toxin are derived respectively from *Vibrio cholera* and *Clostridium tetani*. Some toxins are derived from higher organisms — the deadly *tetrodotoxin*, which blocks nerve conduction, is derived from the liver and ovaries of the puffer fish. Yet others are of fungal origin, such as the liver toxic substance aflatoxin, from a fungus which grows on groundnuts. A.W.C.

See IMMUNIZATION; MICROORGANISMS; POISONS; TOXICOLOGY.

Tracheostomy An opening in the trachea (*stoma*: Greek for 'mouth'). The operation which creates the opening is *tracheotomy* (*tome*: Greek for 'incision'); it involves slitting open the trachea (windpipe), to enable the patient to breathe when the upper respiratory tract is obstructed either by a foreign body or as a result of disease or injury.

It is an operation with an ancient history, reportedly first thought of by Asculaepius in 100 BC when he was, according to GALEN, trying to devise a way of relieving patients suffering from 'those species of quinsies in which there is great danger of suffocation'. There is evidence that the operation was used occasionally in antiquity, and with increasing frequency from the Renaissance. In this simple form, however, it afforded the patient only brief relief, since the artificial opening rapidly closed itself. It was only with the invention of the cannula — a hollow tube which permits the draining of fluids — around 1600, that more extended opening could be practised. The invention of the double cannula in the late eighteenth century was an important improvement: it allowed for the tube to be cleared and cleaned without inconveniencing the patient.

Despite these improvements, tracheostomy was only rarely performed before the mid

nineteenth century, most notably in attempts to revive the hanged. It then achieved greater — and increasing — prominence as more virulent strains of diphtheria emerged in Western Europe in the 1850s. Diphtheria is an acute INFECTIOUS DISEASE characterized by the development of a membrane across the back of the throat, which may threaten SUFFOCATION, although death is usually due to the effects of the toxin released into the patient's system by the infecting organism. Diphtheria was first identified as a specific disease by Pierre Bretonneau in 1824, and it was his pupil, Armand Trousseau, who established tracheostomy as a treatment option through his work at the Paris Childrens' Hospital in the 1830s and 1840s.

With the spread of the virulent form of diphtheria after 1855, doctors across Europe became increasingly familiar with the operation, and its technique was gradually refined. It was the only operation which, it was said, every practising doctor had to be prepared to perform. By the turn of the century, however, American hospital practitioners had begun to use intubation (passing a tube into the trachea via the mouth) in preference to tracheostomy, and this development gradually influenced European practice. Despite the introduction of anti-toxin therapy in the 1890s, diphtheria remained a public health problem in the twentieth century until the development and application of active immunization in the interwar period, and for as long as the disease was present, tracheostomy remained a treatment option, notably in Britain, where it continued to be the intervention of choice for threatened obstruction. By 1950, however, diphtheria had all but vanished as a public health problem in the West.

Meanwhile tracheostomy was beginning to be applied not to relieve obstruction to the airway, but to assist the use of ARTIFICIAL VENTILATION, for example in cases of paralytic poliomyelitis, head injuries, chest injuries, and barbiturate poisoning.

Tracheostomy remains a routine procedure in intensive therapy units when prolonged connection to an artificial ventilator is required. In other instances, permanent tracheostomy allows a person to breathe for himself after operation for cancer of the LARYNX. ANNE HARDY

Transfiguration The transfiguration is a concept in Christianity which is central to the understanding of Christ as joining the human and the divine. The notion of transfiguration marks the historical event when God became present in Christ's body, which occurred as Christ left his followers to pray. Both because of its theological importance and because of the centrality that it had in narratives of Christ's life, the transfiguration was heavily glossed within the early Church. It is the only time in the Gospels where Christ's divinity is revealed to the apostles.

The notion of transfiguration gained centrality in Christian religion because it marks

both the appearance of Christ's divine form in his human body and the time when God names him as the Messiah. On the road to Jerusalem, Christ left the apostles Peter, James, and John to pray (Matthew 17: 1–8; Mark 9: 2–8; Luke 9: 28–36). As he did so, his body underwent METAMORPHOSIS in which his 'face shone like the sun and his clothes became white as light' (Luke 9: 29). For the first time in the gospels, God spoke to the apostles, recognizing his son (Matthew 17: 1–8). Christ appeared in conversation with Elijah and Moses, two figures before whom God had revealed himself in the *Old Testament*, confirming his divinity. Christ told the apostles not to speak of this event until after he had risen from the dead; they offered little description of the event, although the narrative significance in the gospels is implicit: the event strengthened the apostles for the coming passion, and prepares the reader for Christ's resurrection.

Because the passage describes the simultaneous presence of humanity and divinity in one body, it was the subject of extensive exegesis for early Christians. Church Fathers returned to the event as an explanation of the difference of flesh and spirit, and an illustration of the humanity of God. The feast of the transfiguration was commemorated within the Church, and Mt. Tabor became a colony of religious orders and a site of pilgrimage. As an occasion of transcending the physical body it gained metaphorical significance in daily religious practice in Greek Orthodox, Catholic, and Protestant religion. The metaphorical use of transfiguration extends from the Christic narrative to explain the revelation of religious truth. Catholic theologians describe the partaking of Christ's body as an occasion of individual transfiguration, and speak metaphorically of the transfiguration of the Church to mark its spiritual invigoration. Transfiguration gains the quality of a prophetic reading, and extends to the entire Church, as, in taking the sacrament, the Christian prepares for the final revelation of the second coming.

The concept of religious transfiguration gained different significance as a revelation of religious truth in Catholicism, Greek Orthodox, and Protestant churches. In the Byzantine church, images of the transfiguration were among the most common that were used to decorate reliquaries, vessels that contained body parts that joined the spiritual and physical worlds; their popularity suggests the strong link drawn between the transfiguration and the elevation from the body in the Last Judgment. The long tradition of images of the transfiguration that existed in the Greek Orthodox church was paralleled in the West; from the fourteenth century, Italian artists returned to the transfiguration as a dramatic revelation of the glory of Christ. This tradition culminates in Raphael Sanzio's *Transfiguration*. The dramatic construction of the transfiguration in Raphael's fresco returns both to the duality of the Christian god and the confirmation of his divinity through his transcendence of physical form; depicting the concept of transfiguration indeed posed the significant pictorial challenge of illustrating transcendence of the body. Raphael depicted Christ flanked by the Old Testament figures of the prophet and lawgiver, bathed in divine light. Raphael's conflation of Christ's curing an epileptic child with the metamorphosis of his own body juxtaposes an uncontrolled body with transcendence of physical form. The scene was returned to so often because it illustrates a central concept of Christianity: the physical juncture of Christ's humanity and divinity, the human manifestation of God's presence in the world.

The concept of transfiguration gained new significance as a revelation of religious truth to the individual in the reformed churches. The reformer Martin Luther appropriated the concept of transfiguration to emphasize the power of the written word, rather than transfiguration of the worldly body, and linked the concept to the power of individual prayer and inner reflection, to join man and God without mediation. But if transfiguration became the end of an interior journey of self-exploration among Protestant groups, the metaphorical significance of the transfiguration often remained embedded in the transcendence of the bodily form. Protestant theologians often use the metaphor of transfiguration of the individual to draw attention to the embodied state of a man who receives grace; transfiguration becomes a conceit for describing a physical relation to the written word. If the transfiguration of the individual was linked by Catholics to partaking of Christ's flesh or as a spiritual invigoration of the Church, Protestant orders describe a physical preparation as a precondition to transfiguration through reading of the Scriptures. Pietism and Puritanism emphasize disciplining the body in preparation to reading the Scriptures.

The religious concept of transfiguration has broad significance as it illustrates the relation of the physical world to the revelation of divine truth.   DANIEL A. BROWNSTEIN

Further reading
Brown, F. B. (1983). *Transfiguration: poetic metaphor and the legacies of religious belief.* University of North Carolina Press, Chapel Hill, North Carolina.

Carlston, C. F. Transfiguration and resurrection. *Journal of Biblical Literature*, **80**, 233–40.

McGuckin, J. A. (1986). *The Transfiguration of Christ in scriptures and tradition.* Lewiston, New York.

See also CHRISTIANITY AND THE BODY.

Transgenics is the transfer of genetic information that is not normally present into the genome of a species. To create a transgenic species the relevant gene (*transgene*) is introduced into STEM CELLS, which are in turn introduced into a *blastocyst* (the product of the early cell division of a fertilized egg). If the resulting progeny have the transgene in their GERM CELLS then transgenic species can be derived by breeding. The new

characteristics of the resulting animals (their altered PHENOTYPE) reveal or confirm the function of the transgene. By introduction of genetic material to disrupt a gene into a species, such as mice, accurate models of human genetic diseases can be created. These so called 'knockout' animals are essential for formulating approaches to the treatment of human genetic disease.   A.W.C.

See GENETICS, HUMAN; STEM CELLS.

Transplantation Routine success with transplantation of human organs was not obtained until the mid 1960s, in spite of its ancient appeal. Prior to this, SKIN and ENDOCRINE gland grafting had often been attempted from one human to another, but the reports on the outcome were confusing and the observations uncritical.

The groundwork for the new science of *transplantation immunology* was laid by Medawar and other British biologists in the 1940s. They showed that rejection of tissue transferred from one person or animal to another was invariable, except for grafts between identical TWINS, or a few special cases (e.g. cornea). In the 1950s they further showed that this tissue rejection was a response of the IMMUNE SYSTEM, rather than a biochemical or physiological 'misfit'. But since an antibody could not be identified, a new form of immunity was sought and found. Suspicion fell on the small lymphocytes. These, with their relatively huge nucleus and minimal cytoplasm, had always been suspected of some important role in the body, but since they had shown no capability to multiply nor to act as PHAGOCYTES, they had not been taken seriously. Soon, however, these lymphocytes were found in fact to be capable of division and enlargement when suitably provoked by foreign cells or particular proteins. So this previously neglected cell type became recognized as the key player in the exquisite differentiation of foreign material from the 'self', particularly of cells only slightly different from the body's own cells. The recognition of this mechanism explained the rejection of grafts. Although understandably seen as existing to frustrate transplant surgeons, this 'cell-mediated' immune mechanism clearly had a wider, fundamental role, as yet not fully understood.

Human grafts
In the 1950s, surgeons in Boston, led by Joseph Murray, established that a KIDNEY graft, from one healthy human twin to the other who had terminal chronic kidney failure, could reverse all the features of the disease, even though the donor kidney had no nerve supply and was placed in an unnatural position in the patient's pelvis. About this time, Medawar showed that the immune response in adult mice to experimental grafts could be abolished by prior injection of the donor cells at birth — tolerance had been induced.

The first attempts at reducing the human immune response to kidney grafts employed crude total body irradiation to depress the bone marrow and lymphocyte activity. These attempts

largely failed. By 1960 the strategy was to use the newer anti-cancer drugs (notably 6-mercapto-purine and related substances, derived from the military poison gas nitrogen mustard). In cancer patients such drugs were known to suppress the immune response. One such agent, *azathioprine*, was shown by the British surgeon Roy Calne to have a promising effect on cell-mediated immunity against grafts, without serious side-effects of general toxicity or liability to infection. In Paris and Boston, the first medium-term kidney graft survivals were obtained using this drug alone. A major advance followed when Starzl in Denver found that STEROID hormones, previously shown to have no effect on graft survival if given alone, combined with azathioprine to give powerful immunosuppression.

Rapid progress
This unpredicted innovation led to a drug regimen which was to be the core treatment for the next 20 years, establishing kidney transplantation as an acceptable form of treatment. Indeed, from 1963 onwards there was a period of optimism that routine organ grafting of all kinds would soon follow. This was encouraged by the concurrent rapid progress in immunology. The key role of circulating lymphocytes was now known, but the similar cells in the THYMUS gland were apparently inactive; the absence of any demonstrated effect of removing the adult thymus seemed to relegate it to the status of an evolutionary vestige, in spite of its size and prominence in early life. The puzzle was solved in the UK in 1960 by Jacques Miller's serendipitous discovery that immediate removal of the thymus in new-born mice caused profound and lasting absence of cell-mediated immunity, allowing permanent acceptance of a skin graft — but also liability to some types of infection. Clearly the thymus was vital in the maturation of some circulating lymphocytes. Soon, markers were developed for lymphocytes that neatly classified them into *T-cells* (thymus-derived), responsible for cell-mediated immunity, and *B-cells* (bone marrow-derived), responsible (after maturation into plasma cells) for antibody production.

Around this time also, tissue typing methods emerged for identification of antigens on body cells, similar to red blood cell grouping but more complex. This gave the hope that any human organs donated could be matched closely to a potential recipient. Better methods for organ storage and the construction of perfusion machines allowed preservation and even long-distance transport of kidneys to patients with a good match. In this growth period of human transplantation, with the hopes that a final solution was at hand, even monkey kidneys were transplanted to human patients — and some of them were not rejected immediately.

Kidney failure
Meanwhile, from 1960 onwards, patients with renal failure were successfully treated with long-

term DIALYSIS on the artificial kidney. This back-up was crucial before and after transplantation. At this time kidneys were taken a little while after the donor's heart had stopped and death had been pronounced. These kidneys were slightly damaged by the intervening lack of oxygen and did not usually work immediately, but since kidney tissue shows powers of revival and can pick up later, the artificial kidney could be used during this shut-down time. However, when the first human LIVER transplants were attempted in the optimistic mid 1960s, the result was disastrous, not only because of the formidable new surgical challenge, but also because the liver was more sensitive to lack of oxygen after the death of the donor. Since there was no artificial liver or heart equivalent to the artificial kidney, if these transplanted organs did not function immediately, death was inevitable. This created pressure for donor organs to be as fresh as possible, and some cautious initiatives were taken, notably cooling the donor at the time of death, to reduce the oxygen requirement of the organs.

Coincidentally with this need within the service of transplantation, the success of resuscitation and ARTIFICIAL VENTILATION for critically-ill patients in intensive care had thrown up the problem of patients who survived with irreparable brain damage, who had otherwise good physiological function but could no longer breathe for themselves. In these circumstances it was pointless to continue artificial ventilation. The first formal discussion of possible criteria for diagnosis of irreversible coma was by the Harvard Committee of 1968, and the pioneer Boston transplant surgeons unwisely involved themselves in their discussions. Shortly afterwards in that same year, Christian Barnard carried out the first human HEART transplant. He was praised at first for his daring innovation, but others, experienced in transplantation or otherwise, followed his lead with poor results, which were publicly revealed. There was professional criticism of such adventures worldwide, and increasing hostility from the public and media over many aspects, notably the tasteless publicity attaching to the patient and donor. The public were also uneasy when, for the first time, the details of the diagnosis of BRAIN DEATH and 'heart-beating' ORGAN DONATION were revealed. It seemed to some that these reasonable criteria for death had been introduced to help transplant surgeons, whereas they were required primarily in order to avoid pointless persistence with artificial ventilation.

Hesitant times

The consequences of that 'year of the heart' were a loss of confidence inside and outside the small world of organ transplantation, a virtual moratorium on human organ grafting apart from kidneys, and a rise in ethical debates on biomedical matters, with the emergence of a cadre of biomedical ethicists. Worthy government committees embargoed the transport of donors, and declared that death should be decided by

'traditional means', but they did encourage kidney transplantation with supportive publicity and donor card drives, attempting to incorporate organ donation into a respectable routine. This was not unconnected with the emergence of kidney transplantation as a more cost-effective treatment for chronic renal failure than regular dialysis.

In the late 1960s, one new agent, *anti-lymphocyte serum* (ALS), was prepared and had spectacular success in experimental grafting. This encouraged the restart of human liver transplantation by two pioneers, Starzl in Denver and Calne in Cambridge, and evaluation of heart transplantation was funded at a centre under Shumway in Stanford. Such transplants were widely regarded as experiments without hope — a last resort for the most hopeless of patients — but the results of all organ grafting improved slowly, with or without the new ALS and its successors playing a supporting role in immunosuppression. The 1970s were a time of numerous small improvements in the surgical detail of kidney transplantation and post-operative management. The still rapidly-increasing understanding of immunology made little impact on clinical transplantation at this time. Better tissue typing methods appeared, but they did not fulfil the earlier promise (except in bone marrow transplantation).

Innovation resumes

By 1976 it was thought appropriate to formalize the criteria for brain death. These were duly agreed, and issued by medical bodies and governments, separating the matter carefully from the needs of transplantation. In Britain, fully ten years after Barnard, one heart transplant unit was cautiously approved, funded and controlled. Other nations took similar steps. Though there were critics, their objections centred largely on the cost of high technology medicine in a world of simple need. With tasteless publicity avoided, the new heart transplant units soon reported good results.

After the cautious growth of the mid 1970s, organ transplantation moved forward rapidly again with the introduction, in 1978, of a new immunosuppressive agent. This innovation came neither from basic immunology, nor from cancer chemotherapy, but from the routine mass-testing of soil samples in the search for microorganisms producing antibiotics or substances with anti-cancer or immunosuppressive effects. A Norwegian fungus was found to make, in its struggle for survival, a useful product later called *cyclosporine A* (CsA), which had a powerful, safe, inhibitory action on lymphocytes, and which showed promise in animal transplantation. Reluctantly the company concerned prepared CsA for sale, but only as a prestige product, since the transplantation market was judged too small at that time for profitable investment. CsA proved to be a tricky agent to use, and animal testing had failed to reveal its toxicity for human kidneys, but once the art — rather than the science — of its use was mastered, it changed the

history of transplantation. Steroids were still necessary as a partner for the new drug, and the new regimen was so powerful that it overrode the need for precise tissue typing. Results of kidney transplantation improved with its use, and rejection crises were rarer and less dramatic. But the main effect was to make liver and heart transplantation possible and widely accepted, and these became routine medical practice worldwide. In America, liver grafting became the single most expensive standard procedure in the world of surgery. Other pharmaceutical companies noticed the new, expanding potential market, and in the 1990s a steady stream of new products emerged; again they were obtained by synthetic chemists' changes to anti-cancer drugs, and rivals to cyclosporine came from other fungi from Easter Island and Japan. This success in countering rejection, as well as further experience in day-to-day management, meant better graft survival with fewer complications and deaths. Those patients considered eligible for organ transplants increased, and the upper and lower age limits moved steadily apart. Patients with major additional abnormalities, notably diabetes or serious vascular disease, were no longer automatically excluded.

But this success carried with it a crisis in the supply of organs in the 1990s. While candidates for kidney transplant could survive and grow older on dialysis while waiting for an organ, suitable liver and heart patients soon died. This shortage also led to concerns from professionals and patients' organizations about the traditional allocation of scarce organs based on tissue typing matching alone, since this now had only a minor role in the cyclosporine age. New ethical questions were aired. Were those with rare blood and tissue types now unfairly excluded? Was it fair to let older or sicker patients wait as long as younger, fitter ones? Should organs be given to those known to be feckless and likely to default from their medication and follow-up? Was it acceptable to offer cadaver organs to those from ethnic minorities and religious groups opposed to becoming cadaveric donors themselves, but who nevertheless would accept organs if living in countries with well-developed donation and sharing schemes?

As the service of transplantation also expanded out from its origins in the Western, developed nations, it moved from a base in Western academic medicine to become a service available in countries with different cultural assumptions. A remarkable variety of patterns of development was seen. In well-off nations, transplantation and dialysis spread quickly as a routine, but even there divergent views on organ donation were seen — some, such as Norway, used large numbers of living, related donors, and some, such as Eire, used none. Some countries, like Japan, had deep cultural hostility to interfering with the body after death, and no cadaveric donations occurred. Previously poor nations, such as those with new wealth from oil, at first sent even their poor citizens abroad in the 1970s, with their families, for living donor transplantation; then in the 1980s their governments set up transplant units at home, usually with expatriate surgical staff who often trained local professionals and handed over to them in the 1990s. Lastly, in very poor nations with limited facilities and no cadaveric donation, the vast majority of patients with chronic renal failure remained untreated and died, usually unaware of the diagnosis, and certainly having no expectation of cure. In these nations the wealthy or the élite could purchase treatment in private clinics and could easily induce poor people to part with a kidney, for money.

New shortages

In spite of every effort, the attempts to increase cadaveric donors in the developed world were not successful and new initiatives to deal with this shortage were numerous. These included the acceptance of less-than-perfect organs, the increasing use of living, related kidney donors, and even the surgical removal of parts of the liver and pancreas or a lobe of the lung from living donors, with encouragement of emotionally-involved genetically unrelated donors, such as spouses, to come forward. Whilst payment for kidneys from unrelated donors in other lands was officially deplored in the countries in which the science and surgery of transplantation had developed, this practice occurred; if the greed of intermediary brokers could be dealt with, the arrangement was locally accepted as reasonable.

The organ shortage meant a new look at the use of *xenograft* organs — from other species. It had always been assumed that monkeys, with their closeness to man, would be the first source of such organs, but by the 1990s monkeys had powerful human friends, their use in medical research was stringently controlled, and many species were declared to be protected. Pursuit of this 'concordant' source seemed less necessary when another scientific discipline began to impinge on transplantation and even began to supplant immunology from its traditional role as the tissue grafter's essential laboratory partner. Genetic engineering began to provide a range of new techniques which could alter the nature of donor tissue and reduce the violent antibody and cell-mediated attack on xenograft tissue. Selected genes could be inactivated in the donor; gene insertion could add new proteins that would neutralize the reaction to antibody; cloned animals could be raised by transfer of cell nuclei from adult animals to embryos, after suitably engineering the nuclei. All this meant that the use of species 'discordant' with man could be contemplated. The animal turned to was the easily bred, non-violent pig, an animal possessing conveniently human-sized organs, and one already used for food and lacking unpleasant diseases — except one possible retrovirus. After studies had shown no passage of this organism to humans, regulatory bodies gave a careful blessing to the development of xenotransplantation.

Organ transplantation has come far in one generation and those involved continue as before to travel hopefully, with the usual mix of help from both basic science and industry, as well as good luck and serendipity.   DAVID HAMILTON

Further reading
Ginns, L. C., Cosimi, A. B., and Morris, P. J. (1999). *Transplantation*. Blackwell, Oxford.
Starzl, T. E. (1992). *The puzzle people*. University of Pittsburgh Press.

See also BRAIN DEATH; DIALYSIS; IMMUNE SYSTEM; LIFE SUPPORT; ORGAN DONATION; PHAGOCYTES; STEM CELLS; THYMUS.

Transport
In a physiological sense transport generally means the movement of substances across the membranes of CELLS. This is an important process as, without transport, products of digestion would be unable to move from the alimentary tract into the body. Clearly the bounding membranes of cells cannot be generally permeable to all bodily substances, otherwise important cellular components would be able to leak out. Some substances, such as weak acids or bases in their undissociated form, are soluble in lipids and will dissolve in the lipid bilayer of the CELL MEMBRANE. Later the substances may dissociate from the membrane, but statistically more molecules will move by DIFFUSION across the cell membrane from a high concentration to a lower one, than in the reverse direction. This process is known as *non-ionic diffusion*. However many important substances, such as SUGARS, AMINO ACIDS, and IONS, are completely insoluble in cell membranes, and cross them by specialized processes. Many cell membranes contain a number of specialized molecules which combine specifically with one of the substances to be transported. Such a molecule is called a *carrier*, and the complex resulting from the combination can cross the membrane and release the substrate. As with non-ionic diffusion, more carrier–substrate complexes cross the membrane in a direction such that the substrate moves from high to low concentration. This carrier-mediated transport process is known as *facilitated diffusion*.

Neither non-ionic diffusion nor carrier-mediated diffusion require the expenditure of energy, relying simply on the concentration gradients existing across the cell membranes. However, some transport processes require the 'uphill' movement of substances. An example here will be useful, by considering how the body maintains a constant internal environment. We take a small amount of SALT (sodium chloride) in the diet to replace that lost in the urine, sweat, saliva, and other secretions. To move salt from a low concentration in the gut, into the blood where it is at high concentration, means that the movement is up a concentration gradient, and therefore cannot occur by diffusion. The body deals with this by using a two-stage process in which sodium ions are actively transported. The first stage is the movement of sodium ions from the gut cavity across the face of the cells lining the gut; since the concentration of sodium ions inside these cells, as in all cells, is low, movement is by diffusion using specific sodium ION CHANNELS. The second stage is the movement of the sodium ions from these lining cells, across the membrane on their opposite face, away from the gut, into the tissue fluid, where the sodium ion concentration is high. This is achieved using a molecular pump, called the *sodium pump* (otherwise known as sodium–potassium ATPase: a protein molecule that spans the cell membrane). The pump causes a net movement of sodium ions, along with the expenditure of energy, yielded by the hydrolysis of ATP. This transfer of sodium ions across the gut epithelium results in the transfer of positive charge to the outer side of the cells. Because the pump transfers electrical charge in this way, it is said to be electrogenic. The transfer of positive charges provides the driving force for the movement of the negatively-charged chloride ions across the gut lining; thus the transfer of salt is achieved.

Similar two-stage active transport processes are responsible for the absorption or secretion of other salts, as well as sodium chloride, across many epithelial membranes. They occur in glands (such as salivary glands, the pancreas, and sweat glands) in organs such as the kidneys and the liver, as well as in epithelial membranes over the cornea and covering the brain.

Transport processes are also involved in other homeostatic processes, such as the regulation of cellular pH. Here carrier-mediated processes are used which, for instance, exchange a sodium ion for a proton (hydrogen ion) or exchange a chloride anion for a bicarbonate anion. These carriers are said to facilitate exchange-diffusion. As well as the sodium pump described above there are other molecular pumps which consume energy (obtained by the hydrolysis of ATP); for example, the calcium pump maintains low levels of calcium ions inside cells, and the proton pump is involved in generating the hydrochloric acid secreted into the stomach.

Although we refer to 'the sodium pump' and others in the singular, a single cell may have for example, hundreds of thousands of sodium pumps, with the number varying to suit local conditions. The body's energy requirement for these active transport processes accounts for at least a fifth of the metabolic rate of the whole body at rest.

Thus *carriers, exchangers, pumps,* and *ion channels* are the molecular machines which drive the body's transport processes.

ALAN W. CUTHBERT
See also CELL MEMBRANES; DIFFUSION; ION CHANNELS.

Transvestitism
Cross-dressing in the CLOTHES of the other GENDER is a practice dating back into pre-history, though it can only occur in a culture in which the sexes dress in distinctively different fashions. Ritual transvestitism has been associated with MAGIC and shamanism, and also with the more general disguise, and

inversion of conventional roles, of the carnivalesque. There is a long theatrical tradition of travesty in many cultures: the classical Greek and Japanese drama relied on male actors to incarnate often powerful female roles, and the women's parts in the drama of the age of Shakespeare were, of course, played by boys. With the entry of actresses into the profession, the 'breeches part' became a titillating device, though there is some perhaps anecdotal evidence to indicate that women as well as men found the woman masquerading as male alluring. The British pantomime, with its male caricature of mature femininity in the 'Dame', and the traditionally female 'Principal Boy', perhaps draws at a distant remove from the midwinter *Saturnalia* carnival.

Developing definitions

These overt and culturally accepted traditions, however, are a rather different matter from the private and sexual practice of cross-dressing. Reports on the phenomenon in early sexological literature, such as Krafft-Ebing's *Psychopathia Sexualis*, deemed all transvestites to be 'sexual inverts' or homosexual, in keeping with nineteenth-century concepts of homosexuality as due to a pronounced feminine component within the male (and vice versa in the female). However, both Havelock Ellis and Magnus Hirschfeld found that many of the cases which they encountered were heterosexual in general sexual orientation. Ellis additionally suggested that 'Eonists', as he termed them (after the eighteenth-century French cross-dresser, the Chevalier d'Eon), were characterized by a low sexual drive and were often somewhat indifferent to sexual relations.

A number of phenomena are conflated under the general term of transvestitism. There became in the late twentieth century perhaps a clearer distinction than in earlier times between the *transsexual* — who believes him or herself to have been born into a body of the wrong gender, and may seek surgical and hormonal gender reassignment — and the *transvestite*, who cross-dresses but does not desire to change his or her physical body. However, since the possibility of transsexuality has only been created by developments in endocrinology and reconstructive surgery, it is dubious to what extent one can really speak of 'transsexuals' before the mid twentieth century.

Gender differences

There are a number of cases recorded in history of women passing as men. It is debatable whether their motivation was sexual (either lesbian or a fetishistic fascination with male dress), due to existential dissatisfaction with their own gender, or economic and practical. When certain professions were closed to women, and there were considerable differences between male and female wage-scales, some women dressed as men to pursue an occupation either more congenial or better paid than they could have aspired to in a skirt. There are instances in which women even married other women, who were reported as

being unaware of their 'husband's' true gender (this may reflect levels of sexual ignorance, or the furtive, concealed way in which any conjugal rights took place).

For some men wearing female clothes is a form of FETISHISM: the clothes are experienced as sexually arousing; this form of cross-dressing is a specifically sexual act, either leading to masturbation, or being a requirement for successful intercourse. The converse is seldom the case in women. Other (male) transvestites lead a double life as normal heterosexual males, with an alternative identity dressing and passing as women. There are also homosexual transvestites who cross-dress, but in such cases there is often an element of deliberate impersonation and even caricature ('drag queens'): this can be deployed as a critique of existing gender norms but can also be an expression of misogynistic hostility.

There is little evidence that for women transvestism involves the sensuous and erotic response to the garments of the other sex that is reported in many male transvestites. However, whilst it has become increasingly acceptable in Western societies for women to wear trousers in a wide variety of social settings, social custom is still hostile to men wearing skirts, unless they are Highlanders in full kilted regalia. Male clothing is often perceived as a practical choice for the active woman in modern life, whereas female dress tends to be coded as impractical, decorative, and constricting — factors which are often sources of gratification to the male cross-dresser.

Possible explanations

The aetiology of transvestitism is complex. Because it has been recorded in most societies (and in some cultures is even a recognized social role), and throughout history, it has been hypothesized that there must be some innate biological component. While there may be some predisposing endocrine or neurological mechanism involved, the research findings are extremely ambiguous, and no factor has been found to account adequately for its development. The influence of social and cultural factors is more marked: cross-cultural research indicates that discomfort with biological gender is more common in societies with rigid expectations about appropriately gendered behaviour. Thus the inability of the accepted male role to incorporate qualities perceived as 'feminine' may lead to various forms of identifying with the appurtenances of femininity.

However, it would appear that individual psychological factors also play a significant part in the development of quirks in gender identity. Boys who later become transvestites or transsexuals may manifest 'feminine' behavioural characteristics from early childhood. In a significant minority of cases, being cross-dressed as a child by a parent or other relative seems to play a part. What is not clear is why in some cases this 'feminisation' leads to the development in the adult male of a homosexual identity, in other

cases to transvestitism with heterosexual orientation, and in others to full transsexualism.

As with many categories of sexual behaviour, 'transvestitism' as a classification is a lumping together of diverse phenomena, not only in the different sexes, but among members of the same sex obeying different biological, social, or psychic imperatives resulting in phenomena which are only apparently similar. LESLEY A. HALL

See also SEX CHANGE; SEXUAL ORIENTATION.

Tremor With sensitive recording systems it can be shown that all parts of the living body are vibrating; the only time when we are truly still is when we are dead! Most of these micro-vibrations cannot, however, be seen by the naked eye. For most studies of tremor, the motion is recorded by the use of small devices sensitive to acceleration taped onto the fingers. Such instability may often be seen in normal people when they hold out their arms with their fingers gently separated and straight. The oscillation that may then be seen is called physiological tremor. There is a very wide degree of variation in the size of this, and a range of about a hundred-fold has been observed. Heavily pressurized students may have particularly high levels; also, there are statistical variations in the amount of tremor according to occupation.

The extent to which the fingers shake varies with the person's psychological circumstances; there are many references in the Bible and in Shakespeare to the association with fright and strong EMOTION. This is due to the liberation of the hormone ADRENALINE at these times. Musicians and others making public appearances may suffer from stage fright, and excessive tremor is then often seen. High levels have been observed in air squadron cadets learning to fly light aircraft, and unusually high levels have been observed after bungee jumping.

Physiological tremor is usually rhythmic, the peak of the oscillations being at about 10 cycles per second. Whilst its size may vary widely from moment to moment, the rate remains much the same. Each muscle is controlled by the nerve impulse activity in a number of nerve fibres, each of which is responsible for controlling the contraction of a number of individual muscle fibres. The number of muscle fibres controlled by a single nerve fibre (forming a *motor unit*) varies considerably in different muscles. In those of the trunk it is large, but is smaller in the small muscles of the hand where high precision of control is needed. The nerve impulses occur usually at a rate of 5–20 cycles per second. This is not fast enough to cause the muscle elements to produce a smooth contraction; these facts about the behaviour responsible for our posture and its disturbances have been established by animal and human experiments. Our POSTURE is thus based on many small, jerky sources of force. We are not usually aware of these discontinuities, because the different motor units are operating out of step with one another so that overall there is a large measure of smoothing in the force acting through the tendons. An analogue would be soldiers falling out of step when marching over a bridge. These bumpy forces are applied across our joints.

In general, limbs are under-damped, that is, they oscillate preferentially at a certain rate: the resonant frequency. It so happens that the resonant frequency of the human wrist is about 10 cycles per second for small movements — close to the rate of discharge of the nerve fibres to the muscles of the arm. It is the combination of these two factors which is mainly responsible for physiological tremor.

In disease the discharges of the individual nerve fibres may become unusually closely timed to one another; they are then said to be synchronized. There is then a prominent tremor. This is the situation in pathological tremors such as that seen in Parkinsonism. This lower frequency tremor at 4–6 cycles per second can be widespread, involving the forearms and even the head and trunk.

After a STROKE, the foot on the affected side may at times jerk rhythmically, in response to ankle displacement, in a powerful and disturbing manner. Strictly speaking this is classed as *clonus* rather than tremor.

Movements and posture are regulated by the CEREBELLUM. This part of the brain is responsible for organizing the motor programmes. The correct timing of the multiplicity of muscle actions needed in performing everyday tasks is a problem of great magnitude. If the cerebellum or its pathways are not capable of fully normal action, as in *Freidrich's Ataxia*, movements will be poorly co-ordinated and there will be an 'intention tremor': when picking something up, the hand may oscillate to and fro at the end of the motion, under-reaching and over-reaching, instead of coming to rest neatly in the correct position. These pathways are also after impaired in *multiple sclerosis*.

Some people, who are otherwise quite healthy, have unusually prominent shaking. This is called *essential tremor*. Sometimes it is hereditary. In northern Sweden the population moved little for hundreds of years, and very good church records exist. From this region and certain other areas very extensive family trees have been prepared, which show the mode of inheritance of some forms of the condition. If severe, essential tremor can be a serious disability as it interferes with skilled movements such as writing. This can be socially embarrassing, and the person may falsely be believed to be an alcoholic — whereas small amounts of alcohol may actually suppress tremor. Tremor associated with ALCOHOLISM occurs the morning after rather than at the time of the drinking. With excessive intake the person may show widespread shaking, the Latin name for this being *delirium tremens* — a very serious condition. Many other drugs also can give rise to shaking. Adolph Hitler had a prominent tremor, perhaps due to the stimulant amphetamine (purple hearts), which he was taking. Some people find that coffee brings out tremor; this is

due to the presence of CAFFEINE, which is an excitant; these effects are not, however, universal.

As to treatment, there is no panacea. For tremors associated with anxiety, drugs which block the action of adrenaline can be of use, but there may be side actions. Very severe and incapacitating tremors are sometimes treated by surgical operations on the brain. Important and interesting human and animal research is currently being conducted on tremor mechanisms and the possibilities of refining treatment.

E. GEOFFREY WALSH

Further reading
Walsh, E. G. (1992). *Muscles, masses and motion.* Mackeith/Cambridge University Press.

See also CEREBELLUM; MOVEMENT; SKELETAL MUSCLE.

Tuberculosis
is caused by the MICRO-ORGANISM *Mycobacterium tuberculosis*, or tubercle bacillus. It was in 1882 that Robert Koch, among his many historic contributions to bacteriology, identified this as the cause of the disease, thus firmly establishing for the first time its infective nature. It has been estimated that one-third of the world's population has been infected by *M. tuberculosis* but only a minority, probably about 10%, go on to develop disease. Disease manifests in any number of ways, almost all of them chronic, involving practically any part of the body. The most common site involved is the LUNGS, where cavities are produced. When this occurs patients have a COUGH with sputum (which sometimes contains blood), weight loss, and FEVER. Those with this type of disease are the most infectious, because of the presence of the bacillus in the sputum. Animals also carry the disease; although Koch had denied the possibility, it was later realized that the bovine strain of the organism, *Mycobacterium bovis*, could cause human infection from cow's milk.

Historically, tuberculosis has long ranked among the most feared of diseases. Such dread is reflected in some of its alternative names, including John Bunyan's 'Captain of all these Men of Death', and Charles Dickens' 'dread disease' which capture something of the prevalence of the disease in their times. Other names conjure up images of the disease process: the term 'consumption' describes what happened to an individual — a progressive emaciation and wasting away. Still other terms, such 'the King's Evil' describe the lottery of survival (cure arising from the king's touch in medieval England). Yet tuberculosis is not only a disease of the past. Keats' 'death warrant' continues to haunt us. Historically tuberculosis conjures up romantic images of pale, wraith-like artists suffering lingering deaths. Literature, art, and music have all recorded and been transformed by the disease. Those who have succumbed to the disease form a veritable who's who of the artistic and political worlds and notions persist that those with artistic leanings are at greater risk from tuberculosis. As Susan Sontag noted in *Illness as Metaphor,*

'tuberculosis was thought to come from too much passion, afflicting the reckless and sensual.' Gradually, however, perceptions changed. In the US, for example, Katherine Ott noted in *Fevered Lives* that this 'most flattering of all diseases' of the 1870s was transformed, as awareness of the social associations grew in the 1880s, into a disease which was seen as the consequence of either acquired or inherited degeneracy and later came to mirror ethnic and racial fears and prejudices. Yet by the turn of the century the enthusiasm for pointing the finger at individual weaknesses was tempered by an increasing awareness that society's strictures were in part responsible. In truth, in past centuries tuberculosis was a frequent killer of people from all walks of life, not only the famous and infamous, the artistic and notorious. Those living in poverty and squalor were always most susceptible.

The *sanatorium movement*, which promoted wholesome rest and genteel exercise in pleasant surroundings, took off in the second half of the nineteenth century. In Britain, which borrowed the idea from Germany, the first sanatoria opened in the 1890s. Although many sanatoria in Europe catered for a select, affluent, cosmopolitan clientele (an image which persists in the popular imagination conjured up by establishments such as those at Davos in Switzerland), sanatorium treatment also, by the 1920s, became available for those unable to pay, and the average duration of stay shortened. However a decline in the sanatorium movement started with the onset of World War I and was hastened by the Depression which followed. Although there were still thousands of tuberculosis sufferers receiving care in sanatoria by the mid 1940s, the availability of effective drug treatment meant that they soon became obsolete. Removal of infectious sufferers from the community had contributed to a decrease in incidence of the disease, but for the patients in sanatoria or specialized hospitals there was no specific cure. Recovery was sometimes assisted by causing collapse of an infected lung by the introduction of air into the chest (*artificial pneumothorax*) or by an operation that 'caved-in' the overlying ribs (*thoracoplasty*).

The advent of drug treatment followed the discovery, by Selman Waksman in the US in 1944, that *streptomycin* was effective, and other drugs shortly followed. When CHEMOTHERAPY from then on resulted in cure for most tuberculosis sufferers, contemporary commentators told stories largely of hope, of medicine's conquest of nature, and reflected less on societal hindrances to medicine's application. An optimistic faith in the benefits of science shone through such that it seemed merely a matter of time before this ancient scourge would be eradicated. At the time this optimism seemed well-founded: mortality rates in England and Wales, which had been falling by about 1% annually since the 1860s, declined dramatically from the mid 1940s. Death rates for respiratory tuberculosis in England and Wales were about 125/100 000 at the turn of the century, and by the 1960s had fallen to below

10/100 000. Preceding the advent of chemotherapy there had been improvements in social conditions and better identification of those with active disease, along with advances in bacteriology and in X-RAY diagnosis. From the 1920s there were attempts to control bovine infection, first by certifying tuberculin tested (TT) herds, and later by heat treatment to kill bacteria in milk. Although this *pasteurization* had been considered as early as 1913, Britain lagged behind much of Europe and the US by more than a quarter of a century in putting it into consistent effect. A further preventative measure was the introduction in the 1950s of the BCG (Bacille Calmette Guérin) vaccination programme.

Despite the remarkable success in controlling tuberculosis in the West, the overriding optimism which followed the development of effective antituberculosis drugs in the 1940s and 1950s was somewhat premature. The disease continues to target those most marginalized and vulnerable. Each year more than 8 million people acquire tuberculosis (most of them in the developing world), and about 3 million die, including about 100 000 children, annually. In England and Wales there was concern as to why this should be, why Keats' death warrant should still be received by so many, given that we have had at our disposal for over fifty years drugs which are effective in curing the disease? The answer was known half a century ago.

'Tuberculosis is a social disease, and presents problems that transcend the conventional medical approach. On the one hand, its understanding demands that the impact of social and economic factors on the individual be considered as much as the mechanisms by which tubercle bacilli cause damage to the human body. On the other hand, the disease modifies in a peculiar manner the emotional and intellectual climate of the societies that it attacks.' Rene Dubos who, with his wife Jean, wrote these words in 1952, was one of the giants of twentieth-century medicine. As well as being a major figure in the development of antibacterial drugs in the US in the 1920s and 1930s, which led to the later successful antituberculous drugs, he was able, unlike so many, to see the place of tuberculosis in society and to recognize the limits of modern medicine. His words resonate through the years and perhaps are more pertinent now than ever. In 1993 the World Health Organization officially called the global threat of tuberculosis an 'emergency'. New drug-resistant strains of the organism are spreading and modern medical approaches are failing to cure patients. In England and Wales there was a 20% increase in incidence of the disease between 1987 and 1990, weighted towards the underprivileged. Overcrowding, poverty, social alienation, increased incarceration rates in prisons, homelessness, and AIDS (the 'deadly alliance') are combining to overwhelm uncoordinated and under-resourced public health responses.

Perhaps nowhere have the consequences of contemporary public health failures been more obvious than in New York City. In the late 1980s and early 1990s an epidemic of this ancient disease killed hundreds of people, forcing politicians to rethink their approaches to those living on the margins of society, and provoking a response which has cost millions of dollars. As Rene Dubos knew all along, tuberculosis is as much a social and political disease as it is a medical condition.   RICHARD COKER

Further reading

Coker, R. (2000). *From chaos to coercion: detention and the control of tuberculosis*. St Martins Press, New York.

Dormandy, T. (1999). *The White Death: a history of tuberculosis*. The Hambledon Press, London.

Ott, K. (1996). *Fevered lives: tuberculosis in American culture since 1870*. Harvard University Press, Cambridge MA.

Ryan, F. (1992). *Tuberculosis: the greatest story never told*. Swift publishers, Bromsgrove, Worcestershire.

Sontag, S. (1978). *Illness as metaphor*. Farrar, Straus and Giroux, New York.

See also INFECTIOUS DISEASES; IMMUNIZATION.

Tumour Any abnormal growth in or on the body, arising from some particular tissue or cell type. A tumour may be harmless (benign), remaining at its site of origin and becoming a problem only cosmetically or by its size; or cancerous (malignant), invading surrounding tissues, and seeding elsewhere (metastasizing) via the lymphatic or blood vessels. The technical term for a tumour of whatever varity is 'NEOPLASM'.   S.J.

See CANCER.

Twins are of two types: *monovular* (identical), from the union of one sperm and one ovum, and *binovular* (non-identical) resulting from the fertilization of two separate ova. The cell produced by fertilization is called a *zygote* (from the Greek for 'yoked'), so they are also known as *monozygotic* and *dizygotic*. Dizygotic twins are physically and genetically as dissimilar as any siblings. Monozygotic twins, having resulted from the cleavage of a single 'conceptus' — the splitting and separation of an early embryo — are therefore, with rare exceptions, genetically identical.

The incidence of multiple pregnancies varies in different racial groups. To quote 'Hellin's law' (1895): 'twins occur in 1/89 births, triplets 1/(89)^2, quadruplets 1/(89)^3 and so on'. The formula is roughly correct, although twins occur in Caucasians 1/80 to 1/90, in Asiatics 1/150 or less, and black Africans 1/50 with the highest incidence of twinning amongst the Yoruba people of Nigeria for whom 1 in 25 births are of twins. It is the rate of non-identical (dizygotic) twinning that varies around the world: identical (monozygotic) twins occur at a similar rate of 1 in 300 births in all populations. These statistics are based on clinical findings in viable pregnancies. However the initial 'hidden' twinning rate is probably higher: with increasing use of ultrasound in early pregnancy it is found that before 12 weeks one of the twins may die and be absorbed leaving an apparent singleton. In Australia the rate of twinning has increased approximately 25% over the past 20 years, partly due to a significant increase in the percentage of births to women aged 35 and over, and partly to the treatment of infertility by ovulation stimulation or assisted conception by gamete intra-fallopian transfer (GIFT) or in-vitro fertilization (IVF).

Twin PREGNANCY is more prone to complication than single pregnancies and possible hazards of premature birth and poor growth in the womb necessitate increased antenatal surveillance. If twins are identical and they share a single PLACENTA, one baby can steal blood from the other, causing a condition known as 'Twin–twin transfusion syndrome'.

Multiple pregnancies carry a greater risk of losing a baby before, during, or after birth than singleton pregnancies: multiple pregnancies overall account for more than 10% of all perinatal deaths; the greater the number, the greater the risk. CEREBRAL PALSY in survivors is six times more common in twins than singletons.

The birth of twins has been a source of fascination in many cultures throughout history and the twin image has been incorporated in myths, folklore, and religions. The Old Testament of the Bible tells of Isaac's wife, Rebekah, who eventually conceived after nineteen years of marriage. Twin boys were born. The first was red and hairy, and he was named Esau, meaning 'red'. His brother was born holding Esau's heel and so he was called Jacob, meaning 'he who grasps the heel'. Ancient Rome was founded, according to legend by Romulus and Remus, the twin progeny of Mars, god of war, and a mortal princess. In some African communities, twins were regarded with great favour; in others, with great suspicion. The Yoruba in Nigeria were well aware of the high mortality associated with twinning in the past, and they made small wooden sculptures, 'ibeji' that had spiritual significance if one of twins died.   JIM NEILSON

See also ASSISTED REPRODUCTION; PREGNANCY.

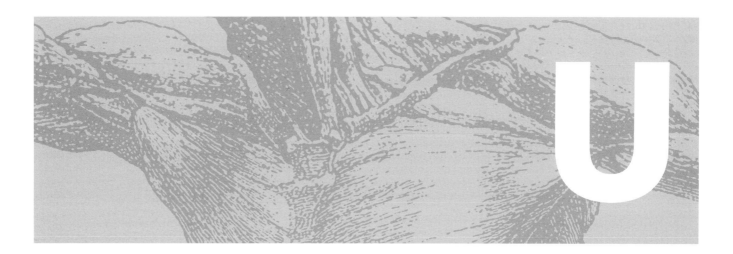

Ugliness The etymology of the word indicates what is at stake: 'ugly' is a Middle English (1150–1475) term meaning 'frightful' or 'repulsive', and is derived from the Old Norse term *uggligr*. *Uggligr* is in turn formed by *uggr*: fear or horror, and the suffix *-ligr*: like. An ugly body is thus a physical body that induces horror in us. This element of fear is evident in the ugly bodies *par excellence*: the monster, the grotesque body, and the FREAK.

Ugliness is conventionally seen as the opposite of BEAUTY, but its modern use contrasts more directly to normalcy. Even though most of us cannot fulfil ideals of beauty, we can still be considered good-looking, pretty, or nice. If we were considered plain-looking or even unattractive, we would hardly be ugly, since we are still within the range of normalcy.

Normalcy as a concept and social standard arose in the early nineteenth century in Europe, and was linked to the development of statistics and the modern, administrative institutions of the state. Until the mid eighteenth century 'normal' meant 'perpendicular'. By 1840 'normal' had become current in the English language as indicating conformity to, and not deviance from, a standard or the usual. 'Normality' and 'normalcy' appeared respectively in 1849 and 1857.

The French statistician Adolphe Quetelet (1796–1847) contributed considerably to the concept of 'the average man', which he defined as 'an individual who epitomized in himself, at a given time, all the qualities of the average man and who would represent at once all the greatness, beauty, and goodness of that being'. Deviations from the mean constituted, Quetelet observed, ugliness of the body, vice in morals, and sickness in regard to constitution.

An important reinterpretation of statistical distribution was made by Sir Francis Galton (1822–1911). Where Quetelet considered any deviation from the average an error, Galton saw this as mere difference from the mean. The total variation of these differences in the height of individuals in a population, for example, was defined as the normal distribution, also known as the 'bell curve'. This way, extremes that Galton saw as positive — intelligence, tallness, fertility etc. — would not be judged as errors as they had been by Quetelet. Variation could be ranked.

The statistics founded by Galton and others enabled the rising state bureaucracies to compile inventories of their citizens' different characteristics and to assess the number of able-bodied persons available for the work force, military purposes, etc. Through the concept of the average and the ranking of the variations, the sound body of the population was defined, thus enabling the state to initiate policies that could further soundness and isolate incurably unsound elements — disabled persons, CRIMINALS, demented persons — in suitable institutions.

The ugly body is thus a body whose difference from the normal body is turned into deviance. Ugliness can be seen as a kind of *stigma* — a term originally used by the ancient Greeks for marks made on the bodies of person who were considered unusual, such as slaves and criminals. 'Stigma' is now also used medically to indicate visible evidence of a disease. Other kinds of stigma, not all resulting in typecasting a person as ugly, are: disability, membership of an ethnic group, and criminality.

Criteria for specifying which bodies are normal, maybe even beautiful, and not ugly, vary from society to society and over time. Should the body be symmetrical? Should the skin be smooth, scarred, or tattooed? Should the teeth be filed? Western societies celebrate the untouched, natural body, but at what point disfiguration becomes ugliness is uncertain. Is squinting ugly? Is a harelip, a person with eyes of two colours, a missing arm, an abnormal arm ugly? Among various peoples in Africa, scars forming patterns covering large parts of the body are basic to the beautiful body. Another criterion for beauty is found in how the body is cared for, and often concerns HEALTH, HYGIENE, or aesthetics. Is the skin to be oiled or to be painted or neither? How often should it be washed and with what (water, soap, disinfectant)? Should scents be applied? The extent and range of non-compliance necessary for a person to be considered not only not-beautiful, but also not-normal, and therefore ugly, varies.

In Euro-America, which for long has been dominated by the standards and culture of white, Anglo-Saxon, Protestant males, a wide range of groups of people have over time been called ugly: for example aboriginal Australians, Africans, disabled persons, Hottentots, Jews, and wrinkled old women (significantly called 'witches').

A protest against the enforcement of normalcy can be found in the use by punk and other movements of 'disfigurement' of the body — for example by TATTOOING which is extensive or in unusual places; piercing of eyebrows, tongues, and noses; and atypical hairstyling. These efforts can be seen as attempts to create an aesthetic of the ugly in protest against conventional standards of beauty.   CLAUS BOSSEN

Further reading

Goffman, E. (1963). *Stigma. Notes on the management of spoiled identity.* Penguin Books, Harmondsworth.

Halprin, S. (1995). *Look at my ugly face. Myths and musings on beauty and other perilous obsessions with women's appearance.* Viking Penguin, New York.

See also BEAUTY; BODY IMAGE; BODY SHAPE.

Ulcer An erosion of an epithelial surface — the SKIN, or any of the internal linings (MUCOUS MEMBRANES) that are in continuity with the skin at the body orifices. Damage may be physical, chemical, due to failure of blood supply or to infection. *Peptic ulcer* may be *gastric* or *duodenal* — affecting the mucous membrane of the stomach or of the duodenum, attributed to the effects of stomach acid, either when it is in excess, or when the normal defences against damage from it are lacking; now known to be linked with infection by *Helicobacter pylori*. *Oesophageal* ulcer is related to reflux of stomach contents. Underlying BLOOD VESSELS can be eroded, with consequences that can be either insidious, or catastrophic in the case of peptic ulcers; bleeding is readily evident if blood is vomited (*haematemesis*), but less immediately so if it moves on down the gut to appear (in an altered state) in the faeces (*melaena*). Less dramatic bleeding can be detected by a test for *occult blood* in the stool. At worst erosion may penetrate right through the wall — most commonly of the duodenum — causing a perforated ulcer, and escape of gut contents leads to peritonitis.

Ulceration of the skin can occur on the legs as a complication of VARICOSE VEINS, or of poor circulation due to arteriosclerosis. Bedsores are ulcers caused by prolonged pressure and immobility. Some types of skin cancers or other skin diseases can form ulcers. *Aphthous ulcers* are small painful erosions of the mucous membrane in the mouth. Without the protection of an intact surface, ulcers from any cause can become deeper due to INJURY or INFECTION.

SHEILA JENNETT

Ultrasound Waves of higher frequency than audible sound waves. Reflection of ultrasound waves was applied to underwater detection during World War II, and subsequently to imaging the body. The harmless waves (>100 Mhz) are aimed at the part to be examined, and reflections are detected from tissue components in proportion to their acoustic impedance. These signals can be processed to create two- or three-dimensional images. The most common use is for viewing the FETUS in early PREGNANCY, but there are also many other diagnostic applications.

Treatment by ultrasound (*ultrasonics*) is widely used by physiotherapists, particularly for soft tissue injuries but also for a variety of more chronic conditions, with a view to promoting healing and relieving pain. Most commonly frequencies of 1–3 MHz are used. There are differences of opinion and practice, related to whether the intended action should be primarily thermal or non-thermal, but there is a lack of controlled trials on the efficacy of the different methods used.
J. K. D.
S. J.

See IMAGING TECHNIQUES; SONOGRAM.

Umbilical cord When the embryo first embeds itself in the lining of the UTERUS it is small enough for adequate exchange of dissolved gases, nutrients, and waste across its surface. Then as part of very early growth and reshaping, a short stalk is formed of its own tissue. Blood vessel loops grow into this stalk along with the development of the heart and circulation. The stalk lengthens as the fetus develops within its amniotic sac, and at the uterine end the blood vessels become part of the developing PLACENTA. Thus the fetus grows its own umbilical cord, containing its own blood vessels: two arteries and a single vein. As these vessels grow they form intertwining spirals, embedded in a simple 'jelly' with a thin outer covering, so that the mature cord resembles a soft, twisted rope. The fetal heart pumps its own blood via the umbilical arteries to the placenta, where their finest branches lie bathed in the mother's blood; they are drained by the tributaries of the umbilical vein which takes it back in the cord to the fetus, to flow back to the heart. Thus 'used' blood is pumped through arteries and 'refreshed' blood is returned to the heart by veins (comparable to the flow to and from the lungs after birth).

By full term, the cord is about 50 cm long, looped within the amniotic sac, allowing freedom of movement of the mature fetus. During LABOUR, the cord is occasionally a hazard: it can prolapse and be compressed by the descending head against the mother's pelvis, obstructing the blood flow, or it may encircle the baby's neck and need to be loosened by the midwife. It is of course the custom to cut the cord, between two clamps, as soon as the infant is born. Attention can then be given separately to the infant, and to the mother for delivery of the placenta. But there are also natural mechanisms that promptly reduce the blood flow in the umbilical arteries. The start of breathing alters the mechanics of the heart and circulation such that blood now flows preferentially through the lungs to become oxygenated. Various chemical changes, as well as stretching and cooling of the cord, can contribute to close-down, by constriction of the smooth muscle of the umbilical vessels.

The cord shrivels and separates from the navel within a week or two.
SHEILA JENNETT

See also ANTENATAL DEVELOPMENT; BELLY BUTTON; GROWTH AND DEVELOPMENT: BIRTH AND INFANCY; PLACENTA.

Ureter The tube of SMOOTH MUSCLE which carries URINE from the KIDNEY to the BLADDER. The ureter starts as the outlet from the 'pelvis' in the centre of the kidney — the receptacle for the urine leaving thousands of microscopic tubules. The two ureters enter the upper part of the bladder symmetrically on the two sides. Between them, they deliver urine on average at a rate of about 1 ml min. The ureters can be a source of pain (colic) if kidney stones fragment and pass down them.
S. J.

See KIDNEYS; PLATE 8.

Urethra The passage from the bladder to the outside world. Short in the female, and nothing more nor less than an exit for urine. Long and tortuous in the male, and with a dual role: the vas deferens on each side joins the duct from the seminal vesicle to form the ejaculatory duct; this enters the urethra where it passes through the PROSTATE GLAND; the next part, the penile urethra, is thus the channel for either urine or

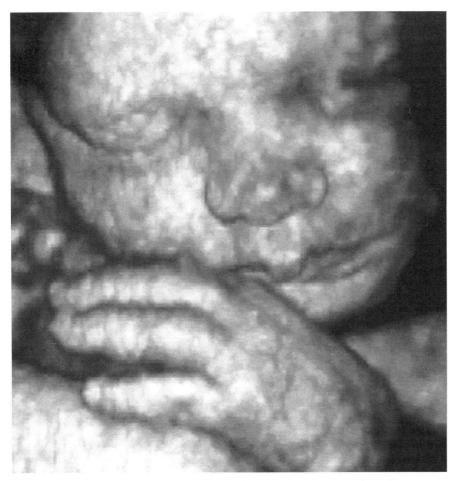
Three-dimension ultrasound scan of the face and hand of a fetus. Bernard Benoit/Science Photo Library.

seminal fluid; reflex contraction of the muscular sphincter around the bladder exit prevents backflow into the bladder during EJACULATION. (There is no special mechanism to prevent urine from entering the vasa — the anatomical arrangements and the less forceful nature of urination are sufficient.)   s.j.

See PLATE 8.

Urine is the fluid excreted by the KIDNEYS. It consists of water, carrying in solution the body's waste products such as urea, uric acid, creatinine, organic acids, and also other solutes such as Na$^+$, K$^+$, Ca^{2+}, Mg^{2+}, Cl$^-$, the body fluid concentrations of which are regulated by the kidneys.

After being produced by the kidneys, urine passes along the *ureters* to be stored in the BLADDER, until it is allowed to flow out of the body through the urethra, in the process of *micturition* (urination). The smooth muscle of the bladder forms an internal sphincter at its junction with the urethra, and further along the urethra is the voluntary-control external sphincter. The bladder begins to contract (micturition reflex), and produces the desire to urinate, when its volume exceeds about 200 ml. However, if we do not relax the external sphincter, the contractions subside, but return with increasing force and frequency as the bladder continues to fill. When the bladder volume is about 500 ml the micturition reflex may force open the internal sphincter and lead to a reflex relaxation of the external sphincter, so that urination occurs involuntarily.

Voluntary urination involves relaxation of the external sphincter and tensing of the abdominal muscles to increase abdominal pressure and compress the bladder, to initiate bladder contraction and relaxation of the internal sphincter.

Most people excrete about 1.5 litres of urine per day, but the volume can range (in healthy adults) from 400 ml up to about 25 litres, depending on fluid intake. In renal failure, there may be no urine production, and in the rare condition of untreated *diabetes insipidus*, the urine volume is consistently 25 litres/day. Urine is termed 'dilute' if its solute concentration (osmolality) is lower than that of the blood plasma, and 'concentrated' if its solute concentration is greater than that of the plasma.

Humans who are maximally conserving water — when their kidneys are reabsorbing as much as possible — can produce urine with a solute concentration (osmolality) about five times that of blood plasma. Many other animals can conserve water much more effectively. For example, cats, dogs, and rats can produce urine of ten times the plasma osmolality, and gerbils twenty times!

When voided, urine is normally sterile and clear, although it has a yellow colour due to the presence of pigments. However, small amounts of particulate matter such as epithelial cells and lipids may be present; these are 'casts'. Protein is not normally filtered from the blood plasma by the kidneys, so protein in the urine — *proteinuria* — is generally indicative of damage to the glomeruli, at the blind inner ends of the kidney tubules, where filtration occurs. The urine may also appear to contain blood (*haematuria*). This may be due to haemolysis in the bloodstream (breakdown of red cells) so that some haemoglobin is released from them and excreted, or it may be due to the presence of whole red cells, as a result of bleeding in the kidneys or urinary tract.

Investigation of urine composition (urinalysis) is a normal part of diagnostic medicine and can indicate the presence of many different illnesses.   CHRISTOPHER LOTE

See also BLADDER; BODY FLUIDS; IONS; KIDNEYS; WATER BALANCE.

Uterus The uterus has three major functions: to prepare a bed for a fertilized ovum, to nourish the developing embryo during PREGNANCY, and to expel the fetus. Shaped like an upside-down pear, and tilted forwards, it lies within the pelvis and is held in place, along with its two extensions, the FALLOPIAN TUBES, by ligaments and folds of the peritoneum. The cervix forms the lower third, connected by a narrow isthmus to the main muscular body of the uterus. The non-pregnant uterus weighs 45–60 g and is 7–8 cm long but its weight increases more than ten-fold by the end of pregnancy.

The main bulk of the uterus is made up of SMOOTH MUSCLE fibres known as the myometrium. The inner layer of muscle fibres is arranged in a circular pattern and the outer layer in a longitudinal pattern with a middle layer of interlacing oblique fibres. Inside the muscle is a cellular lining with a glandular (secretory) surface — the endometrium. While the myometrium is responsible for contractions of the uterus (obviously particularly important during LABOUR), it is the endometrium which develops in every cycle to prepare for an embryo, and which is shed during MENSTRUATION. Thus during reproductive years the uterus is a highly dynamic organ, its functions being controlled by oestrogen and PROGESTERONE secreted by the OVARIES and by other hormones associated with pregnancy and labour.

At the time of puberty, when oestrogen secretion from the ovaries begins to rise, there is an increase in both the size of the uterus and the blood flow which it receives. When MENSTRUAL CYCLES are established both the myometrium and the endometrium show cyclical, hormone-dependent changes in structure and function. These change again after implantation of an embryo, during pregnancy, and at delivery.

In the first half of the menstrual cycle the uterus prepares to receive and transport SPERM from the cervix to the *oviducts* (FALLOPIAN TUBES). Under the influence of oestrogen secreted by the ovaries, the myometrium becomes more excitable and begins to contract sporadically. Meanwhile the cells under the surface of the endometrium begin to proliferate (hence the term proliferative phase of the uterine cycle) and those on the surface grow projections into the cavity of the uterus and invade the deeper layer underneath. Thus, from a relatively smooth surface at the beginning of each cycle, the endometrium not only thickens but becomes a highly indented structure, with the epithelial glands secreting a watery fluid. Spiral arteries grow up into the projections.

Towards mid-cycle, as ovulation approaches, the uterus is primed to bind progesterone. Thus, in the second half of the menstrual cycle, when progesterone production by the ovaries is high, the progestogenic or secretory phase of the uterine cycle begins. Progesterone stimulates the glandular cells of the lining to produce a thick secretion rich in proteins, sugars, and amino acids, and the whole endometrium thickens. The spiral arteries become fully developed and show rhythmic dilatations and constrictions. Progesterone also causes an increase in the size of the smooth muscle cells of the myometrium, but, in contrast to oestrogen, progesterone reduces excitability and so contractions are quietened. So the uterus prepares itself for an embryo, with an endometrium about 5 mm thick and well supplied with blood. It is important to note that these actions of progesterone will only occur if the uterus has been primed with oestrogen during the first half of the cycle.

If fertilization does not occur, the corpus luteum begins to degenerate and its hormone secretions begin to wane. The uterus loses its hormonal support, blood flow to the endometrial tissue is reduced, and consequently this lining layer dies. However, there is some bleeding from the spiral arteries into the disintegrating endometrium, and thus blood and dead cells are shed through the cervix and vagina. At the end of menstruation the endometrium is only about 0.5 mm thick — the change in thickness has been ten-fold.

The cervix also shows cyclical changes with each menstrual cycle. In the first half of the cycle, under the influence of oestrogen, the tissue becomes more vascular, the muscle relaxes and the lining becomes more secretory. In the second half of the cycle when progesterone production is elevated secretion is reduced and the tissue becomes firmer. However, the most important changes seen in the cervix are in the composition and properties of mucus secreted by its lining. Tests on cervical mucus are important since a hostile, impenetrable mucus can reduce FERTILITY. As ovulation approaches the water and salt content of the mucus increase and it becomes less viscous, allowing for easier penetration of sperm. If mucus is taken from a cervical smear at this stage of the cycle and allowed to dry on a glass slide, a characteristic fern-leaf pattern of crystallization occurs, known as *ferning*. One can also draw this mucus out into long threads — a property known as *spinnbarkheit*. In contrast, mucus obtained in the second half of the cycle is thick, and strands of mucus cannot be stretched far before they break — a low *spinnbarkheit*. Thus the ability of sperm to penetrate cervical mucus is high at ovulation but low during the luteal phase when progesterone secretion is elevated. Indeed, the effects of progesterone on cervical mucus are such that low-dose progestogenic contraceptives given throughout the cycle can suppress sperm penetration through the cervix even at the time of ovulation when oestrogen levels are high.

In pregnancy the increase in size of the uterus is impressive: its walls remain thick despite the distension, because of the dramatic growth of its muscle fibres. The size and number of the blood vessels which supply it increase, carrying a twenty-fold increase in blood flow by full term. After delivery it shrinks rapidly, although taking some weeks to return to its previous size.

SAFFRON WHITEHEAD

See also LABOUR; MENSTRUAL CYCLE: PREGNANCY.

Uvula The pendular downward projection from the middle of the soft palate which helps to close off the back of the nasal cavity above it, during the complex movements of SWALLOWING. S.J.

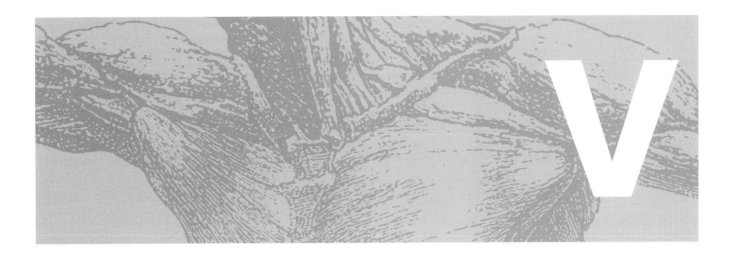

Vagina is the Latin word for 'sheath', which makes an interesting comparison with the alternative word for a condom. From this same root, the term 'invaginated' means ensheathed, or turned in on itself, like the finger of an empty glove introverted into the space for the hand. Comparably, the vagina is a tube which can be considered as part of the outer surface of the body that has been introverted, forming a passage to and from the uterus and lined with an epithelium continuous with that of the vulva, which is in turn continuous with the skin.

The opening of the vagina at the VULVA is initially partly covered by a thin fold of membrane known as the HYMEN. This normally has a central perforation, which is extended when torn by tampon use or during the first sexual intercourse. Once torn the hymen becomes an irregular ring of tissue round the vaginal opening. From the opening, the vagina extends upwards and backwards for about 10 cm and joins the cervix of the uterus at right angles so that the front wall is shorter than the back wall. The passage is roughly H-shaped in cross section, with the walls normally in close contact with each other. Around the epithelial cell lining the wall is formed of CONNECTIVE TISSUE and MUSCLE. The muscle coat is rather thin but is nevertheless very strong. The wall is folded; this allows for expansion and stretching during sexual intercourse, and much more so in childbirth. The vagina is also richly supplied with blood vessels which become engorged during sexual arousal, assisting the opening of the passage.

While the vagina helps to support the uterus it also provides a receptacle for the penis, an entrance for sperm, and an exit for menstrual flow and for the products of conception. Because the vagina is in continuity with the inside of the uterus and in turn with the FALLOPIAN TUBES, which lead to the peritoneal cavity, an important function is the prevention of infection from the outside world. Living in the vagina are *Döderlein's bacilli* (named after a German gynaecologist). These are quite normal inhabitants and ferment the glycogen (which provides glucose)

in the vaginal wall to lactic acid. Thus the vaginal environment is acidic, a pH of 3.8–4.5 compared with the normal pH of 7.4 found in most body tissues. This highly acidic environment helps to prevent the growth of many microorganisms which could otherwise invade the upper parts of the reproductive tract. As a consequence, when the number of these bacilli is reduced, or the availability of glucose changes, a woman becomes susceptible to vaginal infections which cause inflammation and discharge — vaginitis. For example, antibiotics can kill off the friendly bacteria in the vagina so that it becomes an ideal environment for the fungus, *candida albicans*, to flourish. Candidiasis (thrush) develops. Diabetes and SEX HORMONES can alter the amount of glucose available in the vagina and so disturb the acidic environment. Thus oral contraceptives and PREGNANCY, for example, can make women prone to vaginal infections.

Sex hormones not only alter the acidic environment of the vagina but also alter the activity of the vaginal epithelium. When oestrogen levels are high the epithelial cells become keratinized or cornified, an effect reversed by progesterone. The same hormones can alter the proportions of the organic aliphatic acids produced by the vaginal wall which are responsible for the characteristic smells of normal vaginal secretions; in many animals, and maybe even in humans, the odours (PHEROMONES) produced by vaginal secretions can increase the sexual attractiveness of the female around the time of ovulation.

SAFFRON WHITEHEAD

See also COITUS; UTERUS; VULVA.

Vagus nerves 'Vagus' means 'wanderer' — and that is indeed what these nerves are. Attached to the BRAIN STEM, and emerging through the base of the SKULL into the neck, the right and left vagus nerves innervate through their branches a widespread range of body parts, from the head down to the abdominal organs.

These nerves contain fibres that are both incoming to the CENTRAL NERVOUS SYSTEM (the majority) and outgoing from it. Sensory

information comes from the external ear and its canal, and from the back of the throat (pharynx) and upper part of the LARYNX. Longer fibres travel in the branches of the vagi from the organs in the chest and in the abdomen: from the LUNGS and the HEART, and from the alimentary tract, including the oesophagus and right down to half way along the colon. The incoming signals lead to many reflex responses, mediated at cell stations in the brain stem, and entailing either autonomic or somatic motor responses. For example: irritants in the airways stimulate vagal sensory nerve endings and lead to a COUGH reflex; information on the state of inflation of the lungs causes modification of the BREATHING pattern; distension of the stomach leads to reflex relaxation of its wall.

The outgoing, motor fibres in the vagus nerves represent most of the cranial component of the parasympathetic division of the AUTONOMIC NERVOUS SYSTEM. Vagal stimulation slows the heart beat, and excessive stimulation can stop it entirely. When Otto Loewi first showed, in 1921, that stimulation of the vagus nerve to a frog heart caused something to be released that could slow down another heart that was linked to the first only by fluid perfusion, he called the unknown factor *Vagusstoff*. We know now that vagal nerve endings act on the heart's pacemaker by the release of the transmitter ACETYL-CHOLINE; this modulation of the heart rate is continuous, counterbalancing the action of the sympathetic nerves at the same site. The vagus nerves also provide a pathway for reflex reduction of the cardiac output if the BLOOD PRESSURE tends to rise. In the lungs, they stimulate the SMOOTH MUSCLE in the wall of the bronchial tree, tending to increase the resistance to airflow (by causing *bronchoconstriction*), again counterbalancing the sympathetic effect which tends towards relaxation. In the alimentary tract they stimulate smooth muscle in the walls of the stomach and of the intestines, acting through the nerve networks between the layers of smooth muscle, but they have the opposite action on the smooth muscle sphincter that tends to prevent

703

the stomach contents from moving on. They stimulate glandular secretions of stomach acid and of the digestive enzymes that are released into the stomach and intestine, and the ejection of bile from the gall bladder. They also influence the release from the pancreas of the hormones that promote the storage of absorbed nutrients. All these effects add up to support of activity in the alimentary system during and after eating, when the parasympathetic effects predominate over the opposite quietening effects of the sympathetic nerve supply.

The term *'vaso-vagal' attack* refers to FAINTING, when — from a variety of causes ranging from emotional shock to the pain of injury — there is a strong parasympathetic outflow in the vagus nerves, causing slowing of the heart that leads to a fall in blood pressure sufficient to cause unconsciousness. SHEILA JENNETT

See also ALIMENTARY SYSTEM; AUTONOMIC NERVOUS SYSTEM; CRANIAL NERVES; VISCERAL SENSATION.

Vampire The predatory aristocrat whose blood-lust leads him to drain the blood of peasants, usually young women, is the stock figure of the vampire as represented by the cinematic Nosferatu, John Polidori's Lord Ruthven, and Bram Stoker's Count Dracula. For the 'undead', this exsanguination is a reproductive act, that conflates both food and sex. The most effective means of reproduction for the vampire, however, has been textual. Novels such as Sheridan Le Fanu's *Carmilla* (1872), Stoker's *Dracula* (1897), and Prest's *Varney the Vampire* (1847) have perpetuated an image that continues to replicate itself throughout our culture rather like a virus. Vampirism is encoded within popular culture through a complex nexus of literature, folklore, and fantasy.

Traditionally the *revenant*, or *undead*, is a mouldering CORPSE dragging itself out of graves to feed off the life-blood of the living. Premature burial arising from times of plague is one explanation for the prevalence of the vampire phenomenon at certain periods in history. The mecca for vampires is Eastern Europe. The word itself is believed to be of Magyar origin, possibly derived from the Turkish *uber*, meaning witch. The term was first used in English in 1734, according to the *Oxford English Dictionary*, where vampires are described as 'The bodies of deceased persons, animated by evil spirits, which come out of the graves in the night-time, suck the blood of many of the living, and thereby destroy them'.

In contrast, Stoker's eroticized and glamorous cloaked Count is a hybrid of the Wandering Jew and his hypnotic gaze, the libertine Lord Ruthven, who is based on Byron, and at least two notorious historical figures, whose careers were drenched in the blood of Eastern European peoples. These were Vlad Tepes, impaler and Romanian Prince, and Elizabeth Báthory, a Hungarian aristocrat, who was known as the Blood Countess of Cachtice. A sixteenth-century mass murderer whose sadomasochistic practices included biting off the flesh of her victims, Báthory's cruelties towards her servants escalated into capturing women and young girls who were then tortured and killed. Estimates of the numbers range from from thirty to over seven hundred. Their blood was drained for the Countess's rejuvenating bloodbaths, by such torturous contraptions as the cruelly spiked Iron Maiden. The horrors of Báthory's necro-sadism were written out of criminal history into fairy-tale, where she is represented as the wicked queen in *Snow White*, who contemplates her beauty at her looking-glass for hours on end. As this pathological behaviour suggests, vampirism can be a clinical phenomenon within which folklore, fantasy, and deviant behaviour converge.

The ingestion of blood can complement NECROPHILIA, which consists largely of sexual satisfaction derived from physical contact with a dead body. *Auto-vampirism* can include self-induced bleeding, or *auto-haemofetishism*, which is a condition whereby sexual pleasure is derived from the sight of blood.

The most well-known association of pathological conditions with vampires and WEREWOLVES was with the rare group of diseases called *porphyrias*. Caused by the body's overproduction of porphyrins — a normal component of haemoglobin (due in fact to an inborn error of metabolism), one type of this condition caused George III to produce blue urine and to collapse, foaming at the mouth. More obviously vampiric forms of the illness present themselves as an intolerance to light, wherein the skin cracks and bleeds, the gums and upper lip recede, and there is redness of the eyes, teeth, and skin. Seclusion from daylight and, ironically, drinking blood were prescribed remedies.

ANAEMIA has also been attributed to the vampire. During the nineteenth century, sufferers on this side of the grave were treated with animal blood, which they were expected to imbibe. In Joseph-Ferdinand Gueldry's painting, *The Blood Drinkers*, of 1898, a line of pale and languid women queue up in an abattoir for a glass of warm ox's blood. It is likely that their anaemia had been caused by menstrual losses.

A link between MENSTRUATION and vampirism is made by Freud in his essay 'The Taboo of Virginity' (1918). Again, among the myriad ways in which *Dracula* may be read is as an anti-menstrual subtext, which pathologizes femininity and constructs female blood as polluted and male blood as pure. From the writings on menstrual taboo of Stoker's contemporary, James Frazer, in *The Golden Bough*, we can infer similarities between vampires and menstruating women. Both are condemned as unclean, agents of pollution, and instigators of corruption. Sharing an avoidance of MIRRORS and crucifixes, they have been barred from many churches, temples, and synagogues. Some pre-industrial societies believed that a man could die from having contact, particularly intercourse, with a menstruating woman — and to make love with a vampire was potentially lethal. In such cultures, after menarche, a young girl would be kept out of the sun lest she, vampire-like, shrivel up into a withered skeleton. Frazer explains that for their own protection these adolescent girls were kept in tenebrous seclusion, where they were suspended between life and death, heaven and earth, until marriage. Likewise, the vampire exists in a bodily state that is between life and death and in a spiritual limbo betwixt heaven and earth. The coffins to which vampires retreat in the day serve, like menstrual huts, as places of seclusion and safety. For both vampires, their victims, and menstruating women, it is normal for blood to flow outside the body. Mythologised as transgressing the natural order, menstruating women in some cultures have a kinship with vampires.

Psychic vampirism is an affliction that, according to the Victorian physician Jules Michelet, affects young girls: 'A hysterical girl is … a vampire who sucks the blood of the healthy people around her.' The female vampire is a species of the *femme fatale*, whose deadly vampiric embrace can be seen as a metaphor for the transmission of syphilis — a potentially lethal, SEXUALLY TRANSMITTED DISEASE. Not just young female patients but also the male doctors, too, who are known as leeches or blood-suckers and who practise blood-letting, partake of the nature of vampires.

In his vampire-hunter's manual, called *Traité sur les Apparitions des Ésprits et sur les Vampires* (Paris 1746), Dom Augustine Calmet provides case histories of how he set out to 'cure' the supposed plague of vampires that was infecting eighteenth-century Europe. His first resort was decapitation, staking out the heart, and then incineration. The overkill of this zealous Benedictine monk was presumably due to the ambivalent attitude towards death which characterized the average vampire. More *apotropaic* methods (techniques for turning evil away) included stuffing objects into the orifices of corpses or confronting the ambulatory bloodsucker with a crucifix. The latest breed of fictional vampires, such as Ann Rice's androgynous vampires in her *Vampire Chronicles*, which began publication in 1976, have proved to be a strain resistant to such apotropaics, while Poppy Z. Brite's vampires are immune to the deleterious effects of religious symbolism. For them vampirism is drained of signification. In *Lost Souls* (1992), which is an appropriate title for the vampire entering post-modernism, the sexual significance of vampirism is no longer a means of reproduction but a sadomasochistic diversion.

The vampire is a sublimation of our fears of death and disease, articulating our resistance to an acceptance of the process of decomposition. Human decay involves discolouration, bloating, and leaking of blood-stained fluid from the mouth and nostrils — which have been misinterpreted as the superfluities of a blood-satiated cadaver. The taboos surrounding putrefaction and funereal rights, which can involve the second burial of the exhumed undead, suggest that it is not until a corpse no longer resembles the living, and only when it resides in its skeletal state as a *momento mori*, that the living can truly rest in peace. MARIE MULVEY-ROBERTS

See also SADOMASOCHISM; TORTURE.

Vanity

Vanity is the short-sighted pursuit of bodily life, its transient pleasures, and achievements. Characterized by a narcissistic pride in personal appearance and temporary accomplishments, vanity thumbs its nose at the inevitability of death and religious lore setting store on an after-life (though it is possible to be vain about seeking martyrdom). One of the greatest poetic celebrations of vanity — a paean in praise of corporeal pleasure — is Edward Fitzgerald's musical translation (1859) of *The Rubaiyat* of Omar Khayyam:

Ah, make the most of what we yet may spend,
Before we too into Dust descend:
Dust into Dust, and under Dust, to lie,
Sans Wine, sans Song, sans Singer, and — sans End!

Conversely, the classical warning against worldly vanity — 'vanity of vanities; all is vanity' — fills twelve chapters of the book Ecclesiastes. Implying a state of spiritual emptiness, vanity inspired, in seventeenth-century Leiden, a genre of still-life painting called the *vanitas*. Essentially an exhortation to repentance, the *vanitas* featured symbols of earthly wealth and enjoyment such as jewellery and wine goblets, alongside *momento mori* like the human skull or a clock and, sometimes, symbols of eternal life. The message is clear: death comes to all mortals.

In secular society, vanity is most readily identified with the sin of pride in bodily appearance, manifesting in luxurious garb and flamboyant ornamentation. Vanity occurs in differing degrees of severity and ridiculousness and has a number of roots, but few human beings are immune from it. On occasion, it derives from a desire to show a particularly splendid, sexually attractive, part of the anatomy in its best aspect. The parson in Chaucer's *The Canterbury Tales*, for instance, inveighed against the vanity of four-teenth-century youths in sporting ludicrously brief tunic skirts: 'some of them show the very boss of the privy member and pushed out parts that look like the hind parts of an ape.' A similar argument might be made (with the appropriate gender, and anatomical, changes) for the 1960s mini skirt. In most cases, however, vanity is concerned with the concealment, and aesthetic amelioration, of bodily inadequacy, imperfection, or weakness. The vanity of the middle-aged man compelled to scrape a few strands of hair across a bald pate, or of the woman who would rather ask a fellow pedestrian her bus number than don spectacles, tends to be regarded with amused indulgence. However, the ostentatious display of garments which unduly expose the body, and so render it sexually provocative, can invoke moral judgement, censure, and severe disapproval.

Women have traditionally suffered (and been prepared to suffer) more than men in the name of vanity. While the male body lends itself less to remoulding, men's evident disinclination to endure pain in the name of beauty is also an expression of centuries of male social dominance. For instance, although some European men have been known from the eighteenth century to wear CORSETS, women's abdomens have consistently been the main target of tight lacing and whale-bone stays. Even after all the fast-changing cultural and GENDER perceptions of the twentieth century, there is little doubt that women are still judged more from the outside in. Culturally constrained by their appearance, women's body image plays a larger part in determining their self-esteem and self-identity. Ironically, women are willing agents within this process as well as victims of a socially dictated, collective vanity.

Corrective surgery for the repair of accidental and trauma-inflicted injury is acceptable vanity. The surgical restoration of NOSES has a history of thousands of years' duration in India. But the growth, during the twentieth century, in elective surgery for purely cosmetic reasons is probably regarded as the ultimate form of dubious vanity. Although still most popular with women, COSMETIC SURGERY increasingly has a market amongst men. Even where surgery is successful, the aesthetic improvements achieved are often ordinary rather than exquisite. The risks are manifold: danger in undergoing anaesthesia; surgical failure; poisoning of the IMMUNE SYSTEM through silicone dispersal from ruptured breast implants or injections to increase muscle-bulk; and permanent disfigurement at the hands of unscrupulous, inadequately-trained surgeons out to make a fast fortune.

There can be a huge divide between relatively harmless 'peacock' posturing and susceptibility to forms of coercive, collective vanity which irreparably damage the body. A particularly inhumane example of the latter is the binding of young girls' feet in China, a custom which persisted into the twentieth century.

Changes in sartorial FASHION are also society's authorization of the human need for collective vanity. The answer for religious sects like the Amish of North America is to shun bodily vanity through anachronistic adherence to the styles of the seventeenth century. But the seventeenth century was hardly immune from the condition. The anonymous author of *England's Vanity: or the Voice of God Against the Monstrous Sin of Pride, in Dress and Apparel* (1683), compared the vanity of the English with the canker of syphilis, since they would accept 'No Cut but a French Taylor's to shape our Cloaths; No Language but the French to serve our Tongues; no Religion but the French to content our Souls; I pray you what will be the end hereof? There is a disease among us called of that Name too, I pray God it be not too Epidemical; if it be not gotten into our Bodies, sure I am tis gotten into our Heads.' FIONA MACDONALD

Further reading
Woodforde, J. (1992). *The history of vanity*. Alan Sutton, Stroud.

Varicose veins

Varicose veins A varix or varicosity is an irregularity or lumpiness. In the body, this means irregularities caused by dilated and distorted veins.

Veins in the legs have valves which normally prevent any backflow of the blood on its way towards the heart. The pressure of the blood tending to distend these veins is greater than in veins elsewhere simply because, for most of most people's waking hours, they are lower than the rest of the body, and vertical. This can put a considerable strain on the valves, each of which supports the column of blood immediately above it, between it and the next valve further up. In ideal normal circumstances the blood is kept moving upwards effectively because of persistent squeezing of veins by actively contracting muscles as we walk about, as well as by other mechanisms which tend continually to draw the blood towards the chest. The superficial veins just under the skin benefit less directly than the deep ones from leg movements — but because they connect to the deep veins, squeezing by the muscles helps to siphon blood from those near the surface, as well as 'milking' it up the deep ones.

Thus gravity does not normally cause an accumulation of weighty blood in our lowest parts, as it would in, say, a liquid-filled bicycle inner tube suspended vertically. But there are less than ideal circumstances which cause relative stagnation, particularly in the superficial unsupported veins; blood then leans more heavily on the valves, and in some cases these become damaged and develop leaks. This can occur if there is an obstruction to blood flow up from the legs (such as a heavily pregnant uterus pressing on the veins in the pelvic cavity) and the problem is exacerbated by sitting or standing still. As for many bodily dysfunctions, there is no doubt a combination of innate propensity (weak veins and valves) and risk factors (flow obstruction and immobility). The leakage of valves in turn leads to the irregular bulges on the veins which are known as varicosities, along with enlargement and distortion. The sluggishness imposed on the circulation to the skin and underlying tissues by back pressure from these veins predisposes to discomfort, ulceration, and OEDEMA.

Applying pressure by support stockings to keep the varicose veins from filling is the first line of treatment. But the veins which are affected are fortunately usually dispensible: if they are removed, blood can flow through alternative deeper channels. Effective surgical treatment involves making cuts only at the top and the bottom of the offending vein, which is then removed by using a 'stripper'. From the top end (say at the knee) a thin flexible rod is passed down the vein to the far end (say at the ankle). The vein is tied around the rod, which has a knob on its end. Pulling from the top then causes the knob to draw the whole length of the vein up before it, 'crumpling' it as it comes. Thus the vein is pulled by the stripper from under the skin and out through the upper incision.

A similar problem can occur at other sites. In the lower end of the oesophagus, 'varices' may result from back pressure associated with liver disease. In the scrotum a 'varicocoele' is a swelling of the veins around the testis. HAEMORRHOIDS represent a comparable condition of the anal veins.   SHEILA JENNETT

See also BLOOD CIRCULATION; BLOOD VESSELS.

Vas deferens
The tube on each side which leads from the TESTIS to the URETHRA, carrying SPERM and some other components of seminal fluid. Each vas ends by joining the duct of a *seminal vesicle*, to enter the urethra (the urinary passage) where that traverses the PROSTATE GLAND. May be closed off by the operation of VASECTOMY, preventing sperm from entering the ejaculate.   S.J.

See PLATE 8.

Vasectomy
is the operation to sterilize the male by dividing the vas deferens on both sides, and thus to interrupt the passage of SPERM.

Vasectomy has been known for some hundred years — the first operation performed specifically for the purpose of STERILIZATION took place in Indiana in 1899. It was initially believed that by suppressing the sperm-making functions of the TESTES, an increase in the SEX HORMONE could be brought about, producing improvements in physical health and sexual vigour. This led to its practice as a 'rejuvenation' operation, known as the 'Steinach' operation after the Viennese professor whose laboratory experiments led to this conclusion. The numbers of men who underwent this operation in the hopes of increasing their sexual powers cannot be known, but Kenneth Walker, the British expert in male sexual disorders, believed that 'uncritical and unprincipled medical men' widely exploited this belief during the 1920s. He himself was sceptical of its benefit in increasing sexual power, attributing any apparent improvement to suggestion.

As a means of CONTRACEPTION, the operation was also, of course, much easier to perform and less drastic than the equivalent operation on the female. However, in spite of the publicity the operation gained in connection with rejuvenation, for many years it was confused in both the lay and the medical mind with CASTRATION. The very legality of such a 'mutilating operation' was in question.

It increased in popularity as a method of contraception during the 1960s, particularly for couples who had completed their families and were reluctant for the wife to continue taking the Pill for an indefinite period. Unlike female sterilization, it tends to be the choice of couples who share responsibility for fertility control.

There are currently various different operative techniques but the method that is gaining popularity is the 'no scalpel' method invented by Professor Li Shungqiang of Sichuan Reproductive Health Institute, Chengdu, Sichuan, P R China, and worldwide this method is now the most commonly used. It is a very minimal technique using specially designed instruments which enable the vas to be divided through a small puncture wound; the ends are then separated by a bit of tissue. It is interesting to note that Professor Li started life as a neurosurgeon but during the cultural revolution he was redirected to work in family planning. Many lesser men would have become very depressed but he immediately set about devising new operations, culminating in his no scalpel technique. It has now been used on hundreds of thousands of men and probably no other living surgeon has influenced the lives of more men.

A question that is commonly asked is 'Where do the sperm go after vasectomy?' The sperm-producing cells are in the seminiferous tubules inside the testicle and sperm exit from the top of the testicle into a softer area, the epididymis. The epididymis to a certain extent acts as a filter, and abnormal sperm and debris associated with cell division are cleared from the ejaculate. After vasectomy the whole sperm production has to be absorbed through the epididymis: an exaggeration of its normal function. Seminal fluid continues to be produced normally by the PROSTATE GLAND and seminal vesicles.

The effect on subsequent sex-life appears to be beneficial in the majority of cases, in spite of the concern often expressed that it may have a deleterious effect on virility (harking back to the old association with castration) — commonly, increased sexual satisfaction and libido has been reported (perhaps substantiating Steinach, or merely reflecting the release from fear of conception). However, this is more likely to occur when the man has deliberately chosen to undertake vasectomy, unlike the case of the Indian men who were persuaded into vasectomy, in return for portable radios, during a drive to reduce the population problem of the subcontinent.

In recent years there has been some concern about the safety of vasectomy. It has been shown that there is no association between vasectomy and heart attacks or vasectomy and testicular cancer, although there have been worries about both. There is still some concern about the association between vasectomy and prostate cancer, but it seems very likely that this apparent association is because of the introduction of new methods to diagnose prostate cancer, and the way statistics are collected, rather than any cause and effect.

Vasectomy is highly reliable provided that an additional method of contraception is employed during the first weeks following the operation, during which live sperm may still be present in the seminal fluid.

The major disadvantage is that it cannot readily be reversed: even with recent developments in microsurgery, the operation to reunite the severed vasa deferens reopens them in 80–90% of cases, but the success rate in terms of achieving pregnancy is at best only 50%. There have been attempts at temporary, reversible blocking or clipping of the tubes, but so far these have failed to achieve a degree of reliability in any way comparable with the permanent operation.

There is a very small late failure rate (approximately 1 in 2000), but vasectomy remains surer than female sterilization. The only more certain method of contraception is complete abstinence.
                    TIM HARGREAVE
                    LESLEY A. HALL

See also CONTRACEPTION; STERILIZATION.

Vection
is the sensation of movement of the body in space produced purely by visual stimulation. Everyone is familiar with the impression of self-motion experienced when watching a moving train through the windows of a stationary train. Powerful experiences of this kind occur when viewing surround cinema (IMAX) and VIRTUAL REALITY displays, which fill much of the visual field. Vection can be *linear* (apparent forward or backward motion) or *angular* (corresponding to angular body motion). The basis of vection lies in the close association between the processing of visual and vestibular motion in the brain. In part, this perceptual response to sustained visual motion has probably evolved as an adaptation to the fact that signals from the vestibular apparatus in the inner ear decay quite quickly during constant rotation or linear movement of the head. The sensation of vection produced purely by visual stimulation tends to build up fairly slowly, in a way that complements the decay of the vestibular sensation of movement. So, when we rotate with respect to a stationary visual world, the vection reinforces the sense that it is we who are moving, not the visual world itself, which we expect to be stable.

                    GRAHAM BARNES
                    COLIN BLAKEMORE

See also VESTIBULAR SYSTEM; VISION.

Vegan
diets comprise only plant foods and exclude all meat, poultry, fish, dairy products, eggs, and honey. Although many poor peasant agriculturalist populations have diets based on plant foods with only small amounts of animal food, there are no traditional societies which follow a completely vegan diet. The word was coined by Donald Watson as 'the beginning and end of vegetarian', and the first vegan society was formed in Britain in 1944.

The reasons for choosing a vegan diet are similar to those for choosing a vegetarian diet, but the philosophy is more logical because dairy foods, which are included in vegetarian diets, cannot be produced efficiently without the slaughter of cattle. To produce milk a cow must give birth to a calf: most of these calves are reared and slaughtered for meat, and the cows themselves are also slaughtered for meat as soon as they fail to conceive or develop other health problems. The production of eggs involves the slaughter of male chicks and of old laying hens.

Unfortified plant foods contain all the nutrients needed by humans except for vitamin B12 and vitamin D. Animals used for meat obtain vitamin B12 from bacteria in the rumen (cattle and sheep), bacteria in the soil (pigs), or by eating their own faeces (rabbits). Vitamin B12 is now synthesized cheaply and added to many foods including breakfast cereals, yeast extracts, and various soya-based foods. Vitamin D is synthesized in the skin in response to sunlight, and is also added to several foods including margarine. Therefore, with fortification and sunlight, vegan diets can supply all the nutrients needed by humans. Vegan diets are usually higher than non-vegetarian diets in some nutrients such as fibre, vitamin C, vitamin E, potassium, and magnesium, and lower than non-vegetarian diets in protein, riboflavin, vitamin B$_{12}$, and calcium. Vegan diets can be low in iodine and selenium, but this depends on the soil in which the plants are grown.

The nutritional status and health of vegans has been investigated in a number of small studies. These have shown that most vegans are adequately nourished and in satisfactory health, and that vegans are thinner and have lower blood cholesterol concentrations than comparable non-vegetarians. Vegan children grow normally provided that they receive well planned diets. There have been some cases of nutritional deficiency in vegans, notably vitamin B12 deficiency in vegans who were not eating foods fortified with this vitamin (or taking a vitamin B12 supplement).

There is little information on the long-term health of vegans. Epidemiological studies of mortality in vegetarians have included some vegans, and the mortality rate of these vegans has been similar to that of the vegetarians, but the total number studied throughout the world is still far too small to be able to draw any firm conclusions. A diet comprised largely or entirely of plants has several potential advantages for health, land use, and ecological impact, and looking further ahead may be the diet of choice for the extended exploration of space. Further scientific research on plant-based diets and the health of vegans is therefore a priority for the future.

TIM KEY

Further reading

Langley, G. R. (1995). *Vegan nutrition*. The Vegan Society, St Leonards-on-Sea.

Vegetarian

diets exclude all meat, poultry, and fish and are based on plant foods. Most vegetarians include dairy products and eggs in their diet; this type of diet is sometimes described as lacto-ovo-vegetarian whereas vegetarians who exclude all animal foods from their diet are termed VEGANS.

There are three major reasons for which people choose a vegetarian diet. The first is aversion to the slaughter of animals; this view is not logically compatible with the consumption of dairy products or eggs, because the production of these foods inevitably involves the slaughter of calves, cows, and chicks (see vegan). The second

major reason for choosing a vegetarian diet is for more efficient land use, because a hectare of good farmland can produce much more plant food than animal food. The third reason is HEALTH, because most of the meat consumed in Western societies is rich in saturated FAT and this increases the concentration of CHOLESTEROL in the blood and therefore the risk of developing ischaemic heart disease.

Well planned vegetarian diets are adequate for normal growth and health. Some Hindus in India have, for religious reasons, followed vegetarian diets for many generations and their diet is clearly adequate for maintaining a viable population. In Western countries the number of vegetarians has increased greatly since the 1960s. Nutritional studies have shown that on average the diets of these people are nutritionally adequate and are closer to current recommendations for maintaining health than average non-vegetarian diets. Epidemiological studies have shown that vegetarians have significantly lower mortality from ischaemic heart disease than comparable non-vegetarians, and are less likely to be obese, but have not established differences in mortality rates from other causes of death.

The proportion of the population who are vegetarian is still rising in many Western countries, and has probably been accelerated by health issues such as the link between 'mad cow disease' (bovine spongiform encephalopathy — BSE) and new variant Creutzfeld–Jacob disease in humans. Future trends in the dietary preferences of populations are difficult to predict, but there is no doubt that a move towards a 'semi-vegetarian' diet low in animal products would allow more people to be fed from less land and could have substantial ecological benefits.

TIM KEY

Further reading

Thorogood, M. (1995). The epidemiology of vegetarianism and health. *Nutrition Research Reviews*, **8**, 179–92.

See also DIETS; HEALTH FOODS; VEGAN.

Vegetative state

This defines the behaviour of a person in whom brain damage has put out of action the CEREBRAL CORTEX — the thinking, feeling part of the BRAIN — but without any lasting effect on the BRAIN STEM. The intact brain stem ensures that there are long periods of eye opening (unlike COMA) and that there is spontaneous breathing (unlike BRAIN DEATH): these are important distinctions, since the three conditions are not infrequently confused by the media when reporting these tragic stories.

With the cerebral cortex either destroyed or disconnected there is no evidence of a working mind — no psychologically meaningful responses to the person's surroundings. No command is obeyed, no single word is uttered, and there is no evidence of awareness. The patient is therefore unconscious although 'awake' and with several reflex responses and activities. During the periods of eye opening the eyes may rove around

randomly, and they may turn briefly with the head towards a sudden loud noise, when there may also be blinking and sometimes stiffening of the whole body. In some vegetative patients the eyes may briefly focus on an object and follow it when it moves. There are often chewing movements and there may be yawning — less often, brief smiling or weeping, but not in response to any appropriate situation. In response to a painful stimulus the spastic limbs may bend or straighten and the face may grimace. Inexperienced staff and family members are apt to interpret some reflex activity as evidence of meaningful responsiveness, when prolonged and careful observation fails to confirm this. However, the observations of family and carers are always taken seriously because they may be reporting the first signs of recovery from the vegetative state.

The vegetative state may result from an acute brain insult — the commonest causes being severe head INJURY or failure of the OXYGEN supply to the brain. This failure can follow cardiac arrest or respiratory obstruction (from strangulation, SUFFOCATION, or NEAR DROWNING), when RESUSCITATION has been in time to save the heart and the brain stem but too late for the more vulnerable cerebral cortex. These acute insults usually lead to coma for 2–3 weeks before the patient 'wakes' to the vegetative state. Some patients with progressive degenerative brain disease, such as Alzheimer's disease, gradually become vegetative after years of deterioration, and some infants with severe congenital abnormalities of the brain, or with chromosomal defects, can become vegetative.

Diagnosis depends on careful clinical observation over many weeks, because there are no laboratory or imaging tests that reliably indicate that a patient is vegetative. Sometimes a patient is mistakenly believed to be in a vegetative state when subtle signs of responsiveness have been overlooked. It is particularly important to be sure that there has not been localized damage to the brain stem with sparing of the cortex, resulting in the 'locked-in syndrome'. In this, the patient is totally paralysed and speechless but is fully conscious; communication may be established using a yes/no code by eye blinks or movements — using the only muscles not paralysed.

Patients are said to be in a *continuing* or *persistent* vegetative state if there is no recovery after one month. Many of them die from respiratory complications over the next few months; some recover consciousness, while the rest remain vegetative. The longer the vegetative state lasts the less likely is there to be recovery of consciousness, and the less likely is there to be a reasonable recovery of other functions even if consciousness is regained. Those who become conscious after many months in a vegetative state are usually left paralysed and totally dependent, sometimes continuing to need tube feeding and not regaining speech. Patients who become vegetative after an episode of cerebral hypoxia very seldom show any recovery after three months, but after head injury some recovery may still occur up to twelve months after injury. After these periods it is usual to declare the vegetative state *permanent.*

Patients who survive for a year in the vegetative state are often quite stable and can survive for many years if tube feeding is continued and infections treated with antibiotics. Some have lived for 20–40 years. It has been argued by doctors, philosophers, and lawyers in several countries that continued survival in this state is not of benefit to the patient — a view often, but not always, shared by the relatives. If that is so then there is no moral or legal obligation to continue the medical treatment of artificial nutrition and hydration. In the USA and several European countries a decision to withdraw such treatment can be made by doctors after consultation with the family, but in the UK permission has to be sought from the High Court.   BRYAN JENNETT

Further reading

Jennett, B. (2001). *The vegetative state: medical facts, ethical and legal dilemmas.* Cambridge University Press.

Jennett, B. and Plum, F. (1972). Persistent vegetative state after brain damage. A syndrome in search of a name. *Lancet*, 1, 734–7.

See also ARTIFICIAL FEEDING; BRAIN DEATH; BRAIN STEM; COMA.

Veil The earliest evidence for veiling is an Assyrian legal text dating from the thirteenth century BCE, requiring women of clearly defined social status to wear veils, and prohibiting prostitutes and slaves from doing so. The veil thus distinguished respectable women from women who were publicly available, protecting the former from the gaze of men and from their advances.

The veiling of women by scarf or hood, and their seclusion, became a mark of honour and social status in cities of the Middle East and Mediterranean world in the centuries before the Common Era. In this context, the apostle Paul called upon Christian women to cover their heads, and in the third century, Tertulian recommended that the Christian women of Carthage veil themselves outdoors. At around this time, the bridal veil became incorporated into the Christian wedding ceremony, adapted from the Roman model, while women who became consecrated to the service of God 'took up the veil' as a symbol of their marriage to Christ, and a sign of their chastity. The earliest clear evidence for the bridal veil in Jewish custom dates from the early Middle Ages as well, although Jewish women had covered their HAIR in public, as an act of MODESTY, since biblical times.

The veiling of women became a feature of Islamic society some time after the Islamic conquests of the eastern Byzantine lands and the domains of the Sassanian empire in the early seventh century. During the Prophet Muhammad's lifetime (d. 632), the revelation of the Qur'an called for modest dress for both men and women, including the cloaking of women outdoors, and the seclusion of the Prophet's wives.

After the Islamic conquests, in an environment in which respectable non-Muslim urban women covered their hair and remained at home, jurists interpreted the general prescriptions of the relevant Qur'anic verses, and the example of the Prophet's wives, to mandate the wearing of a veil or *hijab* for Muslim women. The definition of the *hijab* — for example, whether it must cover the hands and face — was and continues to be a point of difference among legal traditions and individual jurists. Barbara Showalter has shown how Qur'an commentaries from the tenth, thirteenth, and seventeenth centuries suggest a historical trend, among legal scholars, to ever stricter interpretations of the requirements of modesty in the pre-modern period. In practice, socio-economic and regional variations must have always prevailed in the use and form of the veil.

In the modern period, officials of the European imperial empires and other Westerners pointed to the veil as a symbol of the oppression of women and the backwardness of Muslim societies, and Middle Eastern nationalists and reformers, men and women, began to discuss the status of women and the wearing of the veil. Some women, such as Huda Sha'arawi in Egypt, discarded the veil after becoming active in public life, to mark their departure from the world of seclusion and identify themselves as modern women, while others worked for nationalist goals, or to improve opportunities for girls and women, without deeming it necessary to renounce the veil. By the 1930s, however, many women of the upper and middle classes in many of the major cities of the Middle East no longer veiled themselves, with the encouragement of governments, such as the Turkish republic, or by legislation, as in Iran.

The current politicization of the veil has occurred as part of a general reaction in the Islamic world to the political, economic, and social changes of the last century and a frustration with, or rejection of, what have been identified as Western models for the state, society, and economy. The Islamic Revolution in Iran in 1979 called for the foundation of an Islamic state based on Islamic principles and upholding Islamic law, and imposed the full veiling of women as a visible symbol of that commitment. Since then, the veil has become a widely recognized, and ideologically charged, symbol of Islam, taken up by various Islamist movements not necessarily sympathetic to the Iranian Revolution.

Women in different parts of the Islamic world have been forced or pressured to take up the veil, but women have also chosen to take up the veil out of a political or personal commitment to Islamic reform, or as an expression of their rediscovery of their Muslim identity. In some contexts, the veil is associated with the seclusion of women at home, but in other contexts the veiled woman is active in public life. The identification of the veil as a symbol of an Islamic way of life has stirred a new generation to debate the status

of women in Islamic religion, law, society, and culture.

The increased incidence of new veiling may be misinterpreted in some contexts, because the veil has become so closely identified with Islamist movements and anti-Western politics. Arlene MacLeod's study of lower-middle-class women in Cairo who have taken up the *hijab* — here defined as covering clothes (of varying styles) and a head scarf that generally covers the hair, neck, and ears — reveals that many women who take up the veil are not politically active or particularly interested in Islamic revival. The women of her study were often from rural backgrounds and the first in their families to work outside the home; they adopted the veil as a way to secure respect from those they encountered at work, in the course of their day, and from their families. Their veiling facilitated their activity outside the home and represented an accommodation between their economic needs and social circumstances.

For some Muslims living in predominantly non-Muslim societies, the veil has become a contested symbol of ethnic and cultural identity. In France, for example, Muslims have agitated to allow girls to wear a headscarf to school, asserting the principle of freedom of religion and challenging the tolerance of the state and society, while in Germany, Turkish migrants may wear the head scarf as a sign of pride and rejection of assimilation.

The veil has become a potent symbol of Islam and Muslim identity in recent decades and yet its meaning for those who wear it, or see it being worn, for those who advocate the veiling of women, or reject it, is hardly uniform, and often ambiguous.   JANINA SAFRAN

Further reading

Ahmed, L. (1992). *Women and gender in Islam.* Yale University Press, New Haven.

Showalter, B. (1984). The status of women in early Islam. In *Muslim Women*, (ed. F. Hussain), pp. 11–43. Croom-Helm, London.

MacLeod, A. (1991). *Accommodating protest.* Columbia University Press, New York.

See also ISLAM AND THE BODY.

Venom from the Latin *venenem*, meaning poison. Refers to the poisonous fluid secreted by some snakes and spiders and injected into the victim by a bite or sting.   A.W.C.

See POISONS.

Ventilation in the physiological sense (strictly, *pulmonary ventilation*) refers to the volume of air breathed in and out of the LUNGS: typically 5–6 litres per minute for an average-sized person at rest, with the possibility of increasing by up to twenty-fold in EXERCISE. For example, the size of each breath (*tidal volume*) could vary from 0.5 to 3 litres, and the number of breaths per minute from 10 to 40. When for any reason BREATHING stops or becomes inadequate, or if natural breathing is prevented by drug-induced muscle relaxation as an adjunct to ANAESTHESIA, mechanical or ARTIFICIAL VENTILATION (also known as artificial respiration) is necessary. Methods range from mouth-to-mouth breathing to machines which pump gas rhythmically into the lungs   S.J.

See BREATHING; BREATHING DURING EXERCISE.

Venus The goddess Venus represents the ideal of seductive female beauty. In her Greek form, Aphrodite, or as the Roman Venus, she is associated with the seduction of mortals by gods, and with sexual relationships between mortal men and women. In Greek myth Aphrodite emerged from the sea after the castration of Kronos, the Titan. The etymology of the Latin name 'Venus' is unclear, although it may relate to words for both 'charm' and 'poison'; but, before the elision of the Greek and Roman deities late in the third century BC, the Italian goddess Venus seems to have been associated with the fertility of gardens rather than with human sexuality. Her special importance to the Romans was increased by her role as mother of the hero Aeneas, one of the legendary figures associated with the foundation of the city of Rome. Venus mediates between Jupiter, head of the Roman pantheon, and the Roman people.

In the Roman republic, several generals claimed to be under her personal protection, including Sulla, who marched on Rome and took the city in 88 BC. Most famous of these generals was Julius Caesar, whose family claimed direct descent from Venus; he promoted her cult, especially as Venus Victrix, 'she who conquers', and he built a new temple to the goddess. The first imperial dynasty of the Roman Empire, the Julio-Claudians, emphasised both their links to Julius Caesar and their right to rule through their continued emphasis on Venus.

Aphrodite/Venus has been a popular subject in art since the classical period, providing a rationale for showing the naked female body in a variety of poses in periods when it would be considered inappropriate to represent a real woman in this way. A particularly common theme in post-classical art is 'The Toilet of Venus', showing her with Eros, her son by the war-god Ares, holding up a mirror in which she can admire her own beauty. Other standard poses represent her as a modest young woman about to take a bath, rising from the sea, or wringing her hair out on the beach. In many of these poses she is represented as if she thinks she is unobserved; the observer is thus cast as a voyeur. Sometimes she shields her breasts and pudenda as if she has been startled to find that an onlooker is present, in a pose known

as the *Venus pudens* that paradoxically only draws attention to the parts which are concealed.

In the Middle Ages, Venus was used to represent the sin of *luxuria* or sensuality; in battles for the soul, she was invariably lined up on the side of the vices. However, the Italian Neoplatonists saw love as a metaphysical experience transforming the soul and bringing awareness of the divine, so that images of Venus could be used to suggest divine rather than secular love and union.

The damaged marble image of Aphrodite found on Melos in 1820 (the *Venus de Milo*), perhaps the most famous statue in the history of the nude, dates to the second century BC; Man Ray's version, *Venus Restored*, represents her tied with rope. A description of the *Venus de Milo* by the classical scholar L. R. Farnell, written in 1896, shows the lengths to which Victorian writers went in playing down the sexuality of Venus; he claimed that she was 'free from human weakness or passion', 'stamped with an earnestness lofty and self-contained, almost cold'.

Venus remains the ideal of female BEAUTY, and as such she appears in some unlikely places. It is significant that Leopold von Sacher-Masoch chose to call his novel celebrating masochism *Venus im Pelz* (*Venus in Furs*, 1870), while in 1884, under the pseudonym 'Rachilde', Marguerite Eymery, who sometimes dressed as a

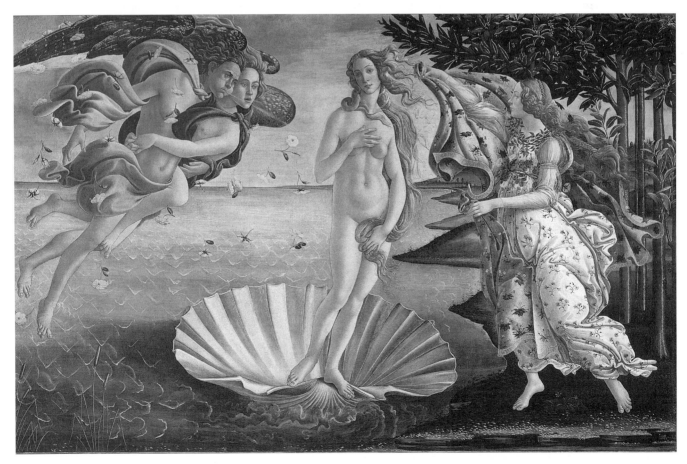

The Birth of Venus, *c.* 1485 (tempera on canvas) by Sandro Botticelli (1444/5–1510). Galleria degli Uffizi, Florence, Italy/Bridgeman Art Library.

man, published her *Monsieur Venus*, the story of a woman who uses the parts of her dead lover to create a male Venus.   HELEN KING

See also BEAUTY; FEMALE FORM; TITANS.

Vesalius
Andreas Vesalius (1514–64) was the Renaissance physician who truly put anatomy on the medical map. In his pathbreaking *De humani corporis fabrica* (*On the fabric of the human body*, 1543), he boldly presented himself as the first to expose the errors of his predecessors: 'How much has been attributed to Galen, easily leader of the professors of dissection, by those physicians and anatomists who have followed him, and often against reason!'

Born Andreas van Wesele, in Brussels, where his father was pharmacist to the Emperor Charles V, Vesalius learned Latin and Greek and enrolled in the Paris Faculty of Medicine, studying under the conservative humanist Sylvius, then Galen's great champion — in later years Sylvius became a scourge of Vesalius, wittily calling him *vesanus* (madman). Vesalius learnt his dissecting skills from Guinther von Andernach, and when in 1536 war forced him to flee Paris, he returned to Louvain, where he introduced DISSECTION; he showed his anatomical zeal by robbing a wayside gibbet, smuggling the bones back home and there reconstructing the SKELETON.

In 1537 he moved to Padua, where he made his anatomical name. Dissection had previously been demonstrated there by surgeons, and had never been mandatory for physicians. The rediscovery of Galen's *On Anatomical Procedures*, and the wider dissemination of his *On the Use of Parts*, however, meant that humanists were beating the drum for the subject, and the appointment of the young physician was one consequence of this. Vesalius's *Tabulae anatomicae sex* (*Six anatomical pictures*, 1538) were amongst the first anatomical illustrations specifically designed for students. The first three sheets were drawn by Vesalius himself and represented the liver and its blood vessels, together with the male and female reproductive organs, the venous system, and the arterial system. He was still viewing the body through Galenic eyes: despite Berengario, he drew the *rete mirabile*; the liver was still five-lobed, and the heart an ape's.

Thereafter Vesalius grew more critical. Familiarity with human ANATOMY as well as Galen's anatomical writings drove him to the unsettling conclusion that the master had dissected only animals, and forced him to see that animal anatomy was no substitute for human. He now began to challenge him on points of detail: for instance, that the lower jaw comprised a single bone, not two, as Galen, relying on animals, had stated. Evidently, human anatomy must be learned from dead bodies, not dead languages.

In 1539 he acquired a larger supply of cadavers of executed criminals and worked on his great masterpiece, the *De humani corporis fabrica*. Finishing it in 1542, he took it to Basel, where the press of Joannes Oporinus published it in 1543

as one of the pearls of Renaissance printing. It presents exact descriptions of the skeleton and muscles, the nervous system, the blood vessels, and the viscera. Though it contains no shattering discoveries, it marks a watershed in the medical understanding of bodily structures, for Vesalius interrogated Galen by reference to the human corpse. Others had criticised odds and ends of Galenic anatomy, but Vesalius was the first to review it systematically. The *Fabrica* gained immensely from the contribution of the artist, Jan Stephan van Calcar, also from the Netherlands, who provided the text with technically accurate drawings displaying the dissected body in graceful, life-like poses. The work also enunciated clear methodological principles: the anatomist–lecturer must perform the dissection

himself, the eye was preferable to authority, and anatomy was the skeleton key to medicine.

Book I of the *Fabrica* began in Galenic fashion with the BONES rather than, as in medieval practice, the internal organs. Various Galenic lapses were corrected — for instance, that the human sternum has not seven but three segments. Book II dealt with the MUSCLES, and included the famous suite of illustrations showing 'musclemen' at different stages of corporeal 'undress'. Book III, on the vascular system, was less accurate because Vesalius still based his descriptions partly on animal material. Book IV described the NERVOUS SYSTEM, following the Galenic classification of the cranial nerves into seven pairs. Book V dealt with the abdominal and reproductive organs, where he corrected Galen's belief in

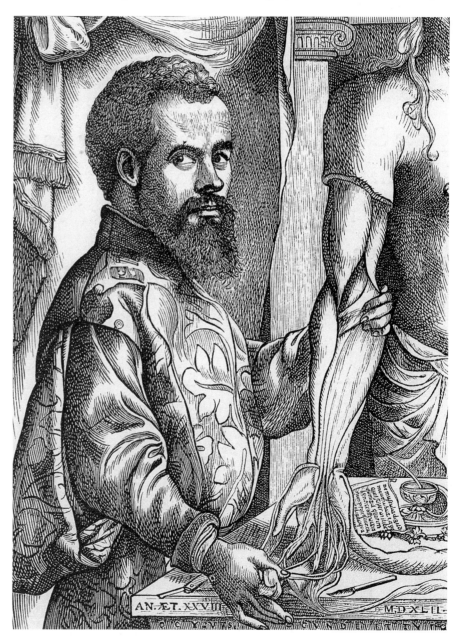

Andreas Vesalius, 1514–64. From *De humani corporis fabrica* (1543) Mary Evans Picture Library.

the five-lobed human liver (a shape characteristic of lower animals). He nevertheless still accepted the Galenic physiological tenet that the liver produced blood from chyle, while denying that the vena cava originated in the liver — an observation that, had Vesalius been more physiologically-minded, might have begun the erosion of the Galenic belief in two distinct vascular systems, the venous, originating in the liver, and the arterial, stemming from the heart.

Book VI was devoted to the thorax. Examining the heart, Vesalius cast doubt on the permeability of the intraventricular septum: 'we are driven to wonder at the handiwork of the Almighty by means of which the blood sweats from the right into the left ventricle through passages which escape the human vision.' In the second edition (1555), that implicit denial of the septum's permeability was made direct. Here lay a milestone of Renaissance anatomy, for it encouraged anatomists like Realdo Colombo to conceive of the pulmonary transit, which was later used by William HARVEY as evidence of the circulation of the blood. Another crucial correction of Galen came in Book VII, on the brain, where Vesalius denied the existence of the *rete mirabile* in humans.

In the end, Vesalius's importance lay in daring to think the unthinkable: that Galen might actually be wrong, and Galen-worship with it. The *Fabrica* thus laid the groundwork for a new, observation-based anatomy, announcing a new principle of fact-finding and truth-testing in anatomy: all anatomical statements were to be subjected to the test of human cadavers.

The frontispiece of the *Fabrica* presents the dreams, the programme, the agenda, of the new medicine. The cadaver is the central figure. Its abdomen has been opened so that everyone can peer in; it is as if death itself had been put on display. A faceless skeleton points toward the open abdomen. Then there is Vesalius, who looks out at us as if he were extending an invitation to anatomy. Medicine would thenceforth be about looking inside bodies for the truth of disease. The violation of the body would be the revelation of its truth.   ROY PORTER

Further reading
O'Malley, C. D. (1964). *Andreas Vesalius of Brussels 1514–1564.* University of California Press, California.

See also GALEN; HARVEY.

Vestibular system
Human beings, in common with other vertebrates, possess a set of SENSE ORGANS that provide information to the brain concerning orientation and motion of the body. They reside in the inner ear and are collectively referred to as the vestibular system. They form a very small part of the human anatomy, the main components being no larger than 10 mm across. Most people are unaware of the vital role they play in everyday life — except when something goes wrong with one of the elements of this system. The vestibular system is deeply embedded in the *temporal bone* alongside the *cochlea* (which

is responsible for HEARING) and it contains two distinct types of sensory organs; the *semicircular canals* and the *otolith organs*.

The semicircular canals respond to rotational movements of the head, whether induced passively during activities such as running or riding a horse or a motorcycle, or actively, as occurs when voluntary head movements are made during visual search. Each canal forms a cavity in the temporal bone and each contains a membranous duct filled with a viscous fluid (*endolymph*). There are three on each side of the head and the plane of each canal is perpendicular to the others, so that between all six of them they can provide information related to rotational acceleration of the head during movement around any axis. During such acceleration in the plane of a particular canal, the endolymph tends to remain stationary because of its inertia, so that there is relative motion of the endolymph within the duct. Motion of the endolymph is resisted by viscous friction at the fluid–duct boundary and by the elasticity of a gelatinous structure inside each canal, the *cupula*. The cupula contains sensory *hair cells* that consequently become deflected, causing stimulation of associated nerve fibres, leading to the transmission of signals to the brain.

The otolith organs respond to linear motion. They lie at the point at which all three semicircular ducts converge. There are two of them on each side of the head, and each contains sensory receptors in a structure known as a *macula*. With the head erect, the macula in each utricle is oriented horizontally, and in the saccule vertically. The base of each macula carries hair cells that project into a gelatinous substrate in which are embedded minute crystals of calcium carbonate (the *otoconia*) forming plaque with an area of only 1.5–2 mm^2; the *otolith* membrane separates this complex from the more fluid endolymph. When linear acceleration occurs in the plane of the macula, the inertia of this dense complex causes it — and therefore the hair cells within it — to be deflected in the direction opposite to that of the movement. These deflections set up trains of nerve impulses, with frequencies proportional to the extent of deflection. In the otolith organs hair cell clusters are tuned to different directions of motion, all directions of motion in the plane of the otolith being represented. The *utricle* can thus send signals to the brain representing a combination of fore–aft and lateral motion of the head, whereas the *saccule* principally conveys information about vertical motion.

Maintenance of visual and postural stability
In general, the function of the vestibular apparatus is (via connections in the brain) to generate activity in various muscle systems, which will compensate for the head and body motion, and result in the maintenance of visual and postural stability. The area in the BRAIN STEM (the *vestibular nucleus*) that receives the output of the canals and otoliths has direct connections with muscles controlling EYE MOVEMENTS and with muscles of the neck and limbs. In the case of the

eyes, the *vestibulo–ocular reflex* generates eye movements that compensate for head motion with a very short delay (around 10 milliseconds).

As we walk or run, the head generally bobs up and down. Stabilization of the eye prevents movement of visual images on the retina, which would otherwise cause images to be blurred. Individuals who have been unfortunate enough to lose the function of the vestibular system (through damage to the inner ear) often experience apparent motion of the visual world (*oscillopsia*) under these circumstances.

Fortuitously, the vestibulo–ocular reflex, 'designed' to deal with maximum running speed, also allows modern man to view stationary objects in the outside world when travelling in high-speed vehicles, where there is often considerable linear and angular vibration. However, sometimes the reflex is inappropriate. Reading a newspaper in a train is often difficult because, when looking at objects within the moving vehicle, the stabilizing reflex is no longer appropriate. To suppress the eye movements we rely largely on the ocular pursuit system, a mechanism that we normally use to track moving objects with the eyes when we are stationary. But ocular pursuit has a very limited range of operation and does not function at frequencies of vibration above about 2 cycles per second. Unfortunately, in moving vehicles frequencies of vibration are frequently much higher — between 2 and 20 cycles per second.

Stabilization mechanisms similar to those for the eye operate for control of the head, limbs, and other postural systems, but they are necessarily more complex than those controlling the eye.

Perception of motion and orientation
As well as controlling actions within the body, vestibular stimulation also engenders powerful sensations of motion and orientation in space. Stimulation of the canals gives a sensation of turning, so that someone who is rotated on a swivelling chair will experience a sensation of rotation even in the absence of any other cues such as vision (i.e. with their eyes closed). However, because the canals are really responsive to angular acceleration, during a constant rate of angular rotation (constant angular velocity) the sensation gradually decays over 10–20 seconds. And when rotation stops, the individual experiences rotation in the opposite direction, even though actual motion has ceased, because the fluid in the canal continues to move when the head has stopped. In everyday life, prolonged rotation is not often encountered, but it does occur frequently when FLYING. Pilots must therefore be aware that they cannot always rely on the sensation of motion, particularly in circumstances where there are no other reference cues such as sight of land (e.g. when flying in cloud).

Stimulation of the otolith organs also gives rise to sensations, but in this case they may be of either linear motion or of orientation with respect to the vertical. When linear acceleration is sustained it causes a continuous deflection of the otoconia. The most common situation in which this occurs is when the head is tilted, when gravitational acceleration causes the otoconia to be deflected in proportion to the degree of tilt. Consequently, application of sustained linear acceleration is usually interpreted as tilt, so that, when accelerating forward in a high-speed vehicle, a sensation of being tipped backwards is experienced. Again, this is particularly important when flying because, on take-off, an aircraft is normally accelerating and climbing at the same time. The combination of vehicle and gravitational accelerations gives rise to a sense of tilt that is greater than it should be, and the pilot must learn not to misinterpret this sensory information.

When linear motion changes frequently, for example during vibration, a true sense of linear motion is normally experienced. This is most sensitive at frequencies close to those of natural head movements (around 2 cycles per second).

In normal circumstances, linear and angular motion stimuli are combined, as when we bend down to tie a shoelace in a moving train. In such circumstances, the sensations can be complex and unexpected as a result of the coriolis components of acceleration that accompany motion in three dimensions. The individual may experience a disturbing sensation of tumbling in these circumstances, which may be sufficient to bring on motion sickness.

Allied to the experience of real linear or angular body motion are similar sensations that may arise from motion of the visual world when the body itself is stationary. These sensations of self-motion are referred to as *linear* or *angular* VECTION respectively.

Disorders of the vestibular system

One of the major consequences of a failure of the vestibular system is the occurrence of *vertigo*, or DIZZINESS, which is experienced by large numbers of individuals. Acute vertigo can occur when the vestibular system on one side of the head suddenly stops working effectively, which can be due to factors such as vestibular neuritis or haemorrhage in the cerebellum or brain stem. In such cases there is sudden onset of a strong sense of rotation, often accompanied by a flicking back and forth of the eyes (*nystagmus*). It generally disappears within hours or days. More persistent vertigo can occur, for example, as a result of the migration of calcite crystals from the otolith organs on to the cupula of the semicircular canal. The cupula then becomes inappropriately sensitive to gravity and a sensation of turning is brought on by a change of head position with respect to gravity. There are other examples of clinical problems arising from vestibular failure, many of which cause great disturbance to the sense of the body in space.   GRAHAM BARNES

See also MOTION SICKNESS; NYSTAGMUS; VECTION.

Violence
Woven into the fabric of most societies, violence exists in many forms and at multiple levels. Whether physical, verbal, sexual, or psychological, whether inflicted by individuals, groups, institutions, or nations, violence threatens the body in numerous and complex ways.

At the microlevel, *personal violence* — acts of aggression or force performed by individuals — may be directed at inanimate objects, animals, one's self, or other bodies. Although some forms of *interpersonal violence*, such as injuries on the SPORTS field or shootings in self-defence, are culturally sanctioned, the more serious forms, like homicide, RAPE, and aggravated assault, are usually criminalized. To understand why individuals commit violence, criminologists and psychologists often focus on the individual's personality type, family background, and possible physiological abnormalities. Sometimes, however, personal manifestations of violence are linked to broader social structures. As numerous feminist scholars have argued, domestic or family violence must be understood in terms of patriarchal family structures, which have traditionally given men the right to control and discipline their wives and children.

True forms of *collective violence* result when individuals engage in violent activities at a group or institutional level. Like personal violence, incidents of group violence such as riots, revolutions, and gang warfare are typically viewed as local events, tied to a specific cause or geographical region. Nevertheless, group violence possesses its own unique dynamics and is generally more destructive than personal violence. Sociologists and psychologists have observed that individual members participating in group violence frequently feel less responsibility for their activities and are willing to commit greater atrocities because they are acting in the name of a higher cause, be it religion, political beliefs, or loyalty to an ethnic group or nation. This process of *deindividualization* is fostered by the military to mobilize individuals for war and other forms of mass destruction like GENOCIDE. In war, not only are soldiers made to feel like cogs in a larger military machine, who 'just follow orders', but enemies are regularly dehumanized through propaganda, allowing for brutal massacres and TORTURE rarely seen in personal, peacetime acts of violence.

Institutional violence — violence that serves or results from institutional objectives — can take extreme forms, like concentration camps or murders committed by totalitarian governments, or it can be part of a socially accepted economic system or religious organization's goals. Various slave systems have, for example, utilized physical, sexual, and emotional violence to deprive slaves of their humanity, while the Catholic Church employed violence in its Crusades, witch burnings, and inquisitions to neutralize perceived threats to its institutional boundaries. As modern industrial work environments like asbestos plants and coal mines demonstrate, however, institutional violence can also be subtle, resulting from acts of omission or deception rather than force.

At the macrolevel, advances in military and media technology have made violence (and the threat of it) *global*. Not only can we annihilate the entire planet through nuclear weapons, but we can transmit, via satellite, war and other public spectacles of violence into homes all over the globe.   CHRISTINA JARVIS

See also GENOCIDE; KILLING; MURDER; WAR AND THE BODY.

Virgin birth
— a woman giving birth without documented involvement of a male figure in the act of conception (attested e.g. by an intact HYMEN) — is a widespread and well-known religious and cultural motif. It belongs to the category of portents and MAGIC signs that announce the extra-ordinary event of a divinity entering into a human body (*theophany*). For example, (*mahayanic*) versions of the life of Buddha recount that his mother conceived him when a white elephant touched her thigh; and the Persian divinity Zoroaster is said to have been born from a virgin. Stories of mythical conceptions, such as the goddess Aphrodite's from the foam of the sea, or that of the hero Perseus, who was conceived by a golden rain emanating from Zeus, are different: here, the act of conception is present, if only metaphorically.

In Christianity, virgin birth assumed a special centrality parallel to the role of VIRGINITY itself. Christ assumed human form, that is became incarnate, when the Word of God penetrated Mary, a virgin, and thus made her fertile. (Mary herself is said to have been conceived without intercourse on the part of her mother Anna; this is the Immaculate Conception and not virgin birth.) Paul mentions only that Jesus was born from a woman (Galatians 4: 4); but the Gospels of Matthew (1: 18–25) and Luke (1: 26–38) emphasize that no human was involved in his conception: God himself, through his Spirit, generated his Son. Interpretations of this phenomenon vary widely, and were subject of many debates throughout the first centuries of Christianity. At stake was, for example, whether or not Mary had been a virgin before, during, or again after her birth; this was relevant in order to ascertain whether Christ had just assumed the form of a human being temporarily, or had fully become human. Since the councils of Ephesos (431) and Chalcedon (451), Mary is seen as *theotokos*, as 'God-bearer', and therefore as having been a virgin at all stages. The great medieval scholar Thomas Aquinas, among many others, re-examined the pro and contra of this definition, and declared that Mary must have been a virgin because of the 'honour of the Father, who sent Christ', and the 'nature of the Son', that is their divinity — however, he did not think that Mary was a virgin while giving birth. Mary's virginity despite her motherhood remained a central and well-liked tenet of faith in Christianity. It was not challenged in the Reformation, though the reform principles considerably lessened its centrality, together with that of Mary herself. However, as a symbol of Christ's divinity, and as such a unique act, his virgin birth retains its theological power.

SUSANNA ELM

See also CHRISTIANITY AND THE BODY; VIRGINITY.

Virginity denotes the state of a person who has not taken part in sexual intercourse. In women, this is ascertained by the physical integrity of the HYMEN. In many cultures, this plays a central role as a prerequisite for MARRIAGE. Prior to genetic testing, only the bride's unbroken hymen could ascertain the husband's paternity, and hence continuity of the family line. Probably as a psychological result of this biological fact, both temporary sexual abstinence and permanent virginity play a fundamental role in most world religions. Virginity represented avoidance of ritual pollution through sexual intercourse and thus was seen as a magic power bestowed upon men and especially women, which predisposed such virgins for specific magic and religious activities. As far as Europe and the Mediterranean world are concerned, permanent virginity, in contrast to temporary abstinence, became a central religious theme only with the rise of Christianity.

Prior to Christianity, virginity was a characteristic of female deities engaged in hunting and fishing, and worshipped as protectors of forests and wildlife. Examples are the Greco-Roman nymphs and the goddess Artemis/Diana, but also Athena/Minerva, the virginal goddess of warfare, early on depicted as the 'goddess of the animals'. Some Near-Eastern mythologies considered virginity a state of primordial innocence terminated by the first sexual experience, which resulted in a fall from grace and a discovery of shameful nakedness. The earliest example is the Gilgamesh epic, a Mesopotamian text as old as *c.* 2000 BCE, which narrates the expulsion of its 'hunter-hero' from the forest. The old Testament book of Genesis is a parallel text, where, it has been argued, the eating of the fruit of knowledge symbolically represents the loss of virginity, and results in expulsion from the 'wilderness of paradise'. Absence of sexual pollution and the resulting magic powers often made virginity a prerequisite for female priesthood. Virgin priestesses were engaged in maintaining fires, easily prone to 'pollution' (the Vestal virgins in Rome, and the virgins in Icelandic lore); functioned as prophetesses (Pythia of Delphi, the Sybills in Rome); or performed acts of magic. Occasionally, virgins were sacrificed as especially potent offerings (seven male and seven female virgins to the Cretan Minotaur, Iphigenia). Male virginity was associated with absence (*congenital* EUNUCHS) or removal of the testicles (CASTRATION), and was also a prerequisite for certain cultic functions. In the Greek world, eunuch-priests served the goddess Artemis of Ephesos, and castrated priests were central to the worship of the Syrian goddess Atagarte as well as to the cult of Cybele and Attis in Asia Minor.

In the history of Israel virginity was always necessary for marriage, but did not appear as a religious theme prior to 200 BCE. Only then, during the so-called apocalyptic period of external pressures, did certain Jewish sects praise virginity as a means to preserve the cohesiveness of their community (Essenes, Qumran). At the same time, those who were 'virgins' by default —

eunuchs and sterile men — or chose to remain chaste, gained acceptance, and were increasingly seen as capable of direct communion with the divine, provided they lived according to the Law.

In Christianity perpetual virginity as a conscious choice of lifestyle, permitting a layperson's complete devotion to God, became a central theme. This notion was present from the beginning. We find it in the Gospels and Paul's writings, but it took several hundred years for the concept of virginity as a form of religious life to develop fully, and equally long to find agreement on ways to practice such a life. One impetus for the later importance of a virginal life was the celibacy of Jesus. Though the Gospels do not discuss his marital status, the life that Jesus led, as an itinerant preacher who moved about announcing the imminent coming of the kingdom of God, implies the absence of a wife and children. Furthermore, certain Gospel passages, especially a controversial saying of Jesus recorded in Matthew 19: 10–12, which mentions those who castrate themselves for the kingdom of heaven, and Luke's references to the virginity of Mary (*virgin birth*), suggest that virginity formed part of the eschatological message of Jesus, the way his teaching relates to the imminent end of the world. Unmarried people increasingly tolerated in the Jewish context of Jesus, were commonplace in the Greco-Roman world of Paul. Stoic philosophy had long since questioned whether or not the truly wise should be married, arguing that marriage was useful but distracting, since it impedes the emotional detachment necessary to serve the Divine truly. Paul takes a similar line in his first Letter to the Corinthians, a text that became fundamental to later Christian developments. What distinguishes Paul's argument from the Stoics or Jewish apocalyptic thinkers is his emphasis: virginity permits complete dedication to the service of God, not only for reasons of ritual purity and emotional detachment, but as a loving gift 'pleasing the Lord'.

Thus, the itinerant lifestyle of Jesus and the apostles merged with Stoic notions to form the basis of a celibate Christian life, which already had a significant following by the second and third centuries CE. In the fourth century, after Constantine had recognized Christianity as a legitimate religion, virginity as a permanent state gained additional popularity because it replaced martyrdom (persecutions had ceased) as a means of gaining a specially revered status within the Christian community. Increasingly, men and women demonstrated their choice to remain virgins dedicated to God not only by remaining unmarried, but also by leaving their families, villages and cities either to roam about as itinerants or to live as desert-dwellers. Both options, that of the wanderer as well as that of the desert-dweller, gave rise to what we now know as monasticism. By the sixth century CE, priests in Western Christianity were expected to be virgins. In the Eastern Church, virginity remains a special choice for monks and nuns, but is not required of priests below the rank of a bishop.

SUSANNA ELM

Further reading

Brown, P. (1988). *The body and society. Men, women and sexual renunciation in early Christianity*. Columbia, University Press, New York.

Rouselle, A. (1988). *On desire and the body in antiquity*. Blackwell, Oxford.

See also ASCETICISM; CHASTITY; FLESH.

Virginity tests Any patrilineal society inevitably values (or over-values) virginity in its females. Tests to detect virginity (or its absence) are as widespread historically as they are unreliable medically. They occur in folklore, in law, in literature, and in medical textbooks, falling into four groups: textile proof of bleeding; gynaecological examination by a jury of women; proof by magical ability on the part of the virgin; and somatic responses to ingested fluid or inhaled fumes. This last is what is usually meant by 'virginity test', and arose in response to the unreliability of the first three.

Mosaic law decreed that the bride's family should display the 'proof of her virginity' (i.e. blood-stained sheets) in public; inability to do so resulted in the bride being stoned to death (Deuteronomy 21: 13–21). The custom was still recognizable in early modern England. Katherine of Aragon kept her wedding sheets for over 30 years, producing them as evidence in the divorce case brought by Henry VIII against her; Shakespeare critics believe that the red-on-white of the strawberry-patterned linen handkerchief in *Othello* emblematizes Desdemona's virginity (hence, her failure to produce the handkerchief results in her death).

This test of the 'first night's bloody napkin' or *pannum menstruatum prima nocte* (Robert Burton's *Anatomy of Melancholy* of 1621) was relatively easy to fake. Farmyard kitchens offered access to chicken blood, and Jacobean drama provides the solution of bed-trick substitution, as in Middleton and Rowley's *The Changeling* (published 1622), where the virgin maid protects her mistress, the unchaste bride, by spending the wedding night with the groom. Unchaste brides could also cheat on a gynaecological test, for the bride had only to wear a veil for modesty's sake, as did Frances Howard, Countess of Essex, in a notorious example in 1613. Her attempt to annul her marriage to Robert Devereux, third Earl of Essex, was controversial, not least because of Frances's reputation for promiscuity. Public opinion held that a veiled substitute submitted to the physical examination on the Countess's behalf, thereby enabling her to pass the test and declare herself *virgo intacta*.

If gynaecological examinations were open to deceit, they were further compromised in that they were carried out by women (allegedly united in conspiratorial mendacity). Folklore offered a third type of virginity-test — MAGIC. Virgins were credited with miraculous herbal healing powers; they could tame savage beasts or calm stinging swarms; they could wear clothing and accessories that would not fit unchaste women (for example, the magic mantle in the King

Arthur legend, the magic girdle in Spenser's *Faerie Queene*). Unsurprisingly, this seems not to have been a prevalent option in real life. Thus the physician's virginity test came into medical prominence.

Essentially this last type of virginity test involves giving the woman a diuretic potion to drink, and seeing if she can contain her urine. Recipes for preparing and administering the potion are found in Pliny the Elder's *History of the World*; recipes in medieval and Renaissance books tend to be translations or derivatives of Pliny. Powdered jet (i.e. black lignite) is a staple ingredient: 'if a woman drink it fasting presently it provoketh urine, if she be [not] a pure virgin'. The medieval *Book of Secrets* by St Albertus Magnus finds tactile contact with the stone sufficient to test virginity: 'if the stone be broken and washed, or be given to a woman to be washed, if she be not a virgin, she will piss soon, if she be a virgin, she will not piss'. Variant ingredients include white amber, purslane seeds, or burdock leaves, the last two administered through inhalation rather than ingestion, but the effect — urination — is consistent.

Clearly such a test owes more to metaphor than to medicine. The vestal virgins were allegedly able to carry water in a sieve. (Like the bloody napkin and the physical examination, this test is not as foolproof as it sounds: one simply anoints the sieve with lanolin to provide a seal.) Queen Elizabeth publicized her status as Virgin Queen in a famous portrait in 1579 in which she holds a sieve in her left hand. Cesare Ripa's *Iconologia* (1611) provides a woodcut illustration of Chastity: she carries a whip in her right hand (presumably to deter Cupid who sits blindfolded at her feet), and, like Queen Elizabeth, she holds a large sieve in her left hand. The paired paintings by Godfried Schalken (1643–1706), *The Wasted Lesson in Morals* and *The Medical Examination* (Mauritshuis, The Hague) use the same iconography to depict the loss of chastity. In the first painting an elderly woman wags her finger at a young woman, cautioning her against opening a casket (symbolizing her virginity). The admonition is evidently unheeded for in the second painting the girl weeps while the doctor examines a flask of her urine. Thus, the chaste woman was sealed, impermeable; the unchaste woman was porous, incontinent. Given the effects on pelvic floor muscles and BLADDER of repeated childbearing and unsophisticated obstetrical instruments, the equation of unchastity with INCONTINENCE was self-fulfilling. A popular Elizabethan proverb held that 'a ship and a woman are ever repairing'.

Renaissance literature frequently refers to virginity tests, and *The Changeling* actually stages one; however, it alters the effect of the potion from micturition to the more stageworthy sneezing, gaping, and yawning. Early modern culture extended the image of the open, unchaste woman as a urinating, leaking vessel to equate the *speaking* woman with unchastity; the logic was that a woman who had the temerity to open

one orifice (her mouth) would readily open another (her vagina). Middleton's *Revenger's Tragedy* compresses the sequence of female speech/sex/virginity-test/urination into two lines: 'Tell but some woman a secret over night, / Your doctor may find it in the urinal i' the morning' (1.3.83–4). The trope is one of containment, with one body part functioning metonymically for another; women cannot control their tongues, their sexual desires, or their bladders.

From here it was an easy step for early modern suspicion to extend to all female bodily fluids: tears, menstruation, lactation. Despite empirical evidence to the contrary, GALEN held that female fluids were related. Breasts and uterus were thought to be connected by tubes (white breast milk was transmuted menstrual fluid), as were tear ducts and bladder (an Elizabethan proverb proclaims, 'Let her cry she'll piss the less'). Thus female leakiness was not just localized proof of loss of virginity but an innate condition signifying the first female transgression in Eden. Incontinence was both proof and punishment — evidence of loss of innocence and chastisement for it.

The virginity test in *The Changeling* is attributed to Antoine Mizauld (*c.* 1520–78), a French doctor who studied medicine in Paris and published many works on medicine, mathematics, and astrology. The play uses his name simply to lend authority to the stage test, which does not correspond, in precise details, with any recipe or experiment in Mizauld's published works, although the broad outlines are authentic in the literature from Pliny onwards. By the seventeenth century the new scientists began to view virginity tests sceptically. Sir Thomas Browne (1605–82), who studied medicine in Leiden and practised in Norwich, wrote: 'I find the triall of

the Pucellage and Virginity of women, which God ordained the Jewes is very fallible' (*Religio Medici*, 1643). He is referring specifically to the proof of the first night's 'bloody napkin', but his suspicion about reliability may be applied to virginity tests in general. Dale Randall points out that by the 1630s plays such as James Shirley's *Hyde Park* (1632) 'endorse a far pleasanter kind of diagnosis', what we might call 'trial by temptation': when asked if he can detect a woman's virginity, the hero replies, 'I'll know't by a kiss, / Better than any doctor by her urine'.

LAURIE MAGUIRE

Further reading

Paster, G. K. (1993). *The body embarrassed*. Cornell University Press, Ithaca NY.

Randall, D. B. J. (1984). Some observations on the theme of chastity in *The Changeling*. *English Literary Renaissance*, **14**, 347–66.

Tilley, M. P. (1950). *A dictionary of the proverbs in England in the sixteenth and seventeenth centuries*. University of Michigan Press, Ann Arbor MI.

See also HYMEN.

Virtual reality

Virtual reality (VR) is a technology that allows people to enter and interact with three-dimensional *computer graphics* worlds. Another term for these worlds is *virtual environments*. When a person uses a virtual world the sensory information that is present in the real world is replaced by computer-generated information, which may be of sufficient fidelity to allow the person effectively to believe that they are in the virtual world.

VR is currently used in applications such as aircraft pilot training, medical rehabilitation, training for surgical procedures, engineering and scientific visualization, manufacturing design,

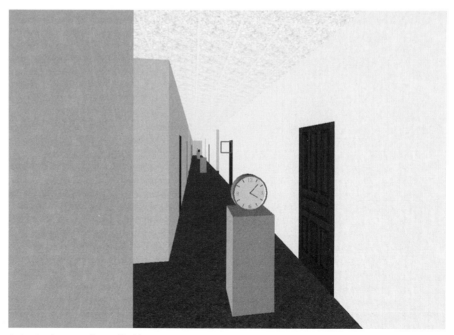

A view inside a typical virtual building.

the control of remote (tele-operated) vehicles, and computer games. Some of the worlds used for these applications are designed to be virtual equivalents of real-world (i.e. physical) environments. Other virtual worlds exist only in their virtual form and for these worlds the term virtual 'reality' is something of a misnomer.

The variety and fidelity of sensory information provided by VR applications varies widely and is typically limited by a trade-off between cost and benefit. A person's sense of presence is one nebulous, subjective measure of the degree to which they feel that they are actually inside a virtual world, and this quantity is influenced by factors that include the size of the visual field of view, the inclusion of auditory information, and the use of head-tracking, where the person's physical movements control their direction of view. Although an increase in presence does not necessarily produce a corresponding increase in the accuracy or speed with which tasks are performed, it does provide a general measure of the degree to which real-world sensory information is replaced by information contained in the virtual world.

Three-dimensional computer graphics allow the shape and form of objects to be perceived, and the use of photo-realistic textures for colour provides detailed visual information. The patterns contained in textures help to increase optic flow and this increases a person's perception of movement as they travel through a virtual world. Technical and cost limitations often restrict a person's field of view to an angle as small as 50 degrees (compared with the 200 degrees or more of normal vision). This effectively means that the person looks at the virtual world using blinkers. The lack of peripheral vision seems to inhibit people's ability to develop mental 'models' of the layout of virtual worlds and frequently causes people to miss events that occur just outside the field of view, but which they would detect in the real world.

Some virtual worlds provide auditory and haptic information. Simple sounds such as a 'bump' can be added to indicate that a person has collided with a 'solid' object. More realistic, spatial sounds can be provided using binaural, stereophonic technology. Force feedback is particularly useful in virtual worlds that are used for pharmaceutical drug research, where it may be used to simulate the powerful forces that are present between different atoms in molecules.

When a person initially navigates a virtual world they tend to become very disoriented but, if they are given sufficient time, they can develop knowledge of the virtual world's layout which is as accurate as the knowledge they develop of the real world environments in which they live and work. The amount of visual detail which is present in a virtual world has an effect on the rate at which a person learns spatial knowledge, because these details are frequently used as landmarks that aid the learning of routes. Other devices such as a compass or a map can also provide effective navigational aids.

In some virtual worlds no interaction is allowed apart from a person's movement (the world is visualized but little else). In more complex worlds each object can have its own behaviour. Thus, doors may be opened, a phone can be used to have a conversation with another person, or a virtual computer can be used to send real electronic mail. Virtual worlds that contain complex object behaviours are time-consuming to develop but are becoming more commonplace. Of course, there is nothing to stop a virtual world redefining the laws of physical reality so that objects can, for instance, 'fall' upwards when they are dropped!

Finally, a significant proportion of people who view virtual worlds using helmet-mounted displays (HMDs) suffer from the side-effects of *VR sickness*, common symptoms of which include eye-strain, nausea, and a loss of balance. VR sickness seems to be related to motion sickness and has many contributory causes. One is the vestibular conflicts which are caused by the (small) time delays that occur between a person's actual bodily movements and the HMD being updated to reflect those movements. Another is the optical quality of the displays themselves. The magnitude of the problems caused by VR sickness is likely to reduced gradually as improvements take place in display and sensor technology, and a better understanding is reached of the factors which contribute toward the sickness.

ROY A. RUDDLE
ROBERT J. SNOWDEN

Further reading
Rheingold, H. (1992). *Virtual reality*. Mandarin, London.

See also ILLUSIONS; MOTION SICKNESS; VECTION.

Virus From the Latin for toxin. These are very tiny MICROORGANISMS not visible with an ordinary microscope but only through electron microscopy. They have a very simple structure, and often consist only of DNA or RNA with a protein coat. They therefore lack some of the chemicals and enzymes needed for replication, so instead they infect other living cells and take over the infected cell's internal 'machinery'. A.P.D.

See MICROORGANISMS.

Visceral sensation Most of the time we go through our daily lives without being consciously aware of the events occurring continuously in our internal organs, or *viscera* — the heart, lungs, stomach, intestines, kidney, etc. These organs contain sensory nerve endings, but the messages that they transmit to the CENTRAL NERVOUS SYSTEM rarely enter into CONSCIOUSNESS. Despite the continuous beating of the heart, and the movements of the stomach and intestines, we are, thankfully, usually unaware of these events. Occasionally we may become conscious of the world inside our bodies, experiencing palpitations of the heart, a throbbing HEADACHE, racing PULSE, abdominal cramps, or colic. And on occasions, such as during STRESS,

we may experience DYSPEPSIA, or vague sensations referred to as 'butterflies in the stomach'. The term 'gut feelings' indicates the overall, vague, unfamiliar, or affective connotations of abdominal sensations.

Visceral sensations and visceral PAIN are often regarded as synonymous; however, not all visceral sensations are painful. Stretch of the walls of the stomach or the bladder can yield two qualities of sensation: an awareness of fullness — which in the case of the stomach may be associated with a pleasant feeling of satiety — or, if the degree of stretch is severe, pain. During childbirth, the midwife asks the mother to report when she feels 'contractions' — the spasmodic pains that wax and wane, associated with contractions of the UTERUS. But some visceral sensations are intensely pleasurable: those associated with contractions of parts of the reproductive organs of both sexes during ORGASM — the climax of sexual sensations.

From the medical perspective, visceral pain is an important symptom of disorders in internal organs. It may arise through a variety of pathological causes: over-distension of a hollow organ; excessive contraction of the muscular walls of hollow organs — particularly against an obstruction; stretch of a region of *mesentery* (the membranous tissue that wraps and holds in place the organs within the abdomen); inflammation of an organ or inadequate blood supply to it; movement of the roughened, inflamed surfaces of viscera over one another; spillage of intestinal contents into the peritoneal cavity through a perforation of the wall of the gut; and internal bleeding.

In SKIN or MUSCLE, pain occurs as a consequence of events that injure or threaten to injure these tissues. In contrast, considerable damage can occur within the viscera without a conscious sensation. The classic investigations of Sir Thomas Lewis in London in the 1930s showed that parts of the intestine may be clamped without eliciting any sensation, whereas the application of similar forces to normal skin would always be painful — and stretching a mesentery always elicits severe pain.

The afferent nerves that innervate the viscera and mesenteries consist of nerve fibres of small diameter, which conduct impulses at relatively slow speeds, because they lack a fatty MYELIN sheath. They have their cell bodies in the *dorsal root ganglia* — swellings on the bundles of nerves, called 'dorsal roots', that enter the spinal cord at each segment along its length. Attempts to analyse the nature of the signals, caused by mechanical and chemical events in internal organs, which give rise to visceral pain, has yielded some controversy. In situations in which pain is the only sensation that arises from an organ, the intensity of that sensation appears to depend on the total number of nerve impulses conducted to the brain along all the sensory nerves from that organ. However, it is less clear how more than one quality of sensation can arise from a single organ.

Many of the small sensory nerve fibres in viscera are *polymodal*: they respond to a variety of forms of stimulation (mechanical, chemical, and possibly thermal). They also respond to — or become more sensitive to other stimuli in the presence of — a cocktail of chemicals in the local environment of their nerve endings. These sensitizing chemicals are generally thought to be inflammatory chemical mediators, released from cells of the IMMUNE SYSTEM or from cells of the tissue itself when injured. Examples of such chemical mediators are PEPTIDES (such as bradykinin, released as a result of the liberation of cellular enzymes); *fatty molecules* (such as eicosanoids, the breakdown products of disrupted CELL MEMBRANES); *intracellular chemicals* (such as potassium, and ATP); and *growth factors* (such as the neurotrophins, which are released from inflamed tissues).

The pain of a HEART ATTACK (*myocardial infarction*), caused by blockage of a main artery in the heart, is often described as a sensation of tightness or heaviness constricting the chest, and may be accompanied by tightness in the throat, and tingling and numbness in the left arm. Why should 'cardiac pain' be associated with such diverse sensory symptoms covering such a wide area of the body? The underlying mechanism that gives rise to such scattered symptoms can be understood if one considers the distribution of the spinal nerves that innervate all of these areas. The segments of the SPINAL CORD that receive sensory fibres from the heart also receive nerves from the throat and parts of the arm and hand. The cells that give rise to these parts of the body all lie close together at early embryonic stages, and they retain nerve connections to the same region of the spinal cord as they migrate away to their ultimate locations in the body.

The common segmental origin of the sensory nerves serving all of the regions involved in the sensation of pain derived from one particular organ is stated in Ruch's Convergence– Projection Theory of Referred Pain. There are many examples of such 'referred pain'. There appear to be no highly specific pathways for visceral sensation in the central nervous system. Rather, information concerning events in the viscera is carried from the spinal cord to the brain by nerve fibres that also carry information from areas of the skin and body musculature innervated by the same segments of spinal cord. Hence there is a potential confusion about the origin of the sensation resulting from the activity of such nerve fibres. Information about the location and nature of abdominal pains is transmitted along busy lines of communication in the spinal cord, usually used for some other purpose. The messages received by the brain are ambiguous, in the sense that the events giving rise to them might have arisen in the viscera, in the skin, or in muscle, and the message can be misinterpreted. No wonder diagnosis of an abdominal pain on the basis of a patient's descriptions can be so unreliable, and so fraught with difficulty. JOHN MORRISON
See also PAIN; SENSATION; SENSORY RECEPTORS.

Vision is the task of understanding the world through our EYES. It is probably the most difficult thing that we do with our brains, yet we do it every waking moment, and it is virtually effortless. Just open your eyes and the universe is there, in all the richness of its shapes and colours, its brightness, distance and movement. But the analysis that underlies seeing involves about one third of the entire human CEREBRAL CORTEX — more than a billion nerve cells. That is one indication of the magnitude of the task of vision.

Using their eyes, most people can thread a needle, recognize thousands of faces, read a newspaper, drive a car, see an orange as orange whatever the colour of the illuminating light. Some people can fly a jet plane at three times the speed of sound, return a tennis ball served at 200 km an hour, distinguish a thrush from a female blackbird at 100 m, or an early Cubist still life by Picasso from one by Braque. Each of these is an accomplishment of staggering complexity. Even the most sophisticated of computer vision systems, which interpret signals from cameras mounted on robots, seem like idiots compared with the genius of normal human vision. This is another indication of the scale of the task of vision.

Vision involves the detection of light — electromagnetic, NON-IONIZING RADIATION, ranging in wavelength from about 400 to about 750 nanometres. The main natural source of light is stars, especially our own sun. Full sunlight appears white, but light consisting of a limited range of wavelengths appears coloured. Short wavelengths look blue, long wavelengths red. Most of the light that enters our eyes does not come directly from the sun but is reflected from the surfaces of objects. Most surfaces (except mirrors and pure white objects) absorb part of the spectrum of light, changing the wavelength composition of the reflected light, thus making the surfaces appear coloured.

Vision has humble origins. In its very simplest form, it probably appeared near the start of life on Earth, with single-celled organisms that produced photopigments — molecules that change shape when they absorb light, and trigger chemical reactions in the cell. The mere detection of light can be useful to organisms, enabling them to regulate their activity according to the time of day or the seasons of the year, and even allowing them to orientate themselves towards or away from the source of light. Eyes — organs for collecting light — exploit the fact that light travels in straight lines. They use a lens, a mirror, or even just a pinhole, to cast an image on to receptor cells containing photopigment (photoreceptors). The crucial feature of an image is that it contains information about individual objects in the scene and their relative positions, thus affording the animal an opportunity to recognize and respond to those objects, as long as it has the apparatus in its head to analyze the information. The other huge value of vision is that it works at a distance, and hence serves to predict the future:

For I dipt into the future, far as human eye could see,
Saw the Vision of the world, and all the wonder that would be.

Alfred, Lord Tennyson, *Locksley Hall*

All vertebrate eyes are built to a common plan. Rather like cameras, they have a lens system that forms an inverted image on a layer of photoreceptor cells in the back of the retina, which lines the eyeball. In front of the receptors are alternating layers of nerve fibres and cells, forming a complex network through which signals from the receptors are passed. Each photoreceptor absorbs light over a particular band of wavelengths, thus providing, between them, a pattern of activity that can be used to retrieve the brightness and colour of light. Essentially, the photoreceptors *pixellate* the information in the image, reducing it to a point-by-point description of intensity and wavelength, rather like that on a computer screen. The grain of photographic emulsion in camera film does much the same. But cameras do not see. Vision depends on the interpretation of the *patterns* of activity from the photoreceptors, across space and time.

Part of the process of interpretation occurs within the retina itself. The essential function of all vertebrate retinas is to reduce the overwhelming flood of information that pours into the eye. In the human eye there are about 120 million *rod* photoreceptors, which work only in dim light, and 6 million *cones,* which respond under brighter conditions and are of three types, sensitive to light in the blue, green or red part of the spectrum. Each photoreceptor produces a signal, dependent on the intensity and wavelength composition of the light that it catches. In computer terminology, this translates into many megabytes of information every second. EVOLUTION, ever the master of tricks and short-cuts to efficiency, has discovered ways in which unneeded information is removed, during processing in the retina, so that only the essential skeleton of the message is transmitted to the brain.

First, the overall number of 'pixels' is dramatically reduced. The signals are passed from the photoreceptors through several connections, to the last retinal cells in the chain, the *ganglion cells*, which cover the inner surface of the retina and whose axons stream out through a hole in the eyeball to form the optic nerve. Each ganglion cell in the *fovea* (the central part of the retina, which we point towards objects when we look directly at them), receives its main input from just one cone photoreceptor, perfectly conserving the fine-grain detail of that part of the image. But, compared with the roughly 125 million photoreceptors, there are a mere 1.5 million or so ganglion cells. Those in the peripheral parts of the retina pool signals from very large numbers of receptors. In effect the output of the retina is like very coarse-grain film for the peripheral parts, and very fine-grain just in the middle. The constant jerky movements of the eye, which occur about 3 times every second, deliver one part of the image after another to the high-resolution fovea.

The second function of the retina is to 'filter' the image in space and in time, through procedures somewhat similar to those used to 'compress' the information of an entire movie on to a DVD. Everyone is familiar with a phenomenon called *dark adaptation*: if you go from a bright environment into a dark room it is initially very hard to see anything, but vision gradually improves, over the course of fully half an hour. In other words, the eye changes its sensitivity over time to suit the average brightness of the scene — rather like having camera film that can constantly change its speed to match the light conditions. On a shorter time-scale, the eye transmits signals only when the image has just changed, for example, after an eye movement. Indeed, if the image is held absolutely stationary on a person's retina (by means of optical or electronic techniques), perception fades out completely within a few seconds.

Our detailed knowledge of the visual system has come largely from the study of animals, and especially from the use of tiny microelectrodes to record impulses from individual nerve cells or fibres. Retinal ganglion cells have been much studied in this way in totally anaesthetized animals (in which the retina, indeed much of the visual pathway, continues, surprisingly, to respond to visual stimulation). Each ganglion cell responds to changes of light intensity over a limited area of the retina, called the cell's *receptive field*, corresponding to the group of photoreceptors that influence the cell, via the network of connections in the retina. Roughly half the retinal ganglion cells respond with a burst of impulses when the centre of the receptive field is illuminated (ON cells). The other half respond to a decrease in illumination (OFF cells). Thus the output of the retina signals the relative brightness and darkness of each point or patch in the visual field.

Horace Barlow discovered (in the frog) and Steven Kuffler (in the cat) that ganglion cells also 'filter' the image in space (as well as in time), to achieve further information-compression. Essentially, the signals from each group of photoreceptors that feed the central part of the receptive field are inhibited by signals from surrounding photoreceptors, a process called *lateral inhibition*. This means that each ganglion cell signals the *difference* of illumination, or *contrast*, between the central and the surrounding part of its receptive field. Any cell whose receptive field happens to view a part of the image with uniform brightness (e.g. the sky on a cloudless day) will be fairly inactive, while those whose receptive fields lie at the boundary of a change of intensity in the image will send strong signals to the brain.

It is almost as if the retina reduces the image to a line drawing of the visual scene. Perhaps this accounts for the fact that simple outlines are so powerful in their ability to evoke rich perception: just think of the how much can be seen in a line drawing or etching by Rembrandt or Matisse.

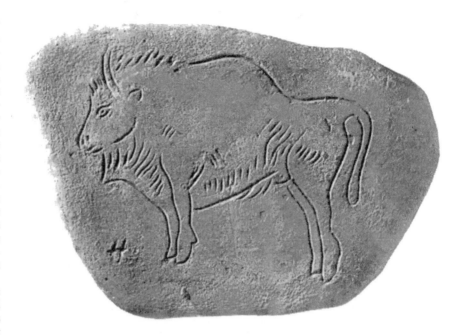

Fig.1 The power of outline to evoke visual perception. A bison drawn between 10 000 and 15 000 years ago on a cave wall in France.

In the retina of old-world monkeys (e.g. rhesus monkeys), assumed to be very similar to the human retina, the ON and OFF classes of ganglion cell can be further sub-divided into two main groups, called P cells and M cells (read on to discover the origin of these terms). P ganglion cells receive the central part of their receptive fields from one, or sometimes two (but not all three) types of colour-selective cone photoreceptors, and thus are *colour-selective* in their responses. M cells, which generally have larger receptive fields, receive input from all cone classes: they are not colour selective but are exquisitely sensitive to contrast and hence to movement of images on the retina. To some extent, this division of function between P and M cells is maintained through the visual pathway, and into the domain of visual perception.

The real business of vision is in the brain. Each optic nerve (the second cranial nerve) passes through a hole at the back of the bony orbit (the cavity in the skull that contains the eyeball), and the two nerves meet to form a distinctive cross-shaped structure, the *optic chiasma*, directly underneath the HYPOTHALAMUS. (Actually, a small number of fibres branch off at this point to provide information about ambient light level to nerve cells of the *suprachiasmatic nucleus*, the heart of the BODY CLOCK mechanism in the brain.)

In the optic chiasma, roughly half the nerve fibres cross over to the opposite side, and the rest continue on to the same side. It was Isaac Newton who first described this anatomical curiosity, and recognized its functional importance:

> Are not the Species of Objects seen with both Eyes united where the optick Nerves meet before they come into the Brain, the Fibres on the right side of both Nerves uniting there, and after union going thence into the Brain in the Nerve which is on the right side of the Head, and the Fibres on the left side going into the Brain in the Nerve which is on the left side of the Head. (*Opticks*, Book 3, Part 1, 14th edition, 1730)

Thus, the arms of the optic chiasma that point towards the brain, called the *optic tracts*, contain a mixture of fibres from geometrically corresponding halves of the two retinas, which, because of optical inversion of the image, view the opposite half of the visual world. Essentially this arrangement splits the representation of the visual field neatly into two. The right side of the field is viewed by the left cerebral hemisphere, the left side by the right. This fits with a general rule, that the left hemisphere is concerned with everything to the right of the body — the skin of right side, control of the muscles of the right side, even sounds coming from the right — while the right hemisphere is devoted to the left side of the body.

This means that damage to the visual pathway on one side of the brain causes blindness or partial blindness in both eyes, on the opposite side of the visual field. Interruption of one optic tract causes total blindness in the opposite half of the visual field — *hemianopia*. Nothing at all is visible to one side of a precise vertical line through the middle of whatever the patient is looking at. Remarkably, patients with this condition are sometimes unaware that they are half-blind: they complain of not being able to read normally, or not being able to drive as well as they used to! This points up a sensible but surprising property of vision — that it is concerned with what we can see, and not with what we cannot see. Think of how indifferent we are to the fact that we cannot see behind our heads. Equally, we are normally unaware that most of the visual field (except that

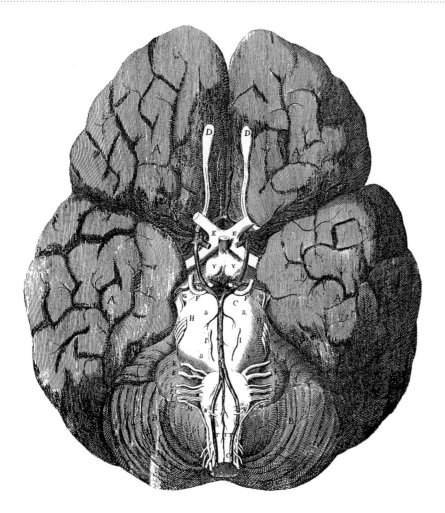

Fig. 2 The base of the human brain (drawn by Christopher Wren) from *Cerebri anatome* (1664) by Thomas Willis showing the optic nerves (E) meeting in the optic chiasm and the optic tracts continuing into the hemispheres of the brain. Wellcome Institute Library, London.

nucleus (the LGN) in the THALAMUS (an egg-shaped mass of GREY MATTER through which virtually all information passes on its way to the CEREBRAL CORTEX). In monkeys, the LGN has six layers. The information from the two eyes remains separate, each eye sending its fibres to three of the layers. The lower two layers are called *magnocellular,* because the nerve cells in them are relatively large. The neurons of the magno-cellular layers receive input from the fibres of the M class of ganglion cells (that is why they are called M cells), and hence they are also sensitive to contrast and motion, but not colour. The upper four, *parvocellular* layers (two for each eye) contain relatively small nerve cells, and receive input (one-to-one connections in some cases) from the axons of P ganglion cells. Hence the parvocellular layers transmit information about colour and fine detail.

The fibres of the roughly 1.5 million cells in the LGN fan backwards and upwards in a bundle of WHITE MATTER called the *optic radiation,* which passes to the back of the hemisphere to reach the region of CEREBRAL CORTEX, called the *primary visual cortex* (or striate cortex, or area 17, or V1). During the First World War, the British neurologist Gordon Holmes examined the visual deficits of soldiers who had suffered shrapnel injuries to this region. If a tiny fragment had entered the back of the skull on one side, there was a corresponding blind patch, a *scotoma,* in the opposite side of the visual field. This implies that there is a kind of 'map' of the retinal image across the surface of the primary visual cortex. Indeed, individual nerve cells in the GREY MATTER receives input, directly or via the net-work of connections in the cortex, from a limited group of cells in the LGN. Thus each cortical cell also has its own receptive field — a patch of reti-na, and hence visual field, through which it responds to appropriate visual stimuli.

Nerve cells in the middle layers of the cortex, where the incoming fibres mainly terminate, respond to brightening or darkening of a par-ticular spot in the visual field, very much like neurons in the LGN. Indeed there are separate sub-layers receiving input from P-type and M-type cells. Input from the two eyes is still kept separate at this point, with axons from the right- and left-eye layers of the LGN terminating in a remarkable alternating pattern. Each eye's input occupies regions that form curving, branching *ocular dominance stripes,* each about 0.3 mm wide, running across the middle layers of the cortex. Alternate stripes are dominated by right eye, then left, forming a pattern similar to a fingerprint impressed on the visual cortex. Neighbouring stripes have input from roughly the same point in the visual field, seen through the two eyes.

Extraordinary things happen as the infor-mation is passed up and down within the grey matter, to the many other neurons in the cortex. David Hubel and Torsten Wiesel won the Nobel Prize in 1981 for their pioneering work on the physiology of the visual cortex. They discovered,

part falling on the fovea) is represented in the brain with very poor detail and colour.

In Dickens' *Pickwick Papers,* Sam Weller says:

> Yes I have a pair of eyes … and that's just it. If they was a pair o' patent double million magnifyin' gas microscopes of hextra power, p'raps I might be able to see through a flight o' stairs and a deal door; but bein' only eyes, you see, my wision's limited.

Indeed, our 'wision' is limited — by the resolu-tion of the optics of our eyes and the structure of the retina, by the range of wavelengths to which our photoreceptors are sensitive, and by the capacity of our brains to fathom, from the mere shadows that flit across the retina, what is there in the outside world. But mercifully we are nor-mally blissfully unaware of those limitations of sight.

This leads to a more general conclusion. Visual experiences are *externalized,* i.e. they happen out-side the body, not inside the head. The visual properties of objects appear to belong to them, not to be the products of the brain. We are hardly even aware of our EYE MOVEMENTS, which cause the image to jerk and slew continuously across

the retina. The task of vision is to inform about the outside world, not about the nature of vision.

The nerve fibres in the optic tract (the axons of retinal ganglion cells) terminate in two main areas of the brain. A minority project to a structure called the *superior colliculus* (the upper little hill), which can be seen as a bump, one on each side, on the roof of the midbrain, as well as to nearby tiny clusters of nerve cells (in the *pretectum*). This general region, the mammalian vestige of the principal visual centre in amphib-ia, reptiles, birds and fish, is concerned mainly with visual reflexes. It contains regions that reg-ulate the size of the pupil of the eye in bright and dim conditions, and that make the eye involun-tarily follow large moving objects. The main function of the two superior colliculi is to con-trol the automatic tendency of the eyes, the head and the body, to turn towards objects of interest — so-called *orienting responses.* They are, in fact, centres for SENSORY INTEGRATION, since they receive input from the ears and the skin as well as the eyes, all helping to guide such reactions.

The bulk of the fibres of the optic nerve reach the *lateral geniculate* (meaning knee-shaped)

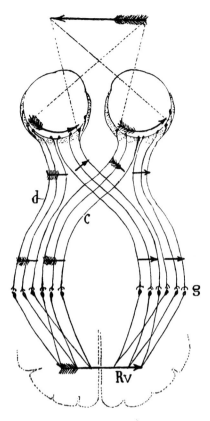

Fig. 3 The visual pathway, depicted by the great Spanish neuroanatomist Ramón y Cajal (1899). Optic nerve fibres from the nasal half of each retina (the half closer to the nose) cross over in the optic chiasma. So, the optic tract contains fibres from corresponding half-retinas of the opposite eye (c) and the eye on the same side (d). The fibres contain nerve cells in the lateral geniculate nucleus (g) whose fibres run up to the primary visual cortex at the back of the hemispheres. The right visual cortex (Rv) views the left side the visual field, the left views the right side.

distribution of the objects that generated the image, 'reversing' the optical process that made the image.

Hubel and Wiesel also discovered that the vast majority of these orientation-selective neurons are also 'binocularly driven': they have receptive fields in roughly corresponding positions on both retinas, and are remarkably similar in their preferences for visual stimuli, whichever eye is open. Thus, in normal viewing conditions, these cells will be stimulated simultaneously through both eyes, by the two images of individual objects in space. This presumably accounts for the fact that we see only one, fused visual world, despite the fact that two eyes are viewing it.

Because our two eyes are horizontally separated in the head, when we view a three-dimensional scene, their retinal images are not absolutely identical. *Binocular parallax*, as it is called, creates tiny differences in the relative positions on the two retinas of the images of individual objects that lie at different distances from the eyes. Sir Charles Wheatstone first described, in 1838, the fact that we can interpret these minute differences between the two retinal images to perceive the solidity of objects and their relative distances in space. This skill, called *stereopsis* or stereoscopic vision, is a wonderful example of inverse optics. The brain has evolved mechanisms for analysing not just the individual retinal images, but also the differences between them, so as to understand the world.

Now, it turns out that, although the two receptive fields of individual visual cortical cells, on average, lie on geometrically corresponding points in the two retinas, there is a little variation in their relative positions. This, combined with the fact that the responses of neurons are often strongly enhanced when both receptive fields are stimulated simultaneously, means that individual such cells respond best to the boundaries of objects at particular distances, behind or in front of whatever the eyes are fixating. Thus, the processing that underlies stereopsis appears to start with the binocular neurons of the primary visual cortex.

first in cats and later in monkeys, that these neurons respond not just to light or dark spots, like the neurons that drive them, but selectively to lines or edges, falling on, or moving over, the receptive field. Each cell prefers a line stimulus, at a particular orientation, and the preferred orientation varies from cell to cell. Somehow, the property of *orientation selectivity* is created by the combination of all the nerve fibres that converge on each cell. These orientation-selective cells are arranged into a beautiful system of *columns*, presumably created by the fact that most connections within the cerebral cortex run up and down radially within the grey matter. The selective neurons within each column, perhaps 0.1 mm across, running from the surface down to the white matter, all prefer the same orientation. And the preferred orientation shifts progressively from column to column, across the cortex.

Orientation-selective neurons remain perhaps the best example of *feature detection* — the notion that sensory neurons are 'programmed' (partly through innate control of the 'wiring' of the pathway, partly through the effects of sensory experience early in life) to respond to particular information-rich features of the sensory world. The primary visual cortex starts the process of 'dissecting' the retinal image, so as to encode its essential structure. In normal conditions, these cells respond to the boundaries of objects in space, or to elements of the texture of surfaces, presumably describing these features to the rest of the brain. This is the beginning of a process that has been called *inverse optics* — inferring from the flat retinal image the true shapes and

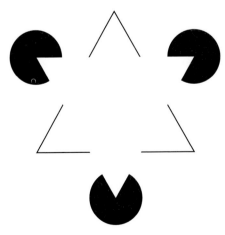

Fig. 4 Vison depends on inference. The bright, white triangle in this illusory figure of Kanizsa is 'invented' by the brain on the basis of the evidence from the other featurer in the image.

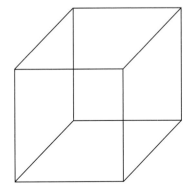

Fig. 5 The brain infers a three-dimensional world from the flat retinal image. But in the case of the Necker cube, it is unable to decide between two equally likely interpretations. The cube spontaneously alternates in depth, depending on which face appears closer.

The existence of a visual area in the back of the cerebral hemispheres was known in the nineteenth century. But at that time, the vast continent of uncharted cortex in between the major sensory and motor regions was thought simply to combine information, in some ill-defined way. It was called *association cortex*. Work on monkeys, starting in the 1960s, has shown that the entire association cortex of the rear part of the hemispheres is in fact devoted exclusively to the analysis of vision. It is divided into a huge patchwork of individual areas, each containing a representation of all or part of the visual field. These are known as *extrastriate* visual areas, to distinguish them from the striate cortex — the primary visual cortex. Virtually all the fibres from the LGN, carrying information from the eyes, reach only the striate cortex, and these other visual areas receive their input mainly from cortico-cortical connections, forming a complex network, with fibres running back and forth linking the striate cortex to the other areas.

While damage to the primary visual cortex leads to blindness in the corresponding area of the visual field, injury in extrastriate areas generally leads to more subtle deficits in perception. It must, however, be said that people rendered clinically blind by damage to the striate cortex can nevertheless sometimes respond unconsciously to a visual stimuli, by moving their eyes towards it, particularly if it moves rapidly or is of very high contrast. Indeed, some can 'guess' reliably the direction of movement of the stimulus and whether a flashed line is vertical or horizontal, even though they deny actually seeing it. This curious residual visual capacity, called 'blindsight', may be mediated by surviving connections from the eyes to other parts of the brain, perhaps via the superior colliculus.

Broadly speaking, the extrastriate areas of the cortex form two broad processing 'streams', both originating in the striate cortex. The 'ventral stream', which runs downwards into the lower parts of the temporal lobe, is dominated by the P-cell system, and thus contains information about colour and fine detail, while the 'dorsal

stream', monopolized by M-cell input, runs up into the parietal lobe, and is concerned with the analysis of movement, and the detection of the position of objects in space. The ventral and dorsal streams have been dubbed 'what' and 'where' systems, although this is an over-simplification.

The ventral stream does seem to be mainly concerned with the recognition of objects, and it feeds signals to parts of the brain, especially the *hippocampus*, thought to be responsible for conscious visual memory. Neurons in some areas within the ventral stream have remarkable properties. In an area called V4, for instance, some cells respond selectively to surfaces of a particular colour, regardless of the spectral composition of the illuminating light. This correlates with the fact that we see the colours of objects as more or less constant, whatever the illumination — a phenomenon called *colour constancy*. To achieve this property, these neurons must somehow take account of the wavelength composition of light reflected from surrounding surfaces, a 'computation' that cannot be done in the primary visual cortex. Further south, in parts of the temporal lobe, are populations of nerve cells that respond selectively to the appearance of monkey or human faces, somehow detecting the combination of features that define a face. Even deeper into the ventral stream cells can 'learn' to respond specifically to one stimulus out of a series of objects or abstract shapes that the animal is shown as part of a memory task. This all suggests that the ventral stream is concerned with identifying and remembering objects.

This work on monkeys has underpinned the recent study of visual areas in the human brain, making use of the new IMAGING TECHNIQUES of Positron Emission Tomography (PET) and functional Magnetic Resonance Imaging (fMRI), which essentially detect the small local changes of blood flow associated with activity in neurons. There may be as many as 50 different extrastriate visual areas in humans, and those occupying the lower part of the occipital and temporal lobes also seem to be concerned with the analysis of colour, faces and the identification of objects.

Damage in these regions, caused, for instance, by STROKE, causes various, selective deficits in visual understanding, such as central *achromatopsia*, a form of COLOUR BLINDNESS, or *prosopagnosia*, the inability to recognize individual faces. In extreme cases, damage of the ventral stream leads to the frightening condition of visual *agnosia*, in which patients simply cannot recognize familiar objects, despite all their basic visual functions being normal.

The dorsal stream in monkeys also has areas with distinctive physiological properties. One, called the middle temporal area (MT) or V5, seems deeply involved in the analysis of motion. Neurons here almost all respond to movement in a particular direction, and they probably also play a part in stereoscopic vision. Neighbouring areas are concerned with analysing the flow of patterns across the retina produced by movements of the head or the whole body through space. Even higher up, in the parietal lobe, cells respond to the positions and movements of objects in ways that imply that they are concerned with guiding hand and eye movements. Again, similar functional areas have been found in the upper parts of the human occipital lobe and the parietal lobe. Damage in these regions can produce such conditions as *akinetopsia* (deficiency in the perception of motion) and visual neglect (failure to attend to objects on the opposite side of visual space).

It has been argued that the dorsal stream is more concerned with unconscious visually-guided reactions, such as manipulating objects with the hands, while the ventral stream underlies the conscious perception of objects. Evidence for this view comes from the fact that some individuals with ventral stream damage, while unaware of the differences between particular objects, can nevertheless shape their hands correctly when asked to pick them up. Equally, some patients with dorsal stream damage make clumsy hand movements when they try to pick up objects that they can recognize perfectly well.

The huge adaptive value of vision has driven its explosive evolution. Its machinery dominates our brains; its impressions dominate our subjective lives. Indeed, for the sighted, it is hard to imagine life without it. Language is full of visual metaphors that bear testimony to the fact that vision is the main route to the mind. 'I see what you mean'; 'A person of vision'; 'My point of view', 'A picture is worth a thousand words'. Moreover, vision not only underpins our understanding of the world around us but also sets the scale of BEAUTY and UGLINESS. The view from a mountaintop, the skyline of New York, sunset in the south of France, Botticelli's *Birth of Venus* (see VENUS). It is seeing that makes those things breathtaking. Vision rules our aesthetic lives.

Vision has been a favourite topic of some of the most eminent individuals in the history of science, including such physicists as Isaac Newton, James Clerk Maxwell, Thomas Young, Hermann von Helmholtz and Ernst Mach. Arguably, we know more about vision than any other high-level function of the brain. Yet much

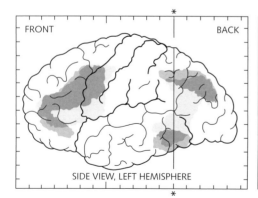
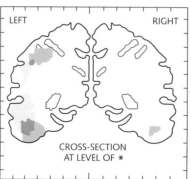

Fig. 6 In the brain of a person imagining the movement of an elephant certain (light grey) areas are active. When imagining the colour of an elephant, separate (dark grey) areas are active. The areas at the back of the brain are those that become active when one actually sees real movement or colour. The activity in the front of the brain is associated with the acts of imagining.

remains mysterious. How does the brain arrive at reliable interpretations of objects? How is the identity of every object we can distinguish represented in the brain? How is the subjective experience of seeing related to, and generated from, the activity of neurons? Indeed, what, if anything, does conscious experience add to the purely computational process of vision?

COLIN BLAKEMORE

Further reading

Gregory, R. L. (2001) *Eye and brain: the psychology of seeing, 5th edition.* Oxford University Press, Oxford.

Hubel, D. H. (1988) *Eye, brain and vision.* Scientific American Library/W.H. Freeman, San Francisco.

Zeki, S. (1999) *Inner vision.* Oxford University Press, Oxford.

See also BLINDNESS; BLINDNESS, RECOVERY FROM; COLOUR BLINDNESS; CONSCIOUSNESS; EYE MOVEMENTS; EYES; ILLUSIONS SENSORY RECEPTORS.

Vitamins In present day Western society, the small print on packets of cereals and of citrus drinks is a ready source of information on the vitamins they provide, the quantity contained therein, and the fraction which that content provides of the *recommended daily allowance* (RDA). In many homes there is also a stock of packaged tablets or bottled syrups, swallowed mostly on the principle that if a little of these stuffs is necessary for health, then more must be better. In some instances this may possibly be so, but by no means to the extent that vitamin supplements are sold and bought. A vitamin is an organic substance that is necessary only in very small amounts (RDAs all less than 200 mg) for normal growth and health and which must be obtained from the diet because it cannot be synthesized by the body. But, as with many original definitions of this sort, exceptions have emerged with the progress of research.

There were three diseases that during the eighteenth and nineteenth centuries began to be linked in some way to the diet. The cure of *scurvy* in a ship's company by provision of citrus fruit dates back to 1754, to a historic, but initially neglected experimental observation: men with the disease were divided into pairs, and each pair given different additions to their rations; those, and only those, who received oranges and lemons recovered. The scurvy was successfully avoided with the issue of fruit and vegetables on Captain Cook's voyages in the 1770s, and official introduction of lemon juice into the Royal Navy diet followed before the end of the century. Understanding of the reason for this was to take more than a century. The occurrence of *pellagra* started to be associated from the mid 1700s with a poor diet of maize-meal without meat or milk in different parts of the world, and this link was still occurring in the US well into the twentieth century. The condition of *beri-beri* was prevalent in nineteenth-century Asian workers who lived mainly on rice that had been 'improved' by

The table shows the main sources of each vitamin, and main features of its deficiency. Most of the names refer to a group of substances with similar action.

Substance(s)	Source	Deficiency effects	SEE ALSO
Fat-soluble vitamins			
A retinol	Carotenes from plants. Animal/fish fats and liver.	Night blindness. Thickened cornea.	VISION
D calciferols	Animal fats. Fish liver oils. Skin and sun.	Bone softening: rickets in childhood, osteomalacia in adult.	BONE, CALCIUM, SKIN, STEROIDS, SUN, TEETH
E tocopherols	Most foods. Vegetable oils.	Wide range proposed; no clear evidence of specific effect.	
K quinones	Plants. Also made by gut flora.	Slow blood clotting, tendency to bleed.	BLOOD
Water-soluble vitamins			
B group			
B_1 thiamin	Grains and pulses. Pork and offal.	*Beri-beri* = 'extreme weakness'; peripheral neuritis, oedema.	DISEASE
B_2 riboflavin	Most foods.	Sore tongue and lips; visual impairment.	
B_6 pyridoxin	Most foods.	Skin lesions, convulsions.	
B_{12} cobalamin	Animal products only. Requires *intrinsic factor* for absorption.	Pernicious anaemia; neurological disorder.	BLOOD ANAEMIA STOMACH
Biotin	Liver, yeast, etc.	No specific syndrome.	
Folic acid	Liver, greens, yeast.	Anaemia. Defective growth. Congenital CNS defects.	ANAEMIA ANTENATAL DEVELOPMENT
Niacin	Meat, liver, grains, pulses.	*Pellagra* = 'rough skin'; nerve, bowel, and mental abnormalities.	
Pantothenic acid	Most foods	General illness; no specific syndrome.	
C ascorbic acid	Fruit and vegetables.	*Scurvy*: bruising and bleeding, impaired healing.	COLLAGEN WOUND HEALING

new machinery which removed the husks; also chickens who ate rice without its husks developed a peripheral nerve abnormality like that in the human disease. It was at first assumed that some toxin had been introduced by the cooking or polishing. But husks — or an extract made from them — were later shown to cure the condition in both people and chickens. Thus the notion gradually arose that diseases might be caused by an *absence* of something, rather than the *presence* of a POISON or INFECTION.

The concept of necessary substances in the diet — in addition to the major energy-providers and MINERALS — whose absence led to disease, entered several minds, and led to many clinical and experimental studies in the early twentieth century. An early pioneer was the British biochemist Frederick Gowland Hopkins, later a Nobel prize winner. He, among others, found that a combination of all known nutrients was

not sufficient to allow young animals to thrive. The word 'vitamine' was invented in 1911 by Funk, a biochemist also working in London, who believed, rightly, that he had isolated a vital dietary constituent from rice husks — and, wrongly, that it was by chemical nature an amine. Such extracts became known as vitamin B, and the original name without the 'e' came to be applied to the family of substances that emerged over the following decades as necessary for health, but required only in very small quantities. In the 1920s 'vitamin B' proved to be more than one substance; B_1 was identified as the anti-beri-beri factor, and others with comparable properties, equally essential, were later added to the group. Knowledge emerged, thanks to a young American physician, William Castle, of a vitamin (B_{12}) necessary for blood cell production, which needed a gastric secretion to allow its absorption — explaining the empirical observation that very large amounts of raw liver were needed to cure pernicious anaemia. Vitamin C — which prevented scurvy — was finally identified in lemon juice in 1932, was found to be readily destroyed by heat, was given the name of ascorbic acid, and became the first vitamin to be artificially synthesized. Meanwhile, some factor in fish oils and egg yolks became recognized as being necessary for growth and health, and was initially called vitamin A. Extracts proved effective against rickets, and this component was separately labelled vitamin D. Thus by the time of World War II the main vitamins had been identified, and their importance recognized; national programmes such as vitamin additions to staple foods and provision of enriched juices for infants and children supported wartime public health; vitamins had also become a major commercial proposition.

Each vitamin is a requisite for some essential metabolic function, and most cannot be synthesized in the body. The exceptions are vitamin D, which can be made in the skin in the presence of sunlight; vitamin A, which need not as such be in the diet, since it can be made from carotenes present in vegetables; and vitamin K, which can be made by bacteria in the gut.

The naming of the vitamins does not appear very logical, for various historical reasons. They are described in two categories — water-soluble and fat-soluble. The significance of this distinction relates to their sources, their absorption, storage, and excretion, and to the manner of their action.

The water-soluble vitamins comprise vitamin C and the 'B group' (see table). Vitamin C is necessary for COLLAGEN synthesis, the basis of CONNECTIVE TISSUE growth and maintenance. Those of the B group act by forming *co-enzymes*, essential for a range of vital, enzyme-dependent cellular processes. These include DNA synthesis, different components of the utilization of nutrients, and the respiratory and energy-releasing processes. Folic acid and B_{12} specifically are essential for the formation of normal red blood cells. B_{12} is unique in requiring the *intrinsic factor* secreted by glands in the stomach to enable it to be absorbed from the intestine, and also in being obtainable only from animal sources.

The fat-soluble vitamins are A, D, E, and K. Fat-solubility means not only that their sources are in fats in the diet, but also that they can be stored in adipose tissue and can have actions on cells by dissolving in the lipid cell membranes. Deficiency may occur not only in malnutrition, but also in any condition that interferes with fat absorption, including liver disease because of the role of BILE. Unlike water-soluble vitamins, their storage means that signs of deprivation are delayed — and also that over-dosage can become toxic.

For many of the vitamins there are distinctive abnormalities related to their deficiency, which can be reversed by an adequate intake. Deficiencies occur in undernourished or malnourished communities or individuals; in ALCOHOLISM,

poverty, and neglect in the aged in any society; and in strict vegetarians. Apart from the treatment of deficiency conditions, the question remains open, and the subject of research, as to whether there is any advantage to be gained from supplements in excess of the minimal adequate amounts. Since the relatively recent understanding of the damaging effect of FREE RADICALS, the counteracting *antioxidant* action of vitamins A, C, and E has been recognized; the fat-soluble and water-soluble vitamins may combine to protect against free radical damage particularly to CELL MEMBRANES, and thus to diminish processes such as arteriosclerosis and others associated with ageing. Some of the B vitamins (folic acid and B12) may have a role in protecting from heart disease. There has been contradictory evidence concerning protection from the common cold or alleviation of its symptoms by large doses of vitamin C. On the other hand, there can be serious ill-effects from overdose of the fat-soluble vitamins and also of vitamin C.

SHEILA JENNETT

Further reading

Carpenter, K. J. (1986). *The history of scurvy and vitamin C.* Cambridge University Press.

Roe, D. A. (1973). *A plague of corn: the social history of pellagra.* Cornell University Press, Ithaca NY.

See also BIOCHEMISTRY; ENZYMES.

Vivisection From the Latin *vivi*, living, and *sectio*, cutting, vivisection, strictly speaking, means cutting live tissues. As such it could be applied to any surgical procedure, including human operations. In practice the word is often used pejoratively as a synonym for experiments on animals, implying cruelty such as the infliction of operative techniques without the use of an anaesthetic, which even if it were not abhorrent to the investigator would be both impracticable and against the law. The term is sometimes used also to refer to any procedure involving laboratory animals — not only operations that are carried out within the law under anaesthetic, but also investigations that do not involve surgery, such as changing diets or giving injections. In the UK all laboratory procedures on vertebrates (and also on the octopus) are regulated by the Home Office, under the 1986 Animals (Scientific Procedures) Act, which superceded the 1876 Cruelty to Animals Act.

E.M.TANSEY

See also ANIMALS IN RESEARCH.

Voice Voice production is dependent on the flow of air from the lungs via the trachea and through the gap between the vocal folds (known more familiarly as *vocal cords*) in the LARYNX and out past the lips. The vocal folds are separated relatively widely during quiet BREATHING, but come closely together during sound production (*phonation*). The position of the vocal folds during speech determines in part the type of sounds produced. Voiced sounds such as vowels

and certain consonants such as b, d, and g require vibration of the vocal folds, while voiceless sounds such as the consonants p, t, and k require the vocal folds to be wide apart. Voiceless sounds are produced by turbulence in the upper vocal tract.

To produce sounds the vocal folds are brought together by the muscles of the larynx. At the same time, the respiratory muscles of the chest wall that assist expiration cause the air pressure immediately below the vocal folds to increase, pushing them apart. As the air escapes between them through the larynx, the pressure below the vocal folds decreases and they come together; the pressure beneath the folds rises again, and the process repeats itself. This rapid opening and closing of the vocal folds produces vibration that we perceive as voice. MARJORIE LORCH

See also LARYNX; SINGING; SPEECH.

Voiceprint An electronic translation of sound into a pictorial or graphical representation; essentially, it is a sonogram of a person's voice. It was first developed in the mid 1960s by Lawrence G. Kersta, an engineer from New Jersey, who researched sound identification for the FBI. According to proponents of the technology, the variations of the human vocal tract ensure that each person's voice is spectographically individual. They compare voiceprints with FINGERPRINTS or footprints in their unique representation of identity.

Law enforcement has long struggled with the admissibility of voiceprints in court, as a means of identifying voices caught on tape. While the US Supreme Court has not ruled on the admissibility of voiceprints, it did, in 1993, set a new standard for the admissibility of expert testimony and scientific evidence; where earlier rules demanded 'general acceptance' of the principles involved, Daubert v. Merrell Dow Pharmaceuticals argued that admissibility of evidence 'rests on a reliable foundation and is relevant to the task at hand.' Thus the admissibility of voiceprints is decided on a case-by-case basis. While proponents argue that voiceprints are analogous to fingerprints, detractors argue that, unlike fingerprints, voices can change due to illness, injury, or age, making voiceprints far less reliable.

With the current explosion of electronic, computer, and telephone commerce, voiceprints are becoming popular as a potential security measure. Defined as a biometric-based signature, voiceprints can be used to identify a speaker positively on the basis of physical characteristics, namely the specific configuration of vocal cavities (throat, naval cavities, and mouth) and articulators (lips, teeth, tongue, and soft palate). Commercial interests are particularly drawn to biometric-based signatures, because they cannot be lost, stolen, or forgotten. Further, one bank, which was using voiceprints experimentally, opined that customers would be likely to accept the idea of voiceprints because they were less intrusive than fingerprints or retina scans, and less likely to be entered in national databases.

While a voiceprint is particularly technological, it extends a previously held idea that one's voice is not simply an identifying marker, like a fingerprint, but is instead the unique expression of one's essential self. In literary studies, this has manifested in the idea that all writers, professional as well as amateur, have an authentic voice that one should be able to identify and strengthen. Movements such as cultural studies, women's studies, and race studies have used the concept to highlight exclusions in various traditions. When a writer, musician, or other artist is hailed as the 'voice of his or her generation', he or she is seen as encapsulating the identity of an age.

JULIE VEDDER

Further reading

Block, E. B. (1975). *Voiceprinting: how the law can read the voice of crime.* David McKay Company, Inc., New York.

Field, R. L. (1997). 'The electronic future of cash: survey: 1996: survey of the year's developments in electronic cash law and the laws affecting electronic banking in the United States.' *The American University Law Review*, April 1997.

See also SPEECH; VOICE.

Vomiting

It would be a rare individual indeed who went through life without experiencing vomiting — the forceful and uncontrollable expulsion of stomach or intestinal contents — whether due to illness, turbulent travel, or extreme disgust.

Vomiting may be preceded by nausea, which is often accompanied by increased AUTONOMIC NERVOUS SYSTEM activity, involving SALIVATION, SWEATING, pallor, and low BLOOD PRESSURE. Just before vomiting occurs there are retrograde contractions in the upper small intestine and in the stomach which propel their contents up the oesophagus and into the mouth.

There is a vomiting 'centre' in the mid-brain which co-ordinates the complex neural reflexes that occur during vomiting. The centre may be activated by incoming fibres in the VAGUS NERVES from the gut, by the VESTIBULAR SYSTEM via auditory nerves, by higher centres in the central nervous system, and also by input from a 'trigger zone' in the brain stem that is responsive to chemical stimulation by DRUGS, acidosis, and HYPOXIA.

Causes, investigation, and management of vomiting

Intestinal infections from food poisoning, particularly that due to *Staphylococcus aureus* and *Bacillus cereus*, produce vomiting soon after ingestion of contaminated food. Other infections can cause vomiting along with DIARRHOEA — particularly acute viral gastroenteritis due to *rotavirus* and bacterial diarrhoeas. There is often a clue to the source of infection, especially if there are several sufferers after a common meal or a sequence of contacts. The diagnosis can usually be made by microbiological examination of faeces. These acute infections are usually self-limiting, although in some instances antibiotics may be appropriate.

Gastrointestinal obstruction The outlet of the stomach may be obstructed, particularly following chronic duodenal ulceration or as a result of gastric cancer, and this often produces vomiting. Gastric emptying may also be impaired when there is nerve damage or muscle damage, such as in the neuropathy associated with DIABETES mellitus. Obstruction of the small bowel can occur as a result of adhesions, fibrotic strictures associated with intestinal inflammation (*Crohn's disease*), or radiation enteritis. Obstruction can usually be confirmed by X-RAY, although more detailed investigation may be required to identify the precise site of the obstruction, and surgery may then be required to relieve it.

Causes arising in the central nervous system Vomiting may be stimulated by excessively unpleasant perceptions — distressing sights, disgusting smells, or extreme ANXIETY are well known causes; MOTION SICKNESS is produced by neural mechanisms involving the vestibular apparatus in the inner ear. Disorders in the brain itself can cause vomiting, for example MIGRAINE, meningitis, and any of the causes of increased intracranial pressure. When the history of the illness and other signs and symptoms indicate raised intracranial pressure, a brain scan is usually required to search for a cause; lumbar puncture and examination of cerebrospinal fluid may be necessary if meningitis is suspected.

Metabolic disorders A variety of produce vomiting, particularly those associated with acidosis, including kidney failure and uncontrolled diabetes with ketoacidosis. These can usually be diagnosed with appropriate blood tests.

Anti-cancer drugs and radiotherapy commonly produce nausea and vomiting, as do other drugs active in the central nervous system, including opiate pain killers (morphine, heroin) and also alcohol. Progress has been made in the development of new anti-emetic drugs (*emesis* = vomiting), particularly the serotonin antagonists which are potent inhibitors of chemotherapy-induced vomiting.

The eating disorders anorexia nervosa and bulimia, are frequently associated with vomiting, usually self-induced.

The vomiting which may accompany early PREGNANCY is a common experience, so far largely unexplained.

Whatever the cause, the effects of vomiting on the body follow from the loss of fluid and of the acid which the gastric juices normally contain. There can therefore be dehydration and disturbance of ACID–BASE HOMEOSTASIS, which have to be corrected if vomiting is persistent or severe.

MICHAEL FARTHING
ANNE BALLINGER

Vulva

In medical terminology the word 'vulva' is used to describe the female external genitalia, namely the mons pubis, the LABIA majora, the labia minora, the CLITORIS, the vestibule, the vestibular bulb, and the greater vestibular gland. The word vulva comes from the Latin *vulva*, which translates as 'a wrapper' (or 'the womb').

By the end of the sixteenth century the vulva no longer meant womb and it had already become an external organ, as described by Vicary in his *Anatomy* when he observed that 'By it goes forth the vrin, or els it should be shed through out at the vulva'. In the early seventeenth century, Crooke in the *Body of Man* described 'The last dissimilar part of the womb is called of some vulva' and Salmon in 1694 in *Bate's Dispensary* advised to 'Anoint the vulva and womb with this mixture.'

Being oestrogen-dependent, the vulva undergoes several physiological changes during the different stages of life. In infancy the vulva is hairless and the labia majora and mons pubis (the central prominence above the labia are composed of fatty subcutaneous tissue which diminishes during childhood, but then appears again at PUBERTY. At this stage the coarse pubic hair grows and covers this area. Then later, after the MENOPAUSE, the vulval skin becomes thinner and much drier. The labia minora shrink, the adipose tissue reduces, and the vaginal orifice becomes smaller. At this stage the labia can often become irritated and this can produce discomfort. This can be a common cause of infection and dermatologic conditions in post-menopausal and elderly women.

The vulval skin suffers from diseases common to all skin such as eczema, psoriasis, contact dermatitis, and malignant lesions such as squamous cell carcinoma or melanoma. LINDA CARDOZO
VIK KHULLAR

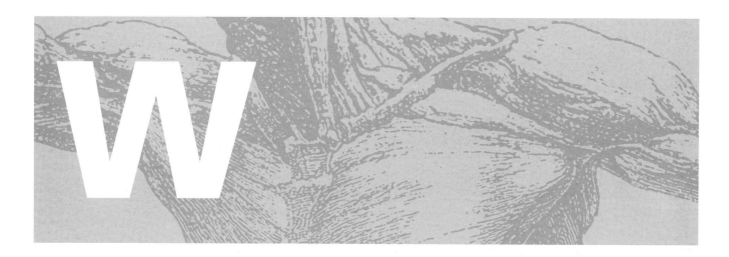

Walking is an activity that we normally take for granted; we consciously start or stop, and give attention to avoidance of obstacles, but otherwise this complex, co-ordinated procedure is seemingly simple and automatic.

Walking, in technical terms, is a form of bipedal (or quadripedal) progression in which there are periods of double support, when both feet are on the ground, alternating with periods of single support. This distinguishes walking from faster gaits in which ground contact is absent for brief periods. Whilst it is commonplace, its mechanics and neurological control are complex. Many neurological disorders affect walking efficiency.

Events in both limbs are essentially identical but are phase shifted. The sequence of events in the right limb begins with heel contact with the ground. At this point the left foot is still on the ground (the first phase of double support). The body moves forward and the centre of gravity passes in front of the left toes. At this point the weight is supported by the right limb alone, the left limb flexes and swings forward. The left limb begins to extend later in the swing phase, causing left heel contact with the ground. This initiates a second period of double support, which is followed by the swing phase in the right limb terminating in right heel contact. The smooth forward movement of the centre of gravity includes lateral movements so that the centre of gravity lies over the right foot during single support on that limb. There are symmetrical leftward sways during left limb stance. In addition, the centre of gravity rises and falls by some 50 mm.

Young adults typically select a range of normal walking speeds of between 80 and 100 metres per minute. This corresponds to a stride length of about 1.4 m, i.e. a step length of 0.7 m, and a stride duration of about 1 second. The duration of the stance phase for each foot is about 0.65 second. The peak vertical force rises to about 120% of body weight during the stance phase.

Limb muscles generally show single bursts of activity during each step. *Extensor* (leg straightening) muscle activity typically begins just before heel contact to prepare the limb for load bearing, whilst *flexor* muscle activity is confined to the swing phase after toe-off, to allow the limb to swing through to its new landing position. The bulk of the forward propulsive force comes from a second short burst of activity in the KNEE and ANKLE extensors just before toe-off.

The patterns of muscle activity during walking are generated by networks of neurons located in the spinal cord and accorded the description *central pattern generator*. These networks, which generate a simple locomotor rhythm, draw upon, and are influenced by, REFLEXES evoked by sensory inputs from the muscles, skin, and joints, particularly the HIP joint. In many animals — the cat, dog, rat, and mouse, for example — and for swimming movements in fish, this locomotor network can express its rhythmic activity entirely independently of control from higher centres in the brain, hence the other name, *spinal locomotor centre*. In the case of the rabbit the movement is a bilaterally synchronous 'hopping' movement. Attempts to demonstrate that such mechanisms can be activated in (spinal man) (when the SPINAL CORD is cut off by injury from the higher parts of the nervous system at a level above the segments that control walking) have however failed. If they could have been elicited it would have facilitated the development of prosthetic devices that could enable spinal man to walk. As it is, even extremely complicated computer control aimed at stimulating muscles with the same pattern as in natural walking has been only partially effective; this emphasizes the importance of the control exerted by the brain despite the automated nature of walking. Nevertheless, it remains likely that when one wishes to walk, or to stop walking, the commands issued from the brain are actually turning on, or off, a spinal pattern generator comparable to that demonstrated in animals.

R. H. BAXENDALE

See also GAIT; MOVEMENT, CONTROL OF; POSTURE.

War and the body There is horror inscribed on the body at war. Otto Dix's *War Triptych* (1932) and Pablo Picasso's *Guernica* (1937) present us with the mutilated, agonized, and contorted flesh of combat. There is no glory here, no hypnotic beating of drums, no braying horses, no clash of sword against sword. Instead, combat has become mechanical slaughter, a silent scream. Even the body has lost its boundaries: guns are 'arms' and radar are 'eyes'. If there is a heroic tale, it is located far behind battle-lines in hospitals where surgeons invest their technical skills and professional acumen in new disciplines in order to reassemble dismembered men. Or it is in research laboratories where scientists concoct gases and viruses to poison enemy bodies more effectively, or in military camps where psychiatrists minister to men's minds in order that their bodies can go forth to kill and be killed. For politicians, military strategists, and many historians, war may be about the conquest of territory or the struggle to recover a sense of national honour, but for servicemen, warfare is more brutal, more bloody, than this.

But these are not the only bodies of war. There is also the glorious flesh of the imagination: the chiselled features of airmen, the muscular bulk of sailors, and the fertile curves of mothers, creators of life in the midst of terrible carnage. These representations of the body at war inspire military fervour. Walter Raleigh, Francis Drake, Robert Clive, Charles Gordon, David Livingston, and T. E. Lawrence are the romantic symbols which preoccupy boys' magazines. Flying aces, such as Germany's Erich Hartmann (who scored 352 hits during World War II), are goals that servicemen dream about. War's emblems include the female sex. Florence Nightingale's nursing zeal in the Crimea; Harriet Tubman's underground railroad during the American Civil War; and female partisans during the Spanish Civil War, and in Yugoslavia and Russia during World War II, encourage women to participate more fully in armed struggles.

Increasingly, female bodies have been drawn closer to the KILLING fields. Of course, they have always been central to the military enterprise by

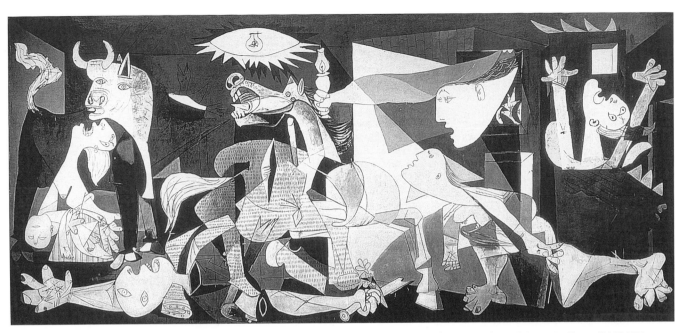

Guernica, 1937 by Pablo Picasso (1881–1973). Museo Nacional Centro de Arte Reina Sofia, Madrid, Spain/Bridgeman Art Library. © Succession Picasso/DACS 2001.

pushing their menfolk into the fray, nursing torn bodies on their return, and creating memorials to the dead. There have always been exceptional women who proved willing to 'sacrifice' their own lives in combat. However, twentieth-century armaments brought physical risk closer to the majority of women. In 1914, for the first time in modern warfare, civilians in countries which were not invaded had bombs rained down upon them. In occupied countries, new, long-distant technologies of war (such as machine guns, artillery, aerial bombers, and atom bombs) could not discriminate between combatants and non-combatants. At Buchenwald, Hiroshima, and My Lai, the chief victims were civilians. 'Body counts' exemplify this sense that individuals are expendable, valueless. So-called 'rules of civilized warfare', embodying the famous principles of discrimination and proportionality, have become absurdly muddled and irrelevant. There is no limit to the damage that can be inflicted upon human bodies.

To focus on dismemberment, however, distorts our understanding of the way war is experienced and imagined within societies. For one thing, in many modern conflicts, and most scandalously during the Crimean War and the Spanish–American War, more men died from DISEASE than from shot and shell. Furthermore, the body is not only decimated by war, it is also moulded by it. From the late nineteenth century, fears that wars were dysgenic because they destroyed the strongest men and left the responsibility for breeding a new generation to 'half-men', stimulated state and private intervention into improving the corporeal well-being of their citizens. From the turn of the twentieth century, the belief that combat effectiveness could be identified by physical examination resulted in mass campaigns in which men were weighed and measured, placed

into their respective 'grades', then sent to the appropriate field of military usefulness. By the time of World War II, such essentialist typologies were being supplemented by psychological testing: as signifiers of military effectiveness, physical prowess and psychological 'balance' became inseparable. In this way, the male body at war is constrained, policed, and disciplined to an extent rarely regarded as acceptable within civilian contexts. Since the soldiers of the Roman army first donned identical military clothing, the experience of men in battle has been one of uniformity. Men are severely punished for infractions of the military code. Repetitive military and physical drill shape men's bodies into similar patterns. Military training unquestionably creates men who are 'harder', more muscular, and 'fitter' than their civilian counterparts.

After war, ex-servicemen's bodies become a site of controversy. Claims for pensions generate some of the most bitter political debates: able-bodied and disabled-bodied servicemen tussle over their respective entitlements, and working-class activists sneer at the so-called 'sacrifices' made by more privileged soldiers. Within a short time, people turn their gaze away from 'suffering warriors', preferring to forget the past and look ahead to the possibility of renewed conflict. Accusations of war's 'brutalizing effect' have been more insidious. Although such insults are expressed after every conflict, they reached a new intensity after the Vietnam War, when the veteran's body came to be portrayed either as 'broken' or as immensely dangerous: victim or executioner. Civilians displace responsibility for social dysfunction from the societies which sent men to war, to combat servicemen themselves.

In death, military bodies had to be reconstructed in the imagination of those left behind. Often, the physical body is absent, lost on some

battlefield or buried at a distance from those who loved it in life. War memorials often scarcely dare to remember their dead in human form, preferring to represent the loss of their young by a simple stone into which the names of the dead are inscribed. Indeed, after World War II, fresh names were often merely added to the bottom of the 1914–18 memorials. The dead soldier disappears, but the nightmare of war continues to be chiselled onto the bodies of those who remain behind, as in Kathe Kollwitz's granite commemoration at the Roggevelde German war cemetery of her young son's death. In this memorial, it is the grieving parents kneeling before their son's grave, their bodies scarcely containing their anguish as they pray for forgiveness for failing to stand against war, who become the lasting representatives of the impact of war on the body.

JOANNA BOURKE

Further reading

Bourke, J. (1996). *Dismembering the male: men's bodies, Britain and the Great War*. Reaktion, London and Chicago.

See also BIOLOGICAL WARFARE; CHEMICAL WARFARE; KILLING; VIOLENCE.

Warts If the artist can flatter with the brush then Sir Peter Lely must have felt that his talents had been neglected when Oliver Cromwell asked him to 'Paint my picture … pimples, warts and everything as you see me.'

Others, both before and after Cromwell, have been rather more concerned about their warts. Hippocratic physicians used the terms *condyloma* and *myrmecia* to describe the 'knuckles' or 'anthills' that were recognizable on the hands and feet of their patients from teenage onwards; whilst according to Galen, warts were composed of 'heterogeneous and unnatural substances, pushed with violence toward the skin by dint of the internal faculties'. Celsus in his *De Medicina* described three sorts of wart according to their size, colour, and shape. This form of taxonomy was continued by David Low in his *Chiropodologia* (1785) with the division of warts or *cutaneous fibrillae* into round, flat, and pendulous types.

Low followed GALEN in suggesting that warts were caused by 'saline, gross and atrabilious humours'. Other authors focused on immorality as a possible cause for warts. MASTURBATION was also picked out, as the 'Medical News' section of the 1849 *Lancet* repeated the assertion that women with 'solitary habits' who gather hens' eggs are likely to catch warts.

Debates dealing with the taxonomy and causes of warts have been matched only by those dealing with cures. From classical times onwards, opinion has been divided over whether to use surgical techniques (cautery, ligature, or incision, or, in the present day, cryotherapy), or external remedies, or simply to leave the wart alone. The Swiss physician Paracelsus (1493–1541) urged practitioners not to employ their 'unfounded arts' of 'caustics and cutting', whilst in his *Pseudodoxia Epidemica* (1646) the English writer Thomas Browne (1605–82) attacked the superstition of 'common female doctrines' such as rubbing one's hands in the moonlight.

Browne's sentiment was in no way universal. His contemporary, Sir Kenelm Digby (1603–65), regarded 'moon beames' as an 'infalliable cure' for warts. Elizabethan and Stuart therapeutics relied heavily on Pliny's folklore-laden *Natural History*, with its suggestion that: 'Warts can be removed by those who, after the twentieth of the month, lie on their backs on a path, gazing upward with their hand stretched over their heads, and rub the wart with whatever they have grasped.'

The line between learned and folk remedies for warts was blurred. The *London Pharmacopoeia* (1696) suggested that given the 'hot and dry' qualities of ants, a 'liquor' could be made which would 'cure the itch, and dissipates corns and warts', whilst David Low assured his readers that given 'a person of knowledge and experience … a real Chiropodist … no mischief [can] flow from the application of a spider's web.' A 'wart-charming' stone in the museum of the Royal College of General Practitioners is testimony to the durability of charms and magic in English medicine.

Until well into the eighteenth century, lay and learned medicine shared a belief in the curing of warts by sympathy or transmission. Moral considerations combined with long held customs and beliefs. Warts could be transferred by rubbing them against the father of an illegitimate child, whilst in Cheshire warts could be 'bought' by reciting the rhyme, 'Ashen tree, ashen tree, Pray buy these warts of me', and sticking a pin into the tree and then into one's warts.

'Wortflower' and 'wortgrass' were local names for buttercup and petty spurge, plants that were believed to cure warts. John Gerard (1545–1612) noted in his *Herball* (1626) that 'wartwort …

taketh awaie all maner of warts, knobs and hard callouses.' The link between the symbolism and the cure of warts has a classical heritage, with the Romans using the term *thymus* to compare the appearance of genital warts to the leaves of the herb, thyme; whilst a popular cure was to kill, boil, and apply the residue from a toad with a comparable number of spots. Similar classifications continued as Linnaeus (1707–78) named the bush cricket *Decticus verrucivorus* after the reputed cure available from its bite.

Present day dermatology classifies over thirty different types of wart according to their structure, location, and relation to a particular virus from the *papova* group; a wart is a *papilloma* — benign tumour of the skin, or more rarely of a mucous membrane, caused by virus infection. Warts usually disappear spontaneously; a variety of treatments can hasten the disappearance, but recurrence is common.

ALEXANDER GOLDBLOOM

See also SKIN.

Water balance

We often drink for social reasons — a coffee break, or an evening in the pub — and yet in spite of this the body weight of a healthy adult on an adequate diet remains remarkably stable from day to day. This stability indicates that the body fluid volume is staying constant — there is a dynamic steady state, in which the fluid output equals the fluid input (Fig. 1).

Water is the most important dietary constituent. We cannot reduce our water losses from the body to less than about 1200 ml per day (the skin, respiratory, and faecal losses, and a minimum urine volume of about 400 ml per day), so survival with no water intake is only possible for a few days.

What determines how much water we need to ingest? Essentially, the simple answer to this question is that it is the concentration of the solutes in the body — the body fluid osmolality. This normally has a value of about 285 milliosmoles/kg H_2O. If the solutes get too concentrated (if the osmolality increases), this indicates that there is insufficient water to keep them at their correct concentration. Conversely, if the solutes are diluted (decreased osmolality), there is an excessive amount of water relative to solute.

The osmolality of the blood supplying the brain is monitored by 'osmoreceptors' in the HYPOTHALAMUS at the base of the BRAIN, and these play a large part in determining our thirst sensation, and in the release of the hormone ADH (antidiuretic hormone, or vasopressin) from its storage site in the posterior PITUITARY GLAND. Water deficit leads to thirst, and to ADH release into the circulating blood. The ADH acts on the kidneys to increase renal water reabsorption (see KIDNEYS). Water excess suppresses thirst and decreases ADH release.

Water deprivation

What happens when our water intake is inadequate? The continuing obligatory water loss from the SKIN and from the LUNGS (Fig. 1) causes a rise in the extracellular fluid osmolality, and this causes water to move from the cells to the extracellular fluid, so that there is water deficiency, and an increased osmolality, in all of the body fluid compartments. The increased osmolality increases ADH release (Fig. 2), and the osmolality and cellular dehydration causes the sensation of thirst.

The normal body fluid osmolality of 285 milliosmoles/kg H_2O is between the osmotic threshold for ADH release (280 milliosmoles/kg H_2O), and that for thirst (290 milliosmoles/kg H_2O), as shown in Fig. 2.

When we are deprived of water, renal mechanisms are activated to conserve water, but, in practice, the situations in which water intake is low are often those in which losses from the lungs

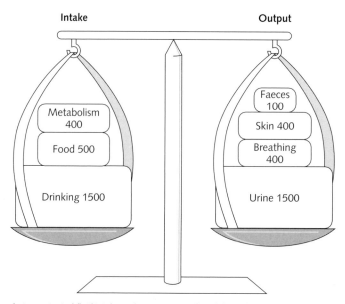

Fig. 1 Balance between typical fluid intake and output in a 70 kg adult. (Values are ml per 24 hours.)

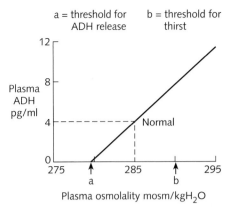

a = threshold for ADH release   b = threshold for thirst

Fig. 2 ADH release from the posterior pituitary, showing effect of plasma osmolality on plasma ADH concentration.

and skin are high (e.g. hot, dry environments). The skin loss shown in Fig. 1 (400 ml) is 'insensible perspiration', and occurs because the skin is not completely waterproof. SWEATING is an additional loss (at up to 5 litres per hour), and is adjusted *not* to the needs of water balance, but to the needs of TEMPERATURE REGULATION. There is no convincing evidence that we humans can 'train' to manage with less water by alterations of our physiological mechanisms, although our behaviour can certainly be modified to conserve water. For example, hard physical work produces metabolic heat, so avoiding such work reduces the need to sweat.

What are the physiological effects of water deprivation? The first sign is the sensation of thirst. This begins when the body fluids have decreased by 2% from the normal volume of about 40–45 litres in a 70 kg person. When the deficit reaches 4%, the mouth and throat feel dry, and functional derangements develop — apathy, sleepiness, impatience. At 8% deficit, there is no longer any salivary secretion; the tongue feels swollen, and speech is difficult. By the time the deficit reaches 12% (4.5–5 litres less water in the body than there should be), the victim is unable to recover without assistance, and is unable to swallow. The lethal limit of water deprivation is about 20%.

Osmoregulation

It is important to appreciate that people can have a water deficit even if they are drinking. This is because there is a maximum possible urine concentration — about 1400 millosmoles per kg H_2O in adults, but only about half of that value in children. So if we ingest hypertonic solution — solutions with a higher solute concentration (osmolality) than the plasma — we may need to excrete more water to remove the solute than we took in with it. For example, if we ingest 1 kg of sea water, of osmolality 2000 millosmoles/kg H_2O, and we can produce urine with a maximum osmolality of 1400 millosmoles/kg H_2O, we need 2000/1400 kg urine (i.e. 1.5 litres) to excrete the solute and we end up dehydrated in spite of the fluid ingested. This is particularly important in infants. Newborn infants have a maximum urine osmolality of only about 600 millosmoles per kg H_2O, so it is very easy to dehydrate them by giving them excessively concentrated drinks.

Volume regulation

The body fluid solute concentration (osmolality) is not the only regulator of our water intake — the BODY FLUID volume is also important. Indeed, sometimes volume regulation and osmoregulation may be in 'conflict'. For example, during prolonged physical activity, sweating leads to a reduction in body fluid volume by loss of salt (NaCl) and water. Drinking water in response to this lowers the body fluid osmotic concentration, which limits thirst. Full restoration of the body fluid volume therefore requires replacement of the lost salt, as well as water.

CHRIS LOTE

Further reading

Lote, C. (1993). The kidneys' balancing act. *Biological Sciences Review*, 5, 20–3.

See also BODY FLUIDS; KIDNEYS; SURVIVAL AT SEA; SWEATING.

Weeping is a physiological process in which some stimulus causes the lacrimal glands of the eyes to emit a salty liquid — tears. Weeping, crying, or shedding tears all refer to a specific type of human behaviour that, although primarily defined as a physiological phenomenon, has also been viewed throughout history as a manifestation of emotion, strongly linked to cultural conceptions of sex, age, and class. While *weeping* is usually considered simply the shedding of tears, the more problematic term *crying* alludes to both the shedding of tears and a vocalization, making crying a much more complex phenomenon that is not an exact synonym for weeping.

Three distinct kinds of tears have been distinguished. Basal tears are shed continually in order to moisten and protect the surface of the eye. Reflex tears cleanse the eye when a foreign object or gas irritates its surface. Emotional tears are the third type. Known also as psychogenic lacrimation, this type of weeping remains rather mysterious. Although many scholars believe that only humans are capable of weeping in response to emotional stimuli, others assert that animals — for example elephants — may do so, and have been seen weeping over the bodies of dead relatives. Tears shed in response to EMOTION have been reported to have a higher protein content than irritant tears. Such findings have led to suggestions that emotional tears are unique, that they might remove substances that accumulate in our bodies during stress; also that this could help to explain how we feel physically exhausted yet emotionally relieved after intense weeping and crying.

Western culture often connects the reasons we weep to what our weeping and tears communicate to others. Views from ancient Greece, medieval and early modern Europe, and modern Western societies involve highly preconceived notions of who should weep, why one weeps, when one weeps, and what weeping communicates to others. Despite the variations in cultures, the one theme that connects these vastly different time periods and their views of weeping is the perception that weeping is a language that enables people to communicate their emotional states without words.

In ancient Greece and Rome some physicians viewed tears as a humour of the body that was emitted when the body was not in balance. One wept copious tears to regulate the body's delicate balance of fluids, assuring good health. In ancient Greece women were also thought to weep more than men, since weeping was perceived to be a sign of emotional and physical weakness. The Greek protagonist Medea, in Euripides' play of that name, laments that women weep so much because they are considered weak creatures. This perception of women weeping more than men because they lack emotional and physical control persists to this day.

In both the Old and the New Testaments, weeping was performed collectively during mourning rituals to communicate sadness and to provide a controlled emotional release so that the community could begin to heal itself after a death. People also wept for their sins, hoping that their god would see and hear their tears and grant them forgiveness. The best known weeping figure in the New Testament is that of a woman weeping silently for her sins at the feet of Jesus, who responded to her tears and forgave her sins.

During the medieval and early modern periods in Western Europe, Christian theologians and other religious figures such as Augustine of Hippo and Bernard of Clairvaux viewed weeping and tears as signs of emotional and devotional states. Weeping was perceived to be the physical manifestation of states such as repentance, love of God, ecstasy and mystical joy, and confession. Medieval religious sources, such as the lives of saints, depict people like Francis of Assisi and Catherine of Siena as weeping during intense prayer or during a mass.

The most famous early modern weeper was the sixteenth-century Spaniard Ignatius of Loyola, whose copious tears filled the pages of his *Spiritual Diary*. He wept every day while praying and recorded all of his weepings to prove his religious devotion as well as to determine the best times during which to provoke his tears. As a good Roman Catholic, Ignatius viewed weeping as a physical sign of sorrow over sin and devotion to God. However, his *Spiritual Exercises* reveal his belief that weeping was not always a spontaneous act but could be learned and perfected in order to promote religious devotion and love of God.

Another sixteenth-century Spaniard, Juan Luis Vives, composed a treatise called *De anima et vita* (*Concerning the Soul and the Life*) in which he describes weeping and tears as the result of passions such as love. Like Ignatius of Loyola, he also considers tears to be gifts from God that demonstrate sorrow and compel others to have compassion for the weeper.

In his *Les Passions de l'âme* (*Passions of the Soul*) Descartes, like Vives, saw tears and weeping as the result of the passions. Unlike Vives, Descartes applied a more mechanistic explanation to the process of weeping in response to emotion. He viewed tears as a liquid that is formed from vapours in the eyes when one is agitated, just as sweat is a liquid that forms on the body when one exercises. He saw only two causes of tears when weeping. The first is when something enters the eye, causes pain, and thus changes the shape of the pore from which tears emanate, allowing more tears to flow. The second cause is sadness followed by love or joy. The initial sadness cools the blood but the subsequent joy or love sends more blood through the arteries, causing an increase in the amount of vapours in the eyes. Descartes thus envisioned a precise process in which the eyes react to the physical sensation of emotion within the body.

In eighteenth-century France both men and women were believed to weep in public while reading or seeing plays in the theatre. According to one modern scholar, their tears communicated the pleasure and pain they experienced, but also their desire to display publicly their heightened literary sensibilities. Physicians in eighteenth-century England believed that women's bodies were wetter than men's, causing them to emit more liquids, particularly tears. Weeping was still associated more with women than with men and this explanation provided a more 'scientific' reason for their penchant for weeping.

In his *Expression of Emotion in Man and Animals*, Charles Darwin used his observations of weeping children to assert that the tears they wept were due to the contraction of the muscles surrounding the eyes. Although he believed that strong emotions of any kind can cause these muscles to contract, generating tears, he did acknowledge that sometimes this happens without the presence of an emotion and can occur as a natural reflex action, as when coughing, vomiting, or when a foreign object enters the eye.

Darwin also included in his research popular nineteenth-century views of weeping. Men, he claimed, are much less likely to weep due to bodily pain since weeping is seen as a weak and unmanly behaviour. Furthermore, the insane weep very easily because they lack restraint. True to the cultural perceptions of his time, Darwin believed that weeping expresses pain and suffering in humans yet he also acknowledged that other cultures give a variety of meanings to this behaviour that do not conform to Western ideas. He saw this behaviour as both a physiological and a cultural phenomenon, and acknowledged that some animals may have the potential to weep tears due to strong emotions.

In its anatomical detail, the *lacrimal apparatus* is intricately suited to its function. The tear-secreting cells of the main *lacrimal glands* form structures described as about the size and shape of an almond, tucked into a recess of bone behind the outer side of each upper eyelid. The fluid flows thence through ducts to reach the conjunctival surface. There are also multiple smaller glands, which back up the function of the main one. Drainage is through two pores, one at the inner end of each eyelid, leading to the lacrimal sac, which drains in turn into the NOSE. In addition to this provision for continual wetting and drainage, any tendency for fluid to overflow is countered by the secretion from a row of 'tarsal glands' embedded in both upper and lower eyelids, that spreads along their edges, with an anti-wetting effect. The lacrimal glands receive nerve fibres from both the sympathetic and parasympathetic branches of the AUTONOMIC NERVOUS SYSTEM, providing pathways for the control of basic and reflex secretion, and the link to the BRAIN and the emotions.

LYN A. BLANCHFIELD
SHEILA JENNETT

Further reading
Frey, W. H. (1985). *Crying: the mystery of tears*. Winston Press, Minneapolis.

Vincent-Buffault, A. (1991). *The history of tears: sensibility and sentimentality in France*, (trans. T. Bridgeman). St Martin's Press, New York.

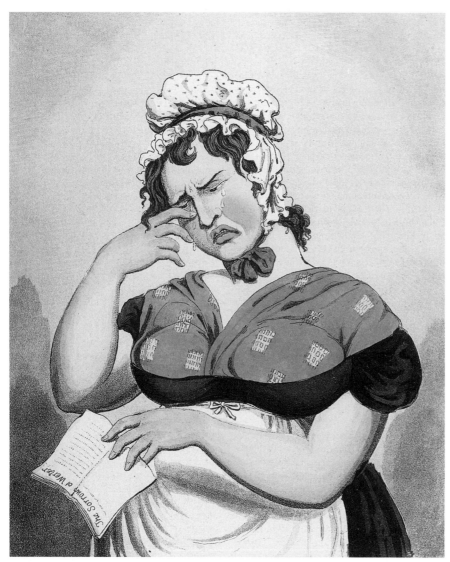

A woman reduced to tears on reading Goethe's *The sorrow of Werther*, c. 1800. Mary Evans Picture Library.

Weightlessness The condition in which a mass possesses no weight, as in the absence of gravitational or accelerative forces, or when the vector sum of opposing forces or fields acting upon it is zero. The state is produced during space flight when the accelerative force due to gravity is exactly balanced by the tangential and inertial forces associated with the motion of the spacecraft through space.

Weightlessness — or microgravity, as it is frequently termed — has major effects on the movement of man in space and upon his physiology. The condition can be produced for only very short periods of time on earth. It exists during the initial stages of free fall through the atmosphere and can be generated for 12–40 second during parabolic flight in an aircraft. J.E.

See FLYING; G AND G-SUITS; SPACE TRAVEL.

Werewolf The werewolf (Old English: *wer*, a man + *wulf*, a wolf) or lycanthrope is one of the most familiar monsters of European mythology. It has stalked the popular imagination from antiquity through to modern times. In classical literature, the werewolf was usually depicted as the victim of a divine or hereditary curse. In Plato's *Dialogues*, King Lykaos of Arcadia was changed into a wolf by Zeus after he attempted to trick the gods into eating human flesh. When Pausanias repeated this tale in the second century AD this curse had been transformed into a racial characteristic. He believed that Arcadia was a nation of werewolves, whilst Virgil and Herodotus identified the Neurians of north east Europe as a lycanthrope tribe.

This early conception of the lycanthrope as a victim of heredity left the monster in a morally ambiguous position. The werewolf could be a benign individual, trapped within a bestial frame. In the Eastern and Celtic churches, St Christopher was often portrayed as a dog-headed convert, a representative of Cynocephali who inhabited the mountain ranges of Northern India. In the medieval romances of *William and the Werewolf* by Guillaume de Palerne and *Laide Bisclaveret*, by Mavie de France, the werewolves appear as noble favourites of the king, tricked into a wolf form by their adulterous wives, and later redeemed into humanity through royal kindness. As late as the seventeenth century the belief that werewolves could serve as 'dogs of God' persisted amongst the Russian and Baltic peasantry. The Italian historian Carlo Ginzburg has reconstructed the trial of one Livonian werewolf, Thiess, who claimed he and his werewolf companions travelled annually to the underworld to protect the harvest from the Devil and sorcerors.

For the most part however, werewolves have been depicted as malign and demonic creatures. The Paschal imagery of Christ as the Lamb of God encouraged the wolf's satanic associations. In post-Reformation Europe, the werewolf was largely seen as a male counterpart of the witch, obtaining his power through a pact made with the devil. Peter Stump, the most notorious werewolf of the sixteenth century, began his lycanthropic career of mass murder, rape, and incest after Satan presented him with a magical wolf skin. His crimes were apparently emulated by thousands of others. Recent authors have claimed that there were 30 000 recorded cases of werewolves between 1520 and 1630 in France alone. Such high estimates must be questioned in light of the recent revisionist historiography of the witch craze.

Post-reformation Europe also saw a growing attempt to medicalize the werewolf. Physicians such as Simon Goulart, Johannes Schrenk von Graftenberg, and Robert Burton claimed that lycanthropy was a form of delusional insanity brought about through an excess of black bile. The condition was epitomized by the madness of Duke Ferdinand in John Webster's *Duchess of Malfi*. Ferdinand is apprehended clutching a human leg and howling at the MOON. As his captors explain, the Duke '[s]aid he was a wolf,

only the difference/Was a wolf's skin was hairy on the outside/His on the inside'. Similar attempts to explain lycanthropy as a delusion rooted in illness have been repeated throughout the twentieth century. Authors have variously suggested congenital hypertrichosis (abnormal HAIR growth), *rabies canina*, and ergot poisoning as possible pathological causes. More recently, Dr Lee Illis, of Guy's Hospital, London, has claimed that werewolves may be victims of porphyria, a disease which results in photosensitivity, reddening of the teeth, and nervous disorders.

With the appearance of novels such as George Reynolds' *Wagner the Werewolf* (1857) or Dudley Costello's *Lycanthropy in London or the Wehrwolf of Wilton Crescent* (1859), more psychological accounts of the werewolf emerged. In these works, the wolf-man emerges as a kind of romantic anti-hero, torn between social mores and carnal desire. These moral struggles were repeated in the Hollywood B-movies of the 1950s. Films such as American International's *I was a Teenage Werewolf* (1957) or Royal's *Werewolf in a Girls' Dormitory* (1962), presented the lycanthrope as a sympathetic character, led into a life of unbridled lust after attending beat gatherings and bongo parties. This model of the werewolf as a figure in which adolescents could identify their own awkward passions persists to this day. The title track of Michael Jackson's *Thriller* (1983), the world's best selling pop album, focused on the emotional and sexual difficulties of a pubescent lycanthrope.

Through its popular associations with SEX and VIOLENCE, the werewolf has become a rich symbol for man's bifurcated human nature. Modern academics see lycanthropy as a fantasy which reveals fundamental aspects of modern personality. The Jungian anthropologist, Robert Eisler, thought that werewolves emerged through an ancestral memory of man's transition from fruit-gatherer to hunter. Man's identification with carnivorous animals, Eisler claimed, was a psychic operation that allowed him to conquer his disgust at killing. This identification could still be seen in hunting groups such as the leopard men of East Africa, Operation Werewolf (a post-war Nazi resistance organization), and British Guards Regiments who continue to decorate themselves with leopard pelts and bearskins.

Sigmund Freud offered a much more reductionist explanation for man's lupine identification. In his study of Wolf-Man, a young Russian whose childhood had been tormented by dreams of wolves that beckoned him from beyond his bedroom window, Freud suggested that the fantasy must be rooted in a primal scene of parental or animal sex. The French philosophers Gilles Deleuze and Felix Guattari contested this interpretation of the dream. They argued that the lupine fantasy could be seen as a fundamental challenge to Western notions of subjectivity. It was a dream in which man cast off his atomic individuality, as the lycanthrope surrendered to the multiplicity of the wolf pack.

RHODRI HAYWARD

Further reading
Douglas, A. (1992). *The beast within: man, myths and werewolves*. Chapmans, London.
Woodward, I. (1979). *The werewolf delusion*. Paddington press, New York and London.

See also VAMPIRE.

Wet-nursing means breastfeeding an infant that is not one's biological offspring. For infants whose mothers cannot or will not suckle them, wet-nursing offers the greatest chance for survival and thus wet-nursing practices influence infant mortality rates and consequently the demographic and economic structure of societies. Wet-nursing customs reflect social arrangements and cultural values, illustrating how individuals, families, communities, and the state respond to the needs of infants and the biological capacities of women.

There are, essentially, four types of wet-nursing arrangements. Informal wet-nursing ranges from the occasional nursing of another woman's child to a private arrangement to suckle a baby whose mother is ailing or who has died. Such practices are hard to document and quantify, but undoubtedly informal wet-nursing was historically the most widespread and most common arrangement. In these cases women may have nursed their own babies along with the suckling. A second form of unpaid wet-nursing involved the use of slave women. Slaves suckled the offspring of patrician families at the height of the Roman Empire, and they suckled the children of plantation owners in the Americas in the eighteenth and early nineteenth centuries.

Commercial wet nurses received remuneration from individual employers. There are references to these arrangements in the Code of Hammurabi, in the Biblical story of *Exodus* (where the daughter of Pharaoh sends her slave to hire a wet nurse for the baby Moses and ends up hiring the child's own mother — so not a true instance of wet-nursing), and in the *Koran*, which forbade marriage among individuals described as milk-kin. Evidence of commercial wet-nursing also appears in laws and contracts, as well as in medical books, and together these sources document the extensive employment of wet nurses in Europe in the sixteenth to the nineteenth centuries — the heyday of the commercial wet nurse. In some cases, families sent their infants to live with wet nurses in the country — but sucklings might not survive if the wet nurses favoured their own babies. In other instances, wet nurses abandoned their own infant and went to live in the home of their employer — and it was then the wet nurses' infants who paid the highest price. As the heroine of George Moore's 1894 novel *Esther Waters* noted of wet nurses 'It is our babies that die, it is life for a life.'

The fourth type of wet-nursing developed when the Church and the State employed wet nurses to suckle foundlings in institutions created for saving souls and lives. Often the women were not paid, but were themselves the recipients of charity or welfare — receiving room and board in return for their suckling of abandoned babies as well as their own offspring. Generally these arrangements failed, at least in terms of saving infant lives. The women coerced into wet-nursing had little incentive to save the lives of the sucklings they were forced to care for, and perhaps little ability to do so, given the harsh conditions under which they lived and the meagre diets they received.

The failures of congregate wet-nursing and the high cost of private commercial arrangements encouraged the search for alternatives. Artificial infant foods — most commonly milk from animals — had always been an alternative, but only in the nineteenth century did relatively safe, digestible products become widely marketed. The use of commercial infant formulae undermined the custom of wet-nursing in much of the developed world and later would lead to a decline of breast-feeding in the developing world. Other factors also played a role in this transition, among them changes in medical practice, evolving customs of infant care, the growth of non-domestic employment opportunities for women, and the recognition of the high mortality rate of the wet nurses' infants. Since the late twentieth century, infants in Western nations who have needed breast milk to survive and who could not obtain it from their mothers have received relief in the form of bottled human milk supplied by a milk bank, stocked by mothers who have had milk to spare. Wet-nursing as a form of service labour has been replaced by milk selling and/or milk donation, a transaction in which human milk has become a commodity.

JANET GOLDEN

Further reading

Fildes, V. (1988). *Wet nursing: a history from antiquity to the present*. Basil Blackwell, Oxford.

See also BREASTS; INFANT FEEDING.

Whistling is familiar as the production of a series of high-pitched sounds that form a simple melody or tuneful sequence. Together with humming it may be presumed to be the simplest form of music making, in particular for self amusement, and as such revealing the emotional state of mind of the whistler. The sound of the human whistle, like that in the most primitive instrumental forms — a whistle fashioned from a hollow tube of wood or straw — is made by the turbulence generated in an airstream at the narrow orifice formed by pursing the lips. The pitch and harmonic content of the sound is modulated by the relative position and shape of the tongue and its relation to the lower teeth. And for a particularly loud whistle used as a call, the lips are braced firmly against the teeth, and the tongue deeply arched so that airflow is directed across the sharp edges of the teeth and through the narrow, stiffened aperture at the lips. Unlike vocalization, the whistle is generated by inspiratory as well expiratory flows of air, allowing legato-like sounds to be produced without interruption.

Whistling appears to be a male-dominated activity, perhaps deriving from ancient forms of the 'wolf whistle' denoting sexual attraction; this is just one example of the use of the whistle as a call sign, with its obvious links to ancestral 'call' signals in lower species, and its 'imitative' value in hunting or for summoning a trained hound. The whistling of an improvised or familiar tune by a contented man or woman at work, even of the Seven Dwarfs who proclaim 'we whistle while we work', can be contrasted to the variety of other whistles, expressing incredulity, surprise, or appreciation. The latter communicate information about the emotional state solely through the sound pattern, while the former carry the additional symbolic meaning relating to the words in the whistled song, thus encompassing both the mental and the emotional life of the whistler.

TOM SEARS

See also SINGING; SPEECH.

White matter That part of the NERVOUS SYSTEM which is composed mainly of the fibres or *axons* of nerve cells, most of which are covered by whitish, fatty sheaths (composed of MYELIN), hence appearing white in freshly-cut BRAIN or SPINAL CORD. The axons in the white matter are responsible for conducting information from and to the nerve cell bodies that are concentrated in the GREY MATTER.

L. J. G.

See MYELIN; NERVES.

Witchcraft can be roughly defined as the power of a person to do harm or influence nature through occult means. It has been believed in by most known cultures. Indeed, the fact that belief in witchcraft and magic has largely been rejected in post Enlightenment Europe and North America could be seen as one of the distinguishing features of the cultures of those continents in modern times.

In its historical dimension, witchcraft is most familiar in the light of the period of the witch persecutions in western and central Europe, between 1450 and 1750. Gaps in records preclude precision, but the best current estimates suggest that some 40 000 people, perhaps 80% of them women, were executed for witchcraft between these dates. (The claim that there were nine million witch executions is now rejected as a wild over-estimate.) Witchcraft as a historical phenomenon continues to attract wide interest, and has also attracted a high degree of serious scholarly attention.

This interest and attention has created a plethora of approaches to and interpretations of witchcraft, but it is only very recently that these have overtly addressed issues related to the history of the body. Certainly, there has been a degree of interest in the medical aspects of witchcraft. Physicians were frequently called in to attend the suspected victims of bewitchment, and a number of them wrote tracts on the subject. Perhaps the most famous was Johann Weyer, court physician to the Duke of Cleves, who in 1563 published *De*

Praestigiis Daemonum, a tract which, while not denying the existence of witchcraft, argued that most cases of supposed witchcraft were, in fact, the outcome of natural causes or of trickery. More recently, writers within the women's movement of the 1970s argued that the witch-persecutions of the late medieval and early modern periods were the outcome of an emergent male-dominated medical profession attacking female healers in general or, more particularly, midwives. This interpretation has been discredited, but the broader issue of the interface between medical practice and witchcraft remains largely unexplored.

Perhaps the key to placing witchcraft within the history of the body will be provided by the investigation of two sets of problems. The first of these is the question of the source of the power of the witch and where it was thought to reside; the second is the rather better documented phenomenon of the physical sufferings supposedly undergone by victims of witchcraft and, more particularly, of witchcraft-induced demonic possession.

Certainly, the research carried out by anthropologists on witchcraft has provided ample evidence of beliefs which locate the power to bewitch in the physical body of the witch. Perhaps the fullest description of this phenomenon came with a famous early study, E. E. Evans-Pritchard's analysis, based on three periods of fieldwork carried out between 1926 and 1930, on witchcraft, magic, and oracles among the Azande, a people living in the Sudan. The Azande thought, as did many other peoples in western and central Africa, that witchcraft existed physically as a substance in the bodies of witches. The exact details of this substance and its location varied, but it was most commonly held that it took the form of an oval brackish swelling or 'bad' that was joined to the edge of the liver of the witch. Thus proof that a person was a witch might take the form of a public autopsy of the suspect's body after death, performed in the presence of the deceased's relatives and, blood-brothers, and important members of the local community.

This type of evidence is less overt in historical materials, and at present much of the thinking on this range of issues remains speculative. It is clear that witchcraft was in some ways conceived of as a form of power which ran between the body of the witch and her victim, and thus notions about witchcraft in this period were connected with ideas about the body, and especially the female body. The medical theory of the day, with its attachment to the importance of humours, made it easy to see the body as a type of vessel in which there might be forces which could get out of hand, were the humoural balance to be upset.

Perhaps these forces were at their most unruly when the witch changed her shape, as many cultures believed was possible. Many early accounts of witchcraft touch on this (and there is the connected issue of *lycanthropy*, the form of witchcraft in which humans were supposed to assume the form and nature of wolves). It was a recurrent theme when, in the nineteenth century, folklorists collected tales of witchcraft. In England, in particular, it was still held at that time that witches were able to change themselves into hares. Other witchcraft beliefs demonstrate the importance of the body of the witch. The counter measures aimed at combating witchcraft often involved sympathetic magic that was aimed at hurting the witch physically. Perhaps the most striking example of this was the witch cake. This was typically made of some sort of flour (and sometimes other substances) mixed with the urine of the person supposedly suffering from witchcraft, and thrown onto a fire. The idea was that the process would cause unbearable pain in the urinary system of the witch, who would reveal her identity by coming to destroy the source of her discomfort. It was also widely held that the witch's victim would gain relief by scratching the witch on the face and drawing blood.

The body of the witch was meant to carry the witch's mark. This normally took the form of an excrescence or area of skin that was insensible to pain, or a supernumerary teat from which the witch's familiar spirit, which normally took an animal form, was thought to suck blood. Thus the body of the witch might be subjected to penetration by bodkins or needles as the insensible spot was sought, or to searches for the teat, which was generally expected to be located on the suspected woman's genitals or anus.

If the body of the witch showed peculiar manifestations, so too, on the evidence of some of the better documented cases, did the body of the witch's supposed victim. We have numerous descriptions of the sufferings allegedly caused by bewitchment, descriptions that, for the most part, await analysis by modern doctors or psychiatrists. These descriptions are especially rich, and the symptoms they record especially puzzling for the modern reader, when contemporaries thought the problem involved the POSSESSION of the body of the sufferer by demons sent into them by the witch. Many modern readers will be familiar with such celebrated incidents as the possession of a whole convent of young nuns at Loudun in France in the 1630s, or the crucial role played by a group of supposedly possessed young girls in the witch-scare at Salem, Massachusetts, in 1692. But these are merely two well-known examples of a phenomenon which was widespread in Europe in the sixteenth to eighteenth centuries. In England, for example, the possession of several children at Warboys in Huntingdonshire, which resulted in the execution of three witches in 1592, created a model of possession through witchcraft that survived for at least another century. The possessed demonstrated clear symptoms: convulsions, contortions, trances, vomiting of foreign bodies (notably pins), speaking with the voice of the possessing demons, and becoming unnaturally strong or unnaturally heavy.

Perhaps the deepest analysis of such possessions has been carried out by the historian Lyndal Roper, on sixteenth-century materials relating to the German city of Augsburg. Here the crucial issue was the changes in attitudes which the Reformation had created towards the relationship between the FLESH and the spirit, with both Catholics and Protestants developing rival theologies of the body. Protestantism weakened the links between the physical and the divine, and therefore forced a revision of the theological understanding of the body. The exorcism of people thought to be possessed by demons, frequently at the instigation of the witch, therefore became an area of dispute between the two sides in the local religious struggle. The fact that most of the supposedly possessed were women added another dimension: the possessed women, as they contorted in their beds as a result of the attentions of male demons, bore strong resemblance to women lost in lust. Analysis of such cases, therefore, introduces medical, theological, and wider cultural attitudes towards the body through the inherently dramatic (and usually public) phenomena of possession and exorcism.   J.A. SHARPE

Further reading
Roper, L. (1994). *Oedipus and the Devil: witchcraft, sexuality and religion in early modern Europe.* Routledge, London and New York.

See also POSSESSION; WITCH DOCTOR; WITCH'S TIT.

Witch doctor In the genre of African colonial literature, the 'witch doctor' — Gagool in Rider Haggard's *King Solomon's Mines*, for example — serves as an allegory for the dark, sinister, forces of barbarism.

This is a gross distortion of the actual situation in Africa; where folk healers are highly respected, are linked to the benevolent ancestors, and work to ensure the well-being of their clients. In fact, the term 'witch doctor' is a misnomer. These functionaries neither doctor witches nor practice witchcraft, though they may occasionally act as witch-finders who smell out the secret workers of death and destruction. The term 'folk healer' is thus more appropriate.

In many parts of Africa the practice of folk healing incorporates two roles — that of the diviner and that of the herbalist.

Diviners
Diviners are experts in DIAGNOSIS who are called to the profession by the ancestors. Their calling is made manifest by the onset of persistent symptoms, which only yield once she or he undergoes formal initiation. To do so the person becomes an apprentice of an established diviner, and learns to trance so that the ancestors can speak through her or him. Though divination processes are diverse, set routines are followed. The diviner's body can become a vehicle for communication through spirit possession. Otherwise, some type of device is employed, from a simple sliding object to the myriad of symbolic items in a diviner's basket. A common method involves using divination dice. When thrown to the ground their combinations reveal specific meaning. Divinatory consultations occur in times of crisis, when there is insufficient practical information available to cope with life's hazards. In these situations diviners enable people to acquire otherwise inaccessible information by generating a shift to a contrary, paranormal, mode of cognition. Because the language of divination is cryptic, all revelations are translated and discussed. During this dialogue between the diviner and client, known facts are scrutinized in the light of a different perspective and old elements are reorganized into new arrangements. Diviners indicate the cause of misfortune, locate stolen property, identify witches, and recommend specific therapies. Sensitivity to the dynamics of personal relationships greatly enhances a diviner's success. While people are often sceptical of individual practitioners, most believe that the revelations of some diviners are true. People frequently consult more than one diviner, especially in cases of suspected witchcraft.

Herbalists
Herbalists undergo a more extensive apprenticeship, and have a vast knowledge of flora and fauna. Early in the twentieth century Shona healers used five hundred different medicinal plants, and also parts of animals, birds, insects, snakes, and fish. Herbalists deal with a wide range of medical, psychological, and social problems. Many therapies are based on practical knowledge, gained through experimentation. Southern African herbalists apply milk of the euphorbia to draw out deep-lying thorns and use wooden splints for broken limbs. They remove ritual pollution through BLOOD-LETTING, ENEMAS, and emetics. Other therapies follow the logic of symbolic association. For example, parts of scorpions are used to heal scorpion stings, and a tree with lumps on its trunk to treat patients with mumps. Medicines not only cure disorders of the body, but also protect babies from illness, ensure good luck, and help workers find employment. Folk healers among the Ndembu of Zambia aim to heal ruptured social relationships. In therapeutic rituals patients become the centre of social concern, kin and neighbours are encouraged to confess their feelings of ill-will, and events are related to wider cosmological frameworks. Zimbabwean healers appease the spirits of a murdered man by negotiating for the family of the slayer to pay a fine of cattle, or a young woman, in compensation for his death.

Studies show very high levels of patient satisfaction with treatment outcomes of folk healers, but have produced inconclusive results on the biomedical efficacy of folk healing. It is suggested that certain medicinal substances have positive pharmacological reactions. The bitter *ithethe* root, used by Zulu healers, is listed in the *British Pharmacopoeia* as an expectorant for chronic chest ailments. Researchers have found that Kenyan *wanganga* successfully cure 33% of patients who suffer from barrenness. This is seen as due to sound advice about sexual intercourse, the use of herbs which may relax the tubal musculature, and the performance of rituals that reduce stress which serves as an impediment to conception. On the other hand, purgatives used in folk healing have been shown to have deleterious side-effects. Existing research on this topic is clearly inadequate. It has proved difficult to extrapolate the findings of laboratory research to actual work on patients; longitudinal observation studies are based on too small sample sizes; and few studies have used randomized, blinded, controlled trails.

Folk healers continue to play a vital role in contemporary Africa, especially in societies undergoing rapid transition. Greater access to biomedicine has not undermined folk healing, since Africans view different types of healers as complementary resources. Illness may initially be explained in non-mystical terms, but if treatment fails, the diagnosis may change to witchcraft or to the ancestors, and recourse can be made successively to a biomedical doctor, diviner, and herbalist. According to one estimate there were some 10 000 *isangoma* in the South African city of Johannesburg in 1985, who were consulted at least occasionally by 85% of all black households. Some postcolonial states have legally recognized folk healers. In Zimbabwe, the Zimbabwe National Traditional Healer's Association (ZINATHA) supervises the practice of folk healing. ZINATHA has 312 branches, and some 24 000 registered 'traditional medical practitioners' and 'spirit mediums'. The Association cooperates with the Health Ministry, organizes workshops on primary health care and AIDS, cultivates medicinal plants, and runs schools for the study of traditional medicine. Similarly, the Rwandan state has pursued a policy of revalorizing 'traditional medicine' and has funded Clinics of Popular Medicine where patients consult folk healers of various specialities. In eastern Cameroon state courts have convicted witches, who are perceived as a threat to development, on the basis of testimony provided by diviners.

I. NIEHAUS

Further reading

Chavunduka, G. L. (1994). *Traditional medicine in modern Zimbabwe*. University of Zimbabwe Publications, Harare.

See also HEALING; HERBAL MEDICINE; SHAMANS.

Witch's tit

The 'witch's tit' or 'witch's mark' was considered proof of the witch's profession during the sixteenth and seventeenth centuries, when between 60 000 and 100 000 were condemned to death as witches by both Catholic and Protestant courts. In England and Scotland, it was common to appoint a man to search the suspect's body for the witch's tit, which was thought to be an extra teat from which an imp or devil, known as a 'familiar', presumably sucked the witch's blood as a form of nourishment. The 'witch pricker' was supposed to recognize a witch if she showed no feeling when he pricked the presumed teat with a pin or if this 'unnatural' protuberance did not bleed.

Trial records often included the depositions of witch prickers, who sometimes reported teats not only on the chest but elsewhere on the woman's body, including her genitals. The 'witch's tit' may have been merely a mole or a wart, a freckle or a blemish, or even a supernumerary NIPPLE, which occurs in approximately one out of two hundred women; but for susceptible minds, it was an aberrant breast, the sign that she had consorted with the devil and that she was a true witch.

Men, too, could be witches, but those accused of witchcraft were overwhelmingly female (80%), and predominantly old and poor. The witch-hunt was, according to historian Margaret King, a war waged by men against women, and what better symbol for that mysogynistic enterprise than the female breast, deformed and vilified under the rubric of the 'witch's tit'?

Witches' breasts — real or imagined — were often subject to humiliating and excrutiating treatment. They were commonly exposed at public whippings and mutilated in some of the more brutal cases. The case of Anna Pappenheimer, member of an outcast family of gravediggers and latrine cleaners in Bavaria around 1600, presents one of the most shocking examples. Tortured into confessing sexual relations with the devil and then condemned as a witch, she and three members of her family were burned at the stake. But before the final ordeal, Anna's breasts were cut off and forced into her mouth and then into the mouths of her two grown sons.

Witches' breasts are usually depicted in art as flat, hanging dugs; they represent the underside of Western EROTICISM, with its glorification of firm, youthful bosoms. The 'witch's tit', while not pictured in art works, has its own mythical lore, as found in old religious treatises, popular expressions, and even medical records. In the case of Anne Boleyn, Henry VIII's ill-fated wife accused of adultery, the rumour that she possessed a third breast — with its implications of witchcraft — was subsequently recorded in books of medical anomalies. To this day, the expression 'cold as a witch's tit' is still used to convey the hostility some men feel toward the female breast when it is not a source of pleasure or nurturance.

MARILYN YALOM

Further reading

King, M. L. (1991). *Women of the Renaissance*. University of Chicago Press, Chicago and London.

Barstow, A. L. (1994). *Witchcraze: a new history of the European witch hunts*. Pandora/HarperCollins, San Francisco.

Wolf-child

Interest in whether the essentials of being human are given to us by nature or by nurture has a long pedigree. So does a concern with distinguishing the human from the bestial. The Greek historian Herodotus, writing in the fifth century BC, told the story of twins brought up in isolation as an experiment to determine which language would be spoken 'naturally' by a child. One of the foundation myths of Rome, dating at least to the fourth century BC, claims that the twins *Romulus and Remus*, fathered by Mars, the god of war, were left to die by their wicked uncle, but were suckled by a wolf before being discovered by a herdsman and going on to establish the city of Rome. In Roman culture the wolf was sacred to Mars, and the cave of the she-wolf at the foot of the Palatine hill became a sacred place associated with the festival of the Lupercalia, which concerned fertility and ritual purification and survived until the end of the fifth century AD, when it was transformed into the feast of the Purification of the Virgin.

Romulus and Remus were destined to rule, and the story of their exposure to die is one of many in which the abandoned child comes back from the animal world to show that destiny cannot be averted. The myth did not, however, deal with the wider issue of whether our essential humanity can be lost. But many stories exist of children who spent years living with wild animals before being brought back into human civilization, where they needed to be taught to speak, to walk upright, to wear clothes, and to eat cooked foods. Interest in such events peaked in the eighteenth century; Wild Peter of Hanover was discovered in 1724, and Jean-Jacques Rousseau used the wolf-boy of Hesse, who lived in the wild for four years before being found in 1344, as the model for his 'natural man'. Carl Linnaeus included *Homo sapiens ferus* as a subdivision of *Homo sapiens* in later editions of his classification of living beings. In 1801 the physician Jean-Marc Itard published the case of the wild boy of Aveyron, later named 'Victor', who — as the chosen name suggests — successfully conquered the wildness of his habits and learned to walk and to speak. Itard used Victor to study the development of the senses. The famous case of two girls, Kamala and Amala, who were supposed to have been discovered living with wolves by the Revd Joseph Singh near Midnapore in the 1920s, remains controversial; with the anthropologist Robert Zingg, Singh published *Wolf-Children and Feral Man* (1942), but the loss of most of Singh's diary has fuelled speculation that although Kamala and Amala may have lived in the wild, they were not in fact raised by wolves. Singh and Zingg claimed that the wolf-children used parts of the body which are no longer used by 'civilized' people; for example, Kamala's ears are said to have trembled when she was afraid. Stories of feral children may be a way of accounting for autistic behaviours: Bruno Bettelheim has also argued that these stories show our wish to believe in a beneficent nature which cares for all creatures.

Other animals are alleged to have brought up human children; these include bears, sheep, pigs, cattle, and even leopards. Among fictional accounts, the most famous are Edgar Rice Burroughs' stories of *Tarzan*, which generated a series of films beginning with *Tarzan of the Apes*

(1918). For sixteen years, Tarzan was played by the Olympic swimming champion Johnny Weissmuller. An English aristocrat brought up by apes to become lord of the jungle, the original Tarzan shows that the natural superiority of the English upper classes even triumphs in the wild; in most of the Tarzan movies, however, he is a simple, gentle, and child-like man baffled by the unnecessary trappings of civilization. Here too, then, the motif of the child raised by animals can be used either to show the victory of human characteristics or to suggest the moral superiority of the animal kingdom.   HELEN KING

Work and the body

One need only look at the toll that industrialization has taken in the form of disease and injury during periods of massive industrialization to understand the destructive relationship between work and the body. As one observer noted in 1907, 'to the unprecedented prosperity … there is a seamy side of which little is said … Thousands of wage earners, men, women, and children, [are] caught in the machinery of our record breaking production and turned out cripples. Other thousands [are] killed outright,' he reported. 'How many there [are] none can say exactly, for we [are] too busy making our record breaking production to count the dead.' No discussion of the relationship between the body and work can begin without recognizing that the human body has long been conceived of as the basic production unit that has created wealth and capital. Hence, the creation of modern capitalism has led to attempts both to exploit the body through work and to maximize its potential as a producer of capital.

In very real ways, the methods and costs of production have been concretely mapped on to the human body. Broken limbs, crushed skulls, and crippling are, perhaps, the most obvious reflections of the costs of speed-ups, long hours of work, poor lighting, fatigue, 'red hot furnaces', and unsafe machinery. Early in the twentieth century it was estimated, for example, that 'A greater number of people are killed every year by so-called accidents than are killed in many wars of considerable magnitude.' The profound social effort to devalue the life of the industrial worker came at a time when traditional humanistic valuation of life and limb had placed a huge cost on producers, who found civil courts imposed harsh judgements for injury and death on the job. The 'death toll from industry' had become viewed as part of a the 'untold costs of progress', and part of a larger class struggle between workers and their employers. Especially in the first decades of this century, as the deaths and injuries in steel, mining, construction, foundries, and other modern American firms increased, the degrading of human life by measuring its worth in dollars and cents had the practical impact of lowering the costs of production. During World War II, more people were injured in the production of war materials than were injured at the front.

But injury is only one manifestation of the way that work is documented on the bodies of workers. Diseases, both acute and long-term, also reflect the changing methods of production and shifting threats created by new forms of social organization or work processes. For example, if EPIDEMIC diseases, borne by water, air, human contact, or insect vectors, were paradigmatic of nineteenth-century urban life, then short-term industrial POISONINGS and long-term industrially related illnesses were emblematic of the twentieth century's industrialization efforts. Devastating lung conditions such as silicosis, for example, gained in prevalence among working-class populations as high-speed pneumatic drills and jack hammers, sand-blasting equipment, and dynamite replaced the pick and shovel, hand polishing, and black powder in mining, milling, foundry work, granite cutting, and construction during the course of the twentieth century. Increase in the incidence of angiosarcoma of the liver, bladder cancers, and brain tumours among workers in the growing plastics and petrochemical industries during the course of the past half century may be attributable to exposure to toxic substances. The diseases we die from, to a significant degree, are a product of the work environment we create.

The horrendous cost of work to the human body has been rationalized to varying extents by materialist theories, explaining the body as little more than a mechanical entity which can be replaced through new hiring, easier immigration laws, or higher wages. Since at least the eighteenth century, there has been a growing popularity of mechanical metaphors describing complex biological and sociological processes, reducing them to physical interactions of springs, levers, molecules or, most recently, genes. In 1748, Julien Offray de la Mettrie conceptualized the human body as 'a machine which winds its own springs.' Seeking to impose a mechanistic schema on older theological and vitalistic understandings, he maintained that the body could be understood as a series of intermeshed gears, springs, and motors that, together, created a living organism. This type of reductionism has been a marker in Western biology and has been a continual point of contention.

Mechanistic ideas gained credibility as an explanatory model with the coming of the industrial age. The technological revolutions spurred a common belief that all forms of complex biological processes could ultimately be understood by reducing them to their molecular and physical levels. Similarly, the creation of a body of literature that supported a reductionist view of humans themselves lent increasing social legitimacy to this understanding of life. In 1911, for example, Frederick Winslow Taylor published his famous work on *The Principles of Scientific Management*, the highly influential manifesto that posited that all work could be broken down into discrete, interchangeable tasks and that workers could be taught to perform these specific discrete tasks efficiently. In effect, scientific management sought to reduce workers' bodies to interchangeable parts of machinery that could be replaced when broken. Challenging the prevailing system of production in which skilled labour itself controlled the speed and methods of production, Taylor, and the industrialists who adopted his scheme, sought to replace the brain of the worker. '[U]seful results have hinged upon (1) the substitution of a science for the individual judgement of the workman; (2) the scientific selection and development of the workman, after each man has been studied, taught, and trained, and one may say experimented with, instead of allowing the workmen to select themselves and develop in a haphazard way …' The implication of scientific management was that the common labourer was viewed at best as a beast of burden, one whose body was to be fitted to the industrial task, and, at worst, as a mechanical part of the production process that could be replaced at the behest of management: 'Now one of the very first requirements for a man who is fit to handle pig iron', Taylor maintained, '… is that he shall be so stupid and so phlegmatic that he more nearly resemble in his mental make-up the ox than any other type … [T]he grinding monotony of work of this character' would only utilize men 'unable to understand the real science of doing this class of work.'

By degrading work itself, and promoting a popular image of the workers as little more than an interchangeable part, management sought to win important political battles in its war with labour. The creation of a workers' compensation system that identified the value of lost limbs, lost eyes, and lost hearing provided further evidence of the way the body at work became a commodity. The adjustments of compensation in court cases according to age and potential earning capacity of the injured worker also tended to link the value of the human body to the work place. Finally, the linkage of private health insurance and Medicare to the workplace and employment history further undercut the autonomy of the body from work.

The body is a map of the insults foisted upon it by the workplace. It is also conceptually tied to mechanistic images borrowed from industrial production. The view of the liver as a filter, or the heart as a pump, the intestines as plumbing, or the brain as a computer all tend to reinforce the metaphor of man as a machine in service to machines.   DAVID ROSNER

Further reading

Markowitz, G. and Rosner, D. (2002) *Deceit and Denial: The Deadly Politics of Industrial Pollution*. University of California Press.

Proctor, R. N. (1991) *Cancer wars: how politics shapes what we know and don't know about cancer*. Basic Books, New York.

Rosner, D., and Markowitz, G. (ed) (1987) *Dying for work: workers' safety and health in twentieth century America*. University of Indiana Press, Bloomington.

See also ENVIRONMENTAL TOXICOLOGY; ERGONOMICS; PROTECTIVE CLOTHING; STRESS.

Wound healing You have a small cut on your face. The cut bleeds for a moment. After the bleeding stops, you can see a clot on the wound. In a few days, the wound is gradually surrounded by a reddened area, which then subsides in a week or so. The scab on the wound eventually sloughs off, exposing a regenerated area of the skin. This is a typical episode of wound healing in the SKIN.

Based on extensive studies of tissue INJURY and current knowledge of growth factor biology, four distinct phases of wound healing can be identified: inflammatory, migratory, proliferative — and late.

The *inflammatory phase* occurs in the first 24 hours. Platelets immediately form a plug by adhering to the COLLAGEN exposed by damage to blood vessels. The wound is then filled by a blood clot containing platelet aggregates, red blood cells, and white blood cells trapped in a fibrin meshwork. During blood clotting, aggregated platelets release chemicals that initially constrict blood vessels and prevent further bleeding. Subsequently, local blood vessels dilate, increasing the blood supply to the wound, bringing in the neutrophils — the white blood cells, which remove bacteria or other foreign materials. This acute INFLAMMATION hastens healing and is seen as reddening, swelling, and warmth around a wound.

In the *migratory phase*, fibroblasts and macrophages infiltrate the wound to initiate reconstruction. Polypeptide growth factors released from platelets stimulate the proliferation of fibroblasts at the site of a wound; these make the new fibres of collagen which will bridge the gap and form the scar. Macrophages begin to digest the blood clot. Under the influence of epidermal growth factor (EGF), epithelial cells advance across the clot to form a scab. It is interesting that the submandibular salivary glands are a major source of EGF. This provides a scientific basis for the expression 'licking one's wounds'.

In the *proliferative phase*, activated macrophages release substances including growth factors which stimulate sprouting from nearby capillary blood vessels. The capillary sprouts eventually join together to form a new network, with arterioles supplying them and venules draining them. This process is of prime importance to the success of wound healing, as it contributes to the metabolic demands of the damaged tissue; delivering nutrients, allowing gaseous exchange, and disposing of waste products.

In the *late phase*, fibroblasts continue to produce new and stronger collagen to remodel the scar while the epithelium on the surface heals. Excessive fibrous tissue formation in a healing skin wound may form a raised and ugly scar, known as *keloid*, especially if the edges of a wound have not been held together effectively.

In normal situations new blood vessel growth (angiogenesis) stops after completion of wound repair, and the new vessels may regress. However, inadequate or excessive angiogenesis often leads to problems. It can be inadequate for example, in limbs with poor circulation, where wounds may lead to gangrene and eventual amputation. In cancer, excessive angiogenesis enables tumours to grow and to metastasize to other parts of the body. For this reason, tumours have been coined 'wounds that never heal'.

There appear to be quantitative and qualitative differences in the angiogenic response in health and disease. It is possible that inadequate or excessive angiogenesis is the result of an imbalance between the production of angiogenic inducers and inhibitors, or due to differential expression of receptors for these molecules. Researchers are currently working to determine if there are indeed such differences. If so, these differences may provide future targets for pharmacological manipulations to enhance angiogenesis in chronic wounds or heart attacks. Conversely, it would be possible to suppress excessive angiogenesis in cancer and rheumatoid arthritis.

The powers of healing or regeneration vary from one tissue to another. The skin epithelium is not as efficient as the epithelia of the mucous membranes that line the gut and airways. For a skin injury, scar tissue is covered by epidermis, but specialized structures such as hair follicles and sweat glands are not regenerated. In contrast, complicated glandular structures of the stomach lining can and do regenerate after injury. In chronic septic ulcers, however, the damaged gastric epithelium does not heal — unless drug treatment is given to reduce gastric acid secretion, thus allowing growth factors to promote the healing process.

The liver is an exceptional organ, in that it can undergo complete and rapid regeneration in response to surgery or disease. A specific growth factor for liver cells is thought to stimulate their vigorous proliferation. Remarkably, after removal of 75% of the liver, the original mass can be restored in about two weeks. However, in chronic alcoholism or serious liver infections, excessive fibrous repair (*cirrhosis*) often outweighs regeneration, dividing the liver up into irregular islands. Such cirrhosis can lead to liver failure.

Wound healing can be affected by many factors, including medications and the state of health. Malnutrition delays healing; in particular, if the supply of vitamin C (ascorbic acid) is inadequate. Certain drugs (STEROIDS or anti-cancer drugs for example) can adversely affect the process. Kidney or liver failure, and poor circulation owing to arteriosclerosis, all delay healing. A high blood glucose concentration in diabetic patients can impair healing and predispose wounds to infection.   TAI PING FAN

See also BLOOD; INJURY; SCARS; SKIN.

Wrestling The modern sportive form of wrestling, an individual weaponless combat activity, probably developed in prehistory from survival fighting, when it became convenient to replace death or serious injury with a more symbolic victory. There is considerable evidence that wrestling existed in all early civilizations, although it was in ancient Greece that it really developed into a sport, and was included in the Olympic Games in 704 BC.

There is not one form of wrestling which is common throughout the world, but several different styles, which can be categorised into three basic types: *belt-and-jacket* styles, in which the clothing of the wrestlers — belt, jacket, or trousers — is used for grips; *catch-hold* styles, in which the wrestlers are required to grip each other prior to, and usually throughout the contest; and *loose styles*, in which the wrestlers, who can take any grip, apart from on clothing, are separated prior to the contest.

Wrestling styles can also be categorised according to five basic criteria required for a win. *Break-stance* involves forcing an opponent to relinquish a position; *toppling* involves forcing an opponent to touch the ground with a part of the body apart from the feet; *touch-fall* involves forcing an opponent into a specified position, usually supine, for a brief period; *pin-fall* involves holding an opponent, once thrown, in a specified position for a certain period of time; and *submission* involves forcing an opponent to admit defeat.

There are a number of notable national and local styles of wrestling. *Glima*, from Iceland, and *schwingen*, from Switzerland, are both belt styles, requiring toppling for victory; *kushti*, from Iran, is a catch-hold style, requiring a supine touch-fall; *yagli*, from Turkey, is a loose style requiring a supine touch-fall; *sumo*, from Japan, is a loose style requiring toppling; *Breton wrestling*, from Brittany, is a jacket style requiring a touch-fall. In Britain there are two notable local styles. *Cornish wrestling* is a jacket style requiring a touch-fall; *Cumberland and Westmorland wrestling* is a catch-hold style requiring toppling.

In international competition, there are only three styles of wrestling recognized by the Federation Internationale des Luttes Amateurs (FILA). Both *freestyle* and *Graeco-Roman* wrestling, which are the only styles fought in the Olympic Games, are loose styles requiring a touch-fall for victory. They differ in that the former allows any fair hold, throw, or trip, whereas the latter does not permit wrestlers to hold below the hips, nor to grip with the legs. There are ten weight divisions in both styles for international competition; light flyweight, flyweight, bantamweight, featherweight, lightweight, welterweight, middleweight, light heavyweight, heavyweight, and super heavyweight. The third style recognised by FILA is a synthesis of styles native to the former Soviet Union called *sambo*; the word is composed of the first three letters of the word *samozash-chita* (self defence) and the initial letters of *bez oruzhiya* (without weapons). It is a combination of loose and jacket styles requiring a submission for victory.

There are two further styles of wrestling worthy of note. *Inter-collegiate wrestling*, which is practised only in American colleges, is broadly similar to the freestyle and Graeco-Roman styles, apart from the points system. *Professional wrestling*, based on freestyle, is more accurately defined as a form of entertainment, rather than a sport, owing to its 'choreographed' moves.

M. TRIPP

Further reading

Arlott, J. (1976). *The Oxford companion to sports and games*. Oxford University Press, Oxford.

See also BOXING; MARTIAL ARTS; SPORT.

Wrinkles are folds and creases in the SKIN. In ageing skin, the normal process of proliferation and organization of skin cells breaks down, the skin thins, and the tidy columns of cells characterizing the young, healthy EPIDERMIS (outer skin) become disarrayed. COLLAGEN fibres, which are found in the *dermis* and which help to maintain the integrity of the skin, decrease in density, number, and organization, while the smooth and ribbon-like *elastin fibres*, which are also found in the dermis and which enable the skin to regain its normal shape after stretching, become coarser, denser, and less resilient.

Wrinkles have *intrinsic* and *extrinsic* causes. The intrinsic cause is a genetically-programmed senescence in which the skin reaches a point when MEMBRANE RECEPTORS in the cells no longer respond to growth factors stimulating DNA replication and cell division. Thus, with age, skin cells lose their ability to proliferate, and generation time lengthens. There is no way to prevent these developments. Extrinsic causes include exposure to *smoking* and *sunlight*. Premature wrinkling increases with cigarette consumption. UVB light damages amino acids (the building blocks of the proteins, enzymes, and nucleic acids), affects various kinds of skin cells, and can cause any single cell to become a high-energy 'singlet' which releases energy that may break chemical bonds, initiating skin damage within 3 minutes of exposure of previously unexposed skin. Sun screens and the general avoidance of sunlight help to prevent *photo-ageing*.

People have considered wrinkles highly undesirable for millennia. An ancient Egyptian treatment for wrinkles was a mixture of incense, wax, olive oil, *cyperus*, and milk, applied for 6 days. A 1713 recipe book advised a distillation of a blend of the flowers of elder, Fleur-de-lis, mallows, and beans, added to the pulp of melon, honey, and the white of eggs, to remove wrinkles, Not so safe were treatments such as an arsenic complexion wafer and an arsenic soap to treat skin blemishes,

wrinkles, and sallow skin, advertised in *Vogue* in 1908. It is doubtful that any of these treatments had lasting success — so women, and sometimes men, resorted to cosmetics. In the sixteenth, seventeenth, and eighteenth centuries in particular, some women concealed wrinkles with thick paint that often contained poisonous substances such as mercury and white lead.

Modern treatments for wrinkles range from *alpha-hydroxy-acid creams*, which promote the shedding of the outer skin layer, to surgical face lifts, which smooth wrinkles through tightening and removing excess skin. One promising skin application is *retinoic acid*, a synthetic derivative of vitamin A, which reduces fine wrinkles, sloughs off outer layers, and causes collagen to reaccumulate, thickening the moisture-conserving skin fibres. Though collagen molecules in creams are too large to be absorbed, collagen may be injected into the skin to smooth wrinkles.

KRISTEN L. ZACHARIAS

Further reading

Corson, R. (1972). *Fashions in makeup from ancient to modern times*. Universe Books, New York.

See also AGEING; SKIN; SUN AND THE BODY.

Wrist The joint between the end of the forearm and the hand. Confusion can arise because a 'wrist' watch is actually worn above the wrist (it would be both inconvenient and uncomfortable

to wear a watch over the joint itself). Movements occur in two planes — flexion/extension and adduction/abduction (inward/outward). This is a relatively complex joint as it is an articulation between the lower end of the long bones of the forearm (*radius* and *ulna*) and the eight small bones of the hand (*carpal bones*). These carpal bones are connected to one another by ligaments so that they form an arch, concave towards the palm, with its ends connected by a fibrous tissue band. Through this 'tunnel' run long tendons which control the fingers and, more importantly, the median nerve which carries the nerve supply to some muscles of the hand and to the skin of some of the fingers. This arrangement can present problems; the sheaths of the tendons can become inflamed and swollen thereby compressing the median nerve, leading to loss of sensation of the thumb, index, and middle fingers and loss of fine co-ordinated movements of the thumb (*carpal tunnel syndrome*). This can result from repetitive movements when using machinery, and the condition has become recognized as a form of industrial injury. Because of the reflex protective outstretching of the hand during a fall, the wrist is a common site of injury, often sprains. Fractures of the ends of the radius and ulna also occur (*Colles fracture*), particularly in elderly women with OSTEOPOROSIS.

WILLIAM R. FERRELL

See also HANDS; JOINTS; SKELETON.

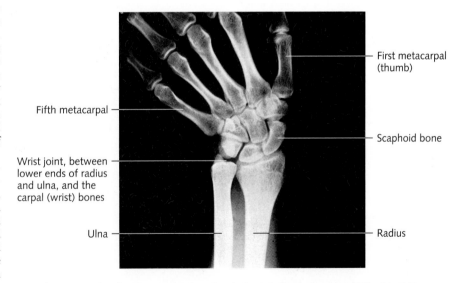

X-ray of wrist. Reproduced, with permission, from *Cunningham's textbook of anatomy* (12th edn), OUP.

First metacarpal (thumb)

Fifth metacarpal

Scaphoid bone

Wrist joint, between lower ends of radius and ulna, and the carpal (wrist) bones

Ulna

Radius

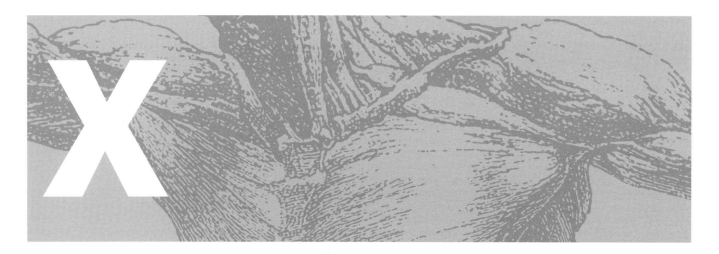

X

X-rays Wilhelm Conrad Röntgen, Professor of Physics in Wurzburg, Bavaria, accidentally discovered X-rays in November 1895 while studying cathode rays in a low pressure gas discharge tube. Alone in his laboratory on a Friday evening, he placed his hand in the path of the invisible rays which he was investigating, and saw an image of the bones on the screen beyond. Later, using a photographic plate instead of a screen, he made the first X-ray photograph — of his wife's hand, her wedding ring clearly visible. This was a highly significant breakthrough in the history of medicine because it made so many other things possible. It opened a window to what goes on in our bodies and in our heads. While news flashed round the world and most read of the discovery in the newspapers, Röntgen sent copies of his

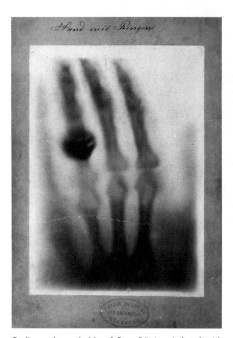

Radiograph, probably of Frau Röntgen's hand with a ring taken by Röntgen on 22 December 1895. Wellcome Institute Library, London.

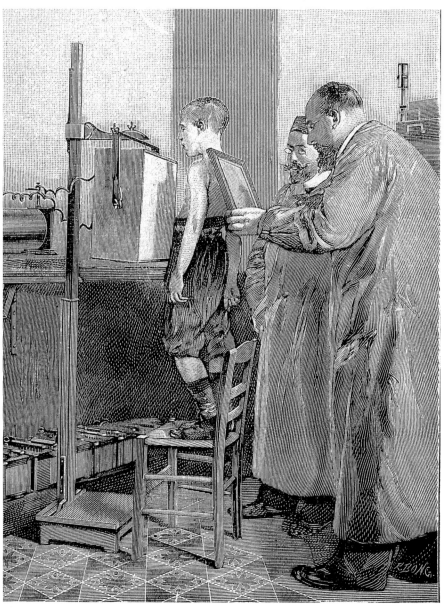

Röntgen examines a patient. From a German popular scientific book of 1896. Mary Evans Picture Library.

scientific paper to only two people in Britain: Lord Kelvin in Glasgow, for whom he had the highest esteem, and Professor Shuster in Manchester. Kelvin passed his copy to Dr John Macintyre, 'Medical Electrician' at the Glasgow Royal Infirmary. Like many others — physicists, electrical engineers, and doctors — in those early hectic days, and perhaps the most energetic of all the medical pioneers, Macintyre quickly grasped the significance of this 'new light' as it was then known. His X-ray department was up and running by March 1896 — one of the first radiological departments in the world. He subsequently had many other 'firsts': an X-ray of a kidney stone, a halfpenny in the gullet of a child, and, most spectacular, a 'cineradiogram' showing movements of a frog's legs. He probably did not produce the first medical radiograph in Britain: this is attributed to another Scot, Campbell Swinton, electrician and photographer in London, who also gave the first public demon-

stration of X-rays to the Royal Photographic Society in February 1896 — just one day before an open-air demonstration by a Birmingham GP, Hall-Edwards; he was also one of the first to apply X-rays to diagnosis: in that same month he took a photograph which located a needle in a woman's hand. There followed a distinct move to treat these new rays as public entertainment, but while some treated Röntgen's discovery with a certain hilarity and scepticism, like a freak show, the medical profession quickly recognized its potential. In the months following the news, scientists and doctors on both sides of the Atlantic were among the earliest pioneers working feverishly to reproduce X-rays and *radiographs* (medical X-ray photographs). Among the first medical radiologists, along with John Macintyre, were Sidney Rowland, who demonstrated X-rays to the Medical Society of London, and greatly advanced the cause whilst an undergraduate scholar in 1896 at St Bartholomew's Hospital;

and Francis H. Williams in Boston, MA, who published a book in 1902 on the diagnostic and therapeutic use of X-rays, and in the 1920s wrote of his reminiscences as a pioneer.

The X-rays were also called 'skiagrams' (coined by Rowland) or 'shadows' at that time. When Röntgen observed the 'new light' he called it an X-ray, because it had been unknown; the name has persisted, although the deservedly eponymous alternative, Röntgen ray, is also used.

During the first two decades, the use of X-rays spread widely, mainly to define fractures and foreign bodies such as bullets — first in the Boer War and later in World World War I. Screening, or *fluoroscopy* (allowing the doctor to view the patient under X-ray, without taking a 'still' photograph), was a frequent alternative to radiographs. At that time electricity supplies were unstable and, before examining the patient, radiologists, or their technical assistants, radiographers, would place their own hands in the X-ray

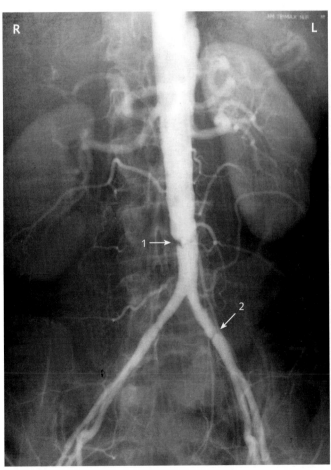 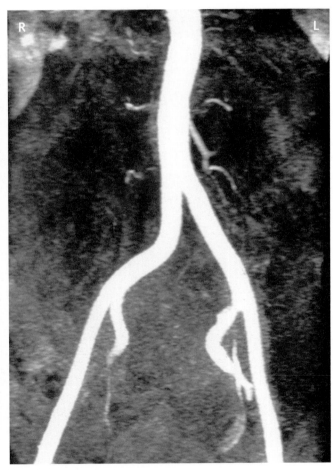

(Left) Aortic arterial disease revealed by X-ray (angiogram). Contrast medium has been injected through a fine catheter passed up the artery from the right groin. The X-ray of the contrast medium outlining the central arteries shows arterial disease at the bifurcation of the aorta (where the supply to the two legs separates): there is a shelf of *atheroma* both in the aorta (arrow 1) and in the left common iliac artery (arrow 2). The area between these is also diffusely diseased. Whilst such disease is common in cigarette smokers, this particular pattern is typical in women who develop arterial disease around the time of the menopause. **(Right) MRI scan of a normal aorta, for comparison.** A magnetic resonance scan that shows no disease around the bifurcation. This technique avoids using X-rays and invasive catheters to demonstrate the arteries. MRI also uses contrast medium to image the blood vessels: a paramagnetic agent is injected into an arm vein and is detected by the MRI scanner as it passes through the arteries (see IMAGING TECHNIQUES). (Courtesy of Dr Allan W. Reid, Glasgow Royal Infirmary.)

beam as a test for optimum exposure. Little was appreciated of the dangers of X-rays and protection was unknown, but the hazards all too soon became apparent. Frequent exposure led to radiation burns, loss of fingers, and fatal skin cancers. A Martyr's Memorial was erected in Hamburg in 1936 by the German Röntgen Society, inscribed with the names of 169 X-ray and radium martyrs from 15 countries who by then had died; the highest tolls recorded were 14 British, 20 German, 39 American, and 40 French. Twenty-eight more British names were later added. It was not until the 1920s that any protective requirements became obligatory, although some steps had been taken earlier — notably, the London Hospital in 1908–9 was among the first to provide protection for operators.

While the specialty of RADIOLOGY has undergone incredible changes and now incorporates a wide range of IMAGING TECHNIQUES, X-rays remain the cornerstone, accounting for a least 60–80% of all diagnostic imaging examinations. In all such systems X-rays are produced in a glass vacuum tube by electrons striking a tungsten target. The resulting beam of X-rays, invisible to the eye, directed at the part being examined, passes through the patient's body. Various structures absorb the X-ray photons differentially: bones more than soft tissues; other organs and tissues such as muscle producing shadows of varying intensity. The image is recorded by a detection device, either a fluorescent screen (*screening*) or photographic film (*radiography*). However, using X-rays alone it is not possible to distinguish between soft tissues of the same density, and to do this various liquid or gaseous *contrast media* are used. The American physiologist Walter Cannon (1871–1945) was a pioneer in this field who devised this way, now in routine diagnostic use, of examining the internal workings of the body without recourse to surgical interference. He utilized the newly discovered X-rays to examine the passage of food which had been mixed with a radio-opaque substance through the gut of humans and experimental animals. He was initially interested in the mechanisms of SWALLOWING, but subsequently, using a range of foods, he analysed the mechanical properties of every region of the gut. Pictures of the 'J' shape of the stomach and pylorus during gastric emptying were originally traced onto lavatory paper held over the Röntgen screen: they are still the classic illustrations used in many textbooks.

Barium is used by mouth to outline the stomach (BARIUM MEAL), or per rectum to outline the large bowel (barium enema). Water-soluble contrast media can be injected into BLOOD VESSELS or the chambers of the HEART to produce an *angiogram* (see figure), or to be excreted by the kidneys, giving an image of the urinary tract: an *intravenous urogram*. With such techniques it is possible to investigate virtually any part of the body by X-ray, to give information not only about structure but also about function. These contrast studies, along with X-rays of bones and of the chest, form a very large component of the practice of radiology.

X-ray tomography is a further technique used to define deep internal structures more clearly. In 'linear tomography' the X-ray tube, emitting a beam of X-rays, moves in a straight line while the X-ray film moves in the opposite direction. In this way most structures are blurred by the movement but the image is focussed at a particular plane, so giving greatly improved definition. More complicated variations include circular and multidirectional tomography, producing even sharper images. This type of tomography was widely used in the past to define bones, kidneys, or the inner ear, but has now largely been supplanted by *computed tomography* (see IMAGING TECHNIQUES).

With so many patients having X-ray examinations, protection from the dangers of radiation has become of paramount importance. X-ray tubes are encased in lead shields and fully protected and equipment is regularly calibrated. Staff are required to wear lead aprons and to remain behind protective screens during exposures, and their radiation dose is monitored by a device contained in a 'badge' which they wear all the time. Likewise patients must be properly supervised and protected. Gonad protection is essential especially in women of child-bearing age. There must be 'a clear-cut clinical indication' before any X-ray is requested so that unnecessary tests are avoided. All X-ray examinations must be directed by a properly trained physician, almost always a radiologist. If recognized practice is followed, the dangers from diagnostic X-rays are negligible.

The damaging properties of X-rays have been put to positive use in radiotherapy; already in the early 1900s this was established for the treatment of skin diseases and cancers. Despite the advent of radioisotopes in radiotherapy, X-rays continue to be used for this purpose in appropriate cases.

J. K. DAVIDSON

Further reading

Mould, R. F. (1980). *A history of X-rays and radium.* IPC Business Press Ltd, Sutton, Surrey.

See also IMAGING TECHNIQUES; RADIATION, IONIZING; RADIOLOGY.

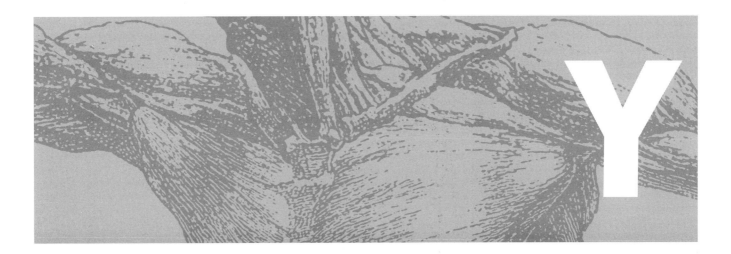

Yoga The word 'yoga' refers primarily to an ancient Hindu spiritual tradition intended to overcome the narrow sense of individual selfhood, though its usage ranges from the very general to the specific and highly technical. The word is probably derived from the Sanskrit root *yuj*, which implies a yoke or harness, invoking the notion that when the ox and the cart are connected via the yoke, the resulting complex is greater than the sum of its parts. In its most general sense, yoga involves harnessing or integrating the forces of *embodiment* (mind, body, and spirit) in order to *transcend* embodiment.

Sometime around 200 BCE, a man named Patanjali developed a system of yoga which ostensibly synthesized previous yogic traditions. It corresponds to a model of the human organism found in the sacred Hindu texts, the Vedas. This model is known as the 'sheath' model, and describes the human organism as a series of concentric sheaths or envelopes, all composed of matter of varying degrees of fineness or subtlety. The spectrum of human material ranges from the most crude or dense, to the most absolutely fine or subtle, and therefore the most 'real.' The goal of Patanjali's yoga is to identify progressively with the finer aspects of one's being until purification leads to identification with the True Self, residing at the core of the sheaths.

Patanjali's yoga, sometimes called *Raja* or 'royal' or 'grand' yoga because of its broadly synthetic ambitions, involves eight steps or stages, of which the first five are considered 'external' and the last three 'internal.' This relates to the sheath model. In Indian medical theory, for instance, which also bases itself in part on the sheath model, disease always begins from the outside and works its way in, so that even mental illness is a form of physical illness that has progressed to the innermost sheaths. Healing, then, must also begin with the physical and proceed to the spiritual.

These eight steps of the yogic path are meant to be accomplished sequentially. That is, one masters the first, and adds the second. When the second is mastered, the third is added, and so on.

The first five or 'external' stages are:

Yama or 'restraint'
The path begins with self-discipline, or the adoption of a basic moral code of non-karmic or 'unselfish' activity. The yogi forsakes stealing, lying, cheating, killing, and other exploitative and self-gratifying behaviours.

Niyama or 'purity'
Purity involves both HYGIENE and diet. In terms of hygiene, radical ablutions or cleansing rituals are performed, such as swallowing a length of gauze and pulling it back out again, in order to scour the intestinal tract. Thus hygiene goes beyond the superficial conception of cleanliness which governs ordinary life. Diet is also important, since the outermost sheaths are composed of the food that we eat. Dense foods such as meat are to be avoided, and subtle, refined foods are to be preferred. Also important are the mode of preparation and the sizes and times of meals. FASTING is also an important purity practice, but is seen as a hygienic concern, and not a dietary one.

Asana or 'postures'
The twisting, bending, and stretching that are commonly associated with the practice of yoga serve a number of purposes. The holding of postures prepares the body to sit for long periods of time in MEDITATION, enables the overcoming of the boredom reflex, and is held to stimulate the endocrine system and thus to be important, since the endocrine system affects our EMOTIONS; this stage of yoga begins to affect the emotional as well as the physical sheaths.

Pranayama or 'breathing exercises'
Prana is the life force which enters the body with the breath and which is metabolized from the foods we eat. Breathing exercises improve the ability of the body to metabolize prana. Also, since breathing affects emotions, breath work helps to regulate and refine the emotional sheath. Finally, breathing also represents a bridge between those physiological functions which we believe we can control (*voluntary*) and those which we cannot (*involuntary*). Adept yogis claim to be able to control metabolism, reflex, and brainwave activity — events slow or virtually stop the heartbeat.

Pratyahara or 'sensory withdrawal'
At this stage, the yogi is able to use the power of concentration to withdraw attention and identification from the outermost, physical, 'external' sheaths. This means that sensory input is blocked out or ignored through an effort of will. The only sound one hears is the pounding of the heart, and this explains why a yogi might want to slow or stop the heartbeat, in order to establish true peace and quiet and facilitate inwardness.

The last three, or 'internal' stages are:

Dharana or 'concentration'
Concentration in this sense involves what is described as *single-pointedness*, that is, the fixation of mind, body, and spirit on a common focal point. Here, the image of the *third eye* is invoked to suggest the strengthening of spiritual vision to the point where it is capable of sustaining a single object for long periods of time, like an eye staring at an object.

Dhyana or 'meditation'
Dhyana refers to meditation, or a sense of radical self-awareness. To return to the metaphor of the third eye, once it has been trained to stare unblinkingly at a single object for a long period of time, it then turns inward upon itself, watching itself watch itself. This awareness takes place without judgment or evaluation, and drives a wedge between our experience and our Self. We watch or 'witness' our own experience as though it were only virtually real, as though it were a drama or play. We cease to identify with it.

Samadhi or 'bliss-trance'
This condition is one of complete effacement of individuality. One no longer identifies with one's body or ego; one's actions are selflessly motivated and non-karmic. This virtually guarantees that liberation will occur with death, which will take place once the consequences of past karmic action have been borne.   ALAN FOX

See also BREATH; BUDDHISM AND THE BODY; THIRD EYE.

Youth No other stage in the life cycle provokes as much debate as the period between childhood and adulthood that embraces PUBERTY. Some historians question whether such a transitional stage has always been recognized in past societies. 'Youth' was, nonetheless, the word usually employed in Western societies to denote how these years were different from the years around them. Jesuit seminaries in fifteenth- and sixteenth-century France, for example, frequently made a distinction between the training of children and the training of youth — suggesting that, for the purposes of religious education at least, these were considered as separate stages of development. Another convincing argument for the recognition of youth as an intermediary stage is the significance attached to it for conversion in religious literature of the period. The early modern definition of 'youth', in so far as one existed, was much broader than the generally accepted meaning of 'adolescence', a concept identified by educational reformers, social scientists, and psychologists only towards the end of the nineteenth century. An extended period of youth became common from the fifteenth to the seventeenth centuries, ranging over a broad age span between the ages of 12 and 25, marked at one end by confirmation (the threshold in Protestant countries between childhood and a new mature status) and at the other by MARRIAGE.

About two-thirds of pre-industrial youths in much of Western and Northern Europe were sent away from their own families and into the households of others as 'servants' or apprentices, in what was almost a 'RITE OF PASSAGE' associated with the onset of puberty, separating them from the lives of their childhood and preparing them for adulthood and citizenship. As apprentices, young men grew accustomed to negotiating with their masters and to being entrusted with adult responsibilities. Young women also left home during their teens, often to large towns as domestic servants, moving from household to household and acquiring a large range of domestic skills by the time they married. This constant mobility of the young was one of the reasons for the relative absence of a distinctive youth culture. In general, the values of the young in the early modern world were not very different from those of their elders because they lacked the peer relations, tastes, or money to become an independent consumer group. Severe constraints were also placed upon relations between the sexes, but the deferment of sexual gratification was accepted by English youth, for example, with surprising equanimity. The rate of illegitimate births was very low considering couples did not normally marry until twelve years or so after puberty because of the difficulty of saving up enough money to set up a separate household. On the other hand, as many as a fifth of seventeenth-century English brides were pregnant at the time of their marriage.

Historical records reveal a certain consciousness of the passage from youth to adulthood. At the close of 1789 John Tennent, apprenticed to a general merchant and grocer in Coleraine, in the Protestant north east of Ireland, demonstrated in his diary a new, Rousseau-like, self-conscious awareness of the transformation he had experienced from the ages of 14 to 17. 'What a wonderful Change have I undergone since 1786 to 1789, I scarce know myself to have been the same person, so alter'd in stature, knowledge and ideas.' As a proper and God-fearing apprentice, John condemns the reading of novels and romances and records the dismissal of a fellow apprentice, 'a very foolish, and careless Boy', for heavy drinking. 'Man is more happy when a child than ever after if I may judge by my own experience', he records lugubriously. 'At twelve years of age I new [sic] very little, at seventeen what I am now rather more and I am emerging into Man.'

A history of growing up in America from the mid-eighteenth to the early twentieth centuries, drawing upon evidence for about 520 individuals of both sexes, testifies that there has never been one common path from childhood to maturity. 'Tried to make up my mind what to do', a young man from Greene City, New York, wrote in his 1851 diary. 'Whether to buy our old farm, teach school, go in a store or study law or go west.' The story of how girls grew up in the nineteenth century away from home is also significant, despite its neglect by historians. Mill work took one young woman from a farm in Epsom, New Hampshire, to the Middlesex Woollen Mills in Lowell in 1843 at age 19. Her journey continued with school teaching from 1845 to 1859, when she married. The combination in late adolescence and early adulthood of work as a mill girl and school teaching was not unusual then, despite crossing middle- and working-class lines. Each was a common experience for American women in this era, and both were routes away from declining opportunities elsewhere. Gender, race, and social class, along with ethnicity, place of residence, and of course age itself, emerge as especially powerful factors in determining the eventual pathway taken to adulthood.　　　　JOHN SPRINGHALL

Further reading

Ben-Amos, I. K. (1994). *Adolescence and youth in early modern England.* Yale University Press.

Graff, H. J. (1995). *Conflicting paths: growing up in America.* Harvard University Press.

See also GROWTH AND DEVELOPMENT: SCHOOL AGE AND ADOLESCENCE; PUBERTY.

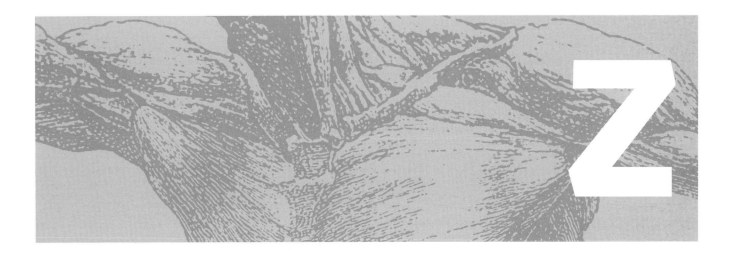

Zen and the body Zen (Chinese: *Ch'an*) Buddhism flourished in China and Japan during the formative period in Tang-era China in the seventh and eighth centuries; during the Sung era from the eleventh to the thirteenth century; and during Kamakura-era Japan in the thirteenth to sixteenth centuries. Zen does not appear to put an emphasis on the body, as it is generally referred to as the '*mind*' school of traditional East Asian philosophy. In its early development in Tang China Zen was closely associated with textual studies of the works of the Yogacara Buddhist school of idealism imported from India, particularly the *Lankavatara Sutra*, which asserted the inseparability of mind and reality, or of subjective response and external phenomena. Later Zen thought, especially in medieval Japan, developed the doctrine of the One Mind (*isshin*), which encompasses all aspects of existence, including humans and nature, being and time, and truth and illusion, by drawing on Mahayana Buddhist conceptions of the universal, primordial Buddha-nature.

However, the very emphasis on the unity or nonduality of mind and reality indicates a focus on the role of the body. In that regard, Zen can be considered a '*body*' school — or a '*mind/body*' school — because it maintains that mind and body do not exist in opposition but are interrelated on every level. The Zen view of body is articulated in several key doctrines, including the oneness of body-mind (*shinjin ichinyo*), just-sitting in *zazen* or meditation-only (*shikan taza*), and the casting off of body-mind (*shinjin datsuraku*). These doctrines concerning the body exerted a strong influence on many other aspects of East Asian culture, including the literary, martial and fine arts.

Zen maintains the inseparability, identity, and equalization of mind and body, which invariably and inextricably interact and interpenetrate one another. To some extent, the Zen view derives from the early Buddhist notion of the unity of cognition and bodily sensations (*nama-rupa*), which stresses that thought formation in the mind is inseparable from the reception of corporeal sense impressions; thus the attachment and ignorance of unenlightenment (*samsara*) stem from the polarity of pleasant or unpleasant sensations, and the freedom and compassion of enlightenment (*nirvana*) are based on neutralizing the extreme response that the sense impressions ordinarily undergo. Zen also builds, however, on the East Asian, especially the Taoist, naturalist view that ultimate reality is manifested in each and every concrete phenomenon, including animate and inanimate beings. It is said that there is no difference between the mind/body of oneself and that of all other aspects of existence. The cycles and images of nature are a macrocosm incorporated in the microcosm of the individual body and reflective of either a disturbed or composed mind.

The Zen doctrine of identity is not merely, or even primarily, intended as an abstract ideological argument. Rather it is firmly rooted in a life of religious praxis in which a specific bodily posture — sitting in *zazen* — takes priority over and serves as the basis of philosophical reflection. The word *zazen* refers to 'sitting meditation' with an emphasis on the somatic component or on composure of the body that fosters the ability to discipline and concentrate the mind. According to the Zen approach, *zazen* is the fundamental, all-encompassing spiritual activity that vitiates the need for following precepts, prayers, ritual, ICONOGRAPHY, and so forth, although many of these elements of religious life are incorporated into the monastic routine. *Zazen* is not merely the act of sitting but is associated with the practice of *gyôjû zaga* (walking, standing, sitting, lying) whereby all gestures and postures of the body throughout the 24-hour daily cycle are considered a form of MEDITATION. Eating is an opportunity for contemplation and the hours of SLEEP are referred to as '*reclining meditation*'. The discipline of *zazen* serves as the basis for the composition of poetry (according to poet and literary critic Fujiwara Teika), the actor's performance in Noh theatre (according to playwright and theorist Zeami), the training of the samurai warrior (according to *bushidô* master Takuan Soho), or the ceremonial etiquette of the tea ritual (according to master Rikyu).

Zen also emphasizes the subitaneous experience of spiritual realization or enlightenment. From this standpoint, the body as well as the mind is a domain that may be inauthentic prior to spiritual pursuit, but is eminently correctible by virtue of partaking of the universal Buddha-nature, and is perfectable through meditative discipline. The sudden enlightenment experience is known as the casting off of (the very distinction) of body and mind, as expressed in the fascicle of the *Shôbôgenzô* on the topic of *Genjôkôan* (Spontaneous Realization) by Japanese Zen master Dôgen (1200–53):

> To study the Buddhist Way is to study the self. To study the self is to forget the self. To forget the self is to be enlightened by the myriad phenomena of the universe. To be enlightened by the myriad phenomena of the universe is to cast off the body-mind of self and the body-mind of others. With this experience, the traces of enlightenment are eliminated and a life of traceless enlightenment is limitlessly renewed.　　STEVEN HEINE

Further reading

Kim, H. J. (1975). *Dôgen Kigen–mystical realist.* University of Arizona Press, Tucson.

Yuasa, Y. (1987). *The body: toward an Eastern mind–body theory.* SUNY Press, Albany.

See also MIND-BODY PROBLEM.

Zombie The word zombie refers to the 'living dead'. In folklore zombies are portrayed as innocent victims who are raised in a comatose trance from their graves by malevolent sorcerers, and led to distant farms or villages where they toil indefinitely as slaves. Zombies are recognized by their docile nature, by their glassy empty eyes, and by the evident absence of will, memory, and emotion. Part of their souls may also be captured by the sorcerers. Zombies can only return to the world of the living upon the death of their masters. Accounts are sometimes cited of actual people who have undergone this ordeal, were declared dead, and later turned up at the homes of their kin in various degrees of health.

Sources indicate that the word is of African origin. The cadaver or spirit of a deceased person is called *zumbi* in the Bonda language, *ndzumbi* in Gabon, and *nzambi* in Kongo. However, the conviction that zombies exist is more widespread. It is encountered not only in sub-Saharan Africa, but also in the Caribbean and in Latin America.

A controversial theory by Wade Davis suggests that there may well be an ethnobiological basis for popular reports of the zombie phenomenon in Haiti. He refers to a case of zombification which had been verified by a team of physicians. In 1962 Clairvus Narcisse was pronounced dead at a hospital, and buried 8 hours later. In 1980 Clairvus reappeared, claiming that he had been made a zombie by his brother because of a land dispute. Davis argues that Clairvus was mistakenly diagnosed as dead, buried alive, and taken from the grave. Among the various preparations of Haitian sorcerers, Davis identified a marine fish containing tetrodotoxin, an extremely potent neurotoxin which induces a complete state of peripheral paralysis and imperceptibly low metabolic levels. He postulates that the Haitian belief in zombies could be based on those rare instances where the individual receives the correct dosage of the poison, is misdiagnosed as dead, and is taken from the grave by a sorcerer. Moreover, Davis argues that zombification is a form of punishment imposed by Bizango secret societies to maintain order in local communities.

Other scholars of Haiti regard the belief in zombies as purely mythical. From a Marxist perspective zombification — the image of people who have lost their minds and souls and are left only with the ability to work — is explained as symbolic comment on the historical process of colonialism.

In many parts of Africa zombies are an integral aspect of witchcraft beliefs; particularly where witchcraft discourses address issues raised by inequalities of wealth and power. For example, among the Bakweri of Cameroon new forms of wealth signalled a transformation in occult forces. When land was alienated for plantations by German and British colonists, the Bakweri were confined to reservations, and the plantations attracted a workforce from elsewhere. In this context a concept of *nyongo* witchcraft emerged. The Bakweri suspected prosperous outsiders of forming witch associations, taking deceased kin from the graves, and of transporting them by lorries to mount Kupe where they used the zombie spirits to work on invisible plantations. Yet the *nyongo* men themselves were in danger. If they were no longer able to sell their intimates to fellow witches, their colleagues would kill them, and reduce them to slavery. Initially these ideas exaggerated ambivalence towards wealth and hindered the emergence of a new elite among the Bakweri. However, when the Bakweri themselves earned much money from the cultivation of bananas, in the 1950s, *nyongo* witches were soon flushed out and brought under control. Hence the ban on individual enrichment was broken.

Similarly, in Malawi, witchcraft discourses constitute an argument about the morality of accumulation. Accumulation is endowed with moral adequacy when entrepreneurs make their constitutive relations visible by supporting their kin financially; and by redistributing wealth through patronage, gift-giving, and feasting. It is perfectly legitimate when entrepreneurs, who are motivated by these concerns, use medicines to protect their businesses and to ensure a steady flow of many customers. By contrast, accumulation which is motivated by individualism and greed is morally despised. In this situation entrepreneurs are said to achieve prosperity at the cost of human lives. Zombies are believed to reside with them, to protect their money, and to affect the minds of customers so that they can come to the business in large numbers. Zombies thus serve exactly the same purposes as medicines, but are an index of morally disputable witchcraft.

In South Africa discourses of zombies capture the illicit desire to dominate and the fear of being dominated. At a symbolic level the image of witches who keep many zombies resonates with the status of white industrialists and farm owners who employ many black labourers. The employment of zombies as servants in a nocturnal 'second world' echoes the daunting experiences of migrant labourers who leave their rural households for alien industrial and mining centres. The tasks of zombies resemble those of domestic assistants and farm labourers. They clean the homes of witches, fetch water and firewood, herd cattle, plough, sow, harvest, and run errands. The unique features of zombies exaggerate some of the less apparent consequences of domination. Zombies are only a metre tall; are similar in appearance; are hypnotized so that they display unquestioning obedience; and their tongues are cut. These features allude to the diminutive, childlike status of African labourers; who are all treated alike by their bosses; and are unable to express themselves. Moreover, zombies are sexless, are devoid of human desires, and are fed a meagre diet of maize porridge — the staple diet of South African labourers. Narratives of zombies also reflect upon the dependence of the dominated. Should witches die, their zombies will wander about endlessly in search of porridge. Being undead, they cannot return to their kin. Persons who aspire to positions of influence; and strong-willed mothers-in-law who command great authority over the wives of their sons, are those most often accused of keeping zombies.

I. NIEHAUS

Further reading
Davis, W. (1988). *Passages of darkness: the ethnobiology of the Haitian zombie.* The University of North Carolina Press, Chapel Hill and London.

See also WITCHCRAFT.

Zygote Derived from the Greek meaning 'yoked', a zygote is the cell that results from fertilization. It is the union of a spermatozoon and an ovum — the mature *germ cells*, known also as the male and female *gametes* (from the Greek for husband and wife). Each of the two gametes is *haploid,* meaning that the nucleus has half the number of chromosomes of normal body cells. Their union results in the *diploid* zygote, with a full set of chromosomes, carrying the combination of genes that will determine all the bodily characteristics of the new individual. When, as a result of this union, matched genes (*alleles*) at particular sites on the newly paired chromosomes are different from each other, the zygote, and hence the resulting individual, is *heterozygous* with respect to those genes. It is *homozygous* if the pairs are identical. Since one of a dissimilar pair of genes can dominate the other, whereas identical pairs can act in unison, this is crucial to the suppression or emergence of the relevant inherited trait.

The zygote carries within its single cell continuing threads in the immemorial lifespan of the human race, as well as the mixed-and-matched microscopic material from which will stem the intricacies common to all human bodies, yet with the remarkable uniqueness of a particular person.

SHEILA JENNETT
COLIN BLAKEMORE

Index

Note: Page numbers in **bold** type are to the main entry for the subject; those in *italic* type, indicate a figure or table (not on the same page as the text referred to).

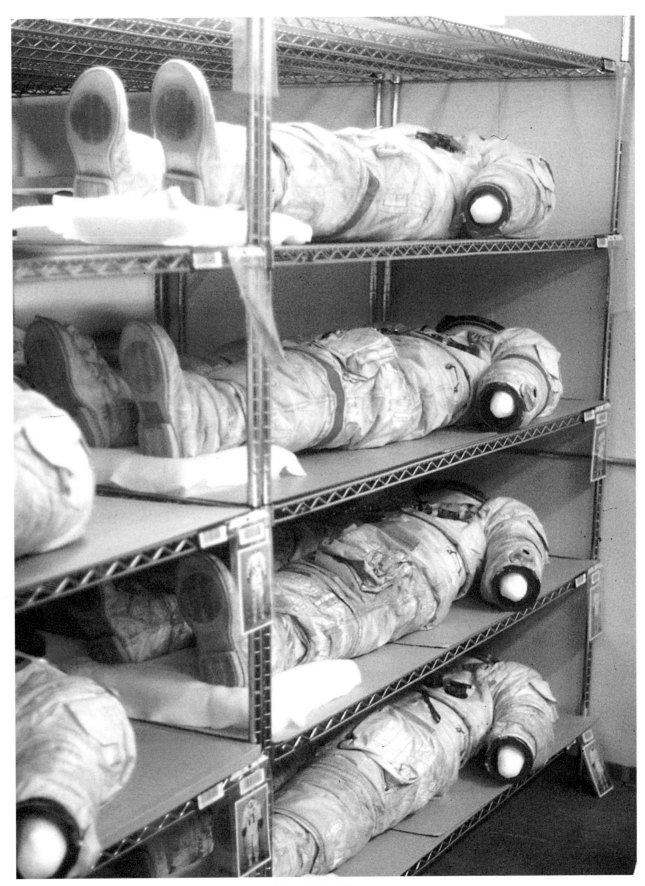

Apollo space suits in storage. Courtesy of Douglas L. Lantry, United States Air Force Museum.

Plate 1 **Alimentary system**

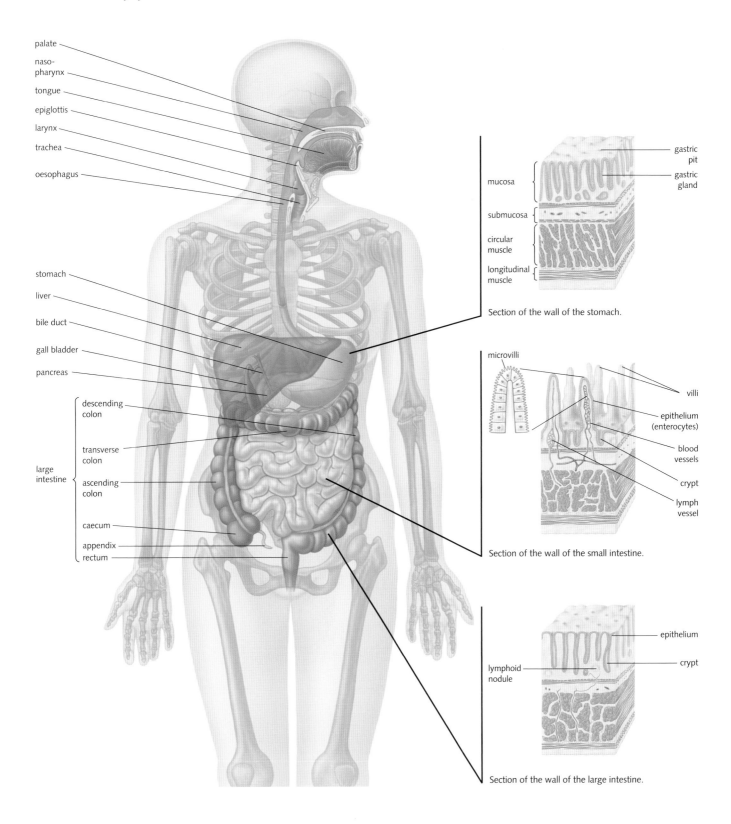

palate
naso-pharynx
tongue
epiglottis
larynx
trachea
oesophagus

stomach
liver
bile duct
gall bladder
pancreas

large intestine
descending colon
transverse colon
ascending colon
caecum
appendix
rectum

mucosa
submucosa
circular muscle
longitudinal muscle

gastric pit
gastric gland

Section of the wall of the stomach.

microvilli
villi
epithelium (enterocytes)
blood vessels
crypt
lymph vessel

Section of the wall of the small intestine.

lymphoid nodule
epithelium
crypt

Section of the wall of the large intestine.

The alimentary tract with associated organs.

Plate 2 **Cardiovascular system**

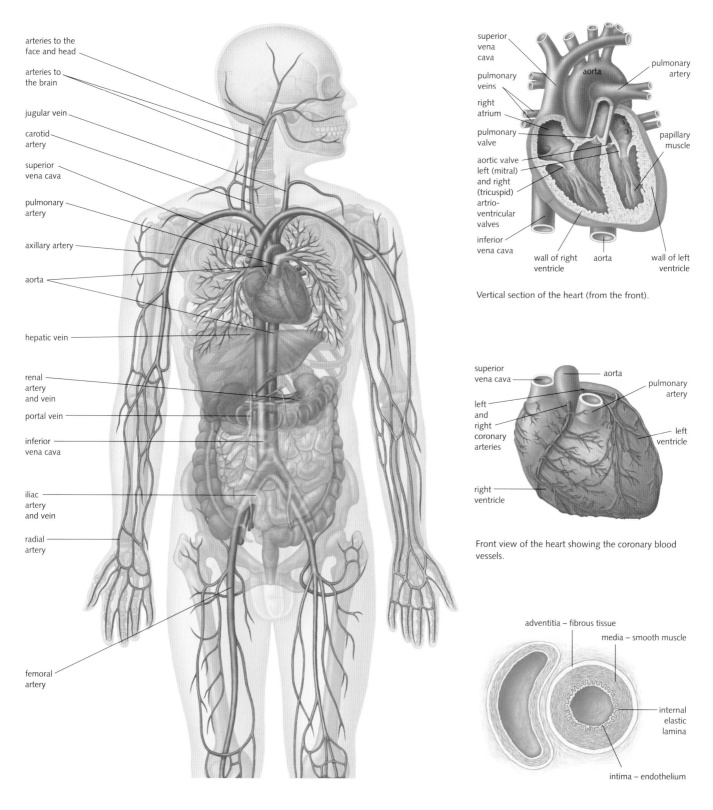

arteries to the
face and head

arteries to
the brain

jugular vein

carotid
artery

superior
vena cava

pulmonary
artery

axillary artery

aorta

hepatic vein

renal
artery
and vein

portal vein

inferior
vena cava

iliac
artery
and vein

radial
artery

femoral
artery

superior
vena
cava

pulmonary
veins

right
atrium

pulmonary
valve

aortic valve
left (mitral)
and right
(tricuspid)
artrio-
ventricular
valves

inferior
vena cava

aorta

pulmonary
artery

papillary
muscle

wall of right
ventricle

aorta

wall of left
ventricle

Vertical section of the heart (from the front).

superior
vena cava

left
and
right
coronary
arteries

right
ventricle

aorta

pulmonary
artery

left
ventricle

Front view of the heart showing the coronary blood
vessels.

adventitia – fibrous tissue

media – smooth muscle

internal
elastic
lamina

intima – endothelium

The heart and main blood vessels of the pulmonary circulation (to and from the lungs) and of the systemic
circulation (to and from the rest of the body). Pulmonary arteries are shown (blue) on the left, and pulmonary
veins (red) on the right of the body, systemic arteries are shown (red) on the right and systemic veins (blue)
on the left.

Cross sections of small vein and artery. The artery is
partially constricted, as shown by folding of the
elastic layer.

Plate 3 **Respiratory system**

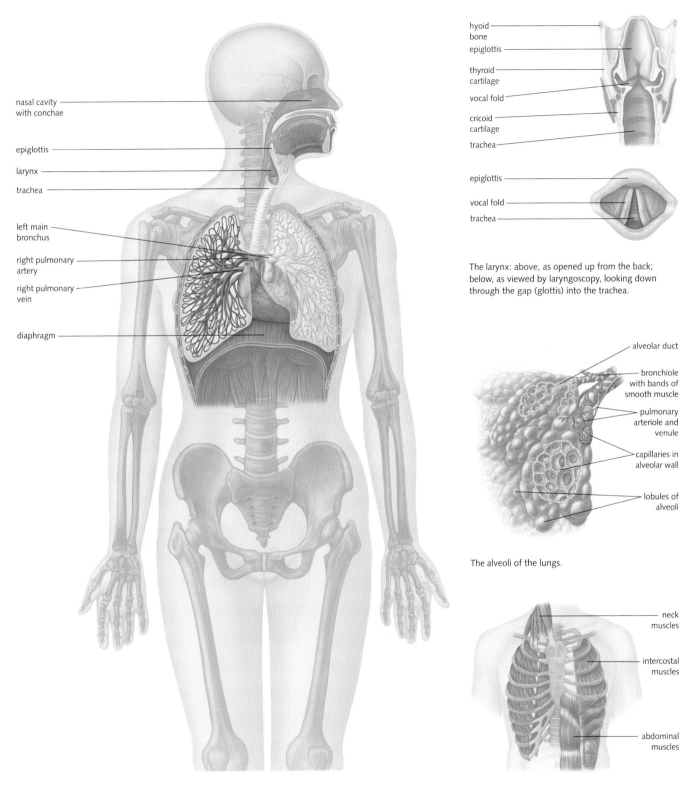

nasal cavity
with conchae

epiglottis

larynx

trachea

left main
bronchus

right pulmonary
artery

right pulmonary
vein

diaphragm

hyoid
bone

epiglottis

thyroid
cartilage

vocal fold

cricoid
cartilage

trachea

epiglottis

vocal fold

trachea

The larynx: above, as opened up from the back;
below, as viewed by laryngoscopy, looking down
through the gap (glottis) into the trachea.

alveolar duct

bronchiole
with bands of
smooth muscle

pulmonary
arteriole and
venule

capillaries in
alveolar wall

lobules of
alveoli

The alveoli of the lungs.

neck
muscles

intercostal
muscles

abdominal
muscles

The respiratory tract from the nose to the bronchial tree (shown in the left lung); the pulmonary blood vessels
are shown in the right lung.

The thoracic cage and muscles (other than the
diaphragm) that are involved in breathing.

Plate 4 **Lymphatic system**

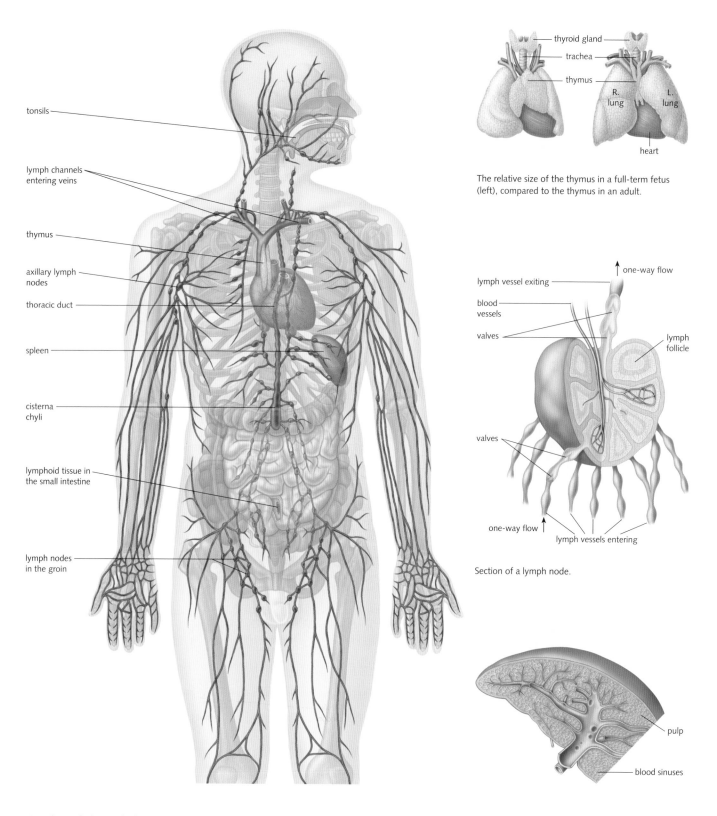

tonsils

lymph channels
entering veins

thymus

axillary lymph
nodes

thoracic duct

spleen

cisterna
chyli

lymphoid tissue in
the small intestine

lymph nodes
in the groin

thyroid gland

trachea

thymus

R.
lung

L.
lung

heart

The relative size of the thymus in a full-term fetus
(left), compared to the thymus in an adult.

one-way flow

lymph vessel exiting

blood
vessels

valves

lymph
follicle

valves

one-way flow

lymph vessels entering

Section of a lymph node.

pulp

blood sinuses

Lymph vessels draining body tissues, via lymph nodes, and finally emptying into veins at the base of the neck.

Section of the spleen. The vein and its tributaries drain
the complex of blood sinuses that form the 'pulp', in
which lymphatic nodules are embedded.

Plate 5 **Musculo-skeletal system**

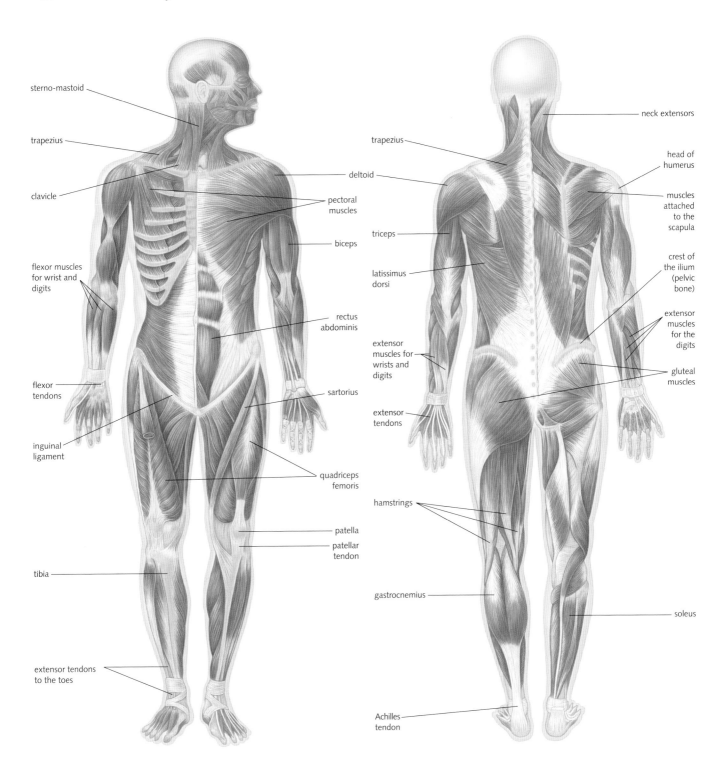

The main skeletal muscles, from the front and back. On the right side of the body in each case the most superficial layer has been removed to show the deeper muscles.

Plate 6 **Nervous system**

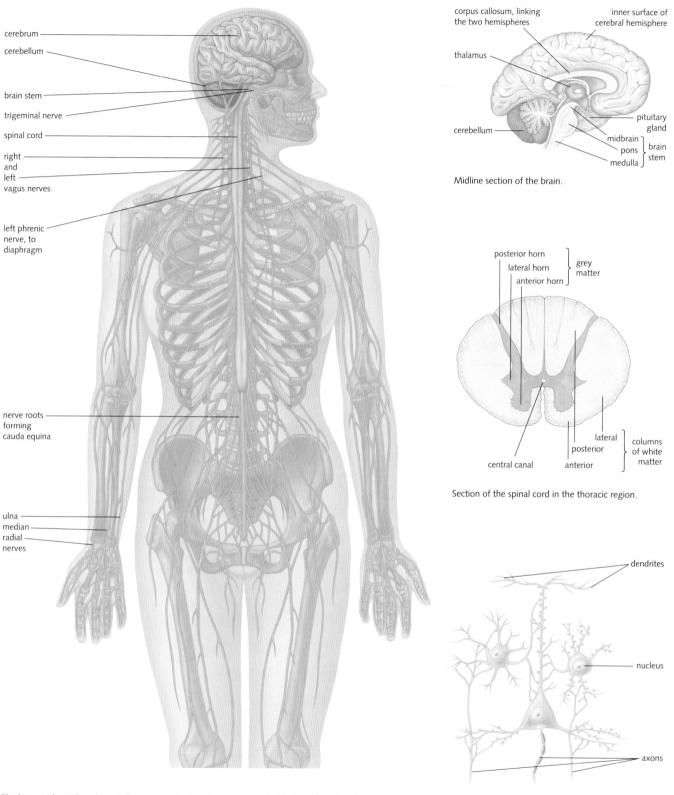

cerebrum

cerebellum

brain stem

trigeminal nerve

spinal cord

right
and
left
vagus nerves

left phrenic
nerve, to
diaphragm

nerve roots
forming
cauda equina

ulna
median
radial
nerves

corpus callosum, linking
the two hemispheres

inner surface of
cerebral hemisphere

thalamus

pituitary
gland

cerebellum

midbrain
pons   brain
medulla   stem

Midline section of the brain.

posterior horn
lateral horn   grey
anterior horn   matter

lateral   columns
posterior   of white
anterior   matter

central canal

Section of the spinal cord in the thoracic region.

dendrites

nucleus

axons

The brain and spinal cord (central nervous system) and nerves connected to them (peripheral nervous system).

Nerve cells.

Plate 7 **Endocrine system**

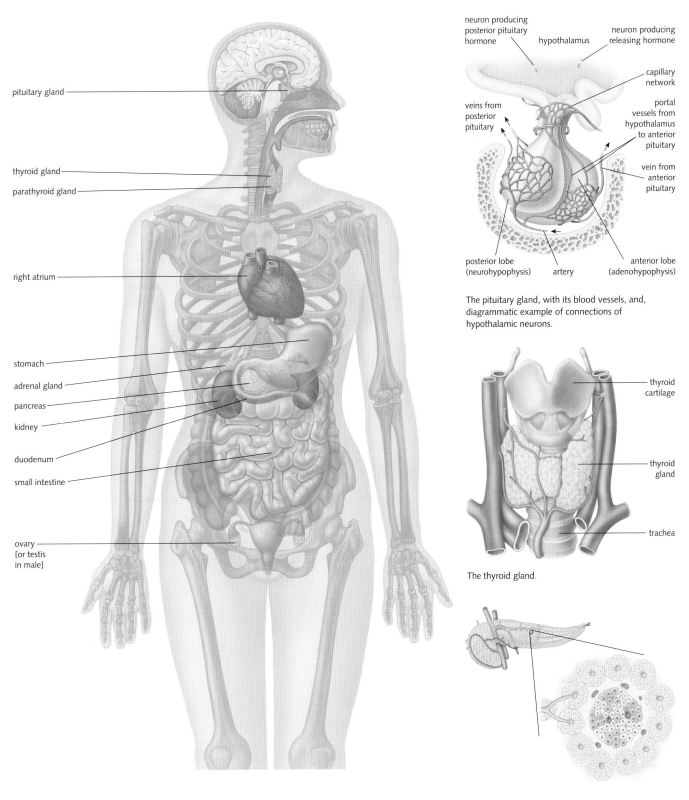

pituitary gland

thyroid gland

parathyroid gland

right atrium

stomach

adrenal gland

pancreas

kidney

duodenum

small intestine

ovary
[or testis
in male]

neuron producing
posterior pituitary
hormone

hypothalamus

neuron producing
releasing hormone

capillary
network

veins from
posterior
pituitary

portal
vessels from
hypothalamus
to anterior
pituitary

vein from
anterior
pituitary

posterior lobe
(neurohypophysis)

artery

anterior lobe
(adenohypophysis)

The pituitary gland, with its blood vessels, and,
diagrammatic example of connections of
hypothalamic neurons.

thyroid
cartilage

thyroid
gland

trachea

The thyroid gland.

Main sites of hormone production by the endocrine glands, and by secretory cells in other organs.

The pancreas, and a diagrammatic section showing a
hormone-secreting 'Islet of Langerhans' surrounded
by enzyme-secreting cells and their ducts.

Plate 8 **Urogenital system**

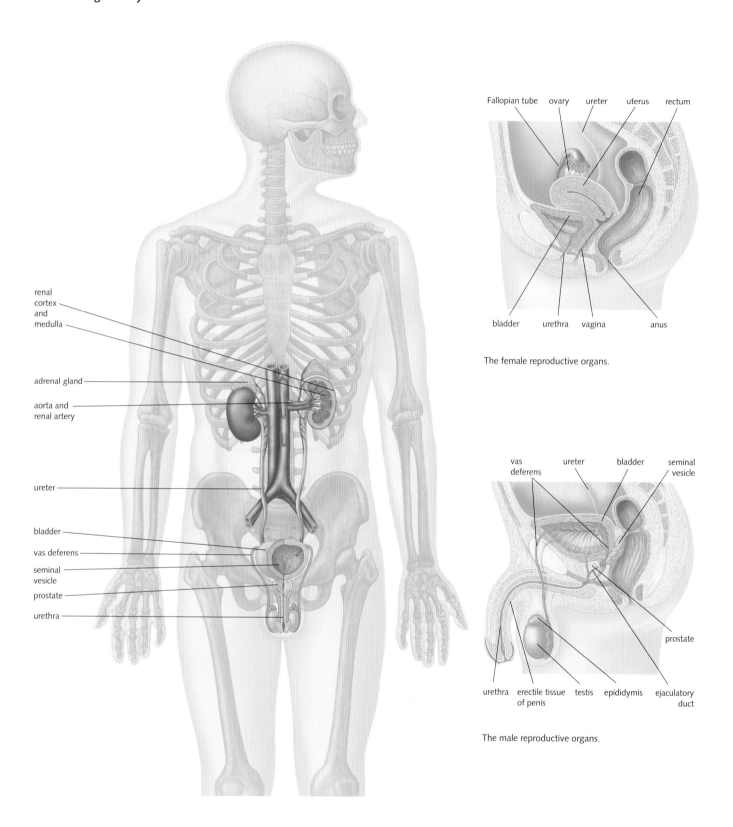

Fallopian tube · ovary · ureter · uterus · rectum

bladder · urethra · vagina · anus

The female reproductive organs.

renal
cortex
and
medulla

adrenal gland

aorta and
renal artery

ureter

bladder

vas deferens

seminal
vesicle

prostate

urethra

vas
deferens · ureter · bladder · seminal
vesicle

prostate

urethra · erectile tissue
of penis · testis · epididymis · ejaculatory
duct

The male reproductive organs.

The urinary tract (kidneys, ureters, bladder and urethra) and the male genital organs. The left kidney is shown
in section.

Phantom limbs, Sleep disorders and Survival at sea. And since the human body is literally the starting point of human culture, it includes discussions of how the body is seen in anthropological contexts, mythology, art, and literature around the globe.

From head to toe, from conception to funeral practices, *The Oxford Companion to the Body* is a wide-ranging, lavishly illustrated reference for the specialist and layman alike.

About the Editors

COLIN BLAKEMORE is Professor of Physiology and Director of the Centre for Cognitive Neuroscience at the University of Oxford. He is also past president of the British Association for the Advancement of Science.

He has published widely on a variety of medical subjects, including mad cow disease, the development of consciousness, the effects of mobile phones, and biomedical ethics.

SHEILA JENNETT is an Emeritus Professor of Physiology at the University of Glasgow, where she was chairperson of the Department of Physiology.